Tachdjian's

PEDIATRIC ORTHOPAEDICS

FROM THE TEXAS SCOTTISH RITE HOSPITAL FOR CHILDREN

Tachdjian's

PEDIATRIC ORTHOPAEDICS

FROM THE TEXAS SCOTTISH RITE HOSPITAL FOR CHILDREN

Fourth Edition

Volume 3

John Anthony Herring, MD

Chief of Staff
Texas Scottish Rite Hospital for Children
Professor of Orthopaedic Surgery
University of Texas Southwestern Medical Center
Dallas, Texas

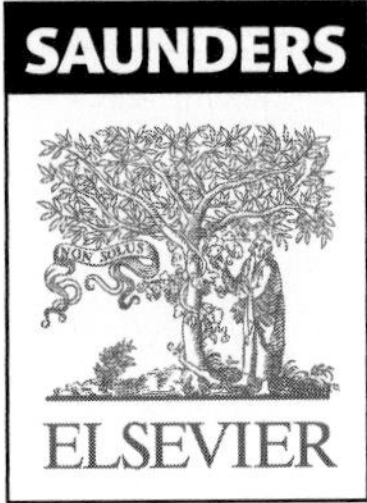

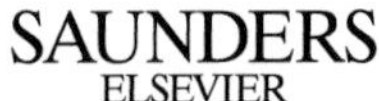

1600 John F. Kennedy Blvd.
Ste 1800
Philadelphia, PA 19103-2899

TACHDJIAN'S PEDIATRIC ORTHOPAEDICS, 4th edition ISBN 978-1-4160-2221-3

Notice

Knowledge and best practice in this field are constantly changing. As new research and experience broaden our knowledge, changes in practice, treatment and drug therapy may become necessary or appropriate. Readers are advised to check the most current information provided (i) on procedures featured or (ii) by the manufacturer of each product to be administered, to verify the recommended dose or formula, the method and duration of administration, and contraindications. It is the responsibility of the practitioner, relying on their own experience and knowledge of the patient, to make diagnoses, to determine dosages and the best treatment for each individual patient, and to take all appropriate safety precautions. To the fullest extent of the law, neither the Publisher nor the Editors assume any liability for any injury and/or damage to persons or property arising out of or related to any use of the material contained in this book.

The Publisher

Library of Congress Cataloging-in-Publication Data (in PHL)

Tachdjian's pediatric orthopaedics / from the Texas Scottish Rite Hospital for Children ; [edited by] John Anthony Herring.—4th ed.
p. ; cm.
Includes bibliographical references and index.
ISBN-13: 978-1-4160-2221-3
1. Pediatric orthopedics. I. Herring, John A. II. Tachdjian, Mihran O. Pediatric orthopedics. III. Texas Scottish Rite Hospital for Children. IV. Title: Pediatric orthopaedics.
[DNLM: 1. Orthopedics. 2. Child. 3. Infant. WS 270 T1173 2007]
RD732.3.C48T33 2007
618.92'7—dc22

2006037519

Vol. 1: 9996004511
Vol. 2: 9996004570
Vol. 3: 9996047482

Acquisitions Editor: Kim Murphy
Developmental Editor: Heather Krehling
Publishing Services Manager: Tina Rebane
Project Manager: Amy Norwitz
Design Direction: Ellen Zanolle

Printed in Canada

Last digit is the print number: 9 8 7 6 5 4 3 2 1

Dedicated with much love to our families

Contributors

John A. Abraham, MD
Fellow in Orthopaedic Oncology
Children's Hospital Boston
Instructor in Orthopaedic Surgery
Harvard Medical School
Staff Surgeon
Center for Sarcoma and Bone Oncology
Dana Farber Cancer Institute
Staff Surgeon, Orthopedic Oncology
Brigham and Women's Hospital
Boston, Massachusetts

Richard C. Adams, MD
Associate Professor of Pediatrics
University of Texas Southwestern Medical Center
Medical Director of Developmental Disabilities
Texas Scottish Rite Hospital for Children
Neurodevelopmental Pediatrician
Parkland Medical Center
Dallas, Texas

John G. Birch, MD, FRCS(C)
Clinical Professor of Orthopedics
University of Texas Southwestern Medical School
Assistant Chief of Staff, Department of Orthopaedics
Texas Scottish Rite Hospital for Children
Dallas, Texas

Peter R. Carter, MD
Professor of Orthopaedic Surgery
University of Texas Southwestern Medical School
Hand Surgeon
Charles E. Seay, Jr. Hand Center
Texas Scottish Rite Hospital for Children
Consulting Surgeon, Department of Orthopaedics
Children's Medical Center
Dallas, Texas

Lawson A. B. Copley, MD
Assistant Professor of Orthopaedic Surgery
University of Texas Southwestern Medical Center
Staff Surgeon, Department of Orthopaedics
Texas Scottish Rite Hospital for Children
Dallas, Texas

Donald R. Cummings, BS, CP
Adjunct Clinical Faculty, Prosthetics and Orthotics Program
School of Allied Heath Sciences
University of Texas Southwestern Medical Center
Director of Prosthetics
Texas Scottish Rite Hospital for Children
Dallas, Texas

Molly E. Dempsey, MD
Medical Director of Radiology
Texas Scottish Rite Hospital for Children
Dallas, Texas

Nancy Noble Dodge, MD, FAAP
Clinical Associate Professor of Pediatrics
Michigan State University
Lansing, Michigan
Neurodevelopmental Pediatrician
Helen DeVos Children's Hospital
Grand Rapids, Michigan

Marybeth Ezaki, MD
Professor of Orthopaedic Surgery
University of Texas Southwestern Medical School
Director of Department of Hand Surgery
Texas Scottish Rite Hospital for Children
Dallas, Texas

Mark C. Gebhardt, MD
Frederick W. and Jane Ilfed Professor of Orthopaedic Surgery
Harvard Medical School
Chief of Orthopaedic Surgery
Beth Israel Deaconess Medical Center
Associate in Orthopaedic Surgery
Children's Hospital Boston
Boston, Massachusetts

John A. Herring, MD
Chief of Staff
Texas Scottish Rite Hospital for Children
Professor of Orthopaedic Surgery
University of Texas Southwestern Medical Center
Dallas, Texas

Charles E. Johnston, MD
Professor of Orthopaedic Surgery
University of Texas Southwestern Medical Center
Assistant Chief of Staff
Medical Director of Research
Texas Scottish Rite Hospital for Children
Dallas, Texas

Lori A. Karol, MD
Professor of Orthopaedic Surgery
University of Texas Southwestern Medical Center
Staff Orthopaedist, Department of Orthopaedic Surgery
Texas Scottish Rite Hospital for Children
Dallas, Texas

Amy Lake, OTH, CHT
Occupational Therapist
Hand Service
Texas Scottish Rite Hospital for Children
Dallas, Texas

Marilyn K. Moody, MD
Assistant Professor of Clinical Radiology
University of Texas Southwestern Medical Center
Staff Pediatric Radiologist
Texas Scottish Rite Hospital for Children
Dallas, Texas

Pamela Nurenberg, MD
Clinical Associate Professor of Radiology
University of Texas Southwestern Medical Center
Staff Pediatric Radiologist
Texas Scottish Rite Hospital for Children
Dallas, Texas

Scott N. Oishi, MD, FACS
Assistant Professor of Plastic and Reconstructive Surgery
University of Texas Southwestern Medical Center
Hand Surgeon
Charles E. Seay, Jr. Hand Center
Texas Scottish Rite Hospital for Children
Dallas, Texas

Karl E. Rathjen, MD
Associate Professor of Orthopaedic Surgery
University of Texas Southwestern Medical Center
Orthopaedic Staff
Texas Scottish Rite Hospital for Children
Chief of Clinical Service, Department of Orthopaedic Surgery
Children's Medical Center
Dallas, Texas

B. Stephens Richards, MD
Professor of Orthopaedic Surgery
University of Texas Southwestern Medical Center
Assistant Chief of Staff
Texas Scottish Rite Hospital for Children
Dallas, Texas

Fay Z. Safavi, MBBS, FFARCS
Associate Professor of Anesthesiology and Pain Management
University of Texas Southwestern Medical Center
Director of Department of Anesthesiology and Pain Management
Texas Scottish Rite Hospital for Children
Dallas, Texas

Eugene G. Sheffield, MD
Clinical Assistant Professor of Radiology
University of Texas Southwestern Medical Center
Dallas, Texas

Daniel J. Sucato, MD
Associate Professor of Orthopaedic Surgery
University of Texas Southwestern Medical Center
Staff Orthopedic Surgeon, Department of Orthopaedic Surgery
Texas Scottish Rite Hospital for Children
Staff Orthopaedic Surgeon, Department of Orthopaedic Surgery
Children's Medical Center of Dallas
Dallas, Texas

Mihran O. Tachdjian, MD*
Former Professor of Surgery
Northwestern University Medical School
Former Head, Division of Orthopaedics
Children's Memorial Hospital
Chicago, Illinois

David C. Wilkes, MD
Staff Radiologist, Department of Radiology
Texas Scottish Rite Hospital for Children
Dallas, Texas

Philip L. Wilson, MD
Assistant Professor of Orthopaedic Surgery
University of Texas Southwestern Medical Center
Staff Surgeon, Department of Orthopaedics
Texas Scottish Rite Hospital for Children
Dallas, Texas

*Deceased

Preface

The fourth edition of *Tachdjian's Pediatric Orthopaedics,* like the third edition, has been prepared by the staff of the Texas Scottish Rite Hospital for Children, with the additional contribution of Dr. Mark Gebhardt.

We have been very pleased and encouraged by the reception for the third edition of *Tachdjian's Pediatric Orthopaedics.* Some have referred to the textbook as the Bible of pediatric orthopedics, and we are very proud that some people consider it so. However, as the knowledge base of our profession seems to change more rapidly every year, it was clearly time for the book to be revised.

The text has been rewritten where necessary to include new concepts, new procedures, and new information developed since publication of the third edition. The extent of change in a number of areas surprised us when we did the review, and it is evident that our profession continues to make important advances. In addition, we have updated the style and readability of the book. We have added many new illustrations and have been able to use color throughout. We hope that these changes will make the book more user-friendly to both the reader seeking a quick overview and the expert who needs to review all the current and pertinent information about a subject.

This work would not exist if not for the effort of many people. First and foremost I want to thank the orthopaedic and medical staff of Texas Scottish Rite Hospital for Children. Each contributor has worked diligently to provide an unbiased review of each subject and to thoroughly review the relevant literature. At the same time, we have added our own preferences for evaluation and management, based on our large clinical experience, which has required a great deal of time and effort by the contributors. Our orthopaedic group prides itself in working as a team, and most major chapters are a product of this teamwork. Treatment alternatives were often discussed by the group before settling on firm recommendations. Out of respect for this process we have chosen not to list chapter authorship. This is in keeping with Dr. Tachdjian's original style, in which extensive consultation from colleagues around the world formed the basis for much that he wrote.

I would like to thank Dr. Mark Gebhardt, whose chapter on malignant tumors is much appreciated. My secretary, Louise Hamilton; Cindy Daniel; and our office manager, Phyllis Cuesta, have put in many hours of very skilled work in pulling the project together. We also want to thank our media department, including Roger Bell, Stuart Almond, Rick Smith, Sandy Carduff, Sarah Tune, Emily Bucholz, and Pat Rogers, for their help with the illustrations and videos. Our president, J. C. Montgomery, Jr.; our administrator, Robert L. Walker; the chairman of our board, The Honorable Jack Hightower; and the entire Board of Directors of the hospital have given us great support, encouragement, and leeway in producing this book.

TONY HERRING

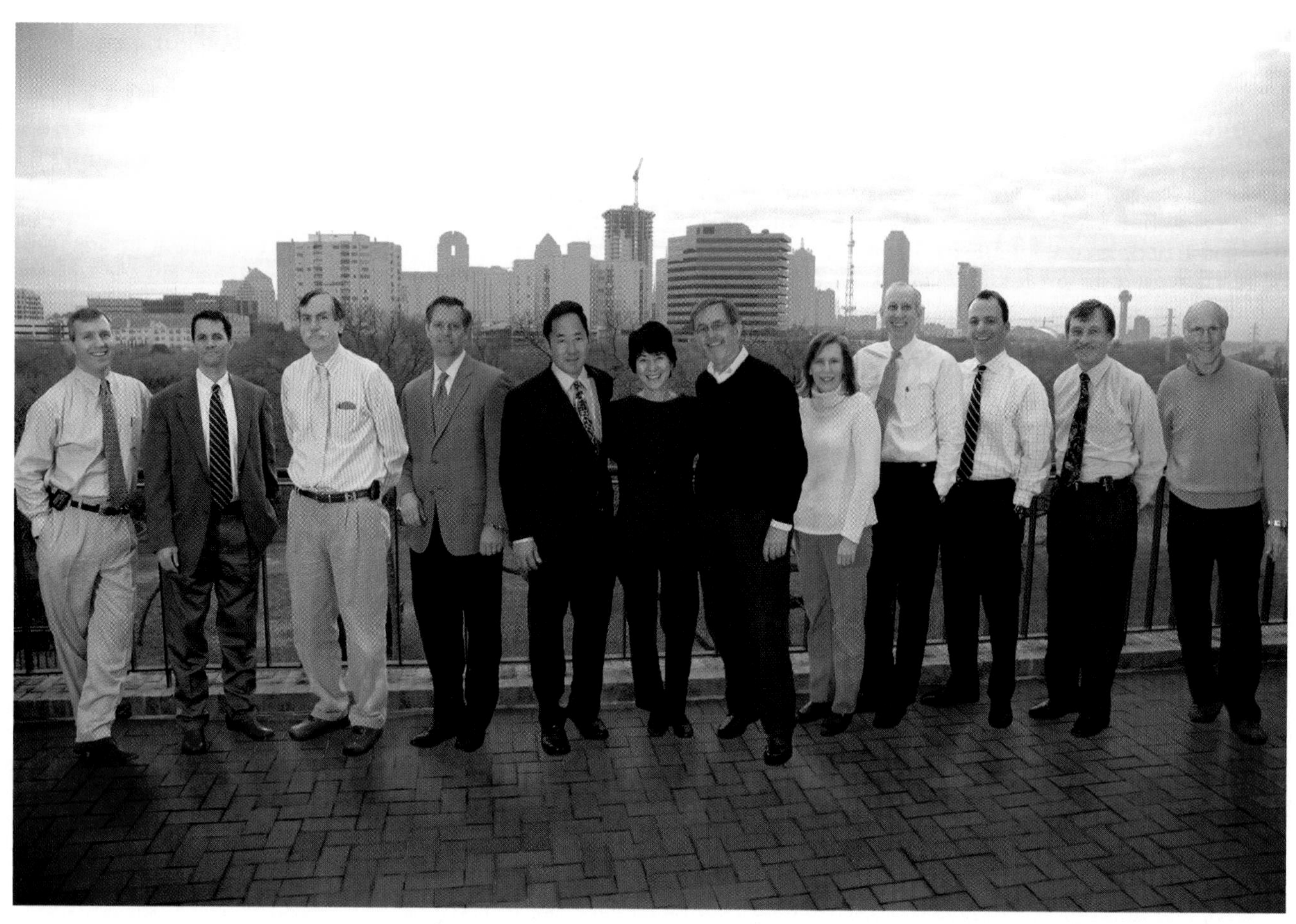

The orthopaedic staff at Texas Scottish Rite Hospital for Children. *From left to right:* Karl E. Rathjen, MD; Philip L. Wilson, MD; Charles E. Johnston, MD; Lawson A. B. Copley, MD; Scott N. Oishi, MD, FACS; Marybeth Ezaki, MD; Peter R. Carter, MD; Lori A. Karol, MD; B. Stevens Richards, MD; Daniel J. Sucato, MD; John G. Birch, MD, FRCS(C); and John A. Herring, MD

Acknowledgments

Editor:

John A. Herring, MD

Managing Editors:

Cindy Godwin Daniel

Louise Nunes Hamilton

Project Manager:

Phyllis Cuesta

Media Production Services:

Stuart Almond

Lilla Tune

Emily Bucholz

Sarah Tune

Paul Jolly

Camera and Video Editor:

Alexander Carduff

Operating Room Video:

Margaret Taylor

Sarah Tune

Medical Librarian:

Mary Peters

Contents

Volume 3

Chapter
32 Metabolic and Endocrine Bone Diseases 1917

ILLUSTRATED PROCEDURES

Chapter 32

Metabolic and Endocrine Bone Diseases

General Pathophysiology

Metabolic bone disease is caused by disturbances in the metabolism of calcium and phosphate. The result is inadequate mineralization of bone matrix. In children, the epiphyseal ends of the bones are the most active in osteogenesis, so the disease is more evident there. A complete understanding of calcium metabolism is needed to understand this group of disorders.[306]

The body is extremely sensitive to serum calcium levels, and a disturbance in calcium balance leads to abnormal irritability, conductivity, and contractility of the cardiovascular and neurologic systems. Almost all of the body's calcium is stored in bone as hydroxyapatite; thus, if extra calcium is needed in the bloodstream to maintain cardiac or neurologic function, bone is the source of the required calcium. Only a very small portion of the body's calcium is present in the bloodstream.

Because of the liver and kidneys' involvement in calcium and vitamin D metabolism, hepatic or renal diseases can lead to metabolic bone diseases. Serum calcium is under the regulation of vitamin D and parathyroid hormone (PTH) (Fig. 32–1).[60,122,123,246,366] Ergosterol (provitamin D) is ingested and absorbed from the small intestine. These precursors of vitamin D must be absorbed from the gut. Because these precursors are fat soluble, gastrointestinal or hepatic diseases that produce steatorrhea result in an inability to absorb vitamin D. Provitamin D undergoes a series of hydroxylation reactions in its transformation to the active form 1,25-dihydroxyvitamin D. The first hydroxylation takes place in the liver. The second hydroxylation, which occurs in the kidney, is stimulated by hypocalcemia and high levels of PTH. The liver also produces 7-dehydrocholesterol (also a provitamin D).

The skin also plays a role in metabolic bone diseases because it is the site of conversion of 7-dehydrocholesterol to vitamin D_3 (cholecalciferol). This change occurs as a result of exposure to ultraviolet light.

The action of 1,25-dihydroxycholecalciferol is to enable absorption of calcium from the small intestine.[367] In a state of vitamin D deficiency, deficient absorption of calcium leads to mild hypocalcemia, which triggers the release of PTH. PTH enables

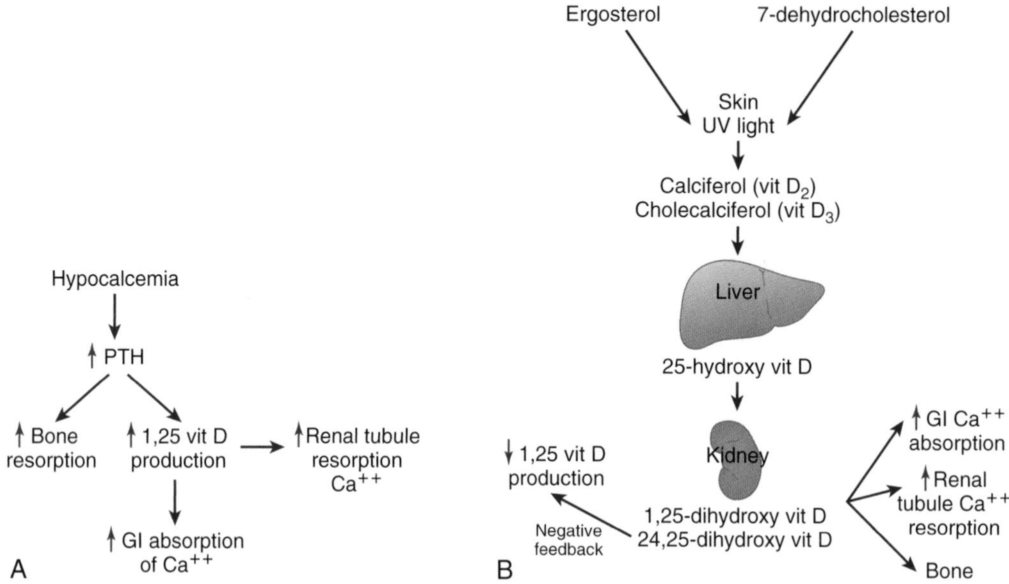

FIGURE 32–1 **A**, Metabolic control of calcium metabolism. **B**, Vitamin D metabolism. GI, gastrointestinal; PTH, parathyroid hormone.

absorption of calcium from the intestines and renal tubules and activates osteoclasts.[530] Calcium is leached out of the bones, and the hypocalcemia is relatively corrected; however, phosphate is excreted from the kidney, which results in hypophosphatemia and poor mineralization of bones.

Nutritional Rickets

Vitamin D deficiency in the diet leads to nutritional rickets. Although this entity is rare in developed countries, it is by no means absent from these areas.[23,483] The dysplasia may result from prolonged breast-feeding and occurs more frequently in children fed a vegetarian diet and in black children.[113,138,235,264,446] Numerous reports suggest an increased frequency of nutritional rickets in the United States in children with dark skin pigmentation who are breast-fed past 6 months of age without vitamin D supplementation.[247,402,413,473,542] In the developed world, rickets is more commonly the result of an inability to absorb vitamin D because of celiac or hepatic disease.[217,260,351,365] Children with either form of rickets are usually first seen between the ages of 6 months and 3 years. Initial findings are listlessness, periarticular swelling, or angular deformities.

In the early 20th century, Hess used a trial of cod liver oil to treat 65 infants with rickets and found that the rickets resolved in 92% during a 6-month course of treatment. This led to development of the first rickets clinic in 1917.[413] Mellanby[336] and Park[381] in the mid-1920s were the first to suggest that rickets could be prevented by adequate vitamin D intake. Since that time, milk and dairy products have been fortified with vitamin D. Thus, it is only in cases of malnutrition and unusual dietary practices that vitamin D–deficiency rickets is seen.

Pathology

In rickets, the primary disturbance in bone is failure of calcification of cartilage and osteoid tissue.[239,311,376,382,488] Normally, the cartilage cells at the provisional zone of calcification proliferate in columns, the most mature of which are calcified, resorbed, and replaced by new bone. In rickets, there is failure of deposition of calcium along the mature cartilage cell columns, followed by disorderly invasion of cartilage by blood vessels, lack of reabsorption at the zone of provisional calcification, and increased thickness of the epiphyseal plate (Fig. 32–2). The chondrocytes multiply normally, but the normal process of maturation of cartilage columns fails to take place.

Osteoblastic activity in both endosteal and periosteal tissues is normal, and abundant osteoid is formed. With defective mineralization, however, osteoclastic resorption of the uncalcified osteoid does not take place. Hence, the overly abundant osteoid produced by normal osteoblasts is laid down irregularly around anything that will serve as a scaffolding. There are widened osteoid seams. The osteoid islets may even persist down into the diaphysis.

In rickets, there is an abnormality in the arrangement of bundles of collagen fibers in compact bone. Instead of running parallel to the haversian canals, they course perpendicularly and are biomechanically inferior.[147]

Grossly, the rachitic bone is soft and becomes misshapen under the force of weight bearing. If the disease remains untreated, angular deformities of the lower extremities and deformities of the thoracic cage and pelvis may develop.

After treatment of rickets with vitamin D, calcium absorption increases and calcification of the cartilage columns and osteoid occurs. Osteoclasts

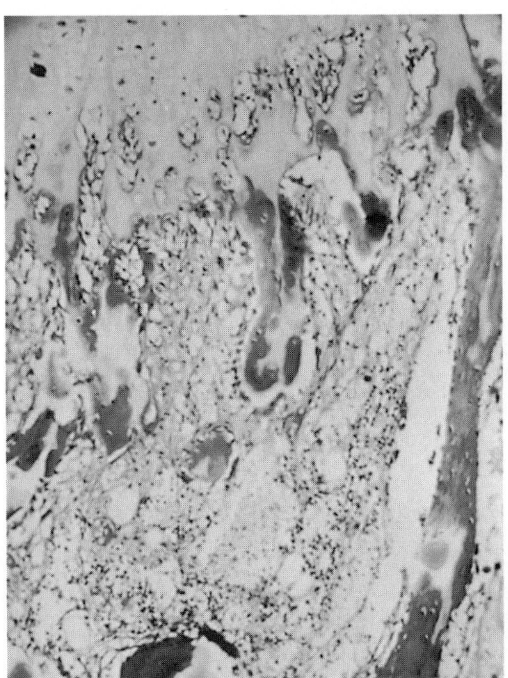

FIGURE 32-2 Histologic appearance of rickets. A photomicrograph through the epiphyseal-metaphyseal junction shows uncalcified osteoid tissue, failure of deposition of calcium along the mature cartilage cell columns, and disorderly invasion of cartilage by blood vessels (×25).

resorb the calcified cartilage, and remodeling of bone follows.[26]

Laboratory Findings

Vitamin D deficiency results in an inability to absorb calcium and phosphorus. PTH is released in response to hypocalcemia, which corrects the serum calcium deficit, but the hypophosphatemia persists. Serum calcium levels are normal to mildly decreased, phosphate levels are low, and vitamin D levels are decreased, but PTH and alkaline phosphatase levels are high (Table 32–1).[190,304,366,412]

Clinical Features

The clinical features of nutritional rickets depend on the severity of the disease and may be subtle. Infants demonstrate generalized muscular weakness, lethargy, and irritability.[466] Sitting, standing, and walking are delayed. The abdomen may appear protuberant.

Early bone manifestations include a slight thickening of the ankles, knees, and wrists. Beading of the ribs, referred to as the "rachitic rosary," is due to enlargement of the costochondral junctions. As the disease continues, the pull of the diaphragm on the ribs produces a horizontal depression known as Harrison's groove. Short stature results from insufficient longitudinal growth. Pectus carinatum is caused by forward projection of the sternum. Closure of the fontanelles is delayed and the sutures are thickened, which leads to a skull appearance described as resembling hot cross buns. The dentition is affected, with delays in appearance of the teeth and defects in the enamel.

As the child begins standing and walking, the softened long bones bow, and it is at this time that the child is usually brought to the orthopaedic surgeon for a diagnosis. In toddlers, bowleg, or genu varum, is one of the most common initial signs.[53] In older children, genu valgum and coxa vara may be initial features. Stress fractures of the long bones may be present.[386] Children may be seen acutely with unexplained fractures suggesting child abuse, tetany, and hypocalcemic seizures.[59] Later, kyphoscoliosis may develop.

Radiographic Findings

Failure of physeal cartilage to calcify leads to elongation of the physis and a hazy appearance of the provisional zone of calcification.[404,501,512] The widened growth plate is particularly suspect for rickets, which differentiates this rare condition from the more common

Table 32-1 Biochemical Abnormalities in Rickets

	Biochemical Abnormality					
Type of Rickets	Calcium	Phosphate	Alkaline Phosphatase	PTH	25 (OH) Vitamin D	1,25 $(OH)_2$ Vitamin D
Nutritional	N1	N1↓	↑	↑	↓↓	↓
Vitamin D–resistant (XLH, RTA, Fanconi's, oncogenic	N1	↓	↑	N1	N1	N1
Vitamin D–dependent type I (inability to hydroxylate)	↓	↓	↑	↑	↑↑	↓↓
Vitamin D–dependent type II (receptor insensitivity)	↓	↓	↑	↑	N1↑↑	↑↑↑↑
Renal osteodystrophy	N1↓	↑	↑	↑↑	N1	↓↓

N1, normal; PTH, parathyroid hormone; RTA, renal tubular acidosis; XLH, X-linked hypophosphatemia.

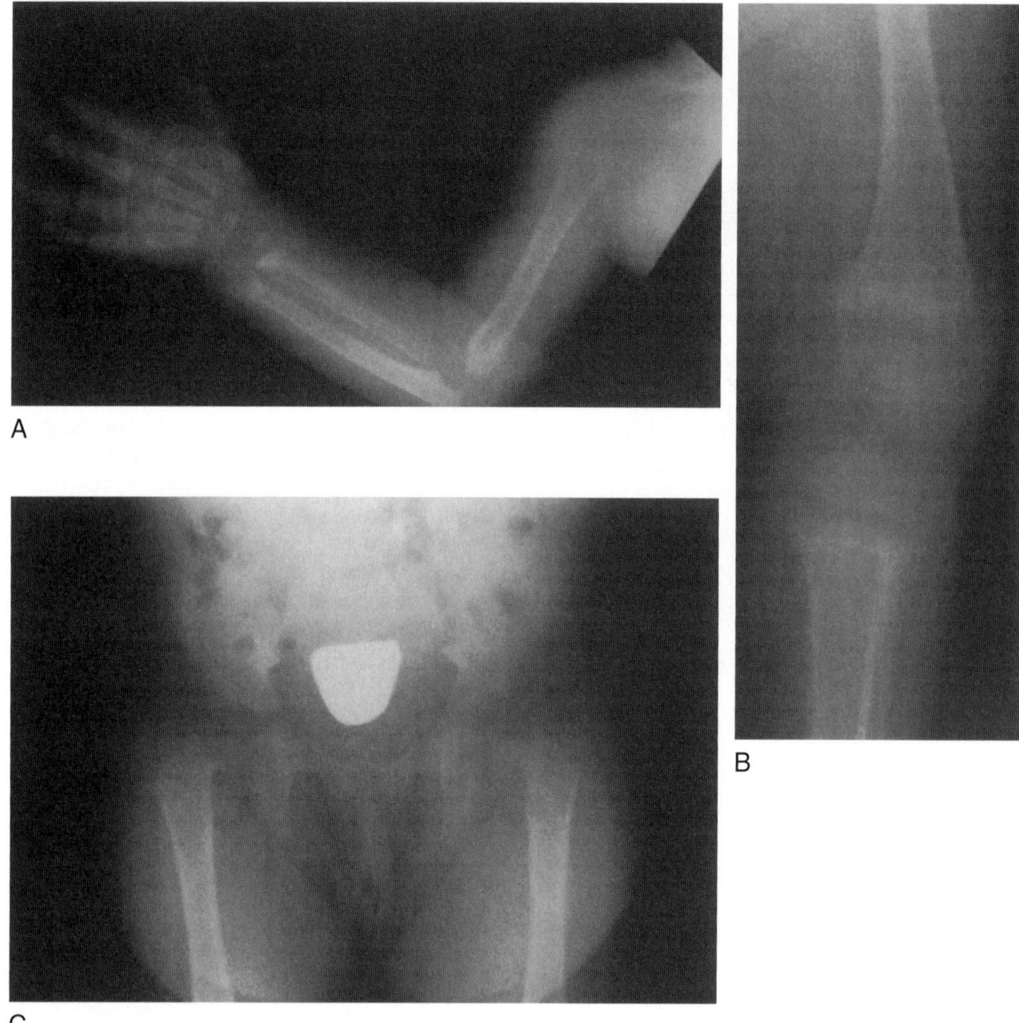

A

B

C

FIGURE 32-3 Radiographs obtained in a 1-year-old black girl with nutritional rickets. All physes are widened and the metaphyses are indistinct. Cupping is most prominent in the metaphysis of the distal radius and ulna and at the knee. See also Figure 32–6.

physiologic angular deformities of the lower extremities (Fig. 32–3).[306] The metaphysis abutting the physis is brushlike in appearance, with islands or columns of cartilage persisting well into the metaphysis (Fig. 32–4). The metaphysis also appears cupped or flared. The bones have an osteopenic appearance overall, with thinning of the cortices.[429] The bony trabeculae are indistinct. Looser's lines, or radiolucent transverse bands that extend across the axes of the long bones, are evident on radiographs in 20% of patients with rickets.[500]

As the rickets continues, deformities of the long bones, ribs, pelvis, and spine develop. Thoracolumbar kyphosis—"rachitic cat back"—may be apparent on radiographs.

Although the diagnosis of nutritional rickets should be made on review of plain films, bone scintigraphy has been used in neonates to confirm the diagnosis and to pick up areas of fractures. Increased uptake is seen.[463]

With treatment, calcification occurs and radiographs become normal. The physis thins and bone density increases (Fig. 32–5).[488,489]

Treatment

Rickets is treated by the administration of vitamin D under the supervision of a pediatric specialist in metabolic bone disease. The usual course of treatment is 6 to 10 weeks. After 2 to 4 weeks, radiographs show improvement in mineralization. Tetracycline labeling shows response to therapy, with new mineralization picking up the drug. (Tetracycline should not be used in young children, however, because of staining of the teeth.[422]) If the child does not respond to vitamin D therapy, vitamin D–resistant rickets should be suspected. Because residual deformity is rare after medical treatment of nutritional rickets, there is no specific orthopaedic treatment of nutritional rickets.

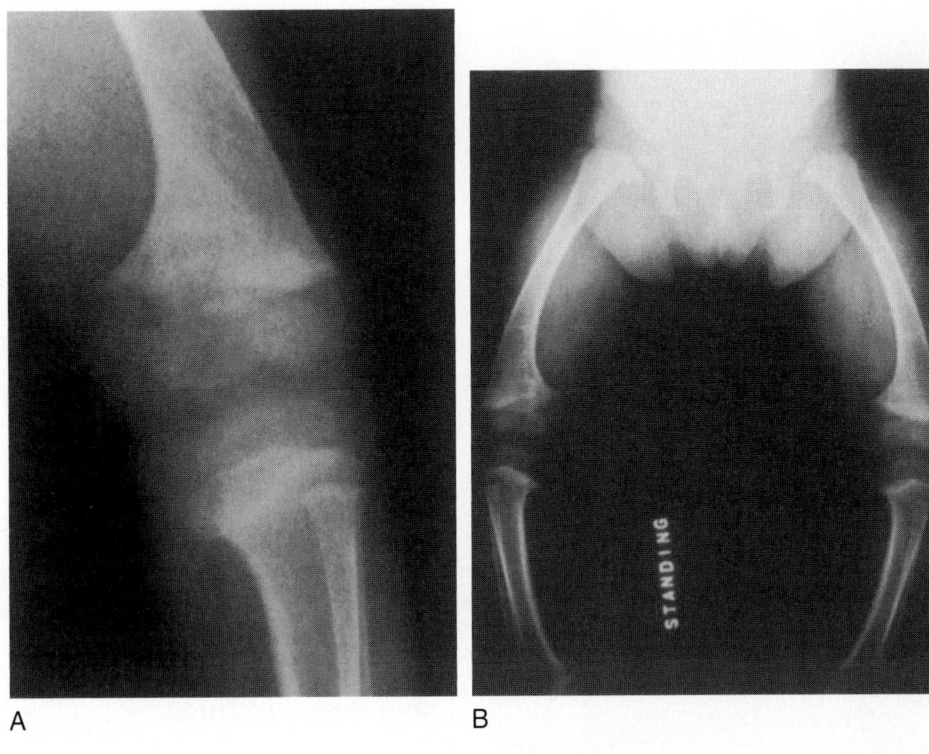

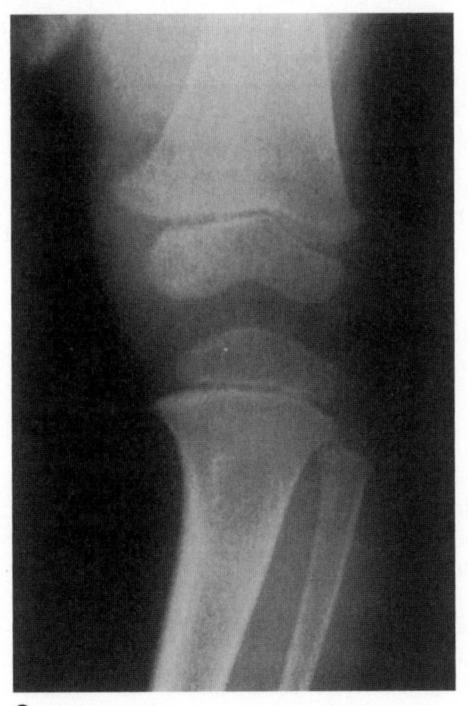

FIGURE 32-4 **A,** Hazy metaphysis with cupping in a young boy with rickets. **B,** Accentuated genu varum is present. **C,** With vitamin D replacement therapy, the bony lesions healed in 6 months.

Rickets of Prematurity

Very premature infants are particularly at risk for the development of nutritional rickets.[64,81,181,376] Risk factors include hepatobiliary disease, total parenteral nutrition, diuretic therapy, physical therapy with passive motion, and chest percussion therapy. These infants are seen with pathologic fractures in the neonatal intensive care unit. With treatment of the rickets, the fractures heal readily with minimal other treatment.[115] Resolution of the rachitic changes and fractures occurs as the infants gain weight.[258]

Drug-Induced Rickets

Certain antiepileptic medications have been known to produce rachitic changes in children.[16,110,348] Seizure

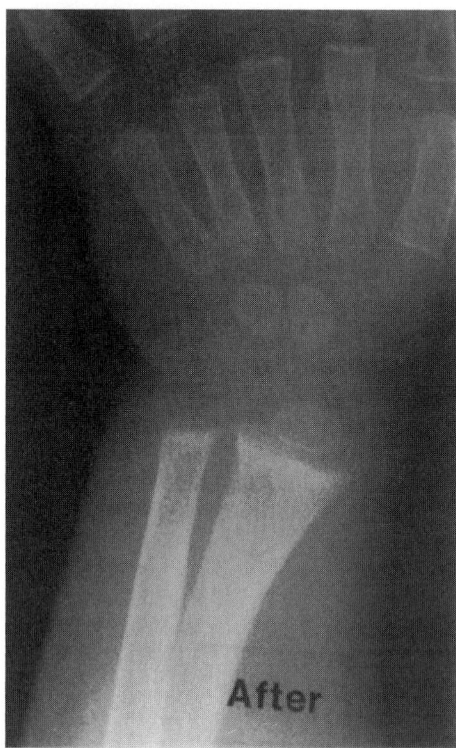

FIGURE 32-5 Radiographic appearance of the wrist of the girl whose radiographs (rickets) appear in Figure 32–4, after 4 months of treatment with vitamin D. The osteopenia has resolved and the physis is narrowed.

medications that affect the liver may induce the P-450 microsomal enzyme system and decrease levels of vitamin D. Hypocalcemia develops, which can aggravate the seizure disorder. Treatment with vitamin D is very helpful. The condition should be suspected in neurologic patients with seizures who begin sustaining frequent fractures.[280,281]

VITAMIN D–RESISTANT RICKETS

Vitamin D–resistant rickets, also known as familial hypophosphatemic rickets, encompasses a group of disorders in which normal dietary intake of vitamin D is insufficient to achieve normal mineralization of bone.[537] There are four major forms, the most common of which is inherited as an X-linked dominant trait, followed in frequency by an autosomal dominant type.[124,537,558] The inherent abnormality in familial vitamin D–resistant rickets is the renal tubule's inability to retain phosphate, which leads to phosphate diabetes and hypophosphatemia.[379] End-organ insensitivity to vitamin D is the cause of autosomal recessive vitamin D–resistant rickets.[70] This form is extremely hard to treat. The third form is characterized by failure of the kidney to perform the second hydroxylation of vitamin D.[124] This type rarely requires orthopaedic intervention because it is easily treated with the administration of dihydroxyvitamin D. Finally, renal tubular acidosis has traditionally been grouped with vitamin D–resistant rickets. In renal tubular acidosis, the kidney excretes fixed base and wastes bicarbonate. This leads to wasting of calcium and sodium as well. The alkaline urine results in precipitation of calcium and severe renal calcinosis.[68,350]

Tubular resorption of phosphate in the kidney is under control of the sodium/phosphate cotransporters located on the tubular cell membranes. Factors that decrease phosphate resorption include a high intake of dietary phosphate, acidosis, PTH, PTH-related peptide, glucocorticoid therapy, calcitonin, and vitamin D. Factors that increase phosphate reabsorption include a low phosphate diet, alkalosis, growth hormone, insulin, insulin-like growth factor I, and thyroid hormones. Recently discovered factors called phosphatonins have been found to cause phosphaturia. These include fibroblast growth factor 23, which was found in patients with tumor-induced osteomalacia and is secreted by the tumor cells. The same factor is also involved in the autosomal dominant form of hypophosphatemic rickets. Other phosphatonins may include matrix extracellular phosphoglycoprotein and secreted frizzled-related protein 4.[273]

Laboratory Findings

Laboratory studies reveal normal or nearly normal levels of calcium. PTH and vitamin D levels are normal, but the serum phosphate concentration is significantly decreased.[303-306,379] Urine assays for phosphate demonstrate an increased concentration of phosphate in urine. The serum alkaline phosphatase concentration is elevated (see Table 32–1).

Molecular Genetics

The gene for hypophosphatemic rickets has been localized. The X-linked dominant form of the disease is attributed to mutations in the *PEX* gene, located at Xp22.1.[230,443] The gene locus for autosomal dominant hypophosphatemic rickets has been located on chromosome 12p13.[140] The locus for an autosomal recessive form has also been identified.[300]

Clinical Features

The disease usually becomes apparent at a slightly older age than nutritional rickets does, with most patients becoming symptomatic between 1 and 2 years of age. Severe hypophosphatemic rickets can be recognized in early infancy, and when the disease is suspected because of the family history, laboratory determination of phosphorus concentrations can lead to the diagnosis in infants as young as 3 months.[343] The usual initial complaints are delayed walking and angular deformities of the lower extremities. In contrast to what is seen in nutritional rickets, systemic manifestations such as irritability and apathy are minimal.

Physical findings in hypophosphatemic rickets include skeletal deformities, which resemble those seen in nutritional rickets but, because of the chronicity of the disease, become far more severe. Once

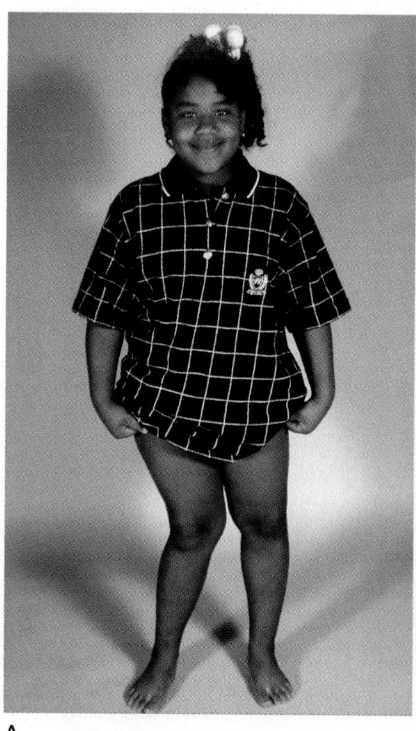
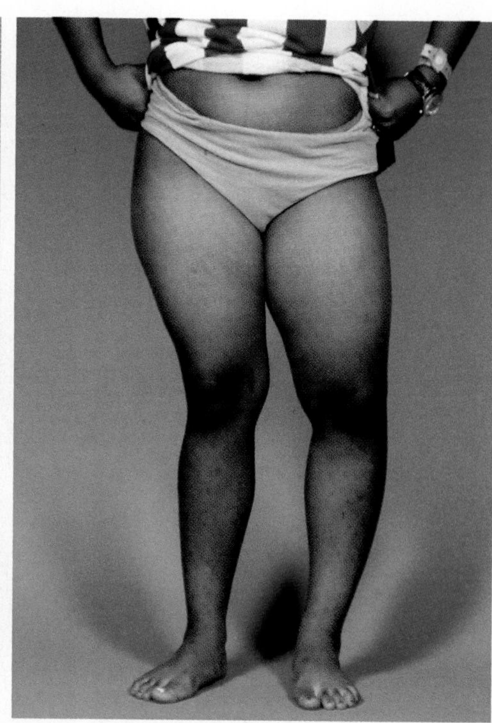

FIGURE 32–6 **A,** Unilateral genu varum in a 12-year-old child with poorly controlled vitamin D–resistant rickets. **B,** Same child at 15 years of age after right medial hemiepiphysiodesis of the femur. Left genu varum is now apparent.

affected children begin to walk, genu varum develops, although genu valgum may occur in some children (Fig. 32–6). Periarticular enlargement is present as a result of widening of the physes and metaphyses. The "rachitic rosary" may also occur.

Short stature is a feature of hypophosphatemic rickets. Height is usually 2 standard deviations below the mean for age in these patients.[499]

Radiographic Findings

The radiographic changes are the same as those seen in nutritional rickets and include physeal elongation and widening and indistinct osteopenic metaphyses. In the lower extremities, genu varum is obvious, and the distal femoral and proximal tibial physes are particularly widened medially (Fig. 32–7). Coxa vara is present, and there may be general anterior and lateral bowing of the entire femur. The varus of the tibia is also generalized, not only present proximally but also producing varus angulation of the ankle.

The upper extremities are involved as well, but to a lesser degree, because of absence of the influence of weight bearing (Fig. 32–8).

Treatment

MEDICAL TREATMENT

Medical treatment of hypophosphatemic rickets is best managed by a pediatric nephrologist with expertise in metabolic bone disease. The usual treatment consists of oral replacement of phosphorus in large doses and the administration of vitamin D.[310,421,546] Nephrocalcinosis is a significant complication of medical treatment.[502] In a recent study, renal calcinosis was present in 79% of treated children with hypophosphatemic rickets, and the severity of the calcinosis correlated with the dose of phosphorus.[533] Because nephrocalcinosis is a significant complication, the decision whether to offer treatment to children with hypophosphatemic rickets has become controversial.[202,275] Studies have shown that longitudinal growth is greater in children who undergo vitamin D treatment.[294,471]

Treatment of children with hypophosphatemic rickets with growth hormone has been shown to increase height and to have beneficial effects on bone density and phosphate retention.[453] Preliminary studies reported that the administration of growth hormone with vitamin D increases the serum phosphate concentration, and it may reduce the incidence of nephrocalcinosis.[385]

Recently, analogs of vitamin D_3 (1,25-dihydroxyvitamin D_3) have been developed and demonstrated to be several hundred times more potent than the original form in treating hereditary vitamin D–resistant rickets.[179,401,510]

ORTHOPAEDIC TREATMENT

The orthotic management of vitamin D–resistant rickets has not been efficacious. If patients are experiencing increasing pain or difficulty walking, surgical correction of angular deformities should be performed. It is important to work closely with the nephrologist or endocrinologist who is managing the medical therapy because calcium levels can suddenly climb in a patient who is immobilized after surgery. Discontinuation of vitamin D before surgery should be discussed.

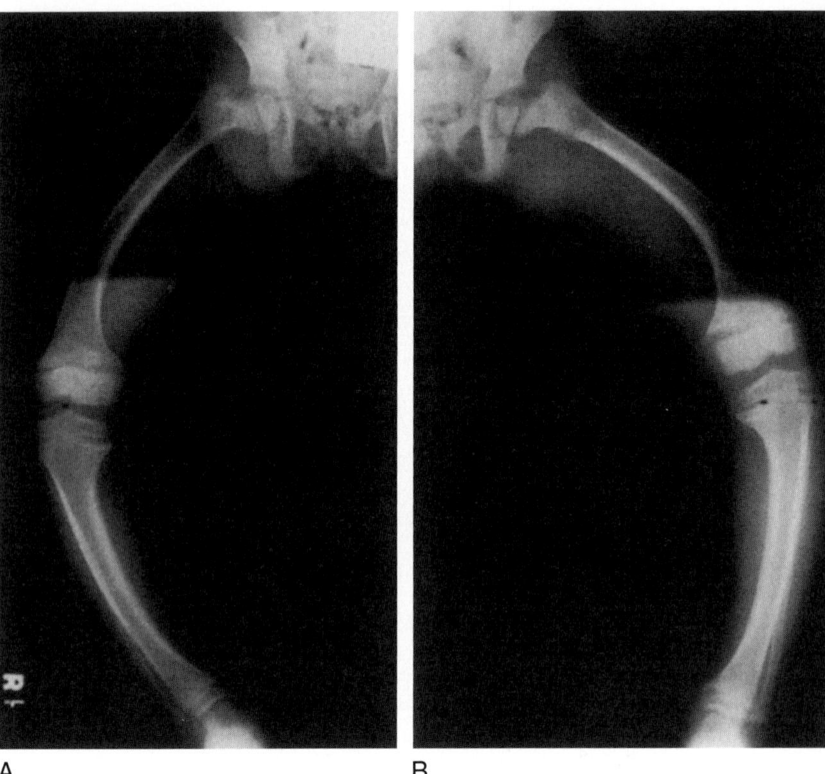

FIGURE 32–7 **A** and **B**, Anteroposterior radiographs of the left and right lower extremities of a standing 7-year-old child with familial hypophosphatemic rickets. Severe genu varum and anterolateral bowing of the femur are evident. The distal femoral and proximal tibial physes are widened medially. See Figures 32–9 and 32–10.

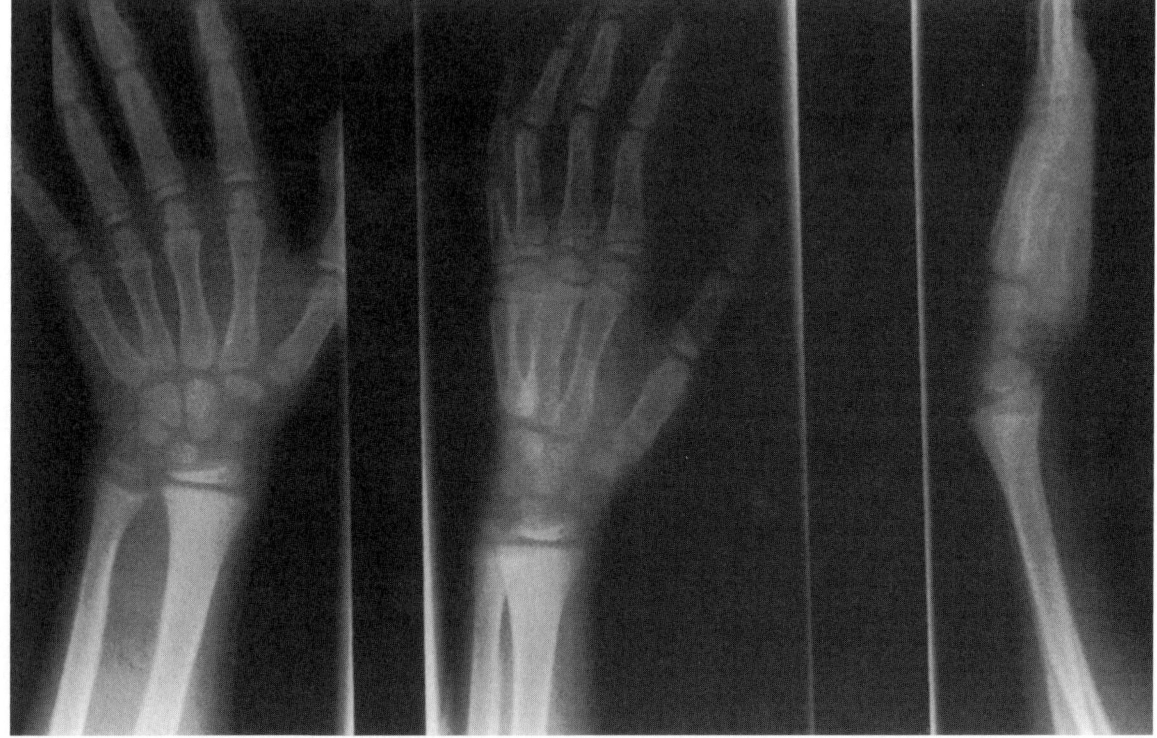

FIGURE 32–8 Physeal widening and metaphyseal cupping of the distal end of the radius and ulna in a 7-year-old child (same as in Fig. 32–8) with vitamin D–resistant rickets.

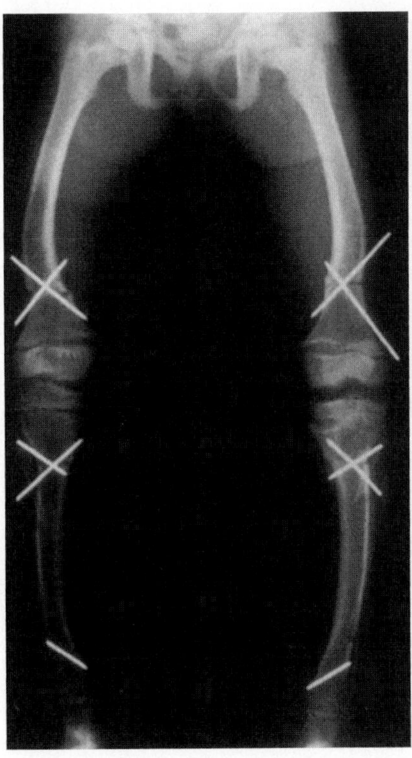

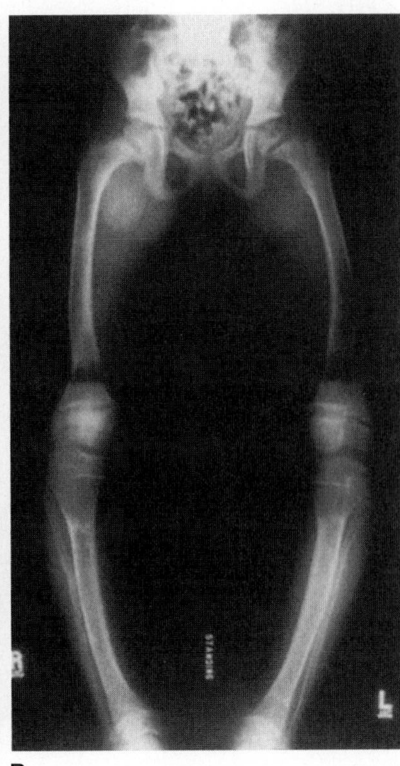

A B

FIGURE 32–9 Postoperative radiographs of the child whose imaging findings are shown in Figures 32–8 and 32–9. **A,** Appearance after distal femoral, proximal tibial, and distal tibial osteotomies for treatment of genu varum. **B,** Varus is recurring 1 year after surgery.

The deformity most commonly seen in patients with hypophosphatemic rickets is a gradual anterolateral bowing of the femur combined with tibia vara. Multilevel osteotomy is generally required to satisfactorily correct the mechanical axis of the limb (Fig. 32–9). The mechanical axis should be mildly overcorrected at surgery. The suggested fixation varies among reports. External fixation allows fine-tuning of the alignment postoperatively, when the patient is able to stand (Fig. 32–10).[245] Others advocate the use of intramedullary fixation or plating (Fig. 32–11).[159,444] Regardless of the type of fixation used, careful preoperative planning of the surgical treatment of these multiplanar deformities is crucial to restoring alignment.

Recurrent deformity is a common sequela of osteotomies in patients with hypophosphatemic rickets.[444] Younger patients have a higher risk of recurrence.[294] For this reason, milder deformities should not be corrected in early childhood. Some children have severe varus at a very young age that leads to thrust during gait. When gait is compromised or symptoms or pain is present, osteotomy should be performed and the alignment monitored for recurrent deformity.

Spinal deformity may be seen in patients with hypophosphatemic rickets. Kyphoscoliosis, Arnold-Chiari malformations, and spinal stenosis have all been described in patients with vitamin D–resistant rickets.[80,563]

Adults with hypophosphatemic rickets are prone to the development of arthritis. Degradation of articular cartilage resembling osteochondritis dissecans has been described. Joint stiffness and bone pain are common complaints.[159]

Tumor-Related Hypophosphatemic Rickets

An association between benign and malignant tumors and hypophosphatemic rickets has been described and termed *oncogenic hypophosphatemic osteomalacia*.[261,262,301,331,442] Conditions such as neurofibromatosis and fibrous dysplasia produce rickets on rare occasion.[320,456] Osteoblastoma, hemangiopericytoma of bone, and skin tumors have produced rachitic changes in bone by disrupting renal tubular resorption of phosphate.[204,279] Certain tumors have been found to secrete phosphatonins, such as fibroblast growth factor 23, that result in phosphaturia.[273] Oncogenic rickets should be suspected in older children with hypophosphatemic rickets because the true genetic form is generally apparent by 2 years of age. The rachitic changes resolve with excision of the tumor.[19,383,456]

Renal Osteodystrophy

As the rate of successful treatment of renal failure in children with kidney transplants has increased, the prevalence of renal osteodystrophy has risen. Manifestations of renal osteodystrophy are present in 66% to 79% of children with renal failure.[157,225] Children in whom renal disease develops in infancy or early childhood are more likely to have osteodystrophy than those who are older when the renal disease develops.[225] Renal failure in children is due to diseases such as chronic pyelonephritis, congenital abnormalities, and polycystic kidney disease. Renal osteodystrophy is more common in renal disease secondary to

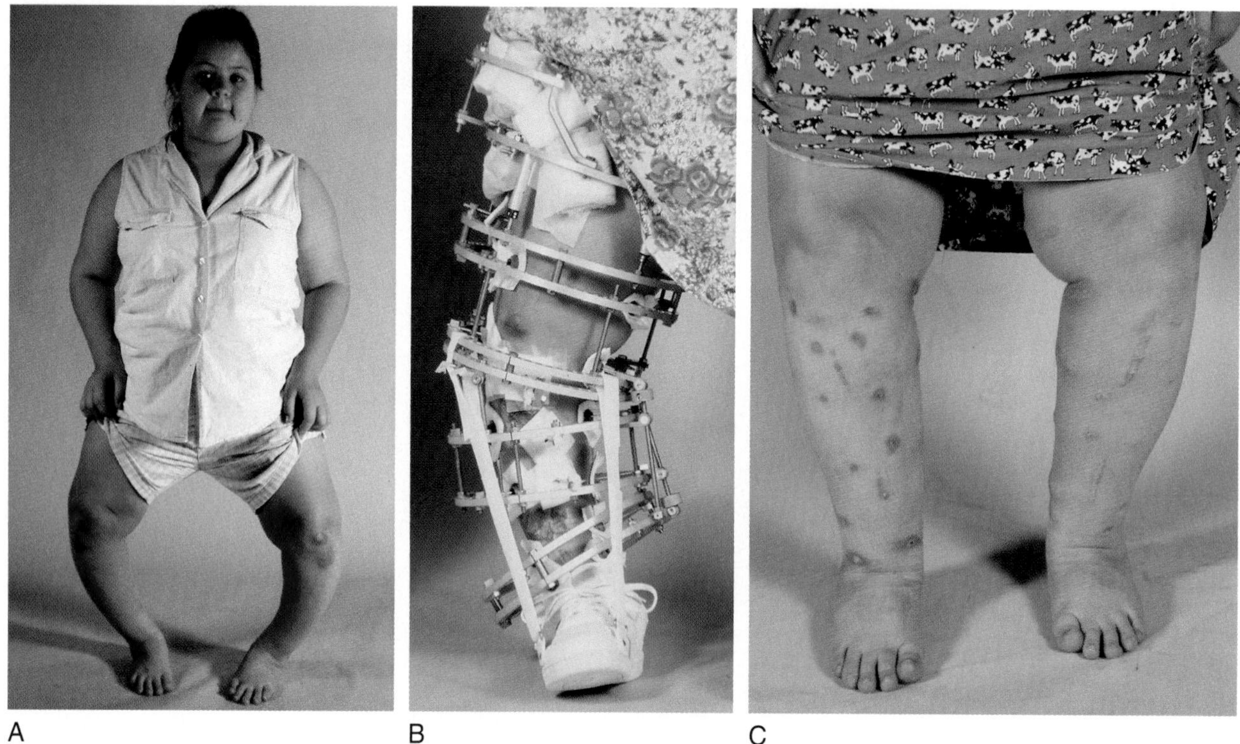

FIGURE 32-10 **A,** Clinical appearance of a 13-year-old girl with severe genu varum secondary to vitamin D–resistant rickets. Calluses on the knees were due to crawling because of knee pain. **B,** Treatment consisted of distal femoral, proximal tibial, and distal tibial corticotomies and gradual correction with the Ilizarov device. Surgery on the two legs was staged because of the extent of the frame. **C,** Clinical appearance of the lower extremities at the end of treatment.

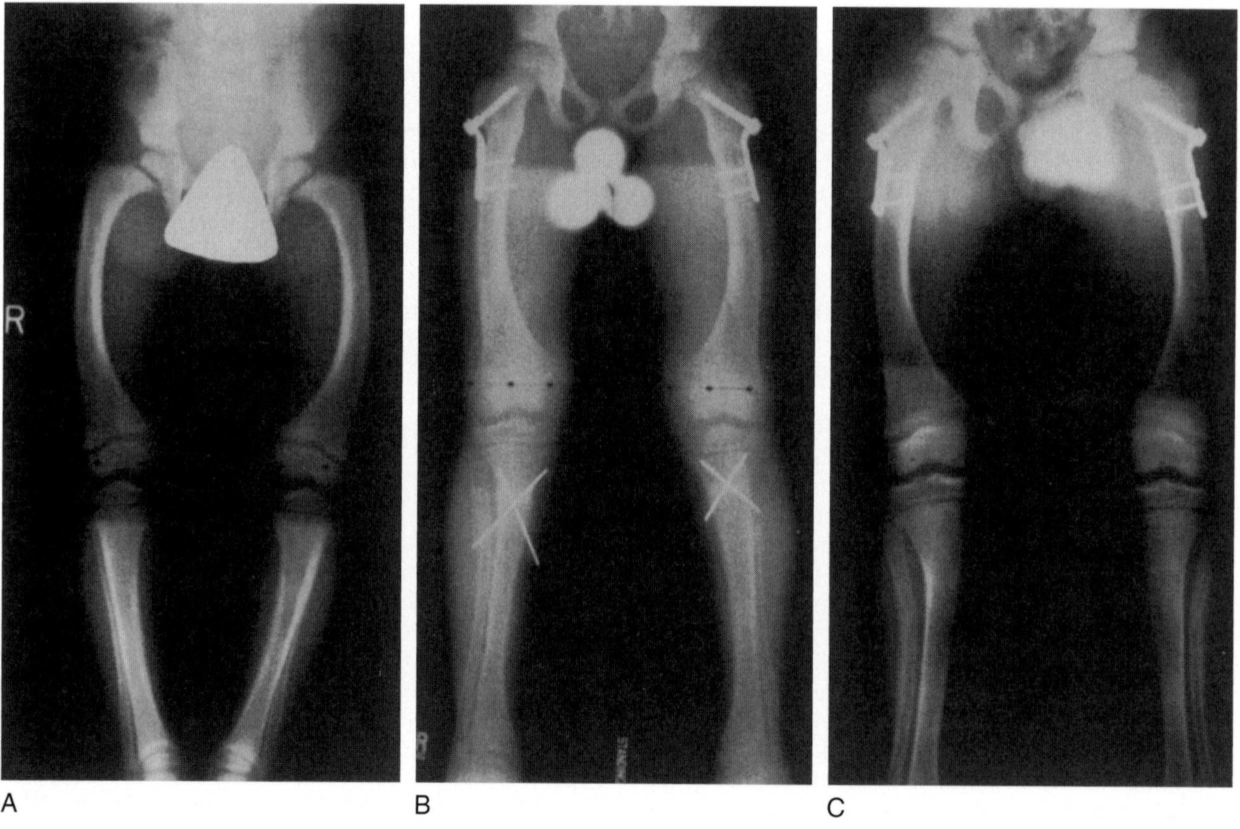

FIGURE 32-11 **A,** Coxa vara and genu varum in a 5-year-old boy with vitamin D–resistant rickets. **B,** Postoperative radiograph obtained after corrective osteotomy with plate fixation of the proximal femora and osteotomy with K-wire fixation of the proximal tibiae. **C,** Alignment remained satisfactory at 2-year follow-up.

congenital or hereditary conditions than in acquired renal failure. Renal osteodystrophy is distinctly different from either nutritional or hypophosphatemic rickets.[305] It is often driven by the presence of secondary hyperparathyroidism, which leads to activation of osteoclasts and resorption of bone. This type of bone involvement is termed *high-turnover disease*.

With improved control of hyperparathyroidism, another form of osteodystrophy termed *low-turnover disease* has been recognized. This adynamic disorder has been attributed to the use of high doses of exogenous calcium, either as phosphate-binding agents or during dialysis, and to aggressive calcitriol therapy. Parathyroidectomy may also contribute to this syndrome.[459,460] In one report, 60% of patients with chronic renal disease had a low-turnover disorder, whereas 40% had high-turnover osteitis fibrosa cystica.[174] Thus, children with renal failure are at risk for both types of metabolic bone disorder.[58] Patients with slowly progressive forms of renal disease such as tubulointerstitial disease are at risk for the hyperparathyroid form of disease. Those with more rapidly progressive diseases such as the glomerular syndromes are more likely to have an adynamic metabolism.[562] It is important to note that the adynamic form may be present with a high parathormone level.[174]

Pathophysiology

The pathophysiology of high-turnover renal osteodystrophy begins with the damaged glomerulus' inability to excrete phosphorus.[305,306,378] Hyperphosphatemia shuts down the production of dihydroxyvitamin D.[88] Calcium absorption from the small intestine is diminished in the absence of vitamin D. Hypocalcemia triggers the release of PTH, which enables demineralization of bone to increase the serum calcium level.[497] The hyperphosphatemia worsens with the release of minerals from bones, thereby leading to a cycle of bony resorption. PTH also acts directly to stimulate osteoclast activity, which worsens the bony changes and leads to osteitis fibrosa.

High levels of serum phosphate are universal in renal failure. In the setting of elevated phosphate levels, calcium may precipitate out and lead to ectopic calcification in tissues. The usual areas for ectopic calcification are the corneas and conjunctivae, skin, blood vessels, and periarticular soft tissues.[46,47,299,378]

Pathology

Features of both rickets and hyperparathyroidism are present in renal osteodystrophy (Fig. 32–12).[497] The rachitic changes consist of failure to replace proliferating cartilage cells by new bone. Physeal cartilage persists into the metaphysis. The physis is widened, and the zone of provisional calcification is irregular as a result of the lack of normal calcification of maturing physeal cartilage. Bony trabeculae have abundant osteoid and widened osteoid seams.

The histologic features of hyperparathyroidism include osteoclastic resorption of bone. Marrow is

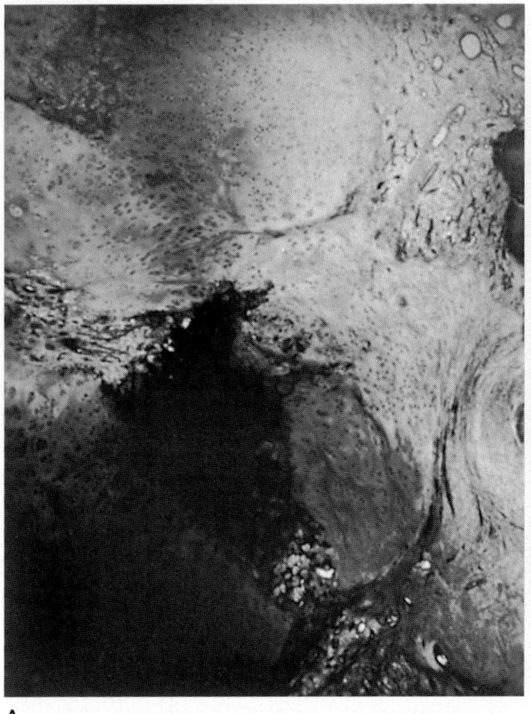
A

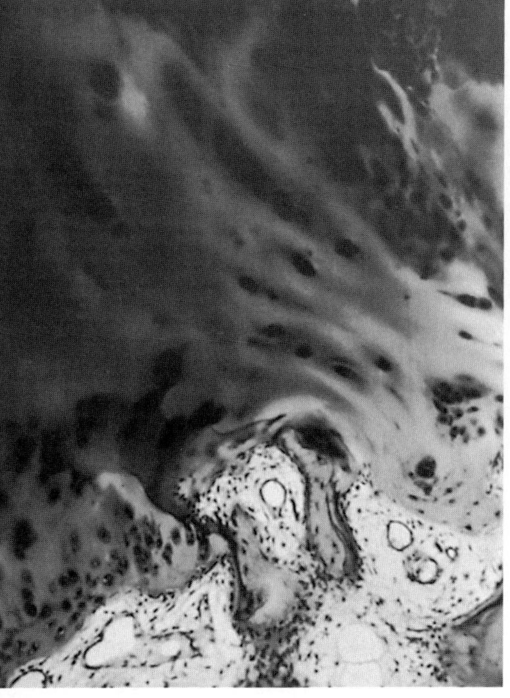
B

FIGURE 32–12 Histologic findings of osteodystrophy secondary to chronic renal insufficiency. **A,** Photomicrograph of a section through the widened physis showing extension of cartilage cells into the metaphysis (×25). **B,** Higher magnification (×100) of the same area. Note the uncalcified osteoid tissue and replacement of normal fatty bone marrow by hyperplastic fibrous tissue.

replaced by hyperplastic fibrous tissue. Patchy formation of new bone leads to areas of osteosclerosis, present in 20% of patients with renal osteodystrophy.

Laboratory Findings

The blood urea nitrogen level is high, as is the serum creatinine concentration. Levels of serum phosphate, alkaline phosphatase, and PTH are elevated. The serum calcium concentration is almost always low, as is the albumin level. Acidosis is present, and vitamin D levels are decreased (see Table 32–1).

Bone biopsy may be necessary for accurate diagnosis and can help guide treatment.[163,323]

Clinical Features

Children with renal osteodystrophy resemble those with rickets.[14] They are short for their age,[201,225] and their bones are fragile.[380] Because of the effects of weight bearing, lower extremity involvement is more severe than upper extremity involvement. Patients may complain of bone pain, and fractures occur easily. Skeletal deformities may consist of genu valgum, periarticular enlargement of the long bones, and slipped capital femoral epiphysis (SCFE).[35,189,208,292,330,475] Gait may be abnormal because of muscular weakness, and a Trendelenburg gait is present in patients with SCFE. Enlargement of the costochondral cartilage may produce a "rachitic rosary," as in nutritional rickets.

Radiographic Findings

Generalized osteopenia is notable, with thinning of the cortices and indistinct bony trabeculae.[12,119,329,543] Overall, the bone looks blurry, like ground glass. The skull takes on a salt-and-pepper appearance because of the coarse granular pattern. The physes are increased in thickness, and the provisional zone of calcification looks uncalcified and indistinct (Fig. 32–13).[195,225] Cupping of the physes is not present, unlike the case in nutritional rickets.

Changes of hyperparathyroidism develop with time.[508] SCFE may be seen, even in young patients (Fig. 32–14).[66] The terminal tufts of the distal phalanges of the fingers resorb, as do the lateral end of the clavicle and the symphysis pubis.[61,177,427,428] Subperiosteal resorption also occurs in the metacarpals and ulna.[262]

Osteosclerosis, when present, is most common at the base of the skull and in the vertebrae.[210,270] The horizontal striped appearance of the spine is called a "rugger jersey" spine.

In severe and prolonged renal failure, peculiar aggressive-appearing lytic areas may develop within the long bones, termed *brown tumors*. The surrounding cortex is thinned, then expands. The margins of a brown tumor are not well defined. Pathologic fracture may result. Radiographically, these lesions mimic malignancy. They are well visualized on magnetic resonance imaging (MRI).[371]

Because many patients with renal failure (and all patients who have undergone kidney transplantation) are treated with steroids, the typical skeletal abnormalities seen with chronic steroid use may develop. Osteonecrosis is common and develops most frequently in the femoral heads (Fig. 32–15).

Treatment

MEDICAL TREATMENT

Treatment of the underlying renal disease is of primary importance. Dialysis and transplantation are extending the life spans of these patients. Medical treatment of osteodystrophy starts with the prescription of vitamin D.[332,431,458] Because the abnormal kidney cannot participate in the hydroxylation of provitamin D, the 1,25-dihydroxy form is given.[347] Serum calcium levels are closely monitored because too much calcium leads to ectopic calcification. The use of high-dose pulsed intravenous, intraperitoneal, and oral calcitriol therapy has significantly decreased serum PTH levels and retarded the progression of osteitis fibrosa.[13,461] Treatment of acidosis with sodium bicarbonate is also important in improving the metabolic bone disease. Phosphate-binding agents have been administered for the management of hyperphosphatemia, but their use is falling out of favor because of problems with aluminum toxicity, which can lead to encephalopathy and worsening of the osteomalacia and osteodystrophy.[31,332,374] Bone biopsy is useful in monitoring response to therapy and in surveillance for such complications.[302] Aluminum toxicity is treated by administering aluminum-chelating agents.

Decreased growth is a significant problem for a child with renal insufficiency, probably because of disturbances in the growth hormone–insulin-like growth factor I axis. Administration of recombinant human growth hormone can restore growth, thus making it possible to achieve normal or improved adult height.[193,201,328,333,459] Growth hormone biomechanically weakens the physis, so vigilance on the part of the treating physician for the development of SCFE or physiolysis must be maintained.

In renal osteodystrophy that is recalcitrant to medical treatment, parathyroidectomy may play a role in control of the bony disease.[148]

ORTHOPAEDIC TREATMENT

Patients with renal osteodystrophy are referred to the orthopaedic surgeon for the treatment of three problems: (1) angular deformity of the lower extremities, (2) SCFE, and (3) avascular necrosis.[86] In the surgical correction of any of the orthopaedic deformities in renal osteodystrophy, the hazards and complications should be carefully weighed because of the increased risks in this patient population. Anemia, hypertension, bleeding tendencies, and electrolyte imbalances are all present in patients with renal failure. The risk for infection is also increased, particularly if the patient has received a transplant and is undergoing immunosuppressive therapy. Despite these potential risks, with careful coordination of surgery and perioperative

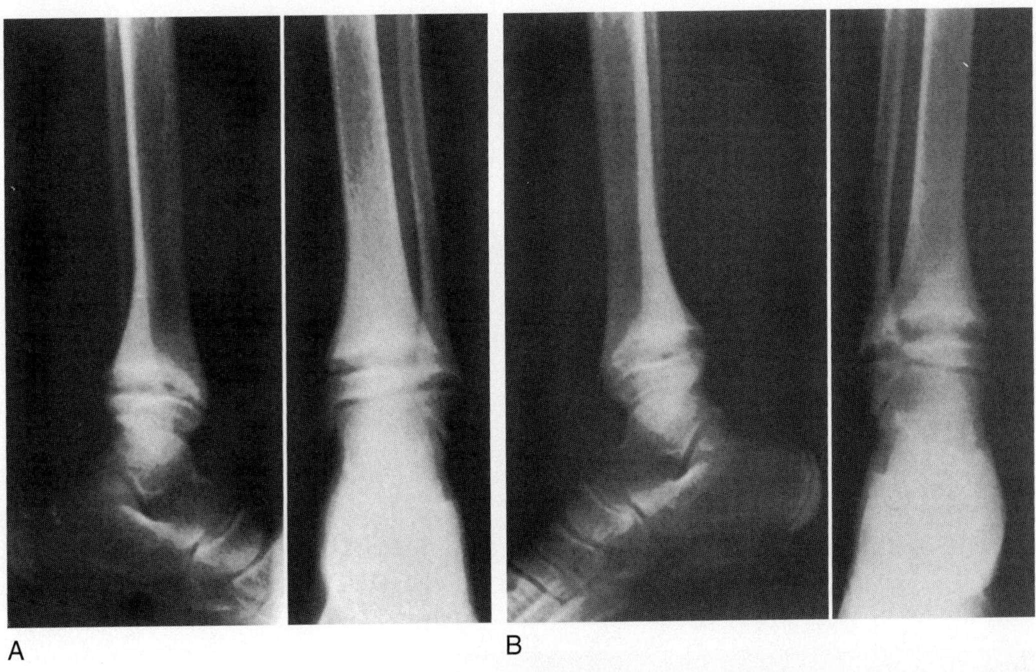

FIGURE 32–13 Osteodystrophy secondary to chronic renal insufficiency in a young girl with progressive slipped capital femoral epiphyses. Anteroposterior **(A)** and lateral **(B)** radiographs of both ankles at the age of 12 years showed increased thickness of the physes and irregularity of the metaphysis at the zone of provisional calcification. **C,** Lateral view of the skull showing a ground-glass appearance. Note the absence of lamina dura of the teeth.

C

management with the pediatric nephrologist, osteotomy can be performed safely.

Angular Deformity

Angular deformity occurs in renal osteodystrophy because the bone is soft, undermineralized, and prone to bend with weight bearing. Genu valgum is the most common deformity,[252] but genu varum may occur in some patients. It has been proposed that if the onset of renal osteodystrophy occurs before 4 years of age, varus deformity may develop because the normal alignment of the leg is in mild varus, which then is accentuated as the bone becomes weak. Likewise, older children are predisposed to the development of genu valgum because of the normal valgus alignment of the lower extremity.[118] Valgus at the ankle may accompany the genu valgum.

Some milder deformities will correct with medical treatment of the renal osteodystrophy.[58] Deformities do not respond well to bracing. If the patient is symptomatic and has had optimal medical management of the osteodystrophy without resolution of deformity, osteotomy is performed.[86] Preoperative assessment of the deformity with long-leg standing radiographs will permit the surgeon to decide where the deformity is and how many osteotomies will be needed to best correct the mechanical axis. Usually, the distal end of the femur is the site of greatest deformity, but some patients also need a proximal tibial osteotomy. Internal or external fixation may be used. Application of the Ilizarov device in metabolic bone disease has met with

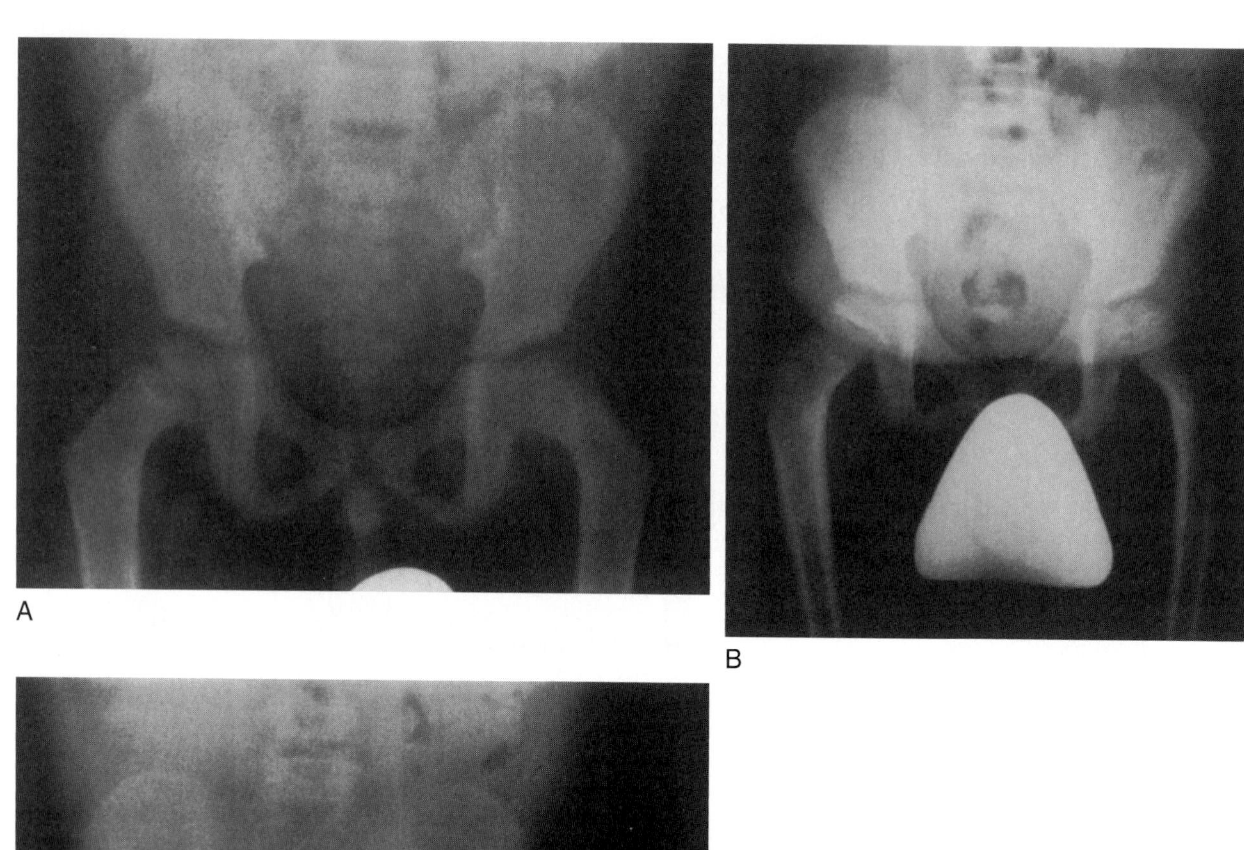

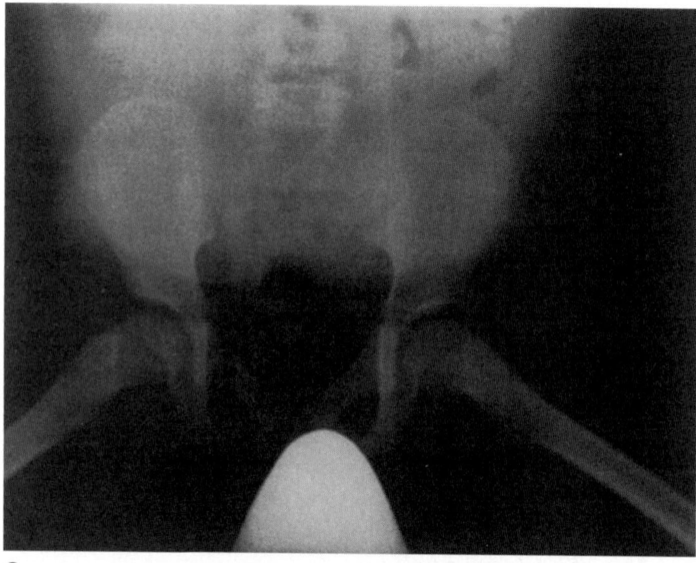

FIGURE 32–14 **A,** Anteroposterior (AP) radiograph of a 7-year-old boy with hip pain. Slipped capital femoral epiphysis is present, osteopenia is obvious, and the physes are wide. AP **(B)** and lateral **(C)** radiographs of the hips after treatment of renal failure with dialysis. The proximal femoral physes have narrowed.

success, although healing was delayed.[498] Recurrence is common in patients with continuing metabolic disease, so medical treatment should be optimized before osteotomy whenever possible. Elevation of the serum alkaline phosphatase concentration above 500 U/L is a good marker of ongoing metabolic bone disease.[118,373] Bone biopsy may be needed to establish that the bone is metabolically healthy before osteotomy.[118] Milder deformity may respond to physeal stapling.[373]

A subset of patients with genu valgum show evidence of a proximal tibial growth disturbance in the form of physeal abnormality in the proximal lateral tibial physis. Oppenheim and associates liken the physeal widening of the lateral physis to that seen in the medial physis in Blount's disease.[375] These patients benefit from tibial osteotomy for realignment.

Slipped Capital Femoral Epiphysis

SCFE is associated with renal osteodystrophy, but the clinical picture of a patient with renal slips differs from the usual clinical scenario.[35,105,189,363] Often the patients are younger than those with idiopathic SCFE, and obesity is not commonly seen. Bilaterality is extremely common. Radiographs show more physeal widening than is usual in SCFE, and osteopenia and blurring of the metaphysis may be obvious.[330] The orthopaedic surgeon should be aware of the radiographic appearance of renal SCFE because on rare occasion patients may seek treatment of hip or groin pain while being unaware of their renal disease. In such cases it is up to the orthopaedic surgeon to make the diagnosis of renal osteodystrophy and promptly refer the child to a nephrologist for appropriate treatment.

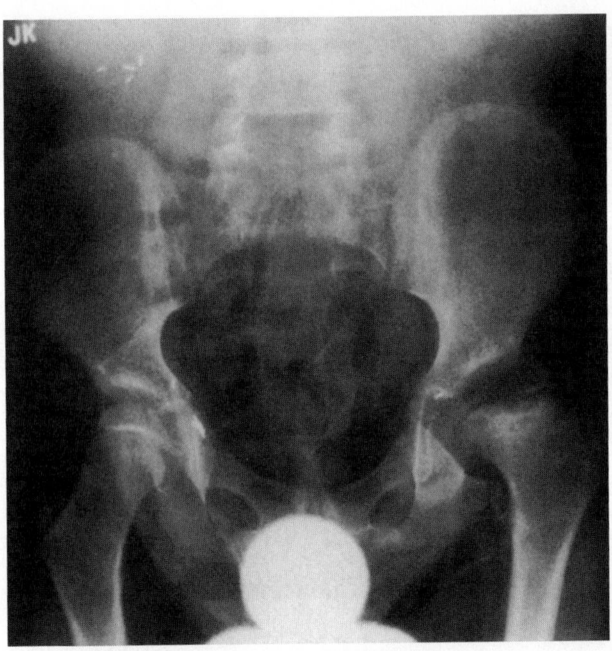

FIGURE 32–15 Avascular necrosis of the left hip in a 7-year-old boy after renal transplantation and steroid therapy.

There are inherent problems in the surgical treatment of SCFE in renal osteodystrophy. The goal of routine treatment of SCFE is to stop proximal femoral physeal growth and thus heal the slip. This may not be a desirable goal in a very young child with renal osteodystrophy. Additionally, physeal healing may be very difficult to achieve in the presence of osteitis fibrosa and metabolic imbalance. Fortunately, in many patients the hip pain resolves and the proximal femoral physis narrows with mineral treatment of the renal osteodystrophy, so surgery is not necessary in every patient with renal SCFE.[292,475] If the slip is displaced or if symptoms persist despite good medical control of the osteodystrophy, surgery may be needed. Fixation with special partially threaded screws to achieve stability and cross but not close the physis has been performed in a small series of patients with renal slips.[208] In an adolescent with SCFE secondary to renal disease, epiphyseal closure with in situ fixation is the treatment of choice once the metabolic bone disease is under appropriate treatment (Fig. 32–16).

Physiolysis has been described in other physes in children with renal osteodystrophy.[515] Sites at which physiolysis has occurred include the distal femur, proximal humerus, and distal radius and ulna (Fig. 32–17). Treatment consists of medical management of the metabolic bone disease and cast immobilization.[18,511]

Avascular Necrosis

Another orthopaedic complication seen in patients with renal failure is avascular necrosis, most commonly of the femoral head.[377] It may be unilateral or bilateral. Prolonged steroid use (commonly needed after renal transplantation) is the probable cause of avascular necrosis in most children, although it has been seen in the hips of some children with renal failure who were not taking steroids. Treatment is symptomatic.

Primary Hyperparathyroidism

Primary hyperparathyroidism results from hyperplasia or adenoma of the parathyroid glands, which leads to increased secretion of PTH.[11,54] The increased PTH stimulates osteoclastic resorption of bone, which produces hypercalcemia. The initial symptoms of hyperparathyroidism are lethargy, bone pain, and abdominal complaints. The diagnosis is usually made late in the course of disease, when the child has abdominal symptoms, toxicity, and a hypercalcemic crisis.[108,257,523] The symptoms of hyperparathyroidism are common and nonspecific, so the diagnosis is frequently missed at initial evaluation.[278] Prolonged hypercalcemia leads to ectopic calcification in tissues and the formation of renal calculi. Abdominal pain and constipation result from the decreased abdominal motility. Hypertension is commonly present. In severe cases, the patient may become obtunded.

In about two thirds of the patients the cause is an adenoma, and in the remainder hyperplasia of the gland is usually found.[112,226,257,418] Patients who have undergone head and neck irradiation are particularly susceptible to the development of parathyroid adenomas.[95,185] Hyperparathyroidism can also be a component of the multiple endocrine neoplasia syndromes, which are inherited and can rarely occur in childhood.[224,403,516,517] There are also very rare genetic forms of hyperparathyroidism,[114] some of which are self-limiting with medical treatment[207,362] whereas others are life-threatening.[254,325] Infants born to parents with familial hypocalciuric hypercalcemia are at risk for the development of severe neonatal hyperparathyroidism as a result of mutations in the calcium-sensing receptor gene.[62,394]

The radiographic findings resemble those of renal osteodystrophy. Bone resorption is seen in the terminal tufts of the phalanges and in the clavicle. The bone appears osteopenic. Angular deformities resembling those seen in rickets can occur.[337]

Laboratory evaluation generally reveals hypercalcemia, hypophosphatemia, and an elevated alkaline phosphatase concentration. Rarely, the calcium and phosphate concentrations are normal. PTH is elevated on direct assays.

Treatment is directed toward correcting the cause of the hyperparathyroidism. In cases of adenoma, tumor resection is performed. Adenomas are imaged with radionuclide scans. It is not uncommon for multiple glands to be involved.[441] Hypercalcemic crisis is treated by hydration, calciuresis, inhibition of bone calcium resorption, and treatment of the parathyroid abnormality.[520,523]

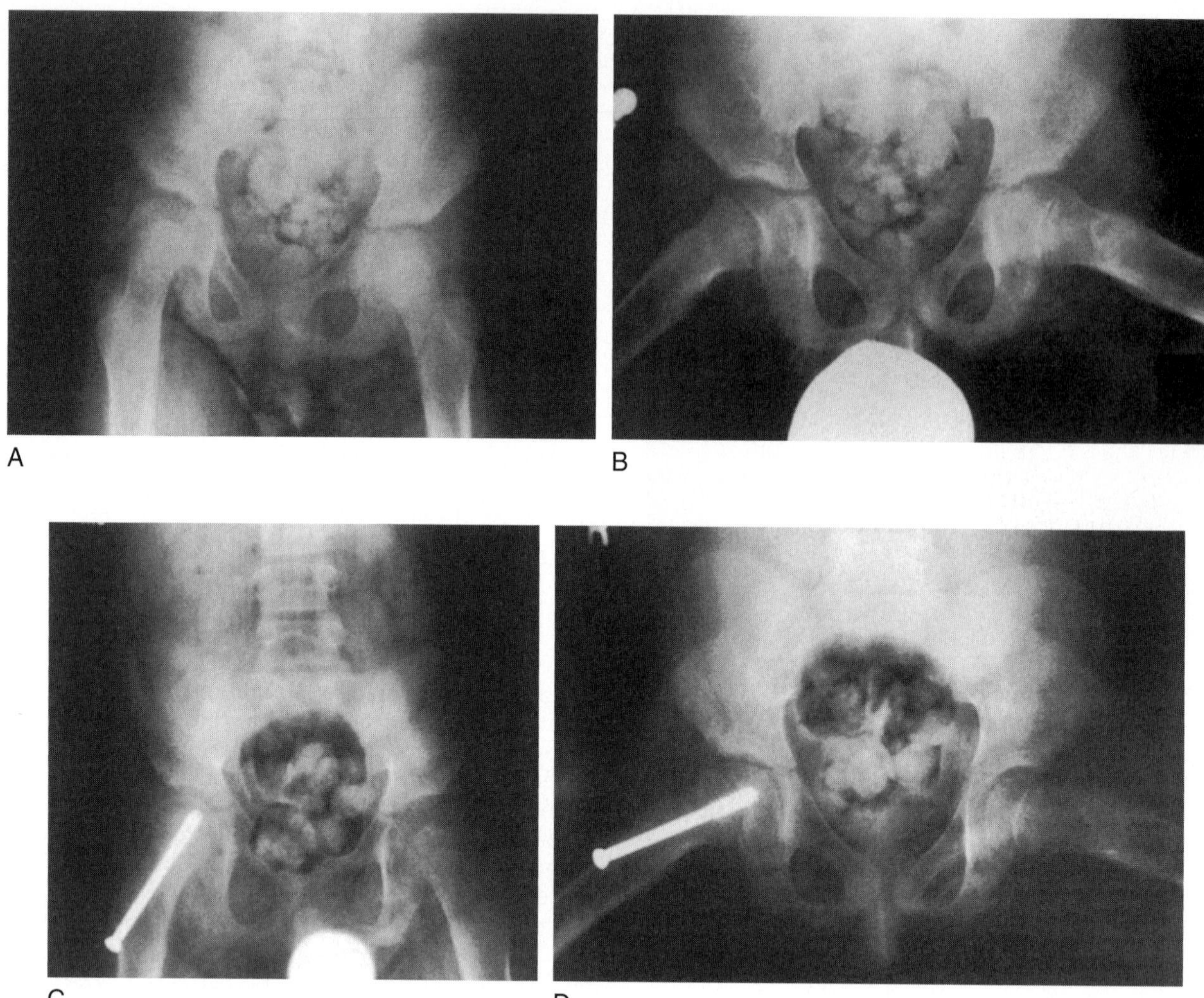

FIGURE 32-16 **A** and **B,** Valgus slipped capital femoral epiphysis in an 11-year-old child after renal transplantation and hypothyroidism. **C** and **D,** In situ fixation was performed.

Idiopathic Hypoparathyroidism

Idiopathic hypoparathyroidism is caused by failure of the parathyroid glands to produce PTH. Inherited forms of hypoparathyroidism exist. An autosomal dominant type is the result of mutations on chromosome 3q13 in the gene encoding for the G protein–coupled Ca^{2+}-sensing receptor, which regulates PTH secretion.[32,120,160] Hypoparathyroidism is also associated with deletions in chromosome 22q11, the gene responsible for DiGeorge's syndrome and cardiac defects.[196,468] Another autosomal dominant syndrome consists of hypoparathyroidism, sensorineural deafness, and renal dysplasia.[209] Other autosomal recessive types are associated with growth retardation, seizures, and severe mental retardation.[316,384,430] Finally, X-linked recessive hypothyroidism has been seen in males.[527,551]

Hypoparathyroidism should be distinguished from pseudohypoparathyroidism, in which production of PTH is increased but the end organs cannot respond to the hormone.

The initial symptoms of hypoparathyroidism are those of hypocalcemia: tetany, paresthesias, and lethargy. The skin is dry, the hair brittle and scanty. The teeth erupt late and fall out early. Cataracts may be present, and papilledema may occur. Mental retardation is seen in very young children.

Laboratory evaluation reveals low serum calcium levels, and the urinary calcium concentration is diminished. Hypoproteinemia should be considered because the serum calcium concentration is normally decreased in patients with decreased albumin concentrations. The serum phosphorus concentration is elevated. If a test dose of PTH is administered, urinary phosphate reabsorption falls and plasma levels of cyclic adenosine monophosphate (cAMP) rise.[265]

Radiographs may be normal or may reveal increased radiopacity of the cortices of the long bones. Soft tissue calcification can occur, including calcification of the basal ganglia.[327]

Treatment is administration of vitamin D and PTH.[22,465] Nephrocalcinosis is a known complication of vitamin D therapy, however.[540] Treatment with inject-

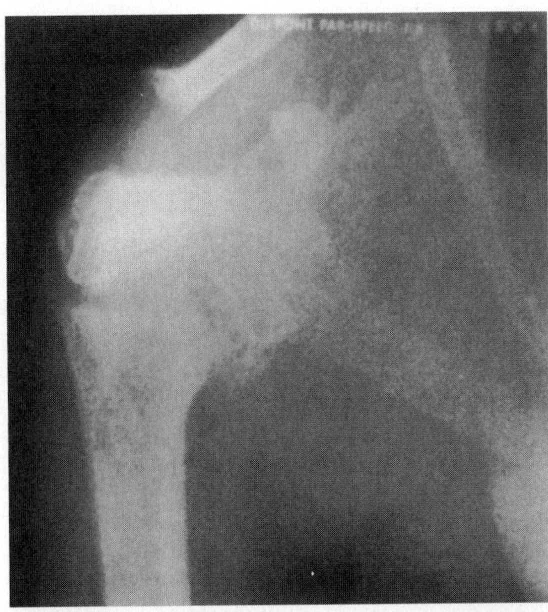

FIGURE 32-17 Osteodystrophy secondary to chronic renal insufficiency in a young girl. An anteroposterior radiograph shows slipping of the humeral head.

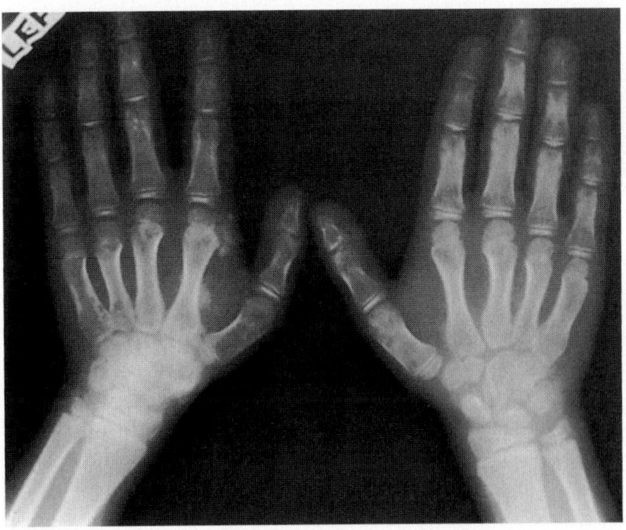

FIGURE 32-18 Pseudohypoparathyroidism. An anteroposterior radiograph of the hands shows shortening (brachydactyly) of the first, fourth, and fifth metacarpals.

able human PTH alone effectively maintains a normal serum calcium level, with less risk for nephrocalcinosis.[556,557] Infants with hypoparathyroidism complicated by tetany may need calcium infusion. Allograft transplantation of parathyroid cells is investigational at present.[521]

There is no orthopaedic treatment specific to the disease.

PSEUDOHYPOPARATHYROIDISM

Pseudohypoparathyroidism is similar to hypoparathyroidism in its clinical and radiographic manifestations but differs in that it does not respond to administration of exogenous PTH. The parathyroid glands are hyperplastic and secrete large amounts of the hormone, but the kidneys are resistant to PTH.[155] Bone changes consistent with hyperparathyroidism occur because the skeleton does respond to the elevated PTH.[149] Thus, findings include hypocalcemia and hyperphosphatemia resembling hypoparathyroidism, as well as osteitis fibrosa cystica resembling hyperparathyroidism.[149,166] The skeletal changes seen in pseudohypoparathyroidism are also termed *Albright's osteodystrophy* because Albright and his associates Burnett, Smith, and Parson were the first to describe the disease.[5]

The etiology is usually genetic. There are four subtypes of pseudohypoparathyroidism: Ia, Ib, Ic, and II. The molecular genetics of type Ia disease is associated with deficient cellular activity of the α-subunit of the guanine nucleotide–binding protein ($G_s\alpha$) that stimulates adenylyl cyclase.[4,490] Many mutations in the $G_s\alpha$ protein gene have been identified.[161,288] Patients with type Ia disease have been found to suffer from multiple endocrinopathies, such as hypothyroidism and growth hormone deficiency.[469]

In type Ib pseudohypoparathyroidism, mutations have been found in chromosome 20q, which contains another stimulatory G protein gene.[244] Yet another genetic association exists between pseudohypoparathyroidism and DiGeorge's syndrome, with mutations present on chromosome 22q11.[104]

The clinical appearance of affected infants is normal, with skeletal changes gradually becoming apparent at 2 to 4 years of age. There is a characteristic shortening of the metacarpals, especially the first, fourth, and fifth, termed *brachydactyly* (Fig. 32–18).[91] When the hands are clenched into a fist, dimples are present at the sites of the knuckles of the fourth and fifth digits, thus giving rise to the mnemonic "knuckle, knuckle, dimple, dimple." Multiple exostoses may be present, and the radius may be bowed. Patients are very short and often obese, and the facies has been described as moon shaped.[372] Heterotopic calcifications occur, especially in the periarticular tissues.[410,467] Intracerebral calcifications have also been described.[478] Sensorineural hearing loss is common.[255]

Pseudohypoparathyroidism may be associated with hypothyroidism, Turner's syndrome, and diabetes. Brachydactyly may also be seen in Turner's syndrome and in myositis ossificans progressiva.

The diagnosis is made by injecting PTH. A patient with pseudohypoparathyroidism is unable to respond to the exogenous hormone, so there will not be a rise in serum calcium or urinary phosphate levels, and plasma cAMP will also not rise.[265,503]

Treatment has been with vitamin D, which has led to problems with nephrocalcinosis.[540]

HYPERVITAMINOSIS D

Hypervitaminosis D is a result of the ingestion of excessive doses of vitamin D.[56,206,236] Patients at risk are those who are taking vitamin D for the treatment of such metabolic bone diseases as vitamin D–resistant rickets and hypoparathyroidism.[465] The elevated vitamin D promotes intestinal absorption of calcium and thereby leads to hypercalcemia. The optimal nutritional requirements for vitamin D in newborns and infants have been established.[334]

Pathology

Histologically, wide osteoid seams are found around the trabeculae, similar to what is seen in rickets.[200] The physis, however, is well calcified and normal in width and length. Metastatic calcification may be found in the kidneys, arteries, thyroid, pancreas, lungs, stomach, and brain. Deposition of calcium salts in the kidneys and degenerative changes in the arteries may produce significant morbidity.

Laboratory Findings

The hypercalcemia can be severe. The serum phosphate concentration is normal with a diminished alkaline phosphatase concentration.[392]

Clinical Features

Anorexia, constipation, nausea and vomiting, polyuria, and thirst are the early manifestations. The child feels very tired. With progression of the intoxication, mental depression and stupor develop. Renal failure and hypertension are common.

Radiographic Findings

Dense metaphyseal bands are seen in the long bones and result from an increase in the proximal zone of calcification. The diaphyses show osteopenia as a result of demineralization. Osteosclerosis is visible at the base of the skull, and there may be premature closure of the sutures. The vertebral end-plates are dense. Metastatic calcifications are seen in soft tissues (Fig. 32–19).[94,221]

Treatment

Treatment is medical and consists of immediate cessation of vitamin D supplements. Diuretics are given, with replacement of volume with saline. Because dehydration can be fatal, serum electrolyte levels must be carefully monitored. Steroids inhibit calcium absorption in the kidney and gut and are helpful in correcting the calcium level.[555] Bisphosphonates inhibit bone resorption and have been useful in treating vitamin D intoxication.[472] Sodium phosphate should not be given because its administration leads to ectopic calcification.

SCURVY

Scurvy is caused by a nutritional deficiency of vitamin C (ascorbic acid).[27,135] The disease is rare and is now most commonly seen in patients who are

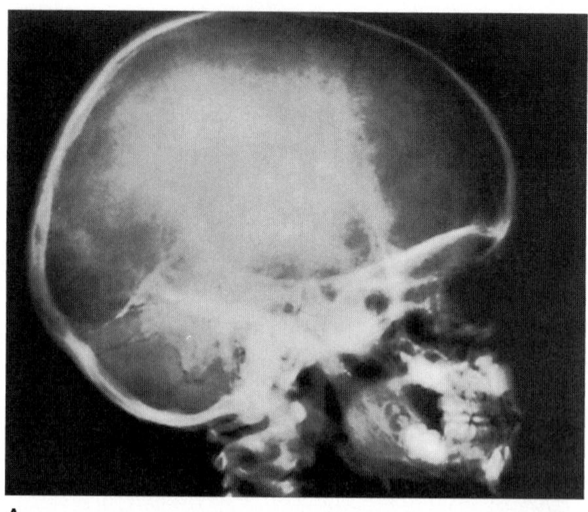

A

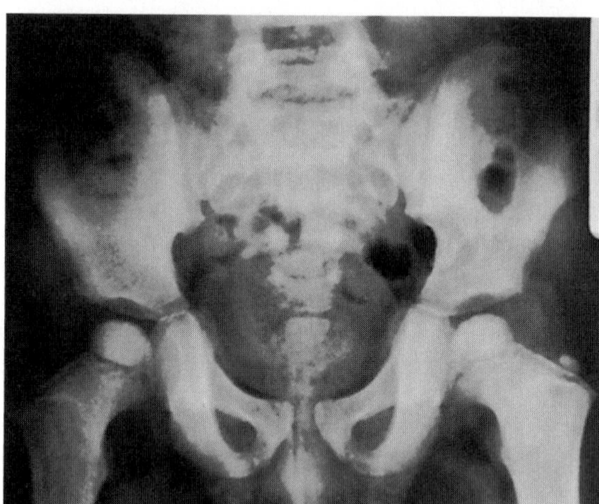

B

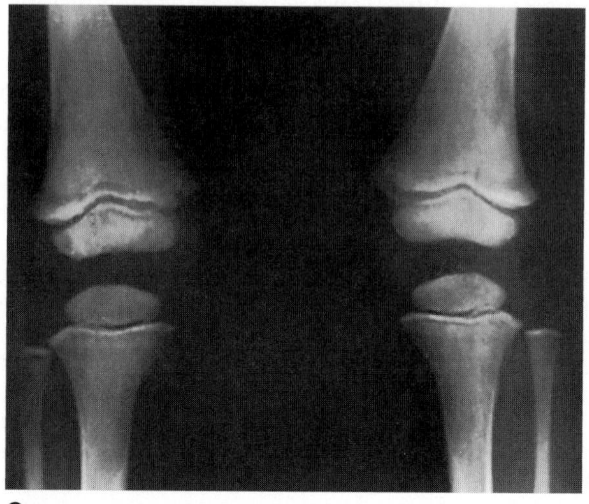

C

FIGURE 32–19 Hypervitaminosis D in a 5-year-old boy who had taken 50,000 IU of vitamin D per day for the past 14 months. **A,** Lateral views of the skull showing metastatic calcification of the cerebral and cerebellar falces. **B** and **C,** Anteroposterior view of both hips and lower limbs. Note the increased radiopacity of the metaphyses.

following extreme diets, such as patients with anorexia nervosa.[326,335] Historically, scurvy was described in sailors whose diets lacked vitamin C during long sea voyages.[518]

Pathology

When vitamin C is deficient, collagen synthesis is impaired.[29,164] Vitamin C is necessary for the hydroxylation of lysine and proline to hydroxylysine and hydroxyproline, two amino acids crucial to proper cross-linking of the triple helix of collagen.[400] The result is primitive collagen formation throughout the body, including the blood vessels, which predisposes to hemorrhage.

Osteoblasts become dysfunctional, with failure to produce osteoid tissue and form new bone. Chondroblasts, however, continue to function normally, and mineralization is unaffected. This leads to persistence of cartilage cells, and calcified chondroid approaches the metaphysis. Radiographically, an opaque white line termed *Frankel's line* is seen at the junction of the physis and metaphysis.

Generalized osteoporosis results from lack of osteoid and new bone. Osteoclasts are normal, but osteoblasts become flattened, with a resemblance to connective tissue fibroblasts. The bone trabeculae and the cortices of the long bones are thin and fragile.

Hemorrhage and fractures are common, but the attempt at repair of these injuries is disorderly. The provisional zone of calcification is weak, which leads to epiphyseal separations.

In the teeth, dentin formation is abnormal because of the defective collagen.

Clinical Features

Scurvy develops after 6 to 12 months of dietary deprivation of vitamin C. For this reason it is not seen in neonates. Early manifestations consist of loss of appetite, irritability, and failure to thrive. Hemorrhage of the gums is common, and they become bluish and swollen. Subperiosteal hemorrhage is a distinctive sign that occurs most commonly in the distal femur and tibia and the proximal humerus.[173] The limbs become exquisitely tender, so much so that the infant screams on movement of the affected areas. The child lies still in the frog-leg position to minimize pain, a posture called *pseudoparalysis.* The limbs are swollen and bruised. Beading of the ribs at the costochondral junctions may occur. Hemorrhage may also develop in the soft tissues, including the joints,[283] kidneys, and gut, and petechiae may be seen.[151,263,559] The hair takes on a coiled appearance.[369] Anemia and impaired wound healing are common. Severe hypertension has been described.[541]

Radiographic Findings

The changes of scurvy are best seen at the knees, wrists, and proximal humeri (Fig. 32–20).[67,69] Osteopenia is the first change seen, with thinning of the cortices.[151] The zone of provisional calcification increases in width and opacity (Fränkel's line) because of failure of resorption of the calcified cartilaginous matrix, and it stands out in comparison to the severely osteopenic metaphyses. The margins of the epiphyses appear relatively sclerotic, a finding termed "ringing of the epiphyses" or "Wimberger's sign." Lateral spur formation at the ends of the metaphysis is produced by outward projection of the zone of provisional calcification. The "scurvy line" or "scorbutic zone" is a radiolucent transverse band adjacent to the dense provisional zone. The corner or "angle" sign of scurvy is a peripheral metaphyseal cleft caused by a defect in the spongiosa and cortex adjacent to the provisional zone of calcification. Epiphyseal separation may occur.[357,486,487]

Subperiosteal hemorrhage most commonly occurs at the femur, tibia, or humerus and is initially seen as an increase in soft tissue density. The hemorrhage becomes radiodense as the scurvy is treated and the lesions calcify.

The development of a physeal bar in a patient with scurvy has been described.[218]

Differential Diagnosis

The most common entity that scurvy is mistaken for is osteomyelitis. The symptoms of pain, tenderness, subperiosteal soft tissue swelling, and pseudoparalysis resemble the symptoms of infection. Because infection is common and scurvy is extremely rare, the condition can be misdiagnosed initially. The sedimentation rate, C-reactive protein level, and white blood cell count are normal in scurvy, however. Other diagnoses to be considered for this clinical picture include polio,[415] leukemia, and purpuric conditions such as Henoch-Schönlein purpura and thrombocytopenic purpura. Syphilis may be suspected[524] but usually occurs earlier.

Serum levels of vitamin C may be difficult to interpret in scurvy. A more reliable test is the absence of vitamin C in the buffy coat of centrifuged blood.

Treatment

Treatment is administration of vitamin C. Rapid recovery is usual, with the pain and tenderness resolving.

Scurvy is prevented by adequate intake of vitamin C, defined as 50 mg/day for infants and children and 75 to 100 mg/day for adults adenylyl cyclase. Intoxication does not occur.

HYPERVITAMINOSIS A

Vitamin A is a fat-soluble vitamin whose primary biologic functions are concerned with skeletal growth, maintenance and regeneration of epithelial tissues, and preservation of visual purple in the retina. It is also necessary for membrane stability. The normal plasma level of vitamin A is 80 to 100 IU/100 mL. Hypervitaminosis A is very rare and usually results from inappropriate use of vitamin supplements.[41,175,464]

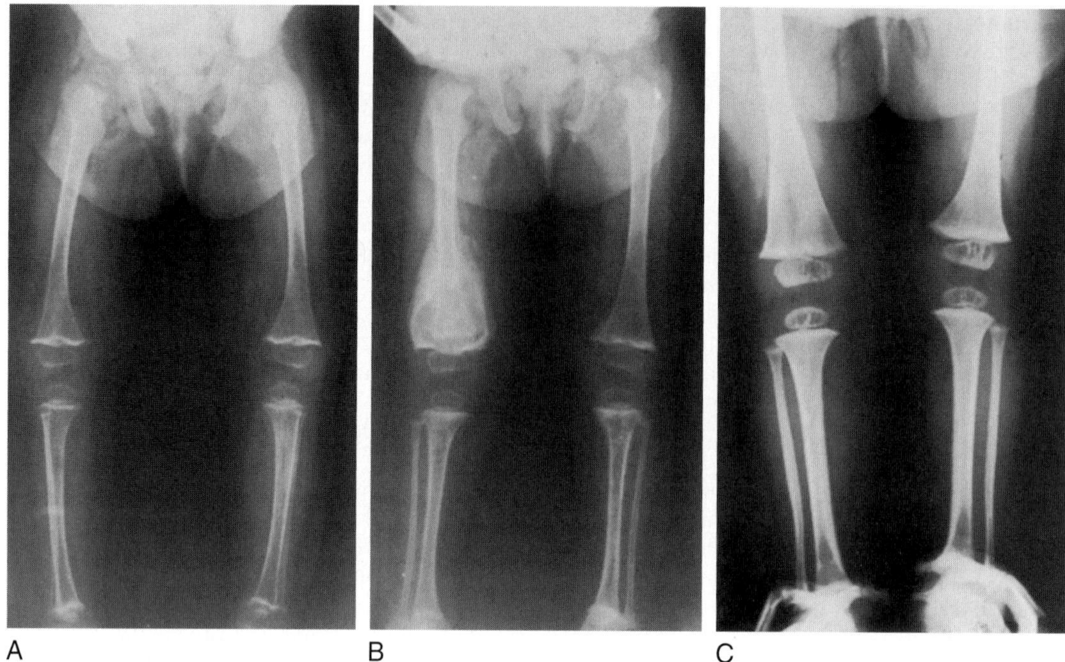

FIGURE 32–20 Scurvy in a 10-month-old infant. **A,** An anteroposterior radiograph of both lower limbs demonstrates early changes in the scorbutic bones. Note the generalized osteoporosis with rarefaction of the spongiosa and atrophy of the cortex. There is relatively increased opacity of the provisional zones of calcification at the ends of the metaphyses and around the margins of the epiphyseal centers of ossification ("ringing of the epiphyses"). **B,** Two weeks after treatment with ascorbic acid, marked calcification of subperiosteal hematoma of the right femur has occurred. Such minimal calcification is also evident in the medial aspects of the distal left femoral shaft and proximal left tibia. Note the multiple metaphyseal spur formation. **C,** Three months later there are further radiographic signs of healing scurvy. The cortices have become thicker and the spongiosa has almost normal density. Note the persistence of rarefaction in the epiphyseal centers.

Retinoids used for acne also contain vitamin A and can lead to toxicity.[45,397,485]

Clinical Features

Clinically, the soft tissues overlying the hyperostotic bones are swollen and tender. Proliferation of basal cells and hyperkeratinization cause dry, itchy skin.[192] Anorexia, vomiting, and lethargy are caused by increased intracranial pressure.[48] The child fails to thrive. Hepatomegaly with cirrhosis-like liver damage or splenomegaly may be present.[153]

Radiographic Findings

The development of bone changes in patients with hypervitaminosis A is slow, so radiographs are normal initially. For this reason, radiographs are normal in children younger than age 1 year. Once changes do occur, there is periosteal hyperostosis and thickening of the cortex of the long bones.[78] The ulna, radius, metacarpals, and metatarsals are particularly affected. The mandible is spared, a fact that distinguishes hypervitaminosis A from Caffey's disease. Subperiosteal new bone formation is seen (Fig. 32–21). Bone scintigraphy shows increased uptake. Premature partial or complete physeal closure may be present.[342,395,445]

Diagnosis

The diagnosis is made by determining the plasma level of vitamin A, which will be elevated 5 to 15 times the normal value. Hypercalcemia can be present.[162,167] Hypervitaminosis A must be differentiated from infantile cortical hyperostosis (Caffey's disease), scurvy, and congenital syphilis.[532]

Treatment

Treatment entails total cessation of administration of vitamin A and eliminating all foods containing vitamin A from the diet. Because of the great body reserves of vitamin A, the hyperostosis will disappear only after a long period, although the systemic symptoms resolve quickly. Growth of the long bones should be monitored because premature physeal closure may not become apparent for years after the initial insult.

HYPOPHOSPHATASIA

Hypophosphatasia is a rare, genetically determined error of metabolism in which a deficiency of alkaline phosphatase in plasma and tissues leads to abnormal mineralization of bone. There is wide variation in the severity of the disease, with the prognosis related to

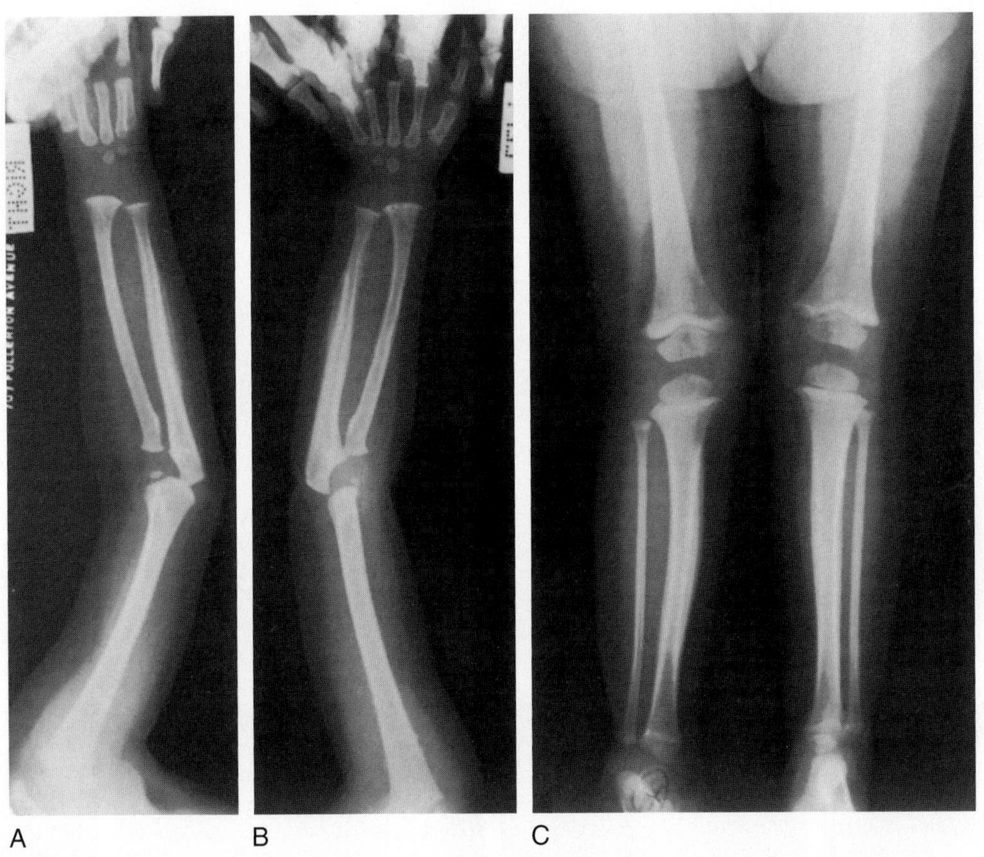

FIGURE 32–21 Hypervitaminosis A in a 2-year-old child. Note the subperiosteal new bone formation and cortical thickening of both tibiae and both ulnae. The mandible and other facial bones are not affected. **A** and **B**, Radiographs of the right and left forearms. **C**, Radiograph of both lower limbs.

the age at onset. Several forms of hypophosphatasia exist—perinatal, infantile, childhood, and adult.[31,414]

Inheritance

The gene for hypophosphatasia is the tissue-nonspecific alkaline phosphatase gene (*TNSALP*), and many different mutations have been described within this gene.[79,194,214] Autosomal recessive inheritance seems to lead to the lethal perinatal form and the infantile type, whereas autosomal dominant transmission produces milder phenotypes. Heterozygous carriers of hypophosphatasia can be detected by abnormally diminished alkaline phosphatase concentrations in plasma.

Pathology

The pathology seen in hypophosphatasia closely resembles that seen in patients with rickets. Osteoid production proceeds unharmed, but without alkaline phosphatase, mineralization of osteoid cannot occur.[548] This leads to widening of the physis with persistence of the provisional zone of calcification (which cannot calcify) and islands of cartilage continuing down into the metaphysis. The normal columnar arrangement of the chondrocytes of the growth plate is disturbed.

If hypercalcemia is present, heterotopic calcification can occur, especially in the kidney.

Laboratory Findings

The hallmark of hypophosphatasia is a decrease or lack of alkaline phosphatase. The enzyme is decreased not only in serum but also in such tissues as the kidneys, bones, leukocytes, and spleen. Serum phosphorus, vitamin D, and PTH levels are normal, but hypercalcemia may be present, especially in young children. Characteristic findings in urine are elevated levels of phosphoethanolamine (which may be elevated in other endocrinopathies) and inorganic pyrophosphate. Pyridoxal-5′-phosphate levels are also increased in hypophosphatasia in relation to disease severity.[231]

Disease carriers have been found to have decreased serum alkaline phosphatase levels and increased urinary pyrophosphate levels.[298]

Clinical Features and Radiographic Findings

PERINATAL HYPOPHOSPHATASIA

The clinical findings vary with the age at which the disease is manifested. In the severe perinatal (or

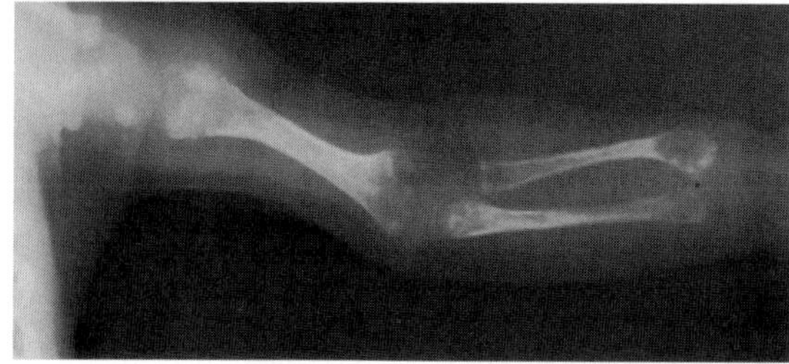

A

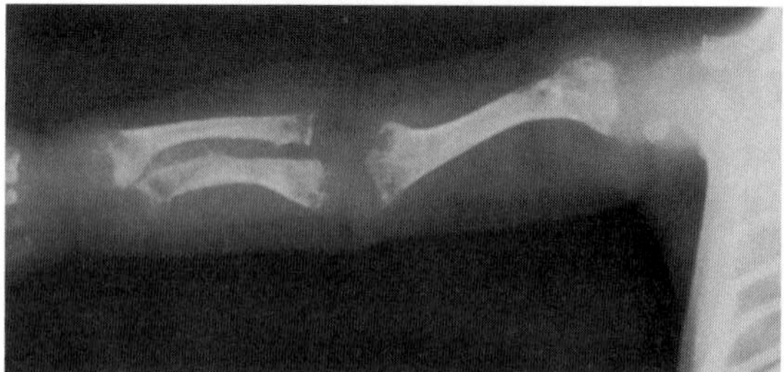

B

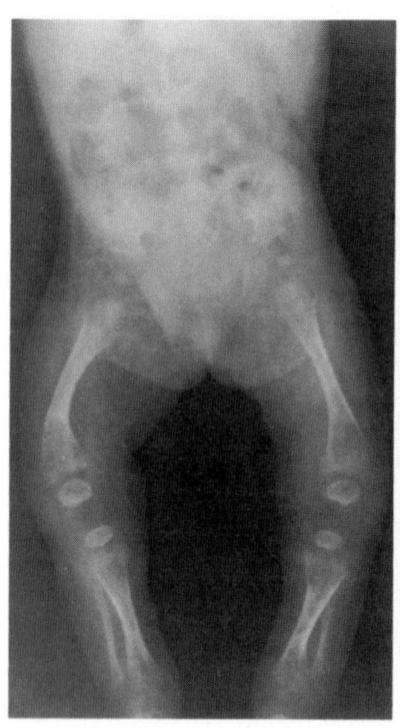

C

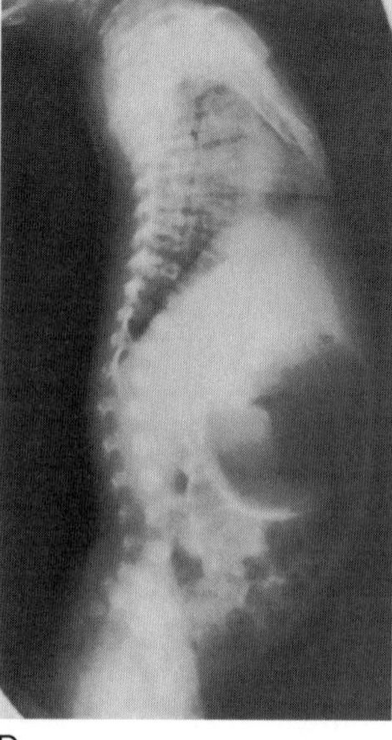

D

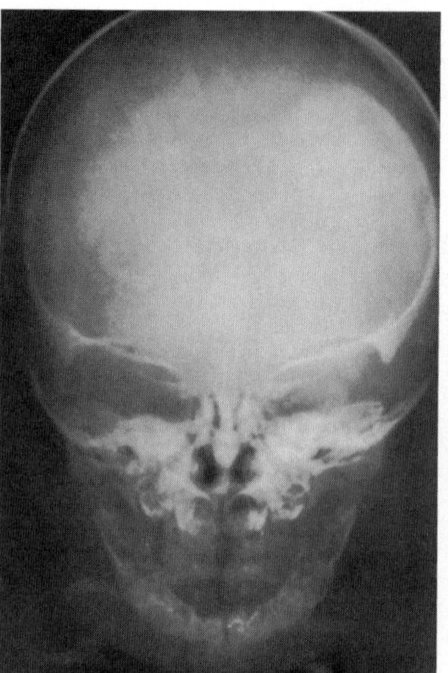

E

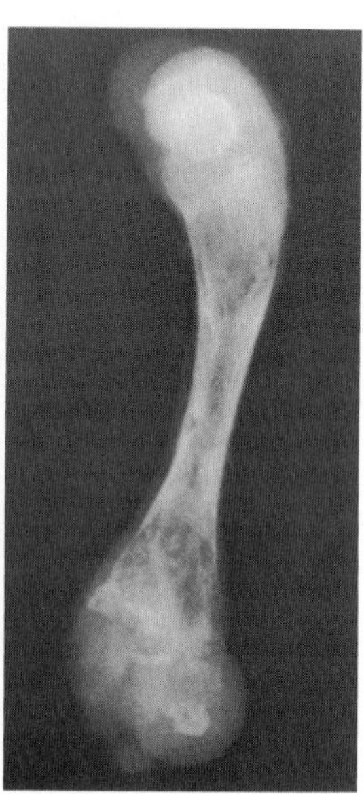

F

FIGURE 32-22 Typical radiographic changes of hypophosphatasia in a 4-month-old infant. **A** and **B**, Both upper limbs. **C**, Lower limbs. **D**, Spine (see text for discussion). **E**, Skull. **F**, Femur, obtained at autopsy (see text for discussion).

congenital) form, the infants may be stillborn. If they survive birth, they usually die from respiratory infections in early infancy.

Radiographs of infants with perinatal hypophosphatasia reveal diffuse, severe demineralization of the entire skeleton (Fig. 32–22). Ossification of the skull is incomplete, and the suture lines are very wide. The ribs are unossified at the ends and slender in the middle. The pelvis is small, soft, and poorly mineralized. The vertebral bodies are paper-thin and the neural arches cannot be seen. The long bones have jagged, rarefied defects extending into the metaphysis.

INFANTILE HYPOPHOSPHATASIA

The onset of symptoms in the infantile form is later in infancy, usually around 6 months of age. Affected children fail to thrive and experience anorexia, vomiting, dehydration, fever, hypotonia, and sometimes seizures.

Demineralization of the bones occurs but is not as marked as in the perinatal form. The bones look rachitic, with widened physes, bossing of the skull, bowing of the ribs, and flaring of the metaphyses of the long bones and costochondral junctions. Lucent streaks in the metaphyses represent nests of unossified physeal cartilage. Fractures and bowing of the extremities are common. The cranial sutures are initially wide but close prematurely, thereby leading to increased intracranial pressure.

Dentition is poor, and the primary teeth fall out very early.[90,539] Hypercalcemia may cause renal calcinosis. Renal failure and hypertension then follow.

Children who survive early infancy tend to improve clinically with time. Stature is normal in the infant, but as the child matures, dwarfism because of lack of normal enchondral bone growth becomes noticeable.

ADULT HYPOPHOSPHATASIA

A rare adult form of hypophosphatasia exists. Clinically, the disease usually becomes apparent with a fracture. Osteomalacia is present.

Prenatal Diagnosis

Hypophosphatasia can be diagnosed in fetuses. Ultrasound shows deficient ossification of the fetal skull.[250] A definitive diagnosis can be established by amniocentesis and molecular genetic testing to search for mutations in *TNSALP* in at-risk infants.[215]

Differential Diagnosis

Hypophosphatasia is most commonly confused with severe type II osteogenesis imperfecta because of the presence of birth fractures and the severe demineralization. Thanatophoric dwarfism and achondrogenesis can also resemble the perinatal form of hypophosphatasia.

Less severe forms of hypophosphatasia should be differentiated from the various types of rickets. In rickets, the alkaline phosphatase concentration is generally increased, whereas in hypophosphatasia, by definition it is decreased or not measurable.

Treatment

Although there is no ordinary medical treatment of hypophosphatasia, successful transplantation of marrow cells with amelioration of the disease has been reported.[550] If the diagnosis of rickets is mistakenly made, treatment with vitamin D can worsen the heterotopic calcification and nephrocalcinosis. Enzyme replacement therapy is not yet available.

Fractures require orthopaedic referral. Healing of fractures is generally delayed in patients with hypophosphatasia. Occasionally, multiple osteotomies with intramedullary fixation, as one would do in cases of severe osteogenesis imperfecta, are needed to correct the bowing and lend structural support to the long bones.

HYPERPHOSPHATASIA

Hyperphosphatasia is an extremely rare bone dysplasia characterized by failure to replace immature woven bone with mature lamellar bone. Biochemically, serum levels of alkaline phosphatase are increased (hence the name *hyperphosphatasia*), as is urinary excretion of hydroxyproline. The disease is transmitted as an autosomal recessive trait, and several genetic loci have been identified.[111,549]

Clinically, the long bones are bowed and prone to stress fractures because of osteopenia and decreased biomechanical strength of the bone.[133] The patient's head is enlarged. Initial complaints are painful swelling of the limbs and bowing. Muscle mass appears diminished, and the limbs may be warm. Affected children are very short.

Radiographic findings include generalized diaphyseal expansion of the bones with subperiosteal new bone deposition.[547,549] Fractures are transverse and usually nondisplaced. The spine and pelvis show patchy areas of sclerosis. The base and vault of the skull are thickened.

Pathologic studies of bone tissue show extensive fibrosis of the marrow with cellular hyperactivity. There is evidence of both increased bone resorption and bone formation resembling fibrous dysplasia.[393,496] There may be a mosaic pattern of cement lines resembling what is seen in Paget's disease.[150]

Conditions from which hyperphosphatasia must be distinguished include Camurati-Engelmann disease, craniodiaphyseal dysplasia, and fibrous dysplasia. Hyperphosphatasia can be differentiated from all these conditions by the distinct elevation in serum alkaline phosphatase.

Treatment previously consisted of administering thyrocalcitonin.[55,136] Recently, successful treatment of the disease has been reported with the use of bisphosphonates such as pamidronate and etidronate.[82,484,491,496]

PITUITARY DWARFISM

A deficiency in somatotropic hormone is due to congenital hypoplasia or aplasia of the eosinophilic cells in about two thirds of cases of hypopituitarism. It is often a hereditary disorder, and four forms exist, with autosomal recessive, autosomal dominant, and X-linked types.[269,399,420] In the remaining cases, cessation of growth results from destructive lesions of the anterior pituitary, most commonly a craniopharyngioma.

Clinical Features

In congenital forms the infant is of normal size, but diminished growth is noted around 2 to 4 years of age. The limbs are of normal proportion in relation to the head and trunk. Intelligence is normal. The condition can be associated with hypogonadism and a delay in or absence of sexual maturation.[191,438]

In the acquired form caused by a pituitary lesion, signs of neurologic deficit such as impaired vision, ocular disturbances, and pathologic sleepiness are present.

Radiographic Findings

In congenital hypopituitarism, skeletal maturation is delayed. The ossification centers are late in both appearance and closure. Osteoporosis of the long bones and the skull is present. The fontanelles close later than normal.

Where there is a lesion in the pituitary, radiographs will reveal enlargement of the sella turcica, the home of the pituitary. Intrasellar or suprasellar calcification suggests craniopharyngioma.

MRI is especially useful in visualizing the pituitary. Enlargement, hypoplasia, or tumor can be seen.[127,396]

Diagnosis

Serum levels of growth hormone will be low or absent. Because low levels are normal in healthy children, a stimulatory test is usually needed to confirm the lack of growth hormone.[289] Insulin or L-arginine is administered to produce hypoglycemia, which stimulates the release of growth hormone. Growth hormone levels do not increase in patients with pituitary dwarfism after the administration of these agents.

Treatment

Pituitary dwarfism is treated by the administration of synthetic growth hormone.[211,440] Such treatment stimulates growth and should be monitored by a pediatric endocrinologist. Patients with growth hormone deficiency after resection of craniopharyngiomas rarely have an isolated deficiency in growth hormone, so additional hormone replacement therapy is necessary, under the guidance of the endocrinologist. In some children with growth hormone deficiency, panhypopituitarism has developed in adulthood, with hypothyroidism and abnormalities in antidiuretic hormone. On rare occasion, referral to an orthopaedic surgeon is needed for treatment of SCFE.

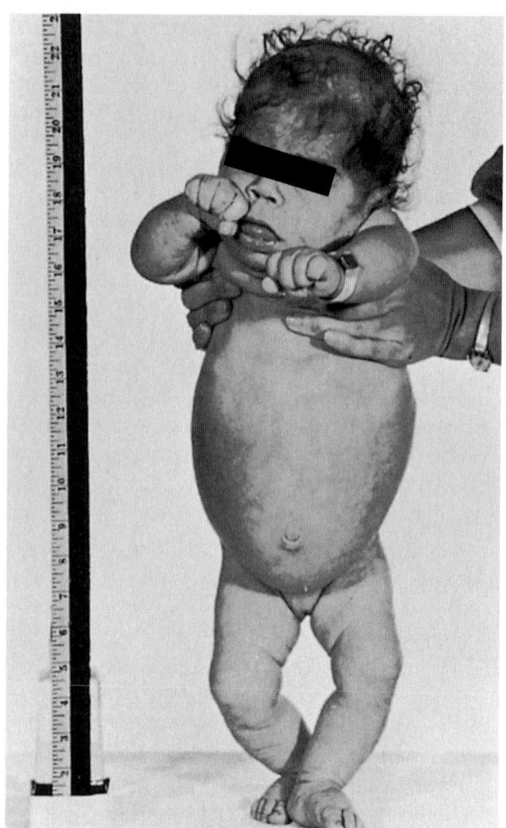

FIGURE 32-23 Typical clinical appearance of congenital hypothyroidism.

HYPOTHYROIDISM

Thyroid hormone deficiency may be congenital or acquired. The degree of deficiency, age at onset, and duration of the deficiency are all factors that determine the severity of disease. Hypothyroidism is fairly common, with an incidence of 1 per 4000 newborns.[268]

Congenital hypothyroidism, previously known as cretinism, is characterized by dwarfism and mental retardation. It is more common in girls than in boys.

Etiology

The usual cause of congenital hypothyroidism is a structural abnormality in the thyroid gland. Abnormalities range from aplasia of the thyroid, hypoplasia, and goiter to ectopic thyroid tissue. Familial forms of hypothyroidism are being delineated through molecular genetic research.[2,132,297,514]

Clinical Features

Symptoms in early infancy include prolonged jaundice, lethargy, sleepiness, feeding difficulties, and constipation. Frequently, these infants are overweight. Other features include dry skin, scanty coarse hair, an enlarged tongue, umbilical hernias, and an expressionless face (Fig. 32–23). Developmental delay is noted. Associated congenital malformations, especially heart defects, are more likely to occur in children with congenital hypothyroidism.[368,477]

In acquired hypothyroidism, which is manifested later in childhood, sluggishness, a slowdown in growth, and worsening school performance are noted.[268] SCFE may occur and lead to groin, hip, or knee pain. Hypogonadism is present, and the children are often overweight.

Radiographic Findings

Thyroid hormone is very important in regulating bone growth and maturation. In patients with hypothyroidism, enchondral bone formation is disturbed. The skeleton is immature for the infant's chronologic age. Appearance of the epiphyses is delayed, and they look irregular and fragmented, which in childhood resembles what is seen in Perthes' disease or multiple epiphyseal dysplasia.[139] *Epiphyseal dysgenesis* was the term used by Reilly and Smyth to describe the ossific nuclei.[425] The physis may be irregular and widened, similar to the radiographic picture in rickets.

The bone age of the patient is delayed. The long bones are abnormally widened as a result of normal intramembranous bone formation in the context of disturbed endochondral ossification.

The head appears large. Radiographically, ossification of the skull is retarded and the base of the skull is shortened. The sella turcica may be enlarged. Closure of the fontanelles is delayed. A delay in the development of normal dentition is common.

Spinal radiographs show a tendency toward thoracolumbar kyphosis. The vertebral body of L2 is wedge shaped and the anterior margin is beaked. L1 and L3 may have a similar appearance. The bony end-plates are convex.

Osteosclerosis develops in some patients as a result of hypercalcemia. Radiographs in these patients show transverse radiopaque bands in the metaphyseal areas and thickened cortices. Metastatic calcification can occur.

MRI has shown enlargement of the pituitary in children with congenital hypothyroidism.[127]

Diagnosis

Great gains have been made in the diagnosis of congenital hypothyroidism. Screening programs are in place to measure thyroid-stimulating hormone (TSH) in the newborn nursery.[10,121,198,228,423] An elevated TSH level is suggestive of congenital hypothyroidism.[538] Further laboratory evaluation of thyroid hormone levels and further imaging studies consisting of radionuclide scintigraphy of the thyroid or thyroid ultrasound are then performed to ascertain the cause of the hormone deficiency.[89,353,529]

Early diagnosis is mandatory because a delay in diagnosis can lead to irreversible mental retardation. The workup of a developmentally delayed child should include laboratory evaluation of thyroid function when the cause of the delay is unknown.[9]

There is an association between Down syndrome and hypothyroidism. One study found that 15% of infants with Down syndrome had congenital hypothyroidism.[238] Another found that 30 of 85 children with Down syndrome had hypothyroidism, and the authors recommended annual screening of these children.[248] Hypothyroidism should be especially considered in children with Down syndrome who have SCFE. In one study, six of eight patients with Down syndrome and slipped epiphyses had hypothyroidism.[63]

Other laboratory findings in children with hypothyroidism may include high serum calcium levels.[534] Patients with panhypopituitarism will have not only hypothyroidism but also the other hormonal deficiencies seen in this disorder, such as growth hormone deficiency.

Treatment

Treatment begins immediately on diagnosis. Hormone replacement therapy with thyroxine is initiated and carefully monitored. If treatment is begun by 24 months of age, subsequent growth has been shown to be normal by 5 years.[17,92] With hormonal replacement therapy, the pubertal growth spurt is normal, and adult height is within normal limits.[129] Long-term thyroxine replacement therapy has not been shown to decrease bone mass and lead to osteopenia.[259] Prompt treatment results in normal intellectual development.[277]

Prenatal diagnosis through cord blood sampling has been achieved, and prenatal treatment of hypothyroidism by means of thyroid hormone injected into amniotic fluid has been successful in experimental settings.[73,398]

If congenital hypothyroidism remains untreated, the mental retardation is progressive, and most children die early of respiratory infection.

Orthopaedic Considerations

In an older child, SCFE may be the first manifestation of hypothyroidism (Fig. 32–24). Loder and associates found that the diagnosis of hypothyroidism was made *after* the patient was seen for treatment of the slip.[293] Screening recommendations range from screening all patients with SCFE for thyroid disease[544] to no routine screening whatsoever. We believe that any patient with SCFE who is younger than usual (<11 years), who has a family history of thyroid abnormalities, or who does not have the typical obese body habitus should be screened for hypothyroidism with a TSH test. Patients with Down syndrome and slips should be considered to have hypothyroidism until proved otherwise.[63] In patients with SCFE secondary to hypothyroidism, contralateral prophylactic pinning should be performed because the incidence of bilateral SCFE in hypothyroidism is 61%.[293]

Idiopathic Juvenile Osteoporosis

Idiopathic juvenile osteoporosis is a rare metabolic bone disease of childhood characterized by a profound reduction in bone mass of unknown cause. The cardinal features of idiopathic juvenile osteoporosis are (1) onset before puberty, (2) compression fractures of the vertebrae and long bones, (3) formation of new but osteoporotic bone, and (4) spontaneous recovery after skeletal maturity.

Etiology

The cause of idiopathic juvenile osteoporosis remains unknown. The disease is not genetically transmitted. The basic mechanism of disease is an imbalance between bone formation and bone resorption. Bone histology generally shows an excess of osteocytes associated with woven bone.[492] In one study, secretion of synthesized collagen by cultured skin fibroblasts in some patients with idiopathic juvenile osteoporosis was reduced, whereas the range of collagen secretion in other patients with the disease overlapped the normal range.[406] Another study found diminished levels of the carboxy-terminal propeptide of type I procollagen in patients with juvenile osteoporosis, again indicating abnormalities in collagen metabolism.[411]

Biomechanical studies are conflicting. Serum calcium and phosphorus levels are normal in these patients. Calcium balance, however, is negative, with poor gastrointestinal absorption of calcium.[220,267] Alkaline phosphatase and urinary hydroxyproline levels

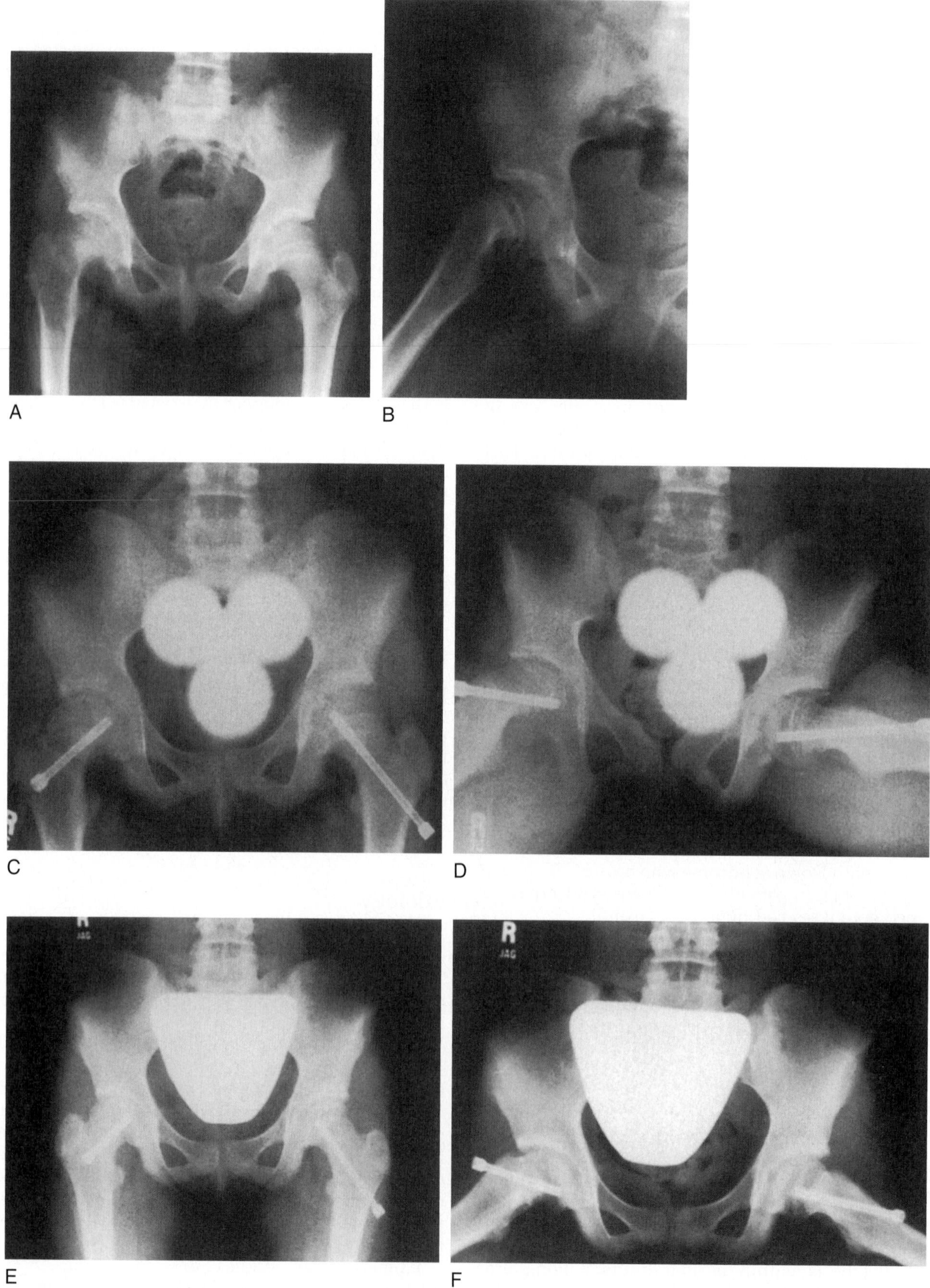

FIGURE 32–24 **A** and **B,** Right slipped capital femoral epiphysis in a 13-year-old girl. Hypothyroidism was diagnosed on initial evaluation. Physeal widening is seen in the asymptomatic left hip. **C** and **D,** In situ fixation was performed bilaterally. **E** and **F,** At 2-year follow-up, the physes were healed.

are usually normal as well. Although most studies report normal vitamin D levels,[233] two studies found low levels of calcitriol (1,25-dihydroxycholecalciferol). Therapy was then directed toward the vitamin deficiency, with improvement in the disease.[309,454] It may be that different forms of the disease have different biochemical profiles.

Clinical Features

The mean age at onset is 7 years, with cases reported in children as young as 1 year.[492] By definition, the disease is always manifested before puberty. There is no sex predilection.

The initial complaints in children with idiopathic juvenile osteoporosis are back and leg pain.[130] Patients may refuse to walk or may have a slow gait or limp.[535] The examining physician should always remember that a limp in children is a common orthopaedic problem, whereas idiopathic juvenile osteoporosis is an extremely rare condition.

Radiographic Findings

Diffuse generalized osteoporosis is seen on radiographs of the spine and limbs (Fig. 32–25). The normal trabecular pattern is markedly decreased and the cortices of the bones are thinned. On lateral radiographs of the spine, a "codfish" appearance is present. Increased thoracic or thoracolumbar kyphosis with anterior wedging of the vertebrae may develop. Vertebral compression fractures may be evident, and scoliosis may be present.

Another radiographic feature is the presence of long-bone fractures in various stages of healing. The fractures are usually metaphyseal and tend to occur in areas of highest stress, such as the femoral neck. Other areas in which stress fractures are common are the distal femur and proximal tibia.

The skull does not have a wormian appearance.

Diagnosis

The diagnosis is one of exclusion. The various known causes of osteoporosis in childhood are listed in Box 32–1. The most difficult distinction to make is between idiopathic juvenile osteoporosis and mild osteogenesis imperfecta. Patients with a positive family history have osteogenesis imperfecta, yet individuals with no affected relatives may have either disease. Other distinguishing features of osteogenesis imperfecta that are not associated with idiopathic juvenile osteoporosis are blue sclerae, dentinogenesis imperfecta, ligamentous laxity, and easy bruising. Patients with juvenile osteoporosis do not sustain fractures in early infancy, and this may help differentiate the two

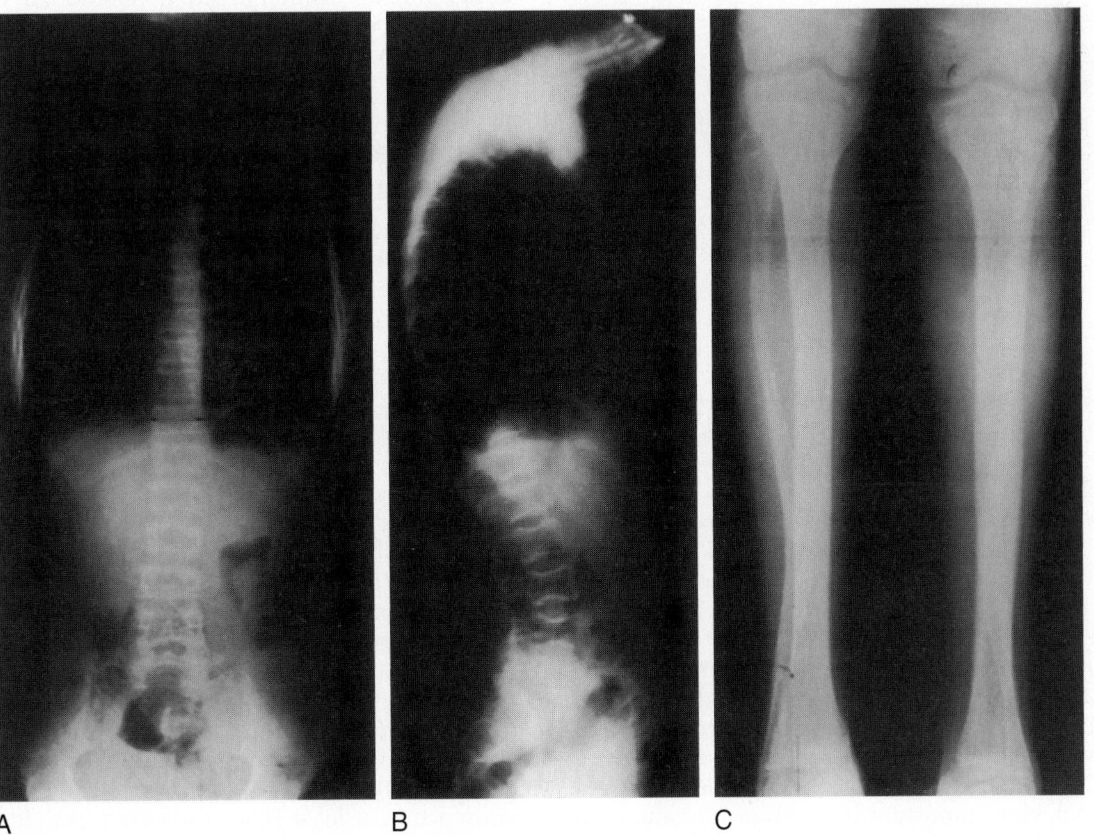

FIGURE 32–25 Idiopathic juvenile osteoporosis. Anteroposterior **(A)** and lateral **(B)** radiographs of the spine showing the severe osteoporosis. Note the compression fractures of the vertebrae in the lumbar region. **C,** AP radiograph of both tibiae. Note the plastic bowing of the fibulae and marked osteoporosis.

Box 32-1

Causes of Osteoporosis in Childhood

- Endocrine disorders
  - Hyperthyroidism
  - Hyperparathyroidism
  - Hypogonadism
  - Glucocorticoid excess—Cushing's syndrome, steroid therapy
- Metabolic disorders
  - Homocystinuria
  - Gastrointestinal malabsorption
  - Idiopathic hypoproteinemia
  - Vitamin C deficiency
  - Rickets of any cause
  - Liver disease
- Renal disease
  - Chronic tubular acidosis
  - Idiopathic hypercalciuria
  - Lowe's syndrome
  - Uremia and regular hemodialysis
- Bone diseases
  - Osteogenesis imperfecta
  - Idiopathic juvenile osteoporosis
  - Idiopathic osteolysis
  - Turner's syndrome (XO chromosome anomaly)
- Malignant diseases
  - Leukemia
  - Lymphoma
- Miscellaneous causes
  - Disuse osteoporosis of paralyzed limbs as in myelomeningocele
  - Generalized osteoporosis of Still's disease, especially after steroid therapy
  - Heparin therapy
  - Anticonvulsant drug therapy

diseases in some patients. Finally, the fracture callus in juvenile osteoporosis is osteopenic.

Fibroblast studies may be of some help in establishing the diagnosis of osteogenesis imperfecta, but overlap of results with normal ranges and with results in idiopathic juvenile osteoporosis may occur in some children.[406]

Bone biopsy is not generally necessary to diagnose either osteogenesis imperfecta or idiopathic juvenile osteoporosis, but when it is performed, increased woven immature bone is seen in osteogenesis imperfecta, whereas increased osteoclastic resorption of bone is seen in idiopathic juvenile osteoporosis.[243]

Another very important distinction to make clinically is that between leukemia and idiopathic juvenile osteoporosis. A child with leukemia may have osteopenia and compression fractures, so urgent referral to a pediatric hematologist is wise in the evaluation of a patient with osteoporosis. Usually, a bone marrow aspirate will be required to definitively rule out leukemia.

Treatment

Treatment of idiopathic juvenile osteoporosis is controversial. Isolated reports of successful medical treatment with calcitonin,[233] calcitriol,[309,454] bisphosphonates,[218] and estrogen[560] have been published. All reported improved bone mineralization and decreased fractures. It appears that when a demonstrable deficiency is found through laboratory testing, treatment aimed toward correcting that deficiency is warranted.

Orthopaedic treatment of the spine is usually conservative. Bracing may relieve back pain and treat the kyphotic deformity. The Milwaukee brace has been used for this purpose, with reported success.[212,242] The role of the brace in accelerating osteoporosis by stress shielding the spine is unknown. Use of the brace should be discontinued gradually as the osteoporosis resolves.

Scoliosis likewise should be managed orthotically when possible. Spinal fusion has been performed in isolated cases, but continued progression of the deformity because of bending of the fusion mass has been described.[37]

Long-bone fractures should be managed by conventional means. Immobilization should be kept to a minimum because prolonged immobilization leads to worsening osteoporosis and may result in a cycle of fractures.

OSTEOGENESIS IMPERFECTA

Osteogenesis imperfecta is a genetic disorder of connective tissue with the trademark clinical feature of bone fragility as evidenced by long-bone fractures. Other major clinical features may include skeletal deformity, blue sclerae, hearing loss, and fragile, opalescent teeth (dentinogenesis imperfecta). Less severe manifestations may include generalized ligamentous laxity, hernias, easy bruisability, and excessive sweating. The spectrum of the presence of the various potential manifestations, their severity, and the age at which these features are manifested is very broad.* The extent of the bone fragility is the best example of this spectrum: fragility can be so severe that the affected infant is born with crumpled ribs, a fragile cranium, and long-bone fractures incompatible with life, whereas at the opposite end of the spectrum, an older child who otherwise appears normal may sustain only a few fractures after a reasonable amount of trauma. The distinction between child abuse (nonaccidental injury) and excessive bone fragility may be difficult to make in these latter circumstances.[21,126,253,388,389,513] It is now known that at least 90% of affected individuals have an identifiable, genetically determined quantitative or

*See references 1, 6, 7, 96, 97, 99, 100, 103, 184, 256, 312, 313, 315, 344, 349, 493, 505, 525, 528.

qualitative defect in type I collagen formation (or both types of defect).* Type I collagen is the major structural protein found in bone and skeletal connective tissue. The disorder may be inherited from a parent in an autosomal dominant fashion, may occur as a spontaneous mutation, or rarely, may be inherited as a homozygous autosomal recessive trait from both parents.[99,100,344]

Historical descriptions of individuals who may have been affected with osteogenesis imperfecta date from Egyptian times. The most colorful description is probably that of "Ivar the Boneless," a Scandinavian prince who led the invasion of Britain during the ninth century.[249,528] He was purportedly carried by his troops into battle on a shield because his limb deformities prevented him from walking. His skeleton is not available for modern substantiation of this diagnosis since his remains were dug up and burned at the direction of William the Conqueror. From a medical perspective, this disorder has been called by a variety of names over the years, including *fragilis ossium, osteopsathyrosis idiopathica, brittle bone disease, Lobstein's disease,* and *Vrolik's disease.* Lobstein[291] described the nonlethal variety in 1835, and Vrolik[536] described the lethal variety manifested as multiple birth fractures in 1849. Vrolik was also the first to use the term *osteogenesis imperfecta.*

Pathophysiology

Extensive molecular genetic and collagen qualitative research has shown that the vast majority (at least 90%) of individuals with osteogenesis imperfecta have an identifiable defect in the genes responsible for encoding type I collagen.† Some understanding of normal collagen formation and errors in that metabolic process that are seen in osteogenesis imperfecta is essential for understanding the pathophysiology and variability of the disorder.

NORMAL COLLAGEN METABOLISM

Collagen is a connective tissue protein with a left-handed triple-helical structure that is found in abundance in many areas of the body. Many specific subtypes have been described that occur in specific parts of the body relatively frequently. The major structural collagen of the skeletal system, including bone, ligament, and tendon, is type I collagen. This type of collagen is composed of three strands of collagen protein: two α_1 (I) strands and one α_2 (I) strand. In a normal fibroblast, precursor subunits for these two types of strands (pro-α_1 [I] and pro-α_2 [I] polypeptide chains) are synthesized in the rough endoplasmic reticulum. These two procollagen polypeptide chains are encoded by two separate genes, *COL1A1* (encoding for pro-α_1 [I]), located on the long arm of chromosome 17, and *COL1A2* (encoding for pro-α_2 [I]), located on the long arm of chromosome 7. Two pro-α_1 (I) chains and one pro-α_2 (I) chain combine to form type I procollagen molecules. Combining of these three chains into the triple helix begins at the carboxy-terminal end and propagates toward the amino-terminal end. An essential feature of the pro-α chains is a recurrent pattern of glycine residues at every third peptide position in the chain, for it is at these residues that cross-linking of the three chains occurs. The type I procollagen molecules are secreted from the cell and are processed extracellularly to type I collagen molecules (Fig. 32–26A).

COLLAGEN METABOLISM IN OSTEOGENESIS IMPERFECTA

In the 90% of patients in whom the nature of the genetic error in type I collagen formation can be determined (to date), that error is of two basic types: qualitative or quantitative. Type I collagen can be assayed from cultures of fibroblasts taken from skin biopsy samples by electrophoresis techniques. First, there can be complete absence of identifiable type I collagen, or a quantitative error. Such patients probably have a stop codon in the affected gene, which leads to absence of the necessary mRNA and in turn results in no collagen formation under the direction of the affected gene. In this circumstance a patient who is heterozygous for the condition will secrete approximately half the normal amount of type I collagen, with no abnormal type I collagen identifiable (Fig. 32–26B). This is the type of defect most commonly identified in type IA osteogenesis imperfecta in Sillence's classification (see discussion under Classification and Heredity).[482] Cole, in a review of the molecular pathology of 200 patients with osteogenesis imperfecta,[100,482] identified rare types that had normal type I collagen, but with even more severe reductions in quantity than the typical type I patients in Sillence's classification, with levels of 20% or less.

Alternatively, there can be an error in substitution or deletion, usually involving a glycine peptide residue somewhere along the polypeptide chain. In such circumstances the affected patient will produce an abnormal, less effectual collagen, generally in reduced amounts. The severity of the disruption in function of the affected collagen is in part related to the location of the glycine residue error. Substitutions at the carboxy end of the polypeptide chains are potentially more serious because cross-linking of the triple helix begins at the carboxy terminal of the chains. This type of defect, both a quantitative and a qualitative one that impairs the function of type I collagen, is the more commonly identified defect in Sillence's types II, III, and IV (discussed later) (Fig. 32–26C). Patients with the most severe or lethal varieties tend to have the coding defect at the carboxy end of either the pro-α_1 (I) or pro-α_2 (I) chains.

Classification and Heredity

Classification of osteogenesis imperfecta has proved troublesome because of variability in the nature, time

*See references 1, 77, 96, 99-101, 103, 141, 344, 359, 509.
†See references 1, 77, 96, 99, 100, 102, 103, 141, 344, 359, 509.

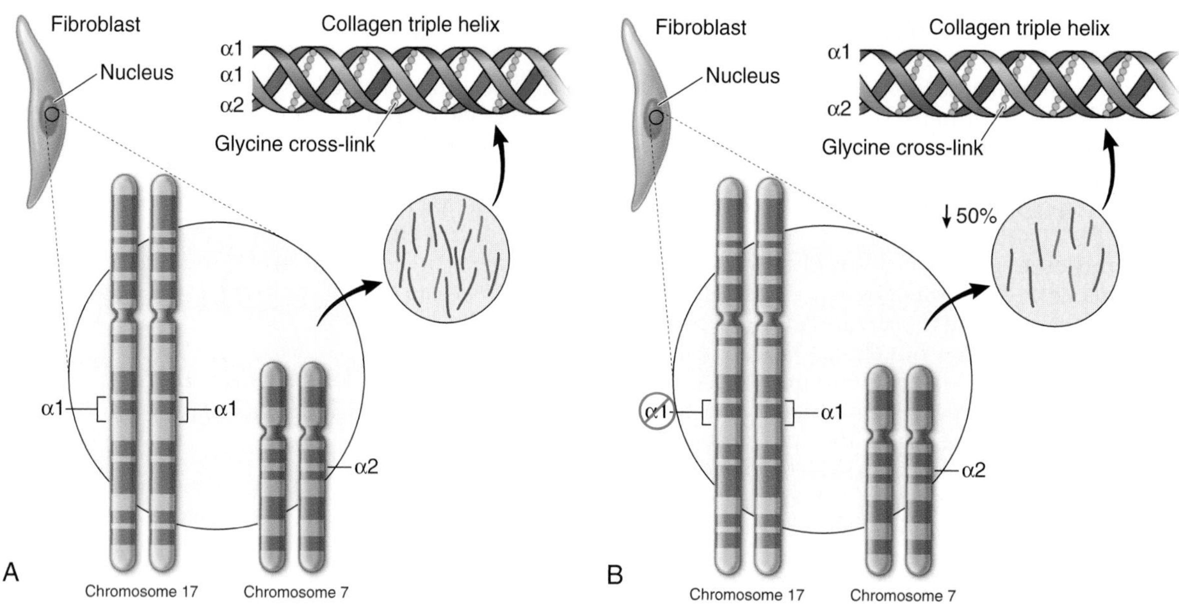

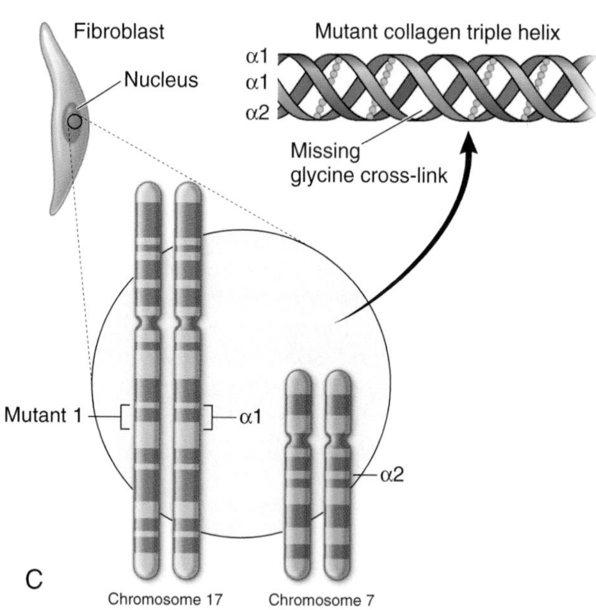

FIGURE 32–26 Schematic representation of normal and abnormal collagen formation. **A,** Normal type I collagen formation. Two pro-α_1 (I) (encoded by *COL1AI* on chromosome 17) and one pro-α_2 (I) (encoded by *COL1A2* on chromosome 7) polypeptide chains form a left-handed triple helix, beginning at the carboxy end and continuing to the amino end. Cross-linking occurs at glycine residues located at every third position in the chains. The procollagen molecule is then secreted from the endoplasmic reticulum into the extracellular matrix, where coalescence into the complete type I collagen fiber continues. **B,** Quantitative defect typified by Sillence's type IA osteogenesis imperfecta. There is a stop codon for one of the *COL1AI* genes, which results in no mRNA from that gene. As a result, normal pro-α_1 polypeptide chains are produced in levels approximately 50% of normal, with the subsequent production of about 50% of the normal amount of type I collagen. The collagen produced is electrophoretically normal, and no abnormal collagen is detectable. **C,** Formation of mutant type I collagen from some defect in either *COL1AI* or *COL1A2.* Skips or substitutions for glycine occur at some point along the polypeptide chains encoding for either pro-α_1 or pro-α_2. The mutant polypeptide chain results in poorer cross-linking. Defects closer to the carboxy terminal are potentially more serious because triple helix formation begins at this end. The mutant procollagen is usually produced in reduced amounts, so there is a qualitative and quantitative deficiency of type I collagen. This type of defect is typical of Sillence's types II, III, and IV osteogenesis imperfecta.

of onset, and severity of the various clinical manifestations of the disorder. The different patterns of inheritance, the relatively high incidence of spontaneous mutations, and the variability in clinical severity, even when the mode of inheritance is known, further compromise the effectiveness of classification schemes. The identification of more than 150 specific locations of disruptions in genetic coding for type I collagen has improved our understanding of the nature and variability of the clinical manifestations but has not simplified the classification process. There are two classification schemes (those of Sillence and associates[100,480-482] and Shapiro[474]) with which orthopaedic surgeons attending to the needs of patients with osteogenesis imperfecta should be familiar.

Sillence and Danks delineated four distinct types of osteogenesis imperfecta based on both clinical and genetic characteristics.[481] Previous classifications did not take genetic modes of transmission into account when delineating types of osteogenesis imperfecta. In the original description of Sillence and Danks, four types were described and identified as either autosomal dominant (types I and IV) or autosomal recessive (types II and III).[481] According to this formulation, type I osteogenesis imperfecta was an autosomal dominant condition characterized by bone fragility and blue sclerae throughout life. This type was subdivided into type IA, without dentinogenesis imperfecta, and type IB, with dentinogenesis imperfecta. Type II was considered a lethal autosomal recessive form characterized by extreme bone fragility and perinatal death. Type III was described as a relatively rare autosomal recessive condition with severe bone fragility and white sclerae. Type IV was described as an autosomal dominant disorder of intermediate severity characterized by white sclerae in adulthood. Type IV, like type I, was subclassified into type IVA, without dentinogenesis imperfecta, and type IVB, with dentinogenesis imperfecta.

More recent work on the nature of type I collagen disorders and the molecular genetic basis for these disorders, however, has elucidated the nature of the genetic defect, and in fact, true autosomal recessive transmission is rare in this condition.[100] Cole has recommended modification of the original Sillence classification based on an extensive review of the collagen defect in 200 patients with osteogenesis imperfecta. The features of Sillence's classification are summarized in Table 32–2.

OSTEOGENESIS IMPERFECTA TYPE I

Osteogenesis imperfecta type I is characterized by generalized osteoporosis with abnormal bony fragility, distinct blue sclerae throughout life, and presenile conductive hearing loss. This is the most common type of osteogenesis imperfecta in most series, and these patients are, in general, the least affected in terms of the incidence of fractures. This type is inherited as an autosomal dominant condition, although spontaneous mutations occur. Molecular genetic studies have revealed that this type is characterized by a quantitative defect in type I collagen.[1,36,99,100,103,141,344,509,526,561] Specifically, one of the inherited *COL1A1* genes in affected patients will not produce effective mRNA for pro-α_1 collagen, so the amount of type I collagen is effectively reduced to approximately 50% of the normal amount, but that 50% is electrophoretically normal, and no "mutant" type I collagen is detectable by electrophoretic techniques.[100] Dentinogenesis imperfecta is present in some of these patients; those without dentinogenesis imperfecta are subclassified as having osteogenesis imperfecta type IA, and those with dentinogenesis imperfecta are classified as having type IB. It is likely that patients with osteogenesis type IB have a mutant collagen present and are biochemically distinctly different from patients with osteogenesis type IA.

OSTEOGENESIS IMPERFECTA TYPE II

Type II osteogenesis imperfecta is characterized by extreme bone fragility leading to death in the perinatal period or early infancy. The long bones are crumbled (accordion femora), and ossification of the skull is markedly delayed; on palpation, the cranial vault feels like numerous small plates of bone. Originally this condition was thought to be inherited as an autosomal recessive trait.[462] However, work on the nature of type I collagen disturbance has revealed that the defect in most cases is a severe disruption in the qualitative function of type I collagen.[1,96,99,100,102,103,141,344,509] In most cases the condition is inherited as a "dominant negative" condition, often as the result of a spontaneous mutation. In the words of Cole, most affected individuals have "their own private mutation," and many different ones have been described.[100]

This pattern of inheritance is more in keeping with the risk of recurrence in subsequent pregnancies of couples with a previously affected fetus. If the condition were inherited as an autosomal recessive trait, the risk in subsequent pregnancies should be on the order of 25% or, if due to spontaneous mutations, essentially zero. In fact, the risk of having a subsequent fetus affected has been estimated at approximately 7%. In these situations, one of the parents has been identified as being "mosaic" for the dominant negative gene, which accounts for the low, but present risk. For a discussion of diagnostic evaluations for identifying an affected fetus, please see Antenatal Diagnosis in the section Prognostication and Parental Counseling.

OSTEOGENESIS IMPERFECTA TYPE III

This variety of osteogenesis imperfecta is also characterized by qualitative and quantitative changes in type I collagen and may be inherited as an autosomal recessive or "dominant negative" trait.[1,99,100,103,344,359] It is characterized by severe bone fragility, multiple fractures and progressive marked deformity of the long bones, and severe growth retardation.[99,100,480,482] The sclerae are bluish at birth but become less blue with age. In adolescents, the sclerae are of normal hue. The most

Table 32-2 Classification of Osteogenesis Imperfecta Syndromes (According to Sillence)

Type	Inheritance	Teeth	Bone Fragility	Deformity of Long Bones	Growth Retardation
IA	Autosomal dominant	Normal	Variable—less severe than other types	Moderate	Short stature, 2% to 3% below mean
IB	Autosomal dominant	Dentinogenesis imperfecta	Variable—less severe than other types	Moderate	Short, 2% to 3% below mean
II	Autosomal recessive	Unknown (because of perinatal death)	Very extreme	Crumbled bone (accordion femora) marked	Unknown (because of perinatal death)
III	Autosomal recessive	Dentinogenesis imperfecta	Severe	Progressive bowing of the long bones and spine	Severe—smallest of all patients with osteogenesis imperfecta
IVA	Autosomal dominant	Normal	Moderate	Moderate	Short stature
IVB	Autosomal dominant	Dentinogenesis imperfecta	Moderate	Moderate	Short stature

severely affected surviving patients often have this type of disease.

OSTEOGENESIS IMPERFECTA TYPE IV

Osteogenesis imperfecta type IV is inherited as an autosomal dominant condition, and most patients, like those with types II and III, have qualitative and quantitative changes in type I collagen. At birth the sclerae are of normal hue; if they are bluish, they become progressively less so with maturation and are normal in adolescence. The osteoporosis, bone fragility, and long-bone deformities are of variable severity. Dentinogenesis imperfecta also occurs in some affected individuals; those with normal dentition are classified as having type IVA disease and those with dentinogenesis imperfecta as having type IVB disease.

One of the problems for the orthopaedic surgeon and the families of patients with osteogenesis imperfecta is the significant variability in the severity of long-bone deformity and fracture frequency within Sillence's classification categories and even within families, whose members presumably share the same genetic defect. Yet these two clinical features have a significant impact on the affected individual's mobility, morbidity, and need for orthopaedic intervention. In general, Sillence's type I patients are the least affected individuals; Sillence's type II patients are almost invariably stillborn or die shortly after birth; and Sillence's types III and IV patients are more severely affected than most type I patients and constitute the majority of patients with severe deformity and frequent fractures; they may require extremity intramedullary rodding and have more difficulty ambulating or are unable to do so. However, within a family, one sibling may have only a few fractures whereas another may have repeated fractures, deformity requiring intramedullary rods, and difficulty ambulating without lower extremity bracing or upper extremity aid. Because of this practical problem, clinical classifications based on the age at onset and the severity of fractures still have prognostic relevance for the orthopaedic surgeon and affected individuals.

The evolution of a useful clinical classification based on the occurrence and severity of fractures is as follows. Looser in 1906[295] classified osteogenesis imperfecta into two types: *osteogenesis imperfecta congenita,* characterized by the presence of numerous fractures at birth, and *osteogenesis imperfecta tarda,* in which the fracture or fractures occur after the perinatal period.[295] Seedorff in 1949[470] subclassified osteogenesis imperfecta tarda into two types: *tarda gravis,* in which the first fracture occurs in the first year of life (severe deformities of the long bones and spine subsequently develop in these children), and *tarda levis,* in which the initial fracture occurs after the first year of life, with the deformity and disability not being so severe in the latter.[439] Falvo and associates[154] noted that age does not always correlate with the severity of the disease and therefore recommended subdivision of osteogenesis imperfecta tarda according to the presence of bowing of the long bones; they subclassified cases with bowing as tarda type I and those without bowing as tarda type II.

Shapiro has recommended a further modification of Looser's classification with respect to prognosis for survival and ambulation based on the evaluation of a large number of patients.[474] This classification, given in Table 32–3, has excellent practical application for the orthopaedic surgeon and the families of affected individuals in regard to prognosis for survival and ambulation. The classification consists of four categories: congenita A, congenita B, tarda A, and tarda B. Shapiro classified patients as having osteogenesis imperfecta "congenita" if they had fractures in utero or at birth, whereas Looser and other later

Presenile Hearing Loss (%)	Prognosis	Sclerae	Spine	Skull	Other	Incidence
40	Fair	Distinctly blue throughout life	Scoliosis and kyphosis in 20%	Wormian bones on radiographs	Premature arcus senilis	1/30,000
40	Fair	Distinctly blue throughout life	Scoliosis and kyphosis in 20%	Wormian bones on radiographs	Premature arcus senilis	1/30,000
	Perinatal death	Blue		Marked absence of ossification		1/62,000 live births
	Nonambulatory, wheelchair bound May die in third decade	Bluish at birth, become less blue with age, white in adult	Kyphoscoliosis	Hypoplastic, more ossified than in type II Wormian bones		Very rare
Low frequency	Fair	Normal	Kyphoscoliosis	Hypoplastic Wormian bones		Unknown
Low frequency	Fair	Normal	Kyphoscoliosis	Hypoplastic Wormian bones		Unknown

Table 32-3 Shapiro's Classification of Osteogenesis Imperfecta*

Type	Description	Positive Family History	Deaths	Ambulatory Status
Osteogenesis imperfecta congenita A	In utero or birth fractures; short, broad, crumpled femora and ribs	0%	15/16 (94%)	One survivor wheelchair bound
Osteogenesis imperfecta congenita B	In utero or birth fractures, normal long bone contours, no chest deformity	4%	2/27 (8%)	59% wheelchair bound; 33% at least household ambulators
Osteogenesis imperfecta tarda A	Fractures after birth but before walking	11%	0/21 (0%)	33% in wheelchair; 67% ambulatory
Osteogenesis imperfecta tarda B	Fractures after walking	76%	0/21 (0%)	100% ambulatory

*Clinical features and prognosis in patients with osteogenesis imperfecta as described by Shapiro. Patients with osteogenesis imperfecta congenita (fractures in utero or at birth) are distinguished by the presence or absence of long bone and rib deformities. Patients with osteogenesis imperfecta tarda (fractures after birth) are distinguished by the onset of fractures before or after walking.

From Shapiro F: Consequences of an osteogenesis imperfecta diagnosis for survival and ambulation. J Pediatr Orthop 1985;5:456.

authors used "congenita" only for in utero fractures. The distinction between the two congenita types is based on the timing of fractures and radiographic features of the affected bones. Patients with *congenita A* are patients who sustain fractures in utero or at birth, with the additional radiographic features of crumpled long bones, crumpled ribs with rib cage deformity, and a fragile skull (Fig. 32–27). These features are incompatible with life, and the patients are almost always either stillborn or die shortly after birth from intracranial hemorrhage or respiratory insufficiency. In Shapiro's series, 15 of 16 patients with congenita A died, whereas 1 survived with wheelchair mobility. Patients with *congenita B* have fractures at birth but are radiographically distinct from congenita A patients in that the long bones, as typified by the femur, are more tubular and have more normal funnelization in the metaphysis, the ribs are more normally formed (although there may be rib fractures), and there is no rib cage deformity. These patients are obviously severely affected, but this type of osteogenesis imperfecta is compatible with survival. In Shapiro's series, only 2 of 27 congenita B patients died, and 9 were able to ambulate in some fashion. Fractures developed in patients with osteogenesis imperfecta tarda only after birth. Patients with *tarda A* have an onset of fractures before walking. In Shapiro's series, 33% were in wheelchairs and 67% were ambulatory. The age at onset of fractures was not prognostic for ambulation within this group. Patients with *tarda B* incur their first frac-

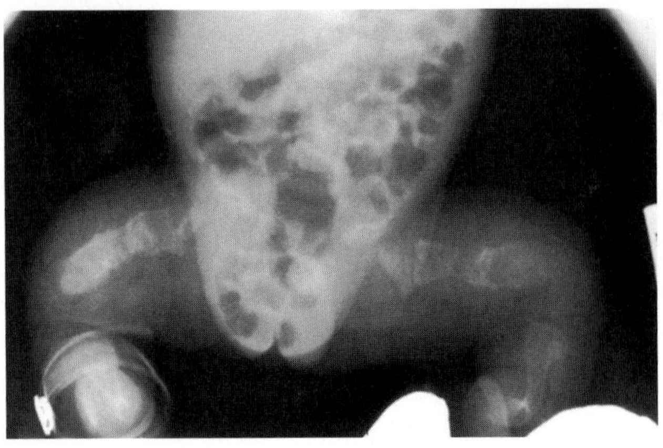

FIGURE 32-27 Radiograph showing crumpled femora and lack of normal funnelization of the long bone in a child with osteogenesis imperfecta, Sillence's type II, and Shapiro's type congenita. This form is virtually universally fatal inasmuch as the child is stillborn or dies in the neonatal period as a result of intracranial hemorrhage or respiratory insufficiency.

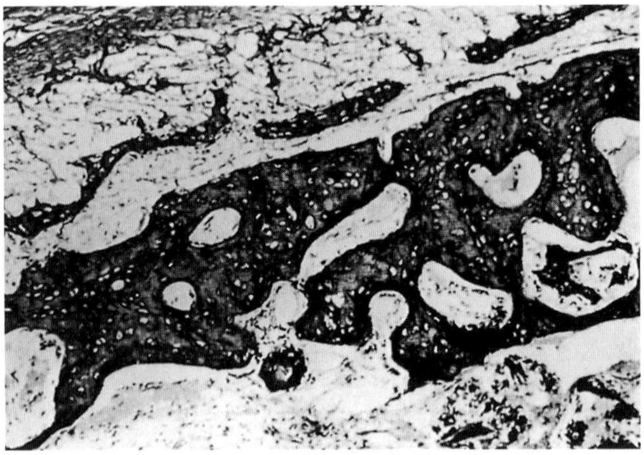

FIGURE 32-28 Histologic appearance in osteogenesis imperfecta. There is a relative abundance of osteocytes with reduced extracellular matrix. Osteoclasts are normal morphologically and normal or increased in number, with an increased number of resorption surfaces.

ture after walking age; in Shapiro's series, all these patients were ambulatory.

Incidence

The exact incidence of the various types of osteogenesis imperfecta is uncertain. The population frequency of type I has been estimated as being approximately 2.35 per 100,000 in Japan, 4.7 per 100,000 in Germany, and 3.4 per 100,000 in Victoria, Australia. The birth incidence of type II has been estimated at 1 per 40,000 to 1.4 per 100,000 live births.[480-482] At present, the exact incidence of type III and type IV is unknown,[528] but these types are less common than type I in most clinical series. In Cole's review of the genetic defect and type I collagen anomaly in 200 patients, 28 patients had type IA (2 had type IB and 1 had IC), 49 had perinatally lethal type II (Cole subdivided this group into three types), 41 had type III, and 79 had type IV.[100]

In Shapiro's review and classification based on clinical severity, 16 patients had congenita A (fractures in utero or at birth, with chest deformity and crumpled ribs and extremities), 27 had congenita B (in utero or birth fractures, without chest deformity but with more normal metaphyseal funnelization), 21 had tarda A (fractures after birth but before walking), and 21 had tarda B (fractures after walking).

Pathology

The fundamental defect in osteogenesis imperfecta is an absolute reduction in the amount of normal type I collagen in bone or its replacement with a poorly functioning mutant collagen (usually also reduced in quantity). That defect is manifested histologically in many ways.[8,33,38,74,75,134,146,322,434] The formation of both enchondral and intramembranous bone is disturbed. Histologic findings vary according to the type of osteogenesis imperfecta. The morphology of the cells and the matrix is not consistent throughout the spectrum of the syndrome. The amount of woven bone is greater than in normal controls, and histometric analyses have shown that in type II, the proportion of primitive osseous tissue with a woven or irregular collagen matrix is significantly higher than in other types.[74,134]

The bone trabeculae are thin and lack an organized trabecular pattern. Fractured spicules of trabeculae may be found. The spongiosa is scanty. The intracellular matrix is reduced, and as a result there is a relative abundance of osteocytes (Fig. 32–28).[75] The osteoclasts are morphologically normal, although they seem to be numerous and have an increased number of resorption surfaces.

Osteoid seams are wide and crowded by plump osteoblasts. The mineralized chondroid lattice is surrounded by wide seams of basophilic substance.[128,134] This large number of osteoblasts and osteoclasts, the large size of the osteoblasts, and the plentiful osteoid tissue covering the thin bone trabeculae indicate increased bone turnover. Tetracycline labeling studies have confirmed the increased bone turnover in osteogenesis imperfecta.[7,33] McCarthy and associates, however, noted normal or (evidence of) decreased bone turnover in eight adult patients with Sillence's type IA osteogenesis imperfecta.[322]

The lamellae in lamellar bone are thin and tenuous. On electron microscopy the collagen fibrils do not aggregate in bundles of normal thickness; instead, they are organized into thin, loosely compacted filaments.[134,506] The compact bone consists of a coarse fibrillary type of immature bone without haversian systems. Periosteum and perichondrium are generally normal, but in one study the periosteum was thickened with a defective microvascular system.[364] The physis is usually broad and irregular, the proliferative and hypertrophic zones are disorganized, and the typical columnar arrangement is lacking. The calcified zone of the growth plates is thinner, and metaphyseal blood vessels permeate the growth plate.[74] Islands of cartilage are present in the juxtaphyseal metaphyseal region. Sanguinetti and associates[462] observed that biopsy specimens from patients with type II osteogenesis imperfecta had a relatively normal appearance of the growth plate, but in specimens from patients with types I and III disease they noted reduced cartilage matrix calcification, thin, newly formed bony trabeculae, and decreased glycosaminoglycan staining within the growth plate.[462]

The primary spongiosa in the metaphysis is sparse, with the osseous tissue almost always of the woven variety. The secondary centers of ossification in the epiphysis are delayed in maturation, and residual islands of cartilage remain in the epiphysis.

When a fracture is present, the endosteal fracture callus is primarily cartilaginous and the periosteal reaction is abundant and consists mainly of woven bone.

Gross anatomic findings consist of porosis (osteopenia), diminution in size, and skeletal deformities secondary to fracture and asymmetric physeal growth disturbance (Fig. 32–29) corresponding to the degree of bone fragility.[75] In severely affected individuals, the long bones are slender and smaller than normal and the cortices are extremely thin, with a paucity of medullary spongy bone and evidence of recent or healed fractures with varying degrees of angular or torsional deformities. The cartilaginous epiphyseal ends of the long bones in general retain a recognizable shape but are disproportionately large and have some irregularity of the articular surface.

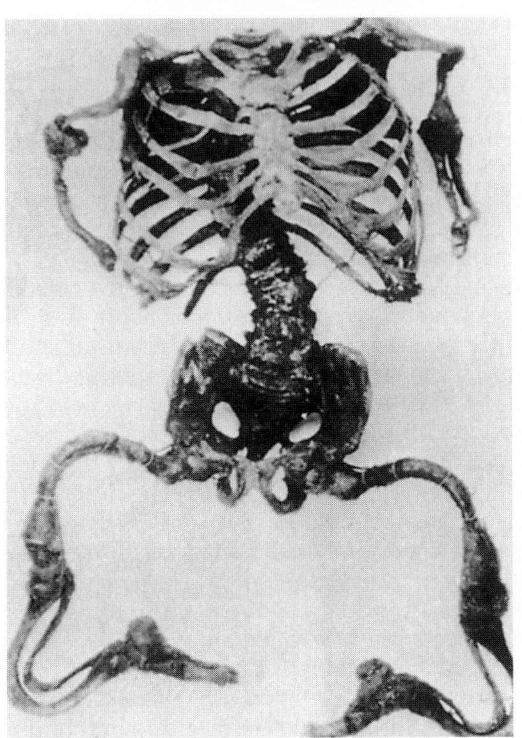

FIGURE 32–29 The skeleton in severe osteogenesis imperfecta.

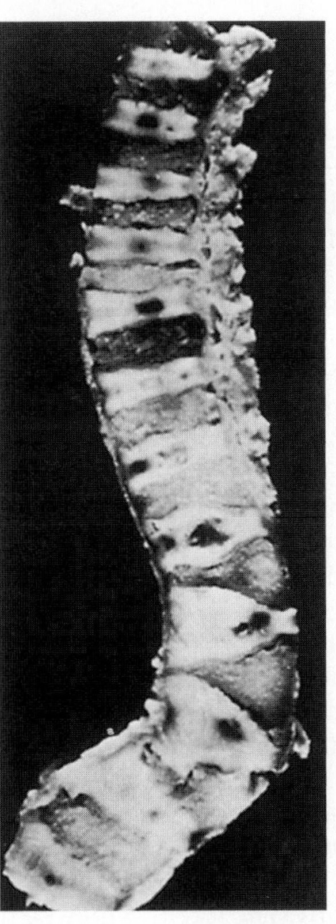

FIGURE 32–30 The spine in severe osteogenesis imperfecta. The vertebral bodies are biconcave and wedge shaped, which has resulted in kyphoscoliosis.

The spine may show varying degrees of deformity, usually scoliosis, often with compression fractures and wedging of the vertebral bodies (Fig. 32–30). Kyphosis may be combined with scoliosis.

In the skull there are multiple centers of ossification, particularly in the occipital region, and wormian bones.

Clinical Features

The clinical picture varies according to the variety of the disease. In the severe congenital form (Sillence's type II or Shapiro's congenita A), multiple fractures from minimal trauma during delivery or in utero cause the limbs to be deformed and short. Crepitation can be demonstrated by palpation at fracture sites. The skull is soft and membranous. This type is usually fatal, with death secondary to intracranial hemorrhage or respiratory insufficiency caused by incompetency of the rib cage; the infant is stillborn or lives only a short time.

In the nonlethal forms of the disease (Sillence's types I, III, and IV), fragility of the bones is the most outstanding feature. In severely affected patients, fractures can occur after the slightest injury. In general, the earlier that fractures occur, the more severe the disease, and according to Shapiro, this has direct prognostic significance for ambulation.[474] The lower limbs are more frequently affected because they are more prone to trauma. The femur is more commonly fractured than the tibia. The pattern of fracture depends on the nature of the trauma, the severity of the bone fragility, and the presence of preexisting deformity acting as a stress concentrator. Any fracture pattern may be seen in osteogenesis imperfecta, and no particular pattern is specifically diagnostic of osteogenesis imperfecta.[126] Fractures heal at a normal rate; nonunion is relatively rare but does occur.[176,345,436] Fracture callus is typically wispy, but on rare occasion it may be very large and hyperplastic, similar to osteogenic sarcoma on radiographs.* A pattern of repeated fractures can develop as the result of a combination of disuse osteopenia, progressive long-bone deformity, and joint stiffness from immobilization. Growth may be arrested by multiple microfractures at the epiphyseal ends. The frequency of fractures declines sharply after adolescence, although it may rise again in postmenopausal women. Bowing results from multiple transverse fractures of the long bones and muscle contraction across the weakened diaphysis. Typically, an anterolateral bow or proximal varus deformity of the femur develops; an anterior or anteromedial bow of the tibia may develop. Acetabular protrusion (Otto's pelvis) may be present; in one reported case this resulted in colonic obstruction.[545] The humerus is usually angled laterally or anterolaterally. The forearm may be in minimal pronation; its rotation is often severely limited. Angulation is generally greater in the upper part of both bones of the forearm. The elbow joint has cubitus varus with flexion contracture.

The forehead is broad, with prominent parietal and temporal bones and an overhanging occiput. The bulging calvaria causes faciocranial disproportion, which gives the face a triangular, elfin shape. The ears are displaced downward and outward. The configuration of the skull in osteogenesis imperfecta has been likened to that of a soldier's helmet and is called "helmet head."

Severe spinal deformity may develop because of the combination of marked osteoporosis, compression fractures of the vertebrae, and ligamentous hyperlaxity.† The resultant scoliosis or kyphosis, or both, may be very severe and disabling. Scoliosis is present in 20% to 40% of patients. The most common type of curve is thoracic scoliosis. In some patients, spondylolisthesis develops as a result of elongation of the pedicles without any actual break in the pars interarticularis. Cervical spinal fractures or instability is relatively rare but does occur,[339,391,447,567] including cases with associated cervical neurologic injury.[391,567] A more commonly reported cervical anomaly is basilar impression.[168,205,229,266,319,409,448] This condition in osteogenesis imperfecta may be due to infolding of the margins of the foramen magnum or upward migration of the odontoid process and results in compression of the brainstem and probably altered cerebrospinal fluid dynamics. Symptoms are highly variable but include headaches, ataxia, cranial nerve dysfunction, and paraparesis. Anterior or posterior decompression (or both) may be required.

Short stature is common. It is due to deformities in the limbs caused by angulation and overriding of fractures, growth disturbance at the physes, and the marked kyphoscoliosis. Hyperlaxity of ligaments with resultant hypermobility of joints is common. Pes valgus is a frequent physical finding. Recurrent dislocation of the patellofemoral joint may occur. The radial head and the hip joint may occasionally be dislocated. Developmental dysplasia of the hip can occur[137]; unfortunately, femoral fractures resulting from screening for the condition have also been reported.[387] Infants suspected of having osteogenesis imperfecta must have their hips examined very gently, and physical examination should be supplemented by ultrasound examination whenever necessary. Adults may be predisposed to rupture of the patellar ligament or Achilles tendon.[125,370]

The muscles are hypotonic, most likely because of the multiple fractures and deformities. The skin is thin and translucent, and subcutaneous hemorrhages may occur. As a rule, surgical scars tend to be wide.

Blue sclerae are one of the best-known manifestations of osteogenesis imperfecta[87] but are not present in all types. In type I they are distinctly blue throughout life, and they are also blue in type II. In type III they may be gray-blue at birth but become less blue with increasing age and are white in adulthood. In type IV they are usually normal. The blueness of the sclera is caused by the thinness of its collagen layer secondary to decreased production of type I collagen. Normal-colored sclerae in patients with osteogenesis imperfecta have normal collagen thickness, but that collagen is, of course, abnormal. The so-called Saturn ring, a frequent finding, is due to a white sclera immediately surrounding the cornea. Hyperopia is frequently present, but vision generally remains unaffected. An opacity in the periphery of the cornea, known as embryotoxon or arcus juvenilis, is common. Retinal detachment may occur.

The teeth are affected in patients with types IB and IVB disease as a result of a deficiency in dentin.[44,285] The enamel is essentially normal because it is of ectodermal, not mesenchymal, origin. Both deciduous and permanent teeth are involved. They break easily and are prone to caries, and fillings do not hold well. Yellowish brown or translucent bluish gray discoloration of the teeth is common (Fig. 32–31). The lower incisors, which erupt first, are the most severely affected. *Dentinogenesis imperfecta* (also called *hereditary opalescent dentin* or *hereditary hypoplasia of the dentin*) can exist as an isolated condition,[39] so the diagnosis of osteogenesis imperfecta must be made on criteria other than the presence of affected teeth alone.

Deafness may occur in osteogenesis imperfecta, usually beginning in adolescence or adulthood.[476] It is present in 40% of those with type I disease and is lower in frequency in type IV disease. Hearing loss may be either of the conduction type, secondary to

*See references 1, 15, 28, 30, 33, 76, 152, 251, 276, 317, 321, 433, 507, 531.

†See references 42, 43, 107, 142, 186, 219, 232, 249, 345, 426, 565.

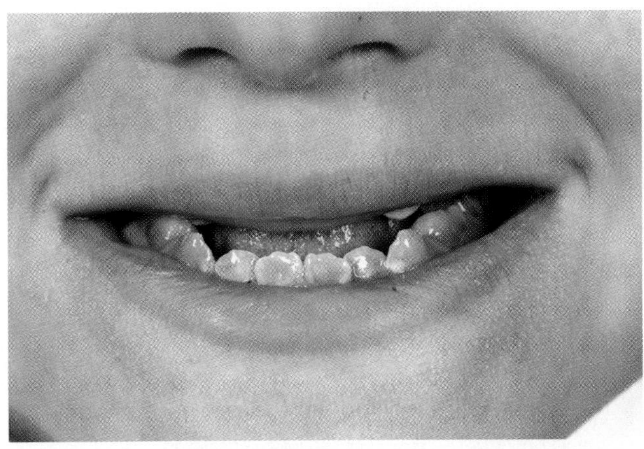

FIGURE 32–31 Dentinogenesis imperfecta. The dentin is opalescent and the teeth are fragile, prone to caries, wearing down, and fractured.

otosclerosis, or of the nerve type, caused by pressure on the auditory nerve as it emerges from the skull. Otosclerosis results from abnormal proliferation of cartilage, which on ossification produces sclerosis of the petrous portion of the temporal bone.[199]

Some patients, particularly those with type III disease, complain of excessive sweating, thought to be due to a resting hypermetabolic state.[109,452] This excessive perspiration is associated with heat intolerance and difficulty tolerating orthoses and can lead to chronic constipation.[213] A related problem is the possible susceptibility of patients to the development of malignant hyperthermia during general anesthesia. The development of increased temperature, metabolic acidosis, and cardiac arrhythmia suggesting this diagnosis has been reported.[287,408,416,450] Porsborg,[408] however, noted that results of the in vitro contracture test for malignant hyperthermia were completely normal in muscle obtained from biopsy in one such affected patient. Both surgeon and anesthesiologist must be aware of the potential for such untoward intraoperative problems.

Radiographic Findings

SEVERE FORM

Radiographic findings in patients with Sillence's type II disease (or Shapiro's congenita A) are striking at birth. The long bones of the limbs are short and wide with thin cortices. The diaphyses are as wide as the metaphyses. Shapiro noted that this appearance is an important distinction from his congenita B type, in which the metaphyses of the femur have more normal funnelization.[474] There are numerous fractures, some recent and others in various stages of healing. Multiple rib fractures and atrophy of the thoracic cage may simulate asphyxiating thoracic dysplasia. The presence of rib cage deformity is the other important radiographic feature distinguishing congenita A from congenita B disease.

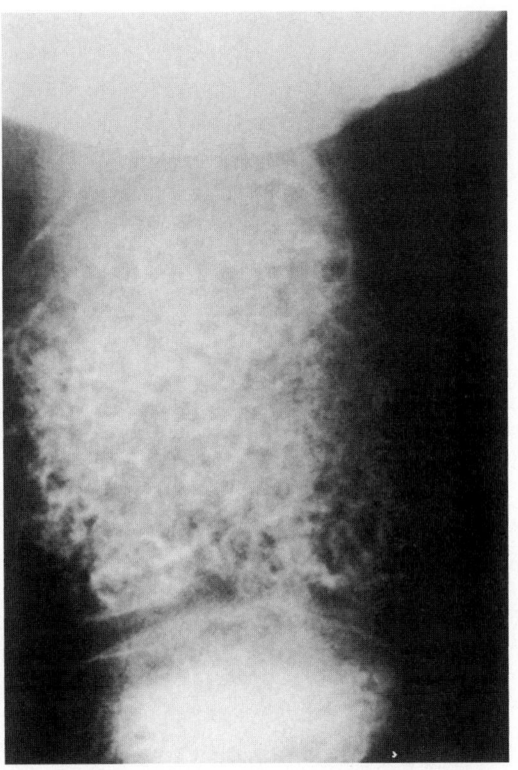

FIGURE 32–32 Appearance of "popcorn" calcifications in the distal femur, as seen in severe osteogenesis imperfecta.

Goldman and associates described "popcorn" calcifications in the metaphyseal and epiphyseal areas of long bones close to the growth plate that appeared as clustered collections of rounded or scalloped radiolucencies, each with a sclerotic margin and some with central radiopacities (Fig. 32–32).[188] These collections have been referred to in the literature as "whorls of radiodensities." They probably represent traumatic fragmentation of the cartilaginous growth plate.[75,188] The popcorn calcifications appear in childhood and usually resolve after the completion of skeletal growth. They are more frequent in the lower than in the upper limbs and more common in the severe congenital type of disease. Their appearance parallels the development of growth plate irregularity. With a growth spurt, popcorn calcifications increase in number. In a severely affected nonambulatory child, as typified by congenita B patients, the lack of normal stress will give rise to a cystic honeycomb pattern in the long bones.

The skull has a mushroom appearance with a very thin calvaria. There is a marked paucity and delay in ossification. Wormian bones (described by a Danish anatomist, Olaus Wormius, in 1643) are a salient radiographic feature of osteogenesis imperfecta.[75] They are detached portions of the primary ossification centers of the adjacent membrane bones. To be significant, wormian bones should be more than 10 in number, measure at least 6 mm by 4 mm, and be arranged in a general mosaic pattern (Fig. 32–33). Cremin and associates[106] studied the skull radiographs of 81 patients with osteogenesis imperfecta and 500 normal children

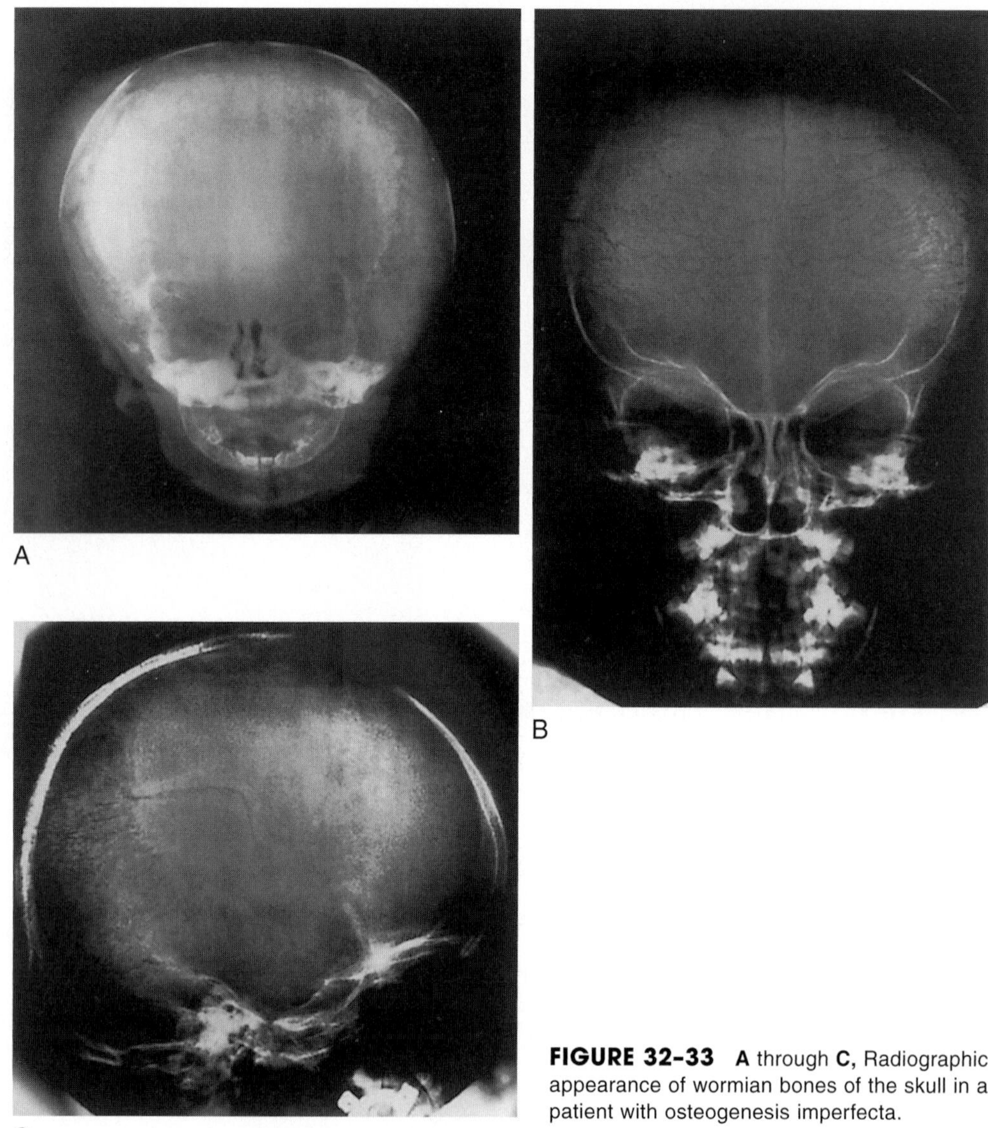

FIGURE 32–33 **A** through **C**, Radiographic appearance of wormian bones of the skull in a patient with osteogenesis imperfecta.

for the presence of significant wormian bones, which they found in all cases of osteogenesis imperfecta but not in the normal skulls.[99] Wormian bones may be present in other bone dysplasias, such as cleidocranial dysplasia, congenital hypothyroidism, pachydermoperiostosis, Menkes' syndrome, and some trisomies,[1] so their presence is not pathognomonic for osteogenesis imperfecta.

The spine shows marked osteoporosis; the vertebral bodies are compressed and become biconcave between bulging disks (Fig. 32–34). Scoliosis and kyphosis eventually develop in the majority of congenital severe forms of osteogenesis imperfecta.

MILDER FORMS

In the milder forms of osteogenesis imperfecta the radiographic picture is that of osteoporosis: the cortices and intramedullary trabeculae are thin. Fractures vary in frequency and age at occurrence. Radiographs may show fractures in various stages of healing. Fractures tend to heal and remodel adequately in less severely affected patients. Plastic bowing of long bones is common and due to microfractures and stress fractures or malunion of fractures. One lower limb may be in valgus deformation and the other in varus deviation. In the hip, coxa vara and acetabular protrusion may be found. The patellar joint, the radial head, or the hip may dislocate. Platyspondyly and biconcave vertebrae are common. Varying degrees of scoliosis and kyphosis develop in up to 40% of cases.

In adolescence or adult life, basilar impression of the foramen magnum into the posterior cranial fossa may develop.[142,168,205,229,249,266,319,409,448]

Laboratory Findings

In osteogenesis imperfecta, the results of routine laboratory investigations are normal. Specifically, serum calcium and phosphorus levels are normal. The alkaline phosphatase level may be elevated.

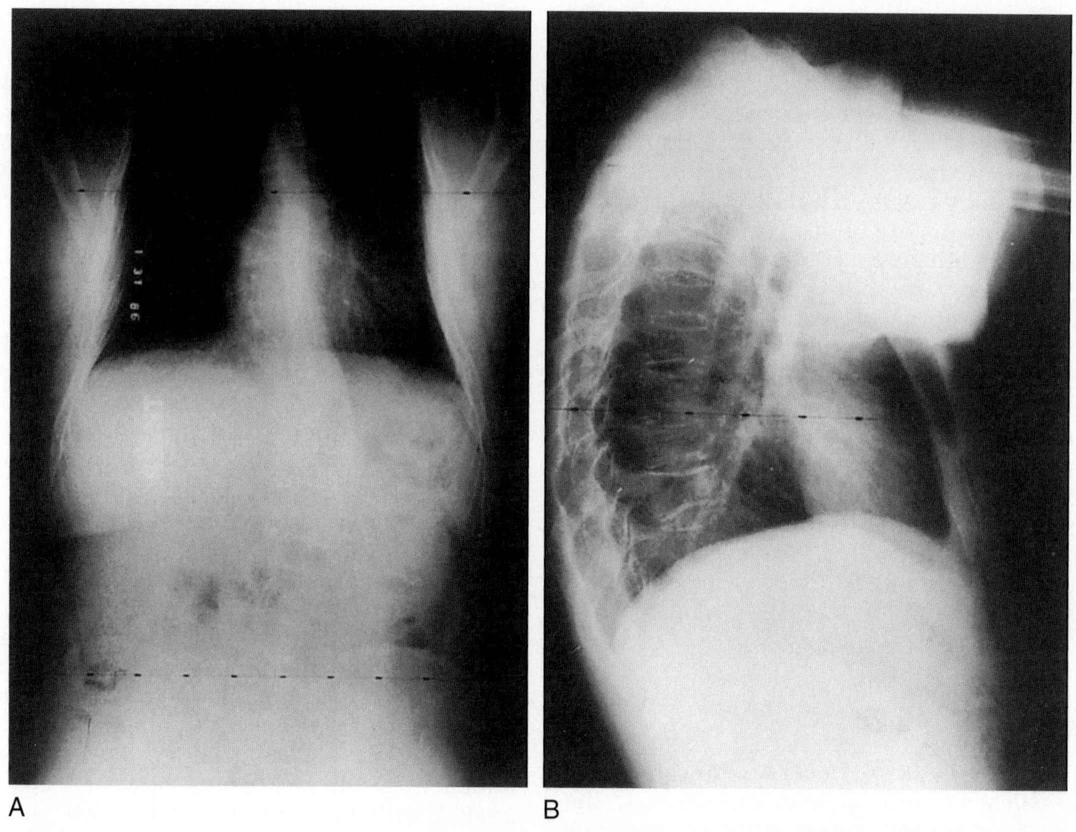

FIGURE 32-34 The spine in an adolescent with osteogenesis imperfecta. Note the structural scoliosis and the collapsed vertebrae. **A,** Anteroposterior radiograph of the spine showing structural scoliosis. **B,** Lateral radiograph of the dorsal spine showing osteoporosis and biconcave vertebrae.

In general, the diagnosis of osteogenesis imperfecta can be made with a positive family history and the presence of typical clinical and radiographic signs of the condition. However, spontaneous mutations in affected individuals, especially in patients who may be mildly affected, with white sclerae, may make the diagnosis more difficult. More than 90% of affected individuals will have a demonstrable quantitative or qualitative defect in type I collagen, or both. A very large number of genetic mutations result in these defects. As a consequence, only a few families have a sufficiently documented specific locus of mutation to allow direct or linkage analysis of the presence of the defective gene in any given individual. Much more commonly, biochemical analysis of type I collagen obtained from fibroblasts cultured from the skin biopsy specimen of the individual in whom the diagnosis is questioned will be required to confirm the diagnosis.

Differential Diagnosis

In the newborn period and in early infancy, Sillence's type II osteogenesis imperfecta should be distinguished from *congenital hypophosphatasia*. In the latter, a lethal affection, laboratory tests will show a low phosphatase level in serum, lack of alkaline phosphatase activity in leukocytes, and excessive excretion of phosphorylethanolamine in urine.

In an infant, osteogenesis imperfecta and *achondroplasia* are frequently confused clinically because an enlarged head and short limbs are common to both conditions. Radiographs will easily distinguish between the two conditions.

Camptomelic dwarfism may be mistaken for osteogenesis imperfecta because of the congenital bowing and angulation of the long bones. Fractures, however, are not a feature of this type of dwarfism.

The presence of osteoporosis and a proclivity to fracture in *cystinosis* may suggest osteogenesis imperfecta.

Patients with *pyknodysostosis* may have a propensity to fracture. Patients with this condition will have bony sclerosis evident on radiographs, persistently wide cranial fontanelles, micrognathism with absence of the mandible, hypoplasia of the clavicles, and osteolysis of the terminal phalanges of the fingers.

The diffuse osteopenia in the early stages of *leukemia,* before the appearance of the typical blood picture, may be mistaken for osteogenesis imperfecta.

Idiopathic juvenile osteoporosis may be very difficult to distinguish from osteogenesis imperfecta; the former is characterized by being a self-limited disorder and by its onset a year or so before puberty. Osteoporosis and compression fractures of the vertebrae may also be caused by prolonged intake of steroids.

An important diagnosis to be considered in patient with fractures is nonaccidental injury, that is, child abuse or battered child syndrome. Accusations of nonaccidental injury in children subsequently proved to have osteogenesis imperfecta, a presumption of osteogenesis imperfecta in abused children, and nonaccidental injury in children with osteogenesis imperfecta are all known to occur.[21,126,253,388,389,513] Therefore, the clinician must carefully assess each child with suspicious fractures. A family history of disease, blue sclerae, or the presence of dentinogenesis imperfecta will make this distinction easy in some patients. The proper diagnosis of milder forms of osteogenesis imperfecta, especially in patients without a family history or obviously blue sclerae (Sillence's type III and IV, Shapiro's tarda A and B), may be more difficult. Other than the very severe multiple fracture patterns, with or without rib and skull deformities, that characterize type II osteogenesis imperfecta, no particular fracture pattern will specifically substantiate or exclude the diagnosis of osteogenesis imperfecta. Because a specific diagnosis is clinically important, skin biopsy for culture of fibroblasts and analysis of type I collagen may be required.[314]

Treatment

There is as yet no specific treatment to correct the basic mutant gene defect in osteogenesis imperfecta. In the past, efforts to medically induce stronger bone less prone to fracture met with limited or no success. Important advances have been made in the medical management of osteogenesis imperfecta, including the use of bisphosphonates to improve bone density. For severe disease, early trials using allogeneic bone marrow transplantation are under way as well.[223] The orthopaedic surgeon will be extensively involved in the care of children with osteogenesis imperfecta in the course of managing individual fractures, repeated fractures, long-bone deformity, spinal deformity, and overall rehabilitation.

MEDICAL TREATMENT

Until recently, efforts to improve bone strength by medical means were largely unsuccessful. The administration of sex hormones,[85] sodium fluoride,[3,49] calcitonin,[84,361] calcium, growth hormone, magnesium oxide, and vitamins D or C were all attempted in the past, generally with no or mixed results.

Considerable experience has been reported in the use of bisphosphonates for children with osteogenesis imperfecta.[20,40,171,187,227,282] These compounds inhibit osteoclastic resorption of bone, an activity that appears to be increased in patients with osteogenesis imperfecta. Aminohydroxypropylidene (pamidronate) has been studied extensively. This medication is administered intravenously in dosages ranging from 15 mg given every 20 days[40] to 7 mg/kg/yr given every 4 to 6 months,[20] with reported improvement in generalized bone pain and a reduced incidence of fractures.[282] In addition, increased bone mineral density as determined by dual-energy x-ray absorptiometry has been noted.[20,40,187,282] Transient fever and increased serum calcium levels can occur during the intravenous administration of this medication. Metaphyseal bands of increased density are seen in radiographs after bisphosphonate treatment.[197]

Oral agents have also been used. Alendronate given over a period of 4 years was associated with reduced frequency of fracture and improved ambulatory or mobility status. Bone mineral density was also improved.[93] Olpadronate treatment was effective in a randomized study in reducing fracture risk and increasing bone mineral density.[455] A study by Dimeglio and coworkers showed equally beneficial effects in children treated with oral versus intravenous bisphosphonates.[131]

Delayed healing of fractures or osteotomies has been reported in children treated with pamidronate. Munns and colleagues found definite delay of healing of osteotomies and possible delay of fracture healing in a study of a large cohort of children.[355] Another study of a small number of children failed to find this effect.[405]

The ideal treatment of osteogenesis imperfecta would be to correct the basic genetic defect by replacing the defective *COL1A1* or *COL1A2* gene with a normal one. That capability, of course, does not yet exist. Horwitz and associates[222] have published preliminary results in three severely affected patients treated with bone marrow harvested from an unaffected sibling after host marrow suppression.[222,223] Subsequent biopsy in the recipients demonstrated exuberant new bone formation, and most hematopoietic cells were of donor origin. Correspondingly, bone density measurements improved, growth velocity increased, and there was a dramatic reduction in the incidence of fractures. However, pulmonary insufficiency and sepsis also developed in one of the three patients during treatment. Thus, these promising preliminary results must be very carefully assessed in the context of the considerable morbidity and potential mortality associated with bone marrow transplantation.

ORTHOPAEDIC TREATMENT

The goal of orthopaedic treatment is to maximize the affected patient's function, prevent deformity and disability resulting from fractures, correct deformities that have developed, and monitor for potential complicating conditions associated with osteogenesis imperfecta. In addition, the orthopaedist should be able to provide realistic expectations of disability and mobility to the family of an affected infant. These goals can be analyzed according to prognostication for future mobility and complications, nonoperative rehabilitation, and the specific management of fractures, long-bone deformity, spinal deformity, and basilar impression.

Orthotic Treatment

The orthopaedist will be called on to assist in the rehabilitation of infants with osteogenesis imperfecta who survive the neonatal period. Infants with birth fractures usually need only careful, supportive handling to prevent further injury. If long-bone fractures are unstable, minimal external splinting may be used to stabilize the affected limb; such fractures will generally heal within a week or two. It is important to avoid excessive or prolonged immobilization at any age because such treatment will aggravate the osteopenia and induce joint stiffness, either of which in turn increases the risk for fracture.

Protective bracing to prevent fractures and aid in ambulation is a mainstay in the conservative management of patients with osteogenesis imperfecta.* Typically, lightweight plastic and metal hip-knee-ankle-foot orthoses (HKAFOs) are required for effective lower extremity bracing in the most severely affected patients. These braces may allow patients to stand or walk, usually with the upper extremity aids of crutches or a walker. In addition, HKAFOs can reduce the incidence of lower extremity fractures as compared with the incidence in unbraced patients.[182,183]

Lightweight air-filled fluted trouser splints have been reported to be an effective simple alternative to HKAFOs for the purpose of allowing severely affected children to stand.[172,284,346] These splints are lighter than conventional orthoses and easier to fit, provided that the child does not have major lower extremity long-bone deformity. However, they are not in common use in North America.

Nonambulatory patients with osteogenesis imperfecta are ideal users of motorized wheelchairs because they have the intelligence to use them effectively and often have upper extremity deformity or weakness that hinders the use of standard wheelchairs. Custom inserts may be required to support the trunk and accommodate the spinal deformity. Such mobility aids should be made available to nonambulatory patients as soon as the child's intellectual development allows safe operation.

Management of Long-Bone Fractures

Management of long-bone fractures depends on the severity of the fracture and the age of the patient. General management principles are based on the observations that most fractures heal, recurrent fractures are common, and inherent osteopenia may be aggravated by prolonged immobilization, thus making the patient even more susceptible to fracture. For these reasons, fractures should be immobilized only until symptoms resolve, with the minimum amount of external immobilization required to provide comfort. Patients should be encouraged to return judiciously to their usual level of activity as soon as feasible. Radiographs are not always required, especially if the fracture is not grossly unstable or does not result in a new deformity. The patient's immobilization should be based on symptoms, and serial radiographs are not generally necessary for minor fractures. Frequently, children have pain suggesting a fracture but radiographs show no evidence of one. Such patients should be immobilized as though a fracture were present (which it almost certainly is). Although technetium 99m–enhanced bone scan, MRI, or follow-up radiographs can demonstrate fracture, these investigations are rarely necessary and are of no help to the patient or physician in management of the fracture. Many times, the parents of a severely affected child will not even seek medical assistance for minor fractures because of the frequency of such fractures and the confidence gained by the parent in treating the infant or child symptomatically.

Fractures in a newborn, if unstable or interfering with normal handling, may be splinted with padded tongue depressors, padded aluminum splints, or plaster splints. Usually, only a week or two of splinting will be required until the fracture has stabilized. Fractures in an older child or adult, particularly when the patient has relatively minor involvement, should be treated by means appropriate to the fracture, including reduction and casting, percutaneous pinning, or internal fixation. The operating surgeon must exercise extreme caution in handling the patient and the fracture to prevent further fracture or fragmentation of the fracture under treatment. As a general principle, intramedullary fixation is preferable to plates and screws whenever possible because of the stress risers produced by the latter. The operating surgeon must be familiar with the techniques and pitfalls unique to the use of intramedullary fixation in patients with osteogenesis imperfecta, as discussed later under Management of Long-Bone Deformity. Presumably, external fixation may also be used in these patients when indicated, and external fixation has been used to correct deformities in patients with osteogenesis imperfecta.[165,271,432] However, the use of external fixation for fractures in patients with osteogenesis imperfecta has not been described in the literature, and the benefits and risks of this technique must be carefully assessed by the treating surgeon.

Other than extreme fragility and the crumpled long-bone deformities seen in severe cases of osteogenesis imperfecta, no specific fracture pattern is unique to these patients.[126] One fracture that occurs commonly, usually in more mildly affected patients with Sillence's type I disease, is a displaced fracture of the olecranon.[128,318,352,506] These fractures often occur bilaterally, though not usually simultaneously.[128,318,506] They can be managed by tension band wiring techniques, with good restoration of function (Fig. 32–35).[482]

Nonunion is an uncommon sequela of fracture or surgery in osteogenesis imperfecta, but it does occur. Gamble and associates reported 12 nonunions in 10 patients; the nonunions occurred most commonly in the femur and humerus, but also in the radius, ulna, and pubis.[176] Nine of the 10 patients had osteogenesis imperfecta type III. Frequent fractures and deformity at the affected site were often associated with the development of nonunion. Eight of the nine fractures that were operated on healed after intramedullary fixation and grafting. Such treatment failed in one

*See references 50-52, 57, 65, 117, 172, 182, 183, 284, 346.

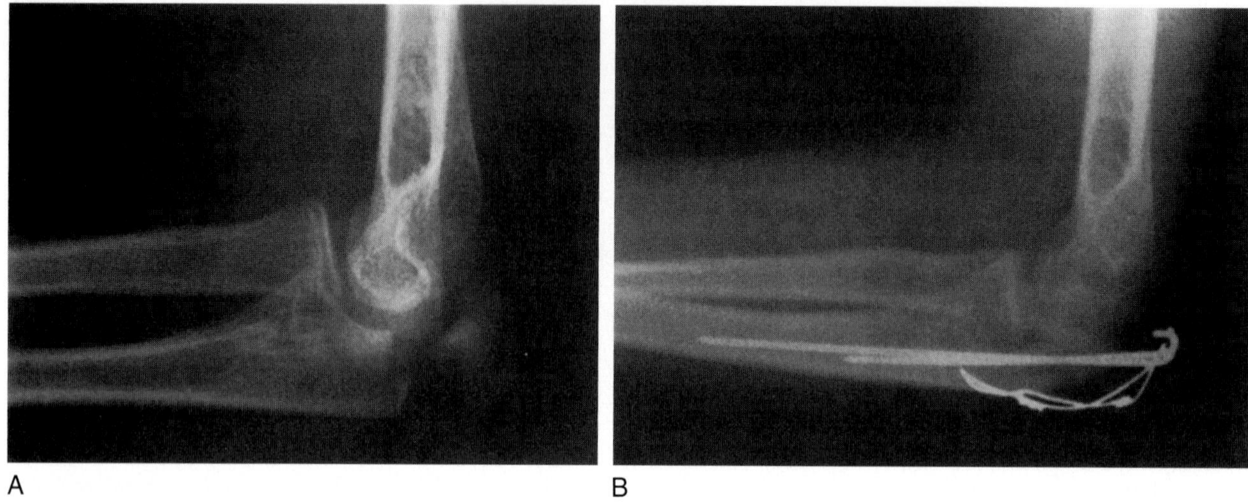

FIGURE 32-35 Olecranon fracture in a patient with mild osteogenesis imperfecta type I. **A,** Preoperative radiograph showing the typical avulsion pattern of this fracture. **B,** Postoperative radiograph after open reduction and internal fixation with a tension band wiring technique.

supracondylar femoral nonunion, and the patient required an amputation for pain relief.

Management of Long-Bone Deformity

Long-bone deformity is one of the most frequent conditions requiring treatment in patients with osteogenesis imperfecta. Its incidence is in general related to the severity of the underlying bone fragility, and thus it is more likely to be seen in Sillence's types III and IV, although this deformity is by no means limited to these types. Long-bone bowing is induced by bone fragility, deforming muscular forces, and repeated fractures and, in turn, results in repeated fractures. Thus, the most important indication for surgical correction of long-bone deformity is repeated fractures induced by the deformity. A further indication for surgery is to remove the deformity to allow bracing either for protection against further fractures or to aid in ambulation. It is not clear from the literature, however, that correction of long-bone deformity alone results in long-term ambulation.[117] Long-bone deformity in infants and children can be corrected by closed osteoclasis without intramedullary fixation,[346] by closed osteoclasis with percutaneous intramedullary fixation,[170,324,340,341,451,479] and by open osteotomy with internal fixation.* In addition, external fixation by the Ilizarov circular fixator with wire fixation and osteotomy has been used to correct long-bone deformity in young adult patients.[165,271,432,457]

Closed Osteoclasis without Internal Fixation. Manual osteoclasis of long-bone deformity has been described[346] and is generally indicated in medically fragile children who may not be able to tolerate the blood loss and other physiologic stresses of a formal open operative procedure but whose deformity creates management difficulties. In essence, the treating physician gently manipulates the deformed bone with the child under adequate sedation or anesthesia and immobilizes the limb until union. This procedure is usually followed by the application of protective bracing to help prevent further fractures and recurrent deformity. The procedure is indicated only when one of the procedures described in the following sections is not possible for any reason.

Closed Osteoclasis with Percutaneous Intramedullary Fixation. This procedure is essentially the same as the previous one, except that in addition to external manual correction of the deformity, the operating surgeon attempts to "splint" the long bone by percutaneously threading a smooth rod (Kirschner wire, Steinmann pin, or Rush rod) in an intramedullary fashion.[170,324,340,341,451,479] This procedure is also indicated for a patient who sustains repeated fractures that interfere with care and in whom formal open fixation is not feasible because of bone fragility. The basic surgical technique is to percutaneously thread a small-diameter smooth rod within the intramedullary canal of an affected bone while simultaneously bending or breaking the bone by external compression to allow the rod to pass within the intramedullary canal. Fluoroscopy and good fortune are required. We prefer to manage patients conservatively until their age, bone size, and medical stability allow them to undergo open osteoclasis with intramedullary fixation.

Open Osteotomy with Intramedullary Fixation (Sofield's Procedure). A procedure entailing multiple diaphyseal osteotomies ("fragmentation") with intramedullary fixation was described for osteogenesis imperfecta by Sofield and Millar.[494] The indications for fragmentation and rodding are a long-bone deformity

---

*See references 24, 25, 72, 98, 116, 117, 143, 169, 178, 180, 240, 272, 296, 307, 308, 338, 356, 358, 360, 407, 435-437, 494, 504, 519, 552-554, 564, 566.

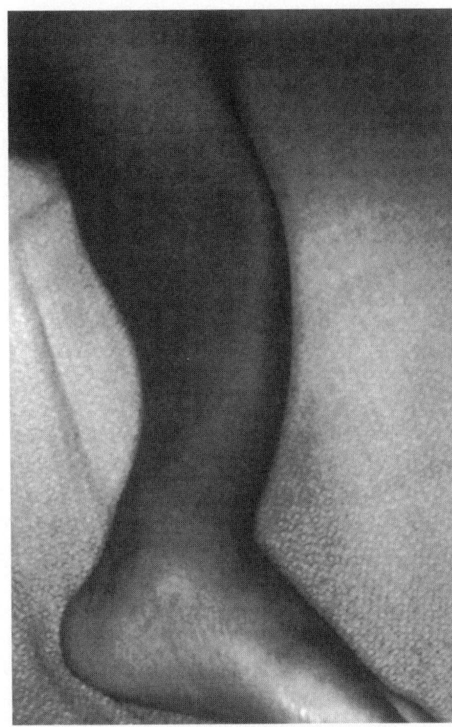
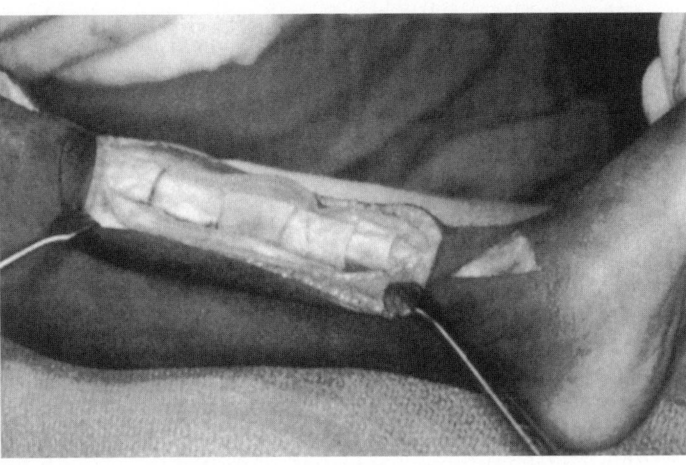

A B

FIGURE 32–36 Sofield's procedure of fragmentation and intramedullary fixation of a long bone. **A,** Preoperative appearance of the long-bone deformity. **B,** Intraoperative photograph showing multiple osteotomies to allow straightening of the bone, with intramedullary fixation of the fragments on a rod (see text).

that interferes with fitting of orthoses and impairs function and repeated fractures. These indications are much more frequent in the lower than in the upper extremity. The basic principle is to expose the deformed bone subperiosteally, make appropriate wedge-shaped osteotomies in the deformed metaphysis and diaphysis to allow straightening of the bone, and fix the fragments on an intramedullary rod of some sort to maintain alignment and provide long-term internal splinting of the fragile bone (Fig. 32–36). A great deal has been written about the technique and the results achieved with different intramedullary devices.* In general, reports are favorable in that deformity is corrected and mobility maintained or achieved.† In a survey of adults, however, Daly and associates were unable to demonstrate that intramedullary fixation had a long-term influence with respect to maintaining the ability to ambulate.[117] Complications of the procedure include nonunion, infection, and rod migration. These complications are nonetheless remarkably uncommon in the context of a procedure that produces multiple devascularized segments of long bone.

Sofield and Millar used a fixed intramedullary rod (a "straight, round steel rod," Rush rod, or Küntscher rod) for internal fixation.[494] Other authors have used Rush rods[296,345,407] or Williams rods.[553,554] The technique of Williams rod insertion is described in Chapter 22, Disorders of the Leg, in the section titled Intramedullary Fixation. When a Williams rod is used in the tibia, the rod is usually left embedded within the tibia itself and not left across the ankle and subtalar joints. This procedure must be undertaken with careful preoperative planning and good communication among the orthopedic surgeon, operating room personnel, and anesthesiologist. All parties must handle the fragile child carefully. Blood pressure cuffs may not be advisable if humeral fragility is extreme. The patient's temperature will often rise during surgery, and the patient should be kept cool. The anesthesiologist must be alert to temperature elevation, metabolic acidosis, the potential for cardiac arrhythmias, and the possible development of true malignant hyperthermia (see Chapter 8, Anesthesiology). Excessive bleeding requiring transfusion is a distinct possibility and must be prepared for. Patients with osteogenesis imperfecta tend to bruise easily, and a bleeding diathesis may develop. The surgeon will probably not be able to use a tourniquet during extremity surgery. Extensive exposure of the deformed bone will be necessary to perform corrective osteotomies, and many trying technical challenges may arise as the surgeon attempts to thread a series of fragile, macaroni-shaped wisps of bone onto an unforgiving rod. Thus, when surgery on both femora or on all four lower limb segments is indicated, the operations may need to be staged to avoid life-threatening hemorrhage.

The operating surgeon and the operating staff must have available a full assortment of lengths and breadths of the intramedullary device to be used, as well as pliers and bolt cutters to modify the device as needed during insertion. Fluoroscopy should be available to

*See references 24, 25, 72, 76, 83, 98, 116, 117, 143, 169, 170, 178, 180, 240, 272, 296, 307, 308, 321, 338, 340, 345, 356, 358, 360, 407, 435-437, 494, 504, 519, 552-554, 564, 566.

†See references 98, 143, 169, 240, 272, 296, 345, 358, 504, 552, 566.

help guide insertion when it is not done under direct vision, such as through the epiphyses.

Extensive exposure of most of the length of the involved bone is almost always required. The femur is approached anterolaterally and the tibia directly anteriorly. Care should be taken to identify the landmarks of the anterolateral approach to the femur, especially the intermuscular septum. Otherwise, excessive bleeding and damage to muscle will result. Once the curved bone is exposed, the surgeon cuts into it with a knife, rongeur, osteotome, or saw, as needed, in as many places as necessary to create a straight diaphysis. Although some authors have recommended preserving as much periosteal insertion in the bone as possible to maintain blood supply to the individual segments,[504,552] in fact, nonunion or infection harbored by devascularized bone is surprisingly infrequent, and such preservation of periosteal insertion may not be important. Straightening the deformed limb will result in soft tissue lengthening, so portions of bone may have to be removed to avoid excessive soft tissue tension.

Intramedullary reaming is frequently required. The surgeon should choose the narrowest bone fragment first and ream with a drill bit of appropriate diameter. There may be no medullary cavity. Beginning at one metaphyseal or epiphyseal end, depending on the rod being used, the rod is then advanced toward the other metaphysis, with the bone fragments threaded on the rod as it is advanced. The rod must be carefully sized for length before it is advanced into the final segment and cut as necessary. In most instances, rotational control of the bone is poor, and the patient should be immobilized in a long-leg or spica cast. Weight bearing in the cast should be encouraged as soon as feasible, and the cast should be replaced with an HKAFO as soon as union is evident radiographically.

Use of Extensible Intramedullary Rods. One of the problems that can develop with the use of a fixed-length intramedullary device in children is growth of the epiphysis beyond the rod. This often results in progressive deformity beyond the limits of the rod, with fracture or protrusion of the rod. Revision of the intramedullary fixation is thus often required, especially if the child was young when the procedure was first performed. To overcome this problem, Bailey and Dubow introduced an extensible intramedullary fixation device to reduce the need for reoperation because of bone overgrowth (Fig. 32–37).[25] The telescoping intramedullary rod consists of an outer tubular sleeve with a detachable T-shaped end and an inner obturator rod with a solid T-shaped end. The inner rod can be entirely telescoped into the sleeve (Fig. 32–38).

The surgical approach to the femur and tibia and the technique of fragmenting and stringing the diaph-

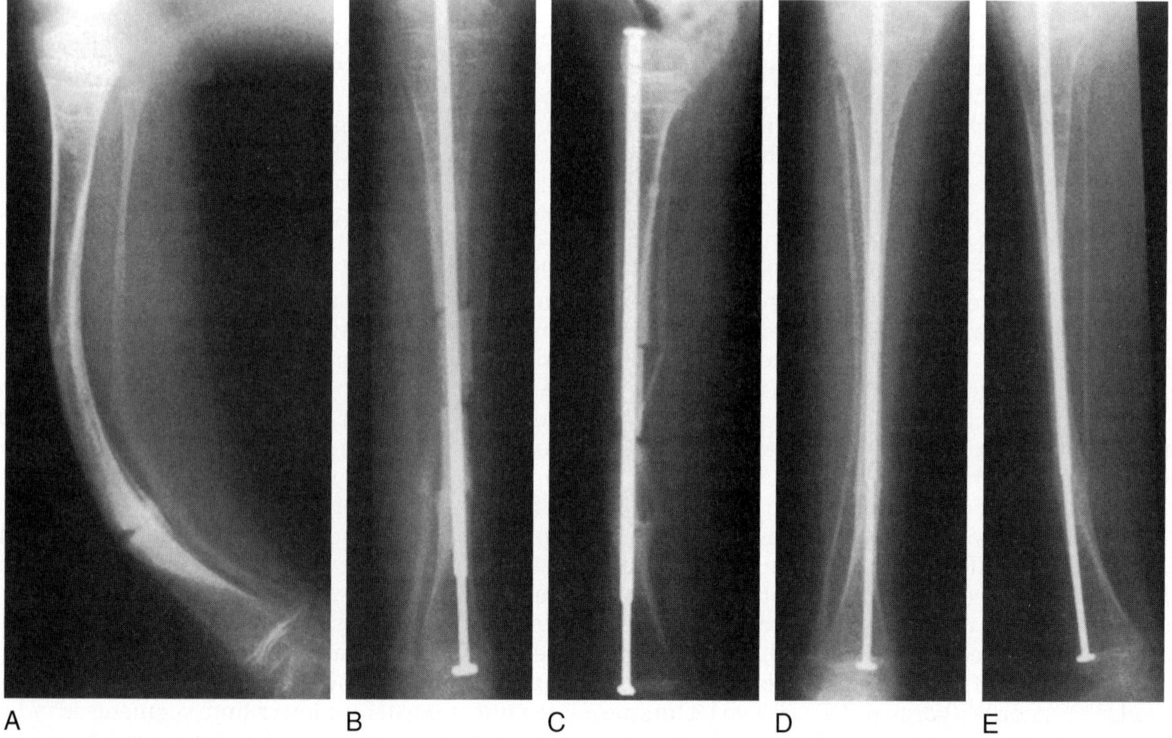

FIGURE 32–37 Use of a Bailey-Dubow extensible rod in the tibia. **A,** Preoperative lateral radiograph of the tibia of a boy with osteogenesis imperfecta type I, repeated fractures, and anterior bowing of the tibial diaphysis. **B,** Postoperative anteroposterior (AP) view of the tibia. Multiple osteotomies of the tibial diaphysis have been performed, with intramedullary fixation of the tibia with a Bailey-Dubow extensible rod. **C,** Postoperative lateral view demonstrating correction of the anterior bow deformity. **D,** AP view of the tibia 2 years later demonstrating extension of the rod. The patient sustained no further fractures of this tibia. **E,** Lateral radiograph demonstrating maintenance of correction of the deformity.

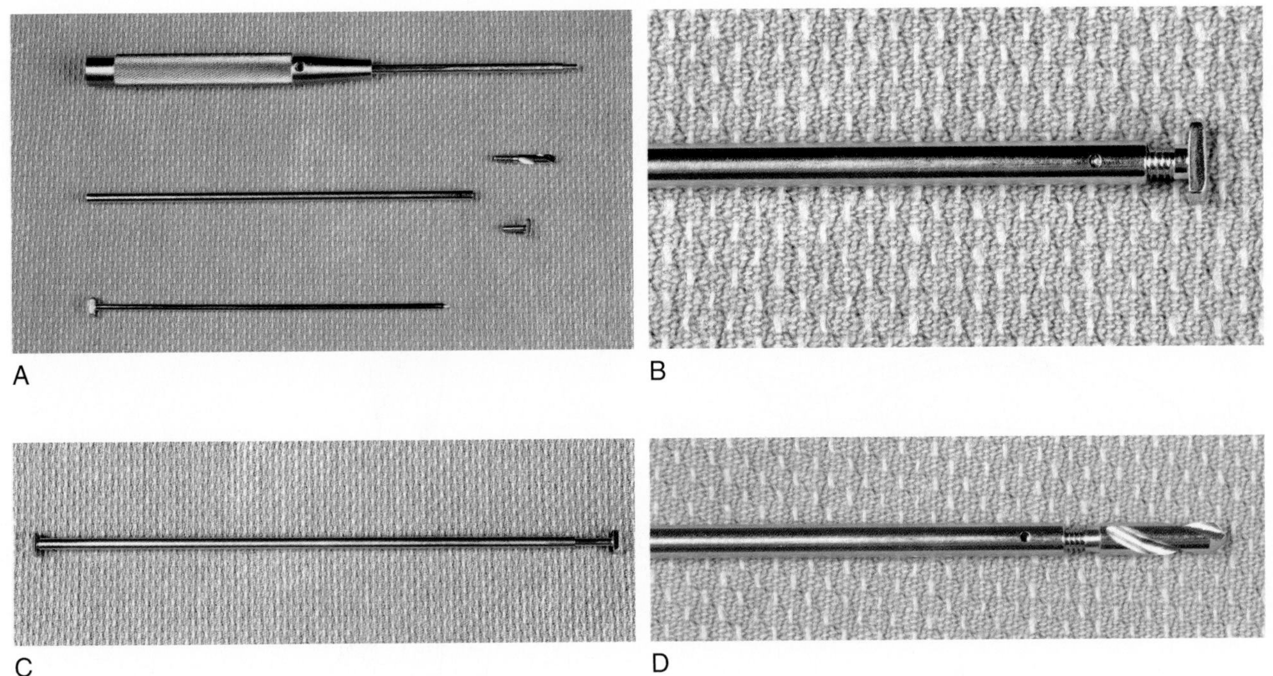

FIGURE 32–38 Bailey-Dubow extensible rod used for intramedullary fixation of a long bone. **A,** The device consists of a hollow outer rod, one end of which is threaded to receive either a like-diameter drill bit or a T-piece; a narrower inner rod with a fixed T-piece; and inserters. **B,** The outer rod has a threaded end to accept the T-piece for fixation into the epiphysis. **C,** The inner rod slides into the outer rod and has a fixed T-piece end. **D,** The outer rod may be inserted by using the removable drill bit, which threads into the end of the rod. See Figure 32–41 for a description of the surgical details.

ysis on the rod are similar to those of Sofield and Millar. The bowed bone is exposed subperiosteally from metaphysis to metaphysis. Additional exposure of the epiphyses is required for insertion of the T-piece for the outer rod and the inner, fixed T-ended rod. In the femur, the intercondylar notch is exposed by knee arthrotomy. Usually, only minimal exposure of the upper end of the femur is required, in the region of the greater trochanter. In the tibia, the tibial plateau is exposed by knee arthrotomy. Access to the distal end of the tibia is gained by arthrotomy and mobilization of the talus. The latter is accomplished by dividing the deltoid ligament, formally osteotomizing the medial malleolus (not generally required or feasible because of bone fragility), or detaching the insertion of the deltoid ligament along with a sliver of medial malleolus with a knife.

The length of the outer rod must be carefully determined. The fragments may be directly measured, or the limb may be gently pulled out to length and the distance between the epiphyses measured. The outer rod should be several centimeters shorter than the total length estimated to be needed, to allow some settling after surgery and to maximize proper rod elongation. The outer rod has a detachable T-piece and a like-diameter drill bit with a threaded base. The drill bit can be threaded onto the outer rod in place of the T-piece to facilitate insertion of the rod during surgery. In the femur, the outer rod is generally placed proximally, where the greater fracture stresses tend to occur. In addition, this T-piece can detach from the rod, and this complication is less of a problem if it occurs at the greater trochanter than in the knee.

After a rod of appropriate length and diameter has been selected, the most effective sequence of rod insertion for the femur is as follows (Fig. 32–39). (1) The drill bit is inserted into the proximal end of the outer rod. (2) Commencing either from the distal end of the lowest metaphyseal fragment (if this is close to the epiphysis) or from the intercondylar region of the distal femur, the surgeon drives the outer rod proximally while threading the segments of bone on the rod as it is advanced. (3) When the rod exits the proximal femur at the greater trochanter or the base of the femoral neck, the outer rod and drill bit are driven further proximally until they tent the skin. (4) A small incision is made over the rod, the drill bit is removed, the T-piece is threaded in place, and the outer rod is crimped over the threads with a pair of pliers to help prevent the T-piece from disengaging from the rod. (5) The outer rod with the T-piece engaged is pushed back into the upper part of the femur, where it is countersunk into the femur. The T-piece should be grasped with small pliers or a similar instrument and rotated 90 degrees to help secure the outer rod within the proximal epiphysis. (6) The obturator is then passed through the intercondylar notch into the outer rod under direct vision or fluoroscopic control. Its T-piece, which is solid on the rod, is likewise countersunk under the distal femoral epiphyseal cartilage and rotated 90 degrees.

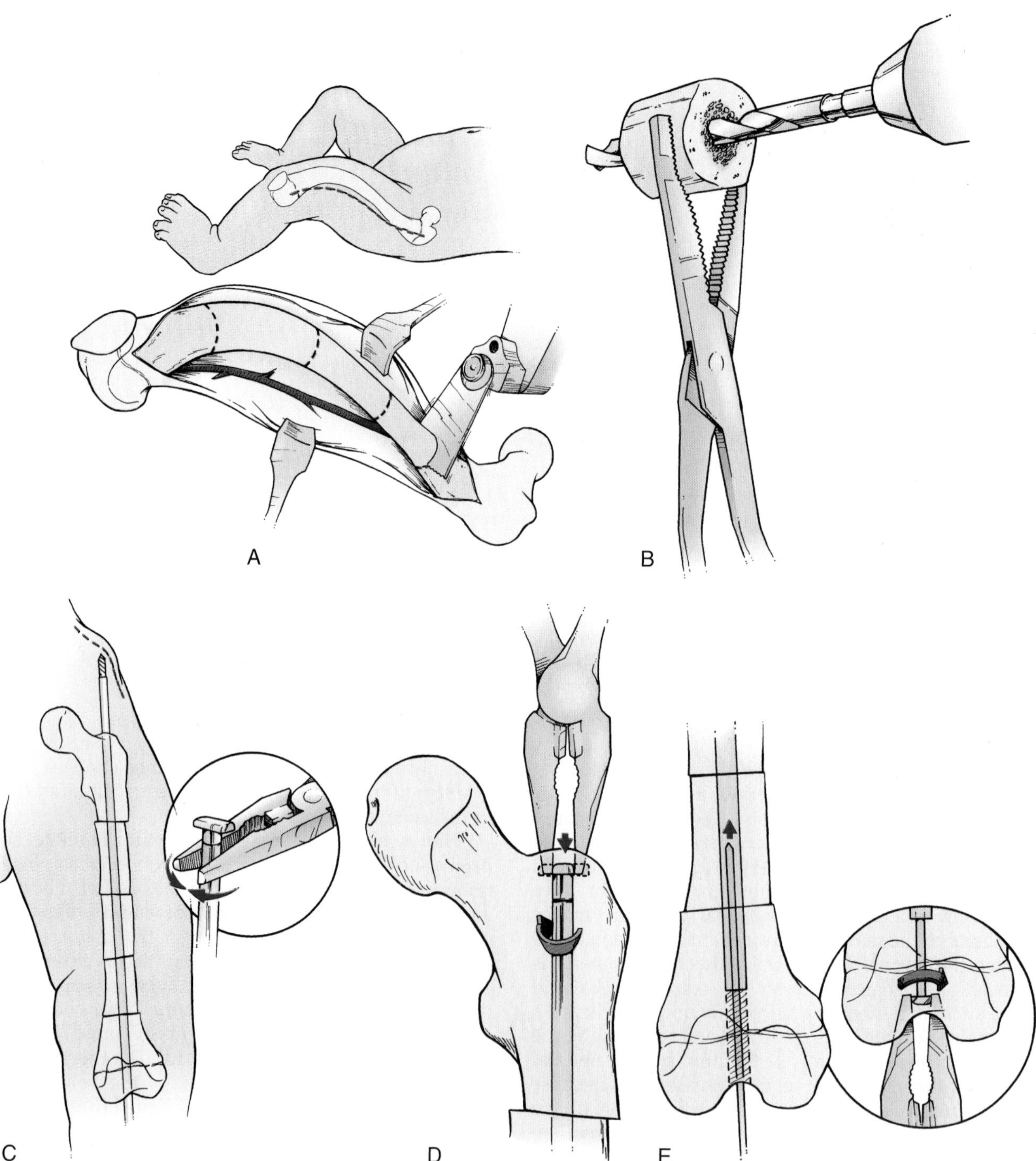

FIGURE 32–39 Surgical technique of insertion of an extensible rod into the femur. **A,** After subperiosteal exposure of the femur from metaphysis to metaphysis, an appropriate number of osteotomies are performed to allow straightening of the bone and fixation on the intramedullary rod. **B,** The individual bone segments are reamed to accept the rod, and the largest-diameter rod is selected based on the reaming. An outer rod of appropriate length is selected either by direct measurement of the fragments or by gently pulling on the limb and measuring from epiphysis to epiphysis. The outer rod should be a few centimeters shorter than this measurement to permit postoperative settling of the fragments and normal telescopic action of the rods. **C,** With the drill bit attached to the proximal end of the selected outer rod, the rod is carefully driven proximally under direct vision or fluoroscopic control. The individual fragments are threaded on the rod as it is advanced. When the rod exits the proximal end of the femur, it is advanced until it tents the skin. The skin is incised at this point, the drill bit is removed, and the T-piece is inserted into the rod. The end of the rod should be crimped over the threaded portion with a pair of pliers before the rod is reinserted to help prevent disengagement of the T-piece. **D,** The outer rod is pushed back to the level of the proximal femur and into the bone. The T-piece is grasped with a small clamp and rotated 90 degrees under the cortex of the bone. This helps prevent proximal migration of the outer rod and keeps the rod in the proximal portion of the femur. **E,** Under direct fluoroscopic guidance, the inner rod is inserted through the intercondylar drill hole into the outer rod. The T-piece of the inner rod is pushed into the distal femoral epiphysis and similarly rotated 90 degrees with a small clamp. The wounds are then closed and the patient is immobilized in a spica cast.

In the tibia, the sequence of steps is similar. Because the detachable T-piece of the outer rod is located intra-articularly, there is no advantageous position for it, in contradistinction to the femur. Gaining access to the distal tibial epiphysis can be awkward, so it may be a little easier to thread the outer rod in a proximal-to-distal direction, remove the drill bit as it exits the distal tibia into the ankle joint, replace it with the T-piece, and then push the rod proximally until the T-piece can be countersunk in the distal tibial epiphysis. However, authors have described both proximal and distal insertion of the outer rod in the tibia. These rods can also be used in the humerus, although the need to correct deformity here is much less frequent than in the femur and tibia. Furthermore, complications related to intramedullary fixation are more common here than in the lower extremity.[98,180,240,308] When used in the humerus, the outer rod is inserted through the upper part of the humerus and exits at the greater tuberosity, and the inner obturator rod is inserted through the lateral epicondyle. These rods are not indicated for use in the radius or ulna.

Although most authors have described burying the T-pieces in the epiphysis and rotating them 90 degrees to help keep them in the epiphysis,* the originators of the device initially described leaving the T-pieces outside the epiphysis.[24,25,436] We agree with the majority of authors on this topic in that we believe that the T-pieces should be buried within the epiphyseal cartilage. Stockley and associates have described a modified version of the original device.[504] The device comes in a broader array of lengths and diameters, the T-pieces are fixed to the end of both rods, and the T-pieces are butterfly-shaped so that they can be more easily grasped for rotation during insertion into the epiphysis.[504,552] Experience with this rod, the Sheffield rod, over a 10-year period has shown significant reduction in the frequency of fractures and improvement in ambulatory status.[354] The procedure may be performed with percutaneous rod placement and small incisions for osteotomies.[286] Another new telescoping device, the Fassier-Duval rod, is implanted through small incisions, with early reports showing good stability and function of the implants.[156] Multiple bone segments can be treated at the same sitting with this procedure, just as with the Bailey-Dubow rod.[145]

Clearly, insertion of these rods is more complex than insertion of fixed devices such as Kirschner wires, Steinmann pins, Williams rods, Rush rods, or other fixed-length rods. Correspondingly, the intraoperative procedure is much more complex and the opportunity for technical problems and rod failure much greater. Complications specific to this device include failure of the rod to elongate, extrusion of the rod into soft tissues (especially the proximal part of the thigh), disengagement of the T-piece of the Bailey-Dubow rod, and bending of the rod with bone fractures at the junction of the outer and inner rods (Fig. 32–40). Other complications of the procedures include infection, nonunion, hypertrophic callus formation, and growth arrest (rarely). These complications are well documented in a number of publications,* in which the reported complication rate varies from 7% to 100%. In addition, several authors have noted that an alarming involution of cortical bone can occur around the rod, with the original bone all but disappearing. Fortunately, no specific clinical problem has been identified with this radiographic finding. On the other hand, when the rods do perform as intended, most publications comparing telescoping rods and fixed-length rods note this advantage when the patient has enough growth remaining to warrant the more complex index procedure. Just what age corresponds to "enough growth remaining" is uncertain, but use of these rods should be strongly considered in children younger than 10 years.

Rodriguez and Wickstrom reported their experience with fragmentation and use of the extensible intramedullary rod; in 13 of the 15 long bones operated on, the telescoping rod proved effective.[437] In the experience of Marafioti and Westin, the use of 47 Bailey-Dubow elongating rods increased the average length of time between replacement operations, yielded a lower removal rate, and showed no additional adverse effects.[307] Reoperation was required three and a half times less often with the telescoping rod than with the solid rod. Jerosch and associates evaluated the results of 107 rods placed in the upper and lower extremities of 29 patients.[240] They reported a 68% complication rate. The most common complication was proximal rod migration into the gluteal region or the knee. The second most common complication was loosening of the T-piece. In addition, there was a 5% infection rate and two nonunions. Additional complications reported with the extensible rod include failure to elongate as desired and bending of the obturator rod at the junction of the two after fracture. Porat and colleagues, however, in a 10-year follow-up comparison of 32 Bailey-Dubow rods and 24 Rush rods used in the lower extremities of 20 patients, found that the overall complication rate was 72% for the Bailey-Dubow rod and 50% for the Rush rod.[407] The authors found that the reoperation rate and time to revision surgery were similar for the two types of rods. Thus, they believed that the results of the Bailey-Dubow rods did not justify the burden of the additional technical challenges that their insertion presents to the surgeon. We recommend the procedure, but the operating surgeon must be alert to and warn families of the relatively high complication rate.

Management of Spinal Deformity

Involvement of the cervical spine, other than basilar impression (see discussion under Basilar Impression), is a relatively uncommon feature of osteogenesis imperfecta.[339,391,447,567] Involvement of the thoracolumbar spine is much more common. Fracture of the

*See references 143, 169, 178, 240, 272, 296, 358, 504, 552, 566.

*See references 72, 76, 116, 142, 169, 178, 180, 240, 272, 296, 307, 321, 358, 407, 435, 436, 504, 552, 566.

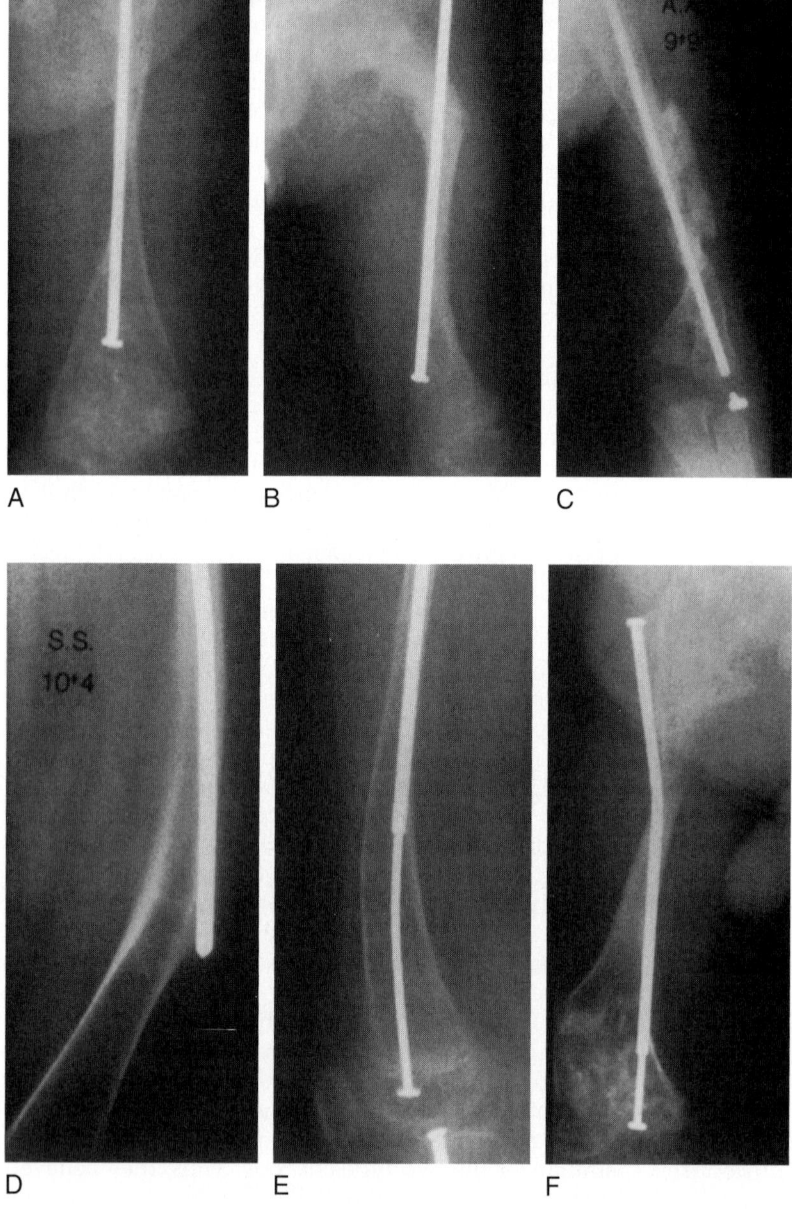

FIGURE 32–40 Complications associated with the Bailey-Dubow extensible rod. **A,** Failure of the rod to elongate. This complication may occur if the inner rod becomes jammed in the outer rod or if anchoring of either T-piece in the epiphysis is inadequate. **B,** Rod migration into soft tissue. This problem also occurs after inadequate fixation of the T-piece in the epiphysis. **C,** Disengagement of the outer rod's T-piece. This complication may be avoided by crimping the end of the rod with a pair of pliers before the T-piece is embedded in the epiphysis. **D,** Rod extrusion from the metaphyseal cortex. This complication is more common with fixed-length rods in growing children. **E,** Resorption of the diaphysis around the rod. Note also bending of the inner rod. **F,** Fracture around a rod, with bending of the intramedullary rod.

vertebral body has been reported,[158,417] as has spondylolisthesis,[203,419] but by far the most common deformity is scoliosis, with or without kyphosis.* The incidence of scoliosis has been reported to be 39% to 100% in this patient population according to Ishikawa and associates.[232] The incidence of scoliosis can be related to the severity of bone fragility, being more common in patients with more severe fragility, and also to vertebral body shape and strength. An inverse correlation with early milestones has been noted, with spinal deformity being more likely to develop in children who are late to achieve sitting.[145] Specifically, both Ishikawa and associates[232] and Hanscom and associates[203] noted that patients with biconcave vertebral bodies and radiographic evidence of osteoporosis were at risk for the development and progression of scoliosis and kyphosis; Ishikawa and associates found that the development of six or more biconcave vertebrae before puberty was a strong risk factor for the development of scoliosis of more than 50 degrees. These radiographic anomalies were more likely to occur in patients with osteogenesis imperfecta congenita B, and these and other authors have found the classifications of Falvo and associates[154] or Shapiro[474] more useful in identifying risk for the development of scoliosis. In

*See references 34, 42, 43, 107, 142, 186, 203, 219, 232, 249, 290, 345, 426, 482, 565.

general, however, scoliosis is more prevalent in patients with Sillence's type III or IV disease.

Conservative management of scoliosis with an orthosis has not generally prevented progression of the deformity and may be detrimental.[42,43,203,565] External pressure applied to the rib cage in an effort to control the spinal deformity may result in secondary compressive deformity of the rib cage itself. Furthermore, the excessive sweating and heat sensitivity often observed in Sillence's type III patients usually make it impossible for the patient to tolerate a spinal orthosis. Thus, use of a corrective spinal orthosis in the management of spinal deformity in osteogenesis imperfecta is rarely indicated.

Spinal fusion has been recommended for the management of severe (>40 or 50 degrees) progressive deformity in patients with osteogenesis imperfecta.[42,43,142,186,203,345,426,565] The specific problems faced by the treating surgeon in completing this recommendation are manyfold. The patients are typically of the more fragile variety and thus are more prone to fractures and other anesthesia-related complications.[495] Intraoperative bleeding tends to be greater than average, presumably related to bone fragility and the bleeding diathesis noted in osteogenesis imperfecta patients in general. Spinal fragility demands very careful surgical exposure and makes instrumentation very difficult. The iliac crest will often serve as only a meager source of autologous bone graft material. Finally, the patient may not tolerate postoperative external immobilization well for the same reasons that spinal orthoses for the prevention of progression are not well tolerated. Thus, when spinal stabilization is deemed warranted, the operating team must be prepared to handle the delicate patient carefully, must be prepared for blood transfusion, and must have allograft bone graft or other bone graft substitutes available to supplement whatever autologous bone can be obtained.

Initially, spinal fusion was performed with in situ techniques or Harrington instrumentation and methylmethacrylate augmentation of hook sites.* However, stable posterior segmental fixation with Luque sublaminar wires or tape appears to be ideally suited to the instrumentation management of these difficult cases (Fig. 32–41).[203] It is not clear that even successful instrumentation and fusion will halt progression of the spinal deformity.[43,203] Halo–gravity traction has been used to gain correction of the deformity, with instrumentation placed in situ to maintain stability.[237] However, these patients are not at high risk for pseudarthrosis after posterior fusion alone, and anterior spinal growth is modest after fusion. Thus, although successful anterior spinal fusion has been described,[203]

*See references 42, 43, 107, 186, 203, 216, 219, 249, 290, 426, 565.

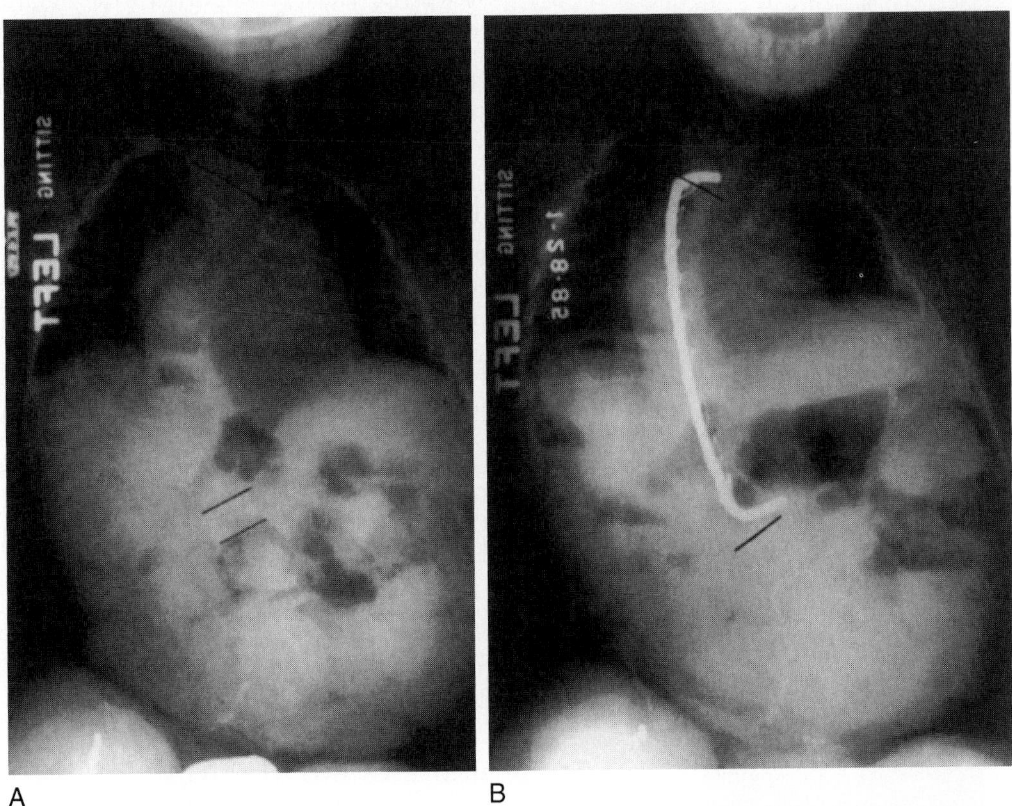

FIGURE 32–41 Scoliosis in osteogenesis imperfecta. **A,** Preoperative radiograph showing the typical deformity in a severely affected patient. **B,** Postoperative radiograph obtained after posterior fusion and instrumentation with the Luque technique. Minimal correction was noted. An allograft was required to supplement the local bone graft.

anterior spinal fusion would seem to be required rarely in these patients.

Complications

HYPERPLASTIC CALLUS FORMATION

Hyperplastic callus formation in patients with osteogenesis imperfecta is a rare but clinically disturbing event.[15,28,30,76,152,276,317,321,433,436,507,531] The clinical scenario is an acute localized inflammation with progressive, often alarming enlargement of the involved limb over a 1- to 3-week period. Hyperplastic callus has been reported to occur as an apparently spontaneous event,[152] after trauma or fracture,[317] and after limb surgery, particularly intramedullary rodding.[76,321,436] The condition appears to be most common in the lower extremities of males with type III or IV osteogenesis imperfecta. An enlarging mass that is painful, warm to the touch, and tender on palpation develops in the involved limb. The overlying skin is tense and translucent, with dilation of the superficial veins. Prolonged low-grade fever is commonly present. In one case, bilateral femoral hyperplastic callus formation after intramedullary rodding led to high-output cardiac failure.[76] Laboratory studies show an elevated erythrocyte sedimentation rate and alkaline phosphatase level. Radiographs show an enlarging, irregular callous mass enveloping the involved bone (Fig. 32–42).

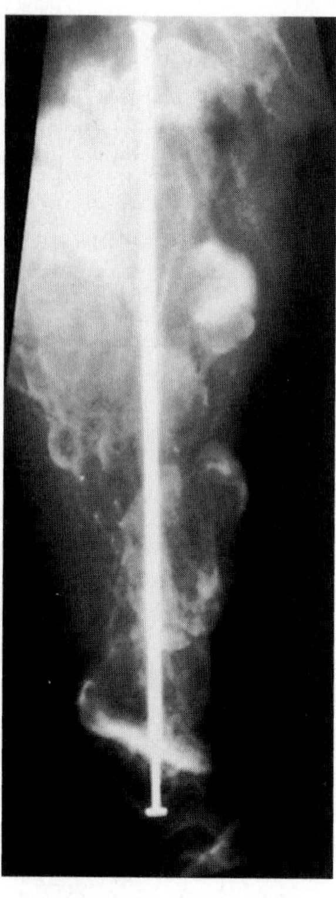

FIGURE 32–42 Hyperplastic callus formation in the femur after intramedullary fixation.

The development of hyperplastic callus is cause for great concern, not only in managing the affected extremity but also because of diagnostic problems in distinguishing hyperplastic callus from osteogenic sarcoma. Banta and associates reported 21 cases of hyperplastic callus.[30] Three of the patients underwent amputation for the presumptive diagnosis of osteogenetic sarcoma, which subsequently proved to be hyperplastic callus. To further complicate the picture, osteogenic sarcoma has been reported in patients with osteogenesis imperfecta,[251,274,424,449] so this is not an idle concern. If there is any doubt in the individual case, a confirmatory biopsy must be performed. Because one postoperative case was associated with initial evidence of deep wound infection,[76] cultures should be performed as well. However, true deep wound infection has not generally been an inciting or intercurrent condition with hyperplastic callus formation.

Histologic examination of the callus shows fibromucoid, cartilage-like tissue, or "chondroid," a transitional form between fibrous, mucoid, and cartilaginous tissue. In contrast, a normal callus consists of a network of woven bone trabeculae lying in fairly dense connective tissue without mucoid or chondroid.[30,126] The peripheral part of the mass shows undifferentiated tissue, whereas the central part is more differentiated, similar to normal callus.

Treatment is symptomatic. The affected extremity is splinted for comfort. Benefit from palliative radiation therapy has been reported in the literature.[30,33,76,285,519] Great caution must be exercised in pursuing this course of treatment, however, because of the risk for development of sarcomatous changes in the irradiated tissue. Diphosphonates have also been tried, but without apparent success.[76]

TUMORS

Osteogenic sarcoma has clearly occurred in patients with osteogenesis imperfecta.[241,251,274,424,449] The treating physician must not only be alert to this possibility but must also consider this diagnosis actively when confronted with a patient in whom hyperplastic callus has formed. The case reported by Jewell and Lofstrom occurred in the pelvis of a 49-year-old man.[241] In most other reported cases the tumor arose from the femur[251,274,449] and the patient died of metastatic disease. Osteogenic sarcoma has been reported in all surviving Sillence types.

Other rare tumor or tumor-like conditions that have been reported in patients with osteogenesis imperfecta include aneurysmal bone cyst in the radius of an 8-year-old girl[234] and unicameral bone cyst of the proximal humerus in three patients.[439]

BASILAR IMPRESSION

Basilar impression is an unusual but well-recognized complicating condition seen in patients with osteogenesis imperfecta.[42,168,205,229,266,319,409,448] Although case reports and reviews of general populations of patients with osteogenesis imperfecta would suggest that this condition is relatively rare, Engelbert and associates found radiographic evidence of basilar impression in 10 of 47 patients with osteogenesis imperfecta.[142] Presumably as a result of pathologic bone softening, the margins of the foramen magnum invaginate into the posterior cranial fossa in affected patients, thereby translocating the upper cervical spine into this depression. This in turn produces direct brainstem compression and, probably, alteration in cerebrospinal fluid flow dynamics, which can result in a wide variety of symptoms, including headaches, facial spasm and numbness, bulbar symptoms (difficulty swallowing and speaking and respiratory depression), and long-tract signs or weakness in the upper and lower extremities. Basilar impression was the confirmed or suspected contributory cause of death in six patients in a study of mortality in patients with osteogenesis imperfecta by McAllion and Paterson.[319] The condition has been reported in all Sillence types except type II. Although basilar impression has been reported in a 3-year-old child,[448] most reported cases have occurred in adults.[168,205,229,266,319,409] More severely affected patients with associated dentinogenesis imperfecta may be more susceptible to the development of basilar impression, and those with ligamentous laxity may be less susceptible, but exceptions to these generalities have been reported.

Diagnosing basilar impression solely on the basis of plain radiographic findings has always been difficult because of difficulty in identifying radiographic landmarks at the foramen magnum and variation in normal measurements in this area. Computed tomography with three-dimensional reconstruction and, even more important, MRI of the upper cervical spine and brainstem greatly simplify the clinician's investigation. These studies should be performed whenever the patient's complaints or physical findings on neurologic examination increase the treating physician's suspicion of this diagnosis.

Relatively short-term relief of symptoms and neurologic signs has been reported after posterior decompression only.[168,229,266,419,448] However, based on the pathophysiology of the deformity, combined transoral anterior decompression and posterior fusion of the occiput to the lower cervical or thoracic spine, as recommended by Harkey and associates, appears to be the most appropriate management of this condition.[205]

Prognostication and Parental Counseling

Parents will need to know the likelihood of survival of the affected infant and, when perinatal death is unlikely, what to expect in the future with regard to ambulation and deformity. They may also want genetic counseling and prenatal screening in future pregnancies. It is important to emphasize to the parents that surviving infants, even if significantly affected by bone fragility, typically have normal intelligence, determination, and excellent social skills that allow them to compensate admirably for their skeletal disability.

SURVIVAL

The most important indicators of survival of an affected infant are the location and severity of the fractures and the radiographic appearance of the skeleton. As pointed out by Sillence[482] and Shapiro,[474] multiple birth fractures or fractures in utero associated with chest wall deformity and crumpled long bones are generally incompatible with life, and if the infant is not stillborn, early death from intracranial hemorrhage or respiratory insufficiency will ensue. On the other hand, multiple fractures at birth without rib cage deformity and with relatively normal funnelization of the femur can be compatible with long-term survival and even walking in some cases.[474]

Patients who are mildly affected (particularly Sillence's type IA patients) often have a normal life span.[319,390] Paterson and associates[390] noted that Sillence's types IB and IV patients had only modestly reduced life spans.[390] More severely affected patients may have their life span shortened by a susceptibility to cardiac or pulmonary insufficiency related to the chest wall deformity or kyphoscoliosis.[319] Paterson and associates noted in their review that of 26 patients with Sillence's type III disease who had died, 19 did so before 10 years of age, so those who survived beyond that age seemed to have a better outlook.[390] More severely affected patients are susceptible to the development of basilar impression and subsequent death. Finally, because of the relative fragility of these patients, deaths have occurred from the consequences of polytrauma after accidents that might otherwise be considered relatively trivial.[319]

AMBULATION

The future ambulatory ability of an affected infant is probably best predicted by Shapiro's classification into the categories of congenita A and B and tarda A and B.[474] Although patients with osteogenesis imperfecta congenita A are unlikely to survive, those with congenita B (fractures at birth or in utero, with normal funnelization and no rib cage deformity) are not only likely to survive, but a third, in Shapiro's experience, also achieved ambulation. Sixty-seven percent of patients who sustained fractures after birth but before walking (tarda A) ultimately were able to walk, by his report, whereas all patients whose initial fracture occurred after walking age remained ambulatory. Prognosis using this classification has been substantiated by Daly and associates, who further found that the age at which the patient achieved independent sitting was also important: 76% of patients who were able to sit independently by 10 months of age achieved ambulation, whereas only 18% of those who were not sitting independently by this age were ultimately able to walk.[117] These authors also found that Sillence's classification was predictive of ambulation. Specifically, in their patient population, nearly all Sillence's type I patients were independent ambulators, all type III patients were wheelchair dependent, and three of seven type IV patients were able to walk. Engelbert and coworkers found that children who could achieve independent sitting or standing, or both, by the age of 12 months were likely to be able to walk.[144]

ANTENATAL DIAGNOSIS

According to Ablin, osteogenesis imperfecta is one of the most common skeletal dysplasias to be diagnosed by fetal ultrasonographic findings.[1] Most cases are Sillence's type II and as such represent an unexpected finding because of the usual absence of a positive family history.

The ultrasonographic features of type II, usually identifiable by the fetal age of 16 weeks, include long-bone deformity (implying fracture), severely reduced femoral length, and decreased echogenicity of the skull, with correspondingly better than usual visualization of the brain.[1,71,522] Rib fractures or chest wall deformity may also be detectable. The prenatal findings of a fetus affected by Sillence's type I, III, or IV disease will vary with the severity of the disease expression and may be normal in mildly affected type I patients.

Couples with a history of a fetus affected by type II osteogenesis imperfecta have a 2% to 7% risk of having another similarly affected fetus because of mosaicism in one parent. In such cases, antenatal diagnosis can be made between 13 and 14 weeks of gestation by DNA analysis of chorionic villous cells obtained by ultrasound-guided chorionic villous sampling.

References

1. Ablin DS: Osteogenesis imperfecta: A review. Can Assoc Radiol J 1998;49:110.
2. Abramowicz MJ, Duprez L, Parma J, et al: Familial congenital hypothyroidism due to inactivating mutation of the thyrotropin receptor causing profound hypoplasia of the thyroid gland. J Clin Invest 1997; 99:3018.
3. Aeschlimann MI, Grunt JA, Crigler JF Jr: Effects of sodium fluoride on the clinical course and metabolic balance of an infant with osteogenesis imperfecta congenita. Metabolism 1966;15:905.
4. Ahmed SF, Dixon PH, Bonthron DT, et al: GNAS1 mutational analysis in pseudohypoparathyroidism. Clin Endocrinol (Oxf) 1998;49:525.
5. Albright F, Burnett CH, Smith PH, et al: Pseudohypoparathyroidism, an example of "sea-bright-bantam" syndrome: Report of three cases. Endocrinology 1942; 30:922.
6. Albright JA: Management overview of osteogenesis imperfecta. Clin Orthop Relat Res 1981;159:80.
7. Albright JA, Grunt JA: Studies of patients with osteogenesis imperfecta. J Bone Joint Surg Am 1971;53: 1415.
8. Albright JP, Albright JA, Crelin ES: Osteogenesis imperfecta tarda. The morphology of rib biopsies. Clin Orthop Relat Res 1975;108:204.
9. al-Qudah AA: Screening for congenital hypothyroidism in cognitively delayed children. Ann Trop Paediatr 1998;18:285.
10. American Academy of Pediatrics AAP Section on Endocrinology and Committee on Genetics, and American Thyroid Association Committee on Public Health: Newborn screening for congenital hypothyroidism: Recommended guidelines. Pediatrics 1993;91:1203.
11. Anast CS: Parathyroid disorders in children. Pediatr Ann 1980;9:376.
12. Andresen J, Nielsen HE: Renal osteodystrophy in non-dialysed patients with chronic renal failure. Acta Radiol Diagn (Stockh) 1980;21:803.
13. Andress DL, Norris KC, Coburn JW, et al: Intravenous calcitriol in the treatment of refractory osteitis fibrosa of chronic renal failure. N Engl J Med 1989;321:274.
14. Apel DM, Millar EA, Moel DI: Skeletal disorders in a pediatric renal transplant population. J Pediatr Orthop 1989;9:505.
15. Apley AG: Hyperplastic callus in osteogenesis imperfecta; report of a case. J Bone Joint Surg Br 1951;33: 591.
16. Aponte CJ, Petrelli MP: Anticonvulsants and vitamin D metabolism. JAMA 1973;225:1248.
17. Aronson R, Ehrlich RM, Bailey JD, et al: Growth in children with congenital hypothyroidism detected by neonatal screening. J Pediatr 1990;116:33.
18. Arvin M, White SJ, Braunstein EM: Growth plate injury of the hand and wrist in renal osteodystrophy. Skeletal Radiol 1990;19:515.
19. Asnes RS, Berdon WE, Bassett CA: Hypophosphatemic rickets in an adolescent cured by excision of a non-ossifying fibroma. Clin Pediatr (Phila) 1981;20:646.
20. Astrom E, Soderhall S: Beneficial effect of bisphosphonate during five years of treatment of severe osteogenesis imperfecta. Acta Paediatr 1998;87:64.
21. Augarten A, Laufer J, Szeinberg A, et al: Child abuse, osteogenesis imperfecta and the grey zone between them. J Med 1993;24:171.
22. Avioli LV: The therapeutic approach to hypoparathyroidism. Am J Med 1974;57:34.
23. Bachrach S, Fisher J, Parks JS: An outbreak of vitamin D deficiency rickets in a susceptible population. Pediatrics 1979;64:871.
24. Bailey RW, Dubow HI: Studies of longitudinal bone growth resulting in an extensible nail. Surg Forum 1963;14:455.
25. Bailey RW, Dubow HI: Evolution of the concept of an extensible nail accommodating to normal longitudinal bone growth: Clinical considerations and implications. Clin Orthop Relat Res 1981;159:157.
26. Bailie JM, Irving JT: Development and healing of rickets in intramembranous bone. Acta Med Scand Suppl 1955;306:1.
27. Baker EM, Hodges RE, Hood J, et al: Metabolism of ascorbic-1-14C acid in experimental human scurvy. Am J Clin Nutr 1969;22:549.
28. Baker L: Hyperplastic callus simulating sarcoma in two cases of fragilitas ossium. J Pathol Bacteriol 1946;58: 609.
29. Banks SW: Bone changes in acute and chronic scurvy: Experimental study. J Bone Joint Surg 1943;25:553.
30. Banta JV, Schreiber RR, Kulik WJ: Hyperplastic callus formation in osteogenesis imperfecta simulating osteosarcoma. J Bone Joint Surg Am 1971;53:115.

31. Bardin T: Renal osteodystrophy, disorders of vitamin D metabolism, and hypophosphatasia. Curr Opin Rheumatol 1992;4:389.
32. Baron J, Winer KK, Yanovski JA, et al: Mutations in the Ca(2+)-sensing receptor gene cause autosomal dominant and sporadic hypoparathyroidism. Hum Mol Genet 1996;5:601.
33. Baron R, Gertner JM, Lang R, et al: Increased bone turnover with decreased bone formation by osteoblasts in children with osteogenesis imperfecta tarda. Pediatr Res 1983;17:204.
34. Barrack RL, Whitecloud TS 3rd, Skinner HB: Spondylolysis after spinal instrumentation in osteogenesis imperfecta. South Med J 1984;77:1453.
35. Barrett IR, Papadimitriou DG: Skeletal disorders in children with renal failure. J Pediatr Orthop 1996;16: 264.
36. Barsh GS, David KE, Byers PH: Type I osteogenesis imperfecta: A nonfunctional allele for pro alpha 1 (I) chains of type I procollagen. Proc Natl Acad Sci U S A 1982;79:3838.
37. Bartal E, Gage JR: Idiopathic juvenile osteoporosis and scoliosis. J Pediatr Orthop 1982;2:295.
38. Bauze RJ, Smith R, Francis MJ: A new look at osteogenesis imperfecta. A clinical, radiological and biochemical study of forty-two patients. J Bone Joint Surg Br 1975;57:2.
39. Beighton P: Familial dentinogenesis imperfecta, blue sclerae, and wormian bones without fractures: Another type of osteogenesis imperfecta? J Med Genet 1981;18: 124.
40. Bembi B, Parma A, Bottega M, et al: Intravenous pamidronate treatment in osteogenesis imperfecta. J Pediatr 1997;131:622.
41. Bendich A, Langseth L: Safety of vitamin A. Am J Clin Nutr 1989;49:358.
42. Benson DR, Donaldson DH, Millar EA: The spine in osteogenesis imperfecta. J Bone Joint Surg Am 1978;60: 925.
43. Benson DR, Newman DC: The spine and surgical treatment in osteogenesis imperfecta. Clin Orthop Relat Res 1981;159:147.
44. Bergman G, Engfeldt B: Studies on mineralized dental tissues. IV. Biophysical studies on teeth and toothgerms in osteogenesis imperfecta. Acta Pathol Microbiol Scand 1954;35:537.
45. Bergman SM, O'Mailia J, Krane NK, et al: Vitamin-A–induced hypercalcemia: Response to corticosteroids. Nephron 1988;50:362.
46. Berlyne GM: Microcrystalline conjunctival calcification in renal failure. A useful clinical sign. Lancet 1968;2: 366.
47. Berlyne GM, Ari JB, Danovitch GM, et al: Cataracts of chronic renal failure. Lancet 1972;1:509.
48. Bhettay EM, Bakst CM: Hypervitaminosis A causing benign intracranial hypertension. A case report. S Afr Med J 1988;74:584.
49. Bilginturan N, Ozsoylu S, Yordam N: Further experiences with sodium fluoride treatment in osteogenesis imperfecta. Turk J Pediatr 1982;24:151.
50. Binder H, Conway A, Gerber LH: Rehabilitation approaches to children with osteogenesis imperfecta: A ten-year experience. Arch Phys Med Rehabil 1993; 74:386.
51. Binder H, Conway A, Hason S, et al: Comprehensive rehabilitation of the child with osteogenesis imperfecta. Am J Med Genet 1993;45:265.
52. Binder H, Hawks L, Graybill G, et al: Osteogenesis imperfecta: Rehabilitation approach with infants and young children. Arch Phys Med Rehabil 1984;65:537.
53. Biser-Rohrbaugh A, Hadley-Miller N: Vitamin D deficiency in breast-fed toddlers. J Pediatr Orthop 2001; 21:508.
54. Bjernulf A, Hall K, Sjogren L, et al: Primary hyperparathyroidism in children. Brief review of the literature and a case report. Acta Paediatr Scand 1970;59:249.
55. Blanco O, Stivel M, Mautalen C, et al: Familial idiopathic hyperphosphatasia: A study of two young siblings treated with porcine calcitonin. J Bone Joint Surg Br 1977;59:421.
56. Blank S, Scanlon KS, Sinks TH, et al: An outbreak of hypervitaminosis D associated with the overfortification of milk from a home-delivery dairy. Am J Public Health 1995;85:656.
57. Bleck EE: Nonoperative treatment of osteogenesis imperfecta: Orthotic and mobility management. Clin Orthop Relat Res 1981;159:111.
58. Blockey NJ, Murphy AV, Mocan H: Management of rachitic deformities in children with chronic renal failure. J Bone Joint Surg Br 1986;68:791.
59. Bloom E, Klein EJ, Shushan D, et al: Variable presentations of rickets in children in the emergency department. Pediatr Emerg Care 2004;20:126.
60. Boden SD, Kaplan FS: Calcium homeostasis. Orthop Clin North Am 1990;21:31.
61. Bonavita JA, Dalinka MK: Shoulder erosions in renal osteodystrophy. Skeletal Radiol 1980;5:105.
62. Bornemann M: Management of primary hyperparathyroidism in children. South Med J 1998;91:475.
63. Bosch P, Johnston CE, Karol L: Slipped capital femoral epiphysis in patients with Down syndrome. J Pediatr Orthop 2004;24:271.
64. Bosley AR, Verrier-Jones ER, Campbell MJ: Aetiological factors in rickets of prematurity. Arch Dis Child 1980;55:683.
65. Bossingham DH, Strange TV, Nicholls PJ: Splints in severe osteogenesis imperfecta. BMJ 1978;1:620.
66. Brailsford JF: Slipping of the epiphysis of the head of the femur: Its relation to renal rickets. Lancet 1933; 1:16.
67. Brailsford JF: Some radiographic manifestations of early scurvy. Arch Dis Child 1953;28:81.
68. Brenner RJ, Spring DB, Sebastian A, et al: Incidence of radiographically evident bone disease, nephrocalcinosis, and nephrolithiasis in various types of renal tubular acidosis. N Engl J Med 1982;307:217.
69. Bromer RS: A critical analysis of the roentgen signs of infantile scurvy. AJR Am J Roentgenol 1943;49:575.
70. Brooks MH, Bell NH, Love L, et al: Vitamin-D–dependent rickets type II. Resistance of target organs to 1,25-dihydroxyvitamin D. N Engl J Med 1978;298:996.
71. Brown BS: The prenatal ultrasonographic diagnosis of osteogenesis imperfecta lethalis. J Can Assoc Radiol 1984;35:63.

72. Brunelli PC, Frediani P: Surgical treatment of the deformities of the long bones in severe osteogenesis imperfecta. Ann N Y Acad Sci 1988;543:170.
73. Bruner JP, Dellinger EH: Antenatal diagnosis and treatment of fetal hypothyroidism. A report of two cases. Fetal Diagn Ther 1997;12:200.
74. Bullough P, Davidson DD: The morphology of the growth plate in osteogenesis imperfecta. Clin Orthop Relat Res 1976;116:259.
75. Bullough PG, Davidson DD, Lorenzo JC: The morbid anatomy of the skeleton in osteogenesis imperfecta. Clin Orthop Relat Res 1981;159:42.
76. Burke TE, Crerand SJ, Dowling F: Hypertrophic callus formation leading to high-output cardiac failure in a patient with osteogenesis imperfecta. J Pediatr Orthop 1988;8:605.
77. Byers PH, Wallis GA, Willing MC: Osteogenesis imperfecta: Translation of mutation to phenotype. J Med Genet 1991;28:433.
78. Caffey J: Chronic poisoning due to excess of vitamin A; description of the clinical and roentgen manifestations in seven infants and young children. Am J Roentgenol Radium Ther Nucl Med 1951;65:12.
79. Cai G, Michigami T, Yamamoto T, et al: Analysis of localization of mutated tissue-nonspecific alkaline phosphatase proteins associated with neonatal hypophosphatasia using green fluorescent protein chimeras. J Clin Endocrinol Metab 1998;83:3936.
80. Caldemeyer KS, Boaz JC, Wappner RS, et al: Chiari I malformation: Association with hypophosphatemic rickets and MR imaging appearance. Radiology 1995; 195:733.
81. Callenbach JC, Sheehan MB, Abramson SJ, et al: Etiologic factors in rickets of very low-birth-weight infants. J Pediatr 1981;98:800.
82. Cassinelli HR, Mautalen CA, Heinrich JJ, et al: Familial idiopathic hyperphosphatasia (FIH): Response to long-term treatment with pamidronate (APD). Bone Miner 1992;19:175.
83. Cassis N, Geldhell R, Dubow H: Osteogenesis imperfecta: Its sociological and surgical implications, with a preliminary report on the use of a telescoping intramedullary nail. J Bone Joint Surg Br 1975;57:533.
84. Castells S, Inamdar S, Baker RK, et al: Effects of porcine calcitonin in osteogenesis imperfecta tarda. J Pediatr 1972;80:757.
85. Cattell H, Clayton B: Failure of anabolic steroids in the therapy of osteogenesis imperfecta: Clinical, metabolic, and biochemical study. J Bone Joint Surg Am 1968; 50:123.
86. Cattell HS, Levin S, Kopits S, et al: Reconstructive surgery in children with azotemic osteodystrophy. J Bone Joint Surg Am 1971;53:216.
87. Chan CC, Green WR, de la Cruz ZC, et al: Ocular findings in osteogenesis imperfecta congenita. Arch Ophthalmol 1982;100:1458.
88. Chan JC, Hsu AC: Vitamin D and renal diseases. Adv Pediatr 1980;27:117.
89. Chanoine JP, Toppet V, Body JJ, et al: Contribution of thyroid ultrasound and serum calcitonin to the diagnosis of congenital hypothyroidism. J Endocrinol Invest 1990;13:103.
90. Chapple IL: Hypophosphatasia: Dental aspects and mode of inheritance. J Clin Periodontol 1993;20:615.
91. Cherninkov Z, Cherninkova S: Two cases of pseudohypoparathyroidism in a family with type E brachydactylia. Radiol Diagn (Berl) 1989;30:57.
92. Chiesa A, Gruneiro de Papendieck L, Keselman A, et al: Growth follow-up in 100 children with congenital hypothyroidism before and during treatment. J Pediatr Endocrinol 1994;7:211.
93. Cho TJ, Choi IH, Chung CY, et al: Efficacy of oral alendronate in children with osteogenesis imperfecta. J Pediatr Orthop 2005;25:607.
94. Christensen WR, Liebman C, Sosman MC: Skeletal and periarticular manifestations of hypervitaminosis D. Am J Roentgenol Radium Ther Nucl Med 1951;65:27.
95. Cohen J, Gierlowski TC, Schneider AB: A prospective study of hyperparathyroidism in individuals exposed to radiation in childhood. JAMA 1990;264:581.
96. Cole DE, Cohen MM Jr: Osteogenesis imperfecta: An update [editorial]. J Pediatr 1991;119:73.
97. Cole WG: Orthopaedic treatment of osteogenesis imperfecta. Ann N Y Acad Sci 1988;543:157.
98. Cole WG: Early surgical management of severe forms of osteogenesis imperfecta. Am J Med Genet 1993; 45:270.
99. Cole WG: Etiology and pathogenesis of heritable connective tissue diseases. J Pediatr Orthop 1993;13:392.
100. Cole WG: The Nicholas Andry Award—1996. The molecular pathology of osteogenesis imperfecta. Clin Orthop Relat Res 1997;343:235.
101. Cole WG, Chan D, Chow CW, et al: Disrupted growth plates and progressive deformities in osteogenesis imperfecta as a result of the substitution of glycine 585 by valine in the alpha 2 (I) chain of type I collagen. J Med Genet 1996;33:968.
102. Cole WG, Dalgleish R: Perinatal lethal osteogenesis imperfecta. J Med Genet 1995;32:284.
103. Cole WG, Jaenisch R, Bateman JF: New insights into the molecular pathology of osteogenesis imperfecta. Q J Med 1989;70:1.
104. Craigen WJ, Lindsay EA, Bricker JT, et al: Deletion of chromosome 22q11 and pseudohypoparathyroidism. Am J Med Genet 1997;72:63.
105. Crawford AH: Slipped capital femoral epiphysis. J Bone Joint Surg Am 1988;70:1422.
106. Cremin B, Goodman H, Spranger J, et al: Wormian bones in osteogenesis imperfecta and other disorders. Skeletal Radiol 1982;8:35.
107. Cristofaro RL, Hoek KJ, Bonnett CA, et al: Operative treatment of spine deformity in osteogenesis imperfecta. Clin Orthop Relat Res 1979;139:40.
108. Cronin CS, Reeve TS, Robinson B, et al: Primary hyperparathyroidism in childhood and adolescence. J Paediatr Child Health 1996;32:397.
109. Cropp GJ, Myers DN: Physiological evidence of hypermetabolism in osteogenesis imperfecta. Pediatrics 1972;49:375.
110. Crosley CJ, Chee C, Berman PH: Rickets associated with long-term anticonvulsant therapy in a pediatric outpatient population. Pediatrics 1975;56:52.
111. Cundy T, Hegde M, Naot D, et al: A mutation in the gene *TNFRSF11B* encoding osteoprotegerin causes an

idiopathic hyperphosphatasia phenotype. Hum Mol Genet 2002;11:2119.

112. Cupisti K, Raffel A, Dotzenrath C, et al: Primary hyperparathyroidism in the young age group: Particularities of diagnostic and therapeutic schemes. World J Surg 2004;28:1153.
113. Curtis JA, Kooh SW, Fraser D, et al: Nutritional rickets in vegetarian children. Can Med Assoc J 1983;128:150.
114. Cutler RE, Reiss E, Ackerman LV: Familial hyperparathyroidism. A kindred involving eleven cases, with a discussion of primary chief-cell hyperplasia. N Engl J Med 1964;270:859.
115. Dabezies EJ, Warren PD: Fractures in very low birth weight infants with rickets. Clin Orthop Relat Res 1997;335:233.
116. Dal Monte A, Manes E, Capanna R, et al: Osteogenesis imperfecta: Results obtained with the Sofield method of surgical treatment. Ital J Orthop Traumatol 1982;8:43.
117. Daly K, Wisbeach A, Sanpera I Jr, et al: The prognosis for walking in osteogenesis imperfecta. J Bone Joint Surg Br 1996;78:477.
118. Davids JR, Fisher R, Lum G, et al: Angular deformity of the lower extremity in children with renal osteodystrophy. J Pediatr Orthop 1992;12:291.
119. Debnam JW, Bates ML, Kopelman RC, et al: Radiological/pathological correlations in uremic bone disease. Radiology 1977;125:653.
120. De Campo C, Piscopello L, Noacco C, et al: Primary familial hypoparathyroidism with an autosomal dominant mode of inheritance. J Endocrinol Invest 1988;11:91.
121. Delange F: Neonatal screening for congenital hypothyroidism: Results and perspectives. Horm Res 1997;48:51.
122. DeLuca HF: Vitamin D: New horizons. Clin Orthop Relat Res 1971;78:4.
123. DeLuca HF: The vitamin D system: A view from basic science to the clinic. Clin Biochem 1981;14:213.
124. Dent CE, Harris H: Hereditary forms of rickets and osteomalacia. J Bone Joint Surg Br 1956;38:204.
125. Dent CM, Graham GP: Osteogenesis imperfecta and Achilles tendon rupture. Injury 1991;22:239.
126. Dent JA, Paterson CR: Fractures in early childhood: Osteogenesis imperfecta or child abuse? J Pediatr Orthop 1991;11:184.
127. Desai MP, Mehta RU, Choksi CS, et al: Pituitary enlargement on magnetic resonance imaging in congenital hypothyroidism. Arch Pediatr Adolesc Med 1996;150:623.
128. DiCesare PE, Sew-Hoy A, Krom W: Bilateral isolated olecranon fractures in an infant as presentation of osteogenesis imperfecta. Orthopedics 1992;15:741.
129. Dickerman Z, De Vries L: Prepubertal and pubertal growth, timing and duration of puberty and attained adult height in patients with congenital hypothyroidism (CH) detected by the neonatal screening programme for CH—a longitudinal study. Clin Endocrinol (Oxf) 1997;47:649.
130. Dimar JR 2nd, Campbell M, Glassman SD, et al: Idiopathic juvenile osteoporosis. An unusual cause of back pain in an adolescent. Am J Orthop 1995;24:865.
131. Dimeglio LA, Ford L, McClintock C, et al: A comparison of oral and intravenous bisphosphonate therapy for children with osteogenesis imperfecta. J Pediatr Endocrinol Metab 2005;18:43.
132. Doeker BM, Pfaffle RW, Pohlenz J, et al: Congenital central hypothyroidism due to a homozygous mutation in the thyrotropin beta-subunit gene follows an autosomal recessive inheritance. J Clin Endocrinol Metab 1998;83:1762.
133. Dohler JR, Souter WA, Beggs I, et al: Idiopathic hyperphosphatasia with dermal pigmentation. A twenty-year follow-up. J Bone Joint Surg Br 1986;68:305.
134. Doty SB, Mathews RS: Electron microscopic and histochemical investigation of osteogenesis imperfecta tarda. Clin Orthop Relat Res 1971;80:191.
135. Dunn PM: James Lind (1716-94) of Edinburgh and the treatment of scurvy. Arch Dis Child Fetal Neonatal Ed 1997;76:F64.
136. Dunn V, Condon VR, Rallison ML: Familial hyperphosphatasemia: Diagnosis in early infancy and response to human thyrocalcitonin therapy. AJR Am J Roentgenol 1979;132:541.
137. du Toit SN, Weiss C: Congenital dislocation of hips associated with osteogenesis imperfecta in male siblings. A case report. Bull Hosp Jt Dis 1969;30:164.
138. Dwyer JT, Dietz WH Jr, Hass G, et al: Risk of nutritional rickets among vegetarian children. Am J Dis Child 1979;133:134.
139. Eberle AJ: Congenital hypothyroidism presenting as apparent spondyloepiphyseal dysplasia. Am J Med Genet 1993;47:464.
140. Econs MJ, McEnery PT, Lennon F, et al: Autosomal dominant hypophosphatemic rickets is linked to chromosome 12p13. J Clin Invest 1997;100:2653.
141. Edwards MJ, Graham JM Jr: Studies of type I collagen in osteogenesis imperfecta. J Pediatr 1990;117:67.
142. Engelbert RH, Gerver WJ, Breslau-Siderius LJ, et al: Spinal complications in osteogenesis imperfecta: 47 patients 1-16 years of age. Acta Orthop Scand 1998;69:283.
143. Engelbert RH, Helders PJ, Keessen W, et al: Intramedullary rodding in type III osteogenesis imperfecta. Effects on neuromotor development in 10 children. Acta Orthop Scand 1995;66:361.
144. Engelbert RH, Uiterwaal CS, Gulmans VA, et al: Osteogenesis imperfecta in childhood: Prognosis for walking. J Pediatr 2000;137:397.
145. Engelbert RH, Uiterwaal CS, van der Hulst A, et al: Scoliosis in children with osteogenesis imperfecta: Influence of severity of disease and age of reaching motor milestones. Eur Spine J 2003;12:130.
146. Engfeldt B, Hjerpe A, Mengarelli S, et al: Morphological and biochemical analysis of biopsy specimens in disorders of skeletal development. Acta Paediatr Scand 1982;71:353.
147. Engfeldt B, Zetterstrom R: Biophysical studies of the bone tissue of dogs with experimental rickets. AMA Arch Pathol 1955;59:321.
148. Esselstyn CB Jr, Popowniak KL: Parathyroid surgery in the treatment of renal osteodystrophy and tertiary hyperparathyroidism. Surg Clin North Am 1971;51:1211.

149. Eubanks PJ, Stabile BE: Osteitis fibrosa cystica with renal parathyroid hormone resistance: A review of pseudohypoparathyroidism with insight into calcium homeostasis. Arch Surg 1998;133:673.
150. Eyring EJ, Eisenberg E: Congenital hyperphosphatasia. A clinical, pathological, and biochemical study of two cases. J Bone Joint Surg Am 1968;50:1099.
151. Fain O: Musculoskeletal manifestations of scurvy. Joint Bone Spine 2005;72:124.
152. Fairbank HAT: Osteogenesis imperfecta and osteogenesis imperfecta cystica. J Bone Joint Surg Br 1948;30: 164.
153. Fallon MB, Boyer JL: Hepatic toxicity of vitamin A and synthetic retinoids. J Gastroenterol Hepatol 1990;5: 334.
154. Falvo KA, Root L, Bullough PG: Osteogenesis imperfecta: Clinical evaluation and management. J Bone Joint Surg Am 1974;56:783.
155. Farfel Z, Brickman AS, Kaslow HR, et al: Defect of receptor-cyclase coupling protein in pseudohypoparathyroidism. N Engl J Med 1980;303:237.
156. Fassier F, Esposito P, Sponseller P, et al: Multicenter radiological assessment of the Fassier-Duval femur rodding. Paper presented at the annual Meeting of the Pediatric Orthopaedic Society of North America, 2006, San Diego, CA.
157. Fassier F, St-Pierre M, Robitaille P: Renal osteodystrophy in children: Correlation between aetiology of the renal disease and the frequency of bone and articular lesions. Int Orthop 1993;17:269.
158. Ferrera PC, Hayes ST, Triner WR: Spinal cord concussion in previously undiagnosed osteogenesis imperfecta. Am J Emerg Med 1995;13:424.
159. Ferris B, Walker C, Jackson A, et al: The orthopaedic management of hypophosphataemic rickets. J Pediatr Orthop 1991;11:367.
160. Finegold DN, Armitage MM, Galiani M, et al: Preliminary localization of a gene for autosomal dominant hypoparathyroidism to chromosome 3q13. Pediatr Res 1994;36:414.
161. Fischer JA, Egert F, Werder E, et al: An inherited mutation associated with functional deficiency of the alpha-subunit of the guanine nucleotide–binding protein Gs in pseudo- and pseudopseudohypoparathyroidism. J Clin Endocrinol Metab 1998;83:935.
162. Fisher G, Skillern PG: Hypercalcemia due to hypervitaminosis A. JAMA 1974;227:1413.
163. Fletcher S, Jones RG, Rayner HC, et al: Assessment of renal osteodystrophy in dialysis patients: Use of bone alkaline phosphatase, bone mineral density and parathyroid ultrasound in comparison with bone histology. Nephron 1997;75:412.
164. Follis RH Jr: Histochemical studies on cartilage and bone. II. Ascorbic acid deficiency. Bull Johns Hopkins Hosp 1951;89:9.
165. Fontanazza C, Razzano M, Mastromarino R: New outlooks in the treatment of osteogenesis imperfecta. An unusual case successfully treated by the Ilizarov method. Ital J Orthop Traumatol 1987;13:67.
166. Frame B, Hanson CA, Frost HM, et al: Renal resistance to parathyroid hormone with osteitis fibrosa: "pseudohypohyperparathyroidism." Am J Med 1972;52:311.
167. Frame B, Jackson CE, Reynolds WA, et al: Hypercalcemia and skeletal effects in chronic hypervitaminosis A. Ann Intern Med 1974;80:44.
168. Frank E, Berger T, Tew JM Jr: Basilar impression and platybasia in osteogenesis imperfecta tarda. Surg Neurol 1982;17:116.
169. Frediani P, Brunelli PC: Corrective femoral osteotomy and telescopic nailing in osteogenesis imperfecta. Ital J Orthop Traumatol 1989;15:473.
170. Frost RB, Middleton RW, Hillier LG: A stereotaxic device for the closed exchange of intramedullary rods, using image-intensified X-rays, in children with osteogenesis imperfecta. Eng Med 1986;15:131.
171. Fujiwara I, Ogawa E, Igarashi Y, et al: Intravenous pamidronate treatment in osteogenesis imperfecta. Eur J Pediatr 1998;157:261.
172. Furey JG, McNamee DC: Air splints for long-term management of osteogenesis imperfecta. J Bone Joint Surg Am 1973;55:645.
173. Gabay C, Voskuyl AE, Cadiot G, et al: A case of scurvy presenting with cutaneous and articular signs. Clin Rheumatol 1993;12:278.
174. Gal-Moscovici A, Popovtzer MM: New worldwide trends in presentation of renal osteodystrophy and its relationship to parathyroid hormone levels. Clin Nephrol 2005;63:284.
175. Gamble JG, Ip SC: Hypervitaminosis A in a child from megadosing. J Pediatr Orthop 1985;5:219.
176. Gamble JG, Rinsky LA, Strudwick J, et al: Non-union of fractures in children who have osteogenesis imperfecta. J Bone Joint Surg Am 1988;70:439.
177. Gamble JG, Simmons SC, Freedman M: The symphysis pubis. Anatomic and pathologic considerations. Clin Orthop Relat Res 1986;203:261.
178. Gamble JG, Strudwick WJ, Rinsky LA, et al: Complications of intramedullary rods in osteogenesis imperfecta: Bailey-Dubow rods versus nonelongating rods. J Pediatr Orthop 1988;8:645.
179. Gardezi SA, Nguyen C, Malloy PJ, et al: A rationale for treatment of hereditary vitamin D–resistant rickets with analogs of 1 alpha,25-dihydroxyvitamin D(3). J Biol Chem 2001;276:29148.
180. Gargan MF, Wisbeach A, Fixsen JA: Humeral rodding in osteogenesis imperfecta. J Pediatr Orthop 1996;16: 719.
181. Gefter WB, Epstein DM, Anday EK, et al: Rickets presenting as multiple fractures in premature infants on hyperalimentation. Radiology 1982;142: 371.
182. Gerber LH, Binder H, Berry R, et al: Effects of withdrawal of bracing in matched pairs of children with osteogenesis imperfecta. Arch Phys Med Rehabil 1998;79:46.
183. Gerber LH, Binder H, Weintrob J, et al: Rehabilitation of children and infants with osteogenesis imperfecta. A program for ambulation. Clin Orthop Relat Res 1990;251:254.
184. Gertner JM, Root L: Osteogenesis imperfecta. Orthop Clin North Am 1990;21:151.
185. Gillis D, Hirsch HJ, Landau H, et al: Parathyroid adenoma after radiation in an 8-year-old boy. J Pediatr 1998;132:892.

186. Gitelis S, Whiffen J, DeWald RL: The treatment of severe scoliosis in osteogenesis imperfecta. Case report. Clin Orthop Relat Res 1983;175:56.
187. Glorieux FH, Bishop NJ, Plotkin H, et al: Cyclic administration of pamidronate in children with severe osteogenesis imperfecta. N Engl J Med 1998;339:947.
188. Goldman AB, Davidson D, Pavlov H, et al: "Popcorn" calcifications: A prognostic sign in osteogenesis imperfecta. Radiology 1980;136:351.
189. Goldman AB, Lane JM, Salvati E: Slipped capital femoral epiphyses complicating renal osteodystrophy: A report of three cases. Radiology 1978;126:333.
190. Goldsmith RS: Laboratory aids in the diagnosis of metabolic bone disease. Orthop Clin North Am 1972;3: 545.
191. Goodman HG, Grumbach MM, Kaplan SL: Growth and growth hormone. II. A comparison of isolated growth-hormone deficiency and multiple pituitary-hormone deficiencies in 35 patients with idiopathic hypopituitary dwarfism. N Engl J Med 1968;278:57.
192. Goskowicz M, Eichenfield LF: Cutaneous findings of nutritional deficiencies in children. Curr Opin Pediatr 1993;5:441.
193. Greenbaum LA, Del Rio M, Bamgbola F, et al: Rationale for growth hormone therapy in children with chronic kidney disease. Adv Chronic Kidney Dis 2004;11:377.
194. Greenberg CR, Taylor CL, Haworth JC, et al: A homoallelic Gly317→Asp mutation in ALPL causes the perinatal (lethal) form of hypophosphatasia in Canadian Mennonites. Genomics 1993;17:215.
195. Greenfield GB: Roentgen appearance of bone and soft tissue changes in chronic renal disease. Am J Roentgenol Radium Ther Nucl Med 1972;116:749.
196. Greig F, Paul E, DiMartino-Nardi J, et al: Transient congenital hypoparathyroidism: Resolution and recurrence in chromosome 22q11 deletion. J Pediatr 1996; 128:563.
197. Grissom LE, Harcke HT: Radiographic features of bisphosphonate therapy in pediatric patients. Pediatr Radiol 2003;33:226.
198. Gruters A: Congenital hypothyroidism. Pediatr Ann 1992;21:15.
199. Hall JG, Rohrt T: The stapes in osteogenesis imperfecta. Acta Otolaryngol 1968;65:345.
200. Ham AW, Lewis MD: Hypervitaminosis D rickets: The action of vitamin D. Br J Exp Pathol 1934;15:228.
201. Hanna JD, Krieg RJ Jr, Scheinman JI, et al: Effects of uremia on growth in children. Semin Nephrol 1996;16:230.
202. Hanna JD, Niimi K, Chan JC: X-linked hypophosphatemia. Genetic and clinical correlates. Am J Dis Child 1991;145:865.
203. Hanscom DA, Winter RB, Lutter L, et al: Osteogenesis imperfecta. Radiographic classification, natural history, and treatment of spinal deformities. J Bone Joint Surg Am 1992;74:598.
204. Hanukoglu A, Chalew SA, Sun CJ, et al: Surgically curable hypophosphatemic rickets. Diagnosis and management. Clin Pediatr (Phila) 1989;28:321.
205. Harkey HL, Crockard HA, Stevens JM, et al: The operative management of basilar impression in osteogenesis imperfecta. Neurosurgery 1990;27:782.
206. Harris LJ: The mode of action of vitamin D: The "parathyroid" theory. Clinical hypervitaminosis. Lancet 1932;1:1031.
207. Harris SS, D'Ercole AJ: Neonatal hyperparathyroidism: The natural course in the absence of surgical intervention. Pediatrics 1989;83:53.
208. Hartjen CA, Koman LA: Treatment of slipped capital femoral epiphysis resulting from juvenile renal osteodystrophy. J Pediatr Orthop 1990;10:551.
209. Hasegawa T, Hasegawa Y, Aso T, et al: HDR syndrome (hypoparathyroidism, sensorineural deafness, renal dysplasia) associated with del(10)(p13). Am J Med Genet 1997;73:416.
210. Haust MD, Landing BH, Holmstrand K, et al: Osteosclerosis of renal disease in children. Comparative pathologic and radiographic studies. Am J Pathol 1964;44:141.
211. Henneman PH: The effect of human growth hormone on growth of patients with hypopituitarism. A combined study. JAMA 1968;205:828.
212. Hensinger RN: Kyphosis secondary to skeletal dysplasias and metabolic disease. Clin Orthop Relat Res 1977;128:113.
213. Hensinger RN: Gastrointestinal problems and osteogenesis imperfecta. J Bone Joint Surg Am 1996;78: 1785.
214. Henthorn PS, Whyte MP: Missense mutations of the tissue-nonspecific alkaline phosphatase gene in hypophosphatasia. Clin Chem 1992;38:2501.
215. Henthorn PS, Whyte MP: Infantile hypophosphatasia: Successful prenatal assessment by testing for tissue–non-specific alkaline phosphatase isoenzyme gene mutations. Prenat Diagn 1995;15:1001.
216. Herron LD, Dawson EG: Methylmethacrylate as an adjunct in spinal instrumentation. J Bone Joint Surg Am 1977;59:866.
217. Heubi JE, Tsang RC, Steichen JJ, et al: 1,25-Dihydroxyvitamin D_3 in childhood hepatic osteodystrophy. J Pediatr 1979;94:977.
218. Hoeffel JC, Lascombes P, Mainard L, et al: Cone epiphysis of the knee and scurvy. Eur J Pediatr Surg 1993;3:186.
219. Hoek KJ: Scoliosis in osteogenesis imperfecta. J Bone Joint Surg Am 1975;57:136.
220. Hoekman K, Papapoulos SE, Peters AC, et al: Characteristics and bisphosphonate treatment of a patient with juvenile osteoporosis. J Clin Endocrinol Metab 1985;61:952.
221. Holman CB: Roentgenologic manifestations of vitamin D intoxication. Radiology 1952;59:805.
222. Horwitz EM, Prockop DJ, Fitzpatrick LA, et al: Transplantability and therapeutic effects of bone marrow–derived mesenchymal cells in children with osteogenesis imperfecta. Nat Med 1999;5:309.
223. Horwitz EM, Prockop DJ, Gordon PL, et al: Clinical responses to bone marrow transplantation in children with severe osteogenesis imperfecta. Blood 2001;97: 1227.
224. Howe JR, Norton JA, Wells SA Jr: Prevalence of pheochromocytoma and hyperparathyroidism in multiple endocrine neoplasia type 2A: Results of long-term follow-up. Surgery 1993;114:1070.

225. Hsu AC, Kooh SW, Fraser D, et al: Renal osteodystrophy in children with chronic renal failure: An unexpectedly common and incapactating complication. Pediatrics 1982;70:742.
226. Hsu SC, Levine MA: Primary hyperparathyroidism in children and adolescents: The Johns Hopkins Children's Center experience 1984-2001. J Bone Miner Res 2002;17(Suppl 2):N44.
227. Huaux JP, Lokietek W: Is APD a promising drug in the treatment of severe osteogenesis imperfecta? J Pediatr Orthop 1988;8:71.
228. Hunter MK, Mandel SH, Sesser DE, et al: Follow-up of newborns with low thyroxine and nonelevated thyroid-stimulating hormone–screening concentrations: Results of the 20-year experience in the Northwest Regional Newborn Screening Program. J Pediatr 1998;132:70.
229. Hurwitz LJ, McSwiney RR: Basilar impression and osteogenesis imperfecta in a family. Brain 1960;83:138.
230. HYP Consortium: A gene (*PEX*) with homologies to endopeptidases is mutated in patients with X-linked hypophosphatemic rickets. The HYP Consortium. Nat Genet 1995;11:130.
231. Iqbal SJ, Brain A, Reynolds TM, et al: Relationship between serum alkaline phosphatase and pyridoxal-5'-phosphate levels in hypophosphatasia. Clin Sci (Lond) 1998;94:203.
232. Ishikawa S, Kumar SJ, Takahashi HE, et al: Vertebral body shape as a predictor of spinal deformity in osteogenesis imperfecta. J Bone Joint Surg Am 1996;78:212.
233. Jackson EC, Strife CF, Tsang RC, et al: Effect of calcitonin replacement therapy in idiopathic juvenile osteoporosis. Am J Dis Child 1988;142:1237.
234. Jacobsen FS: Aneurysmal bone cyst in a patient with osteogenesis imperfecta. J Pediatr Orthop 1996;6:225.
235. Jacobsen ST, Hull CK, Crawford AH: Nutritional rickets. J Pediatr Orthop 1986;6:713.
236. Jacobus CH, Holick MF, Shao Q, et al: Hypervitaminosis D associated with drinking milk. N Engl J Med 1992;326:1173.
237. Janus GJ, Finidori G, Engelbert RH, et al: Operative treatment of severe scoliosis in osteogenesis imperfecta: Results of 20 patients after halo traction and posterior spondylodesis with instrumentation. Eur Spine J 2000;9:486.
238. Jaruratanasirikul S, Patarakijvanich N, Patanapisarnsak C: The association of congenital hypothyroidism and congenital gastrointestinal anomalies in Down's syndrome infants. J Pediatr Endocrinol Metab 1998; 11:241.
239. Jaworski ZF: Pathophysiology, diagnosis and treatment of osteomalacia. Orthop Clin North Am 1972;3:623.
240. Jerosch J, Mazzotti I, Tomasevic M: Complications after treatment of patients with osteogenesis imperfecta with a Bailey-Dubow rod. Arch Orthop Trauma Surg 1998;117:240.
241. Jewell FC, Lofstrom JE: Osteogenic sarcoma occurring in fragilitas ossium. Radiology 1940;34:741.
242. Jones ET, Hensinger RN: Spinal deformity in idiopathic juvenile osteoporosis. Spine 1981;6:1.
243. Jowsey J, Johnson KA: Juvenile osteoporosis: bone findings in seven patients. J Pediatr 1972;81:511.
244. Juppner H, Schipani E, Bastepe M, et al: The gene responsible for pseudohypoparathyroidism type Ib is paternally imprinted and maps in four unrelated kindreds to chromosome 20q13.3. Proc Natl Acad Sci U S A 1998;95:11798.
245. Kanel JS, Price CT: Unilateral external fixation for corrective osteotomies in patients with hypophosphatemic rickets. J Pediatr Orthop 1995;15:232.
246. Kanis JA: Vitamin D metabolism and its clinical application. J Bone Joint Surg Br 1982;64:542.
247. Kaper BP, Romness MJ, Urbanek PJ: Nutritional rickets: Report of four cases diagnosed at orthopaedic evaluation. Am J Orthop 2000;29:214.
248. Karlsson B, Gustafsson J, Hedov G, et al: Thyroid dysfunction in Down's syndrome: Relation to age and thyroid autoimmunity. Arch Dis Child 1998;79: 242.
249. King JD, Bobechko WP: Osteogenesis imperfecta: An orthopaedic description and surgical review. J Bone Joint Surg Br 1971;53:72.
250. Kleinman G, Uri M, Hull S, et al: Perinatal ultrasound casebook. Antenatal findings in congenital hypophosphatasia. J Perinatol 1991;11:282.
251. Klenerman L, Ockenden BG, Townsend AC: Osteosarcoma occurring in osteogenesis imperfecta. Report of two cases. J Bone Joint Surg Br 1967;49:314.
252. Kling TF Jr: Angular deformities of the lower limbs in children. Orthop Clin North Am 1987;18:513.
253. Knight DJ, Bennet GC: Nonaccidental injury in osteogenesis imperfecta: A case report. J Pediatr Orthop 1990;10:542.
254. Kobayashi M, Tanaka H, Tsuzuki K, et al: Two novel missense mutations in calcium-sensing receptor gene associated with neonatal severe hyperparathyroidism. J Clin Endocrinol Metab 1997;82:2716.
255. Koch T, Lehnhardt E, Bottinger H, et al: Sensorineural hearing loss owing to deficient G proteins in patients with pseudohypoparathyroidism: Results of a multicentre study. Eur J Clin Invest 1990;20:416.
256. Kocher MS, Shapiro F: Osteogenesis imperfecta. J Am Acad Orthop Surg 1998;6:225.
257. Kollars J, Zarroug AE, van Heerden J, et al: Primary hyperparathyroidism in pediatric patients. Pediatrics 2005;115:974.
258. Koo WW, Sherman R, Succop P, et al: Fractures and rickets in very low birth weight infants: Conservative management and outcome. J Pediatr Orthop 1989;9: 326.
259. Kooh SW, Brnjac L, Ehrlich RM, et al: Bone mass in children with congenital hypothyroidism treated with thyroxine since birth. J Pediatr Endocrinol Metab 1996;9:59.
260. Kooh SW, Jones G, Reilly BJ, et al: Pathogenesis of rickets in chronic hepatobiliary disease in children. J Pediatr 1979;94:870.
261. Kricun ME, Resnick D: Patellofemoral abnormalities in renal osteodystrophy. Radiology 1982;143:667.
262. Kricun ME, Resnick D: Elbow abnormalities in renal osteodystrophy. AJR Am J Roentgenol 1983;140:577.
263. Kronauer CM, Buhler H: Images in clinical medicine. Skin findings in a patient with scurvy. N Engl J Med 1995;332:1611.

264. Kruger DM, Lyne ED, Kleerekoper M: Vitamin D deficiency rickets. A report on three cases. Clin Orthop Relat Res 1987;224:277.
265. Kruse K, Kracht U: A simplified diagnostic test in hypoparathyroidism and pseudohypoparathyroidism type I with synthetic 1-38 fragment of human parathyroid hormone. Eur J Pediatr 1987;146:373.
266. Kurimoto M, Ohara S, Takaku A: Basilar impression in osteogenesis imperfecta tarda. Case report. J Neurosurg 1991;74:136.
267. Lachmann D, Willvonseder R, Hofer R, et al: A case-report of idiopathic juvenile osteoporosis with particular reference to 47-calcium absorption. Eur J Pediatr 1977;125:265.
268. LaFranchi S: Diagnosis and treatment of hypothyroidism in children. Compr Ther 1987;13:20.
269. Lagerstrom-Fermer M, Sundvall M, Johnsen E, et al: X-linked recessive panhypopituitarism associated with a regional duplication in Xq25-q26. Am J Hum Genet 1997;60:910.
270. Lalli AF, Lapides J: Osteosclerosis occurring in renal disease. Am J Roentgenol Radium Ther Nucl Med 1965;93:924.
271. Lammens J, Mukherjee A, Van Eygen P, et al: Forearm realignment with elbow reconstruction using the Ilizarov fixator: A case report. J Bone Joint Surg Br 1991; 73:412.
272. Lang-Stevenson AI, Sharrard WJ: Intramedullary rodding with Bailey-Dubow extensible rods in osteogenesis imperfecta. An interim report of results and complications. J Bone Joint Surg Br 1984;66:227.
273. Laroche M: Phosphate, the renal tubule, and the musculoskeletal system. Joint Bone Spine 2001;68:211.
274. Lasson U, Harms D, Wiedemann HR: Osteogenic sarcoma complicating osteogenesis imperfecta tarda. Eur J Pediatr 1978;129:215.
275. Latta K, Hisano S, Chan JC: Therapeutics of X-linked hypophosphatemic rickets. Pediatr Nephrol 1993;7: 744.
276. Laurent LE, Salenius P: Hyperplastic callus formation in osteogenesis imperfecta. Report of a case simulating sarcoma. Acta Orthop Scand 1967;38:280.
277. Law WY, Bradley DM, Lazarus JH, et al: Congenital hypothyroidism in Wales (1982-1993): Demographic features, clinical presentation and effects on early neurodevelopment. Clin Endocrinol (Oxf) 1998;48:201.
278. Lawson ML, Miller SF, Ellis G, et al: Primary hyperparathyroidism in a paediatric hospital. Q J Med 1996;89:921.
279. Lee DY, Choi IH, Lee CK, et al: Acquired vitamin D–resistant rickets caused by aggressive osteoblastoma in the pelvis: A case report with ten years' follow-up and review of the literature. J Pediatr Orthop 1994; 14:793.
280. Lee JJ, Lyne ED: Pathologic fractures in severely handicapped children and young adults. J Pediatr Orthop 1990;10:497.
281. Lee JJ, Lyne ED, Kleerekoper M, et al: Disorders of bone metabolism in severely handicapped children and young adults. Clin Orthop Relat Res 1989;245:297.
282. Lee YS, Low SL, Lim LA, et al: Cyclic pamidronate infusion improves bone mineralisation and reduces fracture incidence in osteogenesis imperfecta. Eur J Pediatr 2001;160:641.
283. Leone J, Delhinger V, Maes D, et al: Rheumatic manifestations of scurvy. A report of two cases. Rev Rhum Engl Ed 1997;64:428.
284. Letts M, Monson R, Weber K: The prevention of recurrent fractures of the lower extremities in severe osteogenesis imperfecta using vacuum pants: A preliminary report in four patients. J Pediatr Orthop 1988;8:454.
285. Levin LS: The dentition in the osteogenesis imperfecta syndromes. Clin Orthop Relat Res 1981;159:64.
286. Li YH, Chow W, Leong JC: The Sofield-Millar operation in osteogenesis imperfecta. A modified technique. J Bone Joint Surg Br 2000;82:11.
287. Libman RH: Anesthetic considerations for the patient with osteogenesis imperfecta. Clin Orthop Relat Res 1981;159:123.
288. Lin CK, Hakakha MJ, Nakamoto JM, et al: Prevalence of three mutations in the Gs alpha gene among 24 families with pseudohypoparathyroidism type Ia. Biochem Biophys Res Commun 1992;189:343.
289. Lin T, Tucci JR: Provocative tests of growth-hormone release. A comparison of results with seven stimuli. Ann Intern Med 1974;80:464.
290. Livesley PJ, Webb PJ: Spinal fusion in situ in osteogenesis imperfecta. Int Orthop 1996;20:43.
291. Lobstein J: Lehrbuch der Pathologischen. Anatomie 1835;2:179.
292. Loder RT, Hensinger RN: Slipped capital femoral epiphysis associated with renal failure osteodystrophy. J Pediatr Orthop 1997;17:205.
293. Loder RT, Wittenberg B, DeSilva G: Slipped capital femoral epiphysis associated with endocrine disorders. J Pediatr Orthop 1995;15:349.
294. Loeffler RD Jr, Sherman FC: The effect of treatment on growth and deformity in hypophosphatemic vitamin D–resistant rickets. Clin Orthop Relat Res 1982;162:4.
295. Looser E: Kenntnis der Osteogenesis imperfecta congenita und tarda (sogenannte idiopathische Osteopsathyrosis). Mitt Grenzgebiet Med Cir 1906;15:161.
296. Luhmann SJ, Sheridan JJ, Capelli AM, et al: Management of lower-extremity deformities in osteogenesis imperfecta with extensible intramedullary rod technique: A 20-year experience. J Pediatr Orthop 1998;18: 88.
297. Macchia PE, Lapi P, Krude H, et al: *PAX8* mutations associated with congenital hypothyroidism caused by thyroid dysgenesis. Nat Genet 1998;19:83.
298. Macfarlane JD, Poorthuis BJ, Mulivor RA, et al: Raised urinary excretion of inorganic pyrophosphate in asymptomatic members of a hypophosphatasia kindred. Clin Chim Acta 1991;202:141.
299. Mallick NP, Berlyne GM: Arterial calcification after vitamin-D therapy in hyperphosphatemic renal failure. Lancet 1968;2:1316.
300. Malloy PJ, Feldman D: Hereditary 1,25-Dihydroxyvitamin D–resistant rickets. Endocr Dev 2003;6:175.
301. Malluche HH, Faugere MC: Renal osteodystrophy. N Engl J Med 1989;321:317.
302. Malluche HH, Monier-Faugere MC: The role of bone biopsy in the management of patients with renal osteodystrophy. J Am Soc Nephrol 1994;4:1631.

303. Mankin HJ: Rickets, osteomalacia, and renal osteodystrophy. Part I. J Bone Joint Surg Am 1974;56:101.
304. Mankin HJ: Rickets, osteomalacia, and renal osteodystrophy. Part II. J Bone Joint Surg Am 1974;56:352.
305. Mankin HJ: Rickets, osteomalacia, and renal osteodystrophy. An update. Orthop Clin North Am 1990;21:81.
306. Mankin HJ: Metabolic bone disease. Instr Course Lect 1995;44:3.
307. Marafioti RL, Westin GW: Twenty years experience with multiple osteotomies and intramedullary fixation in osteogenesis imperfecta (including the Bailey expandable rod) at the Shriners Hospital, Los Angeles, California. J Bone Joint Surg Am 1975;57:136.
308. Marafioti RL, Westin GW: Elongating intramedullary rods in the treatment of osteogenesis imperfecta. J Bone Joint Surg Am 1977;59:467.
309. Marder HK, Tsang RC, Hug G, et al: Calcitriol deficiency in idiopathic juvenile osteoporosis. Am J Dis Child 1982;136:914.
310. Marie PJ, Glorieux FH: Stimulation of cortical bone mineralization and remodeling by phosphate and 1,25-dihydroxyvitamin D in vitamin D–resistant rickets. Metab Bone Dis Relat Res 1981;3:159.
311. Marie PJ, Pettifor JM, Ross FP, et al: Histological osteomalacia due to dietary calcium deficiency in children. N Engl J Med 1982;307:584.
312. Marini JC: Osteogenesis imperfecta: Comprehensive management. Adv Pediatr 1988;35:391.
313. Marini JC: Osteogenesis imperfecta—managing brittle bones. N Engl J Med 1998;339:986.
314. Marlowe A, Pepin MG, Byers PH: Testing for osteogenesis imperfecta in cases of suspected non-accidental injury. J Med Genet 2002;39:382.
315. Maroteaux P, Cohen-Solal L, Bonaventure J: Clinical and genetical heterogeneity of osteogenesis imperfecta. Ann N Y Acad Sci 1988;543:16.
316. Marsden D, Nyhan WL, Sakati NO: Syndrome of hypoparathyroidism, growth hormone deficiency, and multiple minor anomalies. Am J Med Genet 1994; 52:334.
317. Massey T, Garst J: Compartment syndrome of the thigh with osteogenesis imperfecta. A case report. Clin Orthop Relat Res 1991;267:202.
318. Match RM, Corrylos EV: Bilateral avulsion fracture of the triceps tendon insertion from skiing with osteogenesis imperfecta tarda. A case report. Am J Sports Med 1983;11:99.
319. McAllion SJ, Paterson CR: Causes of death in osteogenesis imperfecta. J Clin Pathol 1996;49:627.
320. McArthur RG, Hayles AB, Lambert PW: Albright's syndrome with rickets. Mayo Clin Proc 1979;54:313.
321. McCall RE, Bax JA: Hyperplastic callus formation in osteogenesis imperfecta following intramedullary rodding. J Pediatr Orthop 1984;4:361.
322. McCarthy EF, Earnest K, Rossiter K, et al: Bone histomorphometry in adults with type IA osteogenesis imperfecta. Clin Orthop Relat Res 1997;336:254.
323. McCarthy JT, Dayton JM, Fitzpatrick LA, et al: The importance of bone biopsy in managing renal osteodystrophy. Adv Ren Replace Ther 1995;2:148.
324. McHale KA, Tenuta JJ, Tosi LL, et al: Percutaneous intramedullary fixation of long bone deformity in severe osteogenesis imperfecta. Clin Orthop Relat Res 1994;305:242.
325. McHenry CR, Rosen IB, Walfish PG, et al: Parathyroid crisis of unusual features in a child. Cancer 1993;71: 1923.
326. McKenna KE, Dawson JF: Scurvy occurring in a teenager. Clin Exp Dermatol 1993;18:75.
327. McLeod DR, Hanley DA, McArthur RG: Autosomal dominant hypoparathyroidism with intracranial calcification outside the basal ganglia. Am J Med Genet 1989;32:32.
328. Mehls O, Broyer M: Growth response to recombinant human growth hormone in short prepubertal children with chronic renal failure with or without dialysis. The European/Australian Study Group. Acta Paediatr Suppl 1994;399:81.
329. Mehls O, Ritz E, Krempien B, et al: Roentgenological signs in the skeleton of uremic children. An analysis of the anatomical principles underlying the roentgenological changes. Pediatr Radiol 1973;1:183.
330. Mehls O, Ritz E, Krempien B, et al: Slipped epiphyses in renal osteodystrophy. Arch Dis Child 1975;50:545.
331. Mehls O, Ritz E, Oppermann HC, et al: Femoral head necrosis in uremic children without steroid treatment or transplantation. J Pediatr 1981;99:926.
332. Mehls O, Salusky IB: Recent advances and controversies in childhood renal osteodystrophy. Pediatr Nephrol 1987;1:212.
333. Mehls O, Tonshoff B, Haffner D, et al: The use of recombinant human growth hormone in short children with chronic renal failure. J Pediatr Endocrinol 1994;7:107.
334. Mehls O, Wolf H, Wille L: Vitamin D requirements and vitamin D intoxication in infancy. Int J Vitam Nutr Res Suppl 1989;30:87.
335. Mehta CL, Cripps D, Bridges AJ: Systemic pseudovasculitis from scurvy in anorexia nervosa. Arthritis Rheum 1996;39:532.
336. Mellanby E: Experimental rickets: The effect of cereals and their interaction with other factors of diet and environment in producing rickets. Spec Rep Ser Med Res Council 1925;93:48.
337. Menon PS, Madhavi N, Mukhopadhyaya S, et al: Primary hyperparathyroidism in a 14 year old girl presenting with bone deformities. J Paediatr Child Health 1994;30:441.
338. Messinger AL, Teal F: Intramedullary nailing for correction of deformity in osteogenesis imperfecta. Clin Orthop Relat Res 1955;5:221.
339. Meyer S, Villarreal M, Ziv I: A three-level fracture of the axis in a patient with osteogenesis imperfecta. A case report. Spine 1986;11:505.
340. Middleton RW: Closed intramedullary rodding for osteogenesis imperfecta. J Bone Joint Surg Br 1984;66: 652.
341. Middleton RW, Frost RB: Percutaneous intramedullary rod interchange in osteogenesis imperfecta. J Bone Joint Surg Br 1987;69:429.
342. Milstone LM, McGuire J, Ablow RC: Premature epiphyseal closure in a child receiving oral 13-cis-retinoic acid. J Am Acad Dermatol 1982;7:663.
343. Minamitani K, Minagawa M, Yasuda T, et al: Early detection of infants with hypophosphatemic

vitamin D resistant rickets (HDRR). Endocr J 1996; 43:339.

344. Minch CM, Kruse RW: Osteogenesis imperfecta: A review of basic science and diagnosis. Orthopedics 1998;21:558.
345. Moorefield WG Jr, Miller GR: Aftermath of osteogenesis imperfecta: The disease in adulthood. J Bone Joint Surg Am 1980;62:113.
346. Morel G, Houghton GR: Pneumatic trouser splints in the treatment of severe osteogenesis imperfecta. Acta Orthop Scand 1982;53:547.
347. Morii H, Ishimura E, Inoue T, et al: History of vitamin D treatment of renal osteodystrophy. Am J Nephrol 1997;17:382.
348. Morijiri Y, Sato T: Factors causing rickets in institutionalised handicapped children on anticonvulsant therapy. Arch Dis Child 1981;56:446.
349. Moriwake T, Seino Y: Recent progress in diagnosis and treatment of osteogenesis imperfecta. Acta Paediatr Jpn 1997;39:521.
350. Morris RC Jr: Renal tubular acidosis. Mechanisms, classification and implications. N Engl J Med 1969;281: 1405.
351. Moss AJ, Waterhouse C, Terry R: Gluten-sensitive enteropathy with osteomalacia but without steatorrhea. N Engl J Med 1965;272:825.
352. Mudgal CS: Olecranon fractures in osteogenesis imperfecta. A case report. Acta Orthop Belg 1992;58:453.
353. Muir A, Daneman D, Daneman A, et al: Thyroid scanning, ultrasound, and serum thyroglobulin in determining the origin of congenital hypothyroidism. Am J Dis Child 1988;142:214.
354. Mulpuri K, Joseph B: Intramedullary rodding in osteogenesis imperfecta. J Pediatr Orthop 2000;20:267.
355. Munns CF, Rauch F, Zeitlin L, et al: Delayed osteotomy but not fracture healing in pediatric osteogenesis imperfecta patients receiving pamidronate. J Bone Miner Res 2004;19:1779.
356. Murray D, Young BH: Osteogenesis imperfecta treated by fixation with intramedullary rod. South Med J 1960;53:1142.
357. Nerubay J, Pilderwasser D: Spontaneous bilateral distal femoral physiolysis due to scurvy. Acta Orthop Scand 1984;55:18.
358. Nicholas RW, James P: Telescoping intramedullary stabilization of the lower extremities for severe osteogenesis imperfecta. J Pediatr Orthop 1990;10:219.
359. Nicholls AC, Oliver J, Renouf DV, et al: Substitution of cysteine for glycine at residue 415 of one allele of the alpha 1(I) chain of type I procollagen in type III/IV osteogenesis imperfecta. J Med Genet 1991;28:757.
360. Niemann KM: Surgical treatment of the tibia in osteogenesis imperfecta. Clin Orthop Relat Res 1981;159: 134.
361. Nishi Y, Hamamoto K, Kajiyama M, et al: Effect of long-term calcitonin therapy by injection and nasal spray on the incidence of fractures in osteogenesis imperfecta. J Pediatr 1992;121:477.
362. Nishiyama S, Tomoeda S, Inoue F, et al: Self-limited neonatal familial hyperparathyroidism associated with hypercalciuria and renal tubular acidosis in three siblings. Pediatrics 1990;86:421.
363. Nixon JR, Douglas JF: Bilateral slipping of the upper femoral epiphysis in end-stage renal failure. A report of two cases. J Bone Joint Surg Br 1980;62:18.
364. Nogami H, Ono Y, Katoh R, et al: Microvascular and cellular defects of the periosteum of osteogenesis imperfecta. Clin Orthop Relat Res 1993;292:358.
365. Nordin BE: Effect of malabsorption syndrome on calcium metabolism. Proc R Soc Med 1961;54:497.
366. Norman AW: Recent studies on vitamin D and parathyroid hormone regulation of calcium and phosphorus metabolism. Clin Orthop Relat Res 1967;52:249.
367. Norman ME: Vitamin D in bone disease. Pediatr Clin North Am 1982;29:947.
368. Oakley GA, Muir T, Ray M, et al: Increased incidence of congenital malformations in children with transient thyroid-stimulating hormone elevation on neonatal screening. J Pediatr 1998;132:726.
369. Oeffinger KC: Scurvy: More than historical relevance. Am Fam Physician 1993;48:609.
370. Ogilvie-Harris DJ, Khazim R: Tendon and ligament injuries in adults with osteogenesis imperfecta. J Bone Joint Surg Br 1995;77:155.
371. Olmastroni M, Seracini D, Lavoratti G, et al: Magnetic resonance imaging of renal osteodystrophy in children. Pediatr Radiol 1997;27:865.
372. Ong KK, Amin R, Dunger DB: Pseudohypoparathyroidism—another monogenic obesity syndrome. Clin Endocrinol (Oxf) 2000;52:389.
373. Oppenheim WL, Fischer SR, Salusky IB: Surgical correction of angular deformity of the knee in children with renal osteodystrophy. J Pediatr Orthop 1997;17: 41.
374. Oppenheim WL, Namba R, Goodman WG, et al: Aluminum toxicity complicating renal osteodystrophy. A case report. J Bone Joint Surg Am 1989;71:446.
375. Oppenheim WL, Shayestehfar S, Salusky IB: Tibial physeal changes in renal osteodystrophy: Lateral Blount's disease. J Pediatr Orthop 1992;12:774.
376. Oppenheimer SJ, Snodgrass GJ: Neonatal rickets. Histopathology and quantitative bone changes. Arch Dis Child 1980;55:945.
377. Oppermann HC, Mehls O, Willich E, et al: [Osteonecroses in children with chronic renal diseases before and after kidney transplantation (author's transl).] Radiologe 1981;21:175.
378. Parfitt AM: Soft-tissue calcification in uremia. Arch Intern Med 1969;124:544.
379. Parfitt AM: Hypophosphatemic vitamin D refractory rickets and osteomalacia. Orthop Clin North Am 1972;3:653.
380. Parfitt AM: Renal osteodystrophy. Orthop Clin North Am 1972;3:681.
381. Park EA: The etiology of rickets. Physiol Rev 1923; 3:106.
382. Park EA: Observations on the pathology of rickets with particular reference to the changes at the cartilage-shaft junction of the growing bones. Harvey Lect 1938-1939;24:157.
383. Parker MS, Klein I, Haussler MR, et al: Tumor-induced osteomalacia. Evidence of a surgically correctable alteration in vitamin D metabolism. JAMA 1981;245: 492.

384. Parvari R, Hershkovitz E, Kanis A, et al: Homozygosity and linkage-disequilibrium mapping of the syndrome of congenital hypoparathyroidism, growth and mental retardation, and dysmorphism to a 1-cm interval on chromosome 1q42-43. Am J Hum Genet 1998;63:163.
385. Patel L, Clayton PE, Brain C, et al: Acute biochemical effects of growth hormone treatment compared with conventional treatment in familial hypophosphataemic rickets. Clin Endocrinol (Oxf) 1996;44:687.
386. Paterson CR: Vitamin D deficiency rickets simulating child abuse. J Pediatr Orthop 1981;1:423.
387. Paterson CR, Beal RJ, Dent JA: Osteogenesis imperfecta: Fractures of the femur when testing for congenital dislocation of the hip. BMJ 1992;305:464.
388. Paterson CR, Burns J, McAllion SJ: Osteogenesis imperfecta: The distinction from child abuse and the recognition of a variant form. Am J Med Genet 1993;45:187.
389. Paterson CR, McAllion SJ: Osteogenesis imperfecta in the differential diagnosis of child abuse. BMJ 1989; 299:1451.
390. Paterson CR, Ogston SA, Henry RM: Life expectancy in osteogenesis imperfecta. BMJ 1996;312:351.
391. Pauli RM, Gilbert EF: Upper cervical cord compression as cause of death in osteogenesis imperfecta type II. J Pediatr 1986;108:579.
392. Payne WR: The blood chemistry in idiopathic hypercalcemia. Arch Dis Child 1952;27:302.
393. Pazzaglia UE, Barbieri D, Beluffi G, et al: Chronic idiopathic hyperphosphatasia and fibrous dysplasia in the same child. J Pediatr Orthop 1989;9:709.
394. Pearce SH, Trump D, Wooding C, et al: Calcium-sensing receptor mutations in familial benign hypercalcemia and neonatal hyperparathyroidism. J Clin Invest 1995; 96:2683.
395. Pease CN: Focal retardation and arrestment of growth of bones due to vitamin A intoxication. JAMA 1962; 182:980.
396. Pellini C, di Natale B, De Angelis R, et al: Growth hormone deficiency in children: Role of magnetic resonance imaging in assessing aetiopathogenesis and prognosis in idiopathic hypopituitarism. Eur J Pediatr 1990;149:536.
397. Pennes DR, Ellis CN, Madison KC, et al: Early skeletal hyperostoses secondary to 13-cis-retinoic acid. AJR Am J Roentgenol 1984;142:979.
398. Perelman AH, Johnson RL, Clemons RD, et al: Intrauterine diagnosis and treatment of fetal goitrous hypothyroidism. J Clin Endocrinol Metab 1990;71:618.
399. Perez Jurado LA, Argente J: Molecular basis of familial growth hormone deficiency. Horm Res 1994;42:189.
400. Peterkofsky B: Ascorbate requirement for hydroxylation and secretion of procollagen: Relationship to inhibition of collagen synthesis in scurvy. Am J Clin Nutr 1991;54:1135S.
401. Peterson BR: Augmenting vitamin D to combat genetic disease. Chem Biol 2002;9:1265.
402. Pettifor JM: Rickets and vitamin D deficiency in children and adolescents. Endocrinol Metab Clin North Am 2005;34:537.
403. Petty EM, Green JS, Marx SJ, et al: Mapping the gene for hereditary hyperparathyroidism and prolactinoma (MEN1Burin) to chromosome 11q: Evidence for a founder effect in patients from Newfoundland. Am J Hum Genet 1994;54:1060.
404. Pitt MJ: Rachitic and osteomalacic syndromes. Radiol Clin North Am 1981;19:581.
405. Pizones J, Plotkin H, Parra-Garcia JI, et al: Bone healing in children with osteogenesis imperfecta treated with bisphosphonates. J Pediatr Orthop 2005;25:332.
406. Pocock AE, Francis MJ, Smith R: Type I collagen biosynthesis by skin fibroblasts from patients with idiopathic juvenile osteoporosis. Clin Sci (Lond) 1995; 89:69.
407. Porat S, Heller E, Seidman DS, et al: Functional results of operation in osteogenesis imperfecta: Elongating and nonelongating rods. J Pediatr Orthop 1991;11:200.
408. Porsborg P, Astrup G, Bendixen D, et al: Osteogenesis imperfecta and malignant hyperthermia. Is there a relationship? Anaesthesia 1996;51:863.
409. Pozo JL, Crockard HA, Ransford AO: Basilar impression in osteogenesis imperfecta. A report of three cases in one family. J Bone Joint Surg Br 1984;66:233.
410. Prendiville JS, Lucky AW, Mallory SB, et al: Osteoma cutis as a presenting sign of pseudohypoparathyroidism. Pediatr Dermatol 1992;9:11.
411. Proszynska K, Wieczorek E, Olszaniecka M, et al: Collagen peptides in osteogenesis imperfecta, idiopathic juvenile osteoporosis and Ehlers-Danlos syndrome. Acta Paediatr 1996;85:688.
412. Raghuramulu N, Reddy V: Serum 25-hydroxy-vitamin D levels in malnourished children with rickets. Arch Dis Child 1980;55:285.
413. Rajakumar K, Thomas SB: Reemerging nutritional rickets: A historical perspective. Arch Pediatr Adolesc Med 2005;159:335.
414. Ramage IJ, Howatson AJ, Beattie TJ: Hypophosphatasia. J Clin Pathol 1996;49:682.
415. Ramar S, Sivaramakrishnan V, Manoharan K: Scurvy—a forgotten disease. Arch Phys Med Rehabil 1993; 74:92.
416. Rampton AJ, Kelly DA, Shanahan EC, et al: Occurrence of malignant hyperpyrexia in a patient with osteogenesis imperfecta. Br J Anaesth 1984;56:1443.
417. Rao S, Patel A, Schildhauer T: Osteogenesis imperfecta as a differential diagnosis of pathologic burst fractures of the spine. A case report. Clin Orthop Relat Res 1993;289:113.
418. Rapaport D, Ziv Y, Rubin M, et al: Primary hyperparathyroidism in children. J Pediatr Surg 1986;21:395.
419. Rask MR: Spondylolisthesis resulting from osteogenesis imperfecta: report of a case. Clin Orthop Relat Res 1979;139:164.
420. Raskin S, Cogan JD, Summar ML, et al: Genetic mapping of the human pituitary-specific transcriptional factor gene and its analysis in familial panhypopituitary dwarfism. Hum Genet 1996;98:703.
421. Rasmussen H, Pechet M, Anast C, et al: Long-term treatment of familial hypophosphatemic rickets with oral phosphate and 1 alpha-hydroxyvitamin D_3. J Pediatr 1981;99:16.
422. Raubenheimer EJ, Van Heerden WF, Potgieter D, et al: Static and dynamic bone changes in hospitalized patients suffering from rickets—a histomorphometric study. Histopathology 1997;31:12.

423. Ray M, Muir TM, Murray GD, et al: Audit of screening programme for congenital hypothyroidism in Scotland 1979-93. Arch Dis Child 1997;76:411.
424. Reid BS, Hubbard JD: Osteosarcoma arising in osteogenesis imperfecta. Pediatr Radiol 1979;8:110.
425. Reilly WA, Smyth FS: Cretinoid epiphyseal dysgenesis. J Pediatr 1937;11:786.
426. Renshaw TS, Cook RS, Albright JA: Scoliosis in osteogenesis imperfecta. Clin Orthop Relat Res 1979; 145:163.
427. Resnick D, Deftos LJ, Parthemore JG: Renal osteodystrophy: Magnification radiography of target sites of absorption. AJR Am J Roentgenol 1981;136:711.
428. Resnick D, Niwayama G: Subchondral resorption of bone in renal osteodystrophy. Radiology 1976;118:315.
429. Reynolds WA, Karo JJ: Radiologic diagnosis of metabolic bone disease. Orthop Clin North Am 1972;3:521.
430. Richardson RJ, Kirk JM: Short stature, mental retardation, and hypoparathyroidism: A new syndrome. Arch Dis Child 1990;65:1113.
431. Rigden SP: The treatment of renal osteodystrophy. Pediatr Nephrol 1996;10:653.
432. Ring D, Jupiter JB, Labropoulos PK, et al: Treatment of deformity of the lower limb in adults who have osteogenesis imperfecta. J Bone Joint Surg Am 1996;78: 220.
433. Roberts JB: Bilateral hyperplastic callus formation in osteogenesis imperfecta. J Bone Joint Surg Am 1976; 58:1164.
434. Robichon J, Germain JP: Pathogenesis of osteogenesis imperfecta. Can Med Assoc J 1968;99:975.
435. Rodriguez RP: Report of multiple osteotomies and intramedullary fixation by a extensile intramedullary device in children with osteogenesis imperfecta. Clin Orthop Relat Res 1976;116:261.
436. Rodriguez RP, Bailey RW: Internal fixation of the femur in patients with osteogenesis imperfecta. Clin Orthop Relat Res 1981;159:126.
437. Rodriguez RP Jr, Wickstrom J: Osteogenesis imperfecta: A preliminary report on resurfacing of long bones with intramedullary fixation by an extensible intramedullary device. South Med J 1971;64:169.
438. Root AW, Bongiovanni AM, Eberlein WR: Diagnosis and management of growth retardation with special reference to the problem of hypopituitarism. J Pediatr 1971;78:737.
439. Root L: Upper limb surgery in osteogenesis imperfecta. Clin Orthop Relat Res 1981;159:141.
440. Rosenfeld RG, Kemp SF, Gaspich S, et al: In vivo modulation of somatomedin receptor sites: Effects of growth hormone treatment of hypopituitary children. J Clin Endocrinol Metab 1981;52:759.
441. Ross AJ 3rd: Parathyroid surgery in children. Prog Pediatr Surg 1991;26:48.
442. Rowe PS: Molecular biology of hypophosphataemic rickets and oncogenic osteomalacia. Hum Genet 1994;94:457.
443. Rowe PS, Goulding JN, Francis F, et al: The gene for X-linked hypophosphataemic rickets maps to a 200-300 kb region in Xp22.1, and is located on a single YAC containing a putative vitamin D response element (VDRE). Hum Genet 1996;97:345.
444. Rubinovitch M, Said SE, Glorieux FH, et al: Principles and results of corrective lower limb osteotomies for patients with vitamin D–resistant hypophosphatemic rickets. Clin Orthop Relat Res 1988;237:264.
445. Ruby LK, Mital MA: Skeletal deformities following chronic hypervitaminosis A; a case report. J Bone Joint Surg Am 1974;56:1283.
446. Rudolf M, Arulanantham K, Greenstein RM: Unsuspected nutritional rickets. Pediatrics 1980;66:72.
447. Rush GA, Burke SW: Hangman's fracture in a patient with osteogenesis imperfecta. Case report. J Bone Joint Surg Am 1984;66:778.
448. Rush PJ, Berbrayer D, Reilly BJ: Basilar impression and osteogenesis imperfecta in a three-year-old girl: CT and MRI. Pediatr Radiol 1989;19:142.
449. Rutkowski R, Resnick P, McMaster JH: Osteosarcoma occurring in osteogenesis imperfecta. A case report. J Bone Joint Surg Am 1979;61:606.
450. Ryan CA, Al-Ghamdi AS, Gayle M, et al: Osteogenesis imperfecta and hyperthermia. Anesth Analg 1989;68: 811.
451. Ryoppy S, Alberty A, Kaitila I: Early semiclosed intramedullary stabilization in osteogenesis imperfecta. J Pediatr Orthop 1987;7:139.
452. Sadat-Ali M, Sankaran-Kutty M, Adu-Gyamfi Y: Metabolic acidosis in osteogenesis imperfecta. Eur J Pediatr 1986;145:582.
453. Saggese G, Baroncelli GI, Bertelloni S, et al: Long-term growth hormone treatment in children with renal hypophosphatemic rickets: Effects on growth, mineral metabolism, and bone density. J Pediatr 1995;127:395.
454. Saggese G, Bertelloni S, Baroncelli GI, et al: Mineral metabolism and calcitriol therapy in idiopathic juvenile osteoporosis. Am J Dis Child 1991;145:457.
455. Sakkers R, Kok D, Engelbert R, et al: Skeletal effects and functional outcome with olpadronate in children with osteogenesis imperfecta: A 2-year randomised placebo-controlled study. Lancet 2004;363:1427.
456. Salassa RM, Jowsey J, Arnaud CD: Hypophosphatemic osteomalacia associated with "nonendocrine" tumors. N Engl J Med 1970;283:65.
457. Saldanha KA, Saleh M, Bell MJ, et al: Limb lengthening and correction of deformity in the lower limbs of children with osteogenesis imperfecta. J Bone Joint Surg Br 2004;86:259.
458. Salusky IB, Goodman WG: The management of renal osteodystrophy. Pediatr Nephrol 1996;10:651.
459. Salusky IB, Kuizon BG, Juppner H: Special aspects of renal osteodystrophy in children. Semin Nephrol 2004; 24:69.
460. Sanchez CP: Prevention and treatment of renal osteodystrophy in children with chronic renal insufficiency and end-stage renal disease. Semin Nephrol 2001; 21:441.
461. Sanchez CP, Salusky IB: The renal bone diseases in children treated with dialysis. Adv Ren Replace Ther 1996;3:14.
462. Sanguinetti C, Greco F, De Palma L, et al: Morphological changes in growth-plate cartilage in osteogenesis imperfecta. J Bone Joint Surg Br 1990;72:475.
463. Saul PD, Lloyd DJ, Smith FW: The role of bone scanning in neonatal rickets. Pediatr Radiol 1983;13:89.

464. Scherl S, Goldberg NS, Volpe L, et al: Overdosage of vitamin A supplements in a child. Cutis 1992;50:209.
465. Schilling T, Ziegler R: Current therapy of hypoparathyroidism—a survey of German endocrinology centers. Exp Clin Endocrinol Diabetes 1997;105:237.
466. Schott GD, Wills MR: Muscle weakness in osteomalacia. Lancet 1976;1:626.
467. Schuster V, Sandhage K: Intracardiac calcifications in a case of pseudohypoparathyroidism type Ia (PHP-Ia). Pediatr Cardiol 1992;13:237.
468. Scire G, Dallapiccola B, Iannetti P, et al: Hypoparathyroidism as the major manifestation in two patients with 22q11 deletions. Am J Med Genet 1994;52:478.
469. Scott DC, Hung W: Pseudohypoparathyroidism type Ia and growth hormone deficiency in two siblings. J Pediatr Endocrinol Metab 1995;8:205.
470. Seedorff KS: Osteogenesis Imperfecta: A Study of Clinical Features and Heredity Based on 55 Danish Families Comprising 180 Affected Persons. Copenhagen, Munksgaard, 1949.
471. Seikaly MG, Browne RH, Baum M: The effect of phosphate supplementation on linear growth in children with X-linked hypophosphatemia. Pediatrics 1994;94:478.
472. Selby PL, Davies M, Marks JS, et al: Vitamin D intoxication causes hypercalcaemia by increased bone resorption which responds to pamidronate. Clin Endocrinol (Oxf) 1995;43:531.
473. Shah M, Salhab N, Patterson D, et al: Nutritional rickets still afflict children in north Texas. Tex Med 2000;96:64.
474. Shapiro F: Consequences of an osteogenesis imperfecta diagnosis for survival and ambulation. J Pediatr Orthop 1985;5:456.
475. Shea D, Mankin HJ: Slipped capital femoral epiphysis in renal rickets. Report of three cases. J Bone Joint Surg Am 1966;48:349.
476. Shea JJ, Postma DS: Findings and long-term surgical results in the hearing loss of osteogenesis imperfecta. Arch Otolaryngol 1982;108:467.
477. Siebner R, Merlob P, Kaiserman I, et al: Congenital anomalies concomitant with persistent primary congenital hypothyroidism. Am J Med Genet 1992;44:57.
478. Siejka SJ, Knezevic WV, Pullan PT: Dystonia and intracerebral calcification: Pseudohypoparathyroidism presenting in an eleven-year-old girl. Aust N Z J Med 1988;18:607.
479. Sijbrandij S: Percutaneous nailing in the management of osteogenesis imperfecta. Int Orthop 1990;14:195.
480. Sillence D: Osteogenesis imperfecta: An expanding panorama of variants. Clin Orthop Relat Res 1981;159:11.
481. Sillence DO, Danks DM: The differentiation of genetically distinct varieties of osteogenesis imperfecta in the newborn period. Clin Res 1978;26:178.
482. Sillence DO, Senn A, Danks DM: Genetic heterogeneity in osteogenesis imperfecta. J Med Genet 1979;16:101.
483. Sills IN, Skuza KA, Horlick MN, et al: Vitamin D deficiency rickets. Reports of its demise are exaggerated. Clin Pediatr (Phila) 1994;33:491.
484. Silve C: Hereditary hypophosphatasia and hyperphosphatasia. Curr Opin Rheumatol 1994;6:336.
485. Silverman AK, Ellis CN, Voorhees JJ: Hypervitaminosis A syndrome: A paradigm of retinoid side effects. J Am Acad Dermatol 1987;16:1027.
486. Silverman FN: An unusual osseous sequel to infantile scurvy. J Bone Joint Surg Am 1953;35:215.
487. Silverman FN: Recovery from epiphyseal invagination: Sequel to an unusual complication of scurvy. J Bone Joint Surg Am 1970;52:384.
488. Simmons DJ, Kunin AS: Development and healing of rickets in rats. I. Studies with tritiated thymidine and nutritional considerations. Clin Orthop Relat Res 1970;68:251.
489. Simmons DJ, Kunin AS: Development and healing of rickets in rats. II. Studies with tritiated proline. Clin Orthop Relat Res 1970;68:261.
490. Simon A, Koppeschaar HP, Roijers JF, et al: Pseudohypoparathyroidism type Ia. Albright hereditary osteodystrophy: A model for research on G protein–coupled receptors and genomic imprinting. Neth J Med 2000;56:100.
491. Singer F, Siris E, Shane E, et al: Hereditary hyperphosphatasia: 20 year follow-up and response to disodium etidronate. J Bone Miner Res 1994;9:733.
492. Smith R: Idiopathic juvenile osteoporosis: Experience of twenty-one patients. Br J Rheumatol 1995;34:68.
493. Smith R: Osteogenesis imperfecta—where next? J Bone Joint Surg Br 1997;79:177.
494. Sofield HA, Millar EA: Fragmentation, realignment, and intramedullary rod fixation of deformities of the long bones of children: A ten year appraisal. J Bone Joint Surg Am 1959;41:1371.
495. Sperry K: Fatal intraoperative hemorrhage during spinal fusion surgery for osteogenesis imperfecta. Am J Forensic Med Pathol 1989;10:54.
496. Spindler A, Berman A, Mautalen C, et al: Chronic idiopathic hyperphosphatasia. Report of a case treated with pamidronate and a review of the literature. J Rheumatol 1992;19:642.
497. Stanbury SW, Lumb GA: Metabolic studies of renal osteodystrophy. I. Calcium, phosphorus and nitrogen metabolism in rickets, osteomalacia and hyperparathyroidism complicating chronic uremia and in the osteomalacia of the adult Fanconi syndrome. Medicine (Baltimore) 1962;41:1.
498. Stanitski DF: Treatment of deformity secondary to metabolic bone disease with the Ilizarov technique. Clin Orthop Relat Res 1994;301:38.
499. Steendijk R, Hauspie RC: The pattern of growth and growth retardation of patients with hypophosphataemic vitamin D–resistant rickets: A longitudinal study. Eur J Pediatr 1992;151:422.
500. Steinbach HL, Kolb FO, Gilfillan R: A mechanism of the production of pseudofractures in osteomalacia (milkman's syndrome). Radiology 1954;62:388.
501. Steinbach HL, Noetzli M: Roentgen appearance of the skeleton in osteomalacia and rickets. Am J Roentgenol Radium Ther Nucl Med 1964;91:955.
502. Stickler GB, Morgenstern BZ: Hypophosphataemic rickets: Final height and clinical symptoms in adults. Lancet 1989;2:902.
503. Stirling HF, Darling JA, Barr DG: Plasma cyclic AMP response to intravenous parathyroid hormone in pseu-

dohypoparathyroidism. Acta Paediatr Scand 1991;80: 333.
504. Stockley I, Bell MJ, Sharrard WJ: The role of expanding intramedullary rods in osteogenesis imperfecta. J Bone Joint Surg Br 1989;71:422.
505. Stoltz MR, Dietrich SL, Marshall GJ: Osteogenesis imperfecta. Perspectives. Clin Orthop Relat Res 1989; 242:120.
506. Stott NS, Zionts LE: Displaced fractures of the apophysis of the olecranon in children who have osteogenesis imperfecta. J Bone Joint Surg Am 1993;75:1026.
507. Strach EH: Hyperplastic callus formation in osteogenesis imperfecta; report of a case and review of the literature. J Bone Joint Surg Br 1953;35:417.
508. Sundaram M: Renal osteodystrophy. Skeletal Radiol 1989;18:415.
509. Superti-Furga A, Pistone F, Romano C, et al: Clinical variability of osteogenesis imperfecta linked to *COL1A2* and associated with a structural defect in the type I collagen molecule. J Med Genet 1989;26:358.
510. Swann SL, Bergh JJ, Farach-Carson MC, et al: Rational design of vitamin D_3 analogues which selectively restore activity to a vitamin D receptor mutant associated with rickets. Org Lett 2002;4:3863.
511. Swierstra BA, Diepstraten AF, vd Heyden BJ: Distal femoral physiolysis in renal osteodystrophy. Successful nonoperative treatment of 3 cases followed for 5 years. Acta Orthop Scand 1993;64:382.
512. Swischuk LE, Hayden CK Jr: Rickets: A roentgenographic scheme for diagnosis. Pediatr Radiol 1979;8: 203.
513. Taitz LS: Child abuse and osteogenesis imperfecta. Br Med J (Clin Res Ed) 1987;295:1082.
514. Tatsumi K, Miyai K, Amino N: Genetic basis of congenital hypothyroidism: Abnormalities in the TSHβ gene, the PIT1 gene, and the NIS gene. Clin Chem Lab Med 1998;36:659.
515. Tebor GB, Ehrlich MG, Herrin J: Slippage of the distal tibial epiphysis. J Pediatr Orthop 1983;3:211.
516. Teh BT, Kytola S, Farnebo F, et al: Mutation analysis of the MEN1 gene in multiple endocrine neoplasia type 1, familial acromegaly and familial isolated hyperparathyroidism. J Clin Endocrinol Metab 1998;83: 2621.
517. Telander RL, Moir CR: Medullary thyroid carcinoma in children. Semin Pediatr Surg 1994;3:188.
518. Thomas DP: Sailors, scurvy and science. J R Soc Med 1997;90:50.
519. Tiley F, Albright JA: Osteogenesis imperfecta: Treatment by multiple osteotomy and intramedullary rod insertion. Report on thirteen patients. J Bone Joint Surg Am 1973;55:701.
520. Tisell LE, Hedback G, Jansson S, et al: Management of hyperparathyroid patients with grave hypercalcemia. World J Surg 1991;15:730.
521. Tolloczko T, Wozniewicz B, Gorski A, et al: Cultured parathyroid cells allotransplantation without immunosuppression for treatment of intractable hypoparathyroidism. Ann Transplant 1996;1:51.
522. Tongsong T, Wanapirak C, Siriangkul S: Prenatal diagnosis of osteogenesis imperfecta type II. Int J Gynaecol Obstet 1998;61:33.
523. Tonini G, Tato L, Rigon F, et al: Hyperparathyroidism. Minerva Pediatr 2004;56:125.
524. Toohey JS: Skeletal presentation of congenital syphilis: Case report and review of the literature. J Pediatr Orthop 1985;5:104.
525. Tosi LL: Osteogenesis imperfecta. Curr Opin Pediatr 1997;9:94.
526. Trelstad RL, Rubin D, Gross J: Osteogenesis imperfecta congenita: Evidence for a generalized molecular disorder of collagen. Lab Invest 1977;36:501.
527. Trump D, Dixon PH, Mumm S, et al: Localisation of X linked recessive idiopathic hypoparathyroidism to a 1.5 Mb region on Xq26-q27. J Med Genet 1998;35:905.
528. Tsipouras P: Osteogenesis Imperfecta. In Beighton P (ed): McKusick's Hereditable Disorders of Connective Tissues. St. Louis, CV Mosby, 1997, p 281.
529. Ueda D, Mitamura R, Suzuki N, et al: Sonographic imaging of the thyroid gland in congenital hypothyroidism. Pediatr Radiol 1992;22:102.
530. Vaes G: Cellular biology and biochemical mechanism of bone resorption. A review of recent developments on the formation, activation, and mode of action of osteoclasts. Clin Orthop Relat Res 1988;231:239.
531. Vandemark WE, Page MA: Massive hyperplasia of bone following fractures of osteogenesis imperfecta: Report of two cases. J Bone Joint Surg Am 1948;30:1015.
532. Ved N, Haller JO: Periosteal reaction with normal-appearing underlying bone: A child abuse mimicker. Emerg Radiol 2002;9:278.
533. Verge CF, Lam A, Simpson JM, et al: Effects of therapy in X-linked hypophosphatemic rickets. N Engl J Med 1991;325:1843.
534. Verrotti A, Greco R, Altobelli E, et al: Bone metabolism in children with congenital hypothyroidism—a longitudinal study. J Pediatr Endocrinol Metab 1998;11: 699.
535. Villaverde V, De Inocencio J, Merino R, et al: Difficulty walking. A presentation of idiopathic juvenile osteoporosis. J Rheumatol 1998;25:173.
536. Vrolik W: Tabulae ad Illustrandam Embryogenesin Hominis et Mammilium tam Naturalem quam Abnormem. Amstelodami 1849.
537. Walton J: Familial hypophosphatemic rickets: A delineation of its subdivisions and pathogenesis. Clin Pediatr (Phila) 1976;15:1007.
538. Wang ST, Pizzolato S, Demshar HP: Diagnostic effectiveness of TSH screening and of T_4 with secondary TSH screening for newborn congenital hypothyroidism. Clin Chim Acta 1998;274:151.
539. Watanabe H, Umeda M, Seki T, et al: Clinical and laboratory studies of severe periodontal disease in an adolescent associated with hypophosphatasia. A case report. J Periodontol 1993;64:174.
540. Weber G, Cazzuffi MA, Frisone F, et al: Nephrocalcinosis in children and adolescents: Sonographic evaluation during long-term treatment with 1,25-dihydroxycholecalciferol. Child Nephrol Urol 1988;9:273.
541. Weinstein M, Babyn P, Zlotkin S: An orange a day keeps the doctor away: Scurvy in the year 2000. Pediatrics 2001;108:E55.
542. Weisberg P, Scanlon KS, Li R, et al: Nutritional rickets among children in the United States: Review of cases

reported between 1986 and 2003. Am J Clin Nutr 2004; 80:1697S.
543. Weller M, Edeiken J, Hodes PJ: Renal osteodystrophy. Am J Roentgenol Radium Ther Nucl Med 1968;104: 354.
544. Wells D, King JD, Roe TF, et al: Review of slipped capital femoral epiphysis associated with endocrine disease. J Pediatr Orthop 1993;13:610.
545. Wenger DR, Abrams RA, Yaru N, et al: Obstruction of the colon due to protrusio acetabuli in osteogenesis imperfecta: Treatment by pelvic osteotomy. Report of a case. J Bone Joint Surg Am 1988;70:1103.
546. West CD, Blanton JC, Silverman FN, et al: Use of phosphate salts as an adjunct to vitamin D in the treatment of hypophosphatemic vitamin D refractory rickets. J Pediatr 1964;64:469.
547. Whalen JP, Horwith M, Krook L, et al: Calcitonin treatment in hereditary bone dysplasia with hyperphosphatasemia: A radiographic and histologic study of bone. AJR Am J Roentgenol 1977;129:29.
548. Whyte MP: Hypophosphatasia and the role of alkaline phosphatase in skeletal mineralization. Endocr Rev 1994;15:439.
549. Whyte MP, Hughes AE: Expansile skeletal hyperphosphatasia is caused by a 15–base pair tandem duplication in *TNFRSF11A* encoding RANK and is allelic to familial expansile osteolysis. J Bone Miner Res 2002; 17:26.
550. Whyte MP, Kurtzberg J, McAlister WH, et al: Marrow cell transplantation for infantile hypophosphatasia. J Bone Miner Res 2003;18:624.
551. Whyte MP, Weldon VV: Idiopathic hypoparathyroidism presenting with seizures during infancy: X-linked recessive inheritance in a large Missouri kindred. J Pediatr 1981;99:608.
552. Wilkinson JM, Scott BW, Clarke AM, et al: Surgical stabilisation of the lower limb in osteogenesis imperfecta using the Sheffield Telescopic Intramedullary Rod System. J Bone Joint Surg Br 1998;80:999.
553. Williams PF: Fragmentation and rodding in osteogenesis imperfecta. J Bone Joint Surg Br 1965;47:23.
554. Williams PF, Cole WH, Bailey RW, et al: Current aspects of the surgical treatment of osteogenesis imperfecta. Clin Orthop Relat Res 1973;96:288.
555. Winberg J, Zetterstrom R: Cortisone treatment in vitamin D intoxication. Acta Paediatr 1956;45:96.
556. Winer KK, Yanovski JA, Cutler GB Jr: Synthetic human parathyroid hormone 1-34 vs calcitriol and calcium in the treatment of hypoparathyroidism. JAMA 1996;276: 631.
557. Winer KK, Yanovski JA, Sarani B, et al: A randomized, cross-over trial of once-daily versus twice-daily parathyroid hormone 1-34 in treatment of hypoparathyroidism. J Clin Endocrinol Metab 1998;83:3480.
558. Winters RW, Graham JB, Williams TF, et al: A genetic study of familial hypophosphatemia and vitamin D resistant rickets with a review of the literature. 1958. Medicine (Baltimore) 1991;70:215.
559. Wirth PB, Kalb RE: Follicular purpuric macules of the extremities. Scurvy. Arch Dermatol 1990;126: 385.
560. Wright NM, Metzger DL, Key LL: Estrogen and diclofenac sodium therapy in a prepubertal female with idiopathic juvenile osteoporosis. J Pediatr Endocrinol Metab 1995;8:135.
561. Wynne-Davies R, Gormley J: Clinical and genetic patterns in osteogenesis imperfecta. Clin Orthop Relat Res 1981;159:26.
562. Yalcinkaya F, Ince E, Tumer N, et al: Spectrum of renal osteodystrophy in children on continuous ambulatory peritoneal dialysis. Pediatr Int 2000;42:53.
563. Yamamoto Y, Onofrio BM: Spinal canal stenosis with hypophosphatemic vitamin D–resistant rickets: Case report. Neurosurgery 1994;35:512.
564. Yeoman PM: Multiple osteotomies and intramedullary fixation of the long bones in osteogenesis imperfecta. Proc R Soc Med 1960;53:946.
565. Yong-Hing K, MacEwen GD: Scoliosis associated with osteogenesis imperfecta. J Bone Joint Surg Br 1982; 64:36.
566. Zionts LE, Ebramzadeh E, Stott NS: Complications in the use of the Bailey-Dubow extensible nail. Clin Orthop Relat Res 1998;348:186.
567. Ziv I, Rang M, Hoffman HJ: Paraplegia in osteogenesis imperfecta. A case report. J Bone Joint Surg Br 1983; 65:184.

Chapter 33

Limb Deficiencies

EMBRYOLOGY AND GENETICS OF LIMB DEVELOPMENT

Normal Embryology

Normal development of the limbs begins at the end of the fourth week after fertilization, with limb buds forming in the mesoderm along the flank of the embryo (Fig. 33–1).[299] The limb bud is divided into three major regions. The apical ectodermal ridge (AER), in which several fibroblast growth factors are expressed, keeps the adjacent mesenchymal cells in an undifferentiated, rapidly proliferating state. This mesenchyma is known as the progress zone. The third zone is the zone of polarizing activity (ZPA). This region is responsible for anteroposterior polarization as the limb develops. The cells that remain in this region the longest populate the distal portion of the extremity.[123] The limbs develop in a proximodistal direction from the limb girdle to the digits. In embryologic terminology, a limb consists of four segments: a root (the zonoskeleton); a proximal segment (stylopodium) with one bone; a middle segment (zeugopodium) with two bones; and a distal, more complex part (autopodium) with many bones.[123] The proximal bones of the limb girdle and the humerus or femur form before the differentiation of ridge ectoderm, whereas development of the remaining bones and digits depends on the AER.[271,304]

The AER is formed by the thickening of lateral plate mesoderm, which signals the overlying ectoderm to thicken and establish a ridge over the tip of the limb bud. The AER regulates the proximodistal growth of the limbs (Fig. 33–2). Although the AER causes outgrowth of the limbs, the mesenchyma determines the type of limb that will develop.[74,135,355]

The bones and connective tissues of the limbs are formed by lateral plate mesoderm, and the muscles originate from myotome regions of the somitic mesoderm.[268] Forelimb and hind limb development occurs via similar mechanisms, with upper limb growth preceding lower limb growth by 1 to 2 days. By 6 weeks, as the buds extend distally, the terminal parts of the limbs flatten to form hand- and footplates, complete with distal rays, and cartilage begins to appear in the proximal portions of the limbs. During the seventh week, the limbs begin to rotate, with the forelimb turning 90 degrees laterally (positioning the thumb laterally) and the hind limb turning 90 degrees medially (positioning the big toe medially). Digital rays appear in the hand- and footplates. By the eighth week, the limbs have rotated to their final position, and all segments are complete, including the digits. During this time, ossification starts. By 12 weeks, ossification centers are present in all the long bones.[268]

Genetic Regulation of Limb Development

Our present understanding of the genetics involved in the development of human limbs is based primarily on research performed on three experimental models—the fruit fly, the mouse, and the chick.[200]

Fibroblast growth factors (FGFs) play a critical role in limb outgrowth. Recent research has shown that application of FGFs to the flank of chick embryos can stimulate the complete development of extra limbs.[52,120,234] FGFs, which are created by at least eight related genes, act via specific membrane-bound receptors to transmit their signals. FGF-4 and FGF-8, both of which are present in the AER,[137,334] can substitute for an intact ridge when they are applied exogenously to the mesoderm of limb buds.[202,228] When both FGF-4 and FGF-8 are absent in a mouse model, limb

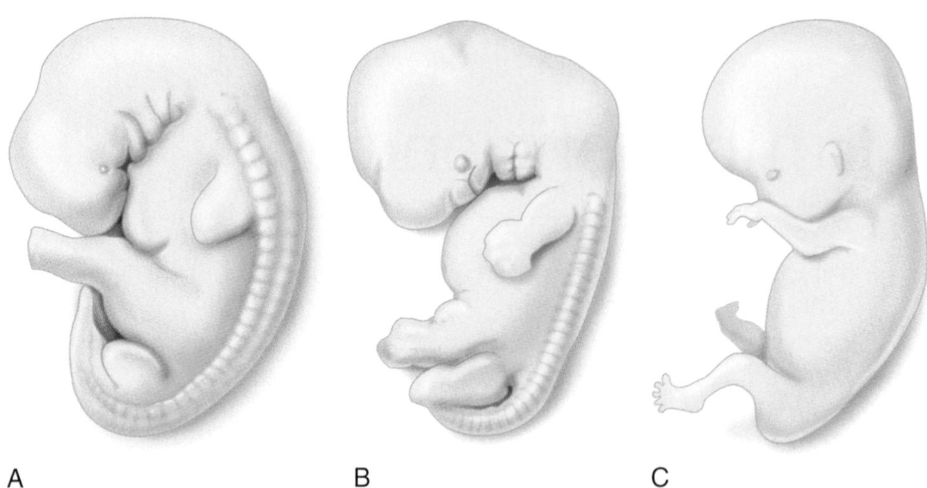

FIGURE 33–1 Limb bud development. **A,** The limb buds appear at the end of the 4th week after fertilization as mesodermal outpouchings on the flank of the embryo. **B,** During the 6th week, the terminal portion of each bud flattens to form the hand- and footplates, complete with digital rays. **C,** By the 12th week, cartilage appears in proximal segments, and ossification centers are present in the long bones.

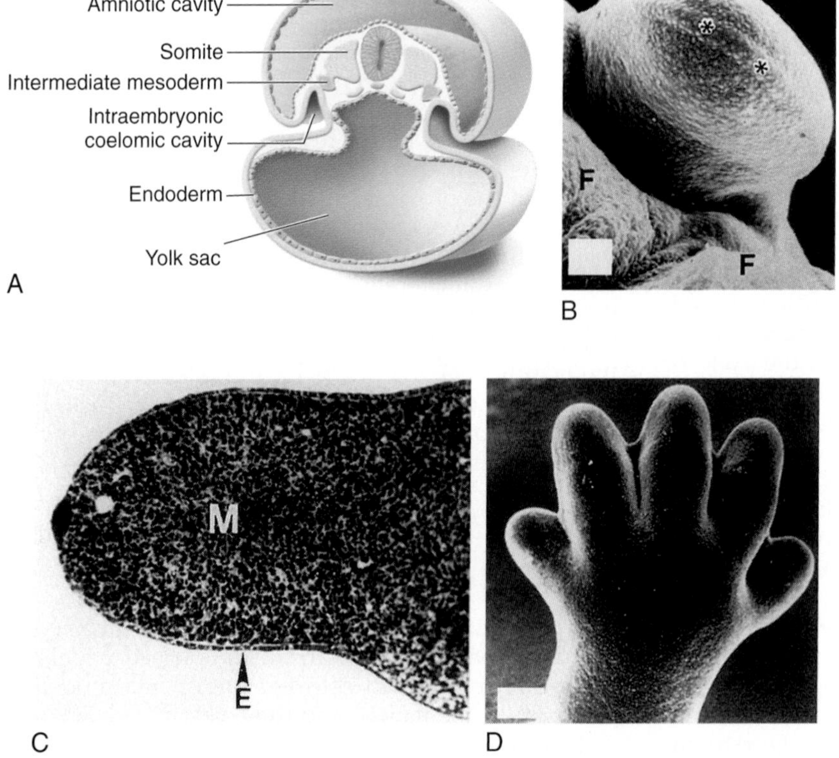

FIGURE 33–2 Limb development. **A,** Cross section through an embryo. The intermediate mesoderm signals the lateral plate mesoderm to initiate limb development. **B,** The early limb bud. *Asterisks* indicate the location of the apical ectodermal ridge (AER), which regulates proximodistal growth of the limb bud. F, flank. **C,** Longitudinal section of the limb bud showing the ectoderm (E) surrounding a core of undifferentiated mesoderm (M). **D,** Digits are forming following programmed cell death in the AER in the spaces between the digits. Each digit then continues to grow under the influence of its own AER. More tissue between the digits will be removed by programmed cell death. (A and C, From Sadler TW: Skeletal development. In Langman's Medical Embryology, 7th ed. Baltimore, Williams & Wilkins, 1995. B and D, From Sadler TW: Embryology and gene regulation of limb development. In Herring JA, Birch JG [eds]: The Child with a Limb Deficiency. Rosemont, Ill, American Academy of Orthopaedic Surgeons, 1998.)

development fails.[306] However, overexpression of FGF-8 in chick embryos can result in limb abnormalities such as truncations, deletions, and extra digits.[334] In some instances, a phenotype similar to achondroplasia is produced, in which limb reductions are associated with shortening of all skeletal elements.

The function of the ZPA, a small block of mesoderm near the posterior edge of the limb close to the body wall, is well known (Fig. 33–3).[268] In normal limbs, as the AER controls distal growth, the ZPA also moves distally as the limb develops, thus maintaining its posterior position near the posterior border of the AER. AER signals promote gene expression in the ZPA. The ZPA is involved in the anteroposterior patterning of the limbs and digits; this was demonstrated when an extra ZPA transplanted to the anterior portion of a

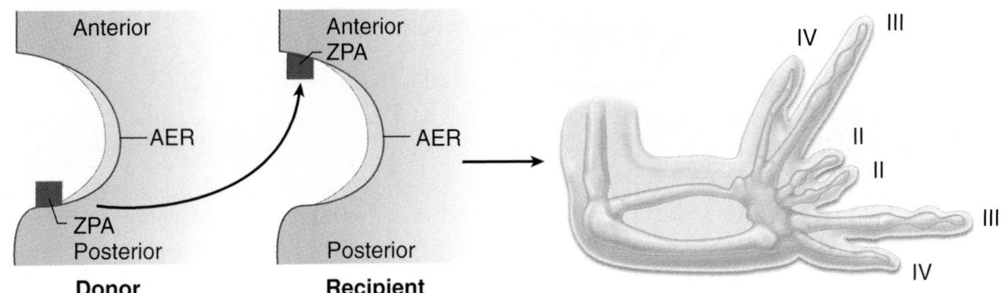

FIGURE 33–3 Regulation of anteroposterior limb development by the zone of polarizing activity (ZPA). The ZPA is a small block of mesoderm near the posterior border of the limb that regulates the anteroposterior patterning of the limb. One of its functions is to cause the digits to appear in proper order. If the ZPA is transplanted into the anterior margin of a normal limb, it will produce a mirror-image duplication of the digits, as shown in the diagram of a chick limb that would normally have three digits. AER, apical ectodermal ridge. (Redrawn from Sadler TW: Embryology and gene regulation of limb development. In Herring JA, Birch JG [eds]: The Child with a Limb Deficiency. Rosemont, Ill, American Academy of Orthopaedic Surgeons, 1998.)

normal chick limb resulted in a mirror-image duplication of the digits.[272,305,316]

The polarizing action of the ZPA is mediated by protein produced by the sonic hedgehog gene (*Shh*).[256] Hedgehog genes, originally described in *Drosophila,* are a multigene family with diverse signaling functions in higher vertebrates.[130] *Shh* is necessary for normal limb development at or just distal to the elbow or knee joints in mouse experiments.[43] *Shh* acts as an inductive signal in the development of several tissues; in the limb bud, it is first seen in the ZPA. The ZPA-inductive signal is encoded by *Shh,* which is expressed in the ZPA. *Shh* induces the expression of a cascade of downstream genes (e.g., *homeobox* genes, bone morphogenetic proteins, *Wnt* genes, *Gli* transcription factors) by binding to its specific receptor, called *patched*.[260] When retinoic acid is placed in the anterior limb mesoderm, it induces the expression of *Shh,* and a new ZPA is created.[337] A decrease in *Shh* activity results in the absence of ulnar and posterior digits, whereas a complete absence of *Shh* results in loss of distal limb structures. Mutations in the human *Shh* gene cause holoprosencephaly (a pleiotropic genetic disorder),[261] indicating the gene's involvement in the myriad stages of human development. Other hedgehog genes play crucial roles during the later stages of limb development,[130] including the *Indian hedgehog (Ihh)* gene, which mediates the rate of cartilage differentiation.[336]

Homeobox (Hox) genes, which are present in all species, act as transcription factors. In the development of the limbs, *HoxA* genes may contribute to proximodistal patterning,[351] and *HoxD* genes may play a role in anteroposterior patterning.[71] A factor known as promyelocytic leukemia zinc finger is a mediator of anteroposterior patterning in the axial and appendicular skeleton and is a regulator of *Hox* gene expression.[19]

In research using the rat model, bone morphogenetic proteins (BMPs) were found to have the property of forming ectopic bone after implantation under the skin or muscle.[146,338] The products of BMPs, which are related to the transforming growth factor-β family of proteins, take part in fracture healing and in the patterning of joint placement. Three BMP genes—*Bmp-2, Bmp-4,* and *Bmp-7*—are expressed within the AER and mesenchyma of developing limb buds.[87,88,182] The role of BMPs in the early developmental stages of limb buds is uncertain; however, the proteins seem to have a function in the ensuing development of digits.[200]

Based on what is currently known about the genetic control of limb development, a relatively small set of genes and gene families appears to be involved in the early stages of formation. The developmental programs differ at the morphologic level from flies to humans[282]; however, there is extraordinary preservation of the molecular pathways in the various animal groups. In general, humans have more genes in a specific gene family, and these genes are used to play variations on a common theme (sometimes in overlapping pathways).[200] The important point is that the molecular theme is maintained from species to species. Continued research on *Drosophila* and transgenic mice will undoubtedly provide further information on this intricate and fascinating process of limb development.

CLASSIFYING LIMB DEFICIENCIES

Frantz and O'Rahilly Classification System

The classification system proposed by Frantz and O'Rahilly in 1961 continues to be widely used as a method of grouping congenital skeletal limb deficiencies (Fig. 33–4).[90,124] Extremity anomalies are categorized as either *terminal deficiencies* or *intercalary deficiencies.* Terminal deficiencies are those in which the entire segment of a limb distal to and in line with the deficit is absent. Intercalary deficiencies are those in which the middle part of a limb is absent but the portions proximal and distal to the affected segment are present. Terminal and intercalary deficiencies may be *transverse,* in which the entire width of the limb is affected (Fig. 33–5), or *paraxial,* in which only the

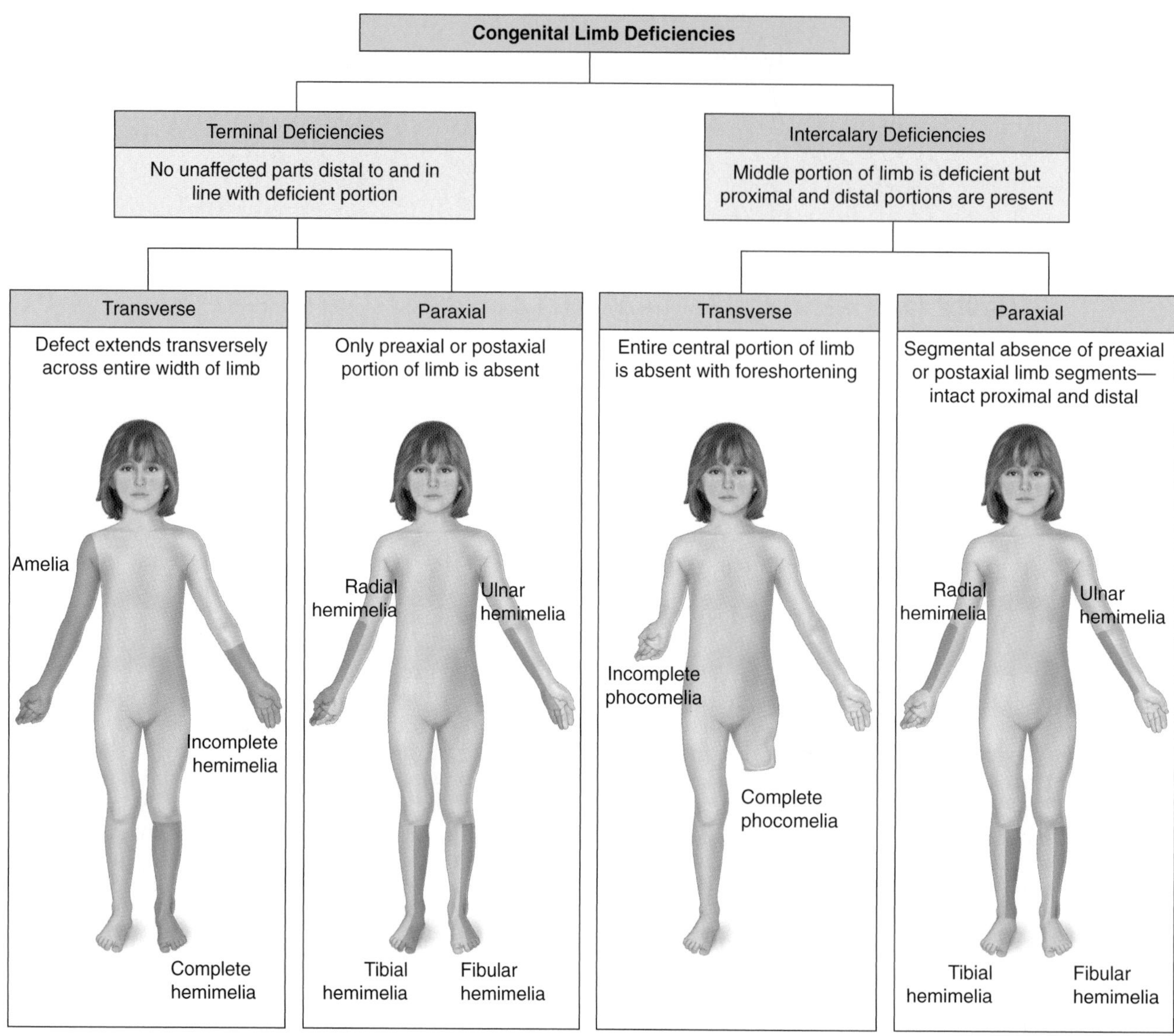

FIGURE 33–4 Frantz and O'Rahilly classification of congenital limb deficiencies.

preaxial or postaxial part of the limb is involved (Figs. 33–6 and 33–7). With transverse terminal deficiencies, the defect extends transversely across the entire width of the limb, whereas with paraxial terminal deficiencies, only the preaxial or postaxial part of the limb is missing. With transverse intercalary deficiencies, the entire middle part of the limb is absent, with foreshortening. With paraxial intercalary deficiencies, only segmental portions of the preaxial or postaxial part of the limb are absent, and the proximal and distal portions are present.

Amelia is the complete absence of a limb. *Hemimelia,* which means half a limb, is used when one of the paired bones of the upper or lower extremity is absent. The terms *complete* and *incomplete* are applied to hemimelias to indicate the absence of all or only part of the affected bone. Deficiencies are designated according to the anatomic part that is absent. For example, when only the tibia is absent, the deficiency is termed *tibial hemimelia,* and it is a paraxial (rather than transverse) defect because only the tibial portion of the limb is affected. If the rays of the foot are also absent, the defect is a terminal deficiency, whereas if the foot is present and normal, the defect is an intercalary deficiency. A glossary of terms associated with limb deficiencies is provided in Box 33–1.

ISO/ISPO International Classification System

An international classification system was proposed in 1991 in an attempt to improve communication among researchers in different countries by standardizing the terminology for congenital deficiencies (Box 33–2; Table 33–1).[65] In the international system, all limb deficiencies are classified as either *transverse* or *longitudinal.* Missing bones are named and described as either *complete* or *partial* in their absence. The authors of this system theorize that there are no true intercalary

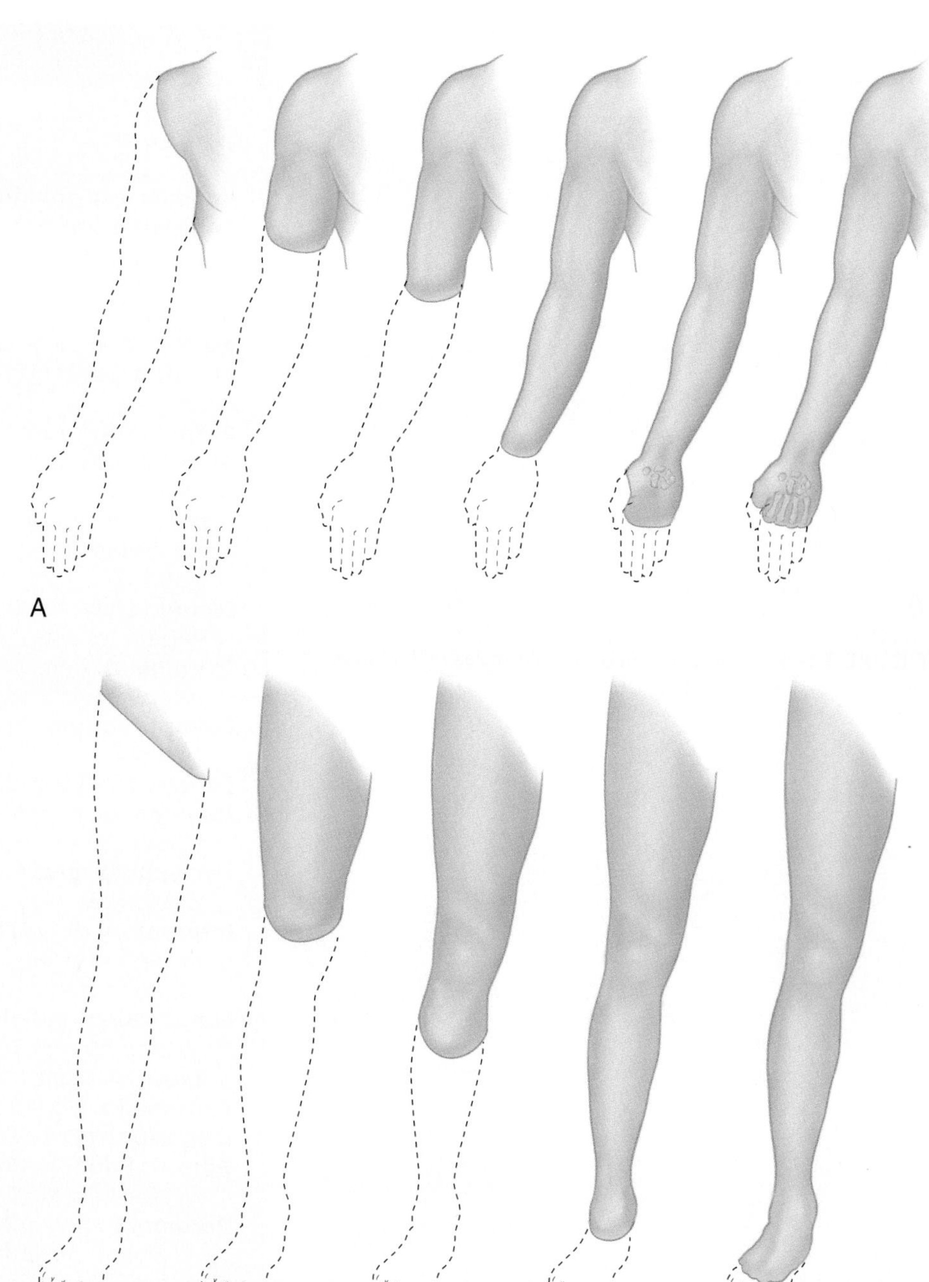

FIGURE 33–5 Spectrum of terminal transverse deficiencies in the upper limb **(A)** and lower limb **(B)**.

deficits, instead treating such deficits as variable degrees of longitudinal deficiencies.

In this international classification system, transverse deficiencies are named according to the level of absence (Table 33–2). Thus, a short congenital below-elbow absence is termed "transverse right Fo (forearm), upper," whereas an elbow disarticulation level is a "transverse right Fo, complete." Longitudinal deficiencies are named for the missing parts, and parts not named are assumed to be present (Table 33–3). For example, a fibular hemimelia is described as a "complete deficiency, Fi (fibula)," implying a normal foot. If the lateral two rays are also missing, one adds "MT (metatarsal) 4, 5, Ph (phalanges) 4, 5" to designate that condition. Although the terminology is laudable for its anatomic accuracy, the lengthy designations have limited its general acceptance.

General Treatment Concepts

Timing of Treatment

The timing of nonsurgical and surgical corrections of limb deficiencies should accord with the child's developmental milestones. For example, at about 6 months of age, most children are able to sit well, put both hands together in the midline, and begin performing two-handed maneuvers. This is the best time to fit a

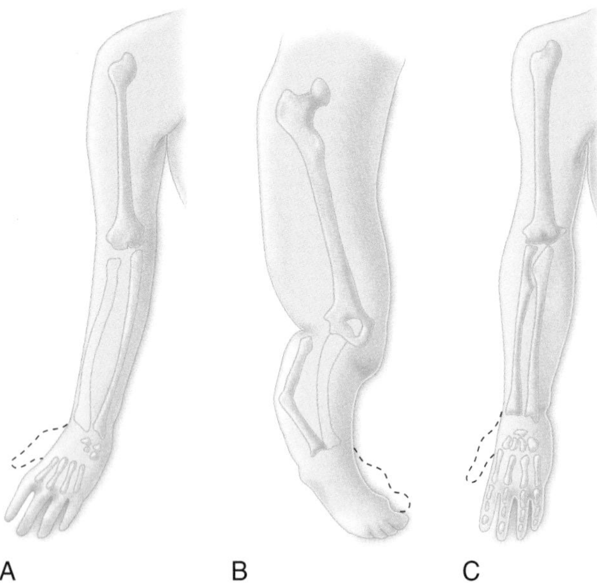

FIGURE 33-6 Preaxial longitudinal deficiencies of the radius **(A)**, tibia **(B)**, and thumb **(C)**.

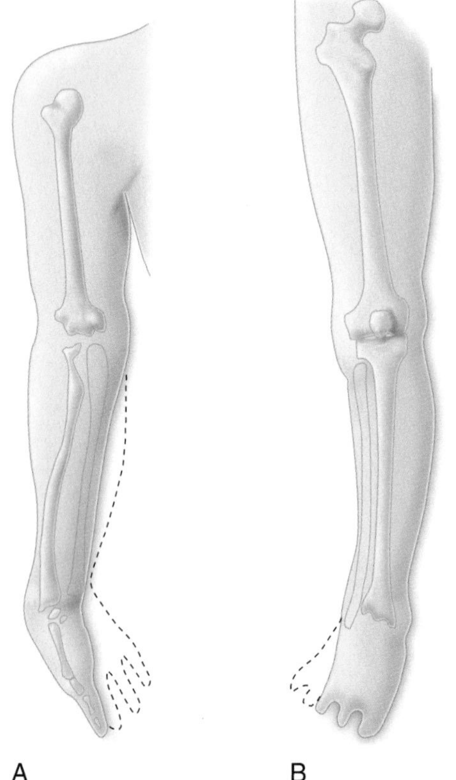

FIGURE 33-7 Postaxial longitudinal deficiencies of the ulna **(A)** and fibula **(B)**.

Box 33-1

Glossary

Acheiria (or achiria): absence of the hand
Acheiropodia: absence of hands and feet
Adactyly (or adactylia): absence of the fingers or toes
Agenesis: absence or no development
Amelia: complete absence of a limb
Amelia totalis: complete absence of all four limbs
Amputation: absence of a distal part of a limb
Aphalangia: absence of phalanges
Aplasia: absence of a specific bone or bones
Apodia: absence of the foot
Ectrocheiria: total or partial absence of the hand
Ectrodactyly: total or partial absence of the fingers
Ectromelia: total or partial absence of one or more long bones or limbs
Ectrophalangia: absence of one or more phalanges
Ectropodia: total or partial absence of the foot
Hemimelia: absence of one of the paired bones of the limbs
Hypophalangia: fewer than normal number of phalanges
Intercalary deficiency: absence of the middle portion of a limb, when proximal and distal portions are present
Longitudinal deficiency: absence of a limb extending parallel to the long axis (may be preaxial, postaxial, or central)
Meromelia: partial absence of a limb
Oligodactyly: absence of some of the fingers
Paraxial deficiency: absence of the preaxial or postaxial portion of a limb
Peromelia: hemimelia, especially hands ending in a stump
Phocomelia: absence of the arm and forearm in the upper limb or the thigh and leg in the lower limb (i.e., the hands or feet sprout directly from the trunk); the deficiency may be proximal (arms or thighs missing) or distal (forearms or legs missing)
Postaxial: pertaining to the ulnar side of the upper limb and the fibular side of the lower limb
Preaxial: pertaining to the radial side of the upper limb and the tibial side of the lower limb
Terminal deficiency: absence of a limb with all portions in line with and distal to the defect involved
Transverse deficiency: absence of the entire width of a limb

Box 33-2

ISO/ISPO Classification of Congenital Limb Deficiency

Transverse Deficiencies

Limb has developed normally to a particular level beyond which no skeletal elements are present, although there may be digital buds

The deficiency is described by naming the segment at which the limb terminates and the level within the segment beyond which no skeletal elements exist

Longitudinal Deficiencies

Reduction or absence of an element or elements within the long axis of the limb in which there may be normal skeletal elements distal to the affected bone or bones

The deficiency is described by naming the bones affected in a proximodistal sequence; any bone not named is present and normal

The affected bone is described as totally or partially absent

For partial deficiencies, the approximate fraction and position of the absent part may be stated

The number of the digit is stated in relation to the metacarpal or metatarsal and phalanges, with numbering beginning from the preaxial, radial, or tibial side

The term *ray* may be used to refer to a metacarpal or metatarsal and its corresponding phalanges

ISO, International Society for Orthotics; ISPO, International Society for Prosthetics and Orthotics.

Table 33-1 Comparison of Standard and ISO/ISPO Terminology for Congenital Limb Deficiencies

Standard	ISO/ISPO
Congenital "Chopart's"	Transverse, tarsal, partial
Congenital absence of forefoot	Transverse, metatarsal, complete
Congenital "Syme's"	Transverse, tarsal, complete
Congenital below-knee, long	Transverse, leg, lower third
Congenital below-knee, short	Transverse, leg, upper third
Congenital knee disarticulation	Transverse, leg, complete
Congenital above-knee, short	Transverse, thigh, upper third
Congenital hip disarticulation	Transverse, thigh, complete
Upper limb amelia, no scapula	Transverse, shoulder, complete
Upper limb amelia, scapula present	Transverse, forearm, upper third
Congenital below-elbow, long	Transverse, forearm, lower third
Congenital wrist disarticulation	Transverse, carpal, complete
Congenital partial hand (with carpals)	Transverse, carpal, partial
Congenital partial foot (with metatarsals)	Transverse, phalangeal, complete
Fibular hemimelia (foot unaffected)	Longitudinal, fibular, complete
Partial fibular hemimelia	Longitudinal, fibular, partial
Tibial hemimelia	Longitudinal, tibial, complete
Absent tibia and first two toes	Longitudinal, tibial, complete; rays 1, 2
Absent radius, ulna (index finger present)	Longitudinal, radius and ulna, complete; carpals, complete; rays 1, 3, 4, and 5, complete
Upper limb phocomelia (hand intact, scapula present)	Longitudinal, humerus, complete; radius and ulna, complete
Clavicle absent, humerus short, radius short, ulna absent, carpals absent, fifth finger absent	Longitudinal, clavicle, complete; humerus, partial; radius, partial; ulna, complete; ray 5

ISO, International Society for Orthotics; ISPO, International Society for Prosthetics and Orthotics.

child with a prosthesis for an upper limb deficiency. The child's ability to adapt to the prosthesis is enhanced because he or she can start using it in apposition with the other hand at an early stage.

For many lower limb deficiencies, surgical interventions should be planned early and completed, if possible, before the child starts to walk. This allows time for the wound to heal properly and for a prosthesis to be fitted when the child starts to walk, which is normally at about 12 months of age. For example, a Syme's amputation for fibular hemimelia is best performed at about 10 months of age, when the child is beginning to stand.

Table 33-2 Identification of Transverse Limb Deficiencies (Congenital Amputations)

Upper Limb (UL)	Lower Limb (LL)	Level of Absence
Arm (Ar) or forearm (Fo)	Thigh (Th) or leg (Le)	Complete, upper third, middle third, or lower third
Carpal (Ca), metacarpal (MC), phalangeal (Ph)	Tarsal (Ta), metatarsal (MT), phalangeal (Ph)	Complete or partial

Table 33-3 Identification of Partial or Complete Longitudinal Deficiencies

Location	Deficiency
Upper Limb (UL)	
Proximal	Humeral (Hu)
Distal	Radial (Ra); central (Ce); ulnar (Ul); carpal (Ca); metacarpal (MC) 1, 2, 3, 4, 5; phalangeal (Ph) 1, 2, 3, 4, 5
Combined	Radial (Ra); humeral (Hu); ulnar (Ul); carpal (Ca); metacarpal (MC) 1, 2, 3, 4, 5; phalangeal (Ph) 1, 2, 3, 4, 5
Lower Limb (LL)	
Proximal	Femoral (Fe)
Distal	Tibial (Ti); central (Ce); fibular (Fi); tarsal (Ta); metatarsal (MT) 1, 2, 3, 4, 5; phalangeal (Ph) 1, 2, 3, 4, 5
Combined	Tibial (Ti); femoral (Fe); fibular (Fi); tarsal (Ta); metatarsal (MT) 1, 2, 3, 4, 5; phalangeal (Ph) 1, 2, 3, 4, 5

The child's developing anatomy is another important factor in the timing of surgical interventions. The correction of some lower limb deficiencies is best maintained with weight bearing, so the surgery should be performed after the child has started walking. An amputation to correct a proximal focal femoral deficiency (PFFD) may be performed when the child is young, but knee fusion is easier once the femoral condyles and proximal tibia have sufficiently ossified (at about 4 to 5 years of age). Alternatively, the child may be treated initially with an equinus prosthesis to allow ambulation, followed by amputation and knee fusion at 3 to 4 years of age. In a patient with a partial tibial hemimelia, fusion of the proximal tibia to the fibula is more easily achieved after the tibial anlage has adequately ossified, rather than when it is still primarily cartilaginous.

Social Factors

For children and adolescents, many important social factors come into play when deciding on interventions to treat limb deficiencies. For example, a young child may discard an upper extremity prosthesis and then request one when starting school. Or, when planning surgery, the surgeon should factor in sufficient recovery time so that the child does not have to enter a new school while still walking on crutches. For an adolescent, every attempt should be made to minimize any embarrassment, such as having to go to school without a prosthesis.

Long-term Planning

Difficult decisions often have to be made regarding the best long-term plans for the child. This is especially true when there is a choice between a prolonged course of multiple corrective procedures and a less involved, early, single intervention such as amputation.

Such a dilemma typically arises in a child with fibular hemimelia.[44] If a Syme's amputation is performed just before the patient starts walking, the child will probably not require any additional operations or hospitalizations for the deformity and will be able to function at a nearly normal level in sports activities. However, the child will have to deal with wearing a prosthesis in place of a foot.

An alternative approach is to use modern limb lengthening techniques to correct the deformity, which will maintain the limb and minimize or eliminate the need for a prosthesis.[342] However, limb lengthening requires that the child endure two or three periods in an external apparatus (each of which may last 6 months or longer) for a successful outcome; the procedures are often difficult and painful, and the social and psychological costs of these interventions can be substantial.[97,103,145,222] Of 56 patients treated by limb lengthening procedures at Texas Scottish Rite Hospital for Children between 1989 and 1996, almost 50% experienced a deterioration in mental status, most of them suffering from depression.[222] Almost half the patients experienced moderate to severe pain at some time during the lengthening process. The medical outcome was compromised in approximately 20% of patients because of a psychological or behavioral factor, particularly noncompliance with exercise and a decline in mental status. In addition to arranging for psychological counseling, the orthopaedist should aggressively treat any pain, sleep, or appetite problems experienced by the patient during lengthening and reconstruction.[222]

Although the anatomic results of lengthening procedures are well known, long-term functional assessments of patients who have undergone such procedures are not available. Thus, Damsin and associates[60] make a good point when they state that "surgeons should remain humble and wise during decision making" and "not yield to the temptation offered by a brilliant equalization procedure." Whenever a choice must be made between amputation and lengthening, the role of the orthopaedist is to make sure that the patient and the parents are fully aware of the risks and benefits of the options available. In that way, informed decisions can be made based on knowledge and realistic expectations, not ignorance or wishful thinking. This may be best accomplished by introducing the child and family to another child and family faced with similar decisions.

CONGENITAL ABSENCE OF LIMBS

Timing of Limb Malformation and Deformation

By 7 weeks of embryonic life, the formation of all parts of the upper and lower limbs is essentially complete. Most limb deficiencies occur early in the period of limb morphogenesis, when there is rapid proliferation and differentiation of cells and tissues. This "sensitive period" of limb formation peaks during the fifth and sixth weeks after fertilization.[268] Thus, major malformations (e.g., absence of a long bone) appear by 7 weeks of fetal development. Major upper limb deficiencies occur at 28 days, major lower limb deficiencies at 31 days, distal upper abnormalities on the 35th day, and distal lower limb deformities on the 37th day.[98] Depending on the timing and severity of the insult, abnormalities develop in a predictable manner.[139] Unlike malformations, deformations—changes in formed structures due to external forces—can occur at any time during fetal development. Distal deformity secondary to a constricting amniotic band is an example of a deformation (Fig. 33–8).

Etiology of Limb Absence

Advances in molecular biology have provided new information about the genes and gene products responsible for coordinating normal limb development. This knowledge has enabled scientists to better identify genes that might be directly responsible for limb defects or indirectly responsible through the effects of teratogens.

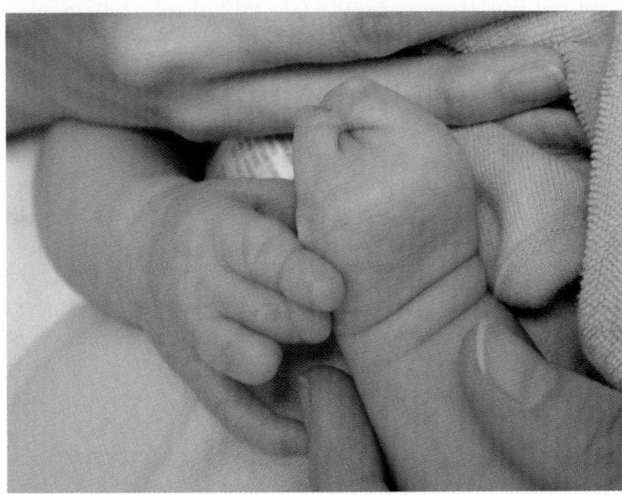

FIGURE 33–8 Amnion disruption caused the ringlike constriction amputations and distal syndactyly in this infant.

At this time, however, the specific cause of congenital limb deficiencies is unknown in most cases. Although there are a few limb abnormalities with genetic bases, most limb deformities develop sporadically, with no identifiable environmental factors, trauma, or familial incidence. Most single-limb anomalies have a very small chance of recurring in subsequent children of the same parents or in the children of the affected person. The incidence of recurrence of the same anomaly is 1% to 3%, only slightly greater than that among the general population.

In a population-based review of birth defects in Norway, Lie and associates reported that in families of children with limb abnormalities, a second child has a significantly greater chance of being born with a similar anomaly compared with the expected rate in the general population.[190] However, they also noted that the risk of a birth defect in subsequent children decreases if the mother moves to another part of the country after the first child is born, which suggests an environmental influence.

Many drugs are known teratogens; however, the only drug specifically identified with a large number of limb abnormalities is thalidomide.[91,92,140,207,220] A possible mechanism of the thalidomide effect is the production of free radicals causing misregulation of limb growth pathways.[132] If the mother took drugs or was exposed to potential teratogens during her pregnancy, a complete history should be obtained to help determine the developmental stage of the fetus during the time of exposure.

Amniotic bands (Streeter band syndrome or congenital constriction band syndrome) are another potential cause of prenatal limb amputation (see Fig. 33–8). Early compression of the embryo is believed to cause early rupture of the amniotic membrane, with subsequent formation of aberrant amnion bands (strands) that can disrupt structures in the craniofacial area, abdominal wall, or limbs.[156] When these bands of tissue form constriction rings around different parts of the limbs, they can impede venous drainage (resulting in edema), remain as deep clefts in the soft tissue, or completely amputate parts of the limb distal to the band. It is uncommon for only one limb to be affected. In most cases, early intrauterine disturbance of the limb bud results in failure of the limbs to develop further.[110] It has been estimated that this syndrome usually occurs at about 6 weeks of fetal development.[164]

Heritable Limb Deficiencies and Associated Anomalies

Upper limb deficiencies are more likely to have associated abnormalities (particularly in patients with genetic disorders), with humeral defects the most predictive of concomitant anomalies.[348]

Poland's syndrome consists of unilateral absence of the pectoralis minor and the sternal portion of the pectoralis major muscles, along with some type of coexisting ipsilateral hand abnormalities, including hypoplasia of the hand and digits with syndactyly, brachydactyly, and reduction deformities.[201]

Patients with thrombocytopenia–absent radius syndrome usually have unilateral or bilateral absence or hypoplasia of the radius, along with a radially clubbed hand, deformed or absent thumb, and hypoplasia of the ulna (Fig. 33–9).[127] Associated anomalies include short stature, strabismus, micrognathia, dislocated hip, clubfoot, congenital heart disease, foreshortened humeri and hypoplastic shoulder girdles, and occasionally lower limb deformities. This syndrome requires prompt diagnosis and treatment in the neonatal period, because hematologic problems may cause central nervous system damage secondary to intraventricular bleeding. Platelet transfusion is often necessary.

In Fanconi's pancytopenia syndrome, dysmorphic and limb reduction defects vary considerably, with skeletal abnormalities including absent or hypoplastic thumbs, hypoplastic radius, and developmental dysplasia of the hip.[109] The patient is born with the limb defects, is relatively small at birth, and usually has patchy brown discoloration of the skin. Some children may have only hematologic disorders (e.g., bleeding, pallor, recurrent infections), which usually manifest between 5 and 10 years of age and can be treated with testosterone and hydrocortisone analog therapy.[280]

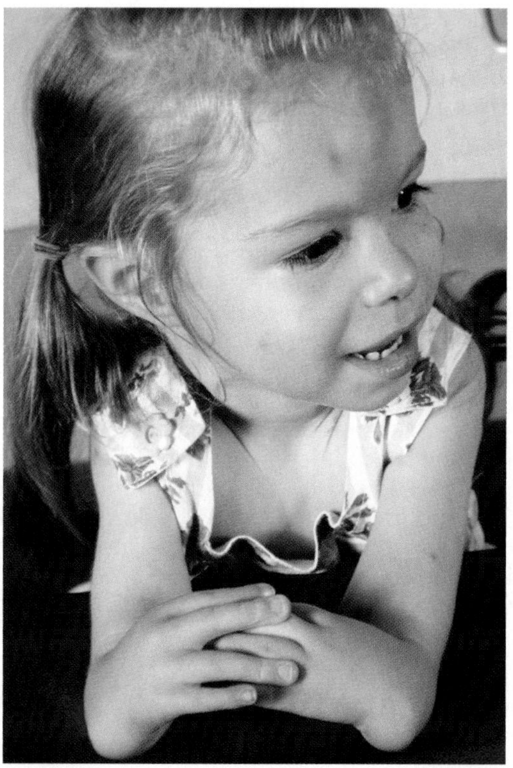

FIGURE 33–9 Patient with thrombocytopenia–absent radius syndrome.

Associated anomalies include cardiac, urogenital, and eye abnormalities and a predisposition to leukemia.

Holt-Oram (hand-heart) syndrome results in upper limb deformities that may consist of partial or complete absence of the thumb or radial aplasia, a radially clubbed hand with or without elbow function, or severe hypoplasia of the forearm and defects of the humerus, clavicle, scapula, or sternum.[147] Associated anomalies include cardiac defects (e.g., atrial septal defect, ventricular septal defect, tetralogy of Fallot) and vertebral defects (e.g., scoliosis, pectus excavatum). The syndrome is usually bilateral but asymmetric.

Anomalies associated with the VATER syndrome include vertebral defects, imperforate anus, tracheoesophageal fistula with esophageal atresia, and radial and renal dysplasia.[249] The more current nomenclature, VACTERL, includes cardiac anomalies and separates renal and limb abnormalities.[280] Patients may also have deficient prenatal growth, a single umbilical artery, and defects of the external genitalia. The cause of this condition is not known, and malformation patterns tend to be sporadic, but a greater frequency has been noted in children of diabetic mothers.[280]

Amelia has been associated with omphalocele and diaphragmatic hernia, and radial ray deficiencies have been associated with cardiac anomalies and imperforate anus.[95-97]

Tibial hemimelia is one of the few lower limb deficiencies in which a heritable pattern is often seen.[168,266] In femoral hypoplasia–unusual facies syndrome (Fig. 33–10), the limb deficiencies can range from a hypoplastic femur to an absent femur and fibula.[289] The humerus may also be affected, producing restricted elbow motion, and deformities may be seen in the lower spine and pelvis. Defects can be unilateral or bilateral. The distinct facial characteristics include a short nose with hypoplastic alae nasi, long philtrum and thin upper lip, micrognathia, cleft palate, and upward slanting of the palpebral fissures. The ulnar-femoral syndrome (a combination of femoral deficiency and ulnar abnormalities) also may be inherited. Some of the more common heritable limb deficiencies are listed in Box 33–3.

Whenever a child has a limb deficiency, the physician should carefully assess the craniofacial, cardiac, gastrointestinal, genitourinary, integumentary, and nervous systems. Peripheral blood cell counts, urinalysis, skeletal radiographs, hearing, visual acuity, and growth should be monitored regularly during infancy and early childhood until it is obvious that the limb deficiency is an isolated event.[348] If there is a family history of an abnormality and the disorder resembles one known to have a genetic cause, the parents should be provided with appropriate genetic counseling.

Hypothesis of Subclavian Artery Supply Disruption Sequence

A vascular cause has been proposed for patients with Poland's, Klippel-Feil, and Möbius' syndromes;

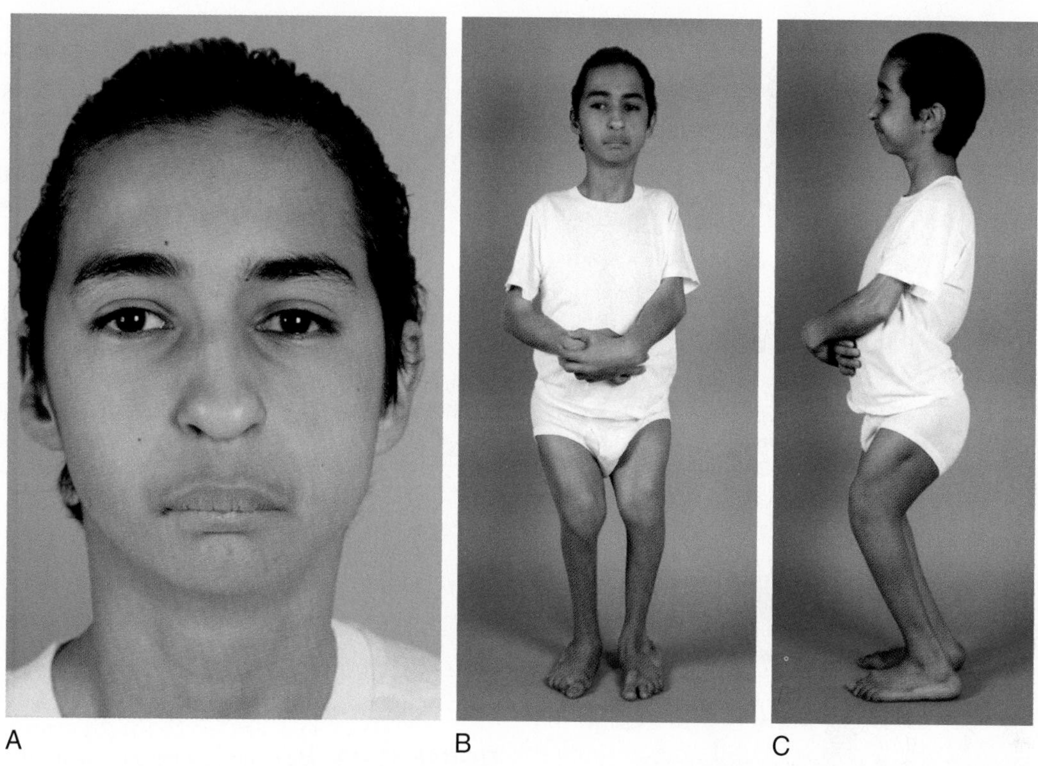

FIGURE 33-10 **A** through **C,** Patient with femoral hypoplasia–unusual facies syndrome.

Box 33-3

Heritable Limb Deficiencies

- Longitudinal deficiencies—preaxial, radial, and tibial
  Fanconi's pancytopenia syndrome (autosomal recessive): upper limb deficiencies of thumb and radius, with occasional developmental dysplasia of the hip; associated anomalies include cardiac, urogenital, and eye abnormalities and a predisposition to leukemia
  Thrombocytopenia-absent radius syndrome (autosomal recessive): radial aplasia or hypoplasia with radially clubbed hand, deformed or absent thumb, and hypoplasia of the ulna; associated anomalies include short stature, congenital heart disease, foreshortened humeri and hypoplastic shoulder girdles, strabismus, micrognathia, dislocated hip, clubfoot, and occasional lower limb deficiency
- Longitudinal deficiencies—postaxial, ulnar, and fibular
  Isolated ectrodactyly (autosomal dominant): deficiency of central rays of both hands and feet; may be difficult to differentiate from autosomal recessive ectrodactyly because of incomplete penetrance
- Longitudinal deficiencies—intercalary, sometimes phocomelic; middle segment
  Holt-Oram syndrome (autosomal dominant): upper limb deficiencies ranging from partial or complete absence of the thumb, radial aplasia, and radially clubbed hand with or without elbow function to severe hypoplasia of the entire forearm and defects of the humerus, clavicle, scapula, or sternum; associated anomalies include cardiac and vertebral defects
- Tibial aplasias
  Tibial absence with polydactyly (autosomal dominant): tibial deficiency with duplications of radial ray; associated anomalies include cardiac defects

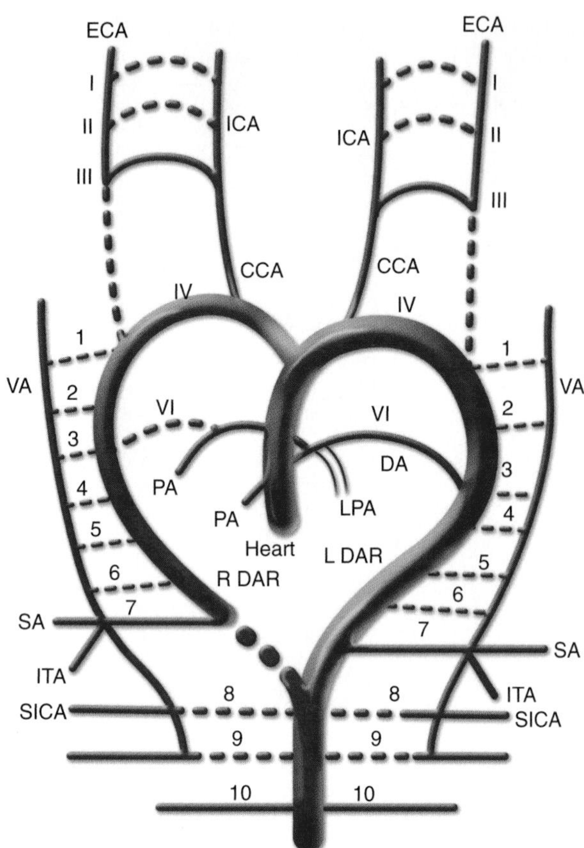

FIGURE 33–11 Schematic diagram of the many components of the aortic arch complex. The *dotted lines* represent vessels that do not persist in the adult. CCA, common carotid artery; DA, ductus arteriosus; ECA, external carotid artery; ICA, internal carotid artery; ITA, internal thoracic arteries; L DAR, left dorsal aortic root; LPA, left pulmonary artery; PA, pulmonary artery; R DAR, right dorsal aortic root; SA, subclavian artery; SICA, superior intercostal arteries; VA, vertebral artery (Redrawn from Bavinck JN, Weaver DD: Subclavian artery supply disruption sequence: Hypothesis of a vascular etiology for Poland, Klippel-Feil, and Möbius anomalies. Am J Med Genet 1986; 23:903. Reprinted by permission of Wiley-Liss Inc., a subsidiary of John Wiley & Sons, Inc.)

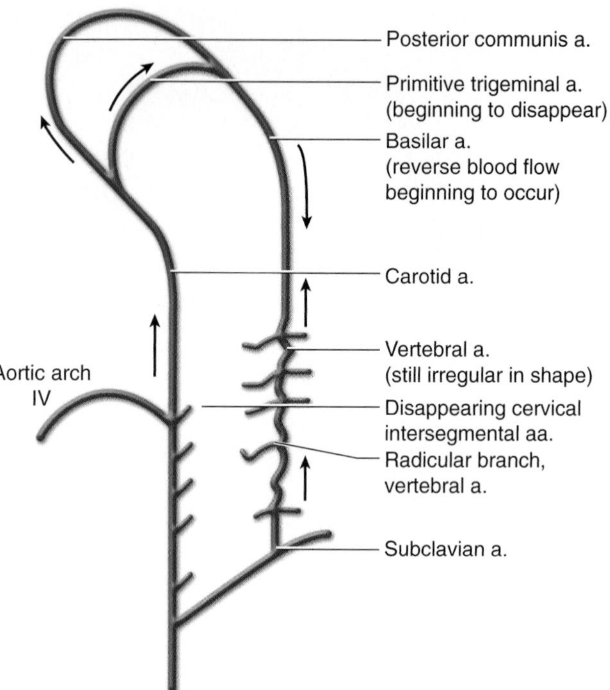

FIGURE 33–12 Major blood supply to the head and neck at 42 days of fetal development. The proximal portions of the first six cervical intersegmental arteries have regressed and disappeared. The subclavian artery has developed from the seven intersegmental arteries. (Redrawn from Bavinck JN, Weaver DD: Subclavian artery supply disruption sequence: Hypothesis of a vascular etiology for Poland, Klippel-Feil, and Möbius anomalies. Am J Med Genet 1986;23:903. Reprinted by permission of Wiley-Liss Inc., a subsidiary of John Wiley & Sons, Inc.)

terminal transverse limb defects; and Sprengel's anomaly.[21] According to this hypothesis, these conditions are caused by interruption of the early embryonic blood supply in the subclavian or vertebral arteries or their branches during the fifth through eighth weeks of fetal development (Figs. 33–11 and 33–12). Vascular disruption in the subclavian artery may be due to internal obstruction of the vessel from edema, thrombi, or emboli or to obstruction secondary to external pressure on the vessel from tissue edema, local hemorrhage, cervical rib, aberrant muscle, amniotic band, tumor, or embryonic intrauterine compression.[21] Exogenous factors (e.g., drugs, chemicals, generalized hypoxia, hyperthermia) may cause premature regression of vessels or a delay in vessel development.

The specific anomaly depends on the blockage site, the extent and timing of the blockage, and the duration of the interruption. Disruptions of specific arteries and their likely subsequent effects are listed in Table 33–4.

Various combinations of obstructions of the subclavian and branch arteries may account for the overlapping clinical features seen in patients with Poland's, Möbius', and Klippel-Feil syndromes; terminal transverse limb defects; and Sprengel's anomalies (Fig. 33–13).[343] The different patterns of vertebral abnormalities associated with Klippel-Feil syndrome may be due to variations in the location and extent of arterial interruption. The pathologic changes seen in Möbius' syndrome may result from ischemia secondary to premature regression of early brain vessels or transient blockage of the basilar or vertebral arteries.[191,293] Interruption of the blood supply from one or more of the internal thoracic arteries during embryonic development could result in the absence or hypoplasia of structures in the upper chest area.

The degree of upper limb deficiency seen in patients with terminal transverse limb defects (as an isolated defect or in association with Klippel-Feil, Poland's, or Möbius' syndromes) varies from very mild (e.g., a slightly smaller hand with no disability) to severe (e.g., a significant reduction in the size of the hand and forearm, with no functional hand). The severity of the defect depends on the timing of the vascular

Table 33-4 Subclavian Artery Supply Disruption Sequence

Obstructed Artery	Subsequent Anomaly
Internal thoracic artery	Ipsilateral absence of costosternal heads of pectoralis major, and hypoplasia or aplasia of breast
Subclavian artery, distal to origin of internal thoracic artery	Isolated terminal transverse limb defects
Subclavian artery, proximal to internal thoracic artery but distal to vertebral artery	Poland's syndrome
At origin or any segment along developing vertebral artery or radicular branches	Klippel-Feil syndrome
One or more early arteries of brain, or basilar or vertebral arteries	Möbius' syndrome
Subclavian, internal thoracic, or supracapsular artery	Sprengel's anomaly—hypoplasia of scapula and lack of development of upper portion of serratus anterior

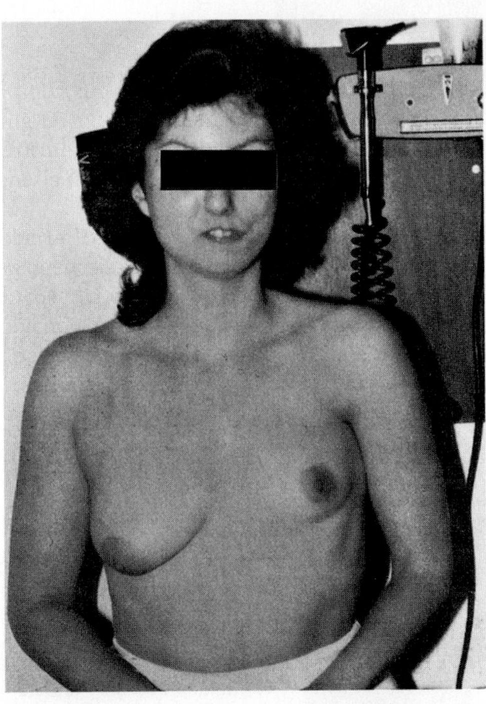

FIGURE 33-13 Woman with Poland's and Möbius' syndromes, probably secondary to a subclavian artery disruption sequence. (From Weaver DD: Vascular etiology of limb defects: The subclavian artery supply disruption sequence. In Herring JA, Birch JG [eds]: The Child with a Limb Deficiency. Rosemont, Ill, American Academy of Orthopaedic Surgeons, 1998.)

interruption—the earlier the occurrence, the more severe the abnormality.[343]

Chorionic villous sampling is typically performed 8 to 12 weeks after the last menstrual period, the same time that limb and hand development takes place. Limb defects related to trauma from the procedure may be due to interruption of the subclavian or other arteries or to some other vascular event.[345]

Poland's syndrome may affect either side but usually is not bilateral, which may lead to death in utero. When the left side is affected, there is about a 10% likelihood of concomitant dextrocardia,[51] which supports the premise that abnormal vascular development is the cause of Poland's syndrome.[343]

Psychosocial Issues

When a child is born with a significant abnormality, such as the absence of one or more limbs, the family experiences a sense of profound loss that normally requires a time of grieving. During this period, the orthopaedist must deal sympathetically with family members and encourage them to work through their feelings of disappointment.[114,264,311,323] In many cases, these early "wounds" are best healed by the child with the abnormality. Children with limb abnormalities are just as responsive and interactive as other children, and most have normal intellects. The degree of limb deficiency has not been found to be associated with depressive symptoms, anxiety, or behavioral problems in children or adolescents.[325-327] Nor does the degree of limb loss affect the general self-esteem of children[322,323]; however, it can adversely affect adolescents' self-esteem.[324,326]

The child's achievement of early developmental milestones helps the family direct its attention to the positive aspects of the child's future. Children with congenital abnormalities do not have a feeling of loss and thus do not require an adjustment period. They are able to make extraordinary adaptations to achieve milestones and perform normal daily activities.[263] Their development of gross motor skills may not follow the "normal" pattern—for example, they may roll early, sit late, and never crawl—but individual modifications should not be misconstrued as evidence of developmental delay.[48] Even those with multiple congenital limb deficiencies may achieve nearly normal physical function by using whatever limb components they have in place of those that are missing (Fig. 33–14).

It is important for the clinician to explain to the parents early on what can and cannot be done to improve their child's situation. Often, the parents' primary concerns are not the same as those of the

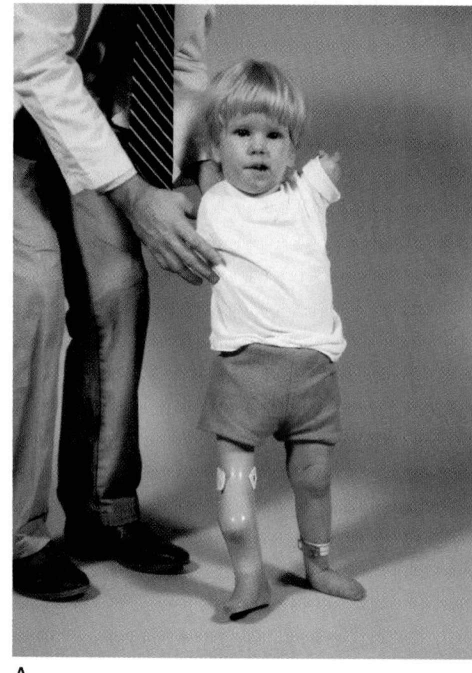

A

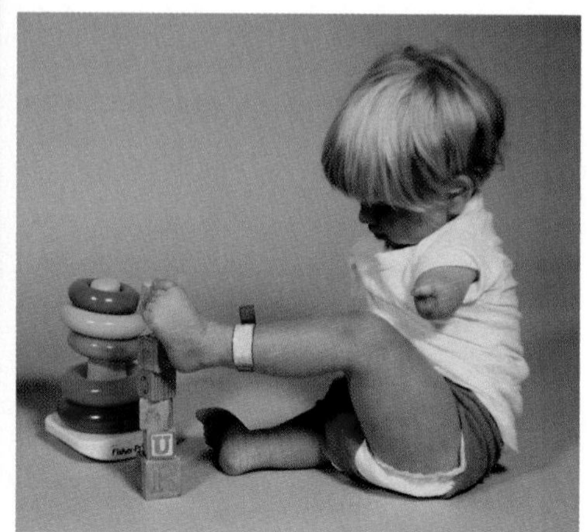

B

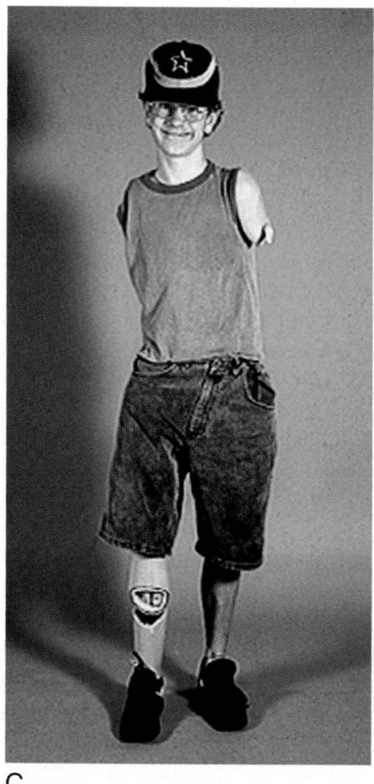

C

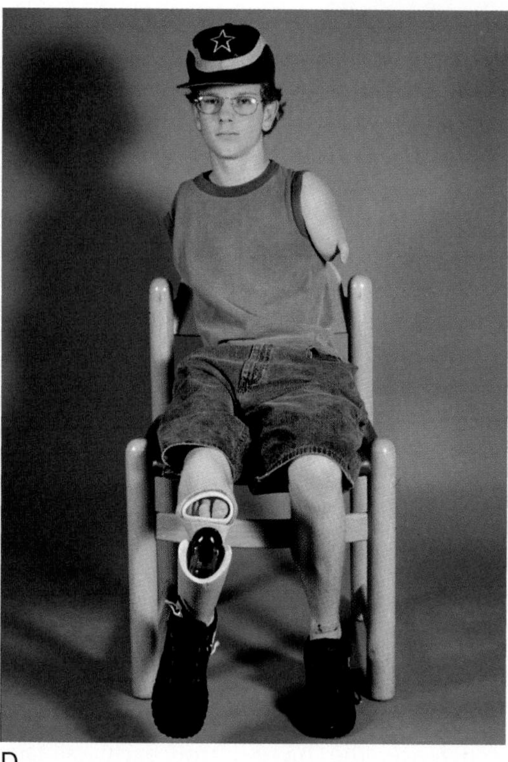

D

FIGURE 33-14 Child with bilateral upper amelia and right proximal focal femoral deficiency. No ablation surgery should ever be considered for such a person. **A,** The boy is able to ambulate at age 2 years with an easily removable prosthesis. **B,** He is ahead of his peers in manual dexterity using his foot at age 2 years. **C,** At age 14, he is using an easily removable equinus prosthesis. **D,** In sitting, the position of the foot is evident.

medical team. Usually, the parents are most anxious about the child's appearance and how others perceive the abnormality, whereas the medical team is concerned with the functional capabilities of the patient.

The possibility of future medical breakthroughs that might benefit the child should be discussed with the parents. The physician needs to help parents distinguish between medical advances that hold promise and impossible hopes. Undoubtedly, nonoperative and operative treatment methods will improve dramatically over the child's lifetime, but the fundamental biologic principles will likely remain the same.

In all cases, the long-term interests of the child must be the primary concern. For instance, if the child has a moderate abnormality, such as partial fibular hemimelia, the foot should be saved and any corrections should be done when the child is older, even though the condition may present a challenge before treatment. In contrast, if there is complete absence of the tibia, with the usual concomitant unstable knee and ankle, trying to save the foot because it might someday be possible to implant a tibial allograft will result in significant developmental delay. In this case, the consequence of delaying appropriate treatment carries too high a price for the child.

CONGENITAL LOWER LIMB DEFICIENCIES

Proximal Focal Femoral Deficiency

Proximal focal femoral deficiency is one of several terms used to describe a deformity in which the femur is shorter than normal and there is apparent discontinuity between the femoral neck and shaft. In many cases, the defect in the proximal femur ossifies as the child grows older. A congenitally short femur without radiographic evidence of an ossification defect is most likely a less severe form of femoral deficiency.[128] In most cases, the cause of the femoral deficiency is unknown. The disorder normally does not have a genetic link, although the combination of femoral deficiency and abnormal facies (femoral hypoplasia–unusual facies syndrome) is believed to be an autosomal dominant malformation.[157]

CLASSIFICATION

Aitken Classification

The Aitken classification system has some clinical relevance and is the most widely used system for classifying femoral deficiencies.[8] PFFDs are categorized as type A, B, C, or D (Figs. 33–15 to 33–17).

In type A PFFD, radiographs of the young child reveal a defect in the upper femur that ossifies as the child matures. The femoral head is present, and the acetabulum is well formed. A pseudarthrosis in the subtrochanteric area normally resolves by the time the patient reaches skeletal maturity. A varus deformity of the upper segment of the femur, which can vary in severity, is usually present, and the shaft of the femur may be positioned above the femoral head.

In type B deficiencies, the femoral portion of the limb is shorter than in type A, a tuft is often present at the proximal end of the femur, and the acetabulum is well formed. At birth, the upper portion of the femur

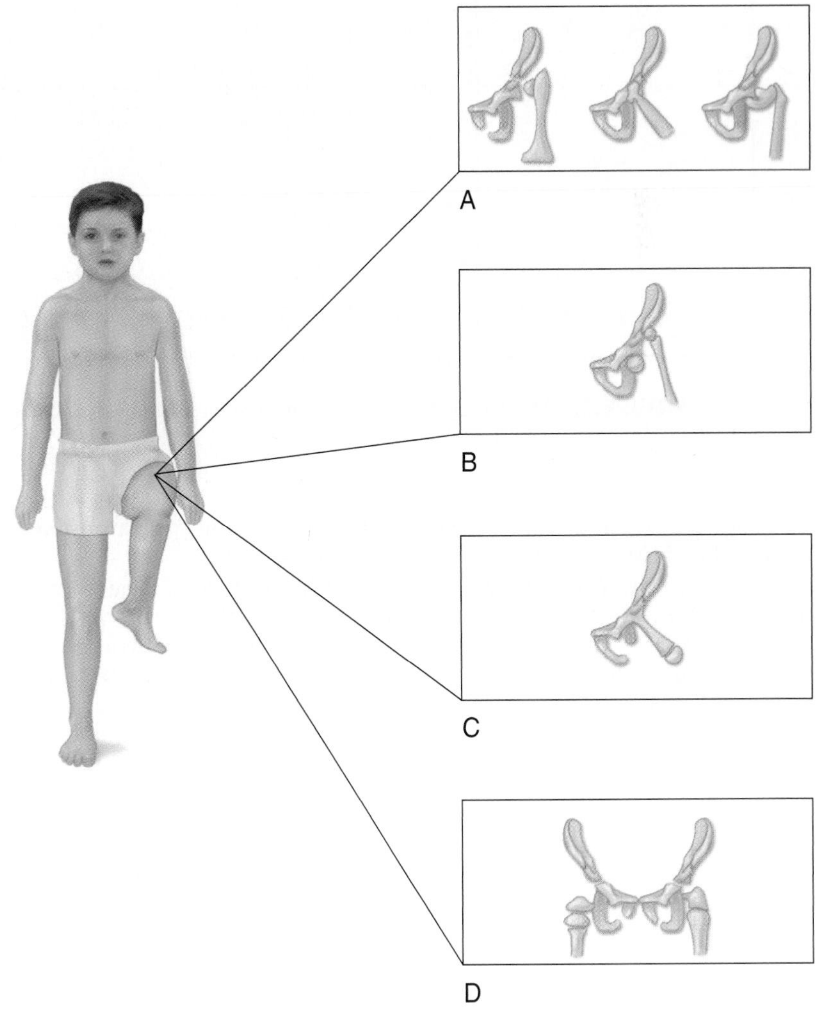

FIGURE 33–15 Schematic illustration of the Aitken classification of proximal focal femoral deficiency.

Type		Femoral Head	Acetabulum	Femoral Segment	Relationship Among Components of Femur and Acetabulum at Skeletal Maturity
A	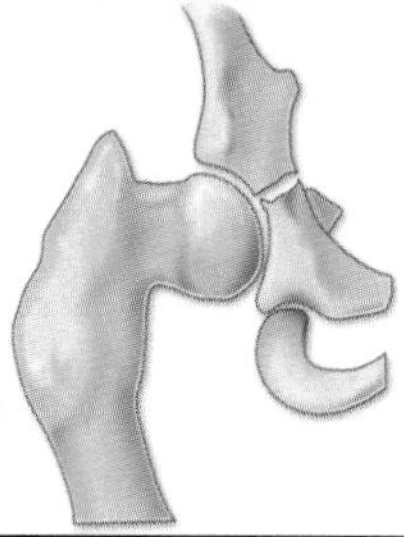	Present	Normal	Short	Bony connection between components of femur Femoral head in acetabulum Subtrochanteric varus angulation, often with pseudarthrosis
B	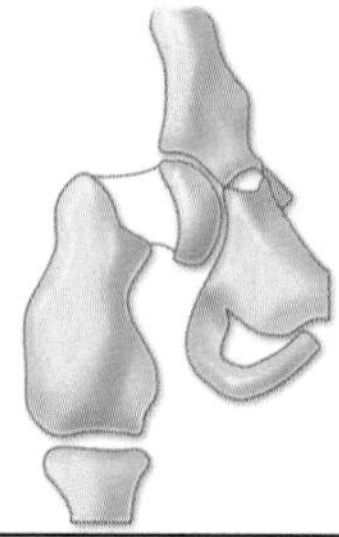	Present	Adequate or moderately dysplastic	Short, usually proximal bony tuft	No osseous connection between head and shaft Femoral head in acetabulum
C	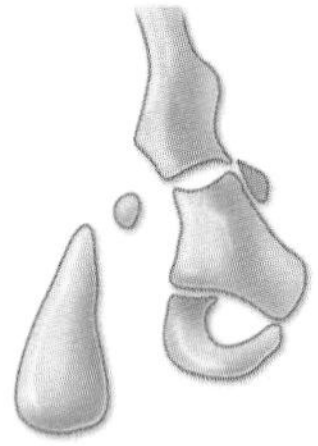	Absent or represented by ossicle	Severely dysplastic	Short, usually proximally tapered	May be osseous connection between shaft and proximal ossicle No articular relation between femur and acetabulum
D	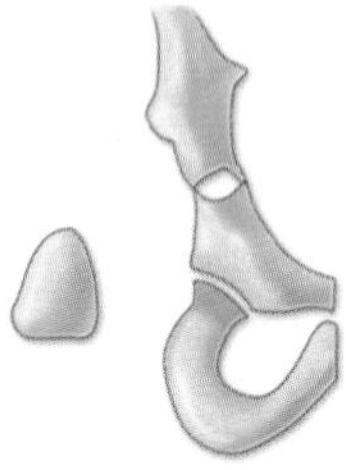	Absent	Absent Obturator foramen enlarged Pelvis squared in bilateral cases	Short, deformed	None

FIGURE 33-16 Description and illustration of the Aitken classification of proximal focal femoral deficiency.

may not be ossified, but as the child matures, the femoral head develops. The proximal end of the femur is usually positioned above the acetabulum, and at maturity, there is no ossific continuity between the femoral shaft and head (a definitive feature of Aitken's type B deformity).

In type C defects, the femoral segment is short, and there is a tuft at the proximal end. There is no ossification of the upper portion of the femur, and the femoral head is missing. The acetabulum is poorly developed or absent. In cases in which there is no acetabulum, the flat, lateral segment of the pelvic wall is seen in its place.

In type D deficiencies, the shaft of the femur is extremely short or absent, there is no femoral head, and the acetabulum is either poorly developed or absent.

Hamanishi Classification

The Hamanishi classification of PFFDs is more comprehensive than the Aitken system, comprising 6 primary groups and 10 subgroups of femoral malformation. There is a category for almost every deformity. The mildest form is a shortened femur with no radiographic defect (grade Ia); the most severe is complete absence of the femur (grade V) (Fig. 33–18).[18] This system supports the premise that limb deficiency is a continuous spectrum representing varying degrees of response to an insult, rather than a group of distinct clinical entities. The severity of the malformation depends on the degree to which growth and development are inhibited. In this classification, isolated congenital coxa vara is considered a separate condition that is not associated with PFFD.

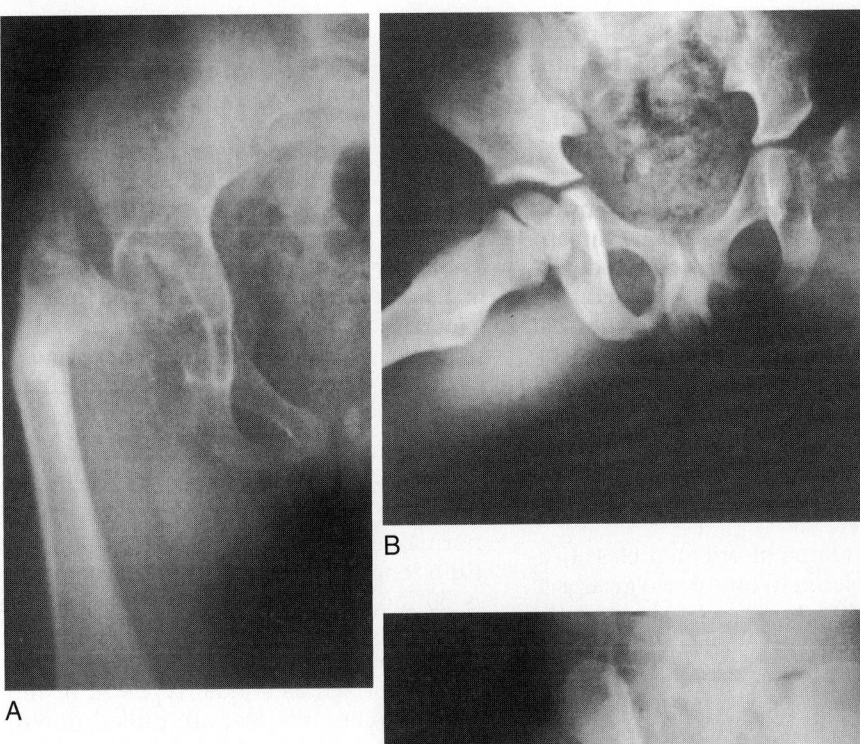

A

B

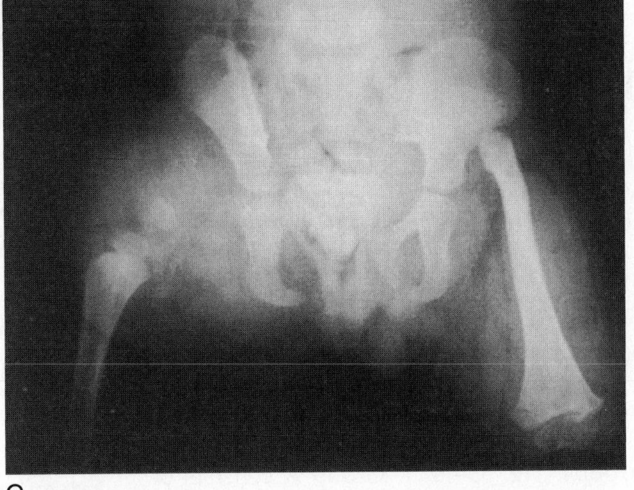

C

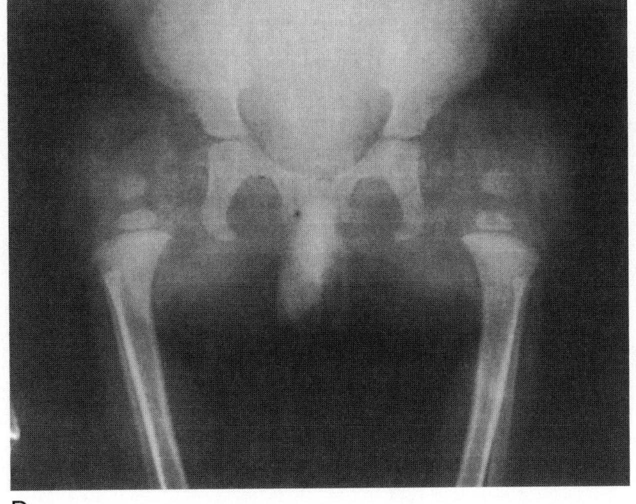

D

FIGURE 33–17 Radiographs showing the four types of proximal focal femoral deficiency according to Aitken. **A,** Type A. **B,** Type B. **C,** Type C. **D,** Type D. (From King RE: Proximal femoral focal deficiency. In Harris DE [ed]: Clinical Orthopedics. Bristol, UK, John Wright, 1983.)

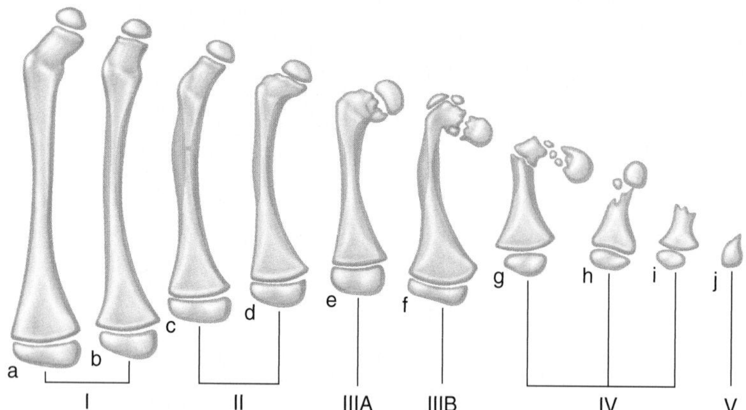

FIGURE 33–18 Hamanishi classification of femoral deficiency.

Gillespie and Torode Classification

In this clinically based, treatment-oriented classification system, patients are placed in one of two groups.[107] In group I, the femur is 40% to 60% shorter than the normal femur, and the hips and knees can be made functional. The foot on the affected side reaches the mid-tibia on the normal side, or lower with the legs extended. These patients are considered suitable candidates for limb lengthening procedures. Group II comprises those patients with more severely shortened femora in which the foot on the affected side reaches above the mid-tibia on the normal side, often being at the level of the normal knee. These patients are best treated with amputation or rotationplasty and prosthetic management.

Gillespie Classification

Gillespie has since proposed a modified clinical classification system that categorizes femoral deficiencies into three groups (Fig. 33–19).[105] Group A consists of deficiencies previously termed *congenital short femur;* in these cases, when the infant's feet are gently pulled down, the foot of the affected limb is positioned opposite the midpoint of the contralateral tibia or lower (indicating that the overall limb length discrepancy is ≤20%). If the femur is at least 60% the length of the normal femur, the patient is considered a candidate for limb lengthening. If the length of the affected femur is 50% or less the length of the contralateral femur, Gillespie recommends a van Nes rotationplasty and prosthetic fitting.[105] The deficiencies in group B would be categorized as Aitken types A, B, and C with true PFFDs. When the feet are pulled down, the affected foot is positioned at the level of the contralateral knee or above, with the overall limb length discrepancy approximately 40%. These patients are best managed with prostheses after surgical conversion (e.g., knee fusion, rotationplasty). In group C, there is a subtotal absence of the femur, similar to Aitken type D. Arthrodesis of the knee is not indicated in group C cases, and these patients should be managed prosthetically. If the femur is extremely short, it may be preferable to retain the foot within the socket to improve suspension and control.[105]

Fixsen and Lloyd-Roberts Classification

This system categorizes PFFDs according to the radiographic appearance of the proximal portion of the shaft of the femur.[84] There are three types of maldevelopment. In type I, the proximal femur is bulbous,

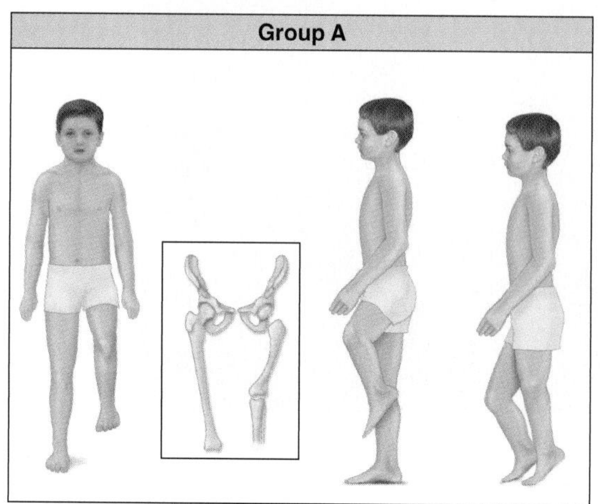

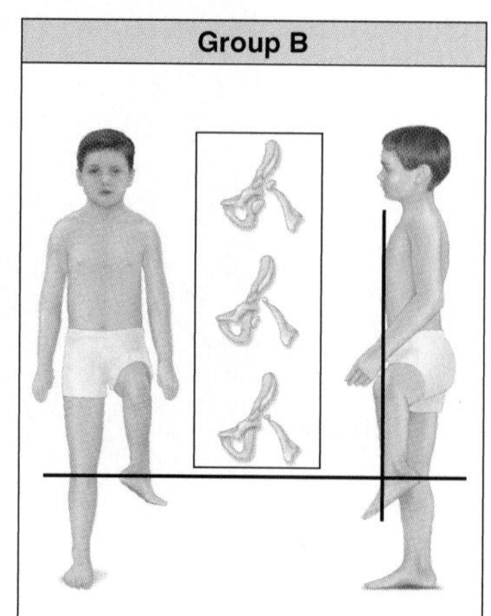

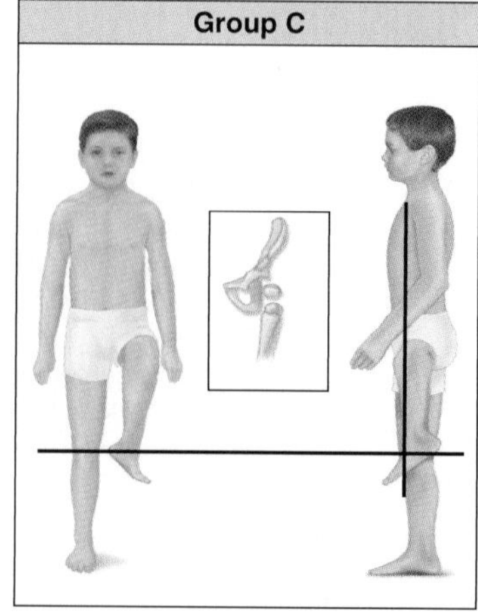

FIGURE 33–19 Gillespie classification of femoral deficiency.

and there is continuity among the femoral head, neck, and greater trochanter. A pseudarthrosis may form distal to the greater trochanter. In type II, there is a tuft or cap of ossification at the proximal end of the femur that is separated from a blunt upper femoral shaft by an area of lucency. A pseudarthrosis is often present, and if it heals, the femoral neck has a varus deformity. The hip is usually unstable. In type III, the femur is blunt or pointed (not bulbous), there is no tuft at the proximal end of the shaft, and an unstable pseudarthrosis is present. The authors of this report recommended surgical stabilization of all unstable pseudarthroses (i.e., types II and III), but recent experience does not support the need to operate on the pseudarthrotic area except in cases of unusual progressive deformities.

CLINICAL FEATURES

Patients with PFFD have a characteristic appearance. The affected thigh is extremely short, the hip is flexed and abducted, the limb is externally rotated, there is often flexion contracture of the knee, and the foot is usually at the level of the contralateral knee (Fig. 33–20). Flexion contractures of the hip and knee make the limb appear shorter than it actually is anatomically. The actual discrepancy can be better determined by comparing the length of the two limbs while the patient is sitting. Although the hip abductors and extensors are present, they are foreshortened and unable to function properly because of the abnormal anatomy of the proximal femur. The knee joint is positioned in the groin and acts as an unstable intercalary segment.[8] In approximately 45% of cases, the patient also has ipsilateral fibular hemimelia of the affected limb, with a short tibia and an equinovalgus deformity of the foot.[166] Lateral rays of the foot may be missing. The disorder may be accurately diagnosed prenatally with sonography.[82]

In patients with congenital shortening of the femur, a disorder related to PFFD, the clinical presentation is more subtle. The affected thigh is shorter than the contralateral thigh, and the lower leg may also be shorter. There is an associated anterolateral femoral bow, along with valgus deformity and external rotation of the knee. Patients often lack the anterior cruciate ligament of the knee, resulting in anteroposterior laxity of the joint. Some patients have shortened hamstrings, which restricts straight-leg raising.[153] Patients with congenital shortening of the femur frequently have an associated ipsilateral fibular hemimelia.

Most children with femoral deficiencies are able to compensate for their deformities and do not experience a delay in achieving developmental milestones. A child who has significant shortening of one lower limb walks by bearing weight on the knee of the normal limb and the foot of the affected leg to equalize the limb length discrepancy (Fig. 33–21). A child with a congenitally short femur walks with the hip and knee of the normal limb flexed and with equinus on the shortened limb to accomplish the same goal. These children usually start walking at the expected age.

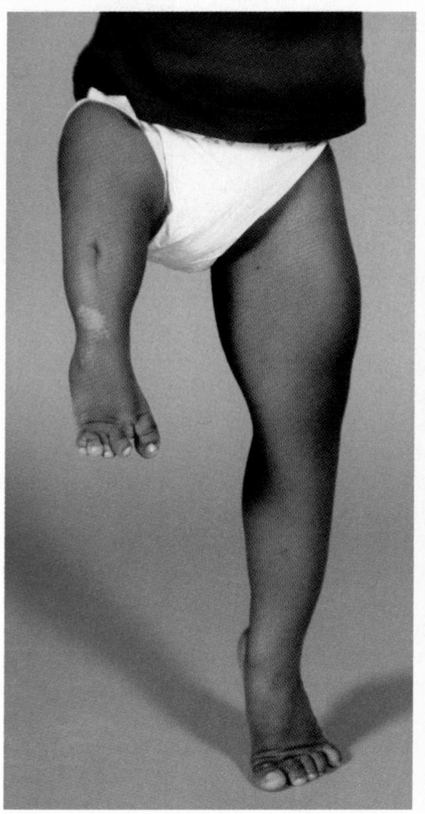

A

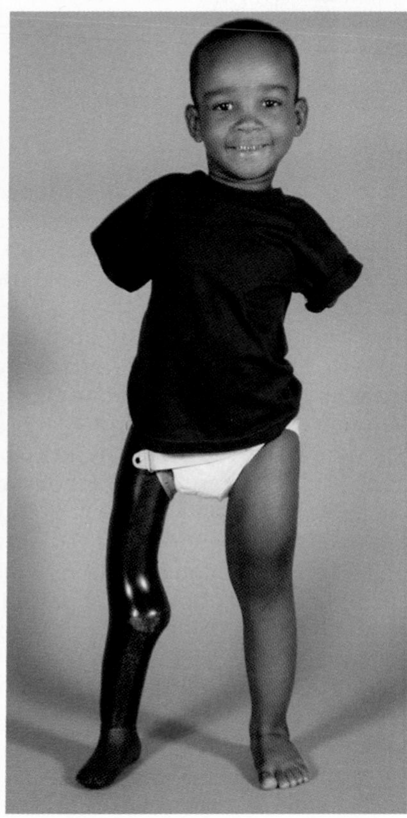

B

FIGURE 33–20 **A,** Typical "ship's funnel" thigh in proximal focal femoral deficiency. **B,** The equinus prosthesis offers good cosmesis.

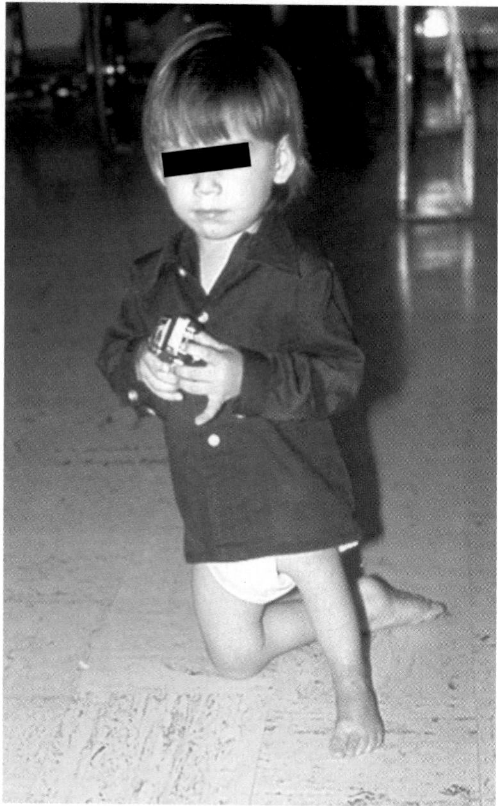

FIGURE 33–21 Child with proximal femoral deficiency walking on the knee of the sound side and the foot of the short extremity. He was treated with a Syme's amputation, knee fusion, and a prosthesis. (From Herring JA, Cummings DR: The limb-deficient child. In Morrissy RT, Weinstein SL [eds]: Lovell and Winter's Pediatric Orthopaedics, vol 2, 4th ed. Philadelphia, Lippincott-Raven, 1996.)

Box 33-4

Surgical Management of Patients with Femoral Deficiencies

Stable Hip

- Predicted length of affected limb at maturity <50% of contralateral limb
  - Knee fusion and Syme's amputation: indicated primarily when the hip is stable and there is a relatively normal relationship between the greater trochanter and the femoral head, and the patient does not wish to have a rotated foot
  - Knee fusion and rotationplasty: indicated when the hip is stable with a good femoral head-to-greater trochanter relationship, and the patient appreciates the value of the rotated foot
- Predicted length of affected limb at maturity >50% of contralateral limb
  - Limb lengthening: additional criteria for lengthening are a predicted discrepancy of <17 to 20 cm and a condition that can be corrected with three or fewer separate limb length equalization procedures

Unstable Hip

- Steel fusion and Syme's amputation: indicated when the hip is unstable and the patient does not desire a rotationplasty
- Steel fusion and rotationplasty: indicated when the hip is unstable and the patient desires the improved function of a rotationplasty
- Brown fusion of femur to pelvis with rotationplasty: indicated as an alternative to the Steel procedure for an unstable hip and for improved knee control and proprioception

TREATMENT

To establish an appropriate treatment plan, the orthopaedist first must determine the child's present limb length discrepancy. The percentage of discrepancy is calculated from measured radiographs. Then, based on the assumption that the relative shortening of the limb will remain consistent throughout the child's growth,[13] the probable discrepancy at maturity is estimated by multiplying the average length of the adult femur by the percentage of the existing discrepancy. The final discrepancy can also be determined by applying the standard methods of Anderson and coworkers[16,17,117] or Moseley,[223,224] with measurements obtained from longitudinal radiographs.

The primary considerations when deciding on a surgical treatment plan for a patient with a significant femoral deficiency are whether the foot should be saved, rotated, or amputated and whether the knee should be fused or the hip stabilized by fusing the femur to the pelvis (Box 33–4). When the hip is stable and the upper femoral anatomy is relatively normal, the two treatment options are (1) knee arthrodesis with a Syme's amputation or (2) knee arthrodesis with a rotationplasty. When the hip is unstable, the current treatment options are (1) a Steel fusion of the femur to the pelvis with either a Syme's amputation or a rotationplasty or (2) a Brown iliofemoral fusion with rotationplasty.

The Syme's amputation has the advantage of being a single procedure that produces satisfactory cosmetic and functional results. A rotationplasty has significant functional advantages, in that the patient can actively control the prosthetic knee with the gastrocnemius and can have proprioception in terms of knee position.[105] The disadvantages of rotationplasty are that the backward foot is a significant cosmetic hurdle for the patient to overcome, and the rotated segment tends to derotate as the patient grows.

Bilateral PFFD is uncommon (Fig. 33–22). The primary functional problems of patients with bilateral PFFD are short stature and a waddling gait. Surgical treatment such as amputation is contraindicated for

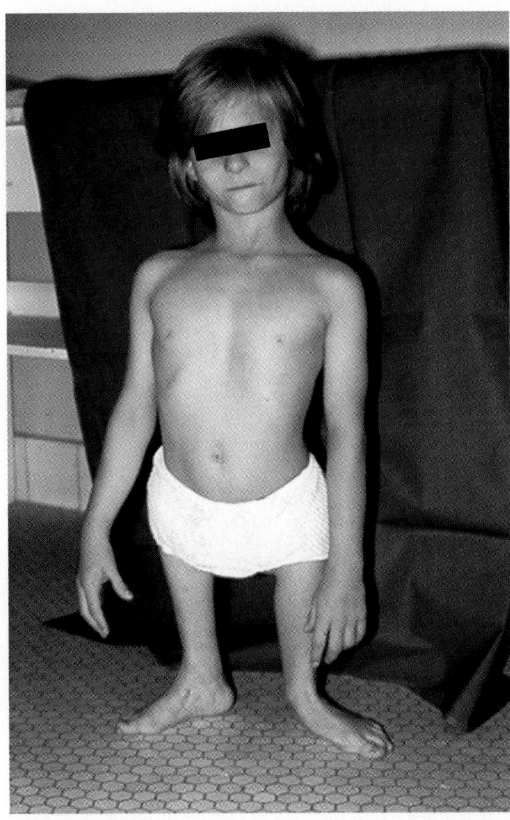

FIGURE 33–22 Girl with bilateral femoral deficiency. Prostheses to increase her height are the only appropriate treatment measures. (From Herring JA, Cummings DR: The limb-deficient child. In Morrissy RT, Weinstein SL [eds]: Lovell and Winter's Pediatric Orthopaedics, vol 2, 4th ed. Philadelphia, Lippincott-Raven, 1996.)

this condition. Treatment is usually limited to the use of a pair of extension, equinus prostheses to enhance the child's height and enable him or her to participate in certain physical activities.[171]

Options

There are at least seven treatment options for children with PFFDs and limb shortening greater than 50%. These children have a predicted final discrepancy of greater than 20 cm and are classified as group II in Gillespie and Torode's classification or group B of the newer Gillespie classification.[106,107] The current options are (1) equinus prosthesis only, (2) ankle disarticulation and prosthetic fitting, (3) ankle disarticulation and knee arthrodesis, (4) ankle disarticulation and femoral-pelvic arthrodesis, (5) rotationplasty and knee arthrodesis, (6) rotationplasty and femoral-pelvic arthrodesis, or (7) limb lengthening and reconstruction, which may be successful in certain cases and are discussed in other chapters.

Treatment decisions are made by the parents and the medical team, and many factors must be considered. Modern prosthetics have made an equinus prosthesis (option 1) a reasonable choice, especially for patients with close to 50% of femoral length. In one study, those treated with the equinus prosthesis were more satisfied than those who had amputation.[161] Option 2, ankle disarticulation, is a simple alternative, but the gait may be substantially improved by adding a knee arthrodesis (option 3). Options 4 and 6 include fusion of the femur to the pelvis to reduce the abductor lurch in the gait; the degree of improvement from such arthrodeses remains controversial. Options 5 and 6, rotationplasty, offer significant gait improvements, but the cosmetic disadvantages must be understood and accepted by the family. If the final predicted discrepancy at maturity is less than 20 cm (which is typical in patients with congenitally short femora), the child may be a suitable candidate for a limb lengthening procedure (option 7). These patients fall into group A of the Gillespie classification system, in which the affected femur is at least 60% the length of the contralateral femur.[106] For femoral lengthening to be successful, the hip and femoral segment must be stabilized.

Techniques

Amputation and Knee Arthrodesis. Amputation of the foot, combined with knee arthrodesis, is a well-documented means of treating significant femoral shortening (Fig. 33–23). Before the knee is fused, the orthopaedist should consider fusing the femur to the pelvis to improve hip stability. Either a modified Syme's amputation or a Boyd's amputation can be performed; both techniques create a residual limb well suited to prosthetic management and weight bearing.[8,162,214,346] However, because migration of the heel pad is rarely a problem following a Syme's amputation, the more difficult Boyd's technique is usually not necessary. After the procedure, the child is able to walk either by using a Syme's-type prosthesis or by bearing weight on the end of the amputated limb and the contralateral knee (i.e., "knee-walking"), thus equalizing the limb length discrepancy without using a prosthesis.

As the child grows, the knee (which is at the upper brim of the prosthesis) flexes with weight bearing, allowing the prosthesis to displace proximally and anteriorly. This instability causes the child to lurch forward and to the side. This problem can be addressed by performing a knee arthrodesis so that the residual limb is straight and the prosthesis is positioned directly below the acetabulum. This surgical approach converts the affected limb to a functional above-knee amputation, usually with the additional advantage of distal loading tolerance. Opinion varies as to when the procedures should be done. Some orthopaedists elect to perform the amputation just before the child starts walking and wait to do the knee arthrodesis until the patient is 3 to 4 years of age. Others perform both procedures simultaneously when the child is 2 to 3 years of age and use an equinus prosthesis in the interim. The patella should be excised, because there are reports of patellofemoral pain when it is retained.[319]

Ideally, after a Syme's amputation and knee arthrodesis, the proximal end of the residual limb lies at least

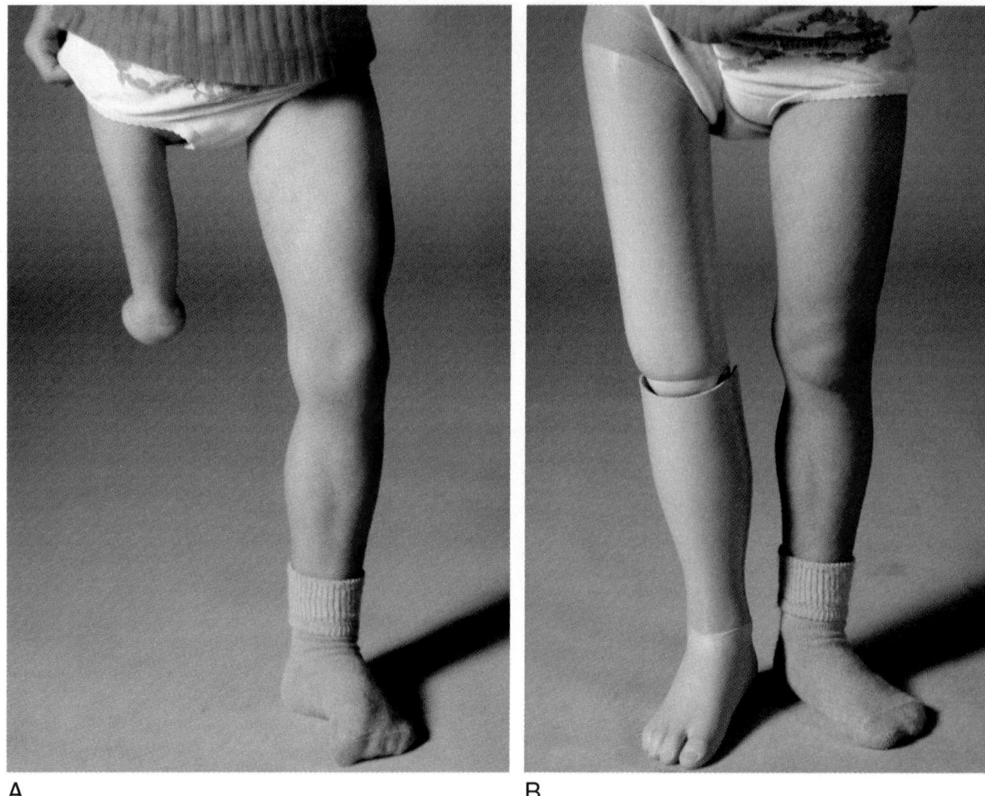

FIGURE 33–23 A and B, Proximal focal femoral deficiency, which was treated with a Syme's amputation and knee fusion.

5 cm (2 inches) above the contralateral knee at skeletal maturity to allow for proper placement of the prosthetic knee. Often, however, the end of the residual limb is at or below the level of the contralateral knee, and the tibial part of the prosthesis has to be shortened to accommodate the mechanism of the prosthetic knee, resulting in a discrepancy in knee heights. This length discrepancy can be minimized by excising the epiphysis of the distal femur at the same time the knee arthrodesis is performed, followed by fusion of the proximal tibial epiphysis to the distal femoral metaphysis (Plate 33–1). If this procedure is performed when the child is 3 to 4 years of age, an acceptable final length discrepancy can usually be achieved. The final discrepancy can be estimated from established growth charts; however, hip and knee flexion contractures before fusion reduce the accuracy of these predictions.

Rotationplasty. Rotationplasty was first described in 1930 by Borggreve, who used the procedure to treat a knee severely damaged by tuberculosis.[32] In 1950, van Nes described his technique of treating congenital femoral deficiencies by rotating the foot of the affected limb 180 degrees so that the toes pointed posteriorly and the ankle and foot were able to control the prosthetic knee (Fig. 33–24).[321]

The goal of the van Nes rotationplasty is to convert the affected limb to a functional "below-knee" amputation in which the rotated foot serves as a knee joint.[163] For optimal prosthetic function, it is essential that the ankle joint of the affected limb be normal and be capable of at least a 60-degree arc of motion after surgery.[315] The ankle should be at the same level as the knee of the contralateral limb, and the ankle joint should be rotated a full 180 degrees.[171] After a van Nes rotationplasty, the gastrocsoleus muscle provides primary motor control to the ankle, which, in essence, is now the "knee" extensor. The sensory feedback from the ankle also allows the patient better proprioceptive control of the prosthetic knee (Fig. 33–25).[126,168,172,321]

In a study comparing the gait mechanics of patients who had undergone van Nes procedures versus those who had undergone Syme's amputations, the van Nes patients demonstrated better prosthetic limb function and fewer compensations with the contralateral normal limb.[236] Data from the van Nes group were closer to normative data for ground reaction forces, forward propulsion, and active knee control. Oxygen cost was lower, and walking speed was higher in the van Nes group.[86] The difference in oxygen cost (0.12 mL/kg per minute) was comparable to the differences reported between below-knee and above-knee amputees.[340]

Despite good initial functional results with the original van Ness procedure,[107] the foot often gradually derotates as the limb grows, making repeated rotationplasties necessary.[107,168] Because of this problem, other techniques have been developed.

PLATE 33-1

Knee Fusion for Prosthetic Conversion in Proximal Focal Femoral Deficiency (King's Method)

King's method converts the proximal focal femoral–deficient limb into a single skeletal lever arm by arthrodesis of the knee in extension and Syme's ankle disarticulation.

Operative Technique

A, With the patient supine, an anterior S-shaped incision is made to expose the anterior aspect of the lower femur and upper tibia. Proximally, the incision is extended laterally to expose the lateral aspect of the upper femur.

B, The capsule and synovium of the knee joint are opened, and the articular cartilage of the upper end of the tibia is excised with an oscillating electric saw until the ossific nucleus of the epiphysis is seen. The distal femoral epiphysis is completely removed.

C, An 8-mm Küntscher or similar nail is inserted retrograde. First it is inserted distally into the tibia, exiting from the sole of the foot.

Section IV Orthopaedic Disorders

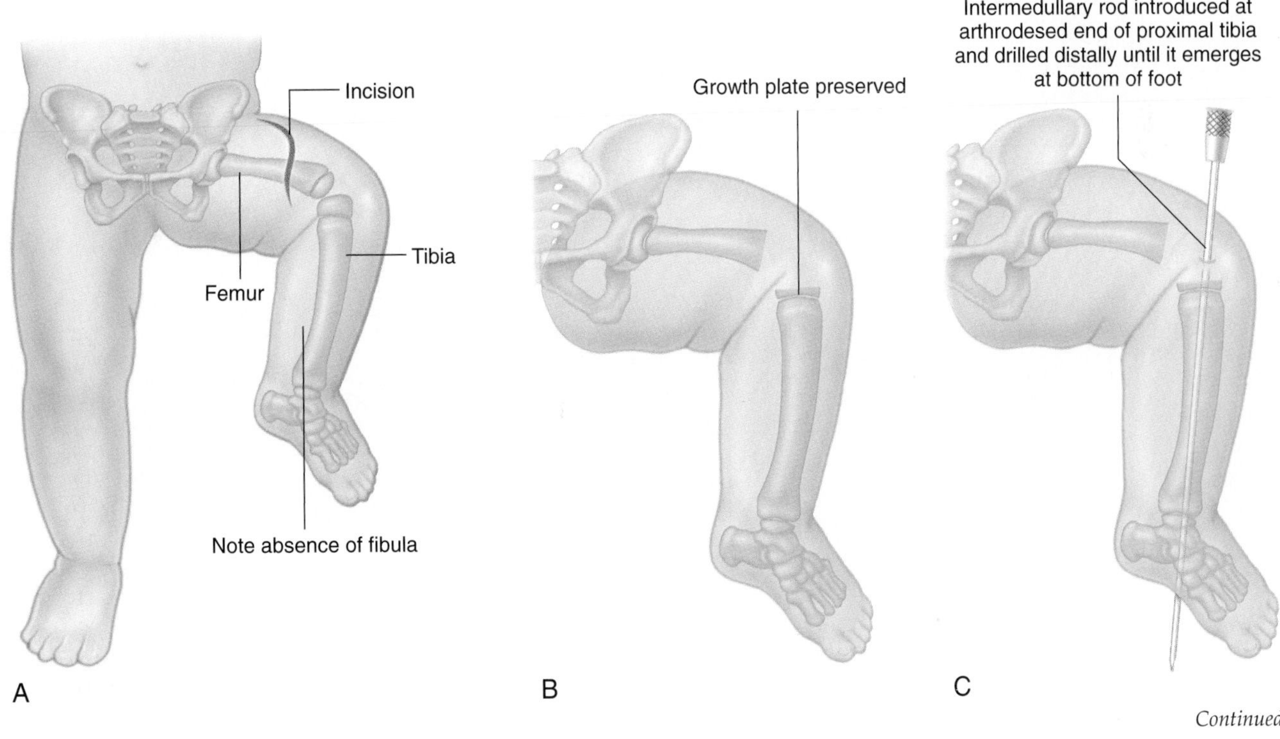

Continued

PLATE 33-1 *(continued)*

Knee Fusion for Prosthetic Conversion in Proximal Focal Femoral Deficiency (King's Method)

D, The nail is then passed proximally into the femur, impacting the lower end of the femur and the upper epiphysis of the tibia in extension. Care is taken to provide proper rotational alignment of the lower limb and ensure that the fused knee is not in flexion. The intramedullary nail should be in the center of the physes of the distal femur and the proximal tibia to avoid growth retardation.

The wound is closed in routine fashion. A one-and-one-half spica cast is applied for immobilization.

E, Six weeks postoperatively, when the intramedullary nail is removed, a Syme's amputation is performed.

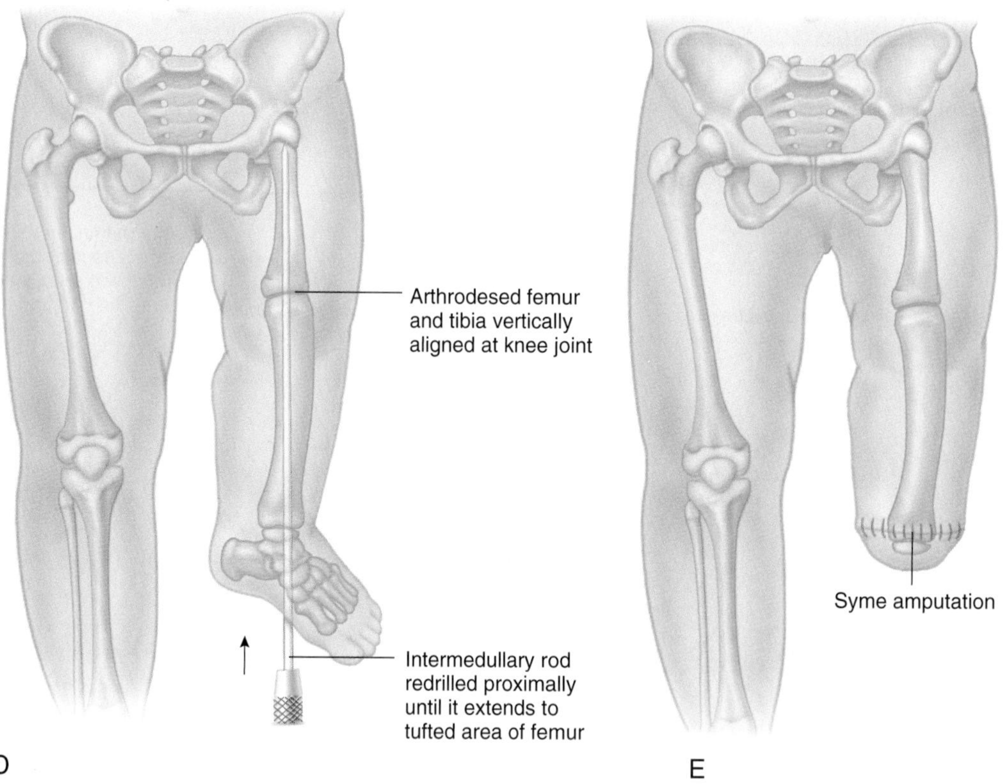

In a technique described by Gillespie and Torode, the tibia is rotated on the femur at the same time that the knee arthrodesis is performed to achieve most of the rotation (approximately 120 degrees); then a tibial osteotomy is done to gain additional rotation.[318] Krajbich further modified the Gillespie-Torode approach such that all the rotation is obtained through the knee, with simultaneous knee arthrodesis.[12,169,170] To prevent late derotation, all the muscles crossing the knee joint are detached (i.e., the medial hamstrings, gracilis, and sartorius from their insertion on the tibia, and the medial head of the gastrocnemius from its origin on the distal femur) and moved into a new position so that they all pull in a straight line across the rotated, arthrodesed knee. The popliteus is divided at the level of the knee joint. Osteotomy is performed about 0.5 to 1.0 cm proximal to the distal femoral growth plate, with the length of the removed segment

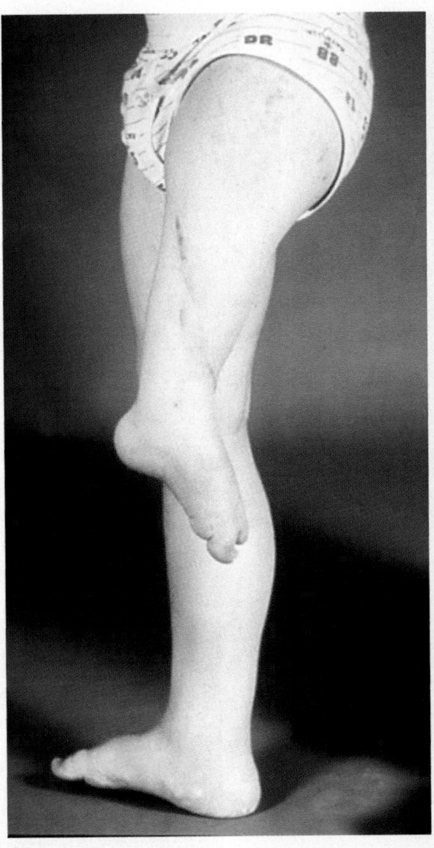
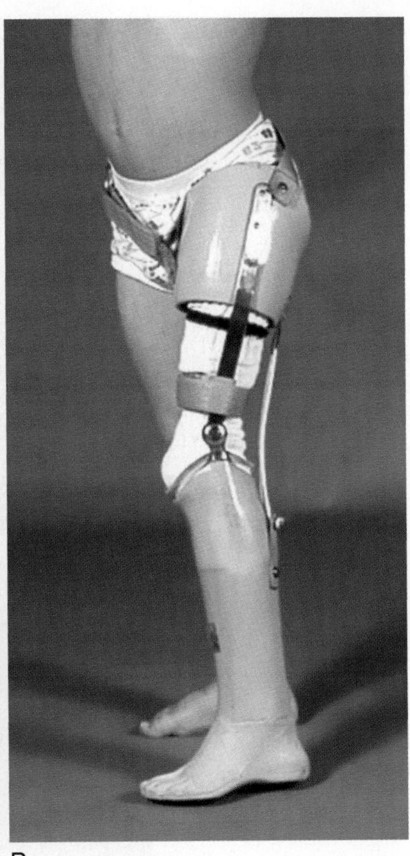

A B

FIGURE 33–24 **A,** Proximal focal femoral deficiency, which was treated with a van Nes rotationplasty. **B,** The ankle provides motor and sensory control of the prosthetic knee. (From Herring JA, Cummings DR: The limb-deficient child. In Morrissy RT, Weinstein SL [eds]: Lovell and Winter's Pediatric Orthopaedics, vol 2, 4th ed. Philadelphia, Lippincott-Raven, 1996.)

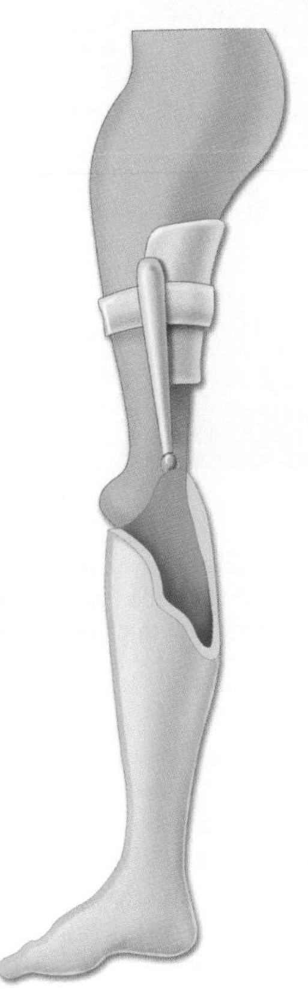

FIGURE 33–25 Rotationplasty for proximal focal femoral deficiency. The ankle and foot are turned 180 degrees to activate the knee of the prosthesis.

based on the goal of making the limb equal to or slightly longer than the contralateral thigh. The distal femoral growth plate is removed in almost every case to prevent the operated limb from growing too long and to obtain adequate shortening so that rotation can be performed without excessive tension on the neurovascular bundle. Adductor tendon insertion division is recommended so that the popliteal vessels can move freely medially and anteriorly. Appropriate prosthetic management follows the surgery.[170] The major drawback to these rotationplasties has been gradual derotation as the child grows. When there is rotational malalignment, overall function deteriorates, and prosthetic management is particularly difficult.

Brown devised a rotational procedure that eliminates the tendency toward derotation.[37] In this variant of a limb salvage procedure, the femur is rotated externally 180 degrees and fused to the pelvis. The muscles of the thigh are excised, isolating the neurovascular structures to allow free rotation of the limb. The femoral segment is fused to the pelvis in a reversed, extended position, with neutral rotation and abduction (see Fig. 33–28). The medial hamstrings are attached to the anterior or lateral muscles of the rotated limb. The gastrocnemius is sutured to the iliopsoas and acts as both a hip flexor and a knee extensor, with the reversed knee joint functioning as a hinged hip joint. As in the van Nes rotationplasty, the retained ankle and foot serve as a knee joint. The procedure is complex and has serious potential complications.

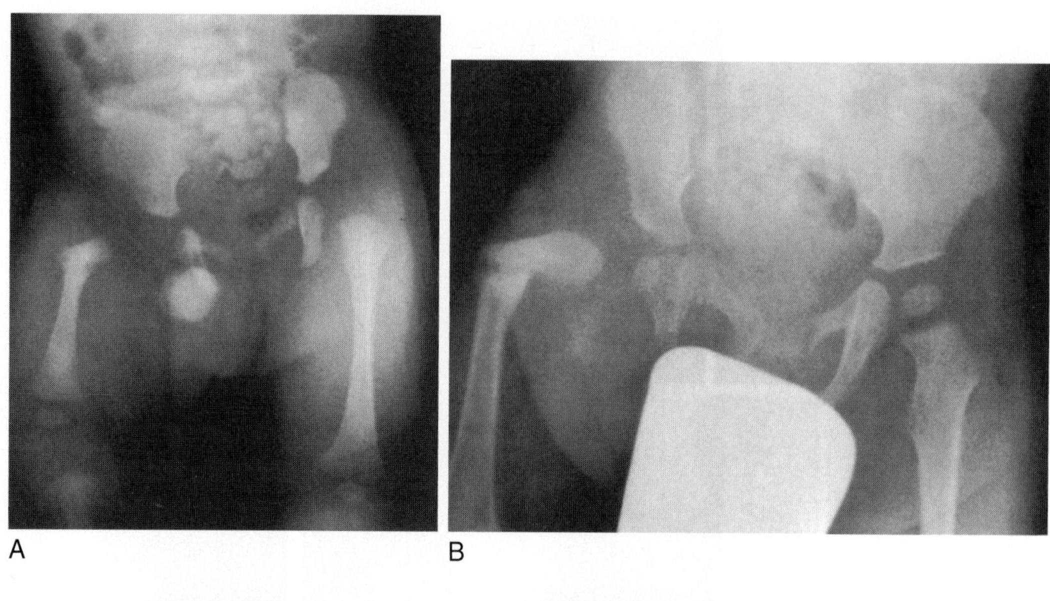

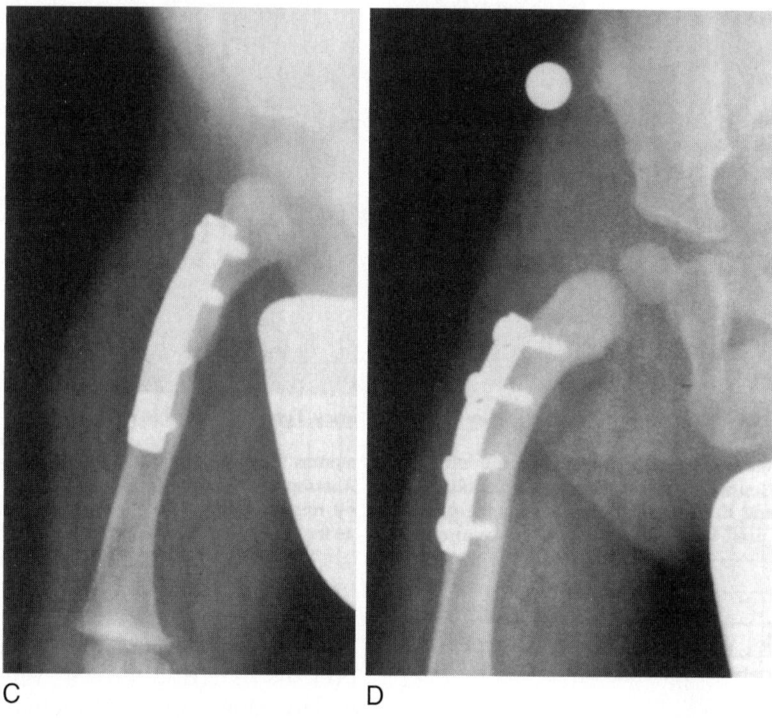

FIGURE 33–26 Proximal focal femoral deficiency type A. **A,** Anteroposterior radiograph of a 1-month-old boy. Note the coxa vara deformity of about 110 degrees, the marked shortening of the femur, and the delay in ossification of the upper end of the femur. **B,** At age 10 months, the coxa vara deformity remains uncorrected. **C** and **D,** Anteroposterior and lateral radiographs after valgus osteotomy.

Femoral Pseudarthrosis Stabilization. The need to stabilize the upper femoral defect is controversial. Although some authors recommend an osteosynthesis when the child is between 3 and 6 years of age,[174,175] most leave the defect alone unless there is progressive deformity or instability. Most upper femoral defects are stable, and surgical intervention is not necessary. An osteosynthesis of the defect is performed only if there is proof of progressive deformity (Fig. 33–26).

Hip Stabilization. Children with major femoral deficiencies who are managed with either amputation or rotationplasty usually have good results and, in most cases, are able to enjoy an active lifestyle. They can walk without aids and, when running, tend to hop twice on the unaffected limb. The primary problem encountered with gait is hip instability.[77] Because of the deformities of the proximal femur (i.e., a short, varus femoral neck combined with abnormalities of the acetabulum), the abductor muscles are unable to support the patient's body weight during the stance phase of gait, resulting in an abductor lurch. In a young child, this condition is often barely discernible and is not a major inconvenience. As the child grows older,

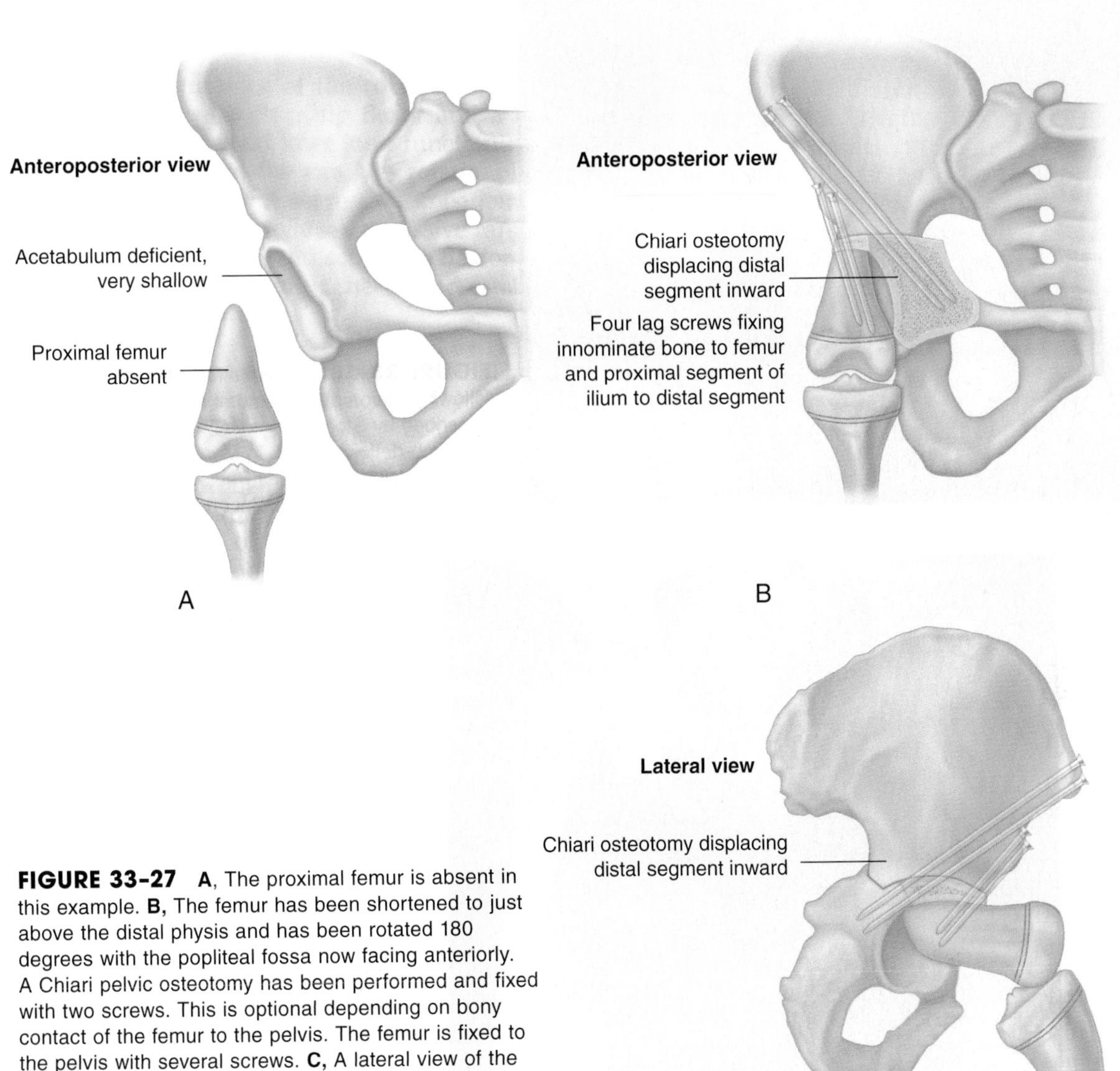

FIGURE 33-27 **A**, The proximal femur is absent in this example. **B,** The femur has been shortened to just above the distal physis and has been rotated 180 degrees with the popliteal fossa now facing anteriorly. A Chiari pelvic osteotomy has been performed and fixed with two screws. This is optional depending on bony contact of the femur to the pelvis. The femur is fixed to the pelvis with several screws. **C,** A lateral view of the final position of the femur. It is important that the femur be shortened as much as possible and that the femoral epiphysis be ablated.

however, the abductor lurch can become a significant functional and cosmetic problem.

A number of different surgical techniques have been developed to try to eliminate the lurch. In one approach, developed by Steel and associates, the femoral segment is fused to the pelvis (iliofemoral fusion) in a flexed position, and the knee functions as a hip joint (Fig. 33–27).[298] This procedure can be done at the same time as a Syme's amputation or a van Nes rotationplasty, adding significant functional advantages to a rotationplasty (Fig. 33–28). Steel[297] described the surgical approach as "a great adventure in the abnormalities of surgical anatomy; i.e., nothing was put together in a normal fashion." The femur needs to be shortened, and the femoral epiphysis must be arrested to ensure that the limb is maintained in line with the patient's body mass. When this technique was first developed, all the patients subsequently underwent revisions because of overgrowth of the femoral segment.[298] Since then, Steel has found that the outcome is greatly improved when femoral growth is stopped at the time of fusion.[297] To avoid the problem of overgrowth, we fuse the femoral condyles to the pelvis after excising the remaining femoral metaphysis and physis. Steel's long-term follow-up of 22 patients found a reduced abductor lurch and improved gait, with only two children having Trendelenburg gaits.[297] After a Steel arthrodesis, there is usually little active hip flexion power, which may cause functional problems.

Another method of preventing derotation and eliminating the abductor lurch in patients with PFFD was developed by Brown.[37] In this variant of a limb salvage procedure, the femur is rotated externally 180 degrees and brought as far proximal as possible for fusion to the pelvis. Excess soft tissue is excised before the femoral segment is fused in a reversed, extended position (Fig. 33–29). The rotated leg is attached in neutral to slight abduction and neutral to slight external rotation. The medial hamstrings are attached to the

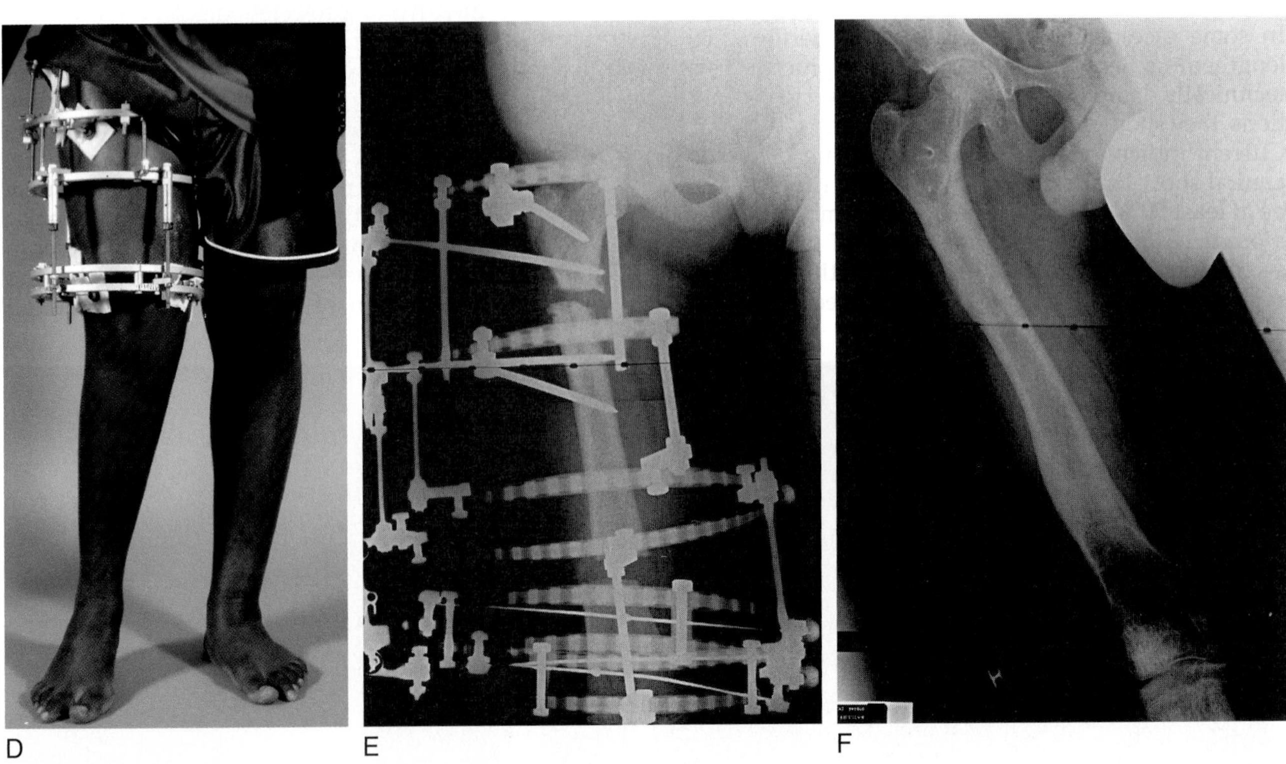

FIGURE 33-31 Child with a Gillespie type A proximal femoral deficiency. **A,** Front view showing a shortened right femur with lateral rotation of the femur and mild genu valgus. **B,** Radiograph obtained at 1 month of age showing varus of the femoral neck, lateralization of the hip, and shortening of the femur. Note that the femur is half as long as the contralateral femur. **C,** Orthoroentgenogram obtained at 6 years of age showing a 12.5-cm limb length discrepancy. The hip appears reduced without treatment. **D,** Patient at age 14 years with a circular fixator in place for femoral lengthening. **E,** Radiograph showing placement of the circular fixator. **F,** Radiograph obtained after femoral lengthening, in which the femur gained 9 cm. The patient also underwent a contralateral epiphysiodesis.

bilevel lengthening may reduce the total time for osteogenesis, the authors advise against this approach, because muscles and nerves appear to respond better to slower rates of distraction.[151,247,269,286,287]

For the same reason, ipsilateral lengthening of the femur and tibia is discouraged in most cases. To prevent translation during lengthening, fixator alignment should be parallel to the mechanical axis. Osteotomies are usually made distal to the midshaft of the femur because of better bone healing at that level. The iliotibial band is released distally when the distal pin is inserted. If contractures start to develop, additional soft tissue releases can be performed.[111] If the adductor magnus is tight, it can be released at the adductor hiatus. The chances of subsequent knee subluxation are minimized by distal pin placement, avoidance of knee flexion movements, and extension splinting for at least 12 hours each day. If knee subluxation occurs, it should be promptly treated by hamstring lengthening or traction and immobilization in extension. Hip subluxation or dislocation should be treated by appropriate soft tissue releases, femoral shortening, extension of fixation across the hip joint, open reduction, or a combination of these procedures.[247]

Paley has proposed a classification of femoral deficiencies to aid in planning reconstructive lengthening procedures (Fig. 33–32).[237] His group 1, which corresponds to congenitally short femur in other classification systems, is the best group for lengthening. He recommends correction of femoral neck varus and acetabular dysplasia before lengthening. He also outlines reconstructive approaches for patellar instability and instability of the knee joint. Paley's group 2a is defined by a mobile pseudarthrosis of the upper femur and a femoral head that is mobile in the acetabulum. The first step in reconstructing these hips is obtaining union of the pseudarthrosis, with subsequent lengthening. Group 2b is defined by a located, immobile femoral head or a dislocated hip; these hips require a pelvic support osteotomy before lengthening. Patient with these more typical femoral deficiencies need to undergo multiple staged lengthenings. Specific indica-

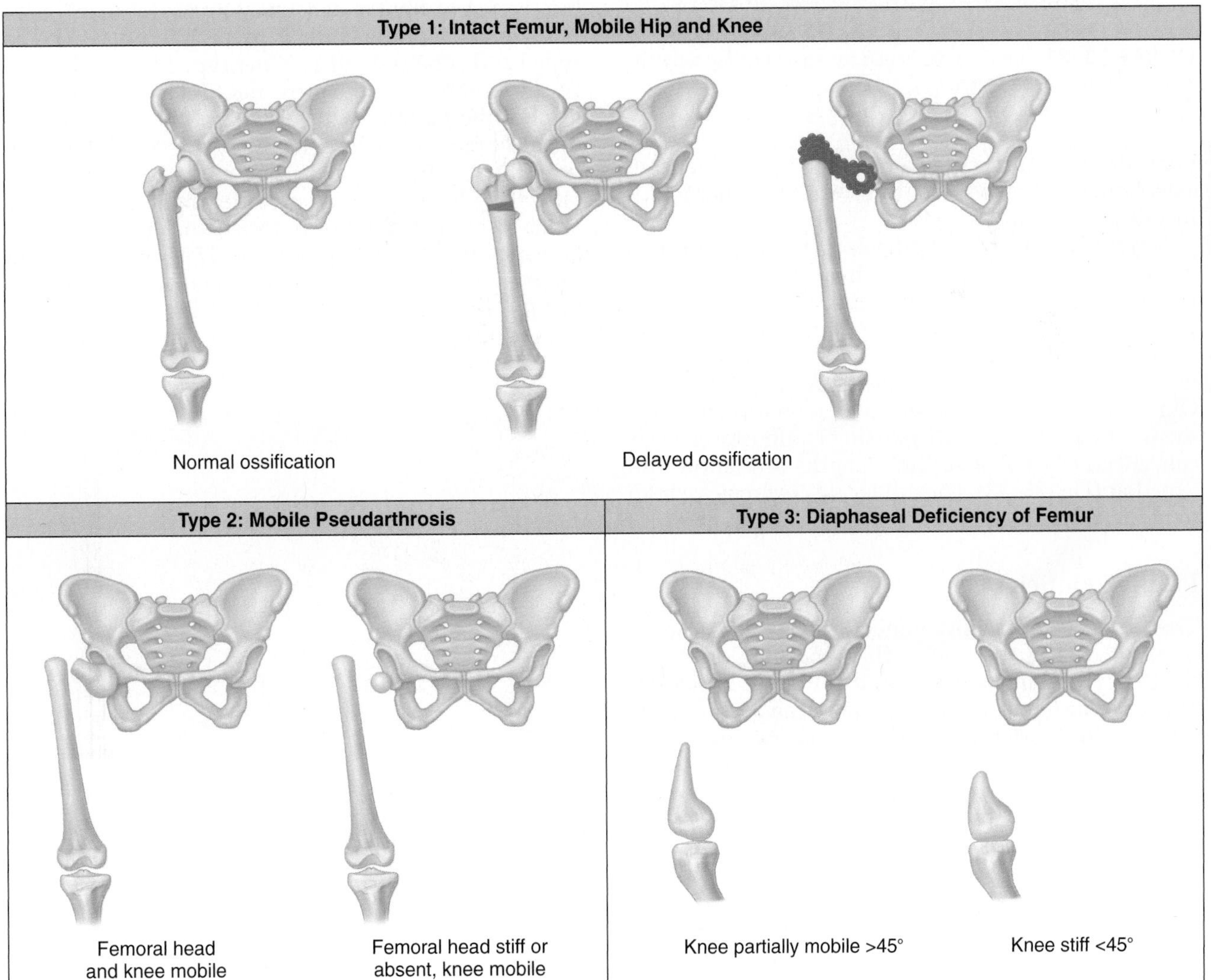

FIGURE 33–32 Paley classification of congenital short femur syndrome, types 1 to 3.

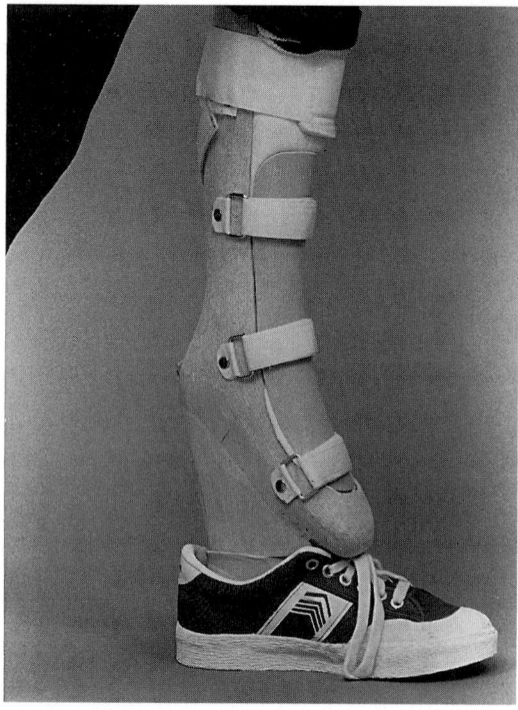

FIGURE 33-33 Equinus prosthesis for equalizing leg lengths in a child with a short femur.

tions for reconstruction await further studies that consider both function and length, as well as the hardships involved.

Normally, femoral lengthening is not performed when the child is young. This means that the orthopaedist must manage the patient so that he or she can participate in normal, everyday childhood activities. In very young children, the shorter limb can be treated with simple extension prostheses or large shoe lifts. Older children find these devices unattractive; for them, a more cosmetically pleasing equinus prosthesis can effectively equalize limb lengths and allow full function (Fig. 33–33). For milder discrepancies, small to moderate shoe lifts can be used.

Fibular Deficiency

The term *fibular deficiency* implies a congenital absence of all or part of the fibula. The syndrome of fibular deficiency encompasses a spectrum of abnormalities affecting the femur, knee, tibia, ankle, and foot. In one form, mild shortening of the fibula, valgus of the knee, anteroposterior instability of the knee, and shortening of the femur are present. In another presentation, the fibula is absent; the tibia is shortened, with a sharp anteromedial bow distally; and the foot is small, with missing rays and a marked equinovalgus deformity.

The precise cause of fibular hemimelia is unknown in most cases, and the deformity normally occurs sporadically. Although 15% of all patients with congenital absence of the fibula have associated deficiencies of the femur,[14] Kruger and Talbott noted that all their fibula-deficient patients with five-rayed feet and 50% of those with fewer rays had shortened femora.[178]

CLASSIFICATION

Frantz and O'Rahilly Classification

Fibular hemimelia may be an intercalary deficiency with a normal foot or a terminal deficiency with absent rays of the foot. The deficiency is always paraxial (i.e., longitudinal).

Coventry and Johnson Classification

This system classifies patients into three groups.[55] Partial absence of the fibula is classified as type I, and complete fibular absence as type II. Type III includes bilateral absence of the fibulae and cases of other skeletal abnormalities associated with unilateral fibular absence.

Achterman and Kalamchi Classification

This system, which is more clinically useful than the preceding ones, classifies fibular hemimelia based on the degree of fibular deficiency present (Fig. 33–34).[2] If any portion of the fibula is present, it is classified as type I and subclassified as either type IA or IB. In type IA, the epiphysis of the proximal fibula is distal to the level of the tibial growth plate, and the physis of the distal fibula is proximal to the dome of the talus. In type IB, the fibula is shorter by 30% to 50%, and distally the fibula does not provide any support at the ankle joint. The authors reported that the tibial discrepancy was 6% in type IA and 17% in type IB, and the total limb length discrepancy at maturity was 12% in type IA and 18% in type IB. If the fibula is completely absent, the deformity is classified as type II.

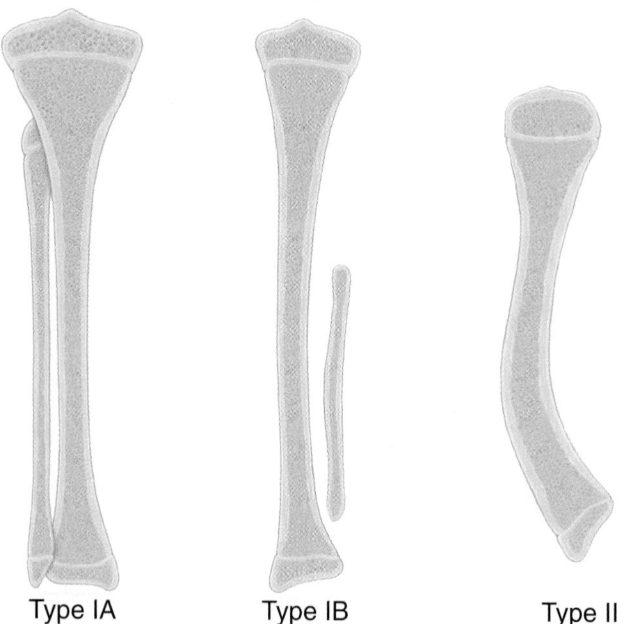

FIGURE 33-34 Achterman and Kalamchi classification of fibular hemimelia.

The tibial discrepancy was 25% and the total limb length discrepancy at maturity was 19% in type II cases.

Birch Classification

This system was developed because the existing classifications of fibular deficiency did not provide satisfactory guidelines for managing the deformities.[25] A major shortcoming of other classification systems is that they do not deal with shortening of the total limb, one of the most important factors orthopaedists must consider when making management decisions.

In a review of children treated for fibular deficiency at Texas Scottish Rite Hospital for Children between 1957 and 1996, approximately 50% of the patients had concomitant shortening of the femur. This study found no direct correlation between fibular length and the severity of the deformity, as implied by other classifications. For example, more than 50% of patients with complete absence of the fibula had a salvageable lower limb with a functional foot. A functional foot was defined as one that was or could be made plantigrade and had three or more rays. A direct correlation was found between the number of rays and the chances of preserving the foot. It was possible to preserve all five-rayed feet, whereas no foot with two or fewer rays was salvageable. Birch's functional classification of fibular deficiency with general treatment guidelines for each group is provided in Table 33–5.

Stanitski Classification

Stanitski and Stanitski proposed a classification based on fibular length, morphology of the distal tibial epiphysis, presence of a tarsal coalition, and number of rays of the foot.[296] They emphasized the need to evaluate all elements of the deformity when making treatment decisions.

Table 33-5 Fibular Deficiency: Birch's Functional Classification and Treatment Guidelines

Classification	Treatment
Type I—functional foot	
IA 0%-5% inequality	Orthosis, epiphysiodesis
IB 6%-10% inequality	Epiphysiodesis ± limb lengthening
IC 11%-30% inequality	One to two limb lengthening procedures or amputation
ID >30% inequality	More than two limb lengthening procedures or amputation
Type II—nonfunctional foot	
IIA Functional upper limb	Early amputation
IIB Nonfunctional upper limb	Consider limb salvage procedure

CLINICAL FEATURES

Children with partial absence of the fibula present with varying degrees of femoral shortening, tibial shortening, valgus of the knee, anterior cruciate ligament deficiency with absence of the tibial spine, and tarsal coalition (Fig. 33–35).[300] The lateral malleolus is proximal in the ankle mortise, and there is a slight valgus of the ankle. Because the deformity affects the entire lower limb, the final limb length discrepancy is due to shortening of both the femur and the tibia and ranges from 12% to 18%.[2] Some patients present with several elements of the fibular hemimelia syndrome but a normal fibula. These manifestations include missing lateral rays of the foot, ball-and-socket ankle with tarsal coalition, clubfoot deformity, and shortening of the tibia.[40,279] When clubfoot is the presenting deformity, tarsal coalition is usually present and may complicate corrective surgery.[40]

Children with complete fibular hemimelia present with anterolateral bowing of the tibia, equinovalgus deformity of the foot, and tarsal coalition. The affected limb is always significantly shorter than the contralateral limb, and there may or may not be additional shortening of the ipsilateral femur (Figs. 33–36 and 33–37).[14,178,349] The articular surface of the distal tibia faces posteriorly and laterally. The distal tibial epiphysis is wedge shaped and narrower on the lateral side, adding to the valgus position of the foot. Choi and colleagues described different degrees of severity of this deformity with relevance to progressive growth.[45] The flat upper surface of the fused talocalcaneus articulates with the tibia in a valgus and equinus position.

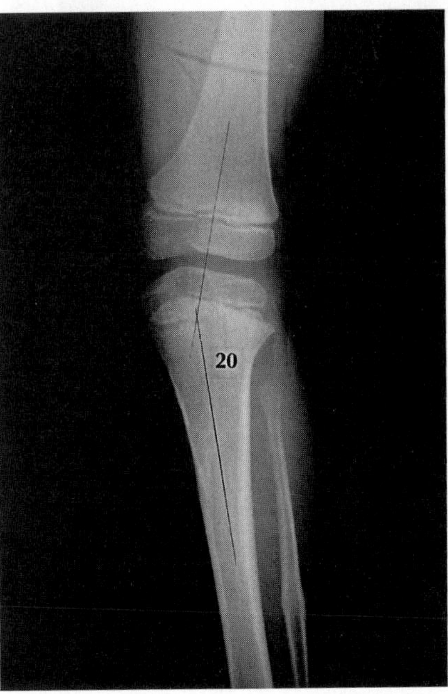

FIGURE 33-35 Typical radiographic appearance of partial fibular hemimelia. (From Herring JA, Cummings DR: The limb-deficient child. In Morrissy RT, Weinstein SL [eds]: Lovell and Winter's Pediatric Orthopaedics, vol 2, 4th ed. Philadelphia, Lippincott-Raven, 1996.)

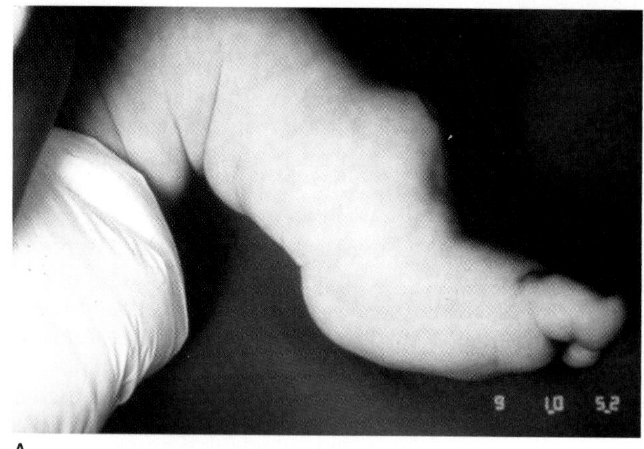

A

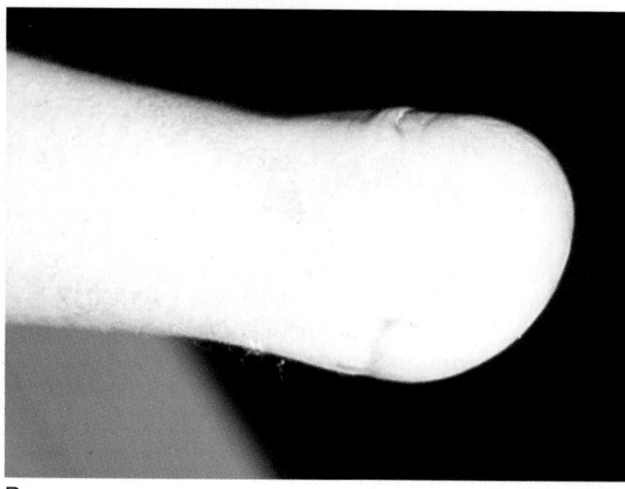

B

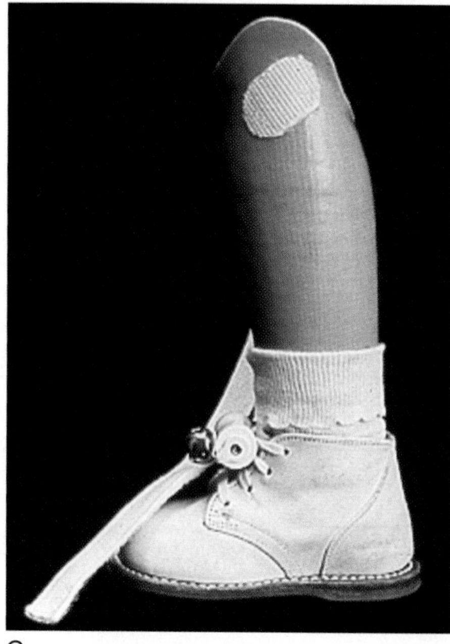

C

FIGURE 33-36 Child with fibular hemimelia treated with a Syme's amputation. **A,** Appearance of the extremity before surgery. **B,** Appearance of the limb after Syme's amputation. **C,** Typical Syme's prosthesis. (From Herring JA, Cummings DR: The limb-deficient child. In Morrissy RT, Weinstein SL [eds]: Lovell and Winter's Pediatric Orthopaedics, vol 2, 4th ed. Philadelphia, Lippincott-Raven, 1996.)

The foot may be missing one, two, or more lateral rays. In milder variants of this type, some fibular remnant is present and there are lesser degrees of shortening and foot deformity.

TREATMENT

Partial Fibular Hemimelia

Amputation or Limb Lengthening. The decision to treat patients with partial fibular hemimelia by amputation or limb lengthening depends on the degree of predicted shortening at maturity and the condition of the foot and ankle of the affected limb.[143] If the predicted discrepancy at maturity is 25 cm or more and there is severe valgus of the ankle with a deformed foot, the patient should be treated with a Syme's or Boyd's amputation and prosthetic management.[26] If the patient has a predicted shortening of 8 cm or less; a functional, plantigrade foot with four or more rays; and a stable, mobile ankle, he or she is a good candidate for a lengthening procedure with or without epiphysiodesis. Realignment of the obliquity of the distal tibial epiphysis may be necessary in this group of patients.[78]

McCarthy and colleagues objectively compared 25 patients who had either limb lengthening or Syme's amputation for fibular hemimelia.[210] The amputation group was more severely affected than the lengthening group. Those with amputations had higher functional scores, less pain, and fewer complications and were more satisfied with their treatment than those whose legs were lengthened. The cost of the amputation surgery was one fourth the cost of the lengthening treatment, although prosthetic costs were not evaluated. It should be noted that 5 of the 11 lengthened patients were treated with the older Wagner method.[238] Naudie and coworkers found that patients lengthened with Ilizarov methods had numerous complications and needed further corrective surgery or required braces or shoe lifts.[227] Two of the 10 lengthened patients

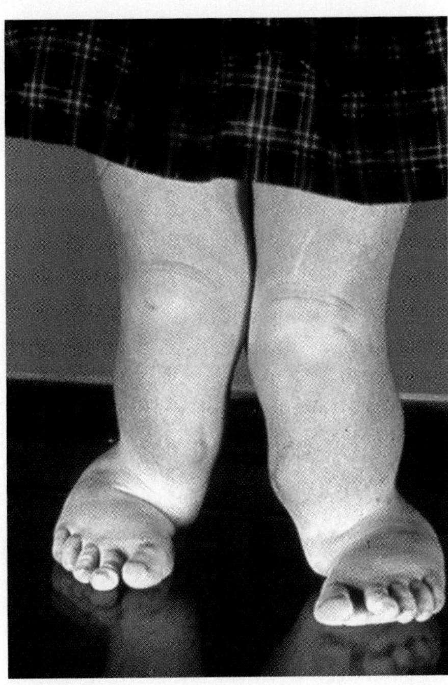

FIGURE 33–37 Clinical presentation of complete, bilateral fibular hemimelia.

underwent later amputation. The patients treated with primary amputation were functioning well with few complications. Choi and associates found that 88% of patients treated with amputation had satisfactory results, compared with 55% of those treated with lengthening using the Wagner technique.[46] Johnston and Haideri compared the function of patients with fibular hemimelia after lengthening versus after Syme's amputation.[155] The lengthened limbs had better power generation at the ankle than the Syme's limbs but had significant loss of dorsiflexion. The Syme's patients were able to generate power similar to that on the normal side by increasing hip power to compensate for decreased ankle power. Actual functional comparisons were difficult to make because the patients who had undergone Syme's amputation had more severely deficient extremities. Birch and colleagues followed a group of patients initially studied as children.[26,145] They found that these young adults treated with Syme's amputation functioned well in terms of walking and running and did not differ from the norm in occupational, recreational, and psychological function.

The choice of amputation or lengthening for children who fall in between the criteria identified earlier must be made on an individual basis. The number of lengthening procedures deemed necessary, the degree of reconstructive difficulty, and the expected functional outcome must be considered. Lengthening procedures can correct deformity and gain significant length, but long-term functional results are not yet available to aid the orthopaedist in making the appropriate decision. It is helpful for parents to consult surgeons experienced in both amputation and lengthening for fibular deficiency and to meet children and families who have undergone the different procedures.

For those patients who qualify, single or staged lengthening with repositioning of the foot may be successful, and the short fibula may be differentially lengthened relative to the tibia to establish a more normal tibial-fibular relation. Most of these patients, however, have a tarsal coalition and an abnormal talotibial articulation, and it is difficult to predict the long-term function of the retained foot and ankle. The frequency of complications of lengthening procedures is directly related to the amount of discrepancy present.

Regardless of which treatment method is used, some patients develop gradually progressive valgus of the knee. This condition is best treated about 1 to 2 years before the patient reaches skeletal maturity, at which time a partial growth arrest procedure may be done. If the degree of valgus is 15 degrees or more and there is at least 2 cm of remaining growth, a medial epiphysiodesis of the proximal tibia or distal femur (based on the site of the valgus) can be performed to gradually correct the deformity.[104] After skeletal maturity, a tibial osteotomy may be necessary for significant deformity. Occasional patients have symptomatic anterior cruciate instability, which can be successfully repaired at skeletal maturity.[99]

Good outcomes have been reported with the use of medial distal femoral physeal stapling to correct the valgus deformity.[28] We prefer not to use staples, however, because they are poorly tolerated under a prosthesis, and the outcome is unpredictable owing to rebound growth after staple removal. Because the deformity may overcorrect into varus following a partial epiphyseal arrest, angular deformity must be closely monitored for the first year after the arrest. When the limb reaches neutral alignment after the procedure and the lateral portion of the physis of the proximal tibia remains open, a lateral epiphysiodesis should be performed to prevent overcorrection.

Complete Fibular Hemimelia

Amputation. In the past, different surgical procedures were performed in an attempt to centralize the patient's foot and lengthen the limb. Today, there is consensus that ankle disarticulation, pioneered by Badgley in the early 1940s, is the best treatment for complete fibular hemimelia.[7,14,80,178,349] The procedure should be done in early childhood, and the patient should be fitted with a Syme's-type prosthesis afterward. Most series in which a modified Syme's amputation was performed have reported good results. Some surgeons prefer the Boyd's amputation, in which the retained calcaneus can be used to stabilize the heel pad, especially for older boys.[174,175] Others have reported good results with both procedures and have found that the best outcomes correlated with central placement of the heel pad.[75] We have found that although migration of the heel pad occasionally occurs following a Syme's amputation, this usually does not create significant problems for the patient or the prosthetist (see Fig. 33–37).[145] Thus, we prefer the Syme's procedure over the Boyd's amputation.

The optimal time to perform the amputation is when the child is just starting to pull up to stand (normally, 9 to 10 months of age). If the operation is done at this time, the child will be able to ambulate in a prosthesis at approximately 1 year of age and will be able to function at a nearly normal level, running and playing all sports.[145] Mild tibial bowing is usually well tolerated, and corrective osteotomy is not necessary. However, if the bowing is marked and there is too great an anterior prominence, the surgeon can perform a tibial osteotomy at the same time the amputation is performed. Distal tibial bowing may recur and occasionally requires osteotomy as the child grows.

Limb Lengthening. Because of improved techniques, there has been renewed interest in using limb lengthening procedures to treat deformities and limb length inequality in children with complete fibular hemimelia (Figs. 33–38 and 33–39).[41,89] Patients whose discrepancies are less than 5 cm at birth and who do not have significant foot deformities may be suitable candidates; however, the specific indications and long-term outcomes of limb lengthening are not well defined at this time. These patients usually must undergo several lengthening procedures and may end up with significant functional deficits because of foot and ankle deformities. Although limb lengthening allows the patient to maintain the foot of the affected limb, this benefit must be weighed against the drawbacks of lengthening procedures.[144] For patients whose limb length discrepancies at birth are greater than 5 cm, and for those who have notable foot deformities, we concur with Kruger that the most appropriate treatment is amputation and prosthetic management.[173-176]

Bilateral Fibular Hemimelia

Amputation. Children with bilateral fibular hemimelia usually have very little length discrepancy between the two lower limbs; however, a major problem is the disproportion between the lengths of the legs and the rest of the body. In a young child this discrepancy may be acceptable, but as the child matures, the difference in femoral and tibial lengths results in an unbecoming "dwarfism" because of the short tibiae. If there is significant shortening of the tibiae, and if the feet and ankles are malformed, the recommended treatment is ankle disarticulation. Bilateral lengthening may at times be appropriate for these individuals.

Limb Lengthening. If tibial shortening is not significant and the feet are well aligned, the feet should be preserved, and lengthening of the tibiae may be considered. Kruger and Talbott concluded that 50% of their patients with bilateral fibular hemimelia should

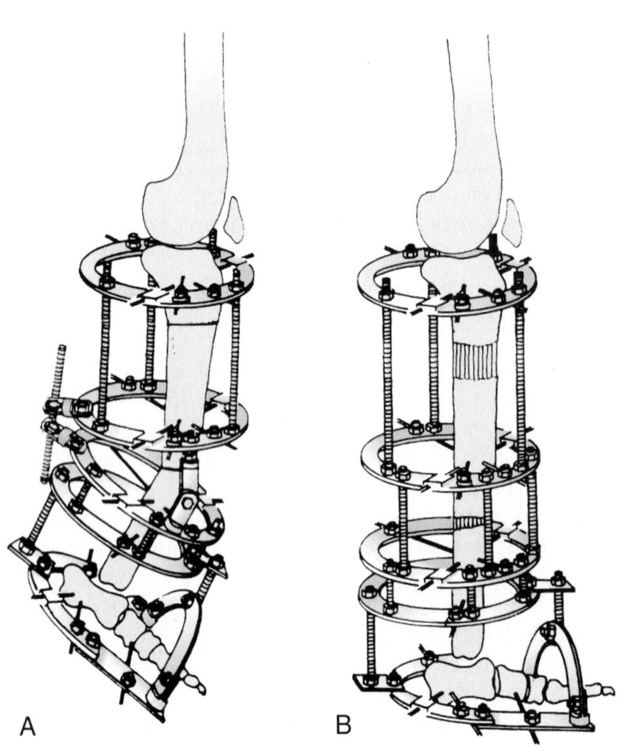

FIGURE 33–38 Ilizarov frame technique for treating fibular hemimelia. **A,** Placement of the frame and osteotomies proximally and at the apex of the deformity. **B,** Position after lengthening and deformity correction. (From Catagni MA: Management of fibular hemimelia using the Ilizarov method. Instr Course Lect 1992;41:431. Reprinted with permission from the American Academy of Orthopaedic Surgeons.)

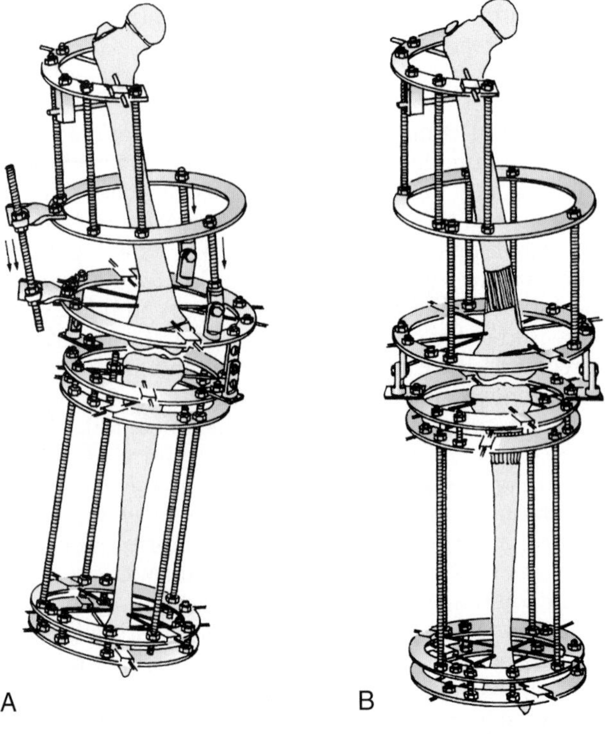

FIGURE 33–39 Femoral-tibial Ilizarov frame for lengthening and deformity correction in a patient with fibular hemimelia and femoral shortening. **A,** Frame placement. **B,** Position after lengthening of the distal femur and proximal tibia and correction of femoral valgus. (From Catagni MA: Management of fibular hemimelia using the Ilizarov method. Instr Course Lect 1992;41:431. Reprinted with permission from the American Academy of Orthopaedic Surgeons.)

have undergone amputation instead of limb salvage procedures.[178] However, this study was conducted before the development of more sophisticated limb lengthening techniques.

Tibial Deficiency

Tibial deficiency, or tibial hemimelia, is a syndrome of partial to complete absence of the tibia at birth. For most children born with tibial hemimelia, the cause is unknown. However, there are a number of heritable forms of the condition that have an autosomal dominant pattern,[49,177,266] and there is at least one report of apparent autosomal recessive inheritance in two brothers.[209,255] In these types of tibial deficiency, the deformity usually involves both limbs, there is duplication of the toes, and the patient may have coexisting anomalies of the hands. Four distinct autosomal dominant syndromes have been identified: tibial hemimelia–foot polydactyly–triphalangeal thumbs syndrome (Warner's syndrome), tibial hemimelia diplopodia syndrome, tibial hemimelia–split hand and foot syndrome, and tibial hemimelia–micromelia–trigonobrachycephaly syndrome.

Many associated abnormalities are seen in these patients, including syndactyly, polydactyly, foot oligodactyly, split hand and foot, five-fingered hand, anonychia, bifid femur, ulnar and fibular reduplication, radioulnar synostosis, radial ray agenesis, micromelia, trigonomacrocephaly, diplopodia, joint hyperextensibility, and deafness.[350] In a retrospective review of patients with tibial deficiency over a 22-year period (1961 to 1983), 79% of patients had associated congenital anomalies, with abnormalities of the hip, hand, or spine occurring alone or in various combinations.[275]

CLASSIFICATION

The Jones system classifies tibial hemimelia into four types, based on radiographic features present during infancy (Fig. 33–40).[156]

Type	Radiologic Description	No. of limbs
1a	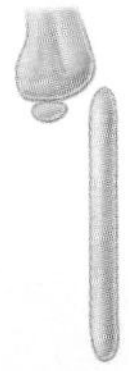 Tibia not seen Hypoplastic lower femoral epiphysis	6
1b	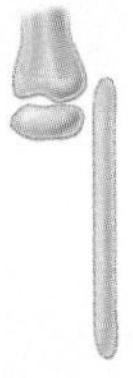 Tibia not seen Normal lower femoral epiphysis	12
2	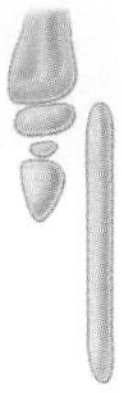 Distal tibia not seen	5
3	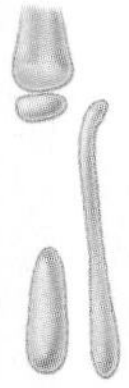 Proximal tibia not seen	2
4	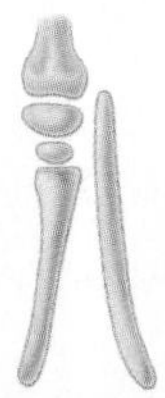 Diastasis	4

FIGURE 33–40 Jones classification of tibial deficiency. (Redrawn from Herring JA, Cummings DR: The limb-deficient child. In Morrissy RT, Weinstein SL [eds]: Lovell and Winter's Pediatric Orthopaedics, vol 2, 4th ed. Philadelphia, Lippincott-Raven, 1996.)

In type 1, the tibia cannot be seen on radiographs at birth. In subtype 1a, the tibia is completely absent, and the ossific nucleus of the distal femoral epiphysis is small or has not appeared. In subtype 1b, the proximal part of the tibia is present, but because it is not ossified at birth, it appears to be absent. In this type, there is normal ossification of the distal femoral epiphysis.

In type 2, the proximal part of the tibia is ossified and visible on radiographs at birth, but the distal tibia is not seen (Fig. 33–41).

In type 3, the distal part of the tibia is ossified and visible, but the proximal portion of the tibia is absent. Often a unique, amorphous osseous structure forms (representative of the shaft of the tibia), and a rudimentary surrogate knee-ankle articulation eventually develops.[274] This is the least common form of tibial hemimelia.

In type 4, the tibia is short, and there is distal tibiofibular diastasis (Fig. 33–42). In these cases (previously referred to as congenital diastasis of the ankle), the distal tibial articular surface is absent, there is proximal displacement of the talus, and the tibia and fibula separate at the ankle.

Other variations of tibial shortening have been described. Tuncay and coworkers described a form of anterolateral tibial bowing with an intact and long fibula.[320] This type resembles tibial pseudarthrosis syndrome and is discussed in Chapter 22, Disorders of the Leg. Two similar cases of shortening of the tibia, one with and one without bowing combined with a relatively longer fibula with fibular subluxation at the

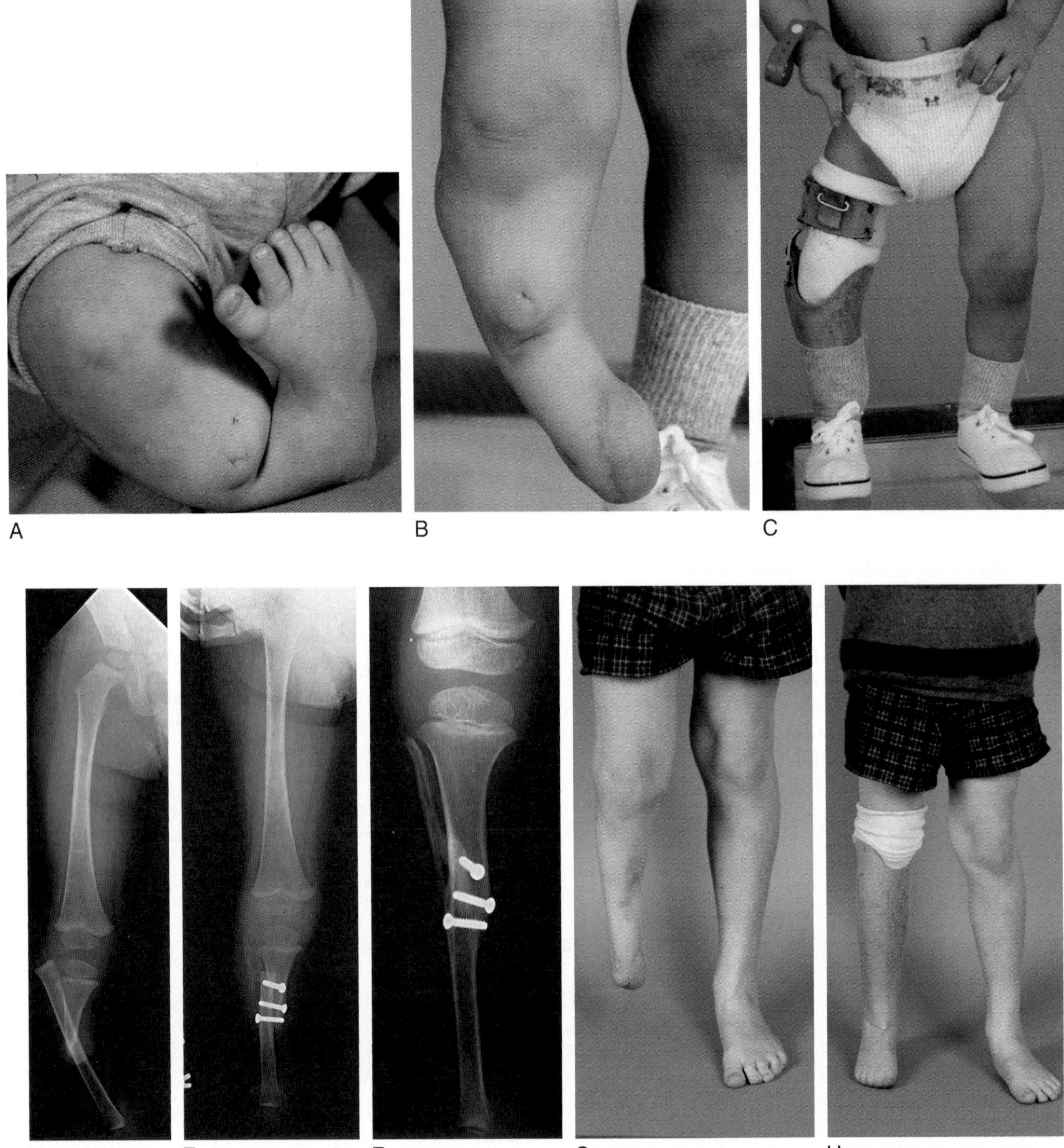

FIGURE 33–41 Child with partial tibial hemimelia, Jones type 2. **A,** In infancy, there was marked varus of the foot. The proximal portion of the tibia could be seen and palpated beneath the dimple. **B,** Appearance after Syme's amputation. The tibial segment was not sufficiently ossified for a synostosis procedure to be performed. **C,** Appearance in a prosthesis with thigh support to control the varus of the lower segment. **D,** Anteroposterior (AP) radiograph obtained at age 5 years showing absence of the tibia below the upper third. **E,** AP radiograph after excision of the upper fibula and synostosis of the fibula to the tibia. **F,** AP radiograph obtained at age 10 years showing solid arthrodesis between the tibia and fibula. **G,** After the synostosis procedure, the limb has excellent alignment and end weight-bearing capabilities. **H,** The simple Syme's-type prosthesis provides excellent functional and cosmetic results.

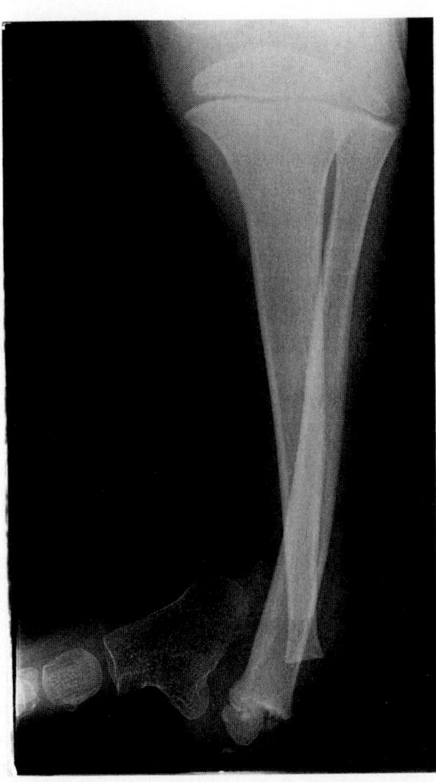

FIGURE 33-42 Tibial hemimelia type 4, with diastasis of the tibia and fibula. Note the severe displacement of the foot.

knee, have been described. Both cases required tibial lengthening.[66]

CLINICAL FEATURES

Patients with complete absence of the tibia (Jones type 1a) have a knee flexion contracture, with the knee positioned proximal and lateral to the femoral condyles (Fig. 33–43). When the tibia is not visible on radiographs, careful examination of the proximal part of the patient's limb may reveal a palpable tibial segment that has not yet ossified. This clinical finding can often be better appreciated on ultrasonography or magnetic resonance imaging.[119] When there is complete absence of the tibia, the child normally has hamstring function but not quadriceps function; the patella is typically absent; and the foot, which is fixed in severe varus, has minimal functional movement.

In patients with Jones types 1b and 2 deformities, in which the proximal part of the tibia is present but the distal portion is absent, hamstring and quadriceps function is normal, and the knee moves normally. The fibular head is displaced proximally and laterally, and the limb is in a varus position, with significant varus instability. At the ankle joint, the foot is displaced medially relative to the fibula and is also in varus.

In Jones type 3 deformity, the knee is unstable, and there are extra digits distally. The tibial shaft is palpable, and there is a severe varus deformity of the leg.

In patients with Jones type 4 deformity, in which there is a diastasis of the distal tibia and fibula, the

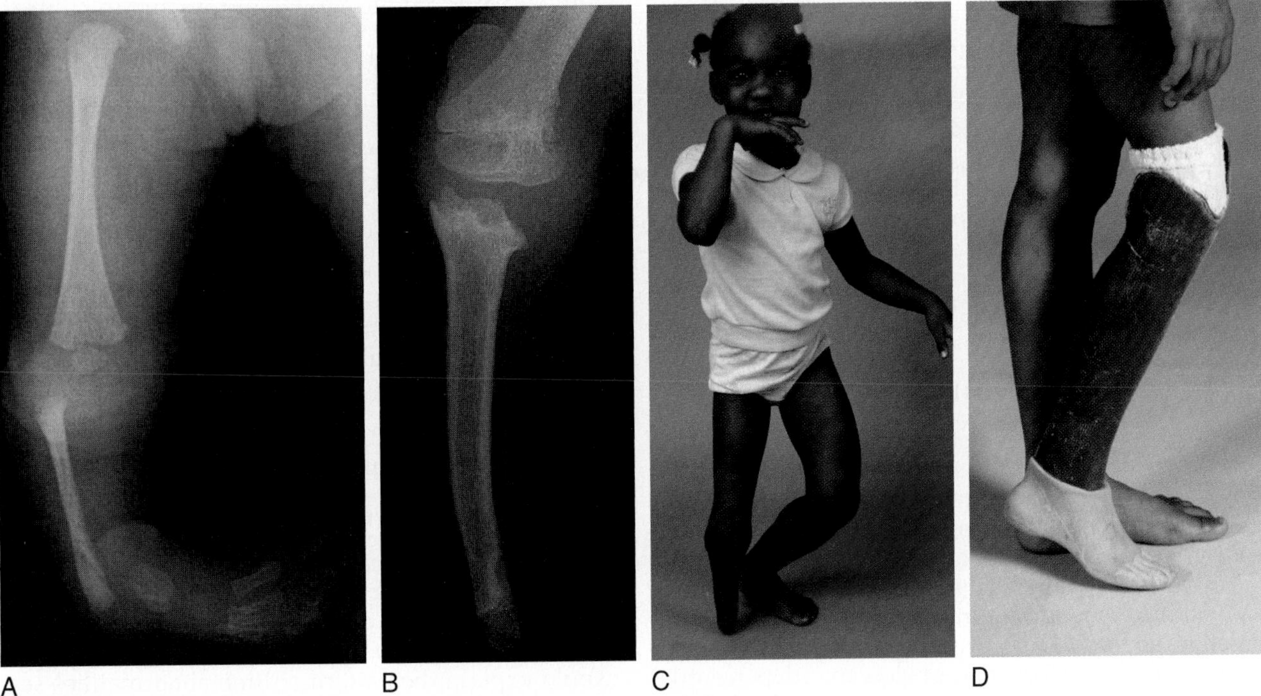

FIGURE 33-43 Girl with complete tibial hemimelia type 1. **A,** Radiograph obtained at age 1 month. **B,** Radiograph of the limb after a Brown centralization procedure. **C,** Clinical appearance after the Brown procedure. **D,** Appearance in the prosthesis. The subsequent development of knee flexion deformity reduced the function of the extremity, and amputation is likely.

limb is moderately short, and the foot is in a severe, rigid varus, positioned between the tibia and the fibula.

TREATMENT

Partial Tibial Hemimelia

For Jones types 1b and 2 deformities, in which the proximal part of the tibia is present, excellent functional results can be obtained by fusing the proximal fibula to the upper part of the tibia (see Fig. 33–41).[9,131,156] In infants, the proximal tibia may be primarily cartilaginous, and fusion cannot be obtained until there is sufficient ossification of the upper tibia to allow for successful synostosis with the fibula. Fusion of the fibula to the tibia may be done in an end-to-end position with intramedullary pin fixation or in a side-to-side position using a screw for fixation. When joining the fibula to the tibia, the surgeon should consider resecting the proximal protruding fibula because, if left intact, it can adversely affect prosthetic fit and function.[274] A Syme's amputation with subsequent prosthetic management is the best treatment for the distal part of the limb because of the severe foot and ankle instability. After the synostosis has healed, these children are able to function as well as other Syme's-level amputees and can participate in normal sports activities.

For a Jones type 4 deformity (see Fig. 33–42), the best treatment is a modified Syme's ankle disarticulation performed when the child reaches walking age. Functional results are usually excellent. Other techniques, such as tibial lengthening and foot repositioning, may make it possible to retain a plantigrade foot, but functional reconstruction is difficult because of talus and calcaneus deformities and the absence of a distal tibial articular surface.[156] New limb lengthening procedures may enable the orthopaedist to treat the diastasis in other ways; however, the long-term results of these techniques are not known.

For the rare Jones type 3 deformity, the limited data available show that these patients function relatively well as below-knee amputees following a Syme's or Chopart's amputation.[274] Some of these patients may be candidates for tibial lengthening, depending on the anatomy of the ankle joint.

Complete Tibial Hemimelia

Most patients with complete tibial hemimelia (Jones type 1a) require knee disarticulation, which usually provides good functional results. In a gait analysis of six children who underwent knee disarticulation, gait velocity averaged 81% of normal, the time for a single gait cycle was 131% of normal, and energy expenditure was within the normal range.[198] As expected, the patients' ability to run was significantly decreased (time for the 50-yard dash was below the 5th percentile for age group). However, the prosthetic knee demonstrated good flexion during the swing phase of gait and no flexion in the stance phase, which allowed patients a stable, extended knee with weight bearing. No residual limb problems developed.

Centralization of the fibula combined with a Syme's amputation (i.e., the Brown procedure) has frequently been used to treat this deformity (see Fig. 33–43)[34,35]; however, this approach is prone to failure, and the patient often requires a subsequent knee disarticulation.[160,198,240,275] Most failures are due to marked knee instability and the progressive development of knee flexion contracture because of unopposed hamstring pull.[275] In one study, 53 of 55 patients with Jones type 1a tibial hemimelia who were treated by the Brown procedure developed flexion contractures that resulted in poor outcomes.[195] Anterior transfer of the hamstrings for active knee extension is impeded because there is no patella or femoral condylar notch. All these factors also make the prosthetic management of these patients very difficult.

Hall has stated that the Brown procedure is indicated only if the patient has a well-developed distal femoral segment; a functioning quadriceps mechanism, preferably a patella; and no evidence of a proximal tibia (by current imaging techniques).[125,284] When these criteria are met preoperatively, the procedure has been reported to be successful.[47] However, patients with type 1 tibial hemimelia rarely have active knee extension. In most cases, there is a gradual decline in knee function, and recurrent deformity often requires repeated surgical revisions and eventual amputation.[174,175] Thus, the Brown procedure is rarely indicated for patients with complete tibial hemimelia. As succinctly stated by Loder,[195] "It is clear from this literature review that the Brown procedure uniformly fails in the treatment of Jones type 1a tibial deficiency. I believe it should not be attempted in the 'hopes that it might work,' because it will always end in failure at long-term follow-up."

Foot Deficiency

Congenital foot deficiencies are most commonly caused by constriction band formation (Streeter bands) (Fig. 33–44). Congenital absence of the complete foot is a rare abnormality. Children with congenital partial foot absences usually do not need surgical intervention, do not develop contractures, and have minimal, if any, functional limitations.[27] A slipper-type prosthesis can allow normal shoe wear and function (Fig. 33–45).

CONGENITAL UPPER LIMB DEFICIENCIES

Transverse Deficiencies

The cause of most transverse upper limb deficiencies is unknown. The subclavian artery disruption sequence has been proposed as a common pathway, but this remains speculative.[21] The resultant vascular insult would explain the pattern of limb abnormalities seen in symbrachydactyly, Poland's and Möbius' syndromes, and transverse deficiencies in which there are small "nubbins." The presence of ectoderm-derived tissues (skin, nails, distal phalangeal tufts) supports the concept of failure of normal mesodermal proliferation.

Limb anomalies range from minimal shortening to a proximal level of absence.

SYMBRACHYDACTYLY

Classification

There are four classes of symbrachydactyly. The short-fingered type is most likely to be associated with Poland's anomaly (absence of the sternal head of the pectoralis major muscle; Fig. 33–46). The other forms are the central defect or split hand type; the monodactylous type, in which the thumb is always preserved; and the peromelic form, which may be proximal.

Treatment

The surgeon must first decide how to treat any existing nubbins, because their presence can result in a number of problems. They may become entangled in hair or strands of thread and become excoriated or dysvascular. Small nails that grow abnormally may become irritated, infected, or difficult to trim. In the split hand form of symbrachydactyly, nubbins may develop on the ridge in the central part of the hand and can be easily traumatized (Fig. 33–47). In this situation, local skin rearrangement and removal of the nubbins can deepen the web and smooth the residual commissure. Some clinicians, though, rarely amputate nubbins (Fig.

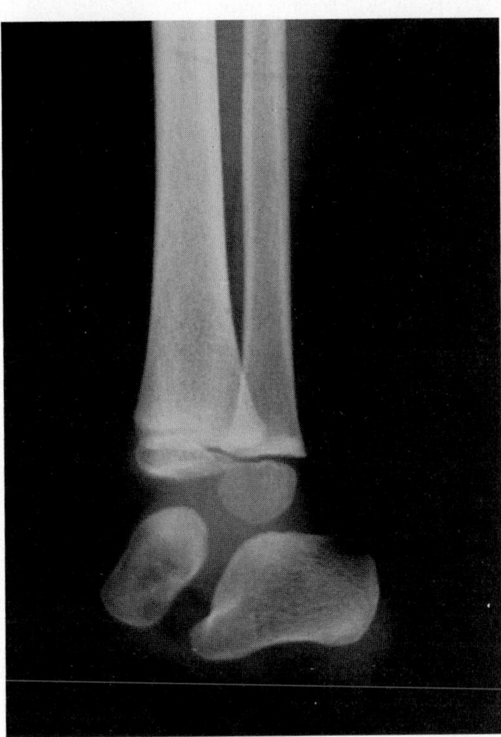

FIGURE 33–44 Congenital absence of the foot distal to the talonavicular calcaneocuboid level. (From Herring JA, Cummings DR: The limb-deficient child. In Morrissy RT, Weinstein SL [eds]: Lovell and Winter's Pediatric Orthopaedics, vol 2, 4th ed. Philadelphia, Lippincott-Raven, 1996.)

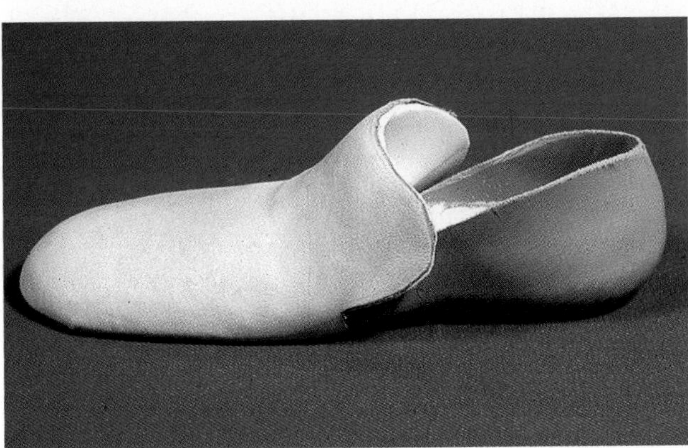

FIGURE 33–45 Slipper-type prosthesis for partial foot absence. (From Herring JA, Cummings DR: The limb-deficient child. In Morrissy RT, Weinstein SL [eds]: Lovell and Winter's Pediatric Orthopaedics, vol 2, 4th ed. Philadelphia, Lippincott-Raven, 1996.)

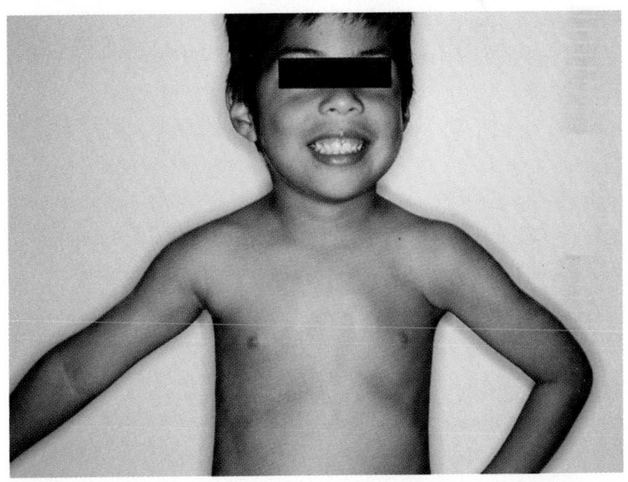

A

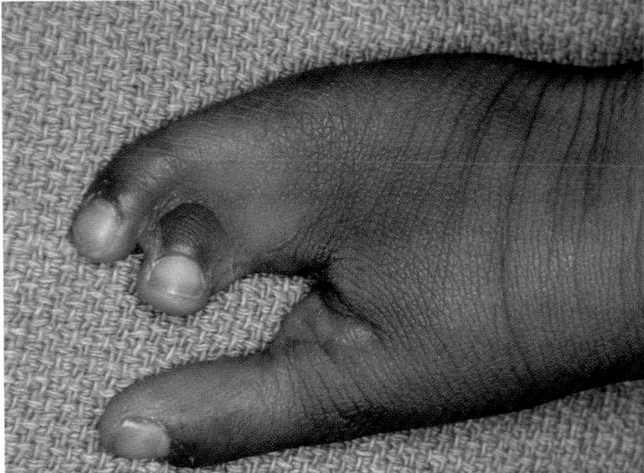

B

FIGURE 33–46 **A** and **B,** Child with the short-fingered type of symbrachydactyly and Poland's anomaly. Note a prior web deepening.

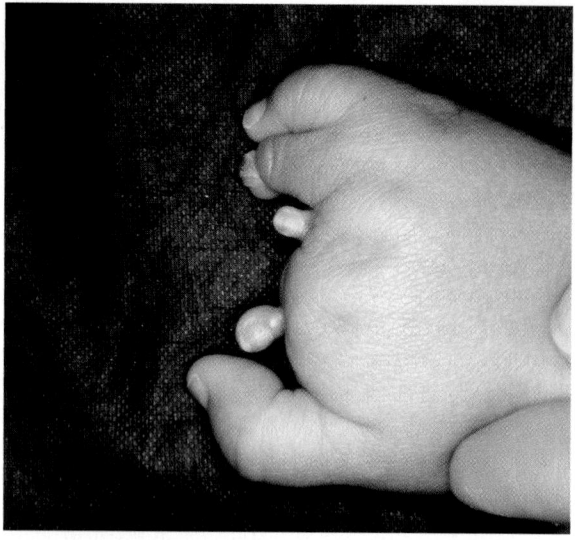

FIGURE 33–47 Split hand form of symbrachydactyly.

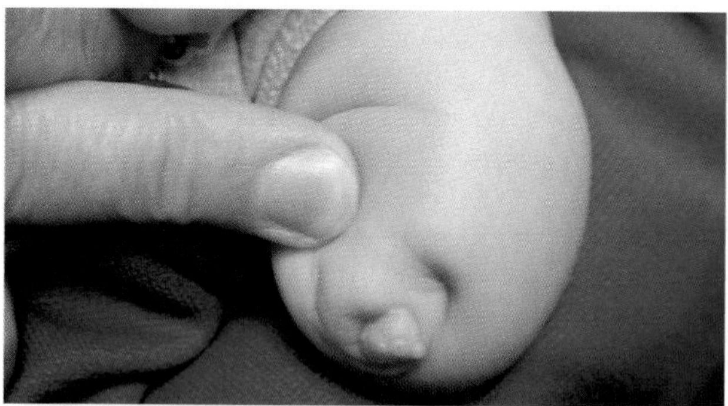

FIGURE 33–48 Residual nubbins in peromelia symbrachydactyly.

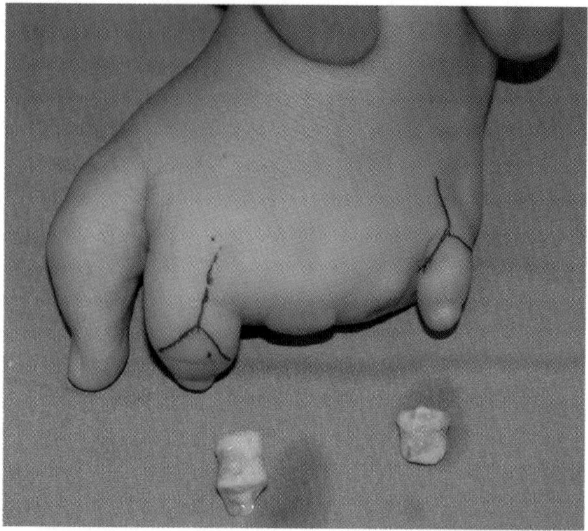

FIGURE 33–49 Augmentation of finger length by the transplantation of nonvascularized phalanges from the patient's toes.

33–48). They report that many children find that these small digits make them feel less abnormal. It is important to keep in mind that some nubbins are functional. Those that are under volitional control or are large enough for possible subsequent soft tissue and bony augmentation should not be removed.[79]

After the nubbins have been appropriately treated, reconstructive surgery to improve limb function is the next step. Children who have some structures distal to the carpus may be candidates for digital reconstruction.

If the digital remnants do not have any bony support and are large enough to permit bone grafting, they can be augmented by the transplantation of nonvascularized toe phalanges (Fig. 33–49). Transplantation must include periosteum and ligamentous support tissue to ensure ready revascularization. To enhance bone stability in the soft tissue sleeve, the surgeon can suture the ligamentous attachments of the phalanx to adjoining bony elements in the finger. The timing of the procedure is debated. Some believe that if the transplantation is performed when the child is young, the epiphysis of the toe (with its periosteum) has a better survival rate and will continue to grow.[38] Others report that if the transfer is done later, the toe phalanges will grow normally on the foot, and there is minimal risk of loss of potential growth after transfer.[79] In either case, the donor toe phalanx will be short and telescoped, similar to the original appearance of the involved finger.

In some patients, digital reconstruction can be performed by repositioning the available bony elements so that they are more functional. For example, an index metacarpal or ray might be transferred to the middle digit position to close a defect. Another option is to transfer metacarpal remnants so that enough bone is "stacked" at a border position in preparation for subsequent lengthening.[79]

Distraction lengthening, however, plays a limited role in treating digital deficiencies. Although the procedure may improve the cosmetic appearance by making the digits longer, there is a risk of functional loss if the digits are thinner, stiffer, and more scarred. Distraction lengthening against atrophic soft tissue can cause ulcerations, so the surgeon will have to augment soft tissue coverage or shorten the digits to an acceptable length. Lengthening in the hand is best done at an intercalary level when there is a normal digit tip (Fig. 33–50).[79]

An option for functional reconstruction of the adactylous hand is microsurgical free toe transfers.[192,329] Most patients with adactylous hands have proximal structures (muscles and tendons for motor function, and nerves for sensation) that permit successful transplantation of toes to the hand. This can improve function significantly; however, the toes will continue to look like toes, despite their new position.

AMNION DISRUPTION SEQUENCE

Transverse deficiencies may also be caused by the early amnion disruption sequence.[164] Disruption of

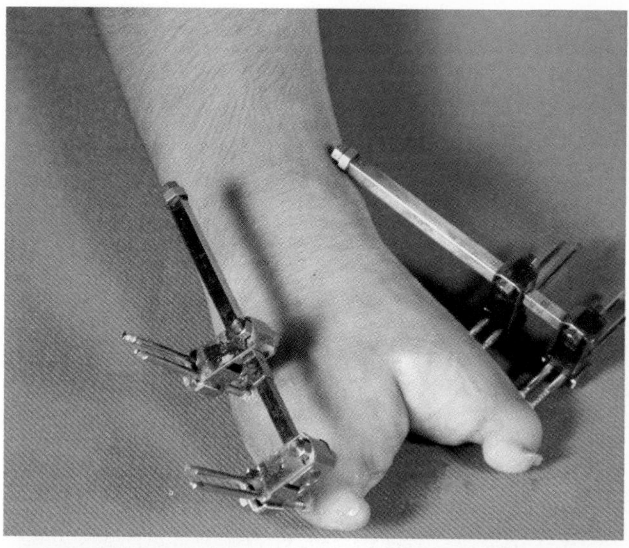

FIGURE 33-50 Lengthening of the hand using external fixators.

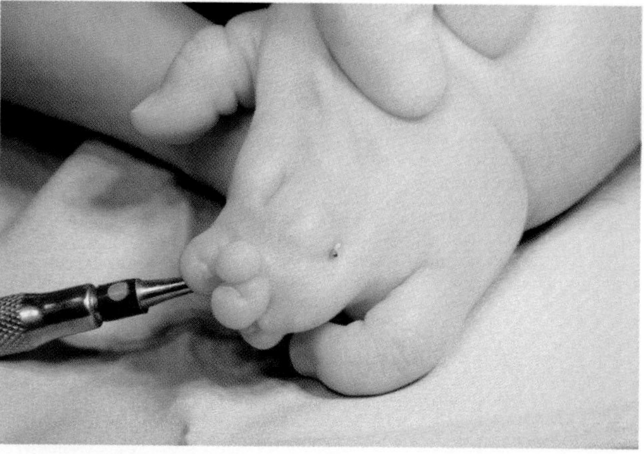

FIGURE 33-52 Fenestrated syndactyly, a hallmark of constriction band formation.

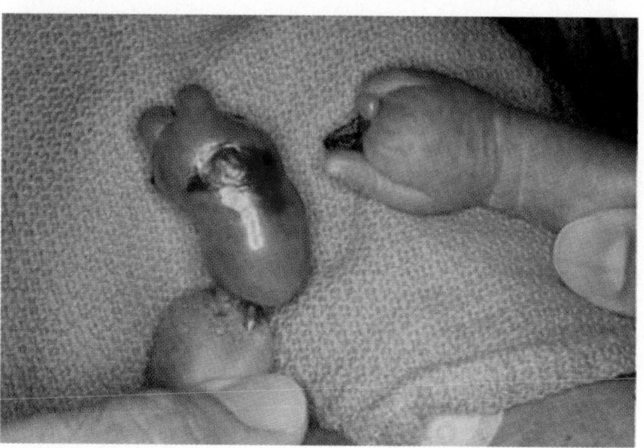

FIGURE 33-51 Near autoamputation due to constriction bands.

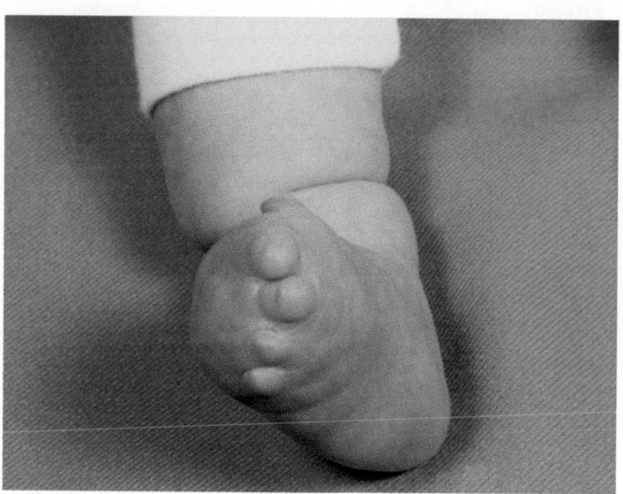

FIGURE 33-53 Severe foot deformity as a result of a constriction band.

upper limb growth is caused by breakdown of the amnion and traumatic lesions of the limbs secondary to constriction by strands of amnion (abnormal amnion bands; Fig. 33–51).[110,158] The digits of the limbs are most often affected, with fenestrated syndactyly (Fig. 33–52) the hallmark of limb involvement (Fig. 33–53). Deep bands can cause a number of problems, including distal edema, injury to nerves, impaired sensation, impeded limb development, amputation of digits or proximal limbs, and bony overgrowth. Late complications associated with band amputations include diaphyseal overgrowth, unstable soft tissue at the proximal end of the residual limb or digit, formation of inclusion cysts at the tip of the limb, and increased susceptibility to infection distal to the band (Fig. 33–54).

Treatment

For limb deficiencies secondary to amnion disruption, early emergent surgery to release the constriction

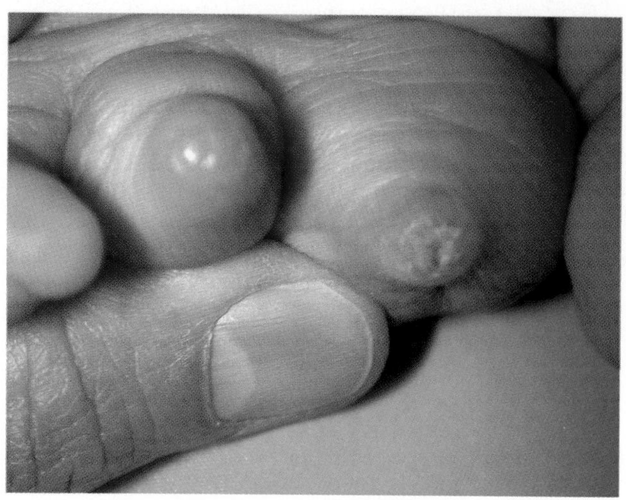

FIGURE 33-54 Late complications of band amputation.

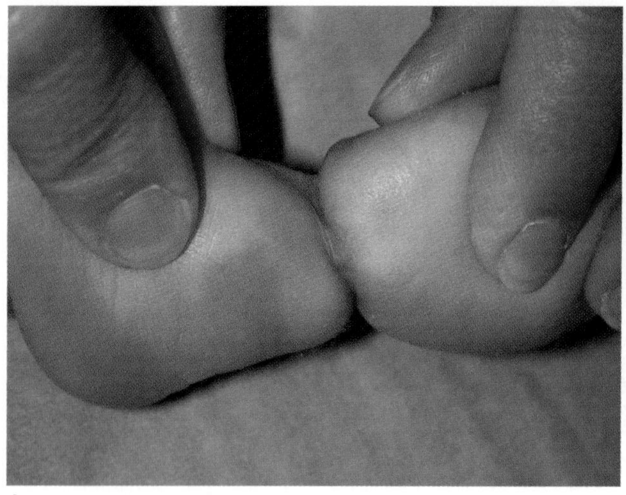

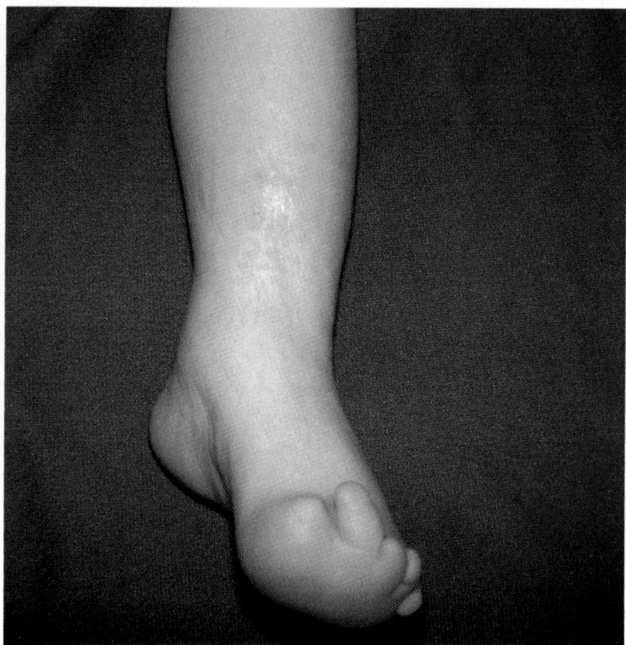

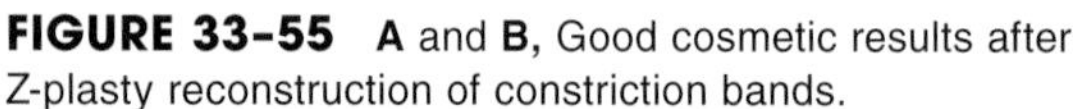

FIGURE 33–55 A and B, Good cosmetic results after Z-plasty reconstruction of constriction bands.

bands is indicated only if there is impending tissue death.[79] For most patients, elective release and Z-plasty of the bands can be performed when the child is older than 6 months and better able to tolerate surgery and anesthesia. The surgeon can circumferentially recontour the constricting defect in one operation by carefully preserving any vessels that are present and releasing impeding fascia (Fig. 33–55).

Digital reconstruction may be performed by syndactyly separation and grafting, augmentation of digits with local skeletal rearrangements, free toe transfer, or digital lengthening.[79] Reconstruction of band syndactyly may be restricted by the presence of epithelialized tracts within the fenestrations; a complex deformity of the bone with fused, entangled digits; or poor tissue quality in the hand. Short digits can be made to appear slightly longer by releasing the transverse intermetacarpal ligament and deepening the interdigital web. During these procedures, the surgeon should be careful to preserve the normal expanse of palmar skin and its sensation.

Free toe transfer (if normal donor toes are available) is indicated in selected cases of band amputation of the digits, especially if the thumb is involved. Because all structures proximal to the constricting band are normal, it is possible to establish motor and sensory function as well as length with toe transplantation. The digits can also be made longer by distraction lengthening; however, results are poor if there is an inadequate digital tip.[79]

Radial Deficiency

Radial deficiency, a relatively common upper limb abnormality, is associated with numerous known genetic and chromosomal conditions as well as with coexisting skeletal, visceral, cardiac, hematologic, renal, and metabolic disorders. This indicates that the regulation of radial development is influenced by a variety of factors. The syndromes of thrombocytopenia–absent radius, VATER, Holt-Oram, and Fanconi present with radial dysplasia.[312] Thus, this anomaly must trigger a search for other significant, potentially life-threatening conditions. Segmentation anomalies of the spine may be associated with tethered cord or other spinal dysraphism.[42]

Treatment decisions for radial deficiencies must take into account the prognosis of any coexisting conditions. In many patients, these associated disorders (e.g., cardiac abnormalities) are successfully treated early in the child's life, leaving the deformity caused by the radial anomaly the major concern of the patient and parents.

CLASSIFICATION

The classification of radial deficiency is based on the amount of residual radius present (Fig. 33–56). In type I, there is a short distal radius. Type II, which is uncommon, consists of a small radius with proximal and distal growth plates. In type III, there is a small proximal radius. Type IV, which is the most common form of radial deficiency, is complete absence of the radius.

TREATMENT

The more severe and common radial deficiencies are first treated by stretching and splinting the hand of the affected limb. The next step is often centralization of the carpus on the ulna, with tendon balancing or "radialization" of the ulna under the carpus. Tendons and muscles across the ulnocarpal articulation are released and transferred so that their forces are rebalanced, and capsulorrhaphy is also performed. Post-

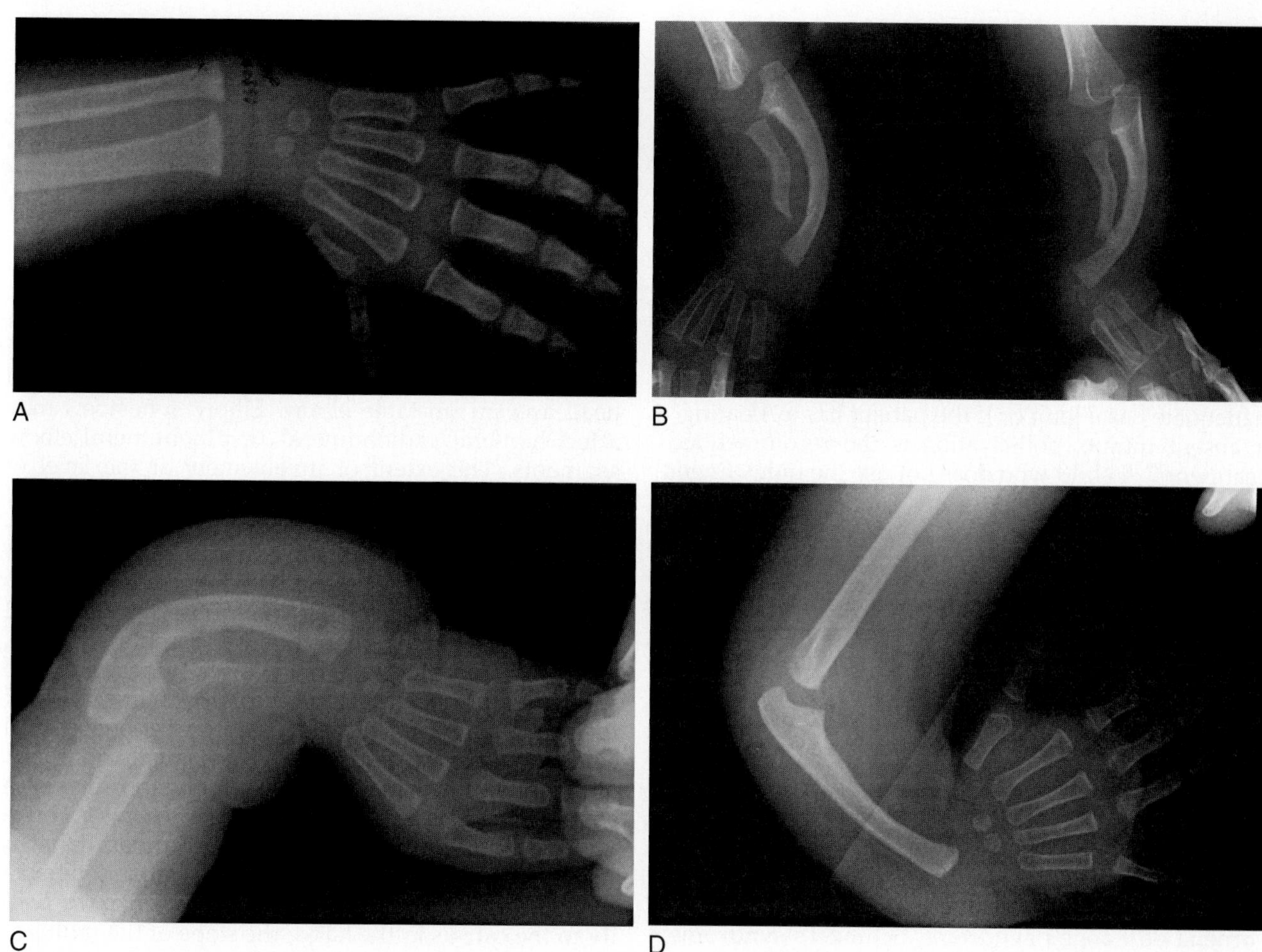

FIGURE 33–56 Classification of radial deficiency. **A,** Type I deficiency, in which there is a short, residual distal radius. **B,** Type II deficiency, in which there is a small radius with proximal and distal growth plates. **C,** Type III deficiency, in which there is a small proximal radius. **D,** Type IV deficiency, in which there is complete absence of the radius.

operatively, prolonged splinting is necessary. The purpose of centralization procedures is to stiffen the ulnocarpal junction and enhance the reach and stability of the musculotendinous units that cross the patient's wrist. However, it is difficult to maintain functional motion at this new "joint" and still provide sufficient stability and tendon balance so that the limb does not become deformed during growth.

A crucial factor when deciding whether to centralize the carpus is the range of motion of the patient's elbow. If the elbow joint is stiff in extension, any surgery that further restricts a patient's ability to reach the face with the hand should not be performed. When a radiocarpal arthrodesis is performed, compensatory motion takes place with rotation of the radioulnar joint. Because patients with radial deficiencies do not have a radioulnar joint, they are not able to rotate the forearm, and compensatory motion is restricted. Their limb strength (and deforming force) is derived from flexion and radial deviation. With current treatment options, it is not possible to establish "normal" alignment and still maintain functional motion. Realignment results in loss of motion, while preservation of motion results in persistence of deformity.[79]

Distraction lengthening of soft tissue may be applicable for radial deficiencies. Lengthening may precede any centralization procedures and does not preclude the performance of other surgical interventions. Factors that may limit the use of lengthening in a particular patient include limb size, proximity of neurovascular structures, risk of infection, and scarring.

A new surgical technique for treating radial clubhand is to restore support on the radial side of the carpus through the use of free metatarsophalangeal joint transfer.[330,331] This procedure is promising but technically demanding.

COMPLICATIONS

Late complications associated with radial deficiency include an inherent reduction in the growth capacity of the ulna, an increased risk of injury to the physis of the distal ulna (with resulting growth disruption), and a substantial risk of recurrent deformity. Patients frequently experience tendon adhesion and subluxation, resulting in decreased dexterity. The risk of recurrence of the deformity is inversely related to the stiffness of the wrist: the stiffer the wrist, the less likely it is that the deformity will recur. To increase wrist stiffness, the surgeon may need to perform an ulnocarpal arthrodesis as a final salvage procedure.[79]

Thumb hypoplasia and marked stiffness and deformity of all the fingers are often associated with radial deficiency. Thumb deformity ranges from mild hypoplasia to complete absence of the digit. Treatment of the thumb depends on the condition of the forearm and the adjoining fingers and on the patient's overall prognosis. If the thumb has a stable carpometacarpal joint, the surgeon can augment the deficient segments by rearranging adjacent tissue, transferring tendons, and reconstructing ligaments. If the thumb has an inadequate basal joint or if the patient has a "floating" or absent thumb, pollicization is the recommended treatment.[79] A child who does not use the index finger in the original position will not use the finger if it is moved to a pollicized position. Currently, no prosthesis exists that can function as an adequate substitute for a thumb.

Ulnar Deficiency

Congenital ulnar deficiencies involve primarily the postaxial or ulnar border of the upper limb. The precise role of genetics and environmental factors in the development of these deformities remains unclear. A recessive inheritance, or X-linked recessive trait, has been reported.[312] A deficient gene at 6q21 may be responsible for some ulnar anomalies.[122,254] Congenital syndromes associated with ulnar deficiency include Cornelia de Lange's syndrome, Schinzel's syndrome, Weyers' ulnar ray oligodactyly syndrome, ulnar mammary syndrome, femoral-fibular-ulnar deficiency syndrome, and ulnar fibula dysplasia.[113,312] Associated cardiovascular abnormalities have also been noted,[67,150] but they are not as frequent as with radial dysplasia. Ulnar deficiencies have been produced in pregnant rats with the administration of busulfan teratologic agents[232] and acetazolamide.[230] Disturbance of the C8 sclerotomes may result in ulnar anomalies.[213] The cause of isolated ulnar hemimelia is not known; cases are apparently sporadic and not genetically induced.

CLASSIFICATION

All the classification systems for ulnar deficiency take into account ulnar and elbow involvement,[53,69,183,219,231,232,258,309] with some also addressing hand abnormalities.[53,183,232] The most commonly used classification is the Bayne system (Fig. 33–57), in which ulnar hypoplasia is classified as type I, partial ulnar aplasia as type II, total ulnar aplasia as type III, and radiohumeral synostosis as type IV. However, this classification system does not address hand or shoulder involvement, nor does it help predict the evolution of the deformity or the outcome of surgical reconstruction.[23]

CLINICAL FEATURES

Longitudinal formation of the ulna is either impaired or completely absent (Fig. 33–58). Patients may have congenital absence of the ulna, longitudinal arrest of ulnar development, paraxial ulnar hemimelia, postaxial deficiency, ulnar dysmelia, ulnar clubhand, or ulnar ray deficiency. With ulnar hemimelia, the radius bows toward the ulnar aspect of the forearm, with the apex of the bow directed radially, creating an apparent ulnar deviation of the hand. Lack of bony development creates a rigid fibrocartilaginous anlage that tethers to the radius and the ulnar carpus.[23] This anlage has been implicated as the underlying cause of significant ulnar deviation of the hand.[258]

If the ulnar deficiency is severe, the patient may have a short proximal ulna, with a dislocated radial head and an unstable elbow. Elbow synostosis may affect humeral, radiohumeral, or ulnohumeral elbow segments. The extent of involvement at the level of the elbow correlates directly with the amount of functional deficit. Proximal limb involvement may produce functional shoulder deficiency.[23] Deformity of the forearm, elbow, and shoulder is aesthetically unappealing and associated with some weakness and loss of dexterity; however, if prehension is possible, good function is often noted in these patients. The anatomic condition of the deformed limb may mislead the clinician into underestimating its functional capabilities.[290]

Some of the anomalies that may be seen include ectrodactyly, carpal hypoplasia, ulnar deviation of the hand, shortening of the forearm with radial bowing, dysplasia of the elbow, and hypoplasia of the entire limb.[85,154,257,258] The radius provides support and stability to the carpus in the hand; the slope of the radius at the distal end tends to flatten to maintain support as the ulnar deformity increases. The entire hand may be involved, and there may be abnormal or absent digits, malrotation of the hand, or symphalangism and syndactyly with abnormality of the thumb and first web.[53] Hand deformities may interfere with prehension, dexterity, and hand strength.

TREATMENT

The primary goal of treatment is to improve functional use of the affected limb. Early casting and splinting (applied at birth and continued until surgery) have been recommended but are not effective.[23] Hand function can be improved by surgical release of syndactyly, web deepening, metacarpal rotational osteotomy, pollicization, and lengthening procedures.[257,309]

Corrective or rotational osteotomies performed at the level of the forearm or the humerus can effectively position the hand in space for function. However, because of dislocation, elbow arthroplasties are not effective in restoring elbow function or correcting radial bowing. Radial head excision may cause further instability of the elbow. Pterygium correction is not beneficial in improving function or appearance.[23]

The establishment of a surgically created single-bone forearm may be helpful in improving stability in unstable forearms[165,244] and elbows.[165,193,257,292,332] However, nonunion and other postoperative complications can be significant, and the results of the proce-

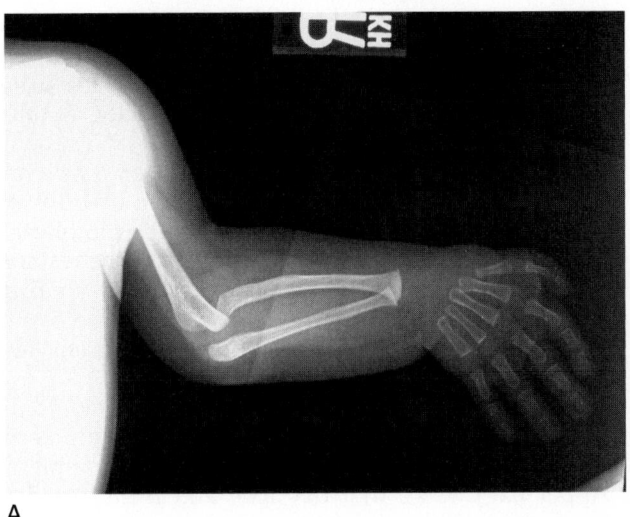

A

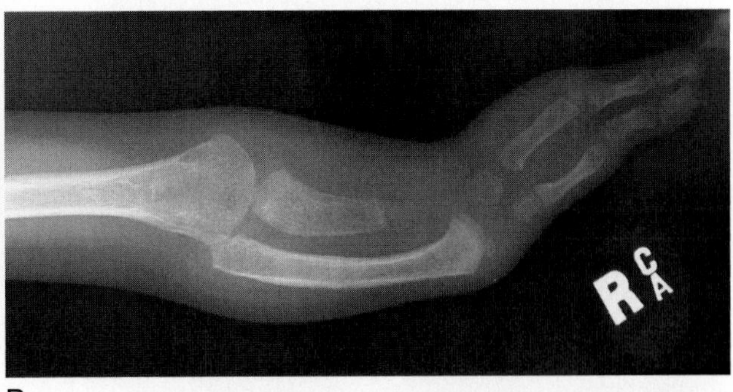

B

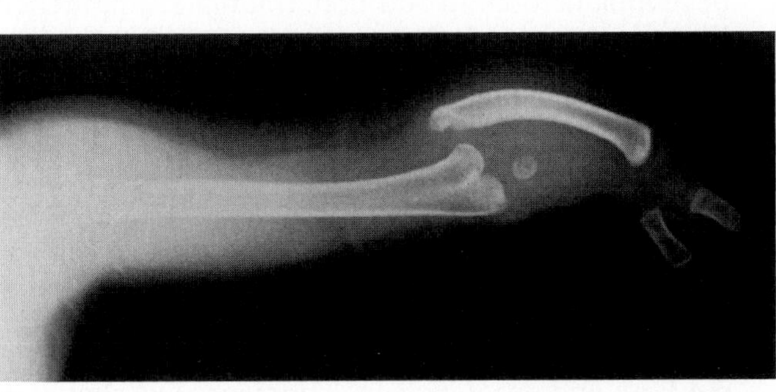

C

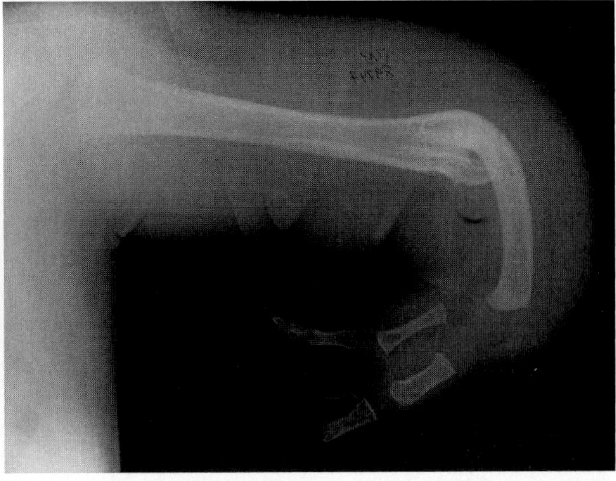

D

FIGURE 33-57 Classification of ulnar deficiency. **A,** Type I ulnar dysplasia, with a short ulna and ulnar deviation of the hand. **B,** Type II ulnar dysplasia, with short ulna and oligodactyly. **C,** Type III ulnar dysplasia, with absence of the ulna and dislocation of the radial head. A tethering ulnar anlage may be present. **D,** Type IV ulnar dysplasia, with a radiohumeral synostosis.

dure may not be as predictable as is indicated in the literature.[23]

Early resection of the fibrocartilaginous anlage at the distal ulna to prevent ulnar deviation of the hand is controversial, with some authors maintaining that the anlage does not create a deviation force.[203,258,341] Resection may be indicated if deviation of the ulna is greater than 30 degrees[203] or if forearm or elbow surgery is being performed at the same time.[23]

Distraction lengthening of the forearm (using the Ilizarov soft tissue and callus distraction procedures) can be used in cases of unilateral ulnar deficiency.[288] Although cosmetic improvement has been noted, long-term follow-up is required to determine whether functional improvement is achieved.

Researchers are also studying the benefits of using free vascularized epiphyseal transfers from the proximal fibula to correct ulnar deficiencies, but this treatment method is still in the experimental stage, and longitudinal growth results are not yet known.[23]

Acquired Limb Absences

Primary Causes and Treatment Principles

TRAUMA

Injuries to children are a major public health problem in North America, and more than 70% of catastrophic injuries resulting in significant morbidity or death are preventable.[184] Trauma is the most common cause of acquired limb amputations in children, with power lawn mowers the main culprit, accounting for 42% of all amputations in children younger than 10 years. The resulting injury is usually extremely severe and very contaminated, making reimplantation impossible. Amputation of a portion of the foot is most commonly seen.[18,73,188] In most cases, the child is riding on the power mower with a parent or grandparent and falls off. Another common cause of traumatic amputation in children is farm machinery accidents.[50,185,187,259,303] A recent report noted successful reimplantation in

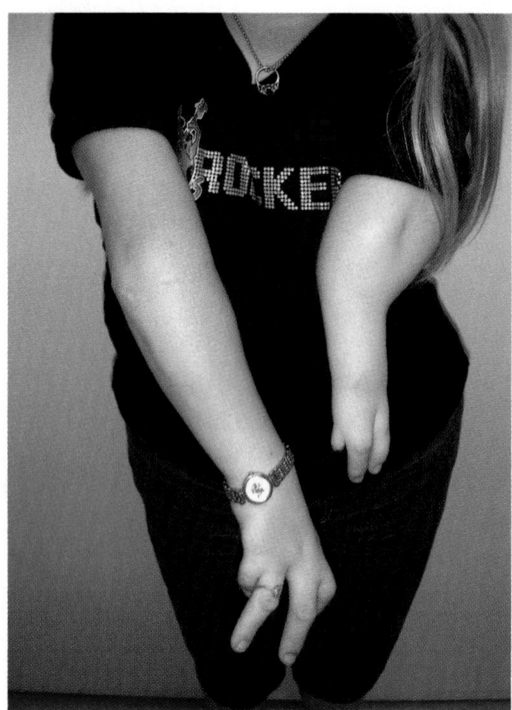

FIGURE 33–58 Bilateral ulnar hemimelia with absence of the ulnar digits.

several farm-related lower extremity amputations and suggested that trauma teams consider this option.[211] Most of these amputations can be prevented with commonsense measures, and orthopaedists should participate in appropriate public education efforts. Loder noted that the ideal time for public awareness campaigns regarding lawn mower safety is March and April, before the peak incidence of injury in June.[196]

Other causes of traumatic amputation include motor vehicle accidents,[70,186,242] gunshot wounds,[302] explosions,[167] and railroad injuries (Fig. 33–59).[281,314,317] Gunshot wounds most commonly involve the fingers and toes. Explosive injuries from fireworks usually cause amputation of the fingers or hands, although higher-level amputations can occur, depending on the power of the explosion. Land-mine explosions in countries previously ravaged by war are a major cause of limb loss in children worldwide.[54,243,301] Males suffer traumatic amputations approximately twice as often as females.[184]

When children require amputation of a severely injured limb, the surgeon must take into account the future growth potential of the child (i.e., the physis), the problem of subsequent overgrowth of the residual limb, the superior healing properties of children (versus adults), and the particular psychosocial issues that affect the rehabilitation of children and adolescents.[72]

In the field, the amputated segment should be wrapped in a sponge slightly moistened with sterile saline, placed in a sterile container (such as a plastic zipper bag) in ice (not dry ice), and transported as soon as possible with the patient to the hospital.[39] These measures improve the chance of a successful reimplantation. The longer the warm ischemic time (the period from injury to initial cooling of the amputated part), the poorer the prognosis for reimplantation.[39] A warm ischemic time longer than 4 hours for a limb and 10 hours for a digit increases the failure rate of reimplantation. In addition, traumatic amputations that are sharp and clean are more successfully reimplanted than those that have crushed or stretched sections. The residual limb is covered with bulky sterile dressings, as are other injured areas. A pressure dressing is used if there is significant bleeding. Clamping or tying vessels or using a tourniquet should be avoided in the field, except as a life-saving measure.

In the hospital emergency department, other surgical specialists (plastic, hand, vascular) should be consulted to deal with particular surgical situations. For medical and legal reasons, photographs should be taken to document the extent of the injury.

All open wounds should be properly debrided and irrigated to minimize the chance of early wound infection. Traumatic amputations should be debrided under tourniquet control. After debridement, the tourniquet is removed and the wound is thoroughly irrigated with sterile normal saline solution or Ringer's lactate solution. Early, aggressive wound *excision* (a term that

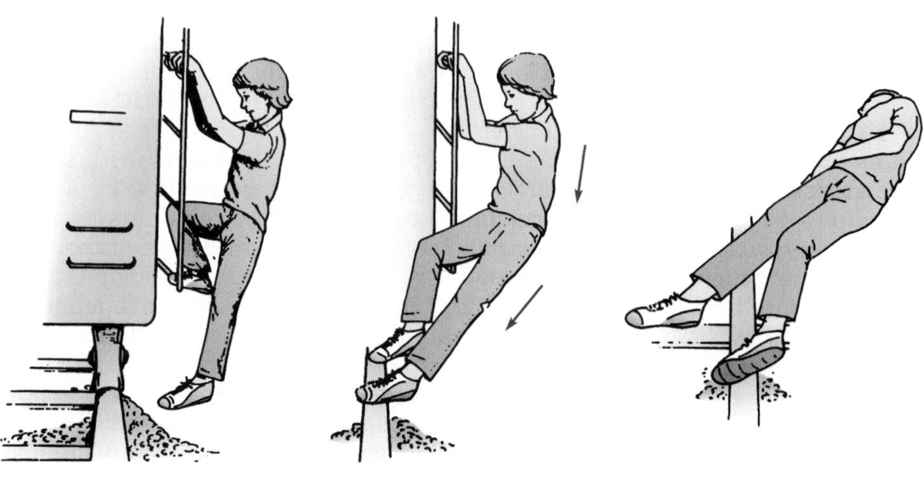

FIGURE 33–59 Mechanism of amputation when a child tries to "hop a freight train." The momentum of the train pulls the legs under the train, often resulting in bilateral amputation. (Redrawn from Thompson GH, Balourdas GM, Marcus RE: Railyard amputations in children. J Pediatr Orthop 1983;3:443.)

some believe should replace *debridement*)[121] and flap coverage within 72 hours of injury result in a significantly lower infection rate compared with delayed reconstruction.[112]

Because of the dynamic healing capabilities of children, more aggressive limb salvage procedures can be attempted than would be feasible in adult patients. The Mangled Extremity Severity Score (MESS) is considered the simplest and most valid method of predicting the success of limb salvage versus amputation (Table 33–6).[68,152] Trials have shown that a MESS score of less than 7 at the time of initial evaluation is highly predictive of successful salvage, whereas a MESS score of 7 or higher indicates the need for amputation.[138,152]

The first priority of the orthopaedist when treating these injuries is to preserve as much limb length as possible, consistent with the appropriate treatment for the particular injury. The epiphysis and growth plate should be maintained whenever possible so that the limb can grow normally, preventing subsequent limb length discrepancies. For example, 80% of femoral growth comes from the distal epiphysis of the femur. Premature loss of that vital growth center in a young child results in a very short femur. To assist in preserving limb length, skin grafts may be used successfully without compromising wound healing or causing subsequent problems with prosthetic management.[6]

It is also important to retain a cartilaginous surface (epiphysis and articular surface) at the distal end of the residual limb to help prevent overgrowth (Fig. 33–60). Traditionally, bony overgrowth has been managed by surgical resection revision.[1,93,159,179,181,262]

Table 33-6 Mangled Extremity Severity Score System

Factor	Score
Skeletal or Soft Tissue Injury	
Low energy (stab, fracture, civilian gunshot wound)	1
Medium energy (open or multiple fracture)	2
High energy (shotgun or military gunshot wound, crush)	3
Very high energy (above plus gross contamination)	4
*Limb Ischemia**	
Pulse reduced or absent but perfusion normal	1
Pulseless, diminished capillary refill	2
Cool, paralyzed, insensate, numb	3
Shock	
Systolic blood pressure always >90 mm Hg	0
Systolic blood pressure transiently <90 mm Hg	1
Systolic blood pressure persistently <90 mm Hg	2
Age (yr)	
<30	0
30-50	1
>50	2

*Double the value if the duration of ischemia is more than 6 hours.

Adapted from Johansen K, Daines M, Howey T, et al: Objective criteria accurately predict amputation following lower extremity trauma. J Trauma 1990;30:568.

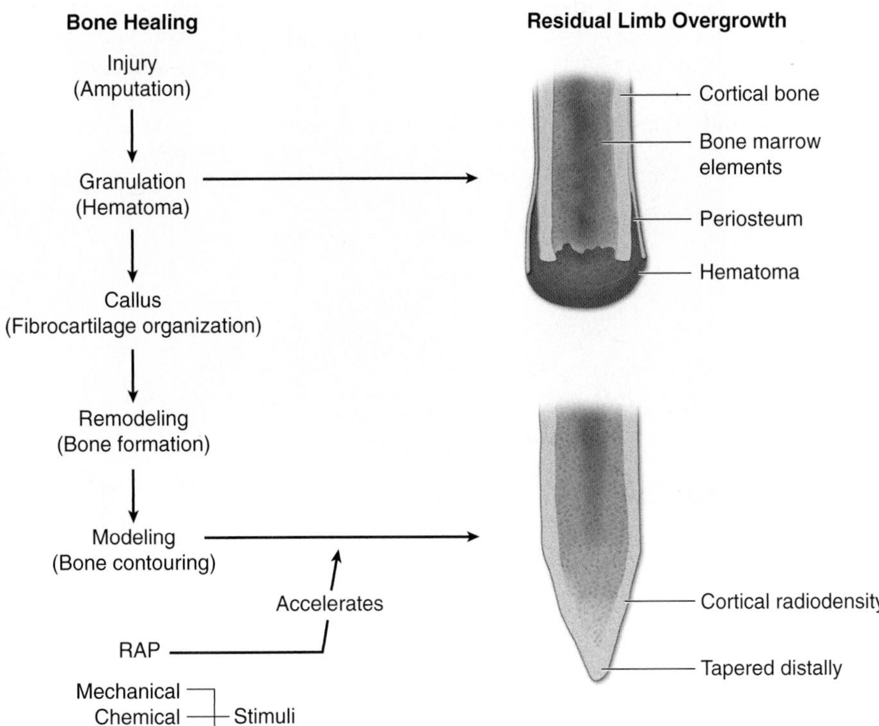

FIGURE 33-60 Mechanism of overgrowth of amputation stumps. RAP, regional acceleratory phenomenon. (Redrawn from Davids JR: Terminal bony overgrowth of the residual limb: Current management strategies. In Herring JA, Birch JG [eds]: The Child with a Limb Deficiency. Rosemont, Ill, American Academy of Orthopaedic Surgeons, 1998.)

Although resection revision is technically simple and can be done quickly, the procedure sacrifices the length of the residual limb, and overgrowth frequently recurs within several years.

To prevent periosteal overgrowth, disarticulation is preferred over a metaphyseal or very short transdiaphyseal amputation in a growing child.[4-6,10] If bony transection is required, prophylactic "biologic capping" (placing a cartilage surface from the amputated segment over the bony stump) may be helpful (Fig. 33–61), particularly in children younger than 12 years.[62]

Based on results from the Ertl procedure, which increases the area of the distal bony surface via a broad synostosis,[221,335] the use of distal tibiofibular synostosis for transdiaphyseal amputations has been reconsidered by some authors (Fig. 33–62).[62,235] The tibia is shortened so that it is 1 to 2 cm proximal to the distal end of the fibula, and a longitudinal osteotomy of the tibia is performed, producing two pillars. A greenstick fracture of the fibula is created, and the distal fibula is displaced medially between the tibial pillars. The fibula is stabilized to the tibia, when necessary, with a nonabsorbable suture. This procedure results in a wide synostosis between the fibula and tibia and creates a biologic cap for the tibia. Early promising outcomes have been reported, but further long-term results are needed to determine the efficacy of this approach.[62]

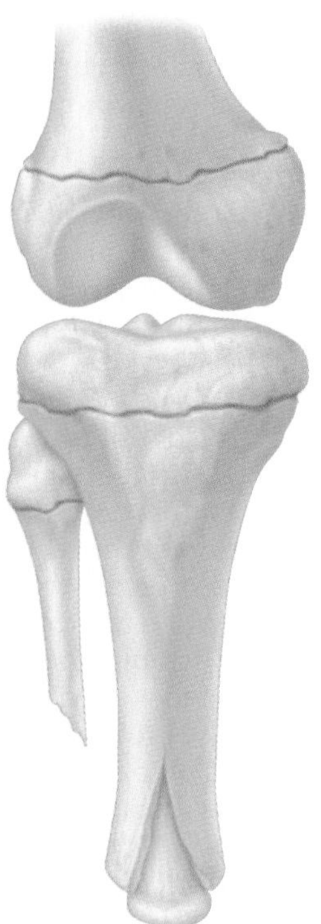

FIGURE 33–61 Use of a bone plug with a cartilage cap to prevent overgrowth of amputation stumps.

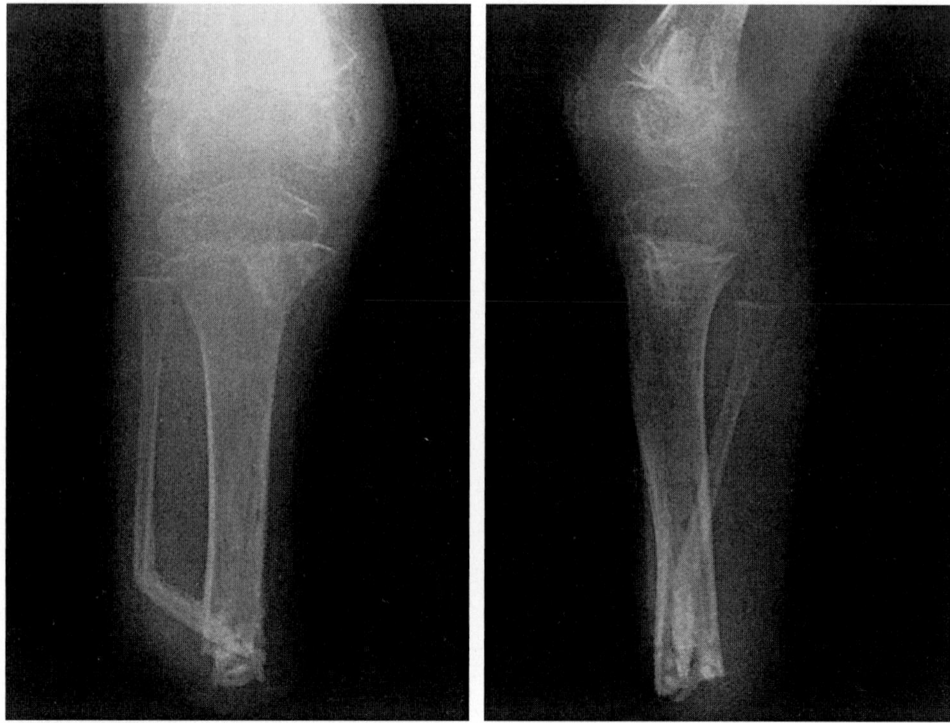

FIGURE 33–62 Ertl procedure to create a distal synostosis between the fibula and tibia. (From Davids JR: Terminal bony overgrowth of the residual limb: Current management strategies. In Herring JA, Birch JG [eds]: The Child with a Limb Deficiency. Rosemont, Ill, American Academy of Orthopaedic Surgeons, 1998.)

When it is possible to maintain the femoral condyles or the distal tibial articular surfaces, full weight bearing is usually possible, even on hard surfaces. In the child's ankle, the medial and lateral malleoli usually are not prominent, and the surgeon should excise them only in patients who are near skeletal maturity when the amputation occurs.[11,93,145]

Traumatic partial foot amputations are commonly seen when children are injured by power lawn mowers. Most children are injured while playing near the lawn mower or when they fall off a riding mower and are run over by the blades.[18,73,188] These amputations are often transverse and are classified based on their level. They can be transmetatarsal, tarsometatarsal (Lisfranc's), or mid-tarsal (Chopart's).

MALIGNANT TUMORS

Malignant musculoskeletal tumors are the second leading cause of acquired amputations in children and adolescents. Surgically, a decision must be made between limb salvage procedures and amputation. The success of chemotherapy in controlling local growth, along with improvements in surgical techniques, has made limb salvage surgery more feasible than in the past.[102] Long-term follow-up comparing the survival of patients treated by limb salvage with the survival of those treated by amputation showed no disadvantage with limb salvage, as long as wide margins were achieved.[265] The authors also found no difference in the psychosocial outcomes in these two patient groups treated for distal femoral tumors. Good functional outcome has been found in both groups as well.[253]

There are a number of specific contraindications to limb salvage. These include the inability to obtain adequate wide excision margins for tumor control, projected significant limb length inequality, an extremely active patient, and inadequate soft tissue coverage. A displaced pathologic fracture may also be a contraindication, although current adjuvant treatments may make limb salvage an acceptable option. In addition, limb salvage should be performed only if the residual limb will be able to function as well as or better than an amputated limb fitted with a well-made prosthesis.[285] Tumors located in the distal two thirds of the tibia are often better treated by amputation than by limb salvage.

Although limb salvage surgery is possible and preferable to amputation when patient survival is not compromised (particularly for upper limbs versus lower limbs), the procedure is complex, and complications often occur. When deciding between limb salvage and amputation, it is critical to remember that the primary goal of surgical treatment is patient survival.

PURPURA FULMINANS

Purpura fulminans, a devastating thromboembolic condition usually caused by meningococcal septicemia, results in high rates of limb gangrene and amputation (Fig. 33–63).[141] Septicemia from other bacteria

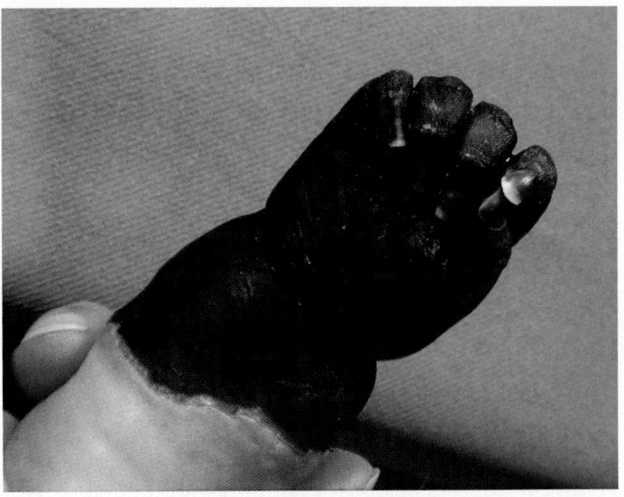

FIGURE 33-63 Necrosis of a hand due to purpura fulminans from meningococcemia.

(e.g., *Haemophilus influenzae*), Kawasaki's disease, toxic shock syndrome, or frostbite may also cause gangrene of the extremities. Intravascular coagulation due to protein S or C deficiency may result in tissue loss.[246] One or all of the upper and lower limbs may be affected. Although purpura fulminans is a devastating, fulminant disease in the acute phase, with good intensive care, almost all patients who survive have no mental impairment and resume age-appropriate development.[347]

The efficacy of surgical intervention in the initial stages of purpura fulminans is controversial. Increased compartment pressures undoubtedly cause additional tissue necrosis, yet the role of fasciotomies is unclear.[64] Additional fluid loss and the increased likelihood of infection from the procedures may increase the overall morbidity of the process. Likewise, the use of tissue plasminogen activator, which may decrease the need for amputation, has been complicated by intracerebral hemorrhage.[354] Early studies with a protein that blocks endotoxin effects (BPI) have shown reduced amputation rates.[189] Artificial skin has been useful in providing coverage for large areas of tissue loss.[118]

These patients frequently have a distinct demarcation of gangrene at the middle of the limb. Vascularized, viable tissue may extend well distal to the proximal edge of the gangrenous skin and subcutaneous tissue eschar. If there is viable muscle and bone beneath the eschar, the surgeon should amputate the limb at the level of deep gangrene, not at the edge of the eschar. This operative approach frequently enables the surgeon to save the patient's knee joint and sometimes the elbow joint. The wound can then be covered with skin grafts, which usually function well, even in weight-bearing areas. Skin grafts and local, regional, and free flaps are used in an appropriate fashion for reconstruction. Skin grafts are used to cover all well-vascularized areas. Extremely well-vascularized tissue is used to cover any exposed bone or joints; local random or pedicled axial subcutaneous or fasciocutaneous flaps are not recommended.[3] Free tissue transfer can be highly beneficial. Microvascular free flaps provide good wound control and have been successfully used to preserve limb length and joints.[3]

Surgical Amputations

UPPER LIMB AMPUTATION

With all upper limb amputations, the surgeon should try to maintain the maximum amount of bone length possible. When small residual carpals and metacarpals are present and successfully lengthened, the patient retains the ability to pinch, a dexterity skill that would otherwise be lost. Periosteal overgrowth is very common after transhumeral amputations and frequently requires multiple surgical revisions. Split-thickness skin grafts are usually adequate for initial coverage, because weight bearing is normally not required of the upper limb.

ABOVE-KNEE AMPUTATION

Some aspects of above-knee amputations are unique to children. The surgeon should retain as long a femoral segment as possible, keeping in mind that there must be sufficient soft tissue coverage at the distal end of the limb. Even extremely short femora should be maintained, because it may be possible to lengthen them in the future.

During the stance phase of gait, the patient's abductor muscles support the rest of the body, and the source of support for the abductors is the femur and its contact with the prosthesis. The longer the femur, the greater its surface contact with the prosthesis. This provides a stable base for abductor function, and the child will have minimal abductor lurch. A child with a short femur and a fatty thigh will ambulate with an abductor limp because the femoral segment is unable to counteract the abduction forces of the abductor muscles.

With transfemoral amputations, the surgeon should shorten the femoral segment just enough so that a muscle flap can be drawn over the distal end. It may be helpful to attach the muscles to the bone. Periosteal bony overgrowth is a common complication after above-knee amputations, particularly in young children, and it may be necessary to perform numerous surgical revisions to correct the problem as the patient matures.

KNEE DISARTICULATION

A knee disarticulation (through-knee amputation) creates a good functional level for pediatric amputees.[197] The distal femoral epiphysis is preserved, bony overgrowth is avoided, a strong femoral lever arm and load-tolerant distal end are maintained, excellent prosthetic suspension and rotational control are provided through the wide femoral condyles and patella (if present), and there is a low energy cost when walking.[245] Children with bilateral disarticulation are usually able to ambulate with full weight bearing at the knees in a prosthesis or when knee-walking.[58]

During amputation, the surgeon should attach the hamstrings to the stump of the cruciate ligaments to provide the patient with better hip extension power.[250] The femur of the amputated limb will grow at a nearly normal rate and will be approximately the same length as the opposite femur, which creates a small problem in the prosthetic management of these patients. Specifically, when the knee mechanism is attached to the prosthesis below the residual limb, the tibial portion of the prosthesis will be shorter than the opposite tibia. To preclude this, the orthopaedist can perform a distal femoral epiphysiodesis several years before the child reaches skeletal maturity so that the femur of the residual limb is 5 to 6 cm shorter than the contralateral femur, thereby providing sufficient room for a prosthesis with a knee.

BELOW-KNEE AMPUTATION

Whenever below-knee amputations are performed, any viable part of the upper tibia should be preserved if the knee joint is intact and soft tissue coverage is possible. Split-thickness skin grafts can be used initially to cover the proximal tibia and can be replaced later with free tissue transfer, if necessary.[174,175] The problem of skin breakdown with prosthetic wear has also been reduced with the availability of new materials and methods for managing sheer forces and pressure within the prosthetic socket.

The Ilizarov and other lengthening techniques have been used successfully to treat extremely short below-knee amputation stumps.[352] These procedures can be difficult for both the surgeon and the patient, but the functional gain achieved from a below-knee amputation compared with a knee disarticulation makes the undertaking well worth the effort (Fig. 33–64). Advantages associated with below-knee amputation include control of the knee, proprioception of knee position, decreased energy expenditure during gait, and less complicated prosthetic devices. For a satisfactory prosthetic fitting, the residual limb should be at least 6 cm long below the knee when the patient is skeletally mature.

Children who undergo below-knee amputations may face some unique problems as they mature. Bony overgrowth of the distal tibia and fibula is common and often requires surgical revision.[7] Recurrent overgrowth of the fibula can be treated by creating a surgical synostosis between the distal fibula and tibia. As the patient gets older, the knee may gradually develop a valgus deformity. This can usually be managed by modifying the prosthesis. Patients may also experience periodic dislocation of the patella, which may be partially associated with the valgus deformity. They can also develop patella alta, which contributes to the instability of the patella.[225] During physical activity, the prosthesis may become twisted, and the medial edge of the prosthesis may cause the patella to dislocate.

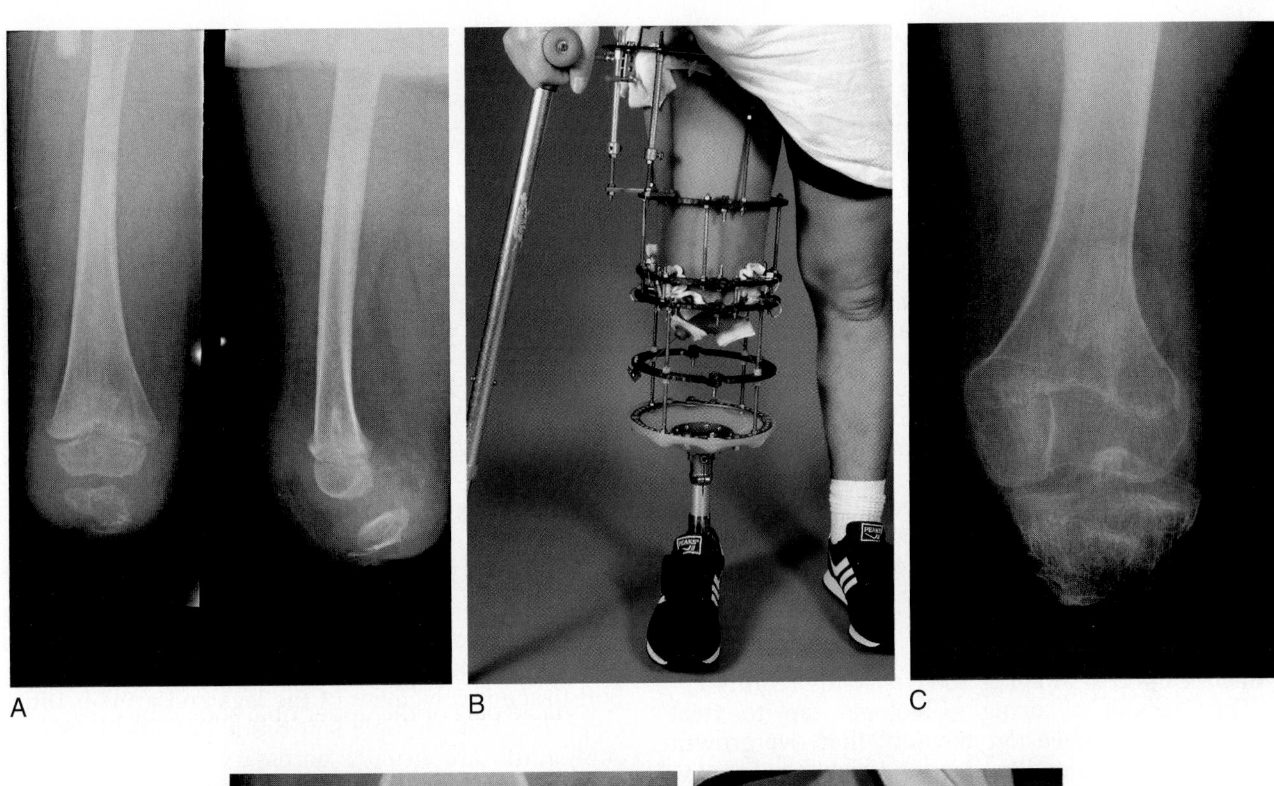

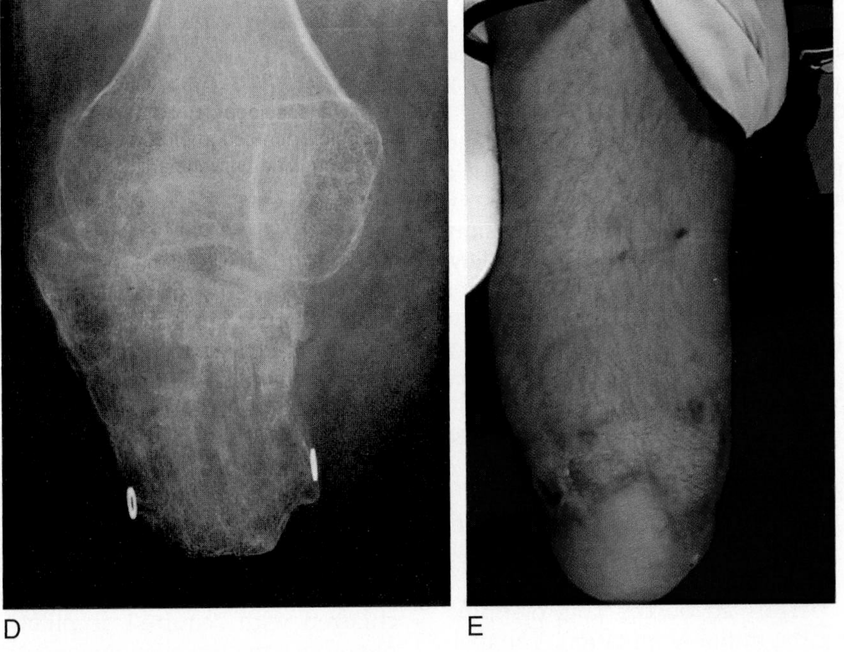

FIGURE 33-64 Boy with a very short residual tibial segment that was lengthened using the Ilizarov device. **A,** Radiograph of the limb with only a proximal tibial epiphysis present. **B,** Patient walking with the lengthening device in place. **C,** Appearance of the limb after the initial lengthening procedure. Because skin coverage was poor, a free flap coverage procedure was performed. **D,** Appearance of the limb after the second lengthening procedure. **E,** Final appearance of the limb. (From Herring JA, Cummings DR: The limb-deficient child. In Morrissy RT, Weinstein SL [eds]: Lovell and Winter's Pediatric Orthopaedics, vol 2, 4th ed. Philadelphia, Lippincott-Raven, 1996.)

Complications

OVERGROWTH AFTER AMPUTATIONS THROUGH LONG BONES

The outcome of amputation through long bone in skeletally immature patients may be compromised by bony overgrowth of the residual limb,[1] which is primarily a consequence of a local biologic phenomenon occurring at the distal portion of the bone.[4,5] The normal wound contracture mechanism may initiate overgrowth by pulling the periosteum into the medullary canal, placing it in contact with the endosteum.[291]

The only stage of normal bone healing unique to children is the modeling phase, which is characterized by the resorption and development of mature lamellar bone, which changes the micro- and macroscopic contours of the bone. The subsequent development of overgrowth is prevented if the medullary canal is occluded with muscle or bone, which impedes the local sealing mechanism of the canal.[16,133]

Overgrowth of bony spicules tends to occur at the distal part of the bone because of periosteal bone formation (not epiphyseal growth), and surgical revision is often necessary to remove the overgrowth. The most common bones in which this occurs are the humerus, fibula, tibia, and femur, in that order.[4,5,291] Over time, a painful bursa develops, and the bone eventually grows through the skin.

Different procedures have been tried to prevent overgrowth—including putting silicone sleeves over the end of the bone or capping the transected bone with autologous cartilage or bone graft—but these attempts have usually failed.[204,215,308] Repeated surgical revisions, sometimes as often as every 2 to 3 years while the child is growing, are frequently required.

The concept of using a biologic cap to treat overgrowth is based on the fact that overgrowth does not occur following disarticulation (see Fig. 33–61).[24,205,206,208] Wang and colleagues and Zaleskey transferred proximal fibular physis or iliac apophysis to the end of the limb to prevent overgrowth, believing that there would be growth of the transferred tissue.[339,353] When it was later recognized that the transfer had little growth potential, Davids and associates used a tricortical iliac crest graft to plug the end of the amputated bone.[63] In a comparison of resection revision, synthetic capping with a high-density polyethylene implant, and biologic capping with an autologous iliac crest bone graft, the authors found that biologic capping was the most efficacious procedure.[63] Subsequently, this group reported successful blocking of overgrowth by capping of the residual limb with a polytetrafluoroethylene felt pad. This procedure increased the time between resection from 3 years 3 months to 7 years 2 months.[313]

A number of authors have recommended a proactive, prophylactic surgical approach for children at risk for overgrowth after an acquired amputation.[22,24,63,206,333] Biologic capping is performed on the tibia or fibula and humerus during the initial amputation. The ipsilateral fibular head, the dome or head of the talus, or the base of the great toe metatarsal can be used as bone graft donor sites.[62]

COMPLICATIONS FOLLOWING BURNS OR PURPURA FULMINANS

If a patient undergoes amputation because of burns or purpura fulminans, the residual limb often is covered with a split-thickness skin graft (Fig. 33–65). These grafts are surprisingly resilient for weight bearing in a prosthesis.[6] With some patients, however, a free tissue transfer must be substituted for the split-thickness skin graft. Free tissue transfers provide excellent coverage of amputated limbs, but they take time to develop protective sensation and may break down if weight bearing is started before this occurs. Soft tissue involvement of the legs and arms is often extensive, and multiple soft tissue debridements and skin grafts are usually necessary for patients who survive the initial onset of meningococcal disease. Meticulous care to maximize limb length and joint function can greatly enhance patient outcome.[3] Neuromas are frequent, owing to extensive loss of overlying skin and subcutaneous tissue.

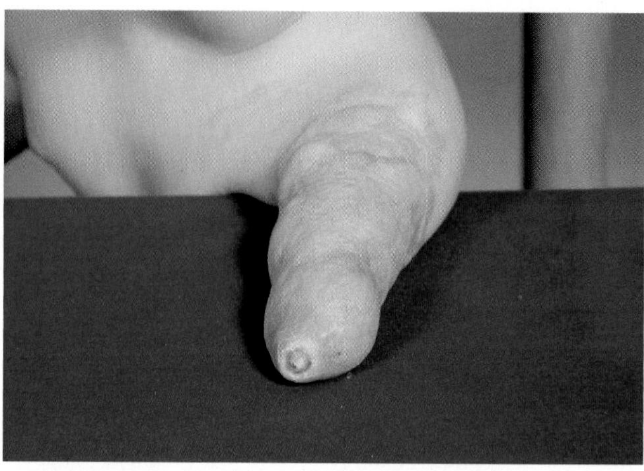

FIGURE 33–65 Limb covered with well-healed split-thickness skin grafts.

IMMEDIATE FITTING OF PROSTHESES IN YOUNG CHILDREN

In young children, immediate fitting of a prosthesis after amputation may be unsafe and can cause wound dehiscence if the child begins full weight bearing prematurely. Because the residual limb rapidly loses size postoperatively, casts tend to fall off. Thus, we elect to use soft elastic bandages to help shape the residual limb after amputation.

PHANTOM PAIN

Phantom pain does not occur in children with congenital limb absences and is uncommon in younger children with acquired amputations. Although older children with acquired amputations may experience phantom pain, the phenomenon usually is not incapacitating. If the condition is painful, the patient can be treated with tactile stimulation, physical therapy, or drug therapy (tricyclic antidepressants such as amitriptyline). The symptoms normally lessen over time. To prevent neuromas from forming, the surgeon should tension the nerves, cut them sharply, and allow them to retract away from the end of the limb during the amputation. Any persistent neuromas may need to be excised and the severed nerve replaced into healthy tissue.

Psychosocial Aspects

Very young children with acquired amputation of one or more limbs because of injury or disease often respond in the same manner as children with congenital limb deficiencies. They experience minimal or no sense of loss, the adjustment period is short, and necessary adaptations are made to meet developmental milestones and participate in activities with their peers. However, older children with acquired amputations experience a sense of loss, and they must be allowed to go through a grieving process as part of the natural course of accepting what has occurred. Limb loss can have a significantly adverse effect on the self-esteem of adolescents.[324,325] A deep-seated wish to be as they were before the amputation may interfere with constructive adaptations.[83] Thus, older children often need more encouragement and positive reinforcement to help them adjust to the reality of their situation. The goals of treatment, as in all limb-deficient patients, are to maximize the individual's functional independence and minimize the psychological impact of the condition.

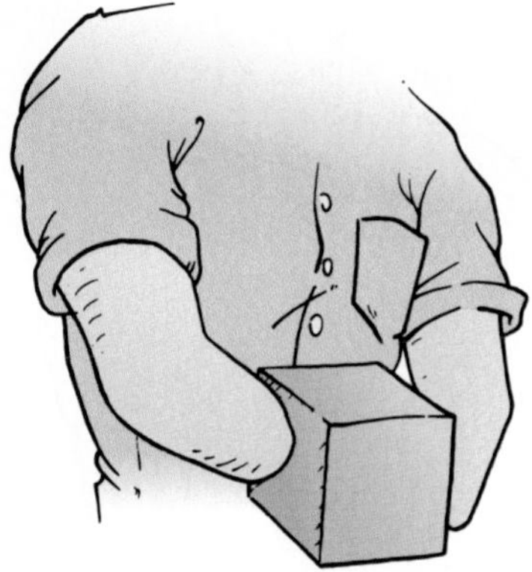

FIGURE 33-66 Children with bilateral below-elbow absences can hold objects very effectively between the two arms. (From Herring JA: Functional assessment and management of multilimb deficiency. In Herring JA, Birch JG [eds]: The Child with a Limb Deficiency. Rosemont, Ill, American Academy of Orthopaedic Surgeons, 1998.)

MULTILIMB DEFICIENCIES

Bilateral Upper Limb Absence

Children who have partial or complete absence of both upper limbs adapt in predictable ways. They may use prostheses at times, but they usually forgo such devices when performing major functional activities, discovering that most of these activities can be better performed using the natural sensory surfaces still available to them.[48] Oddly, it has been found that even though functional need increases as the level of limb absence increases, these patients are the least likely to tolerate prosthetic devices. In most cases, they use the prostheses as tools to assist them in meeting specific functions and then remove them.

There are three primary reasons why children with bilateral upper limb deficiency do not use prostheses.[142] First, the prostheses encase and impede the natural sensory surfaces of the arms. Second, these devices provide only simple and limited functions and are inadequate replacements for the functional sophistication of the hand. Third, and most important, because most of the child's motor and sensory pathways are formed postnatally, they develop the most efficient adaptations for that individual's anatomy. Often the sensory and motor functions of the residual limbs are almost as sophisticated as those of normal hands and arms. Current prosthetic devices cannot improve on these results.

Children with absent hands but mobile wrists use the wrists together for most prehension. Those with bilateral wrist disarticulation have elbows and often movable carpals that have prehensile function. Patients with bilateral below-elbow absence usually function well by using their elbows for prehension and using their residual arms for holding larger objects (Figs. 33–66 and 33–67). Even those with very short forearms have good elbow prehension. The Krukenberg procedure has been recommended for patients with unilateral, long, below-elbow absence[307]; however, we have no personal experience with the procedure.

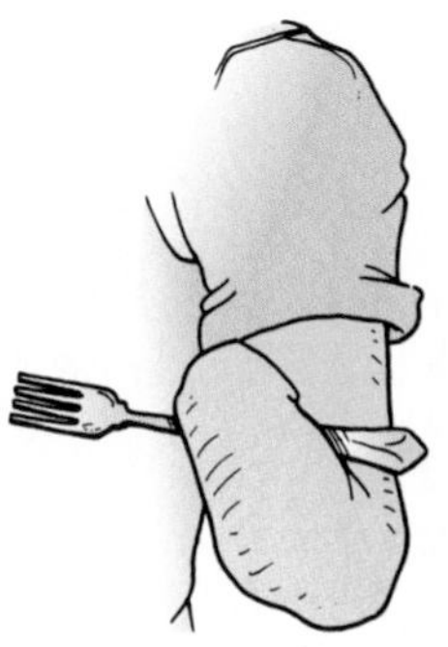

FIGURE 33-67 Children with either unilateral or bilateral below-elbow absences can achieve good prehensile function using the elbow. (From Herring JA: Functional assessment and management of multilimb deficiency. In Herring JA, Birch JG [eds]: The Child with a Limb Deficiency. Rosemont, Ill, American Academy of Orthopaedic Surgeons, 1998.)

Children with bilateral above-elbow absence use the arms together in the midline if the residual limbs are long enough to hold large objects (Fig. 33–68). Children with absence of the limb at the transhumeral level also hold objects against the body with the residual limb, or if the limb is very short, the object may be held against the cheek (Fig. 33–69).

If a child has one limb with a functional elbow and the other limb absent at the distal level of the humerus, the limb with the elbow becomes the dominant extremity. Elbow prehension is used for major functional activities (e.g., writing) and for other fine motor activities, and both limbs are used together (if possible) to maneuver large objects.

If the humeri are extremely short or if there is complete absence of both upper limbs, children usually use their feet to perform most manual and physical activities (Fig. 33–70), including brushing their teeth, writing, and using eating utensils. Most children become adept at using their feet in this manner and are often able to reach just above their heads with their

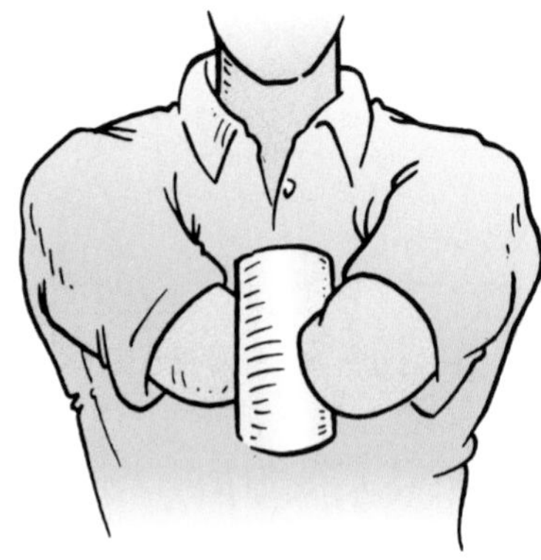

FIGURE 33–68 Children with bilateral above-elbow absences can hold objects with both arms if they are long enough. (From Herring JA: Functional assessment and management of multilimb deficiency. In Herring JA, Birch JG [eds]: The Child with a Limb Deficiency. Rosemont, Ill, American Academy of Orthopaedic Surgeons, 1998.)

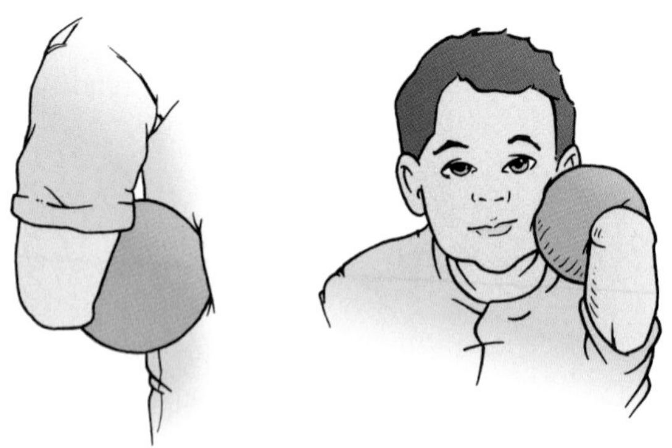

FIGURE 33–69 Children with above-elbow absences use the extremity against the body or face to hold objects or to write. (From Herring JA: Functional assessment and management of multi- limb deficiency. In Herring JA, Birch JG [eds]: The Child with a Limb Deficiency. Rosemont, Ill, American Academy of Orthopaedic Surgeons, 1998.)

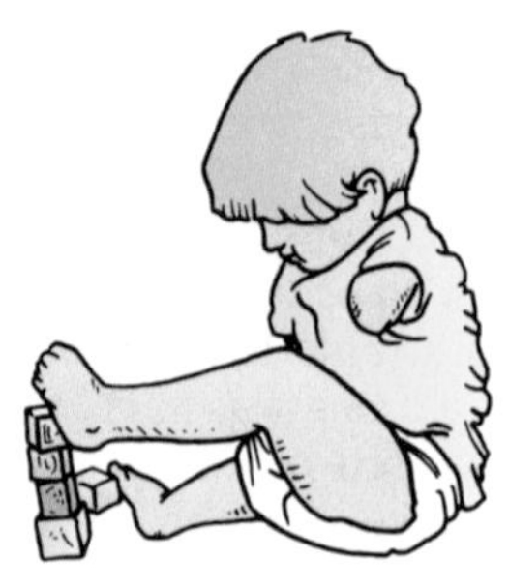

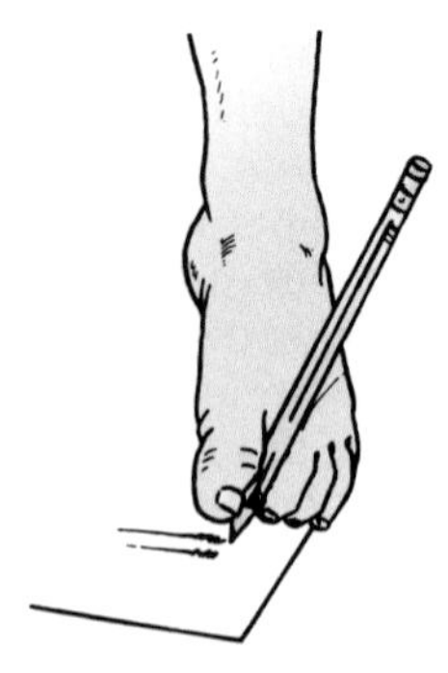

FIGURE 33–70 Children with short or absent upper extremities use the feet for all manual tasks. (From Herring JA: Functional assessment and management of multilimb deficiency. In Herring JA, Birch JG [eds]: The Child with a Limb Deficiency. Rosemont, Ill, American Academy of Orthopaedic Surgeons, 1998.)

feet. Teenagers are able to drive automobiles with automatic shifts. Although toileting can present difficulties, specific bathroom adaptations usually enable the child to overcome these challenges.[94]

For this patient population, prosthetic usage should be viewed as task specific; that is, the devices are worn intermittently, when they can better assist the child with a specific function. Prosthetic choices include body-powered and externally powered devices and hybrid systems that combine body and external power.[48] Hybrid prostheses are often the best option because they are lightweight and allow the patient some degree of proprioceptive feedback via cable-controlled terminal devices or elbows. Components vary depending on the patient's age and developmental status.

Bilateral Lower Limb Absence

Children with bilateral lower limb deficiencies usually try to stand on the ends of the residual limb when they are developmentally ready. If the level of absence is below the knee, prosthetic management is similar to that of patients with unilateral limb deficiencies.[58] However, it may be helpful to make the first pair of prostheses 1 or 2 inches short to assist the child in balancing.

Patients face special problems if the level of the bilateral disarticulation is at the knee. To maintain knee stability after bilateral knee disarticulation, the patient must be able to achieve a strong knee extension at heel strike. Walking on an upward incline or on uneven ground can be challenging. Patients who undergo bilateral above-knee amputations encounter the same compensatory needs and ambulatory difficulties. The child's ability to ambulate depends on the length of the residual limbs. The shorter the limbs, the greater the energy consumption during gait.[340]

In the prosthetic management of these patients, particular attention is paid to a gradual progression in prosthetic height and complexity. The child is first fitted with short, stubby prostheses, which include feet or blocks positioned directly beneath the prosthetic sockets. These prostheses provide the child with a very low center of gravity, which helps him or her to stand. When the child starts to walk, the "stubbies" can be gradually lengthened as needed.[129] In addition, the patient is usually fitted with nonarticulated knees at first; as the child matures, one or both knees may be articulated. Children are often able to function better on the playground with locked knees; however, adolescents usually prefer articulated knees. In these cases, some type of locking knee or stance-phase stabilizer may still be required.

If the limbs are extremely short, walking with full-length legs and articulated knees may be difficult or impossible for the patient. Devices that may enable children to use longer prostheses include manually locking knees, knees with stance-phase braking, polycentric knees, and knee spring-extension assists. Patients with short bilateral above-knee levels may require external support, such as a walker, canes, or crutches, to walk. As bilateral higher-level patients get older, they may opt for wheelchair ambulation, particularly when participating in sports activities, or other means of locomotion.

Bilateral Upper and Lower Limb Absence (Quadrimelic Limb Deficiency)

When a child has bilateral upper and lower limb deficiencies (quadrimelia), the problems are naturally increased. The degree of functional capability depends on the length of the residual limbs. If the level of amputation is below elbow and below knee for all limbs, the child should be able to achieve independent ambulation with the use of lower limb prostheses. For young children, a very short prosthesis ("stubby") is appropriate, whereas for older children, longer prostheses can be used.

If the patient has long above-elbow residual limbs and knee disarticulation or long above-knee limbs, ambulation is usually possible. For young children, very short prostheses are used. As the child matures, longer, nonarticulated devices are employed. The use of articulated knees depends on the patient's level of limb absence and his or her body size and motivation. Some patients choose to stay with nonarticulated prostheses because of the greater stability provided by the rigid knees.

In cases of above-knee amputation of the lower limbs and absent upper limbs, getting up from a seated position is extremely difficult, and using crutches is impossible because the patient lacks forearms to push up with and quadriceps to extend the knees. If the quadrimelic child has below-elbow deficiencies, prosthetic management may be achieved by attaching prosthetic sockets to crutches or a walker. The shorter the upper limbs, the more difficult it is for the child to walk. For these patients, ambulation may be possible only with very short lower limb prostheses.[173] Many of these children choose to use a motorized wheelchair for mobility.

One Upper Limb and One Lower Limb Absence

If the child lacks one upper limb and one lower limb, the deficiencies can usually be managed in the same way as for a single limb absence, with some minor modifications. In some cases, a walking support is needed in conjunction with a lower limb prosthesis. When learning to use the prosthesis, the patient may require a crutch that is specially adapted to the abnormal upper limb or upper limb prosthesis. Many of these patients forgo the use of an upper limb prosthesis, however.

Bilateral Upper Limb and One Lower Limb Absence

Children who lack both upper limbs and also have one deficient lower limb present particularly difficult problems when it comes to managing their lower limbs. Because the lower limb functions as both a hand and a limb for walking, conventional treatments (e.g., amputation for fibular deficiency) are contraindicated. Prosthetic management of the lower limb must maximize function, with the realization that "hand" function takes priority over lower limb function. If both upper limbs and one lower limb are completely absent, the use of a prosthetic leg is extremely difficult because of the lack of support normally provided by the upper limbs. In addition, it is difficult for the patient to remove the prosthesis, because the foot is the only functional "hand." Some of these children use a prosthesis, but others choose to ambulate by hopping on the normal leg.

PROSTHETIC MANAGEMENT

Concepts of Prosthetic Management

GENERAL GUIDELINES

Timing. For children with congenital limb deficiencies, the timing of prosthetic management is usually based on the patient's developmental readiness.[217] Children with upper limb deficiencies are usually fitted with a passive prosthesis when they start to acquire independent sitting balance.[241] Children with lower limb deficiencies are usually fitted when they start trying to stand (normally between 9 and 16 months of age).[30,175,178] Training, prosthetic design, and prosthetic replacement are all matched to the child's developmental state, increasing in complexity as the child matures. A toddler's first transfemoral prosthesis may be nonarticulated or have a lockable knee joint. With proper training, children may be able to use a prosthesis with an articulated knee by 3 to 4 years of age, when they are more physically and intellectually ready to learn how to use it.[233]

Evaluation and Fabrication. During the child's first appointment with the prosthetist, the residual limb is evaluated and measured, and a cast is made. This model is made either by hand casting or with the use of computer-aided design and manufacture equipment.[216] A clear plastic "test" socket is then fabricated over the model and used for the initial evaluation of socket fit. During the patient's next visits, the prosthetist ensures that the prototype socket fits properly and can be adjusted as the child grows. After a suitable socket and suspension system have been made, dynamic alignment of the prosthesis is accomplished. Very young children or recent amputees may require alignment changes over several days, whereas older, more experienced patients may need only a single visit. Final fabrication of the prosthesis occurs after appropriate alignment and design have been determined. Some patients may require additional physical therapy after receiving their prostheses.

Nonstandard Prostheses. A nonstandard prosthesis, often a hybrid between a prosthesis and an orthosis, is used with a limb abnormality that has not been amputated. These prostheses may be used for a variety of reasons, such as when surgical correction of the abnormality has been refused or delayed, during early observation of longitudinal limb deficiencies, or when lower limb abnormalities normally treated by amputation are combined with upper limb deficiencies that require the child to use the feet for hand function.[212] Because of the myriad, diverse anatomic differences among children with congenital deficiencies, many pediatric prostheses can be categorized as "nonstandard."

An equinus, or extension, prosthesis is a common example of a nonstandard prosthesis used for children with congenital deficiencies. To compensate for lower limb length discrepancy, this system incorporates the child's anatomic foot in a position of comfortable equinus above an appropriately aligned prosthetic foot. The socket may be designed similar to an ankle-foot orthosis (AFO), with either an anterior or a posterior opening. If the patient's proximal joints are weak or unstable, the equinus prosthesis may include metal knee joints as well as a plastic thigh cuff. In some cases, ischial weight bearing may be incorporated in the design. An equinus prosthesis enables the prosthetist to make up for significant length discrepancy, avoids the need for a large shoe lift, allows the child to wear conventional shoes and long pants, and enables the child to benefit from the dynamic capabilities of a prosthetic foot.

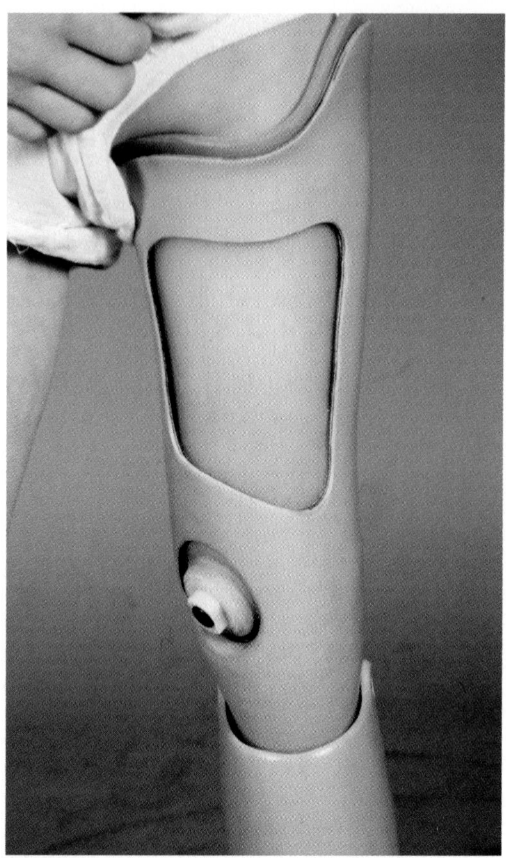

FIGURE 33–71 Open-frame flexible socket for use in amputees when volume changes are anticipated because of chemotherapy or other factors. (From Herring JA, Cummings DR: The limb-deficient child. In Morrissy RT, Weinstein SL [eds]: Lovell and Winter's Pediatric Orthopaedics, vol 2, 4th ed. Philadelphia, Lippincott-Raven, 1996.)

Modifications. As the child grows, the prosthesis may need to be replaced every 12 to 24 months.[83] Growing children are usually examined every 3 to 6 months to ensure that the prosthesis continues to fit and function properly and to make any necessary adjustments. There are some common methods for dealing with changes in the size and length of residual limbs because of growth. Socket liners that allow easy alterations for changes in shape and size can be used. A lower limb prosthesis can initially be fitted over extra socks, which can be removed to accommodate growth. With the use of layered sockets, a thin inner socket can be removed as growth occurs.[101] Removable distal end pads can be replaced with smaller pads as the limb grows. Silicone sockets or other flexible sockets are especially advantageous for patients whose limb volume may fluctuate (Fig. 33–71).[58]

UPPER LIMB PROSTHESES

Children born with partial upper limb deficiencies use the residual portion of the limb, combined with other, often remarkable compensatory strategies, to efficiently meet their functional needs. Because of this adaptation, they often view an upper limb prosthesis as more of an imposition than a benefit. Children with partial transverse amputation of the upper limb generally do not need prostheses for balance, crawling, or achieving other developmental milestones. If they have bilateral involvement (particularly at more proximal levels), the order of gross motor development may be altered in a highly individualized way to meet their unique needs. For example, a child may learn to roll early or develop sitting balance late.[48]

In most cases, a prosthesis is a tool that enables the patient to pinch or grasp an object and then manipulate the object with the intact upper limb. However, the fine manipulative, proprioceptive, and sensory functions of the hand cannot be duplicated by any of today's prostheses, regardless of their sophistication. The reported rejection rate of upper limb myoelectrical prostheses ranges from 0 to 50%.[59,136,180,239,283,344] Often, children (or parents) seek a prosthesis more for cosmetic purposes than for functional needs.

Prosthetic management should correspond to the child's normal developmental milestones.[143] In the past, passive prostheses were fitted when the child had learned to sit independently. In our clinics, we found no benefit from this practice and no longer recommend early fitting. We occasionally fit a passive or active prosthesis in a young child, usually at the parents' request, and the child may use it regularly. The large majority of children, however, prefer not to wear a device and have better function without one. The options include the CAPP (Child Amputee Prosthetic Project, Hosmer, Campbell, Calif) terminal device, body-powered hooks and hands, and cosmetic and myoelectrical hands. School-age children and adolescents often ask for prostheses for specific purposes, such as playing volleyball, riding a bicycle, appearing in a drama, playing the tuba, or performing gymnastic routines. We make every effort to fulfill the request with either an existing device or an improvised one.

Children with below-elbow absences learn to use the elbow for prehensile activities and usually have little functional need for a prosthesis, although they may use one for specific purposes or occasions. Myoelectrical hands are popular because of their "natural" appearance and because they minimize or eliminate harnessing.[148,276] Children as young as age 3 years can be taught to control a hand with a two-site electrode system.[20] With the availability of newer, smaller hands and single-site electrode control systems, some centers have begun training children as young as 20 months of age to use myoelectrical prostheses, and other centers report success in patients as young as 12 to 18 months.[61,276] Cable-operated (or body-powered) hooks can be fitted as soon as the child is amenable to training, which is generally around 24 months. Among these, the CAPP terminal device, which allows for easy visual control, can be adapted specifically for young children. Voluntary opening, as well as voluntary closing, hook terminal devices are the most functional because of their durability, simplicity, and provision of a clear view of the object. However, because of poor grip and high operating forces, voluntary opening cable-operated hands are not appropriate for young children with limb deficiencies.

There are numerous combinations of prosthetic components available for patients with above-elbow limb absences. A passive friction elbow that can be positioned with the other hand is often used first. Later, a body-powered myoelectrical or switch-activated elbow may be tried.[148,276] These complex devices may not be used at all by children with congenital absence of the upper limb because they find it easier to function with their residual limb (or, in the case of bilateral upper limb deficiency, with their feet).[56] With shoulder disarticulation prostheses, the child may not have the excursion or strength needed for a body-powered elbow. For such levels, electrical elbows, combined with body-powered or electrical terminal devices, may be used, but they are seldom used successfully on a long-term basis.

LOWER LIMB PROSTHESES

Because many children with lower limb deficiencies are active and healthy, they can place extreme demands on their prostheses, wearing them out or destroying them during play or sports activities. In addition, as children grow, the close fit of the socket is lost, and periodic adjustments are needed to keep the prosthesis functioning properly. The prosthesis may need to be lengthened every 6 months, and children often outgrow the socket in a year. Thus, prostheses must fit snugly but be easily modified to accommodate growth, be lightweight yet strong, and be durable but reasonably cosmetic. Adolescents often prefer soft, cosmetic covers over modular endoskeletal components, while others prefer to wear exposed components with no cover at all. Still others request patterns, cartoon characters, or other self-expressive designs on their prosthetic covers.

There are a number of different types of prosthetic feet that can be used with lower limb prostheses. The solid ankle-cushioned heel prosthesis is often used with younger children. Older children and adolescents may prefer dynamic-response feet that have a flexible keel, aid propulsion, and enhance the person's running skills and athletic performance. Although multiple-axis ankles are available, they are not recommended for young children because of their complexity, added weight, and lack of durability.

The gait of a person with a lower limb prosthesis is asymmetric, with the degree of asymmetry directly related to the level of the deficiency—the higher the level of loss, the greater the asymmetry.[76] The gait of below-knee amputees is characterized by a longer double-limb support time on the prosthetic side, a longer stance phase on the nonprosthetic side, significantly greater limb loading on the nonprosthetic side, and dominance of the nonprosthetic limb during the gait cycle.[76] With above-knee amputees, comfortable walking speed is reduced, the swing phase is longer on the prosthetic side, energy consumption is greater than in able-bodied subjects, and there is no specific relationship between prosthetic socket design and energy expenditure.[31] Age, general health, fitness, and activity level all play a role in the gait characteristics of amputees.[134] Some of the primary problems associated with gait abnormalities in children who require lower limb prostheses are increased energy expenditure, "whips" (see below), lateral bending of the trunk, excessive adduction of the prosthesis, vaulting, and circumduction.[15,33,252,270]

Increased energy expenditure is seen whenever there is an abnormal gait. It has been estimated that below-knee amputees expend about 60% more energy and above-knee amputees about 100% more energy than normal at comfortable walking speed.[57] In normal subjects, energy expenditure during walking is reduced by minimal excursion of the center of gravity, control of momentum, and the active transfer of energy between limb segments. In amputees, the center of gravity excursion can be minimized by a well-fitted prosthesis, and control over momentum can be maximized by good muscle strength and control of the residual limb. However, transfer of energy between segments of the lower limb prosthesis is not the same as energy transfer in a normal limb.[108,134,273] As a result, amputees expend more energy to walk or run than do able-bodied children.

A whip is a gait abnormality seen during the swing phase in patients with above-knee prostheses. Usually, it is caused by malorientation of the axis of the knee relative to the line of progression. The prosthetic knee is normally rotated externally by 2 to 5 degrees. If the knee axis is excessively rotated internally, the prosthetic shank and foot whip laterally; if the knee is excessively rotated laterally, there is a medial whip. The direction of the whip is always in the opposite direction of the malrotation of the prosthetic knee. The physician can best observe these swing-phase whips from behind during the beginning of the swing phase on the prosthetic side. Whips may also be caused by poor socket fit (either too loose or too tight), or they may develop as the residual limb outgrows the socket. Whips can usually be corrected through prosthetic adjustment or gait training. Exceptions are whips due to hip joint pathology, congenital deformities, or muscular abnormalities.

Lateral trunk bending to the prosthetic side during the stance phase (Trendelenburg lurch) usually occurs when the prosthesis (above- or below-knee) is too short, a situation that can be corrected by simply lengthening the prosthesis. With transfemoral amputees, lateral bending of the trunk may also occur if the lateral socket wall does not comfortably or adequately stabilize the shaft of the femur, if there is excessive pressure on the distal end of the femur, or if there is excess tissue bulging over the upper medial edge of the socket. Patients with weak hip abductors, an unstable hip, or an extremely short residual femoral segment (resulting in a decrease in lateral stabilization) may need to compensate by leaning laterally over the prosthesis. By leaning the trunk laterally, body weight is shifted over the prosthesis, the hip abductors are required to do less work, lateral forces against the femur are minimized, and the patient is better able to balance over the prosthesis. A proper transfemoral amputation (including myodesis of the adductors to maintain anatomic alignment of the femur) may play a greater role in the amputee's ability to stabilize the femur in the prosthesis than the actual design of the socket.[115] If the child has a short residual limb or weak abductors, additional support and stability can be provided by adding a pelvic band and hip joint to the prosthesis.

Excessive adduction of the prosthesis is usually due to developmental changes rather than incorrect prosthetic alignment.[129] When children start to walk, they tend to have a wide-based gait with flexed hips and knees. As the child matures, the base becomes narrower. Thus, a prosthesis fitted before or at the beginning of a child's walking stage will become improperly aligned as the child's gait changes. Because of this, a young child's first prostheses should be changed sooner than subsequent ones.

Vaulting on the normal limb or circumduction of the prosthesis can be seen in children who develop compensatory habits as they learn to use a prosthesis. This is particularly true with new prostheses or above-knee prostheses with knee joint mechanisms. Children quickly adapt their gait patterns to accommodate the prosthesis, often with little regard for gait appearance. Vaulting is characterized by the child's rising on the toe of the normal foot to permit him or her to swing the prosthesis through with minimal knee flexion. In a circumducted gait, there is a swinging of the prosthesis laterally in a wide arc during the swing phase. Vaulting and circumduction may develop because the prosthesis is too long or there is limited knee flexion, the child has an abduction contracture of the residual limb, or the child is afraid to flex the prosthetic knee because of muscle weakness or fear of falling.[134] Physical therapy may be helpful in correcting undesirable gait pattern habits.

GUIDELINES FOR REPLACING PROSTHESES

Prostheses need to be replaced when they wear out—a common occurrence with lower limb prostheses used by active children. Other less obvious indications for replacement include the following: (1) continued prosthetic adjustments cannot reestablish a satisfactory socket fit, (2) weight-bearing surfaces or relief areas in the socket do not conform to the child's anatomy, (3) the patient's weight or activity level is approaching or greater than the maximum values specified for the prosthetic components, (4) developmental changes in gait or posture cannot be accommodated by the prosthesis, and (5) the prosthesis cannot accommodate angular changes of the limb.

Prosthetic Management of Specific Deficiencies

PROXIMAL FOCAL FEMORAL DEFICIENCY

There are a number of prosthetic management options for patients with PFFDs. The first is to do no surgery and simply provide the child with a prosthesis. This approach addresses the common problem of a weak, unstable hip and an extremely proximal knee and foot. The prosthetic socket usually provides the patient with ischial or gluteal weight bearing to offset the piston action of the unstable hip. The knee is normally included in the socket, and the foot is positioned in equinus (mainly for cosmetic purposes). The prosthesis may be suspended by a heel strap or waist belt. As the child matures and approaches adolescence, the limb discrepancy may be great enough to allow for a prosthetic knee joint below the foot. If the discrepancy is not so severe, the child may simply be fitted with an extension prosthesis, with a prosthetic foot placed below the plantar flexed foot. When they are not wearing their prostheses, most children can tolerate walking in equinus on the affected limb.

Another option is the conventional fitting of a Syme's prosthesis following a Syme's amputation. This is appropriate when the femoral segment is long enough to permit the knee to function. The patient usually can bear weight distally, and the prosthesis can be self-suspended over the prominent malleoli. This allows for a good gait, but the patient may have a Trendelenburg lurch if there is an abnormal hip or a short femoral neck. One drawback to this management approach is that a relatively long prosthesis and high knee joint are required because the affected femoral segment is markedly shorter than the contralateral femur and the knee joint is more proximal. Maintaining the anatomic knee provides the child with better function, but the poor cosmesis of the long prosthesis becomes more evident as the child reaches adult proportions.

When a Syme's amputation is combined with knee fusion, a single, straight lever arm is created so that an "above-knee" prosthesis can be fitted and hip flexion contracture can be eliminated or reduced.[162,163] The prosthesis can be fitted when the wound is healed and the patient is developmentally ready to use a prosthesis. To counteract pistoning of the unstable hip, the prosthetic socket usually provides ischial or gluteal weight bearing or containment. In most cases, the prosthesis is suspended by a waist belt for younger children; however, if the malleoli and heel pad are sufficiently bulbous, they may be able to "self-suspend" the prosthesis. Self-suspension can also be achieved by using an expandable inner "bladder" secured above the malleoli that permits the flared distal portion of the limb to pass in or out of the prosthesis.[310] Another approach is to position a compressible suspension pad directly over the residual limb distally. When it is time to add a prosthetic knee joint to the prosthesis, a polycentric "knee-disarticulation" four-bar knee provides good stability and cosmetic appearance.

After a van Nes rotationplasty, the prosthesis typically accommodates the foot in a comfortable equinus position within the socket. Weight bearing is on the plantar (now anterior) part of the foot and calcaneus.[29] Room is provided distally for growth of the toes, and a removable socket liner is fitted between the limb and the prosthesis. Mediolateral stability of the ankle is achieved by extending single-axis joints from the socket up to a rigid, bivalved shell or a leather or plastic cuff around the patient's thigh. If the patient's hip is unstable, the thigh portion of the prosthesis is extended proximally to provide ischial-gluteal weight bearing. If the hip is stable, weight bearing may be through the foot rather than the ischium. A heel strap or waist belt is usually used to suspend the prosthesis. Specific components and alignment are individualized based on the particular needs of the patient. In most cases, it is not possible to achieve a normal gait; the deficient hip joint and musculature usually cause the patient to have a Trendelenburg gait. The degree of functional "knee" control depends on the strength, range of motion, and correct orientation of the rotated ankle.

FIBULAR DEFICIENCY

Prosthetic management following amputation is relatively easy because the limb takes on a cylindrical shape, with only mild enlargement of the distal portion of the leg. Even though the lateral malleolus is usually absent after ankle disarticulation, the child is often capable of full weight bearing on the heel pad. The prosthesis consists of a firm distal pad for protection, combined with a total-contact patellar tendon-bearing socket. If there is anterior tibial bowing, special padding or relief in the socket may be necessary. Soft liners and foam shell designs have eliminated the need for a window in the prosthesis.

The length discrepancy associated with fibular hemimelia often allows for more space in the prosthesis distal to the residual limb in which to place a prosthetic foot, and the prosthetist is not limited to feet specifically designed for a Syme's amputee. For a child who is just beginning to ambulate, the prosthesis usually must be suspended by a cuff above the femoral condyles, a waist belt, or a neoprene sleeve. After the second or third prosthesis, many children are able to keep the device on by actively contracting the heel pad against the contoured inner wall of the socket. Self-suspension may also be attained by using pads or an expandable inner socket liner.[58] The proximal brim of the socket should extend high on each side of the knee to provide rotational control and some mediolateral stability. If knee valgus is present, the prosthesis can be adjusted to allow for medial displacement of the prosthetic foot.

TIBIAL DEFICIENCY

Prosthetic management depends on the type of surgery performed. For a Jones type 2 deformity, in which the proximal tibia has been fused to the upper tibia and a Syme's amputation has been performed distally, a conventional Syme's prosthesis is appropriate. This is also true for a Jones type 4 deformity treated with a modified Syme's ankle disarticulation. If the child's knee is stable and there is good hamstring and quadriceps function, joints and thigh corsets are not necessary.

After a knee disarticulation for complete tibial hemimelia, the patient is fitted with an end-bearing above-knee prosthesis when he or she first attempts to walk. With the first prosthesis, the knee joint usually has a manual lock or is nonarticulated. When the child is approximately 3 years of age, he or she can usually manage well with an articulated knee and should eventually be able to perform at a normal activity level, including running.[198]

For complete tibial hemimelia in which a Brown procedure has been performed (i.e., centralization of the fibula combined with a Syme's amputation), a below-knee prosthesis with knee joints and a thigh corset is used to provide mediolateral knee stability. Prosthetic management is difficult with these patients, however, because the knee is usually extremely unstable (often lacking quadriceps function) and there is a tendency toward progressive knee flexion contracture.

FOOT DEFICIENCY

The prosthetic management of foot deficiencies is generally simple and depends on the degree of congenital deficiency. Some patients may need only a padded toe-filler device to preclude shoe distortion; alternatively, a slipper-type prosthesis (a modified plastic shoe insert) may work well. These systems provide excellent cosmesis and are less restrictive than an AFO. Adequate padding combined with frequent modifications for growth should prevent pressure problems over rudimentary toes. If the residual foot is not long enough to suspend a prosthesis, the child can be fitted with a modified AFO with a partial prosthetic foot. Patients with congenital partial foot deficiencies usually do not have problems with equinus deformity.

FOOT AMPUTATION

The prosthetic management of foot amputations is similar to that for congenital partial foot absence. A patient with a transmetatarsal amputation may need only a toe-filler device. In some cases, however, it may be necessary to use a modified AFO during the early postoperative period to prevent an equinus contracture. Adding a padded cosmetic toe-filler to a polypropylene AFO affords the patient maximum ankle stability, good rotational control, and an extended toe "lever arm." If there is no tendency toward contracture, a less restrictive, flexible, slipper-style prosthesis may be fitted a year or so later. If periosteal overgrowth occurs, the orthopaedist may need to perform revision surgery to excise the sharp ends of the metatarsals. However, this problem may be averted if biologic capping is performed during the initial amputation.[62] Patients with tarsometatarsal and midtarsal amputations function well with a slipper-type prosthesis. After a tarsometatarsal amputation, the foot usually remains in a neutral position if the tibialis anterior and toe extensor tendons are sutured to the talus at the time of the amputation to offset the pull of the Achilles tendon.

AMPUTATION FOR MALIGNANT TUMOR

The prosthetic management of patients who have undergone amputations because of malignancy is often dramatically different from that of patients with traumatic amputations and is influenced by a number of unique factors. Children with malignancies frequently must be fitted with a prosthesis while they are dealing with the emotional trauma of a life-threatening illness and the physical distress caused by chemotherapy and radiation therapy.

Because the child's life span may be attenuated, periods of medical intervention should be minimized, and the child should be mobilized as rapidly as possible. It is important to fit the child with a prosthesis early on to improve his or her body image, keeping in mind that the residual limb will change quickly in size and shape. As the residual limb is maturing, a temporary, easily replaced prosthesis or socket should be used. When patients are receiving chemotherapy, they frequently experience intermittent periods of weight loss that affect the fit of a prosthesis. If changes in limb volume are anticipated, a socket that can be adapted to accommodate these fluctuations should be used (e.g., a flexible above-knee socket with a windowed outer frame or some other mechanism for adjusting for volumetric changes). If the child has multiple tumor sites, prosthetic management may be even more difficult (e.g., the child may not be able to use crutches effectively if he or she has a secondary tumor in the upper limb).

ABOVE-KNEE AMPUTATION

The most commonly used sockets for above-knee prostheses are the quadrilateral socket and the newer ischial containment socket.[199,248,251,267] Ischial containment sockets may provide more control in younger patients without creating uncomfortable pressure as the child grows. This socket may also be preferred by active persons.[277]

For young children, a transfemoral prosthesis is most often suspended by a Silesian belt or a total elastic suspension belt.[278] In most cases, suction suspension should be reserved for patients 6 years or older.[315] If the patient has an extremely short residual limb, weak abductor muscles, or an unstable or painful hip or is obese, the prosthesis may be suspended by a hip joint with a pelvic band and belt.[116] A variety of prosthetic knees are now available for children, including manual locking knees, constant-friction knees, stance-control or weight-activated friction knees, polycentric or four-bar knees, and fluid-controlled knees.[216,218]

KNEE DISARTICULATION

A variety of prosthetic sockets and knee mechanisms have been specifically designed to take advantage of the supracondylar suspension capacity, long lever arm, and end weight-bearing tolerance provided by through-knee amputations.[149] Socket design is often determined by the amount of distal weight bearing the patient can tolerate and the size of the femoral condyles relative to the thigh. If the distal femur is underdeveloped and unable to provide adequate prosthetic suspension, the prosthesis may need to be suspended by suction or by a Silesian or total elastic suspension belt. Almost any knee mechanism can be used with a knee disarticulation prosthesis, but because of the long femoral segment, only a few specifically designed polycentric knees enable the prosthetist to match the knee centers. The choice should be based on the individual patient's goals and needs. If an epiphysiodesis is performed to provide room for the knee, 3 cm should be sufficient for a polycentric knee, and 6 cm can accommodate practically any knee.[229]

BELOW-KNEE AMPUTATION

Socket designs for below-knee prostheses employ some degree of patellar tendon weight bearing, with additional support through the medial flare of the tibia and through total contact. This relieves pressure on the anterior distal tibia and the fibular head. If additional mediolateral stability of the knee is required, the supracondylar design may be used; however, if the collateral ligaments are damaged or absent, greater stability is provided by joints and a thigh corset. Suspension straps are used with young children who have not started walking and are later replaced with the PTS (Portable Technology Solutions, Calverton, New York) socket or with neoprene sleeves. Silicone suspension methods not only suspend the prosthesis but also reduce shear along the socket interface. The most common silicone below-knee device is a pliable silicone sleeve with a ribbed stainless steel pin protruding distally from the sleeve. Silicone suction systems provide excellent suspension and minimize shear as well as up-and-down pistoning of the prosthesis. Replaceable, soft distal pads are used to accommodate longitudinal growth and protect against bony overgrowth.[58] Relative contraindications to silicone suction include fluctuating limb volume, bony overgrowth, neuroma, significant adhesive scar tissue, long residual limb (such as with a Syme's amputation), frequent kneeling or crawling, and physical or mental inability to operate the lock mechanism.[81]

References

1. Abraham E, Pellicore RJ, Hamilton RC, et al: Stump overgrowth in juvenile amputees. J Pediatr Orthop 1986;6:66.
2. Achterman C, Kalamchi A: Congenital deficiency of the fibula. J Bone Joint Surg Br 1979;61:133.
3. Adams W, Hobar P: Surgical treatment of meningococcal-induced purpura fulminans. In Herring JA, Birch JG (eds): The Child with a Limb Deficiency. Rosemont, Ill, American Academy of Orthopaedic Surgeons, 1998, p 447.
4. Aitken G: Overgrowth of the amputation stump. J Assoc Child Prosthet Orthot Clin 1962;1:1.
5. Aitken G: Overgrowth of the amputation stump. Interclin Information Bull 1962;1:1.
6. Aitken G: Surgical amputation in children. J Bone Joint Surg Am 1963;45:1735.
7. Aitken G: Osseous overgrowth in amputations in children. In Swinyard C (ed): Limb Development and Deformity: Problems of Evaluation and Rehabilitation. Springfield, Ill, Charles C Thomas, 1969.
8. Aitken G: Proximal femoral focal deficiency: A congenital anomaly. In Aitken GT (ed): A Symposium on Proximal Femoral Focal Deficiency: A Congental Anomaly. Washington, DC, National Academy of Sciences, 1969, p 1.
9. Aitken G: Tibial hemimelia. In A Symposium on Selected Lower Limb Anomalies: Surgical and Prosthetic Management. Washington, DC, National Academy of Sciences, 1971.
10. Aitken GT: The child amputee: An overview. Orthop Clin North Am 1972;3:447.
11. Aitken GT, Frantz CH: Management of the child amputee. Instr Course Lect 1960;17:246.
12. Alman BA, Krajbich JI, Hubbard S: Proximal femoral focal deficiency: Results of rotationplasty and Syme amputation. J Bone Joint Surg Am 1995;77:1876.
13. Amstutz H: The morphology, natural history, and treatment of proximal femoral focal deficieincy. In Aitken G (ed): A Symposium on Proximal Femoral Focal Deficiency: A Congenital Anomaly. Washington, DC, National Academy of Sciences, 1969, p 50.
14. Amstutz H: Histiocytosis X: Natural history and treatment of congenital absence of the fibula [abstract]. J Bone Joint Surg Am 1972;54:1349.
15. Anderson M, Bray J, Hennessy C: Prosthetic Principles: Above Knee Amputations. Springfield, Ill, Charles C Thomas, 1960.
16. Anderson M, Green W, Messner M: The classic: Growth and predictions of growth in the lower extremities. Clin Orthop Relat Res 1978;136:7.
17. Anderson M, Green WT, Messner MB: Growth and predictions of growth in the lower extremities. Am J Orthop 1963;45-A:1.
18. Anger DM, Ledbetter BR, Stasikelis PJ, et al: Injuries of the foot related to the use of lawn mowers. J Bone Joint Surg Am 1995;77:719.
19. Barna M, Hawe N, Niswander L, et al: Plzf regulates limb and axial skeletal patterning. Nat Genet 2000; 25:166.
20. Baron E, Clarke S, Solomon C: The two stage myoelectric hand for children and young adults. Orthot Prosthet 1983;37:11.
21. Bavinck JN, Weaver DD: Subclavian artery supply disruption sequence: Hypothesis of a vascular etiology for Poland, Klippel-Feil, and Mobius anomalies. Am J Med Genet 1986;23:903.
22. Benevenia J, Makley JT, Leeson MC, et al: Primary epiphyseal transplants and bone overgrowth in childhood amputations. J Pediatr Orthop 1992;12:746.
23. Bennett J, Riordan D: Ulnar hemimelia. In Herring JA, Birch JG (eds): The Child with a Limb Deficiency. Rosemont, Ill, American Academy of Orthopaedic Surgeons, 1998, p 387.
24. Bernd L, Blasius K, Lukoschek M, Lucke R: The autologous stump plasty: Treatment for bony overgrowth in juvenile amputees. J Bone Joint Surg Br 1991;73:203.
25. Birch J, Lincoln T, Mack P: Functional classification of fibular deficiency. In Herring JA, Birch JG (eds): The Child with a Limb Deficiency. Rosemont, Ill, American Academy of Orthopaedic Surgeons, 1998, p 161.
26. Birch JG, Walsh SJ, Small JM, et al: Syme amputation for the treatment of fibular deficiency: An evaluation of long-term physical and psychological functional status. J Bone Joint Surg Am 1999;81:1511.
27. Blanco JS, Herring J: Congenital Chopart amputation: A functional assessment. J Assoc Child Prosthet Orthot Clin 1989;24:27.
28. Boakes JL, Stevens PM, Moseley RF: Treatment of genu valgus deformity in congenital absence of the fibula. J Pediatr Orthop 1991;11:721.
29. Bochmann D: Prosthetic devices for the management of proximal femoral focal deficiency. Orthot Prosthet 1980;12:4.
30. Bochmann D: Prostheses for the limb-deficient child. In Kostuik J, Gillespie R (eds): Amputation Surgery and Rehabilitation: The Toronto Experience. New York, Churchill Livingstone, 1981, p 293.
31. Boonstra AM, Schrama J, Fidler V, et al: The gait of unilateral transfemoral amputees. Scand J Rehabil Med 1994;26:217.
32. Borggreve J: Kniegelenkseratz durch das in der Beilangsachse um 180 degree gedrehte Fussgelenk. Arch Orthop 1930;28:175.
33. Bowker J, Michael J: Atlas of Limb Prosthetics: Surgical, Prosthetic, and Rehabilitation Principles, 2nd ed. St. Louis, Mosby-Year Book, 1992.

34. Brown F, Pohnert W: Construction of a knee joint in meromelia tibia (congenital absence of the tibia): A 15-year followup study. J Bone Joint Surg Am 1972;54: 1333.
35. Brown FW: Construction of a knee joint in congenital total absence of the tibia (paraxial hemimelia tibia): A preliminary report. J Bone Joint Surg Am 1965;47:695.
36. Brown K: Rotationplasty with hip stabilization in congenital femoral deficiency. In Herring JA, Birch JG (eds): The Child with a Limb Deficiency. Rosemont, Ill, American Academy of Orthopaedic Surgeons, 1998, p 103.
37. Brown KL: Resection, rotationplasty, and femoropelvic arthrodesis in severe congenital femoral deficiency: A report of the surgical technique and three cases. J Bone Joint Surg Am 2001;83:78.
38. Buck-Gramcko D: The role of nonvascularized toe phalanx transplantation. Hand Clin 1990;6:643.
39. Buncke H: Microsurgery: Transplantation-Replantation: An Atlas-Text. Philadelphia, Lea & Febiger, 1991.
40. Caskey PM, Lester EL: Association of fibular hemimelia and clubfoot. J Pediatr Orthop 2002;22:522.
41. Catagni M: Mangement of fibular hemimelia using the Ilizarov method. Inst Course Lect 1992;61:431.
42. Chestnut R, James HE, Jones KL: The VATER association and spinal dysraphia. Pediatr Neurosurg 1992;18: 144.
43. Chiang C, Litingtung Y, Harris MP, et al: Manifestation of the limb prepattern: Limb development in the absence of sonic hedgehog function. Dev Biol 2001;236: 421.
44. Choi IH, Kumar SJ, Bowen JR: Amputation or limb-lengthening for partial or total absence of the fibula. J Bone Joint Surg Am 1990;72:1391.
45. Choi IH, Lipton GE, Mackenzie W, et al: Wedge-shaped distal tibial epiphysis in the pathogenesis of equinovalgus deformity of the foot and ankle in tibial lengthening for fibular hemimelia. J Pediatr Orthop 2000;20: 428.
46. Choi IH, Kumar SJ, Bowen JR: Amputation or limb-lengthening for partial or total absence of the fibula. J Bone Joint Surg Am 1990;72:1391.
47. Christini D, Kumar SJ: Fibular transfer in tibial hemimelia: A follow-up study. J Assoc Child Prosthet Orthot Clin 1991;26:8.
48. Clark M, Atkins D, Hubbard S, et al: Prosthetic devices for children with bilateral upper limb deficiencies: When and if, pros and cons. In Herring JA, Birch JG (eds): The Child with a Limb Deficiency. Rosemont, Ill, American Academy of Orthopaedic Surgeons, 1998, p 397.
49. Clark MW: Autosomal dominant inheritance of tibial meromelia: Report of a kindred. J Bone Joint Surg Am 1975;57:262.
50. Cogbill TH, Steenlage ES, Landercasper J, et al: Death and disability from agricultural injuries in Wisconsin: A 12-year experience with 739 patients. J Trauma 1991; 31:1632.
51. Cohen MJ: The Child with Multiple Birth Defects, 2nd ed. New York, Oxford University Press, 1997, p 15.
52. Cohn MJ, Izpisua-Belmonte JC, Abud H, et al: Fibroblast growth factors induce additional limb development from the flank of chick embryos. Cell 1995;80: 739.
53. Cole RJ, Manske PR: Classification of ulnar deficiency according to the thumb and first web. J Hand Surg [Am] 1997;22:479.
54. Coupland RM, Korver A: Injuries from antipersonnel mines: The experience of the International Committee of the Red Cross. BMJ 1991;303:1509.
55. Coventry MB, Johnson EW Jr: Congenital absence of the fibula. J Bone Joint Surg Am 1952;34:941.
56. Crandall RC, Tomhave W: Pediatric unilateral below-elbow amputees: Retrospective analysis of 34 patients given multiple prosthetic options. J Pediatr Orthop 2002;22:380.
57. Crouse SF, Lessard CS, Rhodes J, et al: Oxygen consumption and cardiac response of short-leg and long-leg prosthetic ambulation in a patient with bilateral above-knee amputation: Comparisons with able-bodied men. Arch Phys Med Rehabil 1990;71:313.
58. Cummings D, Kapp S: Lower-limb pediatric prosthetics: General considerations and philosophy. J Prosthet Orthot 1992;4:196.
59. Dalsey R, Gomez W, Seitz WH Jr, et al: Myoelectric prosthetic replacement in the upper-extremity amputee. Orthop Rev 1989;18:697.
60. Damsin JP, Pous JG, Ghanem I: Therapeutic approach to severe congenital lower limb length discrepancies: Surgical treatment versus prosthetic management. J Pediatr Orthop B 1995;4:164.
61. Datta D, Ibbotson V: Powered prosthetic hands in very young children. Prosthet Orthot Int 1998;22: 150.
62. Davids J: Terminal bony overgrowth of the residual limb: Current management strategies. In Herring JA, Birch JG (eds): The Child with a Limb Deficiency. Rosemont, Ill, American Academy of Orthopaedic Surgeons, 1998, p 269.
63. Davids JR, Meyer LC, Blackhurst DW: Operative treatment of bone overgrowth in children who have an acquired or congenital amputation. J Bone Joint Surg Am 1995;77:1490.
64. Davies MS, Nadel S, Habibi P, et al: The orthopaedic management of peripheral ischaemia in meningococcal septicaemia in children. J Bone Joint Surg Br 2000; 82:383.
65. Day HJ: The ISO/ISPO classification of congenital limb deficiency. Prosthet Orthot Int 1991;15:67.
66. Devitt AT, O'Donnell T, Fogarty EE, et al: Tibial hemimelia of a different class. J Pediatr Orthop 2000;20: 616.
67. Di Bella E, Di Stefano G, Romeo M, et al: Upper limb cardiovascular syndrome with ulna agenesis [abstract]. Pediat Radiol 1984;14:259.
68. Dirschl D, Dahners L: The mangled extremity: When should it be amputated? J Am Acad Orthop Surg 1996;4:182.
69. Dobyns J, Wood V, Bayne L, et al: Congenital hand deformities. In Green D (ed): Operative Hand Surgery. New York, Churchill Livingstone, 1982, p 213.
70. Dolan MA, Knapp JF, Andres J: Three-wheel and four-wheel all-terrain vehicle injuries in children. Pediatrics 1989;84:694.

71. Dolle P, Izpisua-Belmonte JC, Falkenstein H, et al: Coordinate expression of the murine Hox-5 complex homoeobox-containing genes during limb pattern formation. Nature 1989;342:767.
72. Dormans J: Management of pediatric mutilating extremity injuries and traumatic amputations. In Herring JA, Birch JG (eds): The Child with a Limb Deficiency. Rosemont, Ill, American Academy of Orthopaedic Surgeons, 1998, p 253.
73. Dormans J, Azzoni M, Davidson R, et al: Major lower extremity lawn mower injuries in children. J Pediatr Orthop 1995;15:78.
74. Dudley AT, Ros MA, Tabin CJ: A re-examination of proximodistal patterning during vertebrate limb development. Nature 2002;418:539.
75. Eilert RE, Jayakumar SS: Boyd and Syme ankle amputations in children. J Bone Joint Surg Am 1976;58:1138.
76. Engsberg JR, Lee AG, Tedford KG, et al: Normative ground reaction force data for able-bodied and below-knee-amputee children during walking. J Pediatr Orthop 1993;13:169.
77. Epps C: Current concepts review: Proximal femoral focal deficiency. J Bone Joint Surg Am 1983;65:867.
78. Exner GU: Bending osteotomy through the distal tibial physis in fibular hemimelia for stable reduction of the hindfoot. J Pediatr Orthop B 2003;12:27.
79. Ezaki M: Upper extremity deficiencies. In Herring JA, Birch JG (eds): The Child with a Limb Deficiency. Rosemont, Ill, American Academy of Orthopaedic Surgeons, 1998, p 381.
80. Farmer A, Laurin C: Congenital absence of the fibula. Am J Orthop 1960;42-A:1.
81. Fillauer C, Pritham CH, Fillauer K: Evolution and development of the silicone suction socket (3S) for below-knee prostheses. J Pediatr Orthop 1989;1:92.
82. Filly AL, Robnett-Filly B, Filly RA: Syndromes with focal femoral deficiency: Strengths and weaknesses of prenatal sonography. J Ultrasound Med 2004;23:1511.
83. Fisk J: Introduction to the child amputee. In Bowker J, Michael J (eds): Atlas of Limb Prosthetics: Surgical, Prosthetic, and Rehabilitation Principles. St Louis, Mosby-Year Book, 1992, p 731.
84. Fixsen JA, Lloyd-Roberts GC: The natural history and early treatment of proximal femoral dysplasia. J Bone Joint Surg Br 1974;56:86.
85. Flatt A: Ulnar deficiencies. In Flatt A (ed): The Care of Congenital Hand Anomalies, 2nd ed. St. Louis, Quality Medical Publishing, 1994, p 411.
86. Fowler E, Zernicke R, Setoguchi Y, et al: Energy expenditure during walking by children who have proximal femoral focal deficiency. J Bone Joint Surg Am 1996;78:1857.
87. Francis PH, Richardson MK, Brickell PM, et al: Bone morphogenetic proteins and a signalling pathway that controls patterning in the developing chick limb. Development 1994;120:209.
88. Francis-West PH, Robertson KE, Ede DA, et al: Expression of genes encoding bone morphogenetic proteins and sonic hedgehog in talpid (ta3) limb buds: Their relationships in the signalling cascade involved in limb patterning. Dev Dyn 1995;203:187.
89. Frankel VH, Gold S, Golyakhovsky V: The Ilizarov technique. Bull Hosp Jt Dis Orthop Inst 1988;48:17.
90. Frantz C: Congenital skeletal limb deficiencies. J Bone Joint Surg Am 1961;43:1202.
91. Frantz C: The increase in the incidence of malformed babies in the German Federal Republic during the years 1959-1962. J Assoc Child Prosthet Orthot Clin 1994;28:62.
92. Frantz C: The upsurge in phocomelic congenital anomalies. J Assoc Child Prosthet Orthot Clin 1994;28:38.
93. Frantz C, Aitken G: Management of the juvenile amputee. Clinl Orthop 1959;9:30.
94. Friedmann L: Toileting self-care methods for bilateral high level upper limb amputees. Prosthet Orthot Int 1980;4:29.
95. Froster UG, Baird PA: Upper limb deficiencies and associated malformations: A population-based study. Am J Med Genet 1992;44:767.
96. Froster UG, Baird PA: Congenital defects of lower limbs and associated malformations: A population based study. Am J Med Genet 1993;45:60.
97. Froster-Iskenius UG, Baird PA: Limb reduction defects in over one million consecutive live births. Teratology 1989;39:127.
98. Fuller D, Duthie R: The timed appearance of some congenital malformation and orthopaedic abnormalities. Instr Course Lect 1974;23:53.
99. Gabos PG, El Rassi G, Pahys J: Knee reconstruction in syndromes with congenital absence of the anterior cruciate ligament. J Pediatr Orthop 2005;25:210.
100. Garca-Cimbrelo E, Curto de la Mano A, Garca-Rey E, et al: The intramedullary elongation nail for femoral lengthening. J Bone Joint Surg Br 2002;84:971.
101. Gazely W, Ey M, Sampson W: Use of triple wall sockets for juvenile amputees. Interclin Information Bull 1964;4:1.
102. Gherlinzoni F, Picci P, Bacci G, et al: Limb sparing versus amputation in osteosarcoma: Correlation between local control, surgical margins and tumor necrosis. Istituto Rizzoli experience. Ann Oncol 1992; 3(Suppl 2):S23.
103. Ghoneem HF, Wright JG, Cole WG, et al: The Ilizarov method for correction of complex deformities: Psychological and functional outcomes. J Bone Joint Surg Am 1996;78:1480.
104. Gibson D: Child and juvenile amputees. In Banjerjee S, Kahn N (eds): Rehabilitation Managment of Amputees. Baltimore, Williams & Wilkins, 1982.
105. Gillespie R: Principles of amputation surgery in children with longitudinal deficiencies of the femur. Clin Orthop Relat Res 1990:29.
106. Gillespie R: Classification of congenital abnormalities of the femur. In Herring JA, Birch JG (eds): The Child with a Limb Deficiency. Rosemont, Ill, American Academy of Orthopaedic Surgeons, 1998, p 63.
107. Gillespie R, Torode IP: Classification and management of congenital abnormalities of the femur. J Bone Joint Surg Br 1983;65:557.
108. Gitter A, Czerniecki JM, DeGroot DM: Biomechanical analysis of the influence of prosthetic feet on below-knee amputee walking. Am J Phys Med Rehabil 1991; 70:142.

109. Glanz A, Fraser FC: Spectrum of anomalies in Fanconi anaemia. J Med Genet 1982;19:412.
110. Glessner J: Spontaneous intra-uterine amputation. J Bone Joint Surg Am 1963;45:351.
111. Glorion C, Pouliquen JC, Langlais J, et al: Femoral lengthening using the callotasis method: Study of the complications in a series of 70 cases in children and adolescents. J Pediatr Orthop 1996;16:161.
112. Godina M: Early microsurgical reconstruction of complex trauma of the extremities. Plast Reconstr Surg 1986;78:285.
113. Goldberg M: The Dysmorphic Child: An Orthopaedic Perspective. New York, Raven Press, 1987.
114. Gonin-Decarie T: The mental and emotional development of the thalidomide children and the psychological reactions of the mothers. J Assoc Child Prosthet Orthot Clin 1994;28:79.
115. Gottschalk F, Sohrab K, Stills M, et al: Does socket configuration influence the position of the femur in above-knee amputation? J Prosthet Orthot 1989;2:94.
116. Gottschalk FA, Stills M: The biomechanics of transfemoral amputation. Prosthet Orthot Int 1994;18:12.
117. Green W, Anderson M: Skeletal age and the control of bone growth. Instr Course Lect 1960;17:199.
118. Greenberg JE, Falabella AF, Bello YM, et al: Tissue-engineered skin in the healing of wound stumps from limb amputations secondary to purpura fulminans. Pediatr Dermatol 2003;20:169.
119. Grissom LE, Harcke HT, Kumar SJ: Sonography in the management of tibial hemimelia. Clin Orthop Relat Res 1990:266.
120. Grossley P, Minowada G, MacArthur C, et al: Roles for FGF8 in the induction, initiation, and maintenance of chick limb development. Cell 1996;84:127.
121. Gupta A, Wolff T: Management of the mangled hand and forearm. J Am Acad Orthop Surg 1995;3:226.
122. Gurrieri F, Cammarata M, Avarello RM, et al: Ulnar ray defect in an infant with a 6q21;7q31.2 translocation: Further evidence for the existence of a limb defect gene in 6q21. Am J Med Genet 1995;55:315.
123. Gurrieri F, Kjaer KW, Sangiorgi E, et al: Limb anomalies: Developmental and evolutionary aspects. Am J Med Genet 2002;115:231.
124. Hall CB, Brooks MB, Dennis JF: Congenital skeletal deficiencies of the extremities: Classification and fundamentals of treatment. JAMA 1962;181:590.
125. Hall J: Borwn's fibula-femur transfer for congenital absence of the tibia. In Herring JA, Birch JG (eds): The Child with a Limb Deficiency. Rosemont, Ill, American Academy of Orthopaedic Surgeons, 1998, p 219.
126. Hall JE: Rotation of congenitally hypoplastic lower limbs to use the ankle joint as a knee. J Assoc Child Prosthet Orthot Clin 1966;6:3.
127. Hall JG, Levin J, Kuhn JP, et al: Thrombocytopenia with absent radius (TAR). Medicine (Baltimore) 1969;48: 411.
128. Hamanishi C: Congenital short femur: Clinical, genetic and epidemiological comparison of the naturally occurring condition with that caused by thalidomide. J Bone Joint Surg Br 1980;62:307.
129. Hamilton E: Gait training. Part 2. Children. In Kostuik J (ed): Amputation Surgery and Rehabilitation: The Toronto Experience. New York, Churchill Livingstone, 1981, p 331.
130. Hammerschmidt M, Brook A, McMahon AP: The world according to hedgehog. Trends Genet 1997;13:14.
131. Hancock C, King R: The one-bone leg. J Assoc Child Prosthet Orthot Clin 1967;7:11.
132. Hansen JM, Harris C: A novel hypothesis for thalidomide-induced limb teratogenesis: Redox misregulation of the NF-kappaB pathway. Antioxid Redox Signal 2004;6:1.
133. Hansen-Leth C: Bone vascularization and bone healing in the amputation stump: An experimental study. Acta Orthop Scand 1979;50:39.
134. Harder J: Gait analysis of the child with a lower limb deficiency. In Herring JA, Birch JG (eds): The Child with a Limb Deficiency. Rosemont, Ill, American Academy of Orthopaedic Surgeons, 1998, p 331.
135. Harrison R: Experiments on the development of the forelimb of *Amblystoma,* a self-differentiating equipotential system. J Exp Zool 1918;25:413.
136. Heger H, Millstein S, Hunter GA: Electrically powered prostheses for the adult with an upper limb amputation. J Bone Joint Surg Br 1985;67:278.
137. Heikinheimo M, Lawshe A, Shackleford G, et al: FGF-8 expression in the post-gastrulation mouse suggests roles in the development of the face, limbs and central nervous system. Mech Dev 1994;48:129.
138. Helfet DL, Howey T, Sanders R, et al: Limb salvage versus amputation: Preliminary results of the Mangled Extremity Severity Score. Clin Orthop Relat Res 1990;256:80.
139. Henkel L, Willert HG: Dysmelia: A classification and a pattern of malformation in a group of congenital defects of the limbs. J Bone Joint Surg Br 1969;51:399.
140. Hepp O: Frequency of congenital defect-anomalies of the extremities in the Federal Republic of Germany. J Assoc Child Prosthet Orthot Clin 1994;28:40.
141. Herrera R, Hobar PC, Ginsburg CM: Surgical intervention for the complications of meningococcal-induced purpura fulminans. Pediatr Infect Dis J 1994; 13:734.
142. Herring J: Functional assessment and management of multilimb deficiency. In Herring JA, Birch JG (eds): The Child with a Limb Deficiency. Rosemont, Ill, American Academy of Orthopaedic Surgeons, 1998, p 437.
143. Herring JA, Birch JG (eds): The Child with a Limb Deficiency. Rosemont, Ill American Academy of Orthopaedic Surgeons, 1998.
144. Herring JA: Symes amputation for fibular hemimelia: A second look in the Ilizarov era. Instr Course Lect 1992;41:435.
145. Herring JA, Barnhill B, Gaffney C: Syme amputation: An evaluation of the physical and psychological function in young patients. J Bone Joint Surg Am 1986;68: 573.
146. Hogan BL: Bone morphogenetic proteins in development. Curr Opin Genet Dev 1996;6:432.
147. Holt M, Oram S: Familial heart disease with skeletal malformations. Br Heart J 1960;22:236.
148. Hubbard S, Kurtz I, Heim W, et al: Powered prosthetic intervention in upper extremity deficiency. In Herring JA, Birch JG (eds): The Child with a Limb Deficiency.

Rosemont, Ill, American Academy of Orthopaedic Surgeons, 1998, p 417.
149. Hughes J: Biomechanics of the through-knee prosthesis. Prosthe Orthot Int 1983;7:96.
150. Inoue G, Miura T: Arteriographic findings in radial and ulnar deficiencies. J Hand Surg [Br] 1991;16:409.
151. Ippolito E, Peretti G, Bellocci M, et al: Histology and ultrastructure of arteries, veins, and peripheral nerves during limb lengthening. Clin Orthop Relat Res 1994; 308:54.
152. Johansen K, Daines M, Howey T, et al: Objective criteria accurately predict amputation following lower extremity trauma. J Trauma 1990;30:568.
153. Johansson E, Aparisi T: Missing cruciate ligament in congenital short femur. J Bone Joint Surg Am 1983;65: 1109.
154. Johnson J, Omar CIJ: Congenital ulnar deficiency: Natural history and therapeutic implications. Hand Clin 1985;1:499.
155. Johnston CI, Haideri N: Comparison of functional outcome in fibular deficiency treated by limb salvage versus Syme's amputation. In Herring JA, Birch JG (eds): The Child with a Limb Deficiency. Rosemont, Ill, American Academy of Orthopaedic Surgeons, 1998, p 173.
156. Jones D, Barnes J, Lloyd-Roberts GC: Congenital aplasia and dysplasia of the tibia with intact fibula: Classification and management. J Bone Joint Surg Br 1978;60: 31.
157. Jones K: Femoral hypoplasia-unusual facies syndrome. In Jones KL (ed): Smith's Recognizable Patterns of Human Malformation. Philadelphia, WB Saunders, 1988, p 268.
158. Jones KL, Smith DW, Hall BD, et al: A pattern of craniofacial and limb defects secondary to aberrant tissue bands. J Pediatr 1974;84:90.
159. Jorring K: Amputation in children: A follow-up of 74 children whose lower extremities were amputated. Acta Orthop Scand 1971;42:178.
160. Kalamchi A, Dawe RV: Congenital deficiency of the tibia. J Bone Joint Surg Br 1985;67:581.
161. Kant P, Koh SH-Y, Neumann V, et al: Treatment of longitudinal deficiency affecting the femur: Comparing patient mobility and satisfaction outcomes of Syme amputation against extension prosthesis. J Pediatr Orthop 2003;23:236.
162. King R: Providing a single lever in proximal femoral focal deficiency: A preliminary report. J Assoc Child Prosthet Orthot Clin 1966;6:23.
163. King R, Marks T: Follow-up findings on the skeletal lever in the surgical management of proximal femoral focal deficiency. Interclin Information Bull 1971;11:1.
164. Kino Y: Clinical and experimental studies of the congenital constriction band syndrome with an emphasis on its etiology. J Bone Joint Surg Am 1969;57:636.
165. Kitano K, Tada K: One-bone forearm procedure for partial defect of the ulna. J Pediatr Orthop 1985;5:290.
166. Koman LA, Meyer LC, Warren FH: Proximal femoral focal deficiency: A 50-year experience. Dev Med Child Neurol 1982;24:344.
167. Kon M: Firework injuries to the hand. Ann Chir Main Memb Super 1991;10:443.
168. Kostuik JP, Gillespie R, Hall JE, et al: Van Ness rotational osteotomy for treatment of proximal femoral focal deficiency and congenital short femur. J Bone Joint Surg Am 1975;57:1039.
169. Krajbich I: Proximal femoral focal deficiency. In Kalamchi A (ed): Congenital Lower Limb Deficiencies. New York, Springer-Verlag, 1989, p 108.
170. Krajbich I: Rotationplasty in the management of proximal femoral focal deficiency. In Herring JA, Birch JG (eds): The Child with a Limb Deficiency. Rosemont, Ill, American Academy of Orthopaedic Surgeons, 1998, p 87.
171. Krajbich I, Bochmann D: Van Ness rotation-plasty in tumor surgery. In Bowker J, Michael J (eds): Atlas of Limb Prosthetics: Surgical, Prosthetic, and Rehabilitation Principles. St. Louis, Mosby-Year Book, 1992, p 885.
172. Kritter AE: Tibial rotation-plasty for proximal femoral focal deficiency. J Bone Joint Surg Am 1977;59:927.
173. Kruger L: The use of subbies for the child with bilateral lower-limb deficiencies. J Assoc Child Prosthet Orthot Clin 1973;12:7.
174. Kruger L: Congenital limb deficiencies. Section II. Lower llimb deficiencies. In Bowker J, Michael J (eds): Atlas of Limb Prosthetics: Surgical, Prosthetic, and Rehabilitation Principles. St. Louis, Mosby-Year Book, 1992, p 522.
175. Kruger L: Lower limb deficiencies. In Bowker J, Michael J (eds): Atlas of Limb Prosthetics: Sugical, Prosthetic, and Rehabilitation Principles. St. Louis, Mosby-Year Book, 1992, p 802.
176. Kruger L: Fibular deficiencies. In Herring JA, Birch JG (eds): The Child with a Limb Deficiency. Rosemont, Ill, American Academy of Orthopaedic Surgeons, 1998, p 151.
177. Kruger L, Adbo R, Schwarts A: Tibial deficiency: A genetic problem. J Assoc Child Prosthet Orthot Clin 1985;20:41.
178. Kruger L, Talbott R: Amputation and prosthesis as definitive treatment in congenital absence of the fibula. J Bone Joint Surg Am 1961;43:625.
179. Kurtz A, Hand R: Bone growth following amputation in childhood. Am J Surg 1939;43:773.
180. Kuyper MA, Breedijk M, Mulders AH, et al: Prosthetic management of children in the Netherlands with upper limb deficiencies. Prosthet Orthot Int 2001;25: 228.
181. Lambert CN: Amputation surgery in the child. Orthop Clin North Am 1972;3:473.
182. Laufer E, Nelson CE, Johnson RL, et al: Sonic hedgehog and Fgf-4 act through a signaling cascade and feedback loop to integrate growth and patterning of the developing limb bud. Cell 1994;79:993.
183. Lausecker H: [Congenital defect of the ulna.]. Virchows Arch 1954;325:211.
184. Letts M, Davidson D: Epidemiology and prevention of traumatic amputations in children. In Herring JA, Birch JG (eds): The Child with a Limb Deficiency. Rosemont, Ill American Academy of Orthopaedic Surgeons, 1998, p 235.
185. Letts R: Farm machinery accidents in children. In Dosman J, Crockcroft D (eds): Principles of Health and

Safety in Agriculture. Boca Raton, Fla, CRC Press, 1986, p 357.
186. Letts RM, Cleary J: The child and the snowmobile. Can Med Assoc J 1975;113:1061.
187. Letts RM, Gammon W: Auger injuries in children. Can Med Assoc J 1978;118:519.
188. Letts RM, Mardirosian A: Lawnmower injuries in children. Can Med Assoc J 1977;116:1151.
189. Levin M, Quint PA, Goldstein B, et al: Recombinant bactericidal/permeability-increasing protein (rBPI21) as adjunctive treatment for children with severe meningococcal sepsis: A randomised trial. rBPI21 Meningococcal Sepsis Study Group. Lancet 2000;356:961.
190. Lie RT, Wilcox AJ, Skjaerven R: A population-based study of the risk of recurrence of birth defects. N Engl J Med 1994;331:1.
191. Lipson AH, Webster WS, Brown-Woodman PD, et al: Moebius syndrome: Animal model–human correlations and evidence for a brainstem vascular etiology. Teratology 1989;40:339.
192. Lister G: Toes to the hand. In Flatt A (ed): The Care of Congenital Hand Anomalies. St. Louis, Quality Medical Publishing, 1994, p 180.
193. Lloyd-Roberts GC: Treatment of defects of the ulna in children by establishing cross-union with the radius. J Bone Joint Surg Br 1973;55:327.
194. Lloyd-Roberts GC, Stone KH: Contenital hypoplasia of the upper femur. J Bone Joint Surg Br 1963;45:557.
195. Loder RT: Fibular transfer for congenital absence of the tibia (Brown procedure). In Herring JA, Birch JG (eds): The Child with a Limb Deficiency. Rosemont, Ill, American Academy of Orthopaedic Surgeons, 1998, p 233.
196. Loder RT: Demographics of traumatic amputations in children: Implications for prevention strategies. J Bone Joint Surg Am 2004;86:923.
197. Loder RT, Herring JA: Disarticulation of the knee in children: A functional assessment. J Bone Joint Surg Am 1987;69:1155.
198. Loder RT, Herring JA: Fibular transfer for congenital absence of the tibia: A reassessment. J Pediatr Orthop 1987;7:8.
199. Long I: Normal shape–normal alignment (NSNA) above-knee prosthesis. Clin Prosthet Orthot 1985;9:9.
200. Lovett M, Clines G, Wise C: Genetic control of limb development. In Herring JA, Birch JG (eds): The Child with a Limb Deficiency. Rosemont, Ill, American Academy of Orthopaedic Surgeons, 1998, p 13.
201. Mace JW, Kaplan JM, Schanberger JE, et al: Poland's syndrome: Report of seven cases and review of the literature. Clin Pediatr 1972;11:98.
202. Mahmood R, Bresnick J, Hornbruch A, et al: A role for FGF-8 in the initiation and maintenance of vertebrate limb bud outgrowth. Curr Biol 1995;5:797.
203. Marcus N, Omar GJ: Carpal deviation in congenital ulnar deficiency. J Bone Joint Surg Am 1984;66:1003.
204. Marquardt E: The multiple limb-deficient child. In Committee on Prosthetics and Orthotics (ed): Atlas of Limb Prosthesis. St Louis, CV Mosby, 1982, p 595.
205. Marquardt E: The multiple limb-deficient child. In Bowker J, Michael J (eds): Atlas of Limb Prosthetics and Rehabilitation Principles. St. Louis, Mosby-Year Book, 1992, p 839.
206. Marquardt E, Correll J: Amputations and prostheses for the lower limb. Int Orthop 1984;8:139.
207. Marquardt E, Fisk J: Thalidomide children: Thirty years later. J Assoc Child Prosthet Orthot Clin 1992; 27:3.
208. Martini A, Marquardt E: Stump plasty on congenital amputations. Garyounis Med J 1980;3(Suppl):83.
209. Matsuyama J, Mabuchi A, Zhang J, et al: A pair of sibs with tibial hemimelia born to phenotypically normal parents. J Hum Genet 2003;48:173.
210. McCarthy JJ, Glancy GL, Chnag FM, et al: Fibular hemimelia: Comparison of outcome measurements after amputation and lengthening. J Bone Joint Surg Am 2000;82:1732.
211. McClure SK, Shaughnessy WJ: Farm-related limb amputations in children. J Pediatr Orthop 2005;25:133.
212. McCoullough N, Trout A, Caldwell J: Non-standard prosthetic applications for juvenile amputations. J Assoc Child Prosthet Orthot Clin 1963;2:7.
213. McCredie J: Neural crest defects: A neuroanatomic basis for classification of mutiple malformations related to phocomelia. J Neurol Sci 1975;28:373.
214. Meyer L, Sauer B: Probelms of treating and fitting the patient with proximal femoral focal deficiency. J Assoc Child Prosthet Orthot Clin 1971;10:1.
215. Meyer L, Sauer B: The use of porous high-density polyethylene caps in the prevention of appositional bone growth in the juvenile-amputee: A preliminary report. J Assoc Child Prosthet Orthot Clin 1975;14:1.
216. Michael J: Reflections on CAD/CAM in prosthetics and orthotics. J Pediatr Orthop 1989;1:116.
217. Michael J: Pediatric prosthetics and orthotics. Phys Occup Ther Pediatr 1990;10:123.
218. Michael J: Prosthetic knee mechanisms. Phys Med Rehabil 1994;8:147.
219. Miller JK, Wenner SM, Kruger LM: Ulnar deficiency. J Hand Surg [Am] 1986;11:822.
220. Minnes P, Stack D: Research and practice with congenital amputees: Making the whole greater than the sum of its parts. Int J Rehabil Res 1990;13:151.
221. Moll J: More on the Ertl osteotomy. Amputee Clin 1970;2:7.
222. Morton A: Psychological considerations in the planning of staged reconstruction in limb deficiencies. In Herring JA, Birch JG (eds): The Child with Limb Deficiency. Rosemont, Ill, American Academy of Orthopaedic Surgeons, 1998, p 195.
223. Moseley CF: A straight-line graph for leg-length discrepancies. J Bone Joint Surg Am 1977;59:174.
224. Moseley CF: A straight line graph for leg length discrepancies. Clin Orthop Relat Res 1978:33.
225. Mowery CA, Herring JA, Jackson D: Dislocated patella associated with below-knee amputation in adolescent patients. J Pediatr Orthop 1986;6:299.
226. Murray DW, Kambouroglou G, Kenwright J: One-stage lengthening for femoral shortening with associated deformity. J Bone Joint Surg Br 1993;75:566.
227. Naudie D, Hamdy RC, Fassier F, et al: Management of fibular hemimelia: Amputation or limb lengthening. J Bone Joint Surg Br 1997;79:58.
228. Niswander L, Martin GR: FGF-4 and BMP-2 have opposite effects on limb growth. Nature 1993;361:68.

229. Oberg K: Knee mechanisms for through-knee prostheses. Prosthet Orthot Int 1983;7:107.
230. Ogden JA, Vickers TH, Tauber JE, et al: A model for ulnar dysmelia. Yale J Biol Med 1978;51:193.
231. Ogden JA, Watson HK, Bohne W: Ulnar dysmelia. J Bone Joint Surg Am 1976;58:467.
232. Ogino T, Kato H: Clinical and experimental studies on ulnar ray deficiency. Handchir Mikrochir Plast Chir 1988;20:330.
233. Oglesby DJ, Tablada C: Prosthetic and orthotic management. In Bowker J, Michael J (eds): Atlas of Limb Prosthetics: Surgical, Prosthetic, and Rehabilitation Principles. St. Louis, Mosby-Year Book, 1992, p 835.
234. Ohuchi H, Nakagawa T, Yamauchi M, et al: An additional limb can be induced from the flank of the chick embryo by FGF4. Biochem Biophys Res Commun 1995;209:809.
235. Okamoto AM, Guarniero R, Coelho RF, et al: The use of bone bridges in transtibial amputations. Rev Hosp Clin Fac Med Sao Paulo 2000;55:121.
236. Oppenheim W, Setoguchi Y, Fowler E: Overview and comparison of Syme's amputation and knee fusion with the van Ness rotationplasty procedure in proximal femoral focal deficiency. In Herring JA, Birch JG (eds): The Child with a Limb Deficiency. Rosemont, Ill, American Academy of Orthopaedic Surgeons, 1998, p 73.
237. Paley D: Lengthening reconstruction surgery for congenital femoral deficiency. In Herring JA, Birch JG (eds): The Child with a Limb Deficiency. Rosemont, Ill, American Academy of Orthopaedic Surgeons, 1998, p 113.
238. Patel M, Paley D, Herzenberg JE: Limb-lengthening versus amputation for fibular hemimelia. J Bone Joint Surg Am 2002;84:317.
239. Patterson D, McMillian P, Rodriguez R: Aceptance rate of myoelectric prosthesis. J Assoc Child Prosthet Orthot Clin 1990;25:73.
240. Pattinson RC, Fixsen JA: Management and outcome in tibial dysplasia. J Bone Joint Surg Br 1992;74:893.
241. Patton J: Developmental approach to pediatric prosthetic evaluation and training. In Atkins D, Meier R (eds): Comprehensive Management of the Upper-Limb Amputee. New York, Springer-Verlag, 1989, p 137.
242. Paulson JA: The epidemiology of injuries in adolescents. Pediatr Ann 1988;17:84.
243. Pearn J: Children and war. J Paediatr Child Health 2003;39:166.
244. Peterson CA 2nd, Maki S, Wood MB: Clinical results of the one-bone forearm. J Hand Surg [Am] 1995;20:609.
245. Pinzur M: Knee disarticulation. In Bowker J, Michael J (eds): Atlas of Limb Prosthetics: Surgical, Prosthetic, and Rehabilitation Principles. St. Louis, Mosby-Year Book, 1992, p 479.
246. Powars D, Larsen R, Johnson J, et al: Epidemic meningococcemia and purpura fulminans with induced protein C deficiency. Clin Infec Dis 1993;17:254.
247. Price C, Noonan K: Femoral lengthening with monolateral half-pin devices. In Herring JA, Birch JG (eds): The Child with a Limb Deficiency. Rosemont, Ill, American Academy of Orthopaedic Surgeons, 1998, p 133.
248. Pritham CH: Biomechanics and shape of the above-knee socket considered in light of the ischial containment concept. Prosthet Orthot Int 1990;14:9.
249. Quan L, Smith DW: The VATER association: Vertebral defects, Anal atresia, T-E fistula with esophageal atresia, Radial and Renal dysplasia: A spectrum of associated defects. J Pediatr 1973;82:104.
250. Rab G: Principles of amputation in children. In Chapman M (ed): Operative Orthopaedics. Philadelphia, JB Lippincott, 1993, p 2469.
251. Radcliffe C: Functional considerations in the fitting of above-knee prostheses. Orthot Prosthet 1955;2:35.
252. Radcliffe C: Prosthetics. In Rose J, Gamble J (eds): Human Walking. Baltimore, Williams & Wilkins, 1994, p 165.
253. Refaat Y, Gunnoe J, Hornicek FJ, et al: Comparison of quality of life after amputation or limb salvage. Clin Orthop Relat Res 2002:298.
254. Reynolds JF, Wyandt HE, Kelly TE: De novo 21q interstitial deletion in a retarded boy with ulno-fibular dysostosis. Am J Med Genet 1985;20:173.
255. Richieri-Costa A, Ferrareto I, Masiero D, et al: Tibial hemimelia: Report on 37 new cases, clinical and genetic considerations. Am J Med Genet 1987;27:867.
256. Riddle RD, Johnson RL, Laufer E, et al: Sonic hedgehog mediates the polarizing activity of the ZPA. Cell 1993;75:1401.
257. Riordan D: The upper limb. In Lovell W, Winter R (eds): Pediatric Orthopaedics. Philadelphia, JB Lippincott, 1978, p 685.
258. Riordan D, Mills E, Alldredge R: Congenital absence of the ulna [abstract]. J Bone Joint Surg Am 1961;43:614.
259. Rivara FP: Fatal and nonfatal farm injuries to children and adolescents in the United States. Pediatrics 1985;76:567.
260. Roberts DJ, Johnson RL, Burke AC, et al: Sonic hedgehog is an endodermal signal inducing Bmp-4 and Hox genes during induction and regionalization of the chick hindgut. Development 1995;121:3163.
261. Roessler E, Belloni E, Gaudenz K, et al: Mutations in the human sonic hedgehog gene cause holoprosencephaly. Nat Genet 1996;14:357.
262. Romano R, Burgess E: Extremity growth and overgrowth following amputation in children. Interclin Information Bull 1966;5:11.
263. Rosenfelder R: Infant amputees: Early growth and care. Clin Orthop Relat Res 1980:41.
264. Roskies E: Abnormality and Normality: The Mothering of Thalidomide Children. Ithaca, NY, Cornell University Press, 1972.
265. Rougraff BT, Simon MA, Kneisl JS, et al: Limb salvage compared with amputation for osteosarcoma of the distal end of the femur: A long-term oncological, functional, and quality-of-life study. J Bone Joint Surg Am 1994;76:649.
266. Russell J: Tibial hemimelia: Limb deficiency in siblings. Interclin Information Bull 1965;14:15.
267. Sabolich J: Contoured adducted trochanteric-controlled alignment method. Clin Prosthet Orthot 1985;9:15.
268. Sadler T: Embryology and gene regulation of limb development. In Herring JA, Birch JG (eds): The Child

with a Limb Deficiency. Rosemont, Ill, American Academy of Orthopaedic Surgeons, 1998, p 3.
269. Saleh M, Hammer A: Bifocal limb lengthening: A premininary report. J Pediatr Orthop 1993;2-B:42.
270. Sanders G: Static and dynamic analysis. In Sanders G (ed): Lower Limb Amputations: A Guide to Rehabilitation. Philadelphia, FA Davis, 1986, p 415.
271. Saunders JJ: The proximo-distal sequence of origin of the parts of the chick wing and the role of the ectoderm. J Exp Zool 1948;108:363.
272. Saunders JJ, Grasseling M: Ectodermal-mesechymal interactions in the origin of limb symmetry. In Fleischmajer R, Billingham R (eds): Epithelial-Mesenchymal Interactions. Baltimore, Williams & Wilkins, 1968, p 78.
273. Schneider K, Hart T, Zernicke RF, et al: Dynamics of below-knee child amputee gait: SACH foot versus Flex foot. J Biomech 1993;26:1191.
274. Schoenecker PL: Tibial deficiency. In Herring JA, Birch JG (eds): The Child with a Limb Deficiency. Rosemont, Ill, American Academy of Orthopaedic Surgeons, 1998, p 209.
275. Schoenecker PL, Capelli AM, Millar EA, et al: Congenital longitudinal deficiency of the tibia. J Bone Joint Surg Am 1989;71:278.
276. Schuch C: Prosthetic principles in fitting myoelectric prosthesis in children. In Herring JA, Birch JG (eds): The Child with a Limb Deficiency. Rosemont, Ill, American Academy of Orthopaedic Surgeons, 1998, p 405.
277. Schuch CM: Modern above-knee fitting practice (a report on the ISPO Workshop on Above-Knee Fitting and Alignment Techniques May 15-19, 1987, Miami, USA). Prosthet Orthot Int 1988;12:77.
278. Schuch CM: Transfemoral amputation: Prosthetic management. In Bowker J, Michael J (eds): Atlas of Limb Prosthetics: Surgical, Prosthetic, and Rehabilitation Principles. St. Louis, Mosby-Year Book, 1992, p 509.
279. Searle CP, Hildebrand RK, Lester EL, et al: Findings of fibular hemimelia syndrome with radiographically normal fibulae. J Pediatr Orthop B 2004;13:184.
280. Setoguchi Y: Medical conditions associated with congenital limb deficiencies. In Herring JA, Birch JG (eds): The Child with a Limb Deficiency. Rosemont, Ill, American Academy of Orthopaedic Surgeons, 1998, p 51.
281. Shapiro MJ, Luchtefeld WB, Durham RM, et al: Traumatic train injuries. Am J Emerg Med 1994;12:92.
282. Shubin N, Tabin C, Carroll S: Fossils, genes and the evolution of animal limbs. Nature 1997;388:639.
283. Silcox DH 3rd, Rooks MD, Vogel RR, et al: Myoelectric prostheses: A long-term follow-up and a study of the use of alternate prostheses. J Bone Joint Surg Am 1993;75:1781.
284. Simmons ED Jr, Ginsburg GM, Hall JE: Brown's procedure for congenital absence of the tibia revisited. J Pediatr Orthop 1996;16:85.
285. Simon MA, Aschliman MA, Thomas N, et al: Limb-salvage treatment versus amputation for osteosarcoma of the distal end of the femur. J Bone Joint Surg Am 1986;68:1331.
286. Simpson AH, Cunningham JL, Kenwright J: The forces which develop in the tissues during leg lengthening: A clinical study. J Bone Joint Surg Br 1996;78:979.
287. Simpson AH, Williams PE, Kyberd P, et al: The response of muscle to leg lengthening. J Bone Joint Surg Br 1995;77:630.
288. Smith AA, Greene TL: Preliminary soft tissue distraction in congenital forearm deficiency. J Hand Surg [Am] 1995;20:420.
289. Smith DW: Recognizable Pattern of Human Malformation. Philadelphia, WB Saunders, 1994.
290. Southwood A: Partial absence of the ulnar and associated structures. J Anat 1927;61:346.
291. Speer DP: The pathogenesis of amputation stump overgrowth. Clin Orthop Relat Res 1981;159:294.
292. Spinner M, Freundlich BD, Abeles ED: Management of moderate longitudinal arrest of development of the ulna. Clin Orthop Relat Res 1970;69:199.
293. St Charles S, DiMario FJ Jr, Grunnet ML: Mobius sequence: Further in vivo support for the subclavian artery supply disruption sequence. Am J Med Genet 1993;47:289.
294. Stanitski DF: The effect of limb lengthening on articular cartilage: An experimental study. Clin Orthop Relat Res 1994:68.
295. Stanitski DF, Rossman K, Torosian M: The effect of femoral lengthening on knee articular cartilage: The role of apparatus extension across the joint. J Pediatr Orthop 1996;16:151.
296. Stanitski DF, Stanitski CL: Fibular hemimelia: A new classification system. J Pediatr Orthop 2003;23:30.
297. Steel HH: Iliofemoral fusion for proximal femoral focal deficiency. In Herring JA, Birch JG (eds): The Child with a Limb Deficiency. Rosemont, Ill, American Academy of Orthopaedic Surgeons, 1998, p 103.
298. Steel HH, Lin P, Betz R, et al: Iliofemoral fusion for proximal femoral focal deficiency. J Bone Joint Surg Am 1987;69:837.
299. Stephens T, Spall R, Baker W, et al: Axial and paraxial influences on limb morphogenesis. J Morphol 1991; 208:367.
300. Stevens PM, Arms D: Postaxial hypoplasia of the lower extremity. J Pediatr Orthop 2000;20:166.
301. Stover E, Keller AS, Cobey J, et al: The medical and social consequences of land mines in Cambodia. JAMA 1994;272:331.
302. Stucky W, Loder RT: Extremity gunshot wounds in children. J Pediatr Orthop 1991;11:64.
303. Stueland D, Layde P, Lee BC: Agricultural injuries in children in central Wisconsin. J Trauma 1991;31: 1503.
304. Summerbell D: A quantitative analysis of the effect of excision of the AER from the chick limb-bud. J Embryol Exp Morphol 1974;32:651.
305. Summerbell D: The zone of polarizing activity: Evidence for a role in normal chick limb morphogenesis. J Embryol Exp Morphol 1979;50:217.
306. Sun X, Mariani FV, Martin GR: Functions of FGF signalling from the apical ectodermal ridge in limb development. Nature 2002;418:501.
307. Swanson AB: The Krukenberg procedure in the juvenile amputee. J Bone Joint Surg Br 1964;46:1540.
308. Swanson AB: Bone overgrowth in the juvenile amputee and its control by the use of silicone rubber implants. J Assoc Child Prosthet Orthot Clin 1969;8:9.

309. Swanson AB: A classification for congenital limb malformations. J Hand Surg [Am] 1976;1:8.
310. Tablada C: A technique for fitting converted proximal femoral focal deficiencies. Artif Limbs 1971;15:27.
311. Talbot D, Solomon D: The function of a parent group in the adaptation to the birth of a limb-deficient child. Interclin Information Bull 1979;17:9.
312. Temtamy S, McKusick V, Bergsma D, et al: The Genetics of Hand Malformations. New York, Alan R. Liss, 1978, p 48.
313. Tenholder M, Davids JR, Gruber HE, et al: Surgical management of juvenile amputation overgrowth with a synthetic cap. J Pediatr Orthop 2004;24:218.
314. Thompson GH, Balourdas GM, Marcus RE: Railyard amputations in children. J Pediatr Orthop 1983;3:443.
315. Thompson GH, Leimkuller J: Prosthetic management. In Kalamchi A (ed): Congenital Lower Limb Deficiencies. New York, Springer-Verlag, 1989, p 210.
316. Tickle C, Summerbell D, Wolpert L: Positional signalling and specification of digits in chick limb morphogenesis. Nature 1975;254:199.
317. Tooms R: Acquired amputations in children. In Bowker J, Michael J (eds): Atlas of Limb Prosthetics: Surgical, Prosthetic, and Rehabilitation Principles. St. Louis, Mosby-Year Book, 1992, p 735.
318. Torode IP, Gillespie R: Rotationplasty of the lower limb for congenital defects of the femur. J Bone Joint Surg Br 1983;65:569.
319. Tsirikos AI, Bowen JR: Patellofemoral arthritis in a fused knee with proximal femoral focal deficiency. J Pediatr Orthop 2003;23:643.
320. Tuncay IC, Johnston CE 2nd, Birch JG: Spontaneous resolution of congenital anterolateral bowing of the tibia. J Pediatr Orthop 1994;14:599.
321. van Ness C: Rotation-plasty for congenital defects of the femur: Making use of the ankle of the shortened limb to control the knee joint of a prosthesis. J Bone Joint Surg Br 1950;32:12.
322. Varni J, Setoguchi Y: Correlates of perceived physical appearance in children with congenital/acquired limb deficiencies. J Dev Behav Pediatr 1991;12:171.
323. Varni J, Setoguchi Y: Psychological factors in the management of children with limb deficiencies. Phys Med Rehabil Clin N Am 1991;2:395.
324. Varni J, Setoguchi Y: Self-perceived physical appearancein children and adolescents with congenital/acquired limb deficiencies. J Assoc Child Prosthet Orthot Clin 1991;26:56.
325. Varni J, Setoguchi Y: Screening for behavorial and emotional problems in children and adolescents with congenital or acquired limb deficiencies. Am J Dis Child 1992;146:103.
326. Varni J, Setoguchi Y: Perceived physical appearance and adjustment of adolescent with congenital/acquired limb deficinecies: A pathanalytic model. J Clin Child Psychol 1996;25:201.
327. Varni J, Setoguchi Y, Rappapport L: Effects of stress, social support, and self-esteem on depression in children with limb deficiencies. Arch Phys Med Rehabil 1991;72:1053.
328. Velasquez R, Bell D, Armstrong P, et al: Complications of the use of the Ilizarov technique in the correction of limb deformities in children. J Bone Joint Surg Am 1993;75:1148.
329. Vilkki SK: Advances in microsurgical reconstruction of the congenitally adactylous hand. Clin Orthop Relat Res 1995:45.
330. Vilkki SK: Distraction and microvascular epiphysis transfer for radial club hand. J Hand Surg [Br] 1998; 23:445.
331. Vilkki SK: Vascularized joint transfer for radial club hand. Techn Hand Upper Extremity Surg 1998;2:126.
332. Vitale CC: Reconstructive surgery for defects in the shaft of the ulna in children. J Bone Joint Surg Am 1952;34:804.
333. Vocke AK, Schmid A: Osseous overgrowth after post-traumatic amputation of the lower extremity in childhood. Arch Orthop Trauma Surg 2000;120:452.
334. Vogel A, Rodriguez C, Izpisua-Belmonte JC: Involvement of FGF-8 in initiation, outgrowth and patterning of the vertebrate limb. Development 1996;122:1737.
335. von Ertl J: The care of amputation stumps by osteomyeloplastic according to v Ertl. Z Plast Chir 1981;5:184.
336. Vortkamp A, Lee K, Lanske B, et al: Regulation of rate of cartilage differentiation by Indian hedgehog and PTH-related protein. Science 1996;273:613.
337. Wanek N, Gardiner DM, Muneoka K, et al: Conversion by retinoic acid of anterior cells into ZPA cells in the chick wing bud. Nature 1991;350:81.
338. Wang E, Roen V, D'Alessandro J, et al: Recombinant human bone morphogenetic protein induces bone formation. Proc Natl Acad Sci U S A 1990;87:2220.
339. Wang GJ, Baugher WH, Stamp WG: Epiphyseal transplant in amputations: Effects on overgrowth in a rabbit model. Clin Orthop Relat Res 1978:285.
340. Waters RL, Perry J, Antonelli D, et al: Energy cost of walking of amputees: The influence of level of amputaion. J Bone Joint Surg Am 1976;58:42.
341. Watson H, Bohne W: The role of the fibrous band in ulnar deficient extremities. J Bone Joint Surg Am 1971; 53:816.
342. Watts H: Lengthening of short residual limbs in children. In Herring JA, Birch JG (eds): The Child with a Limb Deficiency. Rosemont, Ill, American Academy of Orthopaedic Surgeons, 1998, p 281.
343. Weaver D: Vascular etiology of limb defects: The subclavian artery supply disruption sequence. In Herring JA, Birch JG (eds): The Child with a Limb Deficiency. Rosemont, Ill, American Academy of Orthopaedic Surgeons, 1998, p 25.
344. Weaver S: Comparison of myoelectric and conventional prostheses for adolescent amputees. Am J Occup Ther 1988;42:78.
345. Webster W, Lipson A, Brown-Woodman P: Uterine trauma and limb defects. Teratology 1987;35:253.
346. Westin G, Gunderson G: Proximal femoral focal deficiency: A review of treatment experiences. In Aitken G (ed): A Symposium on Proximal Femoral Focal Deficiency: A Congenital Anomaly. Washington, DC, National Academy of Sciences, 1969, p 100.
347. Wheeler JS, Anderson BJ, De Chalain TMB: Surgical interventions in children with meningococcal purpura fulminans—a review of 117 procedures in 21 children. J Pediatr Surg 2003;38:597.

348. Wilson G: Heritable limb deficienceis. In Herring JA, Birch JG (eds): The Child with a Limb Deficiency. Rosemont, Ill, American Academy of Orthopaedic Surgeons, 1998, p 39.
349. Wood WL, Zlotsky N, Westin GW: Congenital absence of the fibula: Treatment by Syme amputation—indications and technique. J Bone Joint Surg Am 1965;47: 1159.
350. Yetkin H, Cila E, Bilgin Guzel V, Kanatli U: Femoral bifurcation associated with tibial hemimelia. Orthopedics 2001;24:389.
351. Yokouchi Y, Sasaki H, Kuroiwa A: Homeobox gene expression correlated with the bifurcation process of limb cartilage development. Nature 1991;353: 443.
352. Younge D, Dafniotis O: A composite bone flap to lengthen a below-knee amputation stump. J Bone Joint Surg Br 1993;75:330.
353. Zaleskey D: Biology of epiphyseal transplantation. In Friedlaender G, Goldberg V (eds): Bone and Cartilage Allografts: Biology and Clinical Applications. Park Ridge, Ill, American Academy of Orthopaedic Surgeons, 1991, p 27.
354. Zenz W, Zoehrer B, Levin M, et al: Use of recombinant tissue plasminogen activator in children with meningococcal purpura fulminans: A retrospective study. Crit Care Med 2004;32:1777.
355. Zwilling E: Ectoderm-mesoderm relationship in the develoopment of the chick embryo limb bud. J Exp Zool 1955;128:423.

Chapter 34

Arthritis

JOINTS

General Considerations

A joint is a connection between bones of the skeleton. Joints can be classified as fibrous, cartilaginous, or synovial. Fibrous joints are represented by the sutures of the skull, whereas an example of a cartilaginous joint is the symphysis pubis; neither of these joint types allows gross motion. Synovial joints, also termed *diarthrodial,* are the movement units of the skeleton and the main consideration of this chapter.

Synovial joints are composed of the ends of bones, which are covered with hyaline cartilage and encased in a fibrous and ligamentous capsule that is lined with synovium. Hyaline cartilage both functions as a shock absorber and provides a smooth gliding surface for motion. The synovium begins at the margins of the articular cartilage but normally does not overlie the cartilage. The ligaments and capsule, along with the muscles and tendons of the area, provide stability for the joint. The synovium secretes synovial fluid, which lubricates and nourishes the articular cartilage.

Every joint contains a small amount of synovial fluid, which is a combination of a dialysate of plasma and hyaluronic acid that is secreted by the synoviocytes. The lubricating qualities of the fluid come from the mixture of viscid hyaluronic acid and water. Coagulation proteins are not present in normal synovial fluid, and consequently it does not clot.[40] The combination of synovial fluid over articular cartilage produces a remarkably friction-free gliding surface. This is especially important because the articular surfaces are not a perfect fit, and the contact areas change in dimension as motion occurs. In adults, all of the cartilage nutrition is derived from synovial fluid, whereas in children there is a smaller contribution from the underlying bone.[24,156,223]

Symptoms arising from a joint are ordinarily associated with motion and with the stresses of standing and walking. Pain is an outstanding feature because joints have numerous nerve endings in the synovial membrane and capsule. Oversecretion of synovial fluid produces distention of the joint capsule. Excess synovial fluid can be easily seen and palpated in superficial joints. In later stages of inflammation, proliferation and general thickening of the synovium can be detected by careful palpation. With joint inflammation, active and passive motion of the joint are limited.

Muscle spasm, a visceromotor reflex response to painful stimuli, usually accompanies joint inflammation. Spasm is more predominant in the flexor muscle groups, producing a flexion deformity. Atrophy of muscles that are antagonists to those in spasm occurs early and lasts for the duration of the joint disease, often persisting after the spasm has resolved. If a weight-bearing joint is affected, the child will walk with an antalgic limp.

Ultrasonography depicts fluid in the joint and distention of the joint capsule.[259] Radiographs show distention of the capsule, and magnetic resonance imaging (MRI) can delineate the synovial hypertrophy or other soft tissue disorders. Later changes include narrowing of the articular space from erosion of articular cartilage. Subjacent bone responds with sclerosis and osteophyte new bone formation, whereas from the cartilage loose bodies may form. The final stage is exposure of cancellous bone with "bone on bone" and fibrous ankylosis of the joint.

Joint Fluid Analysis

Examination of synovial fluid is an important tool in diagnosing joint disease. Joint aspiration should be performed under rigidly aseptic conditions. The area should be surgically prepared and draped to ensure sterility. The examiner wears a mask and gloves, and assistants should be available to control the apprehensive child.

The anatomic approach to aspiration of various joints is illustrated in Figure 34–1. It is best to use an 18-gauge lumbar puncture needle with a stylet inside. A local anesthetic, such 1% lidocaine (Xylocaine) or procaine, is used.

GROSS APPEARANCE

The gross appearance of the joint fluid often yields important information. Normal synovial fluid is clear and colorless or straw-colored. In the course of aspiration, blood vessels may be punctured, and sanguineous streaks may be found in the joint fluid. This uneven distribution of blood in the syringe is distinguishable from the appearance of the fluid aspirated in acute traumatic hemarthrosis, which is entirely sanguineous. In chronic hemarthrosis the fluid may be xanthochromatic. With inflammation, the joint fluid becomes turbid. The greater the degree of inflammation, the more turbid the synovial effusion. The fluid from a pyogenic joint has the creamy or grayish appearance of frank pus. In rheumatoid arthritis the fluid may be clear in the early stages, but as inflammation increases, it becomes turbid. The fluid in acute gout is milky white because of its urate content. In degenerative arthritis, the joint fluid is almost normal in appearance.

VISCOSITY AND MUCIN CLOT

The concentration and quality of hyaluronate are altered in inflammatory states, with resultant changes in the physical characteristics of the synovial fluid. The fluid should be examined at the time of aspiration, with the examiner noting its viscosity by "pulling" it between the gloved fingers and by letting it drop from a syringe. Normal fluid should form a string at least 1 inch in length. Mucin quality can be tested by adding the fluid to either distilled water or 5% acetic acid. The clot that forms is graded as normal; fair, characterized by some loss of clot continuity; poor, in which there are small, friable masses of clot in a cloudy solution; and very poor, characterized by a few flecks in cloudy solution.

MICROSCOPIC EXAMINATION

Synovial fluid may be examined for cellular elements, intracellular inclusions, and crystals. Glucose and protein levels are also determined. Normal synovial fluid has less than 300 white blood cells (WBCs)/mm^3, and the cell types may be determined. Normal fluid has less than 25% polymorphonuclear leukocytes. Specialized microscopy may reveal cytoplasmic inclusions of immunoglobulin, rheumatoid factor (RF), and complement components. Crystals may be seen with polarized light microscopy.

OTHER EXAMINATIONS

It is important to determine glucose levels because the difference between serum and synovial fluid glucose levels increases with more severe inflammation. Septic arthritis lowers the joint fluid glucose level more than other conditions, and this finding is of diagnostic importance. The normal protein content of synovial fluid is about 30% that of serum. The total protein level is usually 1.8 g/dL, 70% albumin and 7% α_2-globulin. Normal values and common abnormalities are listed in Table 34–1. With inflammation, the permeability of the synovium to plasma increases, and the protein content of the joint approaches that of serum. In addition, clotting factors enter the joint, and the inflammatory fluid forms clots.

JUVENILE RHEUMATOID ARTHRITIS

Juvenile rheumatoid arthritis (JRA) is the name applied to a group of disorders characterized by chronic arthritis of one or more joints with a duration of at least 6 weeks. The majority of cases are pauciarticular, with several joints involved, and are often accompanied by uveitis. The polyarticular form is sometimes associated with involvement of other systems with such manifestations as lymphadenopathy, splenomegaly, and fever. Systemic-onset JRA is a severe multisystem disease with arthritis as an accompanying manifestation. In the past, the term *Still's disease* was used to identify these disorders, after G. F. Still, who published a description of 22 cases in 1897.[229] An earlier description by Cornil in 1864 predated Still's paper but lacked its completeness.[46]

Definition and Classification

Diagnosis of JRA is based primarily on clinical findings. There are no specific laboratory tests to confirm the diagnosis. The American College of Rheumatology has established five criteria for the diagnosis of JRA (or JA): (1) age at onset younger than 16 years; (2) arthritis of one or more joints; (3) symptom duration of at least 6 weeks; (4) an onset type, after 6 months' observation, of the polyarthritic form (five or more affected joints), the oligoarthritic form (fewer than five joints affected), or the systemic form with arthritis and characteristic fever; and (5) exclusion of other forms of arthritis. In 1977 the European League Against Rheumatism (EULAR) proposed the term *juvenile chronic arthritis* (JCA) for the same disorder. Their criteria include (1) onset before age 16 years; (2) arthritis in one or more joints; (3) disease duration of at least 3 months; and (4) a pattern of pauciarticular (fewer than five joints affected), polyarticular (more than four joints affected), and RF-negative or systemic arthritis with characteristic fever. They also include juvenile rheumatoid arthritis (more than four joints affected and RF-positive), juvenile ankylosing spondylitis, and juvenile psoriatic arthritis in the classification.

Debate continues regarding the proper terminology for these various disorders. The term *rheumatoid* is considered inappropriate by many authors because so few children carry RF.[67,188]

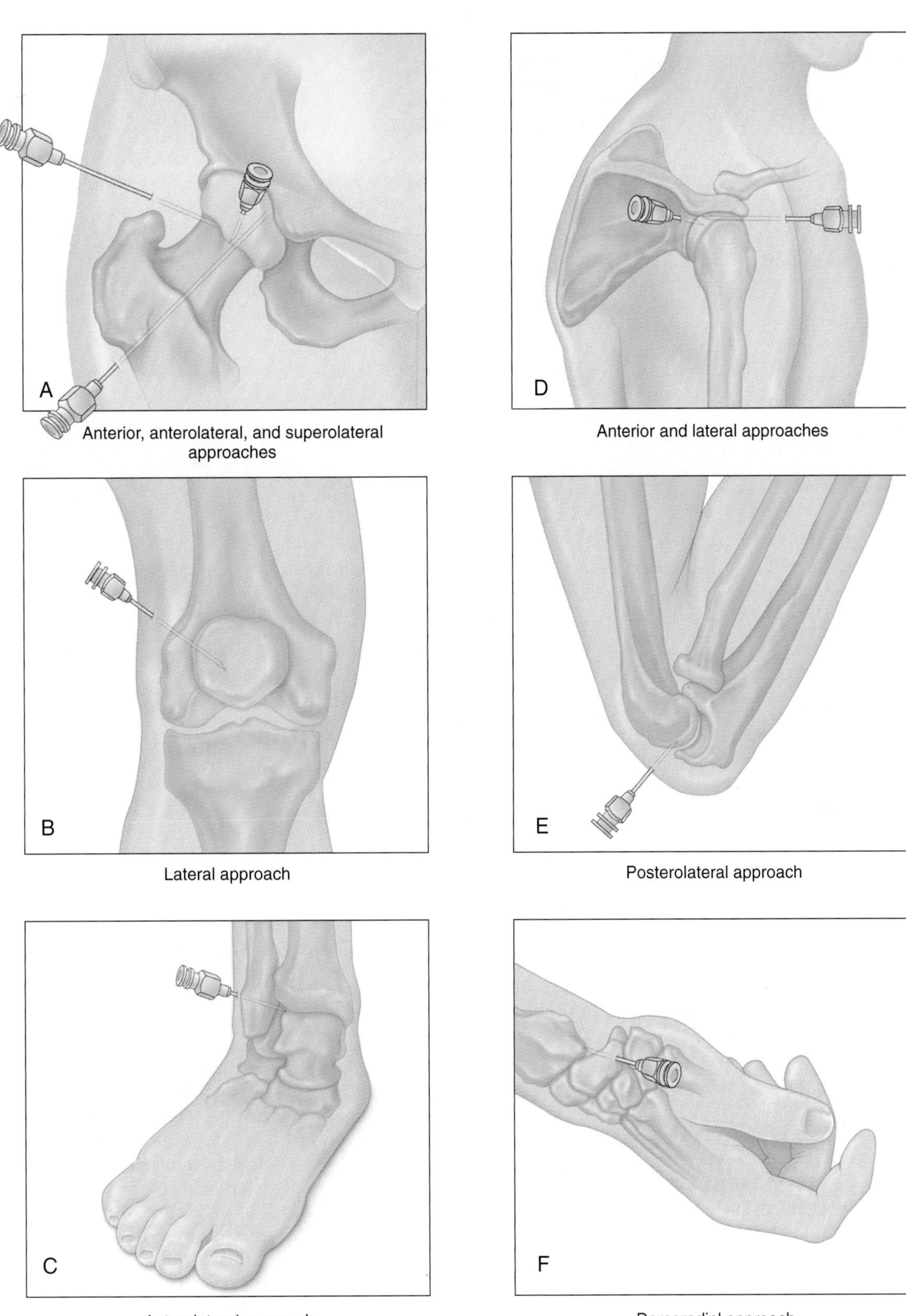

FIGURE 34–1 Routes of aspiration of joints. **A,** Anterior, anterolateral, and superolateral approaches. **B,** Lateral approach. **C,** Anterolateral approach. **D,** Anterior and lateral approaches. **E,** Posterolateral approach. **F,** Dorsoradial approach.

Table 34-1 Synovial Findings in Joint Disorders

	Group I: Noninflammatory			Group II: Noninfectious Inflammatory	
Parameter Measured	Normal	Traumatic Arthritis	Degenerative Joint Disease	Systemic Lupus Erythematosus	Pigmented Villonodular Synovitis
Appearance	Straw or clear yellow	Clear yellow, bloody, or xanthochromatic	Clear yellow	Straw	Xanthochromatic
Clarity	Transparent	Transparent or turbid	Transparent	Slightly cloudy	Turbid
Viscosity	Normal	Normal	Normal	Normal or decreased	Normal
Mucin clot	Good	Good	Good	Good or fair	Good
Total white blood cell count	≤200	≤2000 (few to many RBCs)	≤1000	5000 (10% DNA particles)	≤3000 (some RBCs)
Polymorphonuclear leukocytes	<20%	<20%	<20%	>50%	<20%
Crystals	Negative	Negative	Negative	Negative	Negative
RA or LE cells	Negative	Negative	Negative	LE cells	Negative
Bacteria	Negative	Negative	Negative	Negative	Negative
Glucose—difference between levels in joint fluid and blood	20 mg/mL	20 mg/100 mL	20 mg/100 mL	20 to 30 mg/100 mL	20 mg/100 mL
Total proteins	1.8 g/100 mL	3.3 g/100 mL	3.0 g/100 mL	3.2 g/100 mL	3.0 g/100 mL
Albumin	60%-70%	60%	60%	60%	57%
Gamma-globulin	14%	16%	16%	15%	17%
Immunoglobulin		Normal	Normal	Elevated	Normal
Complement (total and B_1-C)		Normal	Normal	Decreased	Negative
Latex fixation and sensitized sheep cell agglutination	Negative	Negative	Negative	Occasionally positive	Negative

LE, lupus erythematosus; RA, rheumatoid arthritis; RBCs, red blood cells.

Incidence and Prevalence

The reported incidence of JRA ranges from 3 to 13.9 cases per 100,000 per year.[76,248] The prevalence of the disorder is in the range of 113 per 100,000 children (95% confidence limits: 69, 196).[239]

Demographics

The most common age at onset is between 1 and 3 years, and in this age group girls predominate and most often have pauciarticular disease.[47,57,58,84,147] A second peak of onset occurs around age 9 years, and at this age the proportion of boys affected approaches that of girls. Overall, JRA is twice as common in girls as boys. With pauciarticular disease the ratio is 3:1, and with uveitis and arthritis girls outnumber boys by 5:1 or 6:1.[1,41,231,240] It may be that black children are less often affected than white children, but this is uncertain.[92]

Etiology

The etiology of JRA remains unknown, but a number of factors relating to etiology have been reported. The predominant common factors involve the immune system. Children with JRA have altered immune systems, as shown in several studies.[137,143] Specific immunodeficiencies are associated with JRA, and there is much evidence that immune reactions are involved in joint inflammation. T-lymphocyte abnormalities have been reported frequently, but their exact role in pathogenesis has yet to be determined.[14,143,174,206,255] Human leukocyte antigen (HLA) product, T-cell receptor, and an antigen, together called a *trimolecular complex*, play a critical role in JRA pathogenesis.[85]

Heredity may also play a role in the etiology of JRA. The reported familial incidence of the disorder ranges from 23% to 41%,[58,134,205] and twin concordance has been reported.[15,122]

Infection has long been proposed as a factor in the etiology of JRA, and many different hypotheses have been supported. Studies in the late 1960s implicated *Mycoplasma fermentans*, which was isolated from 31 of 79 samples of synovial fluid.[254] More recently, infection with rubella virus has been found in children with rheumatic diseases, with virus isolated from both serum and synovial fluid in 7 of 19 patients.[33]

In addition, infection with *Bartonella henselae* may play a role in the etiology of systemic-onset JRA.[244]

Group II: Noninfectious Inflammatory (cont'd)		Group II: Severe Noninfectious Inflammatory	Group III: Infectious Inflammatory	
Rheumatic Fever	Gout	Rheumatoid Arthritis	Pyogenic Arthritis	Tuberculous Arthritis
Yellow	Yellow to turbid milky	Yellow to greenish	Grayish or bloody	Yellow
Slightly cloudy	Cloudy	Cloudy	Turbid purulent	Cloudy
Decreased	Decreased	Decreased to poor	Decreased to poor	Decreased to poor
Good	Poor	Poor	Poor	Poor
10,000	10,000-14,000	15,000 (1000-60,000)	60,000	20,000
50%	60%-70%	55%	90%	60%
Negative	Urate + (in pseudogout, calcium pyrophosphate)	Negative	Negative	Negative
Negative	Negative	RA cells	Negative	Negative
Negative	Negative	Negative	Positive	Positive
20 mg/100 mL	20 mg/100 mL	≥30 mg/100 mL	30-50 mg/100 mL	30-50 mg/100 mL
3.0 g/100 mL	5 g/100 mL	4.1 g/100 mL	4.2 g/100 mL	4.2 g/100 mL
60%	70%	42%	45%	45%
14%	9%	25%	25%	25%
Normal or slightly elevated	Normal	Elevated	Normal	Normal
Normal	Normal or elevated	Decreased	Normal	Normal
Negative	Negative	Positive	Negative	Negative

Perinatal infection with influenza virus with expression of the disease many years later has also been proposed as an etiology.[190] The infectious agent may supply the antigen that initiates the immune reaction.[191]

Physical and psychological trauma have been associated with the onset of JRA. However, no clear causal relationship has been identified for either type of trauma, and they are considered aggravating factors at best. Barometric changes and weather patterns have anecdotally been associated with disease severity but most likely have no causal role.

Pathology

The histologic changes of the synovium in these disorders are those of chronic inflammation and are not specific to or diagnostic of rheumatoid disorders. The inflamed synovium is hypervascular and infiltrated with small lymphocytes and polymorphonuclear leukocytes in the acute phases (Fig. 34–2). There is excessive synovial fluid, which is thin and watery. Later, the synovium proliferates and forms granulation tissue, which may cover the articular cartilage and is termed a *pannus* (Fig. 34–3). Precipitated fibrin may form small, solid pieces called *rice bodies,* which may float freely in the joint.

Reactions in the bone are secondary to the aggressive inflammation of the synovium. Erosion of bone at the sites of synovial attachments occurs, and subchondral bony resorption is common. Loss of cartilage beneath the pannus is followed by subchondral bony destruction, and this sequence may lead to ankylosis of the joint. Osteopenia may occur and has been noted in 41% of adults with a history of JRA, placing them at increased risk for fracture in later life.[71] Normal bone mineral density, however, is often attained in adulthood by patients in whom JRA is in remission.[96] Delay in linear growth occurs with some children, particularly those with RF-positive polyarticular and systemic JRA.[139]

Clinical Features

PAUCIARTICULAR JUVENILE RHEUMATOID ARTHRITIS

Approximately half of cases of JRA in children are of the pauciarticular form, which by definition includes only cases with fewer than five joints involved.

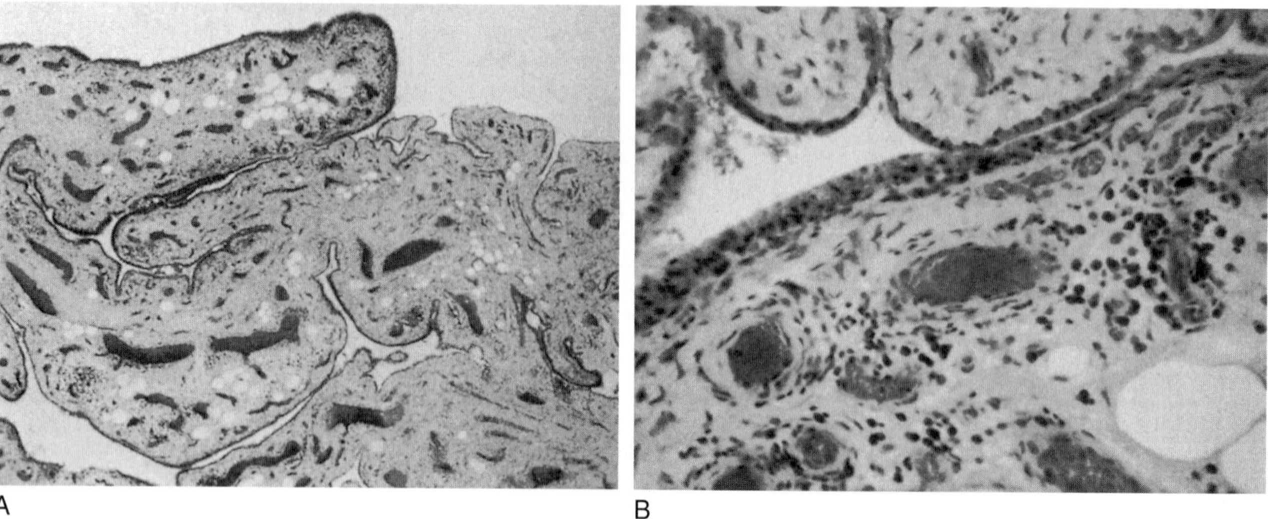

FIGURE 34–2 Histologic appearance of synovium in rheumatoid arthritis. **A,** Original magnification ×100. **B,** Original magnification ×250.

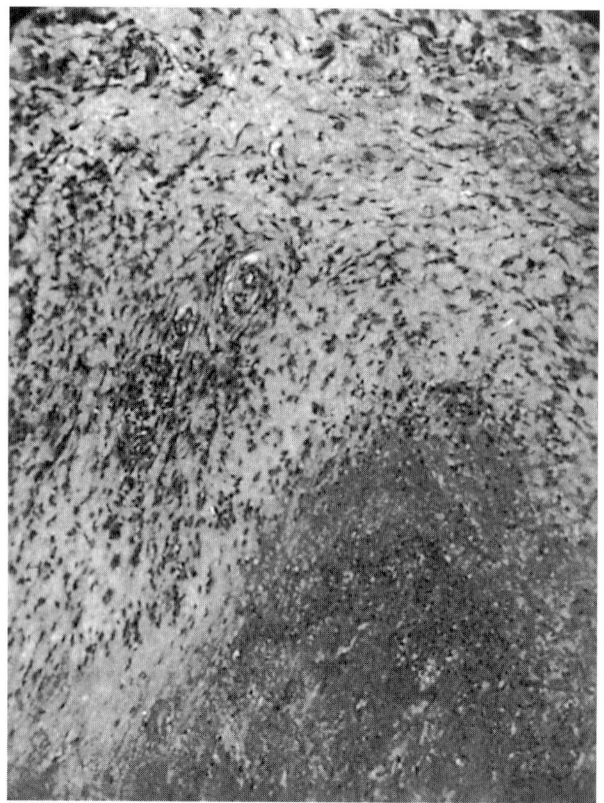

FIGURE 34–3 Microscopic appearance of rheumatoid nodule. Note the focus of fibrinoid degeneration surrounded by fibroblasts arranged in palisade formation.

Girls affected by this variety of the illness outnumber affected boys by a ratio of 7:3. In other words, an affected child is twice as likely to be female than male. The peak period of onset is between 2 and 4 years of age, with half of affected children coming to medical attention before 4 years of age. Approximately 70% of children with pauciarticular JRA demonstrate a positive antinuclear antibody test and will eventually develop iritis.[219] The outlook for remission of pauciarticular JRA is approximately 34% to 54% over the 10-year period after diagnosis.[63,165,219] Among patients with oligoarthritis and late onset of JCA, a lower probability exists for remission among those who are HLA-B27 positive.[165]

Pauciarticular JRA manifests as a low-grade inflammation of one or several joints in an otherwise well child. In about half of patients only one joint is involved. The knee is most often affected, with the ankle–subtalar and elbow joints next in frequency (Fig. 34–4). Hip involvement is unusual and, when present, may raise other diagnostic considerations. The small joints of the hands and feet are usually spared. Cervical spine involvement is extremely rare.[98] On presentation, one or several joints may be involved. Over several months other joints may become inflamed, but in half of the pauciarticular cases only one joint is involved.[32,211]

A history of insidious onset without precipitating trauma is common, although occasionally some traumatic event calls attention to the joint. Morning stiffness is a frequent complaint, with symptoms decreasing during the day as the joint is used. The swelling is persistent; it may gradually increase but usually does not change dramatically from day to day. By convention, a duration of 6 weeks of arthritis is necessary for the diagnosis of JRA to be considered.

The involved joints are usually mildly tender and swollen. The swelling is a combination of synovial thickening and joint effusion. The degree of swelling is often out of proportion to the degree of tenderness or the amount of pain. The joint is warm but usually not erythematous, and there is some loss of range of motion and some pain when the joint is moved. Differential diagnosis includes oligoarticular-onset juvenile psoriatic arthritis (oligo-JPsA) and septic arthritis. Patterns of joint involvement may differentiate oligo-

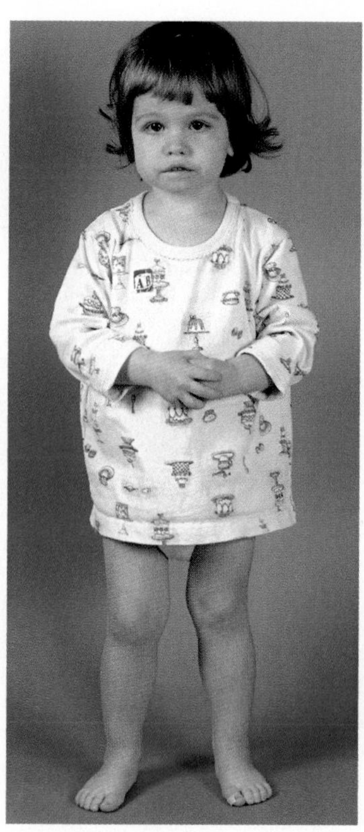

FIGURE 34–4 Typical appearance of a young girl with a swollen knee of pauciarticular juvenile rheumatoid arthritis.

JPsA, with small joint disease of the hands and feet significantly more frequent in oligo-JPsA than in pauciarticular JRA.[109] Patients with septic arthritis typically present with fever and an inability to bear weight, with an erythrocyte sedimentation rate (ESR) of 40 mm/hour, and a WBC count greater than 12,000 cells/mm^3, with larger joints most often involved.[209] Ultrasonographic evaluation confirms the presence of excess fluid in the joints of patients with septic arthritis. Joint aspiration provides relief of symptoms and a specimen for culture, sensitivity, cell count, and differential to facilitate diagnosis.[209] By comparison, a septic joint is exquisitely tender and the limitation of motion is much greater than in the inflamed joint in JRA.

Uveitis is a serious associated problem and may ultimately affect the child's vision. It may be present at onset; in 20% of children it develops over the course of the disease. An early diagnosis can be made on finding increased protein levels and inflammatory cells in the anterior chamber of the eye on slit-lamp examination. Later, posterior synechiae form and tether the iris to the lens, resulting in an irregular and poorly reactive pupil. Band keratopathy and cataracts occur late but eventually may involve 42% to 58% of patients with uveitis.[121,186] Most cases are asymptomatic, and ophthalmologic examination is essential to allow early treatment.

The course of the disease is relatively benign. The arthritis waxes and wanes and is usually responsive to medical control. Over a period ranging from 3 to 11 years, the disease usually resolves. The average duration of disease is 2 years 9 months, and in half of cases it is less than 2 years.[83] In approximately one third of cases there is progressive involvement of more joints, so that the disorder resembles typical polyarthritis with somewhat fewer joints involved (Box 34–1). Regarding indicators of long-term prognosis in JRA, male sex is correlated with increased disability in systemic-onset JRA, but with less disability among patients with RF-negative disease, and with shorter active disease duration in patients with RF-positive polyarticular-onset JRA.[172] The presence of antinuclear antibody correlates with longer active disease duration in patients with pauciarticular-onset JRA.[172] Younger age at disease onset predicts longer active disease duration in patients with pauciarticular and RF-negative polyarticular JRA, and a shorter active disease duration in patients with systemic-onset JRA.[172] Early disease onset and female sex are early indicators of unfavorable outcomes in JRA.[70]

Box 34-1

Pauciarticular Pearls

- Often presents to an orthopaedist
- One or two joints, often knee, subtalar
- Morning stiffness
- Joints swollen, minimally tender
- Erythrocyte sedimentation rate and C-reactive protein level mildly elevated or normal
- Uveitis present

POLYARTICULAR-ONSET JUVENILE RHEUMATOID ARTHRITIS

When five or more joints are involved within the first 6 months of illness, the syndrome is by definition polyarticular JRA.[219] Two peaks of onset exist, the first between 1 and 3 years and the second between 8 and 10 years of age. Girls predominate in the later age group, which may in fact represent early-onset adult rheumatoid arthritis.[219] Remission rate is estimated at 15% to 50% during the 10-year period after diagnosis.[63,165,219] Polyarticular JRA has many characteristics in common with the pauciarticular form. The onset is insidious, the large joints of the lower extremity are often involved, the inflammation is chronic, and pain and swelling are moderate. The small joints of the hands and feet are commonly involved, as are the joints of the cervical spine and the temporomandibular joints (Figs. 34–5 and 34–6). The affected joints are warm, tender, painful on motion, and swollen, with synovial thickening and effusion. Joint range of motion is almost always limited; this is initially caused by protective muscle spasm and later by destruction of articular cartilage and fibrosis. Affected children

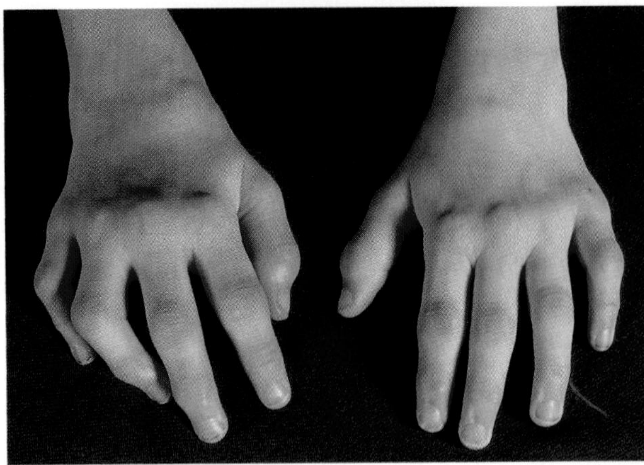

FIGURE 34-5 Swelling of the wrist and metatarsophalangeal and proximal interphalangeal joints of the hand in polyarticular juvenile rheumatoid arthritis.

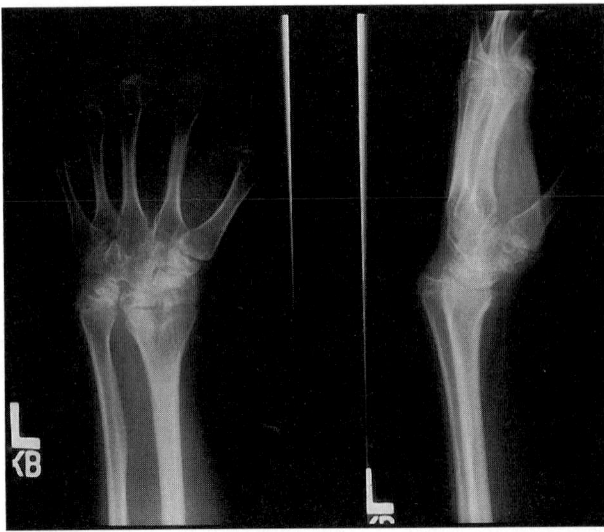

FIGURE 34-6 Radiographic changes of juvenile rheumatoid arthritis of the wrist. Carpal destruction and volar subluxation are common findings.

typically appear apprehensive and guard their painful limbs against movement. Symptoms arising in the temporomandibular joint are often described as "earache," and symptoms arising from the sternoclavicular and costochondral joints are described as "chest pain." On occasion, hoarseness and laryngeal stridor may result from inflammation of the cricoarytenoid joints. Cervical spine involvement with fusion of the apophyseal joints results in limitation of neck motion. Involvement of the temporomandibular joint causes failure of development of the lower jaw and results in a receding chin.

Some systemic manifestations may be present and include low-grade fever, hepatosplenomegaly, lymphadenopathy, and subclinical pleural and pericardial inflammation.

A major distinction is made between children with RF-positive polyarticular disease and those with RF-negative disease. The RF-positive disease in children is in many ways similar to the adult form of rheumatoid arthritis. The children have rheumatoid nodules, erosion of joint surfaces, and a disease course that extends well into adulthood (Fig. 34–7). Children with RF-negative disease have less involvement of the small joints of the hands and feet and do not form nodules.

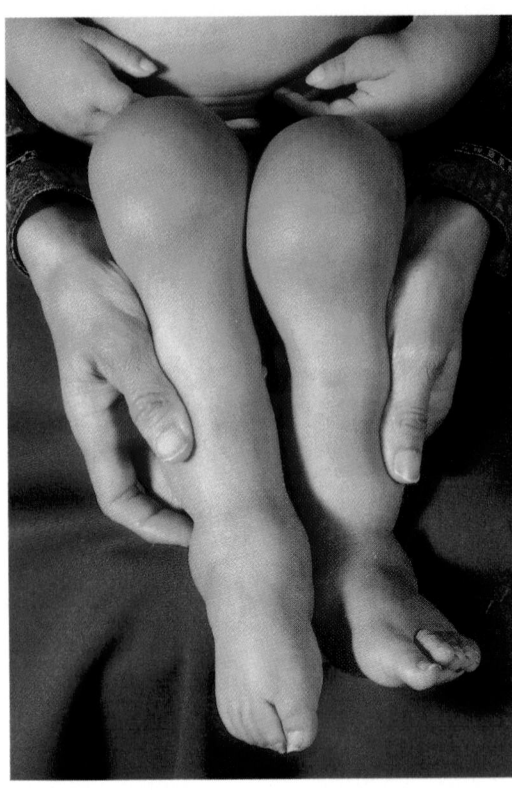

FIGURE 34-7 Arthritis of the knees and ankles in a child with seropositive polyarticular juvenile rheumatoid arthritis.

SYSTEMIC-ONSET JUVENILE RHEUMATOID ARTHRITIS

The systemic form of JRA is a serious disease in which arthritis is only one manifestation of a generalized disorder. It affects 20% of children with JRA and is associated with the worst long-term prognosis, resulting in many cases in severely damaged or destroyed joints.[219] Remission occurs in approximately 29% to 50% of children within 10 years of diagnosis.[63,165,219] Many organs and systems may be involved, including the liver, spleen, pleura, pericardium, and skin. Uveitis is rare. A febrile course with one or two daily spikes from normal to 39°C or 40°C is typical. The temperature spikes most often occur late in the afternoon, and the temperature rapidly returns to baseline. During the febrile periods the children are listless and appear ill but may seem well once they defervesce. The fever usually does not respond to salicylates or nonsteroidal agents.

Affected children usually have a characteristic skin rash with discrete, erythematous maculae 2 to 5 mm in diameter (Fig. 34–8). The skin rash is classically a

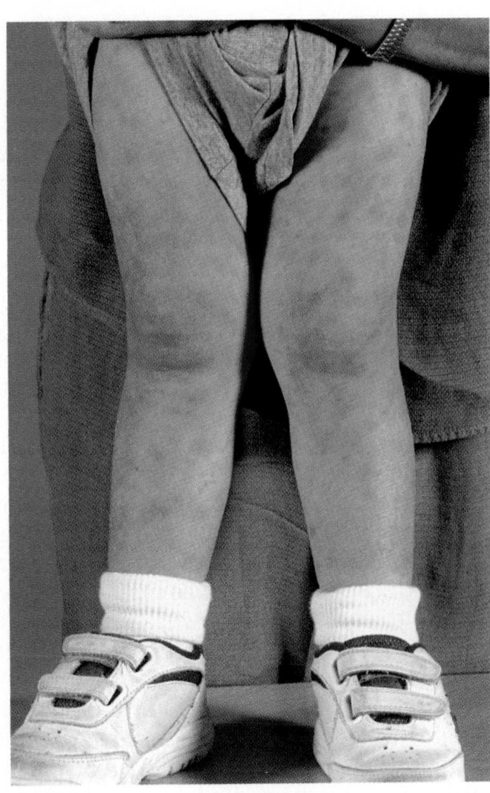

FIGURE 34–8 Typical rash of systemic-onset juvenile rheumatoid arthritis.

salmon color but may be more reddish in the early stage. It is located on the trunk, face, palms, soles, and proximal extremities and tends to migrate fairly rapidly. There is often a clear halo around the maculae, and the larger ones may be clear in the center.

Hepatosplenomegaly and generalized lymphadenopathy are often present. Enlarged, inflamed mesenteric nodes may cause abdominal pain and distention, suggesting an acute surgical abdomen. The enlargement of abdominal organs usually resolves over a few months. Pericarditis and pleural effusions occur in about 10% of those with systemic disease and may manifest with nonspecific chest pain.[80] Electrocardiographic changes are present and the cardiac silhouette is enlarged on the chest radiograph. The cardiac manifestations are usually transient and rarely result in congestive heart failure.[52,140] The presence of pericarditis is not related to the severity of the disease in general or to the joint manifestations.[23]

Amyloidosis is a grave complication that is rare in North America, but in Great Britain it occurs in about 7.5% of cases.[9] It presents with proteinuria and hypertension, and immunoglobulin G and C-reactive protein (CRP) levels are elevated in those who develop amyloidosis. Control of the activity of the inflammatory disease is the mainstay of prevention of amyloidosis.[9]

Laboratory Evaluation

There is no single or definitive test for rheumatoid disease; rather, the diagnosis is made from clinical findings coupled with suggestive laboratory findings. Anemia, leukocytosis, and inflammatory indices generally correspond to the severity of the disease. WBC counts of 30,000 to 50,000/mm^3 may occur in children with systemic disease. Elevation of the platelet count also may accompany severe disease. The elevation of the ESR and CRP level is related to the severity of systemic disease.

Synovial biopsies show villous hypertrophy, vascular endothelial hyperplasia, and infiltration by lymphocytes and plasma cells. These changes are typical of chronic inflammation. Over time, the inflamed synovium forms a pannus of tissue that covers and destroys articular cartilage. Rheumatoid nodules are not seen in children with JRA except for those with the seropositive polyarticular form.[32]

Radiographic Evaluation

Although plain radiography remains the mainstay of radiographic evaluation, ultrasonography and MRI are useful in the early stages of disease to identify joint effusion and synovial hypertrophy.[72,197] The earliest changes seen on plain films include periarticular soft tissue swelling; osteopenia, especially around the joint; and widening of the joint space.

As the disease progresses the radiographic joint space narrows owing to destruction of articular cartilage (Fig. 34–9), and the extent of radiographic damage, especially joint space narrowing, correlates with functional disability.[173] Adjacent osteopenia causes loss of the subchondral bony plate. In late disease, erosive changes produce notching of the bone, especially in the carpals (see Fig. 34–6). Epiphyseal overgrowth

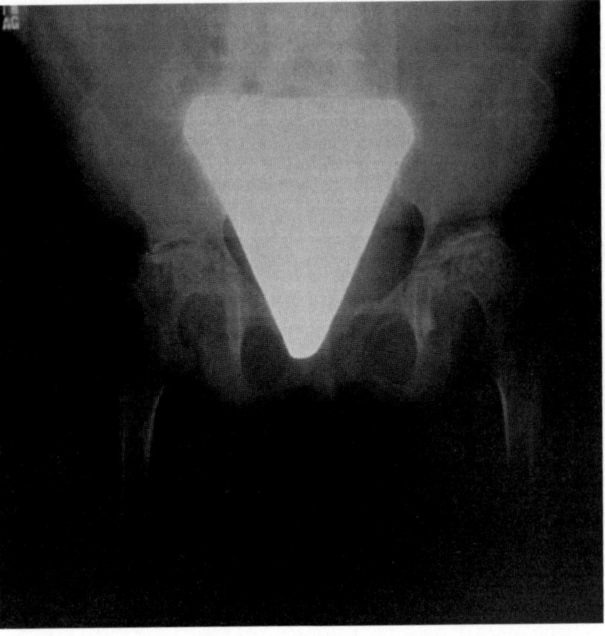

FIGURE 34–9 Bilateral hip involvement with systemic-onset juvenile rheumatoid arthritis. There is almost total loss of joint space on the right. Total hip replacement is usually successful in this situation.

may occur secondary to hyperemia, or disuse may retard growth.

The frequency of abnormal hand and wrist radiographic findings such as periarticular osteopenia, joint space narrowing, and erosion is very high early in the course of polyarticular JRA.[159] In addition, both large and small joints may become subluxated. Most commonly this occurs with volar subluxation of the wrist, posterolateral subluxation of the hip, and ulnar subluxation of the metacarpophalangeal joints. In the final stages, fibrous or bony ankylosis occurs.

Some of the most specific radiographic changes occur in the cervical spine.[65,157] Erosion of the odontoid in a "napkin ring" pattern may be associated with atlantoaxial instability. An atlanto–dens interval greater than 4.5 mm may be seen in 20% of patients but is rarely related to neurologic dysfunction.[62] Fusion between cervical segments is common and most often occurs at C2-3. Cervical spine involvement is rarely present in patients with pauciarticular disease.[98]

Involvement of the temporomandibular joint is also common and may result in mandibular undergrowth. This produces a micrognathia that is characteristically seen in children with long-standing disease.[17]

Treatment

As with other complex disorders, juvenile arthritis is best managed by a specialized team that includes the rheumatologist, orthopaedists, ophthalmologists, physical and occupational therapists, nurses, and social workers.

MEDICAL TREATMENT

The nonsteroidal anti-inflammatory drugs (NSAIDs) are the mainstay of treatment of most patients.[110] Although aspirin was the initial agent of choice, modern agents supply more potency with fewer side effects. Aspirin is given in a dosage of 75 to 90 mg/kg/day, usually in four divided doses with food, seeking a therapeutic salicylate level of 20 to 25 mg/dL. Ibuprofen is given in a dosage of 35 mg/kg/day, again in four doses with food. Naproxen is used at 15 to 20 mg/kg/day twice a day. Tolmetin sodium is given in a dosage of 25 to 30 mg/kg/day in three doses. At this time only these three NSAIDs are approved by the U.S. Food and Drug Administration for use in children.

In more severe disease not responsive to NSAIDs, other, more toxic drugs may be efficacious, although approximately one third of all patients do not respond adequately to methotrexate.[110] Low-dose methotrexate and other cytotoxic drugs may have a rapid effect on resistant disease.[219] Methotrexate is given weekly either orally on an empty stomach or by subcutaneous administration, which is usually well tolerated, although it causes nausea and vomiting in some children and, rarely, hepatic toxicity.[219] Hematologic, hepatic, and pulmonary monitoring is mandatory when these agents are used. A group of agents, the slow-acting antirheumatic drugs (or SARDs), includes antimalarial agents (hydroxychloroquine), parenterally administered gold compounds, and penicillamine. For patients who fail to respond to first-line drugs these drugs may be effective, but they are slow acting, requiring 3 to 6 months for full effect. If significant improvement does not occur within a few months of beginning methotrexate, then sulfasalazine, hydroxychloroquine, or other antirheumatic agents should be added.[219] The tumor necrosis factor (TNF) inhibitor etanercept is also effective and well tolerated by patients with JRA.[110,150,234] An intravenous form of the monoclonal anti-TNF agent infliximab is also available. Use of both these TNF-inhibiting agents is associated with increased infection risk owing to reduced TNF action.

Intra-articular glucocorticoids are indicated and may be effective treatment for recalcitrant joint inflammation. These agents may be administered after joint lavage in refractory disease and typically bring significant clinical improvement within a few days.[222] The average duration of response after each injection is 1 year, and early repeated injections (e.g., three injections over 42 months) may prevent leg length discrepancy by long-term inhibition of synovitis.[219] Intra-articular injections reduce pannus formation and have no detectable deleterious effect on cartilage.[219] Intra-articular injection of glucocorticoids can be performed successfully in children sedated with oral midazolam, although general anesthesia is advisable if several joints must be injected or if the hip or subtalar joint is to be treated.[219] Triamcinolone hexacetonide is the preferred steroid for this purpose because of its long duration of action.[219] Systemic steroids are indicated for life-threatening systemic disease but are not indicated long term because of the side effects of iatrogenic Cushing's syndrome and irreversible growth impairment.[249] Ophthalmic glucocorticoids are used to treat chronic uveitis.

PHYSICAL AND OCCUPATIONAL THERAPY

Physical and occupational therapists should be involved in the clinical team managing children with chronic arthritis. The goals of such therapy are to relieve pain, increase range of motion, improve muscular coordination, and help the patient relearn physiologic functional patterns. Therapists also help children learn about joint protection and self-care. Splinting on a selective basis is useful, and adapted footwear and walking aids may be used.[89] Splinting of the wrists and hands may reduce the tendency toward joint contracture and subluxation. Occasionally, splinting of the knee or ankle at night is indicated to maintain range of motion.

Physical conditioning in children with arthritis is often poor, with decreased aerobic capacity and exercise tolerance in proportion to the severity of the disease.[78,129] Disuse atrophy of muscles, joint contractures, and anemia contribute to deconditioning. Rehabilitation of children with arthritis should include conditioning training in addition to standard physical therapy activities. Conditioning requires that muscles be challenged with repetitive, progressive stress with exercises aimed at specific muscle groups. When joints are acutely inflamed, isometric exercises are recommended. Dynamic exercise can begin when the arthritis is in subacute or chronic stages. A general guideline is to have the child lift the maximum weight he or she can lift for 10 repetitions. That weight is then used for 2 or 3 sets of 2 to 10 repetitions for each muscle to be exercised. That weight is gradually increased. Low-impact sports such as walking, swimming, cycling, or low-impact aerobic dance are more appropriate than highly competitive sports.[130] Although excessive exercise may aggravate an inflamed joint, specific restrictions should be applied only when the management team is relatively certain of a deleterious effect.

Controlled studies of physical therapy interventions with standardized measurement techniques have not shown a positive long-term effect on the arthritic disease,[91,94,228] nor have they shown a negative effect.[88,229] One study reported that children with juvenile arthritis who receive massage therapy from their parents for 15 minutes a day for 30 days showed significant reduction in pain and anxiety and improved activity level compared with a control group of children who engaged in relaxation therapy.[66]

ORTHOPAEDIC TREATMENT

Chronic joint inflammation results in a cycle beginning with muscle spasm to protect the painful joint from motion. If continued, the cycle results in contracture of the muscle and joint capsule and disuse of the extremity, with resultant osteopenia. The orthopaedic management of JRA is concerned with interrupting this cycle. Thus, management emphasizes maintaining joint range of motion and extremity alignment and length, reducing synovial proliferation, observation of cervical spine stability, and ultimately joint replacement as needed. Synovectomy remains a controversial modality. Releases about the hip and knee are sometimes needed; rarely, cervical spine instability requires treatment; and hand and foot deformities are sometimes correctable. All operative procedures in patients with JRA require careful preanesthetic evaluation. Cervical spine stiffness and instability, reduced mobility of the jaw with hypoplasia of the mandible, and coexisting medical conditions may require specialized approaches for intubation and recovery.

Synovectomy may be helpful for severely affected, recalcitrant joints but has not been shown to alter the long-term outcome of joint disease.* Although some studies have shown that after removal of inflamed synovial tissue a new, relatively normal synovial lining regenerates,[73,111] others have reported frequent recurrence of disease.[81,182,194] The results of synovectomy are best in large joints, and the knee is the most common joint so treated. Likewise, the best results with synovectomy are obtained if the procedure is performed early, before significant joint destruction has occurred.[119] Successful synovectomy results in a reduction in swelling and pain.[153] Range of motion is not improved after synovectomy,[153] and care is necessary to avoid losing motion. Arthroscopic synovectomy is associated with less postoperative stiffness and morbidity, and postoperative continuous passive motion may be helpful. Synovectomy is indicated when a trial of medical management for more than 6 months (including intra-articular steroids) has failed.

The development of flexion contractures of the hip and knee results in loss of walking efficiency, with both increased loading on the knee and increased pain.[232] When contractures of the knee exceed 15 to 20 degrees, significant loss of walking ability occurs.[184] Surgical releases of the hip and knee may result in long-term improvement in range of motion and function. Witt and McCullough reported a reduction in flexion deformities of the hip from an average of 35 degrees to 9.5 degrees, with loss of correction to 18 degrees at 3 years. This improvement was maintained in patients followed as long as 12 years.[261] In another study of soft tissue releases of the hip or knee (or both), 10 of 27 patients were able to walk before surgery and 22 could walk after release(s).[167] After 3 years there was some loss of correction. Other authors have reported similar reductions in contracture, with acceptable recurrence rates.[203]

Release of knee flexion contracture is best done with the patient prone. Usually the hamstrings, lateral intermuscular septum, and iliotibial band are released. If necessary, one or both tendinous portions of the gastrocnemius muscles are sectioned and the posterior capsule of the knee is also released. Occasionally the anterior cruciate must be cut to correct posterior tibial subluxation.[42,203] To avoid posterior subluxation, the postoperative cast must be molded to displace the tibia anteriorly as the knee is extended. If full correction cannot be obtained without neurovascular compromise, subsequent cast changes under anesthesia may be required.[42] Postoperative night splinting for up to 6 months is recommended to prevent recurrence.

Flexion contractures of the hip also respond to soft tissue releases. These are indicated when a significant contracture that interferes with ambulation persists after 6 months or more of aggressive medical therapy. Swann and Ansell reported a reduction in flexion contractures after psoas and adductor tenotomy, with improvement still evident 3 years after surgery.[233]

Growth disturbances are most often seen at the knee. When a valgus deformity is present, either an epiphyseal stapling or percutaneous partial epiphysiodesis will correct the deformity without major surgical trauma. The epiphysiodesis approach is preferred because of the minimal incision required. It should be done when growth prediction based on bone age shows 2 to 3 cm of growth remaining at the distal femoral epiphysiodesis. Rydholm and colleagues reported that stapling of the distal femoral epiphysis for valgus was effective in correcting the deformity in 15 of 17 patients so treated. Stapling was also effective in correcting leg length inequality.[202]

Scoliosis occasionally occurs in patients with JRA and may be managed by conventional means.[168]

*See references 10, 60, 61, 68, 73, 106, 113, 140, 157, 176, 201, 204.

Micrognathia due to temporomandibular involvement may be successfully treated by odontoidectomy through the transoral approach using a sagittal split mandibular osteomy.[120]

TOTAL JOINT ARTHROPLASTY

Total joint arthroplasty is an appropriate and effective therapy for adolescents with polyarticular disease and painful, stiff, destroyed joints. Hip disease ultimately develops in 30% to 50% of all children with JRA, although recent aggressive treatment approaches and more effective drug therapy have reduced the proportion of children in whom severe hip disease develops. Consequently, the incidence of hip surgery has decreased, and outcomes of hip arthroplasty have improved.[224] Hip and knee replacements have a well-established role in improving the function and well-being of the patient. Wrist, elbow, and ankle replacements may be useful, but there is less clinical experience behind them.

Total hip or knee arthroplasty is indicated in the adolescent with marked functional impairment or severe disabling pain from advanced structural hip or knee joint involvement[180,216] (see Fig. 34–9). Careful planning with a team approach is essential and should include consideration of high school and college education, use of crutches, medications, and emotional status. Preoperative planning includes procuring miniature or custom-made hip prostheses in up to half of patients. When both hip and knee replacements are necessary, it is best to approach the hip first because it is more difficult to rehabilitate the knee in the presence of a painful, contracted ipsilateral hip. In addition, it is useful at times to manipulate and cast the knee to gain extension at the time of the total hip arthroplasty.[216]

Total hip replacement may be performed in a child with growth remaining. Knee replacement in the setting of open epiphyses is indicated if minimal growth remains. One series of knee replacements with open physes reported no growth disturbances, but all epiphyses had closed within 2 years of replacement.[208]

Total joint replacements are difficult to perform in these patients owing to osteopenia, contractures, and coexisting medical conditions. Cementless arthroplasties are gradually replacing cemented prostheses because of late loosening.

The results of hip and knee replacement are remarkable. Relief of pain is reported in almost all patients after hip replacement and in a high percentage after knee replacement. Improvement in range of motion is excellent at the hip and good at the knee. Most important, functional status improves in a high percentage of patients, often to a remarkable degree.[192] Rates of loosening of hip components range from 12% at 4.5 years to 43% at over 5 years after surgery. Prosthesis survival rates (still functioning) are up to 92% at 10 years and 83% at 15 years.[21,27,31,39,86,87,133,135,138,155,216,256]

There are fewer reports available evaluating replacement of other joints. Connor and Morrey evaluated 19 patients after total elbow replacement and found that 96% had pain relief. Although improvement in motion was less predictable, most patients gained a functionally significant range, including those with ankylosed joints preoperatively.[44] Total ankle replacements are rarely performed in children, and reports in adults are mixed, with a significant number of failures reported.[30,38,114,245,262]

SPONDYLOARTHROPATHIES

The spondyloarthropathies, often termed *seronegative* because of the absence of RF, are a group of disorders that include ankylosing spondylitis, Reiter's syndrome, arthritides associated with inflammatory bowel disease, and psoriasis. Enthesitis, or inflammation of ligament, tendon, and fascial insertions, is a common manifestation of these disorders and is not typical of rheumatoid arthritis. Joints of the axial skeleton as well as peripheral joints are often involved. Iritis, often acute, may occur in any of these related disorders. These entities are uncommon in children. Boys are affected more often than girls. A family history is more likely to be present in these disorders than in rheumatoid arthritis. The familial occurrence is related to the common finding of the HLA-B27 histocompatibility antigen. Remission occurs in approximately 17% to 27% of children with spondyloarthropathies within 10 years of diagnosis.[63,165] Approximately half of all children with these conditions reach adulthood with active arthritis requiring ongoing care.[165]

Clinicians generally agree that psoriatic arthritis represents a discrete subgroup among the spondyloarthropathies, although the exact demarcation between these disease entities and classification criteria for psoriatic arthritis remains controversial.[97] The combination of dactylitis of a toe, heel pain, and oligoarthritis is strongly suggestive of psoriatic arthritis, although ultrasonographic entheseal erosion at the calcaneum suggests either rheumatoid arthritis or psoriatic arthritis. Spinal involvement in psoriatic arthritis may be asymptomatic, and psoriatic spondylitis may occur without sacroiliitis.

Juvenile Ankylosing Spondylitis

Juvenile ankylosing spondylitis is characterized by arthritis of the sacroiliac joint and spine, along with involvement of one or several peripheral joints of the lower extremity. Large joints are more often affected than small. In most series boys predominate, but the apparent male predominance may be misleading because girls may have less symptomatic disease and more peripheral joint involvement.[158,198] Current reports of large series of juvenile cases indicate a male-to-female ratio of 2.7:1, with 73% of patients being male.[82] Ankylosing spondylitis is much less common in children than JRA and usually occurs in adolescence rather than childhood. The HLA-B27 assay is positive in 90% of whites with the disorder.[212,213]

There is often a striking familial occurrence of ankylosing spondylitis.[187] The risk that a parent with

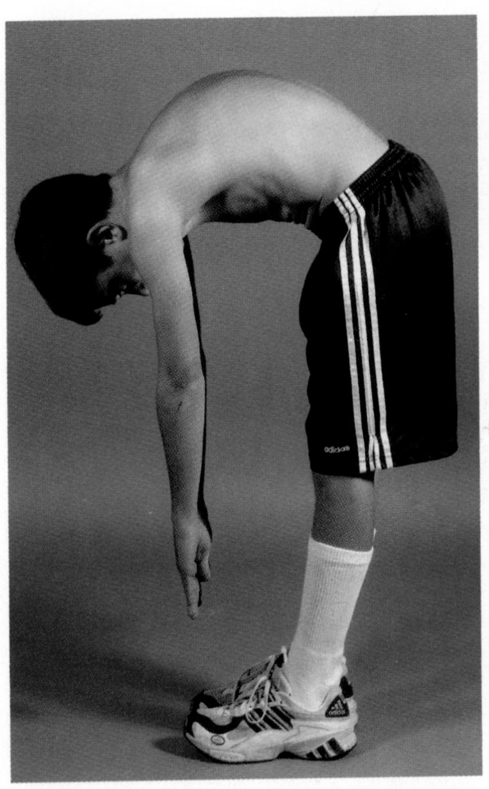

FIGURE 34–10 Limited forward bending with increased kyphosis in a boy with juvenile ankylosing spondylitis.

the HLA-B27 antigen will have a child with the disease is 5% to 10%.[246]

Involvement of the spine and sacroiliac joint is the diagnostic hallmark of ankylosing spondylitis (Fig. 34–10); however, many patients present with other symptoms and develop axial involvement later. Burgos-Vargas and Vazquez-Mellado have shown that enthesopathy, tarsal disease, pauciarthritis, and knee involvement are frequent presenting symptoms and can differentiate this disorder from JRA. In their series, definite spinal and sacroiliac involvement occurred after a mean of 7.3 years of other symptoms.[26]

Patients often are misdiagnosed, and physicians should consider juvenile ankylosing spondylitis when evaluating a patient with chronic pain or joint symptoms. Pain in the buttocks, groin, thigh, heel, or shoulder may be vaguely localized and evanescent. Only 25% of children have definite findings about the spine or sacroiliac joint at presentation. Peripheral joint symptoms predominate and resemble those of JRA. The joints most frequently affected are the knees, the metatarsophalangeal joints of the first toe, and the ankles. Enthesitis is the most distinguishing feature, with tenderness about the patella, tibial tuberosity, calcaneal apophysis, plantar fascia, and metatarsal head or base being most frequent. Occasional tender sites include the greater trochanters, anterior superior iliac spines, pubic symphysis, and ischial tuberosities.

Sacroiliac joint inflammation is noted by tenderness over the joint, pain on compression of the pelvis, and pain on distraction of the sacroiliac joint, known as the Patrick test. Spinal involvement may manifest as loss of lordosis, increased thoracic kyphosis, and a list to the side.

Involvement of the costosternal and costovertebral articulations may manifest as tenderness over those sites. Thoracic cage excursion during inspiration and expiration may be diminished, and a measured excursion of less than 5 cm suggests thoracic cage involvement.

The radiographic diagnosis is definitive when the sacroiliac joint shows widening, sclerosis, or fusion. The widening is termed *pseudo-widening* because it relates to erosions of the joints and disruption of subchondral borders due to inflammation.

The long-term prognosis is relatively good for juvenile-onset ankylosing spondylitis.[210] Flato and coworkers found that 60% of patients reviewed had no disability after 9.7 years of disease, and 60% were in remission. Twenty-five percent had articular erosions and disability, and they tended to have started treatment later in the disease than the others.[69] Affected patients respond well in general to NSAIDs, but not so well to aspirin. Indomethacin (1 to 2 mg/kg/day in three divided doses) is often remarkably effective but may produce significant toxic effects. Sulfasalazine is also useful for treating this disorder.[32]

Orthopaedic management is similar to that for the other arthritides. Spinal extension exercises to prevent loss of lordosis or lumbar flexion may be helpful.

Reiter's Syndrome

Classic Reiter's syndrome is diagnosed by the triad of arthritis, conjunctivitis, and urethritis. It is a postinfectious arthritis with a genetic predisposition, and those affected are usually HLA-B27 positive. In children it usually follows a diarrheal illness.

The arthritis usually affects a few joints. Unlike ankylosing spondylitis, upper extremity joints are often involved. Enthesitis is also frequent, but axial skeletal involvement is less common. Frank urethral discharge is present in 30% of children, and many more have pyuria on urinalysis. In the dysenteric form urethritis is often present as well.

Conjunctivitis is present in two thirds of affected children, and occasionally more severe ocular disease occurs. Characteristic ulcerative oral lesions are seen, as well as keratoderma blennorrhagicum, which is a characteristic skin manifestation with papular eruptions on the soles of the feet. Like the other spondyloarthropathies, Reiter's syndrome is self-limiting and responds to standard treatment regimens.[48,146,170]

Psoriatic Arthritis

Psoriatic arthritis is characterized by arthritis of one or more joints for at least 6 weeks, accompanied by a typical psoriatic rash. The diagnosis can be made in the absence of the typical rash if three of four minor criteria are present: dactylitis, nail pitting or onycholysis, a psoriasis-like rash, or a family history of psoriasis. The family history is positive in 40% of patients.

The disorder is slightly more common in girls than in boys.

Differences from the other entities include the occurrence of dactylitis, in which flexor tendon sheath inflammation produces a sausage-like toe or finger (Figs. 34–11 and 34–12). Large joint involvement and enthesitis are similar to what is found in ankylosing spondylitis, and these children also may have sacroiliac joint involvement. Psoriasis may precede or follow the onset of the other findings.[28,131,142,241] Uveitis occurs in psoriatic arthritis and may be resistant to treatment.

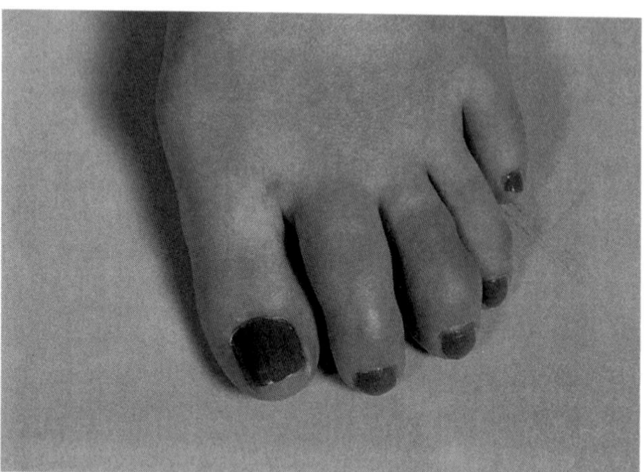

FIGURE 34–11 Sausage dactylitis of the second and third toes in a child with psoriatic arthritis.

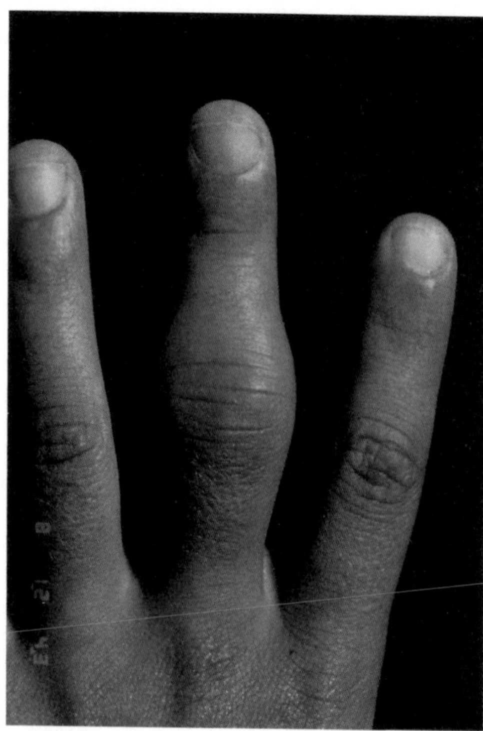

FIGURE 34–12 Sausage dactylitis of the proximal interphalangeal joint of the hand in psoriatic arthritis.

Box 34-2

Other Syndromes with Arthritis

Systemic Lupus Erythematosus
Episodic disease
Inflammation of blood vessels and connective tissues
Antinuclear antibodies
Antibodies to native DNA
Malar (butterfly) rash
Multiple-organ disease
Acute arthritis
Rapid response to steroids

Rheumatic Fever (Jones' Criteria)
Carditis
Polyarthritis (migratory)
Chorea
Erythema marginatum
Subcutaneous nodules
Minor fever (to 39°C), arthralgia
Elevated corrected sedimentation rate, C-reactive protein level
Evidence of prior streptococcal infection

Sarcoidosis
Boggy, nontender synovium
Pulmonary disease (rare in children)
Rash
Iritis
Hepatomegaly

Lyme Disease
Rash
Acute or chronic arthritis
Carditis
Neurologic symptoms
Tick-borne spirochete

Juvenile Dermatomyositis
Inflammation of muscle (weakness and pain)
Inflammation of skin (typical rash)
Calcinosis (late)
Vasculopathy

Treatment guidelines are similar to those for ankylosing spondylitis. The use of low-dose methotrexate was pioneered in psoriatic arthritis, and this drug may be very effective in those with multiple joints involved (Box 34–2).

Acute Transient Synovitis of the Hip

Acute transient synovitis is the most common cause of hip pain in children. It is a self-limiting inflammatory condition of the hip of undetermined etiology that occurs primarily in younger children. Although the disorder itself is benign, it must be distinguished from septic arthritis, which requires emergency treatment. Synovitis of the hip may also be the first symptom of Legg-Calvé-Perthes disease, early juvenile arthritis, or ankylosing spondylitis. Hip irritability also may accompany osteomyelitis in the femur or pelvis, or another bony lesion.

The incidence of transient synovitis in children between the ages of 1 and 13 years is estimated at 0.2% per year. During these childhood years a child has a 3% chance of sometime developing the disorder.[136] After a child has had an episode of synovitis, the annual risk of recurrence for that child is 4%.

The disorder has also been called toxic synovitis, irritable hip syndrome, observation hip, coxitis fugax, and acute transient epiphysitis. The first description given was in 1892 by Lovett and Morse, followed by many subsequent descriptions.[22,62,151,218]

Etiology

The etiology of transient synovitis is unknown. The disorder occasionally follows an upper respiratory tract infection, but the nature of this relationship is unknown. A number of studies have sought evidence of a bacterial or viral etiology, without success.[93,136] In one study, technetium bone scans showed a decrease in isotope uptake in the proximal femoral epiphysis in one fourth of the hips with synovitis. In these hips, a rebound hyperemia was noted on follow-up scan 1 month later. Only one such patient later developed Legg-Calvé-Perthes disease.[95] The significance of this finding is uncertain. Another study found increased levels of proteoglycan antigen in children with both septic arthritis and transient synovitis.[148]

Clinical Features

The usual presentation is a child with the fairly rapid onset of limping and subsequent refusal to walk or bear weight. This sometimes follows a recent upper respiratory tract illness, and parents may report a low-grade fever.

Boys are affected two to three times as frequently as girls.[247] Onset peaks between 4 and 10 years, with a mean age at onset of approximately 6 years.[136,247]

The examiner finds a child in mild distress who will not bear weight or walk or who does so reluctantly and with an antalgic limp. The range of motion of the affected hip is moderately limited by pain and spasm, and the hip is held in flexion. Gentle short-arc motion may be tolerated, but an attempt to extend fully or internally rotate the hip will be resisted. The irritability of the hip is usually several grades less severe than in a child with septic arthritis. There may be low-grade fever.

Diagnostic Studies

The diagnosis of transient synovitis is one of exclusion. The laboratory evaluation may show mild elevations in the WBC count, ESR, and CRP level. Plain radiographs of the pelvis are usually normal or may show slight joint space widening. Capsular distention on plain films, long thought to indicate fluid within the joint, has been shown to be a radiographic artifact due to the positioning assumed by an irritable hip.[25] When there is joint space widening and a smaller femoral ossific nucleus on the involved side, one can make a presumptive diagnosis of early Legg-Calvé-Perthes disease.[136]

Ultrasonography of the hip is useful in documenting the presence of an effusion in the hip joint. Ultrasonography is often performed before hip aspiration to be certain that the clinical findings are accompanied by an effusion. A number of studies have shown that ultrasonography reliably demonstrates fluid in the hip, and a negative study directs attention to other causes of hip pain.[101,161,166,236] One study noted a difference between the fluid present in transient synovitis and the synovial thickening of Legg-Calvé-Perthes disease, but others have not been able to make that distinction sonographically.[74] Another study reported that patients with Legg-Calvé-Perthes disease had cartilage thickening in the femoral head that was detected sonographically.[199] Some have found that the effusion in septic arthritis is more echogenic than the effusion in transient synovitis, but this relative finding does not consistently distinguish the two entities.[166,220]

Differential Diagnosis

The most important diagnosis to exclude is septic arthritis. Classically, there is a clear clinical difference in the presentation of the two, with septic arthritis presenting with more severe pain and marked limitation of motion of the hip due to pain. In practice, however, low-grade septic arthritis is not uncommon. Sometimes a less acute presentation occurs after the child has received antibiotics for another problem such as a respiratory illness. Others, especially older children, have low-grade septic arthritis caused by less virulent organisms. The WBC count, ESR, and CRP level are elevated to a greater degree when there is a septic arthritis. Del Beccaro and coworkers studied the value of laboratory screening combined with degree of temperature elevation and found the values to be useful.[54] Those with septic arthritis had a higher temperature (38.1°C versus 37.2°C), higher mean ESR (44 mm/hr versus 19 mm/hr), and higher mean WBC count (13,200/mm^3 versus 11,200/mm^3). Because of a large degree of overlap in these values, however, a diagnosis could not be based on these findings alone.[54] They recommended aspiration of the hip for diagnosis when the ESR was above 20 mm/hr and the temperature was above 37.5°C.

Other septic processes should be excluded as well. Osteomyelitis of the upper femur or pelvis may produce similar manifestations, including joint effusion, moderate loss of motion, and mild pain on range-of-motion testing. A nearby Brodie's abscess may have similar laboratory characteristics, with minimal elevations in temperature, ESR, CRP level, and WBC count. A psoas abscess may manifest with a subacute course and specific limitation of hip internal rotation. Inflammatory nodes in the groin, avulsion injuries around the pelvis, and trauma may also be confused with transient synovitis.

Arthritis of the hip may be the presenting symptom of JRA or one of the seronegative spondyloarthropathies. In these conditions the arthritis will persist well beyond the 1- or 2-week period of transient synovitis. A careful general physical examination as well as an examination of all joints will clarify the diagnosis.

Legg-Calvé-Perthes disease may present with synovitis before definitive radiographic changes. Radiographic widening of the joint space is more characteristic of Legg-Calvé-Perthes disease than of transient synovitis. Other findings in Legg-Calvé-Perthes disease include a smaller capital femoral ossific nucleus, subtle abnormalities of the contralateral hip, and subsequently an increased density of the femoral epiphysis. Bone scan or MRI can confirm the diagnosis before plain radiographic changes are seen.

Clinical Course

Transient synovitis by definition resolves spontaneously. Usually the child presents when unwilling to walk or when limping severely. The period of nonwalking generally lasts 1 or 2 days. The child then walks with a limp and has reduced range of motion of the hip for another few days to usually not more than 2 weeks before returning to normal. An ultrasonographic study demonstrated that the effusion persisted longer than 1 week in 58% of patients.[233] Other authors found that the effusion was gone by 2 weeks in 73% of patients.[166] Significant deviations from this pattern should prompt further investigation to rule out other causes of synovitis. One must remember that transient synovitis is a diagnosis of exclusion, and septic arthritis can and does present at times with moderate signs and symptoms.

Treatment

Treatment begins almost spontaneously because the child refuses to walk or be moved, and thereby rests the hip. Hip joint aspiration is commonly necessary to rule out septic arthritis and may be beneficial. In one study the degree of capsular distention on ultrasonography was significantly less at 4 days and for the remainder of the follow-up period in children who had undergone joint aspiration than in those who had not.[124] The real purpose of aspiration is diagnostic, and the surgeon should have a low threshold for tapping the hip. Our practice is to aspirate the hip of any child who refuses to walk and has significant limitation of hip motion. When little or no fluid is obtained we perform arthrography to determine that the needle has entered the joint. Considerations that lower the threshold for aspiration even further are elevated infectious indices, significant fever, and leukocytosis.

The child is placed on bed rest until the symptoms and signs are improving. The toddler will pick his or her level of activity and should not be forced to lie down if able to stand. The older child should be allowed gradually increasing activity, as governed by severity of pain and muscle spasm. NSAIDs may be used and often result in rapid improvement. Antibiotics should not be used because the process is not infectious, and antibiotic therapy confuses the picture. In more severe cases, traction can be helpful for a few days.

Hospital admission is appropriate in cases in which septic arthritis remains a possibility or in which other diagnoses have not been eliminated. Close observation is essential and may require hospital admission, especially when the parents are not reliable. Rapid resolution of symptoms and return of range of motion are characteristic of transient synovitis. Worsening symptoms suggest sepsis, and a prolonged course suggests chronic inflammatory conditions such as rheumatoid arthritis and seronegative spondyloarthropathies.

Natural History

No negative long-term effects of transient synovitis have been demonstrated. Coxa magna of the involved hip has been noted in 32% of cases when defined as 2 mm or more enlargement of the involved hip compared to the contralateral hip.[118] Nachemson and Scheller also reported finding coxa magna at follow-up but failed to find any prearthritic abnormalities.[169]

It has been proposed that synovitis of the hip could cause ischemia of the femoral epiphysis by a tamponade effect from increased intra-articular pressure.[258,260] However, a number of studies have shown little or no evidence of a causative relationship.[77,117] The clinical confusion exists because at times synovitis of the hip is the presenting finding in early Legg-Calvé-Perthes disease.[22,151]

Neuropathic Arthropathies

Charcot in 1868 described a bizarre destruction of the knee joints with indolent swelling and instability in patients with tabes dorsalis and proposed that the disease resulted from traumatization of a joint deprived of sensation.[34] Steindler subdivided the condition into the destructive atrophic and the hypertrophic proliferative forms.[227]

Charcot-like changes in joints are seen in patients who have absence or depression of pain and proprioceptive sensation and who engage in extended continuous physical activity. Consequently, their joints sustain repeated trauma. In children, neurologic conditions causing neuropathic arthropathy are congenital insensitivity to pain, peripheral nerve injuries, and diabetic neuropathy, as well as a variety of chronic diseases of the spinal cord that lead to sensory disturbances of the limbs. In myelomeningocele, absence of pain sensation is associated with flaccid paralysis and marked limitation of physical activity; thus, owing to associated severe osteoporosis, the bone and joint changes produce a different picture.

The specific joints involved with neuropathic disease vary with the different etiologic conditions. In congenital insensitivity to pain and diabetic neuropathy, the destructive changes occur primarily in the tarsal and metatarsal joints, less commonly in the ankle, and rarely in the knee. In syringomyelia, the joints involved are those of the shoulder and elbow,[53] whereas in tabes dorsalis, the knee, hip, ankle, and thoracolumbar spine are frequent sites of the disease.

Clinicopathologic Features

When a limb with normal sensation is injured, the joint affected by a severe sprain or hemarthrosis is protected from further trauma by pain. In the absence of pain and proprioceptive sensation, however, the joint continues to be active and is repeatedly injured. Synovial effusion and hemarthrosis are aggravated and, together with the abnormal stresses on the joint, cause extreme stretching and weakening of the capsule and supportive ligaments. Local hyperemia causes bone atrophy and resorption. Cartilage destruction, bone erosion, and minute fractures soon follow. The reparative response results in the formation of callus and metaplastic changes in surrounding traumatized soft tissues. With repeated injury, the joint becomes totally disorganized, subluxation ensues, and severe degenerative changes take place.

Clinically, the affected joints are boggy, tense, swollen, and nontender and have an excessive range of motion, often in abnormal directions. The local triad of swelling, instability, and absence of pain is nearly always suggestive of a Charcot joint.

Radiographic Findings

Computed tomography (CT), MRI, and radionuclide scintigraphy are useful in diagnosing neuropathic arthropathies and may help in distinguishing this condition from septic arthritis and osteomyelitis.[5] The neurotrophic joint shows varying degrees of destructive and hypertrophic changes (Figs. 34–13 and 34–14). Loss of articular cartilage, fragmentation and absorption of subchondral bone, and osseous proliferation of the joint margins also occur. The bony overgrowth may be enormous, bizarre in configuration, and so

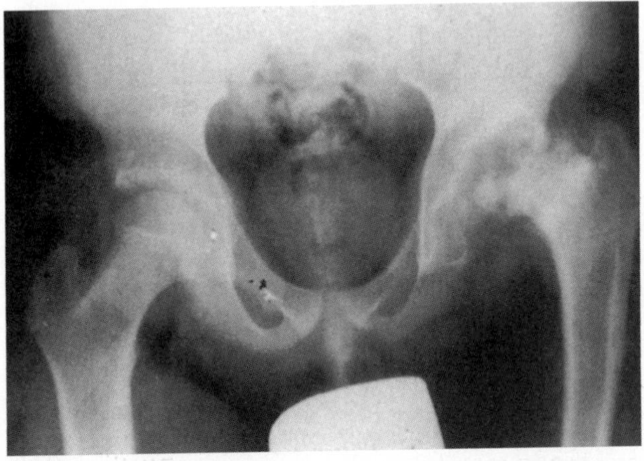

FIGURE 34–13 Pathologic fracture of the neck of the left femur with subluxation of hip in a 10-year-old boy with congenital insensitivity to pain.

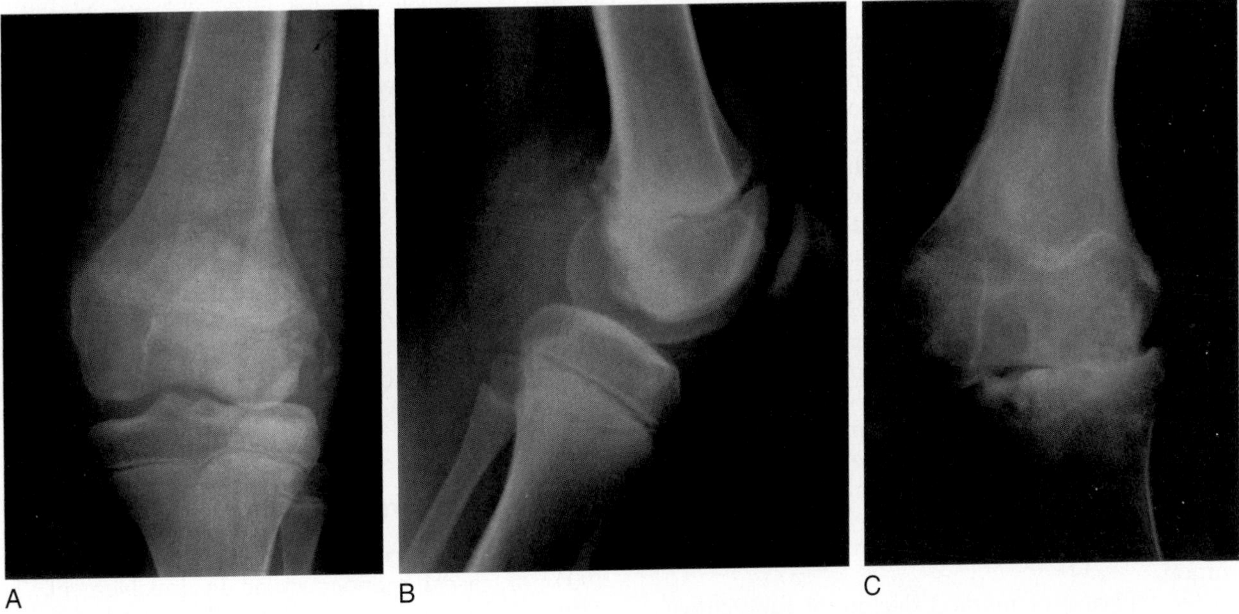

FIGURE 34–14 Progressive Charcot neuropathy in a boy with a demyelinating disease. **A,** Anteroposterior (AP) radiograph of the knee showing early changes. There is lateral subluxation of the tibia and destructive, erosive changes in the lateral femoral condyle. **B,** Lateral radiograph of the knee showing destruction of the posterior portion of the lateral femoral condyle. **C,** AP radiograph of the knee obtained 2 years later. There has been total destruction of the lateral condyle of the femur and tibial plateau with severe subluxation of the knee.

great as to surround the joint as a spongy mass. The periarticular soft tissues are thickened and contain scattered calcifications. Pathologic fractures involving the articular surface are common, as are irregular loose bodies within the joint.

Treatment

The goal of treatment of a neuropathic joint is to reduce the stresses on it to allow healing of the traumatized synovium, ligaments, and cartilage. Immobilization of the joint in a cast or a brace is usually the first line of treatment. When the skin is insensitive to pressure, any form of immobilization carries a risk of severe pressure sores. For the ankle and foot, a well-molded ankle-foot orthosis or cast is appropriate. The knee may be supported with a knee-ankle-foot orthosis, and upper extremity orthoses may also be used. Schon and coworkers have shown that displaced ankle fractures are best managed with open reduction and internal fixation.[214] Forefoot malalignment due to midfoot neuropathy often required operative correction in their series as well to prevent pressure ulceration.[214] Neuropathic arthropathy of the knee may be successfully treated using physical therapy and orthoses.[53]

When joints are more severely involved, gradual destruction of cartilage and underlying bone produces irreversible damage. In these cases arthrodesis is often the only option. Total joint replacement is an alternative but is complex in these patients and has a high likelihood of loosening of components and ultimate failure.[128,181] Arthrodesis is often difficult to achieve in these cases and results in increased stress on adjacent joints.[263]

Tuberculous Arthritis

Tuberculosis of bones and joints is a granulomatous inflammation caused by *Mycobacterium tuberculosis.* It is a localized and destructive disease that is usually blood-borne from a primary focus such as infected peribronchial or mesenteric lymph nodes, typically involving metaphyseal spread of *M. tuberculosis* into the joint.[235] This transphyseal spread is characteristic of tuberculosis and not seen in patients with pyogenic arthritis. This route of infection is particularly prevalent among children younger than 18 months of age, at which time the transphyseal vessels disappear and extension of infection into the epiphysis and joint becomes less common. The infection may be of the human or the bovine type. In countries where raw milk is used extensively, bovine transmission is common, whereas in areas where milk is pasteurized and there is rigid control of dairy herds, the bovine type is extremely rare and the human type is more common.

After a period of marked decline of tuberculosis, especially in North America, a gradual increase in the incidence of the disease has been noted since the late 1980s.[56,152,164,200,226] This increase has been closely associated with the acquired immunodeficiency syndrome (AIDS) epidemic. The incidence of tuberculosis has been projected to increase by 41% between 1998 and 2020 if better prevention is not practiced.[56] Especially alarming is the appearance of drug-resistant strains in various parts of the world.[50,163,185,221,264] Not too long ago, tuberculosis was the most common disease affecting the skeleton; this is still true in certain areas of the world. Even in economically well-developed countries, it is still prevalent. Tuberculosis of bones and joints is more common in children, although it may occur at any age. The invasion of a joint by the tubercle bacillus may occur by direct hematogenous infection of the synovial membrane (synovial tuberculosis) or by indirect spread from a focus in an adjacent bone—for example, in the metaphysis or epiphysis. Tuberculous osteomyelitis is characterized by destruction of bone, with little or no tendency for new bone formation. The tuberculous bone focus spreads centrifugally with increasing destruction of surrounding bone, until finally the joint is breached. The synovial membrane reacts first by secreting excessive fluid and later by proliferation, thickening, studding of its inner surface with tubercles, and fibrosis of its outer surface (Fig. 34–15).

The tuberculous granulation tissue soon covers the hyaline articular cartilage as a pannus that eventually destroys the underlying articular cartilage and subchondral bone. The destruction of articular surfaces is most extensive around the periphery in areas where tuberculous granulations involve the synovial membrane.

With progression of the disease, increasing amounts of caseous necrotic material and tuberculous exudate are produced. Soon, with increasing intraosseous or intra-articular pressure, the bony cortex or joint capsule becomes perforated and the so-called cold abscess forms. These tuberculous abscesses are so named because of the absence of acute inflammation. They spread by dissecting along tissue planes between muscles or between muscle sheaths, being limited by the deep fascia. With increasing tension the deep fascia is perforated and the wall lining the tuberculous abscess becomes subcutaneous. A thick fibrous wall lines the tuberculous abscess, which contains serum along with caseous necrotic tissue, tubercle bacilli, and degenerating leukocytes (see Fig. 34–15). If the original focus remains active and these abscesses remain untreated, they will rupture externally through the skin to form sinuses. The result is the inevitable secondary infection by pyogenic bacteria and complete destruction of the affected joint (Figs. 34–16 and 34–17).

Clinical Features

Tuberculous arthritis is insidious in onset and often (90% of cases) monoarticular in involvement. The affected child appears generally ill, is easily fatigued, and has evident weight loss. A family history of tuberculosis or a personal history of cervical adenitis or pleurisy may be obtained.

If the lesion is in the lower limb, for instance in the hip, the initial symptom may be a slight limp due to

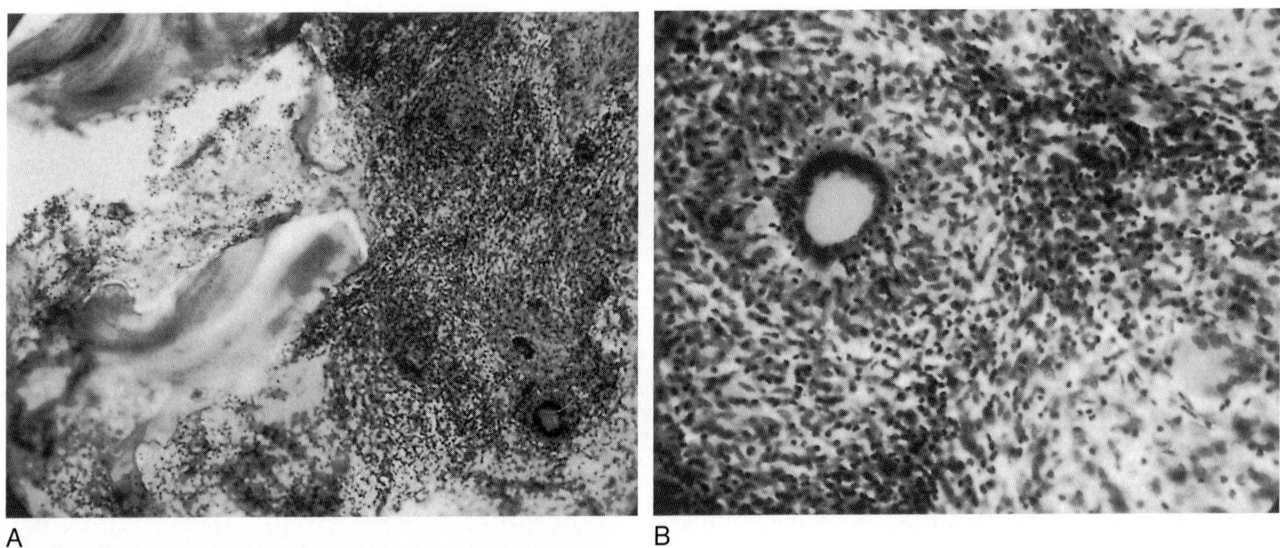

FIGURE 34–15 Microscopic appearance of tuberculous arthritis (hematoxylin-eosin stain). Note the granulomatous inflammation and the Langerhans giant cells. **A,** Original magnification ×100. **B,** Original magnification ×250.

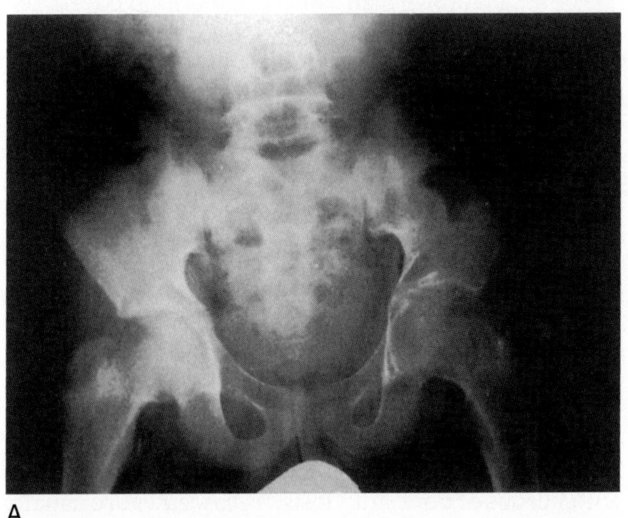

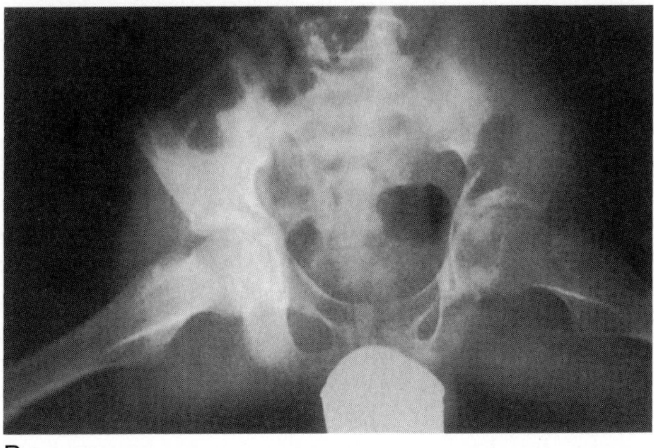

FIGURE 34–16 Tuberculous arthritis of the left hip, anteroposterior **(A)** and frog-leg **(B)** views. Note the regional bone atrophy.

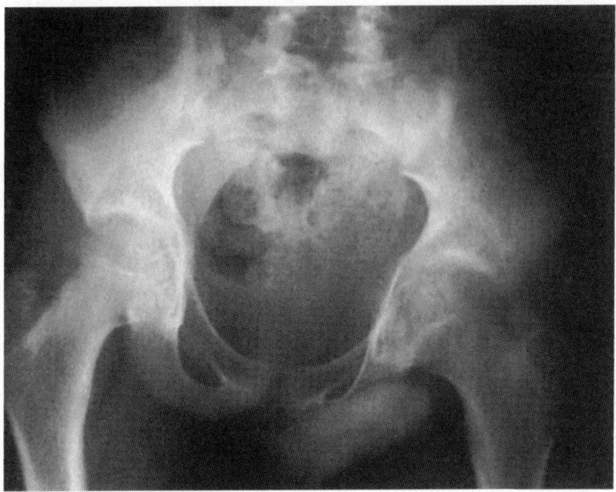

FIGURE 34–17 Tuberculous arthritis of the left hip. Note erosion of the hyaline articular cartilage.

discomfort. The affected joint will be stiff, and soon the "night cries" develop: because irritation from the process is low grade, muscle spasm protects the part satisfactorily during the day, but when the child is asleep the protective action of the muscle is lost, and on motion pain is produced—hence the cry.

Local physical signs vary according to the joint involved. The vertebral column is the most common site involved, the next in order of frequency being the hip, knee, ankle, sacroiliac, shoulder, and wrist joints. Almost any joint can be involved, and small joint involvement, although rare, may be confused with juvenile rheumatoid arthritis.[175,242,243] In tuberculous spondylitis the child usually presents with back pain and stiffness. The affected child walks with a protective gait, keeping the back hyperextended while taking light steps. A kyphosis develops if bone destruction continues and the vertebral bodies collapse. Untreated disease may progress to spinal cord compression with paralysis, which has been termed *Pott's paraplegia.* Caseous material collects in the front of the spine and may track inferiorly, producing a psoas abscess.

In superficial joints, such as the knee or elbow, synovial thickening and effusion present as a fullness or bogginess. This may be difficult to detect in the deep joints such as the hip. Local heat and redness are usually absent, and tenderness is minimal. Muscle atrophy is usually marked and is often present in the early stages. Joint motion is usually limited. Temperature elevation is ordinarily not marked. Although conventional culture methods are often less than useful diagnostically because of poor sensitivity and prolonged culture time, polymerase chain reaction of joint tissue obtained arthroscopically shows some promise in early diagnosis of tuberculous arthritis.[238]

Radiographic Findings

The earliest radiographic findings are regional bone atrophy, soft tissue swelling, and capsular distention (see Fig. 34–16). These changes are due to synovitis and are nonspecific. As a rule, the bony decalcification in tuberculous arthritis is widespread, extending 3 to 5 cm from the joint. Cartilage destruction may not be evident on radiographs in young children, so radiographic visualization of an intact epiphysis should not reassure the clinician regarding severity and progression of the disease.[235]

Because *M. tuberculosis* lacks proteolytic enzymes, the joint space is preserved until late in the course of the disease. Destruction of the hyaline cartilage by the tuberculous granulation tissue is a slow process. Eventually, with progression of the disease, the articular cartilage space gradually narrows, representing one element of the Phemister triad, which also includes juxta-articular osteoporosis and peripheral osseous erosions.[235] This is in contrast to what is seen in suppurative arthritis, in which the destruction of articular cartilage and joint space narrowing occur early in the course of the disease (see Figs. 34–16 and 34–17).

In joints such as the hip, in which there is a congruous and accurate fit of the opposing articular surface, the hyaline cartilage is eroded by the tuberculous granulation tissue in its periphery where there is little or no contact or pressure (see Fig. 34–17). In articulations with incongruous articular surfaces, such as the knee, contact areas are diffusely distributed and the tuberculous granulation tissue destroys articular cartilage wherever the noncontact areas are, centrally or peripherally.

Although tuberculous arthritis is a synovial disease with typical peripheral bony destruction, joints may also be involved when a focus of metaphyseal tuberculous osteomyelitis penetrates into the joint. In these cases the destruction of bone around the joint is more random and does not follow the typical pattern mentioned previously (Fig. 34–18). At times, with tuberculous arthritis, both sides of the joint are involved and the two foci of tuberculosis are directly opposite each other.

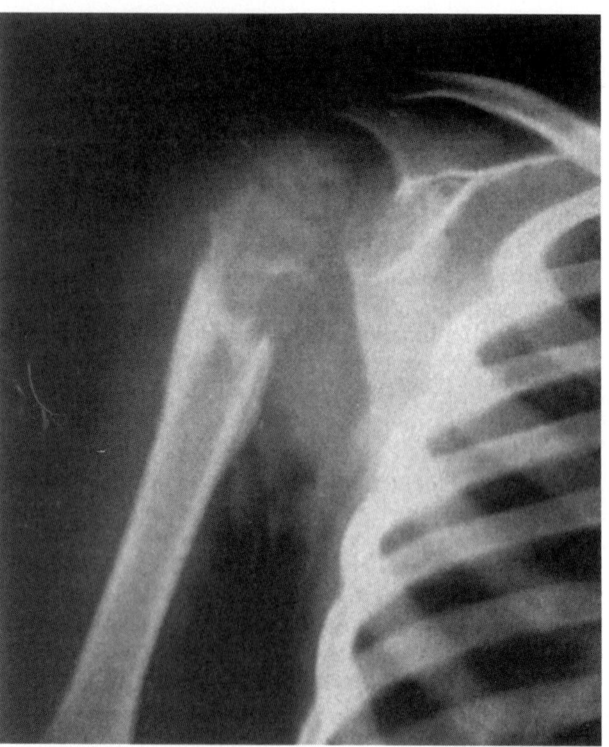

FIGURE 34–18 Tuberculosis of the right shoulder with extensive bone destruction.

Reactive new bone formation is characteristically absent in the early stages of tuberculous arthritis; it is only in the late healing stages that it develops. Sequestra may occasionally be present.

If tuberculous arthritis remains untreated, the entire articular cartilage is eventually eroded and extensive destruction of subjacent bone takes place, resulting in gross deformity of the joint (see Fig. 34–18), often with fibrous or bony ankylosis.[235] Abscesses are usually seen early in tuberculous spondylitis in the form of paravertebral or psoas abscesses.

MRI may be useful in making the diagnosis of tuberculosis of a joint, in differentiating the condition from pyogenic arthritis, and in detecting associated bone marrow and soft tissue abnormalities.[51,107] The diagnosis should be considered when the intra-articular synovial lesions show low or intermediate signal intensity on T2-weighted images.[230] MRI features consistent with tuberculous arthritis include bone marrow edema, cortical erosions, synovitis, joint effusion, tenosynovitis, soft tissue collections, and myositis.[179] Bony erosion is more common in tuberculous arthritis than in pyogenic arthritis, whereas abnormal subchondral marrow signal intensity is seen more often in pyogenic arthritis.[107] On T2-weighted images, no significant difference exists between the synovial lesion signal intensities of tuberculous arthritis and pyogenic arthritis.[107]

The general findings may reflect a chronic illness. Mild anemia is common, and the leukocyte count may be normal or mildly elevated. The ESR and CRP level are almost always elevated. Pulmonary tuberculosis may be detected with chest radiography or CT. Renal tuberculosis may be detected through urinalysis, ultrasonography, or plain radiography.

The synovial fluid shows an elevated leukocyte count, a lowered glucose level, and poor mucin. The leukocyte count usually averages 20,000/mm^3, although it may vary between 3000 and 100,000/mm^3. The differential leukocyte count discloses a predominance of polymorphonuclear leukocytes (60%), with 20% lymphocytes and 20% monocytes. Tubercle bacilli may be seen on microscopic examination of joint fluid sediment. A finding of great help in establishing the diagnosis is the marked reduction in or absence of glucose in the synovial fluid. Results of culture and specific polymerase chain reaction assays usually are positive. The diagnosis is also confirmed by histologic examination of synovium obtained by open or needle biopsy or by biopsy of regional nodes.[112]

Treatment

In the past, patients with tuberculosis were treated with long periods of rest, fresh air, and joint immobilization. As the patient's immune system began to respond, the diseased joint was surgically fused and the disease could be arrested.

Current management is based on early diagnosis and the use of antimicrobial drugs to which the organism is sensitive. It is often necessary to remove diseased synovium by synovectomy and to debride bony lesions. Postoperative immobilization is probably not necessary, and early motion or continuous passive motion may help restore range of motion.

GENERAL MEDICAL TREATMENT

Most patients are not debilitated and may continue reasonable activities while being treated for tuberculosis. Patients with active AIDS and those with visceral disease may need more intensive nutritional and medical management.

ANTITUBERCULOUS DRUGS

The emergence of drug-resistant organisms has prompted a reassessment of treatment protocols.[55,183,195,196,217,225,248] Current recommendations for treating active disease require a total of 6 months of drug administration. Most commonly a three-drug regimen of isoniazid (INH), rifampin, and pyrazinamide is used. One protocol suggests daily doses of all three for 8 weeks, followed by two or three times weekly doses to a total of 6 months. Another approach is to give daily doses for 2 to 3 weeks, followed by doses twice or three times a week to 6 months. Pyridoxine should be given with INH to prevent peripheral neuritis.[193] Streptomycin is the most commonly used fourth drug. Its main adverse effect is cranial nerve VIII deafness, which is most likely to occur when serum concentrations are too high.[59] Ethambutol may be used as a fourth drug but is associated with the serious complication of optic neuritis, which may escape notice in younger children.

If the person who is the source of the infection is known, while awaiting culture results it may be assumed that the child's organism will be susceptible to the same drugs. A resistant organism should be suspected when standard drugs have not controlled the infection. Also, resistance is likely if there has been relapse after a standard course or if there was failure to comply with the initial treatment. Finally, resistance should be anticipated if the organism is acquired in an area in which resistant organisms are indigenous.[59]

Newer trends in management center on more intense, directly observed protocols of shorter duration. Direct observation is proposed to ensure compliance with drug administration. Genetic studies are investigating the genetic basis of drug resistance in the hopes of finding more effective agents.[225] Infections caused by multiple-drug–resistant organisms require four times as long to treat and are more likely to be incompletely controlled. The treatment of resistant cases often involves the use of more toxic drugs.[183]

ORTHOPAEDIC TREATMENT OF THE TUBERCULOUS JOINT

The diagnosis is usually confirmed by joint aspiration and synovial biopsy and a positive tuberculin skin test. Drug treatment is begun once the diagnosis is made and should be continued for 4 to 6 weeks to prevent systemic spread of disease. Synovectomy by either open or arthroscopic technique is then performed to remove the bulk of infected tissue.[237] Bony foci of tuberculous osteomyelitis should be debrided. Early motion is begun; contrary to older teaching, it does not impair the healing process.

Arthrodesis is still occasionally necessary when the disease has destroyed the articular cartilage and underlying bony support. Ordinary techniques of arthrodesis are successful with continued drug treatment for the infection.[6,12,18,29,36,79,99,162] Although there is currently no consensus regarding the best treatment of advanced tuberculous arthritis of the hip in children, hip arthrodesis has produced satisfactory outcomes in adolescents.[178]

Tuberculosis of the Spine

Tuberculosis of the vertebral column* was first described by Percivall Pott as a painful kyphosis of the spine associated with paraplegia.[189] The condition is often referred to as Pott's disease. Skeletal tuberculosis currently represents 10% to 20% of all extrapulmonary tuberculosis, with active pulmonary disease present in less than half of all cases.[235] The spine is the most common site of skeletal tuberculosis, accounting for 50% of cases.[235] Any level of the spine may be involved, the lower thoracic region being the most common

*See references 2, 4, 8, 13, 18-20, 35, 43, 49, 64, 75, 90, 100, 115, 123, 200, 215, 250-253.

segment; next in decreasing order of frequency are the lumbar, upper dorsal, cervical, and sacral regions. A good outcome can be expected if the disease is diagnosed before the appearance of spinal deformity and neurologic symptoms.[7] Tuberculous spondylitis involves the intervertebral disk only late in the disease process, when subligamentous spread of the infection may create multiple levels of vertebral body involvement. The disease may extend into the paravertebral or extradural space.[235] Tuberculous osteomyelitis may manifest as cystic, well-defined lesions; infiltrative lesions; or spina ventosa (a type of tuberculous osteomyelitis in which underlying bone destruction, periosteal reaction, and fusiform expansion of the bone result in creation of cystlike cavities with diaphyseal expansion).[235]

In the past, tuberculous spondylitis was a disease of early childhood, usually affecting children between 3 and 5 years of age. Recently, however, with improved public health measures, this age prevalence has changed, and adults are more frequently affected than children.

Tuberculous spondylitis warrants individual consideration because of certain significant differences between it and tuberculous arthritis of limbs.

Pathology

The initial focus of infection usually begins in the cancellous bone of the vertebral body and only occasionally in the posterior neural arch, transverse process, or subperiosteally, deep to the anterior longitudinal ligament in front of the vertebral body (Fig. 34–19). *M. tuberculosis* is typically deposited through the end arterioles in the vertebral body adjacent to the anterior aspect of the vertebral end-plate, so the anterior portion of the vertebral body is most commonly affected.[235] With progressive infection the cortex is disrupted and infection may spread to the adjacent intervertebral disk and surrounding tissues, commonly forming paravertebral or epidural masses, the latter of which may cause spinal cord compression. Intervertebral disk involvement occurs late in the disease process, so preservation of disk space is an important diagnostic feature; disk space narrowing, when it does occur, is less than that seen with diskitis caused by pyogenic organisms. In the case of cervical spine involvement, paravertebral masses may occur in the retropharyngeal area. The area of infection gradually enlarges and spreads to involve two or more adjacent vertebrae by extension beneath the anterior longitudinal ligament or directly across the intervertebral disk, possibly resulting in a gibbus deformity.[235] Occasionally there may be multiple foci or involvement separated by normal vertebrae, or the infection may be disseminated to distant vertebrae through the paravertebral abscess. Posterior elements are seldom involved, although when these findings are present they are characteristic because they do not occur with pyogenic infections.

The vertebral bodies lose their mechanical strength as a result of progressive destruction under the force of body weight and eventually collapse, with the intervertebral joints and the posterior neural arch intact; the severity of the resulting angular kyphotic deformity depends on the extent of destruction, the level of lesion, and the number of vertebrae involved. The kyphosis is most marked in the thoracic region because of the normal dorsal curvature; in the lumbar area the kyphosis is slight and collapse is partial because of the normal lumbar lordosis, in which most of the body weight is transmitted posteriorly; and in the cervical spine, collapse is minimal, if present at all, because most of the bony weight is borne through the articular processes. Extension of the infection along the iliopsoas muscle creates draining sinus tracts in the buttock, groin, and chest areas.[235]

Healing takes place by gradual fibrosis and calcification of the granulomatous tuberculous tissue. Eventually the fibrous tissue is ossified, with resulting body ankylosis of the collapsed vertebrae.

Paravertebral abscess formation occurs in almost every case. With collapse of the vertebral body, tuberculous granulation tissue, caseous matter, and necrotic

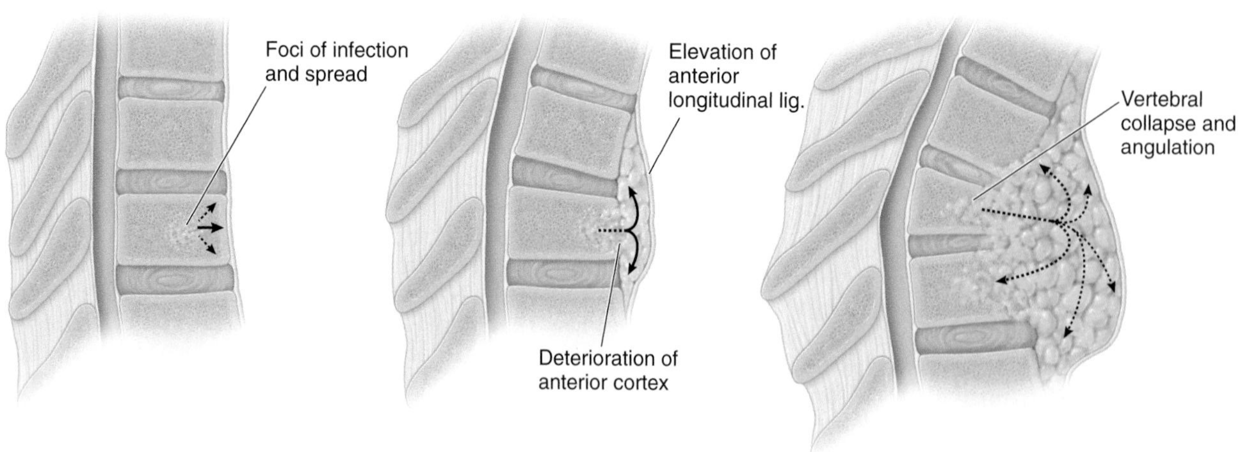

FIGURE 34–19 Pathogenesis of tuberculous spondylitis.

bone and bone marrow are extruded through the bony cortex and accumulated beneath the anterior longitudinal ligament. These cold abscesses gravitate along the fascial planes and present externally at some distance from the site of the original lesion (Fig. 34–20). In the lumbar region the abscess gravitates along the psoas fascial sheath and usually points into the groin just below the inguinal ligament. In the thoracic region the longitudinal ligaments limit the abscess, which is seen on the radiograph as a fusiform radiopaque shadow at or just below the level of the involved vertebra; if under great tension, it may rupture into the mediastinum, where it may be walled off to form the "bird's nest" type of paravertebral abscess. Occasionally, a thoracic abscess may reach the anterior chest wall in the parasternal area by tracking through the intercostal vessels. The prevertebral fascia limits the cervical abscess, which may burst into the retropharyngeal area or gravitate laterally on each side of the neck.

Paraplegia results from compression of the cord by the abscess, by the caseating or granulating mass, or by the posteriorly protruding border of the intervertebral disk or edge of bone. Other contributory factors may be thrombosis of the local vessels and edema of the cord. It occurs most often in the middle or upper thoracic region where the kyphosis is most acute, the spinal canal is narrow, and the spinal cord is relatively large. In the literature it is described as occurring in 6% to 25% of reported cases, but recently, with early diagnosis and effective treatment, the incidence has been greatly diminished.

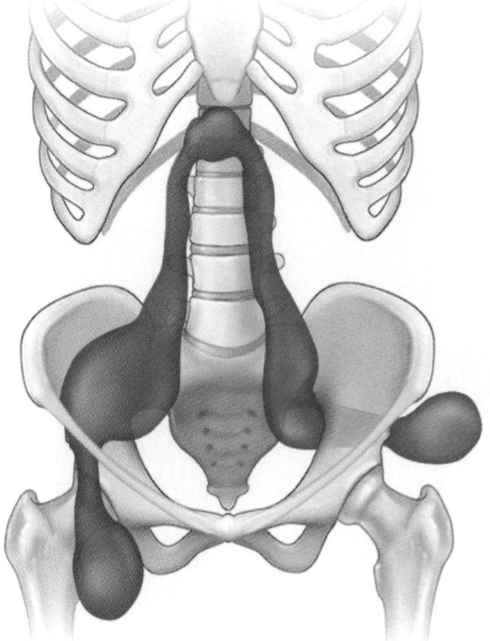

FIGURE 34–20 Abscess formation in Pott's disease. Diagrammed are the various courses a tuberculous abscess arising from the thoracolumbar spine may take.

Clinical Features

Pott's disease is usually characterized by insidious onset and slow evolution. Initial symptoms are vague, consisting of generalized malaise, easy fatigability, loss of appetite and weight, and loss of desire to play outdoors. There may be an afternoon or evening fever. Backache is usually minimal; it may be referred segmentally.

Muscle spasm in the affected region of the spine is a constant finding. The spine is held rigid. When picking an object up from the floor, the child flexes the hips and knees, keeping the spine in extension (Fig. 34–21). Motion of the spine is limited in all directions. Spasm of the paravertebral muscles in the lumbar region is also elicited by passive hyperextension of the hips with the patient prone; this also puts stretch on the iliopsoas muscle, which is in spasm and contracture owing to psoas abscess.

A kyphosis in the thoracic region may be the first noticeable sign. As the kyphosis increases, the ribs crowd together and a barrel chest deformity develops. When the lesion is situated in the cervical or lumbar spine, a flattening of the normal lordosis is the initial finding.

Tenderness is often present on gentle percussion or pressure over the spinous process of the affected vertebrae. The abscesses may be palpated as fluctuant swellings in the groin, iliac fossa, or retropharynx or on the side of the neck, depending on the level of the lesion.

The gait of the child with Pott's disease is peculiar, reflecting the protective rigidity of the spine. The child takes short steps because he or she is trying to avoid any jarring of the back. In tuberculosis of the cervical

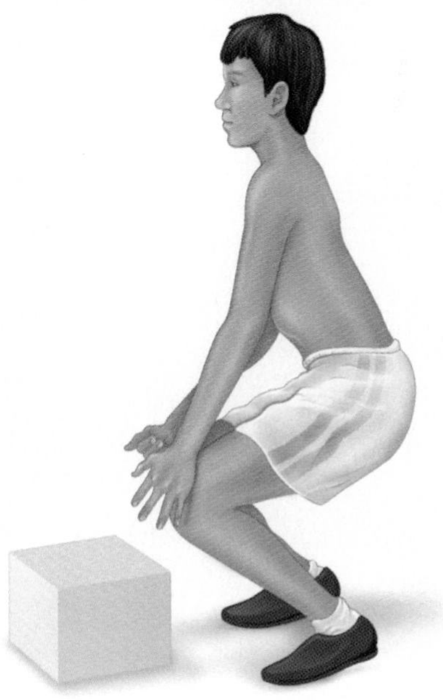

FIGURE 34–21 A child with tuberculous spondylitis. When picking up an object from the floor, because of rigidity of the spine, he flexes his hips and knees, keeping the spine in extension.

spine, the child holds the neck in extension and supports the head with one hand under the chin and the other over the occiput. If the level is in the lumbodorsal area and a psoas abscess is present, the child walks with the knees and hips in flexion and supports the spine by placing the hands over the thighs. If a paraplegia develops, there will be spasticity of the lower limbs with hyperactive deep tendon reflexes, a spastic gait, a varying degree of motor weakness, and disturbances of bladder and anorectal function.

Radiographic Findings

Radiographs are still the mainstay of evaluation of patients with skeletal lesions related to tuberculosis and often are definitive, although it is estimated that bone loss of greater than 50% must occur before changes are visible on plain radiographs.[235] Plain radiographs initially show radiolucency of the vertebral body. As the disease advances, loss of height of vertebral bodies becomes evident, and end-plates, bony erosions, and sequestra become indistinct. With progressive destruction of bone the vertebral body collapses (Figs. 34–22 and 34–23). At first, the intervertebral disk space narrows as disk involvement occurs;

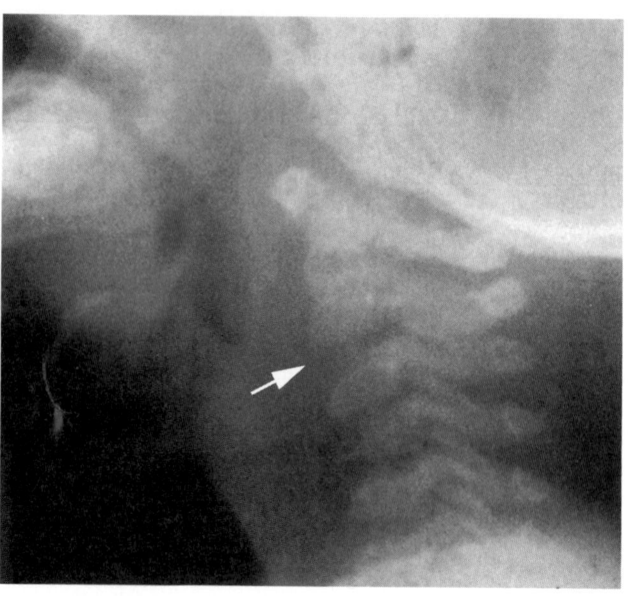

FIGURE 34-22 Tuberculosis of the cervical spine. Note the destruction of the fourth cervical vertebra and the retropharyngeal abscess (*arrow*).

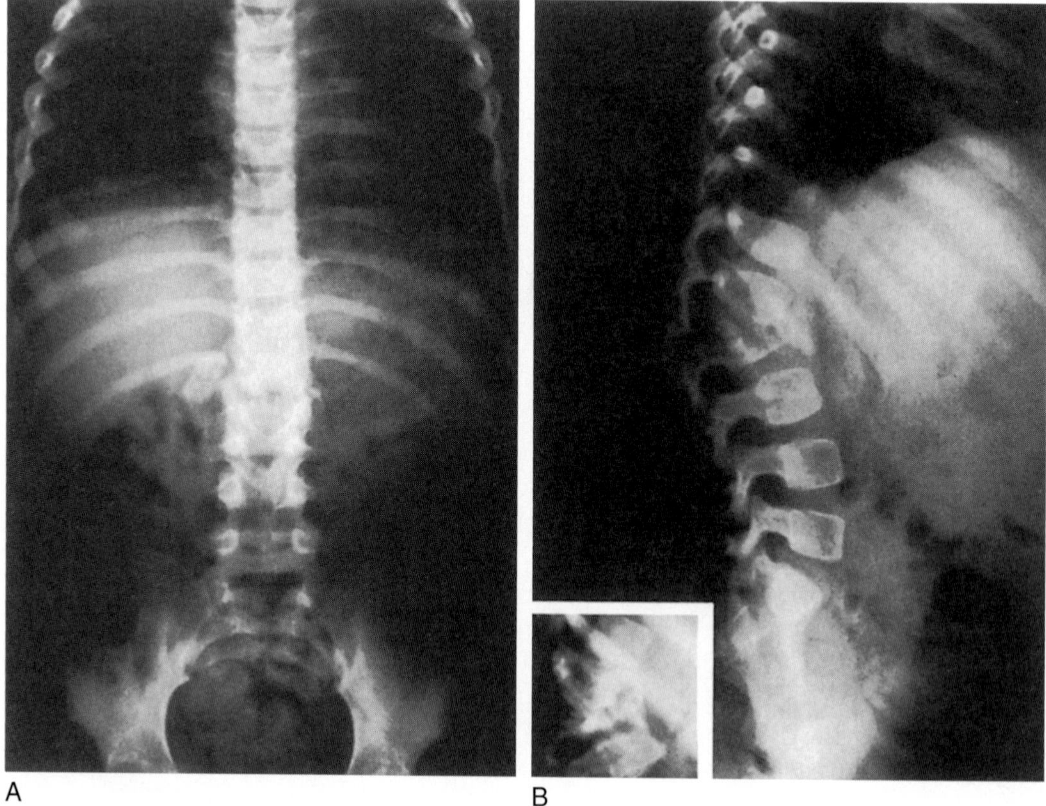

FIGURE 34-23 Tuberculous spondylitis, anteroposterior **(A)** and lateral **(B)** views. First and second lumbar vertebrae are involved. Note collapse of the vertebral bodies, obliteration of intervertebral disk interspaces (*inset*, **B**), and localized kyphosis.

later it is obliterated. Paraspinal abscesses appear as fusiform shadows along the vertebral column on the anteroposterior radiograph and as an anterior soft tissue mass on the lateral radiograph. Late involvement shows a sharply angled kyphosis or gibbus at the level of vertebral destruction.

Various clinical sequelae and complications can occur in the pulmonary and extrapulmonary thorax in patients with treated or untreated tuberculosis.[126] Radiologic manifestations of these complications can be categorized as follows: (1) parenchymal lesions, including tuberculoma, thin-walled cavity, cicatrization, end-stage lung destruction, aspergilloma, and bronchogenic carcinoma; (2) airway lesions, which include bronchiectasis, tracheobronchial stenosis, and broncholithiasis; (3) vascular lesions, including pulmonary or bronchial arteritis and thrombosis, bronchial artery dilatation, and Rasmussen's aneurysm; (4) mediastinal lesions, such as lymph node calcification and extranodal extension, esophagomediastinal or esophagobronchial fistula, constrictive pericarditis, and fibrosing mediastinitis; (5) pleural lesions, which include chronic empyema, fibrothorax, bronchopleural fistula, and pneumothorax; and (6) chest wall lesions, including rib tuberculosis, tuberculous spondylitis, and malignancy associated with chronic empyema. Because radiologic manifestations of these conditions can mimic other disease entities, recognition and understanding of the radiologic findings associated with thoracic sequelae and complications of tuberculosis are important to facilitate correct diagnosis.[126]

Ultrasonography is useful in detecting soft tissue extension of bony lesions and guiding drainage and biopsy procedures.[235] Both CT and MRI are extremely helpful in diagnosis. CT accurately demonstrates bony sclerosis and destruction, especially in areas such as the posterior elements of the vertebral body that are difficult to assess on radiographs. CT can also differentiate between tuberculous and pyogenic spondylitis, tuberculous spondylitis being associated with larger intraspinal extradural abscesses with calcification in about half of cases, and pyogenic spondylitis not being associated with calcification.[154] MRI is the modality of choice in evaluating early marrow involvement and soft tissue extension of the lesion because it detects tuberculosis-related changes of the spine 4 to 6 months earlier than conventional methods.[3,51,132] MRI is also useful in delineating the extent of disease and differentiating it from other types of vertebral osteomyelitis and from pyogenic spondylitis. It is also the modality of choice for identifying the extent of soft tissue involvement of the disease.[116,235] Vertebral and disk destruction and the location of paravertebral abscesses are graphically evident on MRI.[16,127,145] Gadolinium-enhanced studies show rim enhancement of lesions, more typical of tuberculosis than septic conditions.[11,127] More vertebrae are involved and paravertebral abscesses are larger in tuberculosis of the spine than in vertebral osteomyelitis.[11] Brucellar spondylitis may be differentiated from tubercular spondylitis in that brucellosis more commonly involves lumbar vertebrae, whereas tuberculosis more often affects thoracic levels.[45]

A gallium scan may add significant information in the evaluation of a patient with tuberculous spondylitis. In one study, this scan was more likely than a technetium scan to delineate paraspinal abscesses and unsuspected levels of vertebral and other bony and soft tissue involvement.[144]

Entities to be ruled out in the diagnosis of spinal tuberculosis include suppurative spondylitis, leukemia, Hodgkin's disease, eosinophilic granuloma, aneurysmal bone cyst, and Ewing's sarcoma. All of these conditions result in destruction and collapse of the vertebral bodies, narrowing and obliteration of disk spaces, and paraspinal soft tissue swelling.

Treatment

Immobilization and drug therapy are the mainstays of treatment of spinal tuberculosis.[125] Methods for surgical treatment of the condition remain controversial.[37] Anterior spinal stabilization with allograft fibular fusion has demonstrated effectiveness in cases of severe vertebral body destruction, as has fusion with an autogenous anterior iliac tricortical strut bone graft combined with a subsequent autogenous posterior iliac corticocancellous bone graft.[37,177] Video-assisted thoracoscopic surgery using extended manipulating channels placed slightly more posterior than usual appears to be effective and safe in patients with spinal tuberculosis.[108]

Drug therapy is initiated and the patient is placed in a spinal cast or brace as soon as the diagnosis is made. Immobilization itself may enhance healing of the lesion and prevent further bony destruction. In addition, immobilization is helpful in preventing progressive kyphosis. In the lumbar spine it has been recommended that the hips be included in the cast or brace. When there is minimal spinal deformity, nonoperative therapy results in a satisfactory outcome, with solid bony fusion of the spine in 75% of cases.[257]

When there is a large anterior caseous abscess or an unacceptable kyphotic deformity, surgical debridement and stabilization should be considered.[102-105] The surgical approach entails removal of necrotic and caseous material followed by grafting. Autogenous graft is preferred when feasible, and strut grafts may provide anterior stability.[149] Posterior instrumentation and fusion may allow further correction of the kyphotic deformity and may reduce or eliminate the need for postoperative immobilization.

Paraplegia in Tuberculous Spondylitis

Paraplegia is the most serious complication of tuberculosis of the spine. The incidence is reported at between 10% and 29%.[162,207] The current incidence is much lower, owing to better diagnosis and early treatment. Younger children are more likely to become paraplegic.

Hodgson and colleagues classified paraplegia into four types.[105] The first is paraplegia of active disease resulting from external compression of the cord and dura. The compression comes from caseating pus, sequestra of bone and disk, dislocation of vertebrae, and granulation tissue within the spinal canal. Clinically, these patients have varying degrees of spasticity of the lower limbs but do not have involuntary muscle spasms and withdrawal reflex. This type of paraplegia carries a good prognosis for full recovery after decompression and stabilization.

The second type is paraplegia due to direct tuberculous involvement of the spinal cord. In these cases tuberculous meningitis and myelitis are present. These patients have more severe spasticity with involuntary muscle spasm and withdrawal reflex. This type of paraplegia is associated with a poor prognosis for recovery.

The third type of paraplegia occurs after healing and is due to fibrosis of the meninges and granulation tissue causing cord compression.

The fourth type is due to rare causes such as thrombosis of vessels supplying the cord.

When paraplegia occurs, the level and type of lesion are determined by radiography, MRI, and myelography. Spinal fluid cell count and total protein determination determine the extent of intradural infection. Early anterior decompression is strongly recommended, followed by spinal stabilization. Delay in treatment may result in permanent paraplegia.[105]

Gonococcal Arthritis

Gonococcal arthritis is caused by metastatic invasion of the joint by the gonococcus, usually from a recent or inadequately treated gonorrheal urethritis. The arthritis, which usually develops 2 to 4 weeks after the initial infection, may be polyarticular or monoarticular. The knees, ankles, wrists, and sternoclavicular joints are the most frequently affected sites. The disease usually begins as fleeting pains in multiple joints, accompanied by fever and malaise—similar to what is seen at the onset of rheumatic fever. In a few days the obvious infection settles into a single joint, which becomes hot, red, extremely tender, swollen, tense, and very painful on motion. The acute inflammation may spread to the adjacent tendons and bursae. Often there is a history of gonorrheal infection or a concomitant urethritis. In the more chronic cases, systemic reaction is usually minimal and multiple joints are involved. Gonorrheal arthritis may be associated with dermatitis.[141,207]

A mother may have primary gonococcal infection of her genitourinary tract that may be so slight as to go unnoticed. Such maternal infection may be transmitted from mother to infant. When both skin and joint are involved, the condition is referred to as gonococcal arthritis–dermatitis.[171] Gonococcal arthritis–dermatitis may manifest as erythematous papules surrounded by a hemorrhagic or vesiculopustulous lesion that may precede the joint involvement.

Diagnosis is made by bacteriologic study of the aspirated joint fluid and of the urethral or vaginal discharge. The gonococcal organism can often be identified in the joint fluid within the first week of infection; during the course of the disease, however, joint cultures are negative. In such subacute or chronic cases, immunofluorescent methods for the detection of gonococcal antibodies and gonococcal complement fixation tests are of some aid in diagnosis. Gonorrheal arthritis should be distinguished from Reiter's syndrome, which consists of the triad of polyarthritis, urethritis, and conjunctivitis. Reiter's syndrome is rare in childhood; it is a form of nongonococcal urethritis, probably caused by a virus.

In gonococcal arthritis, destruction of articular cartilage is rapid, as shown by the disappearance of articular cartilage space on the radiograph.

Treatment should be instituted immediately to prevent permanent damage to the joint. Penicillin is specific and effective and may be given intravenously or intramuscularly initially, followed by oral administration when the infection is controlled. Unlike in other types of septic arthritis, joint drainage is usually unnecessary.

References

1. Aaron S, Fraser PA, Jackson JM, et al: Sex ratio and sibship size in juvenile rheumatoid arthritis kindreds. Arthritis Rheum 1985;28:753.
2. Adams ZB: Tuberculosis of the spine in children: A review of sixty-three cases from the Lakeville State Sanitorium. J Bone Joint Surg 1940;22:860.
3. Akman S, Sirvanci M, Talu U, et al: Magnetic resonance imaging of tuberculous spondylitis. Orthopedics 2003; 26:69.
4. Alexander GL: Neurological complications of spinal tuberculosis. Proc R Soc Med 1945;46:730.
5. Aliabadi P, Nikpoor N, Alparslan L: Imaging of neuropathic arthropathy. Semin Musculoskelet Radiol 2003; 7:217.
6. Allen AR, Stevenson AW: The results of combined drug therapy and early fusion in bone tuberculosis. J Bone Joint Surg Am 1957;39:32.
7. Alothman A, Memish ZA, Awada A, et al: Tuberculous spondylitis: Analysis of 69 cases from Saudi Arabia. Spine 2001;26:E565.
8. Alpero BJ, Plamer HD: Compression of the spinal cord due to tuberculosis abscess: Report of case of Pott's disease with direct extension from lung to spinal canal. Am J Surg 1934;24:163.
9. Ansell BM: Juvenile spondylitis and related disorders. In Moll J (ed): Ankylosing Spondylitis. Edinburgh, Churchill Livingstone, 1980, p 120.
10. Arden GP: Surgical treatment of juvenile rheumatoid arthritis. Ann Chir Gynaecol Suppl 1985;198:103.
11. Arizono T, Oga M, Shiota E, et al: Differentiation of vertebral osteomyelitis and tuberculous spondylitis by magnetic resonance imaging. Int Orthop 1995;19:319.
12. Badgley CE, Hammond G: Tuberculosis of the hip: A review of seventy-six patients with proved tuberculous

arthritis of seventy-seven hips treated by arthrodesis. J Bone Joint Surg 1942;24:135.
13. Bakalim G: A clinical study with special reference to the significance of spinal fusion and chemotherapy. Acta Orthop Scand Suppl 1960;47:1.
14. Baron K, Lewis D, Brewer E: Cytotoxic anti-T cell antibodies in children with juvenile rheumatoid arthritis. Arthritis Rheum 1984;8:1272.
15. Baum J, Fink C: Juvenile rheumatoid arthritis in monozygotic twins: A case report and review of the literature. Arthritis Rheum 1968;11:33.
16. Bell GR, Stearns KL, Bonutti PM, et al: MRI diagnosis of tuberculous vertebral osteomyelitis. Spine 1990;15: 462.
17. Blasberg B, Lowe A, Petty R: Temporomandibular joint disease in children with juvenile rheumatoid arthritis. Arthritis Rheum 1987:527-530.
18. Bosworth DM: Treatment of bone and joint tuberculosis in children. J Bone Joint Surg Am 1959;41:1255.
19. Bosworth DM, Della Pietra A, Rahilly G: Paraplegia resulting from tuberculosis of the spine. J Bone Joint Surg Am 1953;35:735.
20. Bosworth DM, Levine J: Tuberculosis of the spine: An analysis of cases treated surgically. J Bone Joint Surg Am 1949;31:267.
21. Boublik M, Tsahakis PJ, Scott RD: Cementless total knee arthroplasty in juvenile onset rheumatoid arthritis. Clin Orthop Relat Res 1993;286:88.
22. Bradford E: Treatment of hip disease. Am J Orthop Surg 1912;9.
23. Brewer E Jr: Juvenile rheumatoid arthritis: Cardiac involvement. Arthritis Rheum 1977;20:231.
24. Brower TD, Akakoshi Y, Orlie P: The diffusion of dyes through articular cartilage in vivo. J Bone Joint Surg Am 1962;44:456.
25. Brown I: A study of the capsular shadow in disorders of the hip in children. J Bone Joint Surg Br 1975;57:175.
26. Burgos-Vargas R, Vazquez-Mellado J: The early clinical recognition of juvenile-onset ankylosing spondylitis and its differentiation from juvenile rheumatoid arthritis. Arthritis Rheum 1995;38:835.
27. Cage DJ, Granberry WM, Tullos HS: Long-term results of total arthroplasty in adolescents with debilitating polyarthropathy. Clin Orthop Relat Res 1992;283:156.
28. Calabro J: Psoriatic arthritis in children. Arthritis Rheum 1977;20(Suppl):415.
29. Campos OP: Bone and joint tuberculosis and its treatment. J Bone Joint Surg Am 1955;37:937.
30. Carlsson AS, Montgomery F, Besjakov J: Arthrodesis of the ankle secondary to replacement. Foot Ankle Int 1998;19:240.
31. Carmichael E, Chaplin DM: Total knee arthroplasty in juvenile rheumatoid arthritis: A seven-year follow-up study. Clin Orthop Relat Res 1986;210:192.
32. Cassidy J, Petty R: Pediatric Rheumatology. Philadelphia, WB Saunders, 1995.
33. Chantler JK, Tingle AJ, Petty RE: Persistent rubella virus infection associated with chronic arthritis in children. N Engl J Med 1985;313:1117.
34. Charcot JM: Sur quelques arthropathies qui paraissant dependre d'une lesion du cerveau ou de la moelle epiniere. Arch Physiol Norm Pathol 1868;1:161.
35. Charcot JM: Paraplegie par mal de Pott. Gaz Hop 1883;56:483.
36. Charnley J, Baker SL: Compression arthrodesis of the knee: A clinical and histological study. J Bone Joint Surg Br 1952;34:187.
37. Chen W-J, Wu C-C, Jung C-H, et al: Combined anterior and posterior surgeries in the treatment of spinal tuberculous spondylitis. Clin Orthop Relat Res 2002;398: 50.
38. Cheng YM, Lin SY, Wu HJ: Total ankle replacement: Preliminary report of 3 cases. Kao Hsiung I Hsueh Ko Hsueh Tsa Chih 1993;9:18.
39. Chmell MJ, Scott RD, Thomas WH, et al: Total hip arthroplasty with cement for juvenile rheumatoid arthritis: Results at a minimum of ten years in patients less than thirty years old. J Bone Joint Surg Am 1997;79:44.
40. Cho M, Neuhaus O: Absence of blood clotting substances from synovial fluid. Thromb Diathesis Haemorrh 1960;5:496.
41. Chylack LT Jr: The ocular manifestations of juvenile rheumatoid arthritis. Arthritis Rheum 1977;20:217.
42. Clarke DW, Ansell BM, Swann M: Soft-tissue release of the knee in children with juvenile chronic arthritis. J Bone Joint Surg Br 1988;70:224.
43. Cleveland M, Bosworth DM: The pathology of tuberculosis of the spine. J Bone Joint Surg 1942;24:527.
44. Connor PM, Morrey BF: Total elbow arthroplasty in patients who have juvenile rheumatoid arthritis. J Bone Joint Surg Am 1998;80:678.
45. Cordero M, Sanchez I: Brucellar and tuberculous spondylitis: A comparative study of their clinical features. J Bone Joint Surg Br 1991;73:100.
46. Cornil V: Memoire sur des coincidences pathologiques du rhumastisme articulaire chronique. CR Mem Soc Bio 1864;3:3.
47. Coss JA Jr, Boots RH: Juvenile rheumatoid arthritis: A study of fifty-six cases with a note on skeletal changes. J Pediatr 1946;29:143.
48. Cuttica RJ, Scheines EJ, Garay SM, et al: Juvenile onset Reiter's syndrome: A retrospective study of 26 patients. Clin Exp Rheumatol 1992;10:285.
49. Dalechamps J: Chirurgie Francaise. Paris, 1610.
50. Dawson D: Tuberculosis in Australia: Bacteriologically confirmed cases and drug resistance, 1996. Report of the Australian Mycobacterium Reference Laboratory Network. Commun Dis Intell 1998;22:183.
51. De Vuyst D, Vanhoenacker F, Gielen J, et al: Imaging features of musculoskeletal tuberculosis. Eur Radiol 2003;13:1809.
52. Debre R, Broca R, Lamy M: Forme encarditique de la maladie de Still. Arch Med Enf 1930;33:212.
53. Deirmengian CA, Lee SG, Jupiter JB: Neuropathic arthropathy of the elbow: A report of five cases. J Bone Joint Surg Am 2001;83:839.
54. Del Beccaro MA, Champoux AN, Bockers T, et al: Septic arthritis versus transient synovitis of the hip: The value of screening laboratory tests. Ann Emerg Med 1992; 21:1418.
55. Deol P, Khuller GK, Joshi K: Therapeutic efficacies of isoniazid and rifampin encapsulated in lung-specific stealth liposomes against *Mycobacterium tuberculosis*

infection induced in mice. Antimicrob Agents Chemother 1997;41:1211.

56. Dye C, Garnett GP, Sleeman K, et al: Prospects for worldwide tuberculosis control under the WHO DOTS strategy: Directly observed short-course therapy. Lancet 1998;352:1886.
57. Edstrom G: Rheumatoid arthritis in children: A clinical study. Acta Paediatr 1947;34:334.
58. Edstrom G: Rheumatoid arthritis and Still's disease in children: A survey of 161 cases. Arthritis Rheum 1958; 1:497.
59. Eichenwald H, Stroder J: Current Therapy in Pediatrics. Toronto, BC Decker, 1989.
60. Eyring EJ: The therapeutic potential of synovectomy in juvenile rheumatoid arthritis. Arthritis Rheum 1968;11: 688.
61. Eyring EJ, Longert A, Bass JC: Synovectomy in juvenile rheumatoid arthritis: Indications and short-term results. J Bone Joint Surg Am 1971;53:638.
62. Fairbank H: Discussion of non-tuberculous coxitis in the young. BMJ 1926;2:828.
63. Fantini F, Gerloni V, Gattinara M, et al: Remission in juvenile chronic arthritis: A cohort study of 683 consecutive cases with a mean 10 year followup. J Rheumatol 2003;30:579.
64. Fellander M: Radical operation in tuberculosis of the spine. Acta Orthop Scand Suppl 1955;19:1.
65. Ferguson AB Jr: Roentgenographic features of rheumatoid arthritis. J Bone Joint Surg 1936;18:297.
66. Field T, Hernandez-Reif M, Seligman S, et al: Juvenile rheumatoid arthritis: Benefits from massage therapy. J Pediatr Psychol 1997;22:607.
67. Fink CW: Proposal for the development of classification criteria for idiopathic arthritides of childhood. J Rheumatol 1995;22:1566.
68. Fink CW, Baum J, Paradies LH, et al: Synovectomy in juvenile rheumatoid arthritis. Ann Rheum Dis 1969;28: 612.
69. Flato B, Aasland A, Vinje O, et al: Outcome and predictive factors in juvenile rheumatoid arthritis and juvenile spondyloarthropathy. J Rheumatol 1998;25: 366.
70. Flato B, Lien G, Smerdel A, et al: Prognostic factors in juvenile rheumatoid arthritis: A case-control study revealing early predictors and outcome after 14.9 years. J Rheumatol 2003;30:386.
71. French AR, Mason T, Nelson AM, et al: Osteopenia in adults with a history of juvenile rheumatoid arthritis: A population based study. J Rheumatol 2002;29:1065.
72. Friedman S, Gruber MA: Ultrasonography of the hip in the evaluation of children with seronegative juvenile rheumatoid arthritis. J Rheumatol 2002;29:629.
73. Fujita H: A study of synovectomy of the knee joint in rheumatoid arthritis: Follow-up study of 127 synovectomized joints and histopathological observations on the regenerated rheumatoid synovium. Cent Jpn J Orthop Traumatol 1975;18:1117.
74. Futami T, Kasahara Y, Suzuki S, et al: Ultrasonography in transient synovitis and early Perthes' disease. J Bone Joint Surg Br 1991;73:635.
75. Garceau GJ, Brady TA: Pott's paraplegia. J Bone Joint Surg Am 1950;32:87.
76. Gauchat RD, May CD: Early recognition of rheumatoid disease with comments on treatment. Pediatrics 1957;19:672.
77. Gershuni DH, Hargens AR, Lee YF, et al: The questionable significance of hip joint tamponade in producing osteonecrosis in Legg-Calve-Perthes syndrome. J Pediatr Orthop 1983;3:280.
78. Giannini MJ, Protas EJ: Aerobic capacity in juvenile rheumatoid arthritis patients and healthy children. Arthritis Care Res 1991;4:131.
79. Girdlestone GR, Somerville EW: Tuberculosis of Bone and Joint. London, Oxford University Press, 1952.
80. Goldenberg J, Ferraz MB, Pessoa AP, et al: Symptomatic cardiac involvement in juvenile rheumatoid arthritis. Int J Cardiol 1992;34:57.
81. Goldi I: Pathomorphologic features in original and regenerated synovial tissues after synovectomy in rheumatoid arthritis. Clin Orthop Relat Res 1971;77: 295.
82. Gomez KS, Raza K, Jones SD, et al: Juvenile onset ankylosing spondylitis: More girls than we thought? J Rheumatol 1997;24:735.
83. Griffin PP, Tachdjian MO, Green WT: Pauciarticular arthritis in children. JAMA 1963;184:145.
84. Grokoest AW, Snyder AI, Schlaeger R: Juvenile Rheumatoid Arthritis. Boston, Little, Brown, 1961.
85. Grom AA, Giannini EH, Glass DN: Juvenile rheumatoid arthritis and the trimolecular complex (HLA, T cell receptor, and antigen): Differences from rheumatoid arthritis. Arthritis Rheum 1994;37:601.
86. Gudmundsson GH, Harving S, Pilgaard S: The Charnley total hip arthroplasty in juvenile rheumatoid arthritis patients. Orthopedics 1989;12:385.
87. Haber D, Goodman SB: Total hip arthroplasty in juvenile chronic arthritis: A consecutive series. J Arthroplasty 1998;13:259.
88. Hackett J, Johnson B, Parkin A, et al: Physiotherapy and occupational therapy for juvenile chronic arthritis: Custom and practice in five centres in the UK, USA and Canada. Br J Rheumatol 1996;35:695.
89. Hafner R, Truckenbrodt H, Spamer M: Rehabilitation in children with juvenile chronic arthritis. Baillieres Clin Rheumatol 1998;12:329.
90. Hallock H, Jones JB: Tuberculosis of the spine: An end-result study of the spine-fusion operation in a large number of patients. J Bone Joint Surg Am 1954; 36:219.
91. Hansen TM, Hansen G, Langgaard AM, et al: Long-term physical training in rheumatoid arthritis: A randomized trial with different training programs and blinded observers. Scand J Rheumatol 1993;22:107.
92. Hanson V, Kornreich H, Bernstein B: Prognosis of juvenile rheumatoid arthritis. Arthritis Rheum 1977; 20:279.
93. Hardinge K: The etiology of transient synovitis of the hip in childhood. J Bone Joint Surg Br 1970;52:101.
94. Harkcom TM, Lampman RM, Banwell BF, et al: Therapeutic value of graded aerobic exercise training in rheumatoid arthritis. Arthritis Rheum 1985;28:32.
95. Hasegawa Y, Wingstrand H, Gustafson T: Scintimetry in transient synovitis of the hip in the child. Acta Orthop Scand 1988;59:520.

96. Haugen M, Lien G, Flatø B, et al: Young adults with juvenile arthritis in remission attain normal peak bone mass at the lumbar spine and forearm. Arthritis Rheum 2000;43:1504.
97. Helliwell PS: Relationship of psoriatic arthritis with the other spondyloarthropathies. Curr Opin Rheumatol 2004;16:344.
98. Hensinger RN, DeVito PD, Ragsdale CG: Changes in the cervical spine in juvenile rheumatoid arthritis. J Bone Joint Surg Am 1986;68:189.
99. Hibbs RA: An operation for stiffening the knee joint. Ann Surg 1911;53:404.
100. Hibbs RJ, Risser JC: Treatment of vertebral tuberculosis by spine fusion operation: A report of 286 cases. J Bone Joint Surg 1928;10:805.
101. Hill SA, MacLarnon JC, Nag D: Ultrasound-guided aspiration for transient synovitis of the hip. J Bone Joint Surg Br 1990;72:852.
102. Hodgson AR, Stock FE: Anterior spine fusion. Br J Surg 1956;44:266.
103. Hodgson AR, Stock FE: Anterior spine fusion for the treatment of tuberculosis of the spine. J Bone Joint Surg Am 1960;42:295.
104. Hodgson AR, Stock FE, Fang HS, et al: Anterior spinal fusion: The operative approach and pathological findings in 412 patients with Pott's disease of the spine. Br J Surg 1960;48:172.
105. Hodgson AR, Yan A, Kwon JS, et al: A clinical study of 100 consecutive cases of Pott's paraplegia. Clin Orthop Relat Res 1964;36:128.
106. Holgersson S, Brattstrom H, Mogensen B, et al: Arthroscopy of the hip in juvenile chronic arthritis. J Pediatr Orthop 1981;1:273.
107. Hong SH, Kim SM, Ahn JM, et al: Tuberculous versus pyogenic arthritis: MR imaging evaluation. Radiology 2001;218:848.
108. Huang TJ, Hsu RW, Chen SH, et al: Video-assisted thoracoscopic surgery in managing tuberculous spondylitis. Clin Orthop Relat Res 2000;379:143.
109. Huemer C, Malleson PN, Cabral DA, et al: Patterns of joint involvement at onset differentiate oligoarticular juvenile psoriatic arthritis from pauciarticular juvenile rheumatoid arthritis. J Rheumatol 2002;29:1531.
110. Ilowite NT: Current treatment of juvenile rheumatoid arthritis. Pediatrics 2002;109:109.
111. Ishikawa H, Ziff M: Electron microscopic observations of immunoreactive cells in the rheumatoid synovial membrane. Arthritis Rheum 1976;19:1.
112. Jacobs JC, Li SC, Ruzal-Shapiro C, et al: Tuberculous arthritis in children. Diagnosis by needle biopsy of the synovium. Clin Pediatr (Phila) 1994;33:344.
113. Jacobsen ST, Levinson JE, Crawford AH: Late results of synovectomy in juvenile rheumatoid arthritis. J Bone Joint Surg Am 1985;67:8.
114. Jensen NC, Kroner K: Total ankle joint replacement: a clinical follow up. Orthopedics 1992;15:236.
115. Johnson RW, Jr, Hillman JW, Southwick WO: The importance of direct surgical attack upon lesions of the vertebral bodies, particularly in Pott's disease. J Bone Joint Surg Am 1953;35-A:17.
116. Jung N-Y, Jee W-H, Ha K-Y, et al: Discrimination of tuberculous spondylitis from pyogenic spondylitis on MRI. AJR Am J Roentgenol 2004;182:1405.
117. Kallio P, Ryoppy S, Jappinen S, et al: Ultrasonography in hip disease in children. Acta Orthop Scand 1985;56:367.
118. Kallio PE: Coxa magna following transient synovitis of the hip. Clin Orthop 1988;228:49.
119. Kampner SL, Ferguson AB Jr: Efficacy of synovectomy in juvenile rheumatoid arthritis. Clin Orthop Relat Res 1972;88:94.
120. Kanamori Y, Miyamoto K, Hosoe H, et al: Transoral approach using the mandibular osteotomy for atlantoaxial vertical subluxation in juvenile rheumatoid arthritis associated with mandibular micrognathia. J Spinal Disord Tech 2003;16:221.
121. Kanski JJ, Shun-Shin GA: Systemic uveitis syndromes in childhood: An analysis of 340 cases. Ophthalmology 1984;91:1247.
122. Kapusta MA, Metrakos JD, Pinsky L, et al: Juvenile rheumatoid arthritis in a mother and her identical twin sons. Arthritis Rheum 1969;12:411.
123. Karlen A: Early drainage of paraspinal tuberculous abscesses in children: A preliminary report. J Bone Joint Surg Br 1959;41:491.
124. Kesteris U, Wingstrand H, Forsberg L, et al: The effect of arthrocentesis in transient synovitis of the hip in the child: A longitudinal sonographic study. J Pediatr Orthop 1996;16:24.
125. Khoo LT, Mikawa K, Fessler RG: A surgical revisitation of Pott distemper of the spine. Spine J 2003;3:130.
126. Kim HY, Song KS, Goo JM, et al: Thoracic sequelae and complications of tuberculosis. Radiographics 2001;21:839.
127. Kim NH, Lee HM, Suh JS: Magnetic resonance imaging for the diagnosis of tuberculous spondylitis. Spine 1994;19:2451.
128. Kim YH, Kim JS, Oh SW: Total knee arthroplasty in neuropathic arthropathy. J Bone Joint Surg 2002;84:216.
129. Klepper SE, Darbee J, Effgen SK, et al: Physical fitness levels in children with polyarticular juvenile rheumatoid arthritis. Arthritis Care Res 1992;5:93.
130. Klepper SE, Giannini MJ: Physical conditioning in children with arthritis: Assessment and guidelines for exercise prescription. Arthritis Care Res 1994;7:226.
131. Koo E, Balogh Z, Gomor B: Juvenile psoriatic arthritis. Clin Rheumatol 1991;10:245.
132. Kotevoglu N, Tasbasi I: Diagnosing tuberculous spondylitis: Patients with back pain referred to a rheumatology outpatient department. Rheumatol Int 2004;24:9.
133. Kumar MN, Swann M: Uncemented total hip arthroplasty in young patients with juvenile chronic arthritis. Ann R Coll Surg Engl 1998;80:203.
134. Laaksonen AL: A prognostic study of juvenile rheumatoid arthritis: Analysis of 544 cases. Acta Paediatr Scand 1966:1.
135. Lachiewicz PF, McCaskill B, Inglis A, et al: Total hip arthroplasty in juvenile rheumatoid arthritis: Two to eleven-year results. J Bone Joint Surg Am 1986;68:502.

136. Landin LA, Danielsson LG, Wattsgard C: Transient synovitis of the hip: Its incidence, epidemiology and relation to Perthes' disease. J Bone Joint Surg Br 1987; 69:238.
137. Lang BA, Shore A: A review of current concepts on the pathogenesis of juvenile rheumatoid arthritis. J Rheumatol Suppl 1990;21:1.
138. Lehtimaki MY, Lehto MU, Kautiainen H, et al: Survivorship of the Charnley total hip arthroplasty in juvenile chronic arthritis: A follow-up of 186 cases for 22 years. J Bone Joint Surg Br 1997;79:792.
139. Liem JJ, Rosenberg AM: Growth patterns in juvenile rheumatoid arthritis. Clin Exp Rheumatol 2003;21:663.
140. Lietman PS, Bywaters EG: Pericarditis in juvenile rheumatoid arthritis. Pediatrics 1963;32:855.
141. Lightfoot RW Jr, Gotschlich EC: Gonococcal disease. Am J Med 1974;56:327.
142. Lindsley CB, Schaller JG: Arthritis associated with inflammatory bowel disease in children. J Pediatr 1974;84:16.
143. Lipnick RN, Tsokos GC: Immune abnormalities in the pathogenesis of juvenile rheumatoid arthritis. Clin Exp Rheumatol 1990;8:177.
144. Lisbona R, Derbekyan V, Novales-Diaz J, et al: Gallium-67 scintigraphy in tuberculous and nontuberculous infectious spondylitis. J Nucl Med 1993;34:853.
145. Liu GC, Chou MS, Tsai TC, et al: MR evaluation of tuberculous spondylitis. Acta Radiol 1993;34:554.
146. Lockie GN, Hunder GG: Reiter's syndrome in children: A case report and review. Arthritis Rheum 1971;14:767.
147. Lockie LM, Norcross BM: Juvenile rheumatoid arthritis. Pediatrics 1948;2:694.
148. Lohmander LS, Wingstrand H, Heinegard D: Transient synovitis of the hip in the child: Increased levels of proteoglycan fragments in joint fluid. J Orthop Res 1988;6:420.
149. Louw JA: Anterior vascular rib pedicle graft and posterior instrumentation in tuberculous spondylitis: A case report. S Afr Med J 1987;71:784.
150. Lovell DJ, Giannini EH, Reiff A, et al: Long-term efficacy and safety of etanercept in children with polyarticular-course juvenile rheumatoid arthritis: Interim results from an ongoing multicenter, open-label, extended-treatment trial. Arthritis Rheum 2003; 48:218.
151. Lovett R, Morse J: A transient or ephemeral form of hip-disease, with a report of cases. Boston Med Surg J 1892;127:161.
152. MacIntyre CR, Kendig N, Kummer L, et al: Impact of tuberculosis control measures and crowding on the incidence of tuberculous infection in Maryland prisons. Clin Infect Dis 1997;24:1060.
153. Maenpaa H, Kuusela P, Lehtinen J, et al: Elbow synovectomy on patients with juvenile rheumatoid arthritis. Clin Orthop Relat Res 2003;412:65.
154. Magnus KG, Hoffman EB: Pyogenic spondylitis and early tuberculous spondylitis in children: Differential diagnosis with standard radiographs and computed tomography. J Pediatr Orthop 2000;20:539.
155. Maric Z, Haynes RJ: Total hip arthroplasty in juvenile rheumatoid arthritis. Clin Orthop Relat Res 1993;290: 197.
156. Maroudas A, Bullough P, Swanson SA, et al: The permeability of articular cartilage. J Bone Joint Surg Br 1968;50:166.
157. Martel W, Holt JF, Cassidy JT: Roentgenologic manifestations of juvenile rheumatoid arthritis. AJR Am J Roentgenol Radium Ther Nucl Med 1962;88: 400.
158. Masi AT: HLA B27 and other host interactions in spondyloarthropathy syndromes. J Rheumatol 1978;5: 359.
159. Mason T, Reed AM, Nelson AM, et al: Frequency of abnormal hand and wrist radiographs at time of diagnosis of polyarticular juvenile rheumatoid arthritis. J Rheumatol 2002;29:2214.
160. McCarroll HR, Heath RD: Tuberculosis of the hip in children. J Bone Joint Surg 1947;29:889.
161. McGoldrick F, Bourke T, Blake N, et al: Accuracy of sonography in transient synovitis. J Pediatr Orthop 1990;10:501.
162. McNeur J, Pritchard AE: Tuberculosis of the greater trochanter. J Bone Joint Surg Br 1955;37:246.
163. Mehta JB, Mejia E, Gallemore GH, et al: Drug-resistant tuberculosis of the brain in a two-year-old child. Tenn Med 1998;91:285.
164. Millard FJ: The rising incidence of tuberculosis. J R Soc Med 1996;89:497.
165. Minden K, Kiessling U, Listing J, et al: Prognosis of patients with juvenile chronic arthritis and juvenile spondyloarthropathy. J Rheumatol 2000;27:491.
166. Miralles M, Gonzalez G, Pulpeiro JR, et al: Sonography of the painful hip in children: 500 consecutive cases. AJR Am J Roentgenol 1989;152:579.
167. Moreno Alvarez MJ, Espada G, Maldonado-Cocco JA, et al: Longterm followup of hip and knee soft tissue release in juvenile chronic arthritis. J Rheumatol 1992;19:1608.
168. Moskowitz A: Scoliosis and juvenile rheumatoid arthritis: A case report of surgical treatment. Spine 1990; 15:46.
169. Nachemson A, Scheller S: A clinical and radiological follow-up study of transient synovitis of the hip. Acta Orthop Scand 1969;40:479.
170. Noer H: An experimental epidemic of Reiter's syndrome. JAMA 1966;198:693.
171. Nussbaum M, Scalettar H, Shenker IR: Gonococcal arthritis-dermatitis (GADS) as a complication of gonococcemia in adolescents. Clin Pediatr (Phila) 1975;14: 1037.
172. Oen K, Malleson PN, Cabral DA, et al: Early predictors of longterm outcome in patients with juvenile rheumatoid arthritis: Subset-specific correlations. J Rheumatol 2003;30:585.
173. Oen K, Reed M, Malleson PN, et al: Radiologic outcome and its relationship to functional disability in juvenile rheumatoid arthritis. J Rheumatol 2003;30:832.
174. Oen K, Wilkins J, Drzekotowska D: OKT4:OKT8 ratios of circulating T cells and in vitro suppressor cell function of patients with juvenile rheumatoid arthritis. J Rheumatol 1985;12:321.
175. Ong Y, Cheong PY, Low YP, et al: Delayed diagnosis of tuberculosis presenting as small joint arthritis: A case report. Singapore Med J 1998;39:177.

176. Ovregard T, Hoyeraal H, Pahle J, et al: A three-year retrospective study of synovectomies in children. Clin Orthop Relat Res 1990;259:76.
177. Ozdemir HM, Us AK, Ogun T: The role of anterior spinal instrumentation and allograft fibula for the treatment of Pott disease. Spine 2003;28:474.
178. Ozdemir HM, Yensel U, Cevat Ogun T, et al: Arthrodesis for tuberculous coxarthritis: Good outcome in 32 adolescents. Acta Orthop Scand 2004;75:430.
179. Parmar H, Shah J, Patkar D, et al: Tuberculous arthritis of the appendicular skeleton: MR imaging appearances. Eur J Radiol 2004;52:300.
180. Parvizi J, Lajam CM, Trousdale RT, et al: Total knee arthroplasty in young patients with juvenile rheumatoid arthritis. J Bone Joint Surg Am 2003;85:1090.
181. Parvizi J, Marrs J, Morrey BF: Total knee arthroplasty for neuropathic (Charcot) joints. Clin Orthop Relat Res 2003;416:145.
182. Patzakis MJ, Mills DM, Bartholomew BA, et al: A visual, histological, and enzymatic study of regenerating rheumatoid synovium in the synovectomized knee. J Bone Joint Surg Am 1973;55:287.
183. Peloquin CA, Berning SE: Infection caused by *Mycobacterium tuberculosis.* Ann Pharmacother 1994;28:72.
184. Perry J: Structural Insufficiency: I. Pathomechanics: Principles of Lower Extremity Bracing. New York, American Physical Therapy Association, 1967, p 81.
185. Peter CR, Schultz E, Moser K, et al: Drug-resistant pulmonary tuberculosis in the Baja California-San Diego County border population. West J Med 1998;169:208.
186. Petty RE: Current knowledge of the etiology and pathogenesis of chronic uveitis accompanying juvenile rheumatoid arthritis. Rheum Dis Clin North Am 1987; 13:19.
187. Petty RE: HLA-B27 and rheumatic diseases of childhood. J Rheumatol Suppl 1990;26:7.
188. Petty RE, Southwood TR: Classification of childhood arthritis: Divide and conquer. J Rheumatol 1998;25: 1869.
189. Pott P: Remarks on the kind of palsy of the lower limbs which is frequently found to accompany curvature of the spine and is supposed to be caused by it, together with its method of cure. In Pott P (ed): The Chirurgical Works. London, Lowndes, 1779.
190. Pritchard MH, Matthews N, Munro J: Antibodies to influenza A in a cluster of children with juvenile chronic arthritis. Br J Rheumatol 1988;27:176.
191. Pugh MT, Southwood TR, Gaston JS: The role of infection in juvenile chronic arthritis. Br J Rheumatol 1993;32:838.
192. Rahimtoola ZO, Finger S, Imrie S, et al: Outcome of total hip arthroplasty in small-proportioned patients. J Arthroplasty 2000;15:27.
193. Rakel R: Conn's Current Therapy. Philadelphia, WB Saunders, 1999.
194. Ranawat CS, Straub LR, Freyberg R, et al: A study of regenerated synovium after synovectomy of the knee in rheumatoid arthritis. Arthritis Rheum 1971;14:117.
195. Rastogi N, Goh KS, Horgen L, et al: Synergistic activities of antituberculous drugs with cerulenin and trans-cinnamic acid against *Mycobacterium tuberculosis.* FEMS Immunol Med Microbiol 1998;21:149.
196. Rastogi N, Labrousse V, Goh KS: In vitro activities of fourteen antimicrobial agents against drug susceptible and resistant clinical isolates of *Mycobacterium tuberculosis* and comparative intracellular activities against the virulent H37Rv strain in human macrophages. Curr Microbiol 1996;33:167.
197. Reed M, Wilmot D: The radiology of juvenile rheumatoid arthritis: A review of the English language literature. J Rheumatol 1991;18(Suppl 31):2.
198. Resnick D, Dwosh IL, Goergen TG, et al: Clinical and radiographic abnormalities in ankylosing spondylitis: A comparison of men and women. Radiology 1976; 119:293.
199. Robben SG, Meradji M, Diepstraten AF, et al: US of the painful hip in childhood: Diagnostic value of cartilage thickening and muscle atrophy in the detection of Perthes disease. Radiology 1998;208:35.
200. Rosenheim S: On the pathological changes in the spinal cord in a case of Pott's disease. Johns Hopkins Hosp Bull 1898:240.
201. Rychlicki F, Messori A, Recchioni MA, et al: Tuberculous spondylitis: A retrospective study on a series of 12 patients operated on in a 25-year period. J Neurosurg Sci 1998;42:213.
202. Rydholm U, Brattstrom H, Bylander B, et al: Stapling of the knee in juvenile chronic arthritis. J Pediatr Orthop 1987;7:63.
203. Rydholm U, Brattstrom H, Lidgren L: Soft tissue release for knee flexion contracture in juvenile chronic arthritis. J Pediatr Orthop 1986;6:448.
204. Rydholm U, Elborgh R, Ranstam J, et al: Synovectomy of the knee in juvenile chronic arthritis: A retrospective, consecutive follow-up study. J Bone Joint Surg Br 1986;68:223.
205. Sairanen E: On micrognathia in juvenile rheumatoid arthritis. Acta Rheumatol Scand 1964;10:133.
206. Sakkas LI, Platsoucas CD: Immunopathogenesis of juvenile rheumatoid arthritis: Role of T cells and MHC. Immunol Res 1995;14:218.
207. Sanchis-Olmos V: Skeletal Tuberculosis. Baltimore, Williams & Williams, 1948.
208. Sarokhan AJ, Scott RD, Thomas WH, et al: Total knee arthroplasty in juvenile rheumatoid arthritis. J Bone Joint Surg Am 1983;65:1071.
209. Sauer ST, Farrell E, Geller E, et al: Septic arthritis in a patient with juvenile rheumatoid arthritis. Clin Orthop Relat Res 2004;418:219.
210. Schaller J: The seronegative spondyloarthropathies of childhood. Clin Orthop Relat Res 1979;182:79.
211. Schaller J, Wedgwood R: Pauciarticular juvenile rheumatoid arthritis. Arthritis Rheum 1969;12:330.
212. Schaller JG, Ochs HD, Thomas ED, et al: Histocompatibility antigens in childhood-onset arthritis. J Pediatr 1976;88:926.
213. Schlosstein L, Terasaki PI, Bluestone R, et al: High association of the HLA antigen W27 with ankylosing spondylitis. N Engl J Med 1973;288:704.
214. Schon LC, Easley ME, Weinfeld SB: Charcot neuroarthropathy of the foot and ankle. Clin Orthop Relat Res 1998;349:116.
215. Scott JC: Treatment of tuberculosis of the spine. J Bone Joint Surg Br 1955;37:367.

216. Scott RD: Total hip and knee arthroplasty in juvenile rheumatoid arthritis. Clin Orthop Relat Res 1990;259: 83.
217. Segura C, Salvado M, Collado I, et al: Contribution of beta-lactamases to beta-lactam susceptibilities of susceptible and multidrug-resistant *Mycobacterium tuberculosis* clinical isolates. Antimicrob Agents Chemother 1998;42:1524.
218. Sharwood PF: The irritable hip syndrome in children: A long-term follow-up. Acta Orthop Scand 1981;52: 633.
219. Sherry DD: What's new in the diagnosis and treatment of juvenile rheumatoid arthritis. J Pediatr Orthop 2000;20:419.
220. Shiv VK, Jain AK, Taneja K, et al: Sonography of hip joint in infective arthritis. Can Assoc Radiol J 1990; 41:76.
221. Siddiqi N, Shamim M, Jain NK, et al: Molecular genetic analysis of multi-drug resistance in Indian isolates of *Mycobacterium tuberculosis.* Mem Inst Oswaldo Cruz 1998;93:589.
222. Sornay-Soares C, Job-Deslandre C, Kahan A: Joint lavage for treating recurrent knee involvement in patients with juvenile idiopathic arthritis. Joint Bone Spine 2004;71:296.
223. Soto-Hall R, Johnson LH, Johnson RA: Variations in the intra-articular pressure of the hip joint in injury and disease: A probable factor in avascular necrosis. J Bone Joint Surg Am 1964;46:509.
224. Spencer CH, Bernstein BH: Hip disease in juvenile rheumatoid arthritis. Curr Opin Rheumatol 2002;14: 536.
225. Starke JR: Tuberculosis in children. Curr Opin Pediatr 1995;7:268.
226. Steenland K, Levine AJ, Sieber K, et al: Incidence of tuberculosis infection among New York State prison employees. Am J Public Health 1997;87:2012.
227. Steindler A: The tabetic arthropathies. JAMA 1931; 96:250.
228. Stenstrom CH: Home exercise in rheumatoid arthritis functional class II: Goal setting versus pain attention. J Rheumatol 1994;21:627.
229. Stenstrom CH, Lindell B, Swanberg E, et al: Intensive dynamic training in water for rheumatoid arthritis functional class II: A long-term study of effects. Scand J Rheumatol 1991;20:358.
230. Suh JS, Lee JD, Cho JH, et al: MR imaging of tuberculous arthritis: Clinical and experimental studies. J Magn Reson Imaging 1996;6:185.
231. Sullivan D, Cassidy J, Petty R: Pathogenic implications of age of onset in juvenile rheumatoid arthritis. Arthritis Rheum 1975;18:251.
232. Swann M: The surgery of juvenile chronic arthritis: An overview. Clin Orthop 1990;259:70.
233. Swann M, Ansell BM: Soft-tissue release of the hips in children with juvenile chronic arthritis. J Bone Joint Surg Br 1986;68:404.
234. Takei S, Groh D, Bernstein B, et al: Safety and efficacy of high dose etanercept in treatment of juvenile rheumatoid arthritis. J Rheumatol 2001;28:1677.
235. Teo HEL, Peh WCG: Skeletal tuberculosis in children. Pediatr Radiol 2004;34:853.
236. Terjesen T, Osthus P: Ultrasound in the diagnosis and follow-up of transient synovitis of the hip. J Pediatr Orthop 1991;11:608.
237. Titov AG, Nakonechniy GD, Santavirta S, et al: Arthroscopic operations in joint tuberculosis. Knee 2004;11:57.
238. Titov AG, Vyshnevskaya EB, Mazurenko SI, et al: Use of polymerase chain reaction to diagnose tuberculous arthritis from joint tissues and synovial fluid. Arch Pathol Lab Med 2004;128:205.
239. Tönnis D: Skewfoot [in German]. Orthopade 1986;15: 174.
240. Towner SR, Michet CJ Jr, O'Fallon WM, et al: The epidemiology of juvenile arthritis in Rochester, Minnesota 1960-1979. Arthritis Rheum 1983;26:1208.
241. Truchenbrodt H, Hafner R: Psoriatic arthritis in childhood: A comparison with subgroups of chronic juvenile arthritis. Z Rheumatol 1990;49:88.
242. Tsai YH, Ueng SW, Shih CH: Tuberculosis of the ankle: Report of four cases. Chang Keng I Hsueh Tsa Chih (China) 1998;21:481.
243. Tseng CY, Yang SP, Lee YJ, et al: Tuberculous arthritis of sacroiliac joint with abscess formation: A case report. Chung Hua I Hsueh Tsa Chih (Taipei) 1997;60:168.
244. Tsukahara M, Tsuneoka H, Tateishi H, et al: *Bartonella* infection associated with systemic juvenile rheumatoid arthritis. Clin Infect Dis 2001;32:E22.
245. Unger AS, Inglis AE, Mow CS, et al: Total ankle arthroplasty in rheumatoid arthritis: A long-term follow-up study. Foot Ankle 1988;8:173.
246. van der Linden SM, Valkenburg HA, de Jongh BM, et al: The risk of developing ankylosing spondylitis in HLA-B27 positive individuals: A comparison of relatives of spondylitis patients with the general population. Arthritis Rheum 1984;27:241.
247. Vijlbrief AS, Bruijnzeels MA, van der Wouden JC, et al: Incidence and management of transient synovitis of the hip: A study in Dutch general practice. Br J Gen Pract 1992;42:426.
248. Villarino ME, Ridzon R, Weismuller PC, et al: Rifampin preventive therapy for tuberculosis infection: Experience with 157 adolescents. Am J Respir Crit Care Med 1997;155:1735.
249. Wang S-J, Yang Y-H, Lin Y-T, et al: Attained adult height in juvenile rheumatoid arthritis with or without corticosteroid treatment. Clin Rheumatol 2002;21:363.
250. Weinberg JA: The surgical excision of psoas abscesses resulting from spinal tuberculosis. J Bone Joint Surg Am 1957;39:17.
251. White JF: Case of caries of dorsal vertebrae, with an abscess communicating with the lungs and expectoration of bone. Phila Med Exam 1841;4:213.
252. Wilkinson MC: The treatment of tuberculosis of the spine by evacuation of the paravertebral abscess and curettage of the vertebral bodies. J Bone Joint Surg Br 1955;37:382.
253. Wilkinson MC: Treatment of tuberculosis of the spine. BMJ 1959;2:280.
254. Williams MH: Recovery of mycoplasma from rheumatoid synovial fluid. In Duthie JJR, Alexander WRM (eds): Rheumatic Diseases. Baltimore, Williams & Williams, 1968, p 172.

255. Williams R, Frolich C, Kilpatrick K: T Cell subset specificity of lymphocyte reactive factors in juvenile rheumatoid arthritis and systemic lupus erythematosus sera. Arthritis Rheum 1981;24:585.
256. Williams WW, McCullough CJ: Results of cemented total hip replacement in juvenile chronic arthritis: A radiological review. J Bone Joint Surg Br 1993;75:872.
257. Wimmer C, Ogon M, Sterzinger W, et al: Conservative treatment of tuberculous spondylitis: A long-term follow-up study. J Spinal Disord 1997;10:417.
258. Wingstrand H, Bauer GC, Brismar J, et al: Transient ischaemia of the proximal femoral epiphysis in the child: Interpretation of bone scintimetry for diagnosis in hip pain. Acta Orthop Scand 1985;56:197.
259. Wingstrand H, Egund N: Ultrasonography in hip joint effusion: Report of a child with transient synovitis. Acta Orthop Scand 1984;55:469.
260. Wingstrand H, Egund N, Carlin NO, et al: Intracapsular pressure in transient synovitis of the hip. Acta Orthop Scand 1985;56:204.
261. Witt JD, McCullough CJ: Anterior soft-tissue release of the hip in juvenile chronic arthritis. J Bone Joint Surg Br 1994;76:267.
262. Wynn AH, Wilde AH: Long-term follow-up of the Conaxial (Beck-Steffee) total ankle arthroplasty. Foot Ankle 1992;13:303.
263. Yoshino S, Fujimori J, Kajino A, et al: Total knee arthroplasty in Charcot's joint. J Arthroplasty 1993;8:335.
264. Yoshiyama T: Multidrug-resistant tuberculosis: 3. Epidemiology of drug-resistant tuberculosis in Japan [in Japanese]. Kekkaku 1998;73:665.

Chapter 35

Infections of the Musculoskeletal System

It is difficult to standardize the evaluation and treatment of musculoskeletal infection. Nelson's advice to avoid a "cookbook" approach to these complex and challenging conditions is well respected.[218] A high index of suspicion, careful clinical judgment, and diligent attention to detail are indispensable if one is to avoid the numerous pitfalls that can accompany these infections.

With the wealth of knowledge and experience gained in the latter half of the 20th century, we are now armed with an organized methodology to accurately diagnose and promptly treat most musculoskeletal infections, and we can anticipate complete resolution and excellent clinical outcomes in the majority of children. A recently published clinical practice guideline for the treatment of septic arthritis in children represents the potential to achieve an organized, interdisciplinary, evidence-based approach to the management of musculoskeletal infection.[171] The challenge is to create similar guidelines for the evaluation and treatment of osteomyelitis and to raise awareness of this disease among all physicians who evaluate children; early identification and prompt treatment are necessary to improve the poor outcomes and avoid the permanent sequelae that continue to affect approximately 6% of children with osteomyelitis.[160] Another concern is the emergence of methicillin-resistant *Staphylococcus aureus* (MRSA) as a cause of deep musculoskeletal infection.[22,113,199] However, promising new research may lead to revolutionary ways to identify and respond to genome-specific virulence factors that may be responsible for complications in sequela-prone children.[9,154,199]

Common Conditions

Infections of the musculoskeletal system represent a broad spectrum of conditions with varied manifestations, severities, and responses to treatment. These include osteomyelitis (bone infection), septic arthritis (joint infection), pyomyositis (muscle infection), and other deep soft tissue infections such as septic bursitis, necrotizing fasciitis, abscess, and purpura fulminans. This chapter outlines the epidemiology, pathogenesis, classification, evaluation, treatment, and complications of the most common forms of musculoskeletal infection in children.

Osteomyelitis

There are four discernible types of pediatric osteomyelitis, based on the time of onset, manner of clinical presentation, and response to treatment: acute hematogenous osteomyelitis (AHO), subacute osteomyelitis, chronic osteomyelitis, and chronic recurrent multifocal osteomyelitis (CRMO). In AHO, the child often presents within several days of the rather sudden onset of illness and localized symptoms. In contrast, in subacute osteomyelitis, medical evaluation may not be sought for 2 weeks or longer after the onset of symptoms, which are typically vague and minimized, leading the family or the physician to overlook or discount the child's condition. Chronic osteomyelitis is commonly the consequence of the failure to eradicate AHO, lasting months to years and creating the hallmark clinical findings of dead bone (sequestrum) surrounded by reactive new bone (involucrum). The pathogenesis of CRMO is uncertain, but it typically follows a prolonged, relapsing and remitting course lasting several years and involving multiple sites.

ACUTE HEMATOGENOUS OSTEOMYELITIS

Epidemiology

There is evidence that the epidemiology of musculoskeletal infection is evolutionary and that regional variation exists, making it difficult to extrapolate the reported experience from one institution or region to reliably predict the epidemiology in other areas. Reports from a single health district in Glasgow, Scotland, identified a 44% decrease in the incidence of osteomyelitis (predominantly AHO) between 1990 and 1997 and a 50% decrease between 1970 and 1990.[22,61] In comparison, other authors have reported little change in the incidence of osteomyelitis since the 1970s.[90,160,307]

The estimated annual incidence of AHO in children younger than 13 years is 1 in 5000, with the majority of cases occurring in children younger than 5 years.[160,282]

Staphylococcus aureus is the most commonly identified pathogen in all age groups, accounting for 70% to 90% of culture-positive cases of AHO.* Other organisms responsible for musculoskeletal infection appear to have a proclivity for children of specific age groups in which exposure to the organism is more likely.† Children with underlying disease or injury, such as sickle cell disease or foot puncture wounds, may also be predisposed to infection with specific organisms.[31,40,80,147,236] Infection with obscure or multidrug-resistant organisms may occur under unusual circumstances, including immunocompromise, prolonged hospitalization with multiple invasive procedures, and residence in endemic environments.‡

Certain historical events have had a dramatic impact on the epidemiology of musculoskeletal infection. The introduction of the conjugate vaccine for *Haemophilus influenzae* type b (Hib) in 1987 and its subsequent approval for use in infants starting at 2 months of age in October 1990 led to a dramatic decrease in the incidence of bone and joint infections due to this organism.[25,131,183] Before 1985, nearly 1 in 200 children experienced a major infection such as meningitis, epiglottitis, or pneumonia caused by Hib, and up to 34% of cases of septic arthritis and 13% of cases of osteomyelitis were attributed to this organism.[131,183] Following the advent of widespread vaccination, there has been nearly complete eradication of bone and joint infections caused by Hib in most populations.[25] In a similar manner, the recent development and routine use of the heptavalent conjugate pneumococcal vaccine in infants has reduced the rate of invasive infections from 50 to 100 per 100,000 person-years to 9 per 100,000 person-years in children younger than 2 years.[26,129,146] The continued occurrence of Hib and invasive pneumococcal disease in certain communities may be related to numerous factors, including failure to immunize children in lower socioeconomic groups, lack of immunity in very young children who have not completed the primary series of vaccinations, and infection by other strains of the primary organism not targeted by the immunization.[25,129,183]

Community-acquired methicillin-resistant *Staphylococcus aureus* (CA-MRSA) has recently emerged as a major factor in the changing epidemiology of invasive musculoskeletal infection in many parts of the United States and around the world.[9,113,124,199,206,259,285] Reports from Canada, Australia, New Zealand, Japan, and the United States (Chicago, Atlanta, Houston, and San Antonio) have cited a 28% to 67% incidence of MRSA infections in children with no predisposing risk factors, attesting to the prevalence of MRSA as a community organism.[9,113,124,139,199,200,206,259,285] Although skin and soft tissue infections predominated in the initial descriptions of CA-MRSA infections, more recent reports include invasive infections. Between 2000 and 2002, Texas Children's Hospital in Houston reported CA-MRSA in 31 of 59 children (53%) with deep musculoskeletal infections.[199] This series was the first to suggest an association between bacterial virulence factors and the development of complications associated with musculoskeletal infections caused by *S. aureus*.

Pathophysiology

Acute hematogenous osteomyelitis most commonly affects the metaphyseal region of long bones, with lower extremity locations—femur (27%), tibia (22%), and fibula (5%)—slightly more common than the upper extremity locations—humerus (12%), radius (4%), and ulna (3%).[280] Long-bone infections account for 75% of cases of osteomyelitis; nontubular bone infections occur with a reported incidence of 10% to 11% for pelvic osteomyelitis, 7% to 8% for calcaneal osteomyelitis, 5% for hand involvement, and 2% for vertebral osteomyelitis or diskitis.[69,86,96,140,280] Isolated cases of osteomyelitis in rare locations such as the cuboid, patella, and clavicle have been reported.[185,203,262,263] Bacteria can be introduced into bone by hematogenous spread from bacteremia, local invasion from a contiguous infection, or direct inoculation from penetrating trauma, such as an open fracture or foot puncture wound.

Bacteremia is a common event in childhood; it may be a consequence of other infections such as otitis media, pharyngitis, and sinusitis that gain access to the bloodstream, or it may be related to daily activities such as tooth brushing and Valsalva-type maneuvers.[83] It is presumed that bacteria gain access to the metaphyseal location of long bones via the branches of the nutrient arteries, which ultimately terminate in the regions adjacent to the physis as straight, narrow arterioles that form loops and connect with wider venous sinusoids (Fig. 35–1).[126] Trueta proposed that this anatomy results in a slow, turbulent blood flow in which the circulating bacteria can localize.[299] Gaps in

*See references 22, 54, 68, 90, 145, 160, 208, 272, 280, 307.
†See references 10, 108, 112, 129, 142, 143, 187, 228, 320, 332, 333.
‡See references 21, 32, 139, 190, 211, 244, 291, 292, 313, 319.

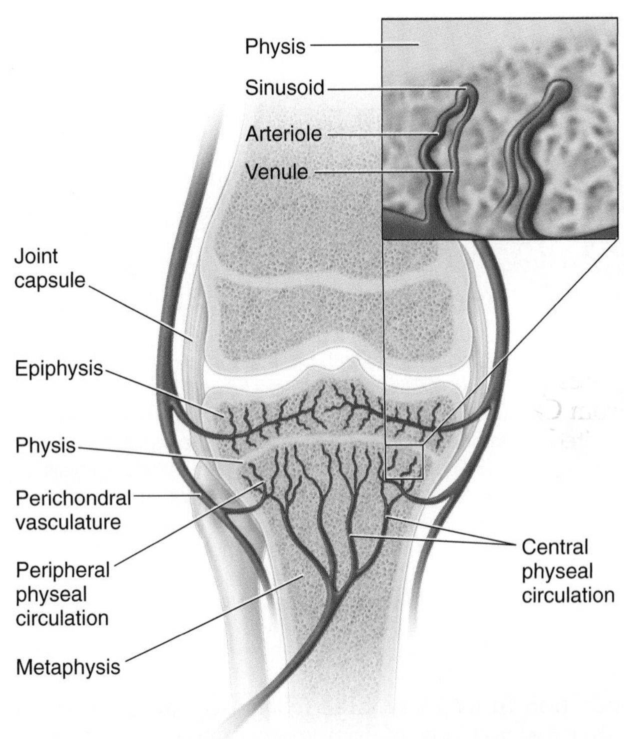

FIGURE 35–1 Metaphyseal circulation of the long bones in children. The nutrient artery terminates in end arterioles, which make a hairpin turn adjacent to the physis and feed into larger venous sinusoids. The resultant turbulent circulation enables bacteria to enter the extravascular space.

the endothelium of metaphyseal vessels in growing children may allow the passage of bacteria from the metaphyseal circulation into the extravascular space.[224,270] These anatomic features differ from those of adults, in whom hematogenous osteomyelitis is rarely identified.[299]

It has long been recognized that the mere presence of bacteria in bone is not enough to cause disease.[157] Numerous investigators have sought to create a model of AHO that resembles the clinical disease, with limited success. Yet one model that originally helped substantiate the effectiveness of antibiotics in the treatment of osteomyelitis was created by injecting sodium morrhuate directly into bone to produce an area of necrosis immediately before injecting the area with bacteria.[223] Hypothesizing that local tissue trauma may be a supplemental causative factor essential to the initiation of osteomyelitis, Morrissy and associates studied the effects of physeal injuries in New Zealand White rabbits before inducing experimental bacteremia and demonstrated a reproducible model resembling AHO.[210,324] In this research, the inflammatory response was consistently confined to the portion of bone beneath the area of injury, in the secondary spongiosa, whereas the bacteria were identified in the primary spongiosa, a relatively acellular area.[210] It is surmised that the lack of phagocytic activity in this vulnerable region in growing children may allow the proliferation of bacteria and the initiation of AHO. Another factor that may influence the localization and proliferation of bacteria, specifically *S. aureus,* is the presence of surface antigens that play a key role in bacterial adherence to type 1 collagen and endotoxins that suppress the local immune response.[62] An extensive glycocalyx may also form around the bacteria and enhance their adherence to other bacteria and metallic implants, which may be protective against antibiotic treatment.[62]

A significant anatomic feature that allows osteomyelitis to gain access to the epiphysis is the continuity of circulation across the physis, which remains open until approximately 18 months of age (Fig. 35–2).[299] Osteomyelitis originating in the metaphysis at an early age can easily spread to the epiphysis and result in the total destruction of both, with profound implications for the subsequent development of the proximal femoral and proximal humeral anatomy.[16,45,78,115,135,196]

Once bacteria have gained access to the extravascular space, local macrophages and monocytes migrate to the foreign stimulus and phagocytize the pathogen, which leads to the production and release of prostaglandins and cytokines. Prostaglandin E production is 30-fold higher in infected bone than in normal bone, and experimental treatment of osteomyelitis in rats with ibuprofen prevents bone resorption and sequestration, despite elevated bacterial counts in the local tissues.[253] The inflammation-associated cytokines include interleukin (IL)-6, IL-1β, tumor necrosis factor α (TNF-α), interferon gamma, transforming growth factor β, and IL-8.[92] IL-6 acts as the chief stimulator of the production and release of most acute-phase proteins by hepatocytes, including C-reactive protein (CRP), fibrinogen, the complement system, and serum amyloid A.[30] CRP acts as an opsonin for bacteria, parasites, and immune complexes and can activate the classic complement pathway, thereby modulating the behavior of several cell types involved in the inflammatory response, including neutrophils, monocytes, natural killer cells, and platelets.[91] The patterns of cytokine production and the acute-phase response may vary in different inflammatory conditions, with the cytokines operating both as a cascade and as a network in stimulating the production of acute-phase proteins.[92] Altogether, the acute-phase response results in physiologic and metabolic alterations, including fever, lethargy, leukocytosis, altered vascular permeability, and changes in hepatic biosynthesis, which act in concert to neutralize the infectious agent and foster the healing of damaged tissues.[150]

Classification

Osteomyelitis can be classified by pathogenesis, anatomic location, extent, duration, and host status. The first classification system for osteomyelitis was described in 1970 by Waldvogel and coworkers; it categorized bone infection as that derived from (1) hematogenous dissemination, (2) contiguous spread from local infection, and (3) an association with vascular insufficiency (predominantly diabetes).[314-316] Although this classification identifies cause, it is not useful for

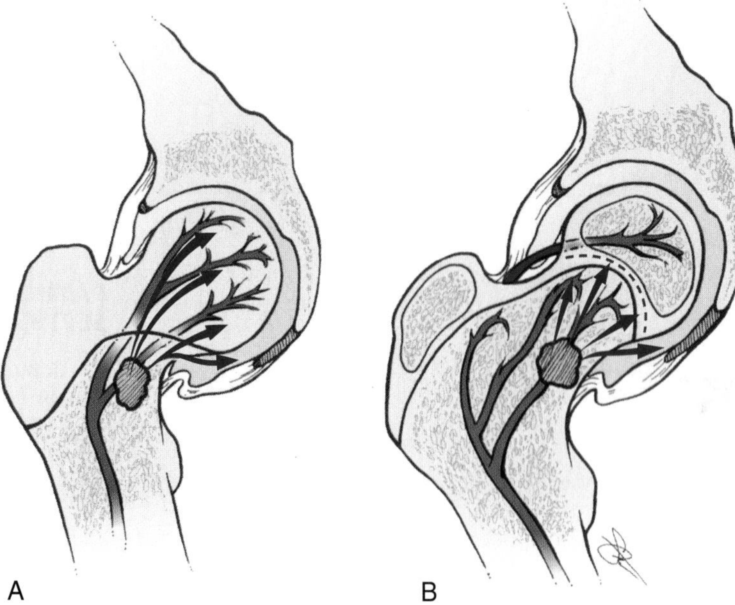

FIGURE 35–2 Vascular anatomy of the proximal femur. **A,** In the neonate, the entire epiphysis shares a blood supply with the metaphysis. Thus, infection in the metaphysis can spread into the epiphysis, producing devastating osteonecrosis of the proximal femur. **B,** After development of the secondary ossification center, the epiphysis and metaphysis have separate blood supplies. Thus, in the older child, the physis prevents the spread of infection into the epiphysis. However, the metaphysis remains intra-articular, and infection may decompress into the joint, producing septic arthritis.

guiding treatment or determining prognosis. The Cierny-Mader classification was proposed in 1984 in an effort to provide comprehensive treatment guidelines for osteomyelitis in adults and children.[49] It is based on anatomic type (medullary, superficial, localized, diffuse) and host status (normal, local compromise, systemic compromise) (Table 35–1). From this classification, the authors developed comprehensive treatment guidelines for 12 stages of infection. Because most children with osteomyelitis are normal hosts with localized osteomyelitis, the Cierny-Mader classification has limited application in pediatric orthopaedics.

A clinically useful subclassification of AHO in children is based on the child's age and development. Ultimately, this may be more helpful in anticipating both the causative organism (and thus guide empirical antibiotic selection) and the clinical manifestations of infection in a given child. There appear to be somewhat distinct age-related periods when certain types of infection have their highest incidence (Table 35–2). Numerous factors may influence this relationship, including exposure to specific organisms during childbirth; loss of maternally conferred immunity; developmental anatomy; exposure to specific organisms during day care, preschool, and school; and the onset of sexual activity during adolescence. These age-related categories are neonatal (birth to 8 weeks), infantile (2 to 18 months), early childhood (18 months to 3 years), childhood (3 to 12 years), and adolescent (12 to 18 years).

Table 35–1 Cierny-Mader Osteomyelitis Staging System

Classification	Description
Anatomic Stage	
1	Medullary osteomyelitis
2	Superficial osteomyelitis
3	Localized osteomyelitis
4	Diffuse osteomyelitis
Physiologic Host Status	
A	Normal host
B	Systemic compromise
	Local compromise
	Systemic and local compromise
C	Treatment worse than the disease

From Mader JT, Shirtliff M, Calhoun JH: Staging and staging application in osteomyelitis. Clin Infect Dis 1997;25:1303.

Neonatal. Neonatal osteomyelitis occurs in two distinct varieties. The first is encountered in infants 2 to 8 weeks of age who are typically discharged from the hospital with their mothers soon after birth, often the product of full-term, spontaneous vaginal delivery. The problem is often identified when parents become concerned about a lack of movement or visible swelling of an extremity in their newborn. Because the clinical features of fever and irritability are usually not present in this age group, diagnosis and treatment may be delayed. These neonates also fail to mount an inflammatory response that could be detected in common laboratory studies, and their radiographic evaluation may be equivocal as well. Because of these issues, a high index of suspicion must be maintained. Aspiration of bone and joint should be performed liberally, and antibiotic therapy should be initiated when infection is identified, followed by appropriate surgical decision making.

S. aureus is the most commonly identified organism in this age group. Other common organisms include those encountered during the childbirth process, such as *Streptococcus agalactiae* (group B streptococcus), enterococci, and Enterobacteriaceae (*Escherichia coli, Proteus* species, *Klebsiella* species).[10,30] Community-

Table 35-2 Causative Organisms and Empirical Antibiotics for Musculoskeletal Infections Based on Patient Age and Risk Factors

Patient Characteristics	Causative Organisms	Empirical Antibiotics
Age Group		
Neonatal (birth to 8 wk)		
Nosocomial infection	*Staphylococcus aureus*, *Streptococcus* species, Enterobacteriaceae, *Candida* species	Nafcillin or oxacillin plus gentamicin or Cefotaxime (or ceftriaxone) plus gentamicin
Community-acquired infection	*S. aureus*, group B streptococcus, *Escherichia coli*, *Klebsiella* species	Nafcillin or oxacillin plus gentamicin or Cefotaxime (or ceftriaxone) plus gentamicin
Infantile (2 to 18 mo)	*S. aureus*, *Kingella kingae*, *Streptococcus pneumoniae*, *Neisseria meningitidis*, *Haemophilus influenzae* type b (nonimmunized)	Immunized: nafcillin, oxacillin, or cefazolin Nonimmunized: nafcillin or oxacillin plus cefotaxime, or cefuroxime
Early childhood (18 mo to 3 yr)	*S. aureus*, *K. kingae*, *S. pneumoniae*, *N. meningitidis*, *H. influenzae* type b (nonimmunized)	Immunized: nafcillin, oxacillin, or cefazolin Nonimmunized: nafcillin or oxacillin plus cefotaxime, or cefuroxime
Childhood (3 to 12 yr)	*S. aureus*, GABHS	Nafcillin, oxacillin, or cefazolin
Adolescent (12 to 18 yr)	*S. aureus*, GABHS, *Neisseria gonorrhoeae*	Nafcillin, oxacillin, or cefazolin; ceftriaxone and doxycycline for disseminated gonococcal infection
Risk Factor		
Sickle cell disease	*Salmonella* species, *S. aureus*, *S. pneumoniae*	Ceftriaxone
Foot puncture wound	*Pseudomonas aeruginosa*, *S. aureus*	Ceftazidime or piperacillin-tazobactam and gentamicin
HIV	*S. aureus*, *Streptococcus* species, *Salmonella* species, *Nocardia asteroides*, *N. gonorrhoeae*, cytomegalovirus, *Aspergillus*, *Toxoplasma gondii*, *Torulopsis glabrata*, *Cryptococcus neoformans*, *Coccidioides immitis*	Broad-spectrum antibiotics per infectious disease recommendations
CGD	*Aspergillus* species, *Staphylococcus* species, *Burkholderia cepacia*, *Nocardia* species, *Mycobacterium* species	Nafcillin, oxacillin, or cefazolin

CGD, chronic granulomatous disease; GABHS, group A beta-hemolytic streptococcus; HIV, human immunodeficiency virus.

acquired osteomyelitis in a neonate should be treated empirically with nafcillin, oxacillin, or a first-generation cephalosporin to cover *S. aureus*, group A and B streptococci, and *Streptococcus pneumoniae*, plus cefotaxime, ceftriaxone, or an aminoglycoside to cover possible gram-negative infection until organism-specific antibiotic therapy can be instituted.[10]

The second form of neonatal osteomyelitis is encountered in the neonatal intensive care unit, typically in low-birth-weight neonates requiring endotracheal intubation, positive-pressure ventilation, intra-arterial or intravenous lines, or umbilical artery or vein cannulation.[139] Multifocal osteomyelitis or septic arthritis is commonly identified in neonates who demonstrate the typical signs and symptoms of sepsis, including temperature instability, poor color and perfusion, abdominal distention, feeding intolerance, bradycardia or apnea, increased oxygen requirements, and tachycardia or tachypnea.[139] Outbreaks of MRSA have been reported in neonatal nurseries in Europe, Asia, the United States, and Australia, making this an important organism for empirical treatment.[139] In one series of 20 cases of musculoskeletal sepsis in an Australian tertiary neonatal unit, all cases were treated with a minimum of 3 weeks of vancomycin therapy, with good short-term results.[139] Other causative organisms in this setting include group B streptococci, Enterobacteriaceae species, *Candida albicans*, and *Staphylococcus epidermidis*. When MRSA is not suspected, the initial parenteral therapy recommended for hospital-acquired neonatal osteomyelitis includes nafcillin or oxacillin plus cefotaxime, ceftriaxone, or an aminoglycoside. Because of the potentially devastating effect on the anatomic development of the proximal femur and humerus, suspicion of large joint infection in these neonates should prompt aspiration and, if positive for infection, surgical drainage. Morrissy even recommends routine aspiration of both hips in all neonates known to have osteomyelitis or septic arthritis at any other site.[209]

Infantile and Early Childhood. Several organisms appear to have the ability to cause deep infection in children between 3 and 36 months of age. This may be due, in part, to the timing of the loss of maternally conferred immunity and the onset of increased exposure to specific organisms in day-care settings. The waning levels of passively transferred maternal antibodies to certain pathogens, such as meningococci, are positively correlated with the highest rates of meningococcemia in young children.[301] During later childhood and early adolescence, the level of bactericidal antibodies rises, and disease associated with these early childhood pathogens declines. Although *S. aureus* remains the most common bacterial isolate in this category, other notable organisms include *Kingella kingae; S. pneumoniae;* group A, B, and C streptococci; Hib (in nonimmunized children); and *Neisseria meningitidis.*[26,146,183,228,320,333] Antibiotic selection in this age group is often single-agent treatment with nafcillin, oxacillin, or cefazolin. Cefotaxime or ceftriaxone should be added in nonimmunized children to cover Hib and *S. pneumoniae.*

It is important to bear in mind that continued vigilance is necessary when treating osteoarticular infections of the large joints in this age category, particularly up to age 18 months, when long-term sequelae from osteonecrosis and growth disturbance may result.[16,45,115,135] For this reason, I endorse early aspiration and surgical debridement of the hip and shoulder whenever sepsis is encountered in early childhood.

Childhood. Among children between 3 and 12 years of age, the most common causative organism of AHO is *S. aureus* (80% to 90%); *Streptococcus pyogenes* (group A beta-hemolytic streptococcus [GABHS]) is next in frequency, accounting for approximately 10% of culture-positive cases.[136,142] The age of children with GABHS AHO is consistent with the peak incidence of GABHS infection in school-age children, with a median age of 36 months reported in one series.[136] Children who experience severe streptococcal infections with multisystem dysfunction are, on average, slightly older, with a median age of 8 years (range, 3 to 11 years).[142] Further evidence of the age specificity of streptococci is noted in varicella-zoster viral infections (chickenpox), which typically occur in children between 5 and 9 years of age. Chickenpox is an associated risk factor in up to 17% of cases of GABHS AHO.[20,108,136,143] Penicillin is the treatment of choice for GABHS infections. However, initial empirical therapy in this age group should include an antistaphylococcal semisynthetic penicillin or first-generation cephalosporin to adequately cover staphylococcal and streptococcal species until a specific organism is identified.

With the recent increase in the incidence CA-MRSA infections, some centers have contemplated the use of empirical clindamycin, because virtually all cases of community-acquired *S. aureus* infections are susceptible to gentamicin, vancomycin, trimethoprim-sulfamethoxazole, clindamycin, and rifampin. At Texas Children's Hospital in Houston, the incidence of CA-MRSA increased from 35% in February 2000 to 67% in January 2002, which prompted a consideration of sequential parenteral-to-oral clindamycin treatment when resistance to a beta-lactam antibiotic was demonstrated.[200] The concern is that if clindamycin were used as empirical therapy, an acquired resistance to this antibiotic might ultimately reduce its usefulness.[200]

Adolescent. Invasive musculoskeletal infection in adolescents is most commonly caused by *S. aureus,* followed by GABHS. Additionally, sexually active adolescents are at risk for the development of disseminated infection with *Neisseria gonorrhoeae* involving the skin, joints, and, rarely, the meninges, heart, and bones.[112] According to the Centers for Disease Control and Prevention (CDC), in 2002, rates of infection among non-Hispanic black females aged 15 to 19 years were the highest of all racial-ethnic or age groups at 3300 per 100,000, compared with only 125 per 100,000 among the general population.[110] Empirical antibiotic treatment of adolescents with AHO is the same as that for older children.

Evaluation

In children, AHO must be differentiated from other conditions that may present with clinical symptoms and signs mimicking this disorder, including extraosseous infection, trauma, and neoplasia. Dedication to a thorough evaluation, taking into account all relevant clinical, laboratory, and radiographic information, should allow a definitive diagnosis in the majority of cases and avoid the pitfalls of an incorrect or delayed diagnosis. When uncertainty persists despite a thorough evaluation in a child with worrisome musculoskeletal complaints, close clinical follow-up is necessary until either the problem resolves or further evidence leads to a specific diagnosis.

Focal pain and decreased use of the affected extremity are the most common presenting signs of infection in all age groups. The acute and systemic nature of AHO is often heralded by additional symptoms such as an abrupt onset of fever and, less commonly, anorexia, irritability, and lethargy. Pain from osteomyelitis may produce restlessness; in contrast, the pain associated with septic arthritis is more likely to result in immobility. Other physical findings in AHO include fever (temperature >38°C), localized tenderness, swelling, warmth, and erythema. A history of antecedent trauma can sometimes obscure the diagnosis. More than one third of patients in Waldvogel and colleagues' original series gave a history of blunt trauma to the area involved in the septic process.[314] The relationship between trauma and infection is upheld by experimental models and is thought to be due to a diminished resistance to infection in injured tissues.[210,324] Despite this belief, there have been relatively few case reports of osteomyelitis complicating closed fractures. Hardy and Nicol in 1985 identified only 16 case examples from a literature review (14 cases) and their own clinical experience (2 cases), demonstrating the rarity of this phenomenon.[119] It is therefore important to ascertain the timing and severity of any injury to ensure that symptoms of infection are not mistakenly attributed to the injury. I occasionally encounter advanced stages of osteomyelitis in children who have been immobilized for 10 to 14 days in a cast or splint for a suspected growth plate injury when the original radiographs failed to demonstrate an obvious fracture.

The evaluation of children who present with clinical signs and symptoms worrisome for musculoskeletal infection begins with radiographic and laboratory studies. High-quality plain radiographs in at least two planes are obtained in all cases to evaluate for deep soft tissue swelling, joint effusions, and skeletal lesions. If the symptoms are thought to originate from the hip, I also obtain a comparative hip ultrasound examination to more carefully evaluate for joint effusion, which is difficult to detect by examination or plain radiographs. Initial laboratory studies include a complete blood count (CBC) with differential, CRP, erythrocyte sedimentation rate (ESR), and blood cultures. Whenever possible, I attempt to aspirate the site of suspected osteomyelitis, using fluoroscopic guidance, in an effort to identify the causative organism before the initiation of antibiotic therapy. This is performed as a two-step procedure by placing an 18-gauge spinal needle adjacent to the bone, removing the stylet, and attempting to aspirate a subperiosteal collection, if present. Next, the stylet is replaced and the needle is driven into the metaphyseal bone. Upon entry, the stylet is again removed, and aspiration is performed. According to the animal research of Canale and associates, this aspiration method should not have an effect on subsequent nuclear imaging.[33] Aspiration has been found to yield positive results in 67% to 93% of AHO cases.[132,208,272,307,314]

In most instances, a supplemental study with bone scintigraphy or magnetic resonance imaging (MRI) is necessary to further clarify the diagnosis and guide the treatment process. In certain locations, such as the pelvis, AHO is difficult to differentiate from septic arthritis or pyomyositis on the basis of the history, physical examination, and laboratory evaluation alone.[72,123,125,138,226,227] Similarly, diagnostic uncertainty often accompanies infections involving the spine and the foot. MRI has proved to be the most useful diagnostic study when seeking to differentiate the cause of worrisome signs and symptoms involving the pelvis, spine, or foot. Bone scintigraphy is useful when infection is suspected but difficult to localize by physical examination in children who are too young to clearly communicate the site of their symptoms. I also use bone scans when multifocal lesions may be present, as in hospital-acquired neonatal infections.

Although numerous conditions may be included in the differential diagnosis, leukemia and neoplasia are the most important to bear in mind.[93,153,177] Leukemia is the most common childhood malignancy. The peak incidence of acute lymphoblastic leukemia (ALL) occurs at approximately 4 years of age, with a range from 3 to 9 years. The skeleton is often the first body system to demonstrate overt manifestations of the acute form of the disease, with bone and joint symptoms reported in 21% to 59% of children.[93,177] The musculoskeletal pain associated with ALL is described as sudden, localized, sharp, and severe in onset and is due to the rapid proliferation of leukemic cells in the medullary canal and under the periosteum.[93] One review of 296 children with ALL found that 65 (22%) had some bone pain, and 52 (18%) had prominent bone pain that overshadowed other manifestations of the disease.[153] The investigators also found that those children with prominent bone pain frequently had nearly normal hematologic values, which often led to a delay in diagnosis.[153] When leukemia is a possibility, I request a manual inspection of the peripheral smear by the pathologist to look for blasts; the automated cell count performed in most laboratories is unable to differentiate blast cells from other white cell lines such as atypical lymphocytes. The ultimate diagnosis of acute pediatric leukemia is confirmed by bone marrow biopsy (Fig. 35–3).

The clinical and radiographic similarities between osteomyelitis and Ewing's sarcoma are well known (Figs. 35–4 and 35–5),[132,217,314] and the pitfall of mistakenly treating Ewing's sarcoma with open irrigation and debridement should be kept in mind.[217] One reasonable recommendation is to obtain a fine-needle bone biopsy at the same time bone is aspirated for bacteriologic examination.[132] This simple procedure, which can be performed with an 11-gauge bone marrow biopsy needle to increase the chance of obtaining diagnostic tissue, helped identify one case of Ewing's sarcoma among 30 children with a presumed diagnosis of osteomyelitis in one series.[132]

Some children with early-stage osteomyelitis are treated empirically with antibiotics, without obtaining a culture specimen. Although it is reasonable to assume that rapid clinical and laboratory improvement with antibiotic therapy is evidence in favor of the diagnosis of osteomyelitis, it is important not to be misled by equivocal improvement and lose sight of other diagnostic possibilities, only to have an unsuspected process declare itself later.

Treatment

Antibiotic Therapy. The management of AHO begins with the intravenous administration of an antibiotic to cover the most likely causative organism until a more specific antibiotic can be chosen based on culture and sensitivity results (see Table 35–2). This decision is frequently based on the age of the child but may also be influenced by the incidence of resistant organisms in a given community.[200] Waldvogel and coworkers reported that after the advent of antibiotics, the mortality rate from osteomyelitis, which had been 15% to 25%, decreased to about 2%.[314] Under most circumstances, the most appropriate initial antibiotic is a semisynthetic penicillin (oxacillin or nafcillin) or a first-generation cephalosporin (cefazolin) to cover *S. aureus*. For children with allergies to these antibiotics, clindamycin is recommended because of its superior intraosseous concentration compared with

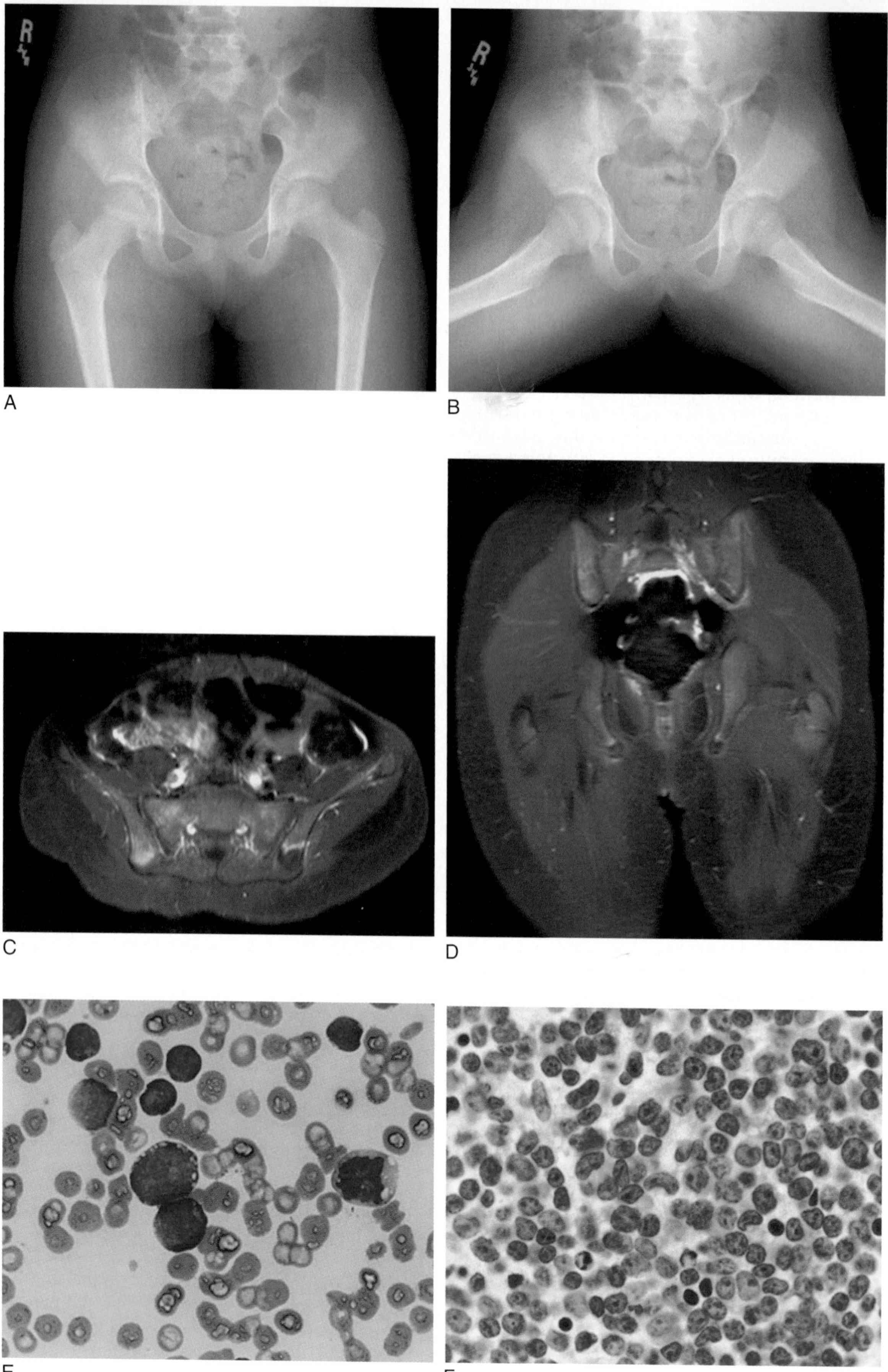

FIGURE 35–3 Eight-year-old girl with 2-day history of left buttock pain and limp. The initial laboratory studies were as follows: C-reactive protein 13.6 mg/dL, erythrocyte sedimentation rate 96 mm/hour, and white blood cell count 2.7 cells/mL, with an automated differential of 54 segmented neutrophils, 7 band neutrophils, 1 monocyte, and 32 lymphocytes. Initial plain films **(A** and **B)** were unremarkable, but magnetic resonance images **(C** and **D)** showed diffuse marrow change within the left ilium, suggestive of infarct. Subsequent manual inspection of the peripheral smear identified 4% blasts **(E).** Bone marrow biopsy was positive for acute lymphoblastic leukemia **(F).**

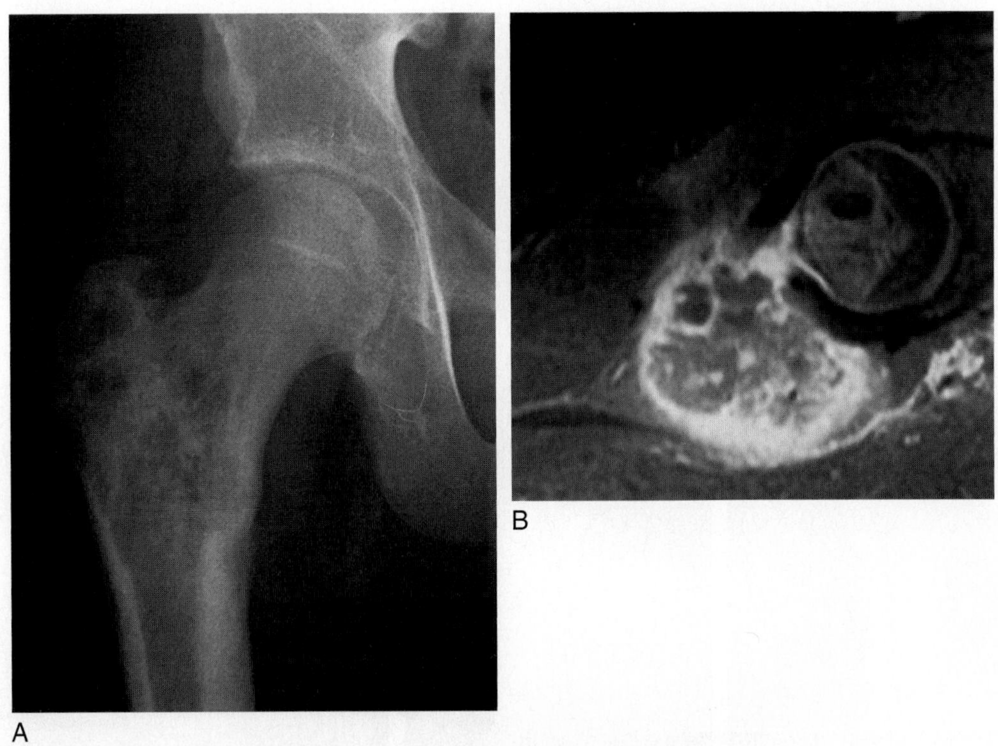

FIGURE 35–4 **A,** Anteroposterior radiograph showing a lytic lesion in the proximal femur. The patient had a 2-month history of pain and an elevated erythrocyte sedimentation rate. The permeative nature of the lesion suggested a neoplastic rather than an infectious cause. **B,** Axial magnetic resonance image of the proximal femur demonstrating a large soft tissue mass posteriorly. Biopsy confirmed the diagnosis of Ewing's sarcoma.

vancomycin. In children younger than 3 years and those with anatomic or functional asplenia, in whom pneumococcal infection is a concern, a third-generation cephalosporin (cefotaxime or ceftriaxone) should be used for empirical therapy. In non–Hib-immunized children, cefuroxime (a second-generation cephalosporin) or a combination of a semisynthetic penicillin and a third-generation cephalosporin would be appropriate empirical therapy.[240,280] Neonatal osteomyelitis requires the addition of an aminoglycoside or the use of a third-generation cephalosporin to cover gram-negative organisms. Culture-negative osteomyelitis can be managed the same as presumed staphylococcal disease and treated with empirical therapy for methicillin-susceptible *S. aureus* (MSSA). Excellent long-term results were reported with this treatment in a series of 40 culture-negative children, despite the fact that more than one third of the 45 culture-positive counterparts in the same series were infected with MRSA.[90]

Antibiotic selection for AHO is based on evidence that the drug penetrates the infected tissues and attains sufficient levels in the bone and pus so that concentrations exceed those minimally necessary to inhibit the pathogen's survival. The antibiotic dosage for osteomyelitis is usually two to three times the standard dose to ensure a peak serum bactericidal titer of 1 : 8 or greater.[221,280,293] Parenteral therapy is continued until an appropriate clinical and laboratory response has occurred, at which time oral antibiotic therapy can be considered. Since the 1980s, sequential parenteral-to-oral antibiotic therapy has been standard for the completion of treatment of uncomplicated osteomyelitis on an outpatient basis.[54,141,160,197,198,219,240,272,307] The duration of the initial intravenous antibiotic therapy varies from 3 to 14 days and is often governed by the normalization of the CRP level.[54,68,145,160,198,219,272,307]

Certain conditions should be satisfied before the transition to oral therapy, including (1) clinical and laboratory improvement toward resolution (near normal), (2) availability of an effective oral agent that is tolerated by the child, and (3) likely compliance with the antibiotic regimen, based on an assessment of familial and social circumstances. Once oral therapy is initiated, peak serum bactericidal titers or serum antibiotic levels can be determined to ensure effective dosing. A peak titer of greater than 1 : 8 constitutes effective dosing.[198,219] Serum bactericidal titers are assessed by drawing blood 60 to 90 minutes after the second or third oral dose of antibiotic, preferably ingested by the child on an empty stomach.[221] Results should be available within 3 to 4 days and can help guide dosing adjustments. A simplified treatment plan, which proposes to dispense with the measurement of serum bactericidal activity, has been successful in two small retrospective series.[198,231] However, a more traditional and conservative perspective is that measuring serum antibiotic concentration or bactericidal activity is neither burdensome nor cost

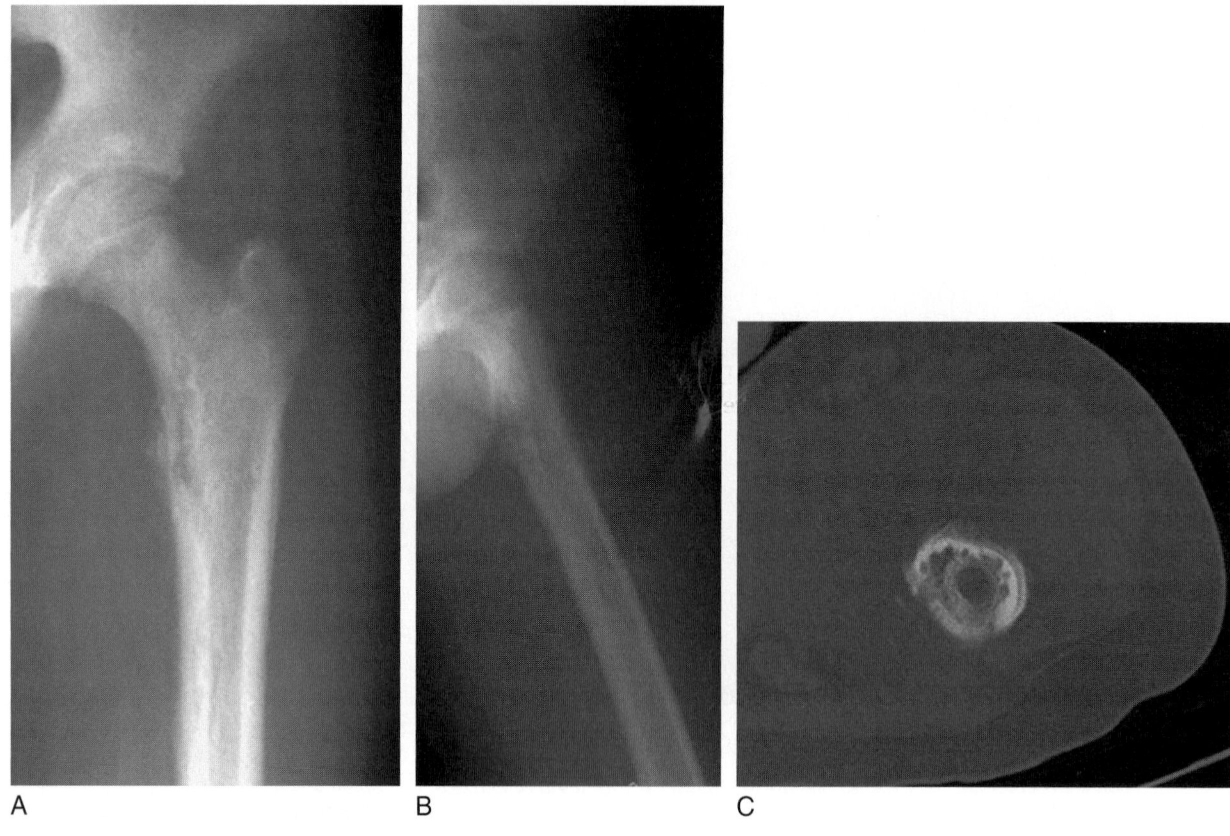

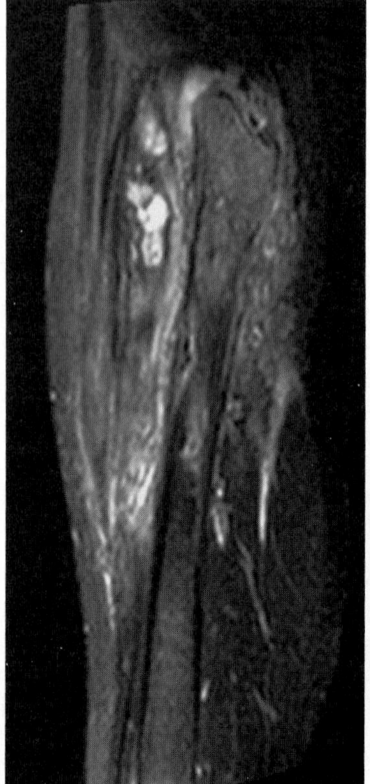

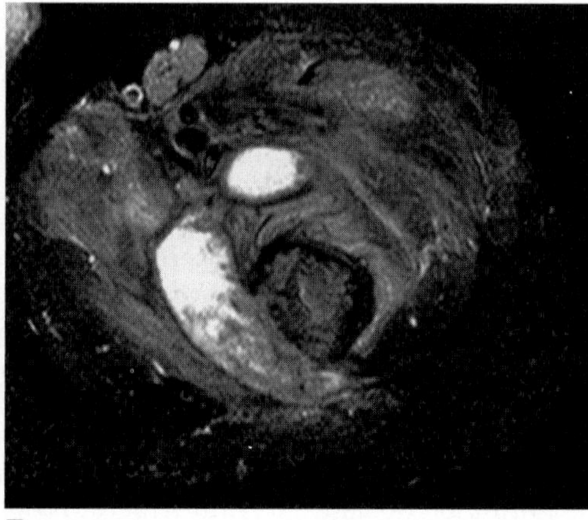

FIGURE 35–5 Fifteen-year-old boy with a 20-pound weight loss and nighttime pain in the left hip of 3 months' duration. **A** and **B,** Plain radiographs show poorly permeative lytic changes in the left proximal femur. **C,** Computed tomography scan of the area of involvement demonstrates permeative cortical erosions with periosteal reaction. **D** and **E,** Magnetic resonance images show diffuse femoral marrow signal changes with a fluid collection adjacent to bone, suggestive of abscess rather than liquefied tumor necrosis. Biopsy and culture confirmed the diagnosis of subacute osteomyelitis with methicillin-resistant *Staphylococcus aureus.*

prohibitive and may reveal the rare child who would benefit from prolonged parenteral therapy.[218]

When oral treatment is not possible, outpatient parenteral antimicrobial therapy (OPAT) is an alternative that allows antibiotic administration for a prolonged period in the child's home at a significantly lower cost compared with conventional in-hospital therapy.[15,104,197,296] OPAT is typically performed with a central venous line or peripherally inserted central catheter; catheter-related complications have been reported in 30% to 50% of children, and complications related to other factors such as adverse drug reactions have occurred in 29% to 32% of children.[104,197] Despite these concerns, the majority of complications are minor and can be resolved without interruption of the antibiotic course. Excellent clinical outcomes have been reported in 93% to 98% of children in whom OPAT is used.[15,104,197]

The end point of antibiotic treatment is difficult to standardize owing to the significant variation in both disease severity and response to treatment among children with AHO. The recommended duration of antibiotics ranges from 4 to 8 weeks, but successful treatment has been reported in uncomplicated cases with a mean duration of only 23 days.[54,145,198,219,231,311] My approach is to aim for a combined intravenous and oral antibiotic duration of 6 weeks, with follow-up laboratory studies performed at approximately 4 to 5 weeks into the course of treatment. In general, the CRP level should normalize long before that point, in contrast to the ESR, which normalizes over several weeks. As long as the ESR has returned to normal by the 4- to 5-week follow-up visit and there has been no secondary rise in CRP, I discontinue antibiotics at 6 weeks. If either the CRP or the ESR is elevated, I continue antibiotics and repeat the laboratory studies every 2 to 3 weeks until normalization of the ESR. If the duration exceeds 12 weeks, I consider MRI to exclude a surgically treatable cause for the slow response to antibiotic therapy.

Surgery. There is considerable difference of opinion regarding the timing, extent, and necessity of surgery to treat AHO.[54,65,202,272,307] The primary problem is the lack of clear and specific indications for surgery. One series reported an aggressive primary surgical protocol in which all 68 children were taken to the operating room for an emergency procedure consisting of extensive open irrigation and drainage of pus, hematoma, and granulation tissue; cortical drilling or fenestration; and curettage of the medullary canal on both sides, with care to avoid the growth plate.[202] Despite this approach, 17% of the children went on to develop chronic osteomyelitis. Other centers have reported a more measured approach to the surgical treatment of AHO, basing the decision on factors that might indicate the failure of antibiotic therapy alone.[54,65,272,307] These factors, which suggest a more advanced stage of AHO, include the presence of a subperiosteal or intra-osseous abscess or a visible metaphyseal lytic cavity on radiographic studies, as well as a limited clinical or laboratory response to an initial course of antibiotics.[54,272,307]

Cole and associates observed that the majority of children with AHO could be cured with a single course of antibiotics and immobilization if treatment were initiated within 1 or 2 days of the onset of symptoms rather than 4 to 5 days, when the condition has advanced to the stage of abscess formation.[54] In a retrospective review, they showed that 92% of 55 children with an early diagnosis were cured by antibiotics alone and less than 1 week of hospitalization, whereas only 25% of 12 children with a delay in diagnosis had a similar outcome; the remainder in the latter group experienced prolonged hospitalization, prolonged duration of antibiotics, and multiple operations. Another series noted that the difference in the rate of chronic infection—12% for the operatively treated group and 4% for the nonoperatively treated group—depended more on the time interval between the onset of symptoms and the beginning of treatment than on other factors.[307] Unfortunately, there are no prospective randomized trials comparing the clinical outcomes of surgical and nonsurgical treatment in groups of children matched by the severity of illness. There is an unavoidably higher failure rate in children subjected to surgical intervention because operations are generally performed when the presence of purulent exudate has already compromised the healing response of local tissues.

Some authors consider surgical intervention to be necessary when the proximal femur is involved, even if the infection is identified early and a discrete abscess is lacking.[65,307] The risk of developing a contiguous septic arthritis or avascular necrosis is high enough that more aggressive intervention is warranted. One report found that 9 of 11 children who had early surgical drilling of the neck of the femur had complete resolution with normal radiographs and examination at follow-up, whereas the remaining 2 children, treated with antibiotics alone, had late clinical and radiographic abnormalities.[65]

Whenever surgery is performed for suspected infection, it is important to follow meticulous biopsy principles and send a specimen to pathology for frozen section before a more aggressive irrigation and debridement procedure is undertaken.[194,195] This may help avoid the pitfall of overlooking a Ewing's sarcoma, which may have a radiographic and gross appearance similar to that of osteomyelitis.[132,217,314]

Complications

The most concerning complications attributed to AHO are chronic infection, avascular necrosis, growth disturbance, deep vein thrombosis, pulmonary embolism, and multisystem involvement.[107,142,235,243,317,336] The likelihood of chronic infection appears to be correlated with the length of antibiotic treatment, with up to 19% of those treated for 3 weeks or less developing this complication, compared with only 2% of children treated for longer than 3 weeks.[243] Avascular necrosis of the proximal femur and proximal humerus appears to be mediated by the delayed recognition and inadequate decompression of contiguous osteomyelitis and septic arthritis in the hip and shoulder.[14,43] Jackson and colleagues identified sequelae in 8 of 13 children with contiguous bone and joint infections, with the worst prognosis in cases involving the hip and shoulder; in contrast, sequelae were identified in only 8 of 41 children with primary joint infection alone.[144] Another series found that the two most important factors associated with poor results in children with hip sepsis were the presence of osteomyelitis of the femur, which was noted in 4 of 7 children with unsatisfactory outcomes, and a delay of longer than 5 days in instituting definitive treatment.[43]

Growth disturbance as a consequence of infection tends to be central and diffuse. This creates a bar that is difficult to resect and may have significant long-term consequences, including major limb length discrepancy when the arrest occurs at an early age.[235] One series noted the difficulty of fully appreciating these growth disturbances until children reach a mean age of 9 years, and the authors recommended follow-up to skeletal maturity to identify this problem.[235]

Deep vein thrombosis and pulmonary embolism are rare in childhood, with an estimated incidence of less than 0.01%.[50] Recent reports have identified a possible association among AHO, deep vein thrombosis, and septic pulmonary embolism as part of a life-threatening clinical syndrome of disseminated staphylococcal disease that requires early recognition and aggressive treatment with antibiotics, surgical drainage, anticoagulation, and assisted ventilation, if needed.[107,317,336] Hematologic values may be normal in these children, which indicates that a prothrombic tendency, which might otherwise be expected, is not essential to the development of thrombosis in the setting of musculoskeletal sepsis.[180,199,317]

There is early evidence that the presence of selected genes encoding certain virulence factors might explain the occurrence of complications such as deep vein thrombosis associated with *S. aureus* infections.[9,199] A recent report noted that the Panton-Valentine leukocidin *(pvl)* gene was encoded in the strains of MRSA and MSSA isolated from all 5 children who developed deep vein thrombosis in a series of 28 children with musculoskeletal infection.[199] The authors also noted a relationship between *pvl*-positive strains and other complications, such as chronic osteomyelitis and prolonged hospitalization.

GABHS disease may manifest as a disseminated infection.[142] This life-threatening clinical syndrome characterized by rash, fever, shock, and multiple organ system dysfunction is analogous to the toxic shock syndrome caused by toxin-producing strains of *S. aureus*. In one report, eight children with severe streptococcal infection demonstrated renal, hepatic, and encephalopathic problems in addition to their musculoskeletal complaints.[142] Up to 87% of children with multisystem GABHS infection have bone or joint involvement.[142] A high index of clinical suspicion and aggressive surgical intervention are recommended to avoid poor outcomes in these children.

Other complications of AHO include functional disability, limb length inequality, deformity, and adverse drug events from antibiotic treatment. Adverse drug reactions developed in 29% of OPAT courses in one series, which prompted early discontinuation of antibiotics in the majority of patients.[104] The most common drug-related complications were neutropenia (13%), rash (12%), hepatitis (5%), and diarrhea, fever, urticaria, anaphylaxis, and ototoxicity (4% combined). The most common antibiotics associated with neutropenia were nafcillin and cefotaxime; oxacillin was associated with rash and hepatitis. Clindamycin may cause pseudomembranous colitis, with a reported incidence of 0.1% to 10%; this complication appears to be unrelated to dosage or duration of therapy.[161]

SUBACUTE OSTEOMYELITIS

Epidemiology

This entity was first described by Brodie in 1836; the descriptive term *subacute* was added by Billroth in 1881.[18,27] Modern experience with subacute osteomyelitis was introduced by Harris and coworkers in 1965,[121] followed by a report from King and Mayo in 1969[168] and the original four-part classification presented by Gledhill in 1973.[103]

Subacute osteomyelitis differs from AHO in that it is more difficult to diagnose because of the lack of characteristic signs and symptoms of infection. The onset is usually insidious, and mild symptoms may be present for more than 2 weeks before medical attention is sought. Laboratory studies may be normal or only mildly elevated in these children. Radiographic features are often suggestive of benign or malignant skeletal neoplasia. Abnormalities that resembled neoplasia were identified on plain radiographs in 50% of cases in one series.[254] For many reasons, diagnostic delay is common, with correct diagnosis taking an average of 3 to 5 months in two separate reports.[105,254]

Subacute osteomyelitis is less common than AHO, with an incidence ranging from 7% to 42% of the combined cases of acute and subacute forms of osteomyelitis.[61,245,254] Recent reports indicate an increasing incidence of subacute osteomyelitis compared with AHO.[22,61,245] The ability to identify the causative organism by culture is more limited in cases of subacute osteomyelitis, with positive results obtained in only 29% to 61% of cases.[117,245,254,260] *S. aureus* is the most commonly identified organism.[117,245,254,260] The location of bone involvement is more diverse than in AHO; diaphyseal and epiphyseal locations are reported with greater frequency in subacute osteomyelitis.[84,254,273] Children with subacute osteomyelitis are also older than those with AHO, averaging 7.5 years of age.[245]

Pathophysiology

Most authors support the theory that subacute osteomyelitis is a consequence of an altered host-pathogen relationship in which there is decreased bacterial virulence, increased host resistance, or a combination of these factors.[105,117,157,245,254,260,273] Some cases are thought to occur secondary to the inadequate or partial treatment of AHO or following the administration of antibiotics for other infections; those children without any antecedent illness or treatment are considered to have primary subacute osteomyelitis.[245,254] One report found that 40% of children with subacute osteomyelitis had recently received antibiotics for other infections, including tonsillitis, acne, or tooth abscess, compared with only 5% of children with AHO.[254] Knowledge of the pathophysiology of this condition is limited. However, one theory is that the bacteria establish a nidus of infection in which only a localized inflammatory response develops. This creates local bone destruction that may or may not stimulate a sclerotic or periosteal reaction through a combination of pressure atrophy and inflammatory granulation tissue.[157]

Classification

A radiographic classification of subacute osteomyelitis was initially proposed by Gledhill and subsequently expanded into a six-part classification by Roberts and colleagues (Fig. 35–6).[103,254] This modification is based on the anatomic location (metaphyseal, diaphyseal, epiphyseal, or spinal), the morphology of the lesion and its surrounding architecture, and the similarity of the lesion to various neoplasms.[254] Type Ia lesions are metaphyseal, have a punched-out appearance, and resemble an eosinophilic granuloma; type Ib lesions differ slightly, having a sclerotic margin and thus resembling a classic Brodie's abscess. Type II lesions erode the metaphyseal cortex and may be difficult to differentiate from osteogenic sarcoma. Type III lesions

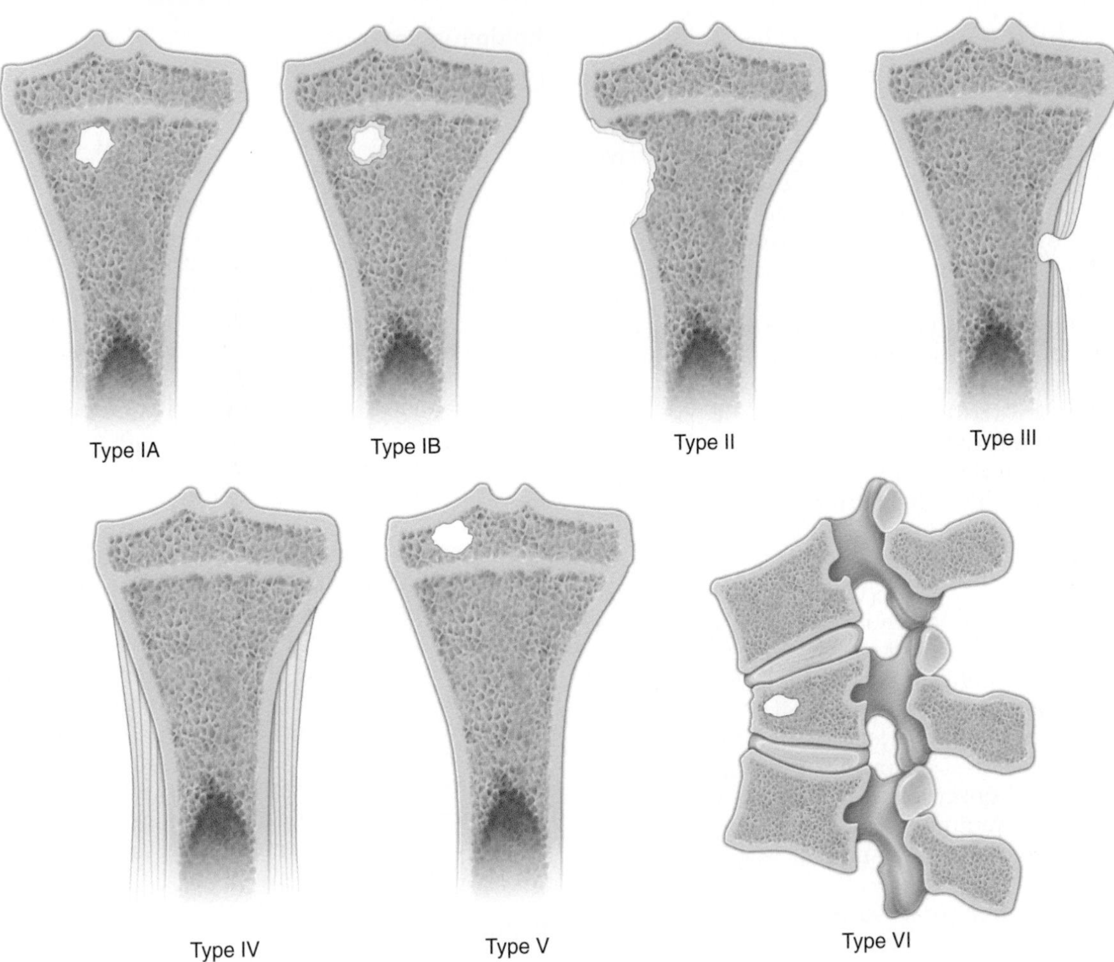

FIGURE 35–6 Radiographic classification of subacute osteomyelitis. This classification system is based on the anatomic location, the response of the surrounding tissue to infection, and the similarity to benign or malignant tumors:
Type IA: Metaphyseal area of radiolucency without marginal sclerosis.
Type IB: Metaphyseal area of radiolucency with surrounding reactive bone, the classic Brodie's abscess.
Type II: Metaphyseal area of radiolucency with cortical erosion (may be misinterpreted as osteosarcoma).
Type III: Localized diaphyseal lesion with periosteal reaction (may be misinterpreted as osteoid osteoma).
Type IV: Diaphyseal lesion with subperiosteal new bone formation (may be misinterpreted as Ewing's sarcoma).
Type V: Epiphyseal lesion.
Type VI: Vertebral lesion (also known as diskitis).
(Redrawn from Roberts JM, Drummond DS, Breed AL, et al: Subacute hematogenous osteomyelitis in children: A retrospective study. J Pediatr Orthop 1982;2:249.)

are localized lucent lesions in the cortex of the diaphysis, with a periosteal reaction that may resemble osteoid osteoma. Type IV lesions are diaphyseal, with an onion-skin periosteal reaction that simulates the appearance of Ewing's sarcoma. Type V lesions are concentric-appearing epiphyseal lucencies; chondroblastoma would be considered in the differential diagnosis. Finally, type VI lesions involve the vertebral body and may produce erosion and destruction in a manner similar to eosinophilic granuloma or tuberculosis.[254]

Evaluation and Treatment

Because of the diagnostic uncertainty in these cases, it is often necessary to perform a more extensive workup before deciding on a course of treatment. At my institution, we frequently obtain a complete laboratory and radiographic evaluation, including CBC with differential, ESR, CRP, and plain radiographs. Subsequent imaging studies may include MRI with and without contrast, three-phase total-body bone scan, and computed tomography (CT) scan with and without contrast. Findings are reviewed with a radiologist to arrive at the most likely differential diagnosis. Plans for biopsy are coordinated with an orthopaedic oncologist to ensure that clear communication is established. In cases with an aggressive and potentially malignant appearance on diagnostic studies (see Fig. 35–4), the orthopaedic oncologist performs the biopsy, whereas in cases without aggressive features (see Fig. 35–5), we perform the biopsy while carefully observing the principles outlined by Mankin and associates.[194,195] A frozen section is obtained and personally reviewed with the pathologist, and intraoperative cultures are obtained for aerobic, anaerobic, fungal, and acid-fast bacterial organisms before initiating antibiotics.

The decision whether to perform a biopsy is controversial. Hamdy and colleagues reported excellent results in 23 of 23 patients who received an appropriate course of antibiotics without biopsy or debridement.[117] In their series, 90% of cases of subacute osteomyelitis showed a benign character upon careful radiographic assessment, reinforcing the decision to forgo biopsy in favor of a 6-week trial of an oral antistaphylococcal antibiotic. This conservative approach has found favor with a few authors,[84,105,260] but most others have expressed a preference for surgical management of these lesions.[100,103,121,128,168,245,254]

Although I agree that surgical debridement is unnecessary from a treatment standpoint, I often biopsy these lesions for the sake of diagnostic certainty and the rare chance that a prolonged course of antibiotics might be avoided if a benign skeletal neoplasm can be definitively diagnosed. Families are often unsettled by the delay in diagnosis that may have already occurred and may be in favor of a biopsy and culture procedure to reach a conclusive diagnosis. On occasion, biopsy results yield unexpected findings that alter the subsequent treatment plan and prevent further delay and frustration for the child and the family (Fig. 35–7).

A 6-week course of an oral antistaphylococcal antibiotic should be used when culture results do not identify a specific organism. These children should be followed long term to ensure the success of treatment.

Complications

Very few complications are reported. For most children with subacute osteomyelitis, the condition resolves following appropriate treatment.[84,105,117,245,254] However, one form of the disease, described as primary chronic sclerosing osteomyelitis, may demonstrate a prolonged course with intermittent symptoms over several years.[95,273] Ultimately, this form may be found to be related to CRMO.

CHRONIC OSTEOMYELITIS

Epidemiology

Chronic osteomyelitis is a consequence of AHO that may lead to extensive bone necrosis, formation of sequestra, and, ultimately, segmental bone defects. The most significant factors in reducing the incidence of chronic osteomyelitis appear to be the early diagnosis of AHO and the prompt initiation of antibiotic therapy with an appropriate duration of treatment.[54,75,314,334] Chronic infection has been reported in 19% of children with AHO who received antibiotics for 3 weeks or less, compared with only 2% of those who received more than 3 weeks of treatment.[75] The prevalence of chronic osteomyelitis is much higher in developing countries as a consequence of delayed diagnosis and undertreatment, whereas this disease is becoming much less common in industrialized nations.[66,214,334]

S. aureus is the most common causative organism in chronic osteomyelitis.[176,214,243,247,334] The most common site of involvement is the tibia; this is likely related to the limited vascularity of this bone, which is further compromised by the extensive periosteal stripping that occurs in advanced AHO.[66] The next most common sites are the femur and humerus. Most children who have chronic osteomyelitis have undergone surgical intervention—often multiple procedures—as part of the treatment of AHO. This may play a role in compromising the soft tissues and skeletal architecture during the treatment process.

Pathophysiology

In children, the metaphyseal cortex is thin, and the periosteum is loosely bound to the underlying bone. If untreated, infection in this region erupts into the subperiosteal space, travels down around the diaphysis, and eventually deprives the bone of its blood supply (Fig. 35–8). The result is dead bone (sequestrum) and granulation tissue, which retard healing and harbor bacteria because neither antibodies nor antibiotics can adequately penetrate these tissues.[157] Certain bacteria, particularly *S. aureus,* adhere to bone by expressing receptors for the components of bone

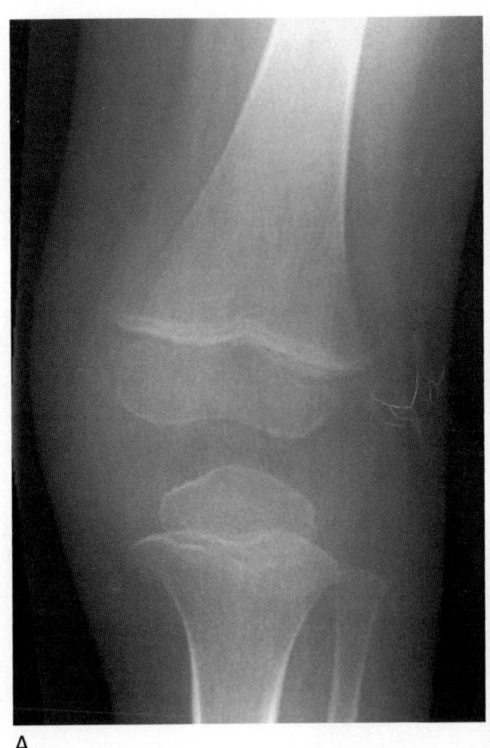

A

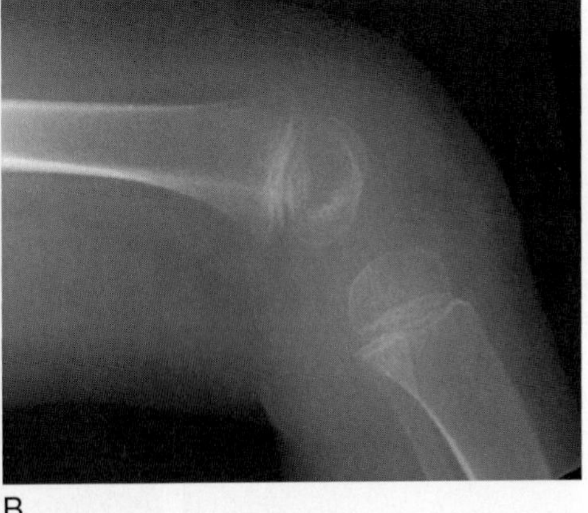

B

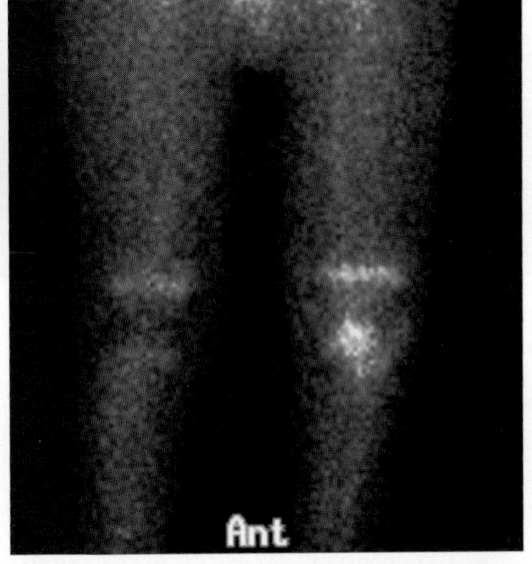

C

FIGURE 35–7 Three-year-old boy with a 3-week history of limp and knee swelling. Plain radiographs **(A** and **B)** show soft tissue swelling without an obvious skeletal lesion. Bone scan **(C)** demonstrates focal uptake in the epiphysis on delayed images.

Continued

matrix and by demonstrating intracellular survival within osteoblasts, which may explain the persistence of infection in chronic osteomyelitis.[243] In response to the sequestrum, the body forms abundant periosteal new bone (involucrum) around the necrotic cortex. In a growing child, involucrum formation can be extensive, creating new bone around the sequestrum from which infection may be reactivated and erupt into draining sinuses.[157]

Classification

Chronic osteomyelitis is often defined as the presence of ongoing bone infection for longer than 1 month in the presence of devitalized bone. The Cierny-Mader classification considers chronic osteomyelitis to be a stage 4B condition, owing to the presence of diffuse osteomyelitis in a host that is compromised either locally or systemically.[49] Authors with experience in the treatment of this condition emphasize the importance of determining the severity of the condition with respect to the presence or absence of sequestrum, involucrum, and bone defects at the time of presentation.[66] Each of these factors has a significant influence on the timing and method of treatment.

Evaluation

Most children with chronic osteomyelitis present with a known diagnosis and a substantial medical history as a consequence of the treatment of AHO. Occasionally, however, the diagnosis is unconfirmed, necessitating a thorough initial evaluation. Laboratory studies should include CBC with differential, CRP, ESR, and blood cultures to assess the ongoing response to the presence of infection and help guide further antibiotic treatment. Most of the time, culture material is obtained at the time of surgical debridement. However, a noninvasive method has been described to obtain cultures in cases that involve draining sinus tracts.[212] First, the sinus orifice is cleansed with povidone-iodine (Betadine). Then, the nozzle of the syringe is placed into the sinus tract, and aspiration is performed while applying deep pressure over the infected region. Using this method, Mousa was able to obtain cultures that were 88.7% sensitive and 95.7% specific for the causative organism from a total of 115 operative isolates.[212]

Radiographic studies should include high-quality plain radiographs to evaluate for sequestrum, involucrum, avascular necrosis, and bone defects. MRI with and without gadolinium may be helpful to

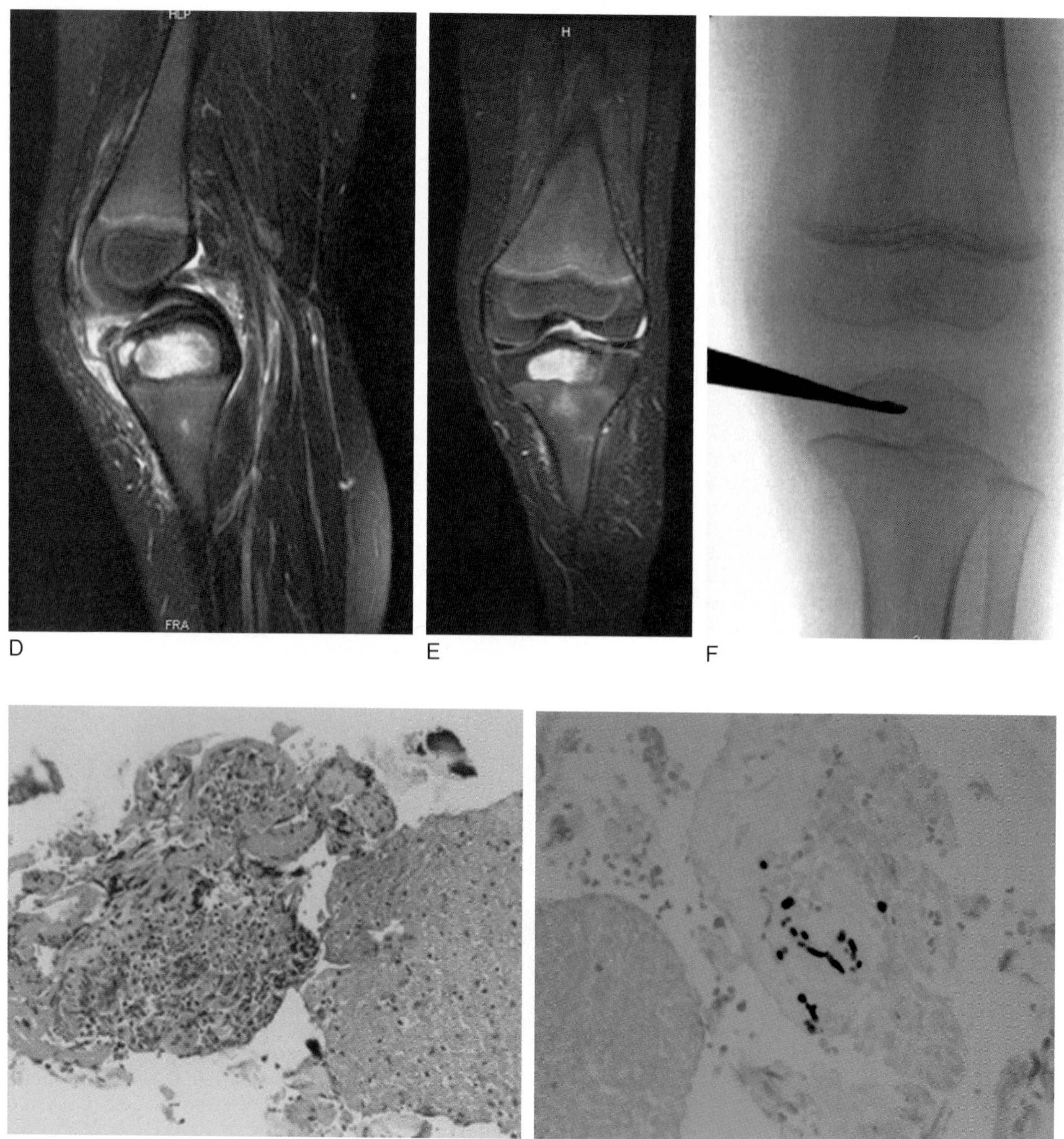

FIGURE 35–7 cont'd Magnetic resonance images **(D** and **E)** identify a well-circumscribed lesion in the upper tibial epiphysis with subtle marrow signal change in the metaphysis, favoring infection over a benign-appearing tumor. Biopsy was performed **(F)**, with pathology demonstrating a mixed granulomatous tissue **(G)** and fungal elements **(H)**. *Candida tropicalis* was cultured from the tissue and traced to a hospitalization more than 1 year earlier when the child had developed line sepsis with *C. tropicalis* in the intensive care unit. Complete clinical resolution was achieved following treatment with amphotericin B.

differentiate areas of bone infarction and sequestrum formation from areas of active osteomyelitis and abscess formation.[239,303] A common pitfall of MRI, however, is the inability to clearly distinguish between acute and chronic osteomyelitis; it is also difficult to interpret the significance of extensive marrow signal abnormalities associated with advanced stages of acute and chronic osteomyelitis (Fig. 35–9).[82] Chronic osteomyelitis can also be imaged with CT, which may help evaluate the nature and magnitude of bone defects.

After radiographic and laboratory studies have been reviewed, unconfirmed chronic osteomyelitis should be cautiously approached with an open biopsy to obtain tissue for frozen and permanent sections, as

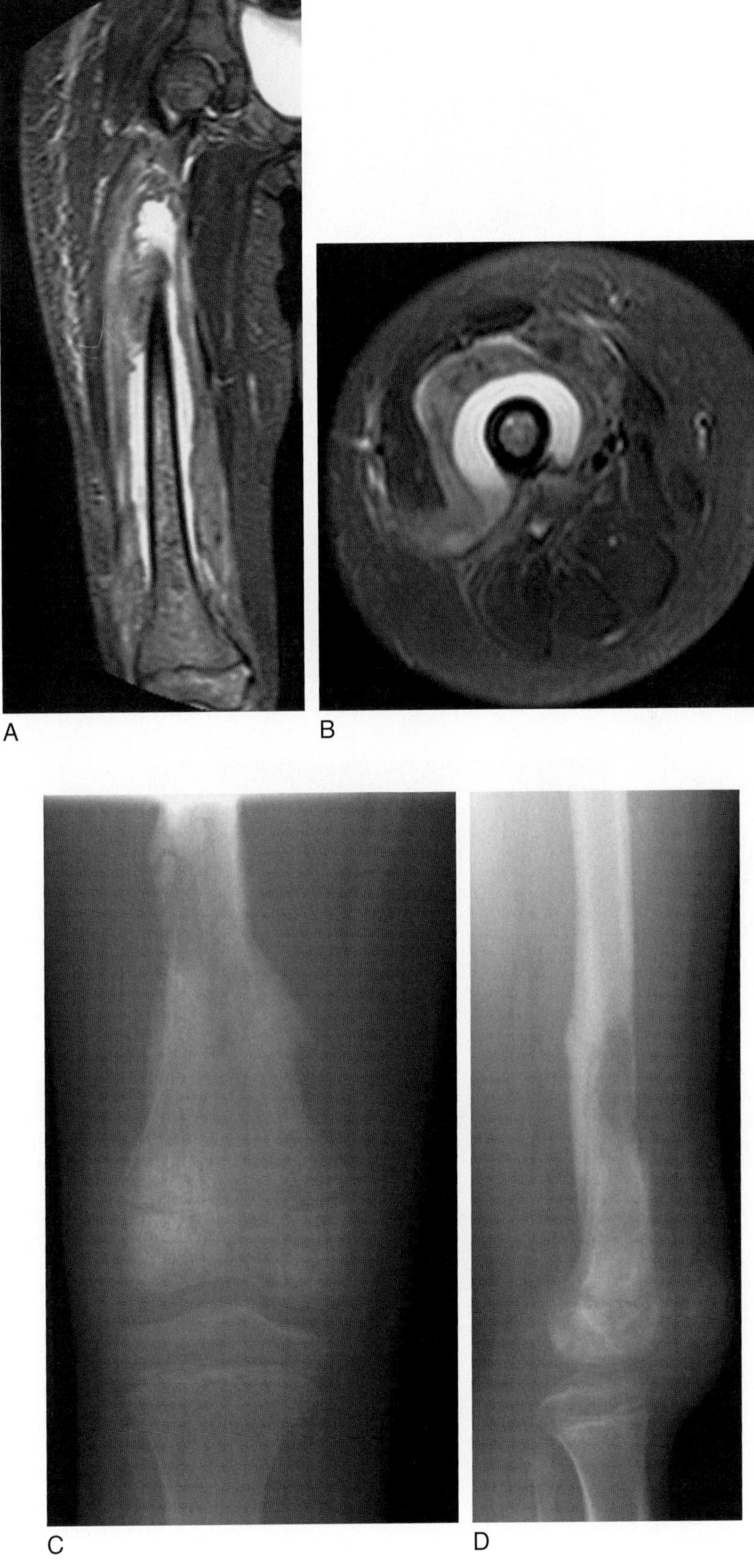

FIGURE 35-8 Magnetic resonance images of a 10-year-old girl with 2 weeks of antecedent knee pain (**A** and **B**). Extensive subperiosteal purulent fluid collection with nearly circumferential stripping of the soft tissues from the femoral cortex is seen on the axial image (**B**). As anticipated, the child developed chronic osteomyelitis and a pathologic fracture through the distal femur secondary to the extensive area of ischemic bone (**C** and **D**).

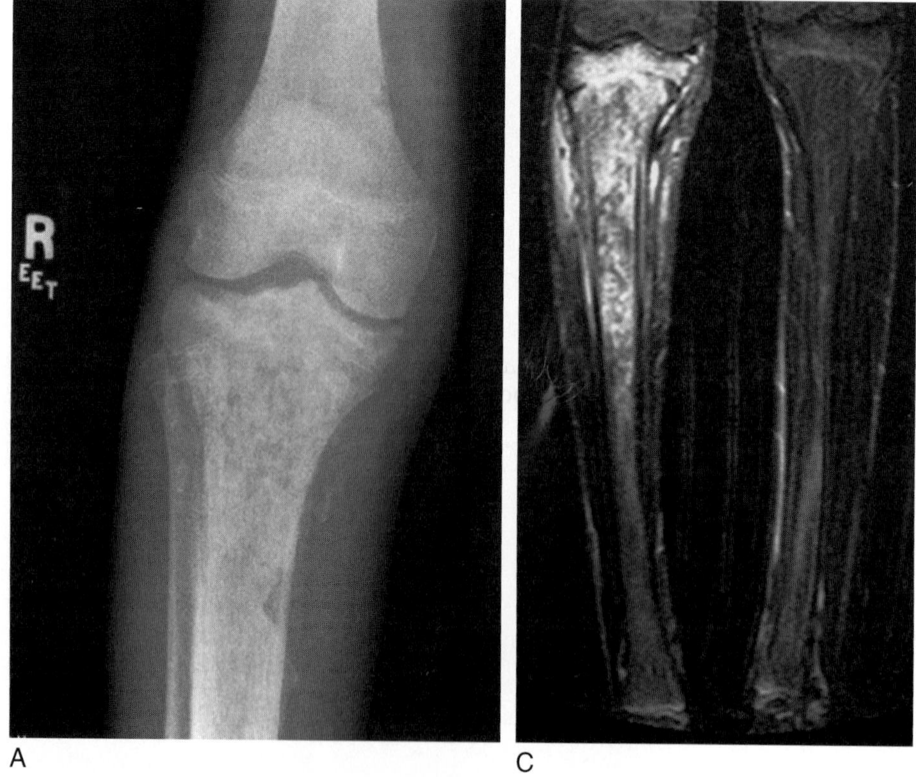

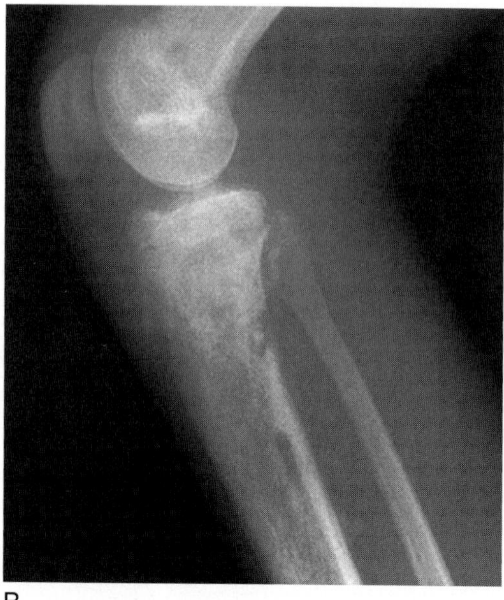

FIGURE 35-9 **A** and **B**, Plain radiographs of chronic proximal tibial osteomyelitis in a 13-year-old boy after 2 months of treatment with intravenous antibiotics and seven surgical debridements. **C**, Magnetic resonance imaging, performed to evaluate a persistent elevation of C-reactive protein (5.0 mg/dL), demonstrates diffuse marrow and periosteal signal changes consistent with healing versus active osteomyelitis, without overt abscess. Ultimately, biopsy was performed, which showed mixed acute and chronic osteomyelitis. The patient was observed and responded to further antibiotic treatment without surgical intervention.

well as a complete set of cultures for aerobic, anaerobic, and fungal organisms and acid-fast bacteria. Osteogenic sarcoma and Ewing's sarcoma have been discovered at open biopsy for suspected chronic osteomyelitis.[214,247,334]

Treatment

The ultimate goals in the treatment of chronic osteomyelitis are eradication of the causative organism, elimination of local inflammatory tissue destruction, and restoration of functional anatomy. Typically, this requires a multidisciplinary effort.

Antibiotic Therapy. In most cases, decisions regarding antibiotic selection, route of administration, and duration of treatment are beyond the expertise of the orthopaedic surgeon and require consultation with an infectious disease specialist. Rifampin is favored as a supplement to first-line antistaphylococcal antibiotics in chronic infection because it achieves intraleukocytic bactericidal action and facilitates the eradication of bacteria from the tissues.[243] Treatment for up to 6 to 9 months may be necessary, and the response should be carefully monitored by serial laboratory, radiographic, and clinical evaluations.

Although most authors would agree that effective treatment of chronic osteomyelitis requires both surgical and medical interventions, some children have been treated solely with antibiotics and demonstrated complete recovery.[176,243,247,334]

Surgery. Debridement surgery is the foundation of osteomyelitis treatment. The major goal of surgery in chronic osteomyelitis is to remove the sequestrum, abscess cavities, and granulation tissue that harbor bacteria and prevent the circulation of systemic antibiotics into the infected tissues.[66,176,243,334] Most children with chronic disease require multiple procedures to achieve this goal, with one series reporting 97 procedures in 30 children, or an average of 3.2 procedures per child.[334] The greatest difficulty lies in determining how extensive the debridement should be; sufficient infected bone and soft tissue must be resected to allow antibiotic therapy to complete the process, but there are no clearly defined guidelines for this decision. Mader and coworkers[192] appropriately suggested that "debridement should be direct, atraumatic, and executed with reconstruction in mind." In general, all devitalized tissues should be excised, with debridement of bone carried down until uniform haversian or cancellous bleeding is visualized (the "paprika" sign).[265] External stabilization is used whenever complete debridement threatens skeletal stability.[192]

Ideally, the dead space is managed by using durable, vascularized tissue and performing complete wound closure whenever possible.[49] Antibiotic-impregnated polymethylmethacrylate (PMMA) beads can be exchanged every 2 to 4 weeks to reduce the dead space while increasing antibiotic levels at the site of infection.[308] Alternatively, implantable drug pumps provide a means of delivering antibiotics locally for extended periods, avoiding the need for repeated exchange of PMMA beads.[234] One group reported the successful use of an antibiotic pump system with infusions sustained for 32 to 40 days (mean, 36 days) in 21 patients, without any unintended increase in systemic antibiotic levels or adverse drug effects such as nephrotoxicity or ototoxicity.[234]

The condition of the periosteum is important to the healing process and is best assessed by the presence of involucrum, which may take 2 to 8 months to form.[66] In the presence of generous involucrum, most children regenerate adequate diaphyseal new bone to avoid the need for bone grafting and reconstructive procedures. Early debridement of the sequestrum is not thought to be detrimental to the subsequent formation of involucrum.[66]

In cases in which extensive debridement, inadequate involucrum, or pathologic fracture results in significant segmental defects, reconstructive procedures must be performed to restore functional anatomy. Choices for reconstruction have included open bone grafting, tibiofibular synostosis, vascularized fibular autograft, soft tissue transfers with gastrocsoleus flaps, and the bifocal method of bone transport using the Ilizarov method. Two groups have reported successful use of the Ilizarov method in the treatment of chronic tibial osteomyelitis.[176,334] Earlier work showed that the method of distraction osteogenesis increases blood flow by 3 to 10 times in the extremity, enhancing local tissue levels of antibiotics.[5] In children, it does not appear necessary to perform bone grafting at the docking site.[176]

Complications

Recurrence of disease within 2 years has been reported in 20% to 30% of children with chronic osteomyelitis, despite treatment with surgical debridement and appropriate antibiotics.[243] More aggressive debridement, such as that performed with the Ilizarov method and oblique wire bone transport (Fig. 35–10), reportedly yields better results, with 80% to 100% good or excellent outcomes.[176,334] Most of the complications reported in the treatment of chronic osteomyelitis are related to the reconstructive procedures; they include osteopenia, joint stiffness, angular deformity, nonunion, proximal tibiofibular joint dislocation, and pin site infections.[176,334]

CHRONIC RECURRENT MULTIFOCAL OSTEOMYELITIS

Epidemiology

CRMO was first described by Giedion and colleagues in 1972, with more than 260 cases subsequently reported in the medical literature in the next 30 years.[99,134] The condition affects predominantly children and adolescents, with a peak age of onset of 10 years and a female-to-male ratio ranging from 1.7:1 to 4:1.[134,271] CRMO is characterized by recurrent inflammation at multiple skeletal sites, most commonly involving the tibia, femur, clavicle, foot, or vertebral body and rarely the pelvis or rib cage.[36,82,94,118,134,255,271] Multifocal distribution has been found in 93% of cases, with a median of three lesions per child detected in one report.[271] Although skeletal lesions may be the most obvious manifestation of this condition, it is frequently associated with other inflammatory disorders, including palmoplantar pustulosis, chronic arthritis, psoriasis, inflammatory bowel disease, pyoderma gangrenosum, Sweet's syndrome, and severe acne.[134,271] Rheumatoid factor has been detected in 8% of patients, and HLA-B27 in 11%.[271] The clinical symptoms and signs of CRMO include multiple episodes of localized redness, pain, and swelling of insidious onset and spontaneous regression. Overall, children demonstrate minimal functional impairment during the episodes.

Pathophysiology

The pathogenesis of this condition remains unexplained. Theories include an autoimmune process or an infection from an as yet unrecognized causative

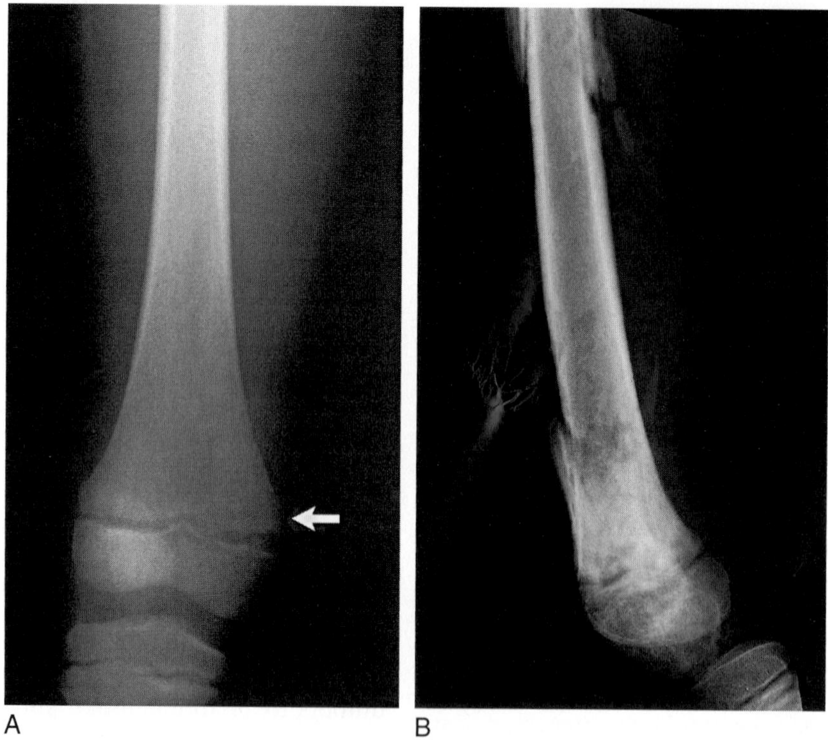

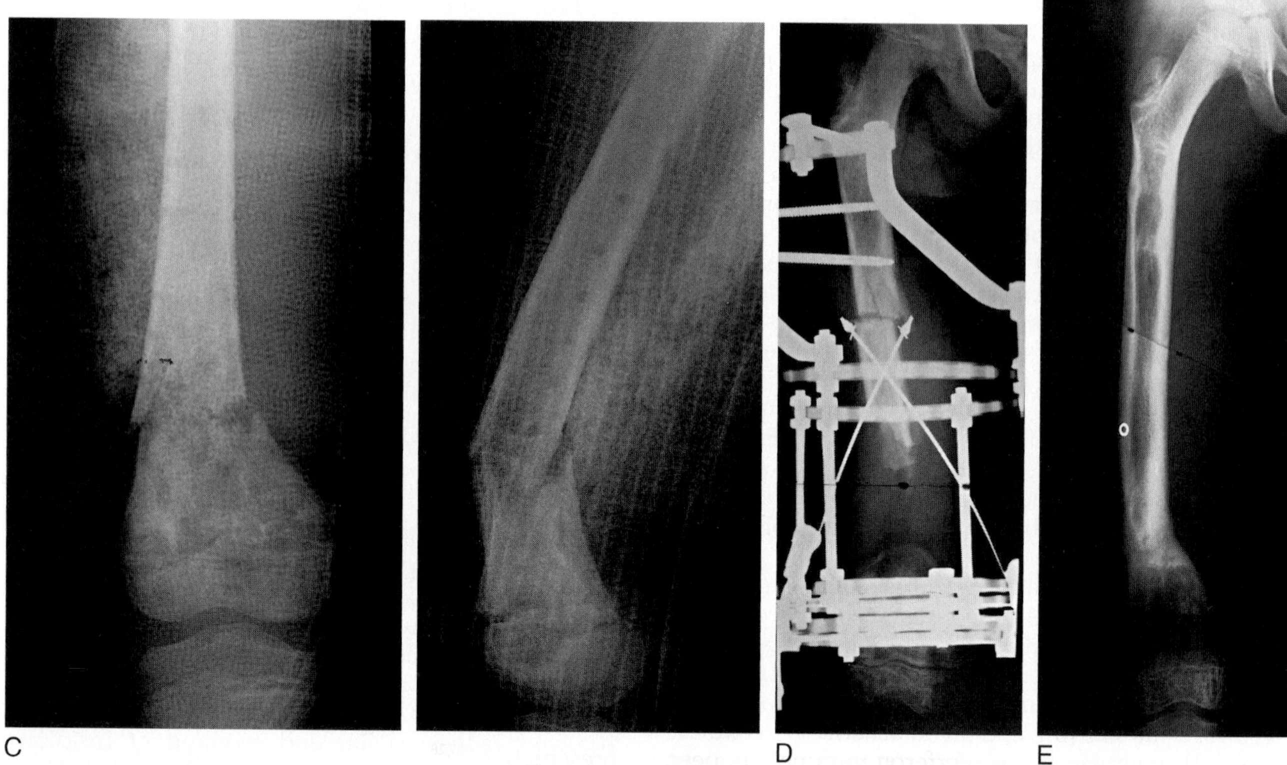

FIGURE 35-10 Progression from acute to chronic osteomyelitis. **A,** Anteroposterior (AP) radiograph of the femur shows subtle lucency in the medial distal femoral metaphysis (*arrow*). **B,** Lateral radiograph of the same patient, untreated, 6 weeks later. Note the periosteal reaction, as well as progression of the radiolucency in the metaphysis. **C,** AP (left) and lateral (right) radiographs obtained after an attempt at surgical decompression without debridement. Note the pathologic fracture at the metaphyseal-diaphyseal junction. The drill holes visible in the lateral view are residua of an attempt to decompress the infection. Adequate debridement of necrotic tissue was not achieved. **D,** AP radiograph obtained after complete debridement and application of an Ilizarov frame for bone transport. **E,** AP radiograph obtained after a successful bone transport.

agent such as *Mycoplasma, Chlamydia,* atypical mycobacterium, or virus. However, most series report negative cultures in nearly all patients.[94,118] *Propionibacterium acnes* has been isolated in a few cases of a related syndrome characterized by synovitis, acne, pustulosis, hyperostosis, and osteitis (SAPHO syndrome) but not specifically in CRMO.[255] One child at the Royal Children's Hospital in Melbourne, Australia, yielded a positive culture of *S. aureus* and responded to flucloxacillin, but subsequent authors from the same institution dismissed the case as an erroneous diagnosis of CRMO.[36,79] A literature review in 1997 found positive cultures reported in 13 of 184 cases, all of which were considered to be contaminants.[271]

Histopathologic examination of lesions may show changes suggestive or diagnostic of osteomyelitis, with numerous neutrophils, bone necrosis, granuloma, and fibrosis with round cell infiltration.[36] Others have described nonspecific inflammation, with a predominance of lymphocytes, plasma cells, histiocytes, and multinucleated giant cells.[271]

Evaluation

The diagnosis of CRMO is essentially one of exclusion. The following criteria have been suggested to avoid the pitfalls of misdiagnosis: (1) protracted clinical course of greater than 3 months' duration, (2) open biopsy results consistent with chronic inflammation, and (3) failure to identify any infectious organism by culture.[271]

The initial evaluation of CRMO should include the same laboratory and radiographic studies performed for any suspected infection. Microbiologic tests of blood and tissue cultures should not be omitted merely because CRMO is suspected. Plain radiographs of each symptomatic area should be obtained and supplemented by bone scintigraphy, because asymptomatic lesions are occasionally identified in this manner.[36,118] Areas of lysis and reactive periosteal sclerosis can mimic conditions such as Ewing's sarcoma, metastatic neuroblastoma, and Langerhans cell histiocytosis.[271] If a malignant neoplasm is being considered in the differential diagnosis, biopsy principles should be followed carefully when obtaining a specimen for histopathology.[195]

Treatment

There is no well-defined treatment for CRMO, although most children are treated with nonsteroidal anti-inflammatory drugs and occasionally corticosteroids. There should be no response to antibiotic treatment. Effective treatment with interferon gamma has been reported in one case, and it is hoped that this method may help circumvent the prolonged, relapsing nature of CRMO. A 13-year-old girl who was treated for 3 months with interferon gamma had no symptomatic episodes in the 15 months immediately after treatment, compared with 11 symptomatic episodes in the $2\frac{1}{2}$ years before treatment.[94] The exact mechanism for the beneficial effect is not known, but the use of interferon gamma in cases of chronic granulomatous disease and in the treatment of intracellular pathogens such as leprosy, *Mycobacterium avium-intracellulare* infections, and leishmaniasis, which are often refractory to standard antimicrobial treatments, may offer indirect support to the theory of an obscure pathogen as the cause of CRMO.

Complications

CRMO is often described as a self-limiting condition of childhood that follows a benign, protracted course without sequelae.[36,118,271] An early diagnosis can avoid complications associated with unnecessary surgical or antibiotic treatment. However, two long-term follow-up studies suggest that the natural history of CRMO is prolonged and associated with adverse sequelae in some individuals.[79,134] In one series, 12 patients were followed to a mean age of 22 years (range, 16 to 31 years); only 2 patients had complete resolution of symptoms, and 7 patients had noticeable deformity.[79] Five patients had limb length inequality of at least 1.5 cm, and one patient had undergone limb lengthening for a discrepancy of 5.5 cm. This finding led the authors to recommend that these individuals be followed until skeletal maturity. The second long-term series reported outcomes at a median of 13 years since initial diagnosis (range, 6 to 25 years).[134] Although 78% of these individuals had no evidence of physical disability or functional impairment, 26% reported residual pain as a result of CRMO. Both reports suggested that overall, most individuals do well both physically and emotionally despite the long-lasting effects of the illness.[79,134]

Septic Arthritis

Epidemiology

Septic arthritis accounts for approximately 0.25% of hospitalizations among children. The condition is thought to be more common than osteomyelitis, with one retrospective review identifying 471 cases of septic arthritis over 26 years, compared with only 258 cases of osteomyelitis in a corresponding 22-year period.[145] The same review noted that the majority of infections (70%) were identified in children from 1 month to 5 years of age, with half of these occurring in children younger than 2 years. Single joint infection was noted in 94% of children, most commonly involving the hip (41%) and knee (23%), followed by the ankle (14%), elbow (12%), wrist (4%), and shoulder (4%). Septic sacroiliitis, though rare, has been reported in children and is often overlooked owing to the vague clinical presentation.[227,287]

The spectrum of causative bacteria and the frequency of occurrence of specific pathogens are similar to those seen in osteomyelitis, with *S. aureus* being the most common organism identified. Certain bacteria appear to have a higher likelihood of causing septic arthritis than of causing osteomyelitis. These organisms include *Brucella melitensis, H. influenzae, K. kingae, N. meningitidis,* and *N. gonorrhoeae.*[112,131,211,320,333]

Septic sacroiliitis is associated with *Mycobacterium tuberculosis.*[227]

Pathophysiology

Hematogenous seeding of the synovium during transient bacteremia is the most common cause of septic arthritis in children. Other foci of infection, such as otitis media or sinusitis, may be present well in advance of the joint infection.[267] Septic arthritis may also arise from a contiguous site of infection, such as adjacent osteomyelitis, or from a penetrating injury with direct inoculation into the joint.[144,233] Joints that are particularly susceptible to the spread of infection from an adjacent osseous source include the knee (31%), hip (23%), ankle (18%), and shoulder (14%); this susceptibility is largely due to the intracapsular location of the metaphysis in these joints (Fig. 35–11).[233]

Bacterial entry into a joint space signals the onset of an inflammatory cascade that, left untreated, may lead to cartilage destruction and loss of normal joint function. The precise pathway of joint degradation is not fully understood. However, research suggests that macrophages, polymorphonuclear leukocytes, and synovial cells release cytokines (IL-1β, IL-6, TNF-α), immunoglobulin G, and lysosomal enzymes into the joint space.[250,278] This results in an early loss of proteoglycan subunits from the cartilage matrix, which may be severe as early as 2 to 5 days after the onset of infection despite the lack of visible cartilage degeneration. In an experimental model of septic arthritis in rabbit knees, *S. aureus* injection resulted in proteoglycan subunit loss of 30% at 48 hours, 50% at 5 days, and 80% at 3 weeks; collagen degradation did not ensue until 3 weeks (28% loss).[278] It remains unclear whether joint cartilage is able to restore normal proteoglycan content after elimination of the bacterial infection and before the onset of collagen loss.

Some strains of *S. aureus* possess a gene encoding for collagen-binding adhesion *(Cna).*[229] Experimental injection of *S. aureus* in mice resulted in septic arthritis in 70% of animals injected with *Cna*-positive strains, versus only 27% of animals when the gene was absent.[154,229]

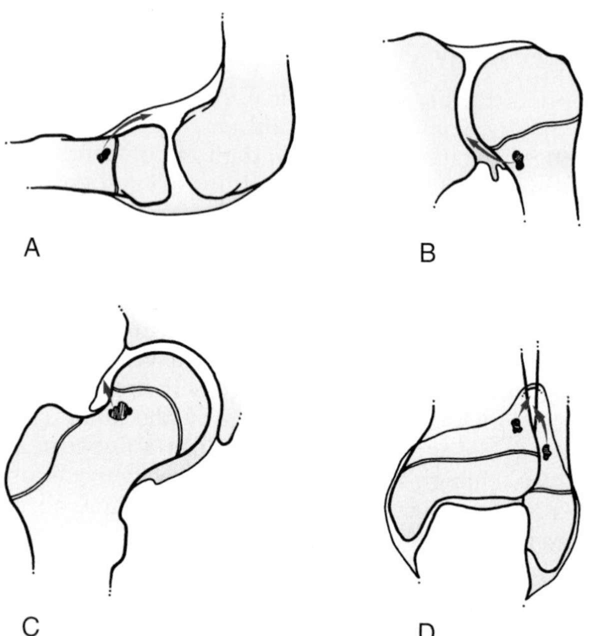

FIGURE 35–11 Metaphyses of the proximal radius **(A)**, proximal humerus **(B)**, proximal femur **(C)**, and distal tibia-fibula **(D)** are intra-articular. Osteomyelitis in these locations may decompress into the joint, producing concomitant septic arthritis.

Evaluation

Septic arthritis should be considered whenever an ill-appearing child with a clinical history of atraumatic limitation of mobility has the physical finding of joint irritability. I use the same initial diagnostic process for septic arthritis as for osteomyelitis: plain radiographs and laboratory studies (CBC with differential, CRP, ESR, and blood cultures). When symptoms are located in the hip region, comparative ultrasonography is performed to evaluate for hip effusion. The differential diagnosis of septic arthritis includes transient synovitis, reactive arthritis, juvenile rheumatoid arthritis, Kawasaki's syndrome, Henoch-Schönlein purpura, rheumatic fever, avascular necrosis, slipped capital femoral epiphysis, trauma, neoplasia, Lyme arthritis, and Legg-Calvé-Perthes syndrome.[2,3,8,19,85,191,205,213,258,302,326] Other infections occurring near a joint, such as osteomyelitis, pyomyositis, septic bursitis, cellulitis, and abscess, can mimic the clinical presentation of septic arthritis. In most cases, it should be possible to significantly narrow the differential diagnosis of an acutely irritable joint following the initial evaluation. Despite all the information that can be obtained with modern laboratory and radiographic studies, it is important not to lose sight of the value of obtaining a complete history and performing a thorough physical examination when dealing with musculoskeletal infections. Morrey and associates[207] noted that "the presence of a warm and tender joint that is painful on even gentle passive motion should differentiate this condition from metaphyseal osteomyelitis, in which . . . gentle passive motion is usually possible without an increase in symptoms."

Frequently, the greatest diagnostic challenge is differentiating between septic arthritis and transient synovitis of the hip. Because of the importance of correctly identifying these two conditions, great attention has been focused on devising an evidence-based clinical prediction strategy.[76,155,172,173,186] Failure to correctly identify septic arthritis may result in poor long-term outcomes.[155,172,173,186] Transient synovitis is one of the most common causes of hip pain in children, responsible for up to 0.9% of pediatric emergency room visits each year, and an early diagnosis can avoid unnecessary invasive procedures and hospitalization for observation.[76]

Kocher and colleagues retrospectively studied 282 children evaluated for an irritable hip at their tertiary care children's hospital between 1979 and 1996.[173] They identified four independent predictors to help differentiate between septic arthritis and transient synovitis: history of fever (oral temperature >38.5°C), history of non–weight bearing, ESR greater than 40 mm/hour, and white blood cell (WBC) count greater than 12,000 cells/mL. Although individual variables alone were not useful in differentiating the two conditions, the authors were able to demonstrate through multiple logistic regression analysis that the predictive probability of septic arthritis in the population studied was 0.2% for zero predictors, 3.0% for one predictor, 40% for two predictors, 93.1% for three predictors, and 99.6% for four predictors.[173] This method was prospectively validated at the same institution by studying 213 children between 1997 and 2002.[172] The authors found that the actual distribution of septic arthritis was 2% for zero predictors, 9.5% for one predictor, 35% for two predictors, 72.8% for three predictors, and 93% for four predictors.

This same clinical prediction algorithm was tested at a separate tertiary care children's hospital in St. Louis by means of a retrospective review of children evaluated for an irritable hip between 1992 and 2000. Using Kocher's criteria, Luhmann and coworkers demonstrated only a 59% predicted probability of septic arthritis when all four independent variables were identified.[186] The authors attempted to select a better model to describe their patient population by choosing three alternative predictors: history of fever, serum WBC count greater than 12,000/mm^3, and a previous health care visit. This combination resulted in a predicted probability of septic arthritis of only 71%. On the basis of this low predictive probability, these authors continue to recommend the use of hip ultrasonography and arthrocentesis as adjunctive diagnostic modalities in the evaluation of an irritable hip.

The valuable work from these two institutions demonstrates the limitations of relying excessively on clinical predictors; they inevitably have diminished performance in a new patient population because they were established to model the original population studied.[172,321,322] However, the presence or absence of multiple independent predictors of septic arthritis in any given patient can be helpful in making the decision whether to observe the patient or aspirate the hip joint in the operating room under general anesthesia. Ultimately, there is no substitute for vigilant surveillance and good clinical judgment.

Many authors consider aspiration of a septic joint to be a significant and indispensable part of the diagnostic process.[14,74,145,170,186,207] Aspiration of the hip joint may be difficult, but a variety of methods can be used to safely access this joint for arthrocentesis, including ultrasound and fluoroscopic guidance.[36] Although blind aspiration based on anatomic landmarks can be attempted, it is not recommended because it is impossible to confirm an intra-articular location in the case of a negative aspirate, as can be done with ultrasonography or an arthrogram (Fig. 35–12).[36] Joint fluid obtained by aspiration should be sent for Gram stain and culture, as well as cell count. Some specialists also obtain joint fluid glucose and protein levels and compare these with serum levels. A WBC count greater than 50,000/mm^3 with a predominance of polymorphonuclear leukocytes, a high protein content, and a low glucose concentration (<33% of serum glucose) are characteristic of septic arthritis. The information obtained from the fluid cell count is important in the diagnostic process because joint fluid may inhibit the growth of certain bacteria and prevent the positive identification of an organism. Although most authors report a low rate of culture-negative septic arthritis

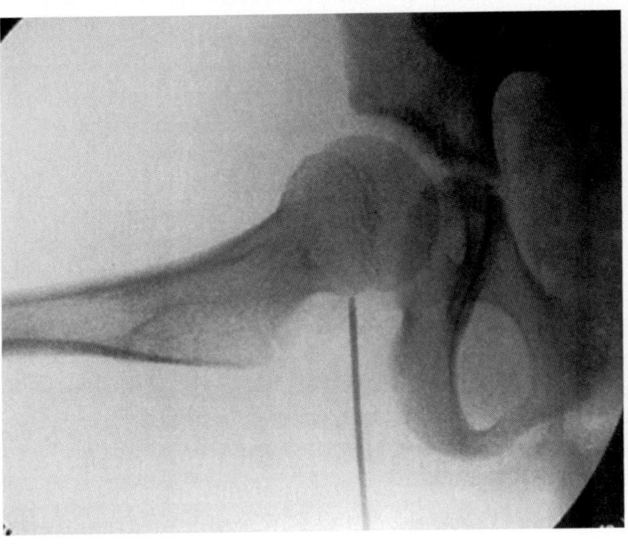
A

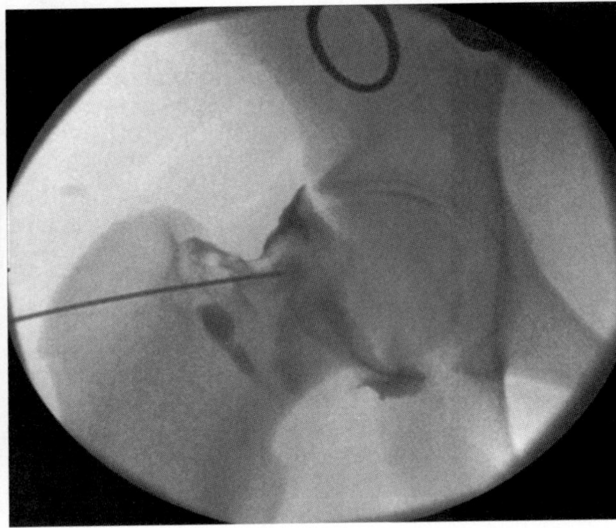
B

FIGURE 35–12 Fluoroscopically guided aspiration of a hip joint **(A)** with an arthrogram **(B)** to confirm the intra-articular location of the aspiration attempt.

(ranging from 18% to 48%), one study reported a rate as high as 70%.[43,145,189,207] *K. kingae* is a fastidious gram-negative coccobacillus that is particularly difficult to isolate in the laboratory, but it is responsible for an increasing number of cases of septic arthritis in children between the ages of 6 months and 3 years.[97,169,228] To facilitate the positive identification of this organism, current recommendations include the immediate inoculation of joint fluid aspirate into aerobic blood culture bottles instead of direct plating on solid media.[97,169,228] This practice was previously recommended by Jackson and Nelson for any joint aspirate, because it was thought that the broth from the blood culture bottle results in dilution of the joint fluid, reducing its inhibitory effects on bacterial culture.[145]

Treatment

Antibiotic Therapy. Empirical antibiotic selection for septic arthritis is similar to that for osteomyelitis. For adolescents suspected of having disseminated gonococcal illness, ceftriaxone should be considered initially. Peak synovial fluid concentrations of commonly used antibiotics have been shown to be greater than 60% of peak serum concentrations, with adequate inhibitory activity against the common organisms that cause septic arthritis.[220] Sequential parenteral-to-oral antibiotic therapy is well established as an effective method of treatment and reduces hospital stay, cost, morbidity, and inconvenience to families.[166,219,221] One series reported an early switch to oral antibiotics after 72 hours of intravenous administration, as long as there was a good response to the initial treatment.[171] In general, the duration of antibiotic therapy for most cases of uncomplicated septic arthritis is approximately 4 weeks, although shorter treatment courses have been described. As in the treatment of osteomyelitis, I decide whether to extend the duration of treatment based on normalization of the ESR.

Surgery. It is commonly agreed that some form of joint decompression with aspiration and lavage, repeated aspirations, arthroscopy, or open arthrotomy should be performed as the initial treatment for septic arthritis, along with the intravenous administration of an appropriate antibiotic.[14,43,145,171,186,189,207] Debate continues over which of these methods is best and the appropriate time frame for the initial invasive intervention. The most conservative approach involves performing a joint aspiration in the emergency room under conscious sedation or in the operating room under general anesthesia, with the expectation that joint arthrotomy will be performed immediately as an emergency procedure if bacteria are present on Gram stain, the joint fluid cell count is greater than 50,000/mm^3, or the clinical suspicion of septic arthritis remains high, regardless of the joint fluid findings. Other methods of treatment have also proved to be successful. Serial joint aspiration, which is well documented for knee and shoulder joint sepsis, was recently studied in the hip joint, with surgery avoided in 24 of 28 patients in one series.[101] The mean number of aspirations in that study was 3.6 per child, and 75% of children resumed walking after 24 hours.

A growing body of evidence attests to the benefits of arthroscopy in the treatment of septic arthritis of the hip, knee, ankle, shoulder, and elbow.[48,51,167,276,284,288,312] Several advantages of this method have been reported, including comprehensive visualization of intra-articular structures; improved ability to assess the severity of sepsis affecting the joint cartilage and synovium compared with limited arthrotomy; capability to remove fibrinous aggregates or advanced synovitis, which may serve as a source of persistent infection if left unattended; allowance of early functional rehabilitation because of the minimally invasive approach; and ease of accurate drain placement through arthroscopic cannulas to ensure thorough postoperative drainage (Fig. 35–13).[51,167,276,284,288,312] In one series of 76 children with arthroscopically treated septic arthritis, 91% were cured by arthroscopic irrigation and antibiotics alone, and open revision was required in only 4%.[288]

Although the necessity of emergent intervention has not been clearly established on the basis of clinical or histopathologic evidence, several studies suggest that early and aggressive intervention is beneficial.[43,276,284,288] Satisfactory clinical results have been reported as long as intervention occurred within 4 days of the onset of symptoms.[43,207] Treatment delay has been associated with fibrinous loculations, synovitis, and pannus formation, which may lead to persistence of infection, further surgery, and prolonged hospitalization.[284]

Clinical Practice Guideline. Based on a systematic review of the best available evidence, an interdisciplinary committee at Children's Hospital in Boston developed a clinical practice guideline for the treatment of septic arthritis of the hip in children.[171] Comparing a historical control group of 30 children with septic arthritis with a similar prospective cohort group, the authors found no significant difference in clinical outcome.[171] However, they noted a significant improvement in the standardization of care for the children treated under the guideline, which resulted in greater compliance with recommended antibiotic therapy (93% versus 7%), faster change to oral antibiotics (3.9 versus 6.9 days), and shorter hospital stay (4.8 versus 8.3 days). Although outcome variables remained unaffected in this limited series, one can only assume that a positive effect would be identified in a larger series, particularly if the guideline could prevent unnecessary delays in treatment or inadequate treatment, which might otherwise occur without evidence-based practice standardization.

Complications

Complications associated with septic arthritis include systemic sepsis, premature arthritis, osteonecrosis of the proximal femur (Fig. 35–14), physeal closure, growth disturbance, synovitis, arthrofibrosis, joint stiffness, and persistent infection. In Morrey and

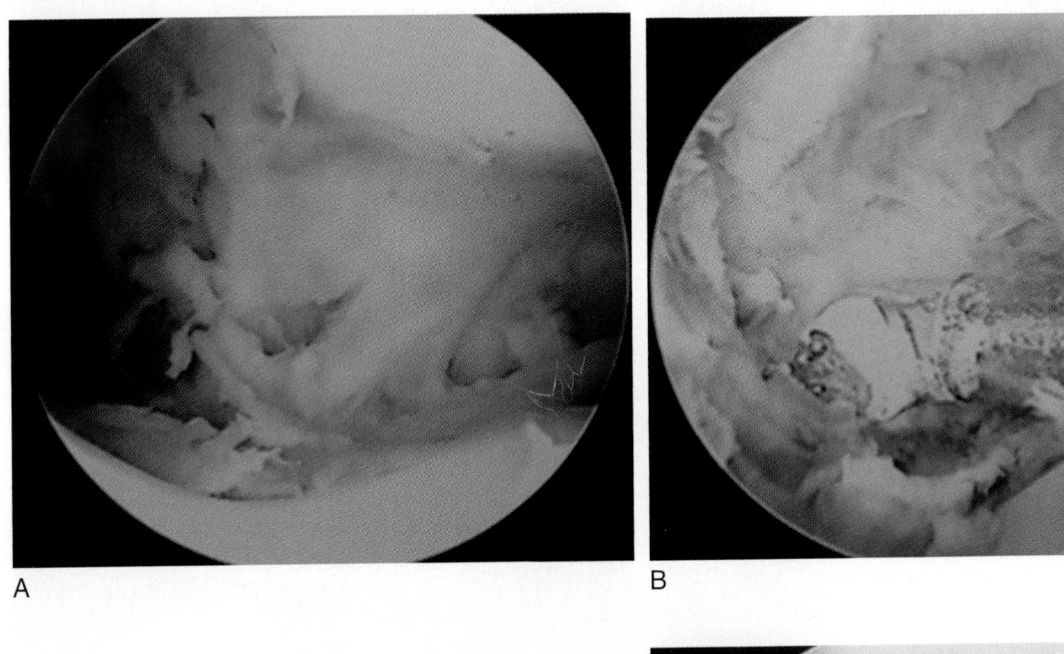

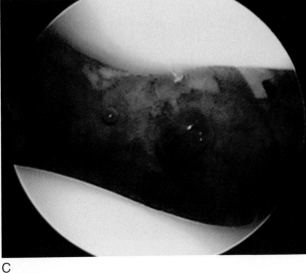

FIGURE 35-13 Arthroscopic image of a knee joint 3 days after arthrotomy, irrigation, and drainage of septic arthritis. The original arthrotomy was through a small incision, with limited visualization of the joint. Lack of a clinical and laboratory response after the initial surgery led to this follow-up procedure. Findings at arthroscopy included a diffuse fibrinous cast of the knee and synovitis involving the suprapatellar pouch and medial and lateral femorotibial gutters **(A).** After arthroscopic debridement **(B** and **C),** the child demonstrated rapid clinical and laboratory improvement.

colleagues' original report on septic arthritis, they noted that a delay in treatment was the single most important factor affecting prognosis in children, and they found no unsatisfactory results if symptoms were present for less than 3 days before treatment.[207] Other prognostic factors include anatomic location of the infection, presence of adjacent osteomyelitis, and adequacy of treatment.[43] It is well recognized that the hip joint is vulnerable to complications, particularly when infection occurs at an early age, when the anatomy allows rapid communication of infection from the metaphysis to the epiphysis and into the joint (see Fig. 35–14).[7,14,43,45,78,115,135,196,329] One review of 33 children with septic arthritis of the hip showed satisfactory outcomes in 89% and identified the two most important factors associated with poor results to be a delay in definitive treatment longer than 5 days and the presence of osteomyelitis of the proximal femur (4 of 7 cases).[43]

Pyomyositis

Epidemiology

Pyomyositis denotes an abscess of skeletal muscle that occurs either spontaneously, as in primary pyomyositis, or secondary to a penetrating injury or local spread from an adjacent infection. This condition, commonly referred to as *tropical pyomyositis,* has been reported predominantly in tropical countries and accounts for approximately 4% of surgical admissions in that setting.[4,111] Pyomyositis is also reported, though less commonly, in temperate climates, where it is called *nontropical pyomyositis;* it occurs during the warmer months in the warmer regions of a country.[109,111,114,130,248,283] One series from southern Texas reported an incidence of 1 per 3000 pediatric admissions.[109]

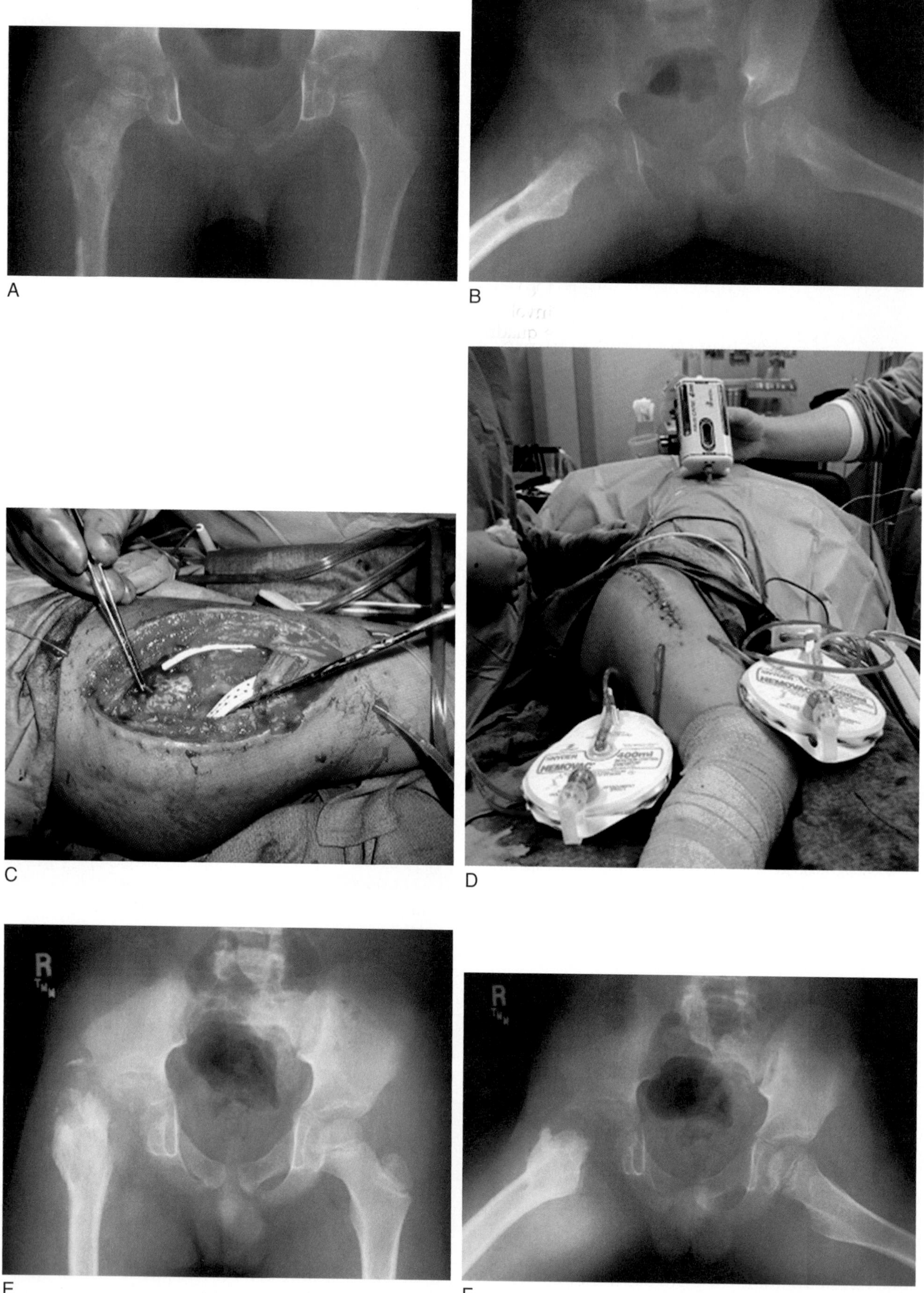

FIGURE 35–14 This 11-year-old boy with a 2-week delay in presentation developed septic arthritis of the right hip and osteomyelitis of the proximal femur. Plain radiographs **(A** and **B)** after nine surgical procedures for irrigation and debridement **(C** and **D)** demonstrate involucrum associated with the proximal femur and a cortical window used for debridement. Radiographs taken 6 months later **(E** and **F)** demonstrate autolytic destruction of the femoral head and loss of the proximal femur.

The condition is most common in the first and second decades of life, with a slight male predominance of 2:1 to 3:1.[44,98,111] The role of injury as a causative factor is unclear. Some authors have reported trauma as a preceding event in 39% to 60% of children in North America, compared with only 25% of children in the tropics.[44,46,98] Other reports have not substantiated this finding, with a history of trauma solicited in less than 5% of reviewed cases.[17] Single muscle involvement is most common. Multiple sites were identified in only 16.6% of cases in a literature review of 676 patients reported between 1960 and 2002.[17] Any muscle group in the body can be involved, but the most common site of infection is the quadriceps muscle, followed by the gluteal and iliopsoas muscles.[44] The presence of infection in a variety of muscles around the pelvis has been reported and can be a diagnostic challenge.[72,123,156,226,230,279,294,295,310,328]

S. aureus is the most common pathogen involved in pyomyositis and has been reported in 50% to 85% of cases in the United States and more than 90% of cases in the tropics.[44,46,98,111,114,156,248] The second most common causative organism is GABHS, which is reported in 25% to 50% of cases in the United States.[111,120,237,248,337] Other notable organisms include *E. coli* (2.4%), *Salmonella enteritidis* (1.5%), and *M. tuberculosis* (1.1%).[17]

Pathophysiology

The cause of pyomyositis is presumed to be hematogenous seeding of a skeletal muscle that has been predisposed to infection by alteration of its normal defenses. The rare occurrence of this condition in comparison to the incidence of bone and joint infections is attributed to the fact that skeletal muscle is inherently resistant to infection, even in the presence of bacteremia. In one study, intravenous injection of sublethal doses of *S. aureus* in laboratory animals was unable to cause pyomyositis until after the muscles were traumatized by pinching, electric shock, or ischemia.[204] The alteration of muscle tissue structure by subclinical parasitic and viral infection has been proposed as a precursor to tropical pyomyositis.[17] However, there does not appear to be a correlation between the geographic distribution of parasitic infections and pyomyositis.[17,44] Further, many patients who present with pyomyositis in tropical countries are free of parasitic disease.[4,17,44] In the United States, nontropical pyomyositis appears to be associated with immune compromise and impaired host bactericidal capabilities, with case reports in patients with diabetes, hematopoietic disorders, cancer, and human immunodeficiency virus (HIV).[46,98,111]

The infection of skeletal muscle evolves through three overlapping stages.[89] Initially, in the invasive stage, the pathogen enters the muscle through the circulation. A cascade of local inflammation develops, resulting in diffuse muscle pain or cramping. No definite abscess is present at this point (Fig. 35–15). Next, during the purulent stage, an abscess accumulates within the skeletal muscle, and more systemic signs and symptoms of infection are identified, including fever, progressive pain, and swelling (Fig. 35–16). This stage occurs approximately 10 to 21 days after the onset of symptoms and is the cause of the initial presentation for medical treatment in more than 90% of children with pyomyositis.[44] Finally, in the late stage, the child presents with signs of systemic toxicity and septic shock, which may occur in up to 5% of children.[44]

Evaluation

The diagnosis of pyomyositis is most commonly based on the clinical examination and imaging studies, which are selected to demonstrate the anatomic and spacial distribution of the infection. Routine laboratory studies, including CBC with differential, ESR, CRP, and blood cultures, are also performed. Although the muscular involvement might be expected to alter the serum creatine kinase level, measurements are commonly normal or only marginally elevated.[111]

Plain radiographs are obtained to exclude skeletal lesions. Ultrasonography and CT may be helpful to aid in the diagnosis and enable percutaneous aspiration and drainage of pyomyositis.[114,156] Ultrasonography is particularly useful in the diagnostic evaluation of a psoas abscess. In one report of 55 children who presented with hip pain and flexion, ultrasonography led to the correct diagnosis in all 36 cases in which it was performed.[156] CT studies should be performed with and without intravenous contrast. Findings characteristically include the presence of a mass and local attenuation within the involved muscle, with ring enhancement of the abscess after the administration of contrast.[114] Unfortunately, CT may fail to reveal the full extent of the diffuse inflammatory changes associated with the early stages of infection and lacks the resolution of MRI.[17,111]

MRI is the most useful diagnostic modality in cases of suspected pyomyositis. It clearly demonstrates muscle inflammation, abscess formation, and significant contiguous infections such as osteomyelitis or septic arthritis, which may alter the method and duration of treatment.[72,123,226,279,294,295,310,328] Findings typically include diffuse muscle enlargement, increased signal intensity on T2-weighted images, and peripheral enhancement, with a central nonenhancing area indicating the abscess on gadolinium-enhanced images.[335] It is believed that MRI with gadolinium enhancement may help differentiate between the invasive and purulent stages of the disease and identify the rare subset of patients who may respond to intravenous antibiotic therapy alone.[283,335] In one series of 40 patients with pyomyositis, the thickness of the enhancing rim of the microabscesses was used as a determinant of the likelihood of response to antibiotics alone.[335] The authors found thin rim enhancement in 9 of 10 patients who were treated solely with antibiotics; all 12 patients with thick rim enhancement required surgery. Because of the diagnostic confusion that often accompanies infections around the pelvis, MRI is considered a

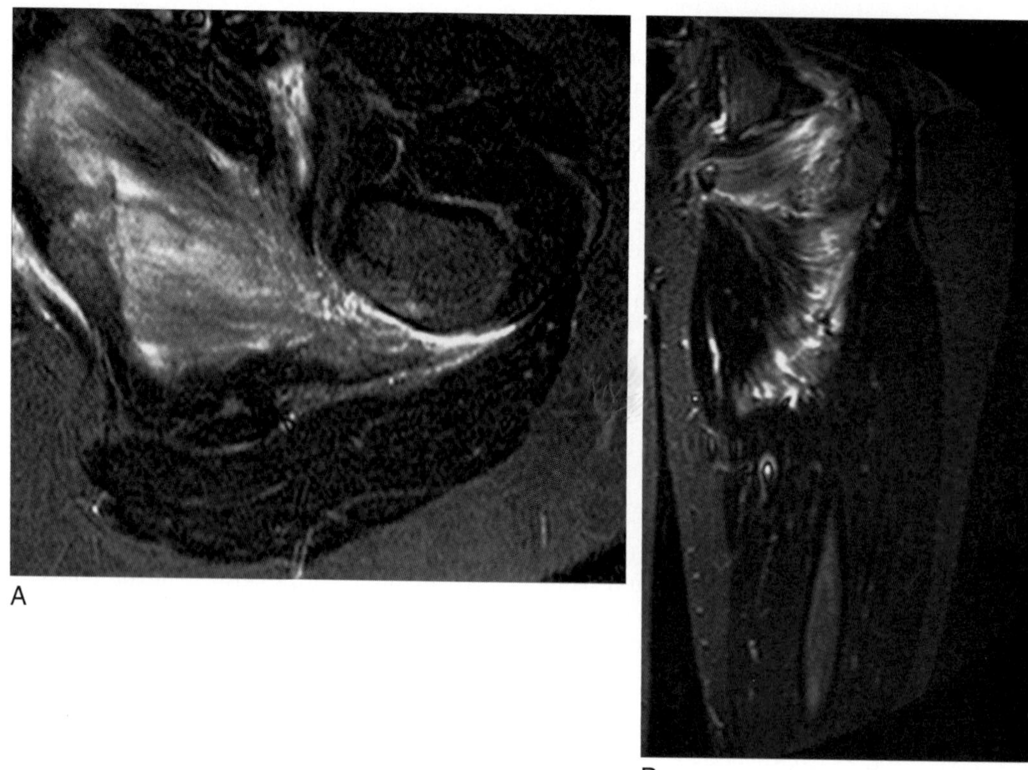

FIGURE 35–15 A and B, Magnetic resonance images demonstrate diffuse inflammatory changes without evidence of a discrete abscess of the piriformis and hip external rotators in this 13-year-old boy with a 3-day history of buttock pain and limp. The initial laboratory results included C-reactive protein 5.2 mg/dL, erythrocyte sedimentation rate 37 mm/hour, and white blood cell count 20,000 cells/mL. Clinical and laboratory improvement followed antibiotic treatment.

necessary part of the diagnostic process, especially if confirmation of the diagnosis of pyomyositis leads to surgery; the detailed imaging provided can help guide the surgical approach.[230,279]

Treatment

Antibiotic Therapy. If antibiotic therapy is initiated early, during the invasive stage, surgery can sometimes be avoided.[111,335] Empirical antibiotic therapy to cover both *S. aureus* and GABHS is recommended owing to the moderate incidence of streptococci as the causative organisms and the high mortality associated with GABHS pyomyositis.[120,337] Because penicillin has a diminished effect in treating streptococcal pyomyositis, the current recommendation is to begin monotherapy with clindamycin.[111,337] Children with invasive streptococcal infection who are treated with clindamycin have better outcomes than those treated with a beta-lactam antibiotic alone.[338] Clindamycin has the added advantage of being effective against most strains of MRSA identified in invasive infections and can continue to be used as specific antibiotic therapy after culture results are obtained in most cases of pyomyositis.[200] The mean duration of antibiotic treatment was 4.3 weeks (range, 2 to 6 weeks) in one series of 16 children in which 8 were managed with antibiotics alone.[111]

Surgery. Surgery is the mainstay of treatment for most children with pyomyositis. Drainage can be performed using image guidance with CT or ultrasonography or by open incision. A report from Children's Hospital of Philadelphia showed successful percutaneous drainage with CT guidance in all five of the children in whom it was attempted.[283] Open surgical drainage is preferred when multiple small abscesses appear to be loculated or when there is concern that the child may be at risk for developing septic shock.[120,337]

Complications

Late-stage pyomyositis, which is reported in up to 5% of cases, can be accompanied by systemic sepsis and shock. Intensive medical resuscitation, along with timely surgical decompression of the focus of infection, is needed in these advanced cases. Streptococcal pyomyositis can be extremely aggressive, with extensive muscle necrosis and rapid progression to multifocal involvement, sepsis, multisystem organ dysfunction, and death.[120,142,337] One case report described the aggressive surgical and medical management needed to stabilize a 5-year-old girl with this condition, including fasciotomies in both legs and one arm for identified compartment syndromes secondary to myonecrosis.[120] The literature indicates

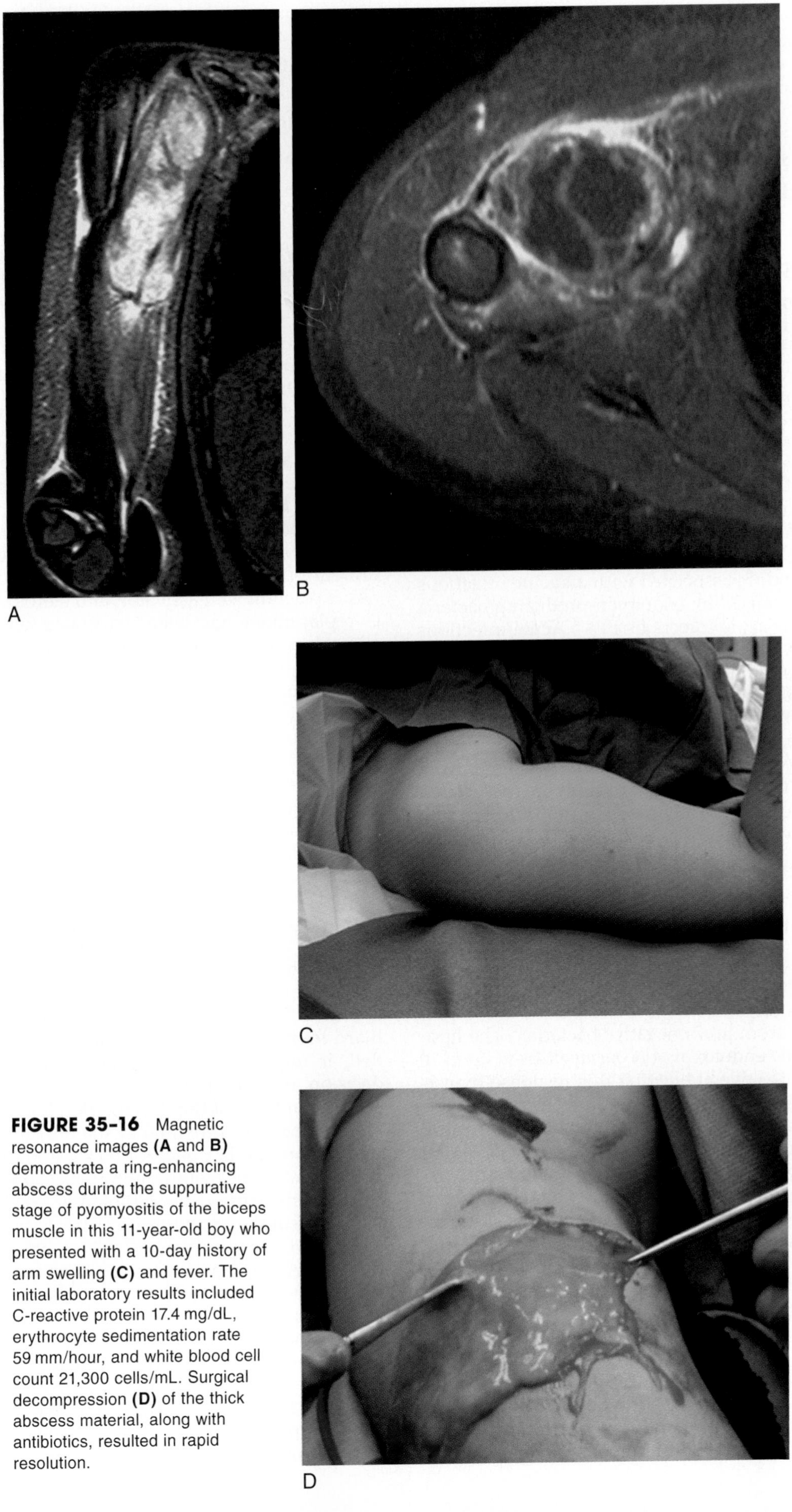

A

B

C

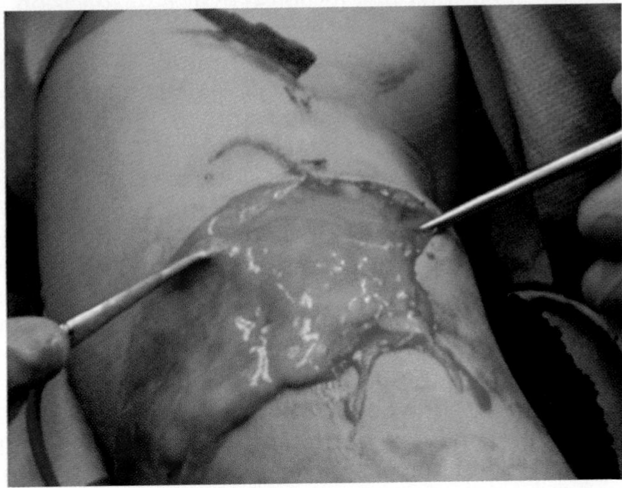

D

FIGURE 35–16 Magnetic resonance images **(A** and **B)** demonstrate a ring-enhancing abscess during the suppurative stage of pyomyositis of the biceps muscle in this 11-year-old boy who presented with a 10-day history of arm swelling **(C)** and fever. The initial laboratory results included C-reactive protein 17.4 mg/dL, erythrocyte sedimentation rate 59 mm/hour, and white blood cell count 21,300 cells/mL. Surgical decompression **(D)** of the thick abscess material, along with antibiotics, resulted in rapid resolution.

a mortality rate of 80% in cases of streptococcal pyomyositis, highlighting the necessity of early surgical intervention and appropriate initial antibiotic treatment with clindamycin.[120,337]

Other Soft Tissue Infections of Orthopaedic Significance

PURPURA FULMINANS

Epidemiology

Purpura fulminans (PF) is classically defined by hemorrhagic skin lesions, fever, septicemia, shock, and disseminated intravascular coagulation (DIC). Previously healthy children are vulnerable to developing a rapidly progressive and sometimes fatal illness that may lead to symmetric gangrene of the distal extremities. PF is noted to occur in three clinical settings: (1) during the neonatal period as a manifestation of inherited protein C or S deficiency; (2) 1 to 2 weeks following a benign antecedent infection with a viral triggering agent such as varicella (chickenpox), rubeola (measles), scarlatina (scarlet fever), or rubella (referred to as idiopathic PF); and (3) associated with an acute infectious illness, often caused by endotoxin-producing bacteria (referred to as acute infectious PF).[67] Acute infectious PF occurs in 10% to 25% of children with meningococcal disease and also rarely occurs in association with systemic pneumococcal infection.[35,53,67,133] One series of pneumococcal sepsis reported PF in 10 of 165 patients (6%).[151]

Previously reported mortality rates ranged from 40% to 80%, whereas recent mortality rates associated with PF in the United States range from 15% to 30%.[67,133] This decrease is thought to be due to an improvement in early diagnosis and critical care.[29,133]

Pathophysiology

The pathogenesis of acute infectious PF is similar to that of the Shwartzman reaction, in which a necrotizing inflammatory lesion is produced by the injection of endotoxin from gram-negative bacteria.[67] The lipopolysaccharide endotoxin of *N. meningitidis* is up to 10 times more effective at eliciting this response than is endotoxin from other gram-negative bacteria.[70] The pneumococcal autolysin is thought to be the purpura-producing agent, because *S. pneumoniae* does not contain endotoxin.[53]

The pathogenesis of PF appears to be related to an inflammatory cascade that is initiated by the stimulating factor (e.g., endotoxin) presented by the triggering agent. This causes increased levels of cytokines—specifically, TNF-α, IL-1, and interferon gamma—which initiate a procoagulant cascade and result in an acquired protein C and S deficiency, as both are rapidly consumed during the coagulation process.[35] The microthrombi that form result in microvascular occlusion and eventually lead to hypoperfusion, ischemia, infarction, and gangrene of the peripheral extremities.[35] Other manifestations of the disease include seizures, hematuria, gastrointestinal hemorrhage, adrenal hemorrhage, pulmonary failure, and renal failure.[29]

Evaluation and Treatment

Owing to the life-threatening nature of this condition, diagnosis and treatment are often performed simultaneously in a critical care setting. Orthopaedic surgeons are rarely involved in the early assessment of children with PF; they usually become involved after skin necrosis has occurred and decisions regarding debridement, reconstruction, and amputation are relevant.

Initial treatment involves resuscitation and administration of intravenous antibiotics. The goals at this stage include maintenance of adequate organ and tissue perfusion to avoid organ failure. The need for invasive monitoring and frequent interventions requires an intensive care setting or burn unit to ensure the best outcome.[29,133] Therapeutic interventions that may be initiated by intensivists include replacement of identified deficiencies of vitamin K–dependent coagulation factors, antithrombin III, protein C, and protein S; selective use of heparin; administration of tissue plasminogen activator; and steroids.[67,133] Protein C replacement has been associated with improved clinical outcomes in nonrandomized trials, with a reduction in the rates of skin grafting, amputation, renal failure, and death.[222,277,325]

Following the resuscitative stage of treatment, attention can be directed to debridement and reconstruction of the extremities. This often requires close communication between orthopaedic and plastic surgeons to determine the best timing and method of intervention. Debate exists whether early aggressive surgical debridement should be performed along with primary closure of all wounds to reduce the risk of wound infection.[29] One study suggested that fasciotomy be considered when compartment pressures exceed 30 mm Hg, reporting positive clinical outcomes with this technique.[29] Other authors advocate delaying amputation until a clear line of demarcation results in the identification of nonviable tissues.[34,133] Canale and Ikard found that once this demarcation line is identified, it remains constant and allows for a prompt decision regarding the level of amputation.[34] They recommended that the skin incision for amputation be placed 1 to 3 cm proximal to the demarcation line. A report from the Hospital for Sick Children in Toronto noted that bone scintigraphy is a useful adjunct, enabling the early differentiation of viable from nonviable tissues in children with extensive peripheral gangrene from fulminant PF.[116] The authors found that the level of amputation was appropriately determined in 13 limbs, and surgical success was achieved in 84% of those limbs.

The final stage of care for these children involves a comprehensive multidisciplinary rehabilitation program with physical and occupational therapists, prosthetists, child life staff, and counselors. Close family support and an aggressive policy of encouraging a return to school are instrumental in the psychological and social readjustment of the child and family following this illness.[29]

NECROTIZING FASCIITIS

Necrotizing fasciitis is an infection involving the skin, subcutaneous tissues, and underlying fascia. It is characterized by widespread skin necrosis, bullae, and crepitation that progress despite treatment with intravenous antibiotics. The condition is frequently associated with systemic toxicity and septic shock. Rapid diagnosis and aggressive surgical management are necessary to reduce the mortality rate, which is reportedly as high as 59% to 73%.[42,184] Intervention within 4 days of disease onset has been shown to reduce mortality to 12%.[175,184]

Diagnosis can be facilitated by ultrasonography, CT, and MRI. Gas may be identified along the fascial planes, and deep fluid collections are noted adjacent to the fascia. Reports indicate that MRI is most useful for differentiating necrotizing fasciitis from cellulitis; it provides a detailed image of the deep fascial thickening, which enhances along with the intramuscular spaces following gadolinium injection.[28,175]

SOFT TISSUE ABSCESS AND SEPTIC BURSITIS

The diagnosis and treatment of soft tissue abscesses are straightforward. Most cases of septic prepatellar bursitis can be diagnosed on clinical examination alone. Occasionally, it is difficult to distinguish among cellulitis, abscess, septic arthritis, and osteomyelitis owing to the extent of soft tissue swelling and limited mobility that may accompany an abscess. In challenging cases, MRI with and without gadolinium enhancement is the preferred method to make the diagnosis and guide treatment.

Soft tissue abscesses typically appear as well-defined fluid collections with low T1 and high T2 signal, with a surrounding rim that enhances while the abscess fluid remains unenhanced following gadolinium administration (Fig. 35–17).[175] MRI confirms that adjacent bone and joint structures are uninvolved.

Abscess treatment is predominantly surgical, with incision and drainage in the most appropriate setting. Small prepatellar abscesses can be drained at the bedside with conscious sedation, whereas more extensive abscesses should be formally debrided in the operating room. Typically, children show rapid clinical and laboratory improvement following surgical decompression of an abscess. Sequential parenteral-to-oral antibiotic treatment is usually of brief duration, with 1 or 2 days of intravenous treatment followed by 2 weeks of oral medication. Antibiotic selection, however, is becoming more challenging in light of the significant increase in the incidence of MRSA in superficial abscesses, which is even higher than that in more invasive infections.[199,200] Oral clindamycin or trimethoprim-sulfamethoxazole has been recommended as empirical therapy for non–critically ill children without evidence of invasive infection in areas where CA-MRSA is commonly identified.[200] Concern exists about the eventual development of strains resistant to clindamycin, which necessitates the continued treatment of MSSA with a beta-lactam antibiotic.[200]

INFECTION IN CHALLENGING LOCATIONS

Spine

PYOGENIC INFECTIOUS SPONDYLITIS

Epidemiology

Infection of a disk space or the adjacent vertebral end-plates is rare in children. One report identified only one to two cases of diskitis per year in a hospital that evaluated 32,500 children annually.[63] Similarly, vertebral osteomyelitis accounts for only 1% to 2% of all cases of osteomyelitis.[75,96] Although these conditions may be defined separately, they likely represent virtually inseparable conditions that occur as a contiguous process in most affected children.[251,252,281] One series, however, reported on comparative differences between diskitis and vertebral osteomyelitis that may allow for their clinical distinction when diskitis is identified during its earliest stages.[86] In an 18-year retrospective review of 57 children with either diagnosis, the authors found that children with diskitis were younger (mean age 2.8 versus 7.5 years) and had symptoms for a shorter duration (22 versus 33 days) than children with vertebral osteomyelitis.[86] Another difference was the presence of fever (temperature >102°F) in 28% of children with diskitis versus 79% of children with osteomyelitis.[86] Regardless of this theoretical distinction, the evaluation and treatment of these processes are the same from the perspective of the orthopaedic surgeon.

The most common area of involvement is the lumbar spine at the L3-4 or L4-5 disk space, followed by the thoracic and cervical spine. *S. aureus* is the most common causative organism, identified in 50% to 67% of cases.[86,96,127] Other organisms associated with spinal infections include *K. kingae, M. tuberculosis, Bartonella henselae,* and *Salmonella* species.[86,127]

Pathophysiology

The pathogenesis of this condition is attributed to the bacterial seeding of either the disk space or the vertebral end-plate during episodes of transient bacteremia. Infants and young children up to age 7 years demonstrate the persistence of blood vessels that penetrate across the vertebral end-plate into the disk space and to the annulus fibrosus.[264] This finding lends support to the theory that younger children may selectively develop infection of the disk space without necessarily having infection of the adjacent vertebral end-plate. The end-organ circulation of the vertebral end-plate is analogous to that of the metaphyseal portion of long bones, whereby low flow through venous sinusoids may result in bacterial access to the extravascular space.[281]

A bacterial cause is suspected, despite positive cultures in only 30% to 50% of cases and the fact that children can recover from this condition without the

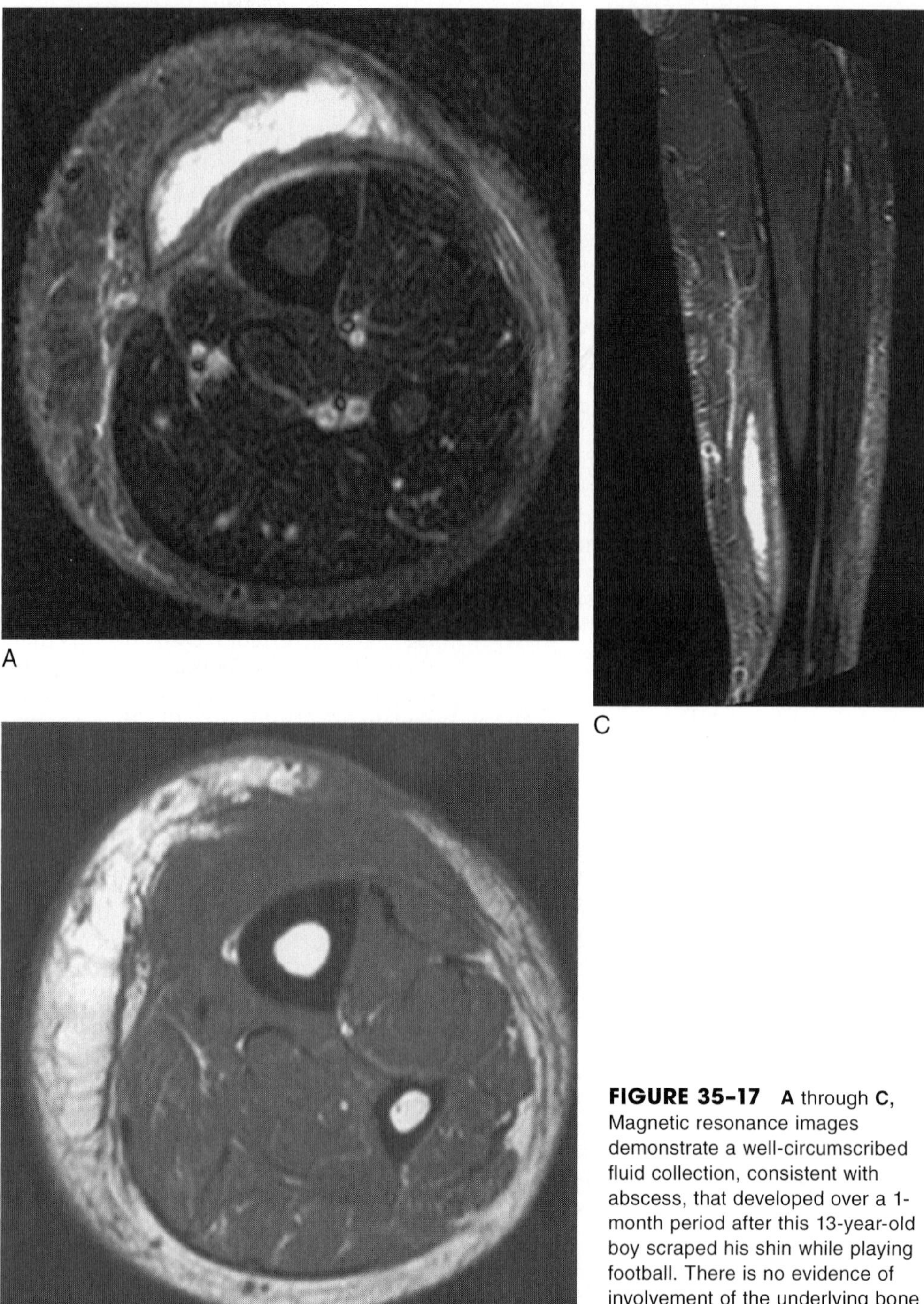

FIGURE 35–17 **A** through **C**, Magnetic resonance images demonstrate a well-circumscribed fluid collection, consistent with abscess, that developed over a 1-month period after this 13-year-old boy scraped his shin while playing football. There is no evidence of involvement of the underlying bone of the tibia.

use of antibiotics.[86,252] In one review of 47 children with pyogenic infectious spondylitis, a prolonged course or recurrence of symptoms was noted in 67% of those who did not receive antibiotics, 50% of those who were treated with oral antibiotics, and 18% of those treated with intravenous antibiotics.[252]

Evaluation

The diagnosis of infectious spondylitis is sometimes delayed owing to vague symptoms, the inability of young children to communicate clearly, and nonspecific physical findings. One series found an average delay of 2 months from the time of symptom onset to the time of definitive diagnosis.[281]

The initial assessment should include laboratory studies (CBC with differential, ESR, CRP, and blood cultures) and imaging. The selection of radiographic studies is influenced by the history and clinical examination (Fig. 35–18). Initially, I obtain plain radiographs of the spine to assess for disk space narrowing, perivertebral soft tissue swelling, and vertebral body

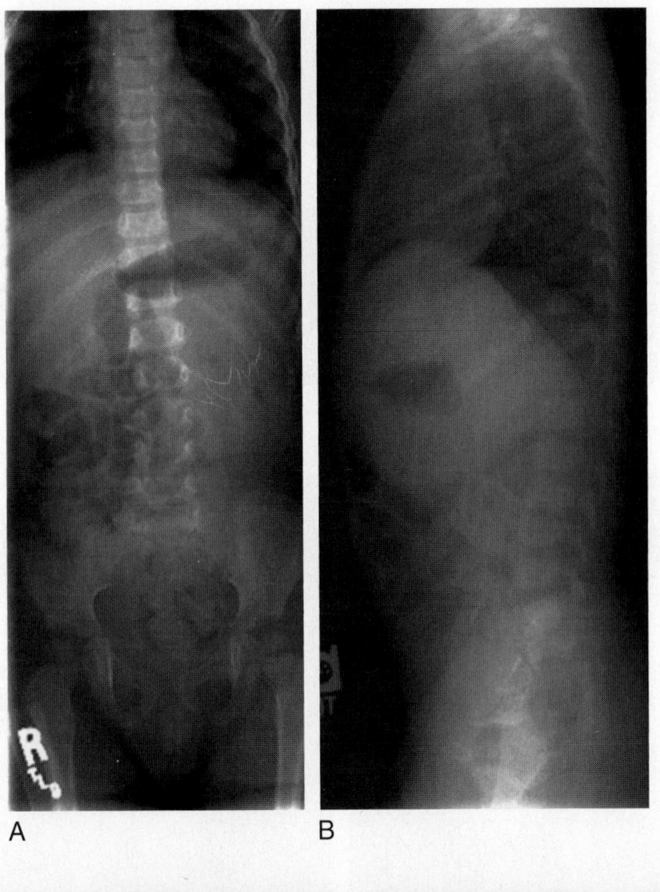

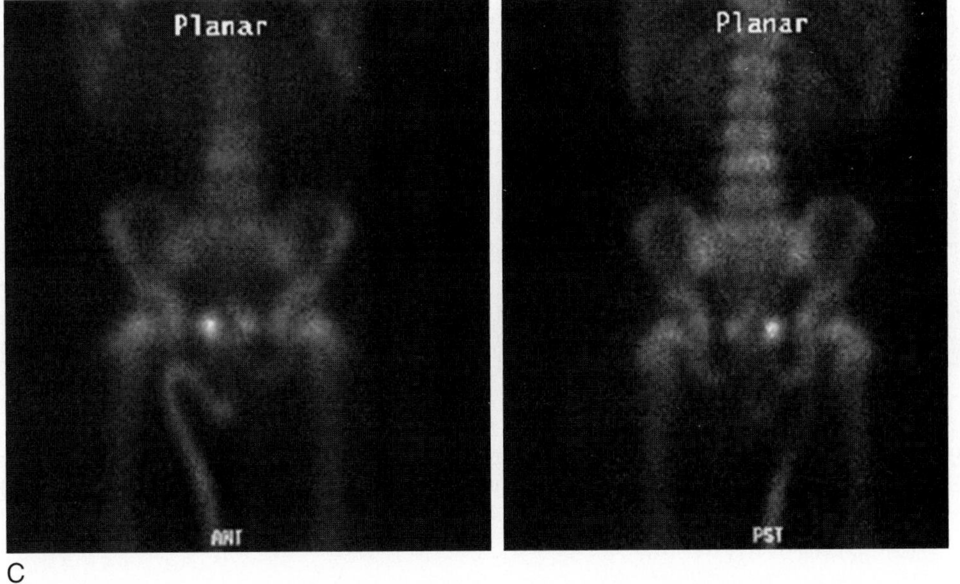

FIGURE 35–18 This 22-month-old girl presented with a 5-day history of refusal to walk and abdominal pain. The initial laboratory evaluation revealed C-reactive protein 1.8 mg/dL, erythrocyte sedimentation rate 43 mm/hour, and white blood cell count 8.2 cells/mL. Initial plain films of the pelvis **(A)** and spine **(B)** were interpreted as negative, although subtle disk space narrowing at L3-4 was noted retrospectively. Nuclear imaging **(C)** was obtained with single-photon emission computed tomography (SPECT) sequences of the spine **(D),** owing to the nonspecific clinical examination and the child's inability to communicate because of her age.

Continued

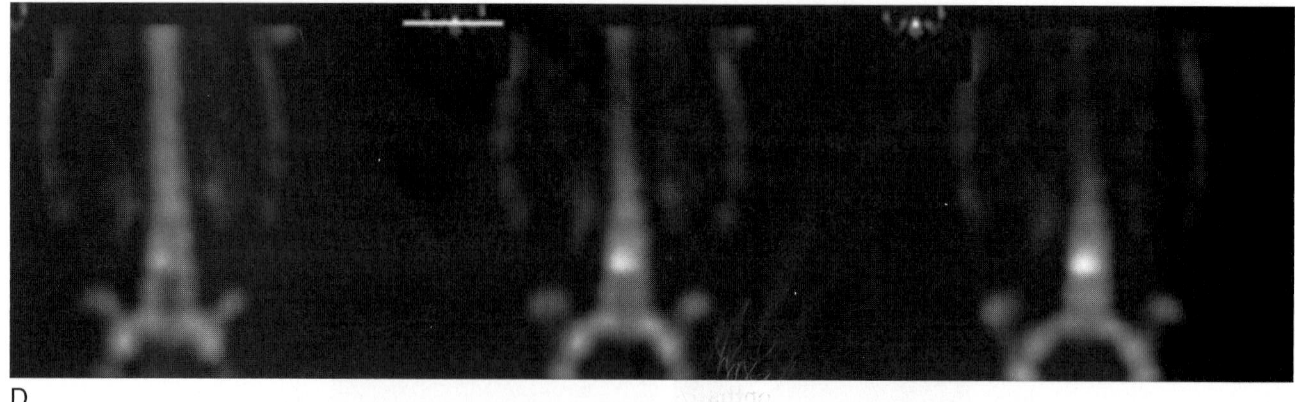

D

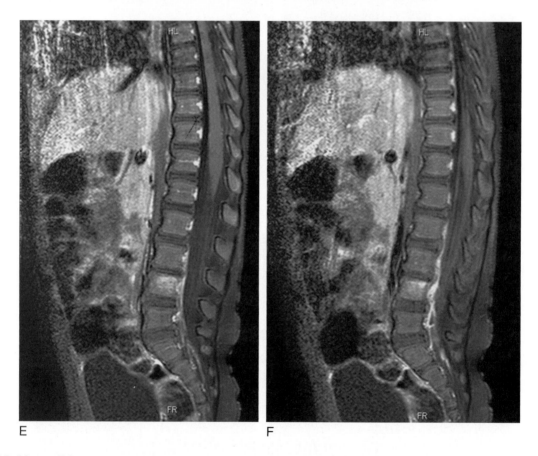

E F

FIGURE 35-18 cont'd The coronal SPECT images **(D)** clearly demonstrate the location of inflammation within the superior end-plate of L4. Magnetic resonance images **(E** and **F)** demonstrate findings consistent with diskitis and vertebral osteomyelitis, with no indication of abscess. The child improved with sequential parenteral-to-oral antibiotics and symptomatic support.

end-plate irregularities. If plain radiographs are negative, the exact location of inflammation is not clear from the physical examination, and infectious spondylitis is still a possibility, I obtain a three-phase total-body bone scan with single-photon emission CT sequences of the spine to enhance the study's diagnostic accuracy. If the overall clinical impression is highly suggestive of infectious spondylitis, I proceed immediately to MRI with and without gadolinium contrast. MRI has a sensitivity of 96% and a specificity of 93% in the diagnosis of vertebral osteomyelitis, which exceeds the overall accuracy of bone scintigraphy.[86,102,165] MRI demonstrates the anatomic and spatial extent of the infection and may rarely reveal intraosseous and perivertebral abscess formation, which might confound antibiotic treatment.

Treatment

Once the diagnosis is confirmed, empirical treatment with an appropriate antistaphylococcal antibiotic is begun. If blood cultures are positive, a more specific antibiotic is chosen based on the sensitivities. Biopsy is not recommended before the initiation of intravenous antibiotic therapy; the limited likelihood of positively identifying the causative organism is outweighed by the risk of the procedure. On rare occasions, when clinical and laboratory improvement is not apparent after a period of observation, CT-guided percutaneous biopsy may be considered.[127] In one report, bacteria were isolated in 22 of 35 specimens taken by needle aspiration of the disk space.[96]

The duration of antibiotic therapy should be approximately 4 to 6 weeks. Although the ESR may normalize within that time frame, prolonged elevation has been reported: up to 3.5 months for cervical, 6 months for thoracic, and 7 months for lumber osteomyelitis.[55] If necessary, the patient can use a removable orthosis to help alleviate symptoms during the acute treatment phase. There is no long-term need or biomechanical requirement for bracing.

Complications

Most children have a complete clinical recovery and return to all functional activities in the short term. Long-term follow-up has documented the persistence of disk space narrowing and vertebral end-plate irregularities that do not appear to reconstitute with time. One series reported frequent or daily backache in 10%, some backache in 22%, and restricted spinal extension in 85% of 35 children an average of 17 years after the treatment of infectious spondylitis.[148] These authors noted 26 cases of intervertebral fusion and 8 cases of marked disk space narrowing.

TUBERCULOUS SPONDYLITIS

Epidemiology

Tuberculous osteomyelitis most commonly involves the spine, with the lower thoracic and upper lumbar areas most commonly affected. The first description of tuberculosis of the spine is credited to Percivall Pott, hence the eponym Pott's disease (Fig. 35–19).[238] Skeletal lesions usually take at least a year to develop after the onset of the primary tuberculosis infection. The most frequent clinical signs and symptoms are low-grade fever, irritability, and restlessness, especially at night.[41] Children with tuberculous spondylitis usually present with back pain and stiffness.[41] They walk with a protective gait, taking light steps and keeping the back hyperextended.

Pathophysiology

The infection usually starts in the anterior third of the vertebral body near the end-plate, where blood perfusion and oxygen concentrations are highest. The

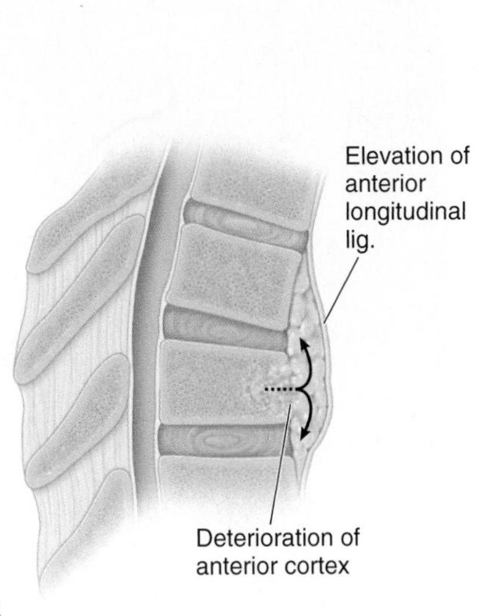

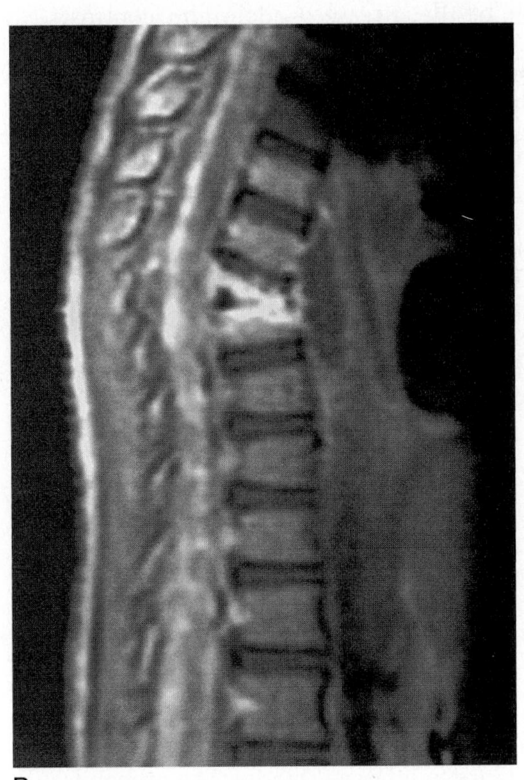

FIGURE 35–19 Pathogenesis of Pott's disease (tuberculosis of the spine). **A,** Infection egressing from bone elevates the anterior longitudinal ligament. **B,** Magnetic resonance image shows collapse of the anterior vertebral bodies and the intervening disk space, as well as abscess formation anteriorly.

formation of an abscess is the hallmark of spinal tuberculosis. Purulent material decompresses through the anterior cortex and spreads under the anterior longitudinal ligament. Often two contiguous vertebral bodies and the intervertebral disk are involved, but the infection may also skip levels. Kyphosis develops if bone destruction continues to the point of vertebral collapse. Untreated, the disease may progress to the point of spinal cord compression and paralysis, referred to as Pott's paraplegia. Caseous material may track along the psoas muscle and create a psoas abscess. Abscesses may also work their way to the skin surface and "point" in the groin or anterior chest wall. Cervical disease and abscess formation can lead to hoarseness (from compression of the recurrent laryngeal nerve), dysphagia, and stridor (Milar's asthma). Epidural abscess is more frequently associated with paralysis, which has been reported in up to 25% of cases.

Evaluation

Plain radiographs initially show radiolucency of the vertebral body. Paraspinal abscesses appear as fusiform shadows along the vertebral column on the anteroposterior radiograph and as an anterior soft tissue mass on the lateral radiograph. Late involvement is characterized by a sharply angled kyphosis or gibbus at the level of vertebral destruction. MRI is useful in differentiating tuberculous spondylitis from other types of vertebral osteomyelitis and in delineating the extent of the disease. Gadolinium contrast shows rim enhancement of the vertebral abscesses, which are more common and larger than those found in pyogenic infectious spondylitis.

The diagnosis of tubercular infection of the spine can be made by identifying acid-fast bacilli on Ziehl-Neelsen stain, by growing *M. tuberculosis* in culture, or by identifying the characteristic caseating granulomas on histologic examination. The tuberculin skin test is reactive in 80% to 90% of cases. Chest radiographs should be obtained whenever the skin test is positive. Surgical biopsy or CT-guided percutaneous biopsy of the area of spinal involvement is usually necessary to establish the diagnosis.

Treatment

Antibiotic Therapy. The first line of treatment is medical. Mycobacteria replicate slowly and can remain dormant in the body for prolonged periods. Subpopulations of drug-resistant organisms occur naturally in large bacterial populations, and the tubercle bacilli can be killed only while replicating during periods of metabolic activity.[286] For these reasons, single antimicrobial drugs cannot cure tuberculosis. Fortunately, resistance to a given antibiotic does not affect the likelihood of resistance to other antibiotics. The probability that a population of *M. tuberculosis* has natural resistance to two drugs simultaneously is virtually nonexistent. Children with spinal tuberculosis are usually treated with at least two drugs because they most likely have medium-sized populations in which significant numbers of drug-resistant organisms may be present.

The trend over the last 2 decades has been to develop antibiotic regimens that are increasingly intense and short. The American Academy of Pediatrics has endorsed a regimen of 6 months of isoniazid and rifampin supplemented during the first 2 months by pyrazinamide as the standard for pulmonary tuberculosis in children. Spinal tuberculosis, however, is associated with a higher failure rate when 6-month chemotherapy is used, especially if surgical intervention has not been performed. The American Academy of Pediatrics recommends at least 12 months of effective chemotherapy for skeletal tuberculosis, consisting of isoniazid, rifampin, pyrazinamide, and streptomycin for the first 2 months, followed by isoniazid and rifampin for the remaining 10 months of therapy.[249]

Surgery. The Medical Research Council Working Party on Tuberculosis of the Spine reported early bony fusion and less kyphosis when radical debridement and bone grafting were performed for spinal tuberculosis.[87] However, this group also acknowledged that ambulatory chemotherapy has yielded very good results and recommended this course of treatment if adequate surgical facilities were lacking.[60,88] Most investigators agree that surgical decompression should be reserved for new or progressive neurologic deficits, marked spinal instability, and failure of medical treatment (Fig. 35–20). When surgery is necessary, I

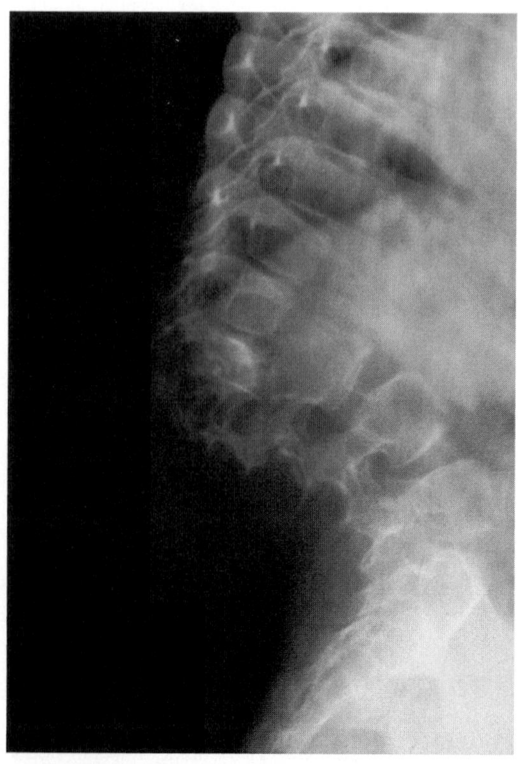

FIGURE 35–20 Kyphotic deformity of the lumbar spine secondary to tuberculosis.

perform the operations under the "umbrella" of optimal chemotherapy. I prefer an anterior approach for decompression of spinal lesions, with adequate autogenous grafting. If the infection does not extend to the posterior spinal elements, the addition of posterior spinal fusion with instrumentation can be helpful in treating extensive spinal lesions and those associated with spinal instability. Laminectomy should be avoided, particularly in the cervical spine, because the procedure is associated with increasing kyphotic deformity and progressive neurologic deterioration.

Pelvis

A variety of infections may involve the pelvic region, including osteomyelitis of the ilium, ischium, or pubis; osteomyelitis of the ischiopubic synchondrosis; septic arthritis of the hip or sacroiliac joint; and septic bursitis involving the iliopsoas bursa or the greater trochanteric bursa.[69,125,138,215,227,287,289] Pyomyositis has been reported in several pelvic muscles, including the adductors, gemelli, gluteus maximus, iliacus, psoas, obturator internus, and piriformis.[72,123,226,230,279,294,295,310,328] Pelvic osteomyelitis accounts for 2.5% to 6.3% of all cases of osteomyelitis.[138,215] Chiedozi reported that the gluteus muscles are the second most common site of involvement, accounting for 35 of 205 cases of pyomyositis.[44] Other pelvic infections, though considered rare, have been noted in an accumulation of case reports, making it difficult to estimate their overall incidence.

The ischiopubic synchondrosis, though not commonly infected, has received attention owing to its peculiar features and various patterns of asymmetric ossification, which may be mistaken for trauma, tumor, or infection (Fig. 35–21). Because the bone in this region resembles a metaphyseal equivalent, with end-arterial circulation leading to sharp loops and venous sinusoids, the site is ideal for hematogenous osteomyelitis.[138] Further, because several pelvic muscles, including the adductors and the perisciatic muscles, originate in this area, infection can rapidly involve them.[123] The synchondrosis usually closes at 9 to 11 years of age, with irregular ossification most frequently noted between 5 and 8 years of age—corresponding to the peak age of incidence of osteomyelitis in this location.[138]

The diverse presentation of pelvic infections and the deceptive nature of symptoms frequently lead to diagnostic confusion and delay. Physical findings may be suggestive of other more common problems around the hip, such as transient synovitis or septic arthritis. The clinical presentation of pelvic osteomyelitis can be divided into three common patterns or syndromes. The lumbar syndrome results from irritation of the lumbosacral plexus and manifests as pain in the back, hip, or thigh. The gluteal syndrome results from a subgluteal abscess and creates buttock pain. Finally, the abdominal syndrome, which mimics an acute abdomen, results from irritation of the peritoneum near a site of iliac inflammation.[69] One series of 64 children with pelvic osteomyelitis found the lumbar syndrome in 51 (80%), the gluteal syndrome in 8 (13%), and the abdominal syndrome in 3 (5%).[69]

Most authors agree that an infection suspected of having a pelvic origin should be evaluated early with MRI to yield the greatest likelihood of an accurate diagnosis.[72,123,138,226,230,287,294,310,328] MRI with and without gadolinium can be essential in guiding treatment as well. In one case, MRI identification of ischiopubic osteomyelitis associated with pyomyositis involving the obturator internus and piriformis guided my surgical approach to decompress the abscess, which was not easily reached, and supported the decision for a longer duration of antibiotics to resolve the osteomyelitis, which would not otherwise require surgical debridement.

Pyogenic infection of the sacroiliac joint is more common in late childhood. Children may complain of pain in the back, hip, or leg. Physical findings include a positive Patrick or FABER test (pain with flexion, abduction, and external rotation of the hip). *S. aureus* is the most common organism, but *M. tuberculosis* and *Brucella* species have also been identified. Most authors report successful results with a 3- to 6-week regimen of antibiotics alone. Surgical decompression is reserved for cases in which an abscess or sequestrum is present. Long-term sequelae are rare, even though most patients have residual radiographic "sclerosis" of the sacroiliac joint.[287]

Foot

Infections of the foot may be challenging to evaluate and manage. Diagnostic delay is common and may lead to adverse outcomes. Two common infections encountered in the foot are hematogenous calcaneal osteomyelitis and infections derived from puncture wounds.

HEMATOGENOUS CALCANEAL OSTEOMYELITIS

The calcaneus accounts for approximately 8% of all cases of osteomyelitis in children, with up to 63% occurring secondary to hematogenous seeding.[140,318] There appears to be an even distribution of cases among children 1 to 14 years of age.[241] Bacteria selectively lodge in the metaphyseal-equivalent region of the posterior tuberosity of the calcaneus adjacent to the apophysis, where the vascular anatomy mimics that of the metaphysis of a long bone. One review of 63 cases found that the most common causative organism was *S. aureus* (48%), followed by GABHS and other *Streptococcus* species (11%); no organisms were identified in 35% of cases.[241]

Diagnostic delay is common owing to unimpressive signs and symptoms and often marginally abnormal laboratory results.[140,241,245,318] Unfortunately, a delay in treatment has been associated with apophyseal plate destruction, with secondary growth arrest and permanent deformity of the involved calcaneus (Fig. 35–22).[140] Cole and associates showed that 92% of children treated within 48 hours of onset were cured; only 25%

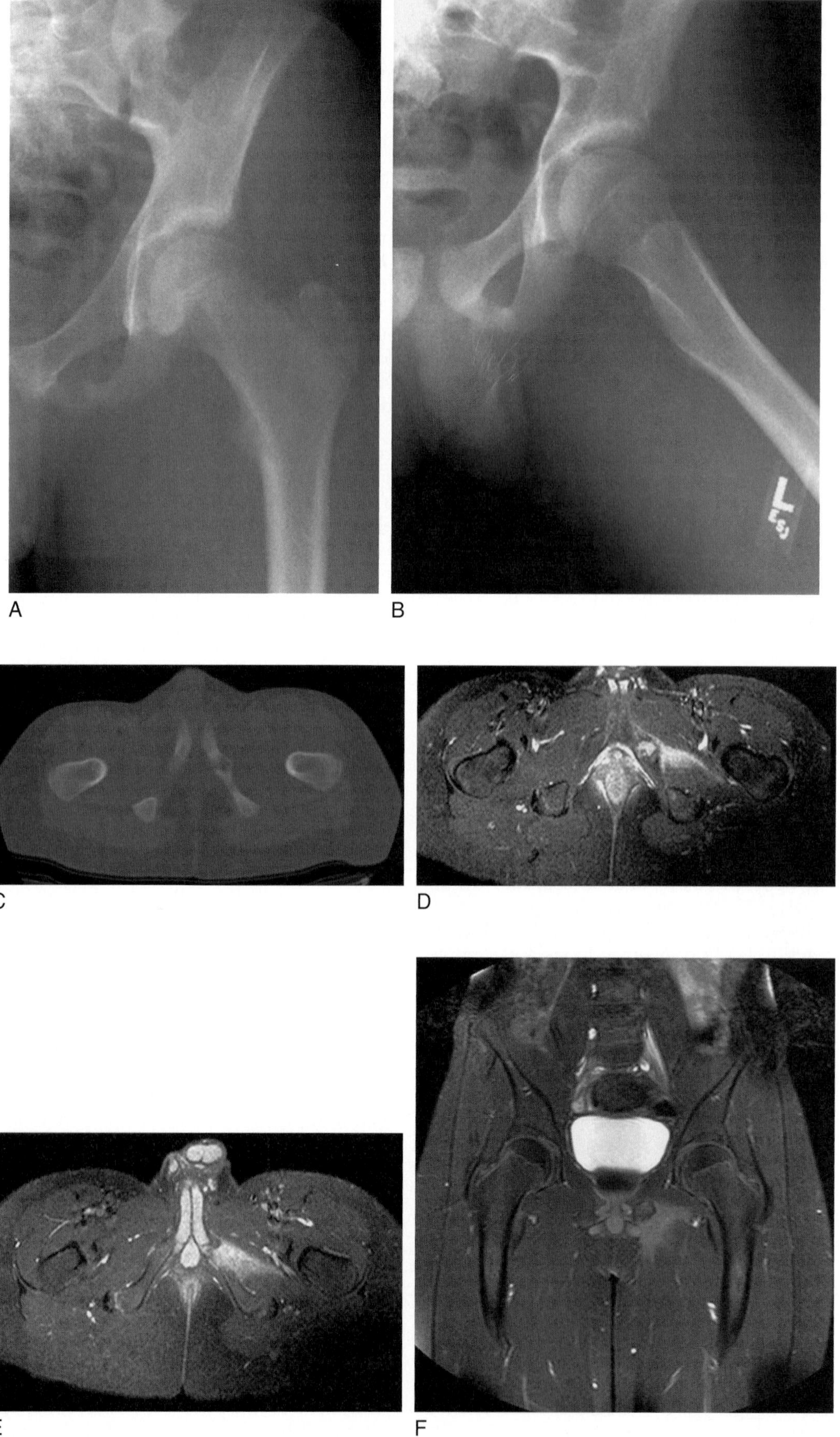

FIGURE 35-21 Thirteen-year-old boy with a 2-day history of left groin and thigh pain, limp, and fever. The initial laboratory evaluation revealed C-reactive protein 5.2 mg/dL, erythrocyte sedimentation rate 37 mm/hour, and white blood cell count 20,000 cells/mL. **A** and **B,** Plain radiographs demonstrate enlargement of the ischiopubic synchondrosis. **C,** Computed tomography scan reveals enlargement and lucency of the ischiopubic synchondrosis, consistent with osteomyelitis. **D** to **F,** Magnetic resonance images reveal osteomyelitis of the ischiopubic synchondrosis with associated myositis.

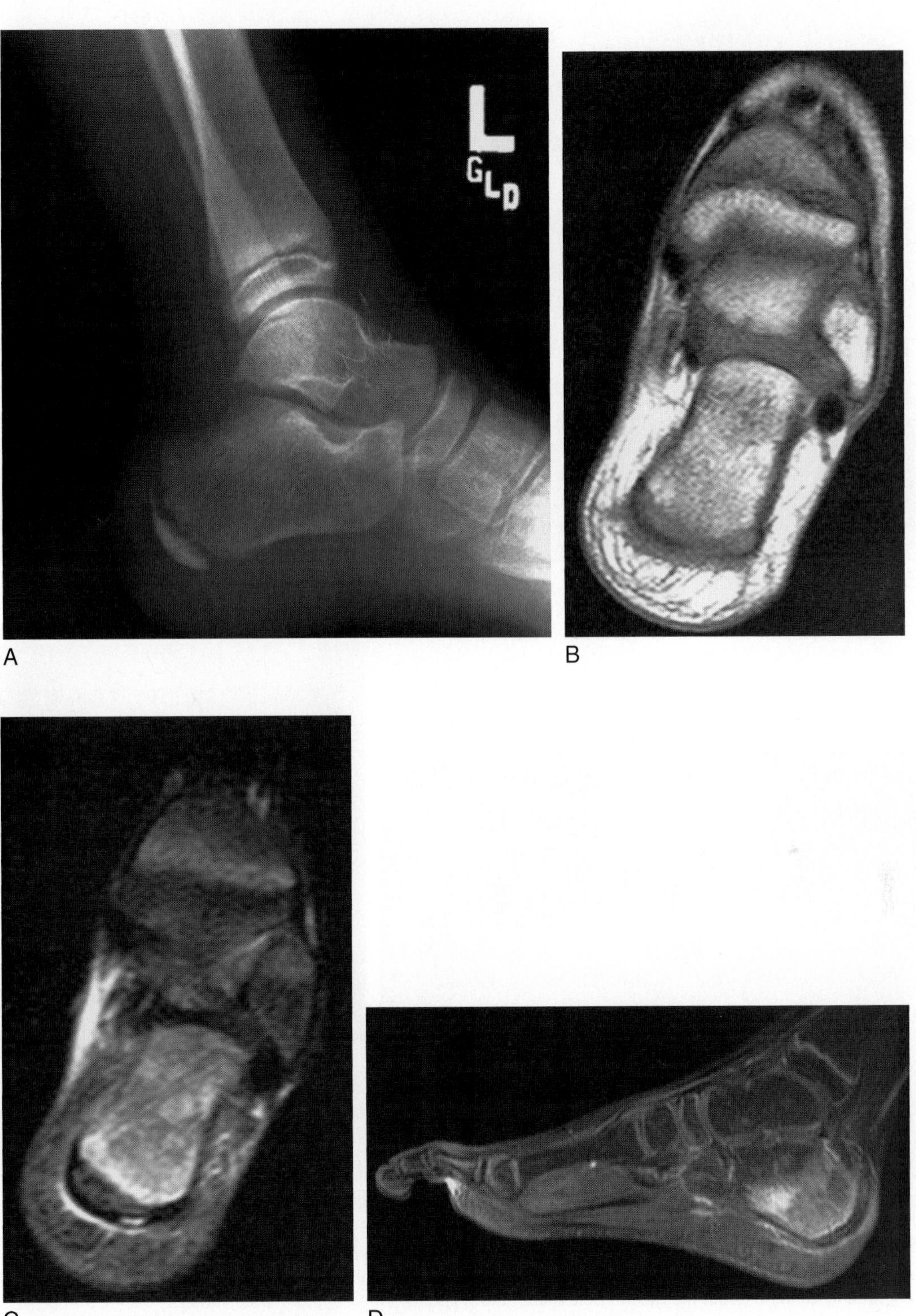

FIGURE 35-22 Seven-year-old girl with a 7-day history of foot pain and limp. The initial laboratory evaluation demonstrated C-reactive protein 6.7 mg/dL, erythrocyte sedimentation rate 72 mm/hour, and white blood cell count 8,600 cells/mL. **A,** Initial plain radiograph shows increased radiodensity of the calcaneal apophysis. **B** to **D,** Subsequent magnetic resonance images show marrow signal enhancement adjacent to the calcaneal apophysis, consistent with osteomyelitis, and no abscess. The patient was treated with intravenous and then oral antibiotics and had laboratory improvement.

Continued

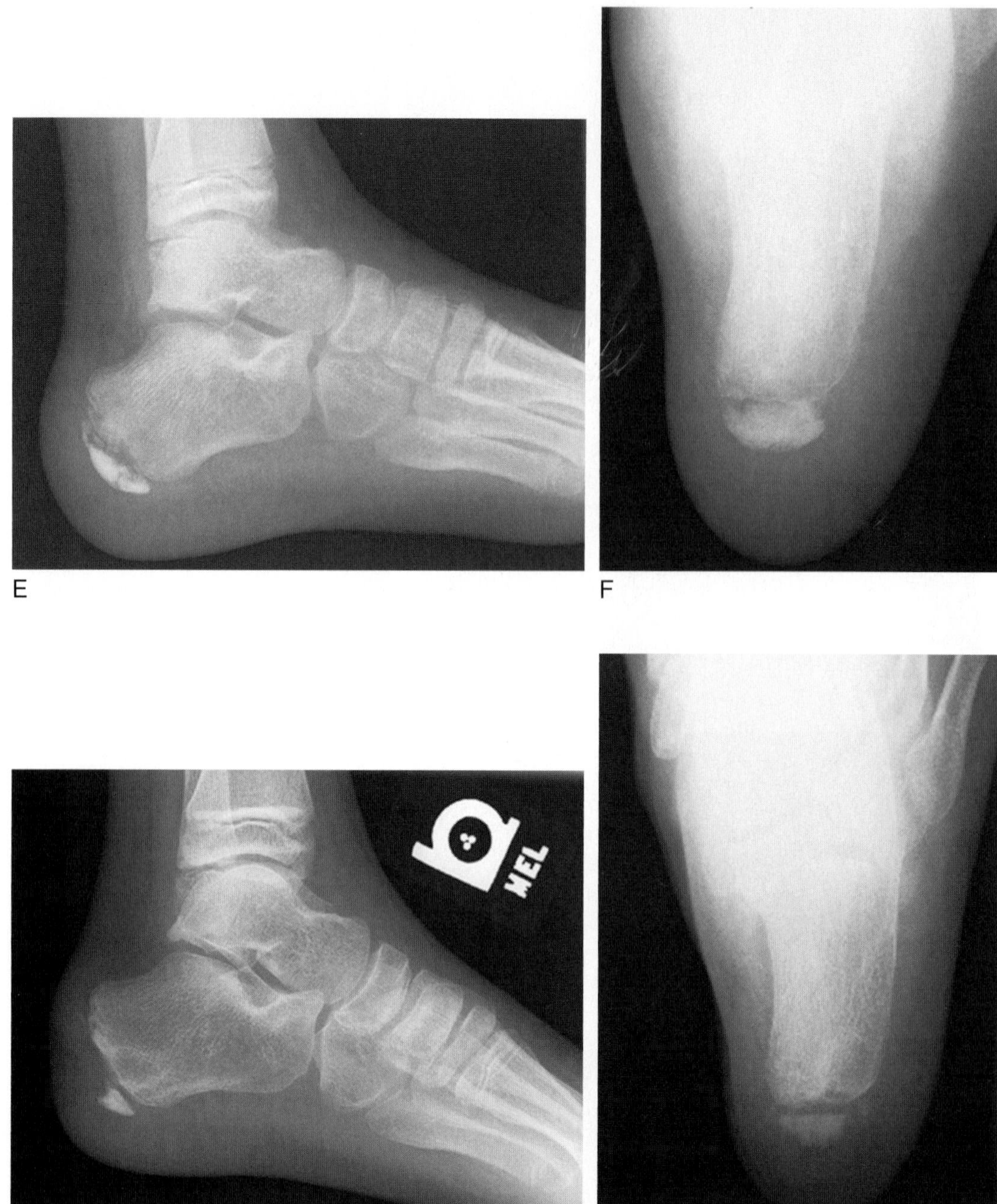

FIGURE 35-22 cont'd **E** and **F**, Clinical examination and follow-up radiographs suggest the presence of an abscess, which required surgical incision and debridement. **G** and **H**, Follow-up radiographs taken 2 months later lead to concern about the growth potential of the posterior tuberosity of the calcaneus.

of children were cured without surgery when the diagnosis was delayed by more than 5 days.[54] Bone scintigraphy is useful to confirm the diagnosis of calcaneal osteomyelitis when plain radiographs are negative but the condition is suspected clinically. Indications for surgery include the identification of abscess, either radiographically or on aspiration, and failure to improve after 24 to 48 hours of appropriate intravenous antibiotics. MRI has proved helpful in identifying abscess formation within the calcaneus, which may prompt early surgical intervention in borderline cases.

PLANTAR PUNCTURE WOUNDS

Puncture wounds of the feet are common in children, accounting for 0.81% of pediatric emergency room visits. The sources of injury include nails (98%), wood, metal, glass, and toothpicks.[80,137] Only a small number of puncture wounds progress to superficial or deep infection. Recommendations for the acute care of puncture wounds range from simple wound care and tetanus prophylaxis to empirical prophylactic antibiotic therapy with an antistaphylococcal drug.

Children in whom superficial or deep infections develop after puncture wounds of the foot typically complain of pain and swelling 2 to 5 days after the injury, at which point in uncomplicated cases symptoms have usually resolved. In one series of 80 children admitted to a hospital because of plantar punctures, 59 had cellulitis, 11 had retained foreign bodies, and 10 had deep infections with osteomyelitis or septic arthritis.[80] A delay in presentation longer than 1 week was associated with deep infection, thought to be related to the depth of initial penetration, and the need for surgery. In children with retained foreign body after a toothpick puncture, the challenge is to identify an object that is not radiographically apparent. Ultrasonography and MRI proved useful in identifying the toothpick in a series of five children who were evaluated for this injury.[137]

Children with cellulitis usually respond to elevation of the foot and antistaphylococcal antibiotics. *Pseudomonas aeruginosa* is the most common pathogen associated with osteomyelitis, osteochondritis, and septic arthritis complicating puncture wounds of the foot.[147] Toothpick injuries have been associated with infection from *Eikenella corrodens*.[137] Children with obvious deep infection and those who fail to improve with empirical antibiotic therapy are treated with surgery. I favor a plantar approach because it allows easier debridement of the puncture tract. After surgical debridement, most cases can be managed successfully with sequential parenteral-to-oral antibiotic therapy.

P. aeruginosa has a predilection to infect cartilage following puncture wounds. Successful treatment in cases of osteochondritis should include surgical debridement followed by 1 to 2 weeks of an antipseudomonal antibiotic.[80,147] The use of oral fluoroquinolone antibiotics (e.g., ciprofloxacin) in children is controversial. For many years, quinolone-induced cartilage toxicity, observed in experiments with skeletally immature animals, was considered a contraindication to the use of these agents in children. However, accruing data indicate the safety and effectiveness of ciprofloxacin in children.[269]

Systemic Diseases Associated with Infection

Sickle Cell Disease

Children with sickle cell disease are more susceptible to osteomyelitis and septic arthritis because of multiple factors, including functional asplenia, frequent tissue infarction, and poor opsonization of polysaccharide antigens from impaired complement activity.[40] The annual incidence of osteomyelitis in sickle cell patients ranges from 0.2% to 5% of those who present with musculoskeletal pain or crisis. In one retrospective review at a pediatric sickle cell clinic with more than 2000 enrolled children, only 10 cases of osteomyelitis and 4 cases of septic arthritis were identified in a 22-year period.[40] The association of sickle cell anemia with *Salmonella* osteomyelitis has been well documented.[13,31,40,64,175,236] A review of the world literature, including nine reported series from 1975 to 1996, clearly established that *Salmonella* is a more common cause of osteomyelitis in patients with sickle cell disease than is *S. aureus*, by an overall ratio of 2.2 : 1.[31] The probable site of entry for *Salmonella* is the intestinal wall, as microinfarctions allow the organism to gain access to the circulation.

Clinical, laboratory, and radiographic findings in children with pain from crisis are often indistinguishable from the findings in those with symptoms from infection. Despite this fact, several recent studies have suggested that improved diagnostic accuracy may be attained by using a variety of radiographic techniques, including ultrasonography, sequential radionuclide bone marrow and bone scans, and gadolinium-enhanced MRI, to distinguish between bone infarct and osteomyelitis in children with sickle cell disease.[23,266,275,303] Ultrasound findings suggestive of infection include subperiosteal fluid collection greater than 10 mm at its thickest point, periosteal thickening, cortical destruction, and intraosseous hypoechoic regions suggestive of abscess.[23,266] Ultrasonography has been used to facilitate aspiration by directing the needle to the area of greatest fluid accumulation, which is likely to yield a suitable sample for culture.[23,266] Sequential bone marrow and bone scanning indicates osteomyelitis when there is normal uptake on the marrow scan but abnormal uptake on the bone scan.[275] This finding helped identify 4 cases of osteomyelitis among 79 children with sickle cell disease who had episodes of acute bone pain.[275] Finally, distinctive findings on gadolinium-enhanced MRI include irregular and geographic marrow enhancement and subtle cortical defects, with traversing signal between the marrow and soft tissue in cases of osteomyelitis, in contrast to the thin, linear rim enhancement in cases of bone infarct.[303]

Because sickle cell patients are approximately 50 times more likely to be in vaso-occlusive crisis than to have infection, and because there are few objective clinical findings or tests to make the distinction, these children should initially be treated for crisis with hydration, analgesics, and oxygen while withholding antibiotics. Laboratory screening is performed for infection, along with serial clinical examinations. If there is no improvement within 24 to 48 hours of conservative observation, all suspected foci should be aspirated, and empirical antibiotics should be initiated. Initial antibiotic therapy should cover both *S. aureus* and *Salmonella* species until cultures confirm the specific organism. *Salmonella* species are responsive to ampicillin, trimethoprim-sulfamethoxazole, and ceftriaxone. Surgery is indicated if gross pus is aspirated or if an abscess is suspected on the basis of radiographic studies. Chambers and colleagues advocated a similar approach but added that an ill appearance, fever higher than 38.2°C, pain, and swelling should prompt early aspiration or biopsy, regardless of other findings.[40]

Recommendations for surgical debridement vary, with some authors reporting improved outcomes with surgery and others reporting good results with nonsurgical management. Because these children have an impaired immune status, they are even more prone to complications when treatment is delayed. Therefore, I perform early surgical intervention when there is no clinical improvement within 24 to 48 hours after the initiation of appropriate antibiotic therapy and aggressive medical management of the underlying sickle cell disease. The use of a tourniquet in patients with sickle cell disease has been considered contraindicated because the ischemia may lead to intravascular thrombosis; however, the safe use of tourniquets during surgery on these children has been reported.[1]

Chronic Granulomatous Disease

Chronic granulomatous disease (CGD) is a rare inherited immunodeficiency disorder in which phagocytic cells are unable to kill catalase-positive bacteria and fungi after ingesting them. Consequently, children with CGD have an increased susceptibility to infection. In October 1992, the Immune Deficiency Foundation began a registry of U.S. residents with CGD to document the prevalence of the condition and the nature and incidence of infectious manifestations in this population; a total of 368 patients were entered into the registry between November 1993 and September 1997.[327] Approximately 14 to 18 infants are born with CGD each year, with an incidence of approximately 1 in 250,000 live births. Patterns of inheritance include X-linked recessive (70%) and autosomal recessive (22%). The majority of patients are diagnosed before 5 years of age (76%), with a greater diagnostic delay reported in the autosomal recessive group.[327]

The most common causative organisms are *Aspergillus* species (41%), *Staphylococcus* species (12%), *Burkholderia cepacia* (8%), *Nocardia* species (7%), and *Mycobacterium* species (4%). The most common types of infection include pneumonia, abscess (subcutaneous, liver, lung, and perirectal), suppurative adenitis, osteomyelitis, and cellulitis. Osteomyelitis was reported in 90 of the 368 registered patients with CGD (24%).[327]

Common treatments include prophylactic antibiotic therapy with trimethoprim-sulfamethoxazole or dicloxacillin, interferon gamma, and granulocyte transfusion. Episodes of infection in children with CGD are treated with standard medical and surgical methods. The mortality of this condition is reportedly greater than 17%.[327]

Human Immunodeficiency Virus

The prevalence of infection in children with HIV in the United States is estimated to be 5.6 per 100,000 population, compared with 125.7 per 100,000 in adults.[110] Children infected with HIV are prone to develop a variety of musculoskeletal disorders, including infection. Sometimes these conditions may be the initial manifestation of the underlying immune deficiency.[292] Characteristic musculoskeletal infections in children who are HIV positive include septic arthritis, osteomyelitis, pyomyositis, bacillary angiomatosis, and tuberculous osteomyelitis.[21,292]

Septic arthritis is the most prevalent form of musculoskeletal infection in HIV-positive patients, followed by osteomyelitis.[292] Although *S. aureus* is the most common bacterium isolated, the spectrum of causative organisms is much broader than in HIV-negative patients, attesting to the opportunistic nature of these infections. The same is true for osteomyelitis, which can be caused by *Salmonella* species, *Nocardia asteroides, S. pneumoniae, N. gonorrhoeae,* cytomegalovirus, *Aspergillus* species, *Toxoplasma gondii, Torulopsis glabrata, Cryptococcus neoformans,* and *Coccidioides immitis.*[292] Osteomyelitis is associated with a mortality rate above 20% in HIV-infected patients. Pyomyositis tends to occur late in the course of HIV infection, with CD4 counts of less than 200 cells/μL.[292]

Bacillary angiomatosis is a multisystem infectious disease caused by *Bartonella henselae* and *Bartonella quintana.*[306] This condition is characterized by vascular proliferation, lymphadenitis, and an associated osteomyelitis in up to one third of individuals.[21,292] The prevalence of tuberculosis is reported to be up to 500 times greater in HIV-infected persons than in uninfected persons.[21,292] The skeletal tuberculosis lesions in immunocompetent children are usually solitary, whereas a multicentric distribution is noted in about 30% of HIV-positive individuals.[122,292] Atypical mycobacterial infections usually produce multifocal musculoskeletal infections during advanced stages of the disease, with CD4 counts of less than 100 cells/μL.[292] *M. avium-intracellulare* complex is the most commonly identified atypical mycobacterial organism among those infected with HIV.[292]

Laboratory Studies

Complete Blood Count

The CBC with differential is a necessary screening study that should be performed in any child with musculoskeletal pain and functional loss suggestive of infection. Kocher and coworkers identified a WBC count greater than 12,000 cells/mL as one of four risk factors for septic arthritis.[172,173] The differential cell count is useful for identifying an increase in the production and release of immature neutrophils (bands), which occurs in the presence of infection. Although only 25% to 35% of children with AHO have elevated WBCs on admission, the study allows an assessment of all three marrow cell lines that may be affected by disorders that interfere with their production, such as leukemia.[153,256] Lymphoblasts may also be detected when the differential is performed manually.[153]

Erythrocyte Sedimentation Rate

The ESR represents the rate at which red blood cells fall through plasma, measured in millimeters per hour. The serum concentration of fibrinogen, an acute phase reactant released by the liver in response to a variety of inflammatory conditions, is the most significant determinant of the ESR.[92] Infection incites an increase in the ESR, which gradually increases to a mean peak value of 58 mm/hour within 3 to 5 days of the onset of infection.[164,304] The value slowly returns to normal within 3 weeks following effective treatment in uncomplicated cases.[164,304] Because the ESR is greatly influenced by the number, size, and shape of erythrocytes, as well as by other plasma constituents, there is significant variation in measured levels, which may be misleading.[92] The ESR should not be significantly elevated in response to trauma.

C-Reactive Protein

C-reactive protein, an acute phase reactant synthesized in the liver, was named for its reaction with the pneumococcal C-polysaccharide in the plasma of patients during the acute phase of pneumonia.[297] Initial laboratory testing, performed in the 1940s and 1950s, could not quantify CRP and was therefore unable to guide treatment decisions.[91] As a result, clinical interest in CRP waned, and ESR became the preferred test for detecting inflammation. However, in the 1970s and 1980s, there was a resurgence in interest in CRP when rapid quantitative measurement techniques became available.[91] With further advances in technology, laser nephelometric assays have enabled the measurement of CRP in the picogram range, within an hour, using only a finger-stick sample of blood.[91,92,150,304,305] Currently, CRP is considered the most sensitive and reliable clinical laboratory test for detecting acute inflammatory reactions or changes in the severity of such reactions.[91,144,305] One study evaluated 77 febrile children (temperature >39°C) who presented to a pediatric emergency department over a 10-month period and found CRP to be superior to WBC count and absolute neutrophil count in detecting children with serious bacterial infection.[242] The authors found that a CRP less than 5.0 mg/dL effectively ruled out serious bacterial infection with a predictive probability of only 1.9%.

In the presence of an inciting infection, CRP levels increase 1000-fold within 6 hours of onset and reach a peak within 36 to 50 hours.[92,304] In one series, CRP values were elevated in 98% of children with AHO at the time of admission, with a mean value of 7.1 mg/dL and a peak value of 8.3 mg/dL, which was reached on day 2.[304] Because of the short half-life of CRP (24 to 48 hours) and constant clearance rate, rapid resolution to normal commonly occurs within 7 days following effective treatment in uncomplicated cases.[305] More recent work showed that a peak CRP level was reached on day 1 (range, 0 to 7 days), with normalization occurring on day 11 (range, 0 to 31 days), in a series of 50 children with bone and joint infections.[164]

Serial CRP determinations combined with repeated clinical evaluations are helpful in identifying sequela-prone children with contiguous septic arthritis and osteomyelitis.[144,256,305] One study found that if the CRP level on the third day of treatment was more than 1.5 times the level at the time of admission, the child was 6.5 time more likely to have a combined bone and joint infection.[305] Given the ease of monitoring CRP and its potential value in altering clinical decision making, it is reasonable to obtain daily or every-other-day serum levels during the early course of treatment to help identify sequela-prone children.

The test characteristics of CRP have been assessed with respect to the ability to differentiate septic arthritis and transient synovitis, with mixed results. A study at Children's Hospital of Philadelphia found CRP to be a better negative predictor than positive predictor of disease, although overall, it is a better independent predictor than ESR.[181] In a series of 133 children with synovial fluid aspiration sent for culture, the sensitivity of CRP ranged from 41% (CRP > 10.5 mg/dL) to 90% (CRP > 1 mg/dL). Even with a normal CRP (<1 mg/dL), the authors found that the probability that the child did not have septic arthritis was only 87%.[181]

Jung and colleagues included CRP greater than 1 mg/dL in a multivariate regression analysis, along with body temperature greater than 37°C, ESR greater than 20 mm/hour, WBC count greater than 11,000/mm^3, and increased hip joint space greater than 2 mm.[155] They reported a 99.1% predictive probability of septic arthritis when all five predictors were present and a 90.9% probability when CRP was less than 1 mg/dL but the other four predictors were positive.

CRP may be elevated in response to surgery and trauma, with the highest response reported in patients with tibia fractures undergoing open reduction and internal fixation with plates, followed by closed intramedullary nailing; the lowest values were reported in those treated conservatively.[159] Despite this phenomenon, Unkila-Kallio and coworkers did not find that surgery had a significant influence on CRP levels in children with osteomyelitis or septic arthritis.[305]

Interleukin-6

Interleukin-6, which is released by local tissue monocytes and fibroblasts in response to infection, is thought to be the cytokine that most influences the hepatic production of CRP.[92,305] It is hypothesized that IL-6 may be detectable in the blood even earlier than CRP during the course of bacterial infection and may thereby enable earlier diagnosis and treatment.[30] Factors that limit the utility of measuring cytokines in the plasma include their short half-lives, the presence of blocking factors and binding proteins, and negative inhibition feedback through an autoregulatory cycle.[30,92] Although high cost, limited availability, and lack of standardization prevent the measurement of plasma cytokine levels in current clinical practice, further research may change this. Buck and colleagues demonstrated the clinical benefit of detecting the presence of IL-6 in newborns with blood culture–positive sepsis, with 100% sensitivity.[30] The authors also found that the presence of IL-6 on admission in this group of septic neonates was more sensitive than the CRP level (73% versus 58%).

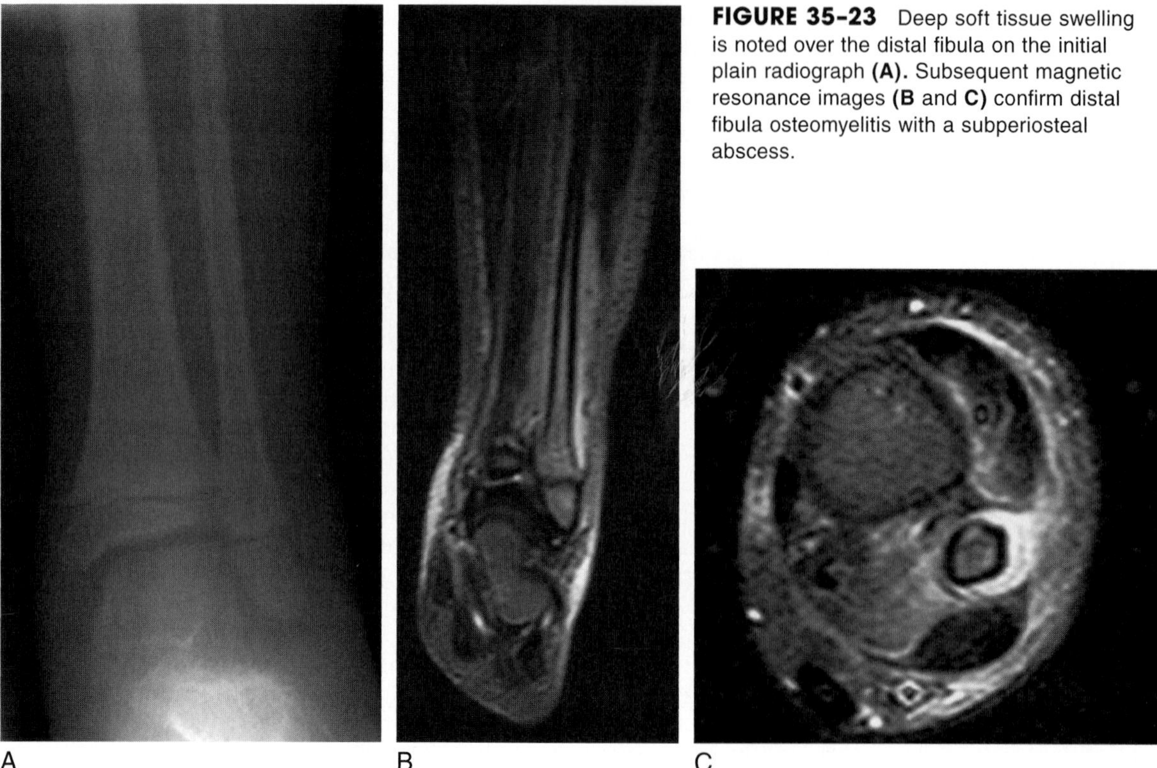

FIGURE 35–23 Deep soft tissue swelling is noted over the distal fibula on the initial plain radiograph **(A).** Subsequent magnetic resonance images **(B** and **C)** confirm distal fibula osteomyelitis with a subperiosteal abscess.

RADIOGRAPHIC STUDIES

Plain Radiography

The greatest value of plain radiographs is to exclude focal disease, such as tumor or trauma, that might otherwise explain the clinical presentation of a child with pain and functional limitation who is suspected of having infection. High-quality plain radiographs in at least two planes are essential and should be obtained with a technique that allows visualization of the deep soft tissues. With modern digital and computerized systems, it is possible to adjust the contrast and intensity on the viewing monitor to more clearly visualize the deep soft tissues and skeletal detail regardless of the method of film acquisition, which is a significant advantage.

Radiographs should be closely inspected for lytic or sclerotic lesions of bone, periosteal elevation or calcification, osteopenia, joint effusions, and cortical disruption. Deep soft tissue swelling is the first radiographic manifestation of musculoskeletal infection (Fig. 35–23).[175,193] Obvious changes within the bone secondary to osteomyelitis may not occur until 10 to 14 days after the onset of infection and after the loss of 30% to 50% of the bone mineral density at the site of infection.

Although plain radiographs are required in all diagnostic evaluations of infection, subsequent studies must be carefully considered in light of the expense, delay in definitive treatment, possible requirement for sedation, radiation exposure, and likelihood of yielding an accurate diagnosis. The decision about which supplemental studies are appropriate should be made in consultation with a radiologist who is knowledgeable of a given facility's capabilities. This practice can also facilitate the interpretation of the selected studies, because the radiologist will be better informed about the child's clinical history.

Ultrasonography

Ultrasonography is most commonly used in the evaluation of septic arthritis of the hip joint (Fig. 35–24). This study may also be used in the setting of vague symptoms related to the pelvic region to assess for the presence of a psoas abscess.[156] Advantages of ultrasonography are its low cost, absence of radiation exposure, noninvasive nature without the need for sedation, and ability to detect and localize fluid collections for aspiration.

The detection of intra-articular fluid often helps guide decision making with regard to the need for aspiration, conservative observation, or further imaging in children with an irritable hip.[12,36,101,186] When a technically adequate study has been performed in a child whose symptoms have been present for at least 24 hours, the false-negative rate of hip ultrasonography is so low as to virtually exclude the diagnosis of septic arthritis.[106] One report noted that 4 of 59 ultrasound studies (7%) were initially interpreted as negative, despite a subsequent diagnosis of confirmed septic arthritis.[106] However, two of the children had inadequate initial ultrasound examinations, and the remaining two children had been symptomatic for less than 24 hours.

The usefulness of ultrasonography is often overlooked in the evaluation of osteomyelitis owing to the

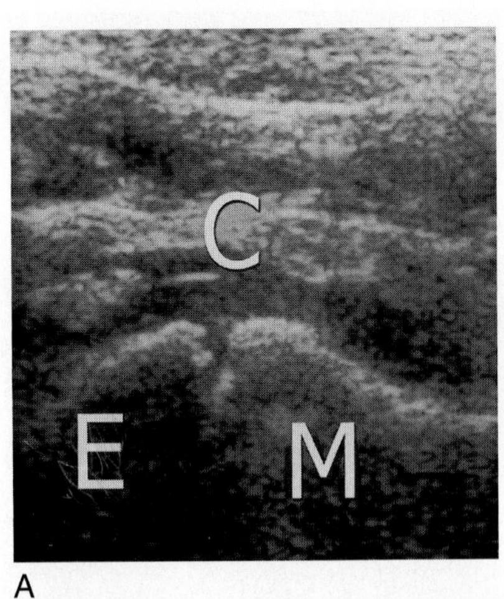

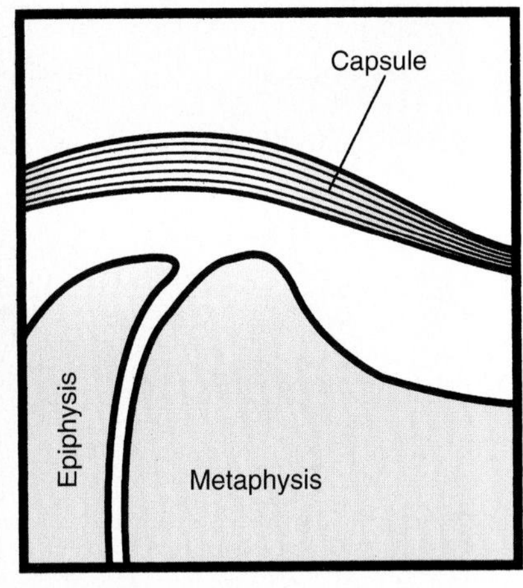

A

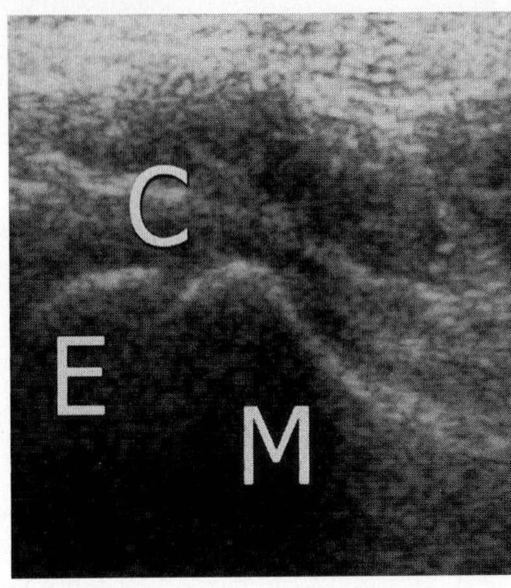

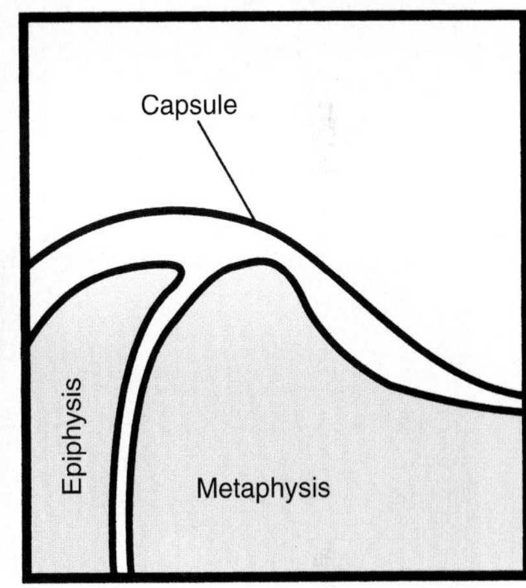

B

FIGURE 35-24 Sonograms with a line drawing of a patient with septic arthritis of the hip. **A,** Intra-articular fluid displaces the capsule into a convex position. The capsule is also thickened. **B,** The capsule on the normal side is concave (following the contour of the metaphysis) and not thickened. C, capsule; E, epiphysis; M, metaphysis.

availability of bone scintigraphy and MRI. However, in isolated communities and developing countries, ultrasonography may prove useful in evaluating and treating bone infection. One study recommended using ultrasonography as a second step, after plain radiographs, in evaluating all patients with suspected AHO of long bones.[158] The ultrasonographic features of osteomyelitis are deep soft tissue swelling, periosteal thickening, subperiosteal fluid collection, and cortical breach or destruction, which typically follows a course of progressive stages based on the duration of the infection.[193] The response to treatment can also be tracked by ultrasonography, and one study found that subperiosteal collections of more than 3 mm resolved completely with antibiotics alone.[158,193]

Nuclear Imaging

Bone scintigraphy has several advantages over the cross-sectional imaging techniques of MRI and CT. It is less expensive, seldom requires sedation, allows for whole-body imaging, and may provide evidence of multifocal involvement in neonatal infections. The method is also useful in assessing a limping toddler when localization of the source of the gait disturbance is not possible by history and physical examination alone.[6] Technetium methylene diphosphonate scanning is the most common nuclear imaging method used to evaluate for infection, although other techniques, including gallium-67 citrate, technetium sulfur colloid, fluorine-18 fluorodeoxyglucose, and indium-111 oxine, have been reported for specific purposes.[73,182,275] Most of these other methods have limited clinical utility and an excessive radiation burden, prohibiting their routine use in children.[24,182,216]

The reported sensitivity of skeletal scintigraphy for the detection of osteomyelitis ranges from 54% to 100%, and the specificity is approximately 70% to 90%, with an overall accuracy of about 90%.[33,56-58,216] In specific locations such as the spine, pelvis, and foot, the sensitivity of bone scintigraphy is reduced. However, with modern techniques of magnified spot views, pinhole collimation, optical or electronic image magnification with camera zoom or computer magnification, and single-photon emission CT, the accuracy of nuclear imaging has been increased above 90%.[56,59,216] The radiology department at Children's Hospital in Boston continues to use skeletal scintigraphy, with the diagnosis of AHO confirmed in 79 of 86 children (92%) without the need for MRI.[57]

A three-phase bone scan consists of the following elements: (1) blood flow or angiogram phase (per-

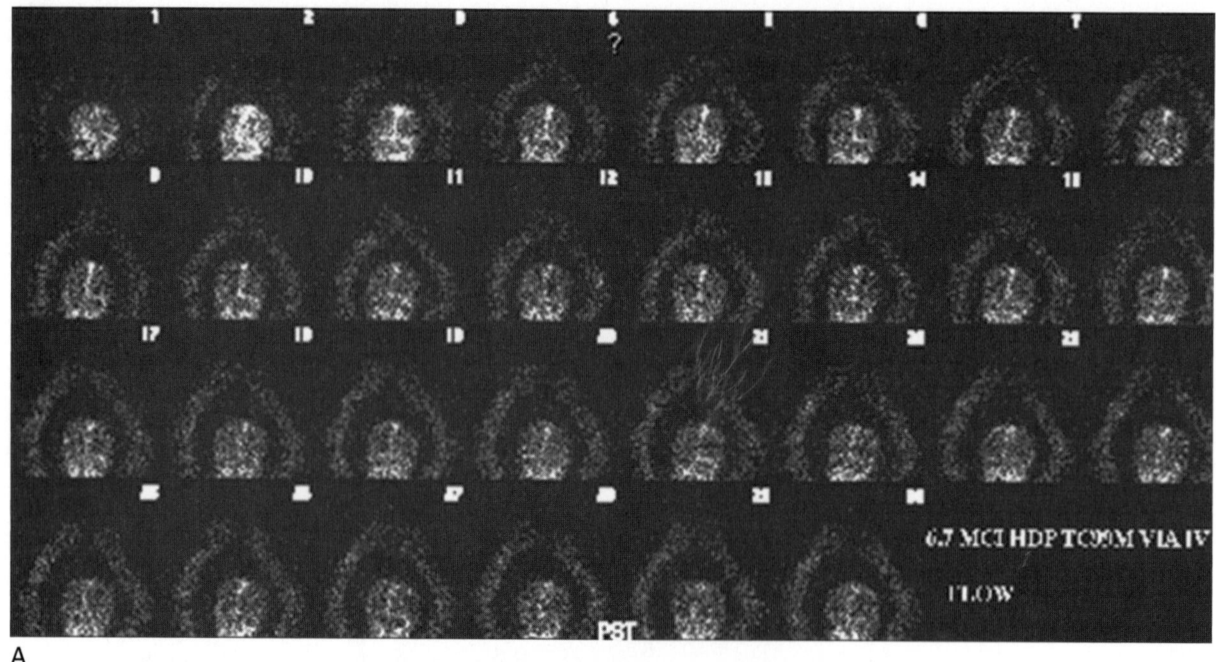

A

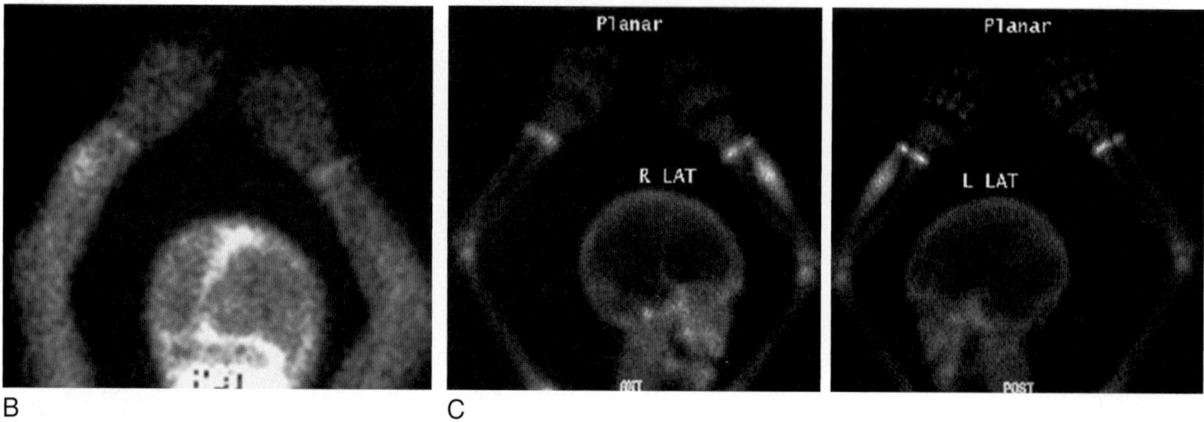

B C

FIGURE 35–25 Components of a three-phase technetium bone scan. Initial **(A)**, blood pool **(B)**, and delayed **(C)** sequences demonstrate increased uptake in all three phases in this 5-year-old boy with subacute osteomyelitis of the left ulna.

formed immediately after injection), (2) blood pool or soft tissue phase (performed about 15 minutes following injection), and (3) delayed or skeletal phase (performed 2 to 3 hours, and may be repeated up to 24 hours, after injection) (Fig. 35–25).[216] Findings in osteomyelitis include focally increased uptake on all three phases of the study. Cellulitis, deep soft tissue abscess, or pyomyositis may appear as diffusely increased soft tissue uptake on the blood flow and blood pool images, with little or no uptake on the delayed images. Septic arthritis is more difficult to diagnose with nuclear imaging. Possible findings include a diffusely increased uptake on both sides of a joint, without focal uptake in bone, or photopenia in the epiphysis on the delayed images.[216] Unfortunately, the reported false-positive (32%) and false-negative (30%) rates limit the value of nuclear imaging for assessing septic arthritis.[290]

Photopenic or "cold" bone scans occur when there is decreased uptake compared with the uninvolved side on the delayed images (Fig. 35–26). This finding has been reported in approximately 8% of cases of osteomyelitis and appears to be associated with an advanced stage of infection in which the microcirculation of the medullary canal is compressed by the intraosseous pressure created by the infection.[232] In one report, 7 of 81 children (8.6%) with AHO were found to have a "cold" defect on bone scan; all 7 patients exhibited septic clinical features, including a mean temperature of 39.9°C, heart rate of 145 beats per minute, and positive blood cultures.[232] The positive predictive value of a "cold" scan was 100% in one study, compared with only 82% for a "hot" scan.[300]

Abnormal uptake at multiple sites or even at a single unexpected axial site may be an indication of a systemic disease, such as leukemia or metastatic

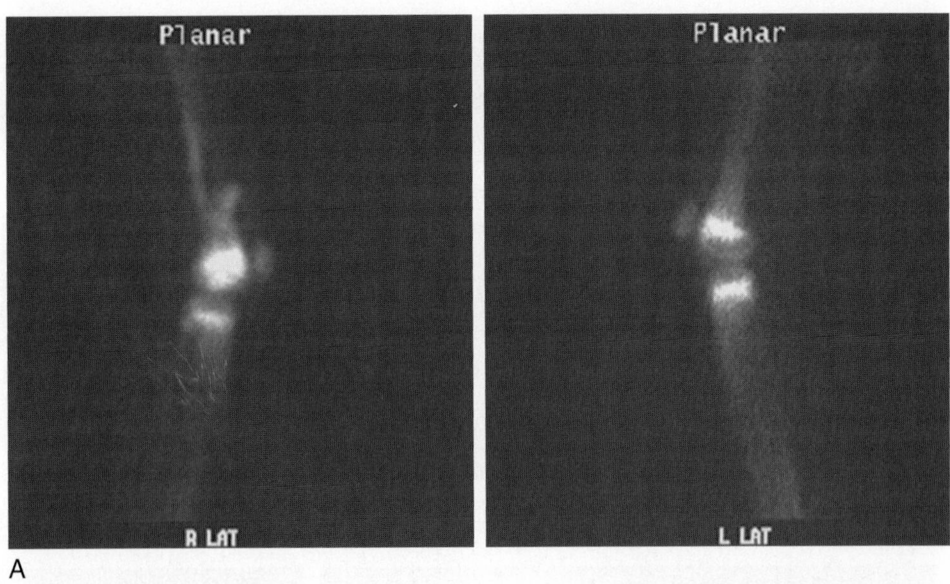

A

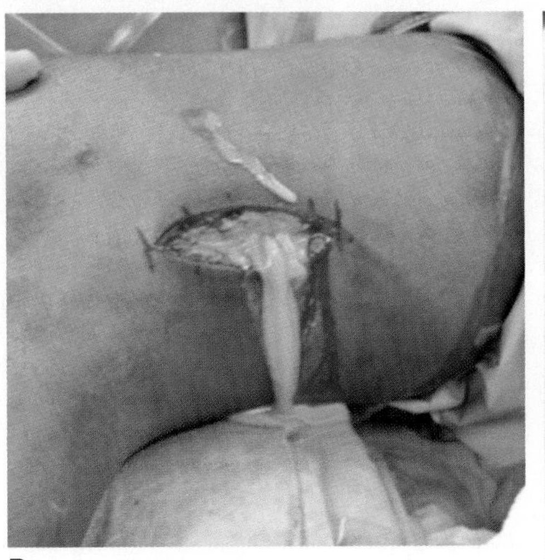

B

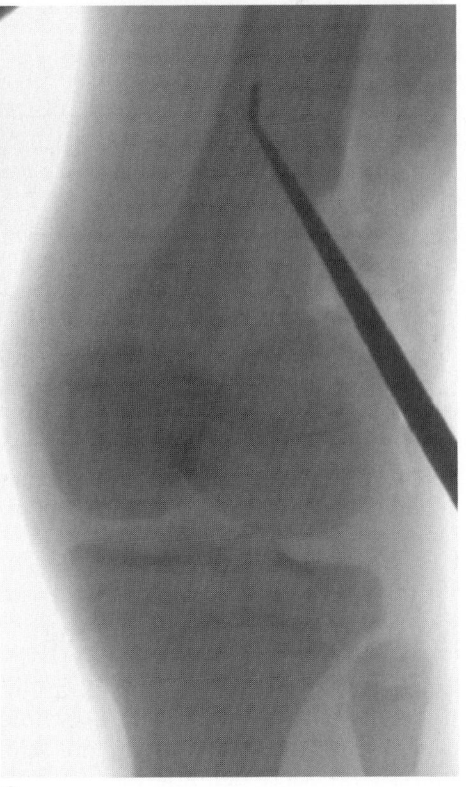

C

FIGURE 35–26 Twelve-year-old boy with a 2-week history of knee pain and fever (39.4°C). The initial laboratory findings included C-reactive protein 12.9 mg/dL, erythrocyte sedimentation rate greater than 140 mm/hour, and white blood cell count 10,400 cells/mL. Bone scan findings were consistent with "cold" osteomyelitis of the distal femur **(A).** Operative findings included a large volume of purulence surrounding the distal femur **(B)** and an extensive area of dead bone of the distal femur **(C).**

neuroblastoma.[56] Uptake by a soft tissue mass and multiple skeletal sites should prompt further investigation for neuroblastoma in an infant or young child. Up to 80% of children with leukemia have skeletal scintigraphic lesions at the time of diagnosis.[52]

Computed Tomography

Although CT is excellent for defining bony pathology, this method has limited application in the diagnosis and management of osteoarticular infections because the bony changes associated with osteomyelitis are usually adequately visible on plain films. CT is useful in the delineation of bony sequestra and segmental defects in chronic osteomyelitis.[239] It may also be helpful in demonstrating soft tissue abscesses of the spine or pelvis. CT-guided percutaneous biopsy is often the preferred method of obtaining tissue from axial locations and placing drains in pelvic abscesses along the inner wall of the ilium (Fig. 35–27).[165]

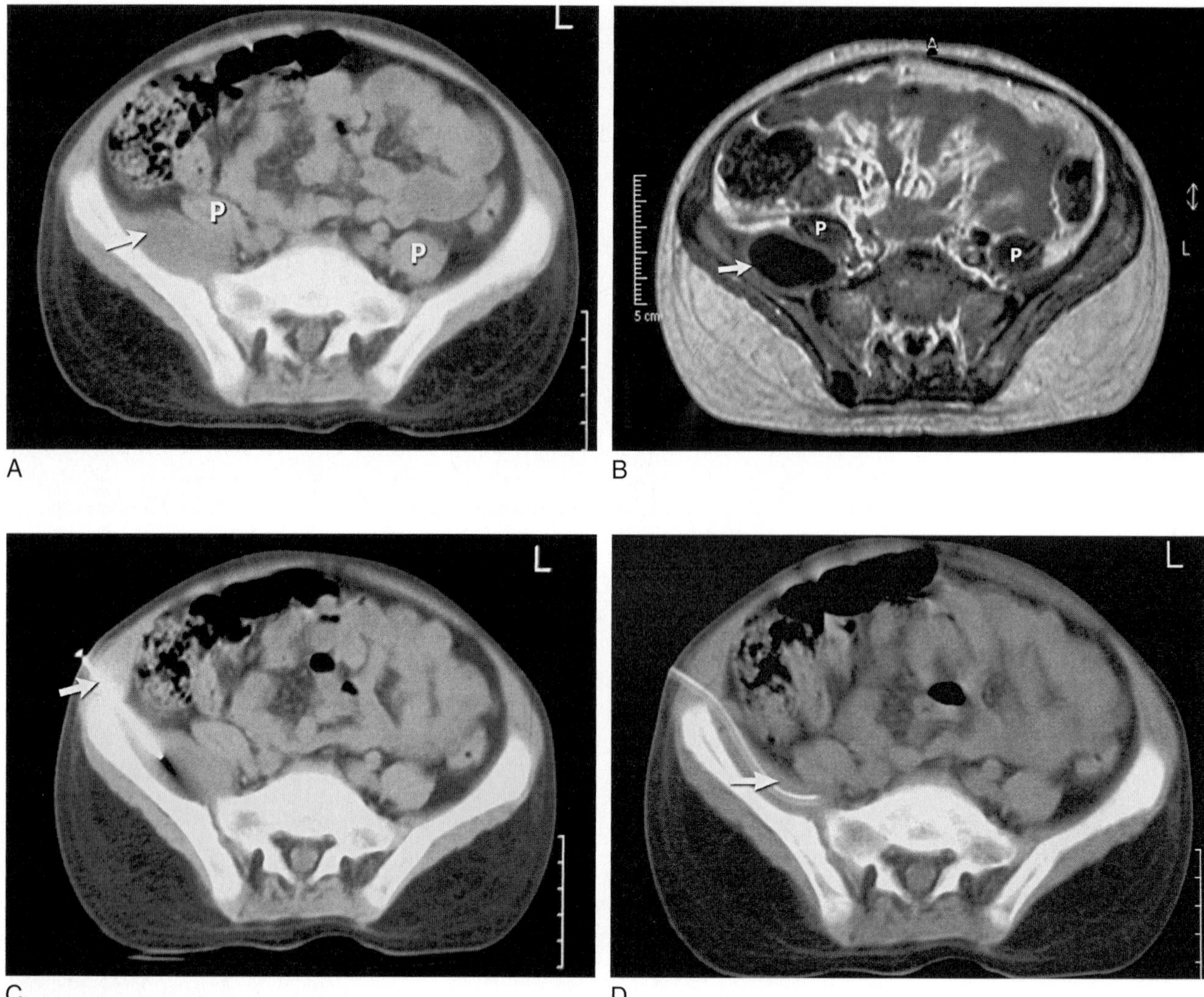

FIGURE 35–27 Computed tomography (CT) scan **(A)** and magnetic resonance image **(B)** demonstrating a psoas abscess (*arrows*) displacing the right psoas muscle (P). CT-guided percutaneous drainage **(C)** was performed, with placement of a drainage tube **(D)**.

Magnetic Resonance Imaging

Magnetic resonance imaging is arguably the most powerful diagnostic imaging technique currently available for the evaluation of musculoskeletal infection. By precisely defining the anatomic location and spatial extent of the inflammatory process, MRI not only helps establish a definitive diagnosis, even in the challenging locations of the spine, pelvis, and foot, but also guides treatment decision making. When surgery is necessary, MRI is useful in determining the appropriate approach when more than one approach is possible. The disadvantages of MRI include the cost, the need for sedation in most children younger than 7 years, and the lack of availability in remote locations.

The sensitivity of MRI has been reported as 97%, with a specificity of 92%, in a narrow subset of children with clinical findings suggestive of AHO.[201] Others have reported that MRI has diminished accuracy when a broader spectrum of pathology is being evaluated. Erdman and colleagues noted a sensitivity of 98% and a specificity of only 75% in their series and advised that certain pitfalls be avoided to help improve the diagnostic accuracy of the study.[82] They found that fracture, infarction, and healing osteomyelitis can mimic the typical features of acute inflammation seen on standard MRI sequences in the presence of active infection. It has been recommended that clinical examination, plain radiography, and scintigraphy be used in cases of diagnostic uncertainty to increase the specificity of MRI and avoid the well-known pitfalls.[82,239]

Characteristics of infection seen on MRI include marrow signal depression on T1-weighted images and increased marrow signal intensity on T2-weighted and short-tau inversion recovery (STIR) images (Fig. 35–28).[47] A complete study should also include fat-suppressed postgadolinium contrast images, which tend to further enhance the intensity of marrow signal changes seen on T1 and T2 images.[149] Abscesses, subperiosteal fluid collections, and joint effusions

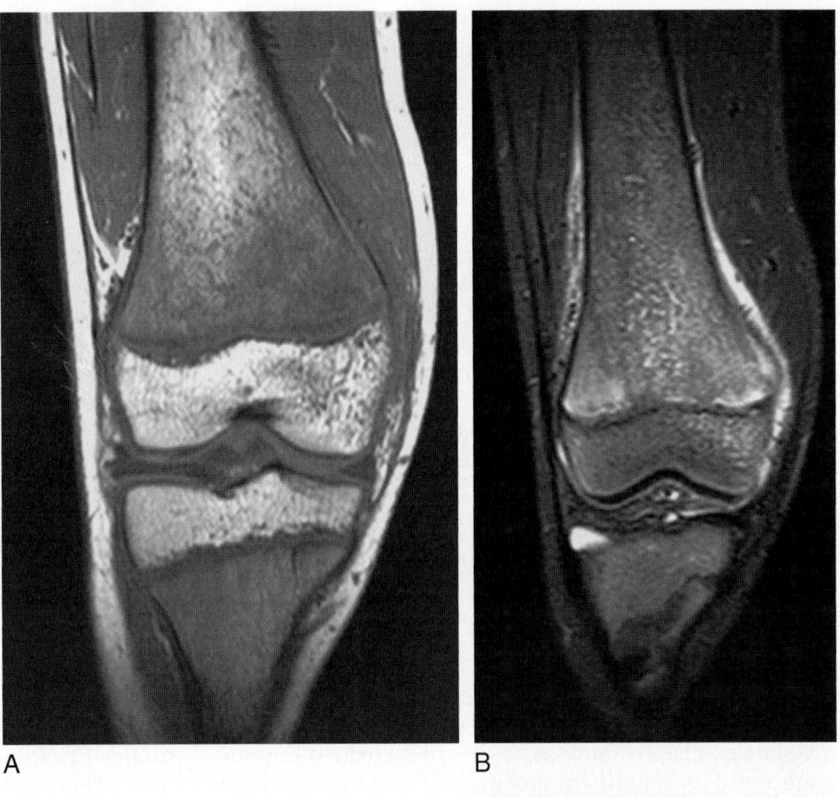

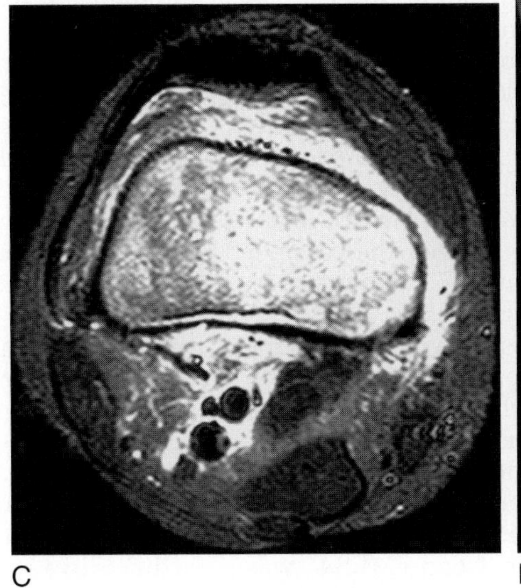

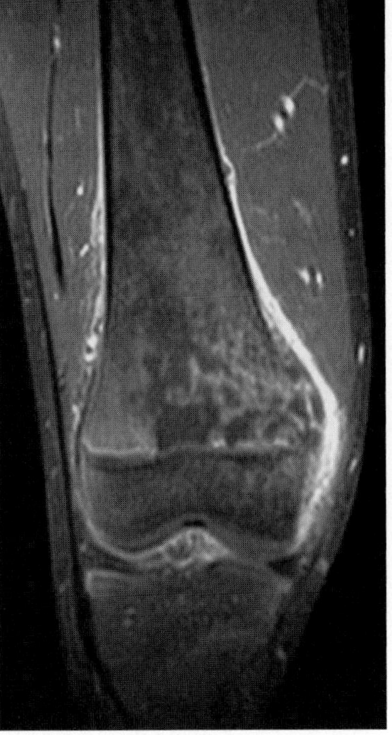

FIGURE 35–28 Magnetic resonance imaging of the distal femur demonstrates decreased marrow signal intensity on T1-weighted images **(A),** increased marrow signal intensity on T2-weighted images **(B)** and short-tau inversion recovery (STIR) images **(C),** and marrow signal enhancement along with synovial enhancement on postgadolinium T2-weighted images **(D).** These findings are consistent with distal femoral osteomyelitis. The possibility of a contiguous septic arthritis is evidenced by the synovial enhancement with contrast compared with the noncontrasted T2-weighted images.

appear as bright and well-demarcated areas on T2 and STIR sequences. Postgadolinium images should result in ring enhancement of abscesses on T1-weighted images.

Septic arthritis results in altered marrow signal intensity of adjacent bone on T1 and STIR images in up to 60% of cases and may be misinterpreted as adjacent osteomyelitis.[82] One study evaluated postgadolinium images and found that the marrow signal alterations in cases of septic arthritis alone were less extensive and limited mainly to an area adjacent to articular surfaces; in contrast, in cases of confirmed contiguous osteomyelitis and septic arthritis, the marrow changes were more extensive and involved the metaphyseal region.[179]

The appearance of chronic osteomyelitis on MRI can be difficult to interpret or even misleading (see Fig. 35–9). Extensive marrow signal changes may encompass an area much broader than the original focus of infection, making it difficult to differentiate active inflammation from persistent infection and reactive bone marrow signal changes from the healing and remodeling process itself. Because of this difficulty, it is important to use good clinical judgment and consider all available information, including the appearance of plain radiographs, the trends of laboratory data, and the clinical appearance of the child, before embarking on further surgical debridement based on MRI findings alone in cases of chronic osteomyelitis.

Causative Organisms

Staphylococcus aureus

With few exceptions, *S. aureus* is the most common cause of musculoskeletal infections of all types in all age groups. The interest focused on the antibiotic resistance of this organism has led to increased knowledge about its genetic composition, which may provide insight into its peculiar ability to cause infections of deep soft tissue, muscle, bone, and joint. It is hoped that future research will also yield improved methods to prevent and treat infections caused by this organism.

The antibiotic resistance of *S. aureus* is rooted in the rise of the antibiotic era. Penicillin was first used to successfully treat a human being in 1941, following its discovery in 1928 by Alexander Fleming. After it was identified as a potential weapon against a variety of bacteria, including *S. aureus,* production of penicillin steadily increased so that it would be available to treat soldiers wounded during World War II, and it rapidly vanquished the high mortality rate associated with infected combat wounds. Subsequently, Andrew Moyer patented an industrial method for the mass production of penicillin, which lowered the cost per dose from $20 in 1943 to $0.55 in 1946. Within a year, resistant bacteria began to emerge.

Penicillin-resistant *S. aureus* first emerged in the 1950s as the most important pathogen in neonatal nurseries.[139] No fully effective therapy was available until the introduction of methicillin in the 1960s.[139] Following this early outbreak of serious nosocomial infections, methicillin-susceptible *S. aureus* emerged in the community as well. Methicillin-resistant *S. aureus* has followed a similar trend. MRSA was reported in Europe in the 1960s, and the first U.S. case was reported in 1968.[11,139] Since then, nosocomial MRSA has become an increasing problem, with the incidence of MRSA isolates in hospitalized patients increasing from 2% in 1974 to approximately 50% in 1997.[39]

Initial reports of community-acquired MRSA were limited to individuals with a history of intravenous drug use and other high-risk patients with serious illness, previous antibiotic therapy, or residence in long-term-care facilities.[200] In the mid-1990s, reports surfaced of CA-MRSA strains that appeared to be different from typical nosocomial MRSA strains, and they were occurring in individuals without established risk factors.[39,124,206,285] Gwynne-Jones and Stott found that 26 of 130 staphylococcal isolates in their pediatric orthopaedic unit (20%) were resistant to methicillin, with all but one acquired in the community.[113] Moreno and coworkers found that 99 of 170 MRSA isolates (58%) were from the community and that no identifiable risk factors differentiated patients with CA-MRSA from those with community-acquired methicillin-susceptible *Staphylococcus aureus* (CA-MSSA).[206] Recent reports have shown a continued rise in the incidence of CA-MRSA, with one institution reporting an increase from 35% in February 2000 to 67% by January 2002.[200] Although skin and soft tissue infections have predominated, increasing numbers of invasive infections in children caused by CA-MRSA have been reported.[199]

Methicillin resistance is usually conferred by the *mecA* gene, which encodes an altered penicillin-binding protein that causes resistance to beta-lactam antibiotics, including cephalosporins.[39] Most nosocomial MRSA strains have acquired resistance to numerous other antibiotic classes through a variety of mechanisms. With one exception, reported in Japan, nosocomial MRSA is still highly susceptible to vancomycin, despite being multidrug resistant.[246] So far, CA-MRSA has also remained susceptible to most other antibiotics (except for beta-lactams), including clindamycin, trimethoprim-sulfamethoxazole, rifampin, and gentamicin.[39,200] However, an inducible macrolide-lincosamide-streptogramin B (MLS_B) resistance to clindamycin has been reported in 6% to 25% of CA-MRSA isolates.[200]

Some clues to the manifestations of infection caused by *S. aureus* are being sought in the virulence factors encoded by its genes.[9,199] Pulsed-field gel electrophoresis of whole-cell DNA from MRSA isolates has been performed to identify these virulence factors, including *pvl, can, fnbB, tst, clfA,* and *mecA.*[199] One group of investigators found that a significantly higher proportion of CA-MRSA strains carried the *pvl* and *fnbB* genes than did CA-MSSA isolates.[199] They also noted that the *pvl* gene may lead to an increased likelihood of complications such as chronic osteomyelitis and deep vein thrombosis in children with *S. aureus* musculoskeletal infections. Another group has isolated the whole genome sequence of two nosocomial MRSA strains (N315 and Mu50), as well as a strain of CA-MRSA (MW2) that caused fatal septicemia and septic arthritis in a 16-month-old girl in North Dakota.[9] They found a total of 19 virulence genes in the MW2 genome. Further work is necessary to understand the significance of these virulence factors and to identify potential methods of combating them.

Invasive musculoskeletal infections caused by *S. aureus* are treated empirically with a first-generation cephalosporin or semisynthetic penicillin that is continued as specific therapy once MSSA has been confirmed or cultures are otherwise negative. Clindamycin is often preferred to treat CA-MRSA unless MLS_B resistance is demonstrated by disk diffusion, which is performed by placing clindamycin and erythromycin disks 15 to 20 mm apart on a culture medium.[200] A D-shaped zone of inhibition around the clindamycin disk, on the side of the erythromycin disk, indicates an inducible MLS_B phenotype.[200] Bactrim and rifampin are suitable oral alternatives under these circumstances. In cases of multidrug-resistant nosocomial MRSA infection, vancomycin is preferred for specific therapy.[139] Because the bone penetration of vancomycin is less effective than that of other antibiotics more commonly used to treat osteomyelitis, rifampin is added to enhance the effects of vancomycin as well as to address intracellular pathogens.

Streptococcus pyogenes

Most cases of GABHS infection occur in school-age children, who have the greatest exposure to the organism. In addition to being the second most common causative organism isolated in pediatric musculoskeletal infection, *S. pyogenes* is associated with other notable conditions. The most serious is a toxic shock–like syndrome characterized by severe local tissue destruction and multisystem organ failure. Musculoskeletal involvement has been noted in up to 87% of cases.[142] During 2002, 986 cases of invasive group A streptococcal infection were reported through the Active Bacterial Core Surveillance Project.[110] Based on this number, the CDC estimates that approximately 9100 cases of invasive GABHS disease and 1350 deaths occurred in the United States in 2002.[110] Affected children often present with fever and a toxic appearance, with evidence of cardiac, hepatic, renal, central nervous system, or hematologic dysfunction.[142] Aggressive resuscitation and medical management are necessary, along with rapid decompression of foci of infection in the musculoskeletal system after a vigilant search for such sites. Involvement of the musculoskeletal system typically manifests as diffuse swelling in one or more extremities, which may raise concern for compartment syndrome as the infection rapidly spreads along fascial planes and creates a diffuse, edematous swelling of the involved muscle groups, as opposed to discrete abscess formation (Fig. 35–29).

Osteomyelitis and septic arthritis caused by GABHS are frequently reported in the aftermath of varicella viral infections in otherwise immunocompetent infants and toddlers.[20,108,143,174] The port of entry seems to be the varicella pocks, with subsequent hematogenous spread to bone or joint. Standard methods of treatment for septic arthritis or osteomyelitis are employed, along with penicillin, which remains the drug of choice for GABHS infections.

Group A streptococcal pharyngitis may be followed by acute rheumatic fever (ARF) or, less commonly, by a poststreptococcal reactive arthritis (PSRA).[2,3,8,19,191,205] These conditions should be considered in the differential diagnosis of warm, erythematous joints in children older than 4 years. The orthopaedic manifestations of ARF classically include a migratory polyarthritis that usually affects the lower extremities first. The modified Jones criteria are useful in establishing a diagnosis. At least two major criteria (carditis, polyarthritis, subcutaneous nodules, erythema marginatum, and chorea) or one major and two minor criteria

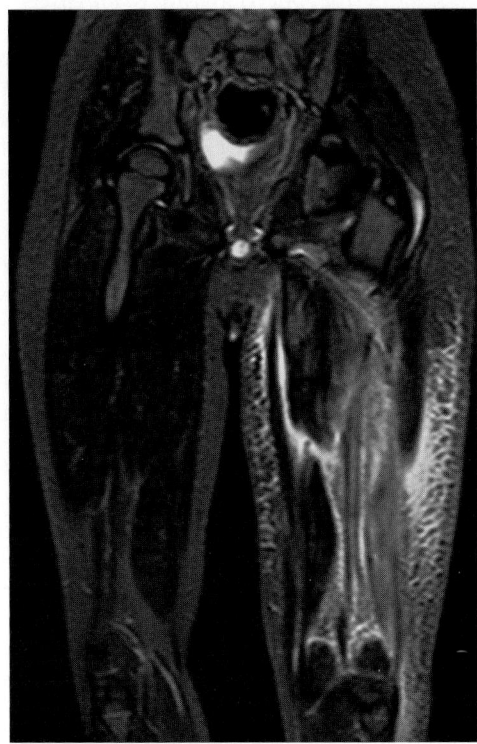
A

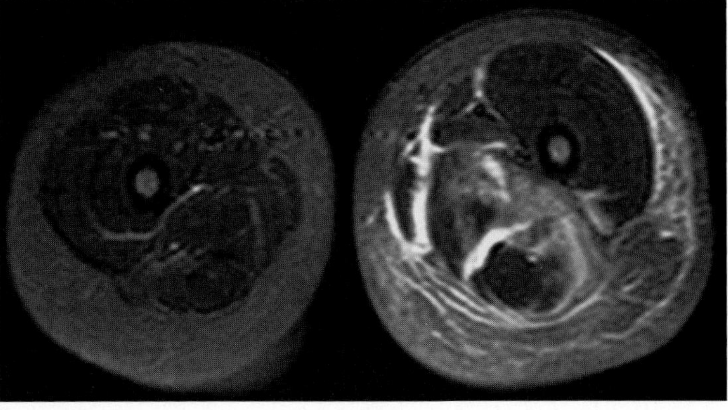
B

FIGURE 35–29 **A** and **B,** Magnetic resonance images of the thigh in a 5-year-old boy with disseminated streptococcal infection and multiorgan system dysfunction. Diffuse edema is noted in the subcutaneous tissues as well as in the deep soft tissues, with extensive perifascial fluid accumulation but no discrete abscess formation. Surgical decompression was performed, with similar findings.

(fever, arthralgia, increased ESR or serum CRP level, and prolonged P-R interval on electrocardiogram), along with evidence of preceding streptococcal infection, are necessary for the diagnosis of ARF.[152] Salicylates and antibiotic treatment followed by lifelong prophylaxis play a significant role in the management and prevention of long-term sequelae in ARF.

PSRA is believed to be a variant of ARF in which the Jones criteria are not otherwise satisfied. It is characterized by a shorter latency period between the inciting streptococcal infection and the onset of arthritis, a higher frequency of involvement of small joints and the axial skeleton, a poor response to nonsteroidal anti-inflammatory drugs, a protracted course, and the absence of other major manifestations of ARF.[8] Approximately 6% of children with PSRA have late-onset carditis, which most commonly manifests as mitral valve disease.[2,8,205] For this reason, the current recommendation is to treat with antimicrobial (penicillin) prophylaxis for a minimum of 5 years or until age 21 years, whichever is longer.[8,205]

Recent studies suggest that the HLA-DRB1*16 allele predisposes to ARF, whereas the HLA-DRB1*01 allele is more commonly associated with PSRA.[2,8,191] In affected individuals, antibodies that develop against group A streptococcus are believed to cross-react with joint synovium at the basement membrane.

The most reliable methods to establish antecedent group A streptococcal infection are to measure antistreptolysin O and antideoxyribonuclease B titers and obtain throat cultures for group A streptococcus.[2,205] The basic workup should also include CBC with differential, ESR, CRP, and blood cultures. If the diagnosis of ARF or PSRA is considered on the basis of the clinical evaluation and laboratory studies, an electrocardiogram, echocardiogram, and pediatric cardiology consultation should be obtained.[19]

Kingella kingae

K. kingae was first identified as a new species by Elizabeth King in 1960.[330] Originally designated *Moraxella kingii*, it was subsequently allocated to the genus *Kingella* after its distinctive properties were characterized in 1976.[77,187] *K. kingae* is a fastidious, aerobic, gram-negative coccobacillus thought to colonize the upper respiratory tract and oropharynx in almost 75% of children between the ages of 6 months and 4 years, which corresponds to the age range of children who contract invasive infections from this organism.[77] The majority of osteoarticular infections have been reported in children between 10 and 24 months of age.[187]

Orthopaedic infections from *K. kingae* were first reported in 1982, with subsequent literature reviews between 1982 and 1998 identifying 58 cases of septic arthritis and 23 cases of osteomyelitis.[71,77,187] A recent report from the CDC established 21 cases of osteoarticular infection (12 septic arthritis and 9 osteomyelitis) between June 2001 and November 2002, suggesting a substantial increase in incidence.[169] Possible explanations for this rise in incidence include an increased awareness of this pathogen in the medical community and improved specimen handling and culture techniques.

Because *K. kingae* is a slow-growing organism with specific culture requirements, it is difficult to isolate from synovial fluid or bone exudates on routine solid media. Recent reports recommend injecting aspirated materials into aerobic blood culture bottles.[97,169,330,333] It is postulated that the dilution of synovial fluid or pus (which may exert an inhibitory effect on the organism's growth) in a large volume of broth decreases the concentration of detrimental factors and facilitates recovery of the organism.[331,332] Solid specimens should be plated immediately onto blood or chocolate agar. One group evaluated the difference between sending the specimen to the laboratory for routine processing versus immediate plating in the operating room.[97] In five of six cases of osteomyelitis, they were able to isolate the organism from the agar plate that was inoculated during surgery, compared with only one of six samples from the same patients that were processed in the laboratory. Several authors believe that these improved methods of organism isolation have been the decisive factor in the increased number of *K. kingae* infections recorded in recent years.[97,169,330]

K. kingae typically demonstrates susceptibility to beta-lactam antibiotics and is covered by the usual empirical treatment given to children in this age group.[333] However, resistance to a variety of antibiotics has been reported, necessitating the use of a third-generation cephalosporin under such circumstances.[77]

Streptococcus pneumoniae

S. pneumoniae is responsible for a small but consistent portion (about 4%) of bone and joint infections in infants and small children, following *S. aureus*, *S. pyogenes*, and *K. kingae* in incidence.[26,261] The organism plays a more dominant role as a cause of bacteremia, meningitis, and respiratory tract infections. The Pediatric Multicenter Pneumococcal Surveillance Study Group (PMPSSG) identified 21 cases of septic arthritis and 21 cases of osteomyelitis caused by pneumococcus in eight pediatric centers across the United States between September 1, 1993, and August 31, 1996.[26] The mean age of infected children was 17 months (range, 11 days to 9 years), with most children being between 3 and 24 months of age.[26,146]

A rising incidence of antibiotic resistance was reported by the PMPSSG, which identified penicillin resistance in 50% of children who had received antibiotics within 4 weeks of hospitalization and 27% of children without previous antibiotic treatment.[26] In 2002, the CDC reported that 11.5% of isolates in the United States were fully resistant to penicillin.[110] Successful treatment has been accomplished using ceftriaxone and clindamycin in those children who cannot be treated with penicillin.[26]

S. pneumoniae has been identified as a cause of purpura fulminans in children. The pneumococcal autolysin is suspected to serve the same role as the endotoxin of *N. meningitidis*.[53] The development of the heptavalent pneumococcal conjugate vaccine, which is recommended for all children aged 2 to 23 months, has had a substantial impact on the epidemiology of invasive pneumococcal disease.[129]

Neisseria meningitidis

N. meningitidis is well known for its role in causing rapid-onset meningitis and severe sepsis with purpura fulminans. The annual incidence of meningococcal disease is 0.6 to 1.4 cases per 100,000 population, and the case-fatality rate is 10% to 20%, with an equal number of survivors sustaining permanent sequelae, including amputation from purpura fulminans.[301,320] Extrameningeal involvement in overt meningococcal disease is well established, with septic arthritis (usually in large joints) reported in 2% of children in a large epidemiologic review in the United States.[320]

A third-generation cephalosporin, such as cefotaxime or ceftriaxone, is the favored treatment for invasive meningococcal infections. Chemoprophylaxis with rifampin, ciprofloxacin, or sulfonamides has been shown to eradicate nasopharyngeal carriage and prevent epidemic outbreaks of invasive disease in close contacts, which typically occur within 5 to 10 days of exposure.[301]

Neisseria gonorrhoeae

Disseminated gonococcal infection (DGI) may occur in children under three circumstances: (1) neonatal infection contracted while passing through the birth canal of an infected mother, (2) pediatric or adolescent infection due to sexual abuse, and (3) adolescent infection through voluntary sexual activity. The onset of disseminated disease may occur anywhere from days to months after the initial infection, with an incidence of 0.5% to 3% in cases of mucosal infection. The most common presenting musculoskeletal complaint is polyarthritis in up to 60% of patients, with involvement of the knee, ankle, or wrist. Associated complaints may include fever, chills, and rash. DGI should be suspected in the presence of dermatitis, tenosynovitis, and migratory polyarthritis. A rash occurs in two thirds of patients and is described as consisting of multiple painless, nonpruritic lesions involving the torso, limbs, palms, and soles.[112]

Although the overall incidence of gonorrhea is higher in males, DGI is four times more common in females.[112] Whenever DGI is suspected, culture specimens should be obtained from the joint fluid, cervix of postpubertal girls, and urethral or prostatic discharge of males, as well as from the vagina, pharynx, and rectum in children suspected of being victimized by child abuse. Because *N. gonorrhoeae* is difficult to culture, special specimen handling instructions are required to increase the chance of positively identifying the organism. Sterile culture specimens are plated on chocolate blood agar, and nonsterile specimens are plated on Thayer-Martin medium, which contains antibiotics to inhibit the growth of oropharyngeal and anorectal flora. Cultures require a 5% to 10% carbon dioxide atmosphere. Gram staining may demonstrate intracellular gram-negative diplococci.

Treatment of DGI involves a 7-day course of intravenous or intramuscular ceftriaxone given once daily or cefotaxime in two divided doses.[112] Doxycycline is also used concurrently in sexually active adolescents to treat chlamydia, which frequently accompanies gonococcal infection. Surgical treatment is rarely indicated except in cases of severe synovitis that is not responsive to conservative treatment, which may require arthroscopic or open synovectomy. Gonococcal osteomyelitis, though rarely reported, may require a longer course of treatment.[298]

Borrelia burgdorferi

Lyme disease is a multisystem infection caused by the spirochete *Borrelia burgdorferi.* It is the most common vector-borne disease in the United States, transmitted by the black-legged or deer tick, *Ixodes scapularis.* A total of 23,305 cases of Lyme disease were reported in 2005.[110] Infection most commonly occurs in children in the northeastern, mid-Atlantic, and north-central regions of the United States. After inoculation, the time before the appearance of systemic manifestations ranges from 2 to 30 days. Because the tick bite and the premonitory erythema migrans rash may go unnoticed, a high level of suspicion is necessary to ensure that the original presenting symptoms, which may involve the musculoskeletal, neurologic, and cardiovascular systems, are recognized without delay. Although this is rarely a problem in endemic areas, physicians outside these locations may not be familiar with the common manifestations of Lyme disease.

Because juvenile arthritis, reactive arthritis, and septic arthritis may be confused with Lyme arthritis, the CDC has established diagnostic criteria, including the presence of a characteristic erythema migrans rash at least 5 cm in diameter or laboratory confirmation of infection and at least one musculoskeletal, neurologic, or cardiovascular manifestation of disease.[188] Erythema migrans is present in 60% to 90% of patients and may occur with other early manifestations, including constitutional symptoms, migratory arthralgia, cardiac conduction defects, aseptic meningitis, and Bell's palsy.[326] Late manifestations of Lyme disease include arthritis, encephalopathy, and polyneuropathy.

The CDC recommends that clinicians use a two-step procedure when ordering antibody tests for Lyme disease: first, an enzyme-linked immunosorbent assay or immunofluorescent assay, and then, if the result is positive or equivocal, an immunoblot (Western blot) test to confirm the screening test result.[188] Antibody tests may not be positive for the first 3 to 6 weeks of infection. In endemic regions, a rapid 1-hour Lyme enzyme immunoassay (EIA) has been used to reduce the incidence of unnecessary surgical intervention in children with Lyme arthritis, owing to the considerable overlap in clinical, radiographic, and laboratory presentations of this condition and septic arthritis.[326]

By using the rapid Lyme EIA, the standard 3- to 5-day period for Lyme serology reporting can be significantly shortened. Willis and colleagues were able to avoid surgery in all 3 children who had the rapid EIA, whereas the remaining 7 of 10 children with subsequently confirmed Lyme arthritis by standard testing were subjected to operative intervention that might have been avoided.[326]

The medical treatment of Lyme disease initially consists of 4 weeks of oral antibiotics (amoxicillin or doxycycline). Children younger than 8 years should not be treated with doxycycline because it may cause permanent discoloration of the teeth. In one series, 88% of children were disease free before the end of 4 weeks, 7% required treatment for 8 weeks, and 5% required treatment for 12 weeks.[258]

A post–Lyme disease syndrome has been described in individuals with long-standing unrecognized Lyme arthritis before antibiotic treatment.[323] This may occur in dark-skinned individuals in whom the erythema migrans rash goes undetected. Some children who continue to have arthritis after antibiotic treatment may have suffered some mechanical damage to the joint structures from the inflammation and synovitis, whereas others may continue to have an autoimmune, or reactive, chronic synovitis following Lyme arthritis.[323] Most patients with suspected post-Lyme syndrome are simply slow responders and will improve with conservative observation and symptomatic support over a 6-month period.

Mycobacterium tuberculosis

During 2005, a total of 14,097 cases of tuberculosis were reported to the CDC.[110] U.S.-born non-Hispanic blacks continue to have the highest tuberculosis rate of any racial or ethnic population, representing 46.5% of cases among U.S.-born persons and about 28% of all cases in the United States.[110] Foreign-born individuals have a case rate more than eight times higher than that among U.S.-born persons.

Extrapulmonary tuberculosis is more common in children younger than 5 years, occurring in approximately 5% to 10% of infected children.[313] Thus, tuberculosis must be included in the differential diagnosis of bone and joint infections in this age group, particularly children who live in high-risk households. Despite the decreasing incidence in the United States, tuberculosis remains prevalent in the developing countries.

Osteoarticular involvement occurs in approximately 1% to 3% of patients with tuberculosis.[81] Aside from spinal involvement (addressed earlier), tubercular infection can manifest as septic arthritis, osteomyelitis of long bones, and dactylitis. This may take the form of spondylitis (50%), peripheral arthritis (30%), osteomyelitis (11% to 19%), and tenosynovitis and bursitis (1%).[244,268] Long bones may not become infected for 1 to 3 years, whereas dactylitis may develop in a few months. A high index of suspicion is needed to diagnose tubercular infection of the bone or joint. Positive culture can be obtained in approximately 80% of children with extrapulmonary disease, but 4 to 6 weeks of incubation may be needed to identify the organism.

Tuberculosis of joints is usually monoarticular, with the knee and hip most frequently affected. The clinical presentation is variable and simulates that of other chronic inflammatory arthritic disorders. Synovitis, effusion, central and peripheral articular erosions, and active and chronic pannus are the most common manifestations.[268] Delay in diagnosis is common. Post-contrast MRI may help differentiate effusion from synovitis and further differentiate acute synovitis from chronic synovitis.[268]

Tubercular osteomyelitis most commonly involves the epiphysis or metaphysis. Unlike in other bone infections, the physeal plate does little to stop the spread of infection. As the infection progresses, the area of skeletal destruction may slowly expand and typically appears on radiographs as a cystic lesion with obscure margins (Fig. 35–30). Because the disease process is almost entirely lytic, there is little periosteal reaction and often no sclerotic margin. Bone lesions often resemble benign or malignant bone tumors or fungal infections.[244] An expansile lesion may form within long bones, associated with periosteal thickening, and give the appearance of a shortened bone filled with air, termed *spina ventosa*.[244]

When bone lesions occur near an involved joint, a biopsy should be taken from the area of involved bone rather than from the synovium alone, because the synovium may show only nonspecific changes.[309] Curettage of the bacilli sequestrated in the necrotic tissue within cavities and bone defects is necessary to exact a cure, because systemic chemotherapeutic agents may not be able to access these locations.[244,319] For tubercular bone and joint involvement, current treatment recommendations include a 12-month regimen of isoniazid, rifampin, pyrazinamide, and streptomycin for the first 2 months, followed by isoniazid and rifampin for the remaining 10 months of therapy.[249]

Nontuberculous Mycobacteria

Nontuberculous mycobacteria are found in many parts of the natural environment, including soil and water. Infections caused by these organisms have been increasingly recognized in immunocompromised and otherwise healthy individuals. Case reports of osteoarticular infections caused by *Mycobacterium fortuitum* and *M. avium-intracellulare* complex illustrate the characteristic features.[32,203] These infections usually present 4 to 8 weeks after penetrating trauma, with a clinical appearance of cellulitis or a draining puncture wound.[32] A recurring cutaneous lesion with scant serous drainage may be noted, and a fistula may form.[203]

Surgical debridement is necessary and may be curative if the infection is well-circumscribed. Otherwise, antimicrobial therapy with a combination of agents is necessary. Commonly used antibiotics include clarithromycin, ciprofloxacin, amikacin, and imipenem.[32,203]

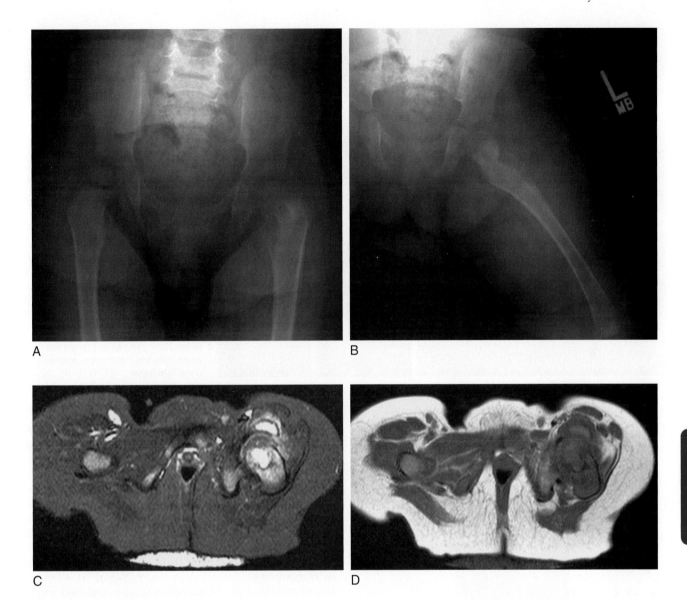

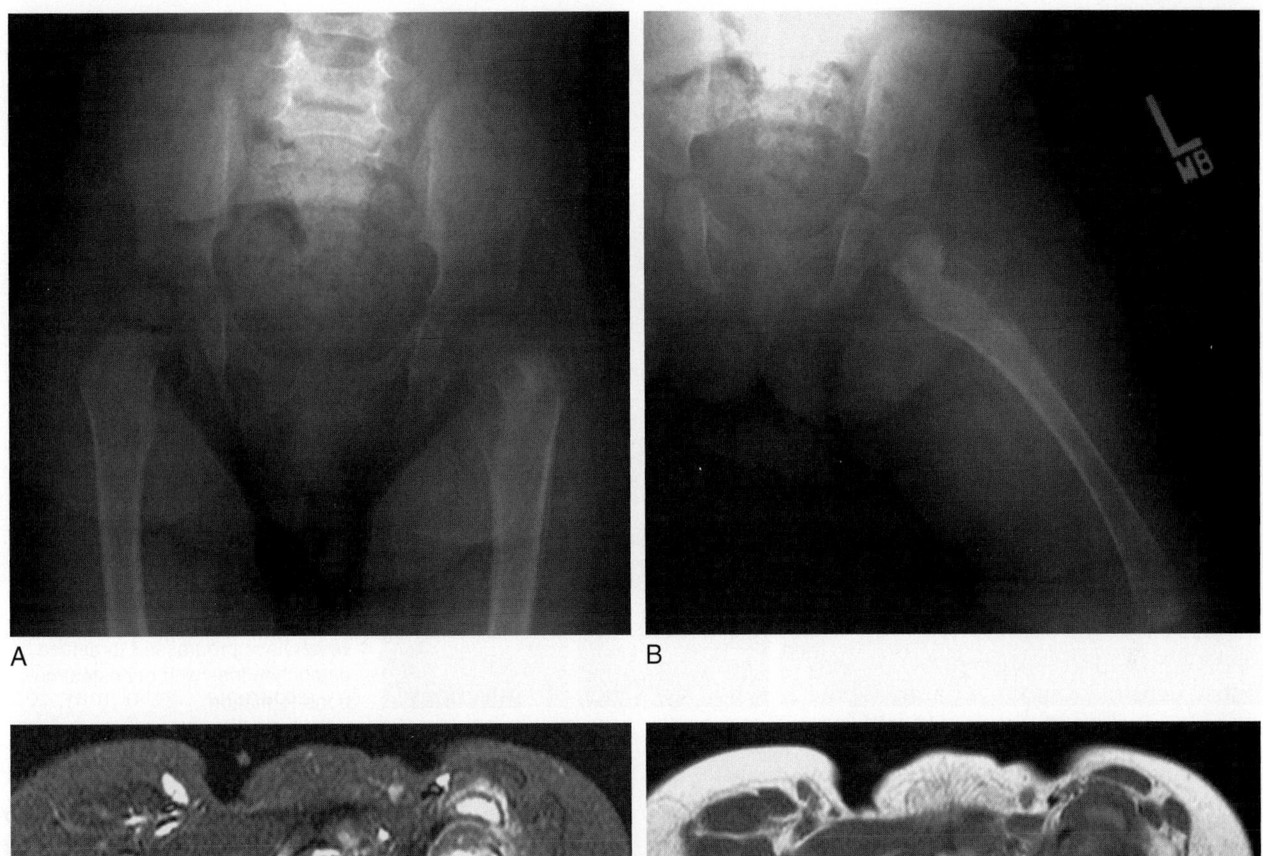

FIGURE 35-30 Fifteen-month-old girl from Ethiopia who had been asymptomatic until 1 day earlier, when she fell from a chair. Plain radiographs (**A** and **B**) demonstrate an expansile lesion in the left proximal femur, with obscure margins and centralized cyst formation without significant periosteal reaction. Magnetic resonance images (**C** and **D**) show the anterior soft tissue component associated with fluid-filled cysts in the bone as well as in the soft tissues. Findings at open biopsy were consistent with extrapulmonary tuberculosis.

Treponema pallidum

With the advent of penicillin, the incidence of syphilis has decreased markedly; however, it remains common in developing countries. Syphilis of bone has been reported in up to 65% of cases of congenital syphilis. During 2002, a total of 412 cases of congential syphilis were reported in the United States, representing a continued sharp decline in recent years.[110]

The organism reaches bone via hematogenous dissemination and can be found in the marrow as early as 36 hours following infection. Pathogens tend to localize in the metaphysis and diaphysis and do not spread to joints. The most common sites of involvement are the tibia, femur, humerus, and cranial bones. Syphilitic metaphysitis is the usual finding in early infancy (Fig. 35–31). Symmetric involvement of multiple bones is characteristic. The physis becomes widened, irregular, and ill-defined. The epiphyses usually are not involved. Pathologic fractures may occur through the weakened metaphyseal area. Necrosis may develop, and frank pus can form if the disease process is not stopped. In later childhood, syphilitic osteoperiostitis produces a dense, circumscribed swelling over the convex side of the bone. In the tibia, the subperiosteal apposition of bone on the anterior cortical surface produces the classic "saber shin" of congenital syphilis (Fig. 35–32).

Brucella melitensis

Brucella melitensis is most commonly transmitted to humans through the consumption of raw milk, a

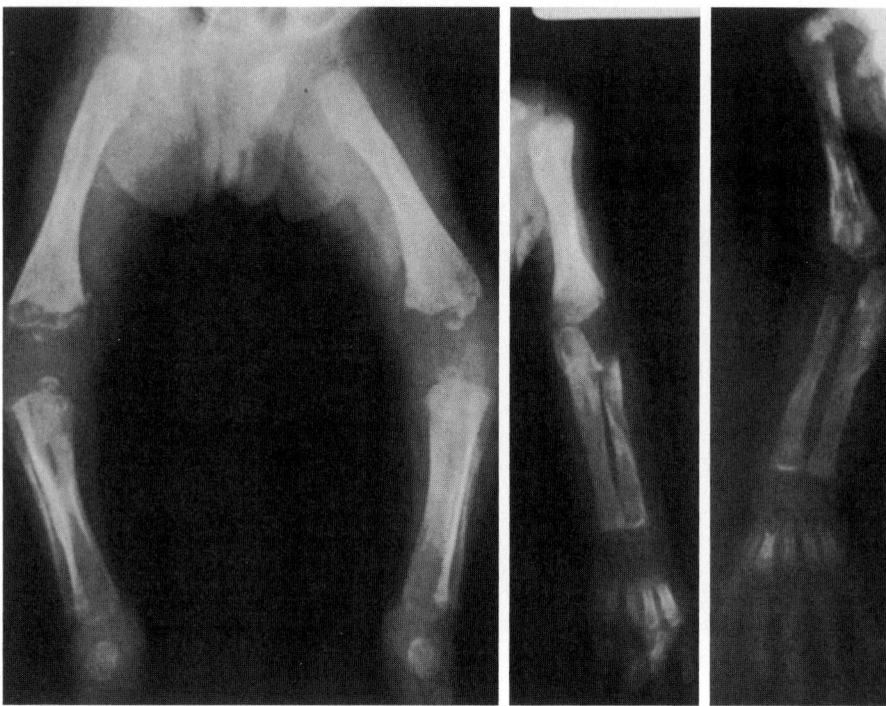

FIGURE 35-31 Congenital syphilis in a 3-month-old girl. Note the characteristic bilateral and symmetric metaphyseal erosions, which have progressed to diffuse osteochondritis with periosteal new bone formation.

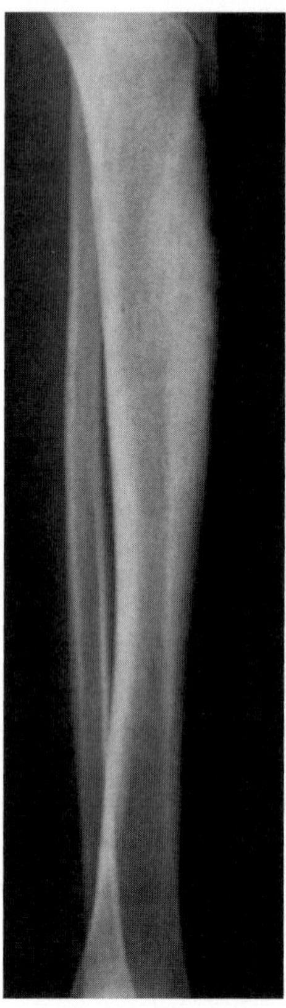

FIGURE 35-32 Classic "saber shin" in an adolescent with untreated congenital syphilis.

practice that is still common among indigenous populations in the Middle East. Other common means of exposure include ingestion of, or contact with, meat from infected animals and contact with the products of conception of infected animals, which may occur in farmers and meat packers. Other reported *Brucella* species include *Brucella abortus* (most common in North America and Europe) and *Brucella suis*.[162] The control program for cattle in the United States has nearly eliminated *B. abortus* infection from U.S. herds; most cases in humans are identified in international travelers or recent immigrants.[110] One of the largest reported series of brucellosis comes from Kuwait, where 452 patients with brucellosis were studied.[211] In that study, 25% of patients were younger than 15 years. Osteoarticular infections occurred in 37.4% (169) of the patients, most commonly manifesting as arthritis (79.8%) followed by spondylitis (6%), osteomyelitis (2.4%), and tendinitis or bursitis (1.2%). The most common sites of arthritis were the hip (53%), knee (36%), sacroiliac (20%), and ankle (15%) joints. Brucellar osteomyelitis is very rare in children, with only one case reported in patients younger than 55 years (a 17-year-old) in this large series.[211]

Because the organism is identified in culture in less than 20% of cases, the diagnosis of brucellosis is often made when a rising antibody titer (or a single titer >1 : 160) is found in the presence of compatible symptoms and a risk of exposure.[211] Treatment is accomplished with a 4- to 6-week course of two-drug therapy using tetracycline and streptomycin, rifampin and tetracycline, or trimethoprim-sulfamethoxazole and streptomycin.[162,211] A relapse rate of 16.6% was reported using either single-drug treatment or only a 2- to 4-week course.[211] Osteomyelitis may require 12 weeks of antibiotic treatment and wide surgical excision.[162]

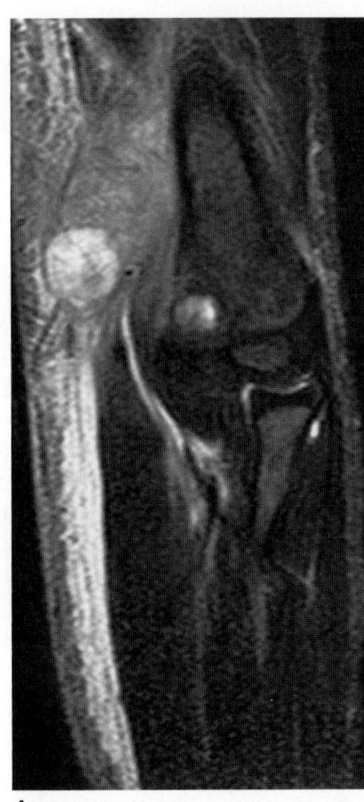

A

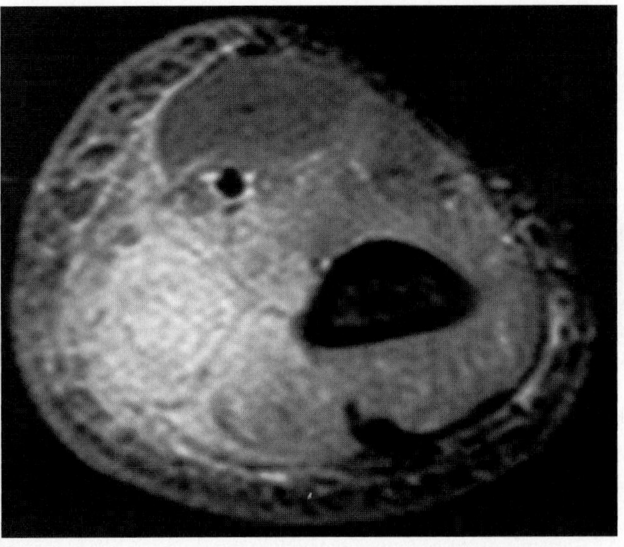

B

FIGURE 35–33 Coronal (**A**) and axial (**B**) magnetic resonance images of the elbow demonstrate an enlarged epitrochlear lymph node in a child with a history of exposure to cats. Enzyme-linked immunosorbent assay serologies were positive for *Bartonella henselae*. Surgical debridement resulted in rapid resolution of her limited elbow motion and pain.

Bartonella henselae

Cat-scratch disease (CSD) is a self-limiting lymphadenopathy caused by *Bartonella henselae* and is most frequently reported in children and young adults. The course of the disease is usually of short duration and benign. Approximately 10% of children with CSD develop complications, however, which may include hepatic granuloma, splenic abscess, encephalitis, or osteomyelitis. Severe systemic disease, which may persist for months, has been described in 2% of patients. Since the first description of CSD in 1954, there have been 22 reported cases of associated osteomyelitis, 19 of them in children.[257]

The diagnosis of CSD is difficult because the clinical presentation and tissue histology are nonspecific. The diagnosis should be considered in children who present with fever and lymphadenitis when a history of contact with cats or kittens is obtained. Tissue specimens typically demonstrate noncaseating granulomas, and organisms may occasionally be identified by Warthin-Starry silver staining.[178] Currently, the diagnosis is made by an enzyme-linked immunosorbent assay or indirect fluorescent antibody test, which demonstrates elevated titers of immunoglobulin G and immunoglobulin M to *B. henselae*.[163,178] Elevated antibody titers are found in less than 5% of the general population who do not have CSD.[178] Polymerase chain reaction assays of pus or tissue have a reported sensitivity and specificity approaching 100%, but this method of testing is not available in most laboratories.[178,257]

Treatment options are controversial. Antibiotic therapy is recommended, but it is uncertain whether the condition may resolve without treatment. A variety of antibiotics have been used with success, including aminoglycosides, azithromycin, cefazolin, and trimethoprim-sulfamethoxazole; however, only aminoglycosides display bactericidal activity against these organisms.[163,178,257] I have occasionally encountered children with such advanced epitrochlear lymphadenopathy that the lymph node architecture was compromised to the point of abscess formation that required surgical debridement (Fig. 35–33).

Mycotic Organisms

Mycotic osteomyelitis and septic arthritis are extremely rare and are often specific to endemic areas (Fig. 35–34). Fungal infections may occur by direct inoculation, as happens with *Aspergillus* species, *Sporothrix schenckii*, and *Scedosporium* species.[291] Alternatively, organisms may infect bone via hematogenous spread from other invasive infectious loci, such as the lungs. This commonly occurs with *Candida* species, *Blastomyces dermatitidis, Coccidioides immitis, Histoplasma capsulatum*, and *Cryptococcus neoformans*.[291] Fungal osteomyelitis is often seen in immunocompromised hosts.[292]

The radiographic features of fungal infections of bone are variable but have been described as similar to those seen in tuberculous osteomyelitis.[190] Fungal infections are often inappropriately treated owing to diagnostic delay. A high level of suspicion is needed to ensure that fungal cultures are sent and a proper biopsy specimen from bone or synovium is obtained for histopathologic evaluation.

Treatment with amphotericin B has been the preferred treatment for fungal infections. More recently,

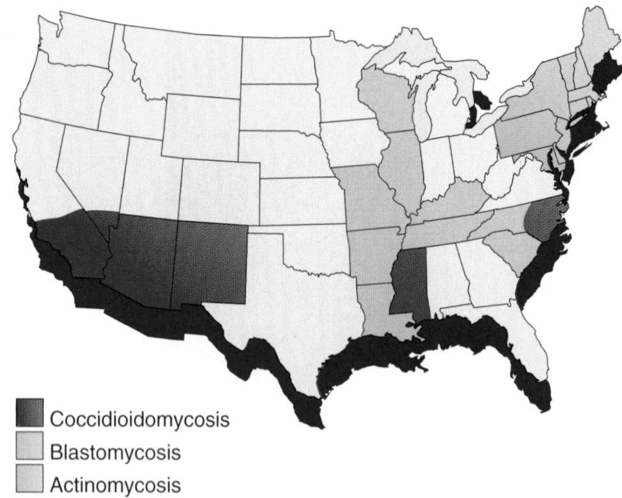

FIGURE 35-34 Endemic areas of fungal infection in the United States. Coccidioidomycosis: southwestern United States, particularly the San Joaquin Valley of California. Blastomycosis: areas extending from Wisconsin to Louisiana and from the Carolinas to Kentucky. Actinomycosis: Mississippi, North Carolina, and the northeastern United States.

the use of ketoconazole, in conjunction with operative treatment, has proved to be effective.[190]

COCCIDIOIDOMYCOSIS

Coccidioidomycosis, a fungal infection caused by *C. immitis,* affects primarily the lungs. Dissemination is rare but may produce skeletal lesions, either solitary or multiple. The diagnosis is made by identifying characteristic spores under the microscope. Serologic and skin tests are not sufficiently specific for diagnosis. The disease is endemic in the southwestern United States, particularly the San Joaquin Valley of California and Arizona. There has been a recent significant increase in the incidence of coccidioidomycosis.[110] A high index of suspicion should be maintained in patients with a flulike illness who live in or have visited areas with endemic disease.

BLASTOMYCOSIS

Blastomycosis affects primarily the skin and lungs. Bone is the third most common location of involvement, with as many as 60% of patients with systemic illness having a skeletal infection.[190] Blastomycosis is endemic throughout the southeastern and south-central United States, along the Mississippi and Ohio River valleys, and in central Canada. The disease is more common in rural areas and among outdoor workers. The diagnosis is made on histologic examination but may also be made by culture of the organism on Sabouraud agar.[190] Curettage and treatment with either amphotericin B or ketoconazole appear to be effective.[190]

ACTINOMYCOSIS

Actinomycosis is a chronic infection caused by the organism *Actinomyces israelii;* it usually involves the soft tissues of the head and neck, followed in frequency by the lungs and intestine.[225,274] Bone becomes involved by direct extension.[274] In North America, actinomycosis is endemic in Mississippi, North Carolina, and the northeastern United States. Patients are treated with long-term administration of penicillin.

SPOROTRICHOSIS

Sporotrichosis is a chronic granulomatous infection caused by the organism *Sporothrix schenckii;* it affects primarily the skin and subcutaneous tissues. Hand involvement is common due to penetrating injury from plant thorns.[37] Skeletal lesions may occur via direct extension from a subcutaneous lesion or, less commonly, through hematogenous spread. Sporotrichosis may be associated with sarcoidosis or tuberculosis.

References

1. Adu-Gyamfi Y, Sankarankutty M, Marwa S: Use of a tourniquet in patients with sickle-cell disease. Can J Anaesth 1993;40:24.
2. Ahmed S, Ayoub EM: Poststreptococcal reactive arthritis. Pediatr Infect Dis J 2001;20:1081.
3. Ahmed S, Ayoub EM, Scornik JC, et al: Poststreptococcal reactive arthritis: Clinical characteristics and association with HLA-DR alleles. Arthritis Rheum 1998; 41:1096.
4. Ansaloni L: Tropical pyomyositis. World J Surg 1996; 20:613.
5. Aronson J: Temporal and spatial increases in blood flow during distraction osteogenesis. Clin Orthop Relat Res 1994;301:124.
6. Aronson J, Garvin K, Seibert J, et al: Efficiency of the bone scan for occult limping toddlers. J Pediatr Orthop 1992;12:38.
7. Aroojis AJ, Johari AN: Epiphyseal separations after neonatal osteomyelitis and septic arthritis. J Pediatr Orthop 2000;20:544.
8. Ayoub EM, Majeed HA: Poststreptococcal reactive arthritis. Curr Opin Rheumatol 2000;12:306.
9. Baba T, Takeuchi F, Kuroda M, et al: Genome and virulence determinants of high virulence community-acquired MRSA. Lancet 2002;359:1819.
10. Baevsky RH: Neonatal group B beta-hemolytic streptococcus osteomyelitis. Am J Emerg Med 1999;17:619.
11. Barrett FF, McGehee RF Jr, Finland M: Methicillin-resistant *Staphylococcus aureus* at Boston City Hospital: Bacteriologic and epidemiologic observations. N Engl J Med 1968;279:441.
12. Bellah R: Ultrasound in pediatric musculoskeletal disease: Techniques and applications. Radiol Clin North Am 2001;39:597.
13. Bennett OM, Namnyak SS: Bone and joint manifestations of sickle cell anaemia. J Bone Joint Surg Br 1990; 72:494.
14. Bennett OM, Namnyak SS: Acute septic arthritis of the hip joint in infancy and childhood. Clin Orthop Relat Res 1992:123.

15. Bernard L, El H, Pron B, et al: Outpatient parenteral antimicrobial therapy (OPAT) for the treatment of osteomyelitis: Evaluation of efficacy, tolerance and cost. J Clin Pharm Ther 2001;26:445.
16. Betz RR, Cooperman DR, Wopperer JM, et al: Late sequelae of septic arthritis of the hip in infancy and childhood. J Pediatr Orthop 1990;10:365.
17. Bickels J, Ben-Sira L, Kessler A, et al: Primary pyomyositis. J Bone Joint Surg Am 2002;84:2277.
18. Billroth N: Clinical Surgery. London, New Sydenham Society, 1881.
19. Birdi N, Allen U, D'Astous J: Poststreptococcal reactive arthritis mimicking acute septic arthritis: A hospital-based study. J Pediatr Orthop 1995;15:661.
20. Bittmann S: Bacterial osteomyelitis after varicella infection in children. J Bone Miner Metab 2004;22:283.
21. Biviji AA, Paiement GD, Steinbach LS: Musculoskeletal manifestations of human immunodeficiency virus infection. J Am Acad Orthop Surg 2002;10:312.
22. Blyth MJ, Kincaid R, Craigen MA, et al: The changing epidemiology of acute and subacute haematogenous osteomyelitis in children. J Bone Joint Surg Br 2001; 83:99.
23. Booz MM, Hariharan V, Aradi AJ, et al: The value of ultrasound and aspiration in differentiating vaso-occlusive crisis and osteomyelitis in sickle cell disease patients. Clin Radiol 1999;54:636.
24. Borman TR, Johnson RA, Sherman FC: Gallium scintigraphy for diagnosis of septic arthritis and osteomyelitis in children. J Pediatr Orthop 1986;6:317.
25. Bowerman SG, Green NE, Mencio GA: Decline of bone and joint infections attributable to *Haemophilus influenzae* type b. Clin Orthop Relat Res 1997:128.
26. Bradley JS, Kaplan SL, Tan TQ, et al: Pediatric pneumococcal bone and joint infections. The Pediatric Multicenter Pneumococcal Surveillance Study Group (PMPSSG). Pediatrics 1998;102:1376.
27. Brodie B: Pathological and Surgical Observations on Disease of Joint. London, Longman, Rees, Orme, Brown, Green, & Longman, 1836.
28. Brothers TE, Tagge DU, Stutley JE, et al: Magnetic resonance imaging differentiates between necrotizing and non-necrotizing fasciitis of the lower extremity. J Am Coll Surg 1998;187:416.
29. Brown DL, Greenhalgh DG, Warden GD: Purpura fulminans: A disease best managed in a burn center. J Burn Care Rehabil 1998;19:119.
30. Buck C, Bundschu J, Gallati H, et al: Interleukin-6: A sensitive parameter for the early diagnosis of neonatal bacterial infection. Pediatrics 1994;93:54.
31. Burnett MW, Bass JW, Cook BA: Etiology of osteomyelitis complicating sickle cell disease. Pediatrics 1998;101:296.
32. Burns JL, Malhotra U, Lingappa J, et al: Unusual presentations of nontuberculous mycobacterial infections in children. Pediatr Infect Dis J 1997;16:802.
33. Canale ST, Harkness RM, Thomas PA, et al: Does aspiration of bones and joints affect results of later bone scanning? J Pediatr Orthop 1985;5:23.
34. Canale ST, Ikard ST: The orthopaedic implications of purpura fulminans. J Bone Joint Surg Am 1984;66: 764.
35. Carpenter CT, Kaiser AB: Purpura fulminans in pneumococcal sepsis: Case report and review. Scand J Infect Dis 1997;29:479.
36. Carr AJ, Cole WG, Roberton DM, et al: Chronic multifocal osteomyelitis. J Bone Joint Surg Br 1993;75:582.
37. Carr MM, Fielding JC, Sibbald G, et al: Sporotrichosis of the hand: An urban experience. J Hand Surg [Am] 1995;20:66.
38. Cavalier R, Herman MJ, Pizzutillo PD, et al: Ultrasound-guided aspiration of the hip in children: A new technique. Clin Orthop Relat Res 2003;415:244.
39. Centers for Disease Control and Prevention: Four pediatric deaths from community-acquired methicillin-resistant *Staphylococcus aureus*—Minnesota and North Dakota, 1997-1999. JAMA 1999;282:1123.
40. Chambers JB, Forsythe DA, Bertrand SL, et al: Retrospective review of osteoarticular infections in a pediatric sickle cell age group. J Pediatr Orthop 2000;20: 682.
41. Chan SP, Birnbaum J, Rao M, et al: Clinical manifestation and outcome of tuberculosis in children with acquired immunodeficiency syndrome. Pediatr Infect Dis J 1996;15:443.
42. Chao HC, Kong MS, Lin TY: Diagnosis of necrotizing fasciitis in children. J Ultrasound Med 1999;18:277.
43. Chen CE, Ko JY, Li CC, et al: Acute septic arthritis of the hip in children. Arch Orthop Trauma Surg 2001; 121:521.
44. Chiedozi LC: Pyomyositis: Review of 205 cases in 112 patients. Am J Surg 1979;137:255.
45. Choi IH, Pizzutillo PD, Bowen JR, et al: Sequelae and reconstruction after septic arthritis of the hip in infants. J Bone Joint Surg Am 1990;72:1150.
46. Christin L, Sarosi GA: Pyomyositis in North America: Case reports and review. Clin Infect Dis 1992;15:668.
47. Chung T: Magnetic resonance imaging in acute osteomyelitis in children. Pediatr Infect Dis J 2002;21:869.
48. Chung WK, Slater GL, Bates EH: Treatment of septic arthritis of the hip by arthroscopic lavage. J Pediatr Orthop 1993;13:444.
49. Cierny G 3rd, Mader JT, Penninck JJ: A clinical staging system for adult osteomyelitis. Clin Orthop Relat Res 2003;414:7.
50. Clark DJ: Venous thromboembolism in paediatric practice. Paediatr Anaesth 1999;9:475.
51. Clarke MT, Arora A, Villar RN: Hip arthroscopy: Complications in 1054 cases. Clin Orthop Relat Res 2003:84.
52. Clausen N, Gotze H, Pedersen A, et al: Skeletal scintigraphy and radiography at onset of acute lymphocytic leukemia in children. Med Pediatr Oncol 1983;11:291.
53. Cnota JF, Barton LL, Rhee KH: Purpura fulminans associated with *Streptococcus pneumoniae* infection in a child. Pediatr Emerg Care 1999;15:187.
54. Cole WG, Dalziel RE, Leitl S: Treatment of acute osteomyelitis in childhood. J Bone Joint Surg Br 1982;64: 218.
55. Collert S: Osteomyelitis of the spine. Acta Orthop Scand 1977;48:283.
56. Connolly LP, Connolly SA: Skeletal scintigraphy in the multimodality assessment of young children with acute skeletal symptoms. Clin Nucl Med 2003;28:746.

57. Connolly LP, Connolly SA, Drubach LA, et al: Acute hematogenous osteomyelitis of children: Assessment of skeletal scintigraphy-based diagnosis in the era of MRI. J Nucl Med 2002;43:1310.
58. Connolly LP, Treves ST: Assessing the limping child with skeletal scintigraphy. J Nucl Med 1998;39:1056.
59. Connolly LP, Treves ST, Connolly SA, et al: Pediatric skeletal scintigraphy: Applications of pinhole magnification. Radiographics 1998;18:341.
60. Controlled trial of short-course regimens of chemotherapy in the ambulatory treatment of spinal tuberculosis: Results at three years of a study in Korea. Twelfth Report of the Medical Research Council Working Party on Tuberculosis of the Spine. J Bone Joint Surg Br 1993;75:240.
61. Craigen MA, Watters J, Hackett JS: The changing epidemiology of osteomyelitis in children. J Bone Joint Surg Br 1992;74:541.
62. Cunningham R, Cockayne A, Humphreys H: Clinical and molecular aspects of the pathogenesis of *Staphylococcus aureus* bone and joint infections. J Med Microbiol 1996;44:157.
63. Cushing AH: Diskitis in children. Clin Infect Dis 1993;17:1.
64. Dalton GP, Drummond DS, Davidson RS, et al: Bone infarction versus infection in sickle cell disease in children. J Pediatr Orthop 1996;16:540.
65. Danielsson LG, Duppe H: Acute hematogenous osteomyelitis of the neck of the femur in children treated with drilling. Acta Orthop Scand 2002;73:311.
66. Daoud A, Saighi-Bouaouina A: Treatment of sequestra, pseudarthroses, and defects in the long bones of children who have chronic hematogenous osteomyelitis. J Bone Joint Surg Am 1989;71:1448.
67. Darmstadt GL: Acute infectious purpura fulminans: Pathogenesis and medical management. Pediatr Dermatol 1998;15:169.
68. Darville T, Jacobs RF: Management of acute hematogenous osteomyelitis in children. Pediatr Infect Dis J 2004;23:255.
69. Davidson D, Letts M, Khoshhal K: Pelvic osteomyelitis in children: A comparison of decades from 1980-1989 with 1990-2001. J Pediatr Orthop 2003;23:514.
70. Davis CE, Arnold K: Role of meningococcal endotoxin in meningococcal purpura. J Exp Med 1974;140:159.
71. Davis JM, Peel MM: Osteomyelitis and septic arthritis caused by *Kingella kingae*. J Clin Pathol 1982;35:219.
72. De Boeck H, Noppen L, Desprechins B: Pyomyositis of the adductor muscles mimicking an infection of the hip. Diagnosis by magnetic resonance imaging: A case report. J Bone Joint Surg Am 1994;76:747.
73. de Winter F, van de Wiele C, Vogelaers D, et al: Fluorine-18 fluorodeoxyglucose-positron emission tomography: A highly accurate imaging modality for the diagnosis of chronic musculoskeletal infections. J Bone Joint Surg Am 2001;83:651.
74. DeLuca PA, Gutman LT, Ruderman RJ: Counterimmunoelectrophoresis of synovial fluid in the diagnosis of septic arthritis. J Pediatr Orthop 1985;5:167.
75. Dich VQ, Nelson JD, Haltalin KC: Osteomyelitis in infants and children: A review of 163 cases. Am J Dis Child 1975;129:1273.
76. Do TT: Transient synovitis as a cause of painful limps in children. Curr Opin Pediatr 2000;12:48.
77. Dodman T, Robson J, Pincus D: *Kingella kingae* infections in children. J Paediatr Child Health 2000;36:87.
78. Dudkiewicz I, Salai M, Chechik A, et al: Total hip arthroplasty after childhood septic hip in patients younger than 25 years of age. J Pediatr Orthop 2000; 20:585.
79. Duffy CM, Lam PY, Ditchfield M, et al: Chronic recurrent multifocal osteomyelitis: Review of orthopaedic complications at maturity. J Pediatr Orthop 2002;22: 501.
80. Eidelman M, Bialik V, Miller Y, et al: Plantar puncture wounds in children: Analysis of 80 hospitalized patients and late sequelae. Isr Med Assoc J 2003;5:268.
81. Engin G, Acunas B, Acunas G, et al: Imaging of extrapulmonary tuberculosis. Radiographics 2000;20: 471.
82. Erdman WA, Tamburro F, Jayson HT, et al: Osteomyelitis: Characteristics and pitfalls of diagnosis with MR imaging. Radiology 1991;180:533.
83. Everett ED, Hirschmann JV: Transient bacteremia and endocarditis prophylaxis: A review. Medicine (Baltimore) 1977;56:61.
84. Ezra E, Cohen N, Segev E, et al: Primary subacute epiphyseal osteomyelitis: Role of conservative treatment. J Pediatr Orthop 2002;22:333.
85. Fendler C, Laitko S, Sorensen H, et al: Frequency of triggering bacteria in patients with reactive arthritis and undifferentiated oligoarthritis and the relative importance of the tests used for diagnosis. Ann Rheum Dis 2001;60:337.
86. Fernandez M, Carrol CL, Baker CJ: Discitis and vertebral osteomyelitis in children: An 18-year review. Pediatrics 2000;105:1299.
87. A 15-year assessment of controlled trials of the management of tuberculosis of the spine in Korea and Hong Kong. Thirteenth Report of the Medical Research Council Working Party on Tuberculosis of the Spine. J Bone Joint Surg Br 1998;80:456.
88. Five-year assessment of controlled trials of short-course chemotherapy regimens of 6, 9 or 18 months' duration for spinal tuberculosis in patients ambulatory from the start or undergoing radical surgery. Fourteenth Report of the Medical Research Council Working Party on Tuberculosis of the Spine. Int Orthop 1999;23:73.
89. Flier S, Dolgin SE, Saphir RL, et al: A case confirming the progressive stages of pyomyositis. J Pediatr Surg 2003;38:1551.
90. Floyed RL, Steele RW: Culture-negative osteomyelitis. Pediatr Infect Dis J 2003;22:731.
91. Foglar C, Lindsey RW: C-reactive protein in orthopedics. Orthopedics 1998;21:687.
92. Gabay C, Kushner I: Acute-phase proteins and other systemic responses to inflammation. N Engl J Med 1999;340:448.
93. Gallagher DJ, Phillips DJ, Heinrich SD: Orthopedic manifestations of acute pediatric leukemia. Orthop Clin North Am 1996;27:635.
94. Gallagher KT, Roberts RL, MacFarlane JA, et al: Treatment of chronic recurrent multifocal osteomyelitis with interferon gamma. J Pediatr 1997;131:470.

95. Garre C: Ueber besondere Formen und Folgezustande d. akuten indekt. Osteomyelitis. Cerh Dtsch Ges Pathol 1893;10:257.
96. Garron E, Viehweger E, Launay F, et al: Nontuberculous spondylodiscitis in children. J Pediatr Orthop 2002;22:321.
97. Gene A, Garcia-Garcia JJ, Sala P, et al: Enhanced culture detection of *Kingella kingae,* a pathogen of increasing clinical importance in pediatrics. Pediatr Infect Dis J 2004;23:886.
98. Gibson RK, Rosenthal SJ, Lukert BP: Pyomyositis: Increasing recognition in temperate climates. Am J Med 1984;77:768.
99. Giedion A, Holthusen W, Masel LF, et al: [Subacute and chronic "symmetrical" osteomyelitis]. Ann Radiol (Paris) 1972;15:329.
100. Gillespie WJ, Moore TE, Mayo KM: Subacute pyogenic osteomyelitis. Orthopedics 1986;9:1565.
101. Givon U, Liberman B, Schindler A, et al: Treatment of septic arthritis of the hip joint by repeated ultrasound-guided aspirations. J Pediatr Orthop 2004;24:266.
102. Glazer PA, Hu SS: Pediatric spinal infections. Orthop Clin North Am 1996;27:111.
103. Gledhill RB: Subacute osteomyelitis in children. Clin Orthop Relat Res 1973;96:57.
104. Gomez M, Maraqa N, Alvarez A, et al: Complications of outpatient parenteral antibiotic therapy in childhood. Pediatr Infect Dis J 2001;20:541.
105. Gonzalez-Lopez JL, Soleto-Martin FJ, Cubillo-Martin A, et al: Subacute osteomyelitis in children. J Pediatr Orthop B 2001;10:101.
106. Gordon JE, Huang M, Dobbs M, et al: Causes of false-negative ultrasound scans in the diagnosis of septic arthritis of the hip in children. J Pediatr Orthop 2002; 22:312.
107. Gorenstein A, Gross E, Houri S, et al: The pivotal role of deep vein thrombophlebitis in the development of acute disseminated staphylococcal disease in children. Pediatrics 2000;106:E87.
108. Griebel M, Nahlen B, Jacobs RF, et al: Group A streptococcal postvaricella osteomyelitis. J Pediatr Orthop 1985;5:101.
109. Grose C: Pyomyositis in children in the United States. Rev Infect Dis 1991;13:339.
110. McNabb SJ, Jajosky RA, Hall-Baker PA, et al: Summary of notifiable diseases—United States, 2005. MMWR Morbidity Mortal Wkly Rep 2007;54(53):2-92.
111. Gubbay AJ, Isaacs D: Pyomyositis in children. Pediatr Infect Dis J 2000;19:1009.
112. Guinto-Ocampo H, Friedland LR: Disseminated gonococcal infection in three adolescents. Pediatr Emerg Care 2001;17:441.
113. Gwynne-Jones DP, Stott NS: Community-acquired methicillin-resistant *Staphylococcus aureus:* A cause of musculoskeletal sepsis in children. J Pediatr Orthop 1999;19:413.
114. Hall RL, Callaghan JJ, Moloney E, et al: Pyomyositis in a temperate climate: Presentation, diagnosis, and treatment. J Bone Joint Surg Am 1990;72:1240.
115. Hallel T, Salvati EA: Septic arthritis of the hip in infancy: End result study. Clin Orthop Relat Res 1978; 132:115.
116. Hamdy RC, Babyn PS, Krajbich JI: Use of bone scan in management of patients with peripheral gangrene due to fulminant meningococcemia. J Pediatr Orthop 1993; 13:447.
117. Hamdy RC, Lawton L, Carey T, et al: Subacute hematogenous osteomyelitis: Are biopsy and surgery always indicated? J Pediatr Orthop 1996;16:220.
118. Handrick W, Hormann D, Voppmann A, et al: Chronic recurrent multifocal osteomyelitis—report of eight patients. Pediatr Surg Int 1998;14:195.
119. Hardy AE, Nicol RO: Closed fractures complicated by acute hematogenous osteomyelitis. Clin Orthop Relat Res 1985:190.
120. Harrington P, Scott B, Chetcuti P: Multifocal streptococcal pyomyositis complicated by acute compartment syndrome: Case report. J Pediatr Orthop B 2001;10: 120.
121. Harris NH, Kirkaldy-Willis WH: Primary subacute pyogenic osteomyelitis. J Bone Joint Surg Br 1965;47: 526.
122. Havlir DV, Barnes PF: Tuberculosis in patients with human immunodeficiency virus infection. N Engl J Med 1999;340:367.
123. Hernandez RJ, Strouse PJ, Craig CL, et al: Focal pyomyositis of the perisciatic muscles in children. AJR Am J Roentgenol 2002;179:1267.
124. Herold BC, Immergluck LC, Maranan MC, et al: Community-acquired methicillin-resistant *Staphylococcus aureus* in children with no identified predisposing risk. JAMA 1998;279:593.
125. Highland TR, LaMont RL: Osteomyelitis of the pelvis in children. J Bone Joint Surg Am 1983;65:230.
126. Hobo T: Zur Pathogenese der akuten haematogenen Osteomyelitis, mit Berucksichtigung der Vitalfarbungslehre. Acta Sch Med Univ Imp Kioto 1921;4:1.
127. Hoffer FA, Strand RD, Gebhardt MC: Percutaneous biopsy of pyogenic infection of the spine in children. J Pediatr Orthop 1988;8:442.
128. Hoffman EB, de Beer JD, Keys G, et al: Diaphyseal primary subacute osteomyelitis in children. J Pediatr Orthop 1990;10:250.
129. Hoffman JA, Mason EO, Schutze GE, et al: *Streptococcus pneumoniae* infections in the neonate. Pediatrics 2003; 112:1095.
130. Hossain A, Reis ED, Soundararajan K, et al: Nontropical pyomyositis: Analysis of eight patients in an urban center. Am Surg 2000;66:1064.
131. Howard AW, Viskontas D, Sabbagh C: Reduction in osteomyelitis and septic arthritis related to *Haemophilus influenzae* type b vaccination. J Pediatr Orthop 1999; 19:705.
132. Howard CB, Einhorn M, Dagan R, et al: Fine-needle bone biopsy to diagnose osteomyelitis. J Bone Joint Surg Br 1994;76:311.
133. Huang DB, Price M, Pokorny J, et al: Reconstructive surgery in children after meningococcal purpura fulminans. J Pediatr Surg 1999;34:595.
134. Huber AM, Lam PY, Duffy CM, et al: Chronic recurrent multifocal osteomyelitis: Clinical outcomes after more than five years of follow-up. J Pediatr 2002;141:198.
135. Hunka L, Said SE, MacKenzie DA, et al: Classification and surgical management of the severe sequelae of

septic hips in children. Clin Orthop Relat Res 1982:30.

136. Ibia EO, Imoisili M, Pikis A: Group A beta-hemolytic streptococcal osteomyelitis in children. Pediatrics 2003;112:e22.
137. Imoisili MA, Bonwit AM, Bulas DI: Toothpick puncture injuries of the foot in children. Pediatr Infect Dis J 2004;23:80.
138. Iqbal A, McKenna D, Hayes R, et al: Osteomyelitis of the ischiopubic synchondrosis: Imaging findings. Skeletal Radiol 2004;33:176.
139. Ish-Horowicz MR, McIntyre P, Nade S: Bone and joint infections caused by multiply resistant *Staphylococcus aureus* in a neonatal intensive care unit. Pediatr Infect Dis J 1992;11:82.
140. Jaakkola J, Kehl D: Hematogenous calcaneal osteomyelitis in children. J Pediatr Orthop 1999;19:699.
141. Jaberi FM, Shahcheraghi GH, Ahadzadeh M: Short-term intravenous antibiotic treatment of acute hematogenous bone and joint infection in children: A prospective randomized trial. J Pediatr Orthop 2002; 22:317.
142. Jackson MA, Burry VF, Olson LC: Multisystem group A beta-hemolytic streptococcal disease in children. Rev Infect Dis 1991;13:783.
143. Jackson MA, Burry VF, Olson LC: Complications of varicella requiring hospitalization in previously healthy children. Pediatr Infect Dis J 1992;11:441.
144. Jackson MA, Burry VF, Olson LC: Pyogenic arthritis associated with adjacent osteomyelitis: Identification of the sequela-prone child. Pediatr Infect Dis J 1992;11:9.
145. Jackson MA, Nelson JD: Etiology and medical management of acute suppurative bone and joint infections in pediatric patients. J Pediatr Orthop 1982;2:313.
146. Jacobs NM: Pneumococcal osteomyelitis and arthritis in children: A hospital series and literature review. Am J Dis Child 1991;145:70.
147. Jacobs RF, Adelman L, Sack CM, et al: Management of *Pseudomonas* osteochondritis complicating puncture wounds of the foot. Pediatrics 1982;69:432.
148. Jansen BR, Hart W, Schreuder O: Discitis in childhood: 12-35-year follow-up of 35 patients. Acta Orthop Scand 1993;64:33.
149. Jaramillo D, Treves ST, Kasser JR, et al: Osteomyelitis and septic arthritis in children: Appropriate use of imaging to guide treatment. AJR Am J Roentgenol 1995;165:399.
150. Jaye DL, Waites KB: Clinical applications of C-reactive protein in pediatrics. Pediatr Infect Dis J 1997;16:735.
151. Johansen K, Hansen ST Jr: Symmetrical peripheral gangrene (purpura fulminans) complicating pneumococcal sepsis. Am J Surg 1993;165:642.
152. Jones T: The diagnosis of rheumatic fever. JAMA 1944;126:481.
153. Jonsson OG, Sartain P, Ducore JM, et al: Bone pain as an initial symptom of childhood acute lymphoblastic leukemia: Association with nearly normal hematologic indexes. J Pediatr 1990;117:233.
154. Josefsson E, Hartford O, O'Brien L, et al: Protection against experimental *Staphylococcus aureus* arthritis by vaccination with clumping factor A, a novel virulence determinant. J Infect Dis 2001;184:1572.
155. Jung ST, Rowe SM, Moon ES, et al: Significance of laboratory and radiologic findings for differentiating between septic arthritis and transient synovitis of the hip. J Pediatr Orthop 2003;23:368.
156. Kadambari D, Jagdish S: Primary pyogenic psoas abscess in children. Pediatr Surg Int 2000;16:408.
157. Kahn DS, Pritzker KP: The pathophysiology of bone infection. Clin Orthop Relat Res 1973;96:12.
158. Kaiser S, Jorulf H, Hirsch G: Clinical value of imaging techniques in childhood osteomyelitis. Acta Radiol 1998;39:523.
159. Kallio P, Michelsson JE, Lalla M, et al: C-reactive protein in tibial fractures: Natural response to the injury and operative treatment. J Bone Joint Surg Br 1990;72:615.
160. Karwowska A, Davies HD, Jadavji T: Epidemiology and outcome of osteomyelitis in the era of sequential intravenous-oral therapy. Pediatr Infect Dis J 1998;17:1021.
161. Kasten MJ: Clindamycin, metronidazole, and chloramphenicol. Mayo Clin Proc 1999;74:825.
162. Kelly PJ, Martin WJ, Schirger A, et al: Brucellosis of the bones and joints: Experience with thirty-six patients. JAMA 1960;174:347.
163. Keret D, Giladi M, Kletter Y, et al: Cat-scratch disease osteomyelitis from a dog scratch. J Bone Joint Surg Br 1998;80:766.
164. Khachatourians AG, Patzakis MJ, Roidis N, et al: Laboratory monitoring in pediatric acute osteomyelitis and septic arthritis. Clin Orthop Relat Res 2003;409:186.
165. Killian JT, Kramer T: Pediatric vertebral osteomyelitis: Diagnosis using computed tomography. J South Orthop Assoc 1997;6:256.
166. Kim HK, Alman B, Cole WG: A shortened course of parenteral antibiotic therapy in the management of acute septic arthritis of the hip. J Pediatr Orthop 2000; 20:44.
167. Kim SJ, Choi NH, Ko SH, et al: Arthroscopic treatment of septic arthritis of the hip. Clin Orthop Relat Res 2003;407:211.
168. King DM, Mayo KM: Subacute haematogenous osteomyelitis. J Bone Joint Surg Br 1969;51:458.
169. *Kingella kingae* infections in children—United States, June 2001-November 2002. MMWR Morb Mortal Wkly Rep 2004;53:244.
170. Klein DM, Barbera C, Gray ST, et al: Sensitivity of objective parameters in the diagnosis of pediatric septic hips. Clin Orthop Relat Res 1997;338:153.
171. Kocher MS, Mandiga R, Murphy JM, et al: A clinical practice guideline for treatment of septic arthritis in children: Efficacy in improving process of care and effect on outcome of septic arthritis of the hip. J Bone Joint Surg Am 2003;85:994.
172. Kocher MS, Mandiga R, Zurakowski D, et al: Validation of a clinical prediction rule for the differentiation between septic arthritis and transient synovitis of the hip in children. J Bone Joint Surg Am 2004;86:1629.
173. Kocher MS, Zurakowski D, Kasser JR: Differentiating between septic arthritis and transient synovitis of the hip in children: An evidence-based clinical prediction algorithm. J Bone Joint Surg Am 1999;81:1662.
174. Konyves A, Deo SD, Murray JR, et al: Septic arthritis of the elbow after chickenpox. J Pediatr Orthop B 2004; 13:114.

175. Kothari NA, Pelchovitz DJ, Meyer JS: Imaging of musculoskeletal infections. Radiol Clin North Am 2001; 39:653.
176. Kucukkaya M, Kabukcuoglu Y, Tezer M, et al: Management of childhood chronic tibial osteomyelitis with the Ilizarov method. J Pediatr Orthop 2002;22:632.
177. Kumar R, Walsh A, Khalilullah K, et al: An unusual orthopaedic presentation of acute lymphoblastic leukemia. J Pediatr Orthop B 2003;12:292.
178. LaRow JM, Wehbe P, Pascual AG: Cat-scratch disease in a child with unique magnetic resonance imaging findings. Arch Pediatr Adolesc Med 1998;152:394.
179. Lee SK, Suh KJ, Kim YW, et al: Septic arthritis versus transient synovitis at MR imaging: Preliminary assessment with signal intensity alterations in bone marrow. Radiology 1999;211:459.
180. Letts M, Lalonde F, Davidson D, et al: Atrial and venous thrombosis secondary to septic arthritis of the sacroiliac joint in a child with hereditary protein C deficiency. J Pediatr Orthop 1999;19:156.
181. Levine MJ, McGuire KJ, McGowan KL, et al: Assessment of the test characteristics of C-reactive protein for septic arthritis in children. J Pediatr Orthop 2003;23: 373.
182. Lewin JS, Rosenfield NS, Hoffer PB, et al: Acute osteomyelitis in children: Combined Tc-99m and Ga-67 imaging. Radiology 1986;158:795.
183. Liptak GS, McConnochie KM, Roghmann KJ, et al: Decline of pediatric admissions with *Haemophilus influenzae* type b in New York State, 1982 through 1993: Relation to immunizations. J Pediatr 1997;130:923.
184. Loh NN, Ch'en IY, Cheung LP, et al: Deep fascial hyperintensity in soft-tissue abnormalities as revealed by T2-weighted MR imaging. AJR Am J Roentgenol 1997; 168:1301.
185. Lowden CM, Walsh SJ: Acute staphylococcal osteomyelitis of the clavicle. J Pediatr Orthop 1997;17:467.
186. Luhmann SJ, Jones A, Schootman M, et al: Differentiation between septic arthritis and transient synovitis of the hip in children with clinical prediction algorithms. J Bone Joint Surg Am 2004;86:956.
187. Lundy DW, Kehl DK: Increasing prevalence of *Kingella kingae* in osteoarticular infections in young children. J Pediatr Orthop 1998;18:262.
188. Lyme disease—United States, 2001-2002. MMWR Morb Mortal Wkly Rep 2004;53:365.
189. Lyon RM, Evanich JD: Culture-negative septic arthritis in children. J Pediatr Orthop 1999;19:655.
190. MacDonald PB, Black GB, MacKenzie R: Orthopaedic manifestations of blastomycosis. J Bone Joint Surg Am 1990;72:860.
191. Mackie SL, Keat A: Poststreptococcal reactive arthritis: What is it and how do we know? Rheumatology (Oxford) 2004;43:949.
192. Mader JT, Shirtliff M, Calhoun JH: Staging and staging application in osteomyelitis. Clin Infect Dis 1997;25: 1303.
193. Mah ET, LeQuesne GW, Gent RJ, et al: Ultrasonic features of acute osteomyelitis in children. J Bone Joint Surg Br 1994;76:969.
194. Mankin HJ, Lange TA, Spanier SS: The hazards of biopsy in patients with malignant primary bone and soft-tissue tumors. J Bone Joint Surg Am 1982;64: 1121.
195. Mankin HJ, Mankin CJ, Simon MA: The hazards of the biopsy, revisited. Members of the Musculoskeletal Tumor Society. J Bone Joint Surg Am 1996;78:656.
196. Manzotti A, Rovetta L, Pullen C, et al: Treatment of the late sequelae of septic arthritis of the hip. Clin Orthop Relat Res 2003:203.
197. Maraqa NF, Gomez MM, Rathore MH: Outpatient parenteral antimicrobial therapy in osteoarticular infections in children. J Pediatr Orthop 2002;22:506.
198. Marshall GS, Mudido P, Rabalais GP, et al: Organism isolation and serum bactericidal titers in oral antibiotic therapy for pediatric osteomyelitis. South Med J 1996; 89:68.
199. Martinez-Aguilar G, Avalos-Mishaan A, Hulten K, et al: Community-acquired, methicillin-resistant and methicillin-susceptible *Staphylococcus aureus* musculoskeletal infections in children. Pediatr Infect Dis J 2004;23:701.
200. Martinez-Aguilar G, Hammerman WA, Mason EO Jr, et al: Clindamycin treatment of invasive infections caused by community-acquired, methicillin-resistant and methicillin-susceptible *Staphylococcus aureus* in children. Pediatr Infect Dis J 2003;22:593.
201. Mazur JM, Ross G, Cummings J, et al: Usefulness of magnetic resonance imaging for the diagnosis of acute musculoskeletal infections in children. J Pediatr Orthop 1995;15:144.
202. Meller I, Manor Y, Bar-Ziv J, et al: Pediatric update #8. Acute hematogenous osteomyelitis in children: Long-term results of surgical treatment. Orthop Rev 1989; 18:824.
203. Miron D, El AL, Zuker M, et al: *Mycobacterium fortuitum* osteomyelitis of the cuboid after nail puncture wound. Pediatr Infect Dis J 2000;19:483.
204. Miyake H: Bietrage zur kentnis der songenannten myositis infectiosa. Mitt Grenzgeb Med Chir 1904;13: 155.
205. Moon RY, Greene MG, Rehe GT, et al: Poststreptococcal reactive arthritis in children: A potential predecessor of rheumatic heart disease. J Rheumatol 1995;22:529.
206. Moreno F, Crisp C, Jorgensen JH, et al: Methicillin-resistant *Staphylococcus aureus* as a community organism. Clin Infect Dis 1995;21:1308.
207. Morrey BF, Bianco AJ Jr, Rhodes KH: Septic arthritis in children. Orthop Clin North Am 1975;6:923.
208. Morrey BF, Peterson HA: Hematogenous pyogenic osteomyelitis in children. Orthop Clin North Am 1975; 6:935.
209. Morrissy R: Bone and joint sepsis. In Morrissy R (ed): Lovell and Winter's Pediatric Orthopaedics, vol 1. Philadelphia, Lippincott-Raven, 1996, p 579.
210. Morrissy RT, Haynes DW: Acute hematogenous osteomyelitis: A model with trauma as an etiology. J Pediatr Orthop 1989;9:447.
211. Mousa AR, Muhtaseb SA, Almudallal DS, et al: Osteoarticular complications of brucellosis: A study of 169 cases. Rev Infect Dis 1987;9:531.
212. Mousa HA: Evaluation of sinus-track cultures in chronic bone infection. J Bone Joint Surg Br 1997;79: 567.

213. Muller G, Cherasse A, Bour JB, et al: Diagnostic usefulness of routine Lyme serology in patients with early inflammatory arthritis in nonendemic areas. Joint Bone Spine 2003;70:119.
214. Museru LM, McHaro CN: Chronic osteomyelitis: A continuing orthopaedic challenge in developing countries. Int Orthop 2001;25:127.
215. Mustafa MM, Saez-Llorens X, McCracken GH Jr, et al: Acute hematogenous pelvic osteomyelitis in infants and children. Pediatr Infect Dis J 1990;9:416.
216. Nadel HR, Stilwell ME: Nuclear medicine topics in pediatric musculoskeletal disease: Techniques and applications. Radiol Clin North Am 2001;39:619.
217. Nance CL Jr, Roberts WM, Miller GR: Ewing's sarcoma mimicking osteomyelitis. South Med J 1967; 60:1044.
218. Nelson JD: Toward simple but safe management of osteomyelitis. Pediatrics 1997;99:883.
219. Nelson JD, Bucholz RW, Kusmiesz H, et al: Benefits and risks of sequential parenteral-oral cephalosporin therapy for suppurative bone and joint infections. J Pediatr Orthop 1982;2:255.
220. Nelson JD, Howard JB, Shelton S: Oral antibiotic therapy for skeletal infections of children. I. Antibiotic concentrations in suppurative synovial fluid. J Pediatr 1978;92:131.
221. Newton PO, Ballock RT, Bradley JS: Oral antibiotic therapy of bacterial arthritis. Pediatr Infect Dis J 1999;18:1102.
222. Nolan J, Sinclair R: Review of management of purpura fulminans and two case reports. Br J Anaesth 2001;86: 581.
223. Norden CW: Experimental osteomyelitis. I. A description of the model. J Infect Dis 1970;122:410.
224. Norden CW: Lessons learned from animal models of osteomyelitis. Rev Infect Dis 1988;10:103.
225. Ogutcen-Toller M, Alkan A, Baris S, et al: An unusual form of actinomycosis of the mandible with a resultant gross sequester in a 4-year-old child: A case report. J Clin Pediatr Dent 2001;25:237.
226. Orlicek SL, Abramson JS, Woods CR, et al: Obturator internus muscle abscess in children. J Pediatr Orthop 2001;21:744.
227. Osman AA, Govender S: Septic sacroiliitis. Clin Orthop Relat Res 1995;313:214.
228. Osteomyelitis/septic arthritis caused by *Kingella kingae* among day care attendees—Minnesota, 2003. MMWR Morb Mortal Wkly Rep 2004;53:241.
229. Patti JM, Bremell T, Krajewska-Pietrasik D, et al: The *Staphylococcus aureus* collagen adhesin is a virulence determinant in experimental septic arthritis. Infect Immun 1994;62:152.
230. Peckett WR, Butler-Manuel A, Apthorp LA: Pyomyositis of the iliacus muscle in a child. J Bone Joint Surg Br 2001;83:103.
231. Peltola H, Unkila-Kallio L, Kallio MJ: Simplified treatment of acute staphylococcal osteomyelitis of childhood. The Finnish Study Group. Pediatrics 1997;99: 846.
232. Pennington WT, Mott MP, Thometz JG, et al: Photopenic bone scan osteomyelitis: A clinical perspective. J Pediatr Orthop 1999;19:695.
233. Perlman MH, Patzakis MJ, Kumar PJ, et al: The incidence of joint involvement with adjacent osteomyelitis in pediatric patients. J Pediatr Orthop 2000;20:40.
234. Perry CR, Davenport K, Vossen MK: Local delivery of antibiotics via an implantable pump in the treatment of osteomyelitis. Clin Orthop Relat Res 1988;226:222.
235. Peters W, Irving J, Letts M: Long-term effects of neonatal bone and joint infection on adjacent growth plates. J Pediatr Orthop 1992;12:806.
236. Piehl FC, Davis RJ, Prugh SI: Osteomyelitis in sickle cell disease. J Pediatr Orthop 1993;13:225.
237. Pong A, Chartrand SA, Huurman W: Pyomyositis and septic arthritis caused by group C streptococcus. Pediatr Infect Dis J 1998;17:1052.
238. Pott P: Remarks on That Kind of Palsy of the Lower Limbs Which Is Frequently Found to Accompany Curvature of the Spine and Is Supposed to Be Caused by It, Together with Its Method of Cure. London, Lowndes, 1779.
239. Poyhia T, Azouz EM: MR imaging evaluation of subacute and chronic bone abscesses in children. Pediatr Radiol 2000;30:763.
240. Prober CG: Current antibiotic therapy of community-acquired bacterial infections in hospitalized children: Bone and joint infections. Pediatr Infect Dis J 1992; 11:156.
241. Puffinbarger WR, Gruel CR, Herndon WA, et al: Osteomyelitis of the calcaneus in children. J Pediatr Orthop 1996;16:224.
242. Pulliam PN, Attia MW, Cronan KM: C-reactive protein in febrile children 1 to 36 months of age with clinically undetectable serious bacterial infection. Pediatrics 2001;108:1275.
243. Ramos OM: Chronic osteomyelitis in children. Pediatr Infect Dis J 2002;21:431.
244. Rasool MN: Osseous manifestations of tuberculosis in children. J Pediatr Orthop 2001;21:749.
245. Rasool MN: Primary subacute haematogenous osteomyelitis in children. J Bone Joint Surg Br 2001;83:93.
246. Reduced susceptibility of *Staphylococcus aureus* to vancomycin—Japan, 1996. MMWR Morb Mortal Wkly Rep 1997;46:624.
247. Reinehr T, Burk G, Michel E, et al: Chronic osteomyelitis in childhood: Is surgery always indicated? Infection 2000;28:282.
248. Renwick SE, Ritterbusch JF: Pyomyositis in children. J Pediatr Orthop 1993;13:769.
249. Report of the Committee on Infectious Diseases. In Peter G (ed): Red Book, vol 24. Elk Grove Village, Ill, American Academy of Pediatrics, 1997, p 541.
250. Riegels-Nielson P, Frimodt-Moller N, Jensen JS: Rabbit model of septic arthritis. Acta Orthop Scand 1987;58: 14.
251. Ring D, Johnston CE 2nd, Wenger DR: Pyogenic infectious spondylitis in children: The convergence of discitis and vertebral osteomyelitis. J Pediatr Orthop 1995;15:652.
252. Ring D, Wenger DR: Pyogenic infectious spondylitis in children: The evolution to current thought. Am J Orthop 1996;25:342.
253. Rissing JP, Buxton TB: Effect of ibuprofen on gross pathology, bacterial count, and levels of prostaglandin

E_2 in experimental staphylococcal osteomyelitis. J Infect Dis 1986;154:627.
254. Roberts JM, Drummond DS, Breed AL, et al: Subacute hematogenous osteomyelitis in children: A retrospective study. J Pediatr Orthop 1982;2:249.
255. Robertson LP, Hickling P: Chronic recurrent multifocal osteomyelitis is a differential diagnosis of juvenile idiopathic arthritis. Ann Rheum Dis 2001;60:828.
256. Roine I, Arguedas A, Faingezicht I, et al: Early detection of sequela-prone osteomyelitis in children with use of simple clinical and laboratory criteria. Clin Infect Dis 1997;24:849.
257. Rolain JM, Chanet V, Laurichesse H, et al: Cat scratch disease with lymphadenitis, vertebral osteomyelitis, and spleen abscesses. Ann N Y Acad Sci 2003;990:397.
258. Rose CD, Fawcett PT, Eppes SC, et al: Pediatric Lyme arthritis: Clinical spectrum and outcome. J Pediatr Orthop 1994;14:238.
259. Rosenberg J: Methicillin-resistant *Staphylococcus aureus* (MRSA) in the community: Who's watching? Lancet 1995;346:132.
260. Ross ER, Cole WG: Treatment of subacute osteomyelitis in childhood. J Bone Joint Surg Br 1985;67:443.
261. Ross JJ, Saltzman CL, Carling P, et al: Pneumococcal septic arthritis: Review of 190 cases. Clin Infect Dis 2003;36:319.
262. Roy DR: Osteomyelitis of the patella. Clin Orthop Relat Res 2001;389:30.
263. Roy DR, Greene WB, Gamble JG: Osteomyelitis of the patella in children. J Pediatr Orthop 1991;11:364.
264. Rudert M, Tillmann B: Lymph and blood supply of the human intervertebral disc: Cadaver study of correlations to discitis. Acta Orthop Scand 1993;64:37.
265. Sachs BL, Shaffer JW: A staged Papineau protocol for chronic osteomyelitis. Clin Orthop Relat Res 1984;184:256.
266. Sadat-Ali M, al-Umran K, al-Habdan I, et al: Ultrasonography: Can it differentiate between vasoocclusive crisis and acute osteomyelitis in sickle cell disease? J Pediatr Orthop 1998;18:552.
267. Saslaw MM, Mishra S, Green M, et al: Suppurative arthritis complicating otitis media. Pediatr Infect Dis J 1999;18:475.
268. Sawlani V, Chandra T, Mishra RN, et al: MRI features of tuberculosis of peripheral joints. Clin Radiol 2003;58:755.
269. Schaad UB, abdus Salam M, Aujard Y, et al: Use of fluoroquinolones in pediatrics: Consensus report of an International Society of Chemotherapy commission. Pediatr Infect Dis J 1995;14:1.
270. Schenk RK, Wiener J, Spiro D: Fine structural aspects of vascular invasion of the tibial epiphyseal plate of growing rats. Acta Anat (Basel) 1968;69:1.
271. Schultz C, Holterhus PM, Seidel A, et al: Chronic recurrent multifocal osteomyelitis in children. Pediatr Infect Dis J 1999;18:1008.
272. Scott RJ, Christofersen MR, Robertson WW Jr, et al: Acute osteomyelitis in children: A review of 116 cases. J Pediatr Orthop 1990;10:649.
273. Segev E, Hayek S, Lokiec F, et al: Primary chronic sclerosing (Garre's) osteomyelitis in children. J Pediatr Orthop B 2001;10:360.
274. Sezer B, Ertugrul F, Gunbay S, et al: Atypical presentations of pediatric actinomycosis: Report of a case. ASDC J Dent Child 2002;69:138.
275. Skaggs DL, Kim SK, Greene NW, et al: Differentiation between bone infarction and acute osteomyelitis in children with sickle-cell disease with use of sequential radionuclide bone-marrow and bone scans. J Bone Joint Surg Am 2001;83:1810.
276. Skyhar MJ, Mubarak SJ: Arthroscopic treatment of septic knees in children. J Pediatr Orthop 1987;7:647.
277. Smith OP, White B: Infectious purpura fulminans: Diagnosis and treatment. Br J Haematol 1999;104:202.
278. Smith RL, Schurman DJ: Comparison of cartilage destruction between infectious and adjuvant arthritis. J Orthop Res 1983;1:136.
279. Song J, Letts M, Monson R: Differentiation of psoas muscle abscess from septic arthritis of the hip in children. Clin Orthop Relat Res 2001;411:258.
280. Song KM, Sloboda JF: Acute hematogenous osteomyelitis in children. J Am Acad Orthop Surg 2001;9:166.
281. Song KS, Ogden JA, Ganey T, et al: Contiguous discitis and osteomyelitis in children. J Pediatr Orthop 1997;17:470.
282. Sonnen GM, Henry NK: Pediatric bone and joint infections: Diagnosis and antimicrobial management. Pediatr Clin North Am 1996;43:933.
283. Spiegel DA, Meyer JS, Dormans JP, et al: Pyomyositis in children and adolescents: Report of 12 cases and review of the literature. J Pediatr Orthop 1999;19:143.
284. Stanitski CL, Harvell JC, Fu FH: Arthroscopy in acute septic knees: Management in pediatric patients. Clin Orthop Relat Res 1989;241:209.
285. Steinberg JP, Clark CC, Hackman BO: Nosocomial and community-acquired *Staphylococcus aureus* bacteremias from 1980 to 1993: Impact of intravascular devices and methicillin resistance. Clin Infect Dis 1996;23:255.
286. Steiner P, Rao M, Mitchell M, et al: Primary drug-resistant tuberculosis in children: Emergence of primary drug-resistant strains of *M. tuberculosis* to rifampin. Am Rev Respir Dis 1986;134:446.
287. Sturzenbecher A, Braun J, Paris S, et al: MR imaging of septic sacroiliitis. Skeletal Radiol 2000;29:439.
288. Stutz G, Kuster MS, Kleinstuck F, et al: Arthroscopic management of septic arthritis: Stages of infection and results. Knee Surg Sports Traumatol Arthrosc 2000;8:270.
289. Sucato DJ, Gillespie R: *Salmonella* pelvic osteomyelitis in normal children: Report of two cases and a review of the literature. J Pediatr Orthop 1997;17:463.
290. Sundberg SB, Savage JP, Foster BK: Technetium phosphate bone scan in the diagnosis of septic arthritis in childhood. J Pediatr Orthop 1989;9:579.
291. Sydnor MK, Kaushik S, Knight TE Jr, et al: Mycotic osteomyelitis due to *Scedosporium apiospermum:* MR imaging-pathologic correlation. Skeletal Radiol 2003;32:656.
292. Tehranzadeh J, Ter-Oganesyan RR, Steinbach LS: Musculoskeletal disorders associated with HIV infection and AIDS. Part I. Infectious musculoskeletal conditions. Skeletal Radiol 2004;33:249.

293. Tetzlaff TR, Howard JB, McCraken GH, et al: Antibiotic concentrations in pus and bone of children with osteomyelitis. J Pediatr 1978;92:135.
294. Thomas S, Tytherleigh-Strong G, Dodds R: Pyomyositis of the iliacus muscle in a child. J Bone Joint Surg Br 2001;83:619.
295. Thomas S, Tytherleigh-Strong G, Dodds R: Adductor myositis as a cause of childhood hip pain. J Pediatr Orthop B 2002;11:117.
296. Tice AD, Hoaglund PA, Shoultz DA: Outcomes of osteomyelitis among patients treated with outpatient parenteral antimicrobial therapy. Am J Med 2003;114:723.
297. Tillett W, Francis TJ: Serological reactions in pneumonia with non-protein somatic fraction of pneumococcus. J Exp Med 1930;52:561.
298. Tindall EA, Regan-Smith MG: Gonococcal osteomyelitis complicating septic arthritis. JAMA 1983;250:2671.
299. Trueta J: [The 3 types of acute hematogenous osteomyelitis]. Schweiz Med Wochenschr 1963;93:306.
300. Tuson CE, Hoffman EB, Mann MD: Isotope bone scanning for acute osteomyelitis and septic arthritis in children. J Bone Joint Surg Br 1994;76:306.
301. Tzeng YL, Stephens DS: Epidemiology and pathogenesis of *Neisseria meningitidis*. Microbes Infect 2000;2:687.
302. Uhl M, Krauss M, Kern S, et al: The knee joint in early juvenile idiopathic arthritis: An ROC study for evaluating the diagnostic accuracy of contrast-enhanced MR imaging. Acta Radiol 2001;42:6.
303. Umans H, Haramati N, Flusser G: The diagnostic role of gadolinium enhanced MRI in distinguishing between acute medullary bone infarct and osteomyelitis. Magn Reson Imaging 2000;18:255.
304. Unkila-Kallio L, Kallio MJ, Eskola J, et al: Serum C-reactive protein, erythrocyte sedimentation rate, and white blood cell count in acute hematogenous osteomyelitis of children. Pediatrics 1994;93:59.
305. Unkila-Kallio L, Kallio MJ, Peltola H: The usefulness of C-reactive protein levels in the identification of concurrent septic arthritis in children who have acute hematogenous osteomyelitis: A comparison with the usefulness of the erythrocyte sedimentation rate and the white blood-cell count. J Bone Joint Surg Am 1994;76:848.
306. Vassilopoulos D, Chalasani P, Jurado RL, et al: Musculoskeletal infections in patients with human immunodeficiency virus infection. Medicine (Baltimore) 1997;76:284.
307. Vaughan PA, Newman NM, Rosman MA: Acute hematogenous osteomyelitis in children. J Pediatr Orthop 1987;7:652.
308. Vecsei V, Barquet A: Treatment of chronic osteomyelitis by necrectomy and gentamicin-PMMA beads. Clin Orthop Relat Res 1981;159:201.
309. Versfeld GA, Solomon A: A diagnostic approach to tuberculosis of bones and joints. J Bone Joint Surg Br 1982;64:446.
310. Viani RM, Bromberg K, Bradley JS: Obturator internus muscle abscess in children: Report of seven cases and review. Clin Infect Dis 1999;28:117.
311. Vinod MB, Matussek J, Curtis N, et al: Duration of antibiotics in children with osteomyelitis and septic arthritis. J Paediatr Child Health 2002;38:363.
312. Vispo Seara JL, Barthel T, Schmitz H, et al: Arthroscopic treatment of septic joints: Prognostic factors. Arch Orthop Trauma Surg 2002;122:204.
313. Vohra R, Kang HS, Dogra S, et al: Tuberculous osteomyelitis. J Bone Joint Surg Br 1997;79:562.
314. Waldvogel FA, Medoff G, Swartz MN: Osteomyelitis: A review of clinical features, therapeutic considerations and unusual aspects. N Engl J Med 1970;282:198.
315. Waldvogel FA, Medoff G, Swartz MN: Osteomyelitis: A review of clinical features, therapeutic considerations and unusual aspects (second of three parts). N Engl J Med 1970;282:260.
316. Waldvogel FA, Medoff G, Swartz MN: Osteomyelitis: A review of clinical features, therapeutic considerations and unusual aspects. 3. Osteomyelitis associated with vascular insufficiency. N Engl J Med 1970;282:316.
317. Walsh S, Phillips F: Deep vein thrombosis associated with pediatric musculoskeletal sepsis. J Pediatr Orthop 2002;22:329.
318. Wang EH, Simpson S, Bennet GC: Osteomyelitis of the calcaneum. J Bone Joint Surg Br 1992;74:906.
319. Wang MN, Chen WM, Lee KS, et al: Tuberculous osteomyelitis in young children. J Pediatr Orthop 1999;19:151.
320. Wang VJ, Kuppermann N, Malley R, et al: Meningococcal disease among children who live in a large metropolitan area, 1981-1996. Clin Infect Dis 2001;32:1004.
321. Wasson JH, Sox HC: Clinical prediction rules: Have they come of age? JAMA 1996;275:641.
322. Wasson JH, Sox HC, Neff RK, et al: Clinical prediction rules: Applications and methodological standards. N Engl J Med 1985;313:793.
323. Weinstein A, Britchkov M: Lyme arthritis and post–Lyme disease syndrome. Curr Opin Rheumatol 2002;14:383.
324. Whalen JL, Fitzgerald RH Jr, Morrissy RT: A histological study of acute hematogenous osteomyelitis following physeal injuries in rabbits. J Bone Joint Surg Am 1988;70:1383.
325. White B, Livingstone W, Murphy C, et al: An open-label study of the role of adjuvant hemostatic support with protein C replacement therapy in purpura fulminans–associated meningococcemia. Blood 2000;96:3719.
326. Willis AA, Widmann RF, Flynn JM, et al: Lyme arthritis presenting as acute septic arthritis in children. J Pediatr Orthop 2003;23:114.
327. Winkelstein JA, Marino MC, Johnston RB Jr, et al: Chronic granulomatous disease: Report on a national registry of 368 patients. Medicine (Baltimore) 2000;79:155.
328. Wong-Chung J, Bagali M, Kaneker S: Physical signs in pyomyositis presenting as a painful hip in children: A case report and review of the literature. J Pediatr Orthop B 2004;13:211.
329. Wopperer JM, White JJ, Gillespie R, et al: Long-term follow-up of infantile hip sepsis. J Pediatr Orthop 1988;8:322.
330. Yagupsky P: Use of blood culture systems for isolation of *Kingella kingae* from synovial fluid. J Clin Microbiol 1999;37:3785.

331. Yagupsky P: *Kingella kingae* infections of the skeletal system in children: Diagnosis and therapy. Expert Rev Anti Infect Ther 2004;2:787.
332. Yagupsky P: *Kingella kingae:* From medical rarity to an emerging paediatric pathogen. Lancet Infect Dis 2004; 4:358.
333. Yagupsky P, Dagan R: *Kingella kingae:* An emerging cause of invasive infections in young children. Clin Infect Dis 1997;24:860.
334. Yeargan SA 3rd, Nakasone CK, Shaieb MD, et al: Treatment of chronic osteomyelitis in children resistant to previous therapy. J Pediatr Orthop 2004;24:109.
335. Yu CW, Hsiao JK, Hsu CY, et al: Bacterial pyomyositis: MRI and clinical correlation. Magn Reson Imaging 2004;22:1233.
336. Yuksel H, Ozguven AA, Akil I, et al: Septic pulmonary emboli presenting with deep venous thrombosis secondary to acute osteomyelitis. Pediatr Int 2004;46:621.
337. Zervas SJ, Zemel LS, Romness MJ, et al: *Streptococcus pyogenes* pyomyositis. Pediatr Infect Dis J 2002;21:166.
338. Zimbelman J, Palmer A, Todd J: Improved outcome of clindamycin compared with beta-lactam antibiotic treatment for invasive *Streptococcus pyogenes* infection. Pediatr Infect Dis J 1999;18:1096.

Chapter 36

Hematologic Disorders

HEMOPHILIA

Hemophilia, a genetically determined disorder, is characterized by abnormal blood coagulation as a result of functional deficiency of a specific factor, namely factor VIII or IX. Since biblical times, the crippling deformities of the musculoskeletal system and death resulting from uncontrolled hemorrhage have been well depicted in the pages of history. Talmudic writings of 200 AD state that a child whose siblings had bled excessively after circumcision was excused from the ritual.[62] Queen Victoria of England transmitted the gene through her daughters to the ruling families of Russia, Spain, and Austria.

The term *hemophilia,* coined by Hopff in 1828, means "blood loving." Wright is credited with being the first to demonstrate the prolonged clotting time in the disorder.[154] The deficient substance was isolated in 1937 by Patek and Taylor, who named it *antihemophilic globulin.*[107]

Modern management of hemophilia has reduced the morbidity of the disease remarkably. The development of human immunodeficiency virus (HIV) infection among those receiving blood products has been a major setback. Better treatment of HIV infection and safer methods of factor preparation are reducing the impact of this unfortunate disease complex.[78] Currently, factors VIII and IX are produced with recombinant DNA methods, which avoids the hazards of blood-borne disease.

Incidence

The incidence of hemophilia is estimated to be 1 per 10,000 male births in the United States and 0.8 per 10,000 male births in England.[5,28] A 1998 study estimated the national prevalence at 13,320 cases of hemophilia A and 3640 cases of hemophilia B, with a U.S. birth prevalence of both A and B of 1 per 5032 live male births.[133]

Classification and Inheritance

The hemophilias may be classified as hemophilia A, hemophilia B, and von Willebrand's disease.

HEMOPHILIA A

Hemophilia A, or classic hemophilia, results from a congenital deficiency in factor VIII (also known as antihemophilic factor or antihemophilic globulin). This type accounts for about 80% of cases and is caused by a gene carried on the X chromosome. Current research has identified at least 58 different mutations that result in a deficiency in normally functioning factor VIII protein.[83]

Hemophilia A occurs in boys and is transmitted by asymptomatic female carriers. A girl could be affected if her mother were a carrier and her father a hemophiliac; this, however, is very rare.

HEMOPHILIA B

Hemophilia B, or Christmas disease, is due to a deficiency in factor IX (plasma thromboplastin component, or Christmas factor). Its clinical manifestations are similar to those of classic hemophilia. The hereditary transmission is also by an X-linked recessive gene. As with hemophilia A, many mutations of the gene responsible for factor IX production have been identified.[103,125] Hemophilia B accounts for about 15% of the cases of hemophilia.

VON WILLEBRAND'S DISEASE

In this bleeding disorder both factor VIII deficiency and platelet functional abnormality are present. It is inherited as an autosomal dominant trait and occurs in both sexes. The bleeding disorder is relatively mild.

Factor VIII, a glycoprotein with a molecular weight of 2000 kD, is composed of subunits of about 200 kD molecular weight. All these subunits contain carbohydrates and are held together by disulfide bonds.[61,113] The precoagulant sex-linked hemophilic defect is located on the lighter protein portion of the glycoprotein, whereas the autosomal dominant von Willebrand's defect is related to the heavier carbohydrate moiety of the molecule.[97]

Clinical Features

HEMORRHAGE

Uncontrolled hemorrhage and repeated episodes of bleeding are the hallmarks of hemophilia. The severity of the disease varies from patient to patient but is constant in any one patient. Clinical manifestations of hemophilia A and B are similar and depend on the blood levels of factor VIII or IX. The level of hemostasis is normal when the blood level of either factor is at least 50% of normal. When the functional plasma level of the factor is 25% to 50% of normal, the hemophilia is *mild,* and excessive bleeding occurs only after major trauma or during surgery. When the plasma level of the factor is 5% to 25% of normal, the hemophilia is *moderate;* severe, uncontrolled bleeding occurs after minor injury or during an operative procedure. When the plasma level of the factor is 1% to 5% of normal, the hemophilia is *moderately severe,* with major hemorrhage occurring after minor injury or unrecognized mild trauma. When the plasma levels of factor VIII or IX are below 1% of normal, the hemophilia is considered *very severe;* clinically there are repeated spontaneous hemorrhages into joints and bleeding into deep soft tissues.

Abnormal bleeding may occur in any area of the body. Joints are the most frequent sites of repeated hemorrhage. The sites next in frequency are muscles and soft tissues. In the patient with severe hemophilia, the abnormal bleeding tendency may manifest in the neonatal period or early infancy. Ordinarily the ecchymosis and soft tissue bleeding are minor, resorb relatively readily, and are not detected by the parents. When the infant begins to crawl and starts bumping into objects, or with standing and falling, abnormal bleeding into joints and soft tissues is noted by the parents. At this stage the infant is usually seen by the pediatrician. It is crucial to have a high index of suspicion for hemophilia to prevent serious consequences or invasive treatment such as aspiration of the joints. Approximately three fourths of episodes of bleeding sustained by hemophilic patients are into a joint, the deep soft tissues, or both.

Hemophilic Arthropathy

Intra-articular hemorrhage is a central clinical hallmark of hemophilia. A single hemarthrosis may precipitate low-grade synovitis, which predisposes the involved joint to recurrent hemarthrosis and a cycle of chronic synovitis, inflammatory arthritis, and progressive arthropathy.[87]

Site of Involvement. The weight-bearing joints are the most common sites of hemophilic arthropathy, with the frequency of involvement being, in decreasing order, the knee, elbow, shoulder, ankle, wrist, and hip.[16] The vertebral column is rarely involved. Any joint, however, may be the site of pathologic change.

Pathophysiology. The pathophysiologic process was initially described by Konig in the late 19th century.[71] There is an initial stage of synovial reaction to the bleeding into the joint, followed by a later stage of cartilage degeneration and joint destruction. After injury, the synovial vessels rupture and the blood accumulates in the joint. Bleeding continues until the intra-articular hydrostatic pressure exceeds arterial and capillary pressure in the synovium. The resultant tamponade of the synovial vessels causes ischemia of the synovium and subchondral bone.

With repeated hemorrhage, hyperplasia and fibrosis of the synovium occur, and a vicious cycle of bleeding–synovitis–bleeding ensues.[119] Pannus formation by the proliferating synovial tissue erodes the hyaline cartilage peripherally, and compression of its opposing cartilaginous surfaces results in degeneration of articular cartilage centrally. Articular cartilage is also degraded by the action of proteolytic enzymes—lysosomal proteases, acid phosphatase, and cathepsin D.[119] Data from animal studies suggest that articular cartilage may be more susceptible to blood-induced damage at younger than at older ages.[122] Prostaglandin levels are also elevated in hemophilic arthropathy. An inflammatory process invades and destroys cartilage. Loss of joint motion and contractual deformity due to the capsular synovial fibrosis follow. Local ischemia causes formation of subchondral bone cysts.

Repeated hemarthrosis causes marked dilation of the capsular and epiphyseal vessels. The resultant hyperemia and increased circulation to the part result in enlargement of the epiphysis and increased length of the limb. Stimulation of growth may be asymmetric, resulting in valgus or varus deformity. Alternatively, shortening of the limb may be produced by early closure of the physis. Osteoporosis and muscle atrophy are common.[118]

Clinical Findings. Clinical findings depend on the severity of hemorrhage and whether the hemarthrosis is acute, subacute, or chronic. In *acute hemarthrosis,* pain and swelling with distention of the joint capsule are the principal findings. A history of injury may not be elicited. With cessation of bleeding, the intensity of the pain decreases. The joint will assume the position of minimal discomfort, which is also the position of minimal intra-articular pressure. The hip joint, for example, is held in 30 to 65 degrees of flexion, 15 degrees of abduction, and 15 degrees of lateral rotation. Extension, wide abduction, and medial rotation of the hip are limited and painful because they increase intra-articular hydrostatic pressure. The knee joint is held in flexion, with range of motion markedly restricted by protective spasm, pain, and the hemarthrosis. Local tenderness and increased heat are present. The overlying skin becomes tense and shiny. The intense pain of acute hemarthrosis subsides rapidly after the administration of factor VIII or IX.

Subacute hemarthrosis develops after several episodes of bleeding into the joint. Pain is minimal. The synovium is thickened and boggy. Joint motion is moderately restricted. Subacute hemarthrosis does not respond rapidly to administration of clotting factor.

Chronic hemarthrosis develops after 6 months of involvement. Progressive destruction of the joint takes place, with the end stage being a fibrotic, stiff, totally destroyed joint.[5]

Differential Diagnosis. A difficult diagnostic challenge is the child with hemophilia and a superimposed joint infection. The diagnosis is often delayed because the symptoms are similar to those of hemarthrosis. In one series, most but not all children with infection had elevated white blood cell counts. Associated risk factors included infected angioaccess catheters, pneumonia, and generalized sepsis. Affected joints should be treated with antibiotics and either repeated aspiration or arthrotomy.[42,115]

Radiographic Findings. Radiographic findings associated with hemarthrosis depend on the stage of the disease, patient age at disease onset, and the joint involved.[68]

Magnetic resonance imaging (MRI) is considered the most accurate imaging modality for assessing hemophilic arthropathy and may significantly affect patient management.[68] Initially, radiographs of an affected joint disclose soft tissue swelling due to distention of the joint capsule. With repeated hemorrhage and resultant chronic synovitis there may be joint effusion, osseous erosion, osteoporosis, enlargement of the epiphysis, subchondral cysts, narrowing of the articular cartilage space, formation of peripheral osteophytes, and other secondary degenerative changes[68] (Figs. 36–1 and 36–2). The final phase of hemophilic arthropathy is fibrous ankylosis (Fig. 36–3). On the basis of radiographic findings and the degree of cartilage destruction, Arnold and Hilgartner classified hemophilic arthropathy into five stages[5] (Box 36–1).

In *stage I* there is soft tissue swelling but no skeletal abnormalities.

Stage II is characterized by overgrowth and osteoporosis of the epiphysis, but joint integrity is maintained—there are no bone cysts and no narrowing of the articular cartilage space. The radiographic stage II parallels the clinical stage of subacute hemophilic arthropathy.

In *stage III* there is minimal to moderate joint space narrowing with subchondral cysts, which occasionally communicate with the joint space. There is widening of the intracondylar notch of the knee and the trochlear notch of the ulna. In the knee there may be squaring of the patella. In stage III the articular cartilage is still preserved, indicating that with treatment, hemophilic arthropathy is still reversible.

Box 36-1

Radiographic Staging of Hemophilic Arthropathy

Stage I

Soft tissue swelling
No skeletal abnormality

Stage II

Overgrowth and osteoporosis of epiphysis

Stage III

Mild to moderate joint narrowing
Subchondral cysts
Patellar squaring
Widening of intercondylar notch of knee and trochlear notch of elbow

Stage IV

Severe narrowing of joint space with cartilage destruction
Other osseous changes very pronounced

Stage V

Total loss of joint space with fibrous ankylosis

From Arnold W, Hilgartner M: Hemophilic arthropathy: Current concepts of pathogenesis and management. J Bone Joint Surg Am 1977;59:287.

In *stage IV* there is destruction of articular cartilage with severe narrowing of the joint space. The other osseous changes found in stage III—subchondral cysts, patellar squaring, and widening of the intercondylar or trochlear notch—are more pronounced.

Stage V is characterized by total loss of joint space with fibrous ankylosis of the joint. There is marked incongruity of the articular structures, with severe, irregular hypertrophy of the epiphysis.

A modified version of the Arnold-Hilgartner system has four grades instead of five (Box 36–2). This modified classification eliminates the original stage II (epiphyseal enlargement and juxta-articular osteoporosis), which is rarely discrete and has no implications for treatment.[87] Osteoporosis frequently accompanies chronic synovitis in patients with stage I arthropathy, and erosions are often present with epiphyseal enlargement.

Soft Tissue Bleeding

After a direct injury, a large hematoma may accumulate in the subcutaneous tissues. The blood usually is absorbed spontaneously; occasionally ulceration occurs, commonly on the forehead, the olecranon process, or the prepatellar area. This type of superficial hematoma usually remains fluid and fluctuant for a long time. Superficial soft tissue hemorrhage in

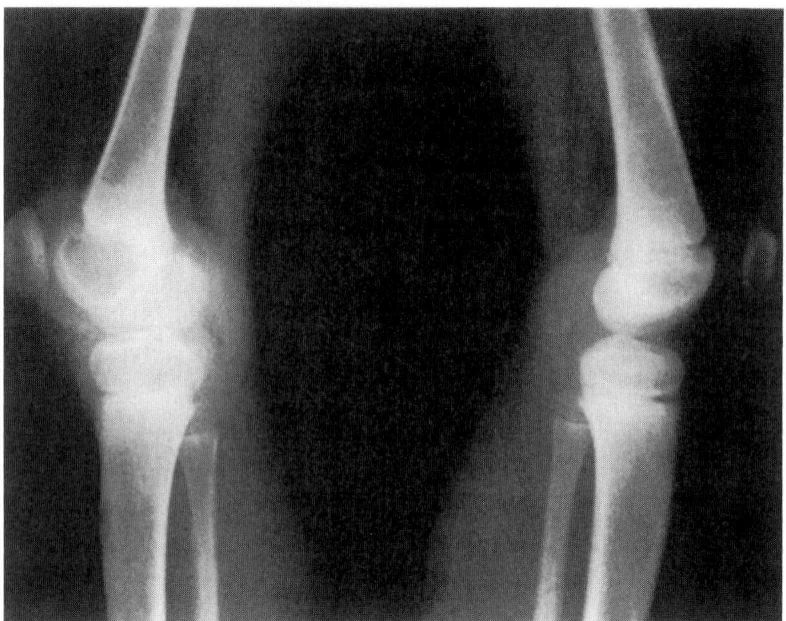

A

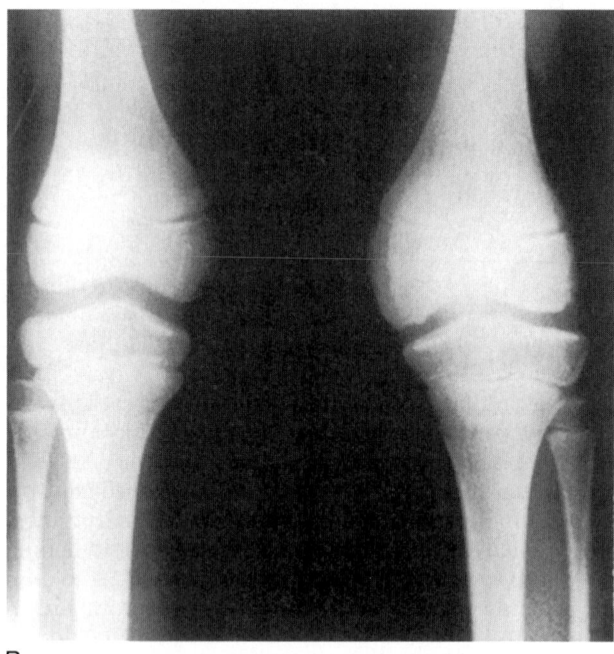

B

FIGURE 36-1 Hemophilic arthropathy of the left knee **(A).** The right knee is provided for comparison **(B).** Radiographs show the chronic synovitis and enlargement of the distal femoral epiphysis.

the form of ecchymosis is common, especially in a subject with severe hemophilia; it is not of clinical significance.

Intramuscular and Intermuscular Hemorrhage

In the lower limb the most common site of bleeding is the quadriceps (44%), followed by the triceps surae (35%), anterior compartment (7%), adductors of the thigh (7%), hamstrings (6%), and sartorius (1%).[6] In the upper limb the most common site of bleeding is the deltoid (24%), followed by the wrist and finger flexors in the forearm (23.5%), the brachioradialis (19.5%), the biceps (14%), the wrist and finger extensors in the forearm (11%), and the triceps (8%).[112] The presenting complaint is pain on movement or at rest.

Hemorrhage in the quadriceps muscle may occasionally be painless and manifest only as "stiffness" or "weakness" of the knee. Physical findings consist of local tenderness and swelling with limitation of motion of the adjacent joints. Bleeding in the deltoid muscle restricts shoulder motion, especially abduction and, to some extent, rotation, flexion, and extension of the shoulder. Bleeding in the forearm flexors restricts motion of the fingers, wrist, or elbow, either individually or in combination.

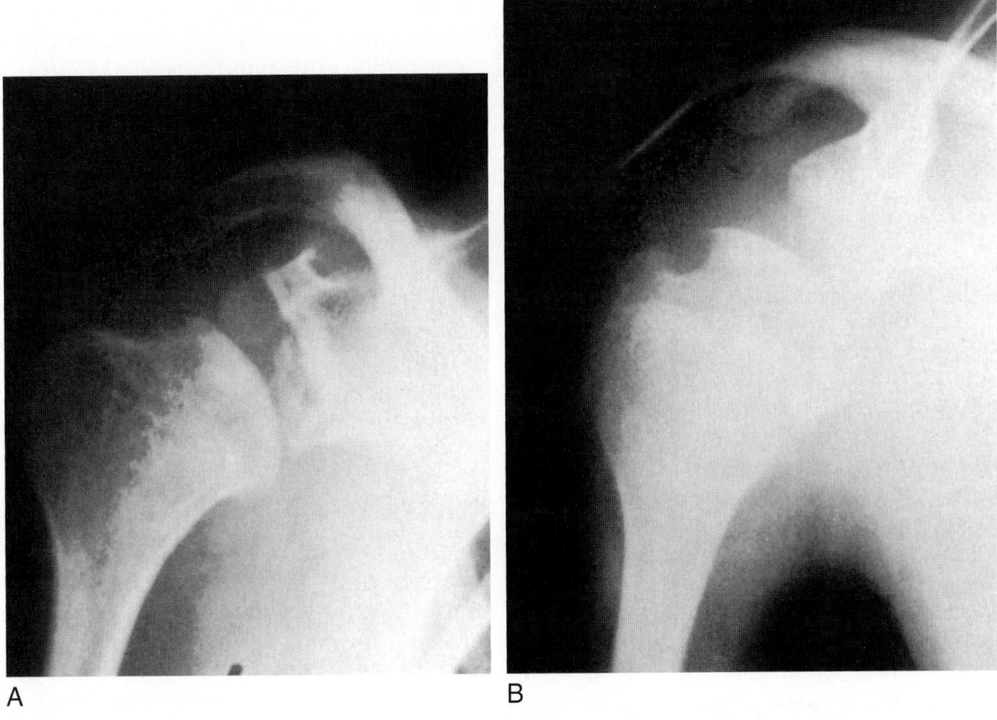

FIGURE 36–2 Two examples of hemophilic arthropathy of the shoulder. **A,** Note the erosive changes of the humeral neck and glenoid. **B,** Note enlargement of the humeral head.

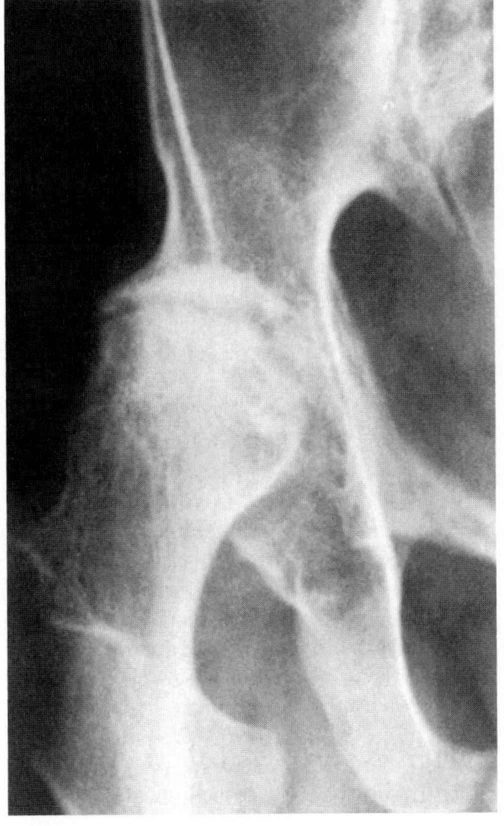

FIGURE 36–3 Fibrous ankylosis of the hip as a result of hemophilic arthropathy.

Box 36–2

Modified Arnold-Hilgartner Arthroplasty Classification

Grade I

Soft tissue fullness indicating effusion and synovial thickening

Juxta-articular osteopenia often present

Grade II

Widened epiphysis, surface irregularity, and small erosions

Normal cartilage interval or joint space

Grade III

Narrowing of cartilage interval with extensive surface erosions

Juxta-articular bony cysts may be present

Grade IV

Same findings as stage III, but with complete loss of cartilage interval and marked surface irregularity

Reactive sclerosis, squaring of the margin of the femoral condyles, and subluxation often present

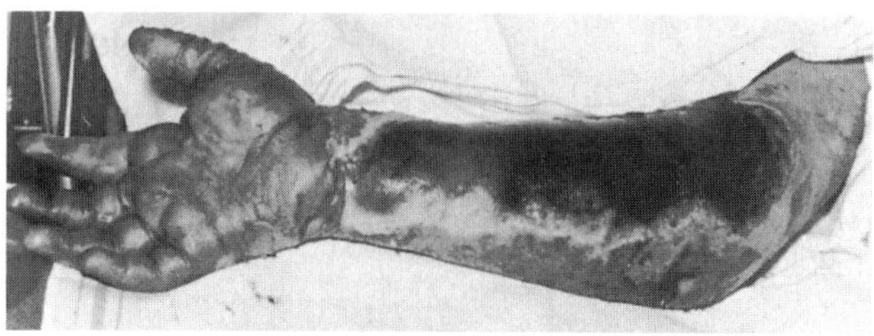

FIGURE 36–4 Volkmann's ischemic contracture of the forearm after fracture of both bones in a hemophilic boy.

Hemorrhage into the iliopsoas muscle or retroperitoneum may mimic a variety of surgical or medical emergencies such as appendicitis or renal colic.

Ischemia and fibrosis of muscles with subsequent myostatic contracture result from bleeding within muscles or among muscles contained in a firm fascial compartment.[75,90,91,100] Hemorrhage within the calf muscles produces fixed equinus deformity. Bleeding in the volar surface of the forearm may produce Volkmann's ischemic contracture with flexion deformity of the digits and wrists (Fig. 36–4).

Diagnostic Ultrasonography

Diagnostic ultrasonography is routinely performed in hemophilic patients in whom hemorrhage into joints or soft tissues is suspected. It is noninvasive and can be performed at the bedside with minimal disturbance of the patient.[11,70,73,98,106,128,147,152,153]

Hemorrhage into superficial joints such as the knee, elbow, ankle, or wrist is readily determined on physical examination. The diagnostic value of ultrasonography is in the identification of bleeding into the hip, shoulder, and deep soft tissues, such as the iliopsoas or retroperitoneum (Fig. 36–5). Effusions into these deep anatomic sites are readily detected on ultrasonography.

The echo pattern varies with the duration and anatomic site of the hemorrhage. In the soft tissues a hematoma initially displays increased echogenicity compared with surrounding soft tissues; within 3 to 4 days, relatively echo-free areas develop in the bleeding site. Ordinarily, in 10 days the established hematoma is relatively echo free. A soft tissue hematoma may be of uniform texture, separating muscle planes, or it may interdigitate with muscle fibers, producing a mottled appearance with poorly defined margins. On follow-up ultrasonographic examination the intramuscular hematoma may have resolved spontaneously or may have progressively liquefied, with decreased internal echoes and the development of well-defined borders. A sudden increase in echogenicity indicates a fresh hemorrhage.

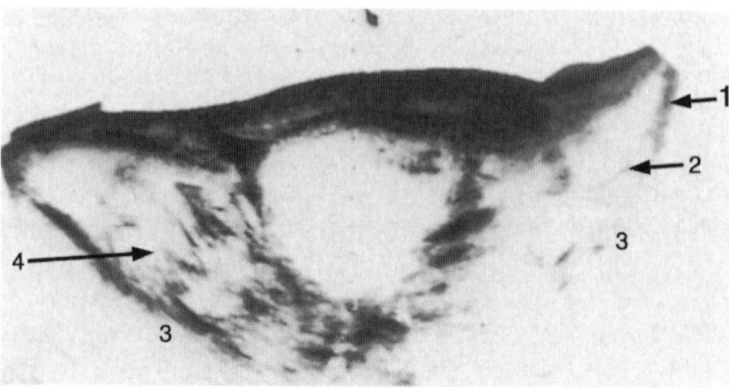

FIGURE 36–5 Ultrasonographic findings in soft tissue bleeding in the iliopsoas muscle. 1, Normal iliopsoas; 2, fascial plane; 3, iliac bone; 4, bleeding in the iliopsoas.

The echo pattern of bleeding into joints shows a mixture of echo-free fluid within the joint and a variable amount of echogenic material floating free. In its initial stage, hemarthrosis is sometimes uniformly echogenic, in contrast to the echo-free appearance of joint effusions from other causes such as toxic synovitis or septic arthritis.

NERVE PALSY

Neurapraxia in hemophilia is primarily due to compression of a nerve from the hematoma. The femoral nerve is most frequently involved because it is in a closed, rigid compartment limited by the iliacus fascia. The psoas sheath is easily distensible. Brower and Wilde reported six cases of femoral nerve palsy,[13] and Goodfellow and associates described 20 cases of femoral nerve compression.[45] The nerve next most frequently affected is the median nerve. The ulnar, radial, sciatic, peroneal, and lateral femoral cutaneous nerves may also be involved.[23]

A history of injury, such as twisting of the limb or strenuous use, may be obtained in some cases. Pain is the presenting complaint and is soon followed by weakness of the affected muscle groups.

In femoral nerve palsy, the hip is held in moderate flexion and some lateral rotation. Extension and medial rotation of the hip are limited and painful. On palpation, a tender mass in the iliac fossa extending to the iliac crest and groin may be present. There will be anesthesia or hypesthesia in the areas of the cutaneous distribution of the femoral nerve. Quadriceps paralysis in varying degrees is often present. Ultrasonography and computed tomography (CT) demonstrate the iliacus hematoma. With adequate factor replacement the natural course is one of gradual and steady recovery, usually within 12 months.[1,2,8,12,24,30,37,49,54,57,89,123,126,135,142]

HEMOPHILIC PSEUDOTUMOR

The term *hemophilic pseudotumor* refers to a progressive cystic swelling involving the musculoskeletal system. It is caused by uncontrolled hemorrhage within a confined space. The hematoma grows and causes pressure necrosis and erosion of surrounding tissues. The subjacent bone is frequently involved.[5]

The entity was first described by Starker in 1918, and since then fewer than 100 cases have been reported.[134] It occurs only in severely affected hemophiliacs who have a functional clotting factor level below 1% of normal. In these patients with severe hemophilia, the estimated incidence is 1% to 2%.

Fernandez de Valderrama and Matthews have described three ways in which such hemophilic cysts

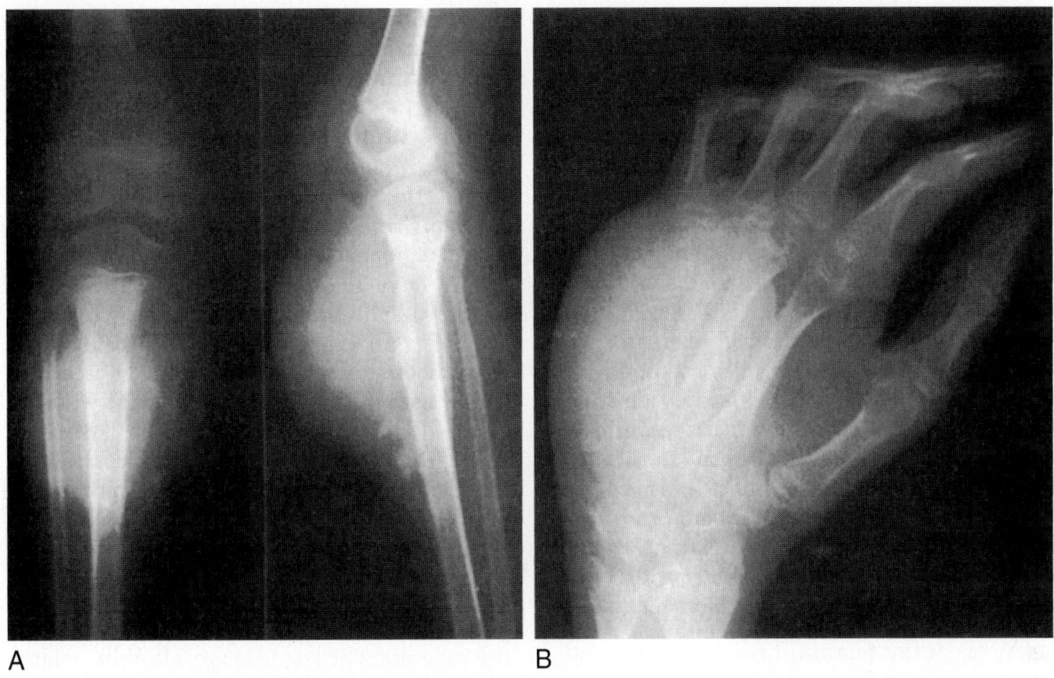

FIGURE 36–6 Hemophilic pseudotumors of the tibia **(A)** and the hand **(B)**.

may develop.[34] The *simple cyst* occurs within the fascial envelope of a muscle or muscles and is confined by the tendinous attachments. No bony changes are seen on radiographs. The cyst usually remains localized under the muscle fascia, although it may extend between muscle and fascia to point internally or through the skin.

The second type of cyst occurs in a muscle with wide and firm fibrous periosteal attachments and may eventually cause cortical thinning because of compressive interference with the periosteal and outer cortical blood supply.

In the third type, the pseudotumor originates as a subperiosteal hemorrhage and progressively strips the periosteum from the cortex until it is limited by the aponeurotic or tendinous attachments. The overlying muscle is raised or destroyed.[141] Most hemophilic pseudotumors are caused by subperiosteal hemorrhage. Occasionally one may arise from intraosseous hemorrhage.[60] In the past, intramedullary bleeding was thought to be a cause of hemophilic pseudotumor.[1,54,60] It was proposed that uncontrolled intraosseous hemorrhage increased the intramarrow pressure and caused necrosis of the marrow and inner cortex of the bone. With progressive bleeding and increasing pressure the cortex would perforate, causing elevation of the periosteum and bone necrosis. Pathologic examination of large hemophilic pseudotumors, however, has failed to demonstrate bone necrosis or resorption of the inner part of the cortex. Trueta[144] cites MacMahon and Blackburn's[89] case of cystic expansion of the metacarpal bone as a pseudotumor that probably had an intramedullary origin.

The most common location of pseudotumors is in the thigh (50% of cases). Next in frequency are the abdomen, pelvis, and tibia[54] (Fig. 36–6A). Pseudotumor may also occur in the hand[8] (Fig. 36–6B). Pseudotumor involving the calcaneus may cause marked erosion of the calcaneal tuberosity.[19,72]

A bone involved by pseudotumor may sustain pathologic fracture. Before adequate factor replacement was available, pseudotumors caused death in the majority of patients; involved limbs were amputated. Fernandez de Valderrama and Matthews observed that the location of these tumors is related to the powerful muscle groups of the quadriceps femoris, triceps surae, gluteus maximus, and iliopsoas muscles, which have firm attachments between their fibers and the periosteum but not to any great extent with the bone itself.[34] These muscles also have profuse vascular connections with the underlying periosteum and bone. Hemorrhage from these injured vessels easily detaches and elevates the periosteum.[34]

Hemophilic pseudotumor is essentially an expanding hematoma. CT demonstrates that the lesion is of fluid consistency and depicts its true extent, bony destruction, and extraosseous abnormality.[108] MRI is also of great value in delineating the nature and extent of the pseudotumor. It is imperative that a hemophilic tumor not be mistaken for a malignant or expanding benign bone tumor. It should not be aspirated, nor should a biopsy specimen be taken for diagnosis, particularly without appropriate preoperative correction of functional factor deficiency.

FRACTURES

Fractures in hemophilia may result from trauma or may occur pathologically after a trivial injury. They are most common in the lower limb, especially in patients with stiff knees, who sustain supracondylar fracture of the femur. Hematomas may be large, especially after femoral fractures. Uncontrolled bleeding into a closed fascial compartment may lead to Volkmann's ischemic contracture (see Fig. 36–5).

DISLOCATIONS

Intra-articular bleeding in the hip stretches the joint capsule and causes subluxation and eventual dislocation of the hip. Floman and Niska reported a 6-year-old boy with hemophilia A who developed a spontaneous posterior dislocation of the hip because of repeated intra-articular bleeding. The prognosis for such dislocation is poor. In this patient, despite immediate reduction, the hip became ankylosed.[36] Other cases of hip dislocation in hemophilia have been reported by Teitelbaum,[141] Driessen,[26] and Boardman and English.[10]

Bleeding in the hip joint is a rare but serious problem in hemophilia. Increased intra-articular pressure, in addition to stretching the joint capsule, causes avascular necrosis (AVN) of the femoral head with eventual joint space narrowing, subchondral irregularity and cyst formation, collapse of the femoral head, osteoarthrosis, and arthrokatadysis.[127,141]

MYOSITIS OSSIFICANS

Ectopic ossification in hemophilia, first described by Hutcheson, develops as a result of intermuscular or intramuscular bleeding.[58] Heterotopic bone formation around the hip joint restricts motion of the hip.[77] In the past it was thought to be a rare complication in hemophilia, but in a radiographic survey by Vas and associates it was found in 15% of patients; in most of their cases the disability was minimal.[145]

MISCELLANEOUS BONE CHANGES

Children with severe hemophilia and hemophilic arthropathy are at risk for reduced bone mineral density related to limitations in weight-bearing exercise and frequent hepatitis C infection.[7] Reduced bone density in childhood is a risk factor for osteoporosis in later life. Because osteoporosis may therefore complicate the future treatment of patients with hemophilia, screening for reduced bone density among young patients with severe hemophilia is recommended. AVN of the talus has also been reported in children with hemophilia.[65]

Treatment

The care of the hemophiliac with musculoskeletal disorders requires a multidisciplinary approach by a team consisting of a hematologist, orthopaedic surgeon, physical therapist, nurse clinician, medical psychologist, social worker, and geneticist. There should be immediate access to a laboratory capable of performing accurate factor VIII or IX assays and detecting factor antibodies. Factor material should be readily available for replacement therapy. The creation of multidisciplinary hemophilia clinics in children's hospitals has simplified the care of hemophilic children.

GENE THERAPY

A number of trials of gene therapy in animals with genetically produced factor deficiencies have been performed, with some success. Most studies have addressed the use of adenoviral vectors to carry the corrected gene into the recipient, with the goal of obtaining long-term therapeutic levels of factor VIII or IX without stimulating an immune response against the transgene product or the vector itself.[44] Host immunity to the adenoviral vector has thus far prevented permanent correction of the factor deficiency, although development of viral vectors devoid of viral genes has allowed reduced immunogenicity and more prolonged expression of factors VIII and IX in investigational settings.[14,32,64,143]

Specific gene therapy methodologies currently under investigation include modification of hematopoietic stem cells to express factor VIII transgene in the megakaryocytic lineage, allowing platelets to store and deliver factor VIII to the site of vascular injury.[116] Permanent therapeutic correction of mutations in the factor IX gene has been reported in a mouse model of hemophilia B without development of host immune reactions.[146] Despite these intriguing developments, gene therapy remains an investigational method with many obstacles to be overcome before it can be reliably used as a treatment for hemophilia.[86]

MEDICAL MANAGEMENT

The objective of medical management is control of bleeding by hemostasis, achieved by intravenous administration of the appropriate coagulation factors. There are two major approaches. The first is treatment on demand, that is, at the onset of any bleeding episodes. The second approach is prophylactic replacement in patients with recurrent hemarthroses.

Treatment on Demand

The most common approach to the treatment of recurrent hemarthrosis is treatment on demand. It is suggested that factor levels of 30 to 50 IU/dL are optimal in controlling an acute hemorrhage. To achieve these levels in a patient with severe hemophilia (plasma levels <1% of normal), 15 to 25 IU/kg of factor VIII and 20 to 50 IU/kg/dL of factor IX are required. Repeated treatments may be required daily for 2 to 3 days to control the hemarthrosis. Aspirin products and nonsteroidal anti-inflammatory medications must be avoided.[114] An investigation into the cost implications of repeated arthrosis among patients with hemophilia A found that the cost of treating a child with on-demand factor VIII more than doubled within 1 year after the development of a target joint (defined as three bleeds into a single joint within a 3-month period).[67] This study, performed among boys an average age of 4.5 years, supports beginning primary prophylactic therapy at younger ages.

Prophylactic Treatment

Several studies have shown that ongoing prophylactic treatment reduces the incidence of hemarthrosis.[48] One study found that starting treatment at 3 years of age resulted in a better outcome than starting at 5 years, but patients with prior repeated hemarthrosis had continued arthropathy despite prophylactic factor replacement.[38] Another study noted reduced bleeding frequency in 41 of 47 patients but an increase in the cost of clotting factors compared with treatment on demand, although a similar investigation identified fewer joint bleeds, less arthropathy, and lower treatment costs among 49 patients receiving factor prophylactically versus on demand.[35,99]

The dosage required to replace a factor deficiency depends on the patient's weight and plasma volume. The hematologist makes the calculation and is in charge of administering the factor. The orthopaedic surgeon, however, should be aware that 20 to 30 minutes after administration of the antihemophilic factor the plasma level will rise. The biologic half-life of factor VIII is 6 to 12 hours, whereas that of factor IX is 8 to 18 hours. In the management of bleeding into joint, muscles, and soft tissue, the dose of factor VIII or IX is calculated to raise the plasma level to 30% of normal. In severe hemarthrosis it may be desirable to raise the plasma level to 40% of normal.

Inhibitors of factors VIII and IX develop as a result of the immunologic response of the human body.[150] A low titer of inhibitors may be circumvented by high-dosage factor VIII infusion. Other methods to overcome this life-threatening problem are the administration of prednisone and cyclophosphamide or the use of concentrations of prothrombin-activated material or use of plasmapheresis. Immune tolerance therapy can eradicate inhibitors but is not uniformly successful. Preliminary data suggest that prophylaxis with activated prothrombin complex concentrates safely reduces the incidence of joint bleeding during immune tolerance therapy and among patients in whom immune tolerance induction fails.[79] Controlled clinical trials are needed, however, to identify whether prophylaxis can prevent joint bleeding and damage and can improve quality of life in patients with inhibitors.

Early Treatment of Bleeding into Muscles and Soft Tissues

Early treatment of bleeding into muscles and soft tissues by self-administration of factor VIII or IX by the hemophiliacs or their parents at home has become effective. The dose of factor is calculated to raise the level to 30% to 40% of normal. The part is splinted in a comfortable neutral position in foam pillows or soft appliances. If the hemorrhage is in the lower limb, weight bearing is restricted by crutches or eliminated by confinement to bed or a wheelchair. As soon as the acute symptoms of pain and muscle spasm have subsided, the affected limb is gradually mobilized under cover of factor replacement. With early treatment (within 2 to 3 hours), the hemorrhage in the muscles usually resolves within 3 to 5 days. Hemorrhages in the quadriceps femoris and biceps brachii take the longest time to resolve.[6,41]

Acute Treatment of Hemarthrosis

Acute bleeding into joints is an emergency requiring immediate attention. With proper education and instructions as to dosage schedules, many patients can be treated at home by themselves or by a family member. Immediate treatment of bleeding into joints results in less arthropathy and minimizes the extent of joint destruction. Home therapy permits factor replacement as soon as a bleeding episode take place. This type of patient self-help, however, has the disadvantages of inadequate follow-up, the possibility of transmission of hepatitis to a family member, and an increased risk of infection because of lack of appropriate sterile technique in handling of materials.[80,81] The parents should be instructed that if the bleeding is severe with marked distention of the joint, the child should be brought to the hospital within 4 hours of the onset of hemorrhage. It cannot be overemphasized that delay in instituting adequate treatment is the primary cause of crippling joint deformity in patients with hemophilia. A minimal or moderate intra-articular hemorrhage may not be so painful at the onset, and the child will continue to use and bear weight on the affected limb, causing continuous or intermittent progressive bleeding into the joint. Within a few days the joint becomes markedly swollen, very painful, and inflamed by reaction to the blood, and it develops fixed flexion contracture. In the event of associated bleeding into the periarticular tissues and muscles, pain and muscle spasm are marked from the onset; the patient is apprehensive of moving the limb and is forced to rest and to seek medical attention.

The affected joint is temporarily immobilized in a molded, well-padded splint in a position of rest and minimum hydrostatic pressure. This position varies with each joint. For example, for the knee it is 35 to 45 degrees of flexion, and for the elbow it is 50 to 60 degrees of flexion. Commercially available semi-flexible splints (such as the Jordan splint) provide partial immobilization and moderate compression.

Compression is effectively achieved by placing a rubber sponge and an elastic bandage over the site of hemorrhage. A second bandage may be applied intermittently over the first one to increase tension. The distal circulation should be carefully watched. Under no circumstances should a circular plaster cast be used, as the swelling underneath will obstruct the blood flow and cause gangrene or compartment syndrome. The limb should be elevated to reduce hydrostatic venous pressure. Cold compresses in the form of ice bags are applied to the affected joint. The clotting defect is corrected by IV administration of antihemophilic factor.

Analgesics

Narcotic analgesics are used with care because in such a chronic disease, addiction can easily become a problem. Also, the course of the bleeding is best assessed by the patient, and under heavy analgesic he or she will be unable to give proper warning of continued bleeding. A diminution in the severity of the pain is the first indication of cessation of hemorrhage. The circumference of the joint is measured at intervals to determine whether there is progressive distention of the joint capsule. Also, analgesic drugs that contain aspirin, guaiacolate, and antihistamines inhibit platelet aggregation and prolong the bleeding time. Giving such medication could produce a secondary bleeding disorder. If the pain is intolerable and does not respond to factor replacement and splinting, the pain medications to be given are propoxyphene (Darvon), acetaminophen (Tylenol), codeine, or methadone.

Aspiration

The need for joint aspiration has been debated. Some authors recommend aspiration only for an extremely tense hemarthrosis and avoid aspiration in ordinary cases, citing the risk of introducing infection, the discomfort to the patient, and the possibility that aspiration will incite more bleeding.[114] Other authors believe that removal of blood is critical to avoiding chronic synovitis and that a large hemarthrosis is much more inviting to infecting organisms than is the sterile aspiration of the joint.[47]

Joint aspiration should be performed under strict aseptic conditions and under local anesthesia. Factors VIII and IX are administered intravenously and reach an effective blood level 20 to 30 minutes later, at which time the joint should be aspirated. Later aspiration, after two to three infusions have been given, will be unsuccessful due to the thickening and clotting of the hemarthrosis. Aspiration is performed with an 18-gauge lumbar puncture needle with a stylet. One or at most two puncture wounds should be made with the needle. The joint is irrigated with normal saline solution until the return is clear. The compression dressing and posterior splint are reapplied.

The appropriate factor is administered for 3 to 7 days after cessation of bleeding. At this time, physical therapy to mobilize the joint is initiated. Isometric muscle exercises are begun and are followed by gentle assisted range-of-motion exercises, first with gravity eliminated and then against gravity. Between exercises the limb is protected in an appropriate splint. The range of motion of the affected joint is progressively increased. Weight-bearing joints are protected with crutches with a three-point gait. Full weight bearing is not permitted for a minimum of 2 weeks, and longer if necessitated by limitation of joint motion and muscle weakness. It is imperative that transition to activity be gradual.

Subacute Hemophilic Arthropathy

Repeated episodes of bleeding into a joint in a relatively short time result in synovial hypertrophy and persistent effusion. This is best managed nonoperatively by immobilization of the joint in a well-padded splint and with factor replacement. Most subacute hemarthroses resolve over a period of 3 to 4 weeks with this regimen. Aspiration is not indicated. Isometric exercises are performed to maintain muscle tone and strength. Initially, passive range-of-motion exercises are not allowed. Partial weight bearing with crutches is permitted. With resolution of the synovitis and effusion, the patient is gradually allowed to return to normal function.

If the subacute hemarthrosis fails to respond to 3 weeks of partial immobilization, physical therapy, and factor replacement, an intra-articular injection of corticosteroid may be given. Prolonged immobilization of the affected joint should be avoided because it will result in marked muscle atrophy and restriction of joint motion. If the knee is involved, quadriceps atrophy will cause joint instability, leading to repeated trauma and bleeding.

Support of the lower limb in orthotic devices is indicated when the motor power of the quadriceps or triceps surae muscle is less than "fair" or when flexion deformity of the knee or equinus deformity of the ankle is present to such a degree that mechanical insufficiency of the lower limb predisposes the child to fall and sustain repeated injury. Rubbing and recurrent trauma to the opposite thigh or leg caused by the medial caliper is a problem, as it will cause soft tissue bleeding. Only a lateral upright is used. A well-padded plastic orthosis should be used whenever possible. When flexion deformity of the knee or equinus deformity of the ankle develops, appropriate splinting is used at night to keep the part out of the position of deformity. Ankle splinting may be done initially with ordinary posterior splints. Recurrent hemarthroses may be prevented by ankle support worn during activities. Air splints, free ankle polypropylene orthoses, and lacers have all been used. Shock-absorbent heel pads have also been shown to reduce the impact on the ankle, with fewer hemarthroses resulting.[50]

During the stage of subacute hemarthrosis, prophylactic factor replacement is administered in conjunction with an intensive physical therapy program. Graduated progressive active resisted and gentle passive range-of-motion exercises are performed immediately after infusion of the factor in the evening and the following morning. The patient is allowed to swim and perform ordinary physical activities of daily living. Contact sports should be avoided.

Chronic Hemophilic Arthropathy

Chronic hemophilic arthropathy can be prevented in most cases by effective and immediate treatment of acute hemarthrosis. The importance of prevention of chronic arthropathy, with its accompanying intra-articular fibrosis, cartilage destruction, and joint stiffness, cannot be overemphasized.

In the management of chronic hemophilic arthropathy, four modalities of treatment are available: physical therapy, orthoses, traction and other corrective appliances, and surgery. The objective is to correct joint deformity and to restore function.

NONSURGICAL TREATMENT OF JOINT DEFORMITY

Nonoperative measures should always be used before surgery. For flexion deformities of the knee and hip, a period of continuous traction is effective in relieving muscle spasm and increasing range of motion. Initially traction forces are in the line of deformity and are gradually altered to achieve correction. Splint Russell traction is effective; the vertical force is exerted by a sling placed under the proximal tibia when the knee is involved; with the hip, the sling support is under the distal thigh. In cases of lateral rotation contracture of the hip, a medial rotation strap is added to the thigh. Houghton and Duthie recommend use of reverse dynamic slings to correct flexion deformity of the knee and elbow.[56]

Prophylactic protection with antihemophilic factor is usually not required for a child in traction. Once a neutral or nearly neutral position is obtained, well-padded plastic splints are used to maintain the part in the corrected position. Active exercises are begun to increase muscle power and range of motion of the joints. It is best to refrain from forceful passive stretching exercises.

If functional range of motion is not achieved after 2 or 3 weeks of traction, a wedging cast is applied. Posterior subluxation of the knee may be prevented by applying an extension-desubluxation hinge; it will lift the proximal tibia anteriorly as the knee is extended.[96,104,105,136] For safety, antihemophilic factor is administered when the cast is wedged. When full knee extension is achieved, the knee is immobilized for 7 to 10 days, a plastic splint is used to maintain the correction, and physical therapy in the form of active exercises is begun. Gradually, partial weight bearing and three-point crutch gait are permitted. If bleeding occurs during this period of training, it is controlled by intravenous administration of antihemophilic factor. Crutch support is discontinued and full weight bearing is allowed when there is functional range of joint motion and a least "fair" strength of the quadriceps muscle.

Management of flexion contracture of the elbow follows the same principles as that of the knee. Equinus deformity of the ankle is treated by a dorsiflexion wedging cast. Forceful manipulation of a joint under general anesthesia is not recommended.

SURGICAL TREATMENT

With early treatment and proper collaboration between the hematologist and orthopaedic surgeon, deformities and crippling in patients with hemophilia can be prevented or corrected. If deformities caused by hemarthrosis cannot be corrected by conservative closed methods, one should not hesitate to perform open operations. In fact, despite increased anesthetic risk, it is sometimes preferable to perform two or three orthopaedic surgical procedures in a single operative session to avoid repetition of surgical procedures and reduce factor consumption.[117]

Hematologic Management

Before surgery is performed, the hematologist determines the factor level and performs tests to rule out the presence of factor inhibitors. During surgery and on the first postoperative day, the factor level should be raised to 100% by infusion of factor concentrate, confirmed by a factor assay before surgery. The patient is then started on a continuous infusion of clotting factor to maintain levels at 60% of normal throughout the operative procedure, with this level of factor maintained until hospital discharge.[87] During the first postoperative week, the factor level is maintained at 50%, and for the next 2 to 4 weeks factor levels are maintained at 30% to 40% of normal by daily home infusion of factor concentrate.

During preoperative evaluation, children with hemophilia are screened carefully for the presence of clotting factor inhibitors. In general, patients with active inhibitors are not candidates for elective surgery but may be considered so after induction of immune tolerance through frequent, regular infusions of clotting factor concentrate.[4] Some patients with active inhibitors respond to the use of factor VIIa as a bypassing agent, although its efficacy in patients undergoing major surgery is controversial.[87] In addition, the half-life of factor VIIa is approximately 2 hours, and the cost of its administration is several times that of recombinant factor VIII.

Treatment of Hemophilic Arthropathy

The most common procedures used to manage hemophilic arthropathy are synovectomy, joint debridement, fusion, and arthroplasty. Despite the medical and surgical complexities of hemophilic arthropathy, these procedures typically result in symptomatic improvement and high levels of patient satisfaction.[87] If equinus deformity is very severe and rigid, Achilles tendon lengthening is indicated. Fractional lengthening of the hamstrings combined with posterior capsulotomy is performed for flexion contracture of the knee. On occasion, one may have to resort to osteotomy of the distal femur, tilting it anteriorly to correct flexion deformity of the knee.[120] Even in cases of marked radiographic joint destruction, corrective osteotomy can give acceptable long-term results and may delay or avoid the need for joint replacement.[148] Osteotomy should be contemplated primarily for patients in whom damage is unicompartmental and accompanied by corresponding axial deviation.

Acute hemarthrosis of the immature hip requires special considerations, including factor replacement and aspiration on an urgent basis to reduce the risk for development of osteonecrosis.[87] Discerning hip hemarthrosis from iliopsoas muscle bleeds can be difficult because the symptoms of these two conditions may be identical. Iliopsoas bleeds may, however, be associated with femoral nerve palsy and numbness in the saphenous nerve distribution, whereas patients with hip hemarthrosis may demonstrate an increased femur-to-teardrop distance on anteroposterior radiographs. CT and MRI reliably differentiate between the two conditions, and high-resolution ultrasonography may also be useful.[87]

Open surgery has become relatively safe, provided that the clotting mechanism is restored to near normal by the administration of antihemophilic factor, which should be continued for 3 weeks, with sutures removed on the 14th to 16th postoperative day. Wounds and bone heal normally in hemophilic patients.

Synovectomy. The objective of synovectomy is to prevent progression of hemophilic arthropathy. The rationale for synovectomy in hemophilic arthropathy is based on the following considerations: Mechanically, the vulnerability to trauma of the highly vascular synovial tissue is diminished by its excision, and biochemically, hemophilic synovial tissue has a high level of fibrinolytic activity that tends to prolong the bleeding episodes.[37,138] Also, the hypertrophic synovial tissue in hemophilia contains increased levels of acid phosphatase and cathepsin D, which are further elevated during bleeding episodes; these proteolytic enzymes destroy hyaline articular cartilage.[52,53,149] The chronic synovial inflammation is perpetuated by the elevated levels of prostaglandin E and polymorphonuclear leukocytes (because of chemotactic properties of the enzymes). Also, hemosiderin deposition in the synovium interferes with the production of collagenase, which may cause death of chondrocytes.

Indications. Synovectomy of peripheral joints, particularly of the knee, is indicated in patients with a history of severe recurrent hemarthrosis (two or three major bleeding episodes per month) and in those whose condition does not respond to aggressive medical management maintained for at least 6 months. Medical management entails a prophylactic factor replacement program that raises factor levels to 30% to 40% of normal (factor replacement is administered every other day in hemophilia A and every third day in hemophilia B). Other indications are failure to respond to orthopaedic nonsurgical treatment consisting of physical therapy and protection with crutches and orthoses, and radiographic stage II or III hemophilic arthropathy (in stages IV and V, synovectomy is ineffective and contraindicated). In the elbow, repeated hemarthroses result in loss of forearm rotation and elbow extension. Limitation of rotation results mainly from hypertrophy of the radial head.[59] A reduction in the incidence of hemarthrosis has been reported after open synovectomy of the elbow with excision of the radial head to improve range of motion. Synoviorthesis with radioactive gold has also been reported to be effective in reducing hemarthroses.[102]

Techniques. Arthroscopic synovectomy, open surgical synovectomy, chemical synovectomy, and radiosynovectomy have all been recommended.

ARTHROSCOPIC SYNOVECTOMY. Although open synovectomy has been used longer than the other methods, it is often complicated by loss of range of motion of the affected joint. Arthroscopic synovectomy, which has now mostly replaced open procedures, is most useful when performed before severe degenerative changes have developed. Several reports have noted a significant reduction in hemarthroses without loss of motion after arthroscopic synovectomy. A cost–benefit analysis of arthroscopic synovectomy identified significant reductions in disease-related costs per month and in the number of hemarthroses reported before and after the procedure ($7500 versus $900, and 71 versus 7 hemarthroses, respectively).[140] Arthroscopic procedures are difficult and often lengthy but avoid some of the motion problems of open approaches.[27,31,88,151] In one study of arthroscopic synovectomy performed in 69 joints in 44 children, subjects experienced 84% fewer hemarthroses compared with control subjects. Range of motion remained stable or improved within 1 year in patients receiving arthroscopic synovectomy, and complications related to the procedure were rare, although radiographic scores of patients treated arthroscopically worsened slightly during the study.[27]

RADIOSYNOVECTOMY. Radiosynovectomy is minimally invasive, does not require hospitalization, necessitates only minimal clotting factor coverage, and preserves range of motion better than does surgical synovectomy.[84,87] This procedure can be accomplished successfully without simultaneous co-injection of corticosteroids.[40,82] Yttrium has been widely used for radiation synoviorthesis, although its use is associated with an unacceptably high rate of reduced range of motion in treated joints.[51] It is therefore suggested that another isotope be used for this purpose and that clinical centers publish their findings in this regard. Radiosynovectomy is highly cost-effective compared with open surgical or arthroscopic synovectomy.[129]

OPEN SYNOVECTOMY. Open synovectomy of the knee is performed under tourniquet ischemia.[101] The surgical approach to the knee is through a long medial parapatellar incision that begins 5 cm above the superior border of the patella and extends to the medial border of the patella and then to the medial border of the proximal tibial tubercle. Throughout the operation, electrocautery is used to maintain strict hemostasis. The subcutaneous tissue, fascia, and capsule are divided and the knee joint is thoroughly inspected. The proliferative synovial tissue is excised first from the suprapatellar pouch, then from the medial and lateral recesses of the knee and intercondylar notch, including that around the cruciate ligaments, and finally from the menisci. The coronary ligaments must be preserved. The synovial tissue on the articular cartilage is removed gently with a moist sponge. Growth of the distal femoral physis must not be disturbed. Next, the joint is copiously irrigated with antibiotic solution, and Gelfoam mixed with a solution of injectable saline and thrombin is applied over the denuded tissues. The wound is packed with moist laparotomy pads, and after several layers of elastic bandages have been applied for compression, the tourniquet is released. Five to 10 minutes later, the wound is inspected and thorough hemostasis is obtained. The previously applied Gelfoam is removed and the wound is closed in layers. Suction drainage is always inserted. A bulky compression dressing is applied, and the limb is immobilized in an above-knee plaster-of-Paris posterior splint. The suction drainage is removed in 2 or 3 days.

Postoperative Care. Isometric quadriceps- and hamstring-strengthening exercises are begun immediately. Active range-of-motion exercises should not be commenced early because they may result in massive hemarthrosis. Seven to 10 days after surgery, gentle active assisted and passive range-of-motion exercises are started. Toe-touch weight bearing with crutch protection is allowed as tolerated. Active range-of-motion exercises are started about 2 weeks after surgery. Passive range-of-knee-motion exercises may also be performed with a continuous passive motion (CPM) machine 14 days after surgery, at first for several hours of the day during waking hours to ensure that there is no bleeding into the joint, then for gradually increasing periods. During the third postoperative week, the limb should be in the CPM machine all night and part of the day. Active exercises are performed intensively to develop quadriceps function. Gradually, full weight bearing is allowed.

Problems and Complications. Postoperative loss of range of joint motion due to adhesions of the patellofemoral and tibiofemoral joints is a common and challenging problem after synovectomy for hemophilic arthropathy. In the series of 13 patients reported by Montane and associates, knee motion was reduced in 11 patients (85%); the average loss of range was 41 degrees. In the younger patients (<11 years of age), the postoperative loss of joint motion was greater owing to lack of motivation and poor cooperation with the postoperative physical therapy program. One of the young patients subsequently required knee arthrodesis.[101] Mannucci and associates reported a marked decrease in joint motion, particularly flexion, in 8 of 15 patients.[93] Kay and associates found decreased knee motion after surgery in nine patients, three of whom required postoperative manipulation under anesthesia; one of these patients sustained a supracondylar fracture of the femur during manipulation, but in the other two patients there was significant improvement of motion.[63] Arnold and Hilgartner recommended manipulation of the knee 2 to 3 weeks after synovectomy if joint motion was lost, and they stressed the importance of increasing factor levels to nearly 100% of normal.[5] The stage of arthropathy, adequacy of control of intra-articular bleeding during and after surgery, degree of quadriceps and hamstring atrophy, and patient's motivation and cooperation are important factors in determining the final range of motion. Intensive, prolonged physical therapy and use of the CPM machine are vital after synovectomy.

Massive bleeding may occur in the joint during the immediate postoperative period after synovectomy or during the rehabilitation phase of treatment. This may require aspiration or surgical arthroscopic evacuation of the hematoma.

Despite these complications, the results reported in the literature indicate that chronic recurrent hemarthrosis and the pain in chronic hemophilic arthropathy can be effectively eliminated after open synovectomy, which also appears to slow the pace of progression of the disease.[15,20,29,63,85,93,95,101,102,110,132,137,138]

Synoviorthesis. A number of methods of synovial ablation using intra-articular radioactive substances have been reported. Children have been infrequently treated in this manner because of unresolved concerns of future oncogenesis. Rifampicin injected intra-articularly has been shown to reduce synovial proliferation and the incidence of hemarthrosis. It seems most effective in younger patients and in smaller joints.[17,18] Radioactive synoviorthesis has been shown to be effective in treating recurrent hemarthrosis in patients with factor inhibitors.[84] Colloidal phosphorus 32 chromic phosphate has also been used to treat hemarthroses. In one series, all patients had a reduced incidence of hemarthrosis. Half of the patients retained range of motion and the other half gradually lost motion. Radiographic scores worsened despite a reduction in the rate of hemarthrosis.[115] A reduction in the incidence of hemarthrosis of the elbow has been reported with synoviorthesis with radioactive gold.[121] Chemical and radioisotope synovectomies have been tried in the treatment of chronic hemophilic arthropathy.[3,33,39,116] The results have been dubious; at present, surgical synovectomy is the procedure of choice.

Total Joint Replacement and Arthrodesis. Deciding between total joint replacement and arthrodesis is difficult, and the decision should be individualized. Disabling pain is the prime indication for surgery.

Total Joint Replacement. In case of bilateral knee involvement, total joint replacement is indicated with stage IV or V arthropathy when persistent knee pain is definitely due to joint derangement; there should be at least 45 degrees of knee motion. Arnold and Hilgartner reported the results of five total knee joint replacements in hemophilic patients; relief of pain was impressive, and functional range of motion was preserved without serious complications.[5] Other encouraging results have been reported by Lachiewicz and associates,[74] London and associates,[85] Magone and coworkers,[92] Marmor,[94] McCollough and associates,[95] and Small and colleagues.[130] Goldberg and associates reported the results of 13 total knee arthroplasties of the semicontainment type in 10 patients with hemophilia A with a follow-up of 2 to 6 years.[43] All patients had severe pain and used crutches with wheelchairs for ambulation before surgery. The results were graded "excellent" or "good" in four, "fair" in eight, and "poor" in one (who required arthrodesis). They recommended total knee arthroplasty, with arthrodesis as the only other alternative.[43]

Total hip replacement is indicated in stage IV or V hemophilic arthropathy when persistent pain with severe disability is not relieved by conservative measures.[25,107] Total joint replacement has been shown to have no adverse effects on the course of HIV infection in patients with hemophilia.[109] Arthroplasty of the elbow has been reported.[131]

Arthrodesis. Arthrodesis of the ankle, subtalar, and mid-tarsal joints in the foot and of the shoulder or knee may be indicated when these joints are destroyed. The surgical technique is the same as in normal patients with the exception that percutaneous pins should not be used in hemophilic patients because they will need factor replacement at moderate levels until the pins are removed.[55,107] Arthrodesis of the hip is considered when the patient has a destroyed hip with little involvement of the other joints. The indication is stronger when the child is unlikely to abide by activity restrictions and likely to overstress a total hip replacement.

Treatment of Neurapraxia

Neurapraxia is treated by factor replacement therapy in doses to attain factor levels of 80% to 100% of normal for 48 hours after onset of hemorrhage; the dose is tapered to maintain a level of 40% for 1 to 2 weeks. The limb is splinted. Gentle physical therapy is performed 7 days after the bleeding episode. Occasionally decompression of the entrapped nerve may need to be performed.[76]

Treatment of Fractures

Fractures usually heal in the normal time.[10,11,21,33,66] Factor replacement should be to the level of 40% to 60% of normal on the day of fracture and the following day; subsequently it should be 20% to 30% for 7 or more days, depending on the degree of associated soft tissue injury.[33] Whenever possible, fractures are treated by closed reduction and immobilization in a cast. Pins should not be used for skeletal traction because the patient will need prolonged factor replacement therapy. External fixators should be avoided. Open reduction and internal fixation is carried out when closed methods are not appropriate.

Treatment of Flexion Contractures

In areas of the world where home infusion of clotting factor is not available, recurrent hemarthrosis is the major source of morbidity, giving rise to joint destruction and flexion contracture. Large-joint contractures have been treated successfully by Ilizarov external fixation under such circumstances, with factor IX levels maintained at 1.0 IU/mL before and after surgery. In one reported case, fixed flexion in the knee joint was reduced from 50 to 5 degrees, and the child walked freely and without pain 4 months after surgery.[69]

Treatment of Pseudotumors

Greene has recommended that pseudotumors be excised whenever they are accessible and believes they will continue to expand if left alone.[46] Before surgical intervention, angiography, CT, and nuclear MRI should be performed to provide accurate anatomic detail of adjacent vessels.[142] The pseudotumor per se is avascular.[139] The surgical extirpation of a hemophilic pseudotumor requires careful preoperative planning and extensive dissection.[49,111,123]

Radiation therapy has been used to control the expanding hematoma of hemophilic pseudotumors; irradiation causes new bone formation and sclerosis of the cystic cavity. Its use may be considered in surgically inaccessible sites. It is important to shield the physis to avoid causing growth disturbance.[82] Amputation of a limb may be indicated when the patient is seen late and in a patient in whom deformity is so severe that the limb is of no use.[9,22,124]

References

Hemophilia

1. Abell J Jr, Bailey R: Hemophilic pseudotumor: Two cases occurring in siblings. Arch Surg 1960;81:569.
2. Ahlberg A: On the natural history of hemophilic pseudotumor. J Bone Joint Surg Am 1975;57:1133.
3. Ahlberg A, Pettersson H: Synoviorthesis with radioactive gold in hemophiliacs: Clinical and radiological follow-up. Acta Orthop Scand 1979;50:513.
4. Aledort LM, Kroner B, Mariani G: Hemophilia treatment. Immune tolerance induction: treatment duration analysis and economic considerations. Haematologica 2000;85:83.
5. Arnold W, Hilgartner M: Hemophilic arthropathy: Current concepts of pathogenesis and management. J Bone Joint Surg Am 1977;59:287.
6. Aronstam A, Browne RS, Wassef M, et al: The clinical features of early bleeding into the muscles of the lower limb in severe haemophiliacs. J Bone Joint Surg Br 1983;65:19.
7. Barnes C, Wong P, Egan B, et al: Reduced bone density among children with severe hemophilia. Pediatrics 2004;114:e177.
8. Bayer WL, Shea JD, Curiel DC, et al: Excision of a pseudocyst of the hand in a hemophiliac (PTC-deficiency): Use of a plasma thromboplastin component concentrate. J Bone Joint Surg Am 1969;51:1423.
9. Blalock A: Amputation of arm of patient with hemophilia. JAMA 1932;99:1777.
10. Boardman KP, English P: Fractures and dislocations in hemophilia. Clin Orthop Relat Res 1980;148:221.
11. Boni M, Ceciliani L: Fractures in haemophilia. Ital J Orthop Traumatol 1976;2:301.
12. Brant EE, Jordan HH: Radiologic aspects of hemophilic pseudotumors in bone. AJR Am J Roentgenol Radium Ther Nucl Med 1972;115:525.
13. Brower TD, Wilde AH: Femoral neuropathy in hemophilia. J Bone Joint Surg Am 1966;48:487.
14. Brownlee GG: Prospects for gene therapy of haemophilia A and B. Br Med Bull 1995;51:91.
15. Bussi L, Silvello L, Baudo F, et al: Results of synovectomy of the knee in haemophilia. Haematologica 1974;59:81.
16. Cahlon O, Klepps S, Cleeman E, et al: A retrospective radiographic review of hemophilic shoulder arthropathy. Clin Orthop Relat Res 2004;423:106.

17. Caviglia H, Galatro G, Duhalde C, et al: Haemophilic synovitis: Is rifampicin an alternative? Haemophilia 1998;4:514.
18. Caviglia HA, Fernández-Palazzi F, Maffei E, et al: Chemical synoviorthesis for hemophilic synovitis. Clin Orthop Relat Res 1997;343:30.
19. Chen YF: Bilateral hemophilic pseudotumors of the calcaneus and cuboid treated by irradiation: Case report. J Bone Joint Surg Am 1965;47:517.
20. Clark MW: Knee synovectomy in hemophilia. Orthopedics 1978;1:285.
21. Coventry M, Owen C Jr, Murphy T, et al: Survival of patient with hemophilia and fracture of femur. J Bone Joint Surg Am 1959;41:1392.
22. Crandon J, Staudinger L Jr, Friedman E: Mid-thigh amputation in a patient with hemophilia. N Engl J Med 1953;249:657.
23. Culver J Jr: Combined posterior interosseous and ulnar nerve compression in a hemophiliac. Bull Hosp Joint Dis 1978;39:103.
24. Cunning H: The surgery of haemophilia cysts. In Biggs R, McFarlane R (eds): Treatment of Haemophilia and Other Coagulation Disorders. Oxford, Blackwell, 1966.
25. D'Ambrosia RD, Niemann KM, O'Grady L, et al: Total hip replacement for patients with hemophilia and hemorrhagic diathesis. Surg Gynecol Obstet 1974;139:381.
26. Driessen A: Arthropathies in Haemophiliacs. Groningen, The Netherlands, Van-Grocum, 1973.
27. Dunn A, Busch MT, Wyly J, et al: Arthroscopic synovectomy for hemophilic joint disease in a pediatric population. J Pediatr Orthop 2004;24:414.
28. Duthie R, Matthews J, Rizza C, et al: The Management of Musculoskeletal Problems in Haemophilias. Oxford, Blackwell, 1972.
29. Dyszy-Laube B, Kaminski W, Gizycka I, et al: Synovectomy in the treatment of hemophilic arthropathy. J Pediatr Surg 1974;9:123.
30. Echternacht A: Pseudotumor of bone in hemophilia. Radiology 1943;41:565.
31. Eickhoff HH, Koch W, Raderschadt G, et al: Arthroscopy for chronic hemophilic synovitis of the knee. Clin Orthop Relat Res 1997;343:58.
32. Fallaux FJ, Hoeben RC: Gene therapy for the hemophilias. Curr Opin Hematol 1996;3:385.
33. Feil E, Bentley G, Rizza CR: Fracture management in patients with haemophilia. J Bone Joint Surg Br 1974; 56:643.
34. Fernandez de Valderrama J, Matthews J: The haemophilic pseudotumor or haemophilic subperiosteal haematoma. J Bone Joint Surg Br 1965;47:256.
35. Fischer K, van der Bom JG, Molho P, et al: Prophylactic versus on-demand treatment strategies for severe haemophilia: A comparison of costs and long-term outcome. Haemophilia 2002;8:745.
36. Floman Y, Niska M: Dislocation of the hip joint complicating repeated hemarthrosis in hemophilia. J Pediatr Orthop 1983;3:99.
37. Fraenkel G, Taylor K, Richards W: Haemophilic blood cysts. Br J Surg 1959;46:383.
38. Funk M, Schmidt H, Escuriola-Ettingshausen C, et al: Radiological and orthopedic score in pediatric hemophilic patients with early and late prophylaxis. Ann Hematol 1998;77:171.
39. Gamba G, Grignani G, Ascari E: Synoviorthesis versus synovectomy in the treatment of recurrent haemophilic haemarthrosis: Long-term evaluation. Thromb Haemost 1981;45:127.
40. Gedik G, Ugur O, Atilla B, et al: Is corticosteroid coinjection necessary for radiosynoviorthesis of patients with hemophilia? Clin Nucl Med 2004;29:538.
41. Ghormley R, Clegg R: Bone and joint changes in hemophilia. J Bone Joint Surg Am 1948;30:589.
42. Gilbert MS, Aledort LM, Seremetis S, et al: Long term evaluation of septic arthritis in hemophilic patients. Clin Orthop Relat Res 1996;328:54.
43. Goldberg VM, Heiple KG, Ratnoff OD, et al: Total knee arthroplasty in classic hemophilia. J Bone Joint Surg Am 1981;63:695.
44. Gómez-Vargas A, Hortelano G: Nonviral gene therapy approaches to hemophilia. Semin Thromb Hemost 2004;30:197.
45. Goodfellow J, Fearn CB, Matthews JM: Iliacus haematoma: A common complication of haemophilia. J Bone Joint Surg Br 1967;49:748.
46. Greene W: Hemophilia. In Weinstein M (ed): Pediatric Orthopedics, vol 1. Philadelphia, Lippincott-Raven, 1996, p 379.
47. Greene WB, McMillan CW: Nonsurgical management of hemophilic arthropathy. Instr Course Lect 1989;38: 367.
48. Greene WB, McMillan CW, Warren MW: Prophylactic transfusion for hypertrophic synovitis in children with hemophilia. Clin Orthop Relat Res 1997;343:19.
49. Hall M, Handley D, Webster C: The surgical treatment of haemophilic blood cysts. J Bone Joint Surg Br 1962; 44:781.
50. Heijnen L, Roosendaal G, Heim M: Orthotics and rehabilitation for chronic hemophilic synovitis of the ankle: An overview. Clin Orthop Relat Res 1997;343: 68.
51. Heim M, Tiktinsky R, Amit Y, et al: Yttrium synoviorthesis of the elbow joints in persons with haemophilia. Haemophilia 2004;10:590.
52. Hilgartner M: Pathogenesis of joint changes in hemophilia. In Committee on Prosthetic Research and Development: Comprehensive Management of Musculoskeletal Disorders in Hemophilia. Washington, DC, National Academy of Sciences, 1973.
53. Hilgartner M: Hemophilic arthropathy. Adv Pediatr 1974;21:139.
54. Horwitz H, Bassen F, Simon N: Haemophilic pseudotumour of the pelvis. Br J Radiol 1959;32:51.
55. Houghton GR, Dickson RA: Lower limb arthrodeses in haemophilia. J Bone Joint Surg Br 1978;60:387.
56. Houghton GR, Duthie RB: Orthopedic problems in hemophilia. Clin Orthop Relat Res 1979;138:197.
57. Hussey HH: Hemophilic pseudotumor of bone [editorial]. JAMA 1975;232:1040.
58. Hutcheson J: Peripelvic new bone formation in hemophilia: Report of three cases. Radiology 1973;109:529.
59. Ishiguro N, Yasuo S, Takamatu S, et al: Hemophilic arthropathy of the elbow. J Pediatr Orthop 1995;15: 821.

60. Ivins J: Bone and joint complications of hemophilia. In Brinkhous K (ed): Hemophilia and Hemophilioid Diseases: International Symposium. Chapel Hill, NC, University of North Carolina Press, 1957.
61. Kass L, Ratnoff O, Leon M: Studies on the purification of antihemophilic factor (factor 8): I. Precipitation of antihemophilic factor by concanavalin A. J Clin Invest 1969;48:351.
62. Katznelson J: Hemophilia with special reference to the Talmud. Hebrew Med J 1958;1:163.
63. Kay L, Stainsby D, Buzzard B, et al: The role of synovectomy in the management of recurrent haemarthroses in haemophilia. Br J Haematol 1981;49:53.
64. Kay MA: Hepatic gene therapy for haemophilia B. Haemophilia 1998;4:389.
65. Kemnitz S, Moens P, Peerlinck K, et al: Avascular necrosis of the talus in children with haemophilia. J Pediatr Orthop B 2002;11:73.
66. Kemp HS, Matthews JM: The management of fractures in haemophilia and Christmas disease. J Bone Joint Surg Br 1968;50:351.
67. Kern M, Blanchette V, Stain A, et al: Clinical and cost implications of target joints in Canadian boys with severe hemophilia A. J Pediatr 2004;145:628.
68. Kerr R: Imaging of musculoskeletal complications of hemophilia. Semin Musculoskelet Radiol 2003;7:127.
69. Kiely PD, McMahon C, Smith OP, et al: The treatment of flexion contracture of the knee using the Ilizarov technique in a child with haemophilia B. Haemophilia 2003;9:336.
70. Kinnas PA, Woodham CH, MacLarnon JC: Ultrasonic measurements of haematomata of joints and soft tissues in the haemophiliac. Scand J Haematol Suppl 1984; 40:225.
71. Konig F: Gelenkerkrankungen bei Bluten mit besonderer Berucksichtigung der Diagnose. Leipzig 1890-1894; 1-25.
72. Krill C Jr, Mauer A: Pseudotumor of calcaneus in Christmas disease. J Pediatr 1970;77:848.
73. Kumari S, Fulco JD, Karayalcin G, et al: Gray scale ultrasound: Evaluation of iliopsoas hematomas in hemophiliacs. AJR Am J Roentgenol 1979;133:103.
74. Lachiewicz PF, Inglis AE, Insall JN, et al: Total knee arthroplasty in hemophilia. J Bone Joint Surg Am 1985;67:1361.
75. Lancourt JE, Gilbert MS, Posner MA: Management of bleeding and associated complications of hemophilia in the hand and forearm. J Bone Joint Surg Am 1977;59:451.
76. Large DF, Ludlam CA, Macnicol MF: Common peroneal nerve entrapment in a hemophiliac. Clin Orthop Relat Res 1983;181:165.
77. Lazerson J, Nagel D, Becker J: Myositis ossificans as a complication of severe hemophilia A. In Committee on Prosthetic Research and Development: Comprehensive Management of Musculoskeletal Disorders in Hemophilia. Washington, DC, National Academy of Sciences, 1973.
78. Lee CA: The natural history of HIV disease in haemophilia. Blood Rev 1998;12:135.
79. Leissinger C: Prevention of bleeds in hemophilia patients with inhibitors: Emerging data and clinical direction. Am J Hematol 2004;77:187.
80. Levine PH: Efficacy of self-therapy in hemophilia: A study of 72 patients with hemophilia A and B. N Engl J Med 1974;291:1381.
81. Levine PH, Britten AF: Supervised patient-management of hemophilia: A study of 45 patients with hemophilia A and B. Ann Intern Med 1973;78:195.
82. Li P, Chen G, Zhang H, et al: Radiation synovectomy by 188 Re-sulfide in haemophilic synovitis. Haemophilia 2004;10:422.
83. Liu M, Murphy ME, Thompson AR: A domain mutations in 65 haemophilia A families and molecular modelling of dysfunctional factor VIII proteins. Br J Haematol 1998;103:1051.
84. Löfqvist T, Petersson C, Nilsson IM: Radioactive synoviorthesis in patients with hemophilia with factor inhibitor. Clin Orthop Relat Res 1997;343:37.
85. London JT, Kattlove H, Louie JS, et al: Synovectomy and total joint arthroplasty for recurrent hemarthroses in the arthropathic joint in hemophilia. Arthritis Rheum 1977;20:1543.
86. Lozier J: Gene therapy of the hemophilias. Semin Hematol 2004;41:287.
87. Luck J Jr, Silva M, Rodriguez-Merchan E, et al: Hemophilic arthropathy. J Am Acad Orthop Surg 2004;12: 234.
88. Luck J, Kasper C: Surgical management of advanced hemophilic arthropathy: An overview of 20 years' experience. Clin Orthop Relat Res 1989;242:60.
89. MacMahon J, Blackburn C: Haemophilic pseudotumour: A report of a case treated conservatively. Aust N Z J Surg 1959;29:129.
90. Madigan RR: Acute compartment syndrome in hemophilia: A case report. J Bone Joint Surg Am 1982;64: 313.
91. Madigan RR, Hanna WT, Wallace SL: Acute compartment syndrome in hemophilia: A case report. J Bone Joint Surg Am 1981;63:1327.
92. Magone JB, Dennis DA, Weis LD: Total knee arthroplasty in chronic hemophilic arthropathy. Orthopedics 1986;9:653.
93. Mannucci PM, De Franchis R, Torri G, et al: Role of synovectomy in hemophilic arthropathy. Isr J Med Sci 1977;13:983.
94. Marmor L: Total knee replacement in hemophilia. Clin Orthop Relat Res 1977;125:192.
95. McCollough N III, Enis JE, Lovitt J, et al: Synovectomy or total replacement of the knee in hemophilia. J Bone Joint Surg Am 1979;61:69.
96. McDaniel WJ: A modified subluxation hinge for use in hemophilic knee flexion contractures. Clin Orthop Relat Res 1974;103:50.
97. McKee PA, Andersen JC, Switzer ME: Molecular structural studies of human factor VIII. Ann N Y Acad Sci 1975;240:8.
98. McVerry BA, Voke J, Vicary FR, et al: Ultrasonography in the management of haemophilia. Lancet 1977;1: 872.
99. Miners AH, Sabin CA, Tolley KH, et al: Assessing the effectiveness and cost-effectiveness of prophylaxis against bleeding in patients with severe haemophilia and severe von Willebrand's disease. J Intern Med 1998;244:515.

100. Moneim MS, Gribble TJ: Carpal tunnel syndrome in hemophilia. J Hand Surg [Am] 1984;9:580.
101. Montane I, McCollough N, Lian E: Synovectomy of the knee for hemophilic arthropathy. J Bone Joint Surg Am 1986;68:210.
102. Nicol RO, Menelaus MB: Synovectomy of the knee in hemophilia. J Pediatr Orthop 1986;6:330.
103. Nielsen LR, Scheibel E, Ingerslev J, et al: Detection of ten new mutations by screening the gene encoding factor IX of Danish hemophilia B patients. Thromb Haemost 1995;73:774.
104. Niemann KM: Surgical correction of flexion deformities in hemophilia. Am Surg 1971;37:685.
105. Niemann KM: Management of lower extremity contractures resulting from hemophilia. South Med J 1974;67:437.
106. Nowotny C, Niessner H, Thaler E, et al: Sonography: A method for localization of hematomas in hemophiliacs. Haemostasis 1976;5:129.
107. Patek A Jr, Taylor FHL: Some properties of a substance obtained from normal human plasma effective in accelerating the coagulation of hemophilic blood. J Clin Invest 1937;16:113.
108. Pettersson H, Ahlberg A: Computed tomography in hemophilic pseudotumor. Acta Radiol Diagn (Stockh) 1982;23:453.
109. Phillips AM, Sabin CA, Ribbans WJ, et al: Orthopaedic surgery in hemophilic patients with human immunodeficiency virus. Clin Orthop Relat Res 1997; 343:81.
110. Pietrogrande V, Dioguardi N, Mannucci PM: Short-term evaluation of synovectomy in haemophilia. BMJ 1972;2:378.
111. Post M, Telfer MC: Surgery in hemophilic patients. J Bone Joint Surg Am 1975;57:1136.
112. Railton GT, Aronstam A: Early bleeding into upper limb muscles in severe haemophilia: Clinical features and treatment. J Bone Joint Surg Br 1987;69:100.
113. Ratnoff OD, Kass L, Lang PD: Studies on the purification of antihemophilic factor (factor VIII): II. Separation of partially purified antihemophilic factor by gel filtration of plasma. J Clin Invest 1969;48:957.
114. Ribbans WJ, Giangrande P, Beeton K: Conservative treatment of hemarthrosis for prevention of hemophilic synovitis. Clin Orthop Relat Res 1997;343:12.
115. Rivard G, Girard M, Belanger R, et al: Synoviorthesis with colloidal ^{32}P chromic phosphate for the treatment of hemophilic arthropathy. J Bone Joint Surg Am 1994;76:482.
116. Rodriguez M, Plantier J, Enjolras N, et al: Biosynthesis of FVIII in megakaryocytic cells: Improved production and biochemical characterization. Br J Haematol 2004;127:568.
117. Rodriguez-Merchan E: Orthopaedic surgery in persons with haemophilia. Thromb Haemost 2003;89: 34.
118. Rodríguez-Merchán EC: Effects of hemophilia on articulations of children and adults. Clin Orthop Relat Res 1996;328:7.
119. Rodríguez-Merchán EC: Pathogenesis, early diagnosis, and prophylaxis for chronic hemophilic synovitis. Clin Orthop Relat Res 1997;343:6.
120. Rodríguez-Merchán EC, Magallón M, Galindo E, et al: Hamstring release for fixed knee flexion contracture in hemophilia. Clin Orthop Relat Res 1997;343:63.
121. Rodríguez-Merchán EC, Magallón M, Galindo E, et al: Hemophilic synovitis of the knee and the elbow. Clin Orthop Relat Res 1997;343:47.
122. Roosendaal G, Tekoppele JM, Vianen ME, et al: Articular cartilage is more susceptible to blood induced damage at young than at old age. J Rheumatol 2000; 27:1740.
123. Rosenthal RL, Graham JJ, Selirio E: Excision of pseudotumor with repair by bone graft of pathological fracture of femur in hemophilia. J Bone Joint Surg Am 1973;55:827.
124. Sancho FG: Experimental model of haemophilic arthropathy with high pressure haemarthrosis. Int Orthop 1980;4:57.
125. Schröder W, Wulff K, Wollina K, et al: Haemophilia B in female twins caused by a point mutation in one factor IX gene and nonrandom inactivation patterns of the X-chromosomes. Thromb Haemost 1997; 78:1347.
126. Schwartz E: Hemophilic pseudotumor of bone. Radiology 1960;75:795.
127. Serre H, Izarn P, Simon L, et al: Les attients de la hanche au cors de l'hemophilie. Mars Med 1969;106:483.
128. Shirkhoda A, Mauro MA, Staab EV, et al: Soft-tissue hemorrhage in hemophiliac patients: Computed tomography and ultrasound study. Radiology 1983;147:811.
129. Silva M, Luck JV Jr, Siegel ME: ^{32}P chromic phosphate radiosynovectomy for chronic haemophilic synovitis. Haemophilia 2001;7(Suppl 2):40.
130. Small M, Steven MM, Freeman PA, et al: Total knee arthroplasty in haemophilic arthritis. J Bone Joint Surg Br 1983;65:163.
131. Smith MA, Savidge GF, Fountain EJ: Interposition arthroplasty in the management of advanced haemophilic arthropathy of the elbow. J Bone Joint Surg Br 1983;65:436.
132. Soreff J: Joint debridement in the treatment of advanced hemophilic knee arthropathy. Clin Orthop Relat Res 1984;191:179.
133. Soucie JM, Evatt B, Jackson D: Occurrence of hemophilia in the United States. The Hemophilia Surveillance System Project Investigators. Am J Hematol 1998; 59:288.
134. Starker L: Knochenusur durch ein Hamophiles, subperiosteles Hamaton. Mit Grezgeb Med Chir 1918-1919; 31:381.
135. Steel WM, Duthie RB, O'Connor BT: Haemophilic cysts: Report of five cases. J Bone Joint Surg Br 1969;51:614.
136. Stein H, Dickson RA: Reversed dynamic slings for knee-flexion contractures in the hemophiliac. J Bone Joint Surg Am 1975;57:282.
137. Storti E, Ascari E: Surgical and chemical synovectomy. Ann N Y Acad Sci 1975;240:316.
138. Storti E, Traldi A, Tosatti E, et al: Synovectomy, a new approach to haemophilic arthropathy. Acta Haematol 1969;41:193.
139. Sundaram M, Wolverson MK, Joist JH, et al: Case report 133: Hemophilic pseudotumor of ilium and soft tissues. Skeletal Radiol 1981;6:54.

140. Tamurian R, Spencer E, Wojtys E: The role of arthroscopic synovectomy in the management of hemarthrosis in hemophilia patients: Financial perspectives. Arthroscopy 2002;18:789.
141. Teitelbaum S: Radiologic evaluation of the hemophilic hip. Mt Sinai J Med 1977;44:400.
142. Thomas ML, Walters HL: The angiographic findings in a haemophilic pseudotumour of bone. Australas Radiol 1977;21:346.
143. Thorrez L, VandenDriessche T, Collen D, et al: Preclinical gene therapy studies for hemophilia using adenoviral vectors. Semin Thromb Hemost 2004;30:173.
144. Trueta J: The orthopedic management of patients with hemophilia and Christmas disease. In Biggs R, McFarlane R (eds): Treatment of Hemophilia and Other Coagulation Disorders. Oxford, Blackwell, 1966.
145. Vas W, Cockshott WP, Martin RF, et al: Myositis ossificans in hemophilia. Skeletal Radiol 1981;7:27.
146. Waddington S, Nivsarkar M, Mistry A, et al: Permanent phenotypic correction of hemophilia B in immunocompetent mice by prenatal gene therapy. Blood 2004;104: 2714.
147. Wallis J, van Kaick G, Schimpf K, et al: Ultrasound diagnosis of muscle haematomas in haemophiliac patients [in German]. Rofo Fortschr Geb Rontgenstr Nuklearmed 1981;134:153.
148. Wallny T, Saker A, Hofmann P, et al: Long-term follow-up after osteotomy for haemophilic arthropathy of the knee. Haemophilia 2003;9:69.
149. Weissmann G, Spilberg I: Breakdown of cartilage protein polysaccharide by lysosomes. Arthritis Rheum 1968;11:162.
150. White GC 2nd, McMillan CW, Blatt PM, et al: Factor VIII inhibitors: A clinical overview. Am J Hematol 1982;13:335.
151. Wiedel JD: Arthroscopic synovectomy of the knee in hemophilia: 10- to 15-year followup. Clin Orthop Relat Res 1996;328:46.
152. Wilson DJ, Green DJ, MacLarnon JC: Arthrosonography of the painful hip. Clin Radiol 1984;35:17.
153. Wilson DJ, McLardy-Smith PD, Woodham CH, et al: Diagnostic ultrasound in haemophilia. J Bone Joint Surg Br 1987;69:103.
154. Wright A: On a method of determining the condition of blood coagulability for clinical and experimental uses. BMJ 1893;2:223.

Sickle Cell Disease

Sickle cell disease is a genetic condition that, in the homozygous state, causes the red blood cells (RBCs) to become distorted into a sickle shape under conditions of low oxygen tension. The affected cells are dysfunctional, which causes a variety of symptoms related to reduced oxygen delivery to tissues. The disorder primarily affects black individuals, although cases in whites have occurred in some countries, including Greece, Turkey, Italy, and India.

Etiology and Pathophysiology

Sickle cell disease is caused by an autosomal dominant gene that results in the production of an abnormal hemoglobin termed *hemoglobin S*. This hemoglobin differs from normal adult hemoglobin by the substitution of valine for glutamic acid in the sixth amino acid position in each of the two β-polypeptide chains.[16] In *sickle cell trait,* the individual receives the abnormal hemoglobin S gene from one parent; sickle cell trait occurs in approximately 10% of black people in the United States. Sickle cell disease is the homozygous state and occurs in 2.5% of the African-American population.

Sickle cell disease also includes conditions in which the abnormal hemoglobin S is combined with other abnormal hemoglobin entities such as C, D, or E.[4] These are referred to as *mixed hemoglobinopathies.* Hemoglobin S may also be associated with other types of hereditary diseases, such as thalassemia, spherocytosis, or ovalocytosis.

Orthopaedic Manifestations and Treatment

BONE INFARCTION

Bone infarction occurs in sickle cell disease when vessels are occluded by the sickled RBCs. Infarction manifests as sudden pain in an extremity with swelling over the affected bone. Other signs of an inflammatory process include local warmth, erythema, and decreased motion of adjacent joints. Fever is uncommon. The most commonly affected bones are the humerus, tibia, and femur. Although bone infarction is more common than osteomyelitis (50 times more common in one study[12]), infection must be ruled out. The erythrocyte sedimentation rate is often mildly elevated. Technetium scans may show increased or decreased uptake, and gallium scans often show increased activity.[12]

The treatment of bone infarction is limited to analgesics and oral or intravenous hydration. Antibiotics are often given until the diagnosis of osteomyelitis is ruled out.[12]

OSTEOMYELITIS

Osteomyelitis is a frequent problem in children with sickle cell disease. In one study the annual incidence for a patient was estimated at 0.36%.[17] Both bone infarction and osteomyelitis are characterized by localized erythema, tenderness, and swelling. Both may also be accompanied by elevation in the erythrocyte sedimentation rate and a high leukocyte count. Both tests are useful in following response to treatment. An ill-appearing patient with fever greater than 38.2°C and localized pain and swelling should prompt the physician to aspirate or sample the area rather than rely on diagnostic studies that may be unreliable in discriminating between these two diseases.[3] Infection is confirmed by aspirating purulent material from the bone or by a positive blood culture.[3,5]

Radiographic studies may help the clinician differentiate between sepsis and infarction, but careful interpretation is essential. The radiographs in the early stages of either condition are negative or show only soft tissue swelling.[5] At about 2 weeks, both conditions exhibit destruction of bone and periosteal reaction.

Technetium and gallium scans may help make the differentiation, but both may be misleading as well.[12,13] A combination of sequential bone marrow and bone scintigraphy may help make the diagnosis based on normal uptake on the bone marrow scan and abnormal uptake on the bone scan at the site of pain.[20] Radionuclide scintigraphy is most useful in locating multiple sites of infection, especially in the pelvis and spine. Gadolinium-enhanced MRI may allow differentiation of bone infarction versus osteomyelitis and recognition of osteomyelitis superimposed on bone infarction, with children with osteomyelitis demonstrating elongated, serpiginous central medullary enhancement with evident periostitis.[21] On ultrasonography, a subperiosteal fluid depth greater than 4 mm is highly suggestive of osteomyelitis, but patients with a subperiosteal fluid depth less than 4 mm require further imaging or aspiration to establish the diagnosis.[22]

The treatment of osteomyelitis must take into account the altered immune status of the patient and the impaired blood flow to the bone. Prompt operative decompression of any abscess is essential, and parenteral antibiotic therapy should be continued for 6 to 8 weeks.[5] The most common organisms causing osteomyelitis in these patients are *Staphylococcus aureus* and *Salmonella* species, with *Salmonella* species being the causative agent in 60% to 80% of cases.[1] Younger patients are more likely to have *Salmonella* osteomyelitis.[5,18] Septic arthritis in this patient group may also be caused by *Salmonella* species.[11] Osteomyelitis due to vancomycin-resistant *Enterococcus faecium* and the anaerobe *Fusobacterium nucleatum* has also been reported.[1,14] In the latter case, infection did not respond completely to antibiotic therapy and resolved only after surgical debridement and hyperbaric oxygen therapy.

HAND-FOOT SYNDROME

Hand-foot syndrome is characterized by swelling and tenderness of the hands and feet of children with sickle cell disease who are younger than 6 years of age (Figs. 36–7 and 36–8). It occurs in up to 58% of children with the disease and may be the presenting symptom. It appears after about 6 months of age, when hemoglobin F has been replaced by hemoglobin S.[9] It does not occur after the disappearance of the hematopoietic marrow from the hands and feet, at around 6 years of age. The clinical findings of hand-foot syndrome

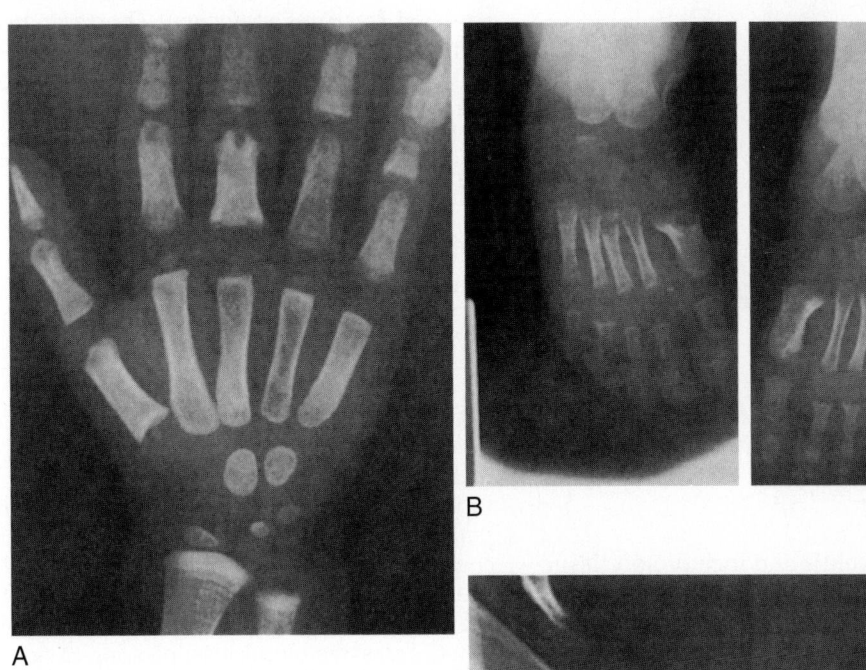

FIGURE 36–7 Hand-foot syndrome in sickle cell disease. The hands and feet were painful and swollen for 2 weeks. **A** and **B**, Radiographs of the right hand and both feet showing patchy areas of bone destruction. **C**, Radiograph of the left foot obtained 2 months later. Repair is taking place by "creeping substitution."

Section IV Orthopaedic Disorders

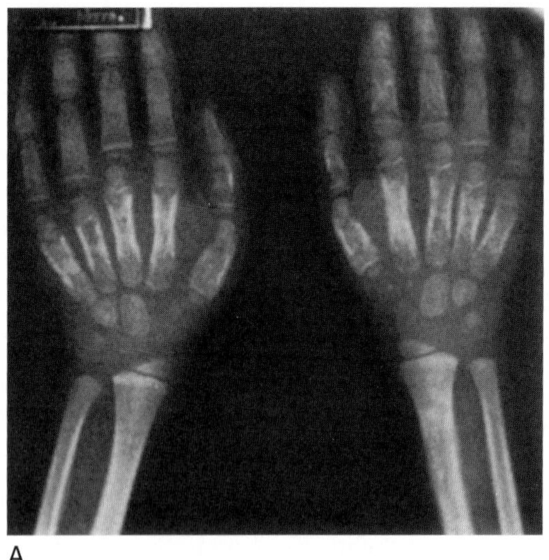

A

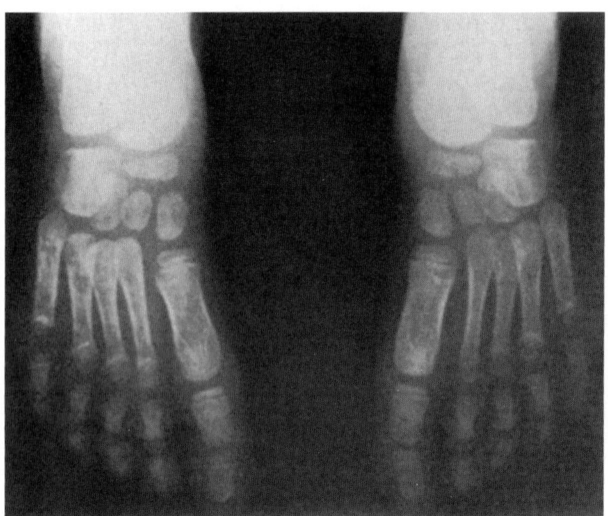

B

FIGURE 36-8 Hand-foot syndrome in sickle cell disease in an 8-month-old infant. Radiographs of the hands **(A)** and feet **(B)** reveal diffuse involvement of the short tubular bones, with patchy areas of destruction and some periosteal reaction.

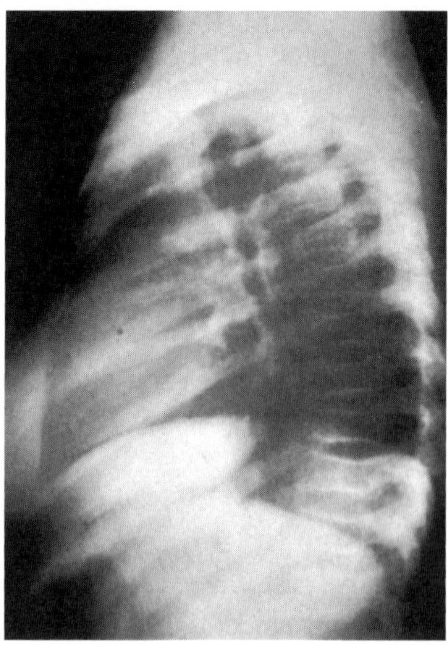

FIGURE 36-9 Sickle cell disease in an 11-year-old girl. Lateral radiograph of the spine shows reduction in the height of the vertebrae.

resemble those of osteomyelitis and include soft tissue swelling, limited motion, tenderness, and pain in the hands and feet of small children.[5,9] Although osteomyelitis is rare in the hands and feet of young children, the disorder must be considered in the differential diagnosis. In both conditions the white blood cell count and infectious indices are elevated. Higher elevations in the presence of significant fever suggest an infection. Blood cultures and aspiration of involved areas may provide the diagnosis. Antibiotic coverage should include coverage for *Salmonella* infection.[9]

VERTEBRAL INVOLVEMENT

Hyperplasia of the bone marrow in response to the hemolytic anemia of sickle cell disease causes radiographic changes in the vertebrae. The height of the vertebrae may be reduced and there may be bulging of intervertebral disks into the bodies (Fig. 36–9). Compression fractures may cause shortening of the trunk or the development of a kyphosis.

Vertebral collapse may be due to AVN of the vertebra.[19] Spinal osteomyelitis must always be considered in the differential diagnosis when spinal symptoms appear. In one center, 24% of patients evaluated for spinal disorders had osteomyelitis of the vertebrae.[19] Surgical decompression and anterior strut grafting are usually required to eradicate infection and preserve spinal alignment.

AVASCULAR NECROSIS

Avascular necrosis of the femoral head eventually occurs in 19% to 31% of patients with sickle cell disease.[7] The humeral head may also undergo AVN, and this is usually better tolerated than AVN in the hip.[23] Total hip replacement is the eventual treatment for most patients with AVN. Unfortunately, the results are compromised by the disease, and complications are frequent.[7] In one series, five of eight arthroplasties required early revision. In addition, the investigators noted excessive blood loss, prolonged hospitalization, and medical or surgical complications in all patients, including those with sickle cell trait. They reported a failure rate of 50% by 5 years after surgery.[10]

SURGICAL COMPLICATIONS

The use of a tourniquet in patients with sickle cell trait or sickle cell disease is considered undesirable by most authors because the hypoxia beyond the tourniquet induces RBC sickling. One author reported using a tourniquet in 19 patients with sickle cell disease. The patients with sickle cell disease had more complications than a control group, and these included bone pain, severe postoperative pain, jaundice, and tissue edema. All complications resolved within 2 weeks.[15]

Autologous blood can be used as well as blood salvaged from the surgical field, but both are difficult to store because of the potential for hemolysis and sickling.[6]

MISCELLANEOUS BONE CHANGES

A lower bone mineral density of between 6% and 21% is usually found in patients with sickle cell anemia.[2] Lucencies in the skull may produce a ground-glass appearance with loss of trabecular pattern. Changes in trabecular patterns of the long bones appear in younger children, corresponding to the location of active bone marrow.[8]

References

Sickle Cell Disease

1. Bibbo C, Patel DV, Tyndall WA, et al: Treatment of multifocal vancomycin-resistant *Enterococcus faecium* osteomyelitis in sickle cell disease: A preliminary report. Am J Orthop 2003;32:505.
2. Brinker MR, Thomas KA, Meyers SJ, et al: Bone mineral density of the lumbar spine and proximal femur is decreased in children with sickle cell anemia. Am J Orthop 1998;27:43.
3. Chambers JB, Forsythe DA, Bertrand SL, et al: Retrospective review of osteoarticular infections in a pediatric sickle cell age group. J Pediatr Orthop 2000;20: 682.
4. Diggs LW: Bone and joint lesions in sickle-cell disease. Clin Orthop Relat Res 1967;52:119.
5. Epps CH Jr, Bryant DD III, Coles MJ, et al: Osteomyelitis in patients who have sickle-cell disease: Diagnosis and management. J Bone Joint Surg Am 1991;73:1281.
6. Fox JS, Amaranath L, Hoeltge GA, et al: Autologous blood transfusion and intraoperative cell salvage in a patient with homozygous sickle cell disease. Cleve Clin J Med 1994;61:137.
7. Garden MS, Grant RE, Jebraili S: Perioperative complications in patients with sickle cell disease: An orthopedic perspective. Am J Orthop 1996;25:353.
8. Golding JS, MacIver JE, Went LN: The bone changes in sickle cell anaemia and its genetic variants. J Bone Joint Surg Br 1959;41:711.
9. Greene WB, McMillan CW: *Salmonella* osteomyelitis and hand-foot syndrome in a child with sickle cell anemia. J Pediatr Orthop 1987;7:716.
10. Hanker GJ, Amstutz HC: Osteonecrosis of the hip in the sickle-cell diseases: Treatment and complications. J Bone Joint Surg Am 1988;70:499.
11. Henderson RC, Rosenstein BD: *Salmonella* septic and aseptic arthritis in sickle-cell disease: A case report. Clin Orthop Relat Res 1989;248:261.
12. Keeley K, Buchanan GR: Acute infarction of long bones in children with sickle cell anemia. J Pediatr 1982;101: 170.
13. Mallouh A, Talab Y: Bone and joint infection in patients with sickle cell disease. J Pediatr Orthop 1985;5:158.
14. Murray SJ, Lieberman JM: *Fusobacterium* osteomyelitis in a child with sickle cell disease. Pediatr Infect Dis J 2002;21:979.
15. Oginni LM, Rufai MB: How safe is tourniquet use in sickle-cell disease? Afr J Med Med Sci 1996;25:3.
16. Pauling L, Itano H, Singer S, et al: Sickle cell anemia, a molecular disease. Science 1949;13:225.
17. Piehl FC, Davis RJ, Prugh SI: Osteomyelitis in sickle cell disease. J Pediatr Orthop 1993;13:225.
18. Sadat-Ali M: The status of acute osteomyelitis in sickle cell disease: A 15-year review. Int Surg 1998;83:84.
19. Sadat-Ali M, Ammar A, Corea JR, et al: The spine in sickle cell disease. Int Orthop 1994;18:154.
20. Skaggs DL, Kim SK, Greene NW, et al: Differentiation between bone infarction and acute osteomyelitis in children with sickle-cell disease with use of sequential radionuclide bone-marrow and bone scans. J Bone Joint Surg Am 2001;83:1810.
21. Umans H, Haramati N, Flusser G: The diagnostic role of gadolinium enhanced MRI in distinguishing between acute medullary bone infarct and osteomyelitis. Magn Reson Imaging 2000;18:255.
22. William RR, Hussein SS, Jeans WD, et al: A prospective study of soft-tissue ultrasonography in sickle cell disease patients with suspected osteomyelitis. Clin Radiol 2000; 55:307.
23. Wingate J, Schiff CF, Friedman RJ: Osteonecrosis of the humeral head in sickle cell disease. J South Orthop Assoc 1996;5:101.

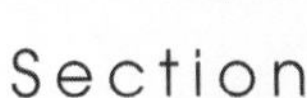

Section

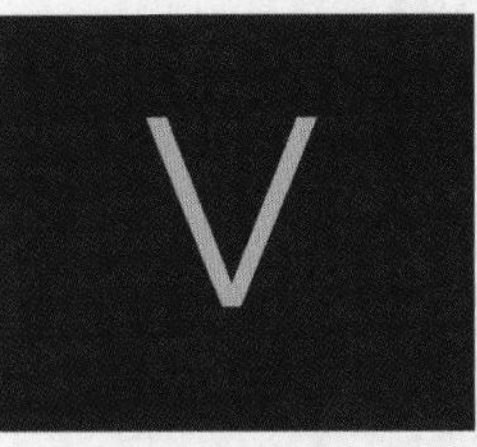

V

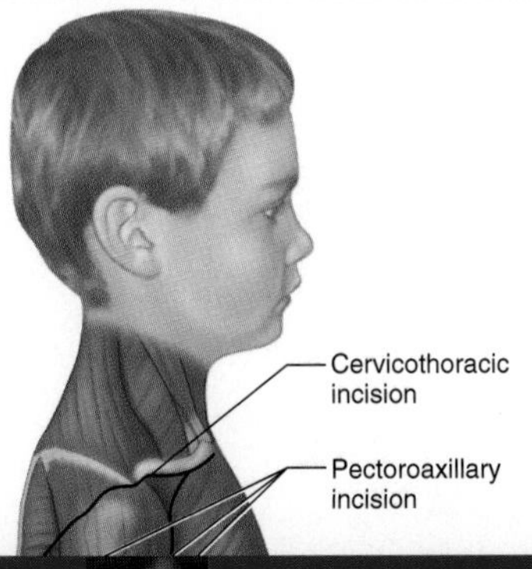

Musculoskeletal Tumors

Chapter 37

General Principles of Tumor Management

TUMORS OF THE MUSCULOSKELETAL SYSTEM

Tumors of the musculoskeletal system present a variety of challenges. Many benign tumors are easily managed by the pediatric orthopaedist with a good outcome, but occasionally serious complications develop. Patients with malignant tumors are best treated by surgeons with specific expertise in oncology. Inexperience may lead to fatal treatment errors even at the stage of primary biopsy. Modern survival rates far exceed those of 20 years ago, largely because of development of the field of orthopaedic oncology and the armamentarium of surgical and adjuvant therapies.

Classification

Benign tumors are classified as latent, active, or aggressive. A latent benign tumor (stage 1) is intracapsular, is usually asymptomatic, and never metastasizes. An active benign tumor (stage 2) is also intracapsular and rarely metastasizes but is actively growing and often symptomatic. An aggressive benign tumor (stage 3) often breaks through its capsule and extends into an adjacent compartment. Rarely, these tumors may metastasize.[18] Oliveira and coworkers have provided an overview of the principles and problems of histologic grading of tumors.[13]

Enneking has classified sarcomas of bone and soft tissue into various stages according to their histologic grade, the location of the tumor relative to anatomic compartments, and the presence of metastases. A low-grade tumor has well-differentiated cells, few mitotic figures, few or no atypical cells, little necrosis, and no vascular invasion. High-grade tumors have frequent mitoses; are poorly differentiated; have atypical cells, necrosis, and little matrix; and show vascular invasion.

The ability to treat malignant tumors successfully with limb salvage depends on understanding sarcoma behavior. As stated by Enneking,[7] "A sarcoma grows centrifugally like a spreading ripple on a pond. However, as it expands it follows the path of least resistance." If a tumor remains within its compartment, either osseous or fascial, it can be removed successfully by resecting the entire compartment. A bone is considered to be a compartment, as is a muscle or a joint. Tumors may invade adjacent compartments and become extracompartmental. The Enneking staging system is shown in Table 37–1.

As tumors grow, they compress surrounding tissues into structures that resemble fibrous capsules. This surrounding tissue contains tumor cells, known as satellites. In addition, there may be tumor cells in surrounding normal tissue, called skips.[7] Within a bone there may also be skip metastases, with intramedullary tumor extending well proximal to the apparent extent of the primary tumor.

Clinical Features

The clinical manifestations in a patient with a musculoskeletal tumor are often a useful clue to the diagnosis. A child with a pathologic fracture and no previous

Table 37-1 Enneking's Classification of Sarcomas of Bone or Soft Tissue

Stage	Grade	Site	Metastases
IA	Low	Intracompartmental	None
IB	Low	Extracompartmental	None
IIA	High	Intracompartmental	None
IIB	High	Extracompartmental	None
III	Low or high	Intracompartmental or extracompartmental	Yes

From Enneking W, Spanier S, Goodman M: A system for the surgical staging of musculoskeletal sarcoma. Clin Orthop Relat Res 1980;153:106.

symptoms most often has a benign lesion of bone that has gradually weakened the cortex and resulted in a fatigue fracture through a cystic lesion. In contrast, a gradually enlarging mass accompanied by increasing pain, especially at night, suggests a diagnosis of primary malignancy. Soft tissue tumors are most often painless and come to medical attention because the patient or parent notices a mass. The more aggressive the tumor, the shorter and more alarming the period of onset.

The presence of a palpable mass is an important finding on physical examination. The examiner should determine its size, consistency, and mobility and whether it is painful on palpation. A rapidly growing lesion is more likely to be malignant than benign. In taking the history, it is helpful to compare the size of the mass with a dime, nickel, quarter, or half-dollar or, if the tumor is larger, with a tennis ball, football, and so on. It is important to measure and record the size of the tumor as accurately as possible for comparison and subsequent examinations.

The consistency of the mass is determined next. Is it firm or soft? Does it feel cystic or bony and hard? A cystic or fluid-filled mass should be examined with a flashlight to determine whether it transilluminates. In general, fluid-filled masses are commonly benign, whereas large, hard masses are more likely to be malignant. Is there a distinct change from normal to abnormal at the margins of the mass? Does the mass have the same consistency as the surrounding normal tissue? Malignant swellings usually invade adjacent tissues. An increase in local temperature is more suggestive of a malignant than a benign lesion.

Mobility of a mass is of great help in ascertaining its nature. When the mass is fixed, it is either attached to bone or intraosseous. An osseous tumor is unaffected by muscle contraction. Intramuscular tumors are usually mobile when the muscle is relaxed and become fixed when the muscle is contracted. Deep, mobile lesions that are unaffected by muscle action are beneath the deep fascia and extramuscular. Tumors that are superficial and can be moved about have not invaded deep fascia and are probably benign.

Tenderness on palpation indicates an active process and is due to an inflammatory response. An abscess or infection is very painful and is usually accompanied by other signs of inflammation, such as erythema, edema, lymphangitis, and adenopathy, whereas moderate tenderness is indicative of an active neoplastic process, and the absence of tenderness suggests a quiescent lesion. One should, however, be wary because rapid growth and necrosis of a malignant tumor may mimic infection. This may be a problem, for example, in distinguishing between Ewing's sarcoma and osteomyelitis. When a rapidly growing malignant tumor is subcutaneous, it may cause vascular dilation, increased local heat, and skin turgor; such a tumor may be mistaken for thrombophlebitis or an infectious process. A neoplastic inflammatory response, however, is characterized by a firmer feeling and lack of local pitting edema, and the cutaneous tissue is not as red as in infection. Point tenderness is indicative of lesions such as osteoid osteoma or a neural or glomus tumor.

Joint range of motion may be limited because of muscle spasm or mechanical interference. There may be reactive synovitis when the lesion is adjacent to a joint or if the joint is directly involved. Muscle atrophy is not uncommon, and an antalgic limp may be present.

A vascular tumor is suspected if elevation or steady, firm pressure causes a diminution in its size, if the size is increased by the use of a venous tourniquet, or if a thrill or palpable pulsation is present. A pathologic fracture may occur in primary or metastatic malignant tumors, or one may complicate a benign process such as a unicameral bone cyst.

Invasion of a nerve will cause neurologic symptoms and signs such as stabbing pain, paresthesia, hypoesthesia, or motor weakness. Pathologically, the nerve may be encased by the lesion or trapped against bone or rigid fascia. Neurologic dysfunction is uncommon except when tumors are in anatomic areas where nerves are unable to move freely, such as the sciatic notch or neural foramina.

Radiographic Findings

Evaluation of the Initial Radiograph

The initial radiographic study of a lesion in bone should be evaluated systematically, with the examiner first considering the character of the lesion itself, the reaction of the surrounding bone, the location of the lesion, and the possibility of lesions in other sites.

Anatomic Site of the Lesion

The location of a bony lesion is an important diagnostic clue (Table 37–2). Epiphyseal lucent lesions are usually chondroblastoma or infection or occasionally eosinophilic granuloma. Epiphyseal lesions after growth plate closure are generally giant cell tumors. The metaphysis is a common site for benign tumors, unicameral cysts, osteoid osteomas, and osteosarcomas. Diaphyseal lesions include fibrous dysplasia, Ewing's sarcoma, and adamantinoma.

The portion of the skeleton involved is of diagnostic importance. Anterior vertebral lesions in children are usually eosinophilic granulomas or infection, whereas posterior element lesions are often aneurysmal bone cysts or osteoid osteomas. Pelvic lesions are frequently Ewing's sarcoma or fibrous dysplasia.

Character of the Lesion

A lesion in bone may be completely radiolucent, suggestive of a cystic disorder; may have soft tissue density; or may have bony or calcific density. Ossification within a lesion has some elements that resemble mature bone, whereas calcifications are usually more haphazard and of greater density. Some lesions, such as fibrous dysplasia, alter the bony architecture so that the cortices become indistinct and the bony trabecular pattern is replaced by a ground-glass appearance. A

Table 37-2 Common Anatomic Sites of Primary Bone Tumors

Location	Bone Tumor
Spine	
Posterior elements (spinous process, lamina, pedicles)	Aneurysmal bone cyst Osteoma Osteoblastoma
Anterior elements (vertebral body)	In a child Histiocytosis X ("vertebra plana") Hemangioma In an adult Metastases Multiple myeloma Paget's disease Hemangioma Chordoma
Long bones (physes open)	
Epiphysis	Chondroblastoma Eosinophilic granuloma (epiphyseal osteomyelitis)*
Metaphysis	Multiple benign lesions such as a unicameral bone cyst Common site for osteogenic sarcoma
Diaphysis	Fibrous dysplasia Histiocytosis X Ewing's sarcoma Osteoblastoma Adamantinoma Lymphoma
Parosteal	Myositis ossificans* Osteosarcoma Chondrosarcoma Enchondroma
Ribs	In children and adolescents Fibrous dysplasia Ewing's sarcoma Metastases In adults Ewing's sarcoma Chondrosarcoma Fibrous dysplasia Multiple myeloma Metastases
Pelvis	In children Ewing's sarcoma Fibrous dysplasia Aneurysmal bone cyst Osteoblastoma In adults Ewing's sarcoma Chondrosarcoma Paget's disease Multiple myeloma Metastases
Scapula	Ewing's sarcoma Osteoblastoma Aneurysmal bone cyst

Continued

Table 37-2 Common Anatomic Sites of Primary Bone Tumors—cont'd

Location	Bone Tumor
Multiple lesions	In children
	Multiple hereditary exostoses
	Fibrous dysplasia (Albright's syndrome)
	Histiocytosis X
	Enchondroma (Ollier's disease)
	Multiple hemangiomatosis
	Metastases—neuroblastoma, hypernephroma
	Lymphoma
	In adults
	Multiple myeloma

*Not a tumor.

soft tissue mass adjacent to a bony lesion suggests malignancy.

Reaction of Surrounding Bone

Often the nature of a bony lesion is clear from the response of the adjacent bony tissue. A benign process such as a unicameral bone cyst has a sharp margin between the cystic cavity and the adjacent bone. The cortex is thinned and expanded, which suggests gradual enlargement from a pressure phenomenon. An irritative lesion such as osteoid osteoma produces a vigorous response of bone formation and cortical thickening in adjacent areas. Eosinophilic granulomas produce punched-out lesions with no host reaction. Malignancies may be permeative without evident margins between the tumor and surrounding bone. When a tumor breaks through a cortex, it elevates the adjacent periosteum, thereby resulting in new bone formation along that cortex. The apex of this elevation is seen as a triangle of periosteal bone formation, the so-called Codman's triangle. A large area of periosteal bone formation is termed a sunburst pattern. These periosteal reactions are indicative of aggressive processes, which may occur with benign tumors and infections, as well as malignancies.

Staging Studies

Staging studies are studies that define the location, extent, activity, and probable treatment of musculoskeletal lesions.[15,21] Obviously, benign lesions (a term to be used cautiously) may be treated on the basis of plain radiographs alone. Examples include unicameral cysts, osteochondromas, and fibrous dysplasia. Any lesion that could be malignant should be staged before biopsy is performed.[18] One reason for this order is that biopsy may alter the findings on later studies. As mentioned previously, the plain radiograph offers the greatest amount of information at the lowest cost and inconvenience, and it should be carefully evaluated before further studies are ordered.

Computed Tomography

Computed tomography (CT) is a vital tool for determining the character and boundaries of bony lesions.[3,6,20] The extent of tumor within the bone may be accurately determined with CT.[16] Soft tissue masses may also be evaluated for size, location, and relationship to bone. Although magnetic resonance imaging (MRI) has supplanted CT for soft tissue imaging, CT remains the best modality for evaluating cortical disruption and fractures. CT-guided biopsies have become a standard approach to many lesions.[24]

Magnetic Resonance Imaging

In the staging of tumors of the musculoskeletal system, MRI is almost indispensable. Soft tissue lesions are demonstrated in exquisite detail, and the relationship of surrounding structures is clearly evident.[14,23] Many of these lesions can be definitively diagnosed by MRI. Other lesions are indeterminate, especially sarcomas, and biopsy is necessary for a definitive diagnosis.[8] In many instances MRI is superior to CT in demonstrating the extent of tumor involvement within a long bone.[4,9,19,25] Skip lesions within the bone might be seen only with MRI. Gadolinium-enhanced imaging is often used to assess tumor necrosis secondary to chemotherapy.[26] Diffusion-weighted imaging has been found helpful in analysis of tumor tissue. Necrotic tumor tissue shows a higher degree of diffusion of water protons than viable tissue does.[2]

Scintigraphy

Technetium scanning is used to detect bone formation and blood flow, and it demonstrates bone lesions nonspecifically. Scintigraphy is more sensitive and more cost-effective for demonstrating bone metastases than plain radiography is. Normal scan findings strongly suggest that a lesion is benign, but an abnormal scan does not distinguish a benign from a malignant lesion.[19] Benign tumors that affect more than one bone may be evaluated with this modality. Benign lesions that are "hot" on scan include osteoid osteoma, osteoblastoma, aneurysmal bone cyst, and fibrous dysplasia. "Cold" lesions include eosinophilic granuloma and myeloma. Intraoperative scintigraphy may be used to locate osteoid osteoma lesions.

Gallium scintigrams are obtained to evaluate soft tissue tumors. Sarcomas usually cause increased uptake of gallium, whereas noninflammatory benign tumors have normal uptake.[11]

Angiography

Angiography is not commonly used in tumor staging today because of the information available noninvasively with MRI. When detailed study of the vasculature is necessary in planning a limb-sparing procedure, angiography may be necessary. In addition, angiography is performed when a lesion is to be embolized before treatment to decrease vascularity. At times angiography is used to instill cytotoxic agents directly into the vasculature of the tumor.

Other Modalities

Positron emission tomography using 2-deoxy-2-fluoro-D-glucose has recently been introduced for the study of tumor tissue. At present it is recommended as a technique that may identify types of cellular components within a tissue. It is not recommended as a method to differentiate between benign and malignant tissue.[1]

Biopsy

A biopsy is required in treating all malignant tumors, and in many cases it is necessary in managing benign lesions. Radiographic diagnoses without biopsy are often made safely for a variety of benign lesions, including unicameral bone cyst, aneurysmal cyst, fibrous cortical defect, fibrous dysplasia, chondroblastoma, osteochondroma, and osteoid osteoma. If malignancy is suspected, a tissue diagnosis is required. When the appearance of the lesion is typical for a certain diagnosis and all staging studies support that diagnosis, a biopsy may be performed as part of the definitive surgical procedure. In all other cases an incisional biopsy before treatment is recommended.

The rules of biopsy for musculoskeletal lesions have been well established for a number of years, yet poorly done biopsies continue to cause harm to patients. In most cases, biopsy of a probable malignant lesion should be deferred to an individual who is capable of definitively treating that patient. Bad biopsies can preclude the use of limb salvage and may increase the risk for tumor recurrence and death. To quote Enneking,[7] "The optimal chance for an adequate local procedure is in the virgin, unbiopsied state."

Needle biopsies are often used, and in centers with appropriate expertise they frequently provide definitive diagnoses. At times they are performed in radiology suites under CT guidance.[24] Fine-needle aspiration cytology is useful in certain tumors and, with proper clinical and radiologic correlation, may approach open biopsy in accuracy.[17] Another technique, needle biopsy with sonographic guidance, has been shown to be reliable in the diagnosis of soft tissue tumors and bone lesions with extraosseous masses in the appendicular skeleton.[22] The volume of tissue obtained is limited, and pathology and radiology consultations should be obtained before biopsy.[12] Welker and colleagues analyzed 173 cases and showed a higher degree of accuracy and lower complication rate with needle biopsy than with open biopsy. Only 7% of patients required open biopsy to obtain more material.[27]

Open incisional biopsies are most often used for bone and soft tissue sarcomas. The incision should be longitudinal and placed so that the incision tract can be completely excised at the time of tumor excision without undue compromise of function. Hemostasis must be meticulous because bleeding into tissues spreads tumor. Retraction must also be gentle; sharp rakes can spread tumor cells. Closure of each compartment should be complete and a bone plug may be reinserted or replaced with methacrylate to seal the bone.[7,12] Before biopsy the surgeon should consult radiologists and pathologists so that the biopsy produces the most diagnostically useful tissue.

Treatment

Treatment of tumors of the musculoskeletal system should be undertaken only by surgeons who possess understanding of and training in the basic principles of tumor management.[5] The margins of excision are vitally important to provide the best chance of curing the disease (Table 37–3).

An intracapsular margin of tumor removal leaves gross tumor behind and is appropriate only for certain benign lesions. An example is curettage of an aneurysmal bone cyst.

A marginal excision is performed by removing the tumor and its pseudocapsule. Because the capsule contains tumor cells, this excision by definition leaves viable tumor in the surrounding local tissues. Marginal excision is inadequate for local removal of a malignancy.

A wide margin is defined as one that is free of tumor. It requires removal of tissue beyond the reactive pseudocapsule so that a cuff of normal tissue surrounds the tumor and capsule. This is sufficient for the primary tumor, but intracompartmental skip lesions may remain.

A radical margin implies removal of the primary lesion and all normal tissue within the compartment. Such surgery ensures removal of the tumor and any skip or satellite lesions.[7]

Whenever possible, limb-sparing procedures are preferred, but the surgeon must adhere to the principles of tumor excision.[10] Amputations often achieve a radical margin and are necessary when limb sparing cannot be safely performed. The principles of compartment involvement and staging apply equally to amputations as to limb salvage surgery.

Table 37-3 Types of Excision of Tumor as Related to Surgical Margins*

Type	Plane of Dissection	Result
Intralesional	Debulking or curettage	Leaves macroscopic disease
Marginal	Pericapsular reactive zone	Likely to leave microscopic disease
Wide	Normal cuff of tissue (intracompartmental)	May leave "skip" or "satellite" disease
Radical	Whole bone or muscle outside compartment (extracompartmental)	No residual

*Needs surgical and pathologic verification.

References

1. Aoki J, Endo K, Watanabe H, et al: FDG-PET for evaluating musculoskeletal tumors: A review. J Orthop Sci 2003;8:435.
2. Baur A, Reiser MF: Diffusion-weighted imaging of the musculoskeletal system in humans. Skeletal Radiol 2000;29:555.
3. Berger PE, Kuhn JP: Computed tomography of tumors of the musculoskeletal system in children. Clinical applications. Radiology 1978;127:171.
4. Bloem JL, Taminiau AH, Eulderink F, et al: Radiologic staging of primary bone sarcoma: MR imaging, scintigraphy, angiography, and CT correlated with pathologic examination. Radiology 1988;169:805.
5. Clarkson P, Ferguson P: Primary multidisciplinary management of extremity soft tissue sarcomas. Curr Treat Options Oncol 2004;5:451.
6. deSantos LA, Goldstein HM, Murray JA, et al: Computed tomography in the evaluation of musculoskeletal neoplasms. Radiology 1978;128:89.
7. Enneking WF: Principles of musculoskeletal oncologic surgery. In Evarts C (ed): Surgery of the Musculoskeletal System. New York, Churchill Livingstone, 1990.
8. Frassica FJ, Khanna JA, McCarthy EF: The role of MR imaging in soft tissue tumor evaluation: Perspective of the orthopedic oncologist and musculoskeletal pathologist. Magn Reson Imaging Clin N Am 2000;8:915.
9. Gillespy T 3rd, Manfrini M, Ruggieri P, et al: Staging of intraosseous extent of osteosarcoma: Correlation of preoperative CT and MR imaging with pathologic macroslides. Radiology 1988;167:765.
10. Hosalkar HS, Dormans JP: Limb sparing surgery for pediatric musculoskeletal tumors. Pediatr Blood Cancer 2004;42:295.
11. Kirchner PT, Simon MA: The clinical value of bone and gallium scintigraphy for soft-tissue sarcomas of the extremities. J Bone Joint Surg Am 1984;66:319.
12. Murray JA, Mankin H: Biopsy technique in musculoskeletal tumors. In Evarts C (ed): Surgery of the Musculoskeletal System, vol 5. New York, Churchill Livingstone, 1990.
13. Oliveira AM, Nascimento AG: Grading in soft tissue tumors: Principles and problems. Skeletal Radiol 2001;30:543.
14. Petasnick JP, Turner DA, Charters JR, et al: Soft-tissue masses of the locomotor system: Comparison of MR imaging with CT. Radiology 1986;160:125.
15. Pommersheim WJ, Chew FS: Imaging, diagnosis, and staging of bone tumors: A primer. Semin Roentgenol 2004;39:361.
16. Schreiman JS, Crass JR, Wick MR, et al: Osteosarcoma: Role of CT in limb-sparing treatment. Radiology 1986;161:485.
17. Shah MS, Garg V, Kapoor SK, et al: Fine-needle aspiration cytology, frozen section, and open biopsy: Relative significance in diagnosis of musculoskeletal tumors. J Surg Orthop Adv 2003;12:203.
18. Simon MA: Diagnostic and staging strategy for musculoskeletal system. In Evarts C (ed): Surgery of the Musculoskeletal system. New York, Churchill Livingstone, 1990.
19. Simon MA, Kirchner PT: Scintigraphic evaluation of primary bone tumors. Comparison of technetium-99m phosphonate and gallium citrate imaging. J Bone Joint Surg Am 1980;62:758.
20. Sundaram M, McGuire MH: Computed tomography or magnetic resonance for evaluating the solitary tumor or tumor-like lesion of bone? Skeletal Radiol 1988;17:393.
21. Temple HT, Bashore CJ: Staging of bone neoplasms: An orthopedic oncologist's perspective. Semin Musculoskeletal Radiol 2000;4:17.
22. Torriani M, Etchebehere M, Amstalden E: Sonographically guided core needle biopsy of bone and soft tissue tumors. J Ultrasound Med 2002;21:275.
23. Totty WG, Murphy WA, Lee JK: Soft-tissue tumors: MR imaging. Radiology 1986;160:135.
24. Tsukushi S, Katagiri H, Nakashima H, et al: Application and utility of computed tomography–guided needle biopsy with musculoskeletal lesions. J Orthop Sci 2004;9:122.
25. Vanel D, Verstraete KL, Shapeero LG: Primary tumors of the musculoskeletal system. Radiol Clin North Am 1997;35:213.
26. Verstraete KL, Lang P: Bone and soft tissue tumors: The role of contrast agents for MR imaging. Eur J Radiol 2000;34:229.
27. Welker JA, Henshaw RM, Jelinek J, et al: The percutaneous needle biopsy is safe and recommended in the diagnosis of musculoskeletal masses. Cancer 2000;89:2677.

Chapter 38

Benign Musculoskeletal Tumors

SIMPLE BONE CYSTS (SOLITARY BONE CYST, UNICAMERAL BONE CYST)

Incidence

Simple bone cysts are benign tumors of childhood and adolescence. They represent approximately 3% of all primary bone tumors sampled for biopsy and nearly always occur during the first two decades of life, most often between 4 and 10 years of age.[339] There is a male predominance, with a 2:1 male-to-female ratio. The majority of cysts occur in the metaphyseal region of the proximal humerus or femur, with approximately 50% of cases involving the humerus and 18% to 27% affecting the femur. The next most common sites are the proximal and distal tibia. Occasionally, cysts may be found in the calcaneus, fibula, ulna, radius, pelvis, talus, lumbar spine, and other parts of the axial skeleton* (Fig. 38–1).

*See references 2-4, 92, 169, 195, 217, 329, 344, 369, 381, 400, 471, 486, 558.

Rarely does more than one cyst occur in an individual, hence the term *solitary bone cyst*. The term *unicameral bone cyst* implies that one chamber exists. Although one large cavity is usually found, a cyst may become multiloculated after a fracture because of the formation of multiple bony septations, thus making the term *unicameral* technically incorrect.

Simple cysts are often categorized as "active" or "latent" based on their proximity to the growth plate.[234,356] A cyst that is juxtaphyseal (less than 0.5 cm from the physis) is considered "active" and possesses greater potential for growth. Epiphyseal involvement is rare, but if present it should be considered an aggressive form of an active lesion.[381] A cyst that has grown away from the plate is considered "latent" and, theoretically, no longer has the capacity for growth (Fig. 38–2). In reality, however, latent cysts continue to have growth potential, as proved time and again by their unexpected recurrence after treatment in the young individual. After skeletal maturity, it is uncommon for the cysts to recur or progressively worsen.

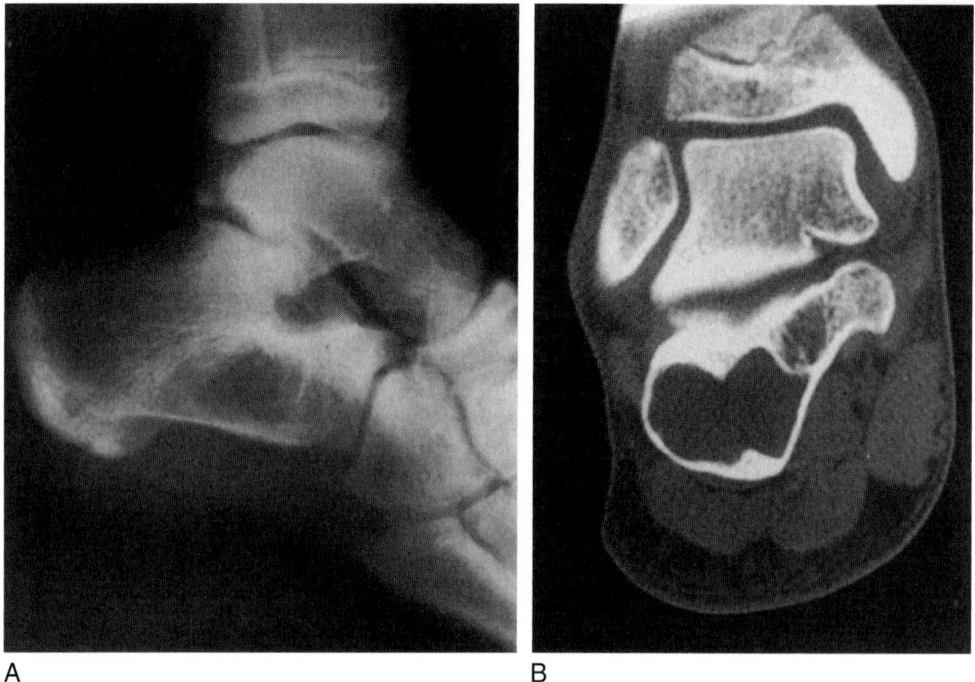

FIGURE 38–1 Imaging findings in a 14-year-old boy with pain in his heel. **A,** Radiograph demonstrating the lucent solitary bone cyst in the calcaneus. **B,** A computed tomography scan showed the extent of the lesion, which is surrounded by a rim of cortical bone.

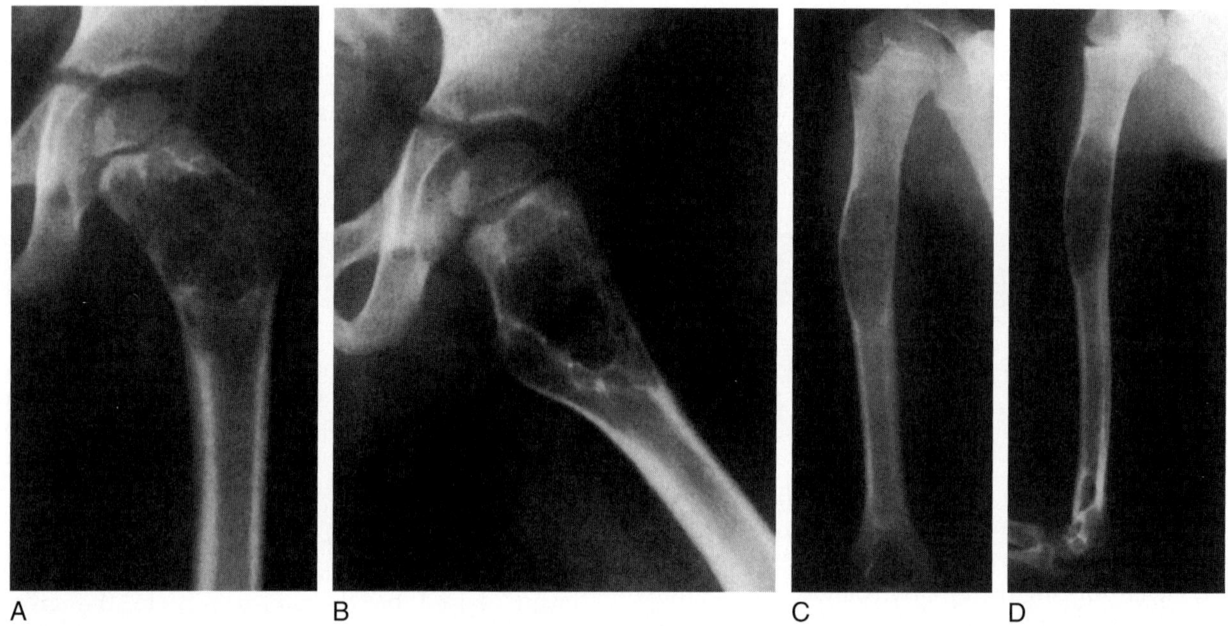

FIGURE 38–2 **A** and **B,** Active solitary bone cyst in the proximal left femur of a 4-year-old boy (D.J.). The cyst is juxtaphyseal. **C** and **D,** A latent solitary bone cyst has grown away from the proximal physis in the right humerus of an 8-year-old boy (D.T.). See Figure 38–4 for post-treatment results.

Etiology

The cause of simple bone cysts remains uncertain. Any theory relating to the etiology of simple bone cysts should be able to explain the following factors: (1) more than 70% are discovered in childhood, (2) more than 95% arise from or involve the metaphysis, (3) most occur in the proximal humerus or femur, (4) a cyst wall and fluid high in protein content are common, and (5) simple bone cysts represent a benign process with a significant recurrence rate after treatment.[339]

Mirra hypothesized an intraosseous synovial cyst in which a small amount of synovial tissue became entrapped in an intraosseous position during early infant development or secondary to trauma at birth.[339] Over time, increased pressure secondary to secretions would lead to expansion within the bone. Jaffe and Lichtenstein postulated that cysts resulted from a localized failure of ossification in the metaphyseal area during periods of rapid growth.[237] Cohen proposed that the cause of the cyst was blockage of the circulation (venous obstruction) and drainage of interstitial fluid in rapidly growing bone. He based this theory on the finding that the chemical constituents of the fluid in simple bone cysts are similar to those of serum.[104,105] Current literature further substantiates this theory of a disturbance in or occlusion of the intramedullary venous circulation.[97,180,268,269,477,542]

Two genetic analyses of simple bone cysts have identified single and multifocal cytogenetic rearrangements associated with the condition.[431,530] These findings emphasize the need for further studies clarifying the frequency and significance of chromosomal anomalies in this type of lesion.

Drilling, trepanation, and reaming of the medullary cavity to open vascular channels between cysts and the intramedullary venous system all have been found effective in healing unicameral cysts. The cyst fluid itself may be both a factor causing cyst formation and an obstacle to healing. Bone-resorptive factors, such as prostaglandins, interleukin-1, and lysosomal enzymes, are found in cyst fluid.[182,268,476] In addition, Komiya and associates reported elevated levels of interleukin-6 and interleukin-1β in cyst fluid and the presence of tumor necrosis factor-α, interleukin-6, and interleukin-1β in cells in the cyst membrane.[267] These findings, along with inducibility of production of nitrate and nitrite from cyst membrane cells in response to cytokine exposure, suggest that conditions within solitary bone cysts may promote production of nitric oxide.[267] Oxygen free radicals, which are cytotoxic and known to be generated under ischemic conditions, have also been found in cysts.[269]

Pathology

Simple bone cysts tend to expand by eroding the cortex, resulting in a localized bulge of the bone. Despite this fact, reactive or periosteal bone formation is not present unless a pathologic fracture occurs. Where the cortical tissue is thinnest, the wall can actually be fluctuant, and a bluish tinge from the underlying fluid can be seen. Once the affected bone has fractured, the cortical wall is thicker, and multiple bony septa may occur throughout the cyst.

The fluid found within simple bone cysts is straw colored or serosanguineous, a feature distinguishing simple bone cysts from aneurysmal bone cysts. Often, significant pressure within the cyst (which can be greater than 30 cm H_2O) is evident when a needle is introduced. After a fracture, however, the cyst may become filled with blood clot, granulation, or fibro-osseous tissues. The most characteristic histopathologic finding is the thin membranous lining of the cyst (Fig. 38–3). Composed primarily of flattened to plump epithelium-like cells, the lining may also possess osteoclast-type giant cells, cholesterol cells, and fat cells. Hemosiderin, fibrin, calcification, and reactive bone may be seen in focal areas of the cyst.

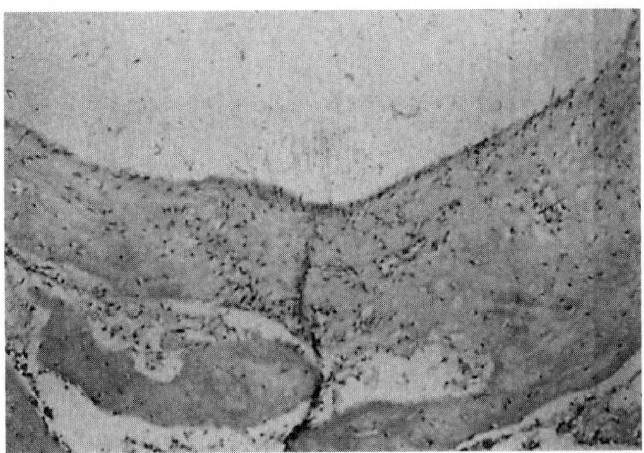

FIGURE 38-3 Histologic appearance of a simple bone cyst (original magnification ×10). The thin membranous lining is composed primarily of epithelium-like cells.

Clinical Features

Clinically, cysts can be asymptomatic and may be discovered incidentally when radiographs, such as a chest film, are obtained for other reasons. More often, though, the cysts are diagnosed because of pain. The pain may be mild and reflective of a microscopic pathologic fracture. More abrupt discomfort occurs when a pathologic fracture occurs after relatively minor trauma, such as a fall.[9] These fractures occur in up to 90% of patients and heal readily, although the cysts do not.[323] After these pathologic fractures, premature physeal closure has been reported in nearly 10% of patients.[314,496]

Radiographic Findings

There are several characteristic radiographic features of simple bone cysts.[85] Approximately 50% occur in the proximal humerus and 18% to 27% in the proximal femur. The cyst is metaphyseal and usually extends to, but not across, the physis. On rare occasions, it crosses the physis into the epiphysis.[194,198] Typically the cyst is symmetrically expansile and radiolucent, with a thin cortical rim surrounding it. Over time, the physis grows away from the cyst, changing from the active to the latent phase. In many newly diagnosed cases there is a pathologic fracture with or without displacement. The one pathognomonic manifestation of a simple bone cyst is the "fallen fragment" sign.[500] This represents a portion of fractured cortex that settles to the most dependent part of the fluid-filled cyst. However, it is seen in less than 10% of cases, and it should not be expected if the cyst has become multiloculated after a previous pathologic fracture.

On magnetic resonance imaging (MRI), simple bone cysts often have a complex appearance because of heterogeneous fluid signals and regions of nodular and thick peripheral enhancement caused by previous pathologic fracture and subsequent healing.[323] MRI may reveal focal, thick peripheral, heterogeneous, or subcortical patterns, with focal nodules of homogeneous enhancement (diameter >1 cm) within the cyst that are associated with areas of ground-glass opacification on plain film. MRI may also detect fluid levels, soft tissue changes, and septations not seen on plain film.

Differential Diagnosis

The diagnosis can usually be established based on the presence of typical radiographic findings. Other lesions to be considered in the differential diagnosis include aneurysmal bone cyst, monostotic fibrous dysplasia, and atypical eosinophilic granuloma. All of these lesions may be radiolucent. Aneurysmal bone cysts and fibrous dysplasia may be expansile and metaphyseal. However, features typically associated with these lesions usually help differentiate them from simple bone cysts.

Treatment

A common misconception in the treatment of simple bone cysts in children is that once the pathologic fracture heals, the cyst also has an excellent chance of spontaneously healing. However, most investigators examining this phenomenon have found that the likelihood of spontaneous healing of the cyst after pathologic fracture is very low, probably less than 5%.[9,172,356] Thus, if treatment of the cyst is deemed necessary, it should be undertaken as soon as the fracture has healed. However, overtreatment in skeletally mature persons should be avoided. In these individuals, if the cyst has a sufficiently thick cortex and is located in the upper extremity, periodic observation may be all that is needed. If the patient is asymptomatic, it may not be necessary to restrict activities.

The treatment approach is more aggressive for all simple bone cysts in younger children and in skeletally mature individuals when the cyst is located in weight-bearing bones of the lower extremities. In these cases, plans should be made for definitive treatment of the cyst to prevent future fractures and possible associated complications (e.g., shortening due to growth arrest and deformity).[314] Findings by Stanton and Abdel-Mota'al suggest that the rate of growth arrest as a complication of simple bone cysts of the humerus approximates 10%, a frequency more common than is generally appreciated.[496]

The preoperative evaluation of patients with simple bone cysts rarely requires more than good-quality radiographs of the lesion. If the diagnosis is equivocal, a bone scan will verify the presence or absence of other abnormal areas. Computed tomography (CT) may be helpful in differentiating simple bone cysts from other lesions, such as aneurysmal bone cysts or fibrous dysplasia. MRI findings of double-density fluid levels and septation associated with low signal on T1-weighted images and high signal on T2-weighted images strongly suggest the presence of an aneurysmal bone cyst rather than a simple bone cyst.[501] The diagnosis is usually confirmed at surgery, when straw-colored fluid is aspirated through a large-bore needle introduced into the cystic cavity.

Treatment modalities include injection of corticosteroids into the cyst, injection of autologous bone marrow, multiple drilling and drainage of the cavity, and curettage of the membranous wall followed by bone grafting. A relatively high recurrence rate has been historically associated with treatment of simple bone cysts.[310] Older forms of treatment, such as subtotal resection with or without bone grafting and total resection, have been associated with increased cyst recurrence and are rarely, if ever, used today.[62]

CORTICOSTEROID INJECTIONS

The successful healing of cysts after injections of methylprednisolone acetate was reported by Scaglietti and colleagues in 1979.[451] They noted favorable results in 90% of lesions and consequently concluded that treatment by curettage was seldom necessary. Healing was believed to have occurred if the cortex thickened and the cystic cavity became radiographically opaque. Filling of the cyst with "bone scar" was considered evidence of healing (Fig. 38–4). Actual remodeling, with complete disappearance of the cystic cavity, often took several years. Subsequent reports have continued to substantiate the effectiveness of injecting steroids into cysts, although the success rates have been lower, ranging from 40% to 80%.[61,77,85,86,154,202,352,444,452] This method continues to be a popular choice for the initial management of simple bone cysts. The antiprostaglandin action of steroids constitutes the rationale for their use in the treatment of cysts.[476]

The patient is given a general anesthetic in the operating room and the procedure is performed using strict aseptic techniques.[188] Fluoroscopy with image intensification is used to locate the margins of the cyst. Two large needles with stylets (at least 14-gauge or Craig biopsy needles) are used. The first needle is introduced percutaneously, the stylet is withdrawn, and fluid is allowed to drip out. The presence of straw-colored (serosanguineous) fluid confirms the diagnosis of simple bone cyst. Vigorous aspiration must be avoided because blood may be returned, making it difficult to distinguish a simple bone cyst from an aneurysmal bone cyst. If straw-colored fluid is returned, contrast material (usually Renografin diluted 1:1 with normal saline) is injected to confirm the presence or absence of intracystic fibrous or osseous septa and loculation. Needles must be introduced into each separate cystic cavity to ensure delivery of the steroid; if the cyst is not filled completely, the incidence of failure of healing increases.[83]

After the contrast material clarifies the structure of the cystic cavity, the second needle is introduced. The cavity is thoroughly flushed with normal

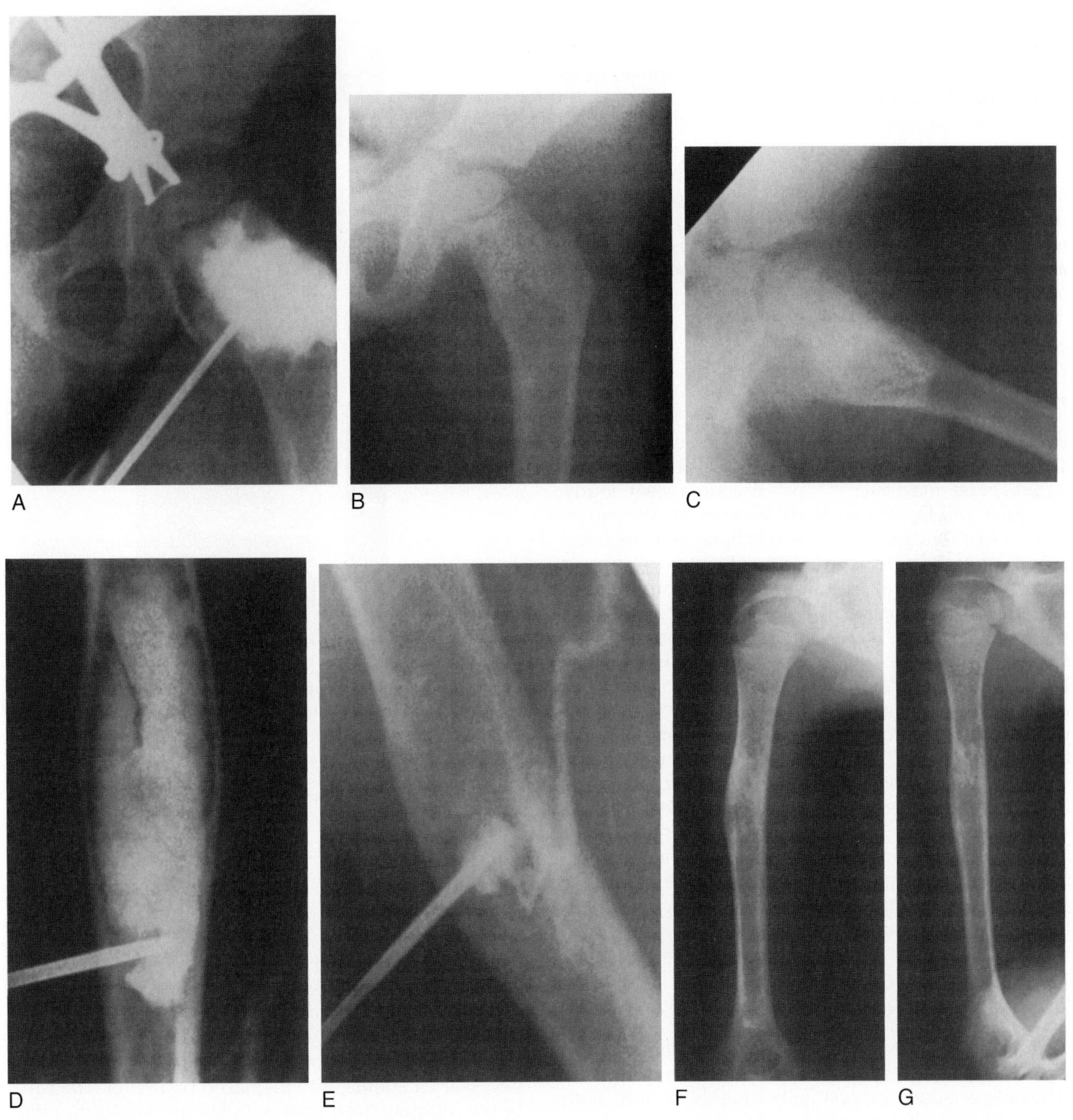

FIGURE 38–4 The patients whose pathologic findings are shown in Figure 38–2 underwent corticosteroid injections into the cysts. In patient D.J., Renografin injected during the first steroid treatment demonstrated filling of the cyst **(A).** Twenty months later, after a total of four injections, the cyst was healed **(B** and **C).** In patient D.T., the entire cyst filled during the first injection **(D).** At the time of the fourth injection 6 months later, minimal cyst cavity was seen **(E).** A venogram was obtained at the time of contrast injection. Eight months after the initial steroid treatment, the cyst had healed **(F** and **G).**

saline solution. The operator should not aspirate when a second needle is in the cyst because air can be aspirated *into* the cyst from the second needle, leading to an air embolus. When lavage with normal saline is completed, the second needle is withdrawn. Through the remaining needle, 40 to 120 mg (1 to 3 mL) of methylprednisolone acetate is introduced into the cyst and a simple compression dressing is applied.

This procedure is usually repeated every 2 months, requiring between two and five injections, with three being the usual minimal number to obtain healing. Radiographic changes usually are not noted in the first 2 to 3 months; thus, radiographs are not needed before then. Subsequently, radiographs are obtained every 2 to 3 months to assess healing. Evidence of healing includes diminution in the size of the cyst, cortical thickening, remodeling of the surrounding bone, and increased internal density (e.g., ground-glass ossification).

Serial steroid injections is the most popular treatment mode because the procedure is simple, injury to the adjacent physis is avoided, the procedure causes a minimal operative scar, there is little morbidity, the patient is able to return promptly to a previous activity level, and the reported results are excellent. A potential disadvantage is a temporary systemic response to the steroid (Cushing's syndrome). It is best not to exceed a total of 120 mg of methylprednisolone during any one injection.

AUTOLOGOUS BONE MARROW INJECTIONS AND OTHER BONE SUBSTITUTES

Recent interest in the injection of other materials to stimulate healing has led to the successful use of autologous bone marrow.[136,309,310,381] In one recent study, Docquier and Delloye reported successful cyst regression in 15 of 17 cases after a single bone marrow injection, with recurrence in 12% of cases during a subsequent 3-year period.[136] Collagen, demineralized bone matrix, and calcium phosphate paste are other injectable materials that are under investigation,[258,283,443] In one small series of 11 patients, Killian and colleagues reported complete cyst healing in 9 patients after primary treatment with demineralized bone matrix, with no recurrences detected during a 2-year follow-up period.[258] Also, using a combination of autologous bone marrow and demineralized bone matrix, Rougraff and Kling noted complete cyst healing in 16 of 23 patients, with 5 recurrences noted during 4 years of follow-up.[443] At our institution, we have been encouraged with the early results using injectable bioresorbable calcium phosphate paste (alpha-BSM), and this is becoming our treatment of choice (Fig. 38–5).

DECOMPRESSION OF CYSTS BY MULTIPLE DRILLING

Multiple percutaneous drilling has been shown to be effective in the treatment of simple bone cysts.[4,268,477] After trepanation, the cyst is thoroughly lavaged with saline. Multiple holes are then created in the cyst wall. Fluid escapes through the drill holes, decreasing the internal pressure in the cyst. When the cysts are drilled with Kirschner wires, the wires are either left in place or removed. Leaving them in place theoretically keeps the holes open and allows for continuous drainage through the cyst wall. However, we have no personal experience with this technique. Successful continuous decompression by insertion of a cannulated screw has been reported, and flexible titanium intramedullary nails can be used to create connections to the medullary canal in several directions through one cortical hole.[4,190] Opening of the intramedullary canal during surgical decompression of the cyst may shorten healing time, and flexible intramedullary nailing has been shown to provide early stability.[69,437,438] Both procedures have been associated with reduced rates of cyst recurrence.[69,437,438]

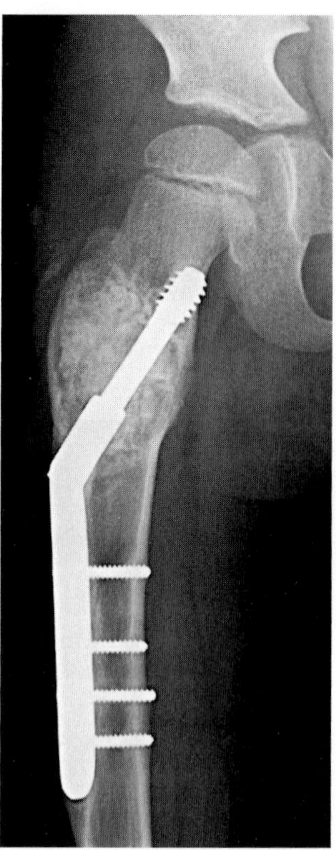

FIGURE 38–5 This 6-year 9-month-old boy underwent cyst injection with calcium phosphate (alpha-BSM) 2 months before this radiograph. He had undergone open reduction and internal fixation of a pathologic femoral neck fracture 2½ years prior, but the cyst failed to heal.

CURETTAGE OF CYSTS FOLLOWED BY BONE GRAFTING

Once the common form of treatment for simple bone cysts, bone grafting was replaced in the late 1970s and early 1980s by steroid injections because of reports of better healing of cysts using methylprednisolone acetate. Nearly 50% of cysts recur after curettage and bone grafting.[154] However, there are some cysts for which curettage followed by bone grafting remains necessary. Patients with displaced pathologic fractures of the hip may need open reduction and internal fixation. At the time of internal fixation, curettage of the cyst and bone grafting is also performed. Materials other than autogenous bone have recently been used with success, including cubes of high-porosity hydroxyapatite and tricalcium phosphate ceramic.[17,225]

ANEURYSMAL BONE CYST

Incidence

An aneurysmal bone cyst is a solitary, expansile, radiolucent lesion usually located in the metaphyseal region of the long bones. Seen much less often than simple bone cysts, they represent 1% of all primary bone tumors sampled for biopsy, with the annual incidence of primary aneurysmal cysts approximating 0.1 per 10^9 individuals.[291,339] Nearly 70% of affected patients are between 5 and 20 years of age, with approximately half occurring in the second decade of life, although the lesion has been reported in infants.[33,129,167,291,339,385,425] There is no sex predilection.[107]

Aneurysmal bone cysts can be found throughout the skeleton and may also arise in soft tissue.[360,540] The most common sites are the femur, tibia, spine, humerus, pelvis, and fibula, with approximately half of reported cases occurring in the long bones of the extremities.[107,425] Although they usually involve the metaphyseal region, aneurysmal cysts may on occasion cross the physis into the epiphysis or may extend into the diaphysis.[392]

Approximately 20% of aneurysmal bone cysts involve the spine.[511] They may occur anywhere between the axis[55,516] and the sacrum[84] and can cause cord compression or spinal deformity.[91,130,176] Within the vertebra itself, the cyst may be found in the body, pedicles, lamina, and spinous process (Fig. 38–6). Involvement of two or more adjacent vertebrae is not uncommon. Aneurysmal bone cysts may also occur in the maxilla, frontal sinus, orbit, zygoma, ethmoid, temporal bone, mandible, sternum, clavicle, hands, and feet.[71,73,211,243,302,304,405,450,462,492,521,531,567]

Etiology

Aneurysmal bone cysts represent either a primary neoplastic condition or a secondary response (arteriovenous malformation) to the destructive effects of an underlying primary tumor.[461] Their presence has been linked to genetic abnormalities involving chromosome segments 7q, 16p, and 17p11-13,[18,35,374-376,391,461] specifically to USP6 oncogene and CDH11 promoter rearrangements.[376] Insulin-like growth factor I may also play a role in the pathogenesis of aneurysmal bone cysts,[289] and the condition may be inherited in some cases.[135,290]

Development of an aneurysmal cyst as a secondary response is supported by the association of aneurysmal cysts with other primary lesions, such as nonossifying fibromas, fibromyxomas, fibrous dysplasia, chondroblastomas, giant cell tumors, simple bone cysts, telangiectatic osteosarcomas, chondrosarcomas, and metastatic disease.[99,272,322] Sixty-five percent of aneurysmal bone cysts have been reported to be primary, with 35% believed to be secondary to other lesions.[53,294] Thus, once the diagnosis of aneurysmal bone cyst is considered, a thorough preoperative evaluation is necessary, adequate tissue must be obtained at the time of surgery, and careful pathologic studies are needed to ensure that the aneurysmal cyst is not secondary to a more serious primary neoplasm.

Pathology

Aneurysmal bone cysts vary considerably in size, with the potential to become large during the rapid, destructive growth phase. On gross inspection, the cyst consists of an encapsulated mass of soft, friable, reddish-brown tissue, usually contained within a thin subperiosteal shell of new bone. At the time of surgery, a large amount of blood may exude from a mesh of honeycomb spaces. In most cases the blood is dark red owing to a slow but continuous circulation. If the circulation to a portion of the aneurysmal cyst has been blocked, the cyst may be filled with serous or serosanguineous fluid or with focal organized blood clots.

Microscopy discloses a variable number of vascular spaces whose walls are lined with tissue composed of fibroblastic cells with collagen, giant cells, hemosiderin, and osteoid (secondary to microfractures; Fig. 38–7). Extensive sampling should be performed to identify possible benign or malignant precursor lesions, as well as to identify transformation into malignant lesions such as malignant fibrous histiocytoma or osteosarcoma.[22,215] The histologic diagnosis of primary aneurysmal bone cyst should be made only after other possible lesions have been excluded. Fibrous tissue, bone, and giant cells are the usual elements seen in most other benign precursor lesions associated with an aneurysmal bone cyst. Any solid area that is 1 cm or greater should raise the suspicion that it may represent another lesion.

Another entity is a solid aneurysmal bone cyst or giant cell reparative granuloma.[42,68,505] This is a solid yet radiolucent lesion that appears grayish-brown and often is friable. Histologic features include fibrous proliferation with giant cells, fibromyxoid areas, and bone production. Characteristically, the giant cells, which are clustered in areas of recent and old hemorrhage, are found throughout the lesion. The solid aneurysmal bone cyst lacks the normally large blood-filled channels (Fig. 38–8). In a review of a large series of aneurysmal bone cysts, the incidence of the solid entity was 7.5%.[42]

Clinical Features

The clinical presentation includes localized pain of several weeks' or months' duration, tenderness, and, if the aneurysmal bone cyst occurs in an extremity, swelling. When the cyst involves the spine, progressive enlargement may compress the spinal cord or nerve roots, resulting in neurologic deficits such as motor weakness, sensory disturbance, and loss of bowel or bladder control. The cysts may also cause other spinal lesions such as vertebra plana.[393] Spinal involvement therefore mandates urgent intervention.

Radiographic Findings

The classic radiographic feature of aneurysmal bone cysts was described by Jaffe as a periosteal "blowout" or ballooned-out lesion that is outlined by a thin shell of subperiosteal new bone formation.[233] In about 80% of cases the cyst involves the metaphyseal region of the long bones and, unlike simple bone cysts, is eccentric in its location. In the spine, it more often involves the posterior elements (spinous process, transverse process, and pedicles) than the vertebral body. In the shorter tubular bones of the feet, the cysts are more central and extend into the diaphysis and subarticular region (this is explained by the smaller size of the bones).

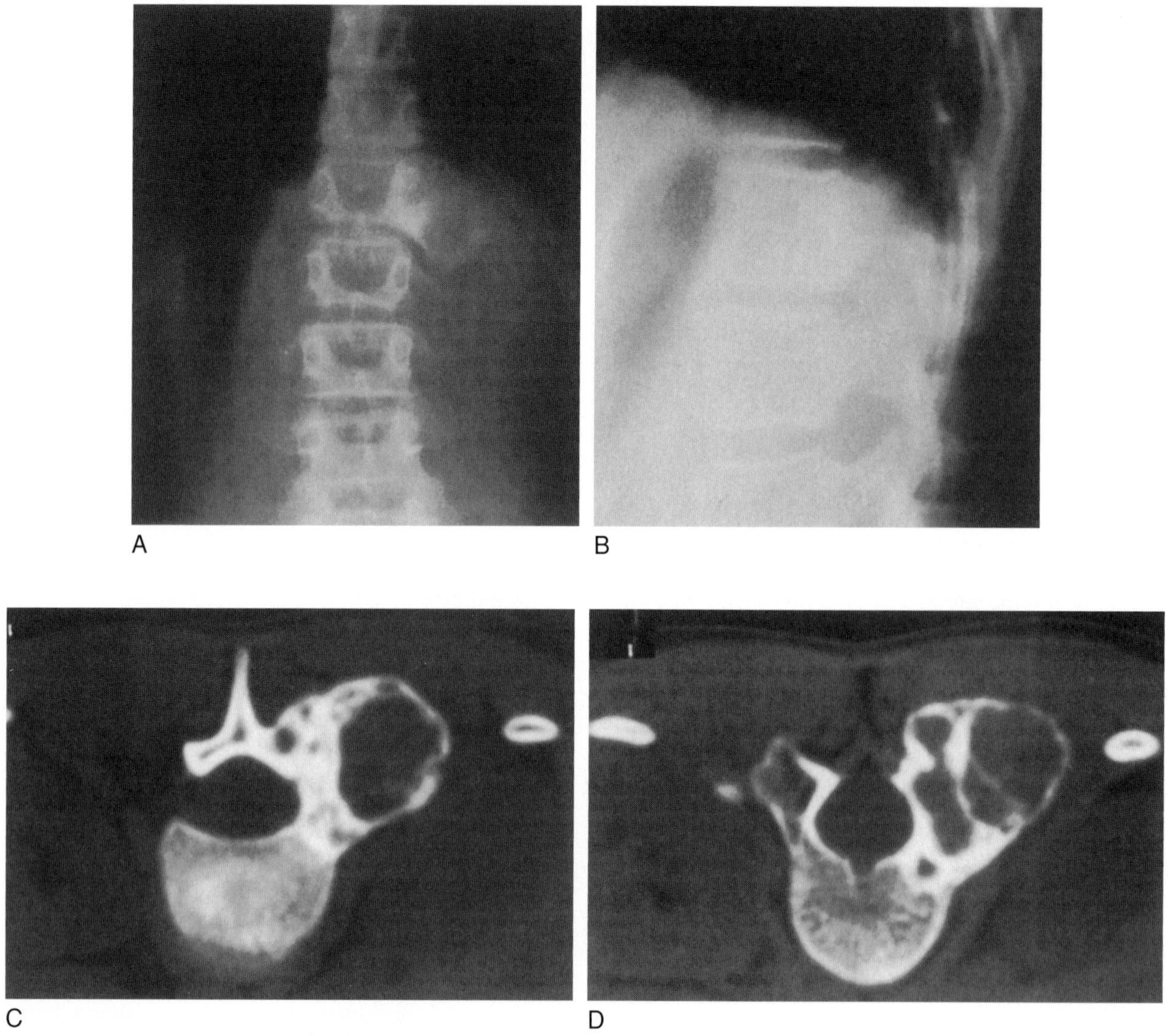

A

B

C

D

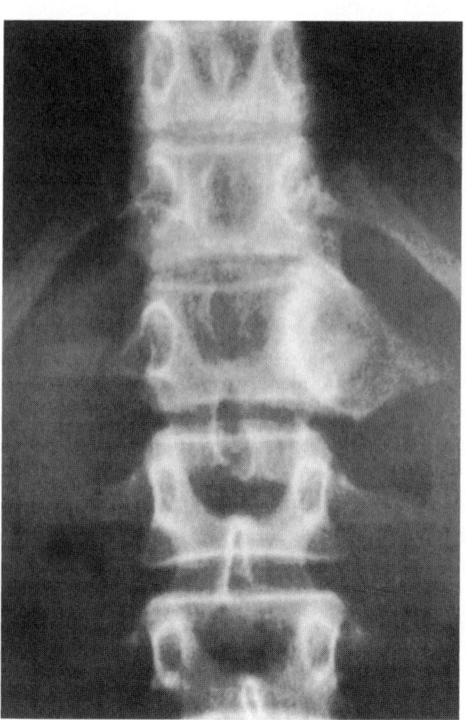

E

FIGURE 38–6 Imaging findings in an 11-year-old girl with moderate back pain in the thoracolumbar spine for 6 months. Anteroposterior **(A)** and lateral spine **(B)** radiographs demonstrated an aneurysmal bone cyst of L1. **C** and **D,** Computed tomography showed that the cyst extensively involved the posterior elements on one side. **E,** Two years after resection and bone grafting, the radiographic appearance still was not normal.

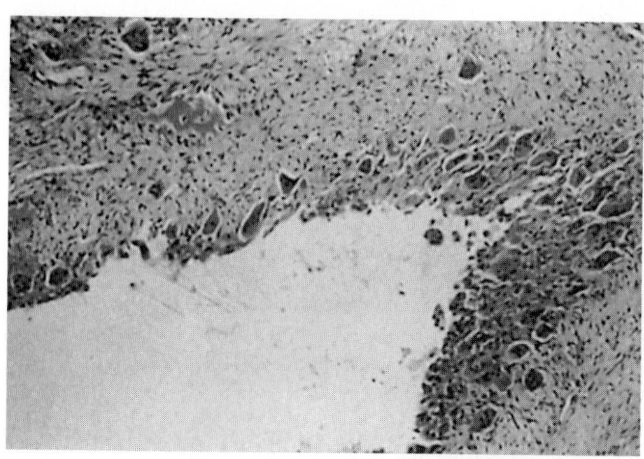

FIGURE 38–7 Aneurysmal bone cyst (original magnification ×10). The wall of the vascular space is lined with giant cells, collagen, and osteoid.

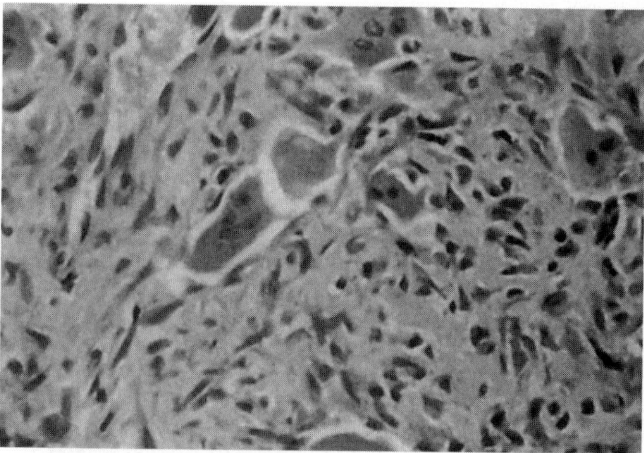

FIGURE 38–8 Solid aneurysmal bone cyst (original magnification ×40). Clusters of giant cells are found throughout the lesion.

Three phases of aneurysmal cysts have been described.[339] The *incipient phase* is characterized by either a small eccentric lucent lesion or a pure lifting off of the periosteum from the host bone without evidence of an intramedullary lesion. Most patients do not present with disease in this phase. Except for focal cortical thinning, the cortex may otherwise be preserved and the periosteum may show no reaction. In this phase, the lesion can be mistaken for a simple bone cyst, nonossifying fibroma, or possibly a lytic osteosarcoma. The *midphase* designates the period of rapid, destructive growth and is characterized by extreme lysis of the bone, focal cortical destruction, and the development of Codman's triangles (periosteal ossification at the corner of the expanded cyst). It is during this phase that the "blowout" appearance is seen on radiographs, and aneurysmal bone cysts can easily be mistaken for an aggressive malignant lesion. In the *late healing* or *stabilization phase,* the lesion grows more slowly, and the periosteum has sufficient time to lay down new bone. The cyst will exhibit eccentric (or possibly concentric), smooth-bordered expansion; a trabeculated or "bubbly" intramedullary appearance; and surrounding host bone sclerosis.

Capanna and colleagues proposed a radiographic classification system that is commonly used today.[84,85,87] *Inactive* cysts have a complete periosteal shell, with the intraosseous margin defined by a sclerotic rim of reactive bone. *Active* cysts have an incomplete periosteal shell and a sharply defined intraosseous border. *Aggressive* cysts show no evidence of reparative osteogenesis, no periosteal shell, and an ill-defined endosteal margin.

Once these lesions are identified on radiographs, the tumor can be better clarified with CT, particularly if it is located in the spine. The extent of involvement of the vertebra and any encroachment of the spinal canal are readily evident. CT also demonstrates the characteristic fluid–fluid levels if the patient is able to lie still long enough for the serosanguineous fluid to separate from the blood within the chambers of the cyst that do not have active circulation. MRI is indicated if there is evidence of spinal cord compression or if the edges of the rapidly expanding cyst cannot be defined with CT. Fluid–fluid levels are readily evident on MRI (Fig. 38–9). MRI is most valuable in differential diagnosis because it can delineate the multicystic appearance, hypointense rim, contrast-enhancing cyst walls, double-density fluid levels, and adjacent soft tissue edema that are typical of this lesion, as well as the extent of the lesions.[51,316,501,552] Gadolinium-enhanced MRI may be helpful for distinguishing the solid variant from conventional aneurysmal bone cyst.[505] Differential diagnosis includes atypical osteosarcoma and telangiectatic osteosarcoma, which may rarely mimic aneurysmal bone cyst radiologically.[447,503]

Treatment

Although spontaneous healing of aneurysmal bone cysts has been reported,[320] it is uncommon. Thus, expectant management should be considered only when the diagnosis has been made with confidence and the lesion is in a location and at a stage that do not entail any risk of fracture or further destruction. More often, when the diagnosis of aneurysmal bone cyst is made, active treatment is recommended.

CURETTAGE AND ADJUNCTIVE THERAPY

Curettage followed by bone grafting of aneurysmal cysts has been the standard treatment for many years[392] (Fig. 38–10). Unfortunately, this tumor has a high incidence of local recurrence (14% to 59%) after curettage,[51,322,339,392,511] although Gibbs and colleagues recently reported rates of local control approaching 90% following curettage with use of a mechanical bur in 40 patients with aneurysmal bone cyst of an extremity.[186] In this series, very young age and open growth plates were associated with increased risk of local recurrence. Overall, however, adjunctive therapy, such as cementation, cryotherapy, or embolization, should be

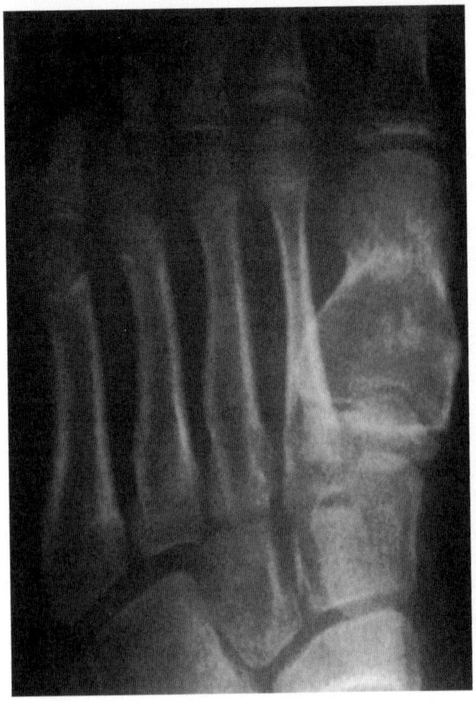

A

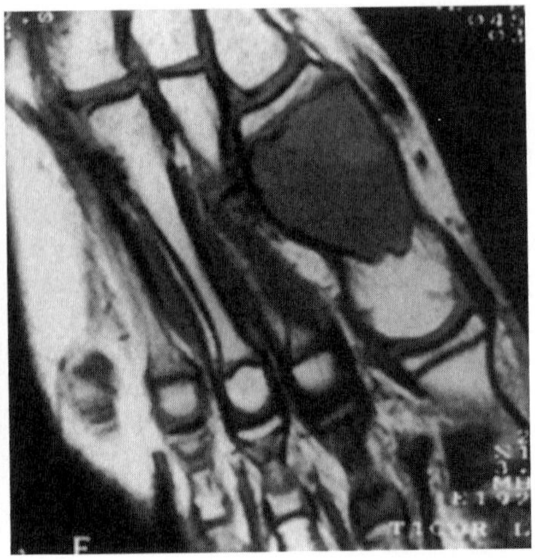

B

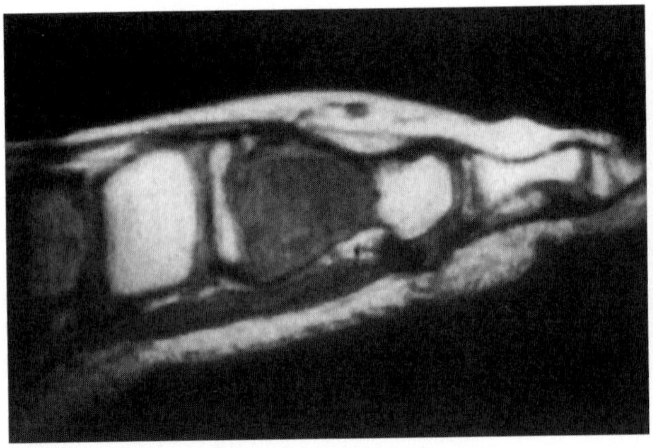

C

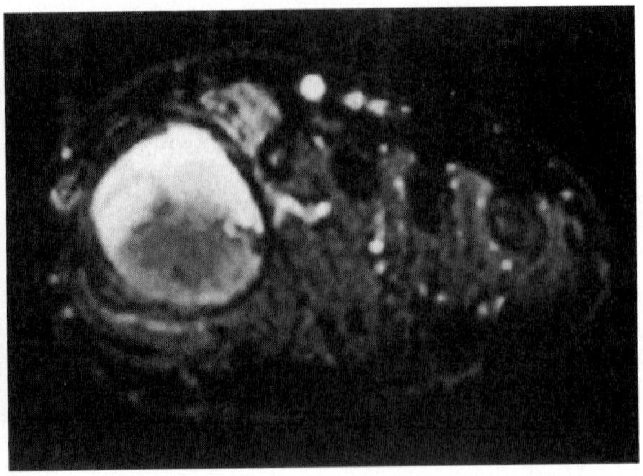

D

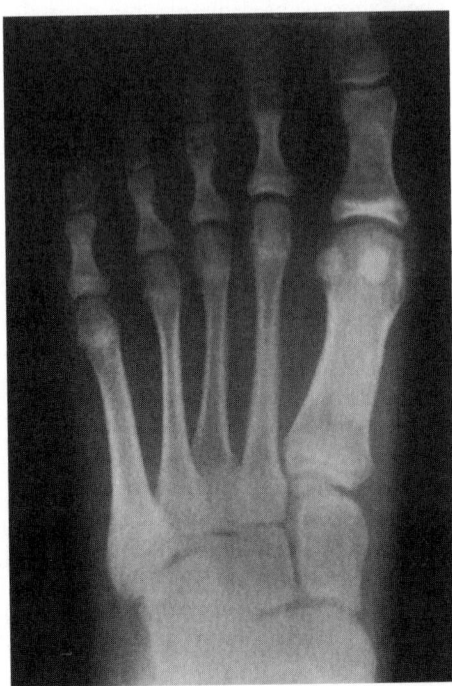

E

FIGURE 38–9 Imaging findings in a 9-year-old girl with a swollen tender first ray of the left foot. **A,** Anteroposterior radiograph demonstrating an expansile well-contained lesion. **B** through **D,** Magnetic resonance images better defined the lesion and showed the layering effect seen with aneurysmal bone cysts. **E,** Three years after curettage and bone grafting, the metatarsal was normal.

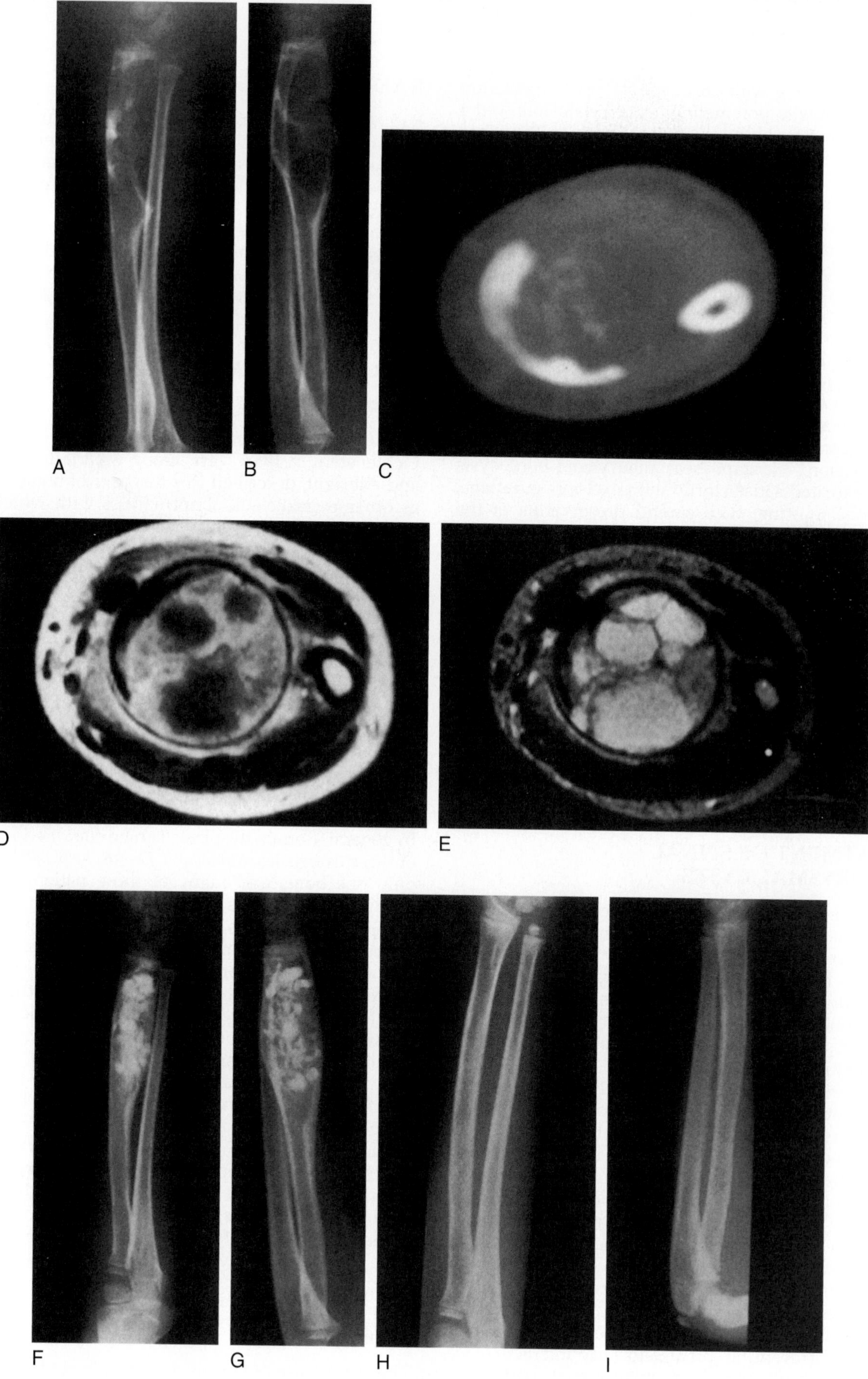

FIGURE 38–10 Imaging findings in a 3-year-old boy who presented with a painful, swollen distal forearm. Anteroposterior **(A)** and lateral **(B)** radiographs demonstrating the "blown-out" appearance of the distal radius. **C,** The edges of the lesion could not be seen well on computed tomography. **D** and **E,** Magnetic resonance imaging demonstrated containment of the lesion. **F** and **G,** After a biopsy confirmed the diagnosis of aneurysmal bone cyst, curettage and bone grafting was performed. **H** and **I,** Three years after surgery, the radius had healed and remodeled.

considered along with curettage.[122,392,394] Cementation of the lesion with polymethylmethacrylate, followed 4 to 6 months later with replacement bone grafting, has been reported to be more effective than curettage and bone grafting alone.[385,386] Cryotherapy as an adjunct to curettage and bone grafting also increases the likelihood of healing.[173,242] Embolization has been used as the sole treatment for aneurysmal bone cysts,[5,101] but it is much more commonly used before surgery to interrupt the vascularity of the lesion. Embolization is useful in treating aneurysmal cysts located in areas of limited access, such as the spine and pelvis,[124,139,185,265,394] although incidences of significant complications including fatal Ethibloc embolization of the vertebrobasilar system have been reported.[404] If the cyst is located in an expendable bone, such as a rib or fibula, the surgeon should consider performing a wide or en bloc excision.[425] Juxtaphyseal aneurysmal bone cysts may be treated satisfactorily with excision, curettage, and bone grafting, with careful preservation of the growth plate.[432]

Anecdotal reports of techniques useful in the treatment of aneurysmal bone cysts include oral dexamethasone (an angiostatic agent),[165] percutaneous intralesional injection with calcitonin and methylprednisolone,[191] endoscopic curettage without bone grafting,[380] and the use of multiple Kirschner pins inserted into the cyst.[396] Garg and colleagues recently reported a significantly reduced rate of recurrence (0/8 cases) when a four-step approach of intralesional curettage, use of a high-speed bur, electrocautery, and bone grafting was used as an alternative to traditional intralesional curettage and bone grafting.[175]

TREATMENT OF SPINAL ANEURYSMAL CYSTS

Aneurysmal cysts in the spine most commonly involve the elements of the posterior column, but the cysts may extend anteriorly into the body.[122] More than one vertebra may be affected. On occasion, neurologic deficit due to compression of the spinal cord by the lesion requires emergency resection. More often, however, time is available to plan the necessary preoperative embolization, surgical approaches, and reconstruction of a surgically destabilized spine.[332,394,523] Treatment for spinal aneurysmal bone cysts remains controversial, but surgical resection, irradiation, and embolization are commonly used.[383] Posterior approaches to spinal cysts may provide insufficient access to lesions that extend anteriorly into the vertebral body and are associated with a higher recurrence rate than when anterior approaches are also used, so intralesional curettage combined with adjuvant therapy such as preoperative embolization is advised.[122] Case series by Ozaki and colleagues[383] and Boriani and associates[57] support radical resection as an optimal method of preventing spinal deformity and recurrence in patients with neurologic involvement, pathologic fracture, technical impossibility of performing embolization, or local recurrence after at least two embolization procedures.

RADIATION THERAPY

Radiation therapy has been used for some aneurysmal bone cysts, especially those that are recurrent, inoperable, or located in areas that are difficult to access, such as the spine.[70,76,155] The dose should be minimized (approximately 3000 and 5000 cGy) to decrease the risk of radiation-induced sarcoma.[76,155] Because of this concern, radiation therapy should be limited to cases of cysts that are inoperable or have become inoperable and to cases in which embolization has failed.[322,394]

FIBROUS DYSPLASIA

Incidence

The term *fibrous dysplasia* was originally proposed by Lichtenstein in 1938.[295] He, along with Jaffe, McCune, and Albright, described this disorder of bone, as well as other extraskeletal abnormalities with which it is occasionally associated.[12,13,298,330] Their descriptions remain among the best for fibrous dysplasia—a benign, nonfamilial disorder characterized by the presence of expanding intramedullary fibro-osseous tissue in one or more bones. The incidence of fibrous dysplasia is not known, but it is not an uncommon primary bone tumor. It occurs more frequently in girls than in boys, particularly the polyostotic form. Although most lesions are probably present in early childhood, they usually do not become evident before late childhood to adolescence.

Classification

In general, fibrous dysplasia can be classified into one of three categories. *Monostotic fibrous dysplasia* involves only one bone, and many of these patients remain asymptomatic unless a fracture or swelling occurs. The *polyostotic form* is more severe, involving multiple bones. Nearly any bone in the body may be affected, including the long bones of the extremities, skull, vertebrae, pelvis, scapula, ribs, and bones of the hands and feet. Often one side of the body (in particular, one of the lower extremities) is more severely affected, resulting in deformity and limb length discrepancy.[339,511] Craniofacial involvement occurs in nearly 50% of patients with polyostotic disease. The third category, *polyostotic form with endocrine abnormalities,* is the least common form. Precocious puberty, premature skeletal maturation, hyperthyroidism, hyperparathyroidism, acromegaly, and Cushing's syndrome can occur in these patients.[1] The triad of precocious puberty (endocrinopathy), café au lait spots, and polyostotic bone involvement is commonly referred to as McCune-Albright (or Albright's) syndrome.

Etiology

The exact cause of fibrous dysplasia is not known. The condition is not believed to be hereditary. Fibrous dysplasia probably results from a failure of maturation from woven to lamellar bone.[307] Recent studies have reported an abnormality of a gene encoding a G protein that is important in the development of bone. Somatic activating mutations of the signal transducer Gs of the alpha chain differentiate fibrous dysplasia (particularly McCune-Albright syndrome) from other lesions, and the mutations may be responsible for the loss of control of local proliferation and growth factor expression.[16,46,80,472] Elevation in the cyclic adenosine monophosphate (cAMP) level induced by the Gs-alpha mutations leads to alterations in the expression of several target genes whose promoters contain cAMP-responsive elements, such as c-fos, c-jun, Il-6, and Il-11. This affects the transcription and expression of downstream genes and results in the alterations of osteoblast recruitment and function in dysplastic bone. These mechanisms provide a cellular and molecular basis for the alterations in bone cells and bone matrix in fibrous dysplasia.[201,312,313,324,397]

Pathology

The outer surface of expanded bone is usually smooth and covered by reactive periosteal bone. The underlying dysplastic tissue is firm and grayish-white, and the proliferative tissue is fibrous. It may feel gritty when palpated, almost like sandpaper. There may be degenerative cystic changes due to cellular necrosis. Islands of hyaline cartilage may be seen.

Histologically, irregular foci of woven (nonlamellar) bone trabeculae are seen in a cellular fibrous stroma[68,537] (Fig. 38–11). Under the microscope, the bony spicules are often described as looking like the letters C, J, or Y or resembling Chinese characters. Osteoclastic resorption may be seen, but osteoblastic rimming of the bony spicules is uncommon. In unusual cases, as much as 95% of the lesional tissue may be fibrous. Cartilage islands, multinucleated giant cells, foamy histiocytes, and callus may be seen if a fracture has occurred. The histologic features of polyostotic lesions are identical to those of monostotic lesions.

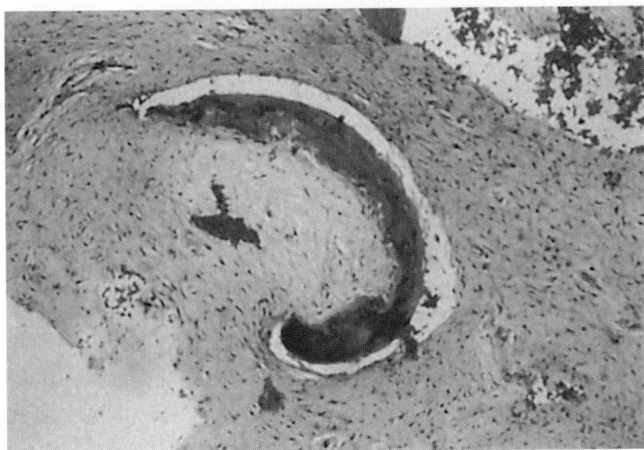

FIGURE 38–11 Histologic appearance of fibrous dysplasia (original magnification ×10). Spicules of woven bone arise from the cellular fibrous stroma.

Clinical Features

The clinical manifestations are usually mild in monostotic fibrous dysplasia. Pain and a limp may be evident when the neck of the femur is involved. Local swelling may be seen when the lesion is in a superficial bone, such as the mandible, skull, or tibia. The skeletal changes are usually more severe in the polyostotic form and may result in pain, swelling, deformity, and limb length discrepancies. The classic example of this is found in the proximal femur.[193] Repetitive microfractures can lead to a "shepherd's crook" deformity with pain, significant varus at the femoral neck, shortening of the femur, an obvious Trendelenburg gait, and limited mobility. Deformity can occur in all of the long bones, but usually not to the degree seen in the femur. In patients with polyostotic disease, the peak incidence of fractures is during the first decade of life, followed by a decrease thereafter.[284] When the facial bones are affected, progressive deformity may become evident to the patient and family. Numerous reports of craniofacial abnormalities are found in the dental and maxillofacial literature[213,252,481] (Fig. 38–12). Spinal lesions and scoliosis may be more common in patients with polyostotic fibrous dysplasia than was previously thought.[285] Dysplastic lesions of the spine, primarily involving the posterior elements, have been reported in 63% of patients, and scoliosis has been reported in 40% of patients. There have also been reports of vertebral collapse, angular deformity, and possible spinal cord compression.[367,418]

The most common nonskeletal manifestation associated with fibrous dysplasia is abnormal cutaneous pigmentation, or café au lait spots. These have irregular borders ("coast of Maine"), are not raised from the surrounding skin, and may be extensive, involving large areas of the trunk, face, or limbs. The café au lait spots can coexist with polyostotic fibrous dysplasia without endocrine changes or precocious puberty, or they may be absent when endocrinopathies accompany fibrous dysplasia. The pigmentation changes usually are not present in monostotic fibrous dysplasia.

When sexual precocity occurs it is most often seen in the female patient secondary to premature ovarian stimulation, and it may occur as early as 1 year of age. Most cases of McCune-Albright syndrome occur in girls and are accompanied by accelerated maturation and advanced skeletal age. In such children, abnormally rapid growth may result in tall stature at a young age. Ultimately, however, their adult stature will usually be below average because of their early maturation.

Malignant transformation of fibrous dysplasia is rare but has been reported.[249]

Radiographic Findings

Fibrous dysplasia can affect any bone.[339] In the long bones, the lesions start in the metaphysis or diaphysis and rarely involve the epiphysis.[363] The flat bones, ribs, jaw, and skull are commonly involved, but the spine is not.

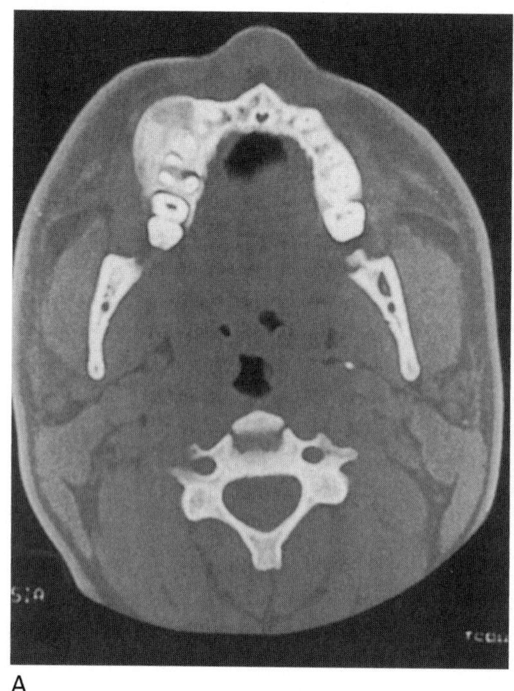

A

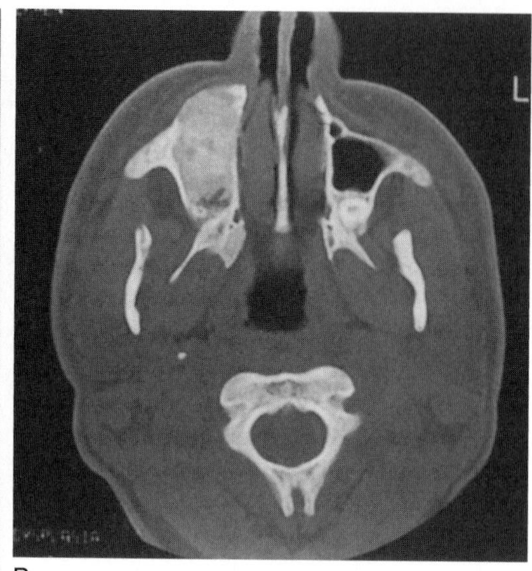

B

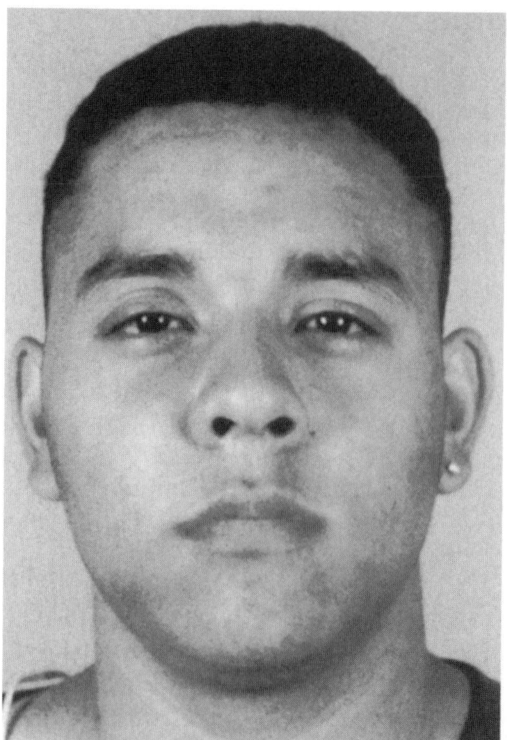

C

FIGURE 38–12 Fibrous dysplasia. Computed tomography scans of the head demonstrate expansion of the maxilla **(A)** and replacement of a normal sinus with fibrous dysplasia **(B).** Slight facial asymmetry is noted because of the affected bone on the right side **(C).**

Some of the smaller lesions of fibrous dysplasia remain confined to the intramedullary region, are often surrounded by sclerosis, and may appear "bubbly" or trabeculated. Normally, however, there is slow replacement of the cortex as expansion takes place. Larger lesions may result in an even or eccentric, smooth-bordered expansion of the bone, but they usually remain confined within a rim of periosteal bone. Angular deformity may occur in the long bones, such as the shepherd's crook deformity in the proximal femur and occasionally in the humerus.[130] This is usually a result of remodeling of the bone after repetitive microfractures or obvious fractures through the dysplastic bone (Fig. 38–13).

The radiographic density of the lesions depends on the amount of woven bone produced and on the amount of cortex replaced. If the lesion is small, has produced little woven bone, or has not replaced cortex, it will appear radiolucent compared with surrounding normal bone. If the cortex is thinned and if the fibrous dysplasia has expanded and replaced most of the normal bone, the characteristic ground-glass

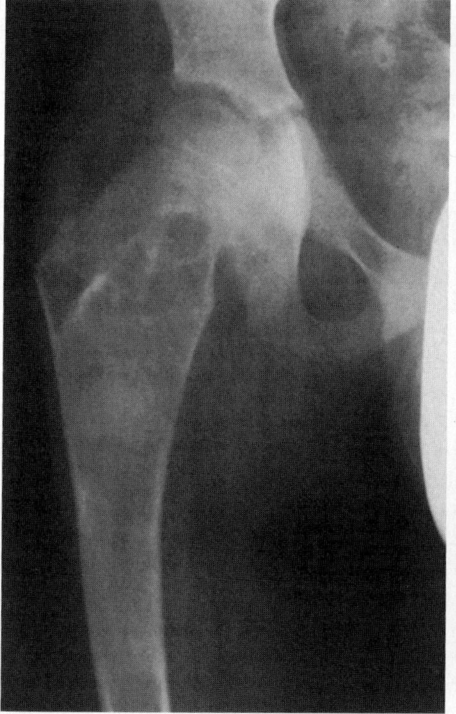
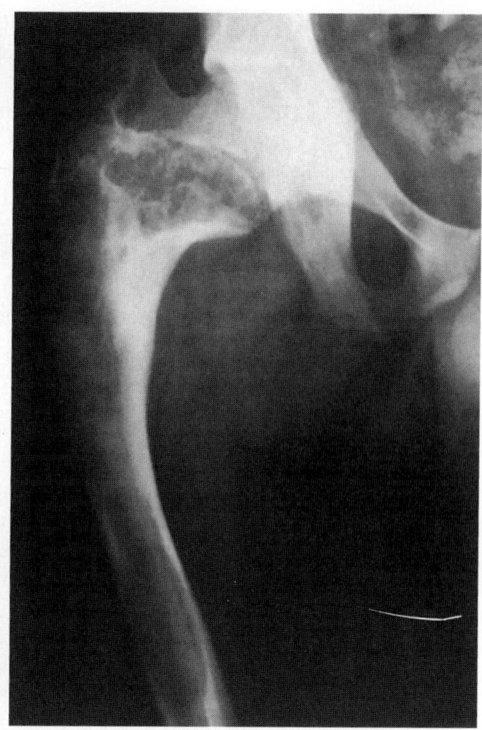

FIGURE 38-13 Imaging findings in a 9-year-old boy with polyostotic disease. **A,** Radiograph obtained at presentation showing fibrous dysplasia of the femur. **B,** Six years later, at 15 years of age, a shepherd's crook deformity had developed as a result of repetitive microfractures of the proximal femur.

appearance is seen. When this feature is extensive, it is nearly pathognomonic of fibrous dysplasia. CT clearly demonstrates this appearance.

A bone scan demonstrates increased uptake throughout the lesion and is helpful in determining the extent of the disorder if radiographs are unable to do so.[482]

Differential Diagnosis

With monostotic fibrous dysplasia, it may be difficult to differentiate small lesions from simple bone cysts on radiographs. Less often, small lesions may be confused with histiocytosis or enchondromas. In these cases a biopsy may be necessary. Larger lesions with cortical thinning and a ground-glass appearance usually do not require a biopsy to confirm the diagnosis. Polyostotic fibrous dysplasia is readily identified on radiographs.

Treatment

NONSURGICAL TREATMENT

The mere presence of fibrous dysplasia in bone is not, in itself, an indication for surgery, and surgical overtreatment should be avoided. For those with bone pain or with lesions that cannot be improved through surgical intervention (particularly in those with McCune-Albright syndrome), the use of bisphosphonates has been shown to be beneficial in controlling pain and improving the quality of life.* Pamidronate, the intravenously administered bisphosphonate, has also been reported to significantly increase bone mineral density.[228,328,398,399]

Although malignancy in fibrous dysplasia is rare, when it does occur the prognosis is poor. Most cases occur in patients who have undergone radiation therapy.[19,94,111,445,562,563] Thus, radiation treatments should be avoided because of the association with malignant transformation. The hormonal abnormalities in McCune-Albright disease should be managed by an endocrinologist.[148,149,173,319,498]

In children, it is nearly impossible to restore dysplastic bone to normal bone after surgery. In the rare case that biopsy is needed to confirm the diagnosis of a monostotic lesion, surgical intervention probably should not be undertaken unless there is a fracture or painful deformity, because simple curettage of the lesion inevitably leads to local recurrence. In addition, the risk of pathologic fracture is increased during the months immediately after surgery. Bone graft used to replace part or even all of the tumorous bone is also predictably resorbed and replaced by the dysplastic bone.[132]

SURGICAL TREATMENT

A proposed exception to the nonoperative approach in children (in the absence of fracture or deformity) is infantile fibrous dysplasia.[21] In these children with polyostotic disease, early surgical treatment to prevent development of skeletal deformities that are difficult to correct later may provide long-term benefit. Prophylactic intramedullary nailing with nails of appropriate size was found to be most effective. In the adult, bone grafting in fibrous dysplasia has been reported to be more successful in healing the dysplastic bone.[189]

*See references 93, 228, 263, 271, 328, 378, 397-399, 410, 456, 571.

Operative intervention is needed when repeated pathologic fractures have occurred, when lesions cause significant or progressive deformity that jeopardizes the integrity of the long bone or that results in unacceptable disfigurement, or when associated pain becomes persistent. Pathologic fractures can occur after mild trauma, they are often minimally displaced, and they heal at a normal rate. Delayed union or nonunion is not a problem, but progressive deformity is. The primary goal of treatment is to realign the deformed bone, particularly in the weight-bearing lower extremities. This objective, along with ready healing of the fracture, can often be achieved with cast immobilization in the young child. If repeated fractures occur in long bones or if a fracture involves the proximal femur, surgical intervention is the preferred treatment approach. Internal fixation maintains proper alignment and can be achieved with intramedullary rods in the long bones or with compression screws with side plates in the proximal femur.[131,226,227,475,488] Before the insertion of internal fixation, osteotomies may be required to achieve satisfactory alignment because bowing of the bone (malunions) is common after fractures. This is particularly true in the proximal femur, in which a shepherd's crook deformity may be present.[193] Intraoperative blood loss may be excessive because of increased vascularity in the bone. In addition, the dysplastic bone may not allow good cortical screw purchase, necessitating alternative plans for internal fixation. Despite the successful use of internal fixation and near-anatomic bone realignment, progressive deformity can still occur, leading to the need for additional surgery.

Some authors advocate attempts to augment bone strength in addition to or in place of internal fixation. Enneking and associates reported that cortical strut grafting was effective in strengthening the bone in the proximal femur[145] (Fig. 38–14). In their opinion, the strength of the bone was greater if cortical rather than cancellous graft was used. Allograft cortical struts avoid the morbidity of harvesting autogenous graft and also appear to slow the resorption process by the dysplastic bone.[464] Ultimately, however, the type of graft used probably does not affect the rate of recurrence.

Osteofibrous Dysplasia of the Tibia and Fibula (Campanacci's Disease)

Incidence

Osteofibrous dysplasia of the tibia and fibula has been described as a variant of fibrous dysplasia.[401] However, molecular investigations have found that the Gs-alpha mutation at the Arg201 codon is present in fibrous dysplasia but is absent in osteofibrous dysplasia.[448] These data suggest that the two disorders have different pathogeneses. Osteofibrous dysplasia may also have a histogenetic relationship to adamantinoma.* Cytokeratin-positive cells are found in the stroma of both osteofibrous dysplasia and adamantinomas, but not in fibrous dysplasia.

The disorder was first reported in the literature in 1921 by Frangenheim,[164] who used the term *congenital osteitis fibrosa*. Other terms for this disorder include *congenital fibrous dysplasia, congenital fibrous defect of the tibia,* and *ossifying fibroma. Osteofibrous dysplasia of the tibia and fibula* was proposed by Campanacci in 1976.[75,78]

Osteofibrous dysplasia differs from the more common fibrous dysplasia with regard to age distribution, site, radiographic features, and clinical course. The lesion is slightly more common in boys. The symptoms almost always appear in the first decade of life. Nearly two thirds of the lesions are noted before 5 years of age,[78] and the disorder has been noted in infants.[20,266] The tibia is almost always involved, and the ipsilateral fibula may be affected. Bilateral involvement has been reported,[220,504] as has involvement of the radius and ulna.[539] Mainly the diaphysis is affected, with localization to the middle third in the tibia. Extension into the proximal or distal metaphysis is seen sometimes. Rarely, there is diffuse involvement of the entire shaft of the tibia. When the disorder is limited to the fibula, the distal third of the bone is affected.

Etiology

The pathogenesis of osteofibrous dysplasia remains unknown[64]; however, several theories have been proposed: (1) it results from excessive resorption of bone with fibrous repair of the defect, (2) it is a congenital lesion or a variant of fibrous dysplasia,[401] and (3) it results from abnormal blood circulation in the periosteum.[266] It has been reported in a family, which may also support a genetic component to its etiology.[220] Recent literature has suggested that the disorder is either a reactive process secondary to adamantinoma or a precursor of adamantinoma.[38,64,204,205,229,279,317,495,525]

Pathology

On gross inspection the periosteum is intact. The affected cortex is thinned and may be perforated. The lesion has been described as either whitish-yellow or reddish.

Histologically, the tissue is similar to fibrous dysplasia, with irregular spicules of trabecular bone and fibrous or collagenous stroma. In contrast to fibrous dysplasia, the spicules are usually lined with osteoblasts (Fig. 38–15). The finding of woven bone with juxtaposed lamellar bone (from osteoblasts) is thought to be characteristic of osteofibrous dysplasia. Immunohistochemical studies have demonstrated isolated cytokeratin-positive cells in the stroma of osteofibrous dysplasia.[38,64,229,244,318,525] These cells are not seen in fibrous dysplasia but are found in adamantinomas. Based on this finding, it is believed that there is a relationship between osteofibrous dysplasia and differentiated adamantinoma; however, it is not certain whether osteofibrous dysplasia represents a possible

*See references 15, 38, 50, 64, 204, 205, 229, 244, 279, 317, 318, 415, 495, 509, 525.

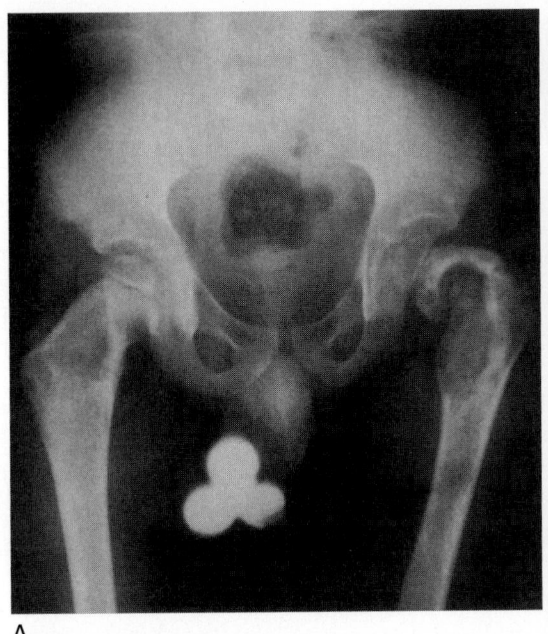

A

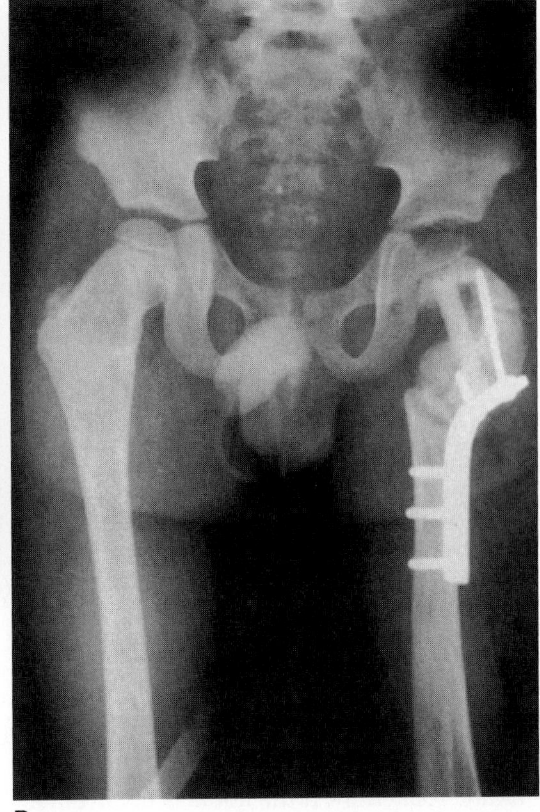

B

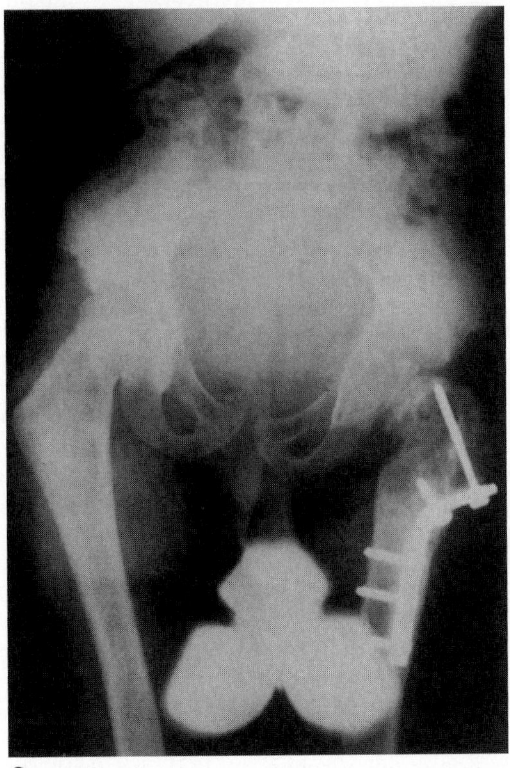

C

FIGURE 38-14 Radiographic appearance in a 7-year-old boy with polyostotic fibrous dysplasia and a painful, progressive varus deformity. **A,** Radiographically, the left hip was found to be involved. **B,** A valgus osteotomy with allograft fibula and internal fixation was performed. **C,** Ten months later, the allograft fibula had been resorbed by the dysplastic bone, and varus of the proximal femur was recurring.

precursor of or is a secondary reaction to adamantinoma. Nests of epithelial cells are a consistent histologic finding in adamantinomas, but they are not found in osteofibrous dysplasia.

Clinical Features

The common presenting complaint is firm swelling localized over the tibia with associated mild to moderate anterior tibial bowing. Osteofibrous dysplasia is usually painless unless there is a coexisting pathologic fracture.

Radiographic Findings

The lesion usually is extensive, involving the anterior cortex of either the diaphysis or the metaphysis of the tibia; the epiphysis usually is not affected.[68] Characteristic eccentric, intracortical osteolysis is found, with moderate or marked expansion of the cortex

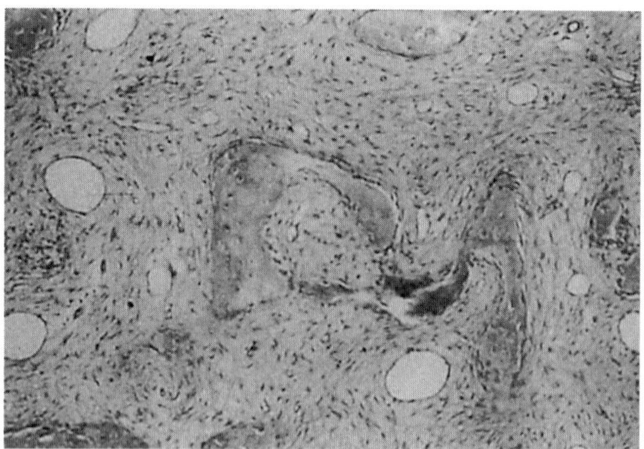

FIGURE 38–15 Histologic appearance of osteofibrous dysplasia (original magnification ×10). The tissue is similar to fibrous dysplasia, with irregular spicules of woven bone. In contrast to the histologic appearance of fibrous dysplasia, the spicules are usually lined with osteoblasts.

(Fig. 38–16). In small areas, the cortex may actually appear absent, and a "bubbled" appearance may be evident. In some areas, the osteolytic areas may have a ground-glass appearance. The tibia may be bowed anteriorly or anterolaterally. If the fibula is involved, it is usually evident in the distal third of the bone, involving nearly the entire circumference of the shaft.

Differential Diagnosis

The two entities that must be distinguished from osteofibrous dysplasia are monostotic fibrous dysplasia and adamantinoma. In contrast to osteofibrous dysplasia, fibrous dysplasia is characterized by the following features: (1) it is usually detected after 10 years of age; (2) it is not routinely associated with anterior or anterolateral tibial bowing; (3) it is noted to be intramedullary on radiographs, with a ground-glass appearance; (4) histologically, the bony trabeculae in the fibrous stroma are rarely surrounded by osteoblasts; and (5) it should have the Gs-alpha mutation at the Arg201 codon. Adamantinomas usually occur in patients older than 10 years of age and contain the epithelial components histologically. In adolescents, an open biopsy is needed to differentiate osteofibrous dysplasia from adamantinoma. This tissue must be carefully evaluated because of the difficulty in distinguishing between the two entities.[495]

Treatment

The natural history of osteofibrous dysplasia varies. The lesion may grow slowly or it may expand rapidly into the entire diaphysis. Spontaneous healing of the lesion has been reported.[526] The most common clinical course is one of steady growth and expansion during the first 5 to 10 years of life. Growth then slows and, after maturity, the lesion stops expanding. Treatment depends on the course of the specific lesion.

In the young child, marginal subperiosteal resection or curettage has been reported to be successful,[384] but this form of treatment is often followed by recurrence of the lesion. A wide extraperiosteal en bloc resection will presumably achieve a cure, but such a radical procedure is rarely, if ever, indicated. Therefore, a conservative approach (observation) is recommended. Bracing, consisting of an ankle-foot orthosis with anterior shell, is indicated if the tibia shows a progressive angular deformity. Cast immobilization of a pathologic fracture is recommended unless angular deformity requires correction; if so, internal fixation may be needed.

Conservative management also is recommended in the treatment of adolescents with osteofibrous dysplasia. If the radiographic appearance is unchanging, the patient should probably be observed indefinitely. If the lesion grows, marginal excision followed by bone transport through distraction osteogenesis has been reported to be successful.[247]

Solitary Osteochondroma

Incidence

Osteochondroma is the most common benign bone tumor, reportedly accounting for 36% to 41% of all such tumors.[114,453] It is characterized by a cartilage-capped osseous projection protruding from the surface of the affected bone. The exostosis is produced by progressive enchondral ossification of the hyaline cartilaginous cap, which essentially functions as a growth plate. More than 50% of solitary osteochondromas occur in the metaphyseal area of the distal femur, proximal tibia, and proximal humerus.[147] Other areas in which solitary osteochondromas may be found include the distal radius, the distal tibia, the proximal and distal fibula, and occasionally the flat bones such as the scapulae, ilium, or ribs. The presence of these solitary lesions within the spinal canal, with resultant neurologic compromise, has received much attention in the recent literature.[63,160,187,275,373,428,470,479]

Etiology

A focal herniation of the medial or lateral component of the epiphyseal plate results in the formation of an aberrant, cartilage-capped, eccentric small bone. Several theories have been proposed to explain this phenomenon. Virchow in 1891 put forth the physeal theory, according to which a portion of the physeal cartilage becomes separated from the parent tissue, rotates 90 degrees, and grows in a direction transverse to the long axis of the bone.[535] However, he did not provide an explanation for the separation and rotation of the detached physeal cartilage. In 1920, Keith proposed that the cause was a defect in the perichondral ring surrounding the physis.[253] Müller in 1913 theorized that the exostoses were produced by small nests of cartilage derived from the cambium layer of the periosteum.[347] By producing osteochondroma using physeal cartilage transplantation, D'Ambrosia and

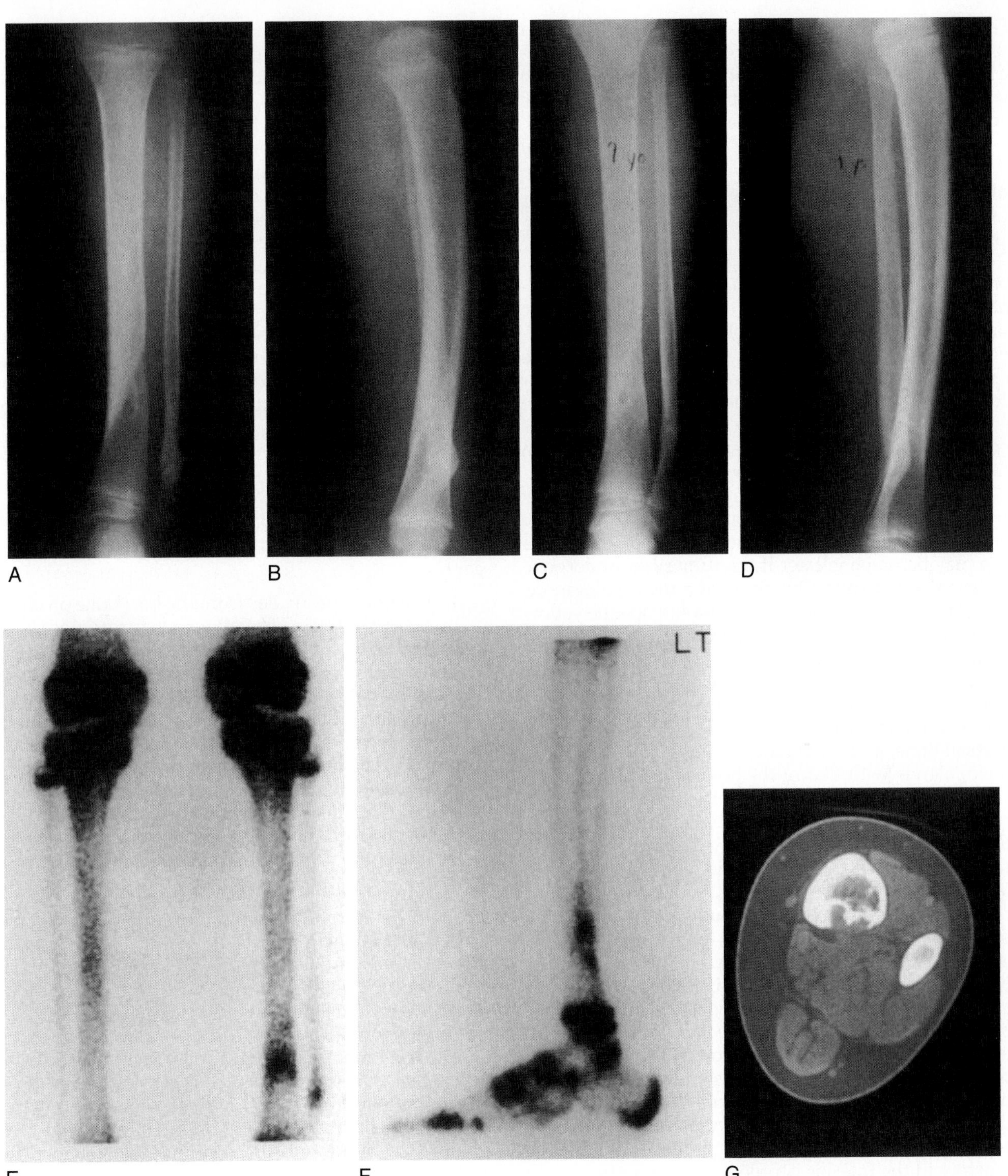

FIGURE 38–16 **A** and **B,** Osteofibrous dysplasia of the tibia and fibula in a 5-year-old girl, associated with mild anterior bowing. **C** and **D,** Radiographs obtained at 9 years of age, when persistent discomfort was present. **E** and **F,** Bone scans showed increased uptake in the area of the lesion. **G,** Computed tomography showed the intracortical osteolysis. Biopsy confirmed the diagnosis of osteofibrous dysplasia.

Ferguson provided support for the physeal plate defect theory.[115] Current thought is that the cause is misdirected growth of a portion of the physeal plate, with lateral protrusions causing the development of the eccentric cartilage-capped bony prominence.

Unlike the more extensive hereditary (autosomal dominant) multiple exostoses, solitary osteochondromas do not appear to be genetically transmitted.

Pathology

Solitary osteochondromas may be sessile (broad-based) or pedunculated (narrow-based). The surface usually is lobular, with multiple bluish-gray cartilaginous caps covering the irregular bony mass. The cartilaginous caps are covered by either thin or comparatively thick perichondrium, which may be adherent to the underlying irregular surface and is continuous with that of the adjacent bony cortex. When this perichondrium is removed, the shiny cartilaginous cap is exposed. The cartilaginous cap is usually 1 to 3 mm thick, but in the younger patient it may be noticeably thicker. The thickness of the cartilaginous cap may be much greater if the tumor has undergone sarcomatous change. On cut section the cartilaginous cap varies in thickness and often has an opaque yellow appearance owing to calcification within the cartilaginous matrix.

The tumor often resembles a cauliflower; however, it may also be flat, hemispheric, or tubular with a prominent end. Its base is contiguous with the normal cortical bone, and the interior of the lesion (spongiosa bone) blends with that of the host bone.

A bursa may develop over the osteochondroma, particularly in larger lesions, where movement of the adjacent soft tissue leads to irritation. This bursal sac may contain mucinous fluid and fibrinous rice bodies.

Histologically, the cartilaginous cap is composed of bland hyaline cartilage. Variable degrees of cellularity are seen, but anaplastic cells are not characteristically evident. Normal enchondral ossification is seen at the cartilage–bone junction. In younger patients, cartilage cores may be present within the subchondral spongiosa near the physes, and these cores may be responsible for recurrence of the lesion should an incomplete resection be performed. Aside from the cartilage cores, the cancellous bone underlying the cartilaginous cap resembles that of the host, although on occasion the marrow in the interior is predominantly fatty.

The appearance of the cartilaginous cap depends on the stage of growth, becoming thinner over time. Remnants of the quiescent cap may persist well into adult life. Should increased thickness of the cartilage become evident in an adult, malignant degeneration must be considered and the lesion should be carefully examined on histologic sections.

Clinical Features

In the majority of affected individuals, the osteochondroma becomes evident between the ages of 10 and 20 years. There is a slight male preponderance. An osteochondroma may be discovered as an incidental radiographic finding or it may be detected on palpation of a protruding bump. Other factors that often draw attention to the osteochondroma include localized pain, growth disturbance of an extremity, compromised joint motion, abnormal cosmetic appearance, or secondary impingement of soft tissues (tendon, nerves, and vessels). Swelling of the lower extremity, accompanied by pain, has been reported due to vascular compression by an osteochondroma at the knee.[449] On occasion, a fracture may occur through a stalk of a pedunculated (narrow-based) lesion after minor trauma. If the patient experiences progressive lower extremity weakness or numbness, MRI evaluation of the neural axis is needed and extradural compression of the spinal cord from an osteochondroma should be given consideration.

Radiographic Findings

There are several pathognomonic radiographic findings associated with an osteochondroma[340] (Fig. 38–17):

1. The lesion protrudes from the host bone on either a sessile (broad-based) or pedunculated bony stalk.
2. It occurs either in the metaphysis or, as the main epiphyseal plate grows away from the lesion, in the diaphysis. It is never found in the epiphysis.
3. The cortex and cancellous bone of the osteochondroma blend with the cortex and cancellous bone of the host. This is the main radiographic finding, and any deviation from this feature should raise suspicion of a more serious lesion.
4. The lesion ranges in size from 2 to 12 cm.

There may be slight metaphyseal widening at the site of the exostosis. Although the cartilaginous cap is not radiographically visible, partial calcification of the cartilage may be seen as small areas of radiopacity.

In the flat bones, such as the ilium or scapulae, exostoses are usually sessile and are located near the cartilaginous ends of the bone. Osteochondromas rarely develop in the carpal and tarsal bones, but they may involve the phalanges. The rare osteochondroma in the spine (occurring primarily in hereditary multiple exostoses) is rarely visualized on plain radiographs. If there is evidence of cord compression, CT and MRI will clearly show the impingement.

Bursal osteochondromatosis overlying an osteochondroma of the rib has been described,[556] and on occasion, ultrasonography may help delineate the extent of the swollen bursa. If there is concern over a progressively enlarging mass, ultrasonography may also help determine the thickness of the cartilaginous cap. Steady growth of the cartilaginous cap is acceptable during childhood and early adolescence, but growth should cease when skeletal maturity is reached. If the cartilaginous cap continues to grow after skeletal maturity, malignant transformation should be considered and the appropriate follow-up studies undertaken.

Differential Diagnosis

Because of their typically distinct radiographic appearance, solitary osteochondromas are usually easily diagnosed. Occasionally they may be confused with a juxtacortical chondroma or, less commonly, with myositis ossificans with a cartilaginous cap. Juxtacortical chondromas usually have a scalloped cortical defect with a sclerotic margin. With myositis ossificans, the apparent tumor does not blend with the cortex and cancellous bone of the host bone, even though it may be attached to the periosteum. This is usually apparent radiographically, thus distinguishing the long-standing lesion of mature myositis ossificans from an osteochondroma. In the skeletally mature individual, enlargement of a solitary osteochondroma (particularly one that is associated with progressive discomfort) must alert the physician to the possibility of malignant degeneration into a chondrosarcoma.

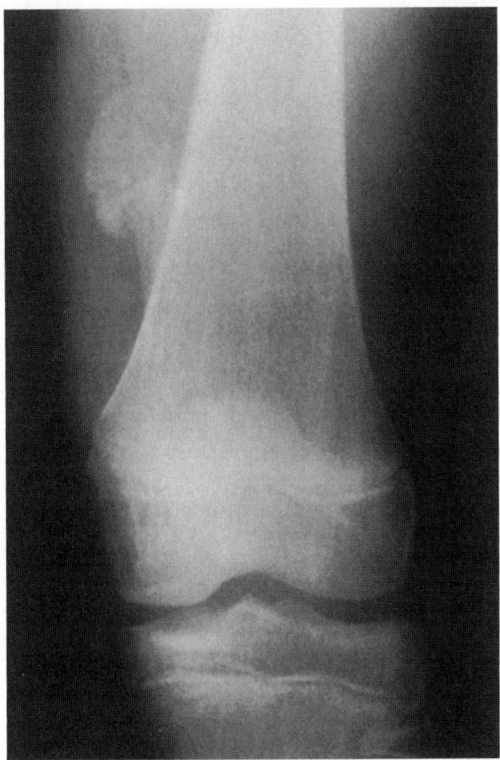

FIGURE 38–17 Anteroposterior radiograph of the distal left femur in a 12-year-old boy with a solitary osteochondroma. The osteochondroma extends medially and proximally on a pedunculated bony stalk. The boy complained of discomfort when the prominence was inadvertently bumped.

Sarcomatous Change

Malignant degeneration of a peripheral solitary osteochondroma leads to chondrosarcoma. However, malignant degeneration of solitary osteochondromas is rare, probably happening in less than 0.25% of lesions. Although Jaffe and Lichtenstein[235] stated that 1% undergo malignant change and Dahlin[113] reported an incidence of 4.1% in solitary osteochondromas treated surgically at the Mayo Clinic, these figures represent select cases referred to oncology centers. Malignant change evolves very slowly, usually occurring in adult life.[6,281,321,421] When malignant changes occur, the lesions become painful and show evidence of growth.

MRI has been found useful in evaluating possible sarcomatous deterioration. The imaging modality delineates extension of the tumor mass into the adjacent soft tissues and allows proper planning of a wide resection of an underlying chondrosarcoma. Scintigraphic imaging with technetium-99m methylene diphosphonate has not been shown qualitatively to differentiate benign active exostoses from chondrosarcoma.[218] Likewise, gallium scans cannot sufficiently distinguish between benign and sarcomatous lesions.[480] Imaging criteria differentiating osteochondroma from chondrosarcoma are provided in Table 38–1.

Biopsy before surgical excision of a presumed chondrosarcoma may be of limited value because there is

Table 38–1 Criteria Differentiating Osteochondroma from Chondrosarcoma

Criterion	Osteochondroma	Chondrosarcoma
Relation to parent bone	Continuity of cortex and medullary cavity with parent bone	Gradual loss of continuity of cortex
External surface of tumor	Distinct, well demarcated	Fuzzy and indistinct
Cartilaginous cap (best visualized on magnetic resonance imaging)	Thin, <1 cm	Thick, >3 cm, lobulated, extending into soft tissues
Matrix pattern	Dense at periphery with solid cortex Normal cancellous bone centrally	Periphery granular in appearance with small areas of rarefaction and disorganized calcification Later, blotchy areas of calcification within center of tumor with streaky densities extending peripherally
Adjacent soft tissue	Normal	Large soft tissue mass containing disorganized areas of calcification

Modified from Kenney PJ, Gilula LA, Murphy WA: The use of computed tomography to distinguish osteochondroma and chondrosarcoma. Radiology 1981;131:129.

a significant chance of a nonrepresentative biopsy and a potential risk of seeding the biopsy tract.[188] The prognosis after excision of a chondrosarcoma is excellent.

Treatment

Because a solitary osteochondroma is a benign tumor, it does not need to be surgically excised if it is asymptomatic. Excision usually is reserved for those lesions that cause pain or symptomatic impingement on neurovascular structures or that interfere with joint function. Pain usually becomes an issue when an osteochondroma is repeatedly bumped on its prominence, if a pedunculated base fractures after trauma, or if a painful bursa develops. Neurovascular impingement may include peroneal nerve compression at the knee, median nerve compression at the wrist, or, rarely, spinal cord compression from a vertebral osteochondroma.[63,160,187,275,373,428,470,479] Sometimes the osteochondroma is considered cosmetically unacceptable and the adolescent will ask to have it removed, preferring a scar to a bump. Finally, surgical excision is indicated any time there is a possibility of malignant transformation of an underlying osteochondroma, as demonstrated by an increase in the size of the lesion or in symptoms after skeletal maturity.

Excision of osteochondromas should, if possible, be postponed until later adolescence, for the following reasons. First, the growth potential of osteochondromas in younger children is unknown, and the full extent of the tumor cannot be appreciated until its growth potential is recognized. Second, because there are small pockets of cartilaginous cores within the spongiosa bone of osteochondromas in young children, the risk of local recurrence after excision is significant. In this situation, if the osteochondroma is removed, the perichondrium and the periosteum along the base of the lesion need to be excised. Finally, because of this dissection, the potential for growth arrest exists if the osteochondroma is very near a physis. In the maturing adolescent, the excision does not need to be quite as extensive because the potential for recurrence is considerably less. Surgical resection can be expected to result in a successful outcome for symptomatic osteochondromas with low morbidity.[58,147]

Occasionally a peripheral nerve (e.g., the peroneal nerve at the fibular head or the radial nerve along the humerus) may be close to the underlying lesion. Preliminary dissection of the nerve above the lesion can help avoid inadvertent injury to the nerve during excision of the osteochondroma. This anatomic situation, however, is more likely to occur with multiple hereditary exostoses than with a solitary osteochondroma.

Hereditary Multiple Exostoses

Incidence

Hereditary multiple exostoses is an autosomal dominant condition affecting numerous areas of the skeleton that have been preformed in cartilage. The overall prevalence approaches 1 in 50,000,[454] which doubles the previously reported prevalence of 1 in 100,000.[207,536] The disorder is known by a variety of terms: multiple hereditary osteochondromas, cartilaginous exostosis, diaphyseal aclasis (stressing abnormality of the modeling process), multiple osteochondromatosis, chondral osteoma, chondral osteogenic dysplasia of direction, deforming chondrodysplasia, hereditary deforming chondrodysplasia, and multiple cancellous exostoses.[406] The term most commonly used today, *hereditary multiple exostoses,* was proposed by Jaffe in 1943.[232]

The median age at the time of diagnosis in affected individuals is approximately 3 years. Hereditary multiple exostoses has a penetrance of 50% by 3 years of age. By the end of the first decade of life, 80% of affected persons will have exostoses. By 12 years of age, nearly all affected individuals have evidence of exostoses because penetrance of the disorder has been found to reach 96% to 100%[287,454,546] (Fig. 38–18). Although some

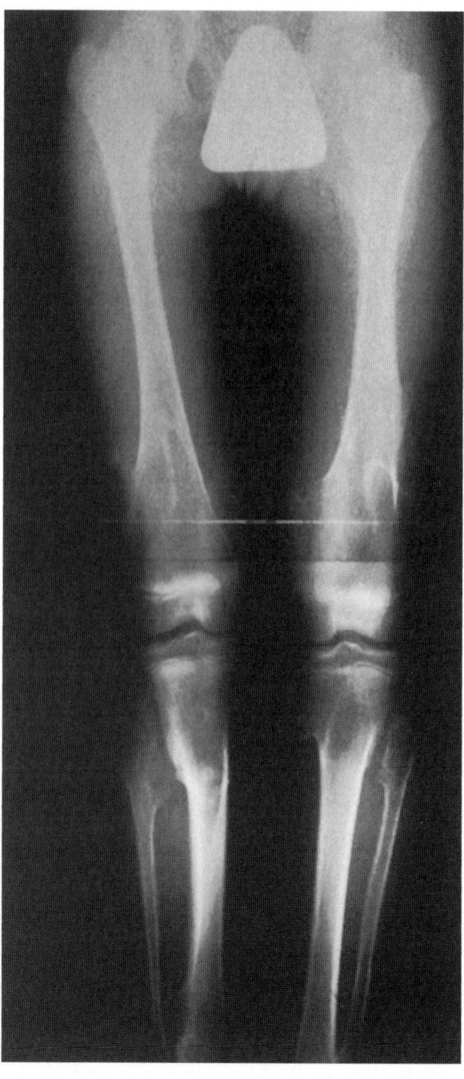

FIGURE 38–18 Hereditary multiple exostoses in a 12-year-old boy. Extensive involvement of the femora, tibiae, and fibulae was evident clinically and radiographically.

studies have reported that incomplete penetrance preferentially affects girls, other investigations have shown no such reduction.[454]

Etiology

The disorder is of autosomal dominant inheritance, with penetrance approaching 96%. If a person whose family is affected by hereditary multiple exostoses has not had an exostosis by 12 years of age, it is unlikely that exostoses will develop later. However, there remains a small risk that a particular individual will have affected children because the gene is nonpenetrant in approximately 4% of carriers. Approximately 10% of affected individuals have no family history of hereditary multiple exostoses.

Numerous genetic studies have found anomalies on chromosomes 8, 11, and 19, making this a genetically heterogeneous disorder.* Specifically, the three loci include 8q23-24.1 (*EXT1*), 11p11-13 (*EXT2*), and 19p (*EXT3*).[162,474] The *EXT1* and *EXT2* genes encode glycosyltransferases involved in the biosynthesis of heparan sulfate proteoglycans.[41,162,206,288,572] These proteoglycans, synthesized by chondrocytes and secreted to the extracellular matrix of the growth plate, play critical roles in growth plate signaling and remodeling necessary for normal endochondral ossification with the growth plate. Mutations of the *EXT1* and *EXT2* genes lead to absence of heparan sulfate (and thus, abnormal cell signaling) in the chondrocyte zones of exostosis growth plates.[206] The chondrocyte disorganization results in the development of the exostoses. The most severe forms of this disorder and malignant transformation of exostoses to chondrosarcomas are associated with the *EXT1* mutations.[162,413] A recent multigenerational study of patients with hereditary multiple exostoses reported a novel mutation, nt112delAT, in the *EXT2* gene.[538] Another gene, *EXTL* (or *EXT-like*), has been identified that shows a striking sequence similarity to both *EXT1* and *EXT2*.

Pathology

The gross pathologic and microscopic features of hereditary multiple exostoses are similar to those described for solitary osteochondromas.

Clinical Features

Multiple exostoses usually manifest during early childhood (although rarely before 2 years of age) with several knobby, hard, subcutaneous protuberances near the joints. Numerous sites can be involved. On presentation, five or six exostoses typically may be found, involving both the upper and lower extremities. The "knobby" appearance of the child is so characteristic that one can usually make the diagnosis by clinical inspection alone. Over time, the upper and lower extremities may appear short in relationship to the trunk. Shortening of the limbs is usually disproportionate. Approximately 10% of affected individuals have a lower limb length inequality. Patients are not considered dwarfs, and the trunk–limb growth difference usually does not become obvious until the pubertal growth spurt. The local presence of osteochondromas is consistently associated with growth disturbance. In particular, an inverse correlation between osteochondroma size and relative bone length exists, suggesting that the growth retardation in this condition may result from the local effects of enlarging osteochondromas rather than a skeletal dysplasia effect.[412,499] On occasion, concerned affected parents may bring in their normal-appearing child for screening. A recent report found that discomfort related to the multiple osteochondromas has been underestimated and that pain is often a problem that needs attention during care of these patients.[117]

For those affected with hereditary multiple exostoses, 70% have involvement of the distal femur, 70% the proximal tibia, and 30% the proximal fibula (Fig. 38–19). The likelihood of involvement near the knee in at least one of these three locations is approximately 94%. The proximal humerus is affected in 50% of cases, the scapula and ribs in 40%, the distal radius and ulna in 30%, the proximal femur in 30%, the phalanges in 30%, the distal fibula in 25%, the distal tibia in 20%, and the bones in the foot in 10% to 25%.[454] Tibiofibular synostosis often develops from chronic apposition of osteochondromas proximally or distally but rarely causes symptoms or functional impairment.

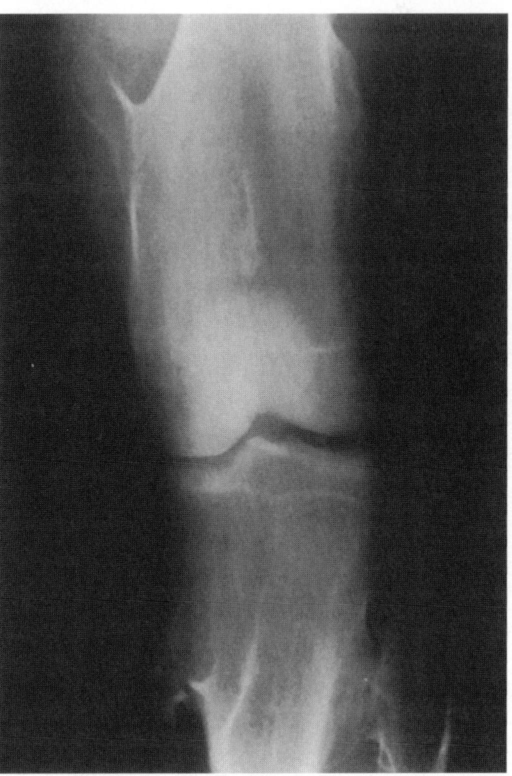

FIGURE 38–19 Osteochondromas are seen involving the femur, tibia, and fibula.

*See references 8, 48, 65, 88, 110, 162, 282, 299, 408, 414, 474, 512, 545, 550, 560, 561.

As the lesions enlarge, they may cause discomfort secondary to pressure on adjacent soft tissues, and they may hinder normal joint mobility.

Osteochondromas of the proximal humerus are often readily palpable but rarely cause neurologic dysfunction (Fig. 38–20). However, because of their proximity to major nerves, great care must be taken if resection is necessary. The scapula is involved in 40% of affected individuals, with osteochondromas located on the anterior or the posterior aspect of the scapula. The presence of osteochondromas on the anterior aspect of the scapula may lead to discomfort during scapulothoracic motion. Winging of the scapula due to the presence of osteochondromas has been described.[116]

Obvious deformity in the forearm is seen in 39% to 60% of patients.[406,454,497] The ulna is shorter than the radius and the radius is bowed laterally, with its concavity toward the short ulna (Fig. 38–21). Often the distal end of the ulna is more severely affected than the distal end of the radius, leading to this discrepancy in length. A mild flexion deformity of the elbow is usually present. Loss of forearm pronation and supination occurs with increasing age.[497] Dislocation of the radial head occurs and is usually associated with a negative ulnar variance. The resulting forearm deformities are usually asymmetric. Often, the patient's main complaint is an undesirable cosmetic appearance. The natural history of these deformities has been described as progressive, with variable weakness,

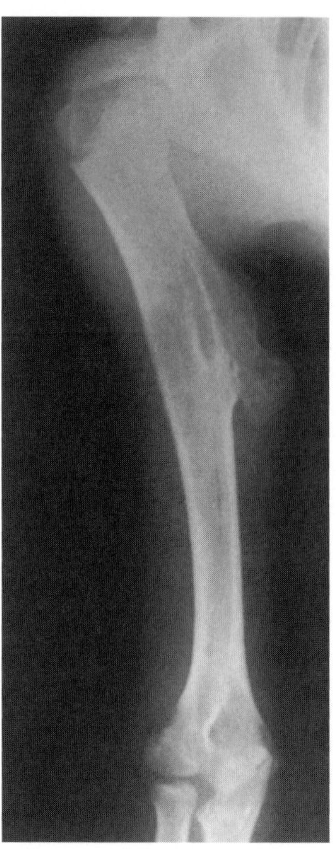

FIGURE 38–20 This exostosis on the medial aspect of the proximal humerus was minimally symptomatic.

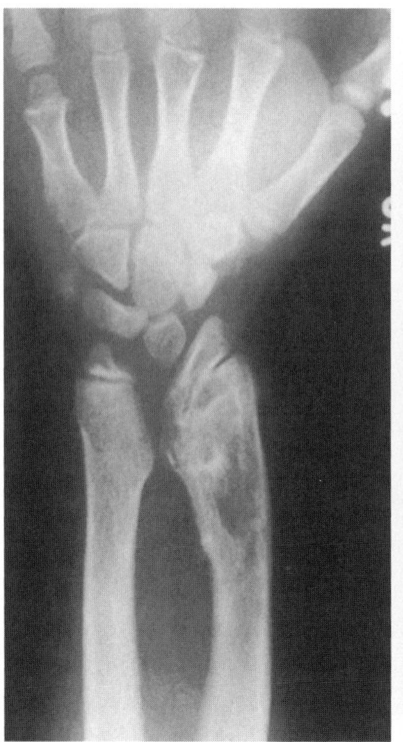

A

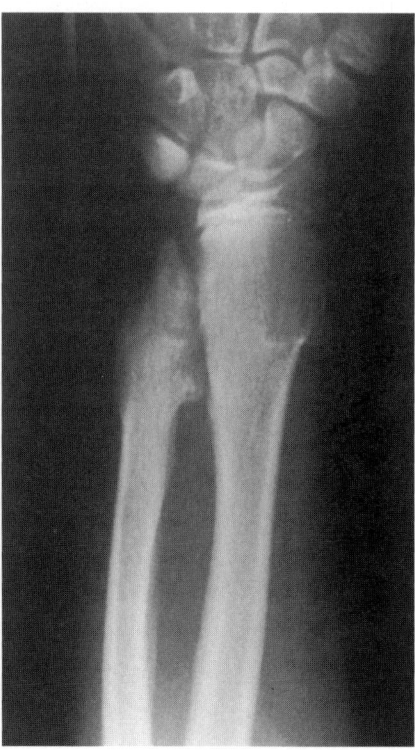

B

FIGURE 38–21 Two wrist deformities in a brother and sister. **A,** In the boy, the distal radius exhibited growth arrest on the ulnar aspect with associated compensation at the wrist joint. **B,** In the girl, the distal ulna was short due to growth arrest.

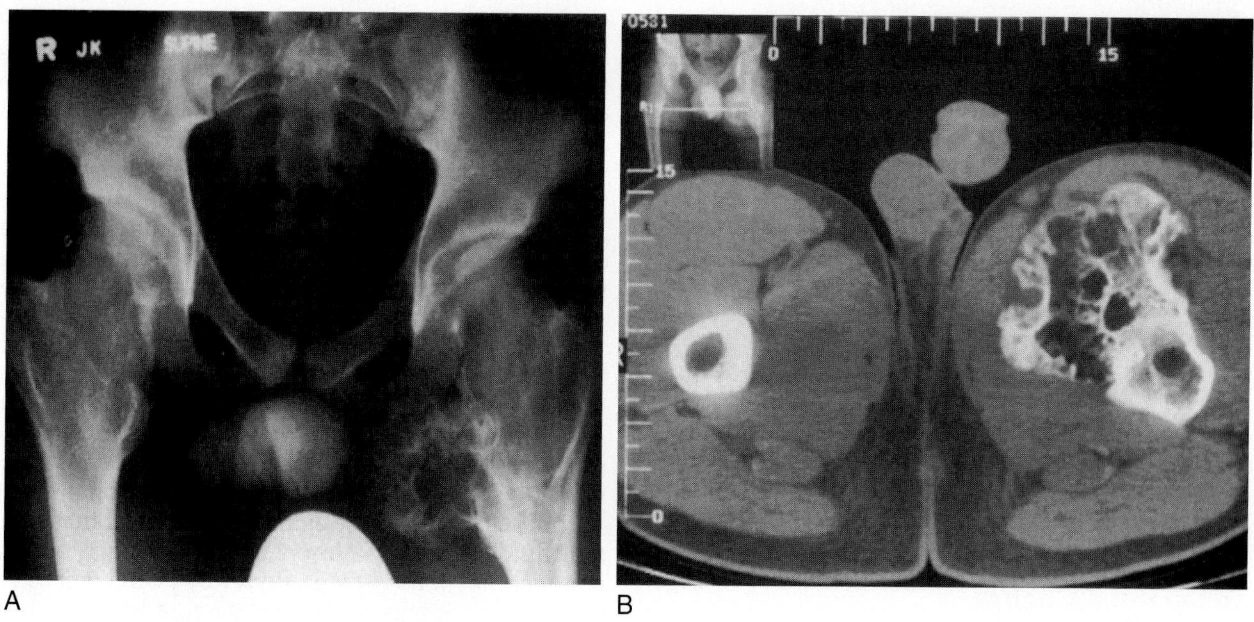

FIGURE 38-22 **A,** Anteroposterior pelvic radiograph showing abnormal proximal femora due to hereditary multiple exostoses. **B,** Computed tomography scans of the hip region clearly demonstrated the 10-cm sessile osteochondroma on the left femur.

functional impairment, and worsening cosmetic deformity of the extremity. Some authors, however, report that the deformities are well tolerated and lead to little loss of function.[497] A recent study evaluating the forearm in untreated adults with hereditary multiple osteochondromatosis found that most were employed in careers of their choice, participated in recreational activities, and were free of pain.[366] Objective measurement of function demonstrated greater disability than that found from subjective reporting.

Deformity of the hand is uncommon. The main area of involvement appears to be around the metacarpophalangeal joint, but the proximal interphalangeal joint is the most common site of deformity. Metacarpal shortening usually does not cause functional problems and does not need to be treated. Angular deformity, although uncommon, does cause problems and requires surgical intervention. There is no evidence that deformity can be prevented by early excision of the osteochondromas.[555]

In the lower extremity, valgus of the proximal tibia is frequently present and is nearly always found in the proximal metaphyseal region of the tibia. The valgus progressively increases during growth spurts. Occasionally there is some angulation distally at the femur, and there may be recurrent dislocation of the patella.[355]

Osteochondromas of the proximal femur may lead to progressive hip dysplasia,[156,411] which occasionally requires corrective varus osteotomy (Fig. 38–22). Adverse effects on femoral growth are less with proximal involvement than with distal involvement.

Although osteochondromas near the ankle are not uncommon, the reported prevalence of ankle deformities ranges widely, from 2% to 54%.[406,454,487] The characteristic ankle valgus deformity is often accompanied by decreased ankle motion. This deformity is caused either by retardation of the normal distal fibular growth or by deficient growth of the lateral half of the distal tibial epiphysis. The severity of the ankle valgus varies, as the distal fibular physis progressively rises in relation to the tibiotalar articular space.[468] A natural history study of the lower extremity in patients with multiple exostoses found measurable decreases in ankle function and suggested that correction/prevention of excessive tibiotalar tilt may be warranted to improve outcome.[365]

There have been numerous reports of spinal cord impingement by vertebral osteochondromas.* The cervical, thoracic, or lumbar region can be affected. Lower extremity discomfort associated with decreased balance, impaired coordination, spastic paraparesis, or other central neurologic dysfunction should raise the consideration of a vertebral osteochondroma. The presence and extent of the lesion are best delineated with CT, whereas MRI of the spinal cord demonstrates the area of spinal cord impingement.

Radiographic Findings

Unlike solitary osteochondromas, hereditary multiple exostoses involve a significantly greater portion of the metaphysis or diaphysis and are generally more irregular in shape. Over time, lesions that begin in the metaphyseal region migrate into the diaphysis of the long bones. The exostoses vary in number, size, and configuration. Like solitary osteochondromas, they may be sessile or pedunculated, cauliflower-like, or

*See references 28, 146, 151, 242, 270, 336, 338, 341, 420, 469.

even narrow with a pointed end. They nearly always point away from the physis. In nearly 95% of cases, evidence of the osteochondroma will be found around the knee. Thus, the disorder can often be confirmed with radiographs of the knee. Irregular zones of calcification may be present, particularly in the cartilaginous cap. In older individuals, however, extensive calcification with changes in the shape of the cartilaginous caps suggests possible malignant degeneration.

Differential Diagnosis

The numerous lesions associated with hereditary multiple exostoses make the radiographic findings pathognomonic of the disorder. If painful growth of an osteochondroma becomes evident in a skeletally mature individual with hereditary multiple exostoses, chondrosarcomatous transformation must be ruled out.

Sarcomatous Change

Transformation of a lesion in hereditary multiple exostoses to chondrosarcoma during childhood is exceedingly rare.[406] In general, transformation in adulthood remains uncommon, with current reports indicating the risk to be 0.9% to 5%.[177,408,454,546] The apparent risk of malignant degeneration may become greater as the duration of follow-up increases. In Schmale and associates' 1994 study, two thirds of the individuals with transformations were younger than 40 years of age when the authors reported an incidence of 0.9%.[454] At this time, the lifetime risk of chondrosarcoma is estimated to be approximately 1% to 2%. The genetic abnormalities found on chromosomes 8 and 11 (*EXT1* and *EXT2*) may play a role in the development of chondrosarcomas.[427] Malignant transformation is more frequently associated with the *EXT1* mutations.[162,413]

The most frequent sign of sarcomatous change is a painful, enlarging mass, usually one of long duration.[334] The relative frequency of chondrosarcomas is reported to be highest with osteochondromas of the pelvis or shoulder girdle.[260] The clinical course of the tumor is slow, and metastasis, usually to the lungs, occurs late.

If the cartilaginous cap of the exostoses exceeds 1 cm in thickness, malignancy should be suspected. Inadequate surgical removal almost always results in recurrence. Patient prognosis is good if metastasis has not occurred. Radiation therapy has no effect on the tumor.

Treatment

The only treatment for hereditary multiple exostoses is surgery. Because the exostoses are numerous and many are asymptomatic, a cautious approach is warranted. The mere presence of an osteochondroma is not an indication for surgery. Reasonable indications include (1) pain from external trauma or irritation of surrounding soft tissues; (2) growth disturbance leading to angular deformity or limb length discrepancy; (3) joint motion compromised by juxta-articular lesions; (4) soft tissue (tendon, nerve, or vessel) impingement or tethering; (5) spinal cord compression; (6) false aneurysm produced by an osteochondroma; (7) painful bursa formation; (8) obvious cosmetic deformity; and (9) a rapid increase in the size of a lesion.[406] During childhood, numerous operations may be necessary, and this prospect should be discussed in detail with the parents soon after the disorder is diagnosed. Life expectancy is normal unless malignant degeneration of an osteochondroma has occurred and metastases have developed.

Osteochondromas involving the forearm frequently lead to surgical intervention. Early excision of the lesions on the radius and ulna does not alter or correct existing deformity, but it may delay progression of the deformity.[407] If ulnar shortening has occurred with bowing of the radius, lengthening of the ulna combined with distal radial hemiepiphyseal stapling has been found effective in correcting the deformity. Ulnar lengthening is best done gradually by distraction osteogenesis.[112,422] Spontaneous regression of an osteochondroma of the radius after lengthening of the ulna has even been reported.[491] Reduction of the ulnar inclination of the radius to normal values by corrective distal radial osteotomy may restore a more physiologic range of motion and decrease wrist pain.[157] Creation of a "one-bone forearm" has been successful as a salvage procedure for severely affected forearms.[435] Deformities of the forearm should be treated early and aggressively in an effort to prevent further progression and to reduce disability. A prominent, symptomatic, dislocated radial head can be safely excised after skeletal maturity.[27]

Marked shortening of the humerus may result from a proximal physeal growth disturbance. If the discrepancy is significant, distraction osteogenesis has been successful in increasing the length of the humerus.

For skeletally mature individuals with significant genu valgum, varus osteotomy of the proximal tibia can result in an improved appearance. However, if an osteochondroma is present in the proximal fibula, any osteotomy of the proximal tibia or fibula carries a significant risk of peroneal nerve palsy.[549] In the skeletally immature patient, stapling along the medial side of the proximal tibial physis or distal femoral physis may be sufficient to correct the valgus. If correction is achieved by this method, the staples should be left in longer (slight overcorrection) to prevent recurrence of the deformity after staple removal.

Ankle valgus is treated either by medial distal tibial physeal arrest in the skeletally immature patient or by a varus corrective osteotomy in the more mature individual[487] (Fig. 38–23). Tibiofibular synostoses frequently occur distally, but there usually are no symptoms or functional impairment from this occurrence and the condition does not need to be surgically treated.

SOLITARY ENCHONDROMA

Incidence

Intramedullary cartilaginous solitary enchondromas are relatively common, accounting for approximately

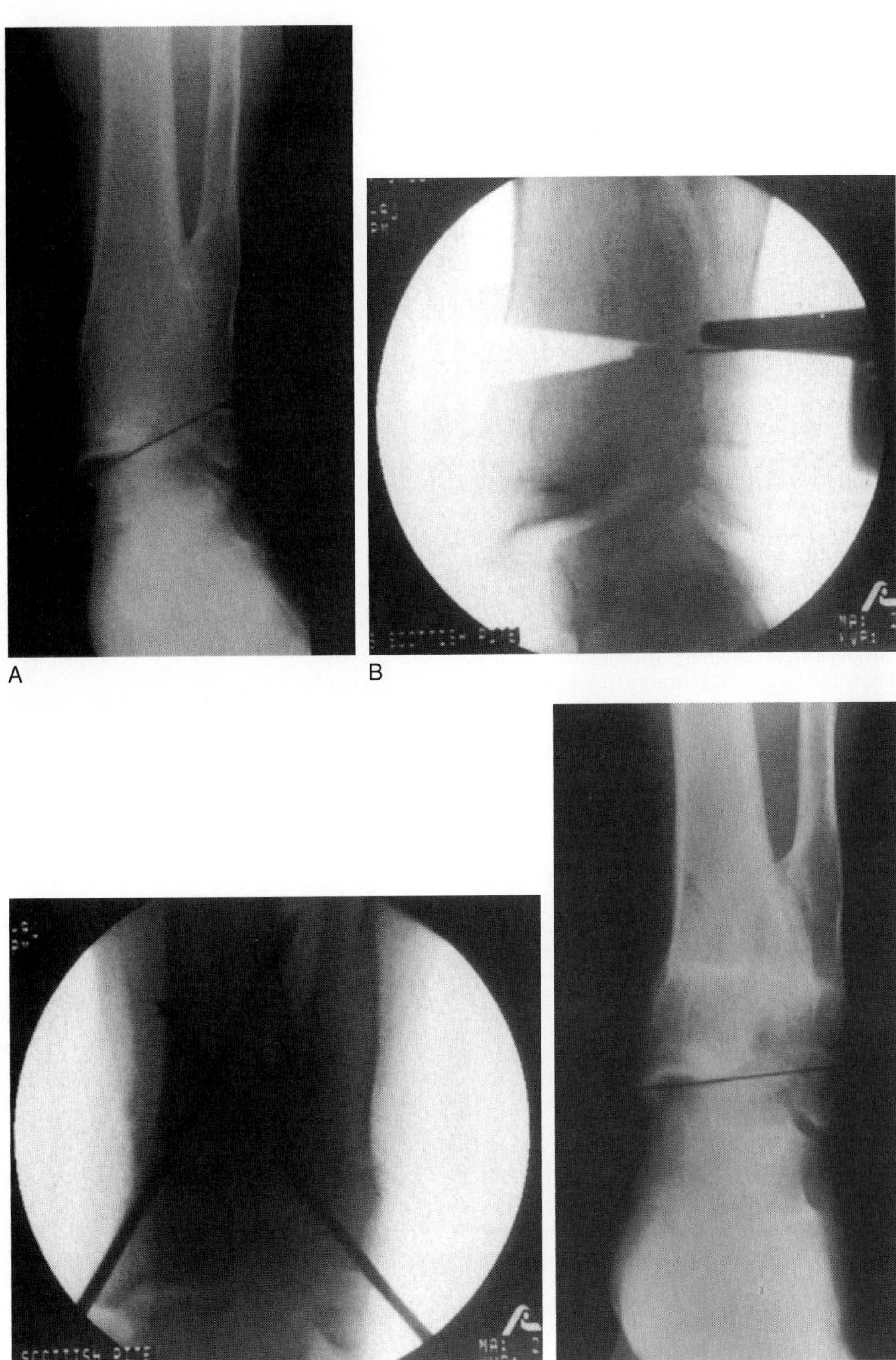

FIGURE 38-23 **A,** Excessive ankle valgus accompanied by a distal tibiofibular synostosis led to discomfort. **B** through **D,** A varus closing wedge osteotomy in the distal tibiofibular region resulted in improved alignment and resolution of the patient's discomfort.

one fourth of all benign tumors. Unlike multiple enchondromatosis, which is frequently diagnosed during childhood, solitary enchondromas are usually diagnosed after the second decade of life.[189] The peak age of presentation is approximately 35 years.

Pathology

Enchondromas appear as glistening white, grayish-white, or pearly tissues that have a gritty feel on palpation owing to the intrinsic calcification.[511] The tumor is easily cut with a knife, as if it were soft chalk.

Histologically, enchondromas are proliferating nests of cartilage cells that lack obvious atypia.[68] Foci of calcification are present. Plates of lamellar bone surround the lobules of cartilage in a partial to complete circumferential manner.[340] Invasive infiltration of the bone marrow spaces is not characteristic of benign solitary enchondromas.

Although mitotic figures within the dysplastic cartilaginous lesions may be found in specimens from growing children, the likelihood of malignancy is low. In the adult, however, it may be difficult to differentiate an enchondroma from a low-grade sarcoma. In general, small peripheral cartilage tumors are usually benign, whereas the large axial tumors in the adult are more likely to be malignant. A malignant change of a solitary enchondroma in childhood or adolescence would be a rare event.

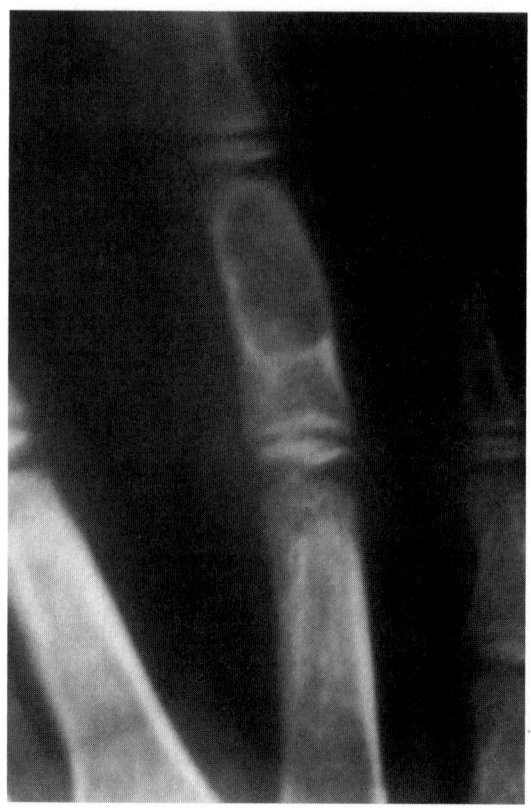

FIGURE 38–24 A solitary enchondroma in the middle phalanx of the ring finger. Radiographs showed a well-delineated lucent lesion with an intact cortical rim. It was noticed because of mild, painless swelling of the digit.

Clinical Features

Nearly 50% of diagnosed solitary enchondromas occur in the hand, involving the phalanges in particular. The carpal bones are occasionally affected.[430] Of the long tubular bones, the femur and humerus are frequent sites of localization. Occasionally the ribs, sternum, innominate bones, and vertebral columns may also be affected.

Clinically, enchondromas in the fingers are usually diagnosed after local trauma. Some patients, however, present with a firm, local swelling in the region of the affected phalanx or metacarpal without a fracture or local pain. Nearly 75% of patients with enchondromas involving the hands or feet have a solitary lesion. The remaining patients have multiple enchondromatosis. When the solitary enchondroma involves the femur or humerus, it is usually quiescent, with no clinical signs evident until adulthood.[293]

Radiographic Findings

Solitary enchondromas usually appear as well-delineated, lucent defects in the metaphyseal region of long bones. In the phalanges of the hand or foot, the entire shaft may be involved. The cortical rim is usually intact unless a fracture has occurred through the weakened bone (Fig. 38–24). Calcification is usually present within the lesion and appears as fine punctate stippling. In the larger long bones, calcification may be more pronounced, which can make the differentiation between enchondroma and bone infarct difficult.[68] Most lesions are 3 to 4 cm, with a range of 1 to 8 cm.[339] There usually is no evidence of focal cortical erosion, scalloping of the cortex, significant cortical thickening, or bone expansion. In the older symptomatic adolescent, cortical thinning and expansion in the larger long bones can be troubling because these radiographic findings may represent features of low-grade chondrosarcoma.

CT is useful for evaluating cartilaginous tumors, especially in the long bones, pelvis, and spine. Technetium bone scanning generally is not necessary when evaluating a child with presumed enchondroma.

Differential Diagnosis

Confusion between an enchondroma and a bone infarct may occur when the radiolucent lesion has a significant amount of calcification. However, in general, the calcification seen with bone infarcts is more peripherally located. In the phalanges of the hand and foot, solitary enchondromas may be difficult to differentiate from epithelial inclusion cysts. In a metacarpal, it may be difficult to distinguish a solitary enchondroma from a small solitary bone cyst, a nonossifying fibroma, or a focus of fibrous dysplasia.

Treatment

For solitary enchondromas in the hand, complete curettage followed by autogenous bone grafting usually results in cure. However, recurrences may occur many years after excision and go undetected until they cause widening or cortical erosion of the phalanx or metacarpal.[179] Similar treatment is undertaken for solitary enchondromas in the long bones, where the recurrence rate remains low. If an en bloc wide excision were performed, the recurrence rate would be even lower. However, the possibly unacceptable postoperative functional deficit makes this more aggressive approach unnecessary.

The risk of malignant degeneration of an isolated enchondroma is rare in childhood.[348] However, these lesions should have regular radiographic follow-up. Enchondromas in the pelvis, scapulae, sternum, vertebrae, and proximal areas of the large long bones have a greater likelihood of malignant transformation in adulthood.

Multiple Enchondromatosis (Ollier's Disease) and Maffucci's Syndrome

Ollier in 1889 described a condition of multiple, typically unilateral enchondromas associated with deformity of the extremity.[377] He referred to the condition as *dyschondroplasia,* implying that it resulted from a developmental defect related to abnormal growth of cartilage.[339]

Pathology

On gross inspection of the lesions, the bones show numerous islands of glistening cartilage, which are usually located in the diaphyseal and metaphyseal regions. Infrequently, abnormal cartilage may also be seen in the epiphyseal region. This close proximity of the tumor to the physis can lead to profound inhibition of growth, resulting in severe limb length discrepancies or angular deformities. As longitudinal growth continues, the abnormal enchondroma cartilage derived near the epiphyseal plate forms long linear masses within the shaft. This phenomenon is seen only in Ollier's disease and explains the pathognomonic "fanlike" metaphyseal septation seen on radiographs. The dense lines represent bone formed by normal enchondral ossification, and the intervening columns of lucency represent the epiphyseally derived areas of abnormal cartilage.[340]

The histologic features in multiple enchondromatosis generally resemble those of a solitary enchondroma. However, in multiple enchondromatosis the appearance might be that of a highly cellular lesion with ominous nuclei mimicking a low-grade chondrosarcoma. Eventual malignant transformation into chondrosarcomas has been reported to occur in 20% to 33% of those affected. Therefore, communication among the surgeon, pathologist, and radiologist is imperative when making the diagnosis in the older adolescent or adult. In general, aggressive histologic findings are likely to represent a benign lesion if the biopsy site is the hand rather than the long bones or the pelvis. Conversely, if the biopsy site is the pelvis or larger bones, suspicion of low-grade sarcomas is higher. The atypical cellular features in Ollier's disease may explain the relatively high incidence of chondrosarcomatous transformation in older individuals who are moderately or severely affected.

Clinical Features

Multiple enchondromatosis is an uncommon, nonhereditary disorder. The physical signs related to this condition commonly begin in childhood and vary with the extent of the lesions and their effect on the weakened bones. The number of bones affected can vary greatly, with the phalanges, femur, and tibia most commonly affected (Fig. 38–25). Because of the tendency toward unilateral involvement, severe lower limb length discrepancies and angular deformities result, with a noted increased incidence of varus angulation in the lower femur.[96] Discrepancies may be in the range of 10 to 25 cm by maturity. Deformity and enlargement of fingers may impair normal function. Forearm abnormalities such as bowing, limited rotation, and ulnar deviation of the hand may be evident.

Maffucci's syndrome is a condition of enchondromatosis associated with multiple hemangiomas involving soft tissue.[7,30,197,246] They may be associated with superficial phleboliths, which can appear on radiographs as roundish opacities in the soft tissues. Hemangiomas have also been noted to occur within internal organs. Because of this, total-body MRI has been recommended to detect asymptomatic lesions that will thus alter the diagnosis to Maffucci's syndrome and change the prognosis.[7] Multiple pigmented nevi and vitiligo are other occasional nonskeletal manifestations. An abnormality in neuropeptides appears to stimulate growth of abnormal blood vessels.[434]

Another related entity, *generalized enchondromatosis,* represents a more severe expression of the disorder. Nearly all of the metaphyseal regions in all of the long and short tubular bones are affected.[403]

Radiographic Findings

Bone abnormalities are usually more extensive than the physical examination would suggest. In the long bones, enchondromatosis is recognized as radiolucent longitudinal streaks that involve the metaphysis and extend down into the diaphysis. Epiphyses are usually not affected but may be involved.[171] The cortex overlying the enchondroma is usually thin, and calcification within the lesion is common. Significant shortening and angular deformity are frequently noted in the involved long bones, whether in the hands, feet, or limbs.

CT is useful for evaluating multiple enchondromatosis, particularly in the long bones and pelvis. CT

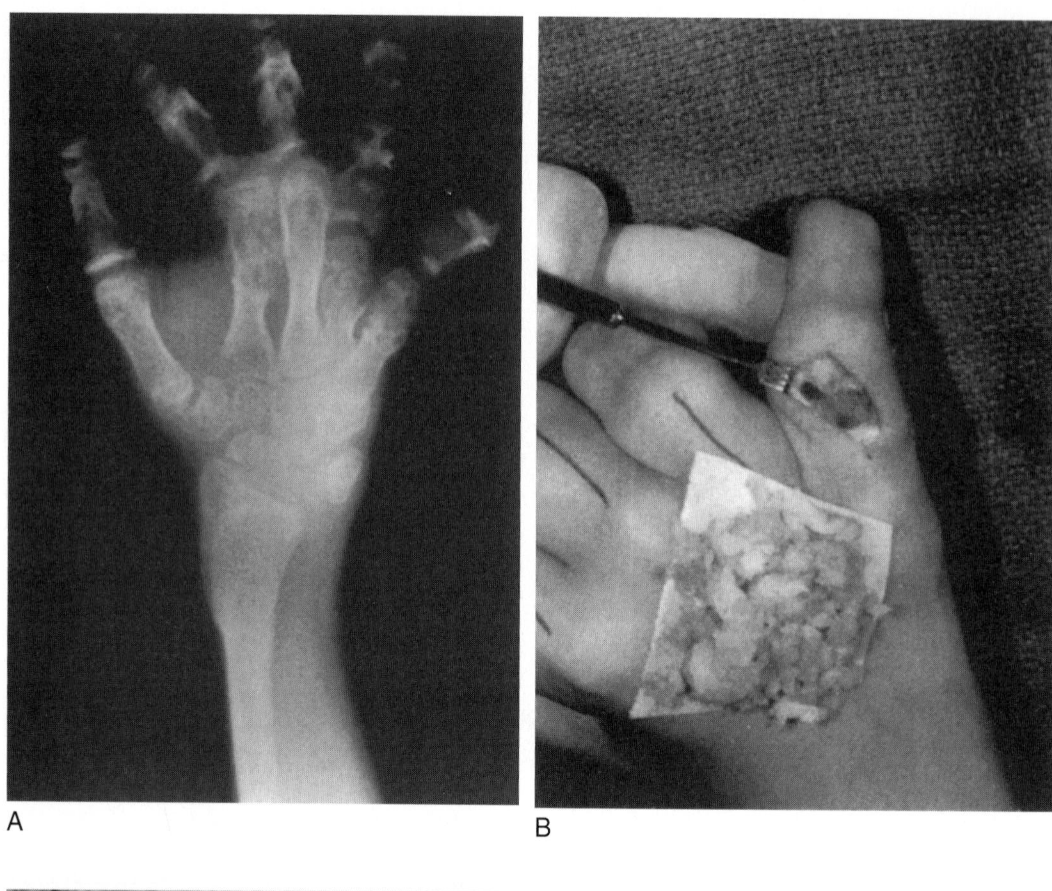

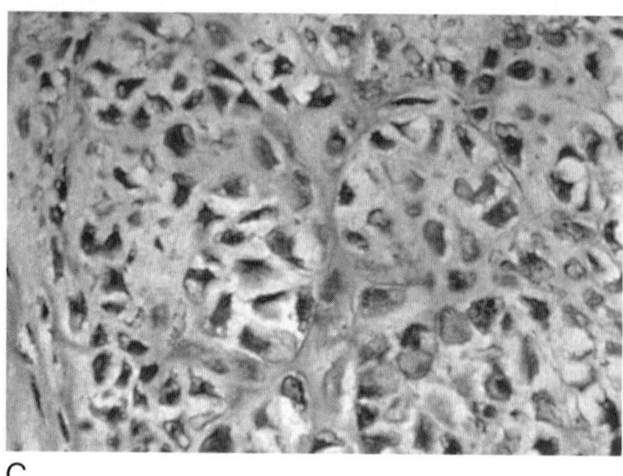

FIGURE 38-25 A young boy with Ollier's disease. **A,** Anteroposterior radiograph. All of the metacarpals and phalanges in the hand were affected. **B,** After curettage of the proximal phalanx of the little finger, glistening white tumor was evident. **C,** Histologic examination demonstrated the proliferative nests of cartilage cells.

clarifies cortical and osteal scalloping better than plain radiography and allows precise comparisons to be made over time.

Sarcomatous Change

The incidence of secondary chondrosarcoma in patients with Ollier's disease is approximately 25% to 30% by 40 years of age.[60,81,303,364,424,460,502] Those patients with Maffucci's syndrome have a similar or higher likelihood of development of malignant degeneration,[11,39] with Schwartz and associates reporting a nearly 100% expectation.[460] Over the long term, periodic surveillance of the brain and abdomen for occult malignant lesions is indicated in patients who have enchondromatosis.[221,333,424] Increased localized growth of a lesion in an extremity accompanied by pain is the hallmark of possible malignancy. In such a situation, biopsy of the lesion is indicated. Hematopoietic malignancies (acute lymphoid leukemia and chronic myeloid leukemia) have been described in association with both Ollier's disease and Maffucci's syndrome.[29,429]

Treatment

Because of the extent of the disease, multiple enchondromatosis cannot be cured by curettage and bone grafting. The numerous deformities that often accompany multiple enchondromatosis require repeated operative interventions over several years to correct the angular deformities and achieve similar limb lengths at maturity.[96,390,467] These procedures include

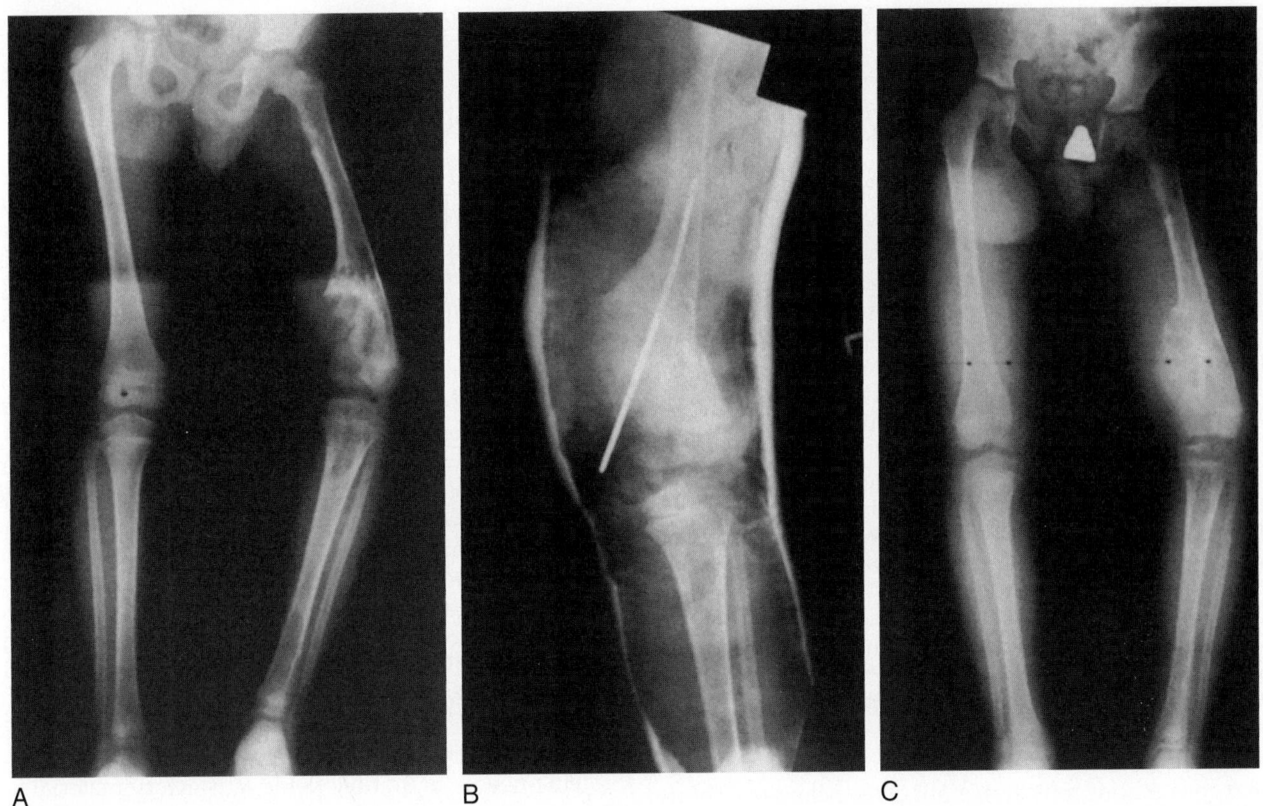

FIGURE 38–26 Findings in a 4-year-old boy with Ollier's disease. **A,** Radiograph demonstrating unilateral left lower extremity involvement. **B,** A valgus osteotomy of the distal femur was performed to correct the notable genu varum. **C,** Two years later, the genu varum recurred, owing to the abnormal growth at the distal femoral physis. Another osteotomy was planned; future limb lengthening will be needed.

osteotomies, limb lengthenings, and epiphysiodeses (Fig. 38–26). Clinicians should be aware of a 0.6-year delay in bone age when planning an epiphysiodesis in children with cartilaginous dysplasias.[306] In the older child, use of the Ilizarov apparatus is the best method to achieve both angular correction and equalization of limb lengths.[106,241,264] Use of multiple wires or half-pins allows sufficient purchase in the enchondromatous bone so that lengthenings can be successfully achieved.

CHONDROBLASTOMA

Incidence

Chondroblastomas are uncommon benign cellular cartilage tumors that are most often located in the epiphyses of the long bone of the extremities.[277,278,423,457] Chondroblastomas are twice as common in male as in female patients. The peak age of occurrence is in the second decade, with the majority of patients presenting before 30 years of age.

Chondroblastoma was first described in detail by Codman in 1931.[103] He called the lesion an *epiphyseal chondromatous giant cell tumor.* Before his description, the tumors were often thought to represent chondrosarcomas. Today, chondroblastomas are still occasionally referred to as Codman's tumor.

Etiology

Jaffe and Lichtenstein conjectured that the lesion arises from cartilage "germ cells" or cells of the epiphyseal cartilage.[235] However, because of reports of the lesion involving the skull or rib (where cartilage "germ cells" would not likely be found), this hypothesis is difficult to confirm.

The biologic nature of chondroblastomas and their histogenetic origin continue to be a matter of debate. Abnormalities in chromosomes 5 and 8 have been reported in chondroblastoma; however, specific locations have not been clearly identified.[507] Cytogenetic and spectral analyses of chondroblastomas have revealed diploid karyotypes with relatively simple karyotypes. Recurrent breakout points have been found at 2q35, 3q21-23, and 18q21.[483] Another study reports that a receptor activator of NF-κB ligand (RANKL), which is a key molecule essential for regulating osteoclast formation and activity, may be involved in the formation of chondroblastomas.[216]

Pathology

Gross specimens obtained at curettage are often characterized by pieces of gray-pink or hemorrhagic tissues intermixed with gritty, calcified, cholesterol-laden

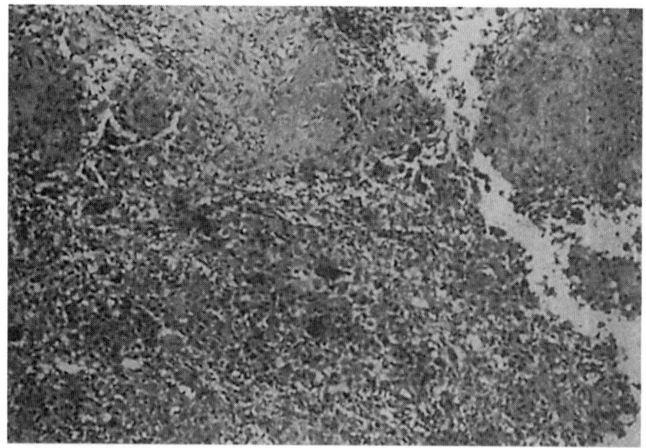

FIGURE 38–27 Histologic evaluation of chondroblastoma shows polygonal cells (chondroblasts), giant cells, islands of chondroid or hyaline cartilage, and "chicken-wire" calcification.

tissues. There may be small islands of bluish to white chondroid. Because chondroblastomas are often found to contain cystic or degenerative areas, the amount of tissue removed may be less than expected based on the radiographic appearance.

Histologically, the tumor is characterized by polygonal cells (chondroblasts), giant cells, islands of chondroid or hyaline cartilage, "chicken-wire" calcification, and nodules of calcification in the stroma[150,170,416] (Fig. 38–27). The chicken-wire calcification results when lacelike deposits of calcium are intermixed on the intercellular chondroid matrix.

A small percentage of chondroblastomas may be primarily cystic or hemorrhagic, making differentiation from aneurysmal bone cysts difficult histologically. Another, more worrisome tumor, clear cell chondrosarcoma, may histologically resemble chondroblastoma. However, clear cell chondrosarcomas occur in adults with closed physes, and their radiographic appearance and clinical presentation would not be consistent with chondroblastomas.

Clinical Features

The most common locations are the proximal humerus, distal femur, and proximal tibia.[423] Chondroblastomas have also been found in the skull, maxilla, temporal bone, ribs, pelvis, hands, patella, talus, calcaneus, and throughout the spine.* Multifocal benign chondroblastomas have been reported. Nonepiphyseal locations in the long bones have been described.[66]

Symptoms usually are mild, consisting of pain and localized tenderness. The discomfort is often present for 6 months to several years before diagnosis. Because the lesion is epiphyseal, the adjacent joint may be swollen and have limited range of motion. If tumor is present in a lower extremity, an antalgic limp may be evident. Pathologic fractures are uncommon. Neurologic deficits can occur if the vertebrae are involved.

*See references 49, 100, 120, 126, 158, 178, 200, 223, 292, 362, 417, 457, 511, 554, 570.

Radiographic Findings

Chondroblastomas are usually located in the epiphyses, but they may extend into the metaphyseal region (Fig. 38–28). They are usually eccentric, involving less than one half of the entire epiphysis. The lesion is rimmed by a border of host bone sclerosis, and small punctate calcifications are present in the tumor. Commonly, the physis adjacent to the lesion is present at the time of diagnosis. If all of these features are present, this radiographic appearance is pathognomonic for chondroblastoma.[339]

CT clearly demonstrates the extent of the lesion within the epiphyseal region and its proximity to the physis or subarticular surface.

MRI findings associated with chondroblastoma have been reported.[382,543,566] Adjacent bone marrow and soft tissue edema, as well as periosteal reactions, are more dramatically demonstrated on MRI than on plain radiographs. Bone marrow edema is common. Knowledge of the MRI findings of chondroblastoma may allow for more accurate diagnosis and help to avoid confusion with infection or aggressive neoplasms.

Fine-needle aspiration yields satisfactory material for interpretation and confirmation of the diagnosis.[153,203,259]

Differential Diagnosis

The differential diagnosis includes giant cell tumors, enchondromas, synovial lesions (e.g., pigmented villonodular synovitis, rheumatoid arthritis), and atypically located eosinophilic granuloma. An epiphyseal osteoblastoma-like osteosarcoma with strong similarities to chondroblastoma has been reported.[54]

Treatment

Complete curettage and excision of the lesion (using a high-speed bur) is often successful.[214,423] The surgeon should avoid interfering with the joint surface or disturbing the physes in the immature skeleton. The defect is filled with either autogenous or allograft bone. Although there is a definite risk of recurrence after intracapsular curettage, one study reported local control in approximately 80% of cases.[522] Preservation of the physis should be considered a secondary concern compared with complete and thorough excision of the chondroblastoma.[90] If the tumor is beneath articular cartilage, adequate excision may occasionally require removal of some of the joint cartilage. Arthroscopy has been used as an adjunct in the excision of lesions in the proximal tibia and proximal femur.[104,515]

Occasional chondroblastomas require wide marginal resection, especially those that have recurred locally. Reconstruction after marginal or wide en bloc resection usually requires a partial or full osteoarticular allograft.

Chondroblastomas have been known to undergo benign pulmonary metastasis.[238,354] When found in the

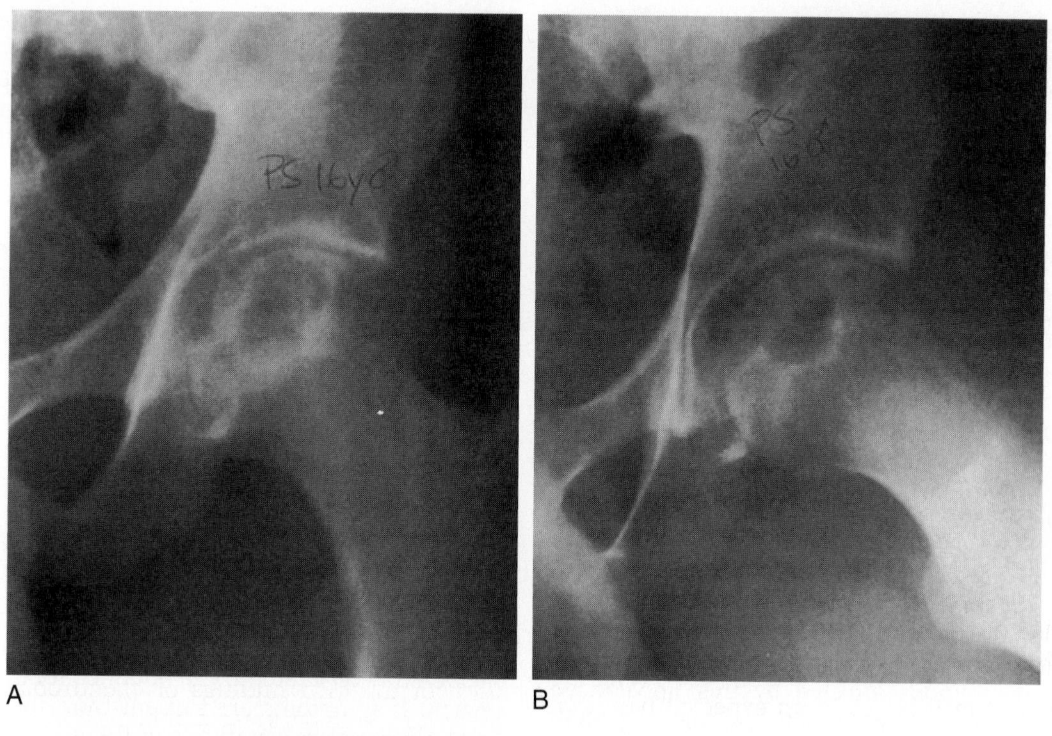

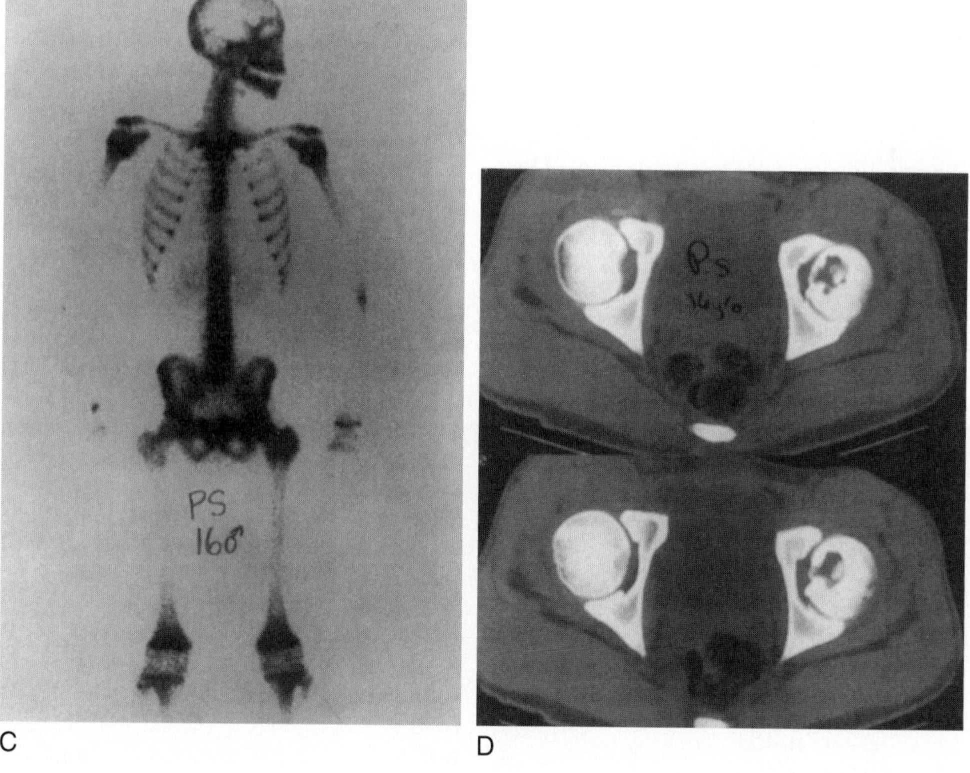

FIGURE 38–28 Chondroblastoma. Anteroposterior **(A)** and lateral **(B)** radiographs of the left hip in a 16-year-old girl showing a subchondral radiolucent lesion in the femoral head (epiphyseal region) that is rimmed by a border of host bone sclerosis. **C,** Bone scan shows significant uptake in the left femoral head. **D,** Computed tomography of the hips shows calcification within the lesion.

lung, these metastases are usually rimmed with bone. When identified, these lesions should be surgically removed to ensure proper diagnosis.

Chondromyxoid Fibroma

Incidence

Chondromyxoid fibromas are rare, benign tumors representing less than 0.4% of primary bone tumors sampled for biopsy.[339,361] They consist mainly of cartilaginous tissue intermixed with areas of myxomatous and fibrous elements. The myxomatous components are probably due to degeneration of chondroid tissue, whereas the fibrous component may result from repair of the degenerated areas.

Etiology

Cytogenetic analysis of chondromyxoid fibromas has found an unbalanced reciprocal translocation between the short arm of chromosome 3 and the long arm of chromosome 6. Two known cartilage-related genes are located in the regions affected by this unbalanced rearrangement. These genes function to control growth and maturation of endochondral bone, the site of origin of cartilaginous tumors.[199] A specific matrix composition, not seen in other mesenchymal neoplasms, has been found in chondromyxoid fibroma.[489]

Pathology

Most chondromyxoid fibromas are less than 5 cm. The tissue is firm, grayish-white, and often covered on the outer surface with a thin rim of bone or periosteum. Cysts or areas of hemorrhage may be found within the lesion (Fig. 38–29). Histologically, chondromyxoid fibromas have a lobulated pattern, with some of these lobules sparsely cellular and others more cellular. Those lobules that have few cells are composed of a myxoid or chondroid matrix.[68,574] Microscopic areas of cystic degeneration may contribute to the myxoid appearance. Other features of a chondromyxoid fibroma include osteoclast-like giant cells, intermixed fibrous tissue, and occasionally cholesterol, hemosiderin, and lymphocytes. Distinct calcification is rare but has been reported.[557,564]

Clinical Features

Chondromyxoid fibromas usually occur in older children and young adults, with individuals most commonly presenting for treatment in the second and third decades of life. Although most of the lesions are found in the tibia, other sites of predilection include the ilium, femur, fibula, metatarsals, and calcaneus.[134,335,368,557] The upper extremities, spine, and sternum are rarely involved.[72,257,490] The sexes are equally affected.

As with other benign bone tumors, it is not uncommon for a chondromyxoid fibroma to be discovered incidentally on a radiograph obtained for an unrelated reason. If symptoms are present from the lesion, the local discomfort usually is mild and intermittent. Swelling of the area and tenderness on palpation are occasionally noted.

Radiographic Findings

Chondromyxoid fibromas are usually ovoid or round. They are slow growing and usually evoke a border of reactive host bone sclerosis.[548] This sclerotic border, most commonly seen in patients younger than 20 years of age, is a useful sign for determining the lesion's benign nature. Many of the tumors have a trabeculated or bubbly appearance, but it is uncommon for calcification of the cartilage to be evident on radio-

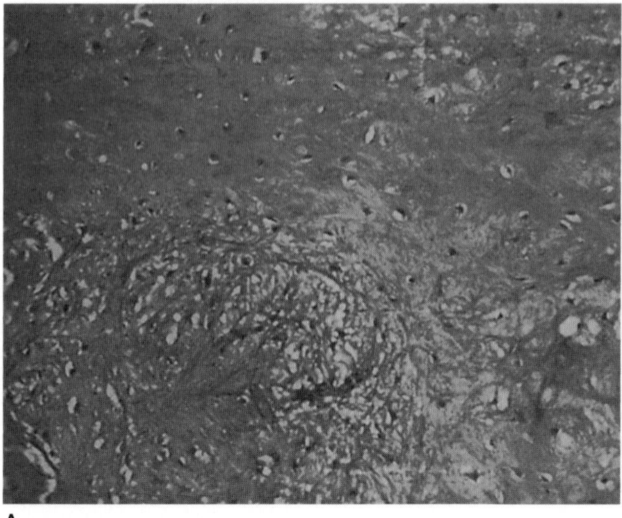

A

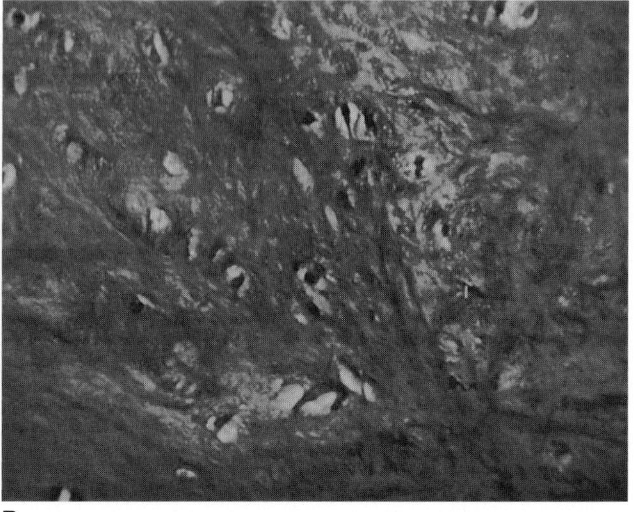

B

FIGURE 38–29 Chondromyxoid fibroma in the neck of the right femur. **A** and **B,** Photomicrographs showing the characteristic histologic picture. Note the ovoid and moderate-sized nuclei of the cells, which are widely separated by myxoid and chondroid matrix.

graphs. Chondromyxoid fibromas appear in the metaphyseal region of the long bones. They are usually eccentric and juxtacortical or even periosteal in location. It may be difficult to differentiate periosteal chondromyxoid fibromas from an aneurysmal bone cyst. In younger children, chondromyxoid fibromas may appear next to the physis, but with growth, the lesions tend to migrate away from the physis.

Differential Diagnosis

The radiographic appearance of a chondromyxoid fibroma can be very similar to that of a nonossifying fibroma. Both lesions are usually metaphyseal, eccentric, surrounded by a border of sclerosis, and trabeculated. Unlike nonossifying fibromas, chondromyxoid fibromas may bulge from the original bony contour. When the chondromyxoid fibroma is notably eccentric and associated with periosteal expansion, differentiation from aneurysmal bone cysts may be difficult. Other lesions to consider include solitary eosinophilic granuloma, enchondroma, simple bone cyst, and, in the older individual, worrisome entities such as chondrosarcoma or myeloma.

Treatment

Fine-needle aspiration cytology can be used to diagnose chondromyxoid fibroma.[203] Many of these lesions have been effectively treated by simple curettage. In younger patients, however, incomplete removal may lead to recurrence, which is estimated to occur in as many as one fourth of patients.[257,557] Therefore, en bloc excision should be considered. Because of the benign nature of this tumor, the surgeon should avoid radical procedures. If the lesion is next to the physis, consideration should be given to delaying surgical intervention until the tumor has grown away from the physeal area. Radiation therapy and chemotherapy are not considered in the management of chondromyxoid fibromas. Chondrosarcomatous transformation is rare.

Osteoid Osteoma

Incidence

Osteoid osteomas were described as a distinct entity by Jaffe in 1935.[231] Earlier reports referred to this entity as sclerosing nonsuppurative osteomyelitis, osteomyelitis of Garré, or localized or cortical bone abscess. Osteoid osteomas are solitary, benign, painful lesions of the bone. They have a nidus, 1.5 to 2 cm, that consists of osteoid, osteoblasts, and variable amounts of fibrovascular stroma.[339] This nidus is surrounded by an area of dense, reactive bone. Osteoid osteomas are relatively common, benign bone lesions, exceeded in incidence only by osteochondromas and nonossifying fibromas.[166] Osteoid osteomas account for approximately 10% to 11% of benign bone tumors and 2% to 3% of all primary bone neoplasms sampled for biopsy. They are characteristically seen in children and adolescents. The male-to-female ratio is approximately 2:1.

Etiology

The etiology of osteoid osteoma remains unknown, but the condition has been reported in siblings.[245]

Pathology

The cortical bone overlying the osteoid osteoma may be mildly pink compared with the surrounding cortex because of the increased local vascularity. The lesion itself is often a small, round or oval, cherry-red or reddish-brown tumor 1 cm or less in diameter. Differentiation between osteoid osteoma and osteoblastoma depends on the size of the lesion: lesions less than 2 cm in diameter are technically classified as osteoid osteomas. The nidus may have a very dense, gritty texture if a significant amount of calcification is present, or it may be soft and granular if it is predominantly vascular with little calcification.

Histologically, osteoid osteomas are characterized by small spicules of immature trabeculae, most often lined by prominent osteoblasts and osteoclasts[68] (Fig. 38–30). In mature lesions, the intervening stroma is sparsely cellular with readily apparent vascular spaces. Cartilage is not present. The demarcation between reactive surrounding bone and nidus is readily apparent microscopically. The pain associated with osteoid osteoma is thought to be caused by the numerous nonmyelinated axons present in the nidus.

Clinical Features

The patient with osteoid osteoma typically presents with a history of dull, aching pain in the region overlying the affected long bone. The pain may have been present for several months before presentation, tends to be worse at night, and is relieved significantly by salicylates or nonsteroidal anti-inflammatory drugs (NSAIDs).

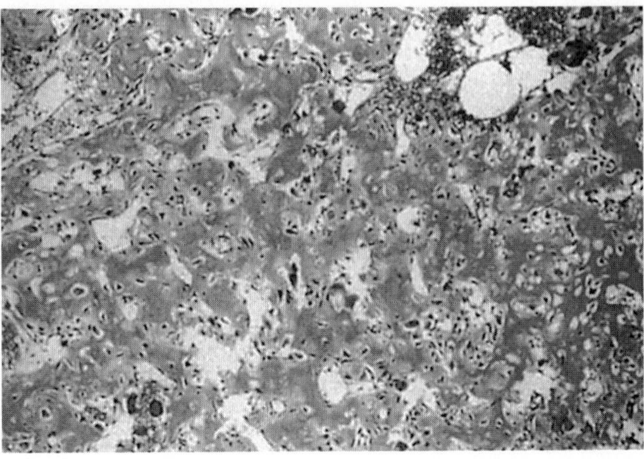

FIGURE 38–30 Osteoid osteoma, histologic appearance. The immature bone in the nidus of osteoid osteomas is lined by prominent osteoblasts and osteoclasts.

The most commonly involved site is the lower extremity, particularly the metaphyseal or diaphyseal region of the femur and tibia. Occasionally the tumor is periarticular, or even intra-articular, in location.[163,510] Less frequent sites of involvement include the humerus, glenoid, elbow, spine, sacrum, foot (talus, calcaneus, and metatarsals), calvaria, maxilla, mandible, clavicle, scapula, ribs, pelvis, and patella.[45,89,109,372,387,541,544,573]

A limp is often noted during evaluation of the patient's gait. Muscle atrophy may be apparent if the lesion has been present for several months and neurologic signs, including weakness and diminished deep tendon reflexes of the affected limb, have been reported.[212] However, direct tenderness, erythema, or swelling is uncommon. If the lesion is in the vertebral column (most commonly in the posterior elements), a secondary painful scoliosis may be evident.[426] The concavity of the curvature is usually on the side of the lesion and is attributed to spasm of the paravertebral muscles.[446] Excision of the nidus in the vertebral column often results in complete resolution of the scoliosis.

Radiographic Findings

The radiographic appearance depends on the location of the osteoid osteoma in the bone. Most of the tumors are intracortical, with the nidus appearing as a radiolucent lesion. This nidus rarely exceeds 1 cm in diameter but may be as large as 2 cm. The dense surrounding reactive sclerotic bone may extend for several centimeters away from the nidus. Less commonly, the osteoid osteoma may be intramedullary, subperiosteal, periarticular, or intra-articular in location.[251] These atypical sites usually do not provoke reactive bone formation around the nidus. Calcification in the central portion of the nidus may be evident on radiographs.

Other radiologic studies may be needed to make a correct diagnosis if the typical radiographic findings are not present or if the lesion is in an atypical location and lacks the associated reactive sclerosis. Technetium 99m bone scan is useful if osteoid osteoma is suspected but the lesion is not clearly demonstrated on plain radiographs. Technetium 99m bone scan nearly always demonstrates an intense focal increase in technetium uptake in the nidus and is of considerable value in evaluating the spine, pelvis, and long bones.[133,433]

Once the general area of the lesion has been localized with bone scan, cross-sectional imaging with CT best demonstrates the well-circumscribed area representing the nidus (Fig. 38–31). Thin sections (1 to 2 mm) may be needed for optimal detail.[565] The reliability of CT diminishes when the nidus is in a cancellous location because of the lack of perinidal density alteration.[493]

MRI demonstrates the soft tissue and bone marrow edema that accompanies osteoid osteomas.[142,569] This imaging modality may be helpful for the identification of osteoid osteomas in cancellous locations (periarticular or intra-articular), but there is potential for missing the diagnosis if MRI is the sole investigation accompanying plain radiographs.[119,210,286] Gadolinium-enhanced MRI demonstrates the lesions better than nonenhanced images.[305]

Differential Diagnosis

The differential diagnosis includes subacute osteomyelitis and osteoblastoma. On radiographs, a quiescent bone abscess may appear very similar to osteoid osteoma.[331] Laboratory studies further assist in distinguishing between the two entities. Local aspiration of subacute osteomyelitis confirms the diagnosis.

Osteoid osteomas are generally differentiated from osteoblastomas by size (osteoblastomas are larger, usually exceeding 2 cm in diameter), degree of sclerosis (osteoid osteomas, in general, have a greater degree of surrounding dense bone), and natural history (osteoblastomas can be more aggressive).

Treatment

Osteoid osteomas are described as self-limiting lesions that may mature spontaneously over the course of several years. The nidus gradually calcifies, then ossifies, and finally blends into the sclerotic surrounding bone. During the maturation period, the local pain gradually diminishes. Knowing this, some clinicians advocate conservative management of osteoid osteomas, with NSAIDs or aspirin recommended for those patients choosing not to undergo operative intervention.[224] In reality, however, very few patients are willing to continue with conservative management because of the intensity of the pain and the favorable outcomes likely with surgery.

NONSURGICAL TREATMENT

Salicylate and NSAIDs are effective in relieving symptoms of pain associated with osteoid osteoma. If the symptoms are moderate and controlled by this treatment program, observation alone is sufficient. Although cyclo-oxygenase-2 (COX-2) inhibitors have been found effective in this condition, their use is precluded owing to the recently identified cardiac-related clinical problems.[59,349] The possibility of spontaneous improvement over the course of several years may make medical management feasible for some patients. However, it is not possible on an individual basis to determine conclusively the ultimate outcome with medical management. Most families understand this and elect a surgical approach to this benign lesion.

SURGICAL TREATMENT

Surgical excision has proved effective in eradicating the pain-producing nidus.[166] Surgery remains the standard treatment when histology of the lesion is in doubt or neurovascular structures are within 1.5 cm, or in repeated failure of any other minimally invasive ablative technique or percutaneous resection.[82] Accurate intraoperative localization of the nidus is crucial for the success of open surgical intervention. Radiography, CT, tetracycline labeling, and bone scintigraphy have all been used for this purpose.[79] More recently,

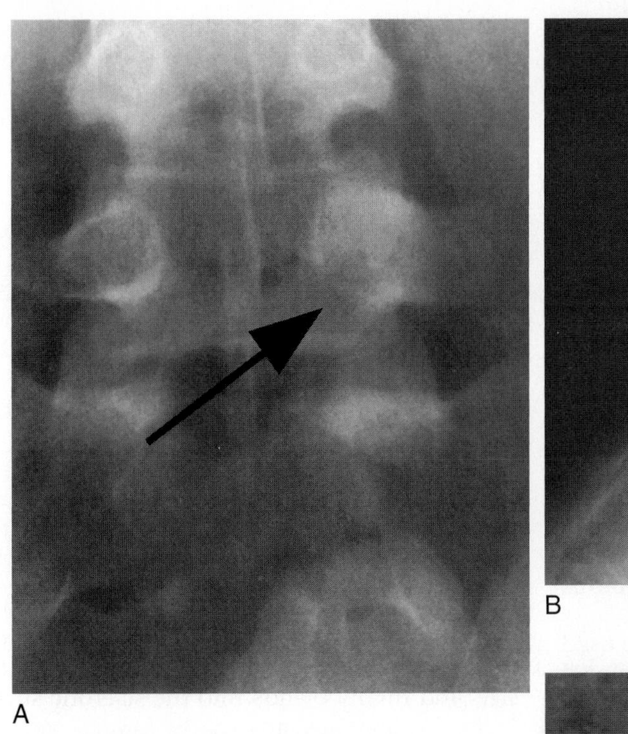
A

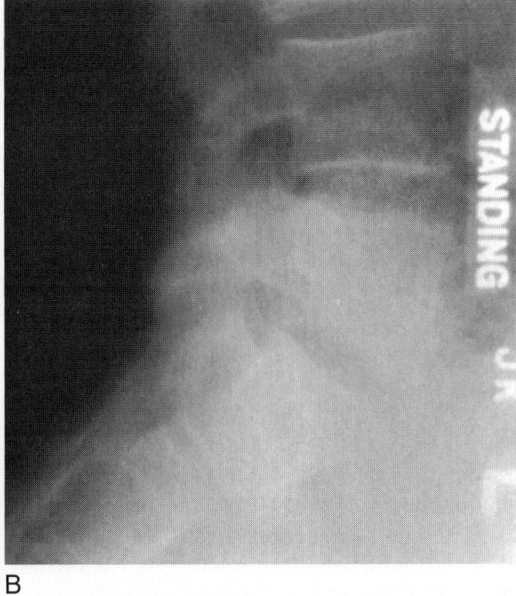

B

C

FIGURE 38-31 Osteoid osteoma. Posteroanterior (**A**) and lateral (**B**) radiographs of the fifth lumbar vertebra demonstrate increased density in the region of the right pedicle (*arrow* in **A**). **C,** Computed tomography clarifies the location and extent of the nidus of the osteoid osteoma.

less invasive percutaneous maneuvers using pinpoint CT-guided localization have become increasingly popular. With either approach (open resection or percutaneous ablation), once the nidus is removed or destroyed, the surrounding sclerotic bone will usually remodel. Relief from the pain is immediate, dramatic, and permanent unless the nidus has been incompletely excised or destroyed. Patients often remark that the incisional pain is far different from the pain of the osteoid osteoma itself.

Numerous recent reports document the usefulness of the less-invasive CT-guided methods such as percutaneous radiofrequency thermocoagulation, percutaneous interstitial laser photocoagulation, and percutaneous excision using a trephine.* The most commonly used CT-guided technique is the percutaneous radiofrequency thermocoagulation. In hard bony areas, a 2-mm drill system is used. In softer areas, an 11-gauge Jamshidi needle can be inserted to allow the passage of a 1-mm radiofrequency probe into the center of the nidus. Radiofrequency ablation is administered at 90° C for 4 to 5 minutes. This directly affects a 1-cm area that should include the nidus. Reports by those who have used this technique indicate that its results are equivalent to those obtained with surgical excision. Its advantages include the fact that it is an outpatient procedure, there is a lower risk of pathologic fracture, and convalescence is rapid. This is rapidly becoming the preferred initial treatment for osteoid osteomas. Occasionally, a second percutaneous procedure is needed if incomplete relief was obtained initially. Failures of this method are usually associated with inaccurate needle placement or lesions

*See references 34, 102, 108, 127, 137, 138, 183, 196, 280, 300, 327, 351, 402, 436, 439-442, 517, 518, 527, 528, 551, 553.

exceeding 10 mm.[528] Multiple needle positions reduce the risk of treatment failure.

Conventional intraoperative radiographs of the excised specimen may help confirm the presence of the nidus. CT-guided exploration, performed under anesthesia in the radiology suite, is helpful in localizing the nidus itself but will be inconclusive regarding the surgical excision of the nidus.[315] Tetracycline labeling can be used in children older than 8 years of age.[31] The risk of permanent staining of the dentin may preclude use of this technique in younger children.[208] A dental consultation may be useful in determining the maturity of the teeth if the use of tetracycline is considered in younger children. Tetracycline, which is avidly taken up by the nidus, is administered orally 1 to 2 days before surgery. Tetracycline fluoresces under ultraviolet light, thus providing an intraoperative method of determining whether the nidus has been removed. With the operating room lights dimmed and a Wood's lamp emitting the ultraviolet light, the nidus can be readily identified in the resected portion.

In a similar fashion, radioactive isotope can be used intraoperatively to assist in identifying the osteoid osteoma.[185] The isotope is administered before surgery and a scintillation probe is used intraoperatively to detect the increased counts per minute in the area of the lesion. However, few centers use this method because of the expense involved and the sometimes equivocal results. We have no experience with this technique.

Open Surgical Techniques

The two most common surgical methods for removing the nidus are en bloc resection and the bur-down technique.[188,485,568] En bloc resection is performed by placing drill bits around the lesion and confirming their placement with fluoroscopy in the operating room. The lesion is then removed en bloc with the margin of reactive bone. This requires a larger resection of bone than the bur-down technique, and therefore either bone grafting or internal fixation may be necessary. With the bur-down technique, the sclerotic reactive bone is burred until the nidus is visible. The nidus is then curetted and the specimen is sent to pathology. The cavity of the lesion is then thoroughly burred. This technique has even been applied arthroscopically in the talus.[524] The advantages of this procedure over en bloc resection include removal of less reactive bone (thus reducing the need for bone grafting) and a decrease in the risk of a postoperative pathologic fracture.

OSTEOBLASTOMA

Incidence

Osteoblastomas have a histologic pattern very similar to that of osteoid osteomas, but they are usually much larger (2 to 10 cm). They are one fifth as common as osteoid osteomas and represent approximately 0.5% of primary tumors sampled for biopsy.[339] Most osteoblastomas occur in persons 10 to 25 years of age, with the peak incidence noted at around 20 years.[311] More than 80% of patients are younger than 30 years of age at the time of diagnosis. The male-to-female ratio is 2:1.

Pathology

On gross pathology, osteoblastomas vary in size from 2 to 10 cm. At surgery, an osteoblastoma is found to consist of hemorrhagic, granular, friable, and calcified tissue.[68] The lesions are gritty on palpation, usually deep red to reddish-brown or pink (reflecting their vascularity), and, if removed intact, often well-circumscribed and surrounded by a shell of cortical bone or thickened periosteum.

Histologically, osteoblastomas are identical to osteoid osteomas, consisting of vascular spindle cell stroma with abundant irregular spicules of mineralized bone and osteoid.[128] Osteoblasts and osteoclasts are readily evident on the edges of the bone spicules (Fig. 38–32). Cartilage is distinctly absent. Because of their similar histologic pattern, osteoblastomas have sometimes been referred to as giant osteoid osteomas.

Occasional osteoblastomas appear aggressive on radiographs, with bone destruction and extension into soft tissues[36,311] (Fig. 38–33). Microscopically, these infrequent lesions may reveal notable cellular atypia with large, plump osteoblasts, making it difficult to differentiate an aggressive osteoblastoma from a low-grade osteosarcoma histologically. Osteoblastomas do not metastasize.[68]

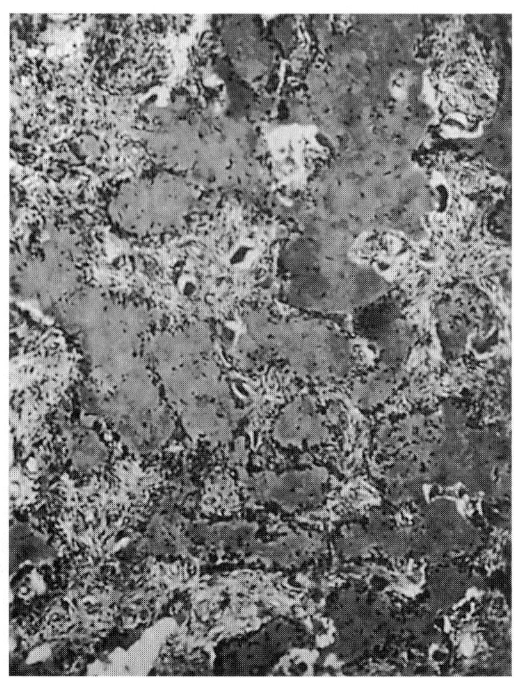

FIGURE 38–32 Benign osteoblastoma, histologic appearance. Note the highly vascularized connective tissue matrix and the trabeculae of osteoid and new bone, with layers of osteoblasts lined against them.

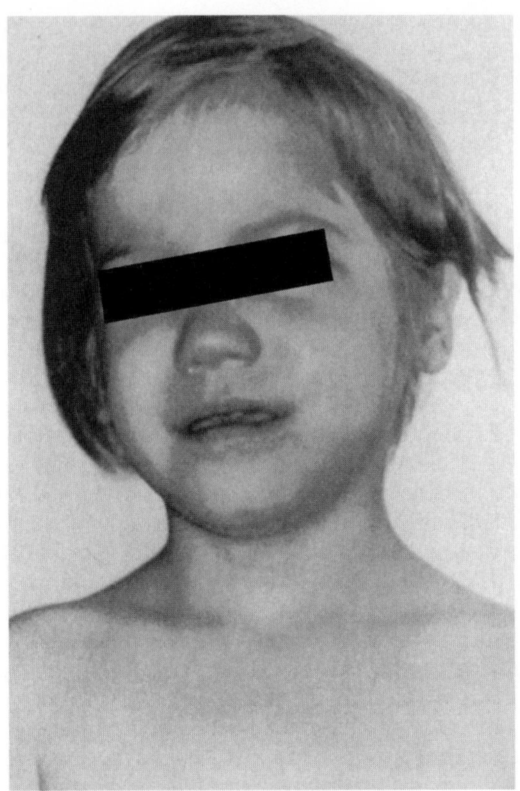
A

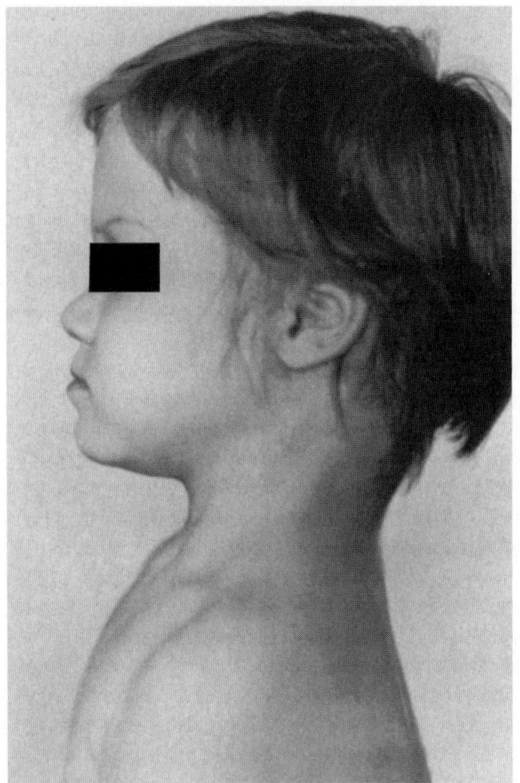
B

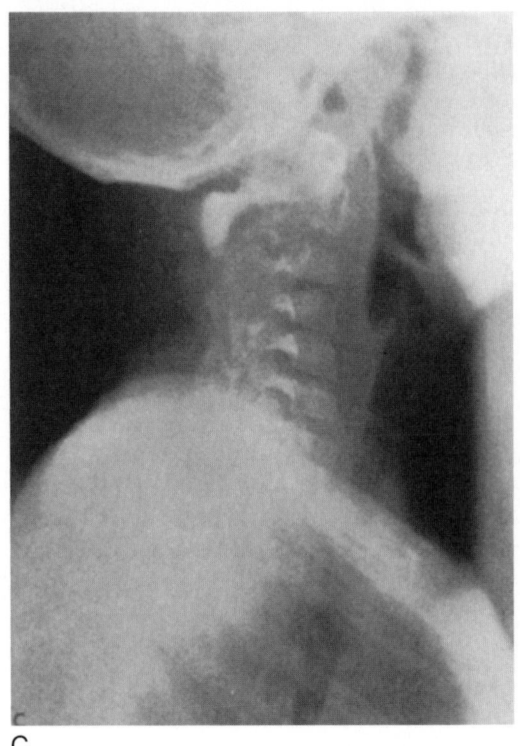
C

FIGURE 38-33 Benign osteoblastoma of the cervical spine in a 6-year-old girl. **A** and **B,** Clinical appearance. The patient presented with a painful torticollis and tender swelling in the left upper neck. **C,** Lateral radiograph of the cervical spine showing the mottled radiolucency of the expanded vertebral bodies of the second and part of the third cervical vertebrae. The posterior processes are also involved. The lesion was surgically excised and bone grafted to fuse the vertebrae from C1 to C4.

Clinical Features

Unlike osteoid osteomas, approximately 30% to 40% of osteoblastomas are found in the spine, where they most often affect the posterior elements, including the spinous and transverse processes, laminae, and pedicles.* Osteoblastomas exceed several centimeters in size, and spinal lesions may extend into the vertebral body. On occasion, the lesion appears to originate from within the vertebral body. All areas of the spine may be involved, from the upper cervical region to the sacrum.[458] The clinical presentation may include myelopathic or radicular symptoms, the risk being higher for osteoblastoma than for osteoid osteoma.[387,389] Progressive painful scoliosis may develop. If the cervical spine is affected, torticollis may be evident.

Other common sites include the long bones, especially the femur and tibia. In the long bones, the osteoblastoma involves the metaphyseal or diaphyseal region. The lesions are centered in the medullary portions of the shaft, unlike osteoid osteomas, which tend to be located in the cortex or subperiosteally.[274,339] Rarely, osteoblastomas may be located on the surface of the cortical bone, so-called periosteal osteoblastomas.[353] Although less often affected than the long bones, the mandible, foot, calvaria, pelvis, scapula, sternum, patella, ribs, clavicle, or hands may be affected.[192] In these nonvertebral locations, pain is usually the prominent complaint. Symptoms may be present for a few months to a year. The pain is less localized than the pain of osteoid osteomas and much less likely to be relieved by salicylates.

Because osteoblastomas are several centimeters in size, physical examination may reveal a palpable mass. Tenderness over the area of the tumor is the most consistent physical finding. If the lesion is located near or within a joint, there may be some loss of joint motion.[26]

Radiographic Findings

Osteoblastomas usually result in a uniform fusiform expansion of the bone. The borders of the lesion are well delineated from the surrounding host bone, and often there is a thin rim of reactive intramedullary bone sclerosis.[274] Most lesions are 3 to 6 cm, although the range is 2 to 10 cm. The reactive bone formation is noticeably less intense and the margins are less defined than those of osteoid osteomas. Although most lesions are metaphyseal or diaphyseal in location, epiphyseal lesions may be seen in the long bones of the hand or foot. The center of the lesion varies: it may be lucent, mixed lucent and blastic, or predominantly blastic.

In the spine, predominantly the posterior elements are affected. Cortical expansion is common and is similar to that seen with aneurysmal bone cysts. Osteoblastomas, however, are usually more radiodense than aneurysmal bone cysts.

Because of the size of the lesion, osteoblastomas can usually be seen on plain radiographs. CT better delineates the extent of involvement, particularly with vertebral lesions. The MRI appearance of spinal osteoblastomas is varied and shows no characteristic features. MRI may also overestimate the extent of the lesion because of extensive reactive changes and adjacent soft tissue masses. CT should continue to be the investigation of choice for the characterization and local staging of suspected spinal osteoblastomas.[466] Radionuclide bone scintigraphy may be helpful in localizing smaller osteoblastomas that are not readily apparent on plain radiographs.

*See references 56, 68, 166, 311, 342, 387, 395, 446, 455, 466, 473, 573.

Differential Diagnosis

Expansile osteoblastomas may be difficult to differentiate radiographically from aneurysmal bone cysts. Clarification, however, is usually obtained with CT. Differences in the size and location of the lesions usually distinguish osteoblastomas from osteoid osteomas.

Up to 10% of low-grade osteosarcomas may have radiographic features that suggest osteoblastoma. As mentioned, an aggressive osteoblastoma may be difficult to differentiate histologically from a low-grade osteosarcoma. In a benign osteoblastoma, however, there is an absence of sarcomatous large, plump connective tissue stromal cells, sarcoma giant cells, and tumor cartilage and bone.

Treatment

Treatment consists of curettage or local excision. The risk of recurrence after such treatment is approximately 10% to 20%. If a spinal osteoblastoma impinges on the spinal cord or nerve roots, surgical decompression is required. Unlike osteoid osteoma, soft tissue extension of an osteoblastoma into the epidural space may become adherent to the dura.[426] Once the tumor is excised, internal fixation of the unstable spine and bone grafting may be necessary. Osteoblastomas located in sites inaccessible to surgical excision have been reported to respond to radiation therapy or chemotherapy.[74] Because of the size of osteoblastoma lesions, CT-guided percutaneous radiofrequency thermocoagulation is not used as it is with osteoid osteomas.

Langerhans Cell Histiocytosis (Histiocytosis X)

The term *Langerhans cell histiocytosis* was introduced in 1973 by Nezelof and associates.[358] It has come to replace the term *histiocytosis X,* which was introduced in 1953 by Lichtenstein to describe a syndrome that consists of a group of clinical pathologic entities: eosinophilic granuloma of bone, Hand-Schüller-Christian disease, and Letterer-Siwe disease.[296] Because these entities are the result of proliferation and dissemination of pathologic histiocyte cells or Langerhans-like cells, the term *Langerhans cell histiocytosis* is used today.

The disseminated forms of the disease (Hand-Schüller-Christian disease and Letterer-Siwe disease) were reported before our understanding of the pathologic entity of eosinophilic granuloma of bone.[533] Alfred Hand, in 1893, Arthur Schüller, in 1915, and

Henry Christian, in 1920, independently described the complex of polyuria, exophthalmos, and defects found in membranous bones. Their descriptions were combined to form what is currently known as Hand-Schüller-Christian disease. Erich Letterer in 1924 and Sture Siwe in 1933 described a generalized disease process with multisystem involvement, including bone. Present in younger children, Letterer-Siwe disease has a poor prognosis. The term *eosinophilic granuloma* was introduced in 1940 and was used to describe solitary bone destruction by large histiocytic cells intermingled with eosinophilic leukocytes.[297,379] Approximately 80% of cases of Langerhans cell histiocytosis are solitary eosinophilic granulomas, 6% are multiple eosinophilic granulomas, 9% are Hand-Schüller-Christian disease, and 1.2% are Letterer-Siwe disease.[188]

The etiology of Langerhans cell histiocytosis is poorly understood.[511] There is speculation that immunologic stimulation of a normal presenting cell, the Langerhans cell, continues in an uncontrolled manner, resulting in these cells' proliferation and accumulation. The cells have been shown to express several antigens, CDla and langerin, together with the monocyte antigens CD68 and CD14.[181] This disorder may not truly represent a neoplasm but instead may be a proliferative lesion that may be secondary to a defect in immunoregulation. In contrast to this theory, a 1994 study reported that this disorder is probably a clonal neoplastic disorder with highly variable biologic behavior.[547] The Langerhans histiocyte is the cell of origin for this spectrum of the disease. No hereditary pattern has been described, although three affected members in one family have been reported.[465]

Langerhans cell histiocytosis can present at any age, from birth to old age. The incidence in children has been estimated at three to four per million, with a 2:1 male-to-female ratio.

Eosinophilic Granuloma: Solitary and Multiple without Extraskeletal Involvement

The mildest, most favorable form of Langerhans cell histiocytosis is an eosinophilic granuloma that is confined to a single bone, or occasionally to several bones, without extraskeletal involvement.[184,339] The lesion is a benign process, and spontaneous healing is common.

PATHOLOGY

Eosinophilic granulomas are usually soft, reddish-brown material. They often show areas of hemorrhage and occasionally cysts.

Histologically, the tissue is characterized by a mixture of eosinophils, plasma cells, histiocytes, and peculiar large mononuclear giant cells (Langerhans cells) with abundant pale-staining cytoplasm and indented or cleaved nuclei[68] (Fig. 38–34). Necrosis, fibrosis, and reactive cells (foamy macrophages) may be evident. There is minimal mitotic activity. The lesions may consist primarily of the histiocytic infiltrates, or there may be a mixture of histiocytes and eosinophils.

Electron microscopy can be used to confirm the diagnosis; the specific pathologic finding is the presence of Birbeck granules in the cell cytoplasm near the nucleus.[14] These granules are rod-shaped structures characterized by central striation and a vesicular expansion resembling the strings of a tennis racket. The origin and function of Birbeck granules are still uncertain[533]; however, when present, these structures are pathognomonic of Langerhans cell histiocytosis.

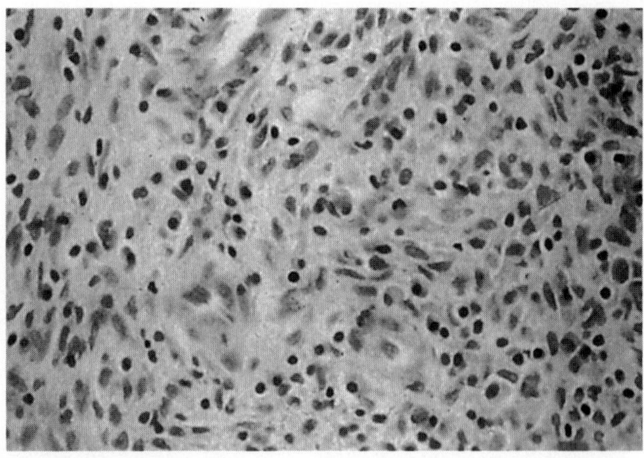

FIGURE 38–34 Eosinophilic granuloma (original magnification ×40). The histologic picture is characterized by a mixture of eosinophils, histiocytes, and Langerhans cells (large mononuclear giant cells with pale-staining cytoplasm).

CLINICAL FEATURES

About two thirds of cases are diagnosed in individuals younger than 20 years of age, with most diagnoses made in the 5- to 10-year-old age group. The first symptom is localizing pain, occasionally accompanied by swelling and low-grade fever. The erythrocyte sedimentation rate may be elevated.

The skull is the most common site of involvement, followed by the femur. Approximately 40% of solitary eosinophilic granulomas are found at one of these two sites, and the skull and femur are also most commonly affected in cases with multiple lesions. Other sites of involvement include the pelvis, ribs, and spine.[32,43,174,230,359,419] The tarsal and carpal bones are rarely affected. In the long bones, the lesions are usually intramedullary and most commonly located in the diaphysis.[230]

RADIOGRAPHIC FINDINGS

A rapidly destructive lytic process occurs in the bone, producing a "punched-out" appearance on radiographs. In the early phases the lesion may be poorly delineated, show a "moth-eaten" pattern of destruction, and exhibit erosions of the cortices. The periosteum may be stimulated, showing some periosteal elevation.[159,339] It is in this phase that the condition most closely mimics osteomyelitis or Ewing's sarcoma. Later, the borders of the lesion become sharp and the contours become round or oval. During the early radiographic phase of the solitary lesion, a biopsy is often necessary to rule out a malignant process (Fig. 38–35). In the skull, the lesion is oval or round, with several satellite lesions sometimes present, making this particular radiographic

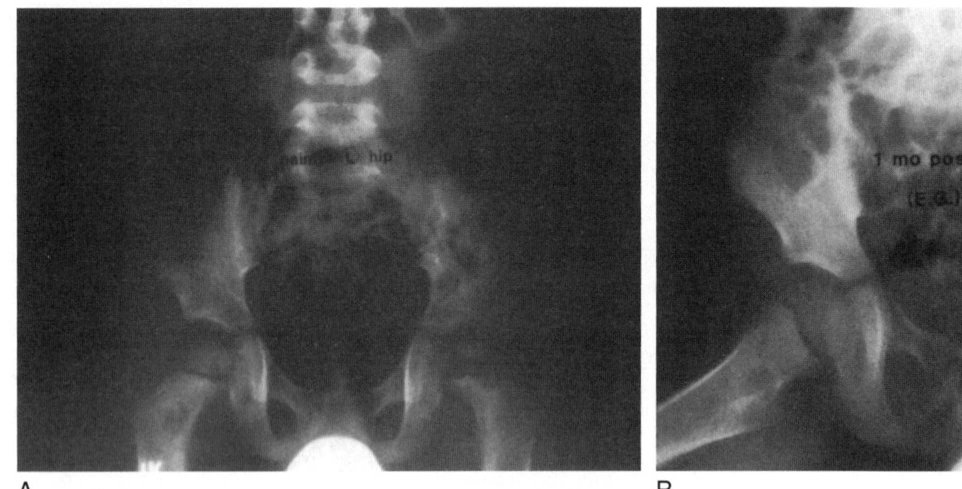

A B

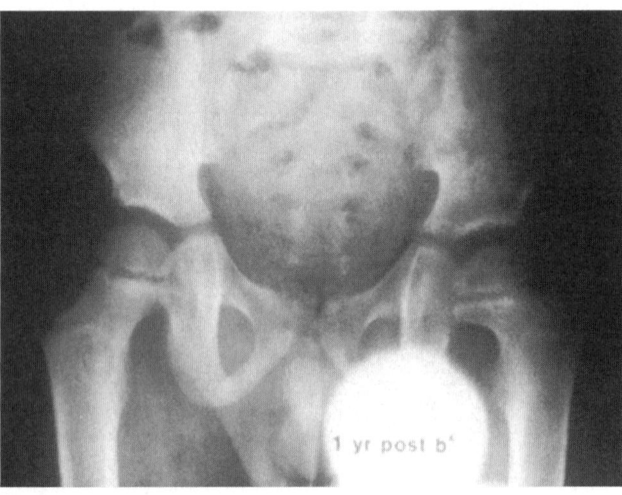

C

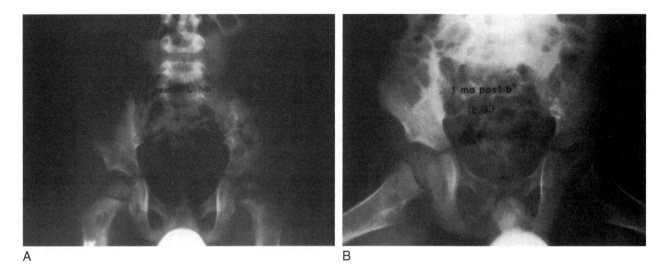

FIGURE 38–35 Eosinophilic granuloma. **A** and **B**, Radiographs of a 4-year-old boy showing lucencies involving the proximal right femoral metaphysis, left femoral periphyseal region, and left iliac bone. Biopsy confirmed the diagnosis of eosinophilic granuloma. **C**, One year later, the multiple lesions had healed.

appearance almost pathognomonic for eosinophilic granuloma. Periosteal new bone formation usually does not occur in the flat bones of the skull or pelvis. Marginal sclerosis during healing can be secondary to treatment or can occur spontaneously.

Another nearly pathognomonic sign of eosinophilic granuloma is the presence of vertebra plana in the spine (Fig. 38–36). This occurs with insidious collapse of the vertebral body, which is eventually compressed into a thin wafer.[534] The patient's neurologic status usually remains intact, although spinal cord or nerve root compression may occur rarely as a result of severe vertebral body destruction.[256,508] With healing, a variable degree of vertebral height is restored in these spinal lesions.

Approximately 10% of patients who initially present with a solitary eosinophilic granuloma develop multifocal lesions with extraskeletal involvement (Hand-Schüller-Christian disease). Nearly any bone other than those in the hands and feet may be affected. Chest radiographs should always be obtained to rule out pulmonary involvement.

CT is used to delineate the extent of the lytic lesions, particularly in the pelvis, spine, and skull. MRI is superior to both radiography and CT in delineating the medullary extent of eosinophilic granulomas and surrounding soft tissue changes[32,37,118,125,343] (Fig. 38–37). The degree of peritumoral edema accompanying an eosinophilic granuloma is less extensive than that seen with Ewing's sarcoma or osteomyelitis.

Radionuclide bone scintigraphy does not consistently demonstrate eosinophilic granulomas. The scans may be completely negative in patients with radiographic evidence of extensive bone involvement. A plain radiographic skeletal survey is superior to scintigraphy for the diagnosis of multiple lesions.

DIFFERENTIAL DIAGNOSIS

The differential diagnosis includes osteomyelitis, Ewing's sarcoma, malignant lymphoma, metastatic disease, and, in the long bones, aneurysmal bone cyst and solitary bone cyst. Unless pathognomonic findings, such as multiple skull lucencies or vertebra plana, are found on radiographic evaluation, biopsy is needed to differentiate the more serious lesions. Fine-needle aspiration yields sufficient material to confirm the diagnosis.[10,144] In osteomyelitis, the fine-needle aspirate

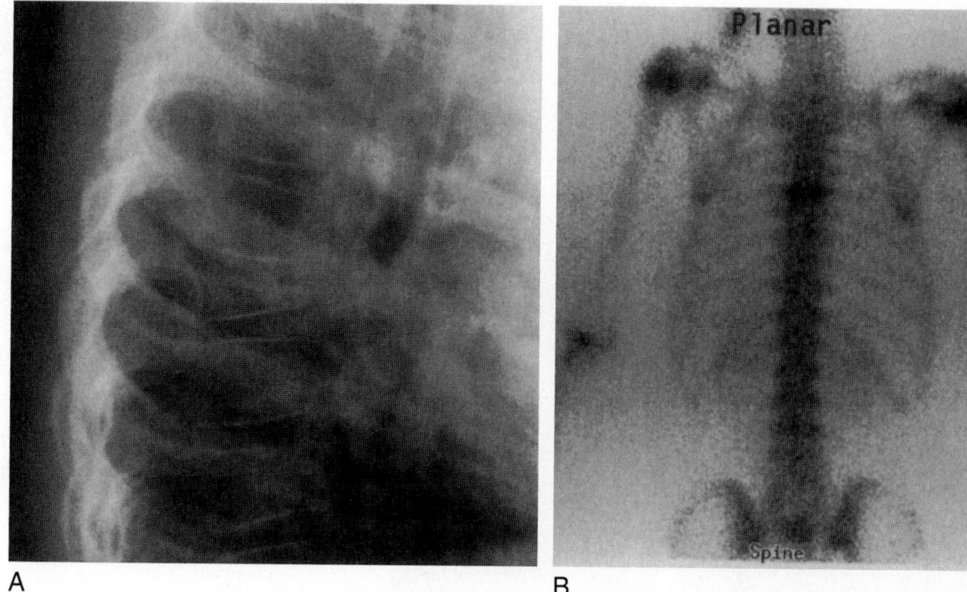

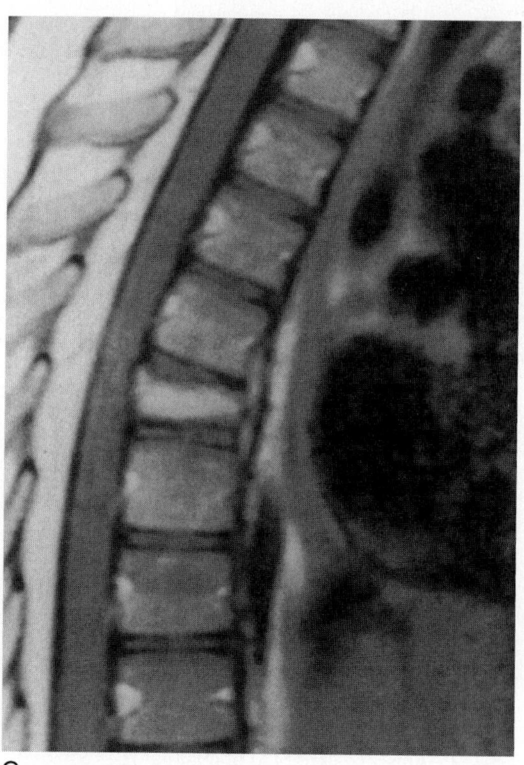

FIGURE 38–36 Imaging findings in a 7-year-old girl with mid-thoracic back discomfort for 6 weeks. **A,** A lateral radiograph of the thoracic spine demonstrated a vertebra plana appearance of T6, consistent with the diagnosis of eosinophilic granuloma. **B,** A bone scan was remarkable for increased uptake at T6, but nowhere else. **C,** Magnetic resonance imaging demonstrated no encroachment on the spinal canal and no significant extension of tumor anteriorly.

contains pus, neutrophils, or organisms. Another benign musculoskeletal tumor, nonossifying fibroma, may also resemble the late healing phase of eosinophilic granuloma. Unlike nonossifying fibromas, however, eosinophilic granulomas usually are diaphyseal and are not distinctly eccentric.

TREATMENT

Patients with solitary eosinophilic granulomas usually have a benign clinical course. They have a good chance of spontaneous remission and a favorable outcome over a period of months to years.[184,350] There is a low rate of recurrence in skeletally immature patients.[409] The single bony lesion usually does not require treatment other than perhaps a biopsy to confirm the diagnosis.[52] At that time, curettage may be performed.[463] Curettage may require augmentation with bone grafting when performed on lesions in weight-bearing bones of the lower extremities that are at risk for spontaneous fracture or on lesions where curettage alone could result in unacceptable deformity. If vertebra plana is identified but the associated back discomfort has resolved, observation alone is sufficient.[43,161,174]

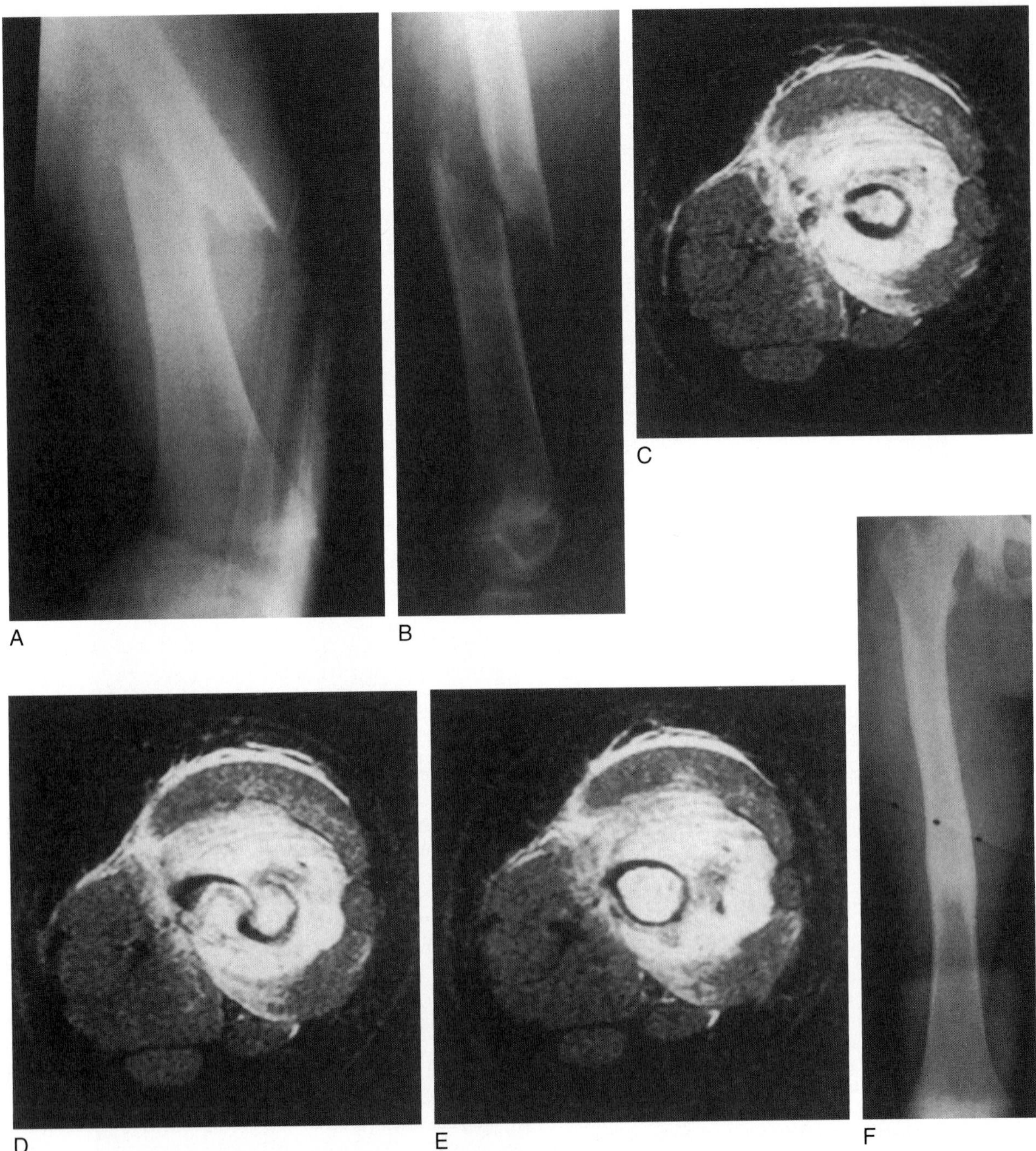

FIGURE 38–37 Anteroposterior **(A)** and lateral **(B)** radiographs demonstrating a displaced pathologic diaphyseal femur fracture through a lucent lesion in a teenage boy. **C** through **E,** Magnetic resonance imaging showed diffuse soft tissue and intramedullary changes near the fracture site. **F,** Eighteen months later, the fracture and the eosinophilic granuloma had healed.

Intralesional infiltration with steroids has been reported to be safe and effective.[511] Although this is a minimally invasive procedure, injections are not needed if the diagnosis is clear.

Lesions can occur in areas where they threaten neurologic function (e.g., the spinal cord or optic nerve) and where local steroid infiltration or surgical resection may not be possible. In these cases, treatment with low-dose radiation may be a good alternative.[143,326] The use of radiation therapy to manage localized bone lesions has decreased considerably, however, because of the favorable natural history (spontaneous remission) and the risk (although low) of development of a secondary malignancy. Chemotherapy has been used with some success in cases of diffuse eosinophilic granuloma and in patients with systemic disease and multiple organ involvement (Letterer-Siwe disease).[184,465,533]

Hand-Schüller-Christian Disease: Multifocal Eosinophilic Granuloma with Extraskeletal Involvement (Chronic Disseminated Type)

The classic description of Hand-Schüller-Christian disease includes multiple eosinophilic granulomas involving bone, diabetes insipidus (due to pituitary gland involvement), and exophthalmos (due to the presence of retro-orbital granulomas). This term is now used to include instances of more chronic evolution, even without the classic findings, that generally occur in children older than 3 years of age with involvement of other systems. In fact, the triad of calvarial defects, exophthalmos, and diabetes insipidus is present in only 10% of cases.[339,511] More than 70% of patients with Hand-Schüller-Christian disease are diagnosed before 5 years of age. In addition to the features just mentioned, fever, hepatosplenomegaly, lymphadenopathy, anemia, and abnormal liver chemistries may be evident. In contrast to solitary eosinophilic granulomas, the bones of the hands and feet may also be affected in Hand-Schüller-Christian disease. Pathologic fractures may occur, particularly in the spine.

In the early phases of the disease, the histologic picture is similar to that of a solitary eosinophilic granuloma. The later phases are characterized by a greater proportion of lipid-laden macrophages and scarring. Significant morbidity is associated with this disorder.

Treatment recommendations in the past have consisted of a combination of low-dose irradiation and corticosteroids. Surgical curettage is occasionally indicated. Currently, chemotherapy consisting of a combination of prednisolone and vinblastine is used primarily in cases with evidence of fever, pain, severe involvement of the skin, failure to thrive, or dysfunction of vital organs.[184] The effectiveness of chemotherapy remains unpredictable. New lesions can occur shortly after chemotherapy is discontinued for a clinically good result.

Letterer-Siwe Disease: Multifocal Eosinophilic Granuloma (Acute Disseminated or Infantile Form)

This acute, disseminated, progressive form of histiocytosis is rare. Characteristically it occurs during the first year of life. All patients are identified before 2 years of age. Visceral involvement is diffuse and severe. The patient may present with fever and debilitating infection secondary to marrow failure. Hepatosplenomegaly, lymphadenopathy, papular rash, bleeding diathesis, anemia, and occasionally exophthalmos and diabetes insipidus may be present. The pulmonary parenchyma may have a granular appearance on chest radiographs. The destructive "punched-out" lesions of the bones, although not a major source of complaint, are identifiable on radiographs.

In the past, Letterer-Siwe disease was considered to be invariably progressive and fatal, with death caused by marrow failure, asphyxia, or septicemia. Today, appropriate treatment with chemotherapy, steroids, and high-dose antibiotics may lead to survival.

Nonossifying Fibroma and Fibrous Cortical Defect

Incidence

Fibrous defects in bone are the most common benign lesions in childhood and are frequently detected incidentally on radiographs taken for an unrelated reason.[44] They are found in the metaphyseal regions of the long bones, particularly the femur and the tibia. Often they are cortical in location, but they can also be found in the cancellous area of bone. In 1942, Jaffe and Lichtenstein reported that when sampled for biopsy, these lesions contained fibrous tissue.[236] They coined the terms *fibrous cortical defect* and *nonosteogenic (nonossifying) fibroma*. Other terms used to describe these fibrous lesions include *fibrous metaphyseal defect* and *fibrous endosteal defect.*

Etiology

Conventional cytogenetic analysis has revealed a reciprocal translocation involving bands 1p31 and 4q34 in one case of a clonally aberrant nonossifying fibroma.[357]

Pathology

Surgical curettage usually reveals soft, friable, yellow or brown tissue. Hemosiderin pigment contributes to the brownish color. The tumor is usually surrounded by ridges of bone septa, which gives it the trabeculated radiographic appearance.

The histologic appearance of all of these lesions is similar. They differ in size and in radiographic appearance, which reflects the varying phases of the development of the same lesion. Histologically, the two basic components are fibroblastic tissue and osteoclast-like giant cells (Fig. 38–38). Foamy pale histocytes, focal hemorrhage, and hemosiderin pigment may also be extensively present. These microscopic findings may cause some confusion with other lesions that contain giant cells, such as solid aneurysmal bone cysts.

Clinical Features

The term *fibrous cortical defect* refers to the small fibrous lesions that occur in young children. These fibrous lesions appear to be developmental defects due to a localized disturbance of bone growth and may not be representative of true neoplasms. Most are eventually obliterated by reparative ossification or by gradual extrusion from the cortex during remodeling at the metaphyseal (growing) end of the bone. In a small percentage of cases, these fibrous cortical defects not only persist but increase in size, penetrate into the medullary canal, and may become symptomatic,

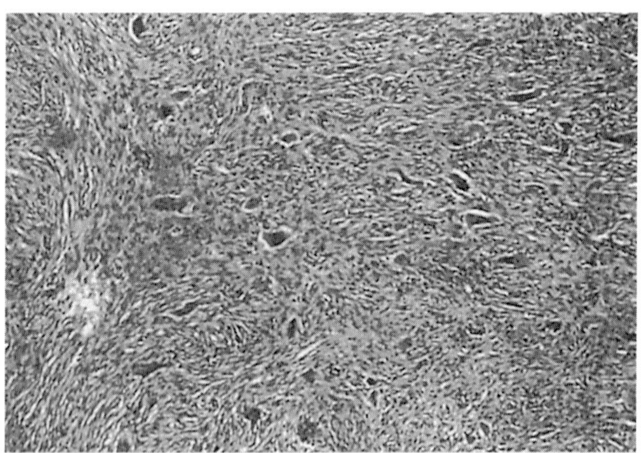

FIGURE 38–38 Nonossifying fibroma (original magnification ×10). The two basic components are fibroblastic tissue and osteoclast-like giant cells.

producing a pathologic fracture. Jaffe and Lichtenstein considered this to be an evolutionary process by which fibrous cortical defects matured into nonossifying fibromas.[236]

Radiographic Findings

Both lesions are sharply delineated, radiolucent, multiloculated, eccentric, and outlined by a sclerotic border[168] (Fig. 38–39). They are usually metaphyseal in location but on rare occasions are found in the epiphyseal region. Nonossifying fibromas have greater extension into the medullary cavity.

The radiographic findings are usually so characteristic of fibrous cortical defect or nonossifying fibroma that further radiologic studies are unnecessary. For those lesions that appear painful but lack evidence of pathologic fracture, better clarification will be obtained with CT. Bone scans may show mild uptake in this isolated lesion and help in differentiating it from other multifocal abnormalities, such as eosinophilic granuloma.

MRI is rarely needed. The MRI features of nonossifying fibroma include hypointensity and septation on T2-weighted images.[24,240] Signal intensity on T1- and T2-weighted MRI and the patterns of contrast enhancement depend on the amounts of hypercellular fibrous tissue, hemosiderin, foamy histiocytes, and bone trabeculae.

Differential Diagnosis

Unicameral bone cysts radiographically resemble nonossifying fibromas more than any other lesions. Other similar benign bone tumors include aneurysmal bone cyst, chondromyxoid fibroma, and eosinophilic granuloma.

Natural History

The fibrous cortical defect usually appears near the physis and then migrates away during its growth. Usually the lesion regresses spontaneously, becoming

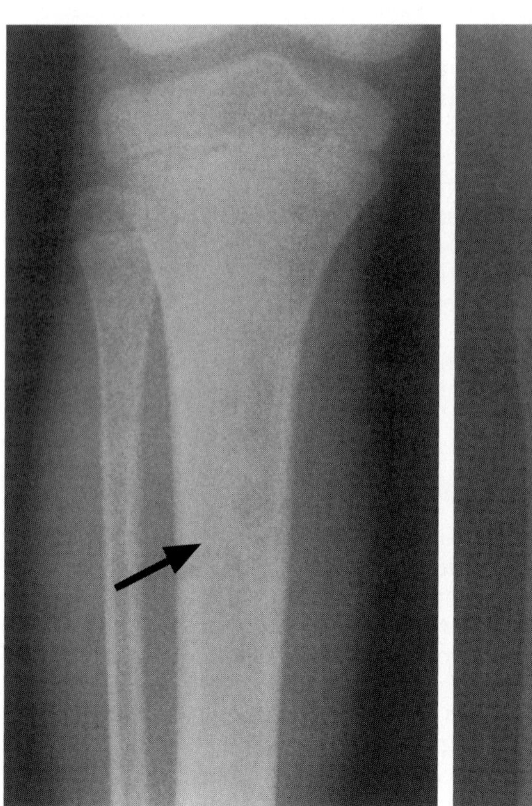

A

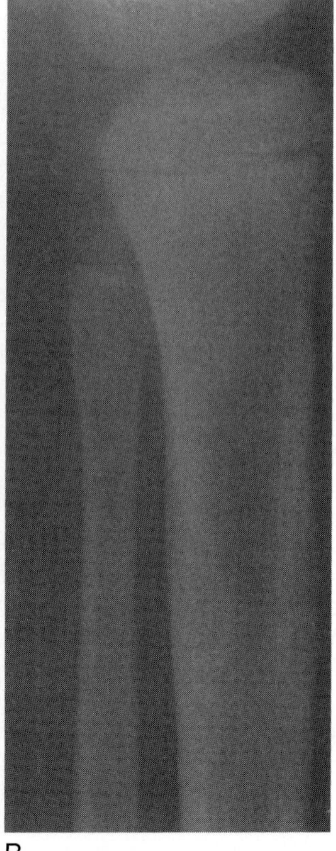

B

FIGURE 38–39 **A** and **B**, This classic-appearing nonossifying fibroma (*arrow* in **A**) is sharply delineated, radiolucent, eccentric, and outlined by a sclerotic border. It requires no treatment.

smaller and less distinct and eventually disappearing. Occasionally the fibrous cortical defect proliferates and increases in size, extending into the endosteum or medullary cavity and involving a greater portion of the width of the bone. At this stage the diagnosis of nonossifying fibroma is made.

Treatment

Most fibrous cortical defects do not require treatment. They usually regress over time. Larger, nonossifying fibromas may lead to some discomfort and possible pathologic fractures.[25] Even so, the majority of patients with nonossifying fibromas can be monitored without surgical intervention, and if fractures do occur, they can be successfully managed nonoperatively.[140,219,325] Biopsy, curettage, and bone grafting are indicated for large lesions that raise concern for impending pathologic fracture, for lesions that have become painful, and for lesions whose characteristics prevent a definitive radiographic diagnosis[44,47] (Fig. 38–40). Local recurrence is rare with this type of treatment, and there is little to no risk of malignant degeneration.

Primary Synovial Chondromatosis

Incidence

Synovial chondromatosis is characterized by the formation of metaplastic and multiple foci of cartilage in the intimal layer of the synovial membrane of a joint.[121,511] The lesion also occurs in bursae and tendon sheaths.[506] The term *synovial osteochondromatosis* is used when the cartilage is ossified.

This benign neoplasm is very rare. It usually occurs in persons older than 40 years of age but occasionally occurs in adolescents. It is twice as common in men as in women.

Etiology

The etiology of primary synovial chondromatosis is unknown, although cytogenetic findings strongly suggest that it is a clonal proliferation.[337] Trauma has been postulated as a possible stimulus of metaplasia of the synovial cells into chondrocytes.[494] Dysregulation of hedgehog signaling is a feature of several benign cartilaginous tumors, including synovial chondromatosis.[209] Blockade of this abnormal signaling may be a potential future treatment for this disorder.

Pathology

Arthrotomy reveals the synovium to be thickened and studded with innumerable small, firm, flat or slightly raised, grayish-white nodules. These cartilaginous or osteocartilaginous foci may become pedunculated and detached from the affected membrane, entering the joint cavity as loose bodies. Histologic studies disclose numerous foci of cartilaginous metaplasia of the synovium, which may be calcified or ossified (Fig. 38–41).

Clinical Features

Clinical complaints consist of pain, swelling, and stiffness of the affected joint; joint locking may also be a symptom when there are loose bodies. Months or years may elapse before a patient seeks treatment. On examination the synovial membrane is noted to be thickened and the joint is limited in its range of motion. Other physical signs that can be elicited are crepitus and palpable loose bodies.

Radiographic Findings

Radiographs reveal multiple areas of stippled calcification in and around the affected joint when the lesion is cartilaginous (Fig. 38–42). In such cases the findings are those of capsular distention and synovial thickening.

Treatment

Treatment consists of simple removal of the loose bodies and partial synovectomy, often performed arthroscopically.[67,239,262,273,308,370,478] Extensive and complete synovectomy is impractical and usually not necessary. The condition has a definite tendency to resolve eventually. Malignant transformation into chondrosarcoma is unusual.[254,559]

Pigmented Villonodular Synovitis and Giant Cell Tumor of the Tendon Sheath

Incidence

Pigmented villonodular synovitis (PVNS) is a benign lesion that develops in joint linings. Giant cell tumor of the tendon sheath (histologically identical to PVNS) develops in the fibrous sheath of tendons.[339]

In addition to diffuse PVNS, a rare localized form of this disorder is characterized by limited involvement of the synovium.[261]

Etiology

Increased expression of the humanin peptide in mitochondria and siderosomes is characteristic of synovial cells from diffuse-type PVNS. Humanin is an antiapoptotic peptide that is encoded in the mitochondrial genome. Mitochondrial dysfunction may be a principal factor in the pathogenesis of diffuse-type PVNS, and humanin peptide may contribute to the neoplastic process in this disorder.[222] In several patients with PVNS, a recent genetic study using comparative hybridization and flow cytometry found abnormalities in the subregions of chromosomal arms 22q, 16p, and 16q.[40]

Pathology

During arthroscopic or open synovectomy, the synovial membrane is found to be diffusely thickened and

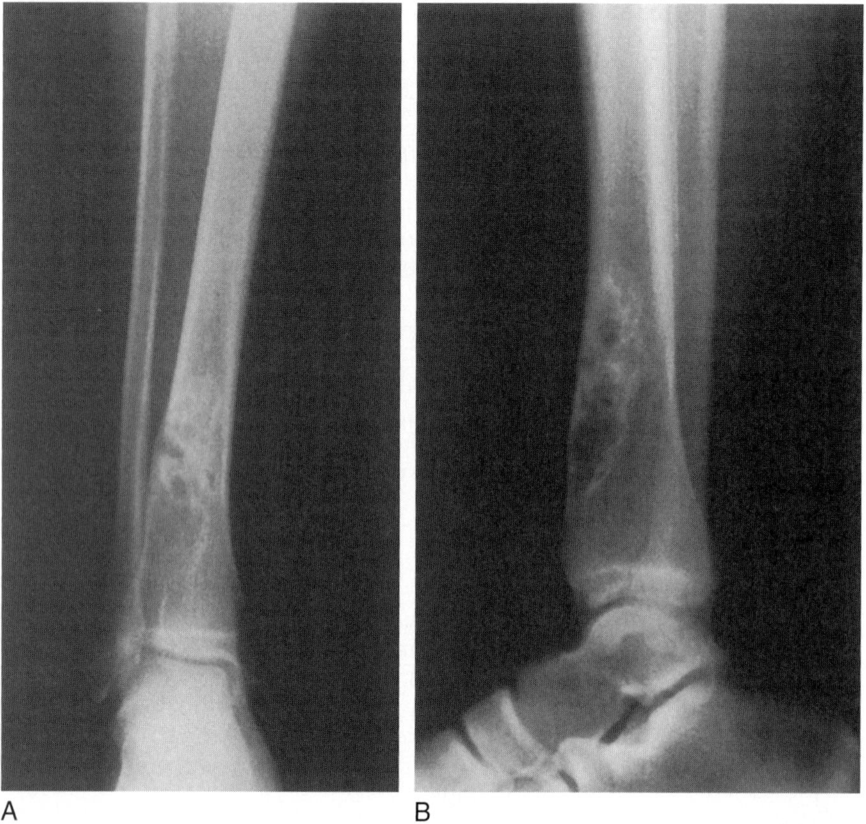

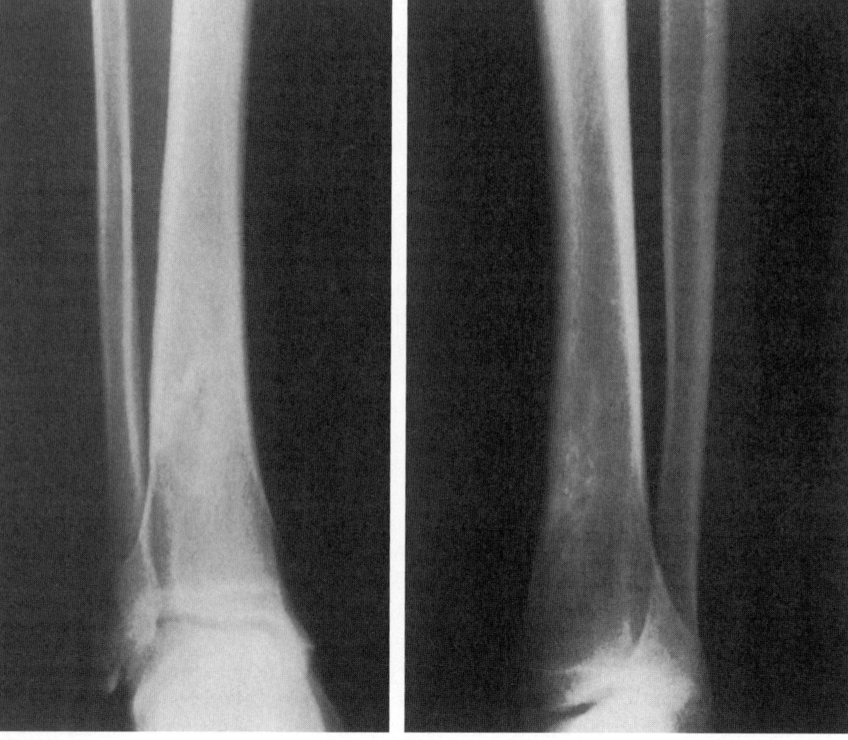

FIGURE 38-40 Imaging findings in a 15-year-old boy with persistent discomfort. **A** and **B,** Radiographs showed a persistent distal tibial nonossifying fibroma. **C** and **D,** Two years after curettage and bone grafting, the lesion had healed.

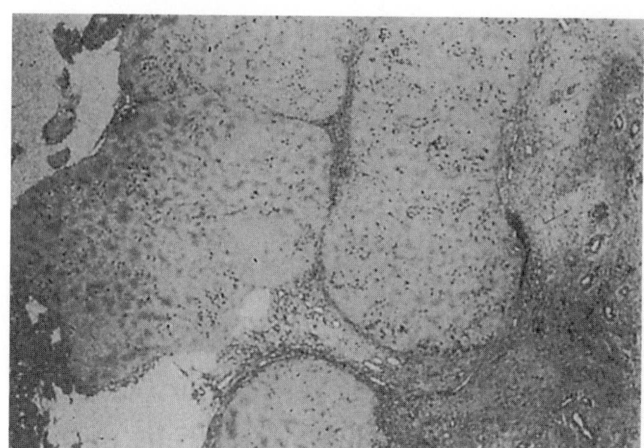

FIGURE 38–41 Synovial chondromatosis. Histologically, the lesion is composed of numerous foci of cartilaginous metaplasia, some of which may be ossified.

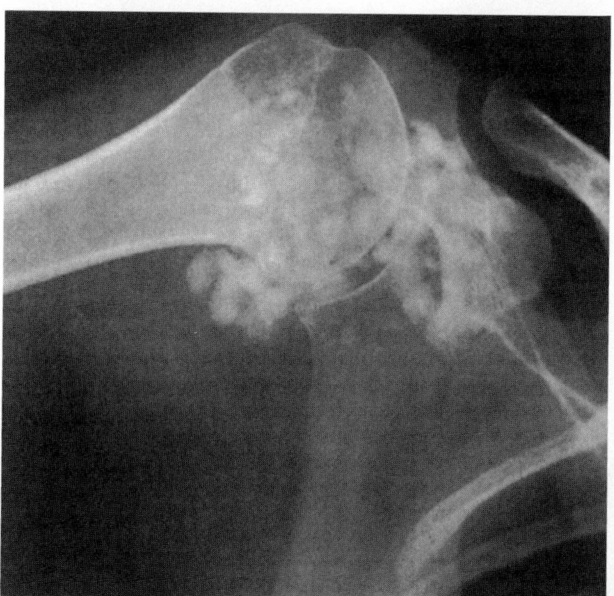

FIGURE 38–42 Synovial chondromatosis of the shoulder. Note the multiple areas of stippled calcification in and around the joint.

tan or brownish-red. Sessile or pedunculated nodules may cover the surface of the synovium. The synovial texture may vary in firmness, depending on how much fibrous tissue is present.[68] Extensive hemosiderin deposition may be evident. In the tendon sheaths of the fingers, the lesion is usually solitary and well circumscribed.

Histologically, the villous nodular appearance of the synovium is characteristic, with tightly packed histiocytes filling the subsynovial tissue (Fig. 38–43). Some of the histiocytes are laden with hemosiderin. Multinucleated giant cells and lipid-laden macrophages are seen in varying numbers. There are few mononuclear cells, lymphocytes, or plasma cells. Histologically, PVNS is similar to the hemosiderotic synovitis that results from multiple episodes of bleeding into a joint, such as seen in hemophilia. Abundant production of collagen may be evident in patients with long-standing disease. Occasionally, cellularity of the lesion may produce a pseudo-sarcomatous appearance.

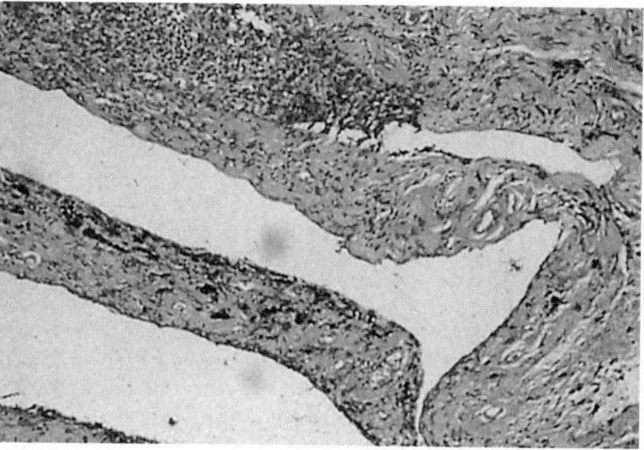

FIGURE 38–43 Pigmented villonodular synovitis (original magnification ×10). The villous nodular appearance of the synovium is characteristic, with tightly packed histiocytes filling the subsynovial tissue.

Clinical Features

Pigmented villonodular synovitis is locally aggressive and almost always monoarticular. Most patients are young to middle-aged adults. The most common sites of involvement are the knee and the tenosynovial region in the hand and wrist.[68,511] Other areas that may be affected include the elbow, spine, foot, ankle, hip, and shoulder.[345,514,529] Multifocal involvement, although rare, has been reported in children.[250,514,532] In these patients, genitourinary and other congenital anomalies may be noted. Multiple sites are involved in less than 1% in reported series of PVNS. The disorder has a slight male predilection.

Patient complaints consist of localized pain and swelling of the affected joint. The proliferated synovial membrane may become caught between the articular ends of the bone, creating a locking within the joint. Range of motion may be limited. Joint aspiration yields a dark brown or serosanguineous fluid. In the absence of trauma to the joint, this finding is of diagnostic significance. PVNS of the knee has presented clinically as a popliteal cyst[513] (Fig. 38–44).

Radiographic Findings

Radiographic findings that are highly suggestive of PVNS include soft tissue (synovial) swelling in the joint and lucent areas involving the epiphyseal (or metaphyseal) ends of two continuous bones across a joint. These radiolucencies may have a border of benign sclerosis. The lytic bone lesions may appear very aggressive, particularly in the femoral head and acetabulum. CT further clarifies involvement on both

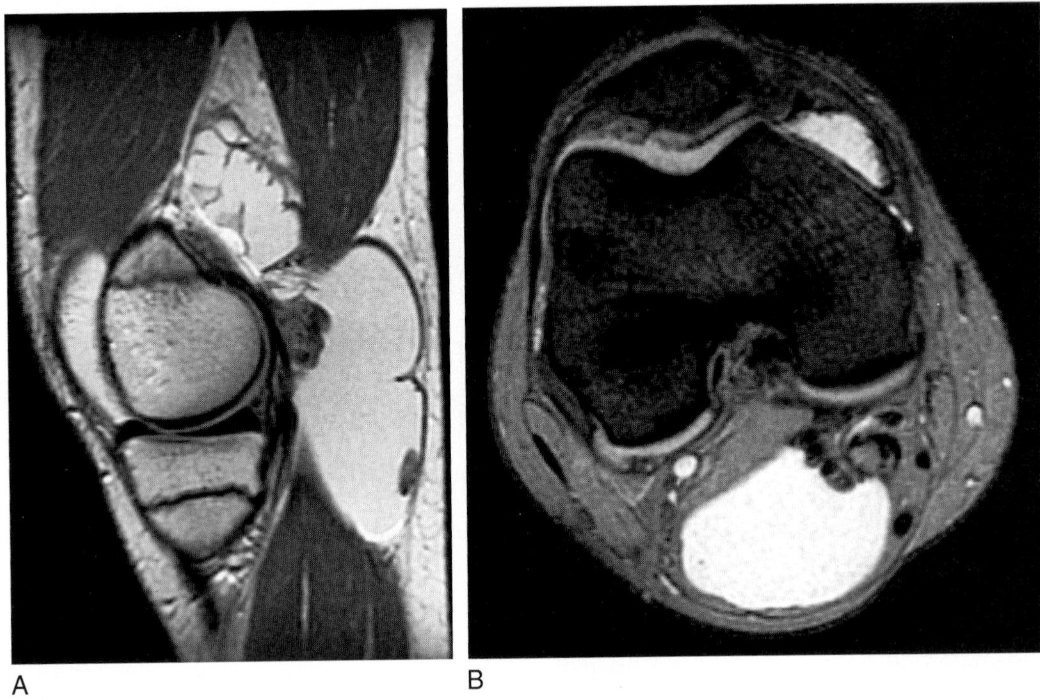

FIGURE 38–44 This 14-year-old boy presented with a large mass behind his right knee and swelling within the knee joint. Plain radiographs were negative. Magnetic resonance imaging showed a large popliteal cyst in the sagittal plane **(A)** and axial plane **(B)**. Pigmented villonodular synovitis tissue is noted within the cyst.

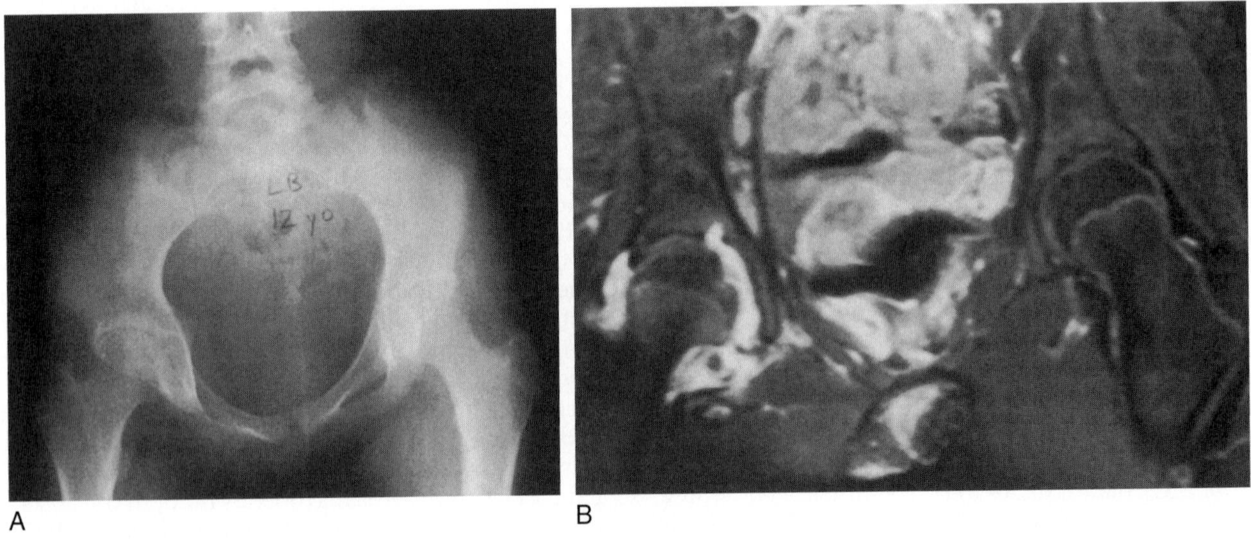

FIGURE 38–45 Imaging findings in a 12-year-old girl with a painful right hip and limited joint range of motion. **A,** Narrowing of the joint space and radiolucencies on the medial aspect of the femoral head and acetabulum are evident. **B,** Magnetic resonance imaging demonstrates an effusion and defect within the acetabulum.

sides of the joint. A marked narrowing of the joint may be present (Fig. 38–45).

MRI findings include scattered areas of low signal intensity that represent hemosiderin deposits in hypertrophied synovium on T2-weighted images and dotted areas of low signal intensity, presumably due to fibrous components of the lesion, on T1-weighted images.[23] Gradient-echo imaging provides superior depiction of the extent of the disease owing to signal decay of hemosiderin-laden thickened synovium in pediatric patients.[95,141] Inflamed synovium with low hemosiderin deposition can be identified on enhanced imaging.

After aspiration of the joint (dark brown or serosanguineous fluid is usually obtained), contrast arthrography reveals multiple filling defects due to the abundant hypertrophic synovium.

Differential Diagnosis

Abnormalities that may affect both sides of a joint are most often considered in the differential diagnosis of PVNS. These abnormalities include chronic monoarticular rheumatoid arthritis, synovial hemangiomatosis, low-grade infection, and, rarely, other inflammatory joint conditions such as tuberculosis. Hemophilia usually is readily diagnosed from its accompanying clinical symptoms, although the histologic findings are similar to those of PVNS.

Treatment

The treatment for PVNS consists of total synovectomy. In the knee, this is best performed arthroscopically.[123,388] Recurrence of PVNS after synovectomy is common, and the patient and family should be made aware of this probability.[371,459]

Radiation synovectomy has been found useful in recurrent cases with extensive bone involvement and joint destruction in the adult patient.[98,248]

DYSPLASIA EPIPHYSEALIS HEMIMELICA (TREVOR'S DISEASE)

Incidence

Dysplasia epiphysealis hemimelica is a rare developmental disorder of epiphyseal osteocartilaginous growth in children, usually in the lower limbs. The lesion consists of osteocartilaginous tissue arising from the epiphysis and usually is hemimelic (either the lateral or the medial part of the ossification centers is involved). Although the incidence has been reported as one per million, it is likely higher than that.

Mouchet and Belot in 1926 first described this as a tarsal bone disorder and used the term *tarsomegalie*.[346] In 1950 Trevor used the term *tarso-epiphyseal aclasis*.[519] In 1956 Fairbank used the now common term *dysplasia epiphysealis hemimelica*.[152]

Etiology

The etiology of dysplasia epiphysealis hemimelica is unknown.[255,276,511] There is no strong evidence to suggest a hereditary component. It has been hypothesized that this condition represents a fundamental defect in the regulation of cartilage proliferation in the affected epiphyses, tarsal bones, or carpal bones.

Pathology

The findings are similar to those described for solitary osteochondromas. The lesion may be a pedunculated mass with a cartilaginous cap, or it may be seen only as an enlarged irregularity of the articular surface.[68] Histologically, the lesion appears similar to benign osteochondromas.

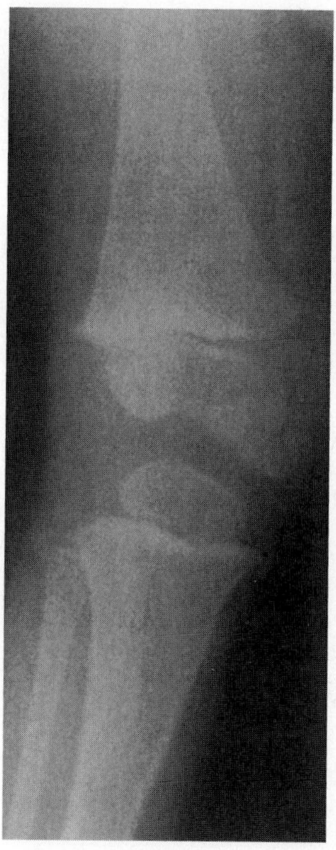

FIGURE 38-46 Dysplasia epiphysealis hemimelica. The lesion on the medial aspect of the distal femur in this 2-year-old boy led to an asymptomatic valgus malalignment.

Clinical Features

The most common sites of involvement are the distal femur, proximal tibia, talus, and tarsal navicular (Figs. 38–46 and 38–47). Other affected areas have included the acetabulum, proximal femur, first cuneiform, scapula, and, infrequently, the upper extremity.[301,484,520] The presenting complaint usually is not discomfort but instead deformity and limited range of motion in the affected joint. Other symptoms include a limp, muscle wasting, and, if long-standing, limb length discrepancy. Angular malalignment of the knee (valgum or varum), ankle, and hindfoot (valgus) may be evident. The affected portion of the epiphysis is enlarged and a mass may be palpable. Articular surface irregularity may lead to early secondary osteoarthritis.

The male-to-female ratio is reported as 3:1, with patients commonly diagnosed between 2 and 14 years of age.

Radiographic Findings

The radiographic findings depend on the patient's age at presentation. With infants or toddlers, radiographs may be negative or may demonstrate minimal metaphyseal widening. As the affected bone matures, a multicentric radiodensity develops adjacent to the

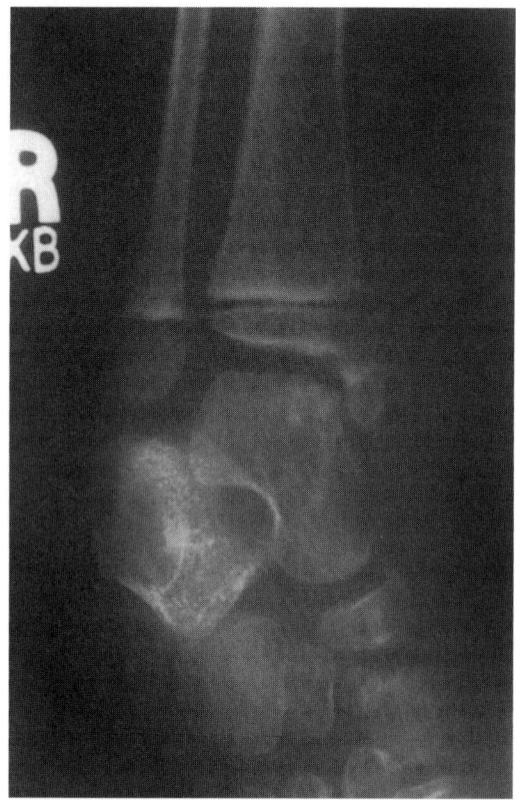

FIGURE 38–47 Dysplasia epiphysealis hemimelica. Multicentric radiodensities are evident along the medial malleolus, talar dome, and tarsal navicular in this radiograph of a 5-year-old boy's foot and ankle.

epiphysis or tarsal bone. In adolescents or adults, the lesion appears as an irregular bony mass, similar to an exostosis. The mass arises from one side of the affected epiphysis, may be single or multiple, and is associated with joint deformity. As the lesion matures and ossifies, it becomes confluent with the underlying bone. Premature physeal closure may occur, with secondary angular deformity and limb length discrepancy.

CT has been useful in accurately demonstrating the relationship between the normal bone and abnormal ossification, particularly at the articular surface. The use of MRI has allowed better imaging of the soft tissue component of the lesion. Most of the recent MRI literature reports a distinct plane of separation between the lesion and the normal epiphyseal bone.[255,276] However, this plane is much more difficult to define during surgery.

Natural History

Dysplasia epiphysealis hemimelica usually stops growing once maturity is reached. Incongruity that occurs in the joint leads to subsequent osteoarthritis. This condition remains benign; malignant transformation has not been reported in dysplasia epiphysealis hemimelica.

Treatment

Observation is warranted if the condition is asymptomatic and has not led to angular deformity or caused significant limitation of joint range of motion. Surgical excision should be undertaken if the lesion is painful, deformity is occurring, or joint function is limited. Recurrence is common, and repeated local excision is often required. Any angular deformities can be treated with corrective osteotomy at the time of lesion excision. Generally, the results are very good after excision of lesions that are juxta-articular. Unfortunately, less successful outcomes are achieved with excision of intra-articular lesions.[276]

References

1. Aarskog D, Tveteraas E: McCune-Albright's syndrome following adrenalectomy for Cushing's syndrome in infancy. J Pediatr 1968;73:89.
2. Abdelwahab IF, Hermann G, Norton KI, et al: Simple bone cysts of the pelvis in adolescents: A report of four cases [see comments]. J Bone Joint Surg Am 1991;73:1090.
3. Abdelwahab IF, Lewis MM, Klein MJ, et al: Case report 515: Simple (solitary) bone cyst of the calcaneus. Skeletal Radiol 1989;17:607.
4. Abdel-Wanis ME, Tsuchiya H, Uehara K, et al: Minimal curettage, multiple drilling, and continuous decompression through a cannulated screw for treatment of calcaneal simple bone cysts in children. J Pediatr Orthop 2002;22:540.
5. Adamsbaum C, Mascard E, Guinebretiere JM, et al: Intralesional Ethibloc injections in primary aneurysmal bone cysts: An efficient and safe treatment. Skeletal Radiol 2003;32:559.
6. Ahmed AR, Tan TS, Unni KK, et al: Secondary chondrosarcoma in osteochondroma: Report of 107 patients. Clin Orthop Relat Res 2003;411:193.
7. Ahmed SK, Lee WC, Irving RM, et al: Is Ollier's disease an understaging of Maffucci's syndrome? J Laryngol Otol 1999;113:861.
8. Ahn J, Ludecke HJ, Lindow S, et al: Cloning of the putative tumour suppressor gene for hereditary multiple exostoses (EXT1). Nat Genet 1995;11:137.
9. Ahn JI, Park JS: Pathological fractures secondary to unicameral bone cysts. Int Orthop 1994;18:20.
10. Akhtar M, Ali MA, Bakry M, et al: Fine-needle aspiration biopsy of Langerhans histiocytosis (histiocytosis-X). Diagn Cytopathol 1993;9:527.
11. Albregts AE, Rapini RP: Malignancy in Maffucci's syndrome. Dermatol Clin 1995;13:73.
12. Albright F: Polyostotic fibrous dysplasia: A defense of the entity. J Med Endocrinol 1947;7:307.
13. Albright F, Scoville B, Sulkowitch HW: Syndrome characterized by osteitis fibrosa disseminata, areas of pigmentation, and a gonadal dysfunction: Further observations including the report of two more cases. Endocrinology 1938;22:411.
14. Aleotti A, Cervellati F, Bovolenta MR, et al: Birbeck granules: Contribution to the comprehension of intra-

cytoplasmic evolution. J Submicrosc Cytol Pathol 1998; 30:295.
15. Alguacil-Garcia A, Alonso A, Pettigrew NM: Osteofibrous dysplasia (ossifying fibroma) of the tibia and fibula and adamantinoma: A case report. Am J Clin Pathol 1984;82:470.
16. Alman BA, Greel DA, Wolfe HJ: Activating mutations of Gs protein in monostotic fibrous lesions of bone. J Orthop Res 1996;14:311.
17. Altermatt S, Schwobel M, Pochon JP: Operative treatment of solitary bone cysts with tricalcium phosphate ceramic: A 1 to 7 year follow-up. Eur J Pediatr Surg 1992;2:180.
18. Althof PA, Ohmori K, Zhou M, et al: Cytogenetic and molecular cytogenetic findings in 43 aneurysmal bone cysts: Aberrations of 17p mapped to 17p13.2 by fluorescence in situ hybridization. Mod Pathol 2004;17:518.
19. Amin R, Ling R: Case report: Malignant fibrous histiocytoma following radiation therapy of fibrous dysplasia. Br J Radiol 1995;68:1119.
20. Anderson MJ, Townsend DR, Johnston JO, et al: Osteofibrous dysplasia in the newborn: Report of a case. J Bone Joint Surg Am 1993;75:265.
21. Andrisano A, Soncini G, Calderoni PP, et al: Critical review of infantile fibrous dysplasia: Surgical treatment. J Pediatr Orthop 1991;11:478.
22. Anract P, de Pinieux G, Jeanrot C, et al: Malignant fibrous histiocytoma at the site of a previously treated aneurysmal bone cyst: A case report. J Bone Joint Surg Am 2002;84:106.
23. Araki Y, Tanaka H, Yamamoto H, et al: MR imaging of pigmented villonodular synovitis of the knee. Radiat Med 1994;12:11.
24. Araki Y, Tanaka H, Yamamoto H, et al: MRI of fibrous cortical defect of the femur. Radiat Med 1994;12:93.
25. Arata MA, Peterson HA, Dahlin DC: Pathological fractures through non-ossifying fibromas: Review of the Mayo Clinic experience. J Bone Joint Surg Am 1981; 63:980.
26. Arauz S, Morcuende JA, Weinstein SL: Intra-articular benign osteoblastoma of the acetabulum: A case report. J Pediatr Orthop 1999;8:136.
27. Arms DM, Strecker WB, Manske PR, et al: Management of forearm deformity in multiple hereditary osteochondromatosis. J Pediatr Orthop 1997;17:450.
28. Atabay H, Kuyucu Y, Korkmaz O, et al: Myelopathy due to hereditary multiple exostoses: CT and MR studies. Clin Neurol Neurosurg 1996;98:186.
29. Au WY, Ooi GC, Ma SK, et al: Chronic myeloid leukemia in an adolescent with Ollier's disease after intensive X-ray exposure. Leuk Lymphoma 2004;45:613.
30. Auyeung J, Mohanty K, Tayton K: Maffucci lymphangioma syndrome: An unusual variant of Ollier's disease, a case report and a review of the literature. J Pediatr Orthop 2003;12:147.
31. Ayala AG, Murray JA, Erling MA, et al: Osteoid-osteoma: intraoperative tetracycline-fluorescence demonstration of the nidus. J Bone Joint Surg Am 1986; 68:747.
32. Azouz EM, Saigal G, Rodriguez MM, et al: Langerhans' cell histiocytosis: Pathology, imaging and treatment of skeletal involvement. Pediatr Radiol 2005;35:103.
33. Balci P, Obuz F, Gore O, et al: Aneurysmal bone cyst secondary to infantile cartilaginous hamartoma of rib. Pediatr Radiol 1997;27:767.
34. Barei DP, Moreau G, Scarborough MT, et al: Percutaneous radiofrequency ablation of osteoid osteoma. Clin Orthop Relat Res 2000;373:115.
35. Baruffi MR, Neto JB, Barbieri CH, et al: Aneurysmal bone cyst with chromosomal changes involving 7q and 16p. Cancer Genet Cytogenet 2001;129:177.
36. Beauchamp CP, Duncan CP, Dzus AK, et al: Osteoblastoma: Experience with 23 patients. Can J Surg 1992;35: 199.
37. Beltran J, Aparisi F, Bonmati LM, et al: Eosinophilic granuloma: MRI manifestations. Skeletal Radiol 1993; 22:157.
38. Benassi MS, Campanacci L, Gamberi G, et al: Cytokeratin expression and distribution in adamantinoma of the long bones and osteofibrous dysplasia of tibia and fibula: An immunohistochemical study correlated to histogenesis. Histopathology 1994;25:71.
39. Ben-Itzhak I, Denolf FA, Versfeld GA, et al: The Maffucci syndrome. J Pediatr Orthop 1988;8:345.
40. Berger I, Rieker R, Ehemann V, et al: Analysis of chromosomal imbalances by comparative genomic hybridisation of pigmented villonodular synovitis. Cancer Lett 2005;220:231.
41. Bernard MA, Hall CE, Hogue DA, et al: Diminished levels of the putative tumor suppressor proteins EXT1 and EXT2 in exostosis chondrocytes. Cell Motil Cytoskeleton 2001;48:149.
42. Bertoni F, Bacchini P, Capanna R, et al: Solid variant of aneurysmal bone cyst. Cancer 1993;71:729.
43. Bertram C, Madert J, Eggers C: Eosinophilic granuloma of the cervical spine. Spine 2002;27:1408.
44. Betsy M, Kupersmith LM, Springfield DS: Metaphyseal fibrous defects. J Am Acad Orthop Surg 2004;12:89.
45. Biagini R, Orsini U, Demitri S, et al: Osteoid osteoma and osteoblastoma of the sacrum. Orthopedics 2001; 24:1061.
46. Bianco P, Kuznetsov SA, Riminucci M, et al: Reproduction of human fibrous dysplasia of bone in immunocompromised mice by transplanted mosaics of normal and Gsalpha-mutated skeletal progenitor cells. J Clin Invest 1998;101:1737.
47. Biermann JS: Common benign lesions of bone in children and adolescents. J Pediatr Orthop 2002;22:268.
48. Blanton SH, Hogue D, Wagner M, et al: Hereditary multiple exostoses: Confirmation of linkage to chromosomes 8 and 11. Am J Med Genet 1996;62:150.
49. Blitch E, Mendicino RW: Chondroblastoma of the calcaneus: Literature review and case presentation. J Foot Ankle Surg 1996;35:250.
50. Bloem JL, van der Heul RO, Schuttevaer HM, et al: Fibrous dysplasia vs. adamantinoma of the tibia: Differentiation based on discriminant analysis of clinical and plain film findings. AJR Am J Roentgenol 1991; 156:1017.
51. Bollini G, Jouve JL, Cottalorda J, et al: Aneurysmal bone cyst in children: Analysis of twenty-seven patients. J Pediatr Orthop B 1998;7:274.
52. Bollini G, Jouve JL, Gentet JC, et al: Bone lesions in histiocytosis X. J Pediatr Orthop 1991;11:469.

53. Bonakdarpour A, Levy WM, Aegerter E: Primary and secondary aneurysmal bone cyst: A radiological study of 75 cases. Radiology 1978;126:75.
54. Bonar SF, McCarthy S, Stalley P, et al: Epiphyseal osteoblastoma-like osteosarcoma. Skeletal Radiol 2004;33:46.
55. Bongioanni F, Assadurian E, Polivka M, et al: Aneurysmal bone cyst of the atlas: Operative removal through an anterolateral approach. A case report. J Bone Joint Surg Am 1996;78:1574.
56. Boriani S, Capanna R, Donati D, et al: Osteoblastoma of the spine. Clin Orthop Relat Res 1992;278:37.
57. Boriani S, De Iure F, Campanacci L, et al: Aneurysmal bone cyst of the mobile spine: Report on 41 cases. Spine 2001;26:27.
58. Bottner F, Rodl R, Kordish I, et al: Surgical treatment of symptomatic osteochondroma: A three- to eight-year follow-up study. J Bone Joint Surg Br 2003;85:1161.
59. Bottner F, Roedl R, Wortler K, et al: Cyclooxygenase-2 inhibitor for pain management in osteoid osteoma. Clin Orthop Relat Res 2001;393:258.
60. Bovee JV, van Roggen JS, Cleton-Jansen AM, et al: Malignant progression in multiple enchondromatosis (Ollier's disease): An autopsy-based molecular genetic study. Hum Pathol 2000;31:1299.
61. Bovill DF, Skinner HB: Unicameral bone cysts: A comparison of treatment options. Orthop Rev 1989;18:420.
62. Bowen RE, Morrissy RT: Recurrence of a unicameral bone cyst in the proximal part of the fibula after en bloc resection: A case report. J Bone Joint Surg Am 2004;86:154.
63. Brastianos P, Pradilla G, McCarthy E, et al: Solitary thoracic osteochondroma: Case report and review of the literature. Neurosurgery 2005;56:E1379; discussion E1379.
64. Bridge JA, Dembinski A, De Boer J, et al: Clonal chromosomal abnormalities in osteofibrous dysplasia: Implications for histopathogenesis and its relationship with adamantinoma. Cancer 1994;73:1746.
65. Bridge JA, Nelson M, Orndal C, et al: Clonal karyotypic abnormalities of the hereditary multiple exostoses chromosomal loci 8q24.1 (EXT1) and 11p11-12 (EXT2) in patients with sporadic and hereditary osteochondromas. Cancer 1998;82:1657.
66. Brien EW, Mirra JM, Ippolito V: Chondroblastoma arising from a nonepiphyseal site. Skeletal Radiol 1995;24:220.
67. Bruggeman NB, Sperling JW, Shives TC: Arthroscopic technique for treatment of synovial chondromatosis of the glenohumeral joint. Arthroscopy 2005;21:633.
68. Bullough P: Orthopaedic Pathology. London, Mosby-Wolfe, 1997.
69. Bumci I, Vlahovic T: Significance of opening the medullar canal in surgical treatment of simple bone cyst. J Pediatr Orthop 2002;22:125.
70. Bush CH, Drane WE: Treatment of an aneurysmal bone cyst of the spine by radionuclide ablation. AJNR Am J Neuroradiol 2000;21:592.
71. Buxi TB, Sud S, Vohra R, et al: Aneurysmal bone cyst of the temporal bone. Australas Radiol 2004;48:251.
72. Cabral CE, Romano S, Guedes P, et al: Chondromyxoid fibroma of the lumbar spine. Skeletal Radiol 1997;26:488.
73. Cakirer S, Cakirer D, Kabukcuoglu F: Aneurysmal bone cyst of the orbit: A case of rare location and review of the literature. Clin Imaging 2002;26:386.
74. Camitta B, Wells R, Segura A, et al: Osteoblastoma response to chemotherapy. Cancer 1991;68:999.
75. Campanacci M: Osteofibrous dysplasia of long bones: A new clinical entity. Ital J Orthop Traumatol 1976;2:221.
76. Campanacci M: Bone and Soft Tissue Tumors. Vienna, Springer-Verlag, 1990.
77. Campanacci M, Capanna R, Picci P: Unicameral and aneurysmal bone cysts. Clin Orthop Relat Res 1986;203:25.
78. Campanacci M, Laus M: Osteofibrous dysplasia of the tibia and fibula. J Bone Joint Surg Am 1981;63:367.
79. Campanacci M, Ruggieri P, Gasbarrini A, et al: Osteoid osteoma: Direct visual identification and intralesional excision of the nidus with minimal removal of bone. J Bone Joint Surg Br 1999;81:814.
80. Candeliere GA, Roughley PJ, Glorieux FH: Polymerase chain reaction-based technique for the selective enrichment and analysis of mosaic arg201 mutations in G alpha s from patients with fibrous dysplasia of bone. Bone 1997;21:201.
81. Cannon SR, Sweetnam DR: Multiple chondrosarcomas in dyschondroplasia (Ollier's disease). Cancer 1985;55:836.
82. Cantwell CP, Obyrne J, Eustace S: Current trends in treatment of osteoid osteoma with an emphasis on radiofrequency ablation. Eur Radiol 2004;14:607.
83. Capanna R, Albisinni U, Caroli GC, et al: Contrast examination as a prognostic factor in the treatment of solitary bone cyst by cortisone injection. Skeletal Radiol 1984;12:97.
84. Capanna R, Albisinni U, Picci P, et al: Aneurysmal bone cyst of the spine. J Bone Joint Surg Am 1985;67:527.
85. Capanna R, Campanacci DA, Manfrini M: Unicameral and aneurysmal bone cysts. Orthop Clin North Am 1996;27:605.
86. Capanna R, Dal Monte A, Gitelis S, et al: The natural history of unicameral bone cyst after steroid injection. Clin Orthop Relat Res 1982;166:204.
87. Capanna R, Springfield DS, Biagini R, et al: Juxtaepiphyseal aneurysmal bone cyst. Skeletal Radiol 1985;13:21.
88. Carroll KL, Yandow SM, Ward K, et al: Clinical correlation to genetic variations of hereditary multiple exostosis. J Pediatr Orthop 1999;19:785.
89. Cassard X, Accadbled F, De Gauzy JS, et al: Osteoid osteoma of the elbow in children: A report of three cases and a review of the literature. J Pediatr Orthop B 2002;11:240.
90. Caterini R, Manili M, Spinelli M, et al: Epiphyseal chondroblastoma of bone: Long-term effects on skeletal growth and articular function in 15 cases treated surgically. Arch Orthop Trauma Surg 1992;111:327.
91. Chan MS, Wong YC, Yuen MK, et al: Spinal aneurysmal bone cyst causing acute cord compression without ver-

tebral collapse: CT and MRI findings. Pediatr Radiol 2002;32:601.
92. Chang H, Park JB, Lee EJ: Simple bone cyst of lamina of lumbar spine: A case report. Spine 2001;26:E531.
93. Chapurlat RD, Hugueny P, Delmas PD, et al: Treatment of fibrous dysplasia of bone with intravenous pamidronate: Long-term effectiveness and evaluation of predictors of response to treatment. Bone 2004;35:235.
94. Cheng MH, Chen YR: Malignant fibrous histiocytoma degeneration in a patient with facial fibrous dysplasia. Ann Plast Surg 1997;39:638.
95. Cheng XG, You YH, Liu W, et al: MRI features of pigmented villonodular synovitis (PVNS). Clin Rheumatol 2004;23:31.
96. Chew DK, Menelaus MB, Richardson MD: Ollier's disease: Varus angulation at the lower femur and its management. J Pediatr Orthop 1998;18:202.
97. Chigira M, Maehara S, Arita S, et al: The aetiology and treatment of simple bone cysts. J Bone Joint Surg Br 1983;65:633.
98. Chin KR, Barr SJ, Winalski C, et al: Treatment of advanced primary and recurrent diffuse pigmented villonodular synovitis of the knee. J Bone Joint Surg Am 2002;84:2192.
99. Choi IH, Chung CY, Cho TJ, et al: Aneurysmal bone cyst arising from a fibrous metaphyseal defect in a toddler. Clin Orthop Relat Res 2002;395:216.
100. Chung OM, Yip SF, Ngan KC, et al: Chondroblastoma of the lumbar spine with cauda equina syndrome. Spinal Cord 2003;41:359.
101. Cigala F, Sadile F: Arterial embolization of aneurysmal bone cysts in children. Bull Hosp Joint Dis 1996;54:261.
102. Cioni R, Armillotta N, Bargellini I, et al: CT-guided radiofrequency ablation of osteoid osteoma: Long-term results. Eur Radiol 2004;14:1203.
103. Codman E: Epiphyseal chondromatous giant cell tumors of the upper end of the humerus. Surg Gynecol Obstet 1931;52:543.
104. Cohen J: Etiology of simple bone cyst. J Bone Joint Surg Am 1970;52:1493.
105. Cohen J: Unicameral bone cysts: A current synthesis of reported cases. Orthop Clin North Am 1977;8:715.
106. Cook A, Raskind W, Blanton SH, et al: Genetic heterogeneity in families with hereditary multiple exostoses. Am J Hum Genet 1993;53:71.
107. Cottalorda J, Kohler R, Sales de Gauzy J, et al: Epidemiology of aneurysmal bone cyst in children: A multicenter study and literature review. J Pediatr Orthop B 2004;13:389.
108. Cove JA, Taminiau AH, Obermann WR, et al: Osteoid osteoma of the spine treated with percutaneous computed tomography-guided thermocoagulation. Spine 2000;25:1283.
109. Crist BD, Lenke LG, Lewis S: Osteoid osteoma of the lumbar spine: A case report highlighting a novel reconstruction technique. J Bone Joint Surg Am 2005;87:414.
110. D' Angelo G, Petas N, Donzelli O: Lengthening of the lower limbs in Ollier's disease: Problems related to surgery. Chir Organi Mov 1996;81:279.
111. Dabska M, Buraczewski J: On malignant transformation in fibrous dysplasia of bone. Oncology 1972;26:369.
112. Dahl MT: The gradual correction of forearm deformities in multiple hereditary exostoses. Hand Clin 1993;9:707.
113. Dahlin D: Bone Tumors. Springfield, Ill, Charles C Thomas, 1978.
114. Dahlin DC, Unni KK: Bone Tumors: General Aspects and Data on 8542 Cases, 4th ed. Springfield, Ill, Charles C Thomas, 1986.
115. D'Ambrosia R, Ferguson AB Jr: The formation of osteochondroma by epiphyseal cartilage transplantation. Clin Orthop Relat Res 1968;61:103.
116. Danielsson LG, el-Haddad I: Winged scapula due to osteochondroma: Report of 3 children. Acta Orthop Scand 1989;60:728.
117. Darilek S, Wicklund C, Novy D, et al: Hereditary multiple exostosis and pain. J Pediatr Orthop 2005;25:369.
118. Davies AM, Pikoulas C, Griffith J: MRI of eosinophilic granuloma. Eur J Radiol 1994;18:205.
119. Davies M, Cassar-Pullicino VN, Davies AM, et al: The diagnostic accuracy of MR imaging in osteoid osteoma. Skeletal Radiol 2002;31:559.
120. Davila JA, Amrami KK, Sundaram M, et al: Chondroblastoma of the hands and feet. Skeletal Radiol 2004;33:582.
121. Davis RI, Foster H, Arthur K, et al: Cell proliferation studies in primary synovial chondromatosis. J Pathol 1998;184:18.
122. de Kleuver M, van der Heul RO, Veraart BE: Aneurysmal bone cyst of the spine: 31 cases and the importance of the surgical approach. J Pediatr Orthop B 1998;7:286.
123. De Ponti A, Sansone V, Malchere M: Result of arthroscopic treatment of pigmented villonodular synovitis of the knee. Arthroscopy 2003;19:602.
124. De Rosa GP, Graziano GP, Scott J: Arterial embolization of aneurysmal bone cyst of the lumbar spine: A report of two cases. J Bone Joint Surg Am 1990;72:777.
125. De Schepper AM, Ramon F, Van Marck E: MR imaging of eosinophilic granuloma: Report of 11 cases. Skeletal Radiol 1993;22:163.
126. de Silva MV, Reid R: Chondroblastoma: Varied histologic appearance, potential diagnostic pitfalls, and clinicopathologic features associated with local recurrence. Ann Diagn Pathol 2003;7:205.
127. DeFriend DE, Smith SP, Hughes PM: Percutaneous laser photocoagulation of osteoid osteomas under CT guidance. Clin Radiol 2003;58:222.
128. Della Rocca C, Huvos AG: Osteoblastoma: Varied histological presentations with a benign clinical course. An analysis of 55 cases. Am J Surg Pathol 1996;20:841.
129. Deo SD, Fairbank JC, Wilson-Macdonald J, et al: Aneurysmal bone cyst as a rare cause of spinal cord compression in a young child. Spine 2005;30:E80.
130. DePalma AF, Ahmad I: Fibrous dysplasia associated with shepherd's crook deformity of the humerus. Clin Orthop Relat Res 1973;97:38.
131. DePalma AF, Dodd PM Jr: Reconstructive surgery in fibrous dysplasia of bone. Clin Orthop Relat Res 1962;19:132.

132. DePalma AF, Smythe VL: Recurrent fibrous dysplasia in a cortical bone graft: A case report. Clin Orthop Relat Res 1963;26:136.
133. DePraeter MP, Dua GF, Seynaeve PC, et al: Occipital pain in osteoid osteoma of the atlas. Spine 1999;24: 912.
134. Desai SS, Jambhekar NA, Samanthray S, et al: Chondromyxoid fibromas: A study of 10 cases. J Surg Oncol 2005;89:28.
135. DiCaprio MR, Murphy MJ, Camp RL: Aneurysmal bone cyst of the spine with familial incidence. Spine 2000;25:1589.
136. Docquier PL, Delloye C: Treatment of simple bone cysts with aspiration and a single bone marrow injection. J Pediatr Orthop 2003;23:766.
137. Donahue F, Ahmad A, Mnaymneh W, et al: Osteoid osteoma: Computed tomography guided percutaneous excision. Clin Orthop Relat Res 1999;366:191.
138. Dussaussois L, Stelmaszyk J, Golzarian J: Percutaneous treatment of an osteoid osteoma of the scapula using a laser under scanner control [in French]. Acta Orthop Belg 1998;64:88.
139. Dysart SH, Swengel RM, van Dam BE: Aneurysmal bone cyst of a thoracic vertebra: Treatment by selective arterial embolization and excision. Spine 1992;17:846.
140. Easley ME, Kneisl JS: Pathologic fractures through nonossifying fibromas: Is prophylactic treatment warranted? J Pediatr Orthop 1997;17:808.
141. Eckhardt BP, Hernandez RJ: Pigmented villonodular synovitis: MR imaging in pediatric patients. Pediatr Radiol 2004;34:943.
142. Ehara S, Rosenthal DI, Aoki J, et al: Peritumoral edema in osteoid osteoma on magnetic resonance imaging. Skeletal Radiol 1999;28:265.
143. el-Sayed S, Brewin TB: Histiocytosis X: Does radiotherapy still have a role? Clin Oncol (R Coll Radiol) 1992; 4:27.
144. Elsheikh T, Silverman JF, Wakely PE Jr, et al: Fine-needle aspiration cytology of Langerhans' cell histiocytosis (eosinophilic granuloma) of bone in children. Diagn Cytopathol 1991;7:261.
145. Enneking WF, Gearen PF: Fibrous dysplasia of the femoral neck: Treatment by cortical bone-grafting. J Bone Joint Surg Am 1986;68:1415.
146. Ergun R, Okten AI, Beskonakli E, et al: Cervical laminar exostosis in multiple hereditary osteochondromatosis: Anterior stabilization and fusion technique for preventing instability. Eur Spine J 1997;6:267.
147. Essadki B, Moujtahid M, Lamine A, et al: Solitary osteochondroma of the limbs: Clinical review of 76 cases and pathogenic hypothesis [in French]. Acta Orthop Belg 2000;66:146.
148. Eugster EA, Rubin SD, Reiter EO, et al: Tamoxifen treatment for precocious puberty in McCune-Albright syndrome: A multicenter trial. J Pediatr 2003;143:60.
149. Eugster EA, Shankar R, Feezle LK, et al: Tamoxifen treatment of progressive precocious puberty in a patient with McCune-Albright syndrome. J Pediatr Endocrinol Metab 1999;12:681.
150. Fadda M, Manunta A, Rinonapoli G, et al: Ultrastructural appearance of chondroblastoma. Int Orthop 1994; 18:389.
151. Faik A, Mahfoud Filali S, Lazrak N, et al: Spinal cord compression due to vertebral osteochondroma: Report of two cases. Joint Bone Spine 2005;72:177.
152. Fairbank T: Dysplasia epiphysealis hemimelica (tarso-epiphyseal aclasis). J Bone Joint Surg Br 1956;38:237.
153. Fanning CV, Sneige NS, Carrasco CH, et al: Fine needle aspiration cytology of chondroblastoma of bone. Cancer 1990;65:1847.
154. Farber JM, Stanton RP: Treatment options in unicameral bone cysts. Orthopedics 1990;13:25.
155. Feigenberg SJ, Marcus RB Jr, Zlotecki RA, et al: Megavoltage radiotherapy for aneurysmal bone cysts. Int J Radiat Oncol Biol Phys 2001;49:1243.
156. Felix NA, Mazur JM, Loveless EA: Acetabular dysplasia associated with hereditary multiple exostoses: A case report. J Bone Joint Surg Br 2000;82:555.
157. Fernandez DL, Capo JT, Gonzalez E: Corrective osteotomy for symptomatic increased ulnar tilt of the distal end of the radius. J Hand Surg [Am] 2001;26:722.
158. Fink BR, Temple HT, Chiricosta FM, et al: Chondroblastoma of the foot. Foot Ankle Int 1997;18:236.
159. Fisher AJ, Reinus WR, Friedland JA, et al: Quantitative analysis of the plain radiographic appearance of eosinophilic granuloma. Invest Radiol 1995;30:466.
160. Fiumara E, Scarabino T, Guglielmi G, et al: Osteochondroma of the L-5 vertebra: A rare cause of sciatic pain. Case report. J Neurosurg 1999;91:219.
161. Floman Y, Bar-On E, Mosheiff R, et al: Eosinophilic granuloma of the spine. J Pediatr Orthop B 1997;6: 260.
162. Francannet C, Cohen-Tanugi A, Le Merrer M, et al: Genotype-phenotype correlation in hereditary multiple exostoses. J Med Genet 2001;38:430.
163. Francesco B, Andrea LA, Vincenzo S: Intra-articular osteoid osteoma of the lower extremity: Diagnostic problems. Foot Ankle Int 2002;23:264.
164. Frangenheim P: Angeborene Ostitis Fibrosa als Ursache einer intrauterinen Unterschenkel Fraktur. Arch Klin Chir 1921;228:22.
165. Fraser RK, Coates CJ, Cole WG: An angiostatic agent in treatment of a recurrent aneurysmal bone cyst. J Pediatr Orthop 1993;13:668.
166. Frassica FJ, Waltrip RL, Sponseller PD, et al: Clinicopathologic features and treatment of osteoid osteoma and osteoblastoma in children and adolescents. Orthop Clin North Am 1996;27:559.
167. Freiberg AA, Loder RT, Heidelberger KP, et al: Aneurysmal bone cysts in young children. J Pediatr Orthop 1994;14:86.
168. Friedland JA, Reinus WR, Fisher AJ, et al: Quantitative analysis of the plain radiographic appearance of nonossifying fibroma. Invest Radiol 1995;30:474.
169. Fujimoto T, Nakamura T, Ikeda T, et al: Solitary bone cyst in L-2: Case illustration. J Neurosurg 2002;97:151.
170. Fukuda T, Saito M, Nakajima T: Imprint cytology of chondroblastoma of bone: A case report. Acta Cytol 1998;42:403.
171. Gabos PG, Bowen JR: Epiphyseal-metaphyseal enchondromatosis: A new clinical entity. J Bone Joint Surg Am 1998;80:782.
172. Galasko CS: The fate of simple bone cysts which fracture [letter]. Clin Orthop Relat Res 1974;101:302.

173. Gallacher SJ, Wilson R, Boyle IT, et al: The hyperthyroidism of polyostotic fibrous dysplasia: A possible autoimmune aetiology. Scott Med J 1989;34:529.
174. Garg S, Mehta S, Dormans JP: Langerhans cell histiocytosis of the spine in children: Long-term follow-up. J Bone Joint Surg Am 2004;86:1740.
175. Garg S, Mehta S, Dormans JP: Modern surgical treatment of primary aneurysmal bone cyst of the spine in children and adolescents. J Pediatr Orthop 2005;25:387.
176. Garneti N, Dunn D, El Gamal E, et al: Cervical spondyloptosis caused by an aneurysmal bone cyst: A case report. Spine 2003;28:E68.
177. Garrison RC, Unni KK, McLeod RA, et al: Chondrosarcoma arising in osteochondroma. Cancer 1982;49:1890.
178. Gaudet EL Jr, Nuss DW, Johnson DH Jr, et al: Chondroblastoma of the temporal bone involving the temporomandibular joint, mandibular condyle, and middle cranial fossa: Case report and review of the literature. Cranio 2004;22:160.
179. Gaulke R, Suppelna G: Solitary enchondroma at the hand: Long-term follow-up study after operative treatment. J Hand Surg [Br] 2004;29:64.
180. Gebhart M, Blaimont P: Contribution to the vascular origin of the unicameral bone cyst. Acta Orthop Belg 1996;62:137.
181. Geissmann F, Lepelletier Y, Fraitag S, et al: Differentiation of Langerhans cells in Langerhans cell histiocytosis. Blood 2001;97:1241.
182. Gerasimov AM, Toporova SM, Furtseva LN, et al: The role of lysosomes in the pathogenesis of unicameral bone cysts. Clin Orthop Relat Res 1991;266:53.
183. Ghanem I, Collet LM, Kharrat K, et al: Percutaneous radiofrequency coagulation of osteoid osteoma in children and adolescents. J Pediatr Orthop B 2003;12:244.
184. Ghanem I, Tolo VT, D'Ambra P, et al: Langerhans cell histiocytosis of bone in children and adolescents. J Pediatr Orthop 2003;23:124.
185. Ghelman B, Thompson FM, Arnold WD: Intraoperative radioactive localization of an osteoid-osteoma: Case report. J Bone Joint Surg Am 1981;63:826.
186. Gibbs CP Jr, Hefele MC, Peabody TD, et al: Aneurysmal bone cyst of the extremities: Factors related to local recurrence after curettage with a high-speed burr. J Bone Joint Surg Am 1999;81:1671.
187. Gille O, Pointillart V, Vital JM: Course of spinal solitary osteochondromas. Spine 2005;30:E13.
188. Gitelis S, MacDonald DJ: Common benign bone tumors and usual treatment. In Simon MA, Springfield DS (eds): Surgery for Bone and Soft Tissue Tumors. Philadelphia, Lippincott-Raven, 1998, p 181.
189. Gitelis S, Wilkins R, Conrad EU 2nd: Benign bone tumors. Instr Course Lect 1996;45:425.
190. Givon U, Sher-Lurie N, Schindler A, et al: Titanium elastic nail: A useful instrument for the treatment of simple bone cyst. J Pediatr Orthop 2004;24:317.
191. Gladden ML Jr, Gillingham BL, Hennrikus W, et al: Aneurysmal bone cyst of the first cervical vertebrae in a child treated with percutaneous intralesional injection of calcitonin and methylprednisolone: A case report. Spine 2000;25:527.
192. Golant A, Lou JE, Erol B, et al: Pediatric osteoblastoma of the sternum: A new surgical technique for reconstruction after removal. Case report and review of the literature. J Pediatr Orthop 2004;24:319.
193. Guille JT, Kumar SJ, MacEwen GD: Fibrous dysplasia of the proximal part of the femur: Long-term results of curettage and bone-grafting and mechanical realignment. J Bone Joint Surg Am 1998;80:648.
194. Gupta AK, Crawford AH: Solitary bone cyst with epiphyseal involvement: Confirmation with magnetic resonance imaging. A case report and review of the literature. J Bone Joint Surg Am 1996;78:911.
195. Ha KY, Kim YH: Simple bone cyst with pathologic lumbar pedicle fracture: A case report. Spine 2003;28:E129.
196. Hadjipavlou AG, Lander PH, Marchesi D, et al: Minimally invasive surgery for ablation of osteoid osteoma of the spine. Spine 2003;28:E472.
197. Haga N, Nakamura K, Taniguchi K, et al: Enchondromatosis with features of dysspondyloenchondromatosis and Maffucci syndrome. Clin Dysmorphol 1998;7:65.
198. Haims AH, Desai P, Present D, et al: Epiphyseal extension of a unicameral bone cyst. Skeletal Radiol 1997;26:51.
199. Halbert AR, Harrison WR, Hicks MJ, et al: Cytogenetic analysis of a scapular chondromyxoid fibroma. Cancer Genet Cytogenet 1998;104:52.
200. Hanna BG, Donthineni R, Dalinka MK, et al: Painful ankle in a 19-year-old man. Clin Orthop Relat Res 2003;415:329.
201. Hannon TS, Noonan K, Steinmetz R, et al: Is McCune-Albright syndrome overlooked in subjects with fibrous dysplasia of bone? J Pediatr 2003;142:532.
202. Hashemi-Nejad A, Cole WG: Incomplete healing of simple bone cysts after steroid injections. J Bone Joint Surg Br 1997;79:727.
203. Hazarika D, Kumar RV, Rao CR, et al: Fine needle aspiration cytology of chondroblastoma and chondromyxoid fibroma: A report of two cases. Acta Cytol 1994;38:592.
204. Hazelbag HM, Hogendoorn PC: Adamantinoma of the long bones: An anatomo-clinical review and its relationship with osteofibrous dysplasia [in French]. Ann Pathol 2001;21:499.
205. Hazelbag HM, Wessels JW, Mollevangers P, et al: Cytogenetic analysis of adamantinoma of long bones: Further indications for a common histogenesis with osteofibrous dysplasia. Cancer Genet Cytogenet 1997;97:5.
206. Hecht JT, Hall CR, Snuggs M, et al: Heparan sulfate abnormalities in exostosis growth plates. Bone 2002;31:199.
207. Hennekam RC: Hereditary multiple exostoses. J Med Genet 1991;28:262.
208. Herzenberg JE, Phillips WA, Hensinger RN, et al: Osteoid-osteoma: Intraoperative tetracycline-fluorescence demonstration of the nidus [letter]. J Bone Joint Surg Am 1987;69:310.
209. Hopyan S, Nadesan P, Yu C, et al: Dysregulation of hedgehog signalling predisposes to synovial chondromatosis. J Pathol 2005;206:143.

210. Hosalkar HS, Garg S, Moroz L, et al: The diagnostic accuracy of MRI versus CT imaging for osteoid osteoma in children. Clin Orthop Relat Res 2005;433:171.
211. Hrishikesh KA, Narlawar RS, Deasi SB, et al: Case report: Aneurysmal bone cyst of the ethmoid bone. Br J Radiol 2002;75:916.
212. Hsich GE, Davis RG, Darras BT: Osteoid osteoma presenting with focal neurologic signs. Pediatr Neurol 2002;26:148.
213. Hsissen MA, Kadiri F, Zamiati S, et al: A case of facial fibrous dysplasia in brothers [in French]. Rev Stomatol Chir Maxillofac 1997;98:96.
214. Hsu CC, Wang JW, Chen CE, et al: Results of curettage and high-speed burring for chondroblastoma of the bone. Changgeng Yi Xue Za Zhi 2003;26:761.
215. Hsu CC, Wang JW, Huang CH, et al: Osteosarcoma at the site of a previously treated aneurysmal bone cyst: A case report. J Bone Joint Surg Am 2005;87:395.
216. Huang L, Cheng YY, Chow LT, et al: Receptor activator of NF-kappaB ligand (RANKL) is expressed in chondroblastoma: Possible involvement in osteoclastic giant cell recruitment. Mol Pathol 2003;56:116.
217. Huch K, Werner M, Puhl W, et al: Calcaneal cyst: A classical simple bone cyst? [in German]. Z Orthop Ihre Grenzgeb 2004;142:625.
218. Hudson TM, Chew FS, Manaster BJ: Scintigraphy of benign exostoses and exostotic chondrosarcomas. AJR Am J Roentgenol 1983;140:581.
219. Hudson TM, Stiles RG, Monson DK: Fibrous lesions of bone. Radiol Clin North Am 1993;31:279.
220. Hunter AG, Jarvis J: Osteofibrous dysplasia: Two affected male sibs and an unrelated girl with bilateral involvement. Am J Med Genet 2002;112:79.
221. Hyde GE, Yarington CT Jr, Chu FW: Head and neck manifestations of Maffucci's syndrome: Chondrosarcoma of the nasal septum. Am J Otolaryngol 1995; 16:272.
222. Ijiri K, Tsuruga H, Sakakima H, et al: Increased expression of humanin peptide in diffuse-type pigmented villonodular synovitis: Implication of its mitochondrial abnormality. Ann Rheum Dis 2005;64:816.
223. Ilaslan H, Sundaram M, Unni KK: Vertebral chondroblastoma. Skeletal Radiol 2003;32:66.
224. Ilyas I, Younge DA: Medical management of osteoid osteoma. Can J Surg 2002;45:435.
225. Inoue O, Ibaraki K, Shimabukuro H, et al: Packing with high-porosity hydroxyapatite cubes alone for the treatment of simple bone cyst. Clin Orthop Relat Res 1993;293:287.
226. Ippolito E, Bray EW, Corsi A, et al: Natural history and treatment of fibrous dysplasia of bone: A multicenter clinicopathologic study promoted by the European Pediatric Orthopaedic Society. J Pediatr Orthop 2003; 12:155.
227. Ippolito E, Caterini R, Farsetti P, et al: Surgical treatment of fibrous dysplasia of bone in McCune-Albright syndrome. J Pediatr Endocrinol Metab 2002;15(Suppl 3):939.
228. Isaia GC, Lala R, Defilippi C, et al: Bone turnover in children and adolescents with McCune-Albright syndrome treated with pamidronate for bone fibrous dysplasia. Calcif Tissue Int 2002;71:121.
229. Ishida T, Iijima T, Kikuchi F, et al: A clinicopathological and immunohistochemical study of osteofibrous dysplasia, differentiated adamantinoma, and adamantinoma of long bones. Skeletal Radiol 1992;21:493.
230. Islinger RB, Kuklo TR, Owens BD, et al: Langerhans' cell histiocytosis in patients older than 21 years. Clin Orthop Relat Res 2000;379:231.
231. Jaffe H: Osteoid-osteoma: A benign osteoblastic tumor composed of osteoid and atypical bone. Arch Surg 1935;31:709.
232. Jaffe H: Hereditary multiple exostoses. Ann Pathol 1943;36:335.
233. Jaffe H: Aneurysmal bone cyst. Bull Hosp Joint Dis 1950;11:3.
234. Jaffe H: Tumors and Tumorous Conditions of the Bones and Joints. Philadelphia, Lea & Febiger, 1958.
235. Jaffe HL, Lichtenstein L: Benign chondroblastoma of bone: A reinterpretation of the so-called calcifying or chondromatous giant cell tumor. Am J Pathol 1942; 18:969.
236. Jaffe HL, Lichtenstein L: Non-osteogenic fibroma of bone. Am J Pathol 1942;18:205.
237. Jaffe HL, Lichtenstein L: Solitary unicameral bone cyst: With emphasis on the Roentgen picture, the pathologic appearance and the pathogenesis. Arch Surg 1942;44: 1004.
238. Jambhekar NA, Desai PB, Chitale DA, et al: Benign metastasizing chondroblastoma: A case report. Cancer 1998;82:675.
239. Jazrawi LM, Ong B, Jazrawi AJ, et al: Synovial chondromatosis of the elbow. Am J Orthop 2001; 30:223.
240. Jee WH, Choe BY, Kang HS, et al: Nonossifying fibroma: Characteristics at MR imaging with pathologic correlation. Radiology 1998;209:197.
241. Jesus-Garcia R, Bongiovanni JC, Korukian M, et al: Use of the Ilizarov external fixator in the treatment of patients with Ollier's disease. Clin Orthop Relat Res 2001;382:82.
242. Johnston CE II, Sklar F: Multiple hereditary exostoses with spinal cord compression. Orthopedics 1988;11: 1213.
243. Kabukcuoglu Y, Kabukcuoglu F, Kucukkaya M, et al: Aneurysmal bone cyst in the hamate. Am J Orthop 2003;32:101.
244. Kahn LB: Adamantinoma, osteofibrous dysplasia and differentiated adamantinoma. Skeletal Radiol 2003; 32:245.
245. Kalil RK, Antunes JS: Familial occurrence of osteoid osteoma. Skeletal Radiol 2003;32:416.
246. Kaplan RP, Wang JT, Amron DM, et al: Maffucci's syndrome: Two case reports with a literature review. J Am Acad Dermatol 1993;29:894.
247. Karita M, Tsuchiya H, Sakurakichi K, et al: Osteofibrous dysplasia treated with distraction osteogenesis: A report of two cases. J Orthop Sci 2004;9:516.
248. Kat S, Kutz R, Elbracht T, et al: Radiosynovectomy in pigmented villonodular synovitis. Nuklearmedizin 2000;39:209.
249. Kaushik S, Smoker WR, Frable WJ: Malignant transformation of fibrous dysplasia into chondroblastic osteosarcoma. Skeletal Radiol 2002;31:103.

250. Kay RM, Eckardt JJ, Mirra JM: Multifocal pigmented villonodular synovitis in a child: A case report. Clin Orthop Relat Res 1996;322:194.
251. Kayser F, Resnick D, Haghighi P, et al: Evidence of the subperiosteal origin of osteoid osteomas in tubular bones: Analysis by CT and MR imaging. AJR Am J Roentgenol 1998;170:609.
252. Kearns D, McGill T, Potsic W: Fibrous dysplasia. Head Neck 1992;14:510.
253. Keith A: Studies on the anatomical changes which accompany certain growth disorders of the human body. J Anat 1920;54:101.
254. Kenan S, Abdelwahab IF, Klein MJ, et al: Case report 817: Synovial chondrosarcoma secondary to synovial chondromatosis. Skeletal Radiol 1993;22:623.
255. Keret D, Spatz DK, Caro PA, et al: Dysplasia epiphysealis hemimelica: Diagnosis and treatment. J Pediatr Orthop 1992;12:365.
256. Kerr R: Radiologic case study: Eosinophilic granuloma of the spine causing neurologic deficit. Orthopedics 1989;12:309.
257. Kikuchi F, Dorfman HD, Kane PB: Recurrent chondromyxoid fibroma of the thoracic spine 30 years after primary excision: Case report and review of the literature. Int J Surg Pathol 2001;9:323.
258. Killian JT, Wilkinson L, White S, et al: Treatment of unicameral bone cyst with demineralized bone matrix. J Pediatr Orthop 1998;18:621.
259. Kilpatrick SE, Pike EJ, Geisinger KR, et al: Chondroblastoma of bone: Use of fine-needle aspiration biopsy and potential diagnostic pitfalls. Diagn Cytopathol 1997;16:65.
260. Kilpatrick SE, Pike EJ, Ward WG, et al: Dedifferentiated chondrosarcoma in patients with multiple osteochondromatosis: Report of a case and review of the literature. Skeletal Radiol 1997;26:370.
261. Kim RS, Kang JS, Jung JH, et al: Clustered localized pigmented villonodular synovitis. Arthroscopy 2005; 21:761.
262. Kistler W: Synovial chondromatosis of the knee joint: A rarity during childhood. Eur J Pediatr Surg 1991;1: 237.
263. Kitagawa Y, Tamai K, Ito H: Oral alendronate treatment for polyostotic fibrous dysplasia: A case report. J Orthop Sci 2004;9:521.
264. Kolodziej L, Kolban M, Zacha S, et al: The use of the Ilizarov technique in the treatment of upper limb deformity in patients with Ollier's disease. J Pediatr Orthop 2005;25:202.
265. Koci TM, Mehringer CM, Yamagata N, et al: Aneurysmal bone cyst of the thoracic spine: Evolution after particulate embolization. AJNR Am J Neuroradiol 1995;16:857.
266. Komiya S, Inoue A: Aggressive bone tumorous lesion in infancy: Osteofibrous dysplasia of the tibia and fibula. J Pediatr Orthop 1993;13:577.
267. Komiya S, Kawabata R, Zenmyo M, et al: Increased concentrations of nitrate and nitrite in the cyst fluid suggesting increased nitric oxide synthesis in solitary bone cysts. J Orthop Res 2000;18:281.
268. Komiya S, Minamitani K, Sasaguri Y, et al: Simple bone cyst: Treatment by trepanation and studies on bone resorptive factors in cyst fluid with a theory of its pathogenesis. Clin Orthop Relat Res 1993;287:204.
269. Komiya S, Tsuzuki K, Mangham DC, et al: Oxygen scavengers in simple bone cysts. Clin Orthop Relat Res 1994;308:199.
270. Korinth MC, Ramaekers VT, Rohde V: Cervical cord exostosis compressing the axis in a boy with hereditary multiple exostoses: Case illustration. J Neurosurg 2004; 100:223.
271. Kos M, Luczak K, Godzinski J, et al: Treatment of monostotic fibrous dysplasia with pamidronate. J Craniomaxillofac Surg 2004;32:10.
272. Kransdorf MJ, Sweet DE: Aneurysmal bone cyst: Concept, controversy, clinical presentation, and imaging. AJR Am J Roentgenol 1995;164:573.
273. Krebs VE: The role of hip arthroscopy in the treatment of synovial disorders and loose bodies. Clin Orthop Relat Res 2003;406:48.
274. Kroon HM, Schurmans J: Osteoblastoma: Clinical and radiologic findings in 98 new cases. Radiology 1990; 175:783.
275. Kulkarni AG, Goel A, Muzumdar D: Solitary osteochondroma arising from the thoracic facet joint: Case report. Neurol Med Chir (Tokyo) 2004;44:255.
276. Kuo RS, Bellemore MC, Monsell FP, et al: Dysplasia epiphysealis hemimelica: Clinical features and management. J Pediatr Orthop 1998;18:543.
277. Kurt AM, Turcotte RE, McLeod RA, et al: Chondroblastoma of bone. Orthopedics 1990;13:787.
278. Kurt AM, Unni KK, Sim FH, et al: Chondroblastoma of bone. Hum Pathol 1989;20:965.
279. Kuruvilla G, Steiner GC: Osteofibrous dysplasia-like adamantinoma of bone: A report of five cases with immunohistochemical and ultrastructural studies. Hum Pathol 1998;29:809.
280. Labbe JL, Clement JL, Duparc B, et al: Percutaneous extraction of vertebral osteoid osteoma under computed tomography guidance. Eur Spine J 1995;4: 368.
281. Lamovec J, Spiler M, Jevtic V: Osteosarcoma arising in a solitary osteochondroma of the fibula. Arch Pathol Lab Med 1999;123:832.
282. Le Merrer M, Legeai-Mallet L, Jeannin PM, et al: A gene for hereditary multiple exostoses maps to chromosome 19p. Hum Mol Genet 1994;3:717.
283. Lee DD, Tofighi A, Aiolova M, et al: alpha-BSM: A biomimetic bone substitute and drug delivery vehicle. Clin Orthop Relat Res 1999;367:S396.
284. Leet AI, Chebli C, Kushner H, et al: Fracture incidence in polyostotic fibrous dysplasia and the McCune-Albright syndrome. J Bone Miner Res 2004;19:571.
285. Leet AI, Magur E, Lee JS, et al: Fibrous dysplasia in the spine: Prevalence of lesions and association with scoliosis. J Bone Joint Surg Am 2004;86:531.
286. Lefton DR, Torrisi JM, Haller JO: Vertebral osteoid osteoma masquerading as a malignant bone or soft-tissue tumor on MRI. Pediatr Radiol 2001;31:72.
287. Legeai-Mallet L, Munnich A, Maroteaux P, et al: Incomplete penetrance and expressivity skewing in hereditary multiple exostoses. Clin Genet 1997;52:12.
288. Legeai-Mallet L, Rossi A, Benoist-Lasselin C, et al: EXT 1 gene mutation induces chondrocyte cytoskeletal

abnormalities and defective collagen expression in the exostoses. J Bone Miner Res 2000;15:1489.
289. Leithner A, Lang S, Windhager R, et al: Expression of insulin-like growth factor-I (IGF-I) in aneurysmal bone cyst. Mod Pathol 2001;14:1100.
290. Leithner A, Machacek F, Haas OA, et al: Aneurysmal bone cyst: A hereditary disease? J Pediatr Orthop B 2004;13:214.
291. Leithner A, Windhager R, Lang S, et al: Aneurysmal bone cyst: A population based epidemiologic study and literature review. Clin Orthop Relat Res 1999;63: 176.
292. Leung LY, Shu SJ, Chan MK, et al: Chondroblastoma of the lumbar vertebra. Skeletal Radiol 2001;30:710.
293. Levy JC, Temple HT, Mollabashy A, et al: The causes of pain in benign solitary enchondromas of the proximal humerus. Clin Orthop Relat Res 2005;431:181.
294. Levy WM, Miller AS, Bonakdarpour A, et al: Aneurysmal bone cyst secondary to other osseous lesions: Report of 57 cases. Am J Clin Pathol 1975;63:1.
295. Lichtenstein L: Polyostotic fibrous dysplasia. Arch Surg 1938;36:874.
296. Lichtenstein L: Histiocytosis X: Integration of eosinophilic granuloma of the bone, Letterer-Siwe disease, and Schüller-Christian disease as related manifestations of a single nosologic entity. Arch Pathol 1953; 56:86.
297. Lichtenstein L, Jaffe HL: Eosinophilic granuloma of bone with report of a case. Am J Pathol 1940;16:959.
298. Lichtenstein L, Jaffe HL: Fibrous dysplasia of bone. Arch Pathol 1942;33:777.
299. Lin X, Wells D: Isolation of the mouse cDNA homologous to the human EXT1 gene responsible for hereditary multiple exostoses. DNA Seq 1997;7:199.
300. Lindner NJ, Ozaki T, Roedl R, et al: Percutaneous radiofrequency ablation in osteoid osteoma. J Bone Joint Surg Br 2001;83:391.
301. Linke LC, Buckup K, Kalchschmidt K: Dysplasia epiphysealis hemimelica (Trevor's disease) of the acetabulum. Arch Orthop Trauma Surg 2005;125:193.
302. Lippman CR, Jallo GI, Feghali JG, et al: Aneurysmal bone cyst of the temporal bone. Pediatr Neurosurg 1999;31:219.
303. Liu J, Hudkins PG, Swee RG, et al: Bone sarcomas associated with Ollier's disease. Cancer 1987;59:1376.
304. Liu JH, Newcomer MT, Murray AD, et al: Aneurysmal bone cyst of the frontal sinus. Am J Otolaryngol 2001; 22:291.
305. Liu PT, Chivers FS, Roberts CC, et al: Imaging of osteoid osteoma with dynamic gadolinium-enhanced MR imaging. Radiology 2003;227:691.
306. Loder RT, Sundberg S, Gabriel K, et al: Determination of bone age in children with cartilaginous dysplasia (multiple hereditary osteochondromatosis and Ollier's enchondromatosis). J Pediatr Orthop 2004;24:102.
307. Logrono R, Kurtycz DF, Wojtowycz M, et al: Fine needle aspiration cytology of fibrous dysplasia: A case report. Acta Cytol 1998;42:1172.
308. Lohmann CH, Koster G, Klinger HM, et al: Giant synovial osteochondromatosis of the acromio-clavicular joint in a child: A case report and review of the literature. J Pediatr Orthop B 2005;14:126.
309. Lokiec F, Ezra E, Khermosh O, et al: Simple bone cysts treated by percutaneous autologous marrow grafting: A preliminary report [see comments]. J Bone Joint Surg Br 1996;78:934.
310. Lokiec F, Wientroub S: Simple bone cyst: Etiology, classification, pathology, and treatment modalities. J Pediatr Orthop B 1998;7:262.
311. Lucas DR, Unni KK, McLeod RA, et al: Osteoblastoma: Clinicopathologic study of 306 cases. Hum Pathol 1994; 25:117.
312. Lumbroso S, Paris F, Sultan C: McCune-Albright syndrome: Molecular genetics. J Pediatr Endocrinol Metab 2002;15(Suppl 3):875.
313. Lumbroso S, Paris F, Sultan C: Activating Gsalpha mutations: Analysis of 113 patients with signs of McCune-Albright syndrome. A European Collaborative Study. J Pediatr Endocrinol Metab 2004;89:2107.
314. Madhavan P, Ogilvie C: Premature closure of upper humeral physis after fracture through simple bone cyst. J Pediatr Orthop B 1998;7:83.
315. Magre GR, Menendez LR: Preoperative CT localization and marking of osteoid osteoma: Description of a new technique. J Comput Assist Tomogr 1996;20:526.
316. Mahnken AH, Nolte-Ernsting CC, Wildberger JE, et al: Aneurysmal bone cyst: Value of MR imaging and conventional radiography. Eur Radiol 2003;13: 1118.
317. Maki M, Athanasou N: Osteofibrous dysplasia and adamantinoma: Correlation of proto-oncogene product and matrix protein expression. Hum Pathol 2004;35: 69.
318. Maki M, Saitoh K, Kaneko Y, et al: Expression of cytokeratin 1, 5, 14, 19 and transforming growth factors-beta1, beta2, beta3 in osteofibrous dysplasia and adamantinoma: A possible association of transforming growth factor-beta with basal cell phenotype promotion. Pathol Int 2000;50:801.
319. Malchoff CD, Reardon G, MacGillivray DC, et al: An unusual presentation of McCune-Albright syndrome confirmed by an activating mutation of the Gs alpha-subunit from a bone lesion. J Clin Endocrinol Metab 1994;78:803.
320. Malghem J, Maldague B, Esselinckx W, et al: Spontaneous healing of aneurysmal bone cysts: A report of three cases. J Bone Joint Surg Br 1989;71:645.
321. Malik R, Kapoor N: Transformation of solitary osteochondroma calcaneum to chondrosarcoma: A case report. Ind J Pathol Microbiol 2004;47:42.
322. Marcove RC, Sheth DS, Takemoto S, et al: The treatment of aneurysmal bone cyst. Clin Orthop Relat Res 1995;311:157.
323. Margau R, Babyn P, Cole W, et al: MR imaging of simple bone cysts in children: Not so simple. Pediatr Radiol 2000;30:551.
324. Marie PJ: Cellular and molecular basis of fibrous dysplasia. Histol Histopathol 2001;16:981.
325. Marks KE, Bauer TW: Fibrous tumors of bone. Orthop Clin North Am 1989;20:377.
326. Martinez-Lage JF, Poza M, Cartagena J, et al: Solitary eosinophilic granuloma of the pediatric skull and spine: The role of surgery. Childs Nerv Syst 1991;7: 448.

327. Mastrantuono D, Martorano D, Verna V, et al: Osteoid osteoma: our experience using radio-frequency (RF) treatment. Radiol Med (Torino) 2005;109:220.
328. Matarazzo P, Lala R, Masi G, et al: Pamidronate treatment in bone fibrous dysplasia in children and adolescents with McCune-Albright syndrome. J Pediatr Endocrinol Metab 2002;15(Suppl 3):929.
329. Matsumoto K, Fujii S, Mochizuki T, et al: Solitary bone cyst of a lumbar vertebra: A case report and review of literature. Spine 1990;15:605.
330. McCune DJ, Bruch H: Progress in pediatrics: Osteodystrophia fibrosa. Am J Dis Child 1937;54:806.
331. McGrath BE, Bush CH, Nelson TE, et al: Evaluation of suspected osteoid osteoma. Clin Orthop Relat Res 1996;327:247.
332. Mehdian H, Weatherley C: Combined anterior and posterior resection and spinal stabilization for aneurysmal bone cyst. Eur Spine J 1995;4:123.
333. Mellon CD, Carter JE, Owen DB: Ollier's disease and Maffucci's syndrome: Distinct entities or a continuum. Case report: Enchondromatosis complicated by an intracranial glioma. J Neurol 1988;235:376.
334. Merchan EC, Sanchez-Herrera S, Gonzalez JM: Secondary chondrosarcoma: Four cases and review of the literature. Acta Orthop Belg 1993;59:76.
335. Merine D, Fishman EK, Rosengard A, et al: Chondromyxoid fibroma of the fibula. J Pediatr Orthop 1989; 9:468.
336. Mermer MJ, Gupta MC, Salamon PB, et al: Thoracic vertebral body exostosis as a cause of myelopathy in a patient with hereditary multiple exostoses. J Spinal Disord Tech 2002;15:144.
337. Mertens F, Jonsson K, Willen H, et al: Chromosome rearrangements in synovial chondromatous lesions. Br J Cancer 1996;74:251.
338. Mikawa Y, Watanabe R, Nakashima Y, et al: Cervical spinal cord compression in hereditary multiple exostoses: Report of a case and a review of the literature. Arch Orthop Trauma Surg 1997;116:112.
339. Mirra JM: Bone Tumors: Diagnosis and Treatment. Philadelphia, JB Lippincott, 1980.
340. Mirra JM, Gold R, Downs J, et al: A new histologic approach to the differentiation of enchondroma and chondrosarcoma of the bones: A clinicopathologic analysis of 51 cases. Clin Orthop Relat Res 1985;201:214.
341. Miyamoto K, Sakaguchi Y, Hosoe H, et al: Tetraparesis due to exostotic osteochondroma at upper cervical cord in a patient with multiple exostoses-mental retardation syndrome (Langer-Giedion syndrome). Spinal Cord 2005;43:190.
342. Mohan V, Sabri T, Marklund T, et al: Clinicoradiological diagnosis of benign osteoblastoma of the spine in children. Arch Orthop Trauma Surg 1991;110:260.
343. Monroc M, Ducou le Pointe H, Haddad S, et al: Soft tissue signal abnormality associated with eosinophilic granuloma: Correlation of MR imaging with pathologic findings. Pediatr Radiol 1994;24:328.
344. Moreau G, Letts M: Unicameral bone cyst of the calcaneus in children. J Pediatr Orthop 1994;14:101.
345. Motamedi K, Murphey MD, Fetsch JF, et al: Villonodular synovitis (PVNS) of the spine. Skeletal Radiol 2005;34:185.
346. Mouchet A BJ: Tarsomegalie. J Radiol Electrol 1926; 10:289.
347. Muller E: Uber hereditare multiple cartilaginare Exostosen and Ecchondrosen. Beitr Pathol Anat 1913;57: 232.
348. Muller PE, Durr HR, Wegener B, et al: Solitary enchondromas: Is radiographic follow-up sufficient in patients with asymptomatic lesions? Acta Orthop Belg 2003; 69:112.
349. Mungo DV, Zhang X, O'Keefe RJ, et al: COX-1 and COX-2 expression in osteoid osteomas. J Orthop Res 2002; 20:159.
350. Muscolo DL, Slullitel G, Ranalletta M, et al: Spontaneous remission of massive solitary eosinophilic granuloma of the femur. J Pediatr Orthop 2003;23: 763.
351. Muscolo DL, Velan O, Pineda Acero G, et al: Osteoid osteoma of the hip: Percutaneous resection guided by computed tomography [see comments]. Clin Orthop Relat Res 1995;310:170.
352. Mylle J, Burssens A, Fabry G: Simple bone cysts: A review of 59 cases with special reference to their treatment. Arch Orthop Trauma Surg 1992;111:297.
353. Nakatani T, Yamamoto T, Akisue T, et al: Periosteal osteoblastoma of the distal femur. Skeletal Radiol 2004; 33:107.
354. Naspinsky S, Siegel A: Chondroblastoma metastasis to lung visualized on bone scan. Clin Nucl Med 2005; 30:110.
355. Nawata K, Teshima R, Minamizaki T, et al: Knee deformities in multiple hereditary exostoses: A longitudinal radiographic study. Clin Orthop Relat Res 1995;313: 194.
356. Neer CS, Francis KC, Johnston AD, et al: Current concepts on the treatment of solitary unicameral bone cyst. Clin Orthop Relat Res 1973;97:40.
357. Nelson M, Perry D, Ginsburg G, et al: Translocation (1;4)(p31;q34) in nonossifying fibroma. Cancer Genet Cytogenet 2003;142:142.
358. Nezelof C, Basset F, Rousseau MF: Histiogenic arguments for a Langerhans' cell origin. Biomedicine 1973; 18:365.
359. Ngu BB, Khanna AJ, Pak SS, et al: Eosinophilic granuloma of the atlas presenting as torticollis in a child. Spine 2004;29:E98.
360. Nielsen GP, Fletcher CD, Smith MA, et al: Soft tissue aneurysmal bone cyst: A clinicopathologic study of five cases. Am J Surg Pathol 2002;26:64.
361. Nimityongskul P, Anderson LD, Dowling EA: Chondromyxoid fibroma. Orthop Rev 1992;21:863.
362. Nishida J, Kato S, Murakami H, et al: Tetraparesis caused by chondroblastoma of the cervical spine: A case report. Spine 2003;28:E173.
363. Nixon GW, Condon VR: Epiphyseal involvement in polyostotic fibrous dysplasia: A report of two cases. Radiology 1973;106:167.
364. Noel G, Feuvret L, Calugaru V, et al: Chondrosarcomas of the base of the skull in Ollier's disease or Maffucci's syndrome: Three case reports and review of the literature. Acta Oncol 2004;43:705.
365. Noonan KJ, Feinberg JR, Levenda A, et al: Natural history of multiple hereditary osteochondromatosis of

the lower extremity and ankle. J Pediatr Orthop 2002;22:120.

366. Noonan KJ, Levenda A, Snead J, et al: Evaluation of the forearm in untreated adult subjects with multiple hereditary osteochondromatosis. J Bone Joint Surg Am 2002;84:397.

367. Oba M, Nakagami W, Maeda M, et al: Symptomatic monostotic fibrous dysplasia of the thoracic spine. Spine 1998;23:741.

368. O'Connor P, Gibbon WW, Hardy G, et al: Chondromyxoid fibroma of the foot. Skeletal Radiol 1996;25: 143.

369. Ogata T, Matsuda Y, Hino M, et al: A simple bone cyst located in the pedicle of the lumbar vertebra. J Spinal Disord Tech 2004;17:339.

370. Ogilvie-Harris DJ, Saleh K: Generalized synovial chondromatosis of the knee: A comparison of removal of the loose bodies alone with arthroscopic synovectomy. Arthroscopy 1994;10:166.

371. Ohnuma M, Sugita T, Kawamata T, et al: Pigmented villonodular synovitis of the knee with lesions of the bursae. Clin Orthop Relat Res 2003;414:212.

372. Okuda R, Kinoshita M, Morikawa J, et al: Tibialis spastic varus foot caused by osteoid osteoma of the calcaneus. Clin Orthop Relat Res 2003;412:149.

373. Okuyama K, Chiba M, Okada K, et al: Huge solitary osteochondroma at T11 level causing myelopathy: Case report. Spinal Cord 1997;35:773.

374. Oliveira AM, Hsi BL, Weremowicz S, et al: USP6 (Tre2) fusion oncogenes in aneurysmal bone cyst. Cancer Res 2004;64:1920.

375. Oliveira AM, Perez-Atayde AR, Dal Cin P, et al: Aneurysmal bone cyst variant translocations upregulate USP6 transcription by promoter swapping with the ZNF9, COL1A1, TRAP150, and OMD genes. Oncogene 2005;24:3419.

376. Oliveira AM, Perez-Atayde AR, Inwards CY, et al: USP6 and CDH11 oncogenes identify the neoplastic cell in primary aneurysmal bone cysts and are absent in so-called secondary aneurysmal bone cysts. Am J Pathol 2004;165:1773.

377. Ollier L: De la dyschondroplasie. Bull Soc Chir Lyon 1900;3:22.

378. O'Sullivan M, Zacharin M: Intramedullary rodding and bisphosphonate treatment of polyostotic fibrous dysplasia associated with the McCune-Albright syndrome. J Pediatr Orthop 2002;22:255.

379. Otani S, Ehrlich JC: Solitary eosinophilic granuloma of bone simulating primary neoplasm. Am J Pathol 1940; 16:479.

380. Otsuka T, Kobayashi M, Sekiya I, et al: A new treatment of aneurysmal bone cyst by endoscopic curettage without bone grafting. Arthroscopy 2001;17: E28.

381. Ovadia D, Ezra E, Segev E, et al: Epiphyseal involvement of simple bone cysts. J Pediatr Orthop 2003; 23:222.

382. Oxtoby JW, Davies AM: MRI characteristics of chondroblastoma. Clin Radiol 1996;51:22.

383. Ozaki T, Halm H, Hillmann A, et al: Aneurysmal bone cysts of the spine. Arch Orthop Trauma Surg 1999;119: 159.

384. Ozaki T, Hamada M, Sugihara S, et al: Treatment outcome of osteofibrous dysplasia. J Pediatr Orthop 1998;7:199.

385. Ozaki T, Hillmann A, Lindner N, et al: Aneurysmal bone cysts in children. J Cancer Res Clin Oncol 1996;122:767.

386. Ozaki T, Hillmann A, Lindner N, et al: Cementation of primary aneurysmal bone cysts. Clin Orthop Relat Res 1997;337:240.

387. Ozaki T, Liljenqvist U, Hillmann A, et al: Osteoid osteoma and osteoblastoma of the spine: Experiences with 22 patients. Clin Orthop Relat Res 2002;397:394.

388. Ozalay M, Tandogan RN, Akpinar S, et al: Arthroscopic treatment of solitary benign intra-articular lesions of the knee that cause mechanical symptoms. Arthroscopy 2005;21:12.

389. Paige ML, Michael AS, Brodin A: Case report 647: Benign osteoblastoma causing spinal cord compression and spastic paresis. Skeletal Radiol 1991;20:54.

390. Pandey R, White SH, Kenwright J: Callus distraction in Ollier's disease. Acta Orthop Scand 1995;66:479.

391. Panoutsakopoulos G, Pandis N, Kyriazoglou I, et al: Recurrent t(16;17)(q22;p13) in aneurysmal bone cysts. Genes Chromosomes Cancer 1999;26:265.

392. Papagelopoulos PJ, Choudhury SN, Frassica FJ, et al: Treatment of aneurysmal bone cysts of the pelvis and sacrum. J Bone Joint Surg Am 2001;83:1674.

393. Papagelopoulos PJ, Currier BL, Galanis EC, et al: Vertebra plana of the lumbar spine caused by an aneurysmal bone cyst: A case report. Am J Orthop 1999;28: 119.

394. Papagelopoulos PJ, Currier BL, Shaughnessy WJ, et al: Aneurysmal bone cyst of the spine: Management and outcome. Spine 1998;23:621.

395. Papagelopoulos PJ, Galanis EC, Sim FH, et al: Clinicopathologic features, diagnosis, and treatment of osteoblastoma. Orthopedics 1999;22:244.

396. Papavasiliou VA, Sferopoulos NK: Aneurysmal bone cyst: A preliminary report on a new surgical approach. J Pediatr Orthop 1990;10:362.

397. Parekh SG, Donthineni-Rao R, Ricchetti E, et al: Fibrous dysplasia. J Am Acad Orthop Surg 2004;12:305.

398. Parisi MS, Oliveri B, Mautalen CA: Effect of intravenous pamidronate on bone markers and local bone mineral density in fibrous dysplasia. Bone 2003;33: 582.

399. Parisi MS, Oliveri MB, Mautalen CA: Bone mineral density response to long-term bisphosphonate therapy in fibrous dysplasia. J Clin Densitom 2001;4:167.

400. Park CK, Cho KK, Lee SW, et al: Simple bone cyst of the axis. Childs Nerv Syst 1997;13:171.

401. Park YK, Unni KK, McLeod RA, et al: Osteofibrous dysplasia: Clinicopathologic study of 80 cases. Hum Pathol 1993;24:1339.

402. Parlier-Cuau C, Champsaur P, Nizard R, et al: Percutaneous removal of osteoid osteoma. Radiol Clin North Am 1998;36:559.

403. Paterson DC, Morris LL, Binns GF, et al: Generalized enchondromatosis: A case report. J Bone Joint Surg Am 1989;71:133.

404. Peraud A, Drake JM, Armstrong D, et al: Fatal Ethibloc embolization of vertebrobasilar system following per-

cutaneous injection into aneurysmal bone cyst of the second cervical vertebra. AJNR Am J Neuroradiol 2004;25:1116.
405. Perrotti V, Rubini C, Fioroni M, et al: Solid aneurysmal bone cyst of the mandible. Int J Pediatr Otorhinolaryngol 2004;68:1339.
406. Peterson HA: Multiple hereditary osteochondromata. Clin Orthop Relat Res 1989;239:222.
407. Peterson HA: Deformities and problems of the forearm in children with multiple hereditary osteochondromata. J Pediatr Orthop 1994;14:92.
408. Philippe C, Porter DE, Emerton ME, et al: Mutation screening of the EXT1 and EXT2 genes in patients with hereditary multiple exostoses. Am J Hum Genet 1997; 61:520.
409. Plasschaert F, Craig C, Bell R, et al: Eosinophilic granuloma: A different behaviour in children than in adults. J Bone Joint Surg Br 2002;84:870.
410. Plotkin H, Rauch F, Zeitlin L, et al: Effect of pamidronate treatment in children with polyostotic fibrous dysplasia of bone. J Clin Endocrinol Metab 2003;88:4569.
411. Porter DE, Benson MK, Hosney GA: The hip in hereditary multiple exostoses. J Bone Joint Surg Br 2001;83: 988.
412. Porter DE, Emerton ME, Villanueva-Lopez F, et al: Clinical and radiographic analysis of osteochondromas and growth disturbance in hereditary multiple exostoses. J Pediatr Orthop 2000;20:246.
413. Porter DE, Lonie L, Fraser M, et al: Severity of disease and risk of malignant change in hereditary multiple exostoses: A genotype-phenotype study. J Bone Joint Surg Br 2004;86:1041.
414. Potocki L, Shaffer LG: Interstitial deletion of 11(p11.2p12): A newly described contiguous gene deletion syndrome involving the gene for hereditary multiple exostoses (EXT2). Am J Med Genet 1996;62:319.
415. Povysil C, Kohout A, Urban K, et al: Differentiated adamantinoma of the fibula: A rhabdoid variant. Skeletal Radiol 2004;33:488.
416. Povysil C, Tomanova R, Matejovsky Z: Muscle-specific actin expression in chondroblastomas. Hum Pathol 1997;28:316.
417. Prohaska DJ, Kneidel TW: Chondroblastoma in a metatarsal. J Foot Ankle Surg 1998;37:63.
418. Przybylski GJ, Pollack IF, Ward WT: Monostotic fibrous dysplasia of the thoracic spine: A case report. Spine 1996;21:860.
419. Puertas EB, Milani C, Chagas JC, et al: Surgical treatment of eosinophilic granuloma in the thoracic spine in patients with neurological lesions. J Pediatr Orthop B 2003;12:303.
420. Quirini GE, Meyer JR, Herman M, et al: Osteochondroma of the thoracic spine: An unusual cause of spinal cord compression. AJNR Am J Neuroradiol 1996;17: 961.
421. Radhi JM, Loewy J: Dedifferentiated chondrosarcoma with features of telangiectatic osteosarcoma. Pathology 1999;31:428.
422. Raimondo RA, Skaggs DL, Rosenwasser MP, et al: Lengthening of pediatric forearm deformities using the Ilizarov technique: Functional and cosmetic results. J Hand Surg [Am] 1999;24:331.
423. Ramappa AJ, Lee FY, Tang P, et al: Chondroblastoma of bone. J Bone Joint Surg Am 2000;82:1140.
424. Ramina R, Coelho Neto M, Meneses MS, et al: Maffucci's syndrome associated with a cranial base chondrosarcoma: Case report and literature review. Neurosurgery 1997;41:269.
425. Ramirez AR, Stanton RP: Aneurysmal bone cyst in 29 children. J Pediatr Orthop 2002;22:533.
426. Raskas DS, Graziano GP, Herzenberg JE, et al: Osteoid osteoma and osteoblastoma of the spine. J Spinal Disord 1992;5:204.
427. Raskind WH, Conrad EU, Chansky H, et al: Loss of heterozygosity in chondrosarcomas for markers linked to hereditary multiple exostoses loci on chromosomes 8 and 11. Am J Hum Genet 1995;56:1132.
428. Ratliff J, Voorhies R: Osteochondroma of the C5 lamina with cord compression: Case report and review of the literature. Spine 2000;25:1293.
429. Rector JT, Gray CL, Sharpe RW, et al: Acute lymphoid leukemia associated with Maffucci's syndrome. Am J Pediatr Hematol Oncol 1993;15:427.
430. Redfern DR, Forester AJ, Evans MJ, et al: Enchondroma of the scaphoid. J Hand Surg [Br] 1997;22:235.
431. Richkind KE, Mortimer E, Mowery-Rushton P, et al: Translocation (16;20)(p11.2;q13): sole cytogenetic abnormality in a unicameral bone cyst. Cancer Genet Cytogenet 2002;137:153.
432. Rizzo M, Dellaero DT, Harrelson JM, et al: Juxtaphyseal aneurysmal bone cysts. Clin Orthop Relat Res 1999; 364:205.
433. Roach PJ, Connolly LP, Zurakowski D, et al: Osteoid osteoma: Comparative utility of high-resolution planar and pinhole magnification scintigraphy. Pediatr Radiol 1996;26:222.
434. Robinson D, Tieder M, Halperin N, et al: Maffucci's syndrome: The result of neural abnormalities? Evidence of mitogenic neurotransmitters present in enchondromas and soft tissue hemangiomas. Cancer 1994;74:949.
435. Rodgers WB, Hall JE: One-bone forearm as a salvage procedure for recalcitrant forearm deformity in hereditary multiple exostoses. J Pediatr Orthop 1993;13: 587.
436. Roger B, Bellin MF, Wioland M, et al: Osteoid osteoma: CT-guided percutaneous excision confirmed with immediate follow-up scintigraphy in 16 outpatients. Radiology 1996;201:239.
437. Roposch A, Saraph V, Linhart WE: Flexible intramedullary nailing for the treatment of unicameral bone cysts in long bones. J Bone Joint Surg Am 2000;82:1447.
438. Roposch A, Saraph V, Linhart WE: Treatment of femoral neck and trochanteric simple bone cysts. Arch Orthop Trauma Surg 2004;124:437.
439. Rosenthal DI, Hornicek FJ, Torriani M, et al: Osteoid osteoma: Percutaneous treatment with radiofrequency energy. Radiology 2003;229:171.
440. Rosenthal DI, Hornicek FJ, Wolfe MW, et al: Percutaneous radiofrequency coagulation of osteoid osteoma compared with operative treatment. J Bone Joint Surg Am 1998;80:815.
441. Rosenthal DI, Marota JJ, Hornicek FJ: Osteoid osteoma: Elevation of cardiac and respiratory rates at biopsy

needle entry into tumor in 10 patients. Radiology 2003; 226:125.
442. Rosenthal DI, Springfield DS, Gebhardt MC, et al: Osteoid osteoma: Percutaneous radio-frequency ablation. Radiology 1995;197:451.
443. Rougraff BT, Kling TJ: Treatment of active unicameral bone cysts with percutaneous injection of demineralized bone matrix and autogenous bone marrow. J Bone Joint Surg Am 2002;84:921.
444. Rud B, Pedersen NW, Thomsen PB: Simple bone cysts in children treated with methylprednisolone acetate. Orthopedics 1991;14:185.
445. Ruggieri P, Sim FH, Bond JR, et al: Malignancies in fibrous dysplasia. Cancer 1994;73:1411.
446. Saifuddin A, White J, Sherazi Z, et al: Osteoid osteoma and osteoblastoma of the spine: Factors associated with the presence of scoliosis. Spine 1998;23:47.
447. Saito T, Oda Y, Kawaguchi K, et al: Five-year evolution of a telangiectatic osteosarcoma initially managed as an aneurysmal bone cyst. Skeletal Radiol 2005;34: 290.
448. Sakamoto A, Oda Y, Iwamoto Y, et al: A comparative study of fibrous dysplasia and osteofibrous dysplasia with regard to Gsalpha mutation at the Arg201 codon: Polymerase chain reaction-restriction fragment length polymorphism analysis of paraffin-embedded tissues. J Mol Diagn 2000;2:67.
449. Sakamoto A, Tanaka K, Matsuda S, et al: Vascular compression caused by solitary osteochondroma: Useful diagnostic methods of magnetic resonance angiography and Doppler ultrasonography. J Orthop Sci 2002; 7:439.
450. Sanchez AP, Diaz-Lopez EO, Rojas SK, et al: Aneurysmal bone cyst of the maxilla. J Craniofac Surg 2004; 15:1029.
451. Scaglietti O, Marchetti PG, Bartolozzi P: The effects of methylprednisolone acetate in the treatment of bone cysts: Results of three years follow-up. J Bone Joint Surg Br 1979;61:200.
452. Scaglietti O, Marchetti PG, Bartolozzi P: Final results obtained in the treatment of bone cysts with methylprednisolone acetate (Depo-Medrol) and a discussion of results achieved in other bone lesions. Clin Orthop Relat Res 1982;165:33.
453. Schajowicz F: Tumors and Tumorlike Lesions of Bone and Joints. New York, Springer-Verlag, 1981.
454. Schmale GA, Conrad EU 3rd, Raskind WH: The natural history of hereditary multiple exostoses. J Bone Joint Surg Am 1994;76:986.
455. Schneider M, Sabo D, Gerner HJ, et al: Destructive osteoblastoma of the cervical spine with complete neurologic recovery. Spinal Cord 2002;40:248.
456. Schoenau E, Rauch F: Fibrous dysplasia. Horm Res 2002;57(Suppl 2):79.
457. Schuppers HA, van der Eijken JW: Chondroblastoma during the growing age. J Pediatr Orthop 1998;7: 293.
458. Schwartz HS, Pinto M: Osteoblastomas of the cervical spine. J Spinal Disord 1990;3:179.
459. Schwartz HS, Unni KK, Pritchard DJ: Pigmented villonodular synovitis: A retrospective review of affected large joints. Clin Orthop Relat Res 1989;247:243.
460. Schwartz HS, Zimmerman NB, Simon MA, et al: The malignant potential of enchondromatosis. J Bone Joint Surg Am 1987;69:269.
461. Sciot R, Dorfman H, Brys P, et al: Cytogenetic-morphologic correlations in aneurysmal bone cyst, giant cell tumor of bone and combined lesions: A report from the CHAMP study group. Mod Pathol 2000;13: 1206.
462. Senol U, Karaali K, Akyuz M, et al: Aneurysmal bone cyst of the orbit. AJNR Am J Neuroradiol 2002;23:319.
463. Sessa S, Sommelet D, Lascombes P, et al: Treatment of Langerhans-cell histiocytosis in children: Experience at the Children's Hospital of Nancy [see comments]. J Bone Joint Surg Am 1994;76:1513.
464. Sethi A, Agarwal K, Sethi S, et al: Allograft in the treatment of benign cystic lesions of bone. Arch Orthop Trauma Surg 1993;112:167.
465. Shahla A, Parvaneh V, Hossein HD: Langerhans cells histiocytosis in one family. Pediatr Hematol Oncol 2004;21:313.
466. Shaikh MI, Saifuddin A, Pringle J, et al: Spinal osteoblastoma: CT and MR imaging with pathological correlation. Skeletal Radiol 1999;28:33.
467. Shapiro F: Ollier's Disease. An assessment of angular deformity, shortening, and pathological fracture in twenty-one patients. J Bone Joint Surg Am 1982;64:95.
468. Shapiro F, Simon S, Glimcher MJ: Hereditary multiple exostoses: Anthropometric, roentgenographic, and clinical aspects. J Bone Joint Surg Am 1979;61:815.
469. Shapiro SA, Javid T, Putty T: Osteochondroma with cervical cord compression in hereditary multiple exostoses. Spine 1990;15:600.
470. Sharma MC, Arora R, Deol PS, et al: Osteochondroma of the spine: An enigmatic tumor of the spinal cord. A series of 10 cases. J Neurosurg Sci 2002;46:66.
471. Shen Q, Jia L, Li Y: Solitary bone cyst in the odontoid process and body of the axis: A case report and review of literature. J Bone Joint Surg Br 1998;80:30.
472. Shenker A, Weinstein LS, Sweet DE, et al: An activating Gs alpha mutation is present in fibrous dysplasia of bone in the McCune-Albright syndrome. J Clin Endocrinol Metab 1994;79:750.
473. Sherazi Z, Saifuddin A, Shaikh MI, et al: Unusual imaging findings in association with spinal osteoblastoma. Clin Radiol 1996;51:644.
474. Shi YR, Wu JY, Hsu YA, et al: Mutation screening of the EXT genes in patients with hereditary multiple exostoses in Taiwan. Genet Test 2002;6:237.
475. Shih HN, Cheng CY, Chen YJ, et al: Treatment of the femoral neck and trochanteric benign lesions. Clin Orthop Relat Res 1996;328:220.
476. Shindell R, Huurman WW, Lippiello L, et al: Prostaglandin levels in unicameral bone cysts treated by intralesional steroid injection. J Pediatr Orthop 1989;9: 516.
477. Shinozaki T, Arita S, Watanabe H, et al: Simple bone cysts treated by multiple drill-holes: 23 cysts followed 2-10 years [see comments]. Acta Orthop Scand 1996; 67:288.
478. Shpitzer T, Ganel A, Engelberg S: Surgery for synovial chondromatosis: 26 cases followed up for 6 years. Acta Orthop Scand 1990;61:567.

479. Silber JS, Mathur S, Ecker M: A solitary osteochondroma of the pediatric thoracic spine: A case report and review of the literature. Am J Orthop 2000;29:711.
480. Simon MA, Kirchner PT: Scintigraphic evaluation of primary bone tumors: Comparison of technetium-99m phosphonate and gallium citrate imaging. J Bone Joint Surg Am 1980;62:758.
481. Simovic S, Klapan I, Bumber Z, et al: Fibrous dysplasia in paranasal cavities. J Otorhinolaryngol Relat Spec 1996;58:55.
482. Sisayan R, Lorberboym M, Hermann G: Polyostotic fibrous dysplasia in McCune-Albright syndrome diagnosed by bone scintigraphy. Clin Nucl Med 1997; 22:410.
483. Sjogren H, Orndal C, Tingby O, et al: Cytogenetic and spectral karyotype analyses of benign and malignant cartilage tumours. Int J Oncol 2004;24:1385.
484. Skaggs DL, Moon CN, Kay RM, et al: Dysplasia epiphysealis hemimelica of the acetabulum: A report of two cases. J Bone Joint Surg Am 2000;82:409.
485. Sluga M, Windhager R, Pfeiffer M, et al: Peripheral osteoid osteoma: Is there still a place for traditional surgery? J Bone Joint Surg Br 2002;84:249.
486. Smith SB, Shane HS: Simple bone cyst of the calcaneus: A case report and literature review. J Am Podiatr Med Assoc 1994;84:127.
487. Snearly WN, Peterson HA: Management of ankle deformities in multiple hereditary osteochondromata. J Pediatr Orthop 1989;9:427.
488. Snetkov AI: Surgical treatment of the polyostotic form of fibrous dysplasia in children and adolescents [in Russian]. Vestn Khir 1988;140:85.
489. Soder S, Inwards C, Muller S, et al: Cell biology and matrix biochemistry of chondromyxoid fibroma. Am J Clin Pathol 2001;116:271.
490. Song DE, Khang SK, Cho KJ, et al: Chondromyxoid fibroma of the sternum. Ann Thorac Surg 2003;75: 1948.
491. Song KS: Spontaneous regression of osteochondromatosis of the radius after lengthening of the ulna: A case report. J Pediatr Orthop 2000;20:689.
492. Sozeri B, Sennaroglu L, Yilmaz T: Aneurysmal bone cyst of the zygoma: A case report and review of the literature. Acta Otorhinolaryngol Belg 2000;54:483.
493. Spouge AR, Thain LM: Osteoid osteoma: MR imaging revisited. Clin Imaging 2000;24:19.
494. Springer KR: Synovial chondromatosis. J Foot Surg 1991;30:446.
495. Springfield DS, Rosenberg AE, Mankin HJ, et al: Relationship between osteofibrous dysplasia and adamantinoma. Clin Orthop Relat Res 1994;309:234.
496. Stanton RP, Abdel-Mota'al MM: Growth arrest resulting from unicameral bone cyst. J Pediatr Orthop 1998;18:198.
497. Stanton RP, Hansen MO: Function of the upper extremities in hereditary multiple exostoses. J Bone Joint Surg Am 1996;78:568.
498. Stanton RP, Montgomery BE: Fibrous dysplasia. Orthopedics 1996;19:679.
499. Stieber JR, Dormans JP: Manifestations of hereditary multiple exostoses. J Am Acad Orthop Surg 2005;13: 110.
500. Struhl S, Edelson C, Pritzker H, et al: Solitary (unicameral) bone cyst: The fallen fragment sign revisited. Skeletal Radiol 1989;18:261.
501. Sullivan RJ, Meyer JS, Dormans JP, et al: Diagnosing aneurysmal and unicameral bone cysts with magnetic resonance imaging. Clin Orthop Relat Res 1999;366: 186.
502. Sun TC, Swee RG, Shives TC, et al: Chondrosarcoma in Maffucci's syndrome. J Bone Joint Surg Am 1985;67: 1214.
503. Sundaram M, Totty WG, Kyriakos M, et al: Imaging findings in pseudocystic osteosarcoma. AJR Am J Roentgenol 2001;176:783.
504. Sunkara UK, Sponseller PD, Hadley Miller N, et al: Bilateral osteofibrous dysplasia: A report of two cases and review of the literature. Iowa Orthop J 1997;17:47.
505. Suzuki M, Satoh T, Nishida J, et al: Solid variant of aneurysmal bone cyst of the cervical spine. Spine 2004;29:E376.
506. Sviland L, Malcolm AJ: Synovial chondromatosis presenting as painless soft tissue mass: A report of 19 cases. Histopathology 1995;27:275.
507. Swarts SJ, Neff JR, Johansson SL, et al: Significance of abnormalities of chromosomes 5 and 8 in chondroblastoma. Clin Orthop Relat Res 1998;349:189.
508. Sweasey TA, Dauser RC: Eosinophilic granuloma of the cervicothoracic junction: Case report. J Neurosurg 1989;71:942.
509. Sweet DE, Vinh TN, Devaney K: Cortical osteofibrous dysplasia of long bone and its relationship to adamantinoma: A clinicopathologic study of 30 cases. Am J Surg Pathol 1992;16:282.
510. Szendroi M, Kollo K, Antal I, et al: Intraarticular osteoid osteoma: Clinical features, imaging results, and comparison with extraarticular localization. J Rheumatol 2004;31:957.
511. Tachdjian M: Pediatric Orthopedics, 2nd ed. Philadelphia, WB Saunders, 1990.
512. Tang Y, Xia JH, Zhou JN, et al: Localization of the gene for 4 hereditary multiple exostoses families [in Chinese]. I Chuan Hsueh Pao 1998;25:1.
513. Tatari H, Baran O, Lebe B, et al: Pigmented villonodular synovitis of the knee presenting as a popliteal cyst. Arthroscopy 2000;16:13.
514. Tavangar SM, Ghafouri M: Multifocal pigmented villonodular synovitis in a child. Singapore Med J 2005; 46:193.
515. Thompson MS, Woodward JS Jr: The use of the arthroscope as an adjunct in the resection of a chondroblastoma of the femoral head. Arthroscopy 1995;11:106.
516. Tokunaga Y, Hirabayashi K, Toyama Y, et al: Aneurysmal bone cyst of the axis treated by laminoplasty with autogenous iliac bone. Spine 1992;17:S57.
517. Torriani M, Rosenthal DI: Percutaneous radiofrequency treatment of osteoid osteoma. Pediatr Radiol 2002;32: 615.
518. Towbin R, Kaye R, Meza MP, et al: Osteoid osteoma: Percutaneous excision using a CT-guided coaxial technique. AJR Am J Roentgenol 1995;164:945.
519. Trevor D: Tarso-epiphysial aclasis: A congenital error of epiphysial development. J Bone Joint Surg Br 1950; 32:204.

520. Tschauner C, Roth-Schiffl E, Mayer U: Early loss of hip containment in a child with dysplasia epiphysealis hemimelica. Clin Orthop Relat Res 2004;427:213.
521. Tuna H, Karatas A, Yilmaz ER, et al: Aneurysmal bone cyst of the temporal bone: Case report. Surg Neurol 2003;60:571.
522. Turcotte RE, Kurt AM, Sim FH, et al: Chondroblastoma. Hum Pathol 1993;24:944.
523. Turker RJ, Mardjetko S, Lubicky J: Aneurysmal bone cysts of the spine: Excision and stabilization. J Pediatr Orthop 1998;18:209.
524. Tuzuner S, Aydin AT: Arthroscopic removal of an osteoid osteoma at the talar neck. Arthroscopy 1998; 14:405.
525. Ueda Y, Blasius S, Edel G, et al: Osteofibrous dysplasia of long bones: A reactive process to adamantinomatous tissue [published erratum appears in J Cancer Res Clin Oncol 1992;118:400]. J Cancer Res Clin Oncol 1992; 118:152.
526. Van Delm I, Fabry G: Osteofibrous dysplasia of the tibia: Case report and review of the literature. J Pediatr Orthop 1999;8:50.
527. Vanderschueren GM, Taminiau AH, Obermann WR, et al: Osteoid osteoma: Clinical results with thermocoagulation. Radiology 2002;224:82.
528. Vanderschueren GM, Taminiau AH, Obermann WR, et al: Osteoid osteoma: Factors for increased risk of unsuccessful thermal coagulation. Radiology 2004;233:757.
529. Vastel L, Lambert P, De Pinieux G, et al: Surgical treatment of pigmented villonodular synovitis of the hip. J Bone Joint Surg Am 2005;87:1019.
530. Vayego SA, De Conti OJ, Varella-Garcia M: Complex cytogenetic rearrangement in a case of unicameral bone cyst. Cancer Genet Cytogenet 1996;86:46.
531. Vedantam R, Crawford AH, Kuwajima SS: Aneurysmal bone cyst of the clavicle in a child. Br J Clin Pract 1996;50:474.
532. Vedantam R, Strecker WB, Schoenecker PL, et al: Polyarticular pigmented villonodular synovitis in a child. Clin Orthop Relat Res 1998;348:208.
533. Velez-Yanguas MC, Warrier RP: Langerhans' cell histiocytosis. Orthop Clin North Am 1996;27:615.
534. Villas C, Martinez-Peric R, Barrios RH, et al: Eosinophilic granuloma of the spine with and without vertebra plana: Long-term follow-up of six cases. J Spinal Disord 1993;6:260.
535. Virchow R: Ueber multiple Exostosen, mit Vorlegung von Praparaten. Klin Wochenschr 1891;28:1082.
536. Voutsinas S, Wynne-Davies R: The infrequency of malignant disease in diaphyseal aclasis and neurofibromatosis. J Med Genet 1983;20:345.
537. Voytek TM, Ro JY, Edeiken J, et al: Fibrous dysplasia and cemento-ossifying fibroma: A histologic spectrum [see comments]. Am J Surg Pathol 1995;19:775.
538. Vujic M, Bergman A, Romanus B, et al: Hereditary multiple and isolated sporadic exostoses in the same kindred: Identification of the causative gene (EXT2) and detection of a new mutation, nt112delAT, that distinguishes the two phenotypes. Int J Mol Med 2004;13:47.
539. Wang JW, Shih CH, Chen WJ: Osteofibrous dysplasia (ossifying fibroma of long bones): A report of four cases and review of the literature. Clin Orthop Relat Res 1992;278:235.
540. Wang XL, Gielen JL, Salgado R, et al: Soft tissue aneurysmal bone cyst. Skeletal Radiol 2004;33:477.
541. Wasserlauf B, Gossett J, Rosenthal DI, et al: Osteoid osteoma of the glenoid: Minimally invasive treatment. Am J Orthop 2003;32:405.
542. Watanabe H, Arita S, Chigira M: Aetiology of a simple bone cyst: A case report. Int Orthop 1994;18:16.
543. Weatherall PT, Maale GE, Mendelsohn DB, et al: Chondroblastoma: Classic and confusing appearance at MR imaging. Radiology 1994;190:467.
544. Weber KL, Morrey BF: Osteoid osteoma of the elbow: A diagnostic challenge. J Bone Joint Surg Am 1999;81: 1111.
545. Wells DE, Hill A, Lin X, et al: Identification of novel mutations in the human EXT1 tumor suppressor gene. Hum Genet 1997;99:612.
546. Wicklund CL, Pauli RM, Johnston D, et al: Natural history study of hereditary multiple exostoses. Am J Med Genet 1995;55:43.
547. Willman CL, Busque L, Griffith BB, et al: Langerhans'-cell histiocytosis (histiocytosis X): A clonal proliferative disease [see comments]. N Engl J Med 1994; 331:154.
548. Wilson AJ, Kyriakos M, Ackerman LV: Chondromyxoid fibroma: Radiographic appearance in 38 cases and in a review of the literature [published erratum appears in Radiology 1991;180:586]. Radiology 1991;179:513.
549. Wirganowicz PZ, Watts HG: Surgical risk for elective excision of benign exostoses. J Pediatr Orthop 1997;17: 455.
550. Wise CA, Clines GA, Massa H, et al: Identification and localization of the gene for EXTL, a third member of the multiple exostoses gene family. Genome Res 1997; 7:10.
551. Witt JD, Hall-Craggs MA, Ripley P, et al: Interstitial laser photocoagulation for the treatment of osteoid osteoma. J Bone Joint Surg Br 2000;82:1125.
552. Woertler K, Brinkschmidt C: Imaging features of subperiosteal aneurysmal bone cyst. Acta Radiol 2002;43: 336.
553. Woertler K, Vestring T, Boettner F, et al: Osteoid osteoma: CT-guided percutaneous radiofrequency ablation and follow-up in 47 patients. J Vasc Interv Radiol 2001;12:717.
554. Wolfe MW, Halvorson TL, Bennett JT, et al: Chondroblastoma of the patella presenting as knee pain in an adolescent. Am J Orthop 1995;24:61.
555. Wood VE, Molitor C, Mudge MK: Hand involvement in multiple hereditary exostosis. Hand Clin 1990;6:685.
556. Wright JM, Matayoshi E, Goldstein AP: Bursal osteochondromatosis overlying an osteochondroma of a rib: A case report. J Bone Joint Surg Am 1997;79:1085.
557. Wu CT, Inwards CY, O'Laughlin S, et al: Chondromyxoid fibroma of bone: A clinicopathologic review of 278 cases. Hum Pathol 1998;29:438.
558. Wu KK: A surgically treated unicameral (solitary) bone cyst of the talus with a 15-year follow-up. J Foot Ankle Surg 1993;32:242.
559. Wuisman PI, Noorda RJ, Jutte PC: Chondrosarcoma secondary to synovial chondromatosis: Report of two

cases and a review of the literature. Arch Orthop Trauma Surg 1997;116:307.
560. Wuyts W, Van Hul W, De Boulle K, et al: Mutations in the EXT1 and EXT2 genes in hereditary multiple exostoses. Am J Hum Genet 1998;62:346.
561. Wuyts W, Van Hul W, Wauters J, et al: Positional cloning of a gene involved in hereditary multiple exostoses. Hum Mol Genet 1996;5:1547.
562. Yabut SM Jr, Kenan S, Sissons HA, et al: Malignant transformation of fibrous dysplasia: A case report and review of the literature. Clin Orthop Relat Res 1988; 228:281.
563. Yalniz E, Er T, Ozyilmaz F: Fibrous dysplasia of the spine with sarcomatous transformation: A case report and review of the literature. Eur Spine J 1995;4:372.
564. Yamaguchi T, Dorfman HD: Radiographic and histologic patterns of calcification in chondromyxoid fibroma. Skeletal Radiol 1998;27:559.
565. Yamamoto K, Asazuma T, Tsuchihara T, et al: Diagnostic efficacy of thin slice CT in osteoid osteoma of the thoracic spine: Report of two cases. J Spinal Disord Tech 2005;18:182.
566. Yamamura S, Sato K, Sugiura H, et al: Inflammatory reaction in chondroblastoma. Skeletal Radiol 1996;25: 371.
567. Yavuz AA, Sener M, Yavuz MN, et al: Aneurysmal bone cyst of the sternum: A case report of successful treatment with radiotherapy. Br J Radiol 2004; 77:610.
568. Yildiz Y, Bayrakci K, Altay M, et al: Osteoid osteoma: The results of surgical treatment. Int Orthop 2001;25: 119.
569. Youssef BA, Haddad MC, Zahrani A, et al: Osteoid osteoma and osteoblastoma: MRI appearances and the significance of ring enhancement. Eur Radiol 1996;6: 291.
570. Yu GV, Sellers CS: Chondroblastoma of the talus. J Foot Ankle Surg 1996;35:72.
571. Zacharin M: Paediatric management of endocrine complications in McCune-Albright syndrome. J Pediatr Endocrinol Metab 2005;18:33.
572. Zak BM, Crawford BE, Esko JD: Hereditary multiple exostoses and heparan sulfate polymerization. Biochim Biophys Acta 2002;1573:346.
573. Zileli M, Cagli S, Basdemir G, et al: Osteoid osteomas and osteoblastomas of the spine. Neurosurg Focus 2003;15:E5.
574. Zillmer DA, Dorfman HD: Chondromyxoid fibroma of bone: Thirty-six cases with clinicopathologic correlation. Hum Pathol 1989;20:952.

Chapter 39

Malignant Bone Tumors

OSTEOSARCOMA

Osteosarcoma (osteogenic sarcoma) is the most common malignant bone tumor in children and adolescents. The neoplasm is composed of a sarcomatous stroma and malignant osteoblasts that directly form tumor osteoid or bone, although fibrous and cartilaginous elements may coexist or even predominate. The classic osteosarcoma develops in the medullary cavity of a bone, usually in the metaphysis of a long bone. There are several variants of the classic high-grade osteosarcoma. Osteosarcomas may also arise from the surface of bones in relation to the periosteum and immediate periosteal connective tissue. These are termed *juxtacortical osteosarcomas* and are less common than central lesions. They may be low-grade fibroblastic osteosarcomas, termed *parosteal osteosarcomas,*[67,455,544] or intermediate-grade chondroblastic osteosarcomas, termed *periosteal osteosarcomas.*[191,202,455,574] Rarely, a low-grade endosteal osteosarcoma variant that arises within bone from the endosteum is encountered.[49] These lesions grow slowly and metastasize later in the course of the disease and less frequently than does high-grade osteosarcoma. Thus, the names of the lesions vary with their location in relation to the bone, but the histologic grade of the sarcoma determines its biologic aggressiveness. Telangiectatic osteosarcoma is a high-grade malignant lesion that shows little evidence of ossification but undergoes cystic and necrotic changes owing to its rapid growth.[29,363] Because the bone is weakened by the rapid destructive osteolytic process, pathologic fracture is common.[145,338,339,352,408,436] Paget's sarcoma is not encountered in children.[160]

Classic Osteosarcoma

Approximately 400 new cases of osteosarcoma are diagnosed in patients younger than 20 years in the United States each year. The second most common bone sarcoma (Ewing's sarcoma or primitive neuroectodermal tumor) is more common than classic osteosarcoma in those younger than 10 years.[93,198] Generally, osteosarcoma occurs between the ages of 10 and 25 years, although it has been found in children as young as 5 years and in the elderly. When osteosarcoma develops in an older person, the possibility of malignant transformation of a preexisting benign bone disease, such as Paget's disease of bone, fibrous dysplasia, or a bone infarct, should be considered.* Osteosarcomas may also arise in bones that have been irradiated for other reasons.† The incidence is almost equal in boys and girls.

The cause of osteosarcoma is unknown, but viral causes have been proposed in a number of studies—most recently, simian virus 40 (SV40), which was a contaminant of the polio vaccine. Although there are plausible mechanisms of how this virus could act to block the activity of *p53* or other tumor suppressor genes, the current thinking is that SV40 is an unlikely cause of osteosarcoma.[72,252,325,472] Trauma has also been proposed, but because of the frequency with which children injure themselves, this is probably only an association. Irradiation is known to cause osteosarcoma in patients irradiated for malignant diseases. Alkylating agents are also associated.

The genetics of osteosarcoma has received much attention. It is known to be a component tumor in familial cancer syndromes such as Li-Fraumeni syndrome, and alterations in genes such as *Rb, p53,* and others are common in these sarcomas.[161] Patients with hereditary retinoblastoma have a high incidence of osteosarcoma, as do those with autosomal recessive

*See references 200, 201, 233, 235, 236, 242, 362, 456, 518, 578.
†See references 18, 61, 143, 160, 162, 204, 239, 298, 412, 485, 538.

Rothmund-Thomson syndrome.[88,306] Patients with Rothmund-Thompson syndrome have been noted to have a mutation in the *RECQL4* gene.[555]

The tumor is usually situated near the metaphyseal region of a long bone, but on occasion it may be diaphyseal in location. The most common sites, accounting for more than 50% of cases, are the lower end of the femur and the upper end of the tibia.[65,354,564] The upper ends of the humerus and the femur are next in frequency. Less commonly, a classic osteosarcoma is encountered in the fibula,[322] pelvic bones,[141,143,186,265] or vertebral column.[152,398,482] Occurrence in the distal part of a limb (hand or foot) is rare.[379,384] However, the tumor has been described in every bone in the body. There are also numerous reports of multiple or multicentric osteosarcomas.[60,91,197,224,257,294,323,324,380,392,479,517]

PATHOLOGY

The tumor ordinarily begins developing in the medullary cavity of a long bone near the metaphysis, but by the time it is recognized, it has already penetrated and extended through the cortex, raising the periosteum (Fig. 39–1).[63,75,94,245,345,454,541,542] In more advanced cases the periosteal barrier may be broken, and a soft tissue tumor mass may be seen invading the adjacent muscle tissue. In general, the central portions of the neoplasm are more heavily ossified than the peripheral areas.

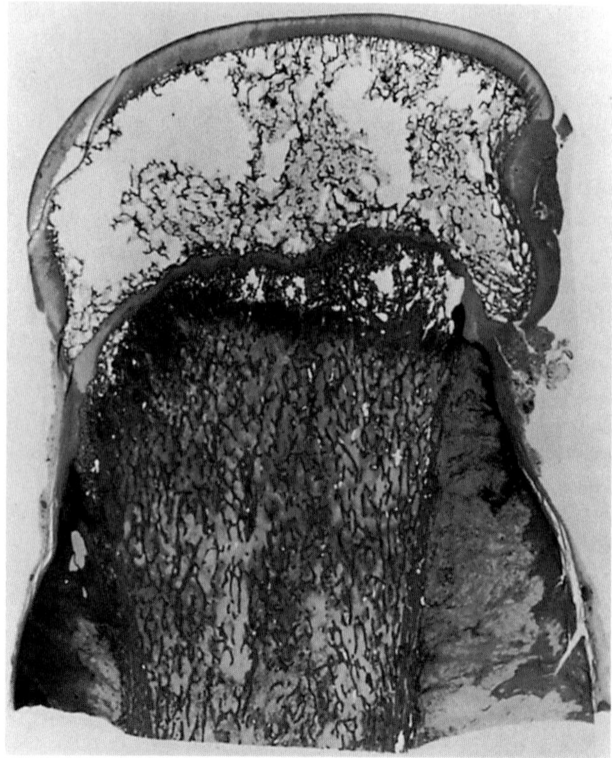

FIGURE 39–1 Osteosarcoma of the proximal humerus. Photomicrograph of a sagittal section of an amputated specimen. The neoplasm is metaphyseal in location; it has perforated the cortex and raised the periosteum. The physis is unbroken; it does not become violated until later in the course of the disease (original magnification ×10).

The ossified portions are of a gritty consistency and have a yellowish appearance; the more cellular areas are softer and tan to whitish. In a sagittal section of an amputated specimen, the boundaries of the epiphyseal end of the tumor are not clearly distinguishable. The physis is less readily violated than the cortical wall and remains unpenetrated until later in the course of the disease. The articular hyaline cartilage serves to block the extension of the neoplasm into the joint. Transepiphyseal extension has been reported,[138,171,385,489] but extension across the articular cartilage does not occur unless there has been a fracture. The tumor may enter the joint, however, by extending along ligamentous and capsular structures (e.g., the cruciate ligaments).[458,491] Toward the diaphyseal end, the advancing tumor presents as a conical plug that marks the limit of growth of the lesion lengthwise along the shaft. Skip metastases (isolated foci of tumor in the same bone, but separated from the main tumor mass by normal marrow) occasionally occur; this is significant when determining the optimal level for resection.[66,137] Skip metastases are usually detectable by bone scans and magnetic resonance imaging (MRI)[299,376] and portend a poorer prognosis, similar to that of a patient with lung metastases.[575]

The histologic findings of osteosarcoma usually show a frankly sarcomatous stroma and direct formation of neoplastic osteoid and bone (Fig. 39–2).* In some pathologic specimens, however, tumor osteoid bone cannot be demonstrated; only collagen strands interwoven with the tumor cells are seen. In anaplastic areas, the neoplasm consists of pleomorphic cells with little intercellular substance. In other tumors, neoplastic cartilage and atypical spindle-shaped cells may be the predominant feature. Aegerter and Kirkpatrick have divided the microscopic picture of osteosarcoma into four types.[5] In the first type, osteoid production is the predominant finding; in the second type, both osteoid and cartilage are formed. In the third type, neither osteoid nor cartilage is produced, but collagen is formed. In the fourth type, there is little or no indication of the presence of these intercellular substances. Attempts to correlate the four histologic types with the clinical manifestations of osteosarcoma have been futile. On the basis of histologic findings alone, one cannot predict the rate of growth, the advent of metastasis, or the duration of survival.[65,96,176,410,520,564] It is important to remember that osteosarcoma may have large areas with little or no bone formation, but if any neoplastic bone is present, it is called osteosarcoma and treated as such. In an adolescent, the diagnosis of chondrosarcoma should be viewed with suspicion, despite the demonstration of only high-grade chondrosarcoma in a biopsy specimen. It is highly likely that examination of the entire specimen of a "chondrosarcoma" in an adolescent will reveal neoplastic bone formation, indicating that it is in fact chondroblastic osteosarcoma.

The pathologist determines the histologic grade of the tumor based on cellularity, atypia, pleomor-

*See references 56, 63, 96, 97, 195, 333, 454, 541, 543, 564.

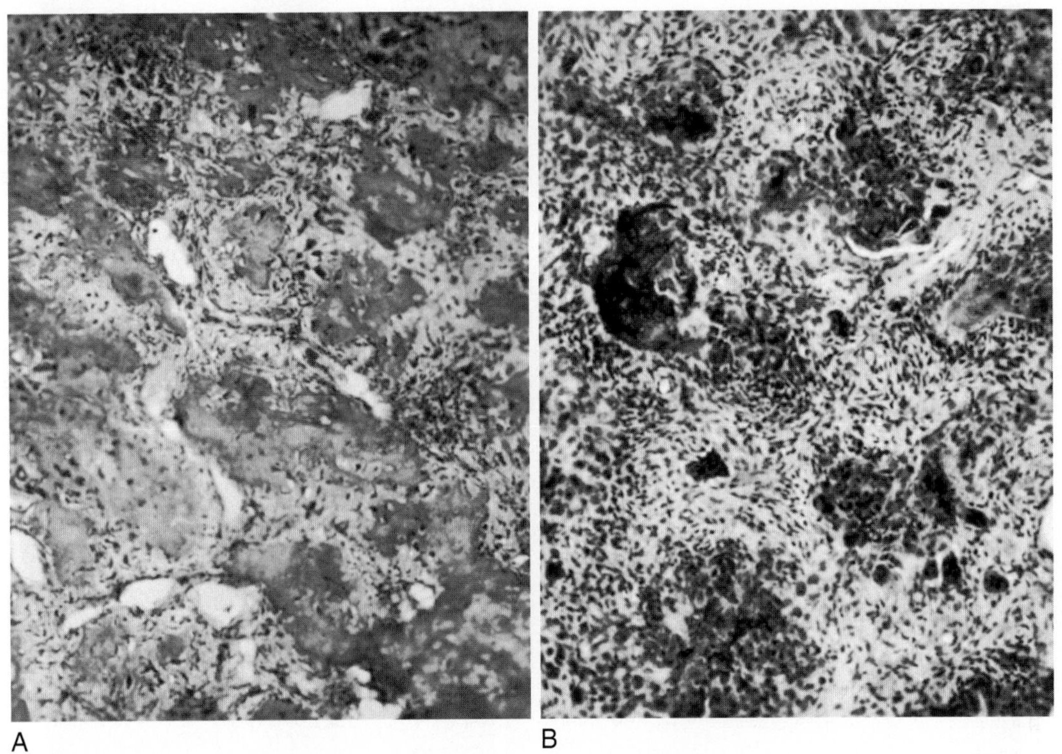

FIGURE 39–2 Histologic findings in osteosarcoma. **A,** Photomicrograph showing the sarcomatous stroma and the direct formation of neoplastic osteoid and bone (original magnification ×100). **B,** Greater magnification (×250).

phism, degree of tumor necrosis, and number of mitoses. A three- or four-grade system is used, depending on the pathologist. The prognostic significance of the number of mitotic figures is uncertain; at best, it is an index of the rate of growth.[349] The histologic grade of the tumor is important, in that a low-grade surface or central osteosarcoma[49,67,283,410] has a much better prognosis than a high-grade (grade 2 or 3) osteosarcoma.[96,352,378,520,564,574]

CLINICAL FEATURES

Local pain in the affected part is the presenting complaint. Initially the pain is intermittent, but within a matter of weeks it becomes severe and constant. There may be a history of trauma that has precipitated discomfort from the tumor. It is often presumed that the trauma caused the tumor, but it is more likely that the injury merely called attention to the affected site. When a lower limb is affected, an antalgic limp may develop. As the condition progresses, a local mass that is hard and fixed to the underlying bone may be palpated (Fig. 39–3A and B). There may also be increased local heat and sensitivity to pressure. The firmness of the tumor varies, depending on the extent of ossification. The tumor may become visible as it enlarges. Limitation of joint motion and disuse atrophy of the muscles are other findings. It is important to recognize that the great majority of patients with osteosarcoma are not "sick." They do not have fever, weight loss, or cachexia, and except for disease at the primary site, they appear to be healthy. This is one reason the diagnosis may be delayed. On rare occasions, however, in a patient with a rapidly growing neoplasm with pulmonary metastases, the patient may exhibit systemic symptoms. At other times, a pathologic fracture through the lesion may be the presenting condition.[2,250,410,469]

RADIOGRAPHIC FINDINGS

Radiography. Osteosarcoma has a typical radiographic picture characterized by destructive and osteoblastic changes (Figs. 39–3C-E, 39–4 through 39–6).[4,74,158,232,445,470] It may be purely radiodense or purely radiolucent, but commonly it is a mixture of both. The neoplasm usually begins eccentrically in the metaphyseal region of a long bone. Bone destruction is evident, with loss of the normal trabecular pattern and the appearance of irregular, ill-defined, poorly marginated, ragged radiolucent defects. New bone formation may be neoplastic or reactive and appears as areas of increased radiopacity. The cortex is invaded by the growing tumor, as evidenced by destruction of the cortical wall and raising of the periosteum. The tumor is large and poorly marginated. There is an incomplete attempt to contain the tumor by periosteum, forming Codman's triangle. The base of Codman's triangle is perpendicular to the shaft and is created by the subperiosteal reactive new bone; it is not diagnostic of osteosarcoma because it is also seen in osteomyelitis and Ewing's sarcoma. The "sunburst"

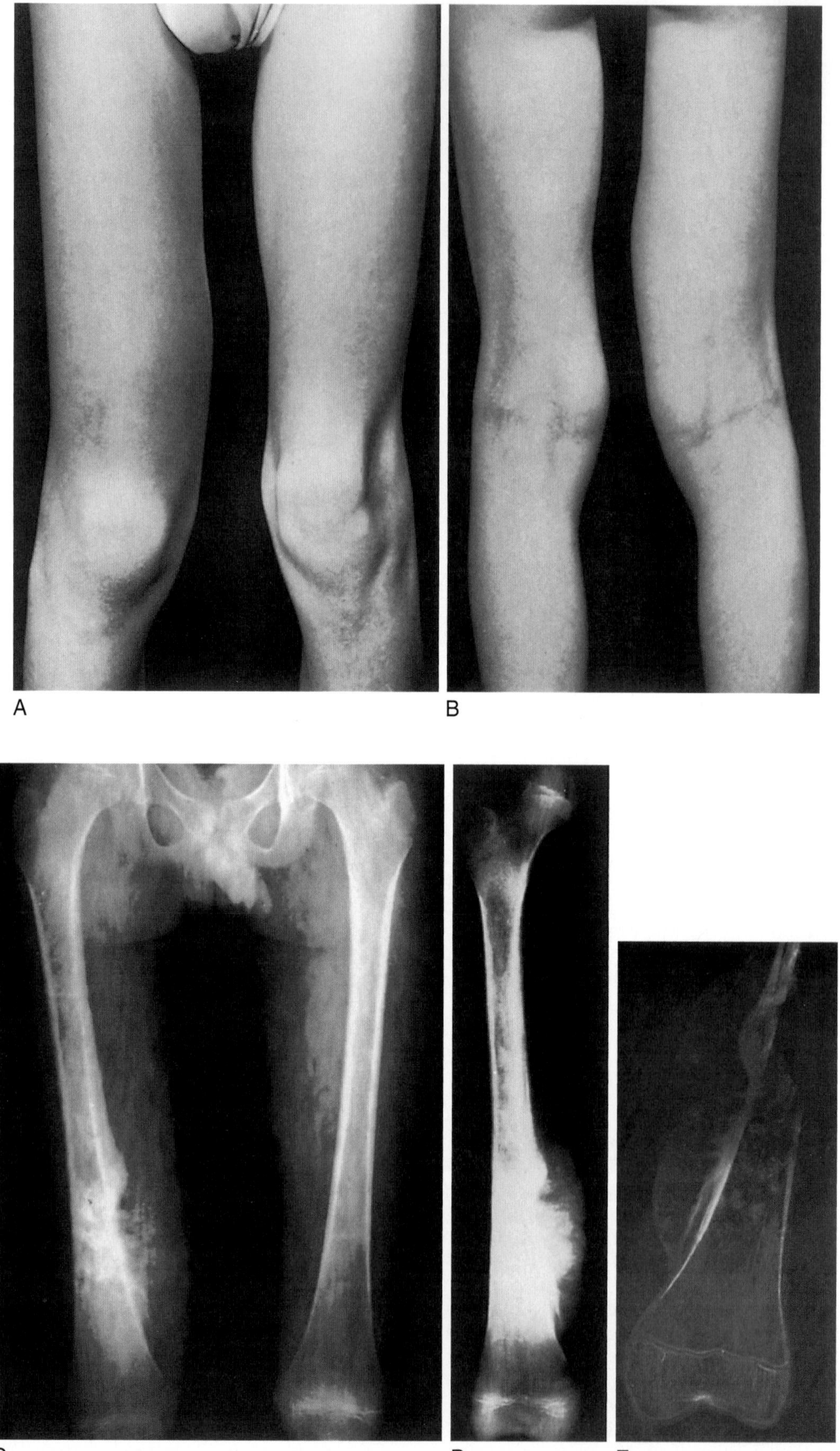

FIGURE 39-3 Osteosarcoma of the right distal femur. **A** and **B,** Clinical appearance, showing swelling of the right lower thigh. **C** and **D,** Radiographs of the femora. Note the "sunburst" appearance and the areas of increased radiopacity (neoplastic bone) and radiolucency (bone destruction). **E,** Radiograph of a gross specimen sectional slab.

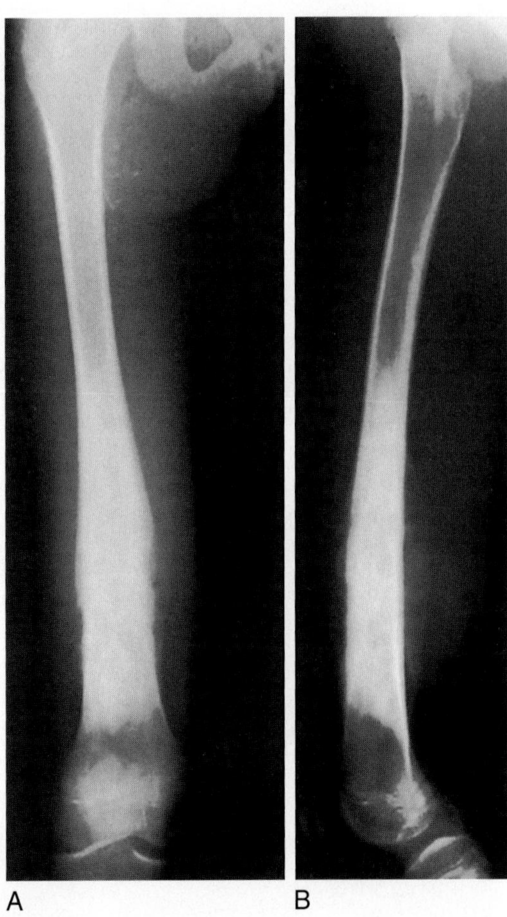

FIGURE 39–4 Osteosarcoma of the distal femur in a 12-year-old girl. **A** and **B,** Radiographs of the femur. The normal trabecular pattern is lost as the neoplastic bone invades the cortex and raises the periosteum. Note the "sunburst" appearance and Codman's triangle. The conical plug of the tumor in the midshaft (best seen on the lateral view) marks the proximal limit of the lesion lengthwise along the shaft.

appearance is produced by the formation of spicules of new bone laid down perpendicular to the shaft along the vessels passing from the periosteum to the cortex. A soft tissue mass is discernible on the radiographs as the tumor advances and transgresses the cortex. Pathologic fracture may occur.

Osteosarcomas do not always exhibit the classic radiographic pattern. They may be subtle in the early stages. They may be radiolucent and diaphyseal, leading one to assume that they are Ewing's sarcoma. We have seen one case detected serendipitously on a comparison radiograph obtained for a suspected fracture. Pathologic fracture (Fig. 39–7) may make the diagnosis difficult, and it is not uncommon for patients to be treated for long-bone fractures, only to have an underlying neoplasm discovered weeks later. Aneurysmal bone cysts can mimic osteosarcomas, and osteosarcomas may have fluid–fluid levels on MRI, adding to the confusion. Clinical suspicion should be raised if a teenager presents with unexplained pain about the knee or shoulder, especially if the pain does not resolve quickly or is present at rest or at night. Radiographs in such cases should be analyzed critically, and if there is any doubt, the patient should be further evaluated by radionuclide scintigraphy or MRI.

Magnetic Resonance Imaging and Computed Tomography. MRI and computed tomography (CT) are of great value in depicting the details of bone destruction and tumor bone production within the lesion. MRI has largely replaced CT as the optimal modality for imaging the primary tumor, and CT is used to evaluate the chest for pulmonary metastases.[231,251,407,513,546,579] On CT, the neoplastic bone appears amorphous and not stress oriented (Fig. 39–8). The areas of cortical erosion by the tumor tissue are well delineated. MRI optimally demonstrates the degree of soft tissue extension and the relationship of the extracompartmental tumor to fascial planes and neurovascular structures. Perhaps the best feature of MRI is its ability to precisely evaluate the extent of tumor in the medullary cavity. Coronal T1-weighted images of the entire involved bone should be included. This is useful when planning limb-sparing resections. The radiologist can measure the extent of the tumor from fixed, palpable landmarks to help the surgeon plan osteotomies. Occult skip metastases of 2 mm or more in long bones are well seen on MRI. MRI is also useful in evaluating the adjacent joint for tumor spread.

Pulmonary metastases 3 to 7 mm or greater in diameter are identified with CT.[397] Conventional radiographs of the chest (dual inspiration and expiration views) show metastatic nodules 10 mm or greater in diameter. The importance of pulmonary CT in the staging of osteosarcoma cannot be overemphasized.[81,82,108,397,549] Approximately 10% to 20% of patients with osteosarcoma present with radiographically detectable metastases at diagnosis. Most of these are in the lungs. Chest CT is superior to plain radiography in demonstrating these metastases, and spiral CT is superior to conventional CT for this purpose.[82,83,220,397,549]

Bone Scan. Bone scan with technetium 99m shows a marked increase in the uptake of the radionuclide in the primary tumor. The increased uptake is due to active formation of new tumor and host bone as well as the vascularity of the lesion (Fig. 39–9). Radionuclide bone scintigraphy is used to look for bony metastases in the involved bone (skip metastases)[66,78,137,470,575] and at other skeletal sites.[33,91,224,257,294,324,415,479,517] Mineralized metastases are more likely to be detected by bone scans than are nonmineralized ones at extrapulmonary sites.[270] The intensity of the uptake increases with the vascularity of the lesion. Ordinarily, the margins of the increased isotope activity mark the extent of the osteosarcoma; this is not absolute, however, because the tumor may extend beyond the margin of increased radioisotope uptake.

Angiography. Angiography is of great value in delineating the extent of soft tissue extension and its relationship to adjacent neurovascular structures, but it is

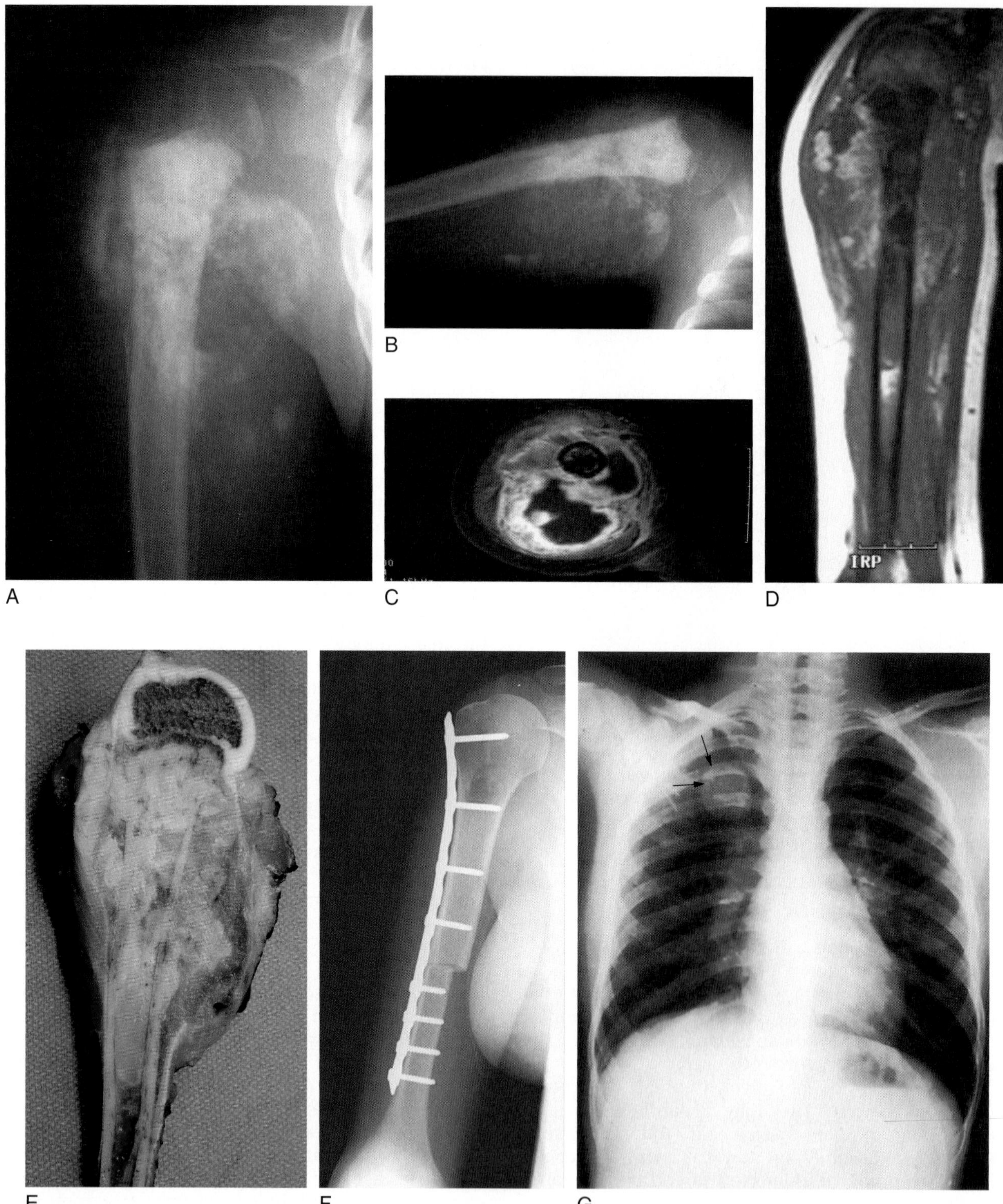

FIGURE 39-5 Osteosarcoma of the right proximal humerus in an 8-year-old boy. The patient presented with pain and a mass in his arm. **A** and **B,** Radiographs demonstrate a large mass in the metaphysis abutting the physis. Periosteal elevation and the corresponding Codman's triangle are seen along the diaphysis. **C** and **D,** Magnetic resonance imaging allows more precise identification of the local extent of the tumor. Areas of necrosis are seen on the axial sections. The extent of the tumor in the medullary cavity can be appreciated on the coronal section. **E,** Resection specimen, demonstrating scattered areas of neoplastic bone. **F,** Example of proximal humeral allograft reconstruction in a different patient. **G,** Example of a lung metastasis (*arrows*).

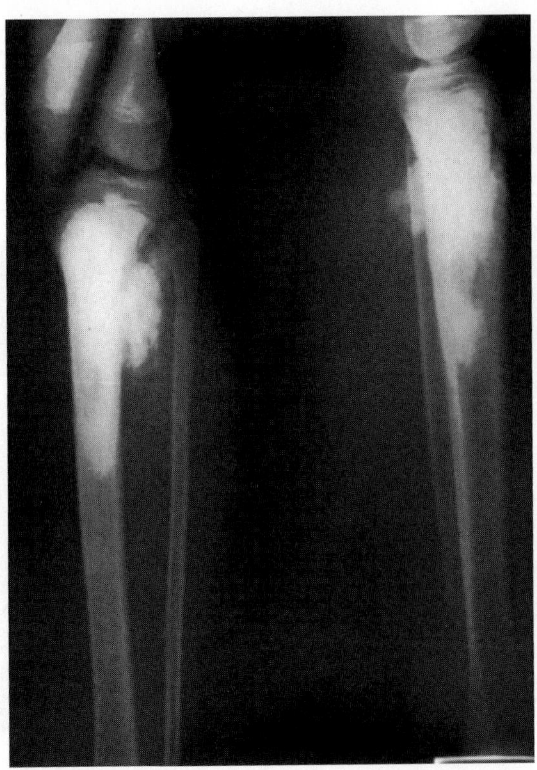

FIGURE 39-6 Initial radiograph showing osteosarcoma of the proximal tibia.

seldom used now because MRI can display this information more easily and less invasively. Angiography is also useful in demonstrating the response to preoperative chemotherapy, but dynamic MRI has replaced it for this purpose as well.[74,230,232,470]

LABORATORY FINDINGS

There are no specific laboratory tests for osteosarcoma. The complete blood cell (CBC) count is usually normal, and although the erythrocyte sedimentation rate (ESR) may be elevated, it is not specific. The serum alkaline phosphatase (ALP) level is usually elevated in osteosarcoma, reflecting osteogenesis in the neoplastic tissue.[24,144,410] The degree of elevation of this enzyme is commensurate with the activity of the neoplastic osteoblasts within the lesion and the size of the tumor. In some studies, an elevated ALP level has been associated with a worse prognosis.[31,148,358] The course of osteosarcoma can be monitored by serial determination of serum ALP levels. Following ablation of the tumor, the enzyme level falls to near normal; it rises with the development of metastases and with recurrence. Clinically, sequential serum ALP levels are used to assess response to chemotherapy. In some studies, the lactate dehydrogenase (LDH) level has been shown to be of prognostic importance. An elevated LDH level is associated with a worse prognosis.[148,310]

DIFFERENTIAL DIAGNOSIS

The primary entity from which osteosarcoma must be differentiated is Ewing's sarcoma, but benign conditions may also mimic osteosarcoma. Exuberant callus of a fatigue fracture, subacute osteomyelitis, active myositis ossificans, aneurysmal bone cyst, and Langerhans cell histiocytosis (eosinophilic granuloma) are some of the benign conditions that may be mistaken for osteosarcoma. Ewing's sarcoma, fibrosarcoma, lymphoma, and metastatic carcinoma are some of the malignant lesions that must be excluded. Age is a major factor in sorting out the various diagnostic possibilities. In a child younger than 5 years of age, histiocytosis, metastatic Wilms' tumor, or neuroblastoma should be considered. In an adolescent, osteosarcoma and Ewing's sarcoma are the most common bone malignancies. Chondrosarcoma is very uncommon in children and adolescents, and most lesions considered to be "chondrosarcoma" by biopsy are really chondroblastic osteosarcoma. Leukemias and lymphomas should also be considered in an adolescent with an aggressive bone neoplasm.

STAGING

Once the diagnosis of osteosarcoma has been made, the disease should be staged. The objectives of the staging workup are to establish the final tissue diagnosis, delineate the local extent of the tumor, and discover any distant metastases. Both radiologic staging and open biopsy should be done by the surgeon who will perform the definitive operation.[43,329,330,402,488,490] The questions to be answered are as follows:

1. Is it a low- or high-grade tumor?
2. Is the tumor limited to the bone (intracompartmental), or has it spread to the adjacent soft tissues (extracompartmental)?
3. Is there evidence of metastatic spread to the lungs or other bones?

Carefully planned imaging of the lesion should precede open biopsy. If a needle biopsy is chosen, the surgeon should direct the placement of the needle in careful discussion with the interventional radiologist. Determining the local extent of disease after biopsy performed elsewhere is difficult and inaccurate because of the disruption of tissue planes, hematoma formation, edema, and wound healing. In choosing the proper surgical procedure, it is vital to know whether there are natural barriers to tumor extension.[136,139,490] Is the lesion intracompartmental (bounded by natural barriers to tumor extension) or extracompartmental (with no proximal, distal, or peripheral barriers to tumor extension)? The vast majority of high-grade osteosarcomas are extracompartmental. During staging, the surgeon should meticulously assess the muscle compartment and the tumor's proximity to neurovascular structures to determine whether limb salvage is feasible. Usually, the final decision is based on postchemotherapy MRI.

In the preoperative staging of osteosarcoma, the following diagnostic tests are performed: complete history and physical examination; CBC count with differential, ESR, and serum levels of calcium, phosphorus, ALP, and LDH; conventional radiographs of the

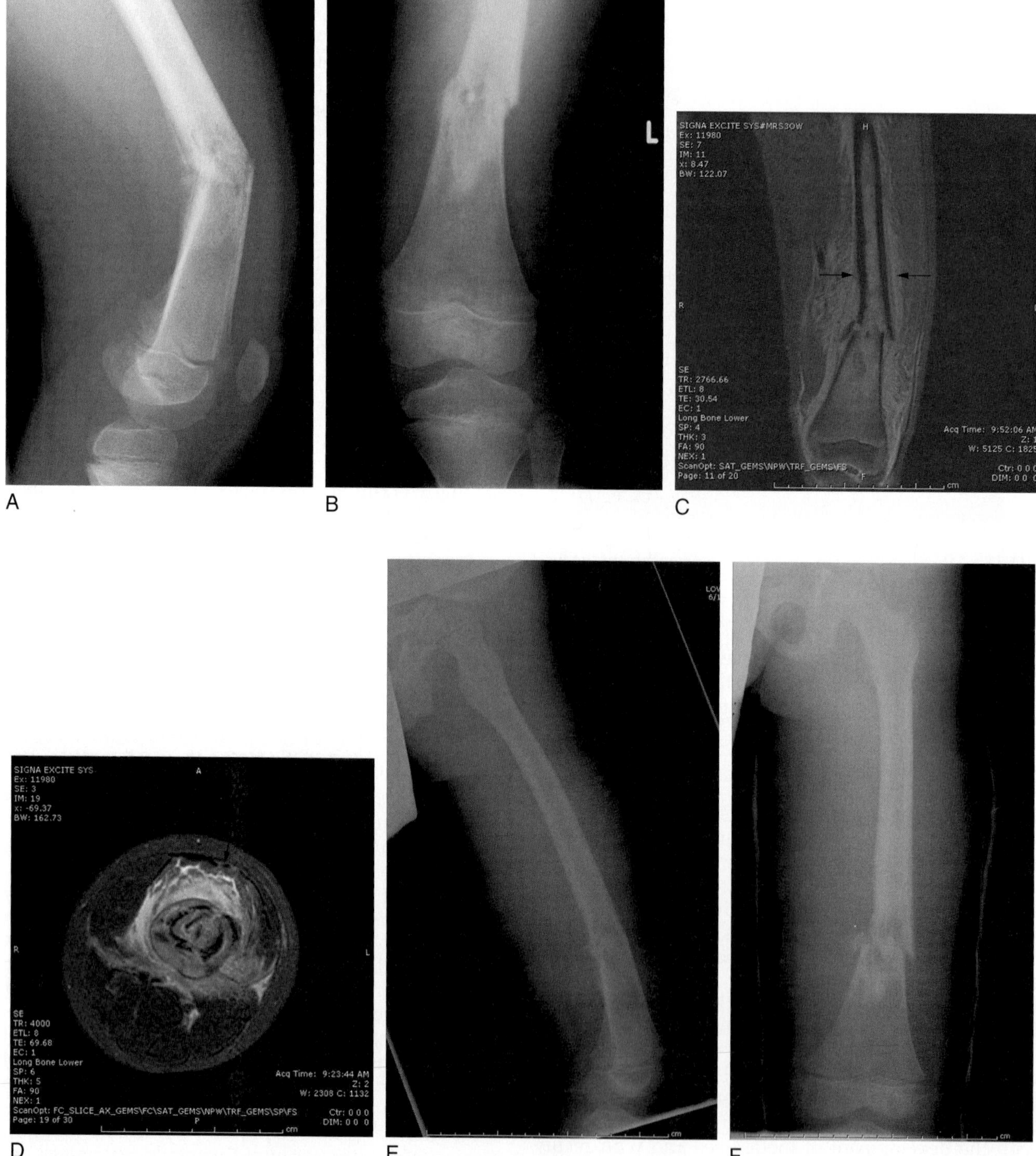

FIGURE 39-7 Pathologic fracture as the presentation of osteosarcoma of the distal femur. **A** and **B,** Radiographs demonstrate a displaced fracture of the distal femur. The medullary cavity immediately distal to the fracture demonstrates mixed radiolucent and radiodense areas. Note the periosteal elevation best seen on the lateral radiograph immediately proximal to the fracture, which is also suggestive of a pathologic fracture. **C** and **D,** Magnetic resonance images demonstrate the tumor mass extending into the soft tissues. Note the extensive edema associated with the fracture (*arrows*). **E** and **F,** At the time of needle biopsy, the fracture was reduced, and the patient was placed in a cast for stabilization of the fracture while the chemotherapy regimen was begun.

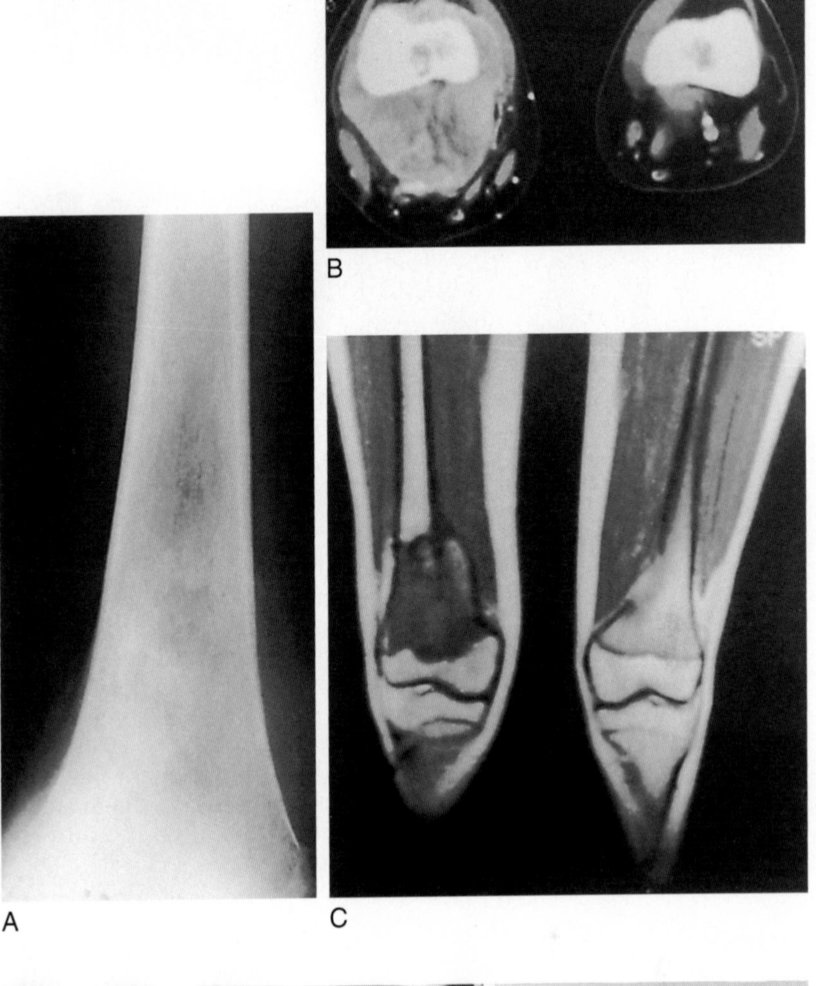

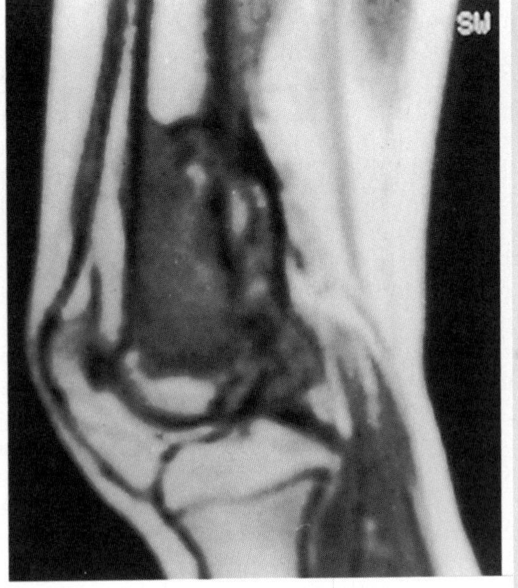

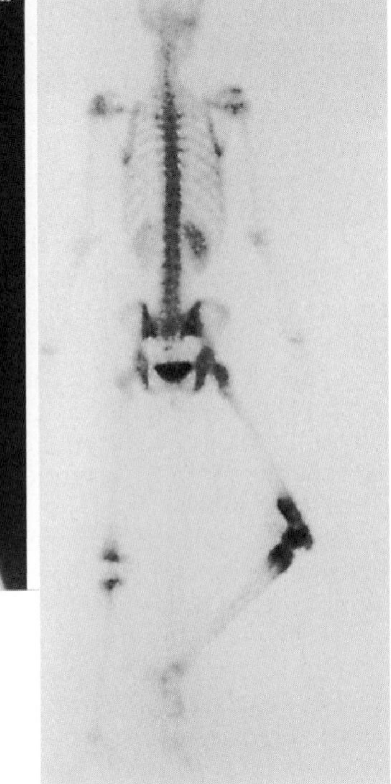

FIGURE 39-8 Osteosarcoma of the left distal femur. **A,** Plain anteroposterior radiograph. Note the distal metaphyseal and lower diaphyseal sclerotic lesion. **B,** Computed tomography scan showing bone-forming tumor. **C** and **D,** Magnetic resonance images showing the extent of the tumor and its relationship to the popliteal soft tissue. **E,** Bone scan with technetium-99m showing increased uptake in the distal femoral metaphyseal region.

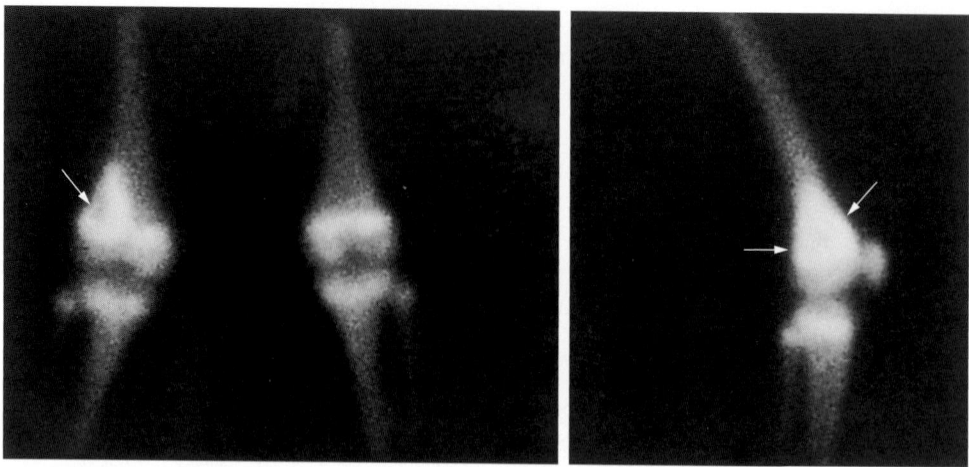

FIGURE 39-9 Osteosarcoma of the right distal femoral metaphysis. Bone scan findings with technetium-99m. Note the increased uptake in the area of the lesion (*arrows*).

tumor site and the chest; scintigraphy with technetium 99m; MRI to assess the intraosseous extent of the tumor, joint involvement, and the relationship of the soft tissue mass to adjacent neurovascular structures; and CT of the chest to rule out metastases.[490]

A pediatric oncologist, radiologist, and pathologist should be part of the treatment team from the beginning, taking part in the staging and subsequent decision making. The management of osteosarcoma requires a multidisciplinary approach, and patients should be treated in medical centers specializing in pediatric oncology.

BIOPSY

Before performing an open biopsy, the surgeon should be knowledgeable in the differential diagnosis and local extent of the lesion; before placing the incision, he or she should be cognizant of the principles of limb salvage surgery and amputation flaps. The surgeon who will perform the definitive operation should perform the biopsy. The technical details of performing a biopsy are presented elsewhere (see Chapter 37, General Principles of Tumor Management). It is crucial to verify the biopsy site with C-arm imaging in the operating room. Frozen sections should be used to ensure that diagnostic tissue has been obtained, and cultures of the tissue specimen should be performed. The pathologist should have the radiographic studies available to review before or during the biopsy. Special stains, cytology, electron microscopy, and immunocytochemistry may be important in establishing the correct diagnosis.

There is always the danger of local tumor spread as a result of an open biopsy. Adequate hemostasis must be obtained. The use of a tourniquet is at the discretion of the surgeon. If a drain is used, it should be placed near and along the direction of the biopsy tract, because it will be excised at the time of primary resection. Core needle biopsies or fine-needle aspirations are used at institutions with experience in these techniques, but not all pathologists are comfortable making the diagnosis from limited tissue.[115,277,402,488,508,565] Although an experienced pathologist might make a correct diagnosis on the basis of a frozen section, immediate definitive wide excision of osteosarcoma is seldom performed at the time of biopsy because most patients receive preoperative (neoadjuvant) chemotherapy. Thus, it is always best to rely on permanent sections for the final diagnosis. If there is uncertainty about the diagnosis, an experienced bone pathologist should be asked to review the slides.

TREATMENT

The treatment of high-grade osteosarcoma occurs in two phases: (1) administration of adjuvant chemotherapy and (2) surgical resection of the tumor.

Chemotherapy

It is important to recognize that osteosarcoma is a systemic disease in most cases. Following amputation alone, metastatic disease, usually in the lungs, occurs in 80% to 90% of patients within the first 2 years.[65,95,180,183,310,345,564] This implies that micrometastatic disease is present from the time osteosarcoma is detected clinically. Because micrometastatic disease is often controlled by adjuvant chemotherapy, it was hypothesized in the 1960s and 1970s that the administration of chemotherapy might prevent the appearance of metastatic disease.[246,515] This hypothesis proved to be true, although the premise was challenged initially.[519] Both randomized and nonrandomized studies have shown a disease-free and overall survival advantage in patients who receive adjuvant chemotherapy.[134,310,519] Before the chemotherapy era, the probability of remaining disease-free after amputation for osteosarcoma was less than 20%.[96,180,182,183,333] Currently, this probability is between 65% and 80%, or perhaps higher.[32,36,163,246,310,311,355,420,438,441,515,572,573]

The standard agents include high-dose methotrexate, doxorubicin (Adriamycin), and cisplatin. These agents have been tested in large series of patients in national trials of the Pediatric Oncology Group and the Children's Cancer Group (now combined as the Children's Oncology Group), providing a good example of how cooperative groups can carry out trials to study the outcomes of therapy for a rare disease. Initially, there was doubt about the effectiveness of chemotherapy. A randomized study definitively addressed this issue and conclusively demonstrated that adjuvant chemotherapy improves the disease-free and overall survival rate of osteosarcoma patients.[310,311] The dramatic improvement in the ability to cure patients with osteosarcoma has come at a price, however. The drugs used are highly toxic, and the adverse effects include infection from neutropenia, cardiotoxicity, renal toxicity, and hearing loss, to name a few.[39,51,131,163,179,247,259,268,276,312,474]

The next advance in treatment was the use of preoperative, or neoadjuvant, chemotherapy. By administering chemotherapy before resection, one can treat the micrometastatic disease earlier, perhaps shrink the tumor to make resection easier, and study the histologic response to the drugs.[27,35,435,570] There was concern, however, that if the patient's tumor did not respond, it might progress during the preoperative period. This also was studied in a randomized trial, and it appears that the outcome is similar regardless of whether chemotherapy is administered both pre- and postoperatively or only postoperatively.[184] This study was difficult to complete, because by the time it was opened, surgeons already had a bias toward preoperative chemotherapy. Because of poor patient accrual, the power to detect a 15% difference in the two groups was only 80%. Nevertheless, preoperative chemotherapy is now standard.[31,151,357]

One of the main advantages of preoperative chemotherapy is that it provides prognostic information. The pathologist can examine the specimen for the percentage of histologic necrosis following resection.[238,258,435,439,448,571] Patients with a higher degree of necrosis (>95%) have a better outcome than those with less necrosis. It seems logical that giving alternative chemotherapy to patients with less tumor necrosis would improve outcome, but this has not been the case in studies addressing the issue. The most recent cooperative trial in the United States studied the results of the addition of a new agent, ifosfamide, and an immunostimulant, muramyl tripeptide (MTP), in a randomized trial to determine whether the addition of either or both of these agents improved the survival of patients with osteosarcoma. It concluded that the addition of ifosfamide in the adjuvant setting did not improve event-free survival compared with the standard combination of cisplatin, doxorubicin, and high-dose methotrexate, but it was confounded by the use of MTP, which appeared to have a beneficial effect in the ifosfamide arm of the study. Further investigation is needed to determine whether this is a reproducible effect.[357]

Many advances have been made in the treatment of osteosarcoma, yet 20% to 40% of patients do not respond to treatment despite similar histology, staging, and other patient characteristics. Just as there are some patients who could benefit from more aggressive chemotherapy, there are others who may need very little or no chemotherapy. It is hoped that more information about the molecular makeup of these tumors will provide insight in this regard and allow us to target therapy more precisely.[45,421,497] This has led to research efforts in drug resistance mechanisms, genetic alterations in these sarcomas, and novel radiographic approaches to detect nonresponders at diagnosis. Multidrug resistance has been demonstrated in osteosarcoma and is a powerful prognostic indicator.[38,77] The P-glycoprotein membrane pump actively exports agents such as doxorubicin out of the cell and can be detected by a variety of immunohistochemical methods.[471,576] The exciting aspect of these findings is that the resistance pump can be blocked by other agents, offering a potential means of overcoming resistance in these patients. Unfortunately, this has not been translated into clinically relevant treatment strategies, and the results of these studies have been mixed, probably because there are multiple resistance mechanisms available to the cancer cell and we are only beginning to understand them.

Genetic alterations in tumor suppressor genes have also been demonstrated in osteosarcomas, and there is some indication that in addition to providing clues to the cause of the tumor, they may be of prognostic and possibly therapeutic import.* Human epidermal growth factor receptor 2 (HER2/erbB-2) appears to be overexpressed in patients with advanced disease (greater expression in metastatic osteosarcomas) in some studies,[149,584] but not in others.[497,526,536] Currently, a monoclonal antibody to HER2/erbB-2, trastuzumab (Herceptin), is being studied to determine its therapeutic value in advanced metastatic disease. Determination of expression is difficult, however, and it is not clear that immunohistochemical techniques are sufficiently accurate.[536] The true importance of HER2/erbB-2 in osteosarcoma awaits further study.

Finally, more aggressive or intensified administration of chemotherapy and novel agents may further improve outcome. Some of these avenues are currently being investigated in cooperative trials.

Surgical Treatment

In addition to advances in the medical management of osteosarcoma, the surgical treatment has improved. Amputation was once the standard of care and remains an important part of the armamentarium of the tumor surgeon, especially in children. Currently, however, most patients who present with osteosarcoma are treated with limb-sparing procedures. There was initial concern about the effect of limb salvage on survival rates, and no randomized studies have been carried out that compare limb salvage and amputation.[66,172,309,427,486,493,503,572] Nonrandomized studies, however, do not show a survival advantage for patients treated with amputation, and the local recurrence rate

*See references 13, 113, 165, 196, 208, 287, 317, 344, 382, 495, 529, 530, 540.

after limb salvage procedures is similar to that after cross-bone amputation.[26,28,151,172,192,431,444,493,559] Some recent studies actually show a worse prognosis for patients treated by amputation, but it is likely that this is due to selection bias (amputations being performed in those with larger, more aggressive tumors or those with pathologic fractures). One large retrospective study of distal femoral osteosarcomas showed a higher local recurrence rate after limb salvage procedures and cross-bone amputation than after hip disarticulation, but the three groups did not differ in overall or disease-free survival.[444,487] It is apparent that achieving a wide margin is important, and doing so, coupled with a good response to chemotherapy, is associated with a low incidence of local recurrence. A less than wide margin or a less than good histologic response dramatically increased the recurrence rate in one study.[28]

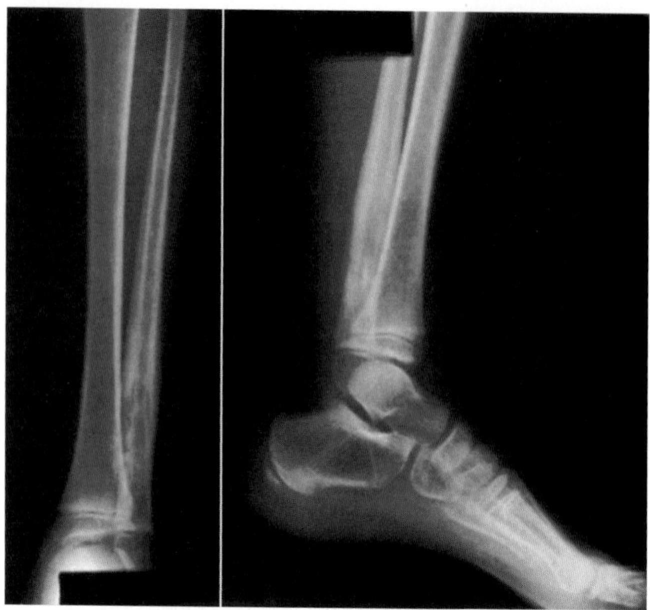

FIGURE 39–10 Osteosarcoma of the distal left fibula in a 5-year-old girl. Initial radiographs of the left leg showed a destructive lesion of the distal metaphysis of the fibula with periosteal new bone formation and soft tissue swelling. Chest computed tomography and bone scan showed no other lesions. Histologic examination of a biopsy specimen disclosed the tumor to be osteosarcoma. Because of the location of the tumor and the age of the patient, she was treated with a below-knee amputation and adjuvant chemotherapy.

Amputation. Irrespective of the method chosen to treat osteosarcoma, the local tumor must be completely excised with negative margins. Although amputation is performed less frequently than in the past, it remains the gold standard of local control, and in the lower extremity, it may be the most functional "reconstruction" in young athletic patients. The primary indications for amputation are very young age, when limb length inequality would be a major problem (lower extremity); displaced pathologic fractures; large soft tissue masses involving neurovascular structures; disease progression during chemotherapy; and local recurrence following limb salvage procedures. In the upper extremity, one usually tries to preserve at least hand function, because prosthetic replacements are not nearly as good as a functional hand. However, in the lower extremity, modern prosthetics are very functional (Fig. 39–10).[263]

The level of amputation is determined by close scrutiny of conventional radiographs, bone scans, and magnetic resonance images. These surgical staging studies should be performed immediately before definitive surgery is undertaken and after completion of preoperative chemotherapy. The entire involved bone should be carefully evaluated by MRI for skip metastases. Most frequently, a wide cross-bone amputation is performed rather than a radical (whole-bone) amputation. Exceptions might be a young child with a tibial osteosarcoma, in whom knee disarticulation or above-knee amputation is performed, or a hindfoot osteosarcoma requiring a below-knee amputation. For distal femoral lesions, a hip disarticulation is seldom performed and is not routinely necessary, as shown by a study from the Musculoskeletal Tumor Society.[444,487] The operative techniques of amputation and disarticulation at various levels in the upper and lower limbs are described and illustrated in Plates 39–1 through 39–9. In very young children, residual limb overgrowth may be a problem. For below-knee amputations, this can be addressed by placing a metacarpal plug in the distal tibial canal if the ipsilateral foot is uninvolved by tumor.[381] Further, in very young children, the predicted length of the residual limb at maturity may be very short if a growth plate is resected. For foot tumors, this can be addressed with a Syme's-type amputation rather than a below-knee amputation[11]; for proximal tibial lesions, a knee disarticulation may be preferable to an above-knee amputation.[42,315,367] These can be revised at maturity if necessary for prosthetic fitting.

Rotationplasty. An alternative to amputation for distal femoral osteosarcomas is the rotationplasty (Fig. 39–11). Young children with high-grade sarcomas of the knee area have limited options for reconstruction following resection of the sarcoma. An above-knee amputation for a distal femoral osteosarcoma in a very young patient leaves the child with a very short lever arm to power a prosthesis, and it becomes relatively shorter as the child grows. The operation described by Borggreve and adapted for congenital defects (e.g., proximal femoral focal deficiency) by van Nes has been applied to tumors and provides a reconstruction option in certain situations.* It can be thought of as an intercalary amputation of the distal femur (or proximal tibia). The reconstruction employs the distal leg, which is rotated 160 to 180 degrees, resulting in a longer lever arm and an active "knee" joint provided by the ankle and foot.

The indications for rotationplasty include a distal femoral or proximal tibial osteosarcoma in a skeletally

*See references 37, 62, 76, 102, 185, 205, 221, 274, 278, 279, 351, 364, 504, 569.

Text continued on page 2311

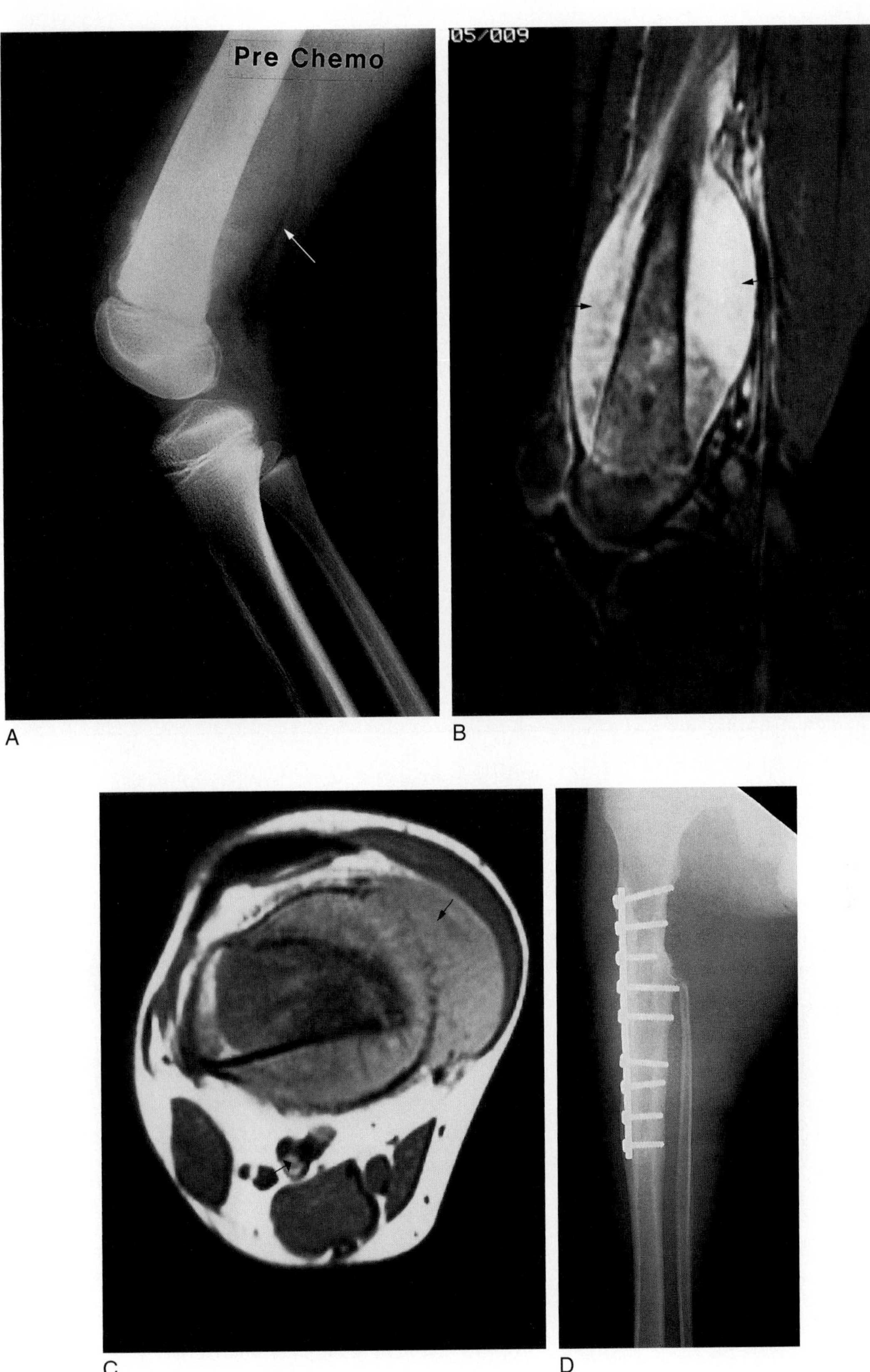

FIGURE 39–11 Osteosarcoma in a 10-year-old boy. **A,** Lateral radiograph of the femur showing a radiodense lesion of the distal femur with a large soft tissue mass. There is a "starburst" type of periosteal reaction of the soft tissue mass (*arrow*). Codman's triangle is seen along the anterior cortex. A biopsy confirmed the diagnosis of osteosarcoma. **B,** Sagittal magnetic resonance image showing the extent of the soft tissue mass and extension into the marrow (*arrows*). Anteriorly, the tumor approaches but does not invade the joint. Posteriorly, the femoral vessels are close to the mass but do not appear to be encased, and the posterior knee capsule is uninvolved. **C,** Axial magnetic resonance image showing that the vessels and nerves are uninvolved (*lower arrow*), and the extent of the soft tissue mass (*upper arrow*). The patient elected to have a rotationplasty because of his age and his desire to play sports. **D,** Radiograph of the lower extremity obtained 1 year later. The boy remains free of disease and fully active 5 years later.

PLATE 39-1

Hemipelvectomy (Banks and Coleman Technique)

The patient lies on the unaffected side and is maintained in position with sandbags and kidney rests, which are placed well above the iliac crests. The underneath normal limb is flexed at the hip and knee and fastened to the table by wide adhesive straps. The uppermost arm is supported on a rest. The perineal area and, in the male, the scrotum and penis are shielded and held out of the operative field with sterile, self-adhering skin drapes. The operative area is prepared and draped so that the proximal thigh, the inguinal and gluteal regions, and the abdomen are sterile. It should be possible to turn the patient onto his or her back and side without contaminating the surgical field.

A, The outlines of the skin flaps, consisting of ilioinguinal, iliogluteal, and posterior incisions, are marked with methylene blue. With the patient placed on his or her back, the ilioinguinal incision is made first. It begins at the pubic tubercle and passes upward and backward parallel to Poupart's ligament to the anterior superior iliac spine and then posteriorly on the iliac crest. Its posterior limit depends on the desired level of section of the innominate bone.

B, The subcutaneous tissue and fascia are divided along the line of the skin incision. The insertions of the abdominal muscles superiorly and the tensor fasciae latae and gluteus medius inferiorly are detached extraperiosteally from the iliac crest.

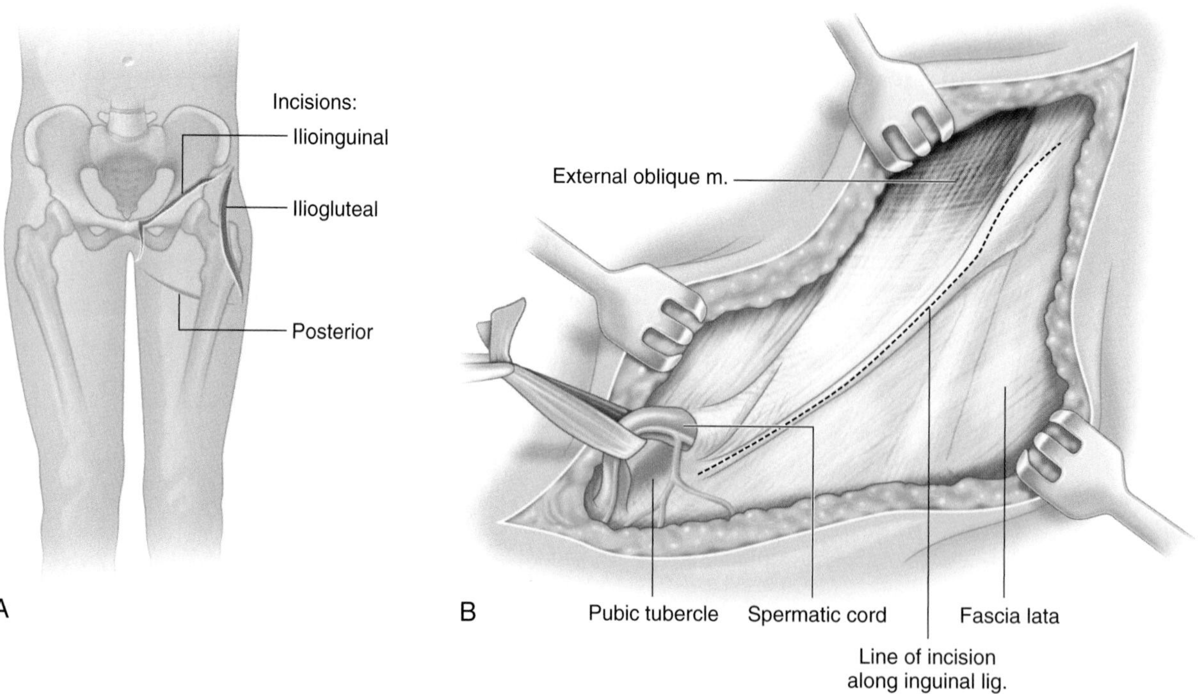

PLATE 39-1 *(continued)*

Hemipelvectomy (Banks and Coleman Technique)

C, The abdominal muscles are detached from the iliac crest and medial wall of the ilium. The tributaries of the deep circumflex vessels are ligated.

D, The inguinal ligament is divided and retracted superiorly, along with the spermatic cord and abdominal muscles. The lower skin flap is retracted inferiorly, and the inner pelvis is freed by blunt dissection. The inferior epigastric artery and lumboinguinal nerve are exposed, ligated, and divided.

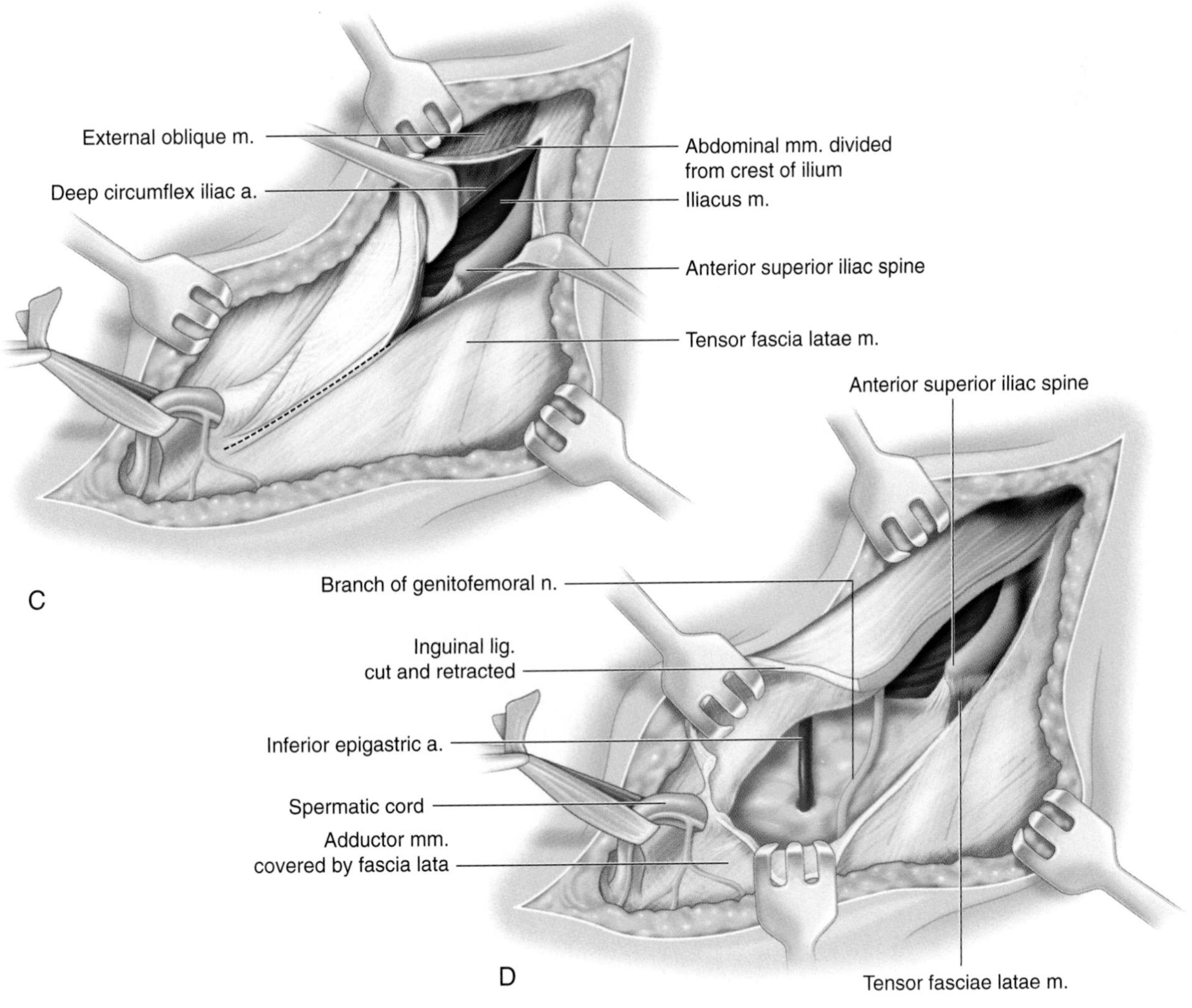

Continued

PLATE 39-1 *(continued)*

Hemipelvectomy (Banks and Coleman Technique)

E, In the loose areolar tissue, the external iliac vessels are dissected, and femoral nerve is divided and dissected. The external iliac artery and vein are individually clamped, severed, and doubly ligated with needle suture 0 silk.

F, The rectus abdominis and adductor muscles are detached from the pubic bone, which is extraperiosteally exposed. The bladder is retracted superiorly. The pubic bone is osteotomized 1.5 cm lateral to the symphysis. Depending on the proximity of the tumor, the osteotomy may have to be made at the symphysis pubis. Injury to the bladder or urethra should be avoided. Any bleeding from the retropubic venous plexus is controlled by coagulation and packing with warm laparotomy pads.

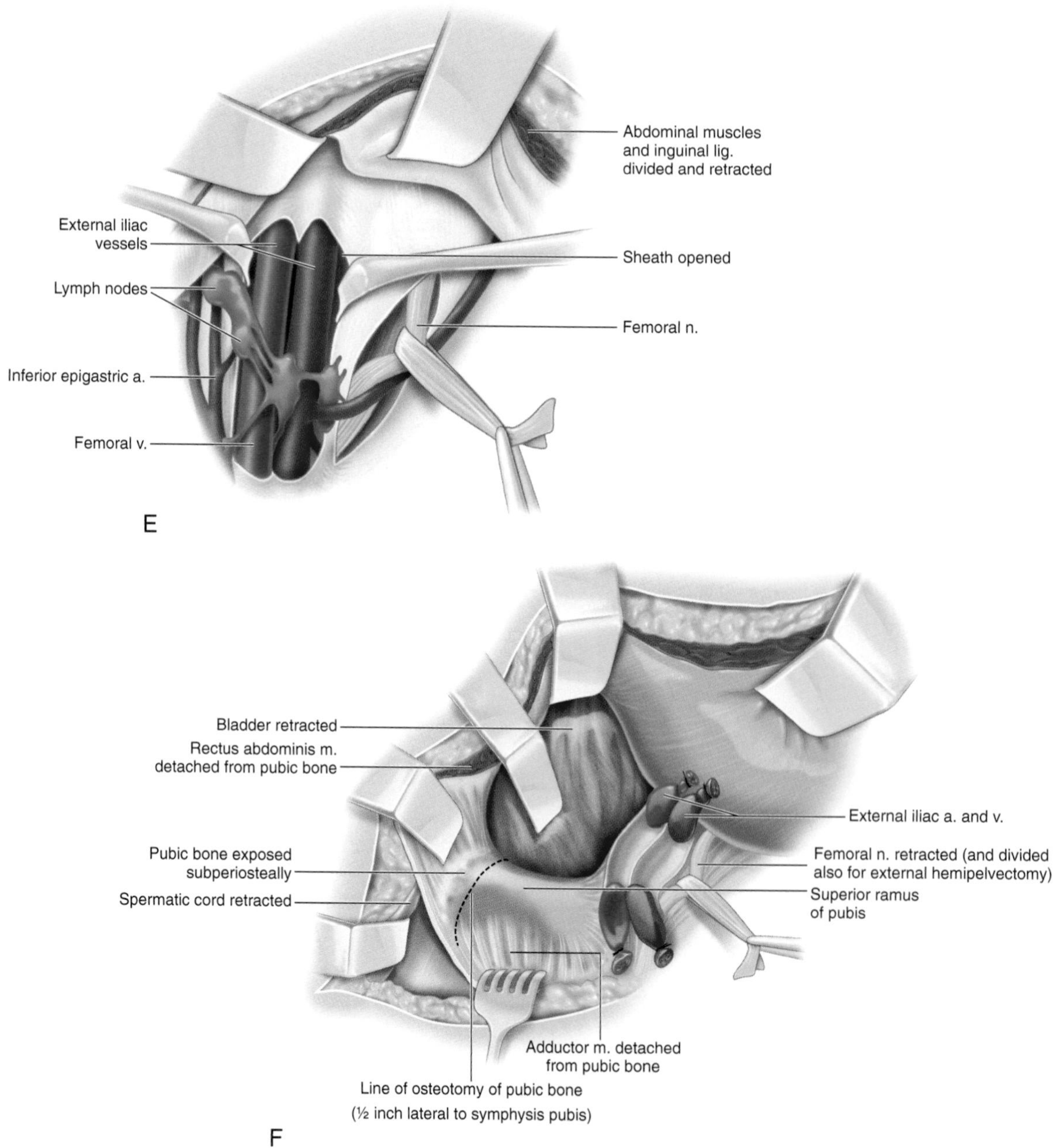

PLATE 39-1 *(continued)*

Hemipelvectomy (Banks and Coleman Technique)

G, The patient is then turned onto his or her side. The drapes are adjusted and reinforced to ensure sterility of the operative field. First the anterior incision is extended posteriorly to the posterior superior iliac spine. From the upper end of the anterior incision, the second or iliogluteal incision is started. It extends to the thigh, curving forward to an area about 5 cm distal to the greater trochanter. It then passes backward around the posterior aspect of the thigh to meet the anterior incision. The subcutaneous tissue and fascia are divided in line with the skin incision.

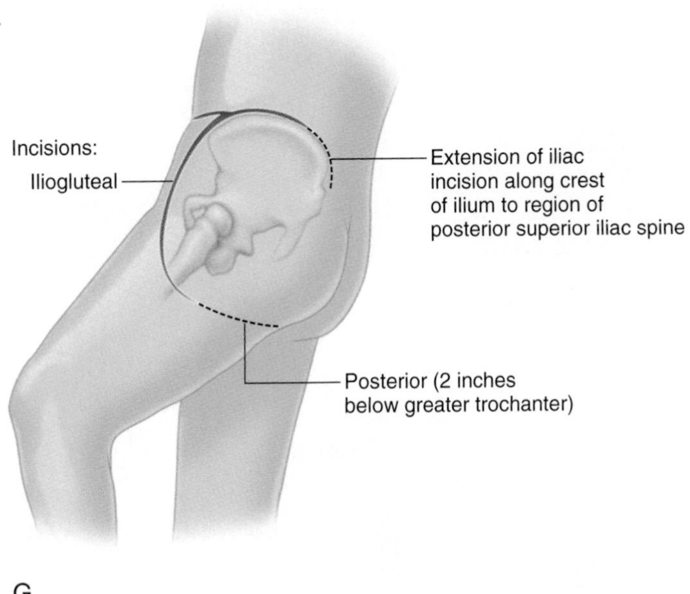

Continued

PLATE 39-1 *(continued)*

Hemipelvectomy (Banks and Coleman Technique)

H, The sciatic nerve is clamped, ligated, and sharply divided distal to the origin of the inferior gluteal nerve. The piriformis, gemellus, and obturator internus muscles are transected near their insertion.

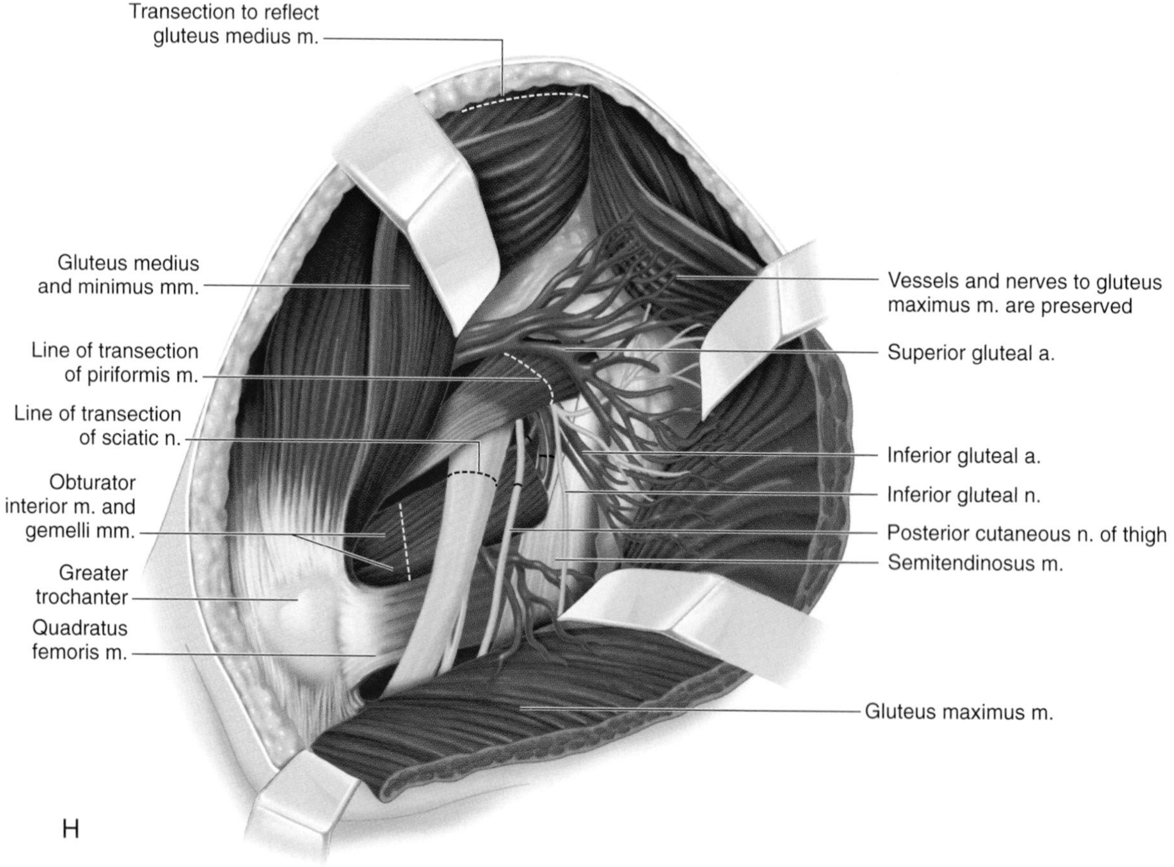

PLATE 39-1 *(continued)*

Hemipelvectomy (Banks and Coleman Technique)

I, The ilium is exposed subperiosteally by elevation and detachment of the latissimus dorsi and sacrospinalis muscles, the posterior portion of the gluteus medius, and the anterior fibers of the gluteus maximus. The inner wall of the ilium is also exposed subperiosteally anterior to the sacroiliac joint. Chandler retractors are placed in the sciatic notch, and, using a Gigli saw, the ilium is osteotomized about 5 cm anterior to the posterior gluteal line. The site of the ilium osteotomy depends on the location of the tumor; it is placed farther posteriorly if the neoplasm is adjacent to the gluteal line.

J, The patient is repositioned on his or her back, and the hip is maximally flexed in some abduction. The posterior incision is completed.

K, The hip is manipulated into maximal abduction and external rotation, laying open the pelvic area and widely exposing the remaining intrapelvic structures to be severed.

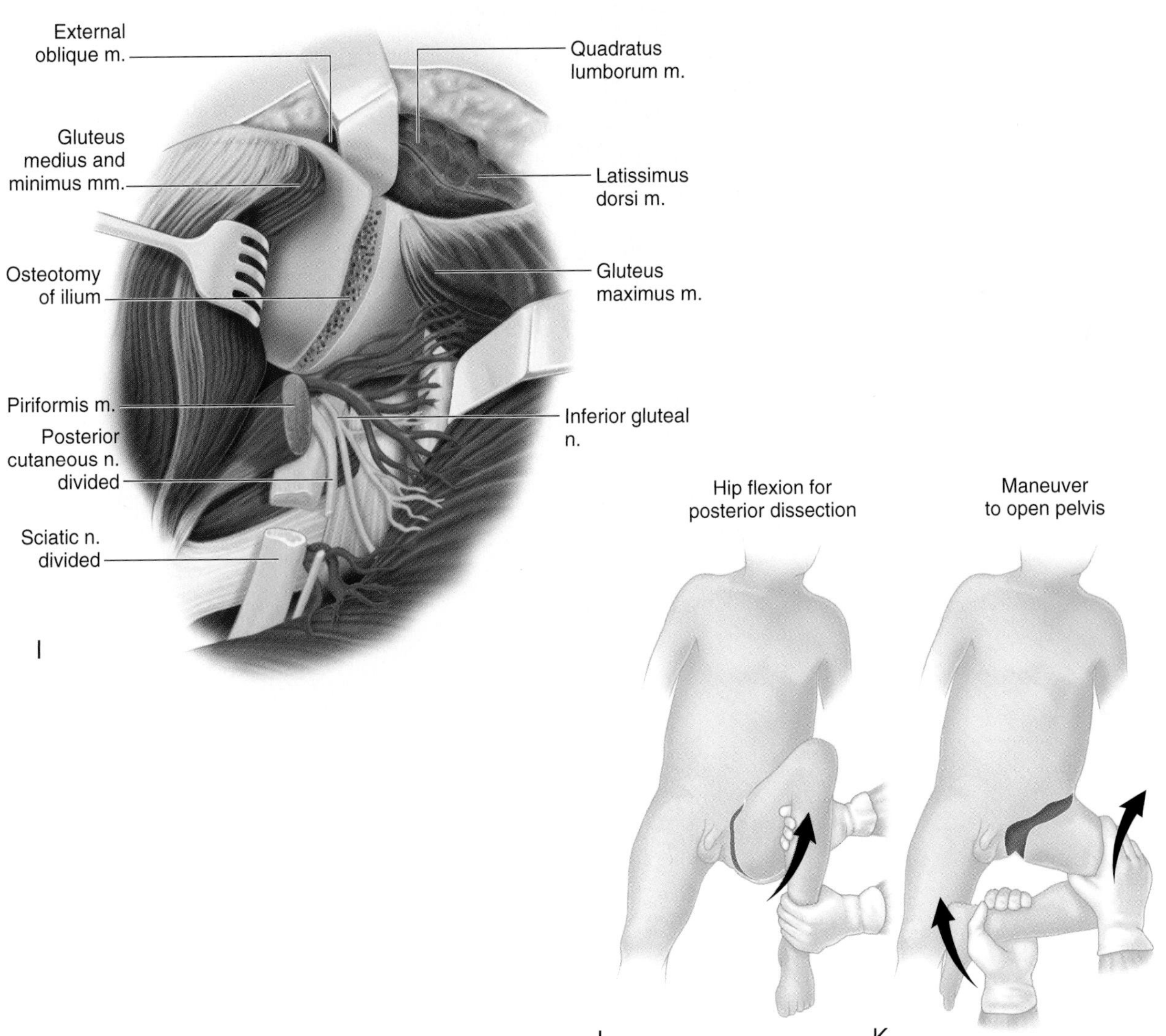

Continued

PLATE 39-1 *(continued)*

Hemipelvectomy (Banks and Coleman Technique)

L, From above downward, the femoral nerve, iliopsoas muscle, obturator vessels, obturator nerve, levator ani, and coccygeus muscles are sectioned. The vessels are doubly ligated before division to prevent troublesome bleeding.

M, Fascia, subcutaneous tissue, and skin are closed in layers in the usual manner. A pressure dressing is applied.

N, The gluteus maximus muscle is sutured to the divided margin of the external oblique muscle and lateral abdominal wall. A couple of perforated silicone catheters are inserted and connected to closed-suction drainage (Hemovac).

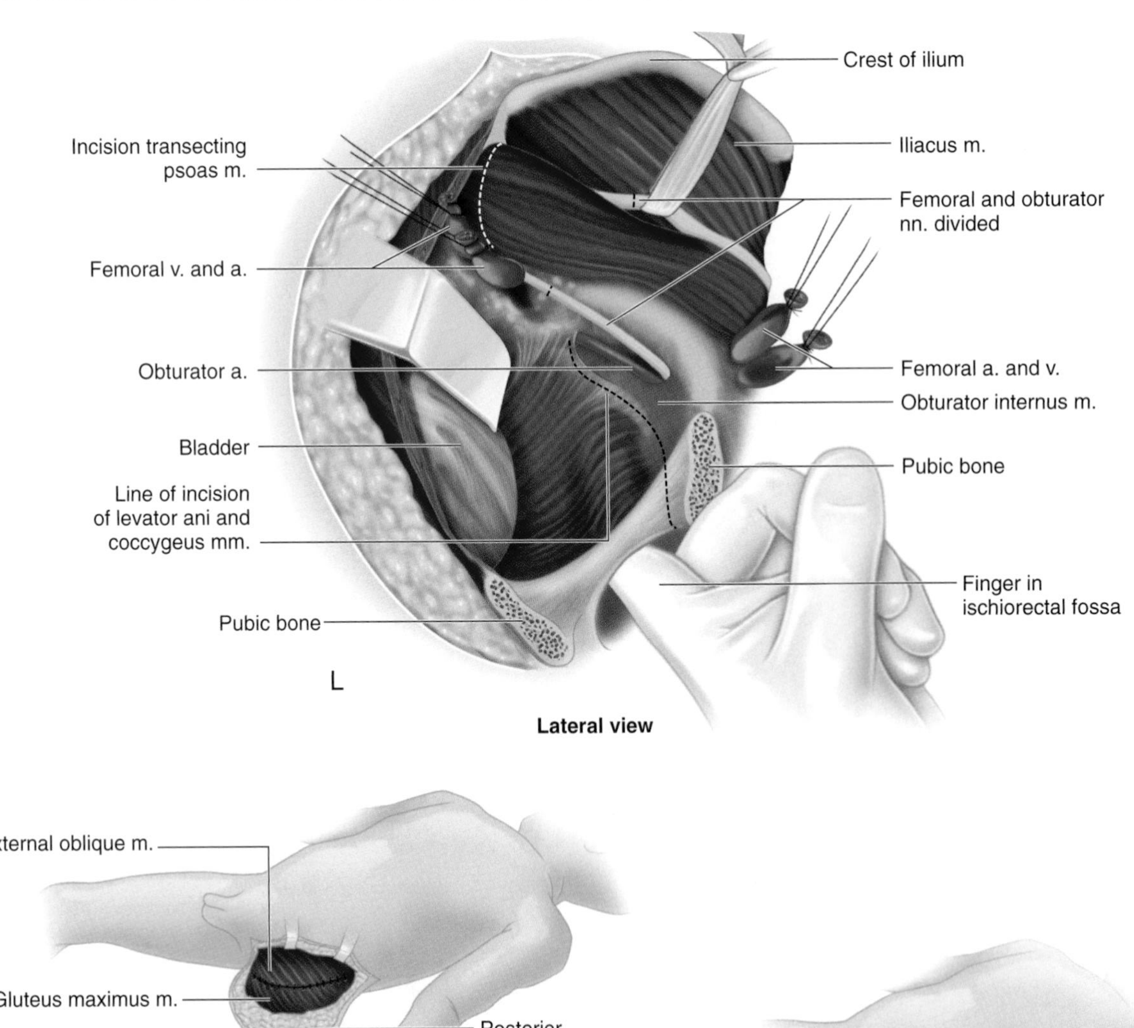

PLATE 39-2

Hip Disarticulation

A, An anterior racquet-type incision is made starting at the anterior superior iliac spine and extending medially and distally, parallel to Poupart's ligament, to the middle of the inner aspect of the thigh about 2 inches distal to the origin of the adductor muscles; it is then continued around the back of the thigh at a level about 2 inches distal to the ischial tuberosity. Next, the incision is carried along the lateral aspect of the thigh about 3 inches distal to the base of the greater trochanter and is curved proximally and medially to join the first incision at the anterior superior iliac spine.

B, The subcutaneous tissue and fascia are divided in line with the skin incision. The long saphenous vein is exposed and ligated, after the operator traces it to its junction with the femoral vein. If lymph node dissection is indicated, it can be performed at this stage. The sartorius muscle is divided at its origin from the anterior superior iliac spine and reflected distally. The origins of the two heads of the rectus femoris—one from the anterior inferior iliac spine and the other from the superior margin of the acetabulum—are detached and reflected distally. The femoral nerve is isolated, ligated with 0-0 silk sutures, and divided on a tongue blade with a sharp scalpel or razor blade just distal to the ligature. The femoral artery and vein are isolated, doubly ligated with 0-0 silk sutures proximally and distally, and severed in between the sutures.

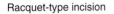

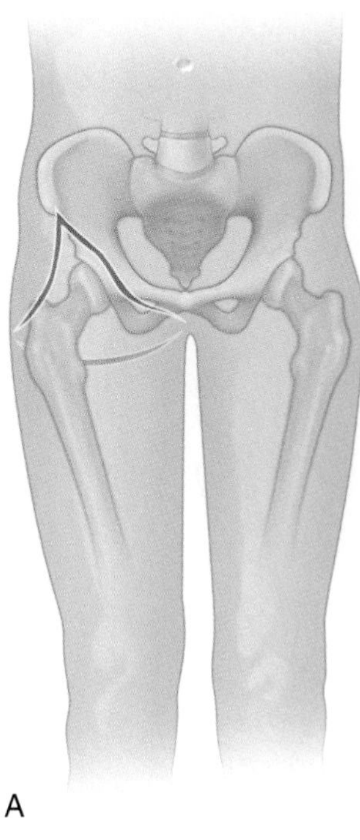

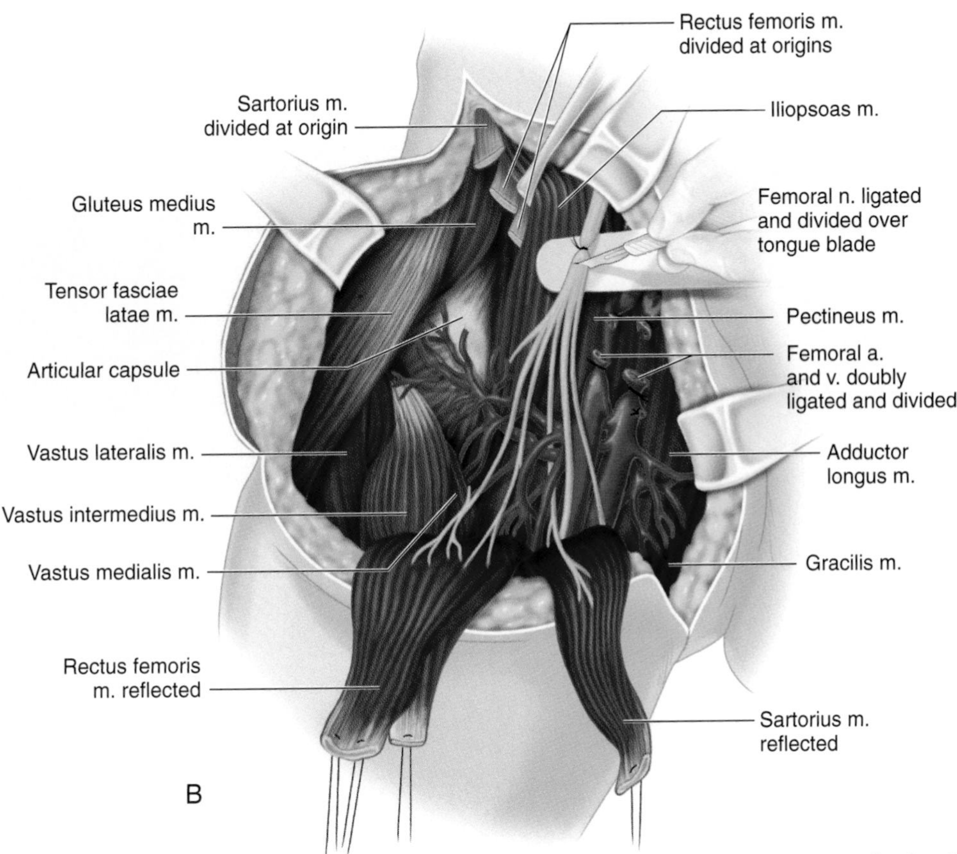

Continued

PLATE 39-2 *(continued)*

Hip Disarticulation

C, The hip is abducted to expose its medial aspect, and the adductor longus is detached at its origin from the pubis and reflected distally. The anterior branch of the obturator nerve is exposed deep to the adductor longus and traced proximally.

D, The adductor brevis is retracted posteriorly. The posterior branch of the obturator nerve is isolated and dissected proximal to the main trunk of the obturator nerve, which is sharply divided. Next, the obturator vessels are isolated and ligated. One should be careful not to sever the obturator artery inadvertently, because it will retract into the pelvis and cause bleeding that is difficult to control.

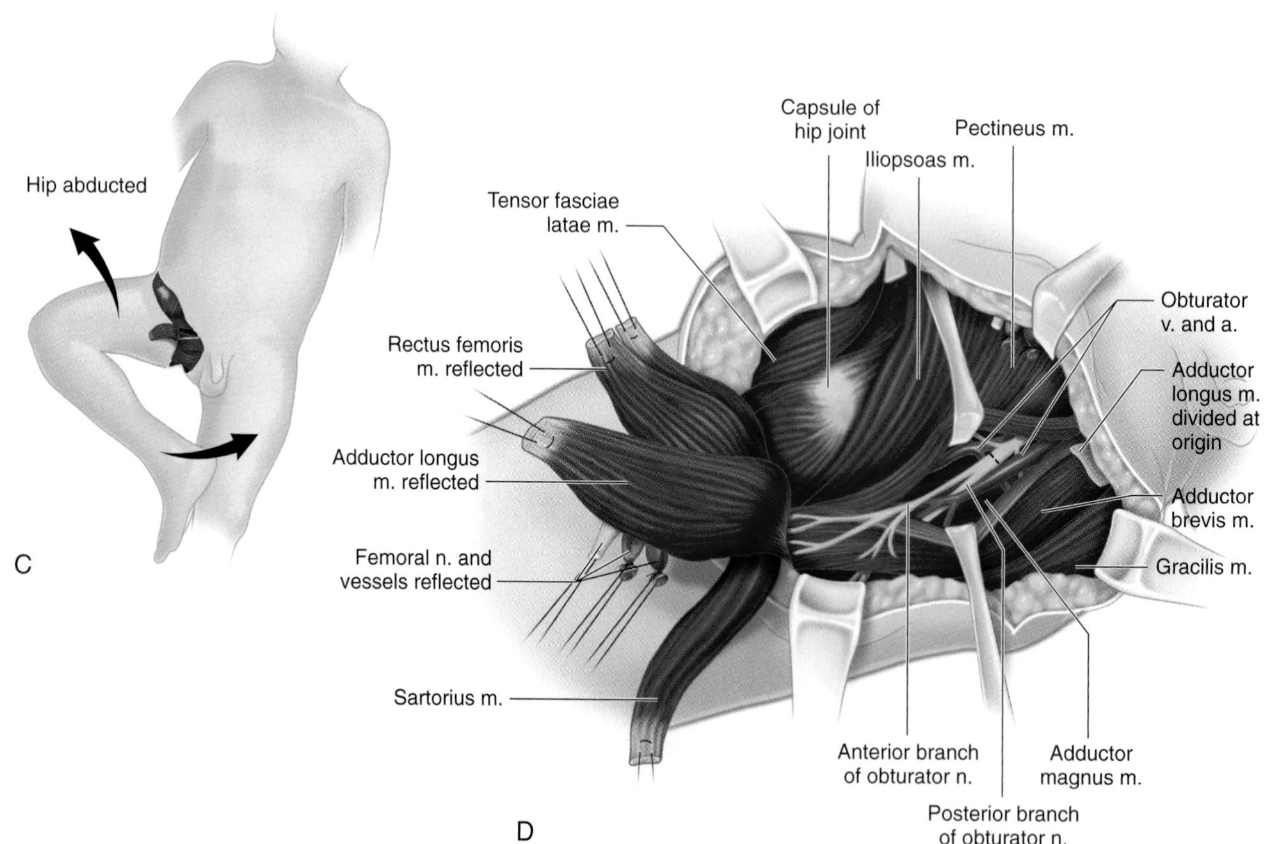

PLATE 39-2 *(continued)*

Hip Disarticulation

E, The pectineus, adductor brevis, gracilis, and adductor magnus are severed near their origins. It is best to use a coagulation knife.

F, The hip is then flexed, externally rotated, and abducted, bringing into view the lesser trochanter. The iliopsoas tendon is exposed, isolated, and divided at its insertion and reflected proximally.

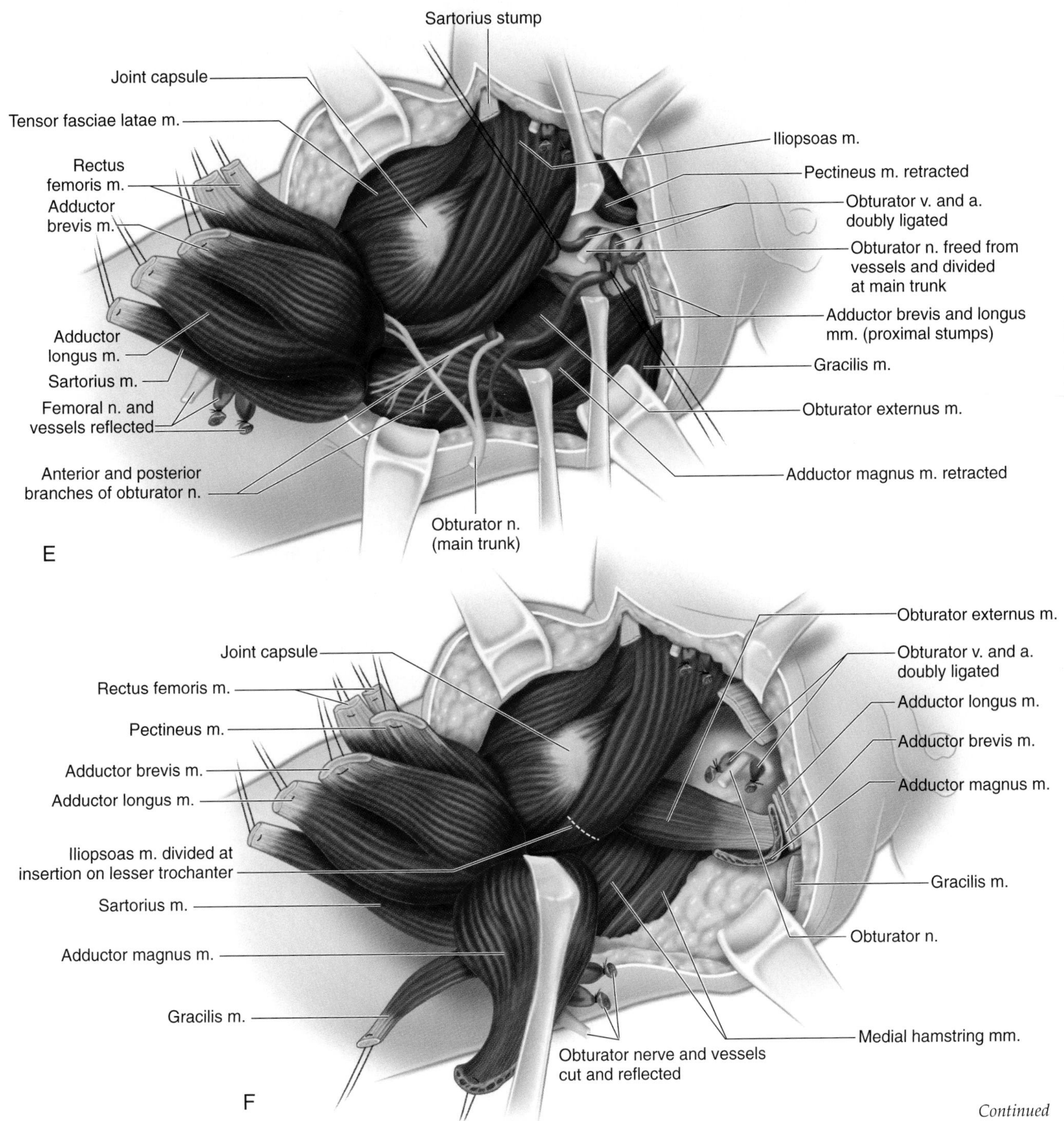

Continued

PLATE 39-2 *(continued)*

Hip Disarticulation

G, To facilitate surgical exposure, a sterile sandbag is placed under the pelvis, and the patient is turned onto the side away from the site of operation. The hip is internally rotated.

H, The gluteus medius and gluteus minimus muscles are divided at their insertion into the greater trochanter and, together with the tensor fasciae latae muscle, reflected proximally. The gluteus maximus muscle is detached at its insertion and retracted upward. The free ends of the gluteus maximus, medius, and minimus muscles and the tensor fasciae latae muscle are marked with 0 silk suture for reattachment.

I, The muscles to be detached at their insertion through the posterior incision are shown. The short rotators of the hip—that is, the quadratus femoris, obturator externus, gemellus, and obturator internus—are detached from their insertion into the femur.

J, The sciatic nerve is identified, dissected free, pulled distally, and crushed with a Kocher hemostat at a level 2 inches proximal to the ischial tuberosity and then ligated with 0-0 silk suture to prevent hemorrhage from its accompanying vessels. Next, it is sharply divided just distal to the ligature.

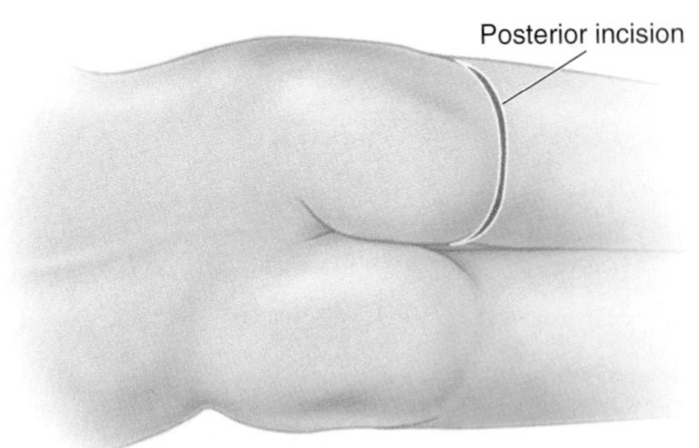

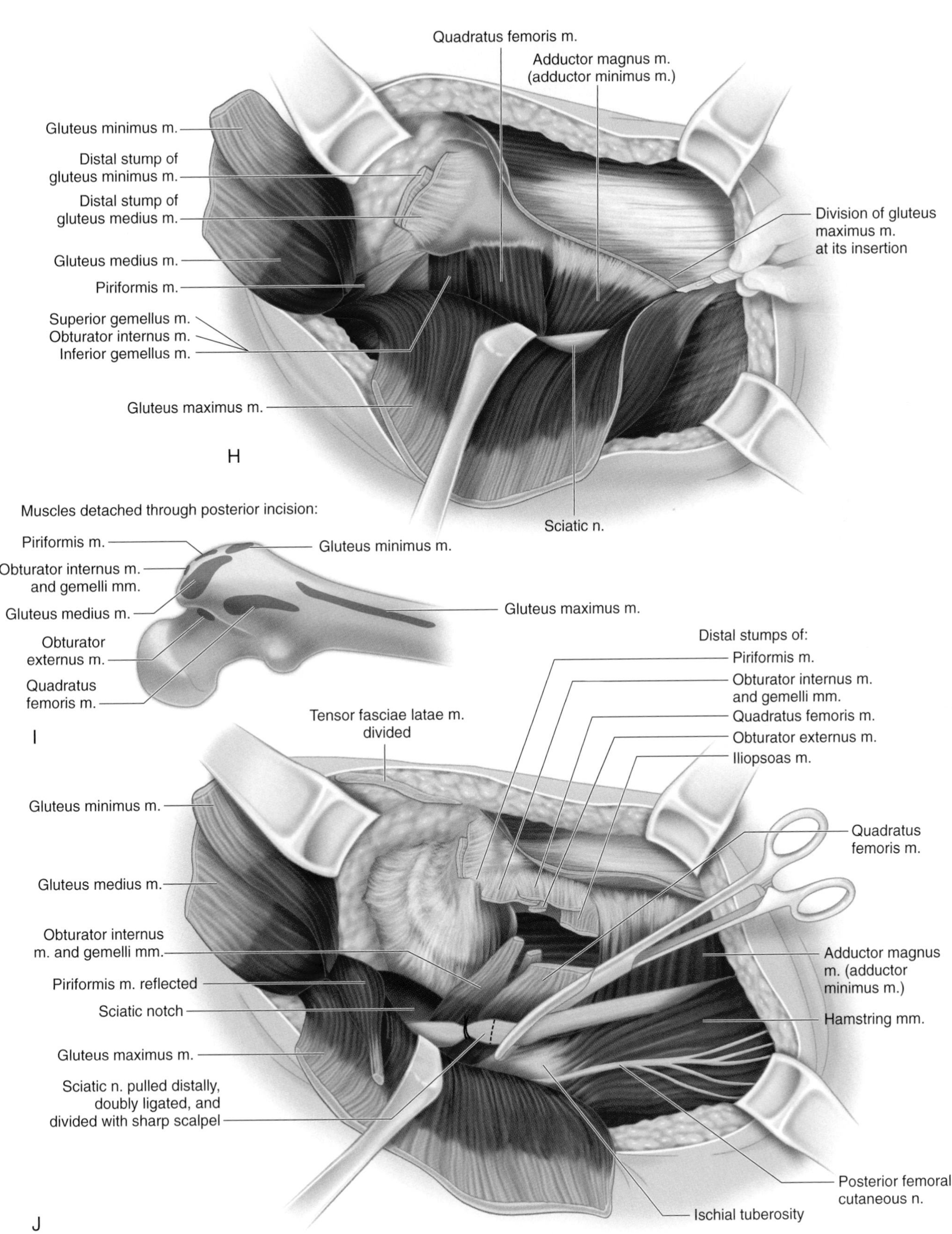

PLATE 39-2 Hip Disarticulation *(continued)*

Continued

PLATE 39-2 *(continued)*

Hip Disarticulation

K, The hamstring muscles are detached at their origin from the ischial tuberosity. The capsule of the hip joint is divided near the acetabulum, and the ligamentum teres is severed, completing the disarticulation.

L and **M,** The gluteal flap is mobilized and brought forward, and the free distal ends are sutured to the pubis at the origin of the adductor and pectineus muscles.

N, The wound is closed in routine fashion. A closed-suction drain (Hemovac) is placed in the inferior portion of the wound. It is removed in 1 to 2 days.

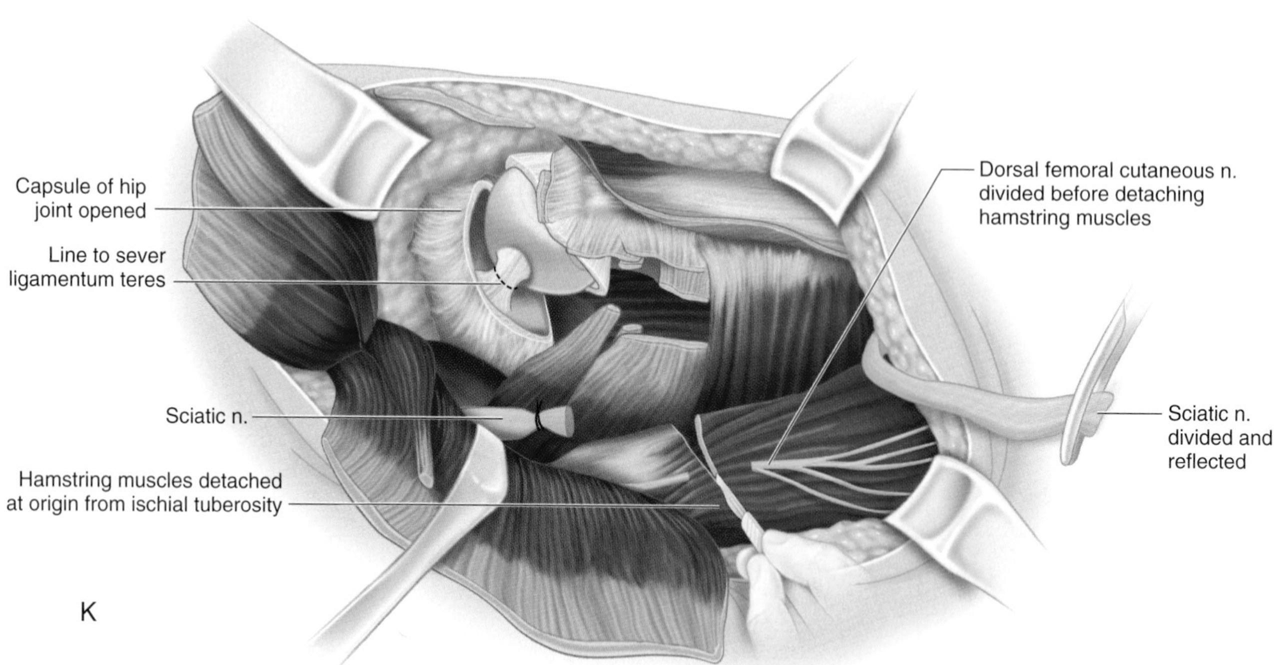

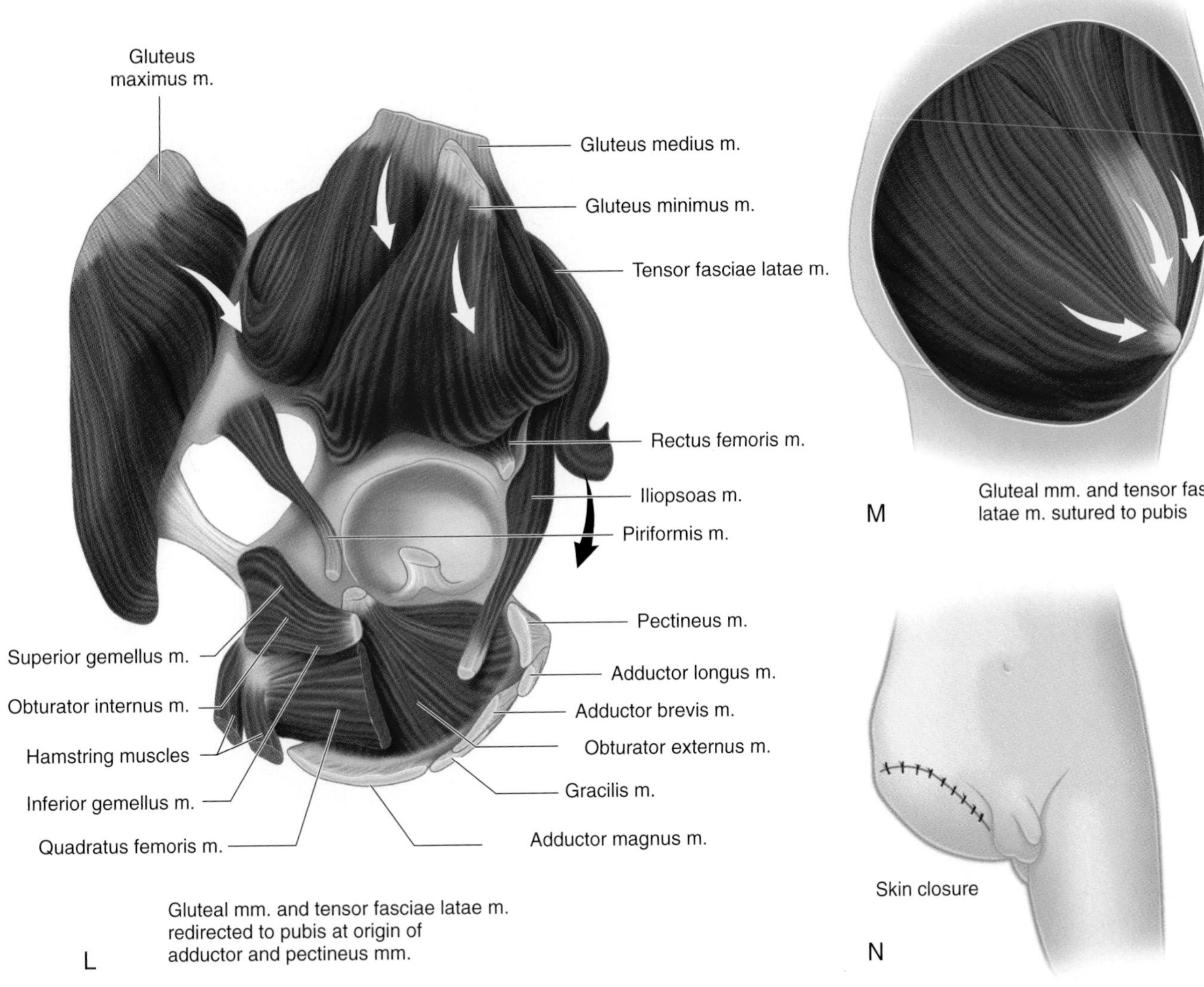
Gluteus maximus m.
Gluteus medius m.
Gluteus minimus m.
Tensor fasciae latae m.
Rectus femoris m.
Iliopsoas m.
Piriformis m.
Pectineus m.
Adductor longus m.
Adductor brevis m.
Obturator externus m.
Gracilis m.
Adductor magnus m.
Superior gemellus m.
Obturator internus m.
Hamstring muscles
Inferior gemellus m.
Quadratus femoris m.
Gluteal mm. and tensor fasciae latae m. redirected to pubis at origin of adductor and pectineus mm.
L
M
Gluteal mm. and tensor fasciae latae m. sutured to pubis
Skin closure
N

PLATE 39-2 Hip Disarticulation *(continued)*

PLATE 39-3

Ischial-Bearing Above-Knee Amputation (Midthigh Amputation)

The level of amputation is determined by measurements made with a Bell Thompson ruler on the preoperative radiographs. Measurements are made from the top of the greater trochanter and from the knee joint line. If the level of amputation permits, a pneumatic tourniquet is employed for hemostasis. A sandbag is placed under the ipsilateral buttock.

The following areas are marked with methylene blue: (1) the intended bone level of amputation, (2) the midpoints of the medial and lateral aspects of the thigh 1 cm above the bony level, and (3) the distal border of the anterior and posterior incisions. The last is determined by a rule of thumb: the combined length of the anterior and posterior flaps is slightly longer than the diameter of the thigh at the intended bone level, and the length of the anterior flap is 2 times the diameter of the posterior flap.

A through **C,** The skin incision begins at the midpoint of the medial aspect of the thigh, gently curves anteriorly and inferiorly to the distal border of the anterior incision, and passes convexly to the midpoint on the lateral aspect of the thigh. The posterior incision starts at the same medial point, extends to the distal margin of the posterior flap, and swings proximally to end at the midpoint on the lateral thigh.

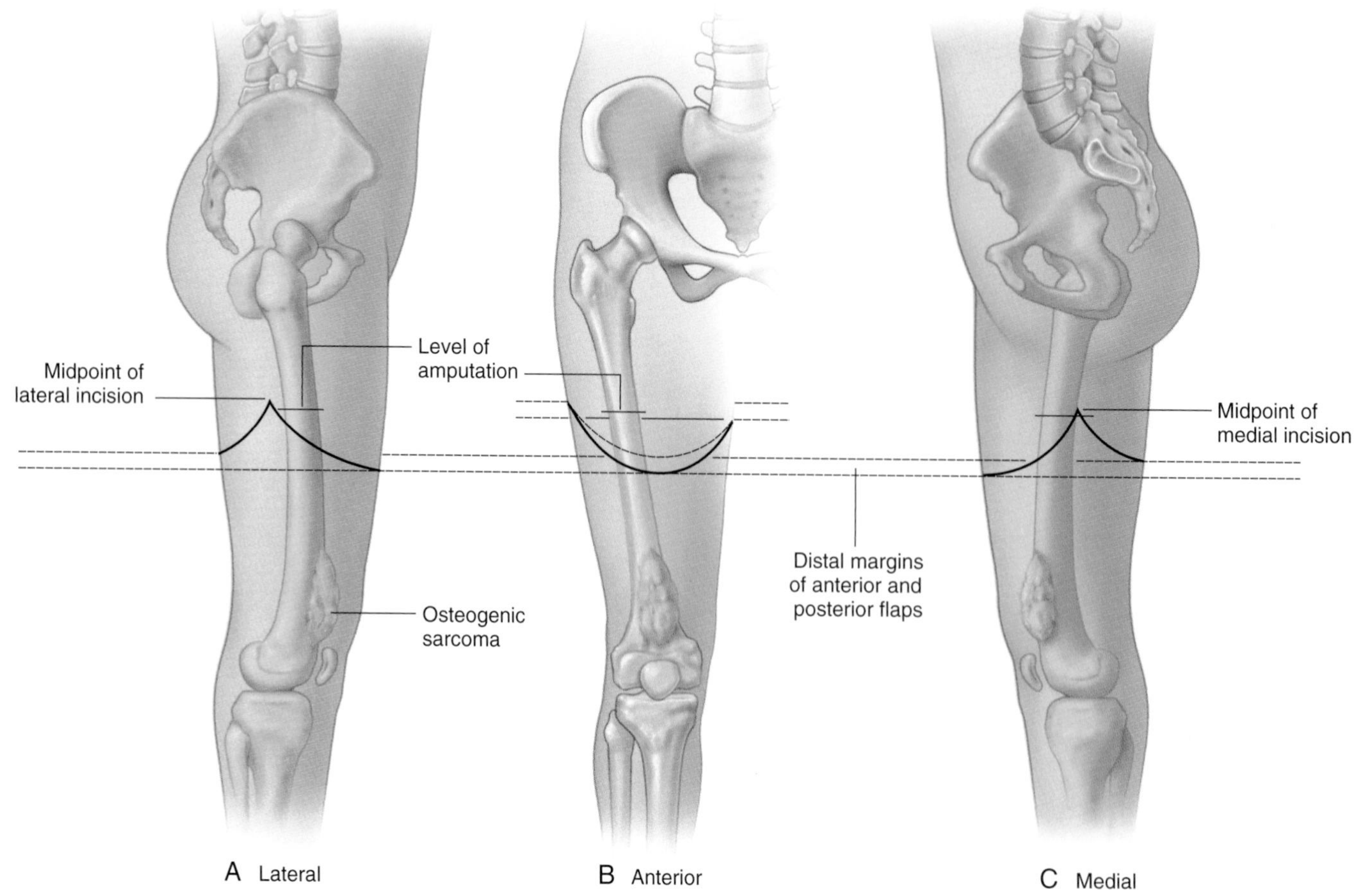

PLATE 39–3 *(continued)*

Ischial-Bearing Above-Knee Amputation (Midthigh Amputation)

D, The subcutaneous tissue and deep fascia are divided in line with the skin incision, and the anterior and posterior flaps are reflected proximally to the amputation level.

E through **G,** The femoral vessels and saphenous nerve are identified. They are located deep to the sartorius muscle, between the adductor longus and the vastus medialis muscles. The deep femoral vessels are found adjacent to the femur in the interval between the adductor magnus, adductor longus, and vastus medialis muscles. There are variations in the origin of the deep femoral artery, as shown in **G.** The femoral artery and vein are isolated, doubly ligated with heavy silk sutures, and divided. The saphenous nerve is pulled distally and divided with a sharp scalpel. If the amputation level is high, the deep femoral vessels may be ligated and divided through this anteromedial approach.

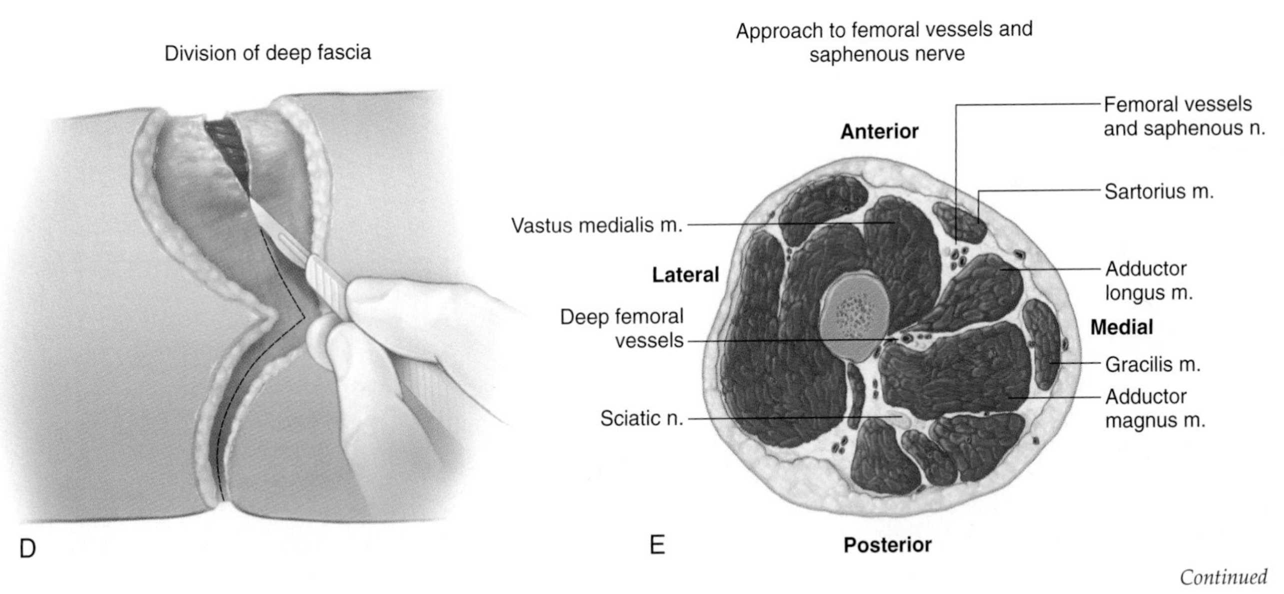

Continued

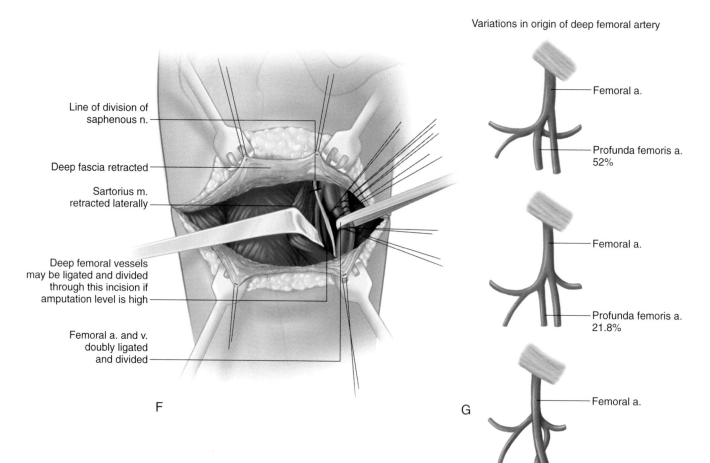

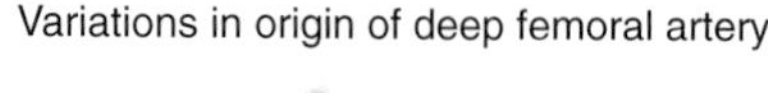

PLATE 39–3 *(continued)*

Ischial-Bearing Above-Knee Amputation (Midthigh Amputation)

H and **I,** The hip is acutely flexed to approach the posterior structures. The sciatic nerve is exposed in the interval between the medial hamstrings medially and the long head of the biceps femoris laterally. The nerve is gently pulled distally, infiltrated with bupivacaine, ligated, and sharply divided over a tongue blade.

J and **K,** Illustrated is the posterior approach to the deep femoral vessels when the level of amputation is distal.

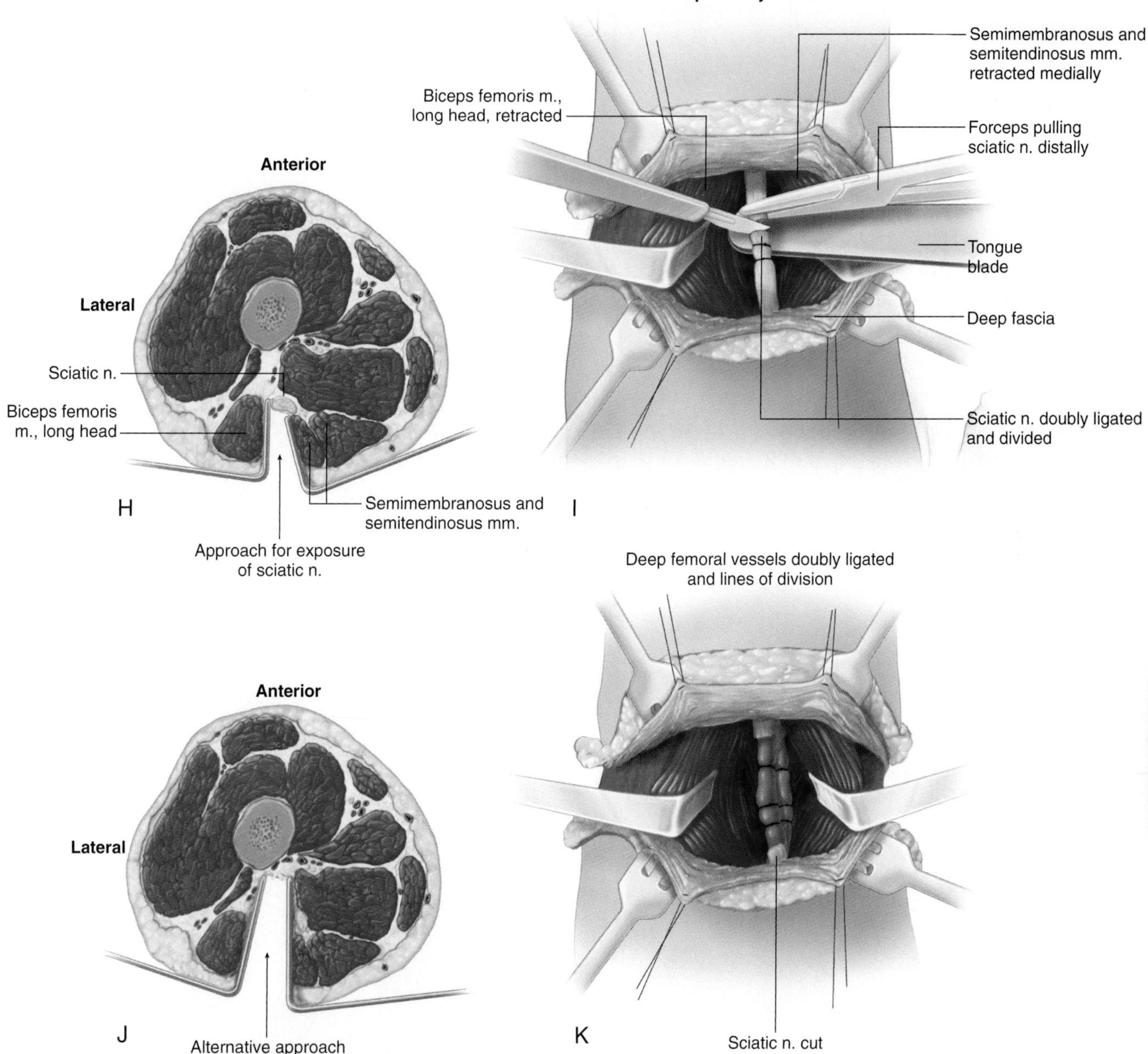

PLATE 39-3 Ischial-Bearing Above-Knee Amputation (Midthigh Amputation) *(continued)*

Continued

PLATE 39–3 *(continued)*

Ischial-Bearing Above-Knee Amputation (Midthigh Amputation)

L, With an amputation knife, the quadriceps and adductor muscles are sectioned and beveled upward to the site of bone division so that the anterior myofascial flap is approximately 1.5 cm thick. The posterior muscles are divided transversely. Muscular branches of the femoral vessels are clamped and ligated as necessary.

M, The proximal muscles are retracted upward with an amputation shield, and the periosteum is incised circumferentially.

N, The femur is sectioned with a saw immediately distal to the periosteal incision.

O, With a rongeur, the prominence of the linea aspera is excised, and the bone end is smoothed with a file. The wound is irrigated with normal saline solution to wash away all loose fragments of bone.

P, Hot packs are applied over the wound, and the tourniquet is released. After 5 minutes, the stump is inspected for any bleeders.

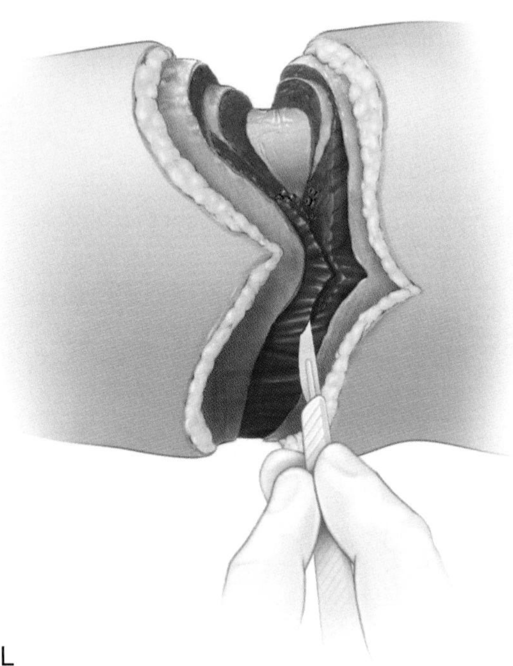

L

Division of muscles

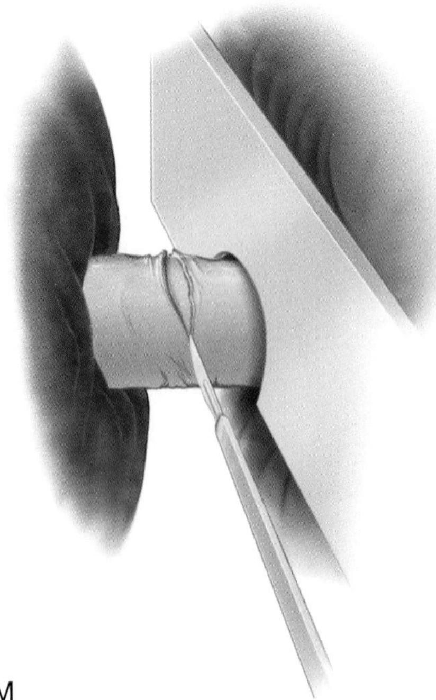

M

Circular incision of periosteum of femur

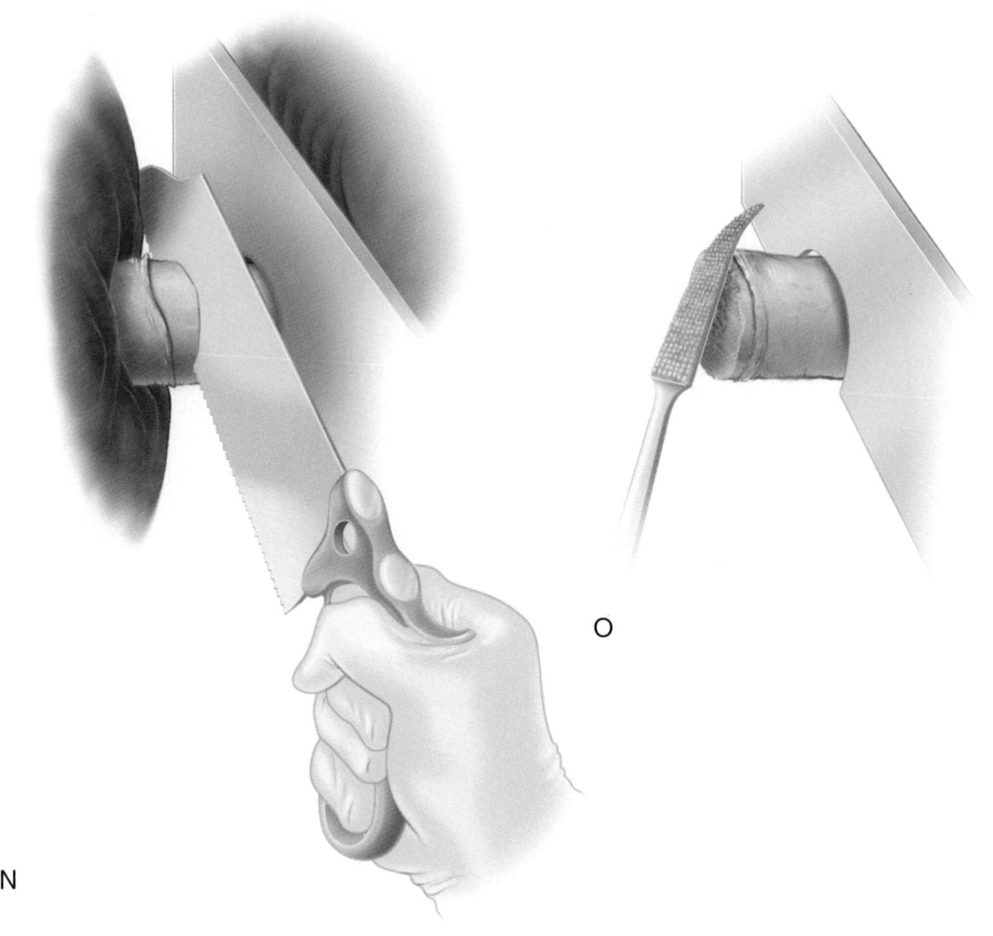

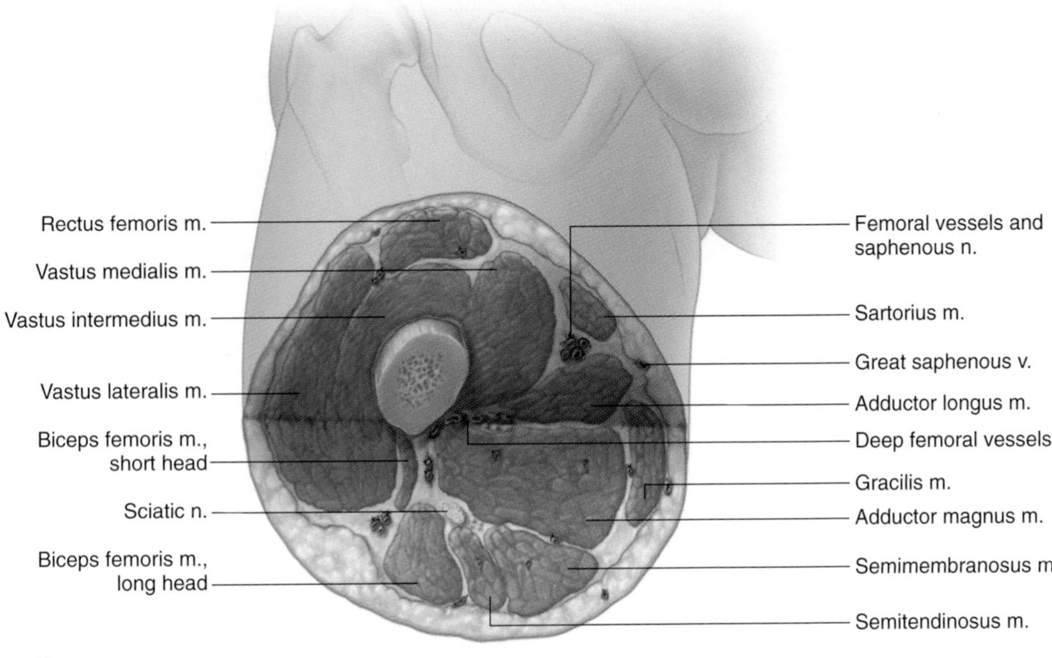

PLATE 39-3 Ischial-Bearing Above-Knee Amputation (Midthigh Amputation) *(continued)*

Continued

PLATE 39-3 *(continued)*

Ischial-Bearing Above-Knee Amputation (Midthigh Amputation)

Q, The anterior and posterior myofascial flaps are pulled distally and approximated with interrupted sutures through their fascial layer. Suction catheters are placed in the wound and connected to a closed-suction drainage evacuator.

R, The subcutaneous tissue and skin are closed in the usual manner. We perform immediate prosthetic fitting in the operating room. The patient is allowed to be ambulatory on the first postoperative day.

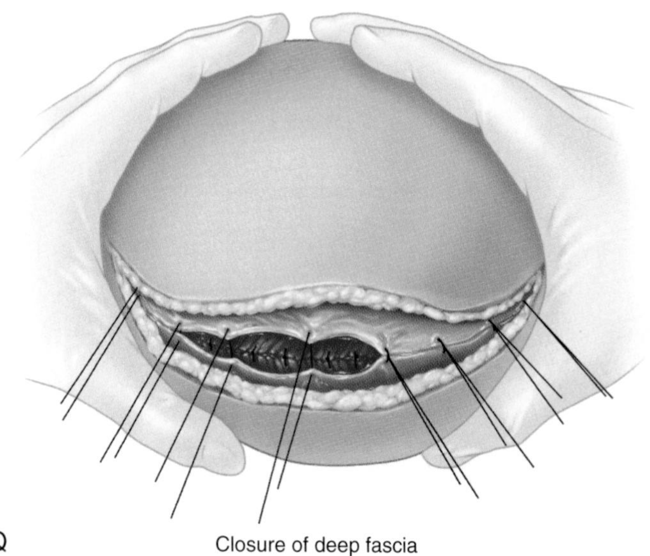

Q Closure of deep fascia

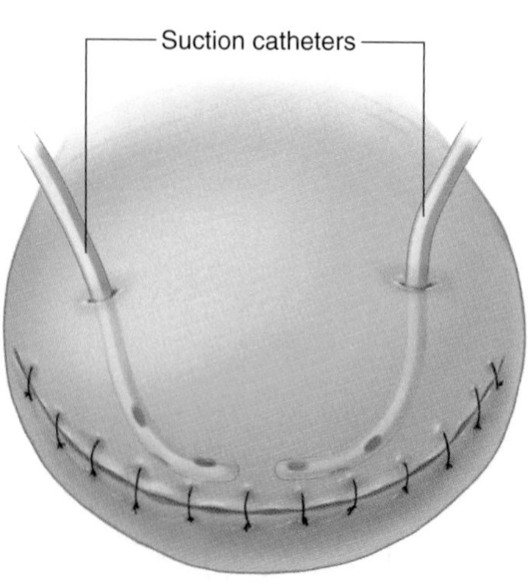

R Skin edges approximated and closed

PLATE 39-4

Disarticulation of the Knee Joint

The patient is placed in a lateral position so that he or she can easily be turned to a supine, prone, or semilateral position. The operation is performed using pneumatic tourniquet ischemia.

A, The skin incisions are placed in such a manner that a long anterior flap and a short posterior flap are provided; thus, the operative scar is posterior and away from the weight-bearing skin. Measuring from the distal pole of the patella to the distal border, the length of the anterior flap is equal to the anteroposterior diameter of the knee, whereas the posterior flap is half the length of the anterior flap. The medial and lateral proximal points of the incisions are at the joint line at the junction of the anterior two thirds and posterior one third of the diameter of the knee. The anterior and posterior wound flaps are raised, including the subcutaneous tissue and deep fascia.

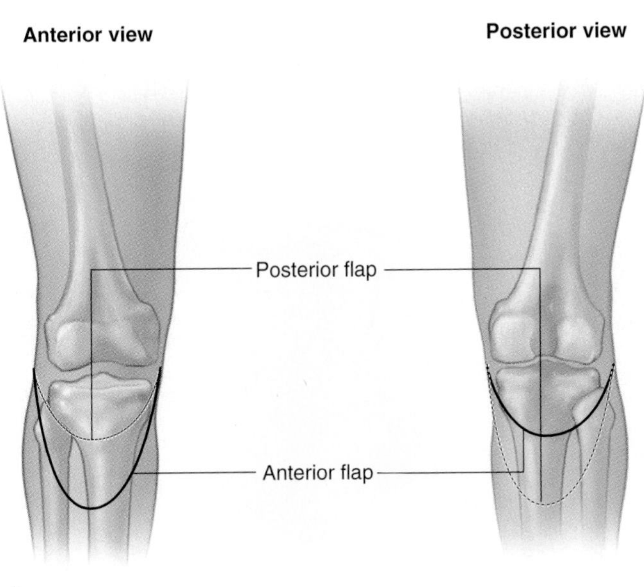

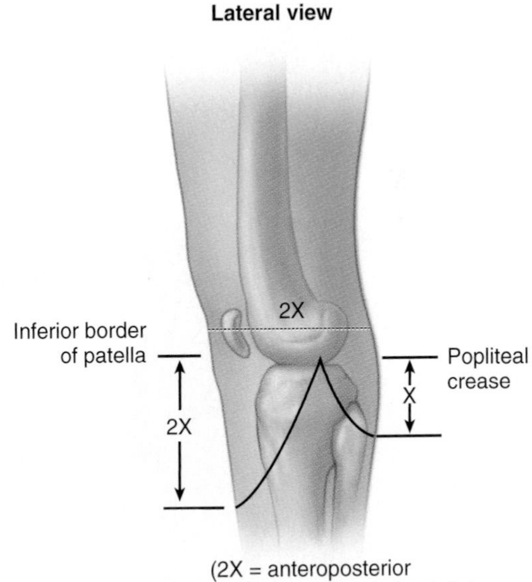

Continued

PLATE 39-4 *(continued)*

Disarticulation of the Knee Joint

B, The medial aspects of the knee joint and the proximal tibia are exposed. Tendons of the sartorius, gracilis, semimembranosus, and semitendinosus muscles are identified and marked with 0-0 silk whip sutures, then sectioned near their insertions on the tibia. The ligamentum patellae is detached at the proximal tibial tubercle. The anterior and medial joint capsule and synovial membrane are divided proximally near the femoral condyles.

C, The lateral aspect of the knee joint is exposed. The iliotibial tract is divided, and the biceps femoris tendon is sectioned from its attachment to the head of the fibula. The lateral part of the joint capsule and synovial membrane is divided above the joint line.

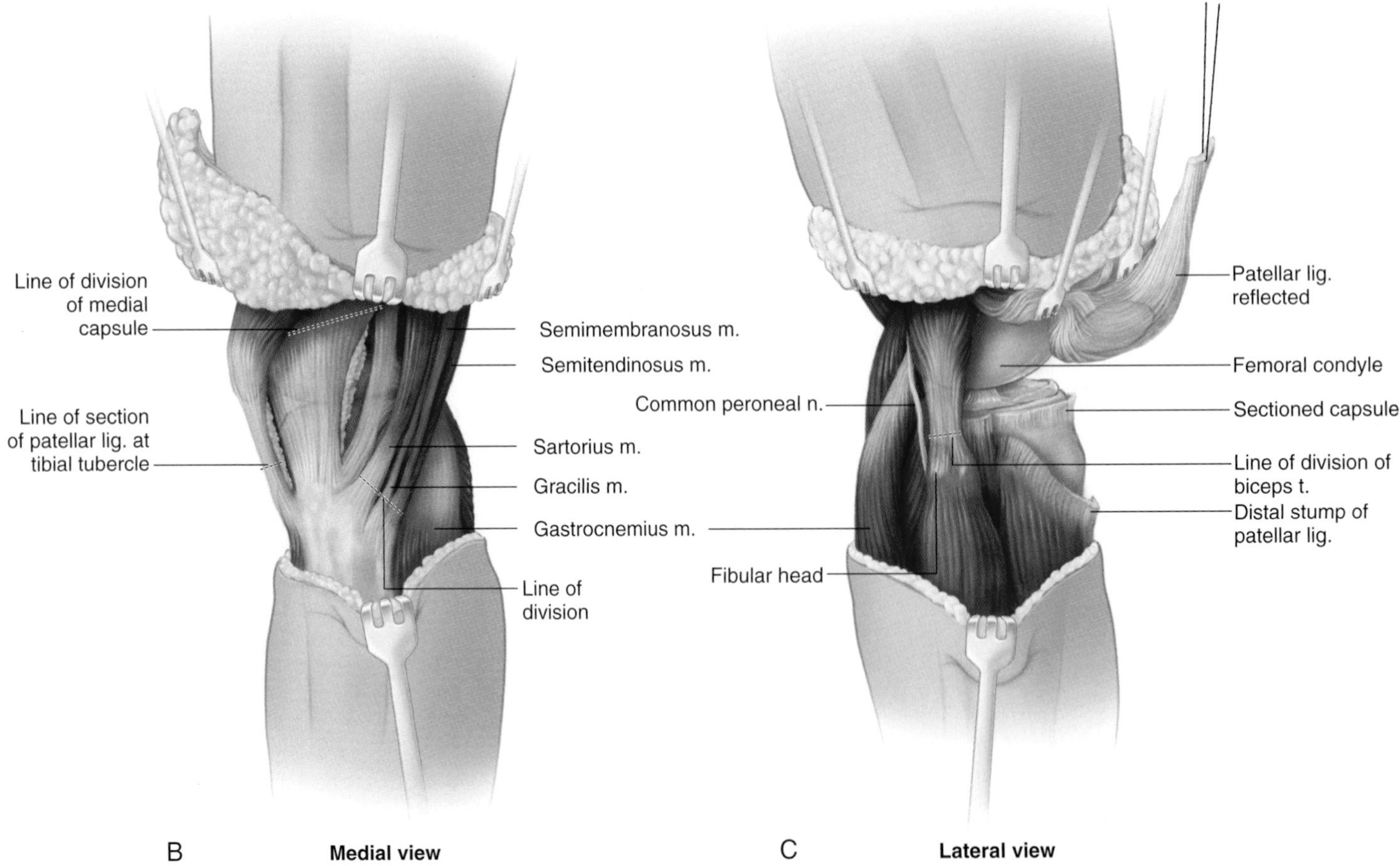

PLATE 39-4 *(continued)*

Disarticulation of the Knee Joint

D, Now the patient is turned to the semiprone position, and the popliteal fossa is exposed. By blunt dissection, the popliteal vessels are identified; the popliteal artery and vein are separately doubly ligated distal to the origin of the superior genicular branches and divided. The tibial nerve and common peroneal nerve are pulled distally, sharply divided with a scalpel, and allowed to retract proximally. The medial and lateral heads of the gastrocnemius are extraperiosteally elevated and stripped from the posterior aspect of the femoral condyles. The distal femoral epiphyseal plate should not be damaged. The plantaris and popliteus muscles, the oblique popliteal ligament, the posterior part of the capsule of the knee joint, and the meniscofemoral ligaments are completely divided.
E, The patient is placed in a semisupine position, and the knee is acutely flexed. The cruciate ligaments are identified and sectioned, completing the amputation. The pneumatic tourniquet is released, and complete hemostasis is secured.

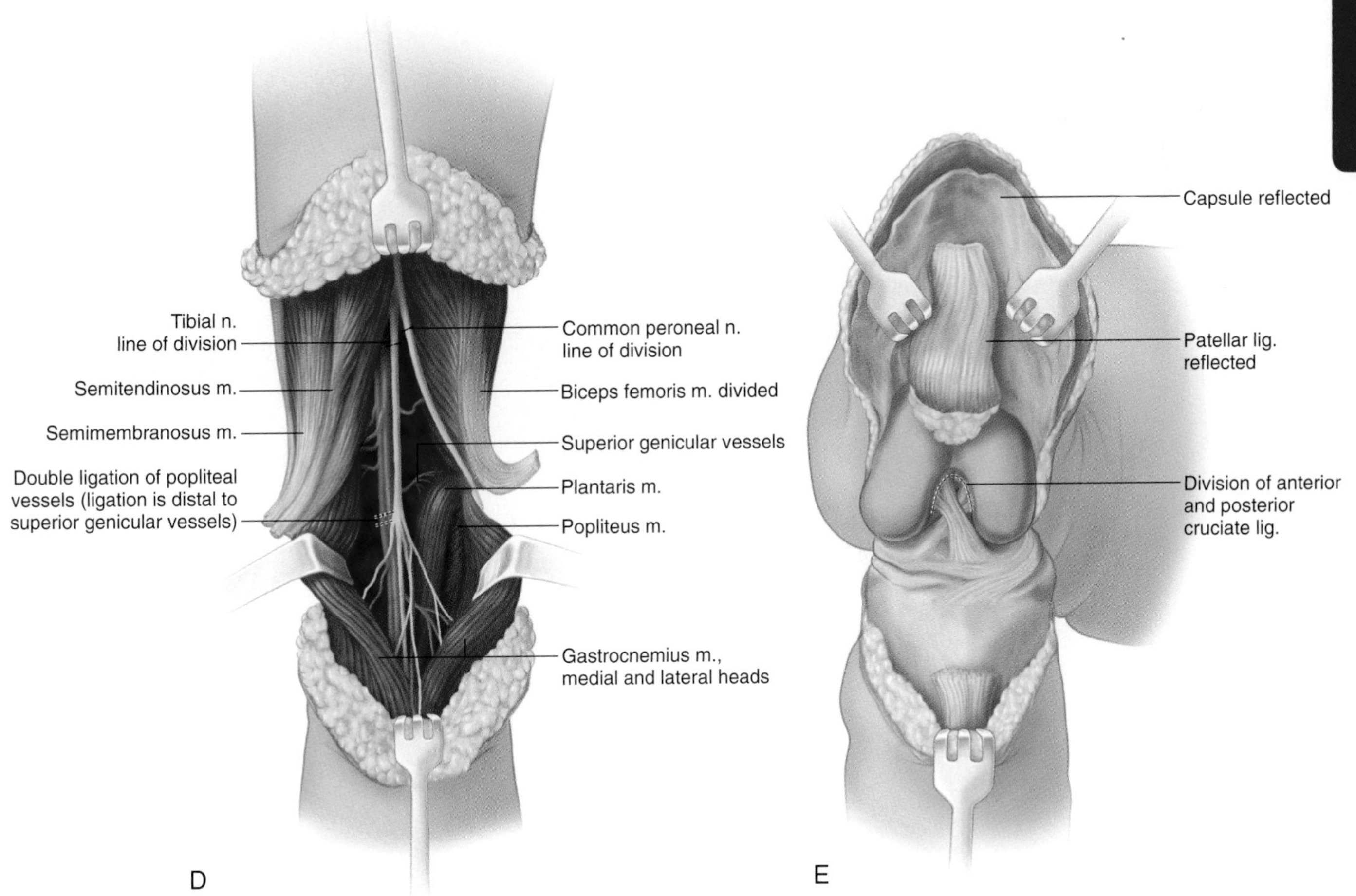

Continued

PLATE 39-4 *(continued)*

Disarticulation of the Knee Joint

F, The patellar ligament is sutured to the medial and lateral hamstrings in the intercondylar notch. In children, the patella usually is not removed, and reshaping of the femoral condyles should not be performed because of the danger of damaging the growth plate. Synovectomy is not indicated.

G, Two catheters are placed in the wound for closed suction. The deep fascia and subcutaneous tissue of the anterior and posterior flaps are approximated with interrupted sutures, and the skin is closed in routine fashion.

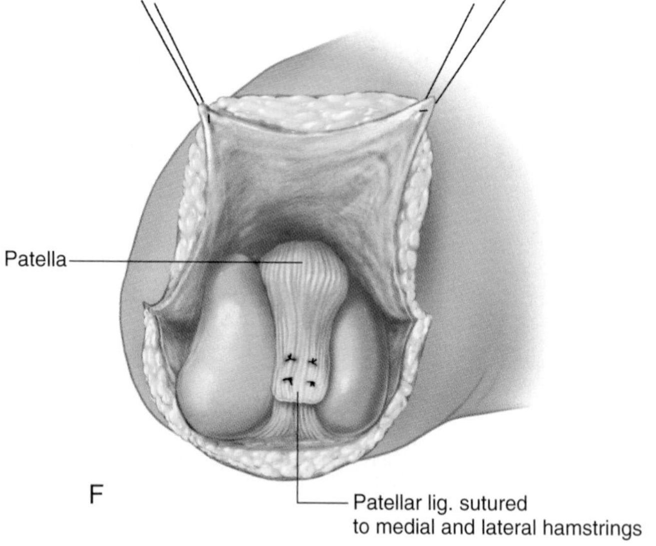

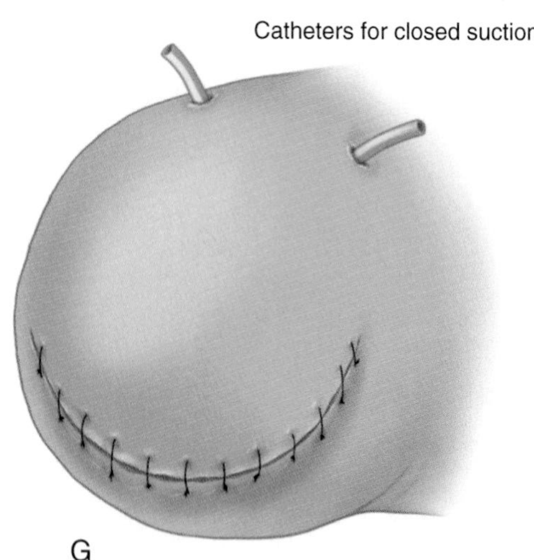

PLATE 39-5

Below-Knee Amputation

The level of amputation is determined preoperatively. With the patient supine, a pneumatic tourniquet is applied on the proximal thigh.

A and **B,** The line of incision for the anterior and posterior flaps is marked on the skin, and the anteroposterior diameter of the leg at the level of bone section is measured. The anterior flap can be fashioned slightly longer than the posterior flap, or they may be of equal length, because the position of the scar is not important in terms of prosthetic fitting. The length of each flap is half the anteroposterior diameter of the leg.

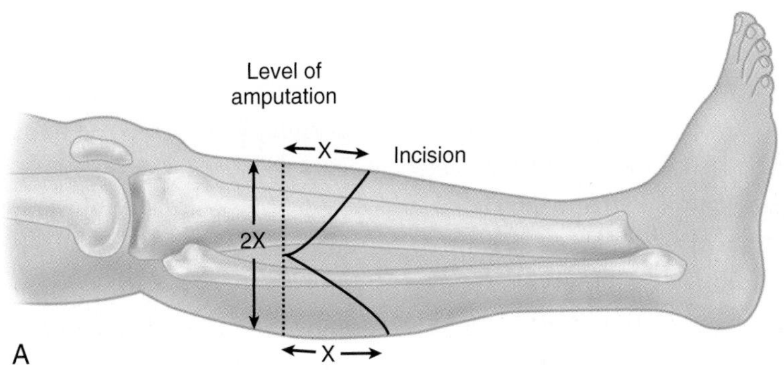

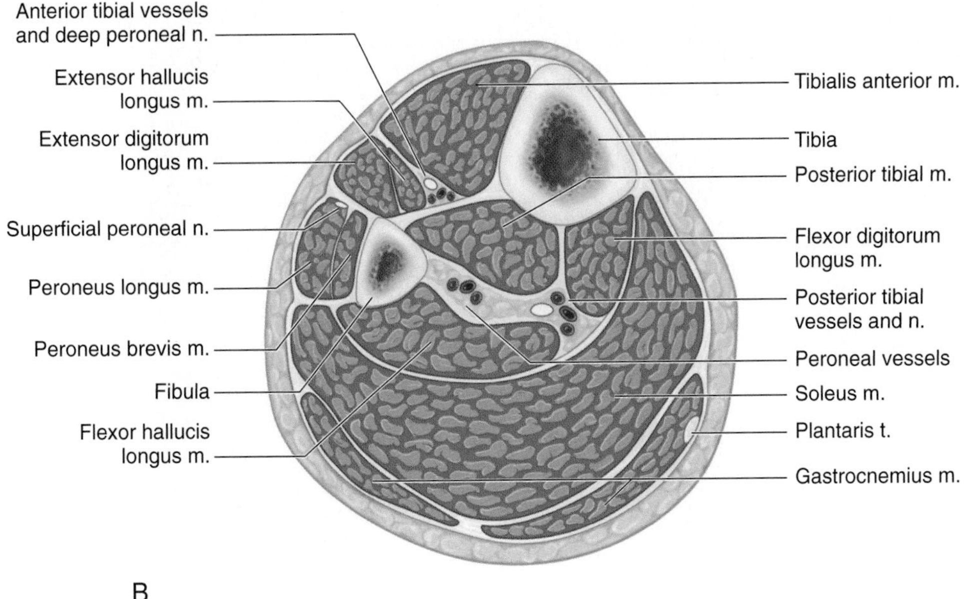

Continued

PLATE 39-5 *(continued)*

Below-Knee Amputation

C and **D,** The incisions are deepened to the deep fascia, which is divided in line with the skin incision. The anterior and posterior flaps are raised proximally in one layer, including skin, subcutaneous tissue, and deep fascia. Over the anteromedial surface of the tibia, the periosteum is incised with the deep fascia, and both are elevated as a continuous layer to the intended level of amputation.

In the interval between the extensor digitorum longus and peroneus brevis muscles, the superficial peroneal nerve is identified; the nerve is pulled distally, sharply divided, and allowed to retract proximally well above the end of the stump.

The anterior tibial vessels and deep peroneal nerve are identified, doubly ligated, and divided.

E and **F,** The muscles in the anterior tibial compartment are sectioned about 0.75 cm distal to the level of bone section. The tibial crest is beveled as follows: beginning 2 cm proximal to the level of amputation, a 45-degree distal oblique cut is made, ending 0.5 cm anterior to the medullary cavity.

G, The tibia is transversely sectioned. The angle of division should be at a right angle to the axis of the bone.

H, The fibula is cleared of surrounding muscle and, using a Gigli saw, sectioned 2 to 3 cm proximal to the distal end of the tibia. The bone ends are smoothed and rounded with a rasp. All periosteal fringes are excised, and the wound is irrigated with normal saline solution to remove bone dust.

Next, the posterior muscles in the leg are sectioned. The posterior tibial and peroneal vessels are carefully identified, doubly ligated, and divided. The tibial nerve is pulled distally and divided with a sharp knife. A fascial flap is developed from the gastrocnemius aponeurosis so that it can be brought forward to cover the end of the stump.

I and **J,** The tourniquet is released following application of hot laparotomy pads and pressure over the cut surfaces of the muscles and bones. After 5 minutes, the pads are removed, and complete hemostasis is secured. The wound should be completely dry. The fascia of the gastrocnemius muscle is brought anteriorly and sutured to the fascia of the anterior compartment muscles. The muscles may be partially excised if they are bulky at the side of the stump. Suction drainage catheters are placed deep to the gastrocnemius fascia. The subcutaneous tissue and skin are closed with interrupted sutures. A nonadherent dressing and a plaster-of-Paris cylinder are applied for immediate prosthetic fitting.

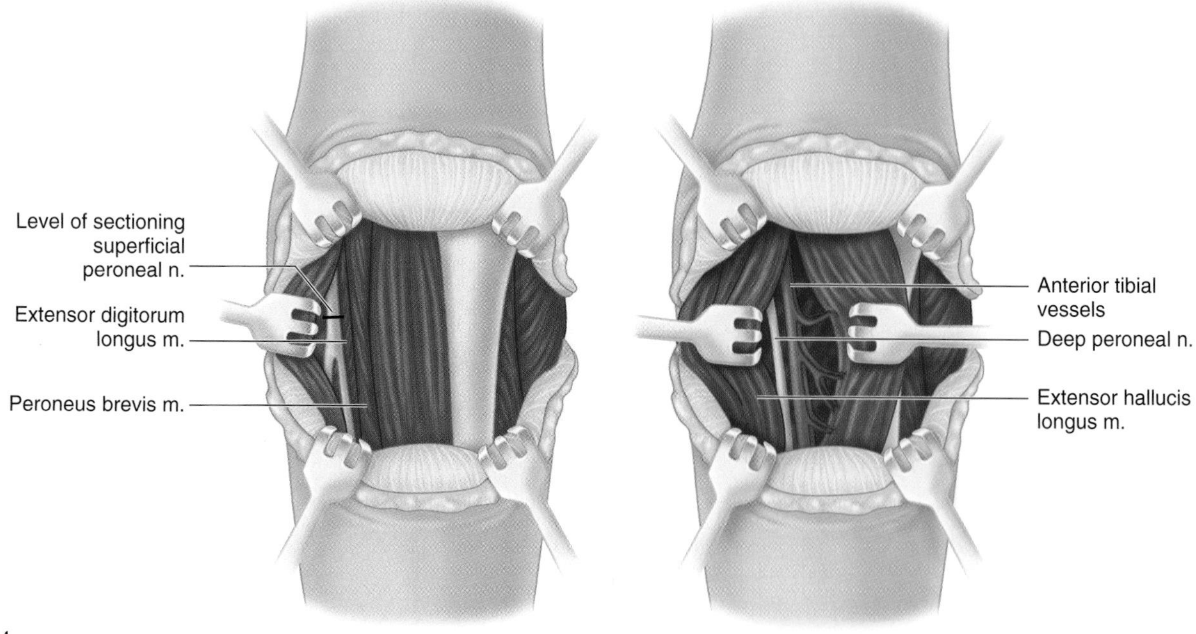

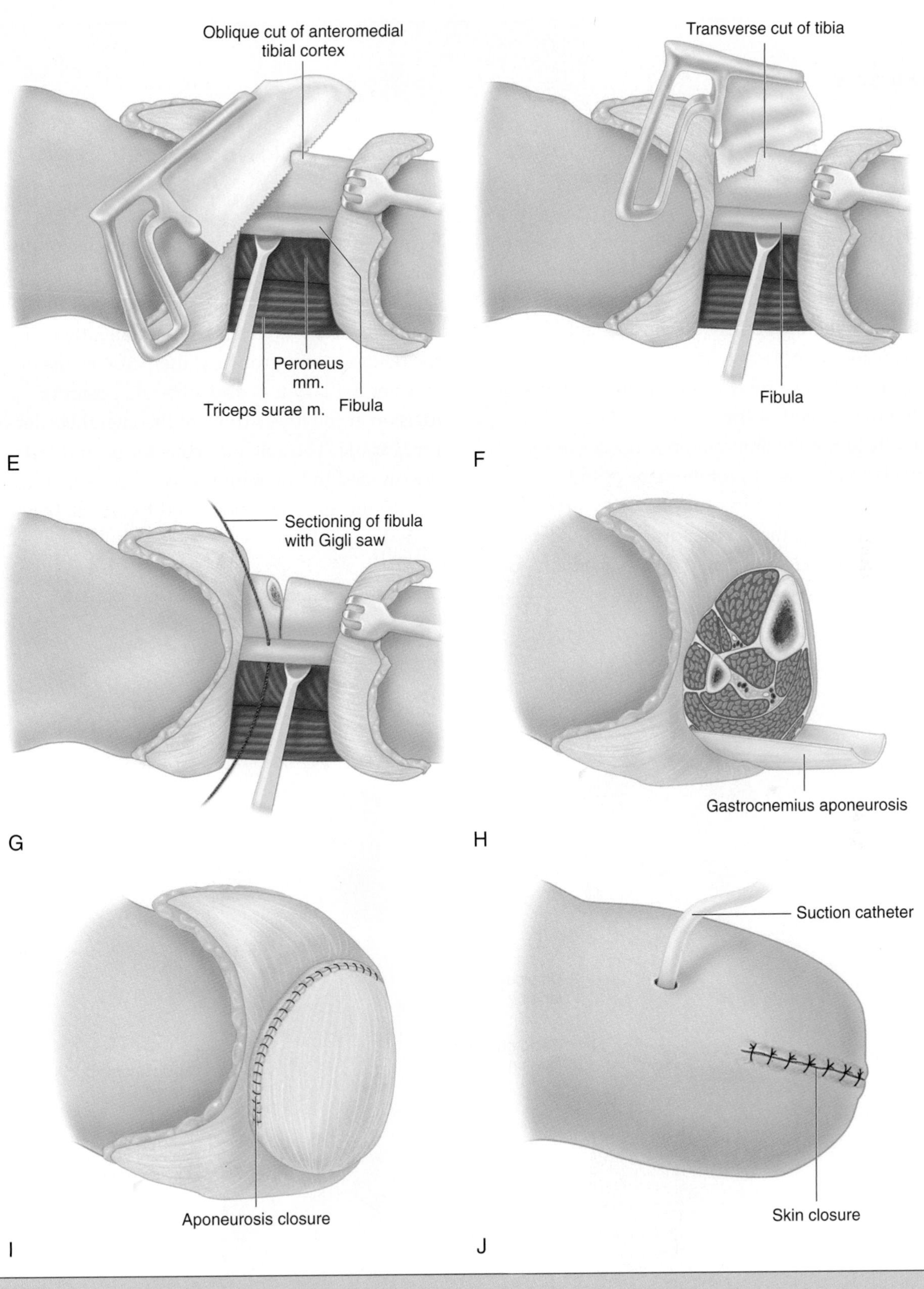

PLATE 39-5 Below-Knee Amputation *(continued)*

PLATE 39-6

Posterior Approach for Forequarter Amputation (Littlewood Technique)

The patient is placed in the lateral position, and the neck, chest, and whole upper limb are prepared and draped. Blood loss is minimal, but adequate whole blood should be available for transfusion if necessary.

A through **C,** The cervicothoracic incision begins at the medial end of the clavicle and extends laterally along the anteroinferior border of the clavicle to the lateral protuberance of the acromion, where it curves posteriorly; then it is continued along the lateral border of the scapula to its inferior angle, where it curves medially to terminate 3 to 4 cm lateral to the midline of the spine.

The pectoroaxillary incision begins at the center of the clavicle and extends inferolaterally along the deltopectoral groove; it then crosses the anterior axillary fold and joins the posterior incision at the lower third of the lateral border of the scapula. The subcutaneous tissue and fascia are divided in line with the skin incision, and the wound flaps are mobilized to expose the underlying muscles.

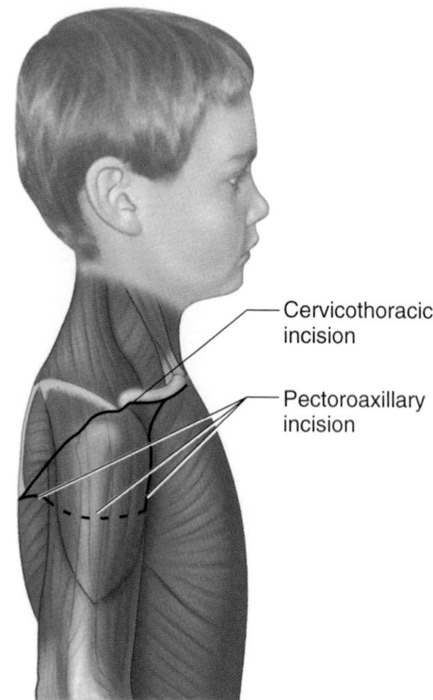

A

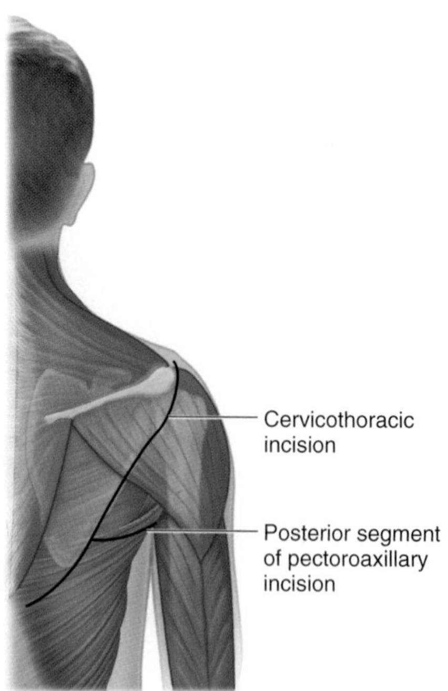

B

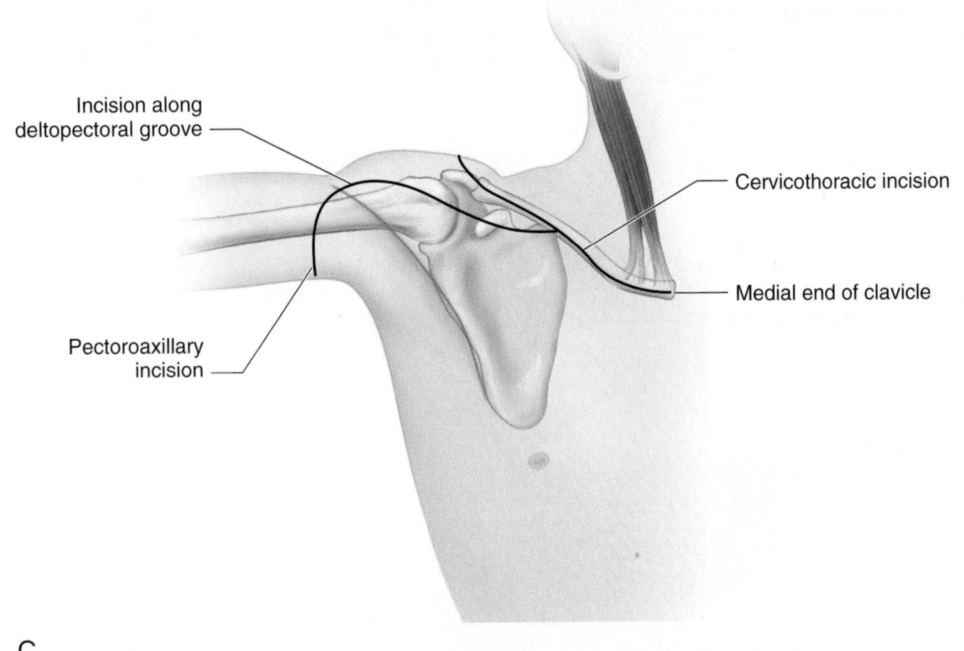

PLATE 39-6 Posterior Approach for Forequarter Amputation (Littlewood Technique) *(continued)*

Continued

PLATE 39-6 *(continued)*

Posterior Approach for Forequarter Amputation (Littlewood Technique)

D and **E,** The muscles connecting the scapula to the trunk are detached from the scapula in layers and marked with silk whip sutures. First the trapezius and latissimus dorsi are divided.

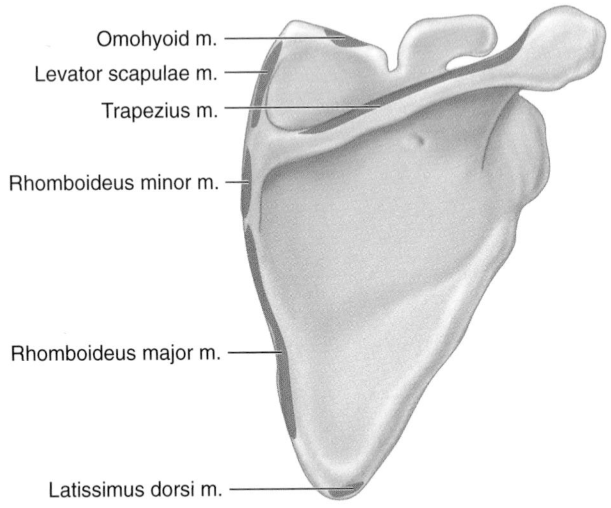

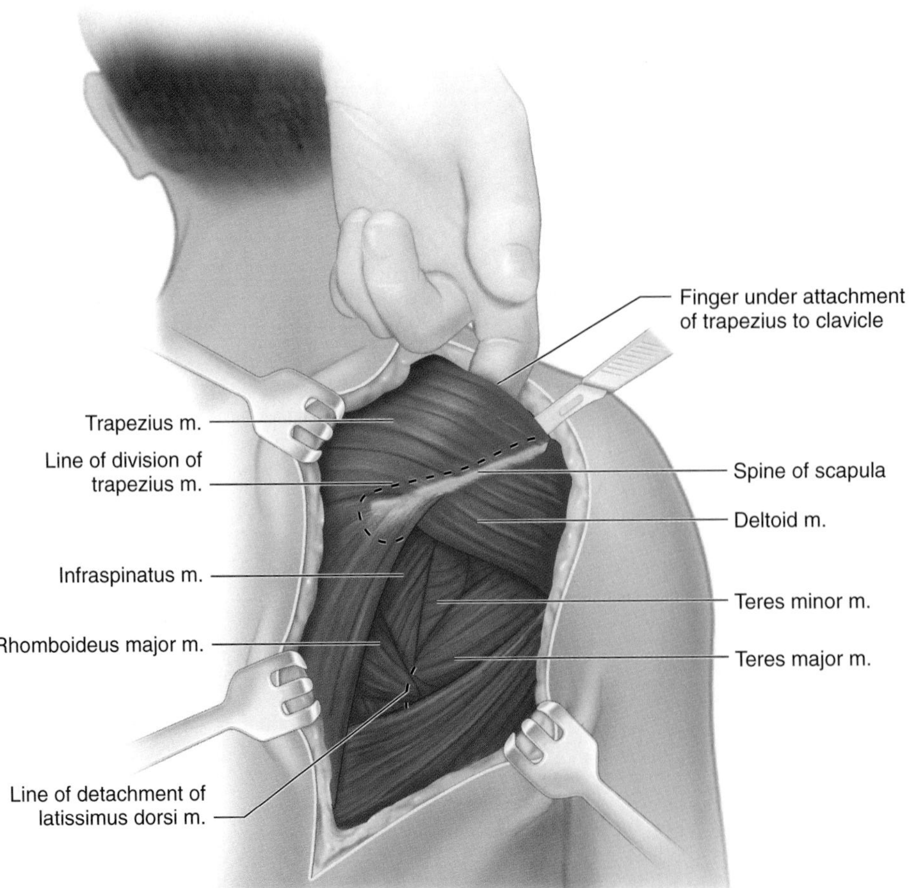

PLATE 39-6 *(continued)*

Posterior Approach for Forequarter Amputation (Littlewood Technique)

F, Next, the omohyoid, levator scapulae, and rhomboid muscles are detached. Transverse cervical and transverse scapular vessels are ligated and divided as dissection proceeds. The cords of the brachial plexus are sectioned with a very sharp scalpel near their origin.

G and **H,** The scapula is retracted forward, and the serratus anterior muscle is sectioned and detached from the scapula.

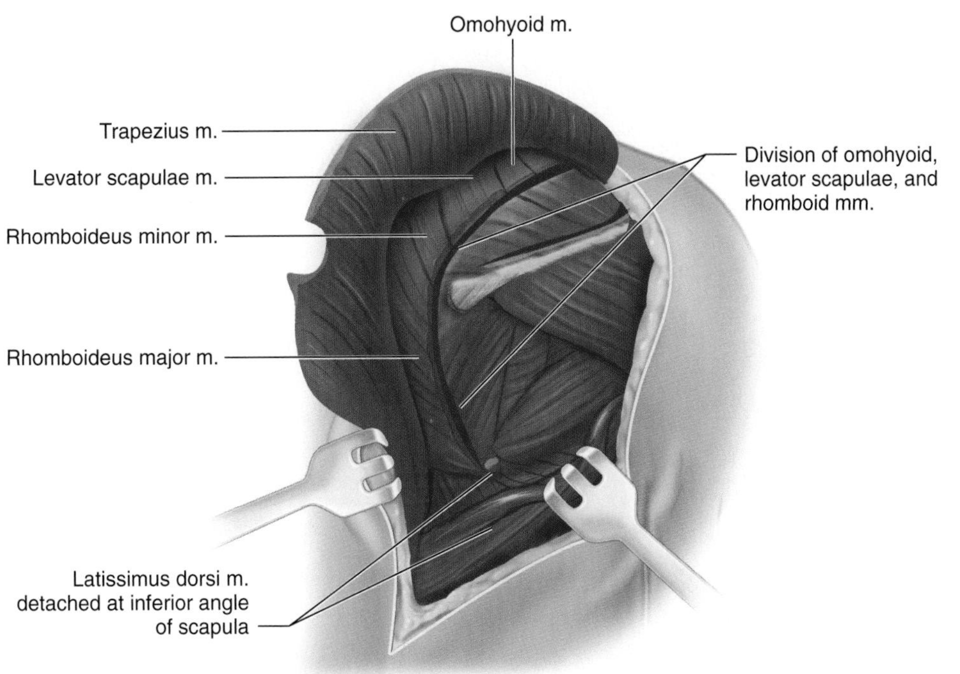

F

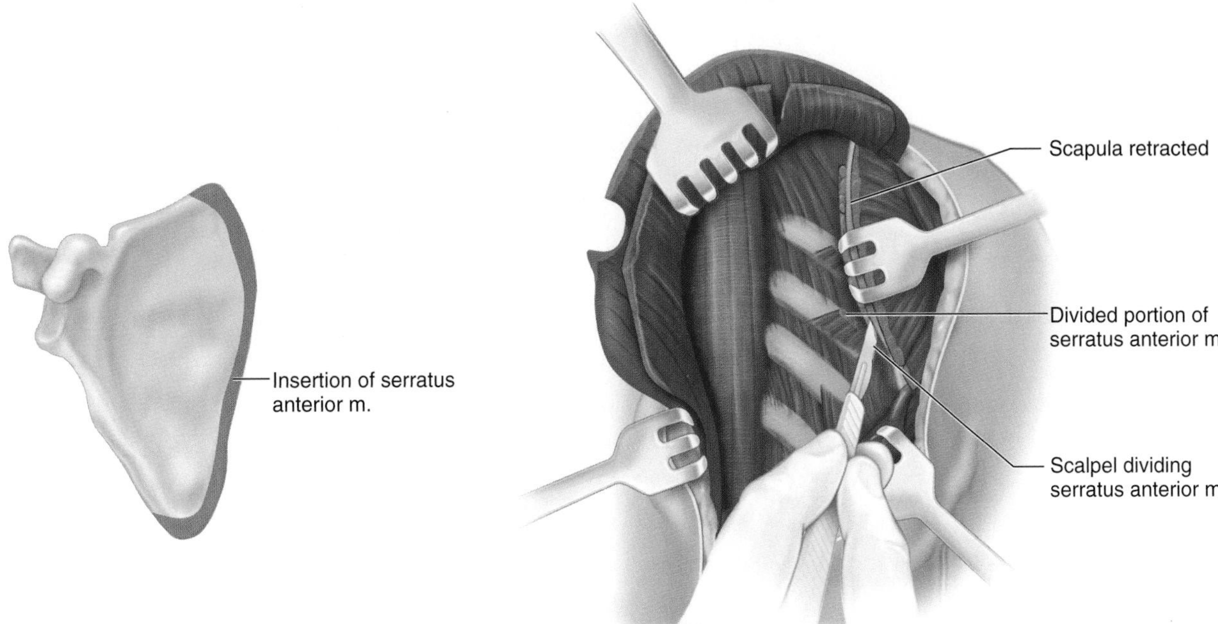

G H

Continued

PLATE 39-6 *(continued)*

Posterior Approach for Forequarter Amputation (Littlewood Technique)

I through **K,** The patient is turned onto his or her back, and the medial end of the clavicle is exposed subperiosteally. Chandler periosteal elevators are placed deep to the clavicle to protect the underlying neurovascular structures. With bone-cutting forceps or a Gigli saw, the clavicle is sectioned near its sternal attachment. The subclavius muscle is divided next.

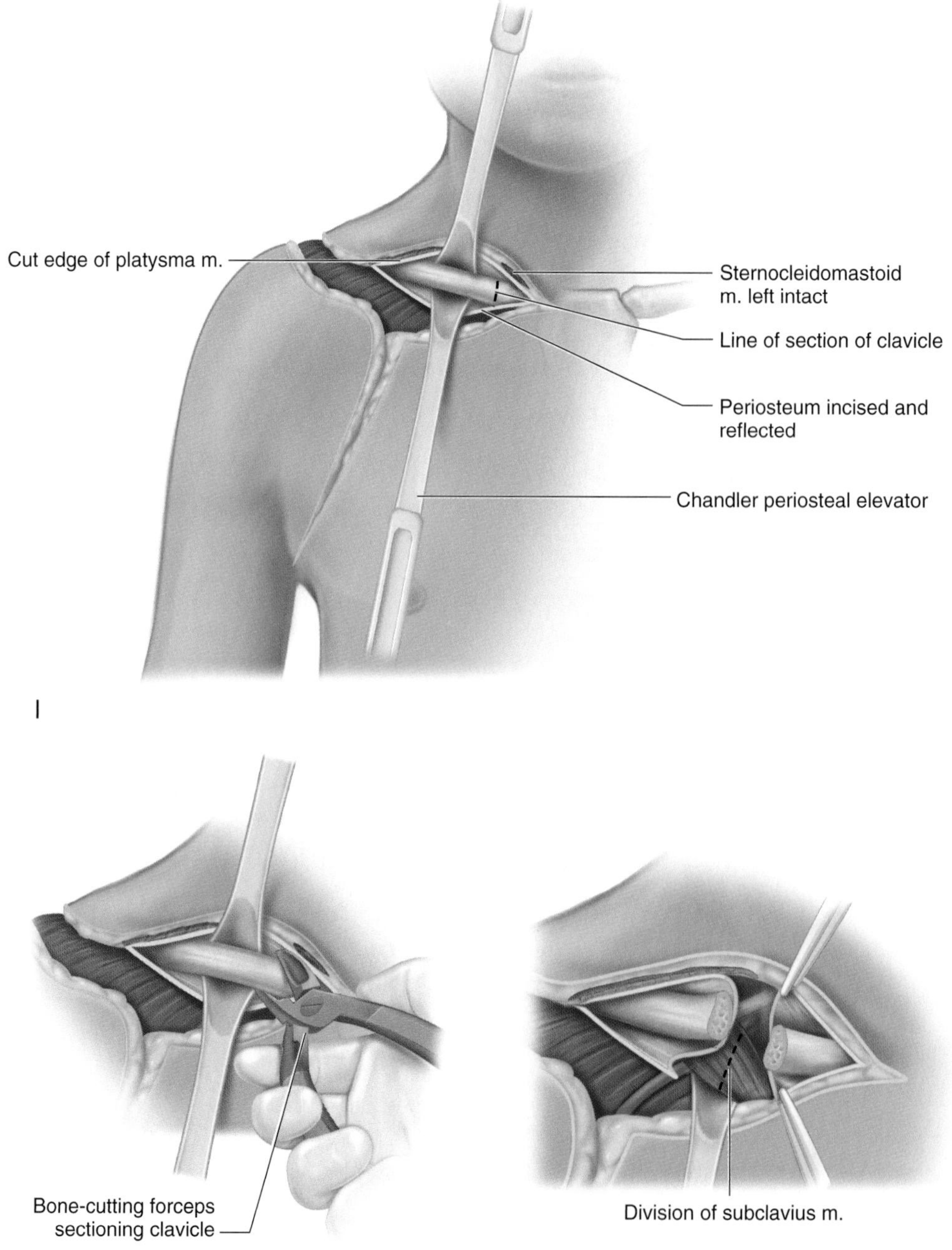

PLATE 39-6 *(continued)*

Posterior Approach for Forequarter Amputation (Littlewood Technique)

L through N, The subclavian vessels and brachial plexus are exposed by allowing the upper limb to fall anteriorly. The subclavian artery and vein are isolated, individually clamped, doubly ligated with sutures, and divided.

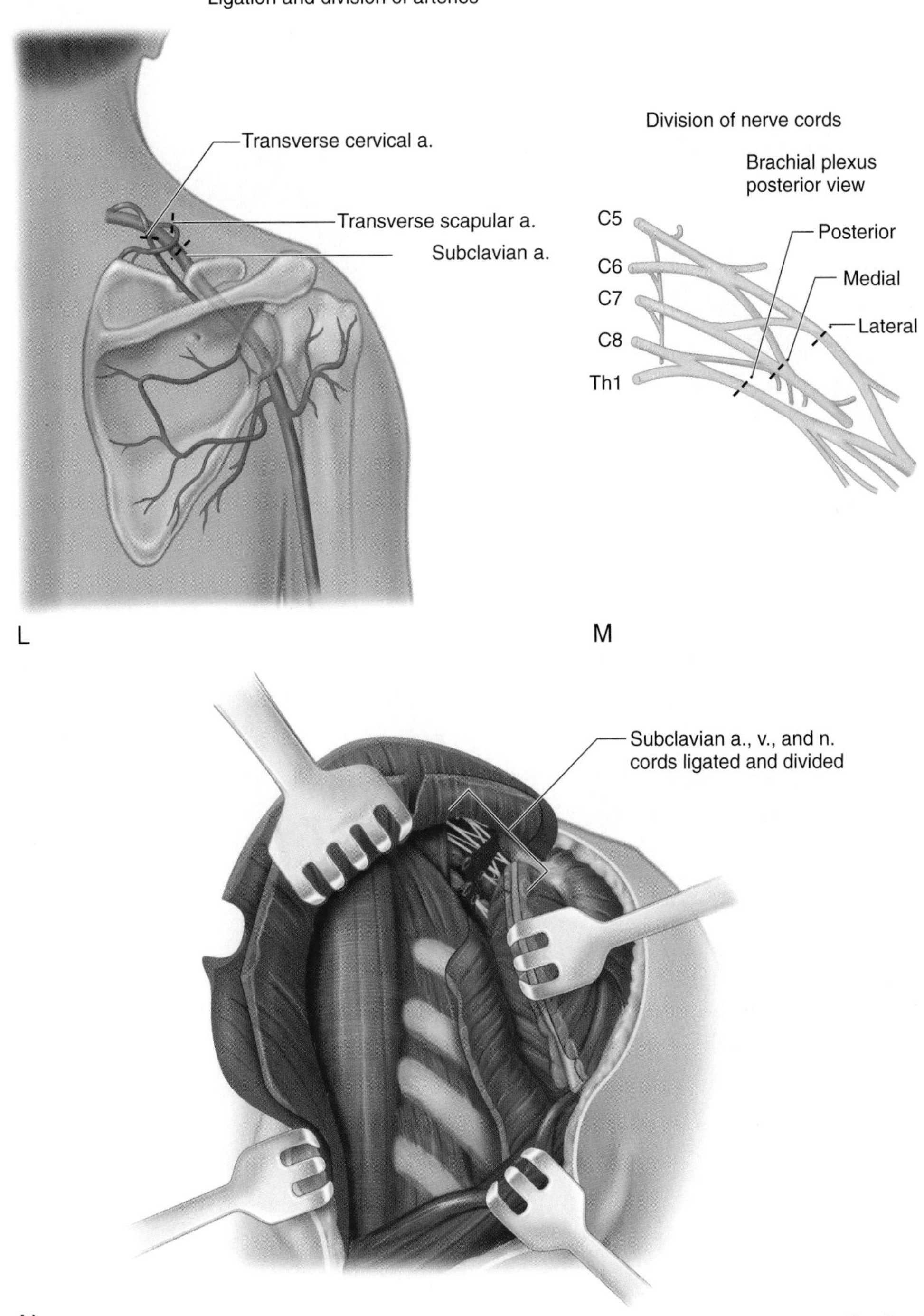

Continued

PLATE 39-6 *(continued)*

Posterior Approach for Forequarter Amputation (Littlewood Technique)

O through **Q,** The pectoralis major and minor, short head of the biceps, coracobrachialis, and latissimus dorsi are sectioned, completing ablation of the limb.

R, The wound flaps are approximated and sutured together. Closed-suction catheters are inserted and connected to an evacuator. A firm compression dressing is applied.

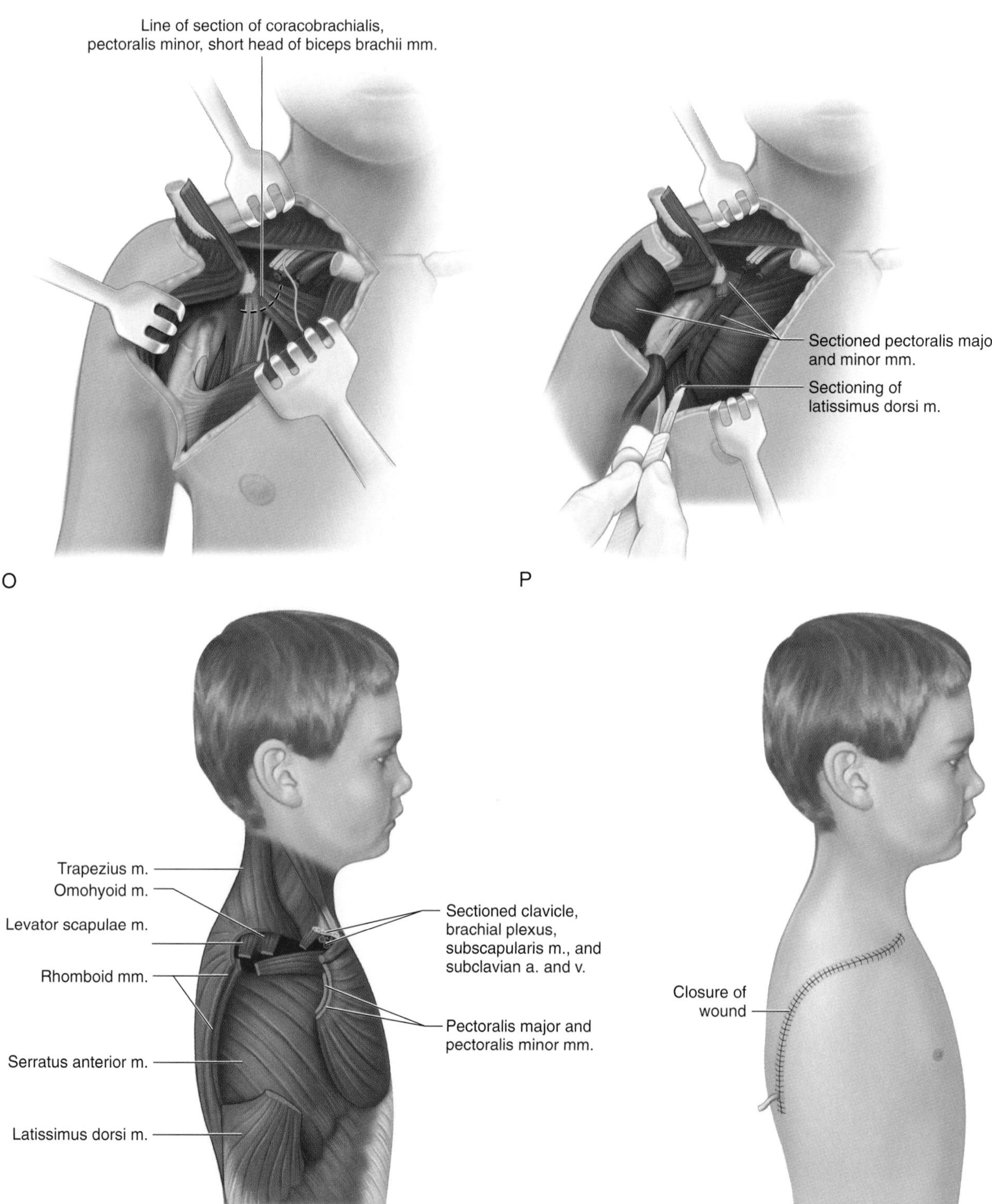

PLATE 39-7

Disarticulation of the Shoulder

The patient is placed in a semilateral position so that the posterior aspect of the affected shoulder, scapula, and axilla and the entire upper limb can be prepared and draped sterilely.

A, The skin incision begins at the coracoid process and extends distally in the deltopectoral groove to the insertion of the deltoid muscle; it then continues proximally along the posterior border of the deltoid muscle to terminate at the posterior axillary fold. A second incision in the axilla connects the anterior and posterior borders of the first incision.

B, In the deltopectoral groove, the cephalic vein is identified, ligated, and excised. The deltoid muscle is retracted laterally to expose the humeral attachment of the pectoralis major muscle, which is divided at its insertion and reflected medially. The coracobrachialis and short head of the biceps are divided at their origins from the coracoid process and reflected distally.

Next, the deltoid muscle is detached from its insertion on the humerus and retracted proximally.

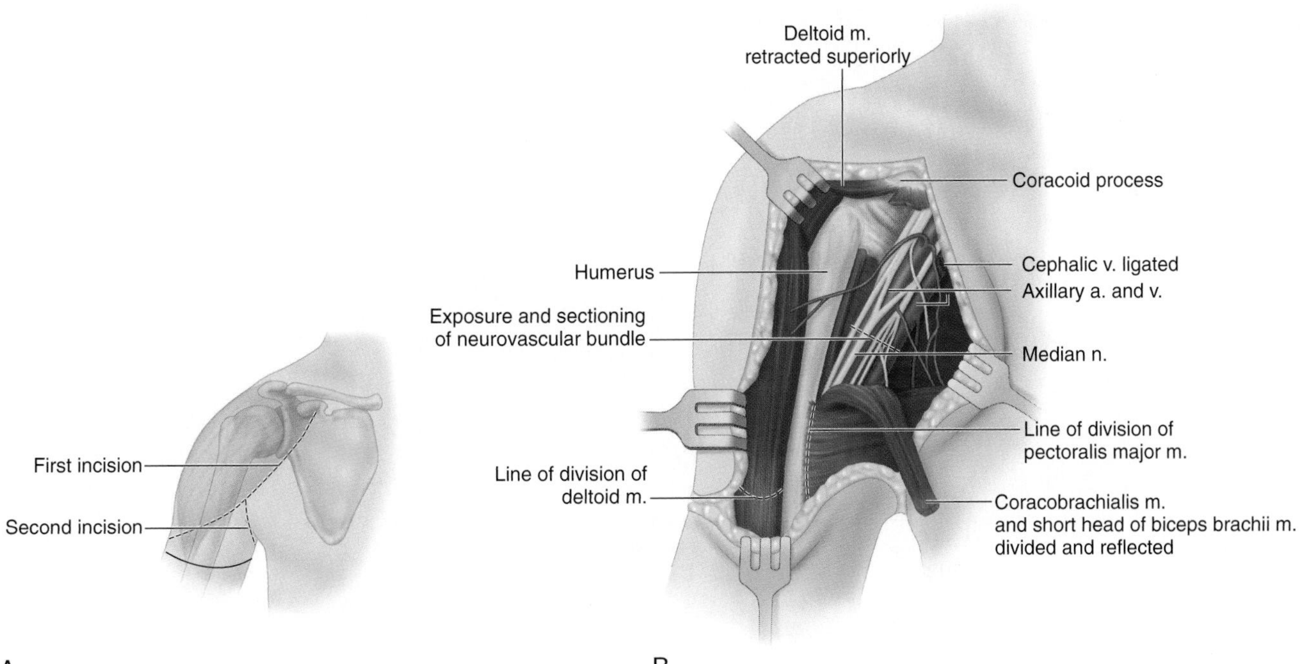

Continued

PLATE 39-7 *(continued)*

Disarticulation of the Shoulder

C, The axillary artery and vein and the thoracoacromial vessels are identified, isolated, doubly ligated with 0 silk suture, and divided. The thoracoacromial artery is a short trunk branching from the anterior surface of the axillary artery. Its origin is usually covered by the pectoralis minor muscle. The median, ulnar, musculocutaneous, and radial nerves are identified, isolated, pulled distally, and divided with a sharp knife, then allowed to retract beneath the pectoralis minor muscle.

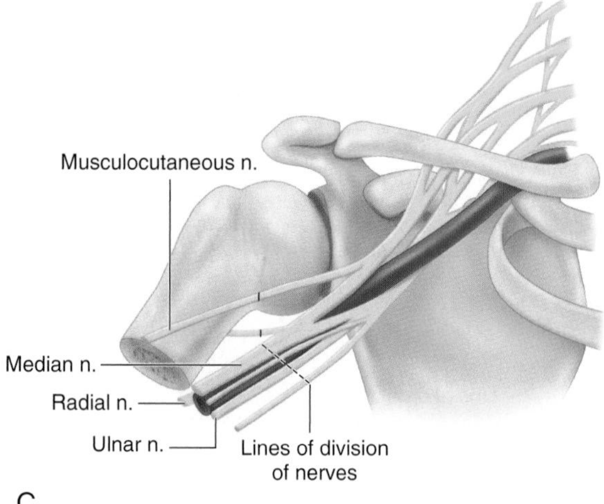

PLATE 39-7 *(continued)*

Disarticulation of the Shoulder

D, The capsule of the shoulder joint is exposed by retracting the deltoid muscle superiorly. Next, the arm is placed in marked external rotation. The subscapularis muscle, long head of the biceps at its origin, and anterior capsule of the shoulder joint are divided. The teres major and latissimus dorsi muscles are sectioned near their insertion to the intertubercular groove of the humerus. The acromion process is exposed extraperiosteally by elevating the origin of the deltoid muscle from its lateral border and superior surface. The acromion process is partially excised with an osteotome to give the shoulder a smooth, rounded contour.

The arm is placed across the chest with the shoulder in marked internal rotation. The supraspinatus, infraspinatus, and teres minor muscles are divided at their insertion. The capsule of the shoulder joint is divided superiorly and posteriorly. The long head of the triceps brachii is sectioned near its origin from the infraglenoid tuberosity of the scapula. The inferior capsule of the joint is divided, completing disarticulation of the shoulder. The hyaline articular cartilage of the glenoid cavity is curetted, exposing cancellous, raw bleeding bone. The cut ends of the muscles are sutured to the glenoid fossa.

E, The deltoid muscle is sutured to the inferior aspect of the neck of the scapula. Suction catheters are placed deep to the deltoid muscle and connected to a suction evacuator. The subcutaneous tissue and skin are closed in layers with interrupted sutures.

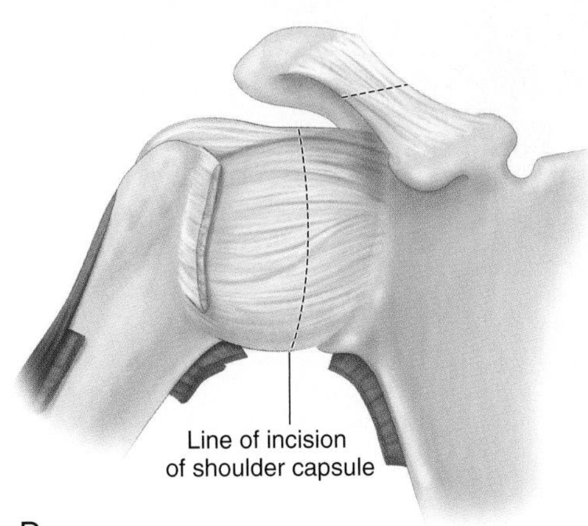

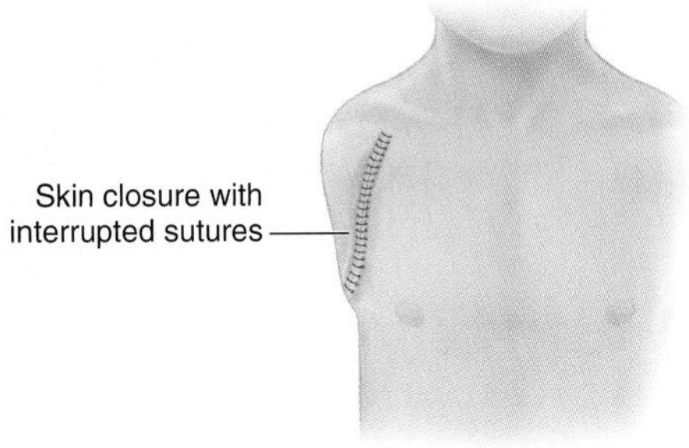

PLATE 39-8

Amputation through the Arm

The patient is placed in a supine position with a sandbag under the shoulder that is to be operated on. A sterile Esmarch tourniquet is applied in the axillary region for hemostasis.

A, Anterior and posterior skin flaps are fashioned so that they are equal in length and 1 cm longer than half the diameter of the arm at the intended level of amputation. The subcutaneous tissue and deep fascia are divided in line with the skin incision, and the wound flaps are retracted.

B and **C,** The brachial artery and vein are identified, doubly ligated, and divided. The median and ulnar nerves are isolated, pulled distally, sectioned with a sharp knife, and allowed to retract proximally. The muscles in the anterior compartment of the arm are divided 1.5 cm distal to the site of bone division, and the muscle mass is beveled distally.

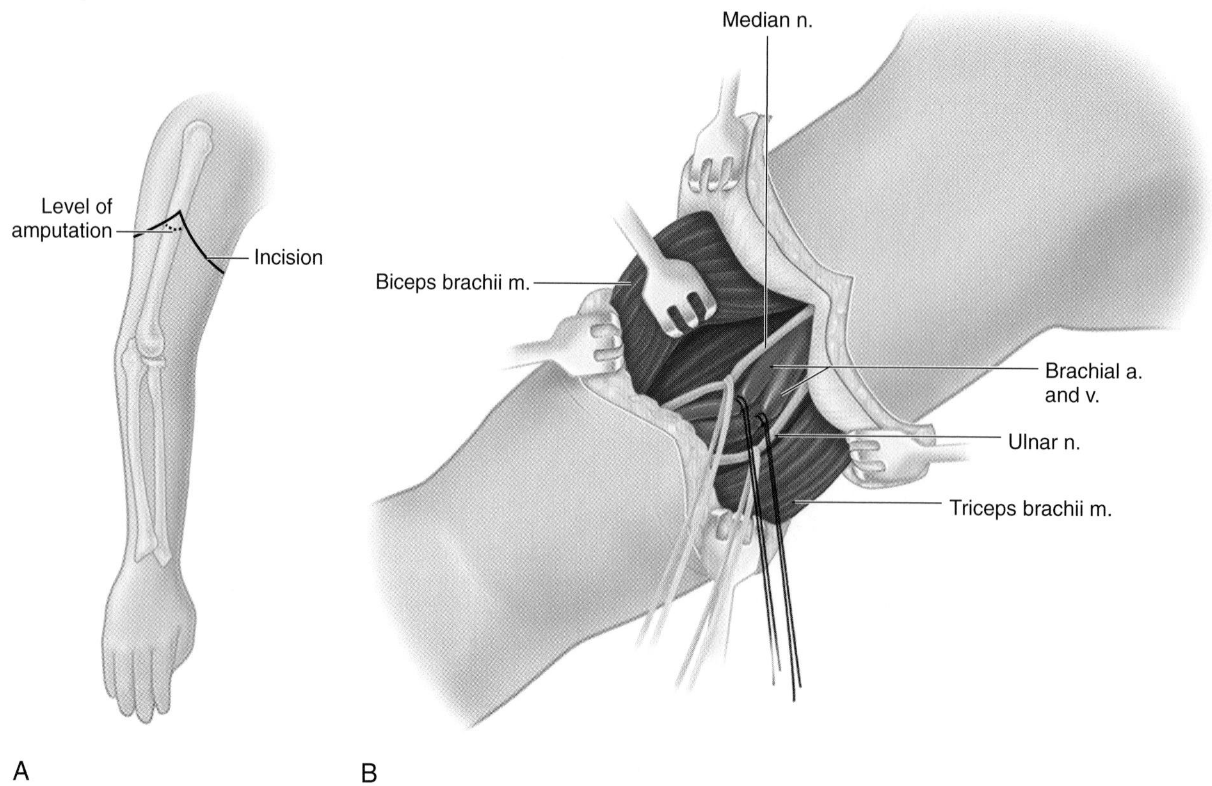

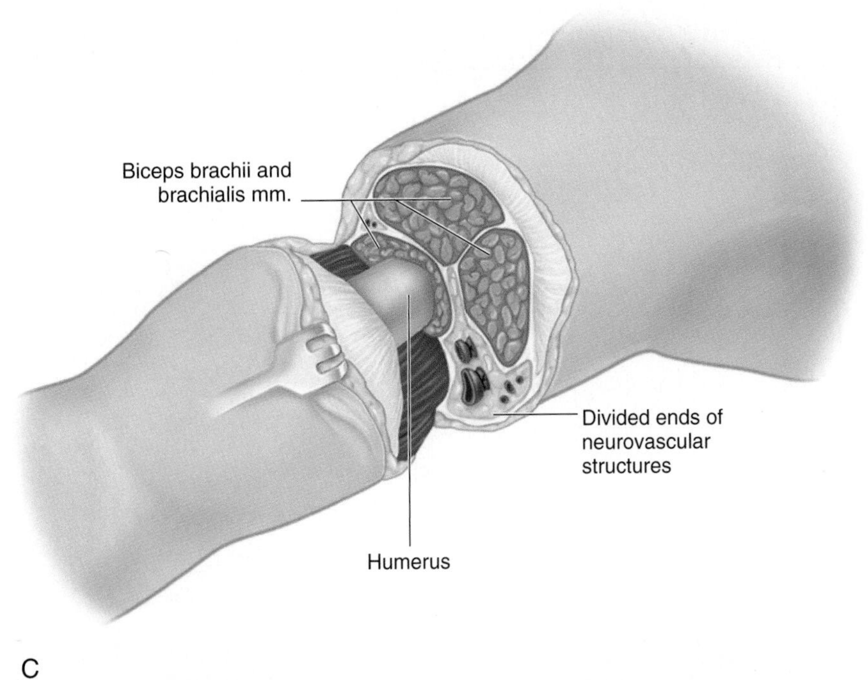

PLATE 39-8 Amputation through the Arm *(continued)*

Continued

PLATE 39-8 *(continued)*

Amputation through the Arm

D, The radial nerve is isolated, pulled distally, and sectioned with a sharp knife. The deep brachial vessels are doubly ligated and divided. The triceps brachii muscle is sectioned 3 to 4 cm distal to the level of the bone section and beveled to form a skin flap.

E, The humerus is divided, and the bone end is smoothed with a rasp.

F, The distal end of the triceps muscle is brought anteriorly and sutured to the deep fascia of the anterior compartment muscles. Catheters are inserted for closed suction, and the wound is closed with interrupted sutures.

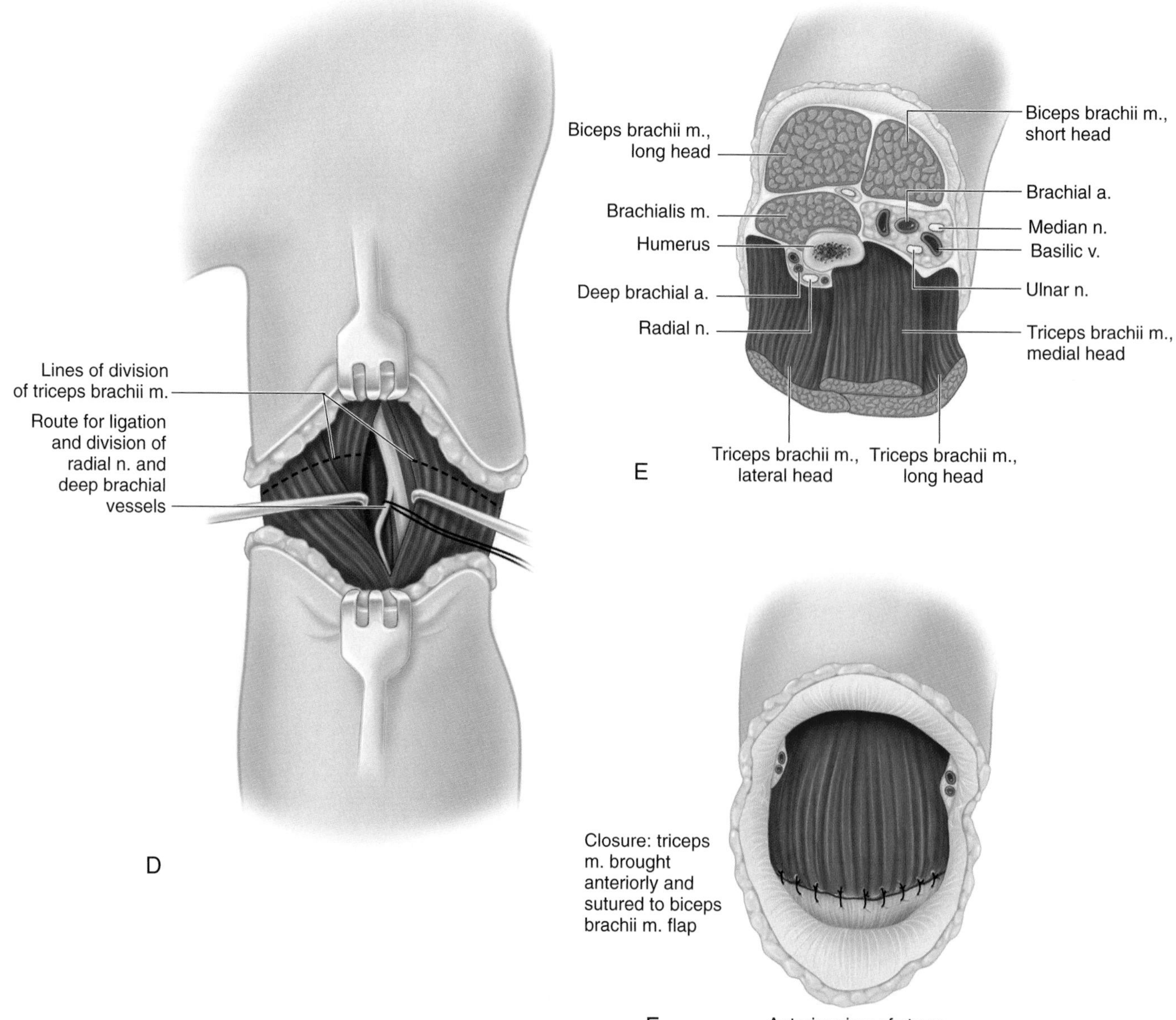

PLATE 39-9

Disarticulation of the Elbow

The operation is performed with a pneumatic tourniquet on the proximal arm.

A, The anterior and posterior skin flaps are fashioned to be equal in length to the medial and lateral epicondyles of the humerus, which serve as the medial and lateral proximal points. The lower margin of the posterior flap is 2.5 cm distal to the tip of the olecranon; the distal margin of the anterior flap is immediately inferior to the insertion of the biceps tendon on the tuberosity of the radius.

B, The wound flaps are undermined and reflected 3 cm proximal to the level of the epicondyles of the humerus. The lacertus fibrosus is sectioned. The common flexor muscles of the forearm are divided at their origin from the medial epicondyle of the humerus, elevated extraperiosteally, and reflected distally.

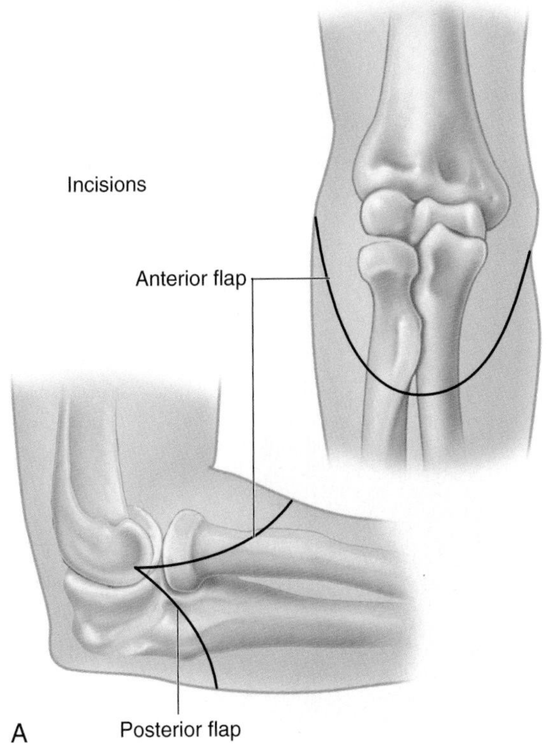

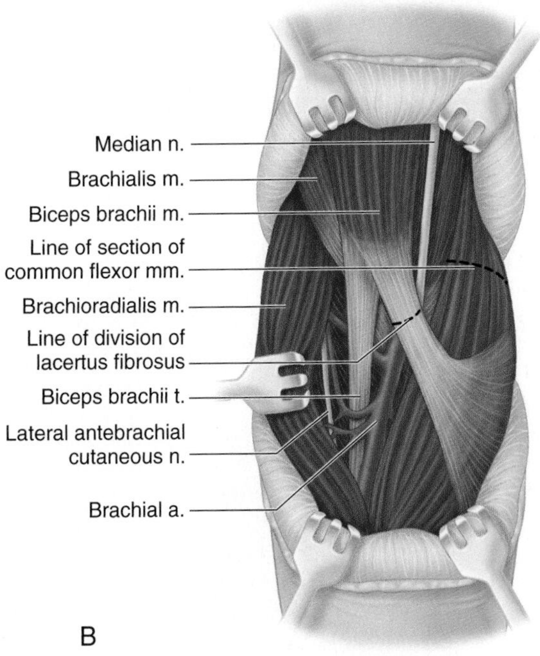

Continued

PLATE 39-9 *(continued)*

Disarticulation of the Elbow

C and **D,** The brachial vessels and the median nerve on the medial aspect of the biceps tendon are exposed. The brachial vessels are doubly ligated and divided proximal to the joint level. The median nerve is pulled distally, divided with a sharp knife, and allowed to retract proximally. The ulnar nerve is dissected free in its groove behind the medial epicondyle, drawn distally, and sharply sectioned. The biceps tendon is detached from its insertion on the radial tuberosity.

The radial nerve is isolated in the interval between the brachioradialis and brachialis muscles. The nerve is pulled distally and divided with a sharp knife. The brachialis muscle tendon is divided at its insertion to the coronoid process.

E and **F,** The brachioradialis and common extensor muscles are sectioned transversely about 4 to 5 cm distal to the joint line. Following detachment of the triceps tendon at its insertion near the tip of the olecranon process, division of the common extensor muscles of the forearm is completed.

G and **H,** The capsule and ligaments of the elbow joint are divided, and the forearm is removed. The tourniquet is released, and complete hemostasis is obtained.

I, The triceps tendon is sutured to the brachialis and biceps tendons. The proximal segment of the extensor muscles of the forearm is brought laterally and sutured to the triceps tendon. The wound flaps are approximated with interrupted sutures. Catheters are placed in the wound for closed suction.

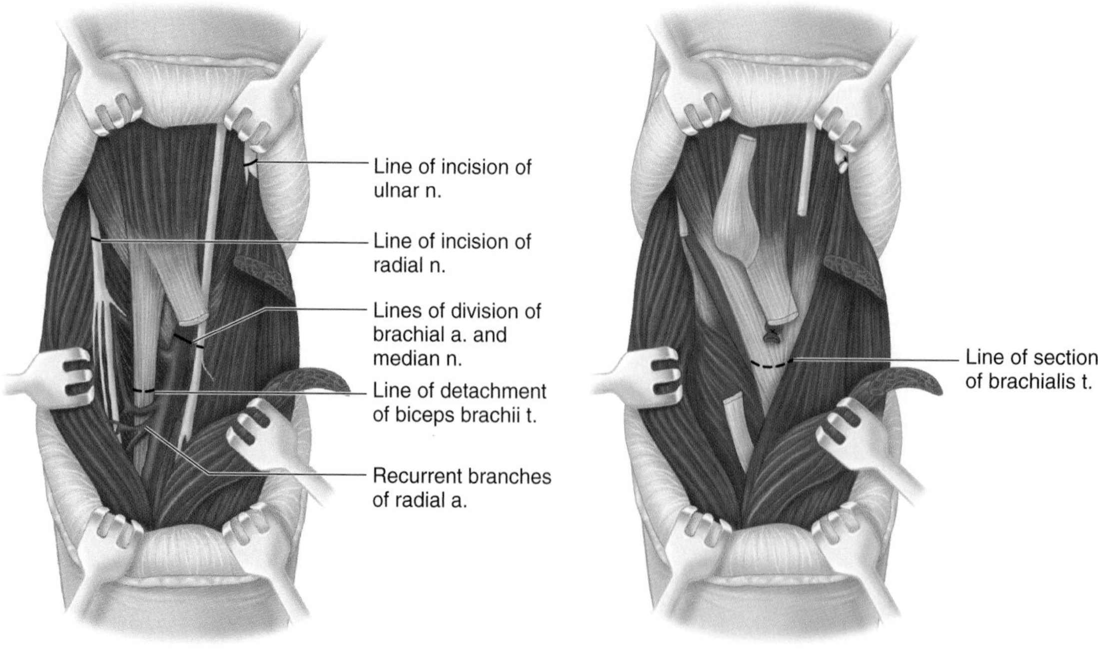

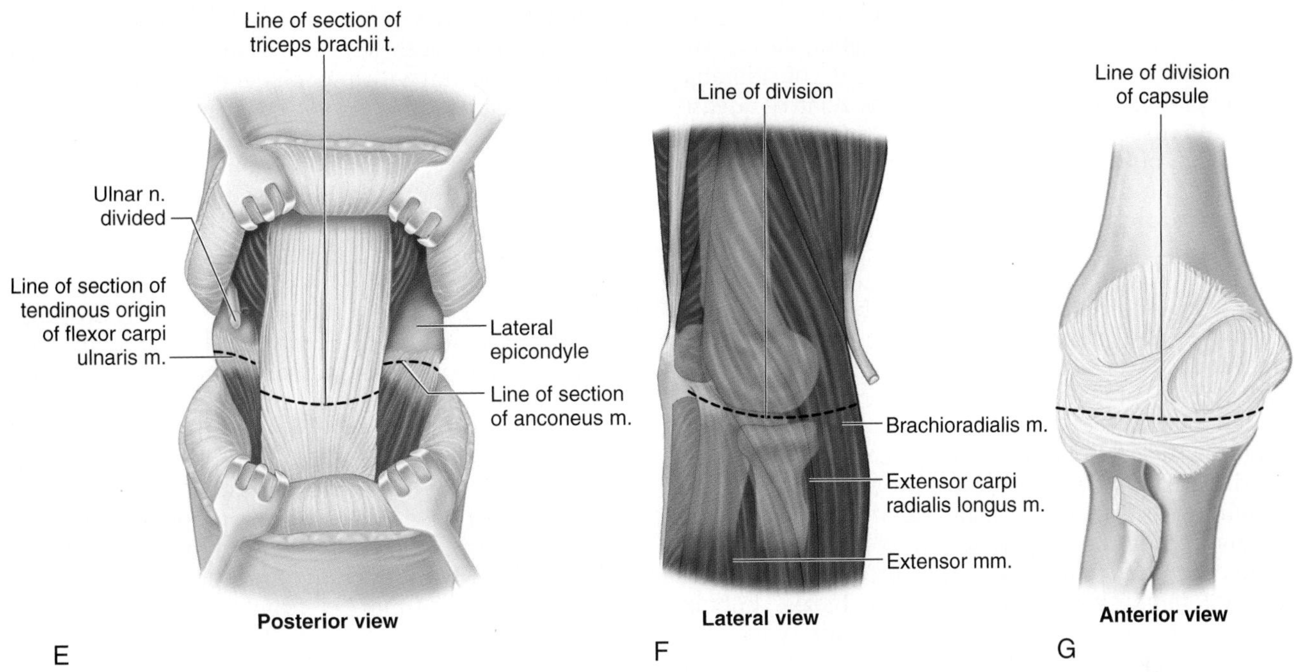

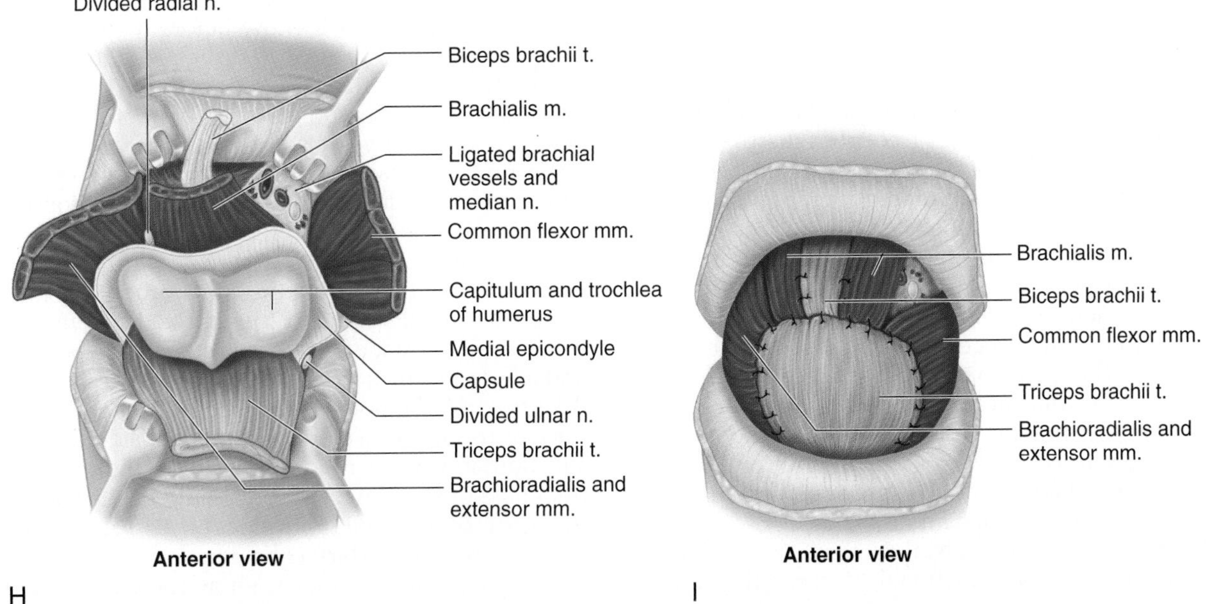

PLATE 39-9 Disarticulation of the Elbow *(continued)*

immature patient or one who wants to continue sporting activities; a failed distal femoral reconstruction; or a pathologic fracture. It must be possible to preserve the sciatic nerve and its branches, although the vessels may be divided and anastomosed to increase the margin if necessary. The advantages of a rotationplasty are the wide margin (which includes the skin, adjacent knee joint, and all thigh muscles), the avoidance of phantom pain, rapid healing of the osteosynthesis site, and a relatively low complication rate. The obvious drawback is the appearance, which some find repulsive. Interestingly, young children usually do not view the procedure as an amputation because the foot remains, and with a good prosthesis, they can function better than and appear similar to standard amputees.

Follow-up studies have not demonstrated any adverse psychological outcomes,[62,221,264,278,347] and in our experience, the patients who have undergone the procedure are quite happy with the results.[351] Preoperative discussions must be honest and complete so that the child and the family are aware of the nature of the procedure and the expected outcome. It is helpful for them to meet with a physical therapist who is familiar with this procedure, view videotapes of patients who have undergone the procedure, and, ideally, meet a patient with a rotationplasty. We employ all these modalities and spend considerable time explaining the rationale and the relative advantages and disadvantages of this and the other options, such as amputation and limb-sparing procedures. Recently, the number of patients willing to undergo this procedure has diminished; many prefer to try a limb-sparing procedure and reserve rotationplasty if that fails.

The procedure itself is well described in the literature.* It is important to plan the skin flaps carefully, and modifications of the rhomboid incision described by Kotz are satisfactory.[279,464] In our experience, there is a tendency to make the thigh long, so that the rotated "knee" appears to be distal to the contralateral knee. It is difficult to accurately predict the amount of growth remaining because the distal tibial physis and the tarsals become analogous to the contralateral distal femoral growth plate. One can attempt to plot the growth remaining using standard tables, but in general, a boy older than 14 years and a girl older than 12 years should probably have the rotationplasty "knee" placed opposite the contralateral knee. For younger patients, placing it 2 to 4 cm more caudal is appropriate. The vessels may be resected with the specimen to increase the amount of normal tissue margin. An anastomosis of the vein and artery can be completed after achieving osteosynthesis. An alternative is to dissect the vessels free from the tumor and loop them carefully back on themselves with the nerves.[279,351] The skin closure is difficult and must be done carefully to avoid postoperative wound complications. The limb is immobilized with the ankle in extension. At 6 weeks, the osteosynthesis is usually healed sufficiently to begin prosthetic wear.

In addition, this procedure has been described for tumors of the proximal tibia, with successful results.[102,205,221,280] Modifications of this procedure have also been described for lesions about the hip or involving a large portion of the proximal femur.[309,568,569] The ilium and distal femur must be preserved for this procedure to provide a "hip" and a "knee."

Rotationplasty for a distal femoral osteosarcoma offers a durable and functional, if cosmetically displeasing, reconstruction option for selected patients. For very young patients with distal femoral lesions, it avoids the repeated surgical procedures necessary to achieve limb length equality and allows the child to run and play exceedingly well. The other useful indication is for a failed limb salvage procedure when amputation is the only alternative.

The child and parents may need psychological support when considering both amputation and rotationplasty. Initially, there is tremendous emotional resistance to ablation of a limb. It is helpful for these patients to see other children with amputations and prostheses before the operation. A physical therapy consultation and a visit to a prosthetist are also valuable. Treatment of these children and adolescents in a children's hospital with a specialized multidisciplinary oncology team is of great value. Fitting with a temporary prosthesis immediately after amputation may also be of psychological benefit, although these temporary prostheses seldom function well. Usually, a permanent prosthesis can be made 6 to 8 weeks after the amputation or rotationplasty.

Limb Salvage. After a complete staging workup, biopsy, and (usually) preoperative chemotherapy, the primary tumor is assessed for response. MRI often shows a reduction in the amount of edema surrounding the tumor, but seldom does the mass decrease in size because of the matrix within the tumor. There is no proven way to accurately judge or predict the histologic response of the tumor preoperatively, but thallium scans, dynamic MRI, dynamic contrast-enhanced MRI subtraction, and position emission tomography (PET) may eventually be useful in this regard.[241,377,423,437,452,533,551] None of these techniques has yet shown a correlation with event-free survival, and it remains to be seen whether earlier evaluation with dynamic MRI or PET can identify poor responders and allow modification of therapy before definitive surgical resection.

Limb salvage is considered if there has been no progression of disease locally or distantly and if the nerves and blood vessels are free of tumor. The most important issue is the ability to completely resect the tumor with wide margins. The adjacent joint and growth plates are assessed for tumor involvement, and the amount of involved muscle is determined. There is no agreement regarding the "safe" amount of normal tissue that must surround the resected specimen, but in general, at least a 3- to 5-cm bone marrow margin and a 5- to 10-mm soft tissue margin are desirable. The thickness of the soft tissue margin depends on the type of tissue. A fascial margin is considered a more substantial barrier to tumor spread than a similar thickness of fat. The resection should be planned with the goal of achieving local control; reconstruction options are a secondary consideration.

In "expendable" bones such as the clavicle, fibula, scapula, and rib, resection without reconstruction can be considered. Lesions of the radius and ulna are rare and can usually be resected with minimal reconstruction or with fibular autografts or allografts used for reconstruction. Lesions of the hands and feet usually require amputation, although ray amputation and partial amputations that preserve some hand or foot function can sometimes be performed. For lesions of the extremities that are deemed resectable, the reconstruction can be complex and depends on the age of the patient and the location of the tumor in reference to joints and growth plates. For most distal femoral and proximal tibial osteosarcomas, an intracompartmental, intra-articular resection can be carried out. The same is usually possible for lesions of the proximal humerus. Reconstruction is achieved either with an osteoarticular allograft or with a metallic prosthe-

*See references 37, 62, 70, 169, 185, 205, 217, 221, 244, 264, 274, 278, 279, 351, 464, 569.

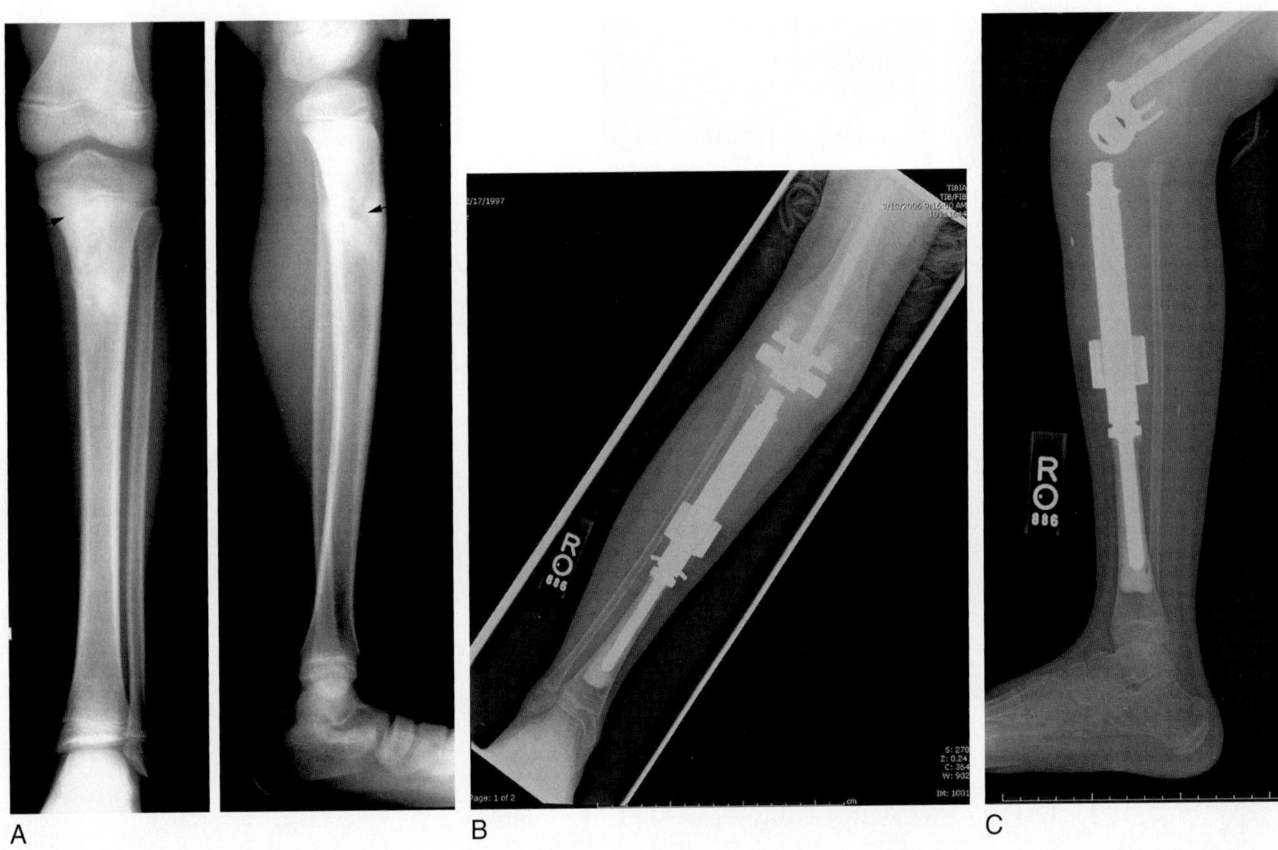

FIGURE 39-12 Expandable prosthesis used to reconstruct the extremity after resection of an osteosarcoma from the proximal tibia of a 6-year-old girl. **A,** Initial radiographs demonstrate a radiodense lesion of the proximal tibia (*arrows*). **B** and **C,** Reconstruction after tumor resection with an expandable prosthesis. Note that the distal femur and its physis are preserved to maximize future growth.

sis. There are no proven advantages of one over the other, and the choice is usually based on surgeon and patient preference. In boys younger than 12 to 14 years and girls younger than 10 to 12 years with lesions about the knee, growth considerations come into play. Limb length is usually not a major concern and can be addressed by standard limb equalization techniques (e.g., epiphysiodesis, limb lengthening, limb shortening) after chemotherapy is completed. Alternatively, a metallic prosthesis that expands as the child grows can be used (Fig. 39–12).[85,130,153,267,457,459,545,558] For older patients with growth remaining, it is usually possible to make the reconstruction 1 to 2 cm longer than the amount resected, resulting in nearly equal limb lengths at maturity.

The choice of metallic prosthesis versus allograft is debatable. The prosthesis is more stable initially and returns the patient to function earlier than an allograft, but there is concern about the longevity of the implant in this young age group. Loosening, particle disease, and metal and polyethylene failure are unsolved problems. We prefer allograft reconstructions in skeletally immature children (Figs. 39–13 and 39–14). Allografts offer the advantage of restoring bone stock but require a longer recuperation period and are associated with relatively high fracture, infection, and nonunion rates.[8,48,121,166,167,319,328,365] The longevity of the articular cartilage is also a concern, and some patients require conversion to a more standard joint replacement over time (Fig. 39–15). One advantage to using osteoarticular allografts in children is the ability to preserve the adjacent growth plate. In the proximal tibia, the ability to reattach the patellar tendon to the allograft tendon is another advantage.[80,225] Similarly, the ability to reconstruct the rotator cuff in the shoulder is an advantage of allografts in that location.[168]

For diaphyseal osteosarcomas, intercalary resections are often possible. These resections allow preservation of the adjacent joints and sometimes the growth plates. The defects can be reconstructed with allografts, vascularized fibulae, or metallic spacers, and because the joints are preserved, function is usually superior to that following osteoarticular resection (Fig. 39–16).[8,365,383] It is critical to accurately assess the magnetic resonance image to plan tumor-free marrow margins. If the growth plate must be sacrificed, standard limb equalization procedures can be used later.

Pelvic osteosarcomas are an extremely difficult challenge. Tumors of the ilium that spare the acetabulum can be resected with little functional loss, but if the acetabulum is involved, there is no adequate reconstruction option, and it is often difficult to achieve tumor-free margins. The adjacent sacrum is frequently involved, making it necessary to sacrifice nerve roots

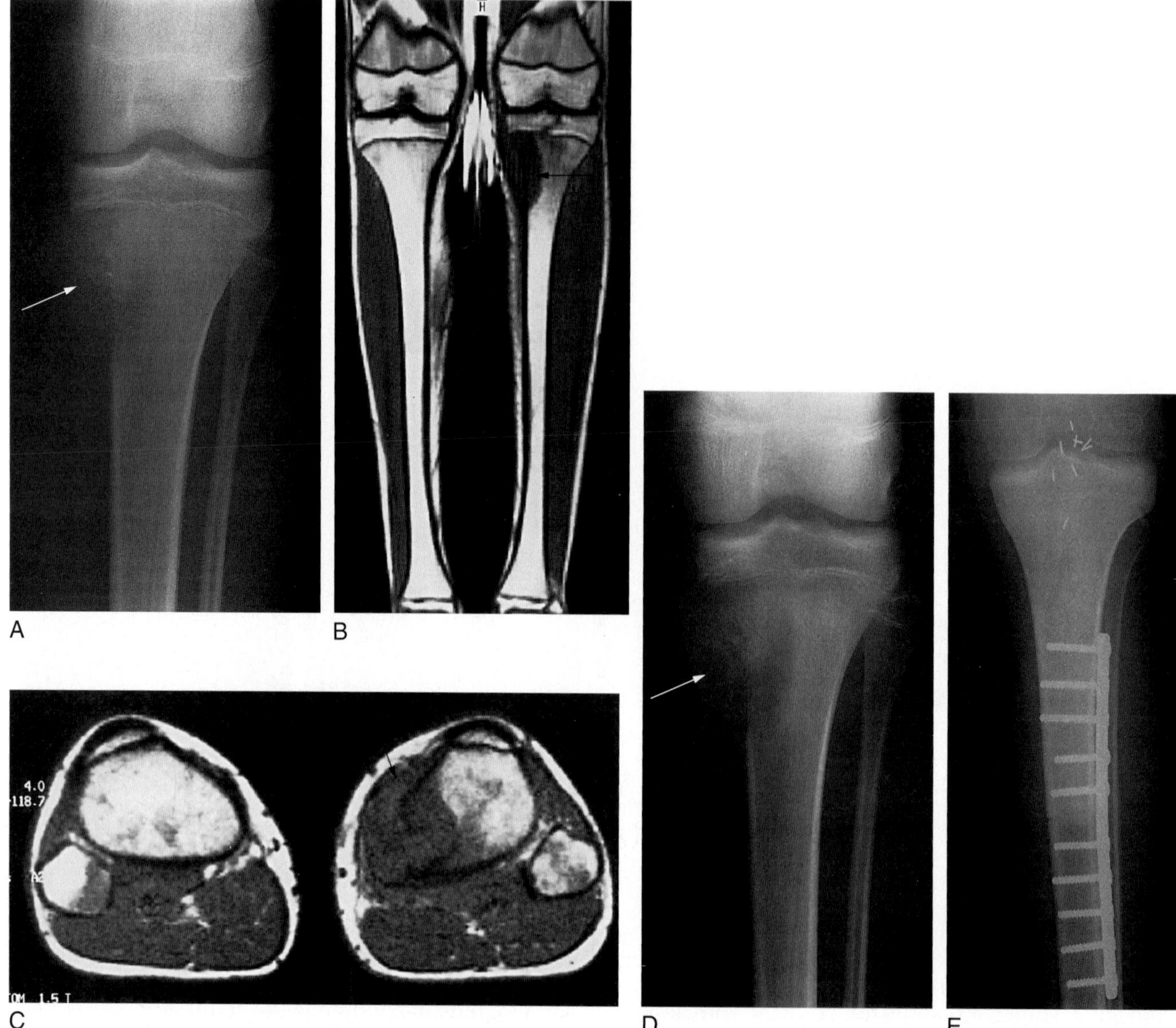

FIGURE 39–13 High-grade osteosarcoma in a 16-year-old boy. **A,** Anteroposterior (AP) radiograph of the tibia. There is a destructive lesion of the proximal metaphysis with internal mineralization (*arrow*). It is poorly marginated and has destroyed the cortex. It appears to stop at the growth plate. At this age, osteosarcoma is the most likely diagnosis. **B,** T1-weighted magnetic resonance image showing the medullary extent of the tumor and the soft tissue mass (*arrow*). The epiphysis appears to be uninvolved except for a linear signal abnormality that may represent a fracture. The adjacent joint appears to be uninvolved. **C,** Axial magnetic resonance image showing the extent of the soft tissue mass and the relationship of the lesion to the popliteal vessels (*arrow*). The vessels are uninvolved. An incisional biopsy showed that the tumor was a high-grade osteosarcoma. **D,** AP radiograph obtained following preoperative chemotherapy. There is mineralization of the tumor and a more complete periosteal shell of bone around the periphery of the lesion (*arrow*). This is considered to be a sign of response to chemotherapy. The patient subsequently underwent an intra-articular wide resection of the osteosarcoma and reconstruction with an osteoarticular allograft. **E,** AP radiograph showing the reconstruction with early healing of the osteosynthesis site 9 months after reconstruction.

at times. Nevertheless, resections of the ilium and acetabulum, even with little or no reconstruction, can result in decent ambulatory function. Options for reconstruction include osteoarticular allografts, allograft arthrodeses, pseudarthroses of the femur to the remaining pubis, or metallic prostheses.[1,44,64,122,141,186] The complication rate is high, and careful attention to soft tissue coverage is required. Adjuvant radiotherapy may be necessary if it is not possible to achieve microscopically negative margins.

Metastatic Osteosarcoma

Patients who present with osteosarcoma are carefully scrutinized for the presence of gross metastatic disease. The most common site is the lung, followed in frequency by bone.[209,356] The prognosis for patients with metastases at diagnosis is much poorer than that for patients with no demonstrable metastatic disease. However, efforts to develop new drugs to treat these

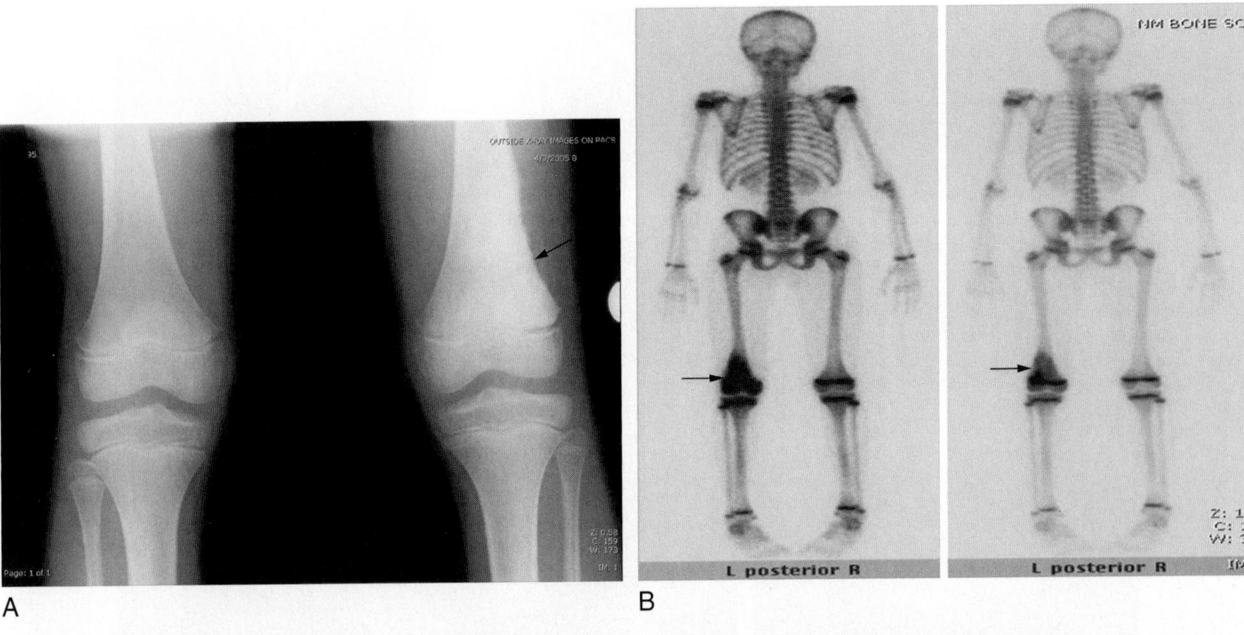

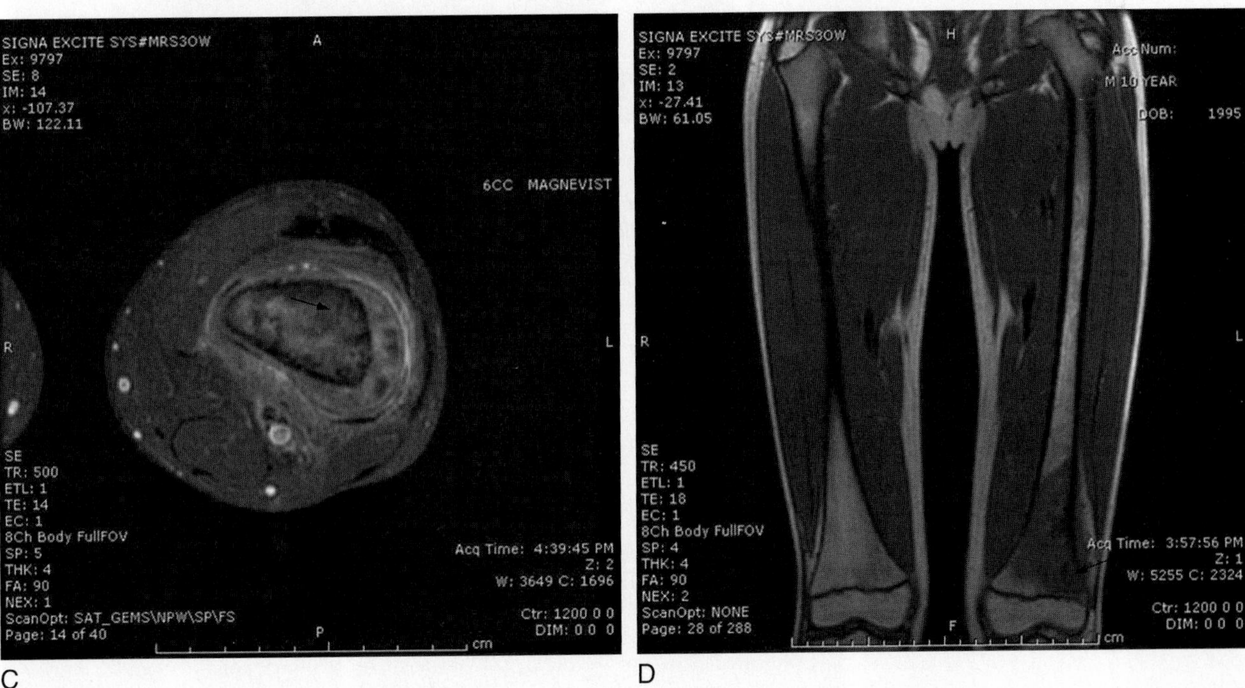

FIGURE 39-14 Allograft reconstruction of a distal femoral lesion. **A,** Radiograph of the lesion in the left distal femur (*arrow*). **B,** Bone scan confirms no other sites of disease (*arrows*). **C** and **D,** Magnetic resonance imaging of the lesion (*arrows*).

Continued

patients are ongoing. Recent studies have shown that if aggressive chemotherapy plus resection of all gross disease can be accomplished, it is possible to achieve long-term survival in about 30% to 40% of patients with metastatic disease at diagnosis.[23,209,356,358] Patients whose disease cannot be completely resected and those with bony metastases usually do not survive. In general, patients with lung metastases are more likely to survive than patients with metastases to other sites. Patients presenting with bony metastases have a dismal prognosis, with few reported survivors, but because they may survive functionally and pain free for long periods, aggressive treatment is warranted.[450]

It is difficult to distinguish a patient with multifocal osteosarcoma from one with metastatic osteosarcoma, and the definitions are somewhat arbitrary. Multifocal osteosarcoma may be synchronous (multiple bony lesions at the time of diagnosis) or metachronous (secondary bone lesions occurring years later).[33,197,249,318,323,324,392,415,479,517]

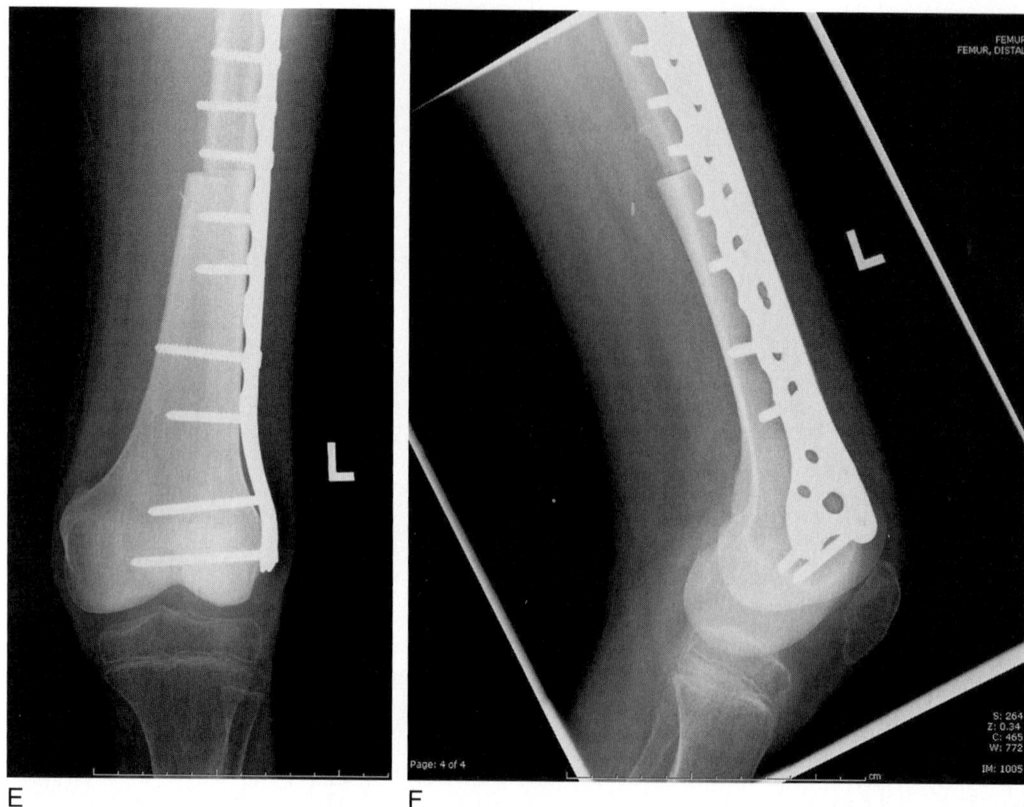

FIGURE 39-14 cont'd E and F, Allograft reconstruction of the distal femur. The reconstructed limb is slightly longer than the contralateral side to minimize limb length discrepancy at skeletal maturity.

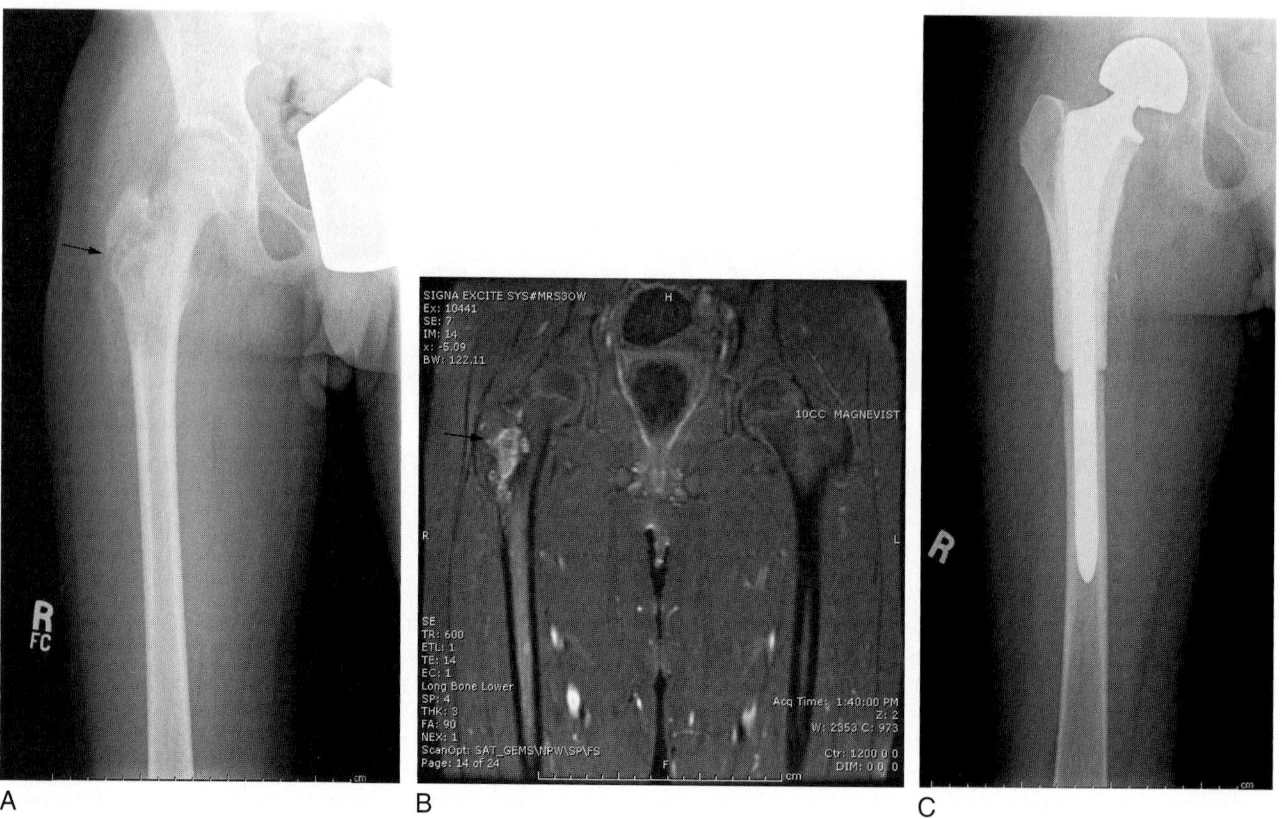

FIGURE 39-15 Sarcoma of the proximal femur in a 13-year-old boy. Appearance of the tumor (*arrows*) on a radiograph (**A**) and magnetic resonance image (**B**). Note the involvement of the abductor insertion on the proximal femur, requiring resection. Allograft prosthetic composite reconstruction (**C**) allows restoration of bone stock and repair of the allograft abductor tendon to the host abductor musculature.

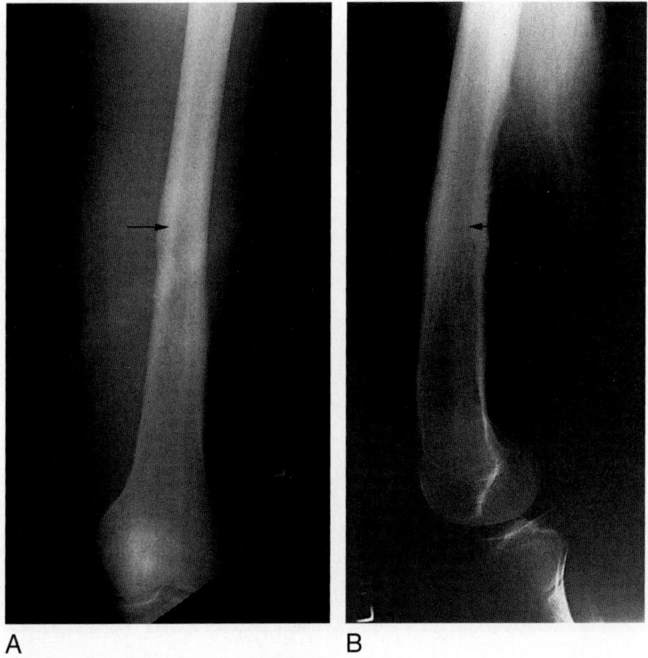

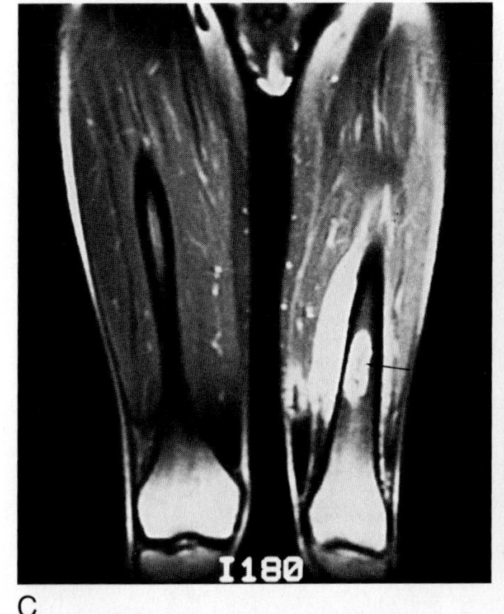

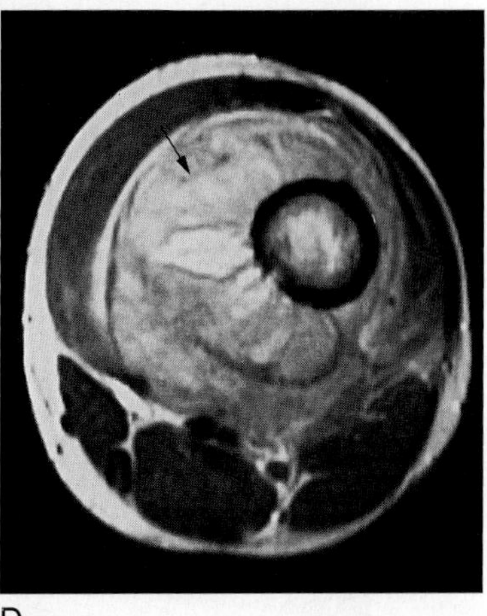

FIGURE 39-16 Ewing's sarcoma or peripheral primitive neuroectodermal tumor (PNET) in a 15-year-old boy. **A,** Anteroposterior radiograph showing a permeative, destructive lesion of the femoral diaphysis (*arrow*). There is a suggestion of a soft tissue mass. **B,** Lateral radiograph. The mass is better seen, and there is erosion of the posterior cortex (*arrow*). **C,** Coronal magnetic resonance image showing the medullary extent of the tumor (*arrow*). **D,** Axial magnetic resonance image showing that a huge soft tissue mass almost completely surrounds the femur (*arrow*). This appearance is typical of Ewing's sarcoma or PNET. Because the tumor does not make tumorous bone or cartilage, there is no mineralization such as that seen in osteosarcoma. A biopsy confirmed the diagnosis of Ewing's sarcoma or PNET.

Continued

Metastatic disease that develops following the completion of chemotherapy usually occurs in the lung. Approximately 30% to 40% of these patients can be salvaged by thoracotomy and resection of the metastases, with or without further chemotherapy.[59,79,135,181,332,492,522,557,573] Sometimes multiple thoracotomies are used with success. More recently, thoracoscopic resections have been performed.[173,266]

Ewing's Sarcoma and Peripheral Primitive Neuroectodermal Tumor

A second primary malignant bone neoplasm in children, composed of primitive, malignant round cells, was named after James Ewing, who first described it as a distinct entity in 1921.[234] He originally named it "diffuse endothelioma" or "endothelial myeloma" in accordance with his belief that it was derived from vasoformative tissue. There has been much debate, however, concerning its pathogenesis. Currently, it is thought that Ewing's sarcoma is part of a family of peripheral primitive neuroectodermal tumors (PNETs) that share a common cytogenetic translocation of chromosomes 11 and 22. There are subtle histologic differences between Ewing's sarcoma and PNET, and both may involve either soft tissue or bone; however, the treatment approaches are the same for both entities. Ewing's sarcoma is poorly differentiated, whereas PNET exhibits definite neural differentiation. There is currently debate about whether one or the other has a better prognosis.[104,199,483] This discussion considers

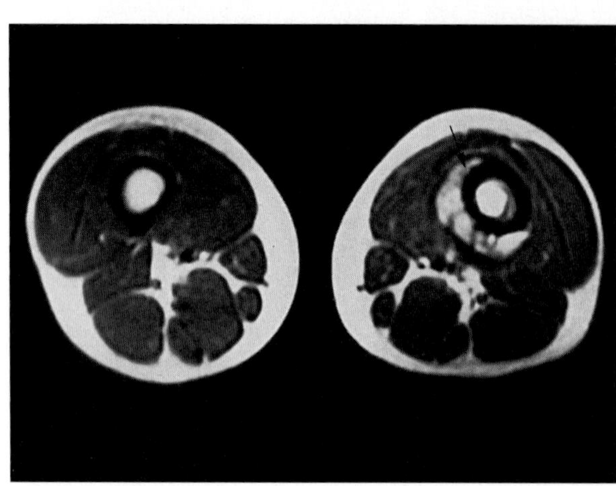
E

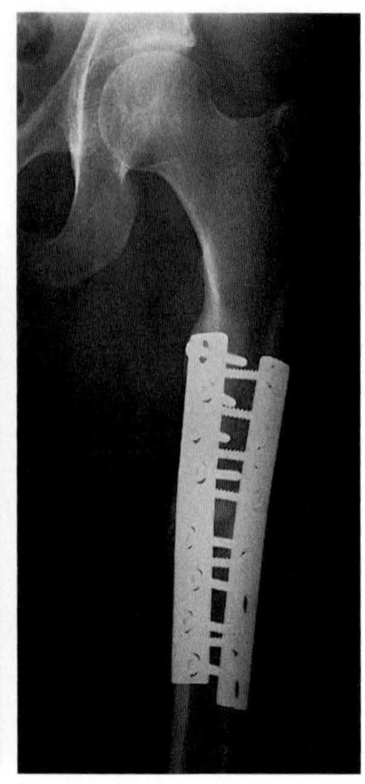
F

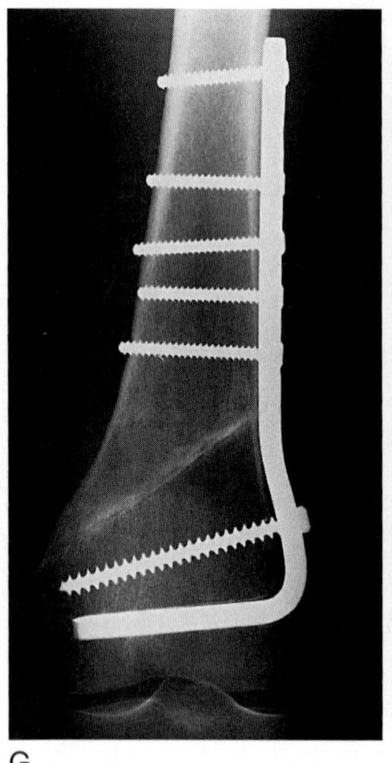
G

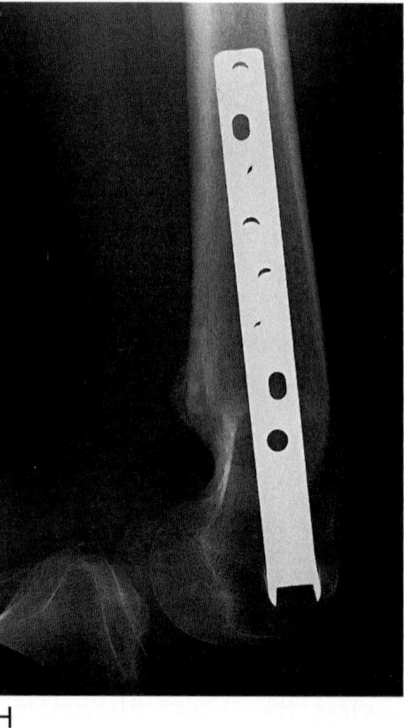
H

FIGURE 39–16 cont'd **E,** Axial magnetic resonance image obtained following induction chemotherapy. There has been considerable reduction in the extent and size of the soft tissue mass (*arrow*). After discussing the alternatives of radiation therapy and surgery for local control, the patient elected to undergo surgical resection. **F** through **H,** Radiographs showing the reconstruction. An intercalary resection with wide margins was performed, and an allograft reconstruction was carried out. Both the hip and the knee joints were preserved. Both osteosyntheses healed, with very good function.

these tumors to be the same entity, although it points out some of the observed differences between them.

Ewing's sarcoma is the second most common primary malignant tumor of bone in children.[188,226,396] It has a predilection for those between 10 and 20 years of age. It is very rarely found in individuals younger than 5 years or older than 30 years. If similar findings are encountered in a child younger than 5 years, neuroblastoma or Wilms' tumor should be considered, whereas if similar findings are encountered in a patient older than the typical age range, lymphoma should be considered. In patients older than 50 years, metastatic carcinoma or myeloma should be considered. Ewing's sarcoma is slightly more common in boys than in girls. It is very rare in black populations in the United States or Africa and in children of Asian origin.[188,226,396]

The most common locations of Ewing's sarcoma or PNET are the pelvis and lower extremity.[273] The sites of disease reported in the large Intergroup Ewing's Sarcoma Study are shown in Table 39–1. The ilium,

Table 39-1 Sites of Ewing's Sarcoma in the Intergroup Ewing's Sarcoma Study

Primary Site	Percentage
Pelvis	20.5
Ilium	12.5
Sacrum	3.3
Ischium	1.7
Pubis	3.0
Lower extremity	45.6
Femur	20.8
Fibula	12.2
Tibia	10.6
Foot	2.0
Upper extremity	12.9
Humerus	10.6
Forearm	2.0
Hand	0.3
Axial skeleton, ribs	11.8
Face	2.3

From Kissane JM, Askin FB, Foulkes M, et al: Ewing's sarcoma of bone: Clinicopathologic aspects of 303 cases from the Intergroup Ewing's Sarcoma Study. Hum Pathol 1983;14:773.

femur, and fibula are common sites; the humerus and tibia are somewhat less so. In the long tubular limb bones, the lesion is more often situated in the diaphysis than in the metaphysis. Ribs are another common site, where the lesion frequently manifests with pneumonia or pleural effusion. Other infrequent sites include the scapula or vertebra. Rarely, the bones of the hands or feet are affected.[84,124,313,480]

PATHOLOGY

On gross inspection, the neoplasm appears as a whitish-gray soft tissue mass that arises in the marrow spaces of the affected bone.[159] Necrotic and hemorrhagic areas in the tumor are frequent. Anatomic involvement of bone is much more extensive than is apparent on radiographs, although MRI reliably demonstrates the extent of bone marrow involvement. The neoplastic tissue destroys and replaces the involved bone. The periosteum is elevated and is often perforated. Nearly always there is a large soft tissue mass extending well beyond the bony boundaries. The tumor is not encapsulated and invades the surrounding muscle. When an innominate bone is involved, the soft tissue mass protrudes into the iliacus, often displacing the pelvic organs toward the midline; laterally, the mass invades the abductor muscles. Not infrequently, the soft tissue mass crosses the sacroiliac joint and invades the adjacent sacrum.

Histologic examination discloses compact sheets of small polyhedral cells with pale cytoplasm and ill-defined boundaries.[103,132,433,481] It is one of a group of tumors referred to as *small round cell tumors.* Ewing's sarcoma or PNET must be distinguished from neuroblastoma, non-Hodgkin's lymphoma, and rhabdomyosarcoma.[535] The nuclei in Ewing's sarcoma are uniform, are round or oval, and contain scattered areas of chromatin (Fig. 39–17). The cytoplasm is scant. There are multiple thin-walled vascular channels among a scant stroma. Reticulin fibers are not a consistent feature of Ewing's sarcoma or PNET. Another distinguishing histochemical finding is the presence of glycogen in the cells of Ewing's sarcoma; in lymphoma, the cells do not contain glycogen. The cytoplasmic material is periodic acid–Schiff positive and diastase digestible, but this finding is not specific for Ewing's sarcoma or PNET. Occasional rosette or pseudorosette formations may be present, and some pathologists view this finding as evidence of PNET.[433]

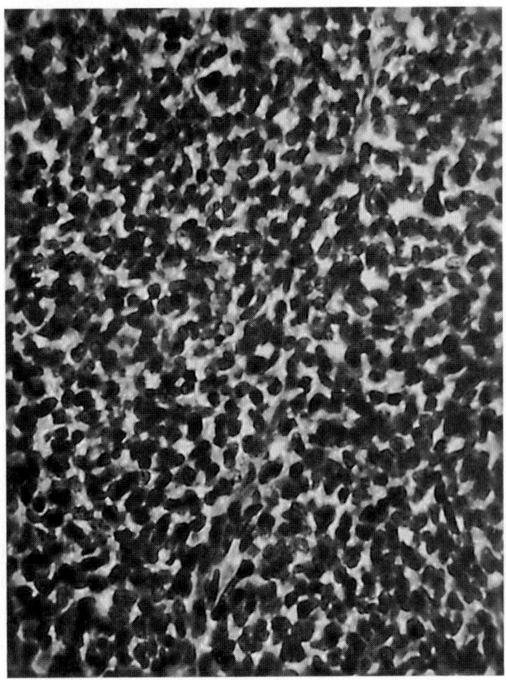

FIGURE 39–17 Histologic findings in Ewing's sarcoma. Photomicrograph shows the round cells, which are polyhedral, with pale cytoplasm and small hyperchromatic nuclei (original magnification ×400).

On light microscopic examination, the cytologic findings may be difficult to differentiate from those of neuroblastoma, lymphoma, or other round cell lesions.[535] Special immunohistochemical stains, electron microscopy, and cytogenetic studies are sometimes necessary to establish the correct diagnosis.* It is important to remember that Ewing's sarcoma is a very primitive tumor and lacks differentiation along any specific mesenchymal lineage, whereas PNET has signs of neural differentiation (S-100, neuron-specific enolase staining, rosettes, and neural elements by electron microscopy).[104] Extensive necrosis may also confuse the picture. Hemorrhage may provoke a

*See references 103, 105, 109, 203, 320, 348, 394, 433, 481, 528, 556.

reparative inflammatory reaction to the tumor, a finding that may be misinterpreted as infection.[129]

Ultrastructural studies have shown small to medium-sized cells, round or polyhedral in shape, with round nuclei, scant membranous organelles, abundant glycogen, absence of filaments, and primitive intercellular junctions.[111,226,229,314]

Monoclonal antibodies (HBA-71 and 12E7) to p30/32MIC2, a cell surface glycoprotein encoded by the *MIC2* gene, have been useful in diagnosing Ewing's sarcoma and PNET.[146] The *MIC2* gene is a pseudoautosomal gene located on the short arms of human chromosomes X and Y. Glycoprotein expression is not specific for these tumors (it is expressed on T cells), but both Ewing's sarcoma and PNET cells express the *MIC2* gene in very high amounts, which helps distinguish them from other round cell tumors.[10] Mesenchymal chondrosarcomas, small cell osteosarcomas, and malignant lymphomas do not routinely express this product. *MIC2* staining should not be relied on as the sole diagnostic criterion because false-negative results can occur in Ewing's sarcoma and related tumors, and positive results can occur in tumors other than PNET.[109,422] In recent studies of Ewing's sarcoma and PNET, 91% to 97% showed a diffuse, strong membranous pattern, suggesting that *MIC2* expression is highly reliable when the results are interpreted in the context of clinical and pathologic parameters.[300,403] Hence, *MIC2* is a useful screen for Ewing's sarcoma and is used routinely in most pathology laboratories.

The most definitive test for Ewing's sarcoma or PNET is demonstration of the chromosomal translocation t(11;22) by karyotyping or reverse transcriptase–polymerase chain reaction (RT-PCR).[19,106,123,156,188,282,300,527] Approximately 80% to 95% of patients with Ewing's sarcoma have a translocation of either chromosomes 11 and 22 or chromosomes 21 and 22.[19,188] The resultant fusion gene is composed of part of the *EWS* gene from chromosome 22 and the *FLY1* gene from chromosome 11 or the *ERG* gene from chromosome 21. The fusion gene is a chimeric transcription factor that retains DNA-binding regions of *FLY1* and allows it to bind to DNA. The resultant gene can transform NIH 3T3 cells in culture, demonstrating that it acts as a dominant oncogene that promotes tumor growth and suggesting that this is a mechanism of carcinogenesis in this tumor.[107,342] The translocation t(11;22) is most common; t(21;22) is the next most common.[498] Rarely, a third translocation, t(7;22), is encountered.[254] Currently, these findings are being used in the diagnosis and staging of Ewing's sarcoma and PNET.[92,539] Rather than performing difficult and time-consuming karyotype analysis, laboratories use RT-PCR to establish the presence of a translocation.[41,156] Correlation with the clinical presentation and with routine histologic and immunohistochemistry studies is necessary, because other tumors may rarely exhibit similar translocations.[499,527]

Interestingly, variability in the presence of these transcripts among patients with Ewing's sarcoma and PNET may be of prognostic significance.[528,560] It is hoped that in the future, vaccines to elicit T-cell immunity with specificity for the tumor-specific fusion peptides in Ewing's sarcoma and PNET can be used as therapy for these tumors and others, such as rhabdomyosarcoma.[19,188,226] Given that these are unique proteins that normal cells do not express, it should be possible to design treatment strategies that target the tumor cell and not the normal cell.

CLINICAL FEATURES

Local pain and swelling are the presenting complaints.[188,226] The pain may be present for months or years before the patient seeks medical attention[25,496]; in one study, 50% of patients had symptoms for 6 months or longer.[419] The delay was less in those with constant symptoms and the presence of a mass, and it did not adversely affect outcome.[496] In the extremities, a tender, local mass is invariably present. Some degree of stiffness of the adjacent joint is common in cases of long-bone involvement, and a limp is usually present. Other symptoms depend on the site of the lesion. When a rib is involved, a pleural effusion may be noted. When the lesion is in the lumbar spine, the nerve roots may be involved, producing symptoms resembling those of disk herniation, such as sciatic pain, tingling sensations, or motor weakness. Rectal and urinary complaints may result when the neoplasm is located in an innominate bone and impinges on pelvic organs or involves the sacral nerve roots. On occasion, the presenting feature is pathologic fracture of an involved femur or tibia.

On physical examination, one can usually palpate a tumor mass (possible in 61% of cases in a Mayo Clinic series)[567] that is tender on pressure. It is larger than the bony lesion seen on radiographs, indicating that the neoplasm has violated the cortex and spread extraosseously into the surrounding soft tissues. In about 20% of cases, the presenting lesion is in some part of the innominate bone.[273] If the pubis or ischium is involved, an irregular globular mass may be palpated on rectal examination; if the ilium is the site of the lesion, a tumor mass may be present in the lower quadrant of the abdomen or in the gluteal region. Pathologic fracture may also be a presenting finding in the case of primary tumor in the long bones (16% in the Mayo Clinic series).[567]

It is important to appreciate that in both osteosarcoma and Ewing's sarcoma or PNET, patients are not systemically ill at presentation and seldom become so until late in the disease. Fever, weight loss, secondary anemia, leukocytosis, and an increase in the ESR are not seen until the disease is advanced. When present, these findings may lead to confusion with osteomyelitis and lymphoma. These findings are hallmarks of a fulminating course and are more likely to be present if there are metastases at diagnosis.[411] LDH levels may be elevated, which was shown to correlate with a worse prognosis in some studies.[177,321]

RADIOGRAPHIC FINDINGS

The radiographic appearance is fairly characteristic but not pathognomonic (see Figs. 39–16A and B, 39–18 to 39–20). It is typically described as a permeative lesion with mottled rarefaction of the medullary cavity and invasion through the overlying cortex, reflecting rapid bone destruction. The bone at the site of the lesion may show some enlargement. Periosteal new bone formation, often of the laminated "onion-peel" type, is common but not specific for Ewing's sarcoma.[5,188,226,245] A soft tissue mass adjacent to the area of bone destruction is frequently seen on radiographs, indicating that the neoplasm has perforated the cortex and spread to the adjacent soft tissues. In the long bones, the lesion is frequently diaphyseal in location, and involvement is extensive. Pathologic fractures are uncommon[567] and may occur at presentation or later in the disease, which portends a poorer prognosis and may suggest recurrence or a second malignancy.[554]

The radiographic findings resemble those of histiocytosis, lymphoma, osteosarcoma, metastatic neuroblastoma, Wilms' tumor, leukemia, and osteomyelitis.[228,245] MRI may only add to the confusion, because the inflammatory reaction around the bone and the medullary extent of histiocytosis may be extensive and mimic the findings of Ewing's sarcoma, although it is usually possible to make the distinction.[206]

STAGING

The staging of Ewing's sarcoma and PNET is similar to that for osteosarcoma, although there are no specific staging systems for the former tumors.[136,139,188,228,490] MRI is useful to determine the extent of the lesion within the bone and adjacent soft tissue (see Fig. 39–16C through E).[54,206,231,240] In general, tumor involvement of the bone marrow is best assessed on T1-weighted sequences, and tumor involvement of the soft tissue is best seen on T2-weighted sequences. Although it may be inferior to CT for assessing cortical destruction, MRI is very helpful in assessing the extent of bone marrow involvement, soft tissue tumor extent, and relationship of tumor to neurovascular structures.[54,251] Because Ewing's sarcoma and PNET may extend throughout the entire medullary cavity, and

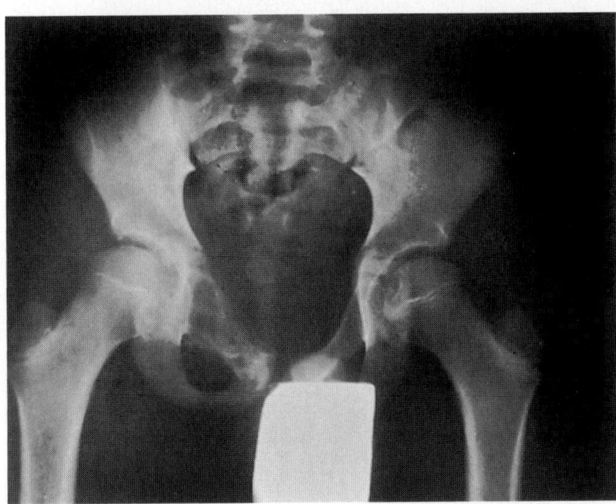

A

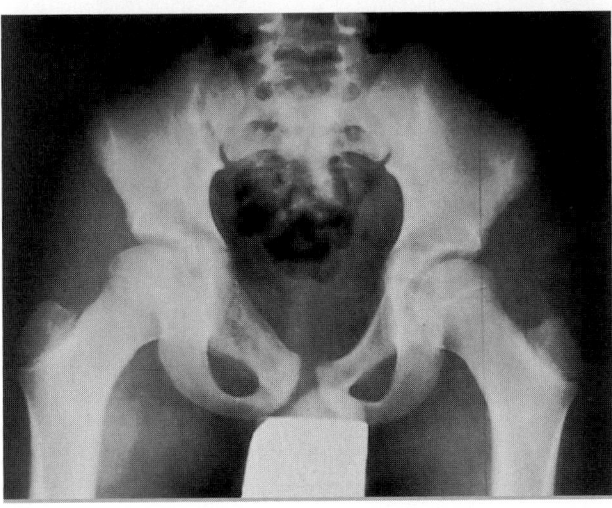

B

FIGURE 39–18 Ewing's sarcoma of the right pubis. **A,** Initial radiograph. Treatment consisted of irradiation and chemotherapy. **B,** Nine months later, some healing is apparent. However, the disease metastasized, and the patient died a year later.

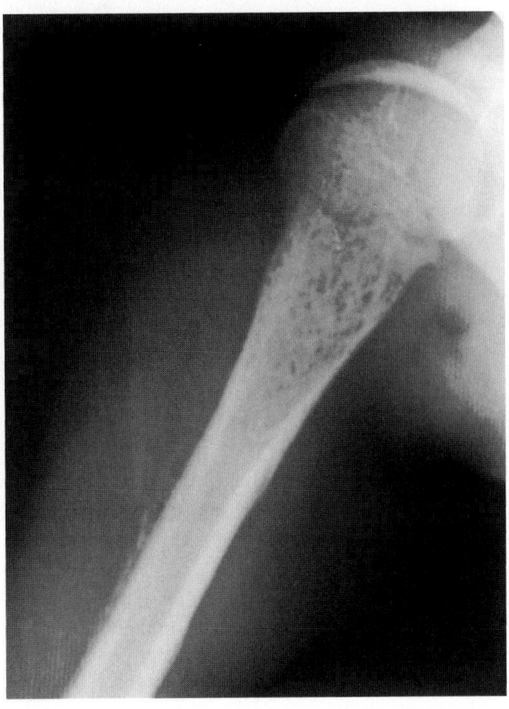

FIGURE 39–19 Ewing's sarcoma of the humerus. Note the mottled areas of rarefaction and subperiosteal reaction.

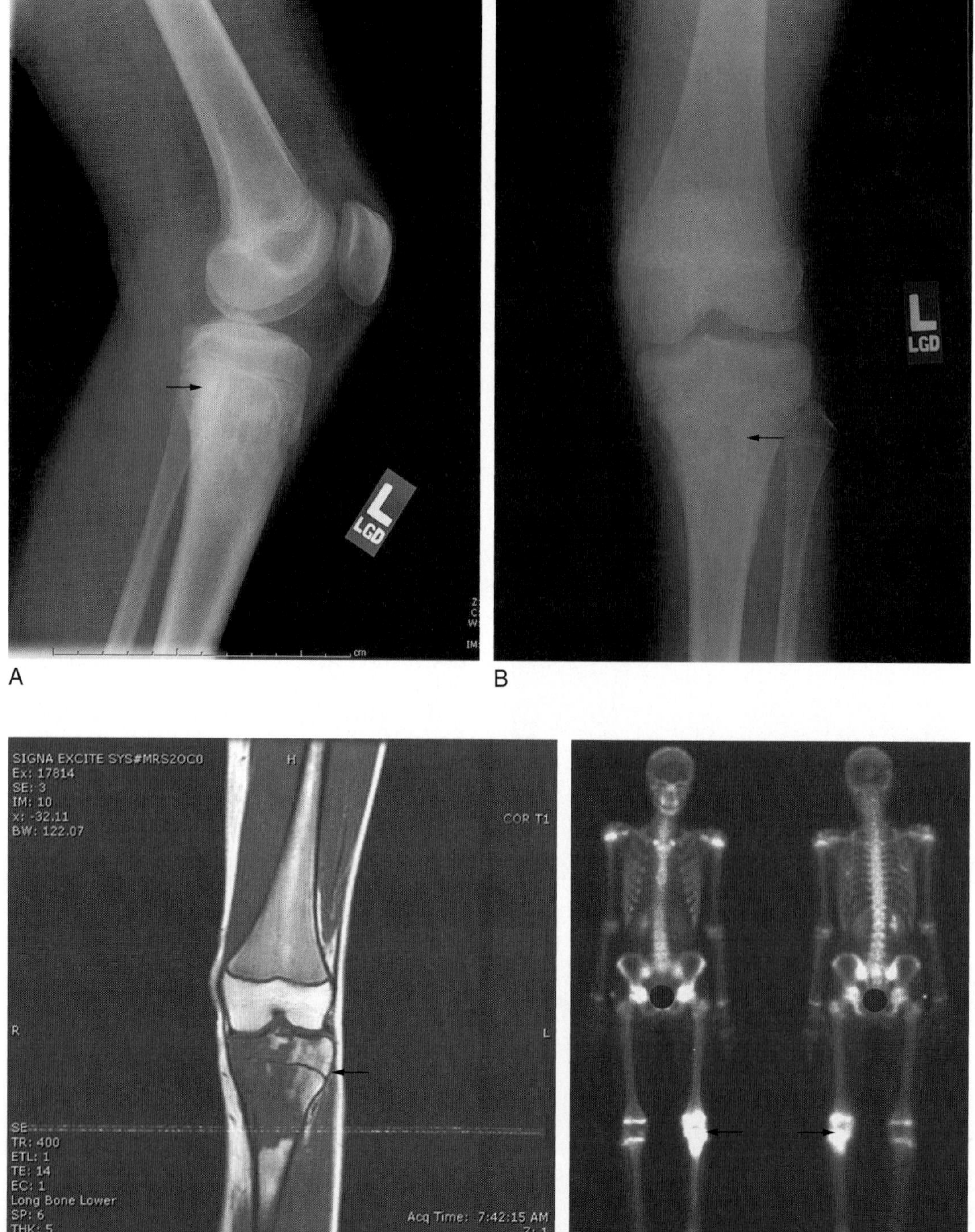

FIGURE 39–20 Ewing's sarcoma of the proximal tibia in a 9-year-old girl. **A** and **B,** Mottled areas of rarefaction are seen in the proximal tibia (*arrows*). **C,** Appearance of the lesion on magnetic resonance imaging (*arrow*), allowing a determination of the bony extent of the tumor. **D,** Bone scan demonstrating uptake in the proximal tibia (*arrows*). In this case, there is uptake in the distal femur as well.

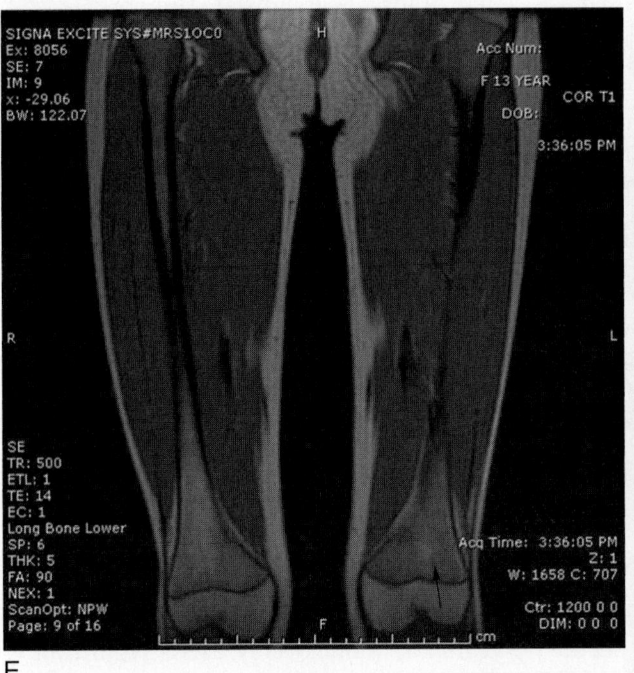

E

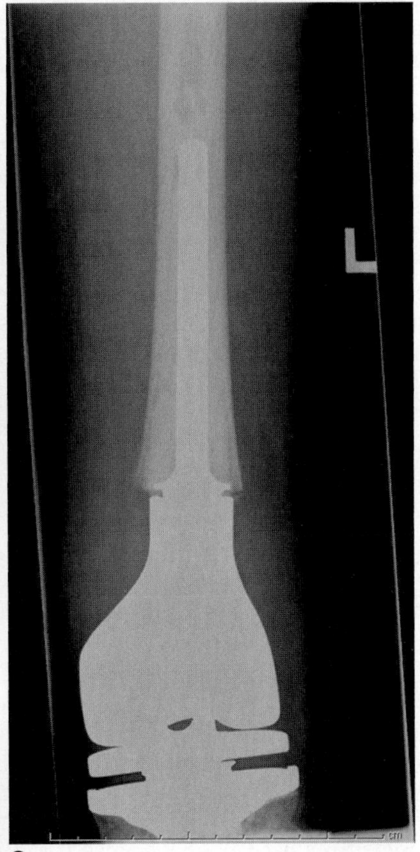

G

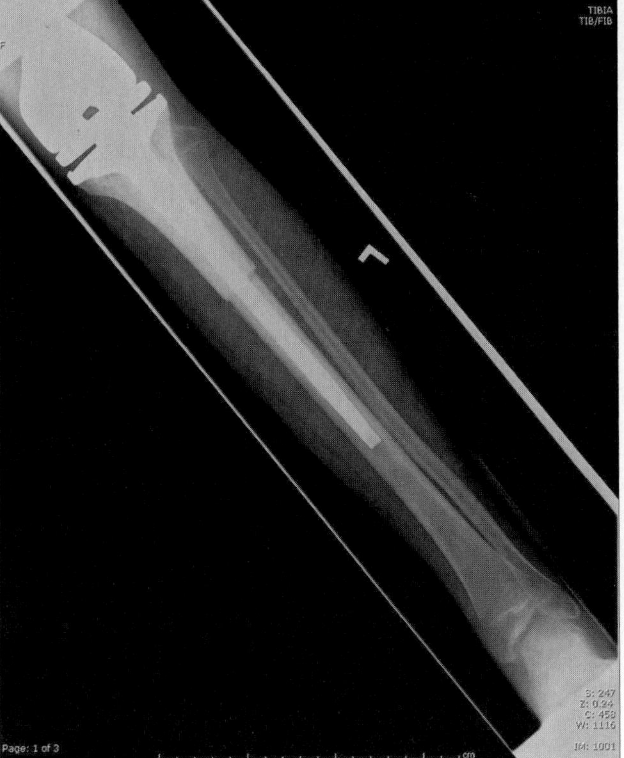

F

FIGURE 39–20 cont'd **E,** Magnetic resonance image demonstrates signal abnormality in the distal femur (*arrow*), corresponding to the uptake seen on the bone scan. **F** and **G,** Allograft prosthetic composite reconstruction allowed resection of the proximal tibia and distal femur and reconstruction of the extensor mechanism with allograft–to–host patellar tendon repair.

skip metastases may rarely be present, the whole bone should be imaged by MRI.[251,514] Subtraction techniques and dynamic MRI have made it possible to use this modality to assess the response to chemotherapy,[207,223,305] although this may not be as predictive of outcome as initial tumor volume.[359]

Metastatic disease is present at diagnosis in approximately 25% of patients.[188,226] Approximately 50% of patients who present with metastases have pulmonary involvement, approximately 25% have bony metastases, and about 20% have bone marrow involvement.[68,409] Liver and lymph node metastases are rare. CT is performed to search for metastatic disease in the chest. A bone scan is obtained to search for other areas of bone involvement or skip metastases. A bone marrow biopsy specimen is obtained to look for detectable disease in the marrow. Most of the time this can be accomplished by light microscopy,[297] but recently, RT-PCR techniques have been used to look for bone marrow and peripheral blood cells that amplify EWS/HumFLI1.[123,560]

BIOPSY

The definitive diagnosis is made from histologic study of tissue sections obtained at open or needle biopsy.[402,488,490] Until recently, an open biopsy was usually done to establish the diagnosis, but needle biopsy or fine-needle aspiration has proved to be useful in many cases.[92,539] When an open biopsy is selected, the usual precautions of avoiding neurovascular structures and creating a longitudinal incision that can be included with the resected specimen are followed. In Ewing's sarcoma, it is best to avoid making a cortical defect in a long bone, because if radiation is chosen for local control, the chances of pathologic fracture are greater.[502] It is crucial that the surgeon obtain a frozen section and review it with the pathologist to ensure that adequate tissue is obtained for histologic, immunohistochemical, and sometimes cytogenetic studies. The histologic differential diagnosis of these small round cell tumors includes neuroblastoma, rhabdomyosarcoma, malignant lymphoma, small cell osteosarcoma, Wilms' tumor, desmoplastic small cell tumor,[484] histiocytosis, and osteomyelitis. Needle biopsy is especially useful in sites that are difficult to access surgically (e.g., vertebral bodies), but adequate amounts of tissue must be obtained for immunohistochemistry, cytogenetics, and culture. Radiographic guidance should be used (unless there is a large palpable mass) to ensure that the specimen is taken from the correct site. Frozen sections are also advisable to ensure that representative tissue has been obtained. Tumor necrosis may make the tissue appear to be a purulent exudate and lead to confusion of Ewing's sarcoma or PNET with osteomyelitis.

PROGNOSIS

In the past, the outlook for patients with Ewing's sarcoma or PNET was uniformly poor, with an overall 10% 5-year survival rate.[34,188,226,419] With the advent of adjuvant chemotherapy and proper local control, the outlook is considerably better, with recent studies showing 5-year and event-free survival rates of approximately 50% to 60%.[188,226] Patients with large central lesions, especially in the pelvis, have a worse outcome than those with distal tumors.[71,99,159,222,308,468,580] The regimen usually includes doxorubicin (Adriamycin), cyclophosphamide (Cytoxan), vincristine, and actinomycin D, although actinomycin D has now been dropped from most treatment protocols, without apparent adverse results, because of concern about toxicity. More recently, it has been shown that a five-drug regimen that adds ifosfamide and etoposide increases the event-free and overall survival in patients with Ewing's sarcoma or PNET. Obviously, patients who present with metastases at diagnosis, especially bony metastases, have a poorer outcome.[14,46,68,399,400,449,525,552] In one large study, the event-free survival rate for patients who presented with metastases 4 years after diagnosis was 27% overall. The site of metastasis affected the outcome; the event-free survival rate was 34% for patients with isolated lung metastases, 28% for those with bone or bone marrow metastases, and 14% for those with combined lung and bone or bone marrow metastases ($P = .005$).[68]

Other factors that portend a poorer prognosis are large tumor volume,[6,222,260,453] size greater than 8 cm,[211] elevated LDH level,[14,177,272,585] and age older than 17 years.[188,201] Controversy exists regarding whether the designation of Ewing's sarcoma versus PNET is related to prognosis. In some studies, PNET had a worse prognosis, whereas in others, it had the same or a better prognosis.[210,461,524]

TREATMENT

Nonmetastatic Ewing's Sarcoma

The treatment of patients with nonmetastatic Ewing's sarcoma consists of the administration of multiagent chemotherapy and efforts to achieve local control.

Chemotherapy. Ewing's sarcoma and PNET tumors are systemic diseases with a very poor prognosis when treated by local measures alone.[34,188,226,419] Beginning in the 1960s, it was shown that adjuvant chemotherapy offered a survival benefit in these patients.[248,272,411,440] The standard chemotherapy regimens include vincristine, doxorubicin, cyclophosphamide, and (in the past) actinomycin D (VDCA)[58,370]; as noted earlier, the addition of ifosfamide and etoposide has been shown to offer an additional benefit in some but not all studies.[188,226,261,374] To test this observation, the Pediatric Oncology Group and the Children's Cancer Group carried out a randomized study comparing the standard VDCA regimen with the standard regimen plus ifosfamide and etoposide. They found that the addition of ifosfamide and etoposide was associated with significantly better 5-year relapse-free survival compared with VDCA alone (69% versus 54%) in patients with nonmetastatic Ewing's sarcoma or PNET.[189] Overall survival was also significantly better among patients in the experimental therapy group than in the standard therapy group (72% versus 61%; $P = .01$). In that study, patients with metastatic disease failed to demonstrate a similar benefit from the additional drugs. A similar outcome was shown with a slightly different regimen in two other single-institution studies.[150,275] Four to six cycles of chemotherapy are given before local control. Clinical response to preoperative chemotherapy is indicated by a decrease in tumor size, drop in LDH level, and tumor necrosis in the resected specimen.[406] Postoperatively, additional cycles of the same treatment are given, and the total duration of therapy is approximately 48 weeks. It is a very toxic regimen, but it offers significant survival benefits to these patients. Recent focus has been on intensifying therapy early in the course of treatment, either by using higher doses of standard drugs or by decreasing the interval between chemotherapy cycles.[432]

Radiation Therapy. Radiation therapy has traditionally been used to treat local disease. This treatment became established partly because the tumor responds to radiotherapy and partly because before chemotherapy was available, physicians were reluctant to perform amputation in patients with such a dismal prognosis. Radiation therapy effectively controls local disease, especially when combined with chemotherapy. The usual dose is 55.8 to 60 Gy to the affected tissues,[117,128,337,511,521,523] and adequate dosages result in local control in 53% to 86% of cases. Attempts to lower the radiation dose when this modality is combined with chemotherapy have not been successful.[211] Initially, it was thought that the entire bone should be irradiated because of the difficulty in judging the medullary extent; however, because MRI can accurately demonstrate the extent of disease, this is no longer the case. A study by the Pediatric Oncology Group showed no difference in local control when the initial tumor volume plus a 2-cm margin was treated compared with whole-bone irradiation.[120] The local recurrence rate in patients with small, distal tumors is reported to be 10% or less, but in those with large, bulky tumors (e.g., pelvic tumors), it may be 30% or more.[17,55,211,429,523] In young children with lower extremity primary tumors, growth is a consideration.[253,307] Irradiation of one or more growth plates in the lower extremity can lead to significant limb length inequality in young children (Fig. 39–21). In patients in whom the biopsy created a hole in the cortex, pathologic fracture may be a significant problem (Fig. 39–22).[100,253,502] Despite internal fixation and bone grafting, union of these fractures is difficult to obtain in irradiated bone. Vascularized fibular grafts may be necessary.[126]

Perhaps the most concerning adverse effect of radiation therapy (combined with alkylating agents) is the late occurrence of a secondary malignancy in the involved bone. This phenomenon was not observed until relatively recently, because most patients died from their disease; however, now that patients are surviving longer, secondary malignancies have become a significant concern. The exact incidence is unknown, but secondary malignancies are believed to occur in 5% to 30% of survivors treated with alkylating agents and radiation therapy.[15,30,187,285,494,509,538]

Surgical Treatment. Concern about secondary neoplasms and the observation in some studies that surgically treated patients have a better prognosis have led treating physicians to reconsider surgical ablation of the primary tumor. Techniques of limb salvage learned from treating osteosarcoma have been applied successfully to patients with Ewing's sarcoma. With adequate chemotherapy, the soft tissue mass usually shrinks considerably (unlike osteosarcoma), making it possible to resect less tissue than might be anticipated at initial presentation (see Fig. 39–16). The obvious advantage is the avoidance of secondary neoplasms. Local control rates appear to be equal to or better than those obtained with radiation therapy. Many studies have shown that the outcome is superior in patients whose primary tumors are resected, but it should be noted that none of these studies were randomized, and patients whose tumors become resectable after preoperative chemotherapy probably have other favorable prognostic factors in addition to the resection.* In other studies, patients who underwent surgical resection did not have a survival advantage when retrospectively compared with patients whose primary tumors were treated by radiation therapy alone.[127,468]

The relative functional results are even more difficult to compare. Each modality has advantages and disadvantages in that regard. Radiation therapy has the advantage of obviating the surgical resection of major bones and muscles, but advances in limb salvage have made it possible to perform resection and functional reconstruction in many of these patients. Resection offers the ability to assess the histologic response to preoperative chemotherapy. As in osteosarcoma, it appears that histologic necrosis following preoperative chemotherapy is a good measure of response and prognosis.[7,14,405,406,547,577]

One area of considerable concern is the pelvis. Resection of the iliac wing with preservation of the acetabulum offers reasonably good function, but when the acetabulum must be resected, a satisfactory functional reconstruction is nearly impossible to obtain. Obviously, if it were clear that the outcome were superior with resection than with irradiation, one would sacrifice function, but the results are not clear. There are no randomized studies of surgery versus radiation therapy in the pelvis or elsewhere. Some studies have shown an improvement with resection of pelvic Ewing's sarcoma or PNET[99,159,580]; others have shown no benefit.[71,468] One recent study from the Children's Oncology Group showed no difference in event-free survival or overall survival when surgery alone or surgery plus radiation was compared with radiation alone for pelvic primary tumors.[581] The local treatment was not randomized, and this was a retrospective review of local control. Thus, the decision of which modality or combination of modalities to use for local

*See references 14, 178, 334, 375, 417-419, 447, 531, 532, 567.

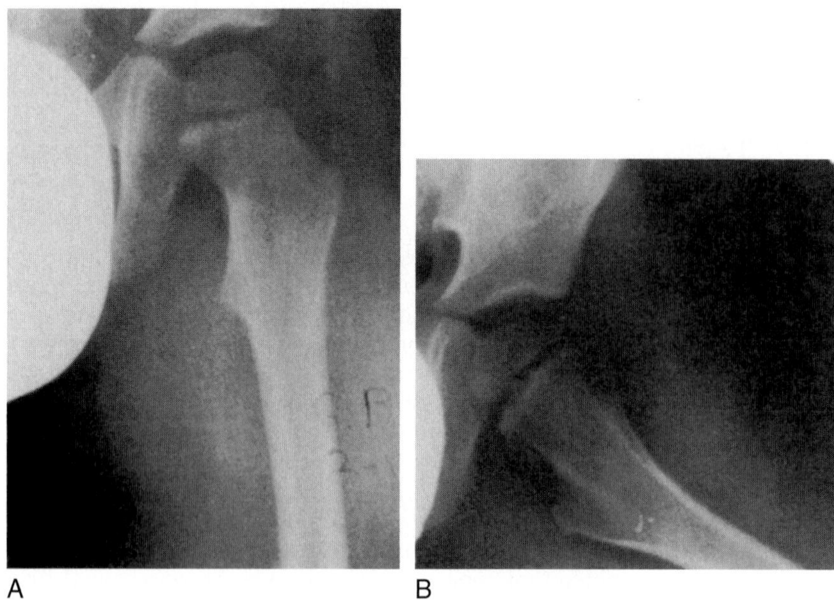

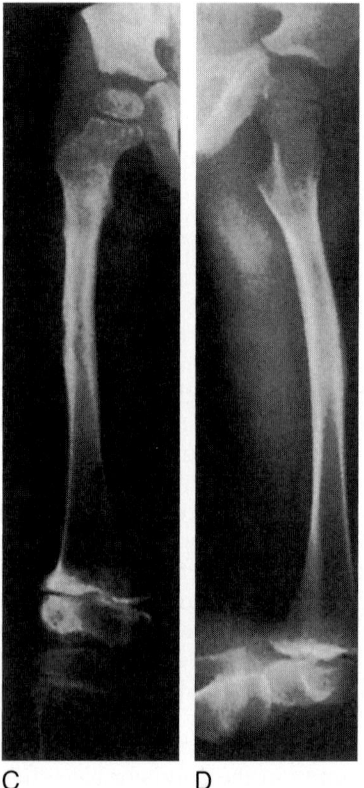

FIGURE 39–21 Ewing's sarcoma of the proximal femur in a 5-year-old boy. Anteroposterior **(A)** and lateral **(B)** radiographs of the proximal femur showing subperiosteal reaction and mottling of the outer cortex. **C** and **D,** Immediate postradiation radiographs.

control of pelvic Ewing's sarcoma or PNET is difficult and requires careful consideration by the treatment team, as well as discussions with the patient and family.

Local control is best delivered after induction chemotherapy, which often decreases the size of the soft tissue mass. Induction chemotherapy may make resection possible or avoid the need for postoperative radiation therapy.[473] The approach used at our institution is to completely restage the patient following the induction phase of chemotherapy. If there has been a good response and if resection can be carried out with a reasonable expectation of negative margins and a good functional result, surgical resection is advised. Both radiation therapy and surgery are discussed with all patients, and they are offered the choice. We believe that the main advantage of resection is the avoidance of secondary malignancies. Margins and histologic

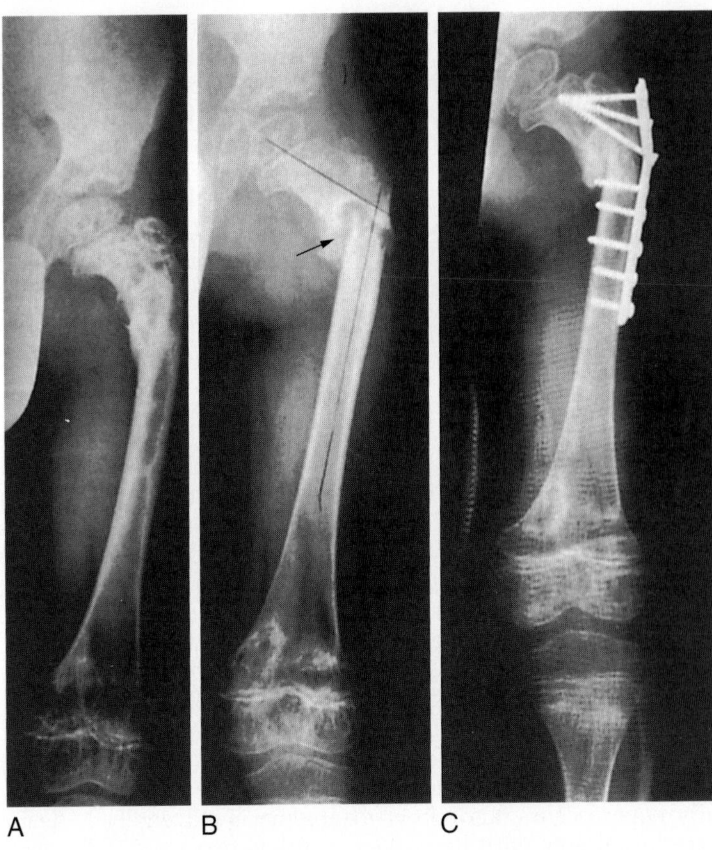

FIGURE 39–22 Subtrochanteric pathologic fracture in Ewing's sarcoma of the proximal femur treated by internal fixation with plate and screws. **A,** Prefracture radiograph showing the sclerosis and radiolucent changes in bone. **B,** Anteroposterior radiograph of the femur showing the subtrochanteric pathologic fracture (*arrow*). **C,** Postoperative anteroposterior radiograph showing internal fixation with plate and screws.

necrosis in the resected specimen are examined, and if the margins are widely negative or negative with a good histologic response, no further local control is advised. If the margin is positive, postoperative radiation therapy is advised, but the dose is lower than if the patient were treated with radiation therapy alone. Patients with tumors in "expendable" bones, such as the fibula, clavicle, and ribs, do not undergo reconstruction. Patients with primary tumors in major long bones undergo reconstructions similar to those used in osteosarcoma patients.

Patients with a poor histologic response, especially those with very close or positive margins, are advised to receive radiation therapy postoperatively. Patients with large, bulky tumors after induction chemotherapy, especially pelvic tumors, are usually advised to receive radiation therapy and are then reassessed for the possibility of resection. Patients with tumors in sites where resection would be functionally devastating or impossible (e.g., sacrum, spine) or those with widespread metastatic disease are usually treated by irradiation for control of the bony disease. Those with periacetabular lesions are often treated by radiation therapy because of the lack of a good reconstruction option for this site and the absence of a demonstrably better outcome with resection.[468]

Amputation is considered in very young patients with lower extremity primary tumors, especially about the knee, where irradiation would result in growth arrest and limb length discrepancy. Other indications for amputation include pathologic fractures and bulky tumors that do not respond to chemotherapy and irradiation.[110,303,510]

Metastatic Ewing's Sarcoma and Peripheral Primitive Neuroectodermal Tumor

Patients who present with metastatic disease have a significantly worse prognosis, with expected survival rates of approximately 25% at 5 years.[46,68,284] Those with isolated pulmonary metastases fare better than those with metastases elsewhere. In a recent study, 120 patients with metastatic Ewing's sarcoma or PNET of bone were entered into a randomized trial evaluating whether the addition of ifosfamide and etoposide to vincristine, doxorubicin, cyclophosphamide, and actinomycin D would improve outcome. Treatment comprised 9 weeks of chemotherapy before local control and 42 weeks of chemotherapy afterward. The event-free survival and survival at 8 years were 20% and 32%, respectively, for those treated with the standard drug regimen, and 20% and 29%, respectively, for those who received ifosfamide and etoposide as well. Patients who had only lung metastases fared better, with event-free survival and survival rates of 32% and 41%, respectively, at 8 years. Thus, adding ifosfamide and etoposide to standard therapy did not improve the outcome in patients with metastases at diagnosis.[46]

Current treatment strategies involve dose intensification of known active drugs, stem cell transplantation, and trials that involve novel chemotherapeutic agents,[20,57,89,409,505,552,562] but the results of these strategies are mixed. The primary tumor is usually treated by irradiation, but when there are pulmonary metastases only and a good response to chemotherapy (i.e., pulmonary metastases disappear), it is not unreasonable to consider resection of the primary tumor if a functional reconstruction is possible. The role of thoracotomy is unclear in these patients,[22,218,290] but pulmonary irradiation appears to play a beneficial role in those with metastatic disease.[128]

CHONDROSARCOMA

Chondrosarcoma occurs primarily in adults; it is encountered rarely in adolescents and almost never in children.[16,237,293,582] The diagnosis of a high-grade chondrosarcoma on frozen section in an adolescent should raise the suspicion of chondroblastic osteosarcoma. There are four types of chondrosarcoma: primary, secondary, mesenchymal, and dedifferentiated.[501] The great majority of cases are primary or secondary chondrosarcoma; the mesenchymal and dedifferentiated types are rare.[90,219] The concern of the pediatric orthopaedist is to distinguish a benign enchondroma or osteochondroma from a secondary chondrosarcoma.[16,164,350] Chondrosarcoma arising from a solitary osteochondroma or enchondroma in childhood virtually never occurs, and chondrosarcoma is extremely rare in patients with hereditary multiple exostosis.[582] The literature is confusing on this subject, however, and the conclusions of pediatric centers differ from those of adult cancer centers in this regard. The reported 25% incidence of malignant degeneration in hereditary multiple osteocartilaginous exostosis is probably a gross overestimation. Malignant transformation is extremely unusual in hereditary multiple exostosis, and several large pediatric series failed to show evidence of this occurrence.[304,460,566] Chondrosarcoma does occur with increased frequency in patients with Ollier's and Maffucci's syndromes but is rare in the pediatric age group.[69,465,512] Maffucci's syndrome patients are also subject to malignancies in other organ systems.

It may be challenging to differentiate benign from malignant cartilage tumors, and there are no fail-safe guidelines, but in general, the clinician should be more concerned about large central lesions and those that enlarge after skeletal maturity. Pelvic cartilage tumors, although rare in childhood, are the most likely to be malignant; in extremity lesions, a metaphyseal cartilage tumor about the knee is the most likely to be malignant. In such cases, the presenting complaint is a dull aching pain in the centrally located chondrosarcoma; the clinical picture of a peripheral chondrosarcoma is a mass or deformity of the limb. Nonetheless, malignant cartilage tumors at any site are rare in children.

PATHOLOGY

On gross inspection, chondrosarcoma has a lobulated appearance and seems to consist of gray, unmineralized cartilage intermixed with chalky white cartilage. It feels firm on palpation. There may be areas of necrosis and degeneration.

The histologic appearance varies with the grade of the lesion and requires the expertise of an experienced bone pathologist.[140,174,237,360,501,582] In low-grade lesions, the cell-to-matrix ratio is low (i.e., relatively more matrix than cells), with the malignant chondrocytes grouped in small clusters among wide areas of chondroid matrix.[327] Malignant chondrocytes with double nuclei are a feature of chondrosarcoma. In high-grade lesions, the cell-to-matrix ratio is high, with no clustering pattern; the hyperchromatic chondrocytes are multinuclear and show numerous mitoses. When a biopsy shows such an area in an enostotic lesion, more tissue should be obtained to look for the presence of neoplastic bone. In the vast majority of cases, a high-grade chondrosarcoma in a child is really a chondroblastic osteosarcoma, and this becomes evident when the entire specimen is available for review. In our opinion, these patients should be treated with adjuvant chemotherapy, as for any osteosarcoma.

RADIOGRAPHIC FINDINGS

Radiographic features of a secondary chondrosarcoma show evidence of the preexisting benign cartilaginous lesion—exostosis or enchondroma. These entities are described elsewhere (see Chapter 38, Benign Musculoskeletal Tumors). In exostotic lesions, sarcomatous proliferation of the cartilage cells occurs from the cartilaginous cap that extends and protrudes into the surrounding soft tissues.[164,373] Calcifications of the cartilaginous cap may be present. Septal enhancement on MRI after the intravenous administration of gadopentetate dimeglumine aids in the characterization of cartilaginous tumors and may assist in distinguishing low-grade chondrosarcoma from osteochondroma.[170] The process is indolent, and the sarcomas are usually of low grade. It is important to understand that benign osteochondromas can become large and grow during the years of skeletal maturity without having malignant features. We do not advise removing a solitary osteochondroma to "prevent" malignancy; rather, they are removed when symptoms occur. An exception may be a pelvic osteochondroma. Enchondromas are much less commonly encountered in children (probably because they are completely asymptomatic).

In the rare exostotic chondrosarcoma, radiographs show an irregular cartilaginous mass with calcification of varying density around the periphery of the exostosis and minimal or no permeative reaction of the underlying cortex. Some authors use the thickness of the cartilaginous cap as a guide to malignancy,[338,373] but it is the histology of the cap, not the thickness, that dictates whether it is a chondrosarcoma. It may be difficult to distinguish a sessile osteochondroma or a periosteal chondroma from a periosteal osteosarcoma or chondrosarcoma. Perhaps the best guideline is that a sessile chondrosarcoma would be very rare in childhood; in addition, it shares a cortex with the underlying bone, and the medullary cavities communicate. A periosteal osteosarcoma does not have these features; the underlying cortex is present, indicating that this is a juxtacortical neoplasm. Similarly, a periosteal chondrosarcoma has an underlying cortex and is a surface lesion. It is sometimes difficult to distinguish a periosteal chondroma from a periosteal osteosarcoma.

A central chondrosarcoma, which may arise in the area of a preexisting enchondroma, has radiographic features indicative of its malignant character.[175,501] These features include medullary radiolucency, poorly marginated bone destruction, and the presence of a soft tissue mass that may be variably mineralized. Endosteal scalloping with gradual erosion or widening and thickening of the cortex occurs. The preexisting enchondroma is usually mineralized, whereas the malignant area is radiolucent. The cortex may respond with endosteal and periosteal thickening, which may mask the malignant nature of the lesion.

MRI and CT are useful in assessing the cartilaginous nature of these lesions and their soft tissue and medullary extent.[442] Osteochondromas with large bursae can mimic chondrosarcoma; MRI is particularly useful in making this distinction.[416,553] A radionuclide bone scan shows increased uptake and is not helpful for the primary lesion,[346] but it does demonstrate other lesions in patients suspected of having Ollier's syndrome or multiple exostoses. Radionuclide scintigraphy is not helpful in distinguishing benign from malignant cartilage neoplasms, but if a patient is followed by sequential bone scans, an increase in uptake may be a worrisome sign.[140] A lesion that does not exhibit marked uptake is a reassuring sign. Chest CT is needed to search for pulmonary metastases from high-grade cartilage tumors, but these lesions are most likely to be chondroblastic osteosarcomas.

TREATMENT

True chondrosarcomas are treated by surgical resection.[140,301,501] For low-grade lesions this should be sufficient, and there is a high probability of cure. There has been some movement recently to consider aggressive curettage, local adjuvants, and graft or cement packing of low-grade chondrosarcomas of the extremity. This less aggressive approach is predicated on the difficulty of distinguishing benign from low-grade malignant cartilage tumors radiographically and histologically.[154] Some believe that we have overtreated these lesions using resection in the past and that a more limited excision runs the potential risk of local recurrence but not metastasis. Clear data to support or refute this concept are lacking, and experience and judgment must be used to decide between these two treatment approaches (curettage versus resection).

High-grade lesions are probably best treated like high-grade osteosarcomas. Limb salvage resection or amputation following neoadjuvant chemotherapy is the proper management. In the very rare case of a true high-grade chondrosarcoma, surgical ablation with wide margins is the most reasonable treatment. The role of chemotherapy in these cases is not well established, but chemotherapy is used in patients with "unresectable" primary lesions or metastatic disease.[16,125,140,269,301]

SOFT TISSUE SARCOMAS

Soft tissue sarcomas in children are much less common than benign soft tissue lesions, but the two can be difficult to distinguish. The most common soft tissue sarcoma in childhood is rhabdomyosarcoma;[19,395,516,561] the other soft tissue sarcomas are much less common than in adults.

Rhabdomyosarcoma

Rhabdomyosarcomas account for 4% of malignant tumors in children 15 years of age or younger. The incidence is between 4 and 7 per 1 million children, and approximately 250 new cases are diagnosed annually in the United States.[281,561] Rhabdomyosarcoma occurs in both the first and second decades of life. Boys are affected slightly more often than girls, and black and Asian children have a lower incidence than white children.[506,507] Rhabdomyosarcoma can occur in all parts of the body, including the head and neck (26% of cases), orbit (9%), mediastinum and abdomen (22%), genitourinary system (24%), and extremities (19%).[391,561] This discussion focuses on extremity rhabdomyosarcoma.

PATHOLOGY

Rhabdomyosarcomas are histologically classified into embryonal, alveolar, botryoid, and pleomorphic types.[116,371,537] Although embryonal rhabdomyosarcoma is the predominant form overall in children, it accounts for only about half of extremity lesions.[371] The other histologic type in the extremity and trunk is alveolar rhabdomyosarcoma. The distinction between alveolar and embryonal rhabdomyosarcoma is difficult but may not be as important as other prognostic factors in extremity lesions.[292] In general, embryonal rhabdomyosarcoma has a much more favorable prognosis than alveolar rhabdomyosarcoma, and the latter is more likely to have lymph node metastases.[213]

On histologic analysis, alveolar rhabdomyosarcomas are round cell tumors with few distinguishing characteristics. Large cells with eosinophilic cytoplasm, some of which may contain muscle striations, are seen. Immunohistochemistry stains reveal the expression of muscle-specific actin and myosin, desmin, myoglobin, Z-band protein, Myo-D, and vimentin to distinguish the muscle phenotype.[116,393,537] Unlike in Ewing's sarcoma and PNET, *MIC2* expression is not seen.[188,386,537]

The alveolar variety of rhabdomyosarcoma is distinguished by its obvious alveolar pattern, similar to alveoli in the lung, but they are lined by large, high-grade tumor cells. The cells are round and densely packed rather than spindled and loosely dispersed in a matrix, as in the embryonal variety.[561] Alveolar rhabdomyosarcoma has been demonstrated to have a translocation of chromosomes 2 and 13, t(2;13)(q35;q14), and, less commonly, t(1;13)(p36;q14), which can be helpful in making the diagnosis.[19,101,390,477] The novel gene products of these translocations are being explored as possible antigens for specific immunotherapy for rhabdomyosarcoma. Other mutations in oncogenes or tumor suppressor genes such as *p53* and overproduction of *IGFII* have been identified and may be of importance in the pathogenesis of rhabdomyosarcoma.[19,561]

Embryonal rhabdomyosarcoma is a spindle cell sarcoma with an abundant myxoid stroma that separates the tumor cells. This histotype has a loss of heterozygosity on chromosome 11 at the 11p15 locus.[19,466,467] The exact significance of this deletion is unclear, but it involves loss of maternal chromosomal information, possibly leading to overexpression of *IGFII* or loss of a tumor suppressor gene.[19,561] DNA ploidy has prognostic significance in this histologic type and in nonmetastatic, unresectable tumors, with DNA diploid tumors having a worse prognosis than hyperdiploid tumors.[476]

CLINICAL FEATURES

Rhabdomyosarcoma presents as a painful or painless deep mass in the extremity. Because the mass is usually deep, redness, warmth, and increased local vascularity are not evident.[212] Symptoms may be present for several months before diagnosis. There are usually no generalized or systemic signs. The parents frequently note a preceding traumatic event that calls attention to the lesion. The mass may be mistaken for a hematoma or a benign neoplasm. Regional lymph nodes may be involved, especially in the alveolar form.[214,326]

RADIOGRAPHIC FINDINGS

Patients who present with deep soft tissue masses should be evaluated for possible sarcomas. This requires a complete history and physical examination; laboratory studies, including CBC count and differential, liver function tests, and determination of electrolyte, calcium, and phosphorus levels; and plain radiographs for extremity and trunk lesions. The differential diagnosis includes nontumorous conditions such as hematoma and myositis ossificans and benign neoplasms such as schwannomas and lipomas. Growth of a painless mass in the absence of trauma should be viewed with suspicion.[561]

A bone scan is obtained to exclude bony metastases, but MRI is more accurate for demonstrating adjacent bone involvement.[475] MRI is also useful for determining the extent of the soft tissue mass and its relationship to surrounding neurovascular structures and bone (Fig. 39–23).[343] Chest CT should be performed to assess for the presence of lung metastases. Unlike in bone sarcomas, regional lymph nodes are involved with tumor in approximately 15% of cases,[296] and this worsens the prognosis.[292,326] One study of extremity sarcomas achieved histologic documentation of lymph node status in 70% of patients, and histologically positive nodes were found in 40%.[292] The regional lymph nodes should be carefully assessed clinically and by MRI.

BIOPSY

If lymph node involvement is suspected, lymph node sampling should be done. Some authors recommend regional lymph node biopsies in all extremity rhabdo-

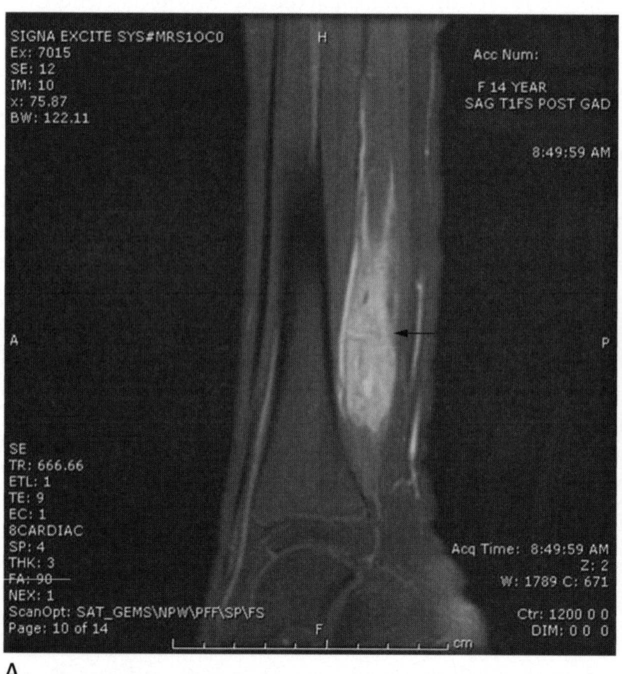

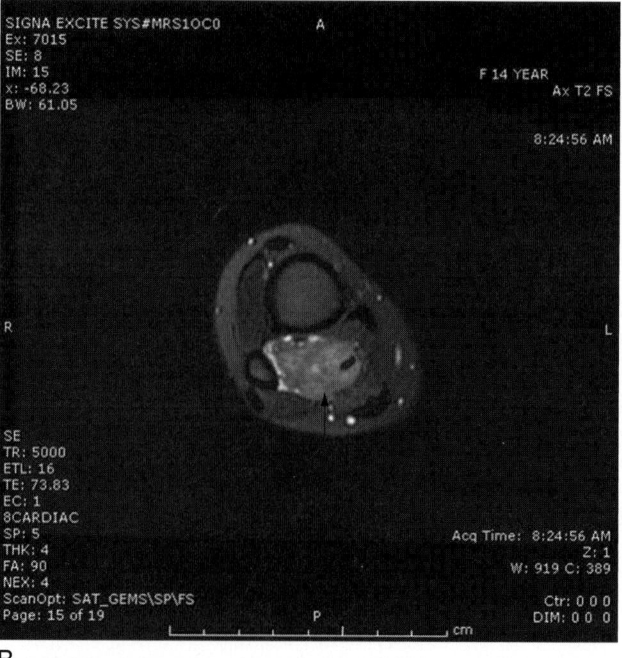

FIGURE 39–23 Rhabdomyosarcoma in the calf of a 14-year-old girl. **A** and **B**, Magnetic resonance images of an alveolar rhabdomyosarcoma (*arrow*) located in the flexor hallucis longus muscle.

myosarcomas.[12] Although routine lymph node dissection is controversial, most investigators do not recommend it as a therapeutic maneuver.[255] The oncologist usually performs a bone marrow aspiration and biopsy to search for bone marrow involvement.

TREATMENT AND PROGNOSIS

The treatment of rhabdomyosarcoma of the extremity is multidisciplinary and involves pediatric oncologists, radiation therapists, and surgical oncologists. In a patient with nonmetastatic disease, the primary tumor is completely excised, and adjuvant chemotherapy is administered.[19,214,215,255,291] The international Intergroup Rhabdomyosarcoma Study (IRS) has documented the value of adjuvant chemotherapy in several large multimodality, sequential trials beginning in the 1970s.[86,112,214,340,341,386,425,426,563] Standard chemotherapy regimens include vincristine, cyclophosphamide, and actinomycin D.[212,561] The details of the sequential trials are beyond the scope of this discussion but are summarized elsewhere.[212,561] These trials have resulted in an increase in the intensity of chemotherapy and have defined prognostic groups and local treatment measures. Outcomes have improved from a less than 20% survival rate with surgical treatment alone to a survival rate of about 60% today.[212,516] Unfortunately, although the survival rate has improved with each successive IRS trial, children with nonmetastatic extremity rhabdomyosarcoma have an estimated 5-year survival rate of only 74%, which is worse than the survival rates from orbital or genitourinary disease.[12]

The prognosis varies with the stage of the disease, and there are a variety of staging systems, including the one used by the Musculoskeletal Tumor Society,[136,139] that can be applied to rhabdomyosarcoma. However, the IRS has traditionally used a clinical grouping of patients based on residual tumor after initial resection for reporting most of its studies (Table 39–2).[12] This system differs from many others in that the initial surgical procedure affects the grouping, and it does not take into account other prognostic factors that might be important based on staging before surgical intervention. One drawback of using this system for extremity lesions is that a lesion of the hand or foot could be classified as group I, II, or III, depending on the surgical procedure, and an extremity tumor of virtually any size could be placed in group I or II if an amputation was performed. Treatment obviously varies in aggressiveness from center to center and from surgeon to surgeon. These groups are clearly predictive of outcome in extremity rhabdomyosarcomas and overall (Table 39–3), but assignment to a group has the disadvantage of depending on the initial surgical procedure. These shortcomings led to the creation of a prospective staging system that is being tested in the IRS-IV protocol and is based on prognostic information identified by Lawrence and Gehan and their colleagues using IRS-I data (Table 39–4).[295] It

Table 39-2 Clinical Grouping System Based on Residual Tumor after Resection

Clinical Group	Description
I	Completely resected tumor
Iia	Microscopic residual tumor, negative nodes
IIb	Positive regional nodes, resected
Iic	Positive regional nodes with microscopic residual margins or nodes
III	Gross residual disease
IV	Distant metastatic disease

From Andrassy RJ, Corpron CA, Hays D, et al: Extremity sarcomas: An analysis of prognostic factors from the Intergroup Rhabdomyosarcoma Study III. J Pediatr Surg 1996;31:191.

Table 39-3 Estimated Five-Year Survival Rates in Patients with Extremity-Site Tumors versus All Patients

	Survival (%)	
Clinical Group	Extremity Site	All
I	95	93
II	67	81
III	58	73
IV	33	30

From Andrassy RJ, Corpron CA, Hays D, et al: Extremity sarcomas: An analysis of prognostic factors from the Intergroup Rhabdomyosarcoma Study III. J Pediatr Surg 1996;31:191.

Table 39-4 Lawrence-Gehan Staging System for Rhabdomyosarcoma

Stage	Description
1	Favorable site (orbit, head and neck, genitourinary; *not* extremity), M0
2	Other site (extremity), any T, a, N0, M0
3	Other site (extremity), any T, b, N0, or N1, M0 or any T, a, N1, M0
4	M1

a, size ≤5 cm; b, size >5 cm; M0, no distant metastases; M1, distant metastases; N0, no regional nodal metastases; N1, regional nodal metastases; T0, no tissue invasion past the muscle of origin; T1, tissue invasion past the muscle of origin.

From Andrassy RJ, Corpron CA, Hays D, et al: Extremity sarcomas: An analysis of prognostic factors from the Intergroup Rhabdomyosarcoma Study III. J Pediatr Surg 1996;31:191.

should be noted that because extremity and trunk sarcomas have a poorer prognosis, they are never included in stage 1 in the Lawrence-Gehan staging system.

A study of 35 extremity rhabdomyosarcomas from a single institution found that tumor invasion beyond the muscle of origin was a prognostic factor at diagnosis on multivariate analysis.[292] Other prognostic factors found to be important in extremity rhabdomyosarcoma on univariate analysis were regional node involvement, alveolar subtype, size of the primary tumor, and complete resection. Amputation and location of the primary tumor were not significant factors.

The local treatment of rhabdomyosarcoma is controversial. Some surgeons prefer to attempt a wide excision at diagnosis. Others prefer to treat patients with preoperative chemotherapy in the hope that the lesion will shrink and become more amenable to resection without the sacrifice of so much normal tissue. Neither approach has been shown to be superior to the other.[12,292] In most cases, radiation therapy is used either before or after surgical resection.[343,563] Novel techniques such as brachytherapy and hyperfractionation may be used to maximize local control and minimize damage to adjacent growth plates.[118,366] Careful review of the staging studies with a radiologist and the treatment team is necessary. If resection would involve loss of major neurovascular structures, radiation therapy alone is indicated. In very young children with lower extremity lesions, amputation may be the optimal method of local control.[194,214] These decisions can be difficult and require detailed discussions among the treatment team and with the parents and the child.

The overall survival rate for extremity rhabdomyosarcoma has improved from 47% in IRS-I to 74% in IRS-III for patients without distant metastases at diagnosis. The outcome varied by clinical group in IRS-III (see Table 39–3).[12] In clinical group III, the type of radiation (hyperfractionated versus conventional) made no difference in IRS-III. The 5-year local failure rate for extremity sarcoma was 7%. The 5-year regional failure rate for extremity tumors was 20%. The 5-year distant failure rate for extremity tumors was 28%.[119] Overall 3-year event-free survival and survival were 77% and 86%, respectively, for the IRS-IV study.[87]

About 20% of patients with rhabdomyosarcoma have metastatic disease at diagnosis, and their prognosis is much poorer. Five-year survival rates are about 20% to 30% overall.[12,19] These patients are treated with more intensive chemotherapy and radiation therapy delivered to the primary tumor. Disease in patients with local relapse should be restaged, and if the recurrence is localized, surgical resection is performed if possible. This is often combined with chemotherapy and radiation therapy. Resection of pulmonary metastases may be appropriate. Patients with local relapse and distant metastases or with distant metastases alone are most often treated with chemotherapy and palliative radiation therapy.[561]

Nonrhabdomyosarcoma Soft Tissue Sarcoma

Soft tissue sarcomas other than rhabdomyosarcoma are rare, collectively accounting for less than half of soft tissue sarcomas in children.[583] For the most part, these lesions appear and behave similarly to adult soft tissue sarcomas, except in the very young. In children younger than 5 years, the histopathology of soft tissue sarcomas is somewhat different, and the biologic behavior is more benign than in adults.

CONGENITAL AND INFANTILE FIBROSARCOMA

Congenital and infantile fibrosarcoma is encountered in neonates.[40,98,414] Fibrosarcoma is one of the more common nonrhabdomyosarcomas in childhood and is the most common soft tissue sarcoma in children younger than 1 year.[500,507] There is a second peak in incidence between 10 and 15 years of age. In general, congenital fibrosarcoma has a more benign clinical course than fibrosarcoma in older children, which behaves more like the adult counterpart.[142,500]

Pathology

The histology is that of a high-grade spindle cell sarcoma arranged in a herringbone pattern intermixed with collagen fibers.[361] It is a very cellular lesion with many mitoses, but despite this appearance, surgical treatment alone is curative in more than 90% of cases.[414] It may be difficult to distinguish congenital fibrosarcoma from congenital fibromatosis, but recently, chromosomal alterations have been identified in congenital fibrosarcoma but not in other fibrosarcomas. The most common alteration is a nonrandom gain of chromosome 11, yielding a trisomy 11.[3,47,98,451] Chromosomal alterations can be demonstrated with fluorescent in situ hybridization techniques on paraffin-embedded tissue and can be helpful in confirming the diagnosis.[155,463] Congenital and infantile fibrosarcomas also have a novel recurrent reciprocal translocation t(12;15)(p13;q25), resulting in the gene fusion *ETV6-NTRK3* (ETS variant gene 6; neurotrophic tyrosine kinase receptor type 3).[478] The use of RT-PCR methods to detect *ETV6-NTRK3* fusion transcripts in archival formalin-fixed paraffin-embedded tissue can help distinguish these tumors from other soft tissue sarcomas.

Clinical Features

Congenital fibrosarcoma presents as a rapidly growing mass at birth or shortly thereafter (Fig. 39–24). It occurs most commonly in the extremities, usually in the distal extremity.[52,500] As is the case for all soft tissue sarcomas, there is nothing in the history or physical examination to alert the physician that this is a malignant process, and congenital fibrosarcomas are frequently mistaken for hemangiomas, lymphangiomas, or lipomas initially.[414] Metastases are present at diagnosis

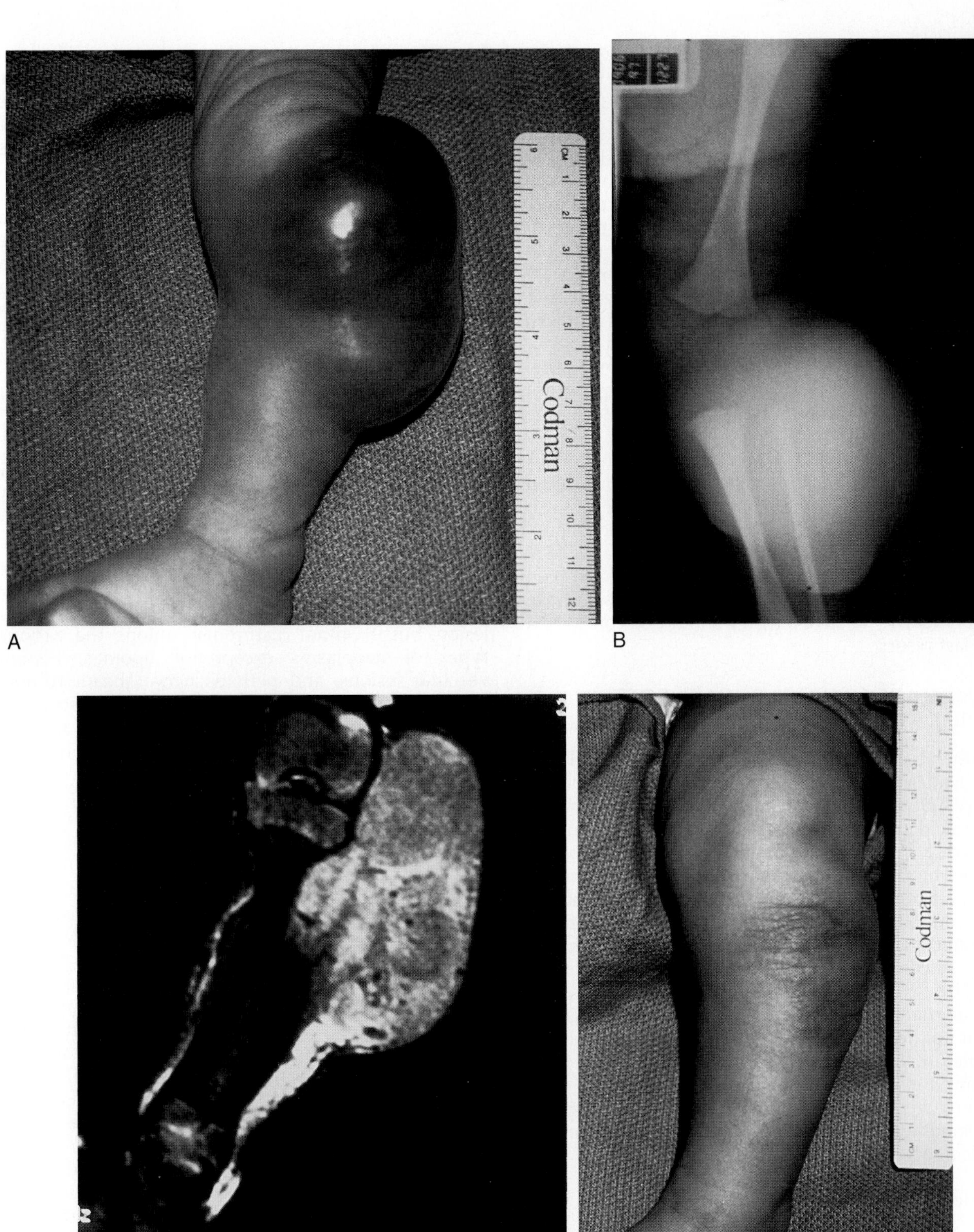

FIGURE 39–24 Congenital fibrosarcoma in a newborn infant. **A,** Clinical appearance at birth. The mass in the left leg increased significantly in the first hours of life. A needle biopsy showed congenital fibrosarcoma. The options of immediate amputation versus adjuvant chemotherapy were discussed, and chemotherapy was begun. **B,** Anteroposterior radiograph of the child's lower extremity showing the soft tissue mass and no definitive evidence of bone involvement. **C,** Magnetic resonance image showing a large soft tissue mass adjacent to the bone and knee joint, with no evidence of bony infiltration. **D,** Appearance of the leg after neoadjuvant chemotherapy. The lesion shrank considerably. Excision of the tumor bed revealed no evidence of recurrent tumor. One year after diagnosis, the child is free of disease, with a normally functioning lower extremity.

in less than 20% of cases and are more frequent for trunk lesions.[368]

Treatment

Treatment is surgical excision whenever feasible, as it frequently is in the extremity, although it may be difficult to achieve wide margins in young children. Local recurrence does not appear to worsen the prognosis, so that limb-sparing procedures that preserve function and avoid amputation are preferred.[361,414] Radiation therapy is generally not used for extremity lesions because of the late effects of irradiating growth plates, although it is occasionally employed in techniques such as brachytherapy that avoid growth plates. If complete resection is achieved, chemotherapy is not needed as an adjuvant, and it is best to avoid the side effects.

For unresectable lesions, treatment with chemotherapy often results in a dramatic response and may even be curative,[190,286,316,372] or it may make subsequent surgical resection possible. The preferred agents are vincristine and actinomycin D because of their relative lack of long-term side effects,[361] but other agents have been used. Rare instances of spontaneous regression have been noted, so ablative surgery should be considered as a last resort.

NONRHABDOMYOSARCOMA SOFT TISSUE SARCOMA IN OLDER CHILDREN

Nonrhabdomyosarcomas are rare in older children and adolescents.[114] They vary widely in their histology and perhaps in their biologic behavior, but in general, they are similar to such soft tissue tumors occurring in adults, although the relative frequency of the histologic subtypes differs. Liposarcoma is rarely encountered in children, whereas in adults it is common. In children, synovial sarcoma, fibrosarcoma, malignant schwannoma, and undifferentiated sarcomas are the most common histologic subtypes.[50,114,147,288,302,335,361,387,428,462] Other subtypes, such as malignant fibrous histiocytoma, are much less frequent but do occur.[424,534] It is beyond the scope of this chapter to discuss each entity, but they have been reviewed elsewhere.[361] Certain histologic types, such as fibrosarcoma and synovial sarcoma, may respond to chemotherapy, but this group of lesions is generally treated surgically.

Clinical Features

The clinical presentation is that of a painless or tender mass of varying size in the extremity or trunk. The mass may compress or arise in association with peripheral nerves, yielding nerve pain, weakness, or sensory findings. Systemic symptoms are absent unless there are widespread metastases.[535] Although benign masses far outnumber malignant ones, they may be difficult to distinguish. In general, a lesion that is enlarging, deep to the fascia, and greater than 5 cm in diameter should be suspected of being malignant until proved otherwise. Unfortunately, vascular malformations, hemangiomas, lymphangiomas, fibromatosis, and nontumorous entities such as myositis ossificans can make the distinction difficult.[53,216] Large lipomas and nerve sheath tumors can mimic sarcomas, and small superficial lesions could be subcutaneous sarcomas (malignant fibrous histiocytoma and synovial sarcoma). It should be noted that up to 15% of patients with neurofibromatosis type 1 develop malignant peripheral nerve sheath tumors.[361] These patients are very difficult to assess because they often have many large neurofibromas, and distinguishing benign from malignant is challenging. Likewise, a patient with a malignant schwannoma should be carefully evaluated for the possibility of unrecognized neurofibromatosis.

Staging and Radiographic Findings

A careful physical examination with particular attention to regional lymph nodes is important. Chest CT is included in the staging workup because the lung is the most frequent site of distant metastases. A bone scan is usually performed in children, because bony metastases are occasionally encountered. MRI is the most useful diagnostic tool to assess the primary lesion, but it cannot distinguish among the various types of neoplasms except for lipomas, benign vascular lesions, and perhaps nerve sheath tumors (Fig. 39–25). MRI may allow the distinction between benign and malignant soft tissue masses, however.[133,289,331,353,401,548,550] MRI is also useful in planning surgical and radiotherapeutic treatment.

Treatment and Prognosis

Treatment of these soft tissue sarcomas in children is similar to that in adults. An open or needle biopsy is essential, following the principles of biopsy discussed in Chapter 37, General Principles of Tumor Management.[330,402,488] Because these neoplasms are difficult to classify, special immunohistochemical stains and cytogenetic studies may be necessary to establish the correct diagnosis. Most important, a pathologist knowledgeable about pediatric soft tissue neoplasms should examine the pathology slides. For small, superficial lesions, an excisional biopsy may be considered, but if malignancy is suspected, wide margins should be achieved, or the excision should be done in such a manner that a wide excision of the tumor bed can be carried out later. Incisions should be longitudinal and not transverse for extremity masses. When in doubt, it is best to perform an incisional biopsy.

Complete surgical resection is the optimal treatment, often in combination with radiation therapy (see Fig. 39–25B).[50,193,194,361,389,404,428] A multidisciplinary approach involving pediatric oncologists, radiation oncologists, and surgeons is necessary to arrive at the appropriate treatment regimen. The staging studies should be carefully reviewed to ascertain the relationship of the mass to surrounding osseous or neurovascular structures. In most cases, a complete excision with wide margins of normal tissue surrounding the

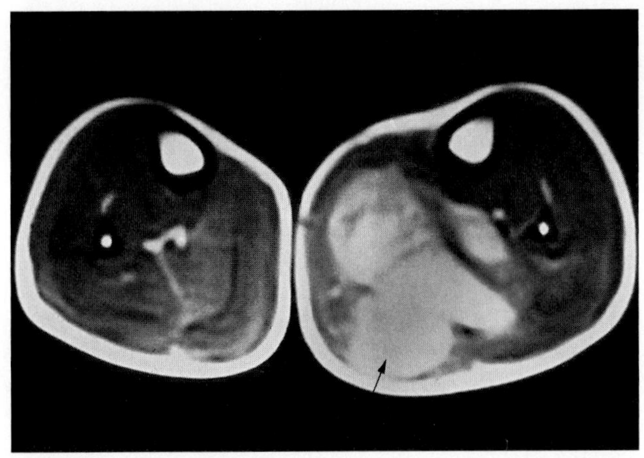

A

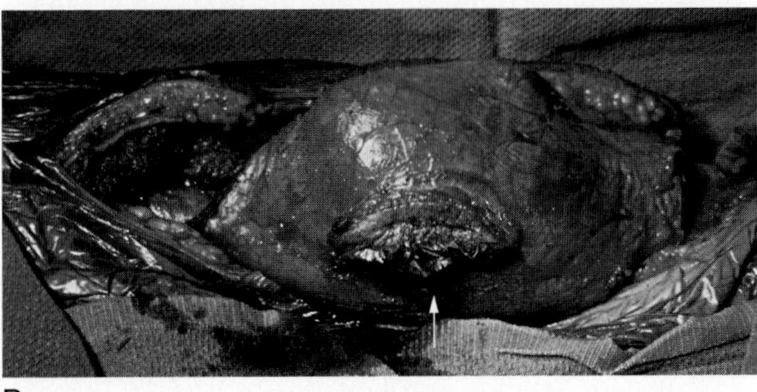

B

FIGURE 39–25 Synovial sarcoma in a 17-year-old boy. The calcified lesion in the leg was initially mistaken for myositis ossificans over a 6-month period. **A,** Magnetic resonance imaging shows extensive involvement of the superficial posterior compartment of the leg. The lesion (*arrow*) is close to the deep posterior compartments and neurovascular bundle but does not involve these structures. An incisional biopsy showed that the lesion was a synovial sarcoma. The patient also had multiple pulmonary metastases, which initially responded to preoperative chemotherapy and radiation therapy. **B,** The patient underwent wide resection of the tumor that included the superficial compartment (the biopsy tract is also visible). *Arrow* shows the biopsy scar. After extensive chemotherapy the patient did well, but he died of metastatic disease 3 years after diagnosis.

tumor is possible. For some lesions, however, this is not possible without sacrificing normal structures. In these cases, preoperative treatment with chemotherapy, radiation therapy, or both may be indicated. It is not necessary to remove entire muscle groups from their origin to insertion (radical excision) unless the muscle is totally involved. If there has been a prior excision of the tumor, the tumor bed should be re-excised to ensure that complete gross and microscopic tumor eradication has been achieved. In the hand or the foot, ray amputations that resect part of the hand or foot and preserve some meaningful function are usually possible.[21,193,194,256,271,384]

Lymph node involvement at diagnosis is not as frequent as in rhabdomyosarcoma (possibly up to 15% in high-grade sarcomas), and, though controversial, routine lymph node dissection is not performed.[428] One study suggested that excision of isolated regional lymph nodes may improve survival in patients of all ages with soft tissue sarcomas.[430] Lymph node dissection may be indicated if lymph node involvement is suspected on clinical grounds. As in patients with bone sarcomas, thoracotomy to resect pulmonary metastases may be indicated if local control has been achieved.[218,243,413,443]

Radiation is useful in cases in which microscopic residual tumor cannot be excised[89,157,271,288,335,336] or extends to the margin of resection. It may also be useful in patients with malignant peripheral nerve sheath tumors and can be combined with chemotherapy in cases of unresectable tumors.[73] If radiation therapy is planned, measures should be taken to avoid growth plates, depending on the location of the lesion and the age of the child. Novel techniques such as brachytherapy or special fields are sometimes employed to minimize the amount of surrounding normal tissue exposed to radiation (Fig. 39–26). The choice of pre-

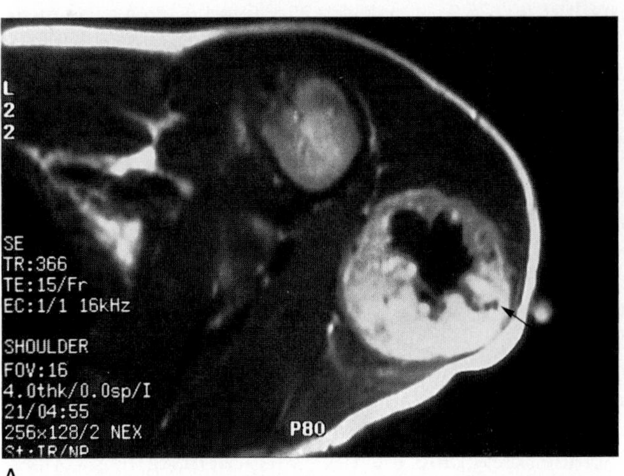

A

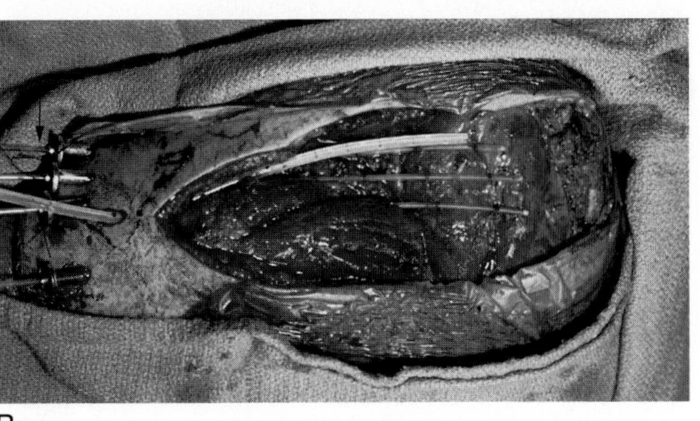

B

FIGURE 39–26 Malignant schwannoma of the left deltoid in a 10-year-old boy. **A,** Magnetic resonance imaging appearance of the schwannoma (*arrow*). Because of the child's age, it was desirable to limit external beam irradiation to the proximal humerus, so he was treated with a modified field preoperatively to avoid the growth plate. **B,** Operative appearance. A wide resection was performed, with a negative but narrow margin and preservation of part of the axillary nerve. Brachytherapy catheters (*arrow*) were placed to deliver focused radiation to the closest margin. The boy remains free of disease 5 years after diagnosis.

operative versus postoperative radiation is controversial; each has advantages and disadvantages.

The role of adjuvant chemotherapy is less well established.[361] No study has definitively documented its value in preventing systemic relapse,[361,387] but chemotherapy is being evaluated in the treatment of high-risk patients (those with high-grade metastatic or unresectable soft tissue sarcomas) by the Pediatric Oncology Group. Recent studies of patients with synovial sarcoma suggest a benefit to adjuvant chemotherapy, but this has not been documented in randomized trials.[147,262,288,387,446] On occasion, responses are noted that make subsequent resection and radiation therapy more feasible. Tumor regression in patients with metastatic or unresectable disease has also been documented with various chemotherapy regimens.[262,361,446]

The outcome for patients with nonrhabdomyosarcomas who present without metastases is generally good. One study showed an 82% 5-year survival rate, with local and systemic recurrence rates of 21%.[361] At our institution, 75% of patients survived 10 years or more following a treatment regimen that included an attempt at resection and, in most cases, radiation therapy.[335] Histologic grade was important, in that 92% of patients with low- to intermediate-grade tumors were free from local recurrence or systemic relapse, whereas 73% of patients with high-grade neoplasms remained relapse free ($P = .09$). The ability to eradicate the local disease is also important. Despite radiation therapy, the local relapse rate was 50% in patients with gross residual tumor remaining, whereas only one patient relapsed locally after complete excision. In another study, 84% of patients remained free of disease after complete removal of the tumor, whereas only 1 of 26 (4%) survived after incomplete excision.[227] Prognostic variables include size, grade, location, surgical margin, and presence or absence of metastases.[9,369,388,428,434]

References

1. Aboulafia AJ, Buch R, Mathews J, et al: Reconstruction using the saddle prosthesis following excision of primary and metastatic periacetabular tumors. Clin Orthop Relat Res 1995:203.
2. Abudu A, Sferopoulos NK, Tillman RM, et al: The surgical treatment and outcome of pathological fractures in localised osteosarcoma. J Bone Joint Surg Br 1996; 78:694.
3. Adam LR, Davison EV, Malcolm AJ, et al: Cytogenetic analysis of a congenital fibrosarcoma. Cancer Genet Cytogenet 1991;52:37.
4. Aegerter E: Diagnostic radiology and the pathology of bone disease. Radiol Clin North Am 1970;8:215.
5. Aegerter E, Kirkpatrick JA: Orthopaedic Diseases. Philadelphia, WB Saunders, 1975.
6. Ahrens S, Hoffmann C, Jabar S, et al: Evaluation of prognostic factors in a tumor volume-adapted treatment strategy for localized Ewing sarcoma of bone: The CESS 86 experience. Cooperative Ewing Sarcoma Study. Med Pediatr Oncol 1999;32:186.
7. Akerman M: Tumour necrosis and prognosis in Ewing's sarcoma. Acta Orthop Scand Suppl 1997;273:130.
8. Alman BA, De Bari A, Krajbich JI: Massive allografts in the treatment of osteosarcoma and Ewing sarcoma in children and adolescents. J Bone Joint Surg Am 1995;77:54.
9. Alvegard TA, Berg NO, Ranstam J, et al: Prognosis in high-grade soft tissue sarcomas: The Scandinavian Sarcoma Group experience in a randomized adjuvant chemotherapy trial. Acta Orthop Scand 1989;60:517.
10. Ambros IM, Ambros PF, Strehl S, et al: MIC2 is a specific marker for Ewing's sarcoma and peripheral primitive neuroectodermal tumors: Evidence for a common histogenesis of Ewing's sarcoma and peripheral primitive neuroectodermal tumors from MIC2 expression and specific chromosome aberration. Cancer 1991;67: 1886.
11. Anderson L, Westin GW, Oppenheim WL: Syme amputation in children: Indications, results, and long-term follow-up. J Pediatr Orthop 1984;4:550.
12. Andrassy RJ, Corpron CA, Hays D, et al: Extremity sarcomas: An analysis of prognostic factors from the Intergroup Rhabdomyosarcoma Study III. J Pediatr Surg 1996;31:191.
13. Andreassen A, Oyjord T, Hovig E, et al: p53 Abnormalities in different subtypes of human sarcomas. Cancer Res 1993;53:468.
14. Aparicio J, Munarriz B, Pastor M, et al: Long-term follow-up and prognostic factors in Ewing's sarcoma: A multivariate analysis of 116 patients from a single institution. Oncology 1998;55:20.
15. Aparicio J, Segura A, Montalar J, et al: Secondary cancers after Ewing sarcoma and Ewing sarcoma as second malignant neoplasm. Med Pediatr Oncol 1998;30:259.
16. Aprin H, Riseborough EJ, Hall JE: Chondrosarcoma in children and adolescents. Clin Orthop Relat Res 1982: 226.
17. Arai Y, Kun LE, Brooks MT, et al: Ewing's sarcoma: Local tumor control and patterns of failure following limited-volume radiation therapy. Int J Radiat Oncol Biol Phys 1991;21:1501.
18. Arlen M, Higinbotham NL, Huvos AG, et al: Radiation-induced sarcoma of bone. Cancer 1971;28:1087.
19. Arndt CA, Crist WM: Common musculoskeletal tumors of childhood and adolescence. N Engl J Med 1999; 341:342.
20. Atra A, Whelan JS, Calvagna V, et al: High-dose busulphan/melphalan with autologous stem cell rescue in Ewing's sarcoma. Bone Marrow Transplant 1997;20: 843.
21. Azouz EM, Kozlowski K, Masel J: Soft-tissue tumors of the hand and wrist of children. Can Assoc Radiol J 1989;40:251.
22. Bacci G, Briccoli A, Picci P, et al: Metachronous pulmonary metastases resection in patients with Ewing's sarcoma initially treated with adjuvant or neoadjuvant chemotherapy. Eur J Cancer 1995;31A:999.
23. Bacci G, Briccoli A, Rocca M, et al: Neoadjuvant chemotherapy for osteosarcoma of the extremities with metastases at presentation: Recent experience at the Rizzoli Institute in 57 patients treated with cisplatin, doxoru-

bicin, and a high dose of methotrexate and ifosfamide. Ann Oncol 2003;14:1126.

24. Bacci G, Dallari D, Battistini A, et al: The prognostic value of serum alkaline phosphatase in osteosarcoma of the limbs. Chir Organi Mov 1992;77:171.
25. Bacci G, Di Fiore M, Rimondini S, et al: Delayed diagnosis and tumor stage in Ewing's sarcoma. Oncol Rep 1999;6:465.
26. Bacci G, Ferrari S, Bertoni F, et al: Long-term outcome for patients with nonmetastatic osteosarcoma of the extremity treated at the Istituto Ortopedico Rizzoli according to the Istituto Ortopedico Rizzoli/osteosarcoma-2 protocol: An updated report. J Clin Oncol 2000;18:4016.
27. Bacci G, Ferrari S, Mercuri M, et al: Neoadjuvant chemotherapy for extremity osteosarcoma—preliminary results of the Rizzoli's 4th study. Acta Oncol 1998;37:41.
28. Bacci G, Ferrari S, Mercuri M, et al: Predictive factors for local recurrence in osteosarcoma: 540 patients with extremity tumors followed for minimum 2.5 years after neoadjuvant chemotherapy. Acta Orthop Scand 1998;69:230.
29. Bacci G, Ferrari S, Ruggieri P, et al: Telangiectatic osteosarcoma of the extremity: Neoadjuvant chemotherapy in 24 cases. Acta Orthop Scand 2001;72:167.
30. Bacci G, Longhi A, Barbieri E, et al: Second malignancy in 597 patients with Ewing sarcoma of bone treated at a single institution with adjuvant and neoadjuvant chemotherapy between 1972 and 1999. J Pediatr Hematol Oncol 2005;27:517.
31. Bacci G, Longhi A, Fagioli F, et al: Adjuvant and neoadjuvant chemotherapy for osteosarcoma of the extremities: 27 year experience at Rizzoli Institute, Italy. Eur J Cancer 2005;41:2836.
32. Bacci G, Picci P, Ferrari S, et al: Primary chemotherapy and delayed surgery for nonmetastatic osteosarcoma of the extremities: Results in 164 patients preoperatively treated with high doses of methotrexate followed by cisplatin and doxorubicin. Cancer 1993;72:3227.
33. Bacci G, Picci P, Ferrari S, et al: Synchronous multifocal osteosarcoma: Results in twelve patients treated with neoadjuvant chemotherapy and simultaneous resection of all involved bones. Ann Oncol 1996;7:864.
34. Bacci G, Picci P, Gherlinzoni F, et al: Localized Ewing's sarcoma of bone: Ten years' experience at the Istituto Ortopedico Rizzoli in 124 cases treated with multimodal therapy. Eur J Cancer Clin Oncol 1985;21:163.
35. Bacci G, Picci P, Pignatti G, et al: Neoadjuvant chemotherapy for nonmetastatic osteosarcoma of the extremities. Clin Orthop Relat Res 1991:87.
36. Bacci G, Picci P, Ruggieri P, et al: Neoadjuvant chemotherapy for the treatment of osteosarcoma of the limbs. Preliminary results in 100 patients treated preoperatively with high doses of methotrexate IV followed by cisplatin (IA) and adriamycin. Chir Organi Mov 1991;76:1.
37. Badhwar R, Agarwal M: Rotationplasty as a limb salvage procedure for malignant bone tumours. Int Orthop 1998;22:122.
38. Baldini N, Scotlandi K, Barbanti-Brodano G, et al: Expression of P-glycoprotein in high-grade osteosarcomas in relation to clinical outcome. N Engl J Med 1995;333:1380.
39. Balis F, Holcenberg J, Poplack D: General principles of chemotherapy. In Pizzo P, Poplack D (eds): Principles and Practice of Pediatric Oncology. Philadelphia, JB Lippincott, 1997, p 215.
40. Balsaver AM, Butler JJ, Martin RG: Congenital fibrosarcoma. Cancer 1967;20:1607.
41. Barr FG, Chatten J, D'Cruz CM, et al: Molecular assays for chromosomal translocations in the diagnosis of pediatric soft tissue sarcomas. JAMA 1995;273:553.
42. Baumgartner RF: Knee disarticulation versus above-knee amputation. Prosthet Orthot Int 1979;3:15.
43. Becker W, Ramach W, Delling G: Problems of biopsy and diagnosis in a cooperative study of osteosarcoma. J Cancer Res Clin Oncol 1983;106(Suppl):11.
44. Bell RS, Davis AM, Wunder JS, et al: Allograft reconstruction of the acetabulum after resection of stage-IIB sarcoma: Intermediate-term results. J Bone Joint Surg Am 1997;79:1663.
45. Benassi MS, Molendini L, Gamberi G, et al: Involvement of INK4A gene products in the pathogenesis and development of human osteosarcoma. Cancer 2001;92:3062.
46. Bernstein ML, Devidas M, Lafreniere D, et al: Intensive therapy with growth factor support for patients with Ewing tumor metastatic at diagnosis: Pediatric Oncology Group/Children's Cancer Group Phase II Study 9457—a report from the Children's Oncology Group. J Clin Oncol 2006;24:152.
47. Bernstein R, Zeltzer PM, Lin F, et al: Trisomy 11 and other nonrandom trisomies in congenital fibrosarcoma. Cancer Genet Cytogenet 1994;78:82.
48. Berrey BH Jr, Lord CF, Gebhardt MC, et al: Fractures of allografts: Frequency, treatment, and end-results. J Bone Joint Surg Am 1990;72:825.
49. Bertoni F, Bacchini P, Fabbri N, et al: Osteosarcoma: Low-grade intraosseous-type osteosarcoma, histologically resembling parosteal osteosarcoma, fibrous dysplasia, and desmoplastic fibroma. Cancer 1993;71:338.
50. Blakely ML, Spurbeck WW, Pappo AS, et al: The impact of margin of resection on outcome in pediatric nonrhabdomyosarcoma soft tissue sarcoma. J Pediatr Surg 1999;34:672.
51. Blatt J, Copeland D, Bleyer W: Late effects of childhood cancer and its treatment. In Pizzo P, Poplack D (eds): Principles and Practice of Pediatric Oncology. Philadelphia, JB Lippincott, 1997, p 1303.
52. Blocker S, Koenig J, Ternberg J: Congenital fibrosarcoma. J Pediatr Surg 1987;22:665.
53. Boon LM, Fishman SJ, Lund DP, et al: Congenital fibrosarcoma masquerading as congenital hemangioma: Report of two cases. J Pediatr Surg 1995;30:1378.
54. Boyko OB, Cory DA, Cohen MD, et al: MR imaging of osteogenic and Ewing's sarcoma. AJR Am J Roentgenol 1987;148:317.
55. Brown AP, Fixsen JA, Plowman PN: Local control of Ewing's sarcoma: An analysis of 67 patients. Br J Radiol 1987;60:261.
56. Bubis JJ: Pathology of osteosarcoma. Prog Clin Biol Res 1982;99:3.

57. Burdach S, Peters C, Paulussen M, et al: Improved relapse free survival in patients with poor prognosis Ewing's sarcoma after consolidation with hyperfractionated total body irradiation and fractionated high dose melphalan followed by high dose etoposide and hematopoietic rescue. Bone Marrow Transplant 1991; 7(Suppl 2):95.
58. Burgert EO Jr, Nesbit ME, Garnsey LA, et al: Multimodal therapy for the management of nonpelvic, localized Ewing's sarcoma of bone: Intergroup study IESS-II. J Clin Oncol 1990;8:1514.
59. Burk CD, Belasco JB, O'Neill JA Jr, et al: Pulmonary metastases and bone sarcomas: Surgical removal of lesions appearing after adjuvant chemotherapy. Clin Orthop Relat Res 1991:88.
60. Cabitza P, Mapelli S: Multicentric osteosarcoma: Presentation of a case and review of the literature. Ital J Orthop Traumatol 1981;7:255.
61. Cahan WG, Woodward HQ, Higinbotham NL, et al: Sarcoma arising in irradiated bone. Cancer 1948;1:3.
62. Cammisa FP Jr, Glasser DB, Otis JC, et al: The van Nes tibial rotationplasty: A functionally viable reconstructive procedure in children who have a tumor of the distal end of the femur. J Bone Joint Surg Am 1990;72: 1541.
63. Campanacci M: Bone and soft tissue tumors. In Bertoni F, Bacchini P, Campanacci M (eds): Bone and Soft Tissue Tumors. New York, Springer-Verlag, 1990.
64. Campanacci M, Capanna R: Pelvic resections: The Rizzoli Institute experience. Orthop Clin North Am 1991;22:65.
65. Campanacci M, Cervellati G: Osteosarcoma: A review of 345 cases. Ital J Orthop Traumatol 1975;1:5.
66. Campanacci M, Laus M: Local recurrence after amputation for osteosarcoma. J Bone Joint Surg Br 1980;62: 201.
67. Campanacci M, Picci P, Gherlinzoni F, et al: Periosteal osteosarcoma. J Bone Joint Surg Br 1984;66:313.
68. Cangir A, Vietti TJ, Gehan EA, et al: Ewing's sarcoma metastatic at diagnosis: Results and comparisons of two Intergroup Ewing's Sarcoma Studies. Cancer 1990; 66:887.
69. Cannon SR, Sweetnam DR: Multiple chondrosarcomas in dyschondroplasia (Ollier's disease). Cancer 1985;55: 836.
70. Capanna R, Del Ben M, Campanacci DA, et al: Rotationplasty in segmental resections of the femur. Chir Organi Mov 1992;77:135.
71. Capanna R, Toni A, Sudanese A, et al: Ewing's sarcoma of the pelvis. Int Orthop 1990;14:57.
72. Carbone M, Rizzo P, Procopio A, et al: SV40-like sequences in human bone tumors. Oncogene 1996;13: 527.
73. Carli M, Ferrari A, Mattke A, et al: Pediatric malignant peripheral nerve sheath tumor: The Italian and German Soft Tissue Sarcoma Cooperative Group. J Clin Oncol 2005;23:8422.
74. Carrasco CH, Charnsangavej C, Richli WR, et al: Osteosarcoma: Interventional radiology in diagnosis and management. Semin Roentgenol 1989;24:193.
75. Carter JR, Abdul-Karim FW: Pathology of childhood osteosarcoma. Perspect Pediatr Pathol 1987;9:133.
76. Catani F, Capanna R, Benedetti MG, et al: Gait analysis in patients after van Ness rotationplasty. Clin Orthop Relat Res 1993:270.
77. Chan HS, Grogan TM, Haddad G, et al: P-glycoprotein expression: Critical determinant in the response to osteosarcoma chemotherapy. J Natl Cancer Inst 1997; 89:1706.
78. Chew FS, Hudson TM: Radionuclide bone scanning of osteosarcoma: Falsely extended uptake patterns. AJR Am J Roentgenol 1982;139:49.
79. Chou AJ, Merola PR, Wexler LH, et al: Treatment of osteosarcoma at first recurrence after contemporary therapy: The Memorial Sloan-Kettering Cancer Center experience. Cancer 2005;104:2214.
80. Clohisy DR, Mankin HJ: Osteoarticular allografts for reconstruction after resection of a musculoskeletal tumor in the proximal end of the tibia. J Bone Joint Surg Am 1994;76:549.
81. Coakley FV, Cohen MD, Waters DJ, et al: Detection of pulmonary metastases with pathological correlation: Effect of breathing on the accuracy of spiral CT. Pediatr Radiol 1997;27:576.
82. Cohen M, Grosfeld J, Baehner R, et al: Lung CT for detection of metastases: Solid tissue neoplasms in children. AJR Am J Roentgenol 1982;139:895.
83. Collie DA, Wright AR, Williams JR, et al: Comparison of spiral-acquisition computed tomography and conventional computed tomography in the assessment of pulmonary metastatic disease. Br J Radiol 1994;67:436.
84. Cook MA, Manfredi OL: Ewing's sarcoma of the hand: A case report. Bull Hosp Jt Dis 1996;55:75.
85. Cool WP, Grimer RJ, Carter SR, et al: Longitudinal growth following a growing endoprosthesis replacement of the distal femur in the skeletally immature. Eighth International Symposium on Limb Salvage, 1995, Florence, Italy.
86. Crist W, Gehan EA, Ragab AH, et al: The Third Intergroup Rhabdomyosarcoma Study. J Clin Oncol 1995; 13:610.
87. Crist WM, Anderson JR, Meza JL, et al: Intergroup Rhabdomyosarcoma Study-IV: Results for patients with nonmetastatic disease. J Clin Oncol 2001;19:3091.
88. Cumin I, Cohen JY, David A, et al: Rothmund-Thomson syndrome and osteosarcoma. Med Pediatr Oncol 1996; 26:414.
89. Czyzewski EA, Goldman S, Mundt AJ, et al: Radiation therapy for consolidation of metastatic or recurrent sarcomas in children treated with intensive chemotherapy and stem cell rescue: A feasibility study. Int J Radiat Oncol Biol Phys 1999;44:569.
90. Dabska M, Huvos AG: Mesenchymal chondrosarcoma in the young. Virchows Arch A Pathol Anat Histopathol 1983;399:89.
91. Daffner RH, Kennedy SL, Fox KR, et al: Synchronous multicentric osteosarcoma: The case for metastases. Skeletal Radiol 1997;26:569.
92. Dagher R, Pham TA, Sorbara L, et al: Molecular confirmation of Ewing sarcoma. J Pediatr Hematol Oncol 2001;23:221.
93. Dahlin D, Unni K: Bone Tumors: General Aspects and Data on 8542 Cases. Springfield, Ill, Charles C Thomas, 1986.

94. Dahlin DC: Pathology of osteosarcoma. Clin Orthop Relat Res 1975:23.
95. Dahlin DC: Osteosarcoma of bone and a consideration of prognostic variables. Cancer Treat Rep 1978;62:189.
96. Dahlin DC, Coventry MB: Osteogenic sarcoma: A study of six hundred cases. J Bone Joint Surg Am 1967;49: 101.
97. Dahlin DC, Unni KK: Osteosarcoma of bone and its important recognizable varieties. Am J Surg Pathol 1977;1:61.
98. Dal Cin P, Brock P, Casteels-Van Daele M, et al: Cytogenetic characterization of congenital or infantile fibrosarcoma. Eur J Pediatr 1991;150:579.
99. Damron TA, Sim FH, Frassica FJ, et al: Ewing's tumor of the pelvis. Orthopedics 1995;18:577.
100. Damron TA, Sim FH, O'Connor MI, et al: Ewing's sarcoma of the proximal femur. Clin Orthop Relat Res 1996:232.
101. Davis RJ, D'Cruz CM, Lovell MA, et al: Fusion of PAX7 to FKHR by the variant t(1;13)(p36;q14) translocation in alveolar rhabdomyosarcoma. Cancer Res 1994;54:2869.
102. de Bari A, Krajbich JI, Langer F, et al: Modified van Ness rotationplasty for osteosarcoma of the proximal tibia in children. J Bone Joint Surg Br 1990;72:1065.
103. Dehner LP: Primitive neuroectodermal tumor and Ewing's sarcoma. Am J Surg Pathol 1993;17:1.
104. Dehner LP: Neuroepithelioma (primitive neuroectodermal tumor) and Ewing's sarcoma: At least a partial consensus. Arch Pathol Lab Med 1994;118:606.
105. Dehner LP: The evolution of the diagnosis and understanding of primitive and embryonic neoplasms in children: Living through an epoch. Mod Pathol 1998; 11:669.
106. Delattre O, Zucman J, Melot T, et al: The Ewing family of tumors—a subgroup of small-round-cell tumors defined by specific chimeric transcripts. N Engl J Med 1994;331:294.
107. Denny CT: Gene rearrangements in Ewing's sarcoma. Cancer Invest 1996;14:83.
108. deSantos LA, Goldstein HM, Murray JA, et al: Computed tomography in the evaluation of musculoskeletal neoplasms. Radiology 1978;128:89.
109. Devaney K, Abbondanzo SL, Shekitka KM, et al: MIC2 detection in tumors of bone and adjacent soft tissues. Clin Orthop Relat Res 1995:176.
110. Dhillon MS, Singh DP, Sur RK, et al: Ewing's sarcoma of the foot bones: An analysis of seven cases. Contemp Orthop 1994;29:127.
111. Dickman PS, Triche TJ: Extraosseous Ewing's sarcoma versus primitive rhabdomyosarcoma: Diagnostic criteria and clinical correlation. Hum Pathol 1986;17:881.
112. Diller L: Rhabdomyosarcoma and other soft tissue sarcomas of childhood. Curr Opin Oncol 1992;4:689.
113. Diller L, Kassel J, Nelson CE, et al: p53 Functions as a cell cycle control protein in osteosarcomas. Mol Cell Biol 1990;10:5772.
114. Dillon P, Maurer H, Jenkins J, et al: A prospective study of nonrhabdomyosarcoma soft tissue sarcomas in the pediatric age group. J Pediatr Surg 1992;27:241.
115. Dodd LG, Scully SP, Cothran RL, et al: Utility of fine-needle aspiration in the diagnosis of primary osteosarcoma. Diagn Cytopathol 2002;27:350.
116. Dodd S, Malone M, McCulloch W: Rhabdomyosarcoma in children: A histological and immunohistochemical study of 59 cases. J Pathol 1989;158:13.
117. Donaldson SS: Ewing sarcoma: Radiation dose and target volume. Pediatr Blood Cancer 2004;42:471.
118. Donaldson SS, Asmar L, Breneman J, et al: Hyperfractionated radiation in children with rhabdomyosarcoma—results of an Intergroup Rhabdomyosarcoma Pilot Study. Int J Radiat Oncol Biol Phys 1995;32:903.
119. Donaldson SS, Meza J, Breneman JC, et al: Results from the IRS-IV randomized trial of hyperfractionated radiotherapy in children with rhabdomyosarcoma—a report from the IRSG. Int J Radiat Oncol Biol Phys 2001;51:718.
120. Donaldson SS, Torrey M, Link MP, et al: A multidisciplinary study investigating radiotherapy in Ewing's sarcoma: End results of POG #8346. Pediatric Oncology Group. Int J Radiat Oncol Biol Phys 1998;42:125.
121. Donati D, Di Liddo M, Zavatta M, et al: Massive bone allograft reconstruction in high-grade osteosarcoma. Clin Orthop Relat Res 2000:186.
122. Donati D, Giacomini S, Gozzi E, et al: Osteosarcoma of the pelvis. Eur J Surg Oncol 2004;30:332.
123. Downing JR, Head DR, Parham DM, et al: Detection of the (11;22)(q24;q12) translocation of Ewing's sarcoma and peripheral neuroectodermal tumor by reverse transcription polymerase chain reaction. Am J Pathol 1993;143:1294.
124. Dryer RF, Buckwalter JA, Flatt AE, et al: Ewing's sarcoma of the hand. J Hand Surg [Am] 1979;4:372.
125. Du YK, Shih HN, Wang JM, et al: Dedifferentiated chondrosarcoma arising from osteochondromatosis: A case report. Changgeng Yi Xue Za Zhi 1991;14:130.
126. Duffy GP, Wood MB, Rock MG, et al: Vascularized free fibular transfer combined with autografting for the management of fracture nonunions associated with radiation therapy. J Bone Joint Surg Am 2000;82:544.
127. Dunst J, Jurgens H, Sauer R, et al: Radiation therapy in Ewing's sarcoma: An update of the CESS 86 trial. Int J Radiat Oncol Biol Phys 1995;32:919.
128. Dunst J, Schuck A: Role of radiotherapy in Ewing tumors. Pediatr Blood Cancer 2004;42:465.
129. Durbin M, Randall RL, James M, et al: Ewing's sarcoma masquerading as osteomyelitis. Clin Orthop Relat Res 1998:176.
130. Eckardt JJ, Safran MR, Eilber FR, et al: Expandable endoprosthetic reconstruction of the skeletally immature after malignant bone tumor resection. Clin Orthop Relat Res 1993:188.
131. Ecklund K, Laor T, Goorin AM, et al: Methotrexate osteopathy in patients with osteosarcoma. Radiology 1997;202:543.
132. Eggli KD, Quiogue T, Moser RP Jr: Ewing's sarcoma. Radiol Clin North Am 1993;31:325.
133. Eich GF, Hoeffel JC, Tschappeler H, et al: Fibrous tumours in children: Imaging features of a heterogeneous group of disorders. Pediatr Radiol 1998;28:500.
134. Eilber F, Giuliano A, Eckardt J, et al: Adjuvant chemotherapy for osteosarcoma: A randomized prospective trial. J Clin Oncol 1987;5:21.
135. Ellis PM, Tattersall MH, McCaughan B, et al: Osteosarcoma and pulmonary metastases: 15-year experience from a single institution. Aust N Z J Surg 1997;67:625.

136. Enneking WF: A system of staging musculoskeletal neoplasms. Clin Orthop Relat Res 1986:9.
137. Enneking WF, Kagan A: "Skip" metastases in osteosarcoma. Cancer 1975;36:2192.
138. Enneking WF, Kagan A 2nd: Transepiphyseal extension of osteosarcoma: Incidence, mechanism, and implications. Cancer 1978;41:1526.
139. Enneking WF, Spanier SS, Goodman MA: A system for the surgical staging of musculoskeletal sarcoma. Clin Orthop Relat Res 1980:106.
140. Eriksson AI, Schiller A, Mankin HJ: The management of chondrosarcoma of bone. Clin Orthop Relat Res 1980:44.
141. Estrada-Aguilar J, Greenberg H, Walling A, et al: Primary treatment of pelvic osteosarcoma: Report of five cases. Cancer 1992;69:1137.
142. Exelby PR, Knapper WH, Huvos AG, et al: Soft-tissue fibrosarcoma in children. J Pediatr Surg 1973;8:415.
143. Fahey M, Spanier SS, Vander Griend RA: Osteosarcoma of the pelvis: A clinical and histopathological study of twenty-five patients. J Bone Joint Surg Am 1992;74:321.
144. Farley JR, Hall SL, Herring S, et al: Skeletal alkaline phosphatase specific activity is an index of the osteoblastic phenotype in subpopulations of the human osteosarcoma cell line SaOS-2. Metabolism 1991;40:664.
145. Farr GH, Huvos AG, Marcove RC, et al: Telangiectatic osteogenic sarcoma: A review of twenty-eight cases. Cancer 1974;34:1150.
146. Fellinger EJ, Garin-Chesa P, Triche TJ, et al: Immunohistochemical analysis of Ewing's sarcoma cell surface antigen p30/32MIC2. Am J Pathol 1991;139:317.
147. Ferrari A, Casanova M, Massimino M, et al: Synovial sarcoma: Report of a series of 25 consecutive children from a single institution. Med Pediatr Oncol 1999;32:32.
148. Ferrari S, Bertoni F, Mercuri M, et al: Predictive factors of disease-free survival for non-metastatic osteosarcoma of the extremity: An analysis of 300 patients treated at the Rizzoli Institute. Ann Oncol 2001;12:1145.
149. Ferrari S, Bertoni F, Zanella L, et al: Evaluation of P-glycoprotein, HER-2/ErbB-2, p53, and Bcl-2 in primary tumor and metachronous lung metastases in patients with high-grade osteosarcoma. Cancer 2004;100:1936.
150. Ferrari S, Mercuri M, Rosito P, et al: Ifosfamide and actinomycin-D, added in the induction phase to vincristine, cyclophosphamide and doxorubicin, improve histologic response and prognosis in patients with non metastatic Ewing's sarcoma of the extremity. J Chemother 1998;10:484.
151. Ferrari S, Smeland S, Mercuri M, et al: Neoadjuvant chemotherapy with high-dose ifosfamide, high-dose methotrexate, cisplatin, and doxorubicin for patients with localized osteosarcoma of the extremity: A joint study by the Italian and Scandinavian Sarcoma Groups. J Clin Oncol 2005;23:8845.
152. Fielding JW, Fietti VG Jr, Hughes JE, et al: Primary osteogenic sarcoma of the cervical spine: A case report. J Bone Joint Surg Am 1976;58:892.
153. Finn HA, Simon MA: Limb-salvage surgery in the treatment of osteosarcoma in skeletally immature individuals. Clin Orthop Relat Res 1991:108.
154. Flemming DJ, Murphey MD: Enchondroma and chondrosarcoma. Semin Musculoskelet Radiol 2000;4:59.
155. Fletcher JA: Cytogenetics of soft tissue tumors. Cancer Treat Res 1997;91:9.
156. Fletcher JA, Kozakewich HP, Hoffer FA, et al: Diagnostic relevance of clonal cytogenetic aberrations in malignant soft-tissue tumors. N Engl J Med 1991;324:436.
157. Fontanesi J, Pappo AS, Parham DM, et al: Role of irradiation in management of synovial sarcoma: St Jude Children's Research Hospital experience. Med Pediatr Oncol 1996;26:264.
158. Forrester DM, Becker TS: The radiology of bone and soft tissue sarcomas. Orthop Clin North Am 1977;8:973.
159. Frassica FJ, Frassica DA, Pritchard DJ, et al: Ewing sarcoma of the pelvis: Clinicopathological features and treatment. J Bone Joint Surg Am 1993;75:1457.
160. Frassica FJ, Sim FH, Frassica DA, et al: Survival and management considerations in postirradiation osteosarcoma and Paget's osteosarcoma. Clin Orthop Relat Res 1991:120.
161. Fuchs B, Pritchard DJ: Etiology of osteosarcoma. Clin Orthop Relat Res 2002:40.
162. Fuchs B, Valenzuela RG, Inwards C, et al: Complications in long-term survivors of Ewing sarcoma. Cancer 2003;98:2687.
163. Fuchs N, Bielack SS, Epler D, et al: Long-term results of the co-operative German-Austrian-Swiss osteosarcoma study group's protocol COSS-86 of intensive multidrug chemotherapy and surgery for osteosarcoma of the limbs. Ann Oncol 1998;9:893.
164. Garrison RC, Unni KK, McLeod RA, et al: Chondrosarcoma arising in osteochondroma. Cancer 1982;49:1890.
165. Gebhardt MC: Molecular biology of sarcomas. Orthop Clin North Am 1996;27:421.
166. Gebhardt MC, Flugstad DI, Springfield DS, et al: The use of bone allografts for limb salvage in high-grade extremity osteosarcoma. Clin Orthop Relat Res 1991:181.
167. Gebhardt MC, Jaffe K, Mankin HJ: Bone allografts for tumors and other reconstructions in children. In Langlais F, Tomeno B (eds): Limb Salvage: Major Reconstruction in Oncologic and Nontumoral Conditions. Berlin, Springer-Verlag, 1991, p 561.
168. Gebhardt MC, Roth YF, Mankin HJ: Osteoarticular allografts for reconstruction in the proximal part of the humerus after excision of a musculoskeletal tumor. J Bone Joint Surg Am 1990;72:334.
169. Gebhart MJ, McCormack RR Jr, Healey JH, et al: Modification of the skin incision for the van Ness limb rotationplasty. Clin Orthop Relat Res 1987:179.
170. Geirnaerdt MJ, Bloem JL, Eulderink F, et al: Cartilaginous tumors: Correlation of gadolinium-enhanced MR imaging and histopathologic findings. Radiology 1993;186:813.
171. Ghandur-Mnaymneh L, Mnaymneh WA, Puls S: The incidence and mechanism of transphyseal spread of

osteosarcoma of long bones. Clin Orthop Relat Res 1983:210.
172. Gherlinzoni F, Picci P, Bacci G, et al: Limb sparing versus amputation in osteosarcoma: Correlation between local control, surgical margins and tumor necrosis: Istituto Rizzoli experience. Ann Oncol 1992; 3(Suppl 2):S23.
173. Gilbert JC, Powell DM, Hartman GE, et al: Video-assisted thoracic surgery (VATS) for children with pulmonary metastases from osteosarcoma. Ann Surg Oncol 1996;3:539.
174. Gitelis S, Bertoni F, Picci P, et al: Chondrosarcoma of bone: The experience at the Istituto Ortopedico Rizzoli. J Bone Joint Surg Am 1981;63:1248.
175. Giudici MA, Moser RP Jr, Kransdorf MJ: Cartilaginous bone tumors. Radiol Clin North Am 1993;31:237.
176. Glasser DB, Lane JM, Huvos AG, et al: Survival, prognosis, and therapeutic response in osteogenic sarcoma: The Memorial Hospital experience. Cancer 1992;69:698.
177. Glaubiger DL, Makuch RW, Schwarz J: Influence of prognostic factors on survival in Ewing's sarcoma. Natl Cancer Inst Monogr 1981:285.
178. Gobel V, Jurgens H, Etspuler G, et al: Prognostic significance of tumor volume in localized Ewing's sarcoma of bone in children and adolescents. J Cancer Res Clin Oncol 1987;113:187.
179. Goorin A, Strother D, Poplack D, et al: Safety and efficacy of l-leucovorin rescue following high-dose methotrexate for osteosarcoma. Med Pediatr Oncol 1995;24:362.
180. Goorin AM, Abelson HT, Frei E 3rd: Osteosarcoma: Fifteen years later. N Engl J Med 1985;313:1637.
181. Goorin AM, Delorey MJ, Lack EE, et al: Prognostic significance of complete surgical resection of pulmonary metastases in patients with osteogenic sarcoma: Analysis of 32 patients. J Clin Oncol 1984;2:425.
182. Goorin AM, Frei E 3rd, Abelson HT: Adjuvant chemotherapy for osteosarcoma: A decade of experience. Surg Clin North Am 1981;61:1379.
183. Goorin AM, Perez-Atayde A, Gebhardt M, et al: Weekly high-dose methotrexate and doxorubicin for osteosarcoma: The Dana-Farber Cancer Institute/the Children's Hospital Study III. J Clin Oncol 1987;5:1178.
184. Goorin AM, Schwartzentruber DJ, Devidas M, et al: Presurgical chemotherapy compared with immediate surgery and adjuvant chemotherapy for nonmetastatic osteosarcoma: Pediatric Oncology Group Study POG-8651. J Clin Oncol 2003;21:1574.
185. Gottsauner-Wolf F, Kotz R, Knahr K, et al: Rotationplasty for limb salvage in the treatment of malignant tumors at the knee: A follow-up study of seventy patients. J Bone Joint Surg Am 1991;73:1365.
186. Gradinger R, Rechl H, Hipp E: Pelvic osteosarcoma: Resection, reconstruction, local control, and survival statistics. Clin Orthop Relat Res 1991:149.
187. Greene MH, Glaubiger DL, Mead GD, et al: Subsequent cancer in patients with Ewing's sarcoma. Cancer Treat Rep 1979;63:2043.
188. Grier HE: The Ewing family of tumors: Ewing's sarcoma and primitive neuroectodermal tumors. Pediatr Clin North Am 1997;44:991.
189. Grier HE, Krailo MD, Tarbell NJ, et al: Addition of ifosfamide and etoposide to standard chemotherapy for Ewing's sarcoma and primitive neuroectodermal tumor of bone. N Engl J Med 2003;348:694.
190. Grier HE, Perez-Atayde AR, Weinstein HJ: Chemotherapy for inoperable infantile fibrosarcoma. Cancer 1985;56:1507.
191. Grimer RJ, Bielack S, Flege S, et al: Periosteal osteosarcoma—a European review of outcome. Eur J Cancer 2005;41:2806.
192. Grimer RJ, Taminiau AM, Cannon SR: Surgical outcomes in osteosarcoma. J Bone Joint Surg Br 2002;84:395.
193. Gross E, Rao BN, Bowman L, et al: Outcome of treatment for pediatric sarcoma of the foot: A retrospective review over a 20-year period. J Pediatr Surg 1997;32: 1181.
194. Gross E, Rao BN, Pappo AS, et al: Soft tissue sarcoma of the hand in children: Clinical outcome and management. J Pediatr Surg 1997;32:698.
195. Grundmann E, Roessner A, Ueda Y, et al: Current aspects of the pathology of osteosarcoma. Anticancer Res 1995;15:1023.
196. Grundmann E, Ueda Y, Schneider-Stock R, et al: New aspects of cell biology in osteosarcoma. Pathol Res Pract 1995;191:563.
197. Gunawardena S, Chintagumpala M, Trautwein L, et al: Multifocal osteosarcoma: An unusual presentation. J Pediatr Hematol Oncol 1999;21:58.
198. Gurney J, Swensen A, Bulterys M: Malignant bone tumors. In Ries SM, Gurney JG, et al (eds): Cancer Incidence and Survival among Children and Adolescents: United States SEER Program 1975-1995. Bethesda, Md, National Cancer Institute SEER Program, 1999, p 99.
199. Gururangan S, Marina NM, Luo X, et al: Treatment of children with peripheral primitive neuroectodermal tumor or extraosseous Ewing's tumor with Ewing's-directed therapy. J Pediatr Hematol Oncol 1998;20:55.
200. Hadjipavlou A, Lander P, Srolovitz H, et al: Malignant transformation in Paget disease of bone. Cancer 1992; 70:2802.
201. Haibach H, Farrell C, Dittrich FJ: Neoplasms arising in Paget's disease of bone: A study of 82 cases. Am J Clin Pathol 1985;83:594.
202. Hall RB, Robinson LH, Malawar MM, et al: Periosteal osteosarcoma. Cancer 1985;55:165.
203. Halliday BE, Slagel DD, Elsheikh TE, et al: Diagnostic utility of MIC-2 immunocytochemical staining in the differential diagnosis of small blue cell tumors. Diagn Cytopathol 1998;19:410.
204. Hamre MR, Severson RK, Chuba P, et al: Osteosarcoma as a second malignant neoplasm. Radiother Oncol 2002;65:153.
205. Hanlon M, Krajbich JI: Rotationplasty in skeletally immature patients: Long-term followup results. Clin Orthop Relat Res 1999:75.
206. Hanna SL, Fletcher BD, Kaste SC, et al: Increased confidence of diagnosis of Ewing sarcoma using T2-weighted MR images. Magn Reson Imaging 1994;12: 559.
207. Hanna SL, Langston JW, Gronemeyer SA, et al: Subtraction technique for contrast-enhanced MR images of

musculoskeletal tumors. Magn Reson Imaging 1990;8: 213.
208. Hansen MF: Molecular genetic considerations in osteosarcoma. Clin Orthop Relat Res 1991:237.
209. Harris MB, Gieser P, Goorin AM, et al: Treatment of metastatic osteosarcoma at diagnosis: A Pediatric Oncology Group Study. J Clin Oncol 1998;16:3641.
210. Hartman KR, Triche TJ, Kinsella TJ, et al: Prognostic value of histopathology in Ewing's sarcoma: Long-term follow-up of distal extremity primary tumors. Cancer 1991;67:163.
211. Hayes FA, Thompson EI, Meyer WH, et al: Therapy for localized Ewing's sarcoma of bone. J Clin Oncol 1989; 7:208.
212. Hays DM: Rhabdomyosarcoma. Clin Orthop Relat Res 1993:36.
213. Hays DM, Newton W Jr, Soule EH, et al: Mortality among children with rhabdomyosarcomas of the alveolar histologic subtype. J Pediatr Surg 1983;18:412.
214. Hays DM, Soule EH, Lawrence W Jr, et al: Extremity lesions in the Intergroup Rhabdomyosarcoma Study (IRS-I): A preliminary report. Cancer 1982;49:1.
215. Hays DM, Sutow WW, Lawrence W Jr, et al: Rhabdomyosarcoma: Surgical therapy in extremeity lesions in children. Orthop Clin North Am 1977;8:883.
216. Hayward PG, Orgill DP, Mulliken JB, et al: Congenital fibrosarcoma masquerading as lymphatic malformation: Report of two cases. J Pediatr Surg 1995;30: 84.
217. Heeg M, Torode IP: Rotationplasty of the lower limb for childhood osteosarcoma of the femur. Aust N Z J Surg 1998;68:643.
218. Heij HA, Vos A, de Kraker J, et al: Prognostic factors in surgery for pulmonary metastases in children. Surgery 1994;115:687.
219. Herman TE, McAlister WH, Dehner LP, et al: Dedifferentiated chondrosarcoma in childhood: Report of a case. Pediatr Radiol 1995;25(Suppl 1):S140.
220. Herold CJ, Bankier AA, Fleischmann D: Lung metastases. Eur Radiol 1996;6:596.
221. Hillmann A, Hoffmann C, Gosheger G, et al: Malignant tumor of the distal part of the femur or the proximal part of the tibia: Endoprosthetic replacement or rotationplasty. Functional outcome and quality-of-life measurements. J Bone Joint Surg Am 1999;81:462.
222. Hoffmann C, Ahrens S, Dunst J, et al: Pelvic Ewing sarcoma: A retrospective analysis of 241 cases. Cancer 1999;85:869.
223. Holscher HC, Bloem JL, Nooy MA, et al: The value of MR imaging in monitoring the effect of chemotherapy on bone sarcomas. AJR Am J Roentgenol 1990;154: 763.
224. Hopper KD, Eggli KD, Haseman DB, et al: Osteosarcomatosis and metastatic osteosarcoma. Cancer Treat Res 1993;62:163.
225. Hornicek FJ Jr, Mnaymneh W, Lackman RD, et al: Limb salvage with osteoarticular allografts after resection of proximal tibia bone tumors. Clin Orthop Relat Res 1998:179.
226. Horowitz M, Malawer M, Woo S, et al: Ewing's sarcoma family of tumors: Ewing's sarcoma of bone and soft tissue and the peripheral primitive neuroectodermal tumors. In Pizzo P, Poplack D (eds): Principles and Practice of Pediatric Oncology. Philadelphia, JB Lippincott, 1997, p 831.
227. Horowitz ME, Pratt CB, Webber BL, et al: Therapy for childhood soft-tissue sarcomas other than rhabdomyosarcoma: A review of 62 cases treated at a single institution. J Clin Oncol 1986;4:559.
228. Horowitz ME, Tsokos MG, DeLaney TF: Ewing's sarcoma. CA Cancer J Clin 1992;42:300.
229. Hou-Jensen K, Priori E, Dmochowski L: Studies on ultrastructure of Ewing's sarcoma of bone. Cancer 1972;29:280.
230. Hudson TM, Enneking WF, Hawkins IF Jr: The value of angiography in planning surgical treatment of bone tumors. Radiology 1981;138:283.
231. Hudson TM, Hamlin DJ, Enneking WF, et al: Magnetic resonance imaging of bone and soft tissue tumors: Early experience in 31 patients compared with computed tomography. Skeletal Radiol 1985;13:134.
232. Hudson TM, Schiebler M, Springfield DS, et al: Radiologic imaging of osteosarcoma: Role in planning surgical treatment. Skeletal Radiol 1983;10:137.
233. Huvos AG: Osteogenic sarcoma of bones and soft tissues in older persons: A clinicopathologic analysis of 117 patients older than 60 years. Cancer 1986;57: 1442.
234. Huvos AG: James Ewing: Cancer man. Ann Diagn Pathol 1998;2:146.
235. Huvos AG, Butler A, Bretsky SS: Osteogenic sarcoma associated with Paget's disease of bone: A clinicopathologic study of 65 patients. Cancer 1983;52:1489.
236. Huvos AG, Higinbotham NL, Miller TR: Bone sarcomas arising in fibrous dysplasia. J Bone Joint Surg Am 1972;54:1047.
237. Huvos AG, Marcove RC: Chondrosarcoma in the young: A clinicopathologic analysis of 79 patients younger than 21 years of age. Am J Surg Pathol 1987; 11:930.
238. Huvos AG, Rosen G, Marcove RC: Primary osteogenic sarcoma: Pathologic aspects in 20 patients after treatment with chemotherapy, en bloc resection, and prosthetic bone replacement. Arch Pathol Lab Med 1977; 101:14.
239. Huvos AG, Woodard HQ, Cahan WG, et al: Postradiation osteogenic sarcoma of bone and soft tissues: A clinicopathologic study of 66 patients. Cancer 1985;55: 1244.
240. Ibarburen C, Haberman JJ, Zerhouni EA: Peripheral primitive neuroectodermal tumors: CT and MRI evaluation. Eur J Radiol 1996;21:225.
241. Imbriaco M, Yeh SD, Yeung H, et al: Thallium-201 scintigraphy for the evaluation of tumor response to preoperative chemotherapy in patients with osteosarcoma. Cancer 1997;80:1507.
242. Ishida T, Machinami R, Kojima T, et al: Malignant fibrous histiocytoma and osteosarcoma in association with fibrous dysplasia of bone: Report of three cases. Pathol Res Pract 1992;188:757.
243. Jablons D, Steinberg SM, Roth J, et al: Metastasectomy for soft tissue sarcoma: Further evidence for efficacy and prognostic indicators. J Thorac Cardiovasc Surg 1989;97:695.

244. Jacobs PA: Limb salvage and rotationplasty for osteosarcoma in children. Clin Orthop Relat Res 1984:217.
245. Jaffe H: Tumors and Tumorous Conditions of the Bones and Joints. Philadelphia, Lea & Febiger, 1968.
246. Jaffe N, Frei E 3rd, Traggis D, et al: Adjuvant methotrexate and citrovorum-factor treatment of osteogenic sarcoma. N Engl J Med 1974;291:994.
247. Jaffe N, Keifer R 3rd, Robertson R, et al: Renal toxicity with cumulative doses of cis-diamminedichloroplatinum-II in pediatric patients with osteosarcoma: Effect on creatinine clearance and methotrexate excretion. Cancer 1987;59:1577.
248. Jaffe N, Paed D, Traggis D, et al: Improved outlook for Ewing's sarcoma with combination chemotherapy (vincristine, actinomycin D and cyclophosphamide) and radiation therapy. Cancer 1976;38:1925.
249. Jaffe N, Pearson P, Yasko AW, et al: Single and multiple metachronous osteosarcoma tumors after therapy. Cancer 2003;98:2457.
250. Jaffe N, Spears R, Eftekhari F, et al: Pathologic fracture in osteosarcoma: Impact of chemotherapy on primary tumor and survival. Cancer 1987;59:701.
251. Jaramillo D, Laor T, Gebhardt MC: Pediatric musculoskeletal neoplasms: Evaluation with MR imaging. Magn Reson Imaging Clin N Am 1996;4:749.
252. Jasani B, Cristaudo A, Emri SA, et al: Association of SV40 with human tumours. Semin Cancer Biol 2001; 11:49.
253. Jentzsch K, Binder H, Cramer H, et al: Leg function after radiotherapy for Ewing's sarcoma. Cancer 1981; 47:1267.
254. Jeon IS, Davis JN, Braun BS, et al: A variant Ewing's sarcoma translocation (7;22) fuses the EWS gene to the ETS gene ETV1. Oncogene 1995;10:1229.
255. Johnson DG: Trends in surgery for childhood rhabdomyosarcoma. Cancer 1975;35:916.
256. Johnstone PA, Wexler LH, Venzon DJ, et al: Sarcomas of the hand and foot: Analysis of local control and functional result with combined modality therapy in extremity preservation. Int J Radiat Oncol Biol Phys 1994;29:735.
257. Jones RD, Reid R, Balakrishnan G, et al: Multifocal synchronous osteosarcoma: The Scottish Bone Tumour Registry experience. Med Pediatr Oncol 1993; 21:111.
258. Juergens H, Kosloff C, Nirenberg A, et al: Prognostic factors in the response of primary osteogenic sarcoma to preoperative chemotherapy (high-dose methotrexate with citrovorum factor). Natl Cancer Inst Monogr 1981:221.
259. Jurgens H, Beron G, Winkler K: Toxicity associated with combination chemotherapy for osteosarcoma: A report of the Cooperative Osteosarcoma Study (COSS 80). J Cancer Res Clin Oncol 1983;106(Suppl):14.
260. Jurgens H, Exner U, Gadner H, et al: Multidisciplinary treatment of primary Ewing's sarcoma of bone: A 6-year experience of a European cooperative trial. Cancer 1988;61:23.
261. Jurgens H, Exner U, Kuhl J, et al: High-dose ifosfamide with mesna uroprotection in Ewing's sarcoma. Cancer Chemother Pharmacol 1989;24(Suppl 1):S40.
262. Kampe CE, Rosen G, Eilber F, et al: Synovial sarcoma: A study of intensive chemotherapy in 14 patients with localized disease. Cancer 1993;72:2161.
263. Kasser JE: Amputations and prosthetics. In Kasser JE (ed): Orthopaedic Knowledge Update, vol 5. Chicago, American Academy of Orthopaedic Surgeons, 1997.
264. Kawai A, Hamada M, Sugihara S, et al: Rotationplasty for patients with osteosarcoma around the knee joint. Acta Med Okayama 1995;49:221.
265. Kawai A, Huvos AG, Meyers PA, et al: Osteosarcoma of the pelvis: Oncologic results of 40 patients. Clin Orthop Relat Res 1998:196.
266. Kayton ML, Huvos AG, Casher J, et al: Computed tomographic scan of the chest underestimates the number of metastatic lesions in osteosarcoma. J Pediatr Surg 2006;41:200.
267. Kenan S, Bloom N, Lewis MM: Limb-sparing surgery in skeletally immature patients with osteosarcoma: The use of an expandable prosthesis. Clin Orthop Relat Res 1991:223.
268. Kharasch VS, Lipsitz S, Santis W, et al: Long-term pulmonary toxicity of multiagent chemotherapy including bleomycin and cyclophosphamide in osteosarcoma survivors. Med Pediatr Oncol 1996;27:85.
269. Kilpatrick SE, Pike EJ, Ward WG, et al: Dedifferentiated chondrosarcoma in patients with multiple osteochondromatosis: Report of a case and review of the literature. Skeletal Radiol 1997;26:370.
270. Kim SJ, Choi JA, Lee SH, et al: Imaging findings of extrapulmonary metastases of osteosarcoma. Clin Imaging 2004;28:291.
271. Kinsella TJ, Loeffler JS, Fraass BA, et al: Extremity preservation by combined modality therapy in sarcomas of the hand and foot: An analysis of local control, disease free survival and functional result. Int J Radiat Oncol Biol Phys 1983;9:1115.
272. Kinsella TJ, Miser JS, Waller B, et al: Long-term follow-up of Ewing's sarcoma of bone treated with combined modality therapy. Int J Radiat Oncol Biol Phys 1991; 20:389.
273. Kissane JM, Askin FB, Foulkes M, et al: Ewing's sarcoma of bone: Clinicopathologic aspects of 303 cases from the Intergroup Ewing's Sarcoma Study. Hum Pathol 1983; 14:773.
274. Knahr K, Kristen H, Ritschl P, et al: Prosthetic management and functional evaluation of patients with resection of the distal femur and rotationplasty. Orthopedics 1987;10:1241.
275. Kolb EA, Kushner BH, Gorlick R, et al: Long-term event-free survival after intensive chemotherapy for Ewing's family of tumors in children and young adults. J Clin Oncol 2003;21:3423.
276. Komiya S, Gebhardt MC, Mangham DC, et al: Role of glutathione in cisplatin resistance in osteosarcoma cell lines. J Orthop Res 1998;16:15.
277. Koscick RL, Petersilge CA, Makley JT, et al: CT-guided fine needle aspiration and needle core biopsy of skeletal lesions: Complementary diagnostic techniques. Acta Cytol 1998;42:697.
278. Kotz R: Rotationplasty. Semin Surg Oncol 1997;13:34.

279. Kotz R, Salzer M: Rotation-plasty for childhood osteosarcoma of the distal part of the femur. J Bone Joint Surg Am 1982;64:959.
280. Krajbich JI: Modified van Ness rotationplasty in the treatment of malignant neoplasms in the lower extremities of children. Clin Orthop Relat Res 1991:74.
281. Kramer S, Meadows AT, Jarrett P, et al: Incidence of childhood cancer: Experience of a decade in a population-based registry. J Natl Cancer Inst 1983;70:49.
282. Kumar S, Pack S, Kumar D, et al: Detection of EWS-FLI-1 fusion in Ewing's sarcoma/peripheral primitive neuroectodermal tumor by fluorescence in situ hybridization using formalin-fixed paraffin-embedded tissue. Hum Pathol 1999;30:324.
283. Kurt AM, Unni KK, McLeod RA, et al: Low-grade intraosseous osteosarcoma. Cancer 1990;65:1418.
284. Kutluk MT, Yalcin B, Akyuz C, et al: Treatment results and prognostic factors in Ewing sarcoma. Pediatr Hematol Oncol 2004;21:597.
285. Kuttesch JF Jr, Wexler LH, Marcus RB, et al: Second malignancies after Ewing's sarcoma: Radiation dose-dependency of secondary sarcomas. J Clin Oncol 1996;14:2818.
286. Kynaston JA, Malcolm AJ, Craft AW, et al: Chemotherapy in the management of infantile fibrosarcoma. Med Pediatr Oncol 1993;21:488.
287. Ladanyi M, Cha C, Lewis R, et al: MDM2 gene amplification in metastatic osteosarcoma. Cancer Res 1993;53:16.
288. Ladenstein R, Treuner J, Koscielniak E, et al: Synovial sarcoma of childhood and adolescence: Report of the German CWS-81 study. Cancer 1993;71:3647.
289. Lang P, Johnston JO, Arenal-Romero F, et al: Advances in MR imaging of pediatric musculoskeletal neoplasms. Magn Reson Imaging Clin N Am 1998;6:579.
290. Lanza LA, Miser JS, Pass HI, et al: The role of resection in the treatment of pulmonary metastases from Ewing's sarcoma. J Thorac Cardiovasc Surg 1987;94:181.
291. LaQuaglia MP: Extremity rhabdomyosarcoma: Biological principles, staging, and treatment. Semin Surg Oncol 1993;9:510.
292. LaQuaglia MP, Ghavimi F, Penenberg D, et al: Factors predictive of mortality in pediatric extremity rhabdomyosarcoma. J Pediatr Surg 1990;25:238.
293. Larsson SE, Lorentzon R: The incidence of malignant primary bone tumours in relation to age, sex and site: A study of osteogenic sarcoma, chondrosarcoma and Ewing's sarcoma diagnosed in Sweden from 1958 to 1968. J Bone Joint Surg Br 1974;56:534.
294. Laus M: Multicentric osteosarcoma. Ital J Orthop Traumatol 1980;6:249.
295. Lawrence W Jr, Gehan EA, Hays DM, et al: Prognostic significance of staging factors of the UICC staging system in childhood rhabdomyosarcoma: A report from the Intergroup Rhabdomyosarcoma Study (IRS-II). J Clin Oncol 1987;5:46.
296. Lawrence W Jr, Hays DM, Heyn R, et al: Lymphatic metastases with childhood rhabdomyosarcoma: A report from the Intergroup Rhabdomyosarcoma Study. Cancer 1987;60:910.
297. Lazda EJ, Berry PJ: Bone marrow metastasis in Ewing's sarcoma and peripheral primitive neuroectodermal tumor: An immunohistochemical study. Pediatr Dev Pathol 1998;1:125.
298. Le Vu B, de Vathaire F, Shamsaldin A, et al: Radiation dose, chemotherapy and risk of osteosarcoma after solid tumours during childhood. Int J Cancer 1998;77:370.
299. Leavey PJ, Day MD, Booth T, et al: Skip metastasis in osteosarcoma. J Pediatr Hematol Oncol 2003;25:806.
300. Lee CS, Southey MC, Waters K, et al: EWS/FLI-1 fusion transcript detection and MIC2 immunohistochemical staining in the diagnosis of Ewing's sarcoma. Pediatr Pathol Lab Med 1996;16:379.
301. Lee FY, Mankin HJ, Fondren G, et al: Chondrosarcoma of bone: An assessment of outcome. J Bone Joint Surg Am 1999;81:326.
302. Lee SM, Hajdu SI, Exelby PR: Synovial sarcoma in children. Surg Gynecol Obstet 1974;138:701.
303. Leeson MC, Smith MJ: Ewing's sarcoma of the foot. Foot Ankle 1989;10:147.
304. Legeai-Mallet L, Munnich A, Maroteaux P, et al: Incomplete penetrance and expressivity skewing in hereditary multiple exostoses. Clin Genet 1997;52:12.
305. Lemmi MA, Fletcher BD, Marina NM, et al: Use of MR imaging to assess results of chemotherapy for Ewing sarcoma. AJR Am J Roentgenol 1990;155:343.
306. Leonard A, Craft AW, Moss C, et al: Osteogenic sarcoma in the Rothmund-Thomson syndrome. Med Pediatr Oncol 1996;26:249.
307. Lewis RJ, Marcove RC, Rosen G: Ewing's sarcoma—functional effects of radiation therapy. J Bone Joint Surg Am 1977;59:325.
308. Li WK, Lane JM, Rosen G, et al: Pelvic Ewing's sarcoma: Advances in treatment. J Bone Joint Surg Am 1983;65:738.
309. Lindner NJ, Ramm O, Hillmann A, et al: Limb salvage and outcome of osteosarcoma: The University of Muenster experience. Clin Orthop Relat Res 1999:83.
310. Link MP, Goorin AM, Horowitz M, et al: Adjuvant chemotherapy of high-grade osteosarcoma of the extremity: Updated results of the Multi-institutional Osteosarcoma Study. Clin Orthop Relat Res 1991:8.
311. Link MP, Goorin AM, Miser AW, et al: The effect of adjuvant chemotherapy on relapse-free survival in patients with osteosarcoma of the extremity. N Engl J Med 1986;314:1600.
312. Lipshultz SE, Lipsitz SR, Mone SM, et al: Female sex and drug dose as risk factors for late cardiotoxic effects of doxorubicin therapy for childhood cancer. N Engl J Med 1995;332:1738.
313. Liu Y, Chen WY: Ewing's sarcoma of the metacarpal bone of the hand: A case report. J Hand Surg [Am] 1998;23:748.
314. Llombart-Bosch A, Contesso G, Peydro-Olaya A: Histology, immunohistochemistry, and electron microscopy of small round cell tumors of bone. Semin Diagn Pathol 1996;13:153.
315. Loder RT, Herring JA: Disarticulation of the knee in children: A functional assessment. J Bone Joint Surg Am 1987;69:1155.
316. Loh ML, Ahn P, Perez-Atayde AR, et al: Treatment of infantile fibrosarcoma with chemotherapy and surgery:

Results from the Dana-Farber Cancer Institute and Children's Hospital, Boston. J Pediatr Hematol Oncol 2002;24:722.
317. Lonardo F, Ueda T, Huvos AG, et al: p53 and MDM2 alterations in osteosarcomas: Correlation with clinicopathologic features and proliferative rate. Cancer 1997; 79:1541.
318. Longhi A, Fabbri N, Donati D, et al: Neoadjuvant chemotherapy for patients with synchronous multifocal osteosarcoma: Results in eleven cases. J Chemother 2001;13:324.
319. Lord CF, Gebhardt MC, Tomford WW, et al: Infection in bone allografts: Incidence, nature, and treatment. J Bone Joint Surg Am 1988;70:369.
320. Lucas DR, Bentley G, Dan ME, et al: Ewing sarcoma vs lymphoblastic lymphoma: A comparative immunohistochemical study. Am J Clin Pathol 2001;115:11.
321. Luksch R, Sampietro G, Collini P, et al: Prognostic value of clinicopathologic characteristics including neuroectodermal differentiation in osseous Ewing's sarcoma family of tumors in children. Tumori 1999;85:101.
322. Lushiku HB, Gebhart M: Osteosarcoma of the proximal fibula: Report of 3 cases. Acta Chir Belg 1997;97:260.
323. Mahoney DH Jr, Shepherd DA, DePuey EG, et al: Childhood multifocal osteosarcoma—diagnosis by 99m technetium bone scan: A case report. Med Pediatr Oncol 1979;6:347.
324. Mahoney JP, Spanier SS, Morris JL: Multifocal osteosarcoma: A case report with review of the literature. Cancer 1979;44:1897.
325. Malkin D, Chilton-MacNeill S, Meister LA, et al: Tissue-specific expression of SV40 in tumors associated with the Li-Fraumeni syndrome. Oncogene 2001;20:4441.
326. Mandell L, Ghavimi F, LaQuaglia M, et al: Prognostic significance of regional lymph node involvement in childhood extremity rhabdomyosarcoma. Med Pediatr Oncol 1990;18:466.
327. Mankin HJ, Cantley KP, Lippiello L, et al: The biology of human chondrosarcoma. I. Description of the cases, grading, and biochemical analyses. J Bone Joint Surg Am 1980;62:160.
328. Mankin HJ, Gebhardt MC, Jennings LC, et al: Long-term results of allograft replacement in the management of bone tumors. Clin Orthop Relat Res 1996:86.
329. Mankin HJ, Lange TA, Spanier SS: The hazards of biopsy in patients with malignant primary bone and soft-tissue tumors. J Bone Joint Surg Am 1982;64:1121.
330. Mankin HJ, Mankin CJ, Simon MA: The hazards of the biopsy, revisited: Members of the Musculoskeletal Tumor Society. J Bone Joint Surg Am 1996;78:656.
331. Marcantonio DR, Weatherall PT, Berrey BH Jr: Practical considerations in the imaging of soft tissue tumors. Orthop Clin North Am 1998;29:1.
332. Marcove RC, Martini N, Rosen G: The treatment of pulmonary metastasis in osteogenic sarcoma. Clin Orthop Relat Res 1975:65.
333. Marcove RC, Mike V, Hajek JV, et al: Osteogenic sarcoma under the age of twenty-one: A review of one hundred and forty-five operative cases. J Bone Joint Surg Am 1970;52:411.
334. Marcove RC, Rosen G: Radical en bloc excision of Ewing's sarcoma. Clin Orthop Relat Res 1980:86.
335. Marcus KC, Grier HE, Shamberger RC, et al: Childhood soft tissue sarcoma: A 20-year experience. J Pediatr 1997;131:603.
336. Marcus RB Jr: Current controversies in pediatric radiation oncology. Orthop Clin North Am 1996;27:551.
337. Marcus RB Jr, Cantor A, Heare TC, et al: Local control and function after twice-a-day radiotherapy for Ewing's sarcoma of bone. Int J Radiat Oncol Biol Phys 1991; 21:1509.
338. Masciocchi C, Sparvoli L, Barile A: Diagnostic imaging of malignant cartilage tumors. Eur J Radiol 1998;27(Suppl 1):S86.
339. Matsuno T, Unni KK, McLeod RA, et al: Telangiectatic osteogenic sarcoma. Cancer 1976;38:2538.
340. Maurer HM, Gehan EA, Beltangady M, et al: The Intergroup Rhabdomyosarcoma Study-II. Cancer 1993;71: 1904.
341. Maurer HM, Moon T, Donaldson M, et al: The Intergroup Rhabdomyosarcoma Study: A preliminary report. Cancer 1977;40:2015.
342. May WA, Gishizky ML, Lessnick SL, et al: Ewing sarcoma 11;22 translocation produces a chimeric transcription factor that requires the DNA-binding domain encoded by FLI1 for transformation. Proc Natl Acad Sci U S A 1993;90:5752.
343. McHugh K, Boothroyd AE: The role of radiology in childhood rhabdomyosarcoma. Clin Radiol 1999;54: 2.
344. McIntyre JF, Smith-Sorensen B, Friend SH, et al: Germline mutations of the p53 tumor suppressor gene in children with osteosarcoma. J Clin Oncol 1994;12:925.
345. McKenna RJ, Schwinn CP, Soong KY, et al: Sarcomata of the osteogenic series (osteosarcoma, fibrosarcoma, chondrosarcoma, parosteal osteogenic sarcoma, and sarcoma arising in abnormal bone): An analysis of 522 cases. J Bone Joint Surg Am 1966;48:1.
346. McLean RG, Choy D, Hoschl R, et al: Role of radionuclide imaging in the diagnosis of chondrosarcoma. Med Pediatr Oncol 1985;13:32.
347. Medcalf A: Van Ness rotationplasty: The psychosocial perspective. Can Oper Room Nurs J 1987;5:12.
348. Meier VS, Kuhne T, Jundt G, et al: Molecular diagnosis of Ewing tumors: Improved detection of EWS-FLI-1 and EWS-ERG chimeric transcripts and rapid determination of exon combinations. Diagn Mol Pathol 1998; 7:29.
349. Meister P, Konrad E, Lob G, et al: Osteosarcoma: Histological evaluation and grading. Arch Orthop Trauma Surg 1979;94:91.
350. Merchan EC, Sanchez-Herrera S, Gonzalez JM: Secondary chondrosarcoma: Four cases and review of the literature. Acta Orthop Belg 1993;59:76.
351. Merkel KD, Gebhardt M, Springfield DS: Rotationplasty as a reconstructive operation after tumor resection. Clin Orthop Relat Res 1991:231.
352. Mervak TR, Unni KK, Pritchard DJ, et al: Telangiectatic osteosarcoma. Clin Orthop Relat Res 1991:135.
353. Meyer JS, Dormans JP: Differential diagnosis of pediatric musculoskeletal masses. Magn Reson Imaging Clin N Am 1998;6:561.
354. Meyers PA, Gorlick R: Osteosarcoma. Pediatr Clin North Am 1997;44:973.

355. Meyers PA, Heller G, Healey J, et al: Chemotherapy for nonmetastatic osteogenic sarcoma: The Memorial Sloan-Kettering experience. J Clin Oncol 1992;10:5.
356. Meyers PA, Heller G, Healey JH, et al: Osteogenic sarcoma with clinically detectable metastasis at initial presentation. J Clin Oncol 1993;11:449.
357. Meyers PA, Schwartz CL, Krailo M, et al: Osteosarcoma: A randomized, prospective trial of the addition of ifosfamide and/or muramyl tripeptide to cisplatin, doxorubicin, and high-dose methotrexate. J Clin Oncol 2005;23:2004.
358. Mialou V, Philip T, Kalifa C, et al: Metastatic osteosarcoma at diagnosis: Prognostic factors and long-term outcome—the French pediatric experience. Cancer 2005;104:1100.
359. Miller SL, Hoffer FA, Reddick WE, et al: Tumor volume or dynamic contrast-enhanced MRI for prediction of clinical outcome of Ewing sarcoma family of tumors. Pediatr Radiol 2001;31:518.
360. Mirra JM, Gold R, Downs J, et al: A new histologic approach to the differentiation of enchondroma and chondrosarcoma of the bones: A clinicopathologic analysis of 51 cases. Clin Orthop Relat Res 1985:214.
361. Miser J, Triche T, Kinsella T, et al: Other soft tissue sarcomas of childhood. In Pizzo P, Poplack D (eds): Principles and Practice of Pediatric Oncology. Philadelphia, JB Lippincott, 1997, p 865.
362. Moore TE, King AR, Kathol MH, et al: Sarcoma in Paget disease of bone: Clinical, radiologic, and pathologic features in 22 cases. AJR Am J Roentgenol 1991;156: 1199.
363. Murphey MD, van Jaovisidha S, Temple HT, et al: Telangiectatic osteosarcoma: Radiologic-pathologic comparison. Radiology 2003;229:545.
364. Murray MP, Jacobs PA, Gore DR, et al: Functional performance after tibial rotationplasty. J Bone Joint Surg Am 1985;67:392.
365. Muscolo DL, Ayerza MA, Aponte-Tinao LA, et al: Partial epiphyseal preservation and intercalary allograft reconstruction in high-grade metaphyseal osteosarcoma of the knee. J Bone Joint Surg Am 2004;86: 2686.
366. Nag S, Grecula J, Ruymann FB: Aggressive chemotherapy, organ-preserving surgery, and high-dose-rate remote brachytherapy in the treatment of rhabdomyosarcoma in infants and young children. Cancer 1993; 72:2769.
367. Neff G: Knee-disarticulation. Acta Chir Belg 1981;80: 253.
368. Neifeld JP, Berg JW, Godwin D, et al: A retrospective epidemiologic study of pediatric fibrosarcomas. J Pediatr Surg 1978;13:735.
369. Neifeld JP, Godwin D, Berg JW, et al: Prognostic features of pediatric soft-tissue sarcomas. Surgery 1985; 98:93.
370. Nesbit ME Jr, Gehan EA, Burgert EO Jr, et al: Multimodal therapy for the management of primary, nonmetastatic Ewing's sarcoma of bone: A long-term follow-up of the first Intergroup Study. J Clin Oncol 1990;8:1664.
371. Newton WA Jr, Soule EH, Hamoudi AB, et al: Histopathology of childhood sarcomas, Intergroup Rhabdomyosarcoma Studies I and II: Clinicopathologic correlation. J Clin Oncol 1988;6:67.
372. Ninane J, Gosseye S, Panteon E, et al: Congenital fibrosarcoma: Preoperative chemotherapy and conservative surgery. Cancer 1986;58:1400.
373. Norman A, Sissons HA: Radiographic hallmarks of peripheral chondrosarcoma. Radiology 1984;151:589.
374. Oberlin O, Habrand JL, Zucker JM, et al: No benefit of ifosfamide in Ewing's sarcoma: A nonrandomized study of the French Society of Pediatric Oncology. J Clin Oncol 1992;10:1407.
375. O'Connor MI, Pritchard DJ: Ewing's sarcoma: Prognostic factors, disease control, and the reemerging role of surgical treatment. Clin Orthop Relat Res 1991:78.
376. O'Flanagan SJ, Stack JP, McGee HM, et al: Imaging of intramedullary tumour spread in osteosarcoma: A comparison of techniques. J Bone Joint Surg Br 1991; 73:998.
377. Ohtomo K, Terui S, Yokoyama R, et al: Thallium-201 scintigraphy to assess effect of chemotherapy in osteosarcoma. J Nucl Med 1996;37:1444.
378. Okada K, Unni KK, Swee RG, et al: High grade surface osteosarcoma: A clinicopathologic study of 46 cases. Cancer 1999;85:1044.
379. Okada K, Wold LE, Beabout JW, et al: Osteosarcoma of the hand: A clinicopathologic study of 12 cases. Cancer 1993;72:719.
380. Olson PN, Prewitt L, Griffiths HJ, et al: Case report 703: Multifocal osteosarcoma. Skeletal Radiol 1991;20:624.
381. O'Neal ML, Bahner R, Ganey TM, et al: Osseous overgrowth after amputation in adolescents and children. J Pediatr Orthop 1996;16:78.
382. Ookawa K, Tsuchida S, Adachi J, et al: Differentiation induced by RB expression and apoptosis induced by p53 expression in an osteosarcoma cell line. Oncogene 1997;14:1389.
383. Ortiz-Cruz E, Gebhardt MC, Jennings LC, et al: The results of transplantation of intercalary allografts after resection of tumors: A long-term follow-up study. J Bone Joint Surg Am 1997;79:97.
384. Ozdemir HM, Yildiz Y, Yilmaz C, et al: Tumors of the foot and ankle: Analysis of 196 cases. J Foot Ankle Surg 1997;36:403.
385. Panuel M, Gentet JC, Scheiner C, et al: Physeal and epiphyseal extent of primary malignant bone tumors in childhood: Correlation of preoperative MRI and the pathologic examination. Pediatr Radiol 1993;23:421.
386. Pappo AS: Rhabdomyosarcoma and other soft tissue sarcomas of childhood. Curr Opin Oncol 1995;7:361.
387. Pappo AS, Fontanesi J, Luo X, et al: Synovial sarcoma in children and adolescents: The St Jude Children's Research Hospital experience. J Clin Oncol 1994;12: 2360.
388. Pappo AS, Pratt CB: Soft tissue sarcomas in children. Cancer Treat Res 1997;91:205.
389. Pappo AS, Rao BN, Cain A, et al: Dermatofibrosarcoma protuberans: The pediatric experience at St Jude Children's Research Hospital. Pediatr Hematol Oncol 1997;14:563.
390. Pappo AS, Shapiro DN, Crist WM: Rhabdomyosarcoma: Biology and treatment. Pediatr Clin North Am 1997;44:953.

391. Pappo AS, Shapiro DN, Crist WM, et al: Biology and therapy of pediatric rhabdomyosarcoma. J Clin Oncol 1995;13:2123.
392. Parham DM, Pratt CB, Parvey LS, et al: Childhood multifocal osteosarcoma: Clinicopathologic and radiologic correlates. Cancer 1985;55:2653.
393. Parham DM, Webber B, Holt H, et al: Immunohistochemical study of childhood rhabdomyosarcomas and related neoplasms: Results of an Intergroup Rhabdomyosarcoma Study project. Cancer 1991;67:3072.
394. Park YK, Chi SG, Park HR, et al: Detection of t(11;22)(q24;q12) translocation of Ewing's sarcoma in paraffin embedded tissue by nested reverse transcription-polymerase chain reaction. J Korean Med Sci 1998;13:395.
395. Parkin DM, Stiller CA, Draper GJ, et al: The international incidence of childhood cancer. Int J Cancer 1988;42:511.
396. Parkin DM, Stiller CA, Nectoux J: International variations in the incidence of childhood bone tumours. Int J Cancer 1993;53:371.
397. Pass HI, Dwyer A, Makuch R, et al: Detection of pulmonary metastases in patients with osteogenic and soft-tissue sarcomas: The superiority of CT scans compared with conventional linear tomograms using dynamic analysis. J Clin Oncol 1985;3:1261.
398. Patel DV, Hammer RA, Levin B, et al: Primary osteogenic sarcoma of the spine. Skeletal Radiol 1984;12: 276.
399. Paulussen M, Ahrens S, Burdach S, et al: Primary metastatic (stage IV) Ewing tumor: Survival analysis of 171 patients from the EICESS studies. European Intergroup Cooperative Ewing Sarcoma Studies. Ann Oncol 1998;9:275.
400. Paulussen M, Ahrens S, Craft AW, et al: Ewing's tumors with primary lung metastases: Survival analysis of 114 (European Intergroup) Cooperative Ewing's Sarcoma Studies patients. J Clin Oncol 1998;16:3044.
401. Peabody TD, Gibbs CP Jr, Simon MA: Evaluation and staging of musculoskeletal neoplasms. J Bone Joint Surg Am 1998;80:1204.
402. Peabody TD, Simon MA: Making the diagnosis: Keys to a successful biopsy in children with bone and soft-tissue tumors. Orthop Clin North Am 1996;27: 453.
403. Perlman EJ, Dickman PS, Askin FB, et al: Ewing's sarcoma—routine diagnostic utilization of MIC2 analysis: A Pediatric Oncology Group/Children's Cancer Group Intergroup Study. Hum Pathol 1994;25:304.
404. Philippe PG, Rao BN, Rogers DA, et al: Sarcomas of the flexor fossae in children: Is amputation necessary? J Pediatr Surg 1992;27:964.
405. Picci P, Bohling T, Bacci G, et al: Chemotherapy-induced tumor necrosis as a prognostic factor in localized Ewing's sarcoma of the extremities. J Clin Oncol 1997; 15:1553.
406. Picci P, Rougraff BT, Bacci G, et al: Prognostic significance of histopathologic response to chemotherapy in nonmetastatic Ewing's sarcoma of the extremities. J Clin Oncol 1993;11:1763.
407. Picci P, Vanel D, Briccoli A, et al: Computed tomography of pulmonary metastases from osteosarcoma: The less poor technique. A study of 51 patients with histological correlation. Ann Oncol 2001;12:1601.
408. Pignatti G, Bacci G, Picci P, et al: Telangiectatic osteogenic sarcoma of the extremities: Results in 17 patients treated with neoadjuvant chemotherapy. Clin Orthop Relat Res 1991:99.
409. Pilepich MV, Vietti TJ, Nesbit ME, et al: Radiotherapy and combination chemotherapy in advanced Ewing's sarcoma—Intergroup Study. Cancer 1981;47:1930.
410. Pochanugool L, Subhadharaphandou T, Dhanachai M, et al: Prognostic factors among 130 patients with osteosarcoma. Clin Orthop Relat Res 1997:206.
411. Pomeroy TC, Johnson RE: Prognostic factors for survival in Ewing's sarcoma. Am J Roentgenol Radium Ther Nucl Med 1975;123:598.
412. Potish RA, Dehner LP, Haselow RE, et al: The incidence of second neoplasms following megavoltage radiation for pediatric tumors. Cancer 1985;56:1534.
413. Potter DA, Kinsella T, Glatstein E, et al: High-grade soft tissue sarcomas of the extremities. Cancer 1986;58: 190.
414. Pousti TJ, Upton J, Loh M, et al: Congenital fibrosarcoma of the upper extremity. Plast Reconstr Surg 1998;102:1158.
415. Pratt CB, Rao BN, Meyer WH: Multifocal synchronous osteosarcoma: The Scottish Bone Tumour Registry experience by Jones et al, 1993. Med Pediatr Oncol 1994;22:428.
416. Prayer LM, Kropej DH, Wimberger DM, et al: High-resolution real-time sonography and MR imaging in assessment of osteocartilaginous exostoses. Acta Radiol 1991;32:393.
417. Pritchard DJ: Indications for surgical treatment of localized Ewing's sarcoma of bone. Clin Orthop Relat Res 1980:39.
418. Pritchard DJ: Surgical experience in the management of Ewing's sarcoma of bone. Natl Cancer Inst Monogr 1981:169.
419. Pritchard DJ, Dahlin DC, Dauphine RT, et al: Ewing's sarcoma: A clinicopathological and statistical analysis of patients surviving five years or longer. J Bone Joint Surg Am 1975;57:10.
420. Provisor AJ, Ettinger LJ, Nachman JB, et al: Treatment of nonmetastatic osteosarcoma of the extremity with preoperative and postoperative chemotherapy: A report from the Children's Cancer Group. J Clin Oncol 1997;15:76.
421. Ragland BD, Bell WC, Lopez RR, et al: Cytogenetics and molecular biology of osteosarcoma. Lab Invest 2002; 82:365.
422. Ramani P, Rampling D, Link M: Immunocytochemical study of 12E7 in small round-cell tumours of childhood: An assessment of its sensitivity and specificity. Histopathology 1993;23:557.
423. Ramanna L, Waxman A, Binney G, et al: Thallium-201 scintigraphy in bone sarcoma: Comparison with gallium-67 and technetium-MDP in the evaluation of chemotherapeutic response. J Nucl Med 1990; 31:567.
424. Raney RB Jr, Allen A, O'Neill J, et al: Malignant fibrous histiocytoma of soft tissue in childhood. Cancer 1986;57:2198.

425. Raney RB Jr, Gehan EA, Hays DM, et al: Primary chemotherapy with or without radiation therapy and/or surgery for children with localized sarcoma of the bladder, prostate, vagina, uterus, and cervix: A comparison of the results in Intergroup Rhabdomyosarcoma Studies I and II. Cancer 1990;66:2072.
426. Raney RB Jr, Ragab AH, Ruymann FB, et al: Soft-tissue sarcoma of the trunk in childhood: Results of the Intergroup Rhabdomyosarcoma Study. Cancer 1982; 49:2612.
427. Rao BN, Champion JE, Pratt CB, et al: Limb salvage procedures for children with osteosarcoma: An alternative to amputation. J Pediatr Surg 1983;18:901.
428. Rao BN, Santana VM, Parham D, et al: Pediatric nonrhabdomyosarcomas of the extremities: Influence of size, invasiveness, and grade on outcome. Arch Surg 1991;126:1490.
429. Razek A, Perez CA, Tefft M, et al: Intergroup Ewing's Sarcoma Study: Local control related to radiation dose, volume, and site of primary lesion in Ewing's sarcoma. Cancer 1980;46:516.
430. Riad S, Griffin AM, Liberman B, et al: Lymph node metastasis in soft tissue sarcoma in an extremity. Clin Orthop Relat Res 2004:129.
431. Rodriguez-Galindo C, Shah N, McCarville MB, et al: Outcome after local recurrence of osteosarcoma: The St Jude Children's Research Hospital experience (1970-2000). Cancer 2004;100:1928.
432. Rodriguez-Galindo C, Spunt SL, Pappo AS: Treatment of Ewing sarcoma family of tumors: Current status and outlook for the future. Med Pediatr Oncol 2003;40:276.
433. Roessner A, Jurgens H: Round cell tumours of bone. Pathol Res Pract 1993;189:111.
434. Rooser B: Prognosis in soft tissue sarcoma. Acta Orthop Scand Suppl 1987;225:1.
435. Rosen G, Caparros B, Huvos AG, et al: Preoperative chemotherapy for osteogenic sarcoma: Selection of postoperative adjuvant chemotherapy based on the response of the primary tumor to preoperative chemotherapy. Cancer 1982;49:1221.
436. Rosen G, Huvos AG, Marcove R, et al: Telangiectatic osteogenic sarcoma: Improved survival with combination chemotherapy. Clin Orthop Relat Res 1986:164.
437. Rosen G, Loren GJ, Brien EW, et al: Serial thallium-201 scintigraphy in osteosarcoma: Correlation with tumor necrosis after preoperative chemotherapy. Clin Orthop Relat Res 1993:302.
438. Rosen G, Nirenberg A: Chemotherapy for osteosarcoma: An investigative method, not a recipe. Cancer Treat Rep 1982;66:1687.
439. Rosen G, Nirenberg A, Caparros B, et al: Osteogenic sarcoma: Eight-percent, three-year, disease-free survival with combination chemotherapy (T-7). Natl Cancer Inst Monogr 1981:213.
440. Rosen G, Wollner N, Tan C, et al: Proceedings: Disease-free survival in children with Ewing's sarcoma treated with radiation therapy and adjuvant four-drug sequential chemotherapy. Cancer 1974;33:384.
441. Rosenberg SA, Cabner BA, Young RC, et al: Treatment of osteogenic sarcoma. I. Effect of adjuvant high-dose methotrexate after amputation. Cancer Treat Rep 1979; 63:739.
442. Rosenthal DI, Schiller AL, Mankin HJ: Chondrosarcoma: Correlation of radiological and histological grade. Radiology 1984;150:21.
443. Roth JA, Putnam JB Jr, Wesley MN, et al: Differing determinants of prognosis following resection of pulmonary metastases from osteogenic and soft tissue sarcoma patients. Cancer 1985;55:1361.
444. Rougraff BT, Simon MA, Kneisl JS, et al: Limb salvage compared with amputation for osteosarcoma of the distal end of the femur: A long-term oncological, functional, and quality-of-life study. J Bone Joint Surg Am 1994;76:649.
445. Rubinstein Z, Morag B: The role of radiology in the diagnosis and treatment of osteosarcoma. Prog Clin Biol Res 1982;99:23.
446. Ryan JR, Baker LH, Benjamin RS: The natural history of metastatic synovial sarcoma: Experience of the Southwest Oncology Group. Clin Orthop Relat Res 1982:257.
447. Sailer SL, Harmon DC, Mankin HJ, et al: Ewing's sarcoma: Surgical resection as a prognostic factor. Int J Radiat Oncol Biol Phys 1988;15:43.
448. Salzer-Kuntschik M, Delling G, Beron G, et al: Morphological grades of regression in osteosarcoma after polychemotherapy—study COSS 80. J Cancer Res Clin Oncol 1983;106(Suppl):21.
449. Sandoval C, Meyer WH, Parham DM, et al: Outcome in 43 children presenting with metastatic Ewing sarcoma: The St Jude Children's Research Hospital experience, 1962 to 1992. Med Pediatr Oncol 1996;26:180.
450. San-Julian M, Diaz-de-Rada P, Noain E, et al: Bone metastases from osteosarcoma. Int Orthop 2003;27:117.
451. Sankary S, Dickman PS, Wiener E, et al: Consistent numerical chromosome aberrations in congenital fibrosarcoma. Cancer Genet Cytogenet 1993;65:152.
452. Sato O, Kawai A, Ozaki T, et al: Value of thallium-201 scintigraphy in bone and soft tissue tumors. J Orthop Sci 1998;3:297.
453. Sauer R, Jurgens H, Burgers JM, et al: Prognostic factors in the treatment of Ewing's sarcoma: The Ewing's Sarcoma Study Group of the German Society of Paediatric Oncology CESS 81. Radiother Oncol 1987;10: 101.
454. Schajowicz F: Tumors and tumorlike lesions of bone. In Sundaram M, Gitelis S, McDonald C (eds): Tumors and Tumorlike Lesions of Bone. Berlin, Springer-Verlag, 1994, p 71.
455. Schajowicz F, McGuire MH, Santini Araujo E, et al: Osteosarcomas arising on the surfaces of long bones. J Bone Joint Surg Am 1988;70:555.
456. Schajowicz F, Santini Araujo E, Berenstein M: Sarcoma complicating Paget's disease of bone: A clinicopathological study of 62 cases. J Bone Joint Surg Br 1983; 65:299.
457. Schiller C, Windhager R, Fellinger EJ, et al: Extendable tumour endoprostheses for the leg in children. J Bone Joint Surg Br 1995;77:608.
458. Schima W, Amann G, Stiglbauer R, et al: Preoperative staging of osteosarcoma: Efficacy of MR imaging in detecting joint involvement. AJR Am J Roentgenol 1994; 163:1171.
459. Schindler OS, Cannon SR, Briggs TW, et al: Use of extendable total femoral replacements in children with

malignant bone tumors. Clin Orthop Relat Res 1998: 157.
460. Schmale GA, Conrad EU 3rd, Raskind WH: The natural history of hereditary multiple exostoses. J Bone Joint Surg Am 1994;76:986.
461. Schmidt D, Herrmann C, Jurgens H, et al: Malignant peripheral neuroectodermal tumor and its necessary distinction from Ewing's sarcoma: A report from the Kiel Pediatric Tumor Registry. Cancer 1991;68:2251.
462. Schmidt D, Thum P, Harms D, et al: Synovial sarcoma in children and adolescents: A report from the Kiel Pediatric Tumor Registry. Cancer 1991;67:1667.
463. Schofield DE, Fletcher JA, Grier HE, et al: Fibrosarcoma in infants and children: Application of new techniques. Am J Surg Pathol 1994;18:14.
464. Schwartz HS, Frassica FJ, Sim FH: Rotationplasty: An option for limb salvage in childhood osteosarcoma. Orthopedics 1989;12:257.
465. Schwartz HS, Zimmerman NB, Simon MA, et al: The malignant potential of enchondromatosis. J Bone Joint Surg Am 1987;69:269.
466. Scrable H, Witte D, Shimada H, et al: Molecular differential pathology of rhabdomyosarcoma. Genes Chromosomes Cancer 1989;1:23.
467. Scrable HJ, Witte DP, Lampkin BC, et al: Chromosomal localization of the human rhabdomyosarcoma locus by mitotic recombination mapping. Nature 1987;329:645.
468. Scully SP, Temple HT, O'Keefe RJ, et al: Role of surgical resection in pelvic Ewing's sarcoma. J Clin Oncol 1995;13:2336.
469. Scully SP, Temple HT, O'Keefe RJ, et al: The surgical treatment of patients with osteosarcoma who sustain a pathologic fracture. Clin Orthop Relat Res 1996:227.
470. Seeger LL, Gold RH, Chandnani VP: Diagnostic imaging of osteosarcoma. Clin Orthop Relat Res 1991: 254.
471. Serra M, Scotlandi K, Reverter-Branchat G, et al: Value of P-glycoprotein and clinicopathologic factors as the basis for new treatment strategies in high-grade osteosarcoma of the extremities. J Clin Oncol 2003;21:536.
472. Shah KV, Galloway DA, Knowles WA, et al: Simian virus 40 (SV40) and human cancer: A review of the serological data. Rev Med Virol 2004;14:231.
473. Shamberger RC, Laquaglia MP, Krailo MD, et al: Ewing sarcoma of the rib: Results of an intergroup study with analysis of outcome by timing of resection. J Thorac Cardiovasc Surg 2000;119:1154.
474. Shamberger RC, Rosenberg SA, Seipp CA, et al: Effects of high-dose methotrexate and vincristine on ovarian and testicular functions in patients undergoing postoperative adjuvant treatment of osteosarcoma. Cancer Treat Rep 1981;65:739.
475. Shapeero LG, Couanet D, Vanel D, et al: Bone metastases as the presenting manifestation of rhabdomyosarcoma in childhood. Skeletal Radiol 1993;22:433.
476. Shapiro DN, Parham DM, Douglass EC, et al: Relationship of tumor-cell ploidy to histologic subtype and treatment outcome in children and adolescents with unresectable rhabdomyosarcoma. J Clin Oncol 1991;9: 159.
477. Shapiro DN, Sublett JE, Li B, et al: Fusion of PAX3 to a member of the forkhead family of transcription factors in human alveolar rhabdomyosarcoma. Cancer Res 1993;53:5108.
478. Sheng WQ, Hisaoka M, Okamoto S, et al: Congenital-infantile fibrosarcoma: A clinicopathologic study of 10 cases and molecular detection of the ETV6-NTRK3 fusion transcripts using paraffin-embedded tissues. Am J Clin Pathol 2001;115:348.
479. Shinozaki T, Chigira M, Watanabe H, et al: Osteosarcoma with multiple skeletal metastases: A case of "nonstochastic" metastasis. Arch Orthop Trauma Surg 1993;112:292.
480. Shirley SK, Askin FB, Gilula LA, et al: Ewing's sarcoma in bones of the hands and feet: A clinicopathologic study and review of the literature. J Clin Oncol 1985;3: 686.
481. Shishikura A, Ushigome S, Shimoda T: Primitive neuroectodermal tumors of bone and soft tissue: Histological subclassification and clinicopathologic correlations. Acta Pathol Jpn 1993;43:176.
482. Shives TC, Dahlin DC, Sim FH, et al: Osteosarcoma of the spine. J Bone Joint Surg Am 1986;68:660.
483. Siebenrock KA, Nascimento AG, Rock MG: Comparison of soft tissue Ewing's sarcoma and peripheral neuroectodermal tumor. Clin Orthop Relat Res 1996:288.
484. Silverman JF, Joshi VV: FNA biopsy of small round cell tumors of childhood: Cytomorphologic features and the role of ancillary studies. Diagn Cytopathol 1994; 10:245.
485. Sim FH, Cupps RE, Dahlin DC, et al: Postradiation sarcoma of bone. J Bone Joint Surg Am 1972;54:1479.
486. Simon MA: Limb salvage for osteosarcoma. J Bone Joint Surg Am 1988;70:307.
487. Simon MA, Aschliman MA, Thomas N, et al: Limb-salvage treatment versus amputation for osteosarcoma of the distal end of the femur. J Bone Joint Surg Am 1986;68:1331.
488. Simon MA, Biermann JS: Biopsy of bone and soft-tissue lesions. J Bone Joint Surg Am 1993;75:616.
489. Simon MA, Bos GD: Epiphyseal extension of metaphyseal osteosarcoma in skeletally immature individuals. J Bone Joint Surg Am 1980;62:195.
490. Simon MA, Finn HA: Diagnostic strategy for bone and soft-tissue tumors. J Bone Joint Surg Am 1993;75:622.
491. Simon MA, Hecht JD: Invasion of joints by primary bone sarcomas in adults. Cancer 1982;50:1649.
492. Skinner KA, Eilber FR, Holmes EC, et al: Surgical treatment and chemotherapy for pulmonary metastases from osteosarcoma. Arch Surg 1992;127:1065.
493. Sluga M, Windhager R, Lang S, et al: Local and systemic control after ablative and limb sparing surgery in patients with osteosarcoma. Clin Orthop Relat Res 1999:120.
494. Smith LM, Cox RS, Donaldson SS: Second cancers in long-term survivors of Ewing's sarcoma. Clin Orthop Relat Res 1992:275.
495. Smith-Sorensen B, Gebhardt MC, Kloen P, et al: Screening for TP53 mutations in osteosarcomas using constant denaturant gel electrophoresis (CDGE). Hum Mutat 1993;2:274.
496. Sneppen O, Hansen LM: Presenting symptoms and treatment delay in osteosarcoma and Ewing's sarcoma. Acta Radiol Oncol 1984;23:159.

497. Somers GR, Ho M, Zielenska M, et al: HER2 amplification and overexpression is not present in pediatric osteosarcoma: A tissue microarray study. Pediatr Dev Pathol 2005;8:525.
498. Sorensen PH, Lessnick SL, Lopez-Terrada D, et al: A second Ewing's sarcoma translocation, t(21;22), fuses the EWS gene to another ETS-family transcription factor, ERG. Nat Genet 1994;6:146.
499. Sorensen PH, Shimada H, Liu XF, et al: Biphenotypic sarcomas with myogenic and neural differentiation express the Ewing's sarcoma EWS/FLI1 fusion gene. Cancer Res 1995;55:1385.
500. Soule EH, Pritchard DJ: Fibrosarcoma in infants and children: A review of 110 cases. Cancer 1977;40:1711.
501. Springfield DS, Gebhardt MC, McGuire MH: Chondrosarcoma: A review. Instr Course Lect 1996;45:417.
502. Springfield DS, Pagliarulo C: Fractures of long bones previously treated for Ewing's sarcoma. J Bone Joint Surg Am 1985;67:477.
503. Springfield DS, Schmidt R, Graham-Pole J, et al: Surgical treatment for osteosarcoma. J Bone Joint Surg Am 1988;70:1124.
504. Steenhoff JR, Daanen HA, Taminiau AH: Functional analysis of patients who have had a modified van Ness rotationplasty. J Bone Joint Surg Am 1993;75:1451.
505. Stewart DA, Gyonyor E, Paterson AH, et al: High-dose melphalan ± total body irradiation and autologous hematopoietic stem cell rescue for adult patients with Ewing's sarcoma or peripheral neuroectodermal tumor. Bone Marrow Transplant 1996;18:315.
506. Stiller CA, McKinney PA, Bunch KJ, et al: Childhood cancer and ethnic group in Britain: A United Kingdom Children's Cancer Study Group (UKCCSG) study. Br J Cancer 1991;64:543.
507. Stiller CA, Parkin DM: International variations in the incidence of childhood soft-tissue sarcomas. Paediatr Perinat Epidemiol 1994;8:107.
508. Stoker DJ, Cobb JP, Pringle JA: Needle biopsy of musculoskeletal lesions: A review of 208 procedures. J Bone Joint Surg Br 1991;73:498.
509. Strong LC, Herson J, Osborne BM, et al: Risk of radiation-related subsequent malignant tumors in survivors of Ewing's sarcoma. J Natl Cancer Inst 1979;62:1401.
510. Sudanese A, Toni A, Ciaroni D, et al: The role of surgery in the treatment of localized Ewing's sarcoma. Chir Organi Mov 1990;75:217.
511. Suit HD: Role of therapeutic radiology in cancer of bone. Cancer 1975;35:930.
512. Sun TC, Swee RG, Shives TC, et al: Chondrosarcoma in Maffucci's syndrome. J Bone Joint Surg Am 1985;67:1214.
513. Sundaram M, McGuire MH, Herbold DR: Magnetic resonance imaging of osteosarcoma. Skeletal Radiol 1987;16:23.
514. Sundaram M, Merenda G, McGuire MM: A skip lesion in association with Ewing sarcoma: Report of a case. J Bone Joint Surg Am 1989;71:764.
515. Sutow WW, Sullivan MP, Fernbach DJ, et al: Adjuvant chemotherapy in primary treatment of osteogenic sarcoma: A Southwest Oncology Group study. Cancer 1975;36:1598.
516. Tabrizi P, Letts M: Childhood rhabdomyosarcoma of the trunk and extremities. Am J Orthop 1999;28:440.
517. Taccone A, Di Stadio M, Oliveri M, et al: Multifocal synchronous osteosarcoma. Eur J Radiol 1995;20:43.
518. Taconis WK: Osteosarcoma in fibrous dysplasia. Skeletal Radiol 1988;17:163.
519. Taylor WF, Ivins JC, Pritchard DJ, et al: Trends and variability in survival among patients with osteosarcoma: A 7-year update. Mayo Clin Proc 1985;60:91.
520. Taylor WF, Ivins JC, Unni KK, et al: Prognostic variables in osteosarcoma: A multi-institutional study. J Natl Cancer Inst 1989;81:21.
521. Tefft M: Treatment of Ewing's sarcoma with radiation therapy. Int J Radiat Oncol Biol Phys 1981;7:277.
522. Temeck BK, Wexler LH, Steinberg SM, et al: Reoperative pulmonary metastasectomy for sarcomatous pediatric histologies. Ann Thorac Surg 1998;66:908.
523. Tepper J, Glaubiger D, Lichter A, et al: Local control of Ewing's sarcoma of bone with radiotherapy and combination chemotherapy. Cancer 1980;46:1969.
524. Terrier P, Henry-Amar M, Triche TJ, et al: Is neuroectodermal differentiation of Ewing's sarcoma of bone associated with an unfavourable prognosis? Eur J Cancer 1995;31A:307.
525. Terrier P, Llombart-Bosch A, Contesso G: Small round blue cell tumors in bone: Prognostic factors correlated to Ewing's sarcoma and neuroectodermal tumors. Semin Diagn Pathol 1996;13:250.
526. Thomas DG, Giordano TJ, Sanders D, et al: Absence of HER2/neu gene expression in osteosarcoma and skeletal Ewing's sarcoma. Clin Cancer Res 2002;8:788.
527. Thorner P, Squire J, Chilton-MacNeil S, et al: Is the EWS/FLI-1 fusion transcript specific for Ewing sarcoma and peripheral primitive neuroectodermal tumor? A report of four cases showing this transcript in a wider range of tumor types. Am J Pathol 1996;148:1125.
528. Thorner PS, Squire JA: Molecular genetics in the diagnosis and prognosis of solid pediatric tumors. Pediatr Dev Pathol 1998;1:337.
529. Toguchida J, Yamaguchi T, Dayton SH, et al: Prevalence and spectrum of germline mutations of the p53 gene among patients with sarcoma. N Engl J Med 1992;326:1301.
530. Toguchida J, Yamaguchi T, Ritchie B, et al: Mutation spectrum of the p53 gene in bone and soft tissue sarcomas. Cancer Res 1992;52:6194.
531. Toni A, Neff JR, Sudanese A, et al: The role of surgical therapy in patients with nonmetastatic Ewing's sarcoma of the limbs. Clin Orthop Relat Res 1993:225.
532. Toni A, Sudanese A, Ciaroni D, et al: The role of surgery in the local treatment of Ewing's sarcoma of the extremities. Chir Organi Mov 1990;75:262.
533. Torricelli P, Montanari N, Spina V, et al: Dynamic contrast enhanced magnetic resonance imaging subtraction in evaluating osteosarcoma response to chemotherapy. Radiol Med (Torino) 2001;101:145.
534. Tracy T Jr, Neifeld JP, DeMay RM, et al: Malignant fibrous histiocytomas in children. J Pediatr Surg 1984;19:81.
535. Triche TJ: Diagnosis of small round cell tumors of childhood. Bull Cancer 1988;75:297.

536. Tsai JY, Aviv H, Benevenia J, et al: HER-2/neu and p53 in osteosarcoma: An immunohistochemical and fluorescence in situ hybridization analysis. Cancer Invest 2004;22:16.
537. Tsokos M: The diagnosis and classification of childhood rhabdomyosarcoma. Semin Diagn Pathol 1994; 11:26.
538. Tucker MA, D'Angio GJ, Boice JD Jr, et al: Bone sarcomas linked to radiotherapy and chemotherapy in children. N Engl J Med 1987;317:588.
539. Udayakumar AM, Sundareshan TS, Goud TM, et al: Cytogenetic characterization of Ewing tumors using fine needle aspiration samples: A 10-year experience and review of the literature. Cancer Genet Cytogenet 2001;127:42.
540. Ueda Y, Dockhorn-Dworniczak B, Blasius S, et al: Analysis of mutant p53 protein in osteosarcomas and other malignant and benign lesions of bone. J Cancer Res Clin Oncol 1993;119:172.
541. Unni K: Dahlin's Bone Tumors: General Aspects and Data on 11,087 Cases. Philadelphia, Lippincott-Raven, 1966.
542. Unni KK: Osteosarcoma of bone. J Orthop Sci 1998;3: 287.
543. Unni KK, Dahlin DC: Osteosarcoma: Pathology and classification. Semin Roentgenol 1989;24:143.
544. Unni KK, Dahlin DC, Beabout JW, et al: Parosteal osteogenic sarcoma. Cancer 1976;37:2466.
545. Unwin PS, Walker PS: Extendible endoprostheses for the skeletally immature. Clin Orthop Relat Res 1996: 179.
546. van der Woude HJ, Bloem JL, Pope TL Jr: Magnetic resonance imaging of the musculoskeletal system. Part 9. Primary tumors. Clin Orthop Relat Res 1998:272.
547. van der Woude HJ, Bloem JL, Taminiau AH, et al: Classification of histopathologic changes following chemotherapy in Ewing's sarcoma of bone. Skeletal Radiol 1994;23:501.
548. van der Woude HJ, Verstraete KL, Hogendoorn PC, et al: Musculoskeletal tumors: Does fast dynamic contrast-enhanced subtraction MR imaging contribute to the characterization? Radiology 1998;208:821.
549. Vanel D, Henry-Amar M, Lumbroso J, et al: Pulmonary evaluation of patients with osteosarcoma: Roles of standard radiography, tomography, CT, scintigraphy, and tomoscintigraphy. AJR Am J Roentgenol 1984;143:519.
550. Varma DG: Optimal radiologic imaging of soft tissue sarcomas. Semin Surg Oncol 1999;17:2.
551. Verstraete KL, Van der Woude HJ, Hogendoorn PC, et al: Dynamic contrast-enhanced MR imaging of musculoskeletal tumors: Basic principles and clinical applications. J Magn Reson Imaging 1996;6:311.
552. Vietti TJ, Gehan EA, Nesbit ME Jr, et al: Multimodal therapy in metastatic Ewing's sarcoma: An Intergroup Study. Natl Cancer Inst Monogr 1981:279.
553. Voegeli E, Laissue J, Kaiser A, et al: Case report 143: Multiple hereditary osteocartilaginous exostoses affecting right femur with an overlying giant cystic bursa (exostosis bursata). Skeletal Radiol 1981;6:134.
554. Wagner LM, Neel MD, Pappo AS, et al: Fractures in pediatric Ewing sarcoma. J Pediatr Hematol Oncol 2001;23:568.
555. Wang LL, Gannavarapu A, Kozinetz CA, et al: Association between osteosarcoma and deleterious mutations in the RECQL4 gene in Rothmund-Thomson syndrome. J Natl Cancer Inst 2003;95:669.
556. Wang M, Nilsson G, Carlberg M, et al: Specific and sensitive detection of the EWS/FLI1 fusion protein in Ewing's sarcoma by Western blotting. Virchows Arch 1998;432:131.
557. Ward WG, Mikaelian K, Dorey F, et al: Pulmonary metastases of stage IIB extremity osteosarcoma and subsequent pulmonary metastases. J Clin Oncol 1994; 12:1849.
558. Ward WG, Yang RS, Eckardt JJ: Endoprosthetic bone reconstruction following malignant tumor resection in skeletally immature patients. Orthop Clin North Am 1996;27:493.
559. Weeden S, Grimer RJ, Cannon SR, et al: The effect of local recurrence on survival in resected osteosarcoma. Eur J Cancer 2001;37:39.
560. West DC, Grier HE, Swallow MM, et al: Detection of circulating tumor cells in patients with Ewing's sarcoma and peripheral primitive neuroectodermal tumor. J Clin Oncol 1997;15:583.
561. Wexler L, Helman L: Rhabdomyosarcoma and the undifferentiated sarcomas. In Pizzo P, Poplack D (eds): Principles and Practice of Pediatric Oncology. Philadelphia, JB Lippincott, 1997, p 799.
562. Wexler LH, DeLaney TF, Tsokos M, et al: Ifosfamide and etoposide plus vincristine, doxorubicin, and cyclophosphamide for newly diagnosed Ewing's sarcoma family of tumors. Cancer 1996;78:901.
563. Wharam MD, Hanfelt JJ, Tefft MC, et al: Radiation therapy for rhabdomyosarcoma: Local failure risk for clinical group III patients in Intergroup Rhabdomyosarcoma Study II. Int J Radiat Oncol Biol Phys 1997;38: 797.
564. Whelan JS: Osteosarcoma. Eur J Cancer 1997;33:1611.
565. White VA, Fanning CV, Ayala AG, et al: Osteosarcoma and the role of fine-needle aspiration: A study of 51 cases. Cancer 1988;62:1238.
566. Wicklund CL, Pauli RM, Johnston D, et al: Natural history study of hereditary multiple exostoses. Am J Med Genet 1995;55:43.
567. Wilkins RM, Pritchard DJ, Burgert EO Jr, et al: Ewing's sarcoma of bone: Experience with 140 patients. Cancer 1986;58:2551.
568. Winkelmann WW: Hip rotationplasty for malignant tumors of the proximal part of the femur. J Bone Joint Surg Am 1986;68:362.
569. Winkelmann WW: Rotationplasty. Orthop Clin North Am 1996;27:503.
570. Winkler K, Beron G, Delling G, et al: Neoadjuvant chemotherapy of osteosarcoma: Results of a randomized cooperative trial (COSS-82) with salvage chemotherapy based on histological tumor response. J Clin Oncol 1988;6:329.
571. Winkler K, Beron G, Kotz R, et al: Adjuvant chemotherapy in osteosarcoma—effects of cisplatinum, BCD, and fibroblast interferon in sequential combination with HD-MTX and adriamycin: Preliminary results of the COSS 80 study. J Cancer Res Clin Oncol 1983; 106(Suppl):1.

572. Winkler K, Bielack SS, Delling G, et al: Treatment of osteosarcoma: Experience of the Cooperative Osteosarcoma Study Group (COSS). Cancer Treat Res 1993;62: 269.
573. Winkler K, Bieling P, Bielack S, et al: Local control and survival from the Cooperative Osteosarcoma Study Group studies of the German Society of Pediatric Oncology and the Vienna Bone Tumor Registry. Clin Orthop Relat Res 1991:79.
574. Wold LE, Unni KK, Beabout JW, et al: High-grade surface osteosarcomas. Am J Surg Pathol 1984;8:181.
575. Wuisman P, Enneking WF: Prognosis for patients who have osteosarcoma with skip metastasis. J Bone Joint Surg Am 1990;72:60.
576. Wunder JS, Bull SB, Aneliunas V, et al: MDR1 gene expression and outcome in osteosarcoma: A prospective, multicenter study. J Clin Oncol 2000;18:2685.
577. Wunder JS, Paulian G, Huvos AG, et al: The histological response to chemotherapy as a predictor of the oncological outcome of operative treatment of Ewing sarcoma. J Bone Joint Surg Am 1998;80:1020.
578. Xu D, Luan H, Zhan A, et al: Spontaneous malignant transformation of fibrous dysplasia. Chin Med J (Engl) 1996;109:941.
579. Yamaguchi H, Minami A, Kaneda K, et al: Comparison of magnetic resonance imaging and computed tomography in the local assessment of osteosarcoma. Int Orthop 1992;16:285.
580. Yang RS, Eckardt JJ, Eilber FR, et al: Surgical indications for Ewing's sarcoma of the pelvis. Cancer 1995; 76:1388.
581. Yock T, Krailo M, Fryer C, et al: Local control in pelvic Ewing sarcoma: Analysis from INT-0091—a report from the Children's Oncology Group. J Clin Oncol 2006; 24:3838-3843.
582. Young CL, Sim FH, Unni KK, et al: Chondrosarcoma of bone in children. Cancer 1990;66:1641.
583. Young JL Jr, Miller RW: Incidence of malignant tumors in US children. J Pediatr 1975;86:254.
584. Zhou H, Randall RL, Brothman AR, et al: Her-2/neu expression in osteosarcoma increases risk of lung metastasis and can be associated with gene amplification. J Pediatr Hematol Oncol 2003;25:27.
585. Zucker JM, Henry-Amar M, Sarrazin D, et al: Intensive systemic chemotherapy in localized Ewing's sarcoma in childhood: A historical trial. Cancer 1983;52:415.

Section 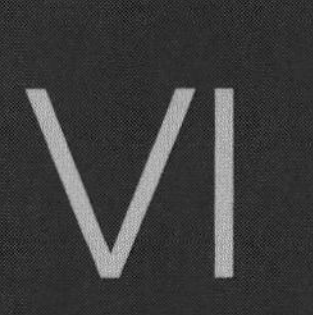

VI

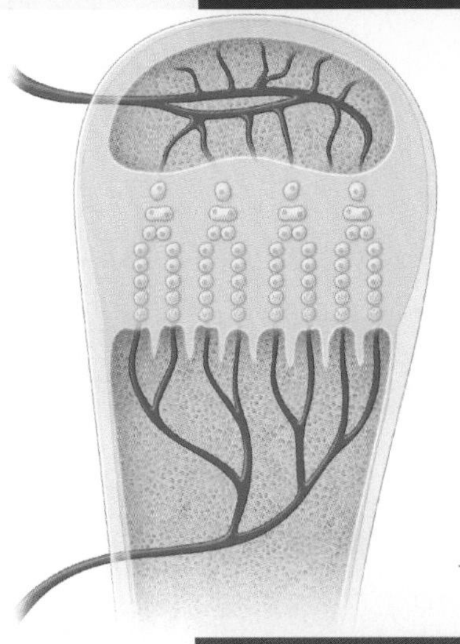

Injuries

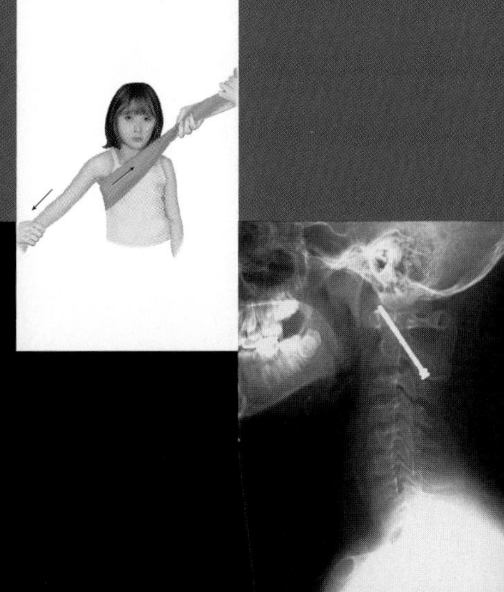

Chapter 40

General Principles of Managing Orthopaedic Injuries

Skeletal injuries are common in children. In a review of over 8000 children's fractures, Landin[184] estimated that over 40% of boys and 25% of girls had sustained a fracture by 16 years of age. Because of the properties of the immature skeleton, these injuries have different characteristics, complications, and management than similar injuries in adults.

A number of studies have examined the epidemiology of fractures in children.[154,184,273,344,352] Most studies have shown a male predominance, particularly in adolescence. Fractures in children younger than 18 months of age are rare and should raise the question of nonaccidental trauma.[352] Combining the data from five large epidemiologic studies reveals fractures of the distal forearm to be the most common fracture in children, accounting for nearly 25% of 12,946 fractures. The clavicle is the next most commonly injured site, representing over 8% of all children's fractures[154,184,273,344,352] (Table 40–1).

Properties of the Immature Skeleton

The immature skeleton has several properties that affect the management of injuries in children. These properties include an increased resiliency to stress, a thicker periosteum, an increased potential to remodel, shorter healing times, and the presence of a physis.

Plastic Deformation

A few studies have compared the mechanical properties of bone in children and bone in adults.[7,78,142,171,330] Currey and Butler found immature bone to be weaker in bending strength but to absorb more energy before fracture.[78] This is a result of the ability of immature bone to undergo plastic (permanent) deformation (Fig. 40–1). Although plastic deformation has been described in adults,[274,300] it is much more common in children. Borden is often credited with the first clinical description of plastic deformation in children.[40] Although plastic deformation is most common in the forearm, particularly the ulna,[41,99,211,237,285,307] Griffith and colleagues have recently described the cross-sectional magnetic resonance imaging (MRI) appearance of plastic deformation of the femur.[116] Although bone in young children may remodel after plastic deformation, most authors recommend reduction of plastic deformation of the forearm if there is more than 20 degrees of angulation or the child is older than 4 years of age and has either a clinically evident deformity or limitation of pronation/supination. Sanders and Heckman were able to reduce an average of 85% of the angulation present before reduction. They used general anesthesia and a fulcrum to apply a steady force at the apex of the deformity for several minutes.[285] Plastic deformation of the ulna has also been reported in a majority of isolated radial head dislocations.[201]

Buckle (Torus) Fractures

Buckle fractures, also called *torus fractures* because of their resemblance to the base of an architectural column, most commonly occur at the transition between metaphyseal woven bone and the lamellar bone of the diaphyseal cortex[200,268] (Fig. 40–2). Buckle fractures represent a spectrum of injuries from mild plastic deformation of one area of the cortex to complete fractures with a buckled appearance.

Table 40-1 Frequency of Fractures at Selected Sites in Children

	Epidemiologic Study					
	A	B	C	D	E	**Total (%)***
Total fractures in series	923	2040	410	291	8682	12,346 (100)
Anatomic site						
Clavicle	58	222	55	45	703	1083 (8.8)
Humerus (proximal end and shaft)	18	81	14	13		126 (1.0)
Distal humerus	71	158	68	287		584 (4.7)
Radial neck	25	45	1	104	175	350 (2.8)
Radius/ulna (shafts)	60	108	23	39	295	525 (4.3)
Distal radius/ulna	330	755	81	80	1971	3217 (26.1)
Hand	136	494	88			718 (5.8)
Femur	18	87	27	13	145	290 (2.3)
Tibia/fibula (shafts)	40	256	19	10	434	759 (6.1)
Ankle	37	61	28	14	478	618 (5.0)
Foot	71	172	28			271 (2.2)

*Because not all fractures are listed, the percentages of fractures do not total 100%.
Modified from Reed MH: Epidemiology of children's fractures. In Letts RM (ed): Management of Pediatric Fractures. New York, Churchill Livingstone, 1994, p 2.

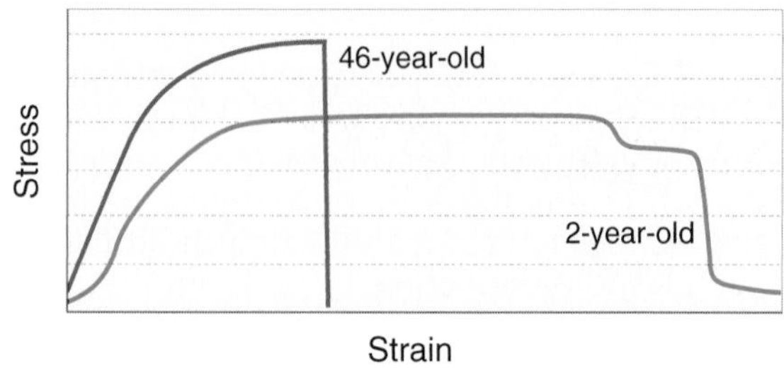

FIGURE 40-1 Stress–strain curves for mature and immature bone. The increased strain of immature bone before failure represents plastic deformation. (Redrawn from Rang M: Children's Fractures. Philadelphia, JB Lippincott, 1983. Originally from Currey JD, Butler G: The mechanical properties of bone tissue in children. J Bone Joint Surg Am 1975;57:810.)

It is not uncommon for torus fractures to be diagnosed several days or even weeks after injury because the pain and swelling may be attributed to a sprain. Although most torus fractures can be managed successfully with minimal symptomatic treatment,[82,339] it is important to identify minimally displaced complete fractures that have a buckled appearance. These complete fractures are potentially unstable and may displace if not managed with a well-molded cast (Fig. 40–3). Although such late displacement is usually mild and remodels with no sequelae, parents are often upset when the fracture is more displaced when the cast is removed than at the time of injury.

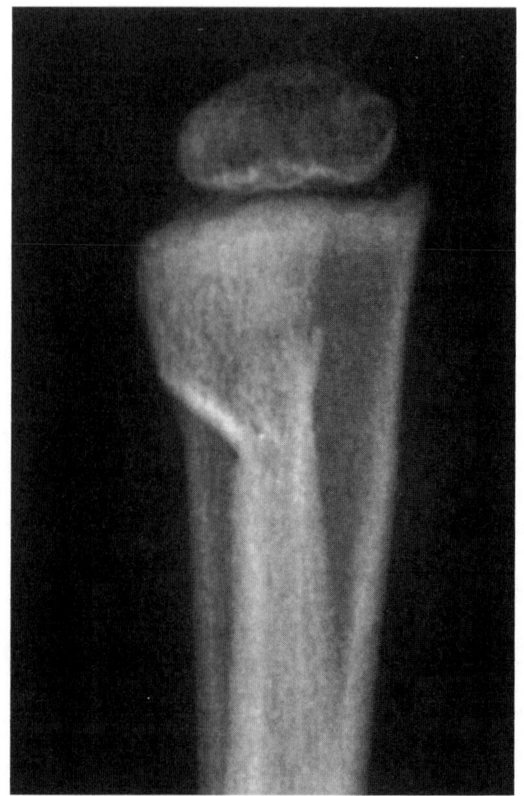

FIGURE 40-2 Lateral radiograph of the distal radius showing a buckle fracture of the dorsal cortex. The volar cortex is uninvolved and the dorsal cortex is not completely fractured.

Greenstick Fractures

Greenstick fractures are unique to children because immature bone is more flexible and has a thicker

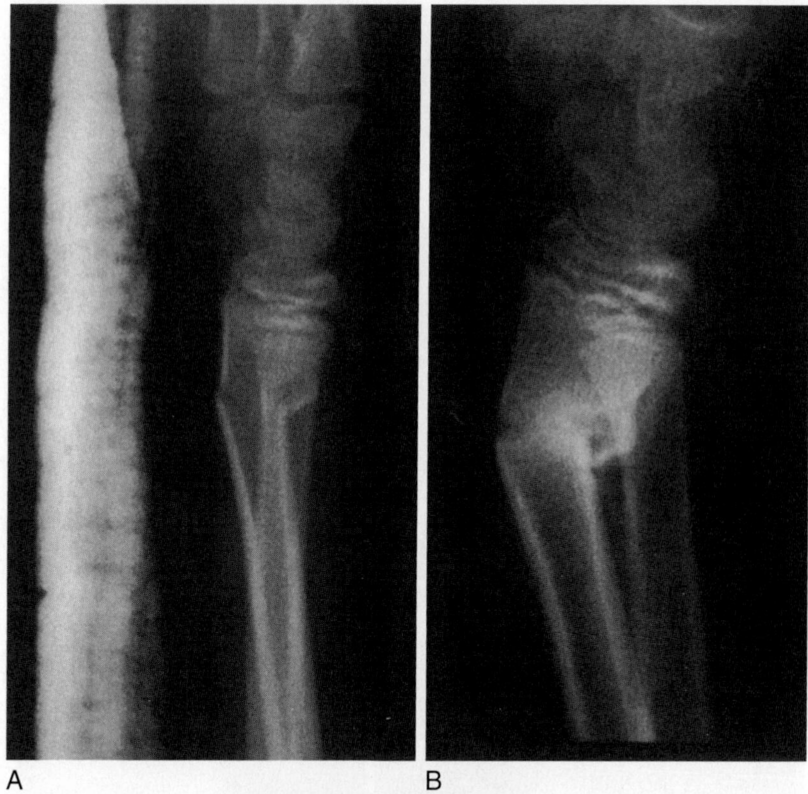

FIGURE 40–3 **A,** Lateral radiograph of a minimally displaced fracture of the distal radial metaphysis. Despite the buckled appearance, both cortices are completely fractured. This fracture was managed in a poorly molded volar splint. **B,** Radiograph obtained after removal of the volar splint, 4 weeks after the injury. Note the increased angulation.

periosteum than mature adult bone. In a greenstick fracture, the cortex in tension fractures completely while the cortex and periosteum in compression remain intact but frequently undergo plastic deformation. It has been said that it is necessary to "complete" the fracture on the intact compression side of greenstick fractures[96,245]; however, this has not been our experience. We believe it is necessary only to achieve an anatomic reduction of a greenstick fracture. To reduce a greenstick fracture, it is usually necessary to "unlock" the impacted fragments on the tension side. This is accomplished by initially exaggerating the deformity and then applying traction and a reducing force. In our experience, whether the fracture is completed during the exaggeration of the deformity has not been important. Because of the intact cortex and periosteum, greenstick fractures are usually stable after reduction (Fig. 40–4). Because greenstick fractures have been reported to have an increased likelihood of refracture,[331] we usually immobilize these fractures for a full 6 weeks and warn the parents that although they are usually simple to reduce, they are more likely to refracture.

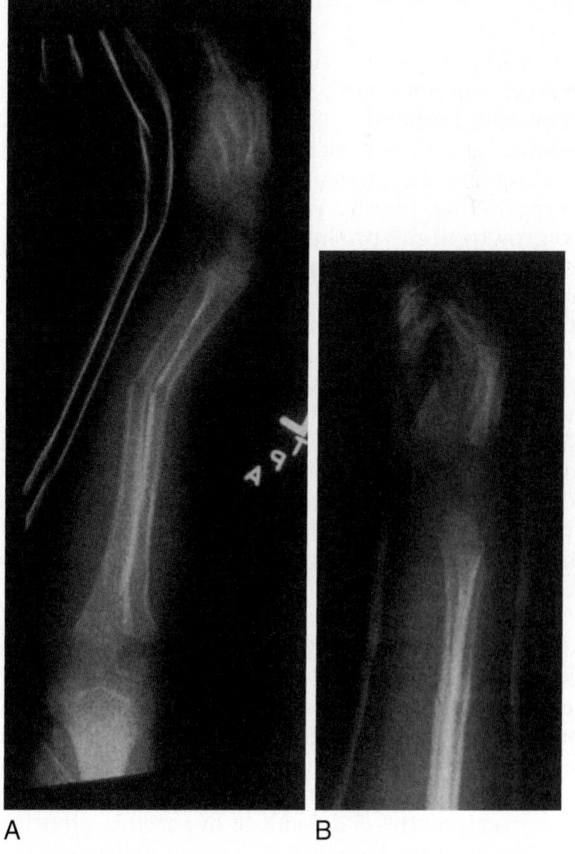

FIGURE 40–4 **A,** Lateral radiograph of a greenstick both-bone forearm fracture. The dorsal cortex angles without completely fracturing (plastic deformation). **B,** Lateral radiograph obtained after reduction.

Remodeling/Overgrowth

Not only do children's fractures heal more rapidly than those in adults, but once healed, they are more likely to remodel residual deformity (Fig. 40–5). Factors that affect the remodeling potential of a deformity include the amount of growth remaining and the plane of the deformity in relation to adjacent joints.[101,102,109,191,331,335,346] The single most important factor

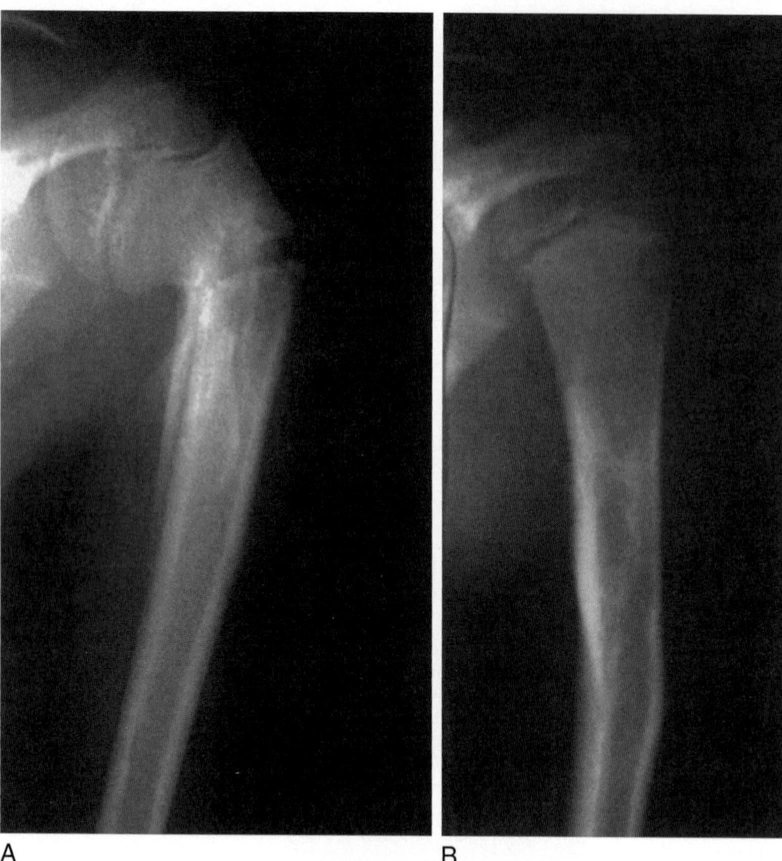

FIGURE 40–5 **A,** Anteroposterior (AP) radiograph of a proximal humerus fracture in an 8-year-old boy. The fracture has healed with significant angulation. **B,** AP radiograph obtained 1 year after injury demonstrates extensive remodeling of the proximal humerus.

determining how much growth will contribute to the remodeling potential of a fracture is the patient's skeletal age. Other factors include the deformity's proximity to the physis and the growth potential of the particular physis. For example, because 80% of the growth of the proximal humerus comes from the proximal physis, deformity associated with proximal humeral fractures is much more likely to remodel than deformity associated with distal humeral fractures.[266]

Wolff's law states that bone remodels according to the stress placed across it.[181,354] It follows that post-traumatic deformity in the plane of motion of a joint will have greater potential to remodel than deformity not in the plane of motion. This fact is demonstrated with fractures of the femoral shaft, which remodel a large amount of sagittal plane deformity, a lesser amount of coronal deformity, and little or no rotational deformity.[80,335]

Another consideration in the management of children's fractures is the potential for accelerated growth of an injured limb. Clinically, this is most frequently seen in diaphyseal femoral fractures. It has long been recognized that fractures of the femoral shaft will spontaneously correct shortening of up to 2 cm.[4,71,109,136,144,157,158] It has been hypothesized that this "overgrowth" is a result of hyperemia associated with the fracture. However, recent evidence casts some doubt on this theory. First, fractures of the radius do not demonstrate this propensity for overgrowth.[56,83] Second, efforts to stimulate blood flow by periosteal stripping do not result in permanent growth increases.[107,162,305,323] Finally, anatomic reduction of femoral shaft fractures treated operatively has not resulted in significant overgrowth.[18,36,47,84,173,180] Thus, there may exist some other, yet to be determined factor that predisposes an injured extremity to return to its normal, preinjury length.

Physeal Injuries

Physeal injuries represent 15% to 30% of all fractures in children.[33,70,212,228,352] The incidence varies with age and has been reported to peak in adolescents.[228,259,261] Physeal injuries involving the phalanges have been reported to account for over 30% of all physeal fractures.[228,261] Fortunately, although physeal injuries are common, growth deformity is rare, occurring in only 1% to 10% of all physeal injuries.[228,259,282]

Although problems arising from physeal injury are rare, they are often predictable and, occasionally, preventable. A basic understanding of the anatomy and physiology of the physis and its response to injury is necessary to manage injuries to the growth plate effectively.

PHYSEAL ANATOMY

It is important to distinguish the physis (also referred to as the *epiphyseal plate, epiphyseal growth plate,* or *epiphyseal cartilage*) from the epiphysis, or secondary ossification center. The physis is connected to the epiphysis and metaphysis by the zone of Ranvier and the perichondral ring of LaCroix (Fig. 40–6). The zone of Ranvier is a wedge-shaped group of germinal cells that is continuous with the physis and contributes to latitudinal, or circumferential, growth of the physis.[152] The zone of Ranvier consists of three cell types—osteoblasts, chondrocytes, and fibroblasts. Osteoblasts form the bony portion of the perichondral ring at the metaphysis; chondrocytes contribute to latitudinal growth; and fibroblasts circumscribe the zone and anchor it to perichondrium above and below the growth plate.[152] The perichondral ring of LaCroix is a fibrous structure that is continuous with the fibroblasts of the zone of Ranvier and the periosteum of the metaphysis. It provides strong mechanical support for the bone–cartilage junction of the growth plate.[164]

The physis consists of chondrocytes in an extracellular matrix. Both the chondrocytes and the matrix are preferentially oriented along the longitudinal axis of long bones. The physis has traditionally been divided into four zones: the resting or germinal zone, the proliferative zone, the zone of hypertrophy, and the zone of enchondral ossification, which is continuous with the metaphysis (see Fig. 40–6). The first two zones have an abundant extracellular matrix and, consequently, a great deal of mechanical integrity, particularly in response to shear forces. The third layer, the hypertrophic zone, contains scant extracellular matrix and is weaker. On the metaphyseal side of the hypertrophic zone there is an area of provisional calcification leading to the zone of enchondral ossification. The calcification in these areas provides additional resistance to shear. Thus, the area of the hypertrophic zone just above the area of provisional calcification is the weakest area of the physis, and it is here that most injuries to the physis occur.[124,133,282] The fact that the cleavage plane through the physis is through the hypertrophic zone implies that after most injuries, the germinal layer of the physis remains intact and attached to the epiphysis. Thus, provided that there is no insult to the blood supply of the germinal layer or development of a "bony bridge" across the injured physis, normal growth should resume after an injury.

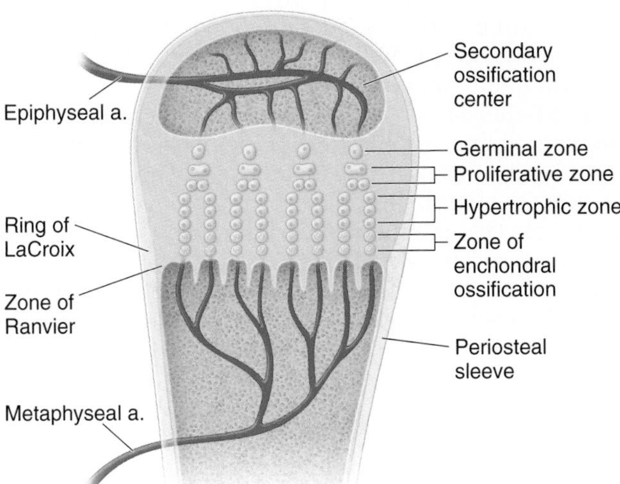

FIGURE 40–6 Anatomy of a physis. Most injuries occur just above the area of provisional calcification within the hypertrophic zone. Subsequently the germinal layer frequently remains intact and attached to the epiphysis.

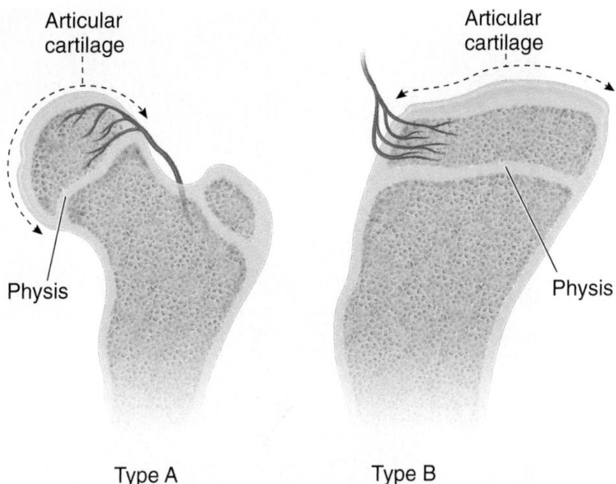

FIGURE 40–7 Two types of epiphyseal blood supply as defined by Dale and Harris. In type A, the epiphysis is nearly entirely covered by articular cartilage. Consequently, the blood supply traverses the metaphysis and may be damaged on separation of the metaphysis and epiphysis. In type B, the epiphysis is only partially covered by articular cartilage. Because the blood supply enters through the epiphysis, separation of the metaphysis and epiphysis will not compromise the blood supply to the germinal layer. (Redrawn from Dale GC, Harris WR: Prognosis of epiphyseal separation: An experimental study. J Bone Joint Surg Br 1958;40:116.)

The blood supply to the germinal zone of the physis was studied in a classic set of experiments in monkeys by Dale and Harris.[79] They described two types of epiphyseal vascularization (Fig. 40–7). Type A epiphyses are nearly entirely covered by articular cartilage. In these epiphyses, the blood supply enters the periphery after traversing the perichondrium. Consequently, the blood supply is vulnerable to damage if the epiphysis is separated from the metaphysis. Type B epiphyses are only partially covered by articular cartilage. Their blood supply enters from the epiphyseal side and is protected from vascular injury during separation. The proximal femur and proximal radius are the only two type A epiphyses. Dale and Harris confirmed their theory that type B epiphyses were protected from vascular injury by studying the histologic changes that occurred after separation of the distal radial epiphysis in rabbits. They noted that by 3 weeks after separation it was nearly impossible to distinguish the injured epiphysis from the control.[79]

HARRIS GROWTH ARREST LINES

Harris is credited with the first radiographic observation of "bony striations" in the metaphysis of long bones.[131] These "Harris growth arrest lines" are transversely oriented condensations of normal bone and are thought to represent slowing or cessation of growth.

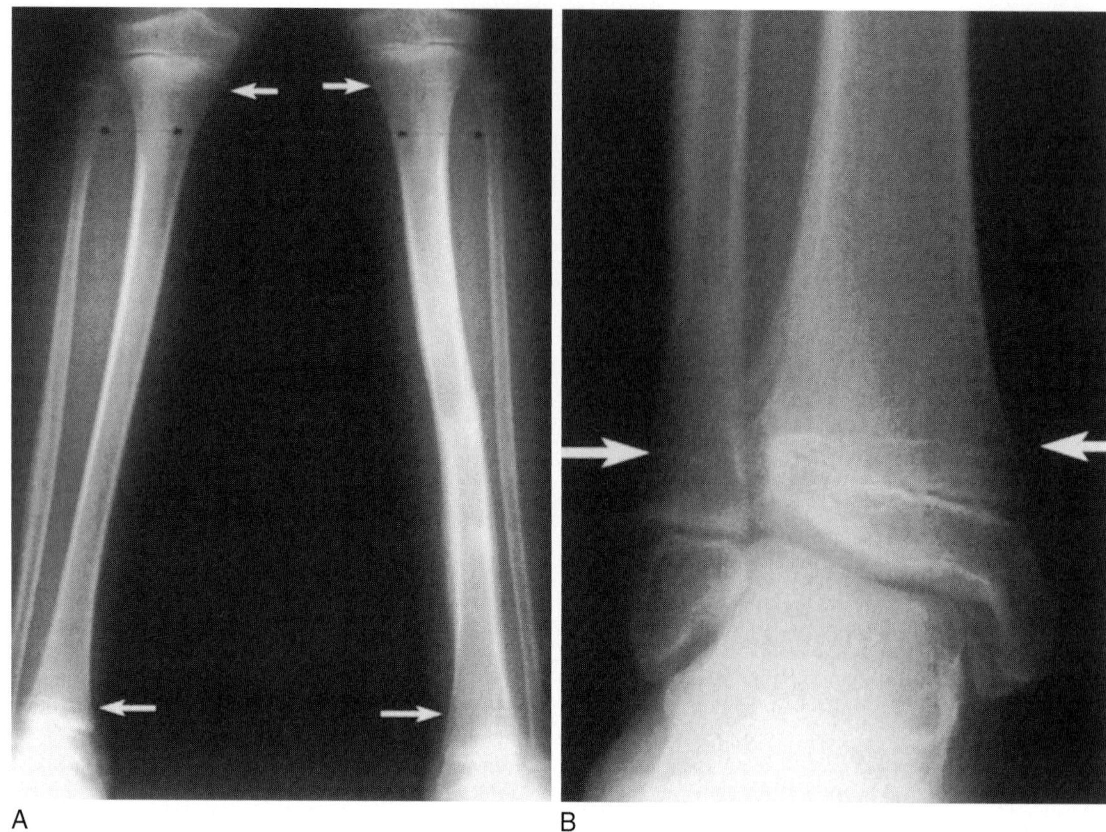

FIGURE 40–8 Harris growth arrest lines. **A,** Bilateral, symmetric, transverse growth arrest lines (*arrows*) in the proximal and distal tibias of a 7-year-old boy 1 year after a vehicle–pedestrian accident in which the boy sustained multiple injuries. Note the healed left tibial fracture. On the left side, both the proximal and distal growth arrest lines have migrated farther from their physes, probably as a result of the fracture. **B,** Asymmetric growth arrest line in the distal tibia (*arrow*). Although the line appears perpendicular to the tibial shaft, it is not parallel to the physis. There has been medial growth but no lateral growth; thus, the growth arrest line appears "tethered" to the physis laterally. Note the normal growth arrest line in the fibula (*arrow*).

They may be present in a single bone after an isolated traumatic injury or in all long bones after a significant systemic illness.[131,151,246,247] When present after a physeal injury, they serve as an effective representation of the health of the physis.[151] If the growth arrest line is transverse and parallel to the physis, the physis can be assumed to be growing normally. If there has been a partial injury to the physis, the growth arrest line will be asymmetric. There will be no growth arrest line if there has been no growth following a total physeal injury (Fig. 40–8). Harris growth arrest lines may also be seen on MRI.[357]

CLASSIFICATION OF PHYSEAL INJURIES

Over the years, a number of classification systems for physeal injuries have been described, including those by Foucher, Poland, Aitken, and Ogden.[1-3,100,249,250,263] However, the most widely used system is that of Salter and Harris[283] (Fig. 40–9).

A Salter-Harris type I injury is a separation of the epiphysis from the metaphysis occurring entirely through the physis. It is rare and seen most frequently in infants or in pathologic fractures, such as those secondary to rickets or scurvy. Because the germinal layer remains with the epiphysis, growth is not disturbed unless the blood supply is interrupted, as frequently occurs with traumatic separation of the proximal femoral epiphysis.

In a Salter-Harris type II injury the fracture extends along the hypertrophic zone of the physis and at some point exits through the metaphysis. The epiphyseal fragment contains the entire germinal layer as well as a metaphyseal fragment of varying size. This fragment is known as Thurston Holland's sign. The periosteum on the side of the metaphyseal fragment is intact and provides stability once the fracture is reduced. Growth disturbance is rare because the germinal layer remains intact.

In a Salter-Harris type III injury, the fracture extends along the hypertrophic zone until it exits through the epiphysis. Thus, by definition, type III fractures cross the germinal layer and are usually intra-articular. Consequently, if displaced, they require an anatomic reduction, which may need to be achieved open.

Salter-Harris type IV injuries extend from the metaphysis across the physis and into the epiphysis. Thus, the fracture crosses the germinal layer of the

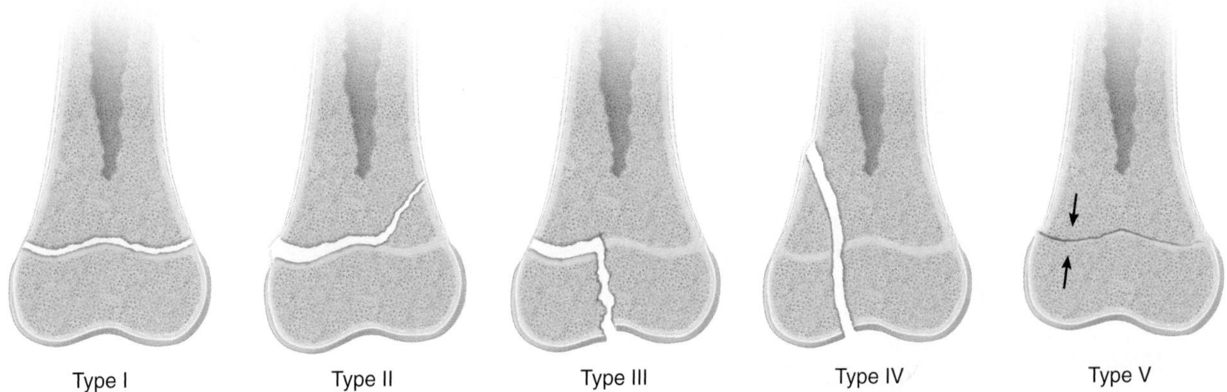

FIGURE 40–9 Salter-Harris classification of physeal fractures.

physis and usually extends into the joint. As in type III injuries, it is important to achieve an anatomic reduction to prevent osseous bridging across the physis and to restore the articular surface.

A Salter-Harris type V injury is a crushing injury to the physis from a pure compression force. It is so rare that Peterson and Burkhart have questioned whether such an injury can occur.[260] Those authors who have reported Salter-Harris type V injuries have noted a poor prognosis, with almost universal growth disturbance.[283,304]

Although the Salter-Harris classification of physeal fractures is by far the most widely used system, there are a few physeal injuries that do not fit into this classification scheme. The first is an injury to the perichondral ring. Salter's colleague Mercer Rang termed this a type VI physeal injury[249,250] (Fig. 40–10). (This injury is also included in Ogden's classification.) Basing his system on a review of 951 fractures, Peterson purposed a new classification scheme[259] (Fig. 40–11). Although this classification system has many similarities to the Salter-Harris scheme, its important addition is the Peterson type I fracture—a transverse fracture of the metaphysis with extension longitudinally into the physis. Clinically, this fracture is seen commonly in the distal radius. Peterson also described a type VI injury, which is an open injury associated with loss of the physis.

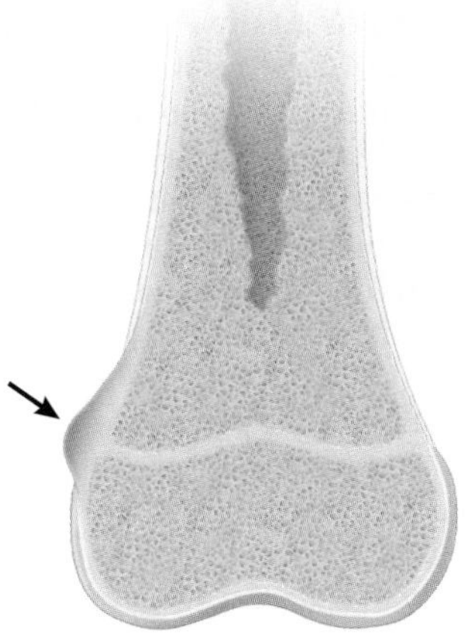

FIGURE 40–10 Rang's type VI physeal injury. This represents an injury to the perichondral ring (*arrow*).

TREATMENT OF PHYSEAL INJURIES

In general, the principles involved in the treatment of physeal injuries are the same as those involved in the treatment of all fractures, although there are a few important caveats. As with all traumatic injuries, before an injury to the physis is treated, the patient must be thoroughly assessed using the ABCs of trauma (see subsequent discussion under Care of the Multiply Injured Child).

Once the child has been stabilized and all life- and limb-threatening injuries identified, a treatment plan can be developed. It is important to remember that physeal fractures can and often do coexist with neurovascular or open injuries.[138] When this occurs, the physeal fracture is treated after appropriate management of the soft tissue injuries.

The goal in treating physeal fractures is to achieve and maintain an acceptable reduction without subjecting the germinal layer of the physis to any further damage. The most subjective of these goals, and perhaps the most important, is determining the limits of an acceptable reduction. A number of factors must be considered when assessing a "nonanatomic" reduction. These include the amount of residual deformity, the location of the injury, the age of the patient, and the amount of time that has elapsed since the injury. The location of the injury and the patient's age are determining factors in the bone's remodeling potential. Obviously, more deformity can be accepted if the potential to remodel is high. Both Rang[270] and Salter[282] have stressed the importance of avoiding damage to the germinal layer of the physis during reduction. They recommend accepting *any* displacement in type I or II injuries after 7 to 10 days, believing it is safer to perform an osteotomy later than to risk injuring the

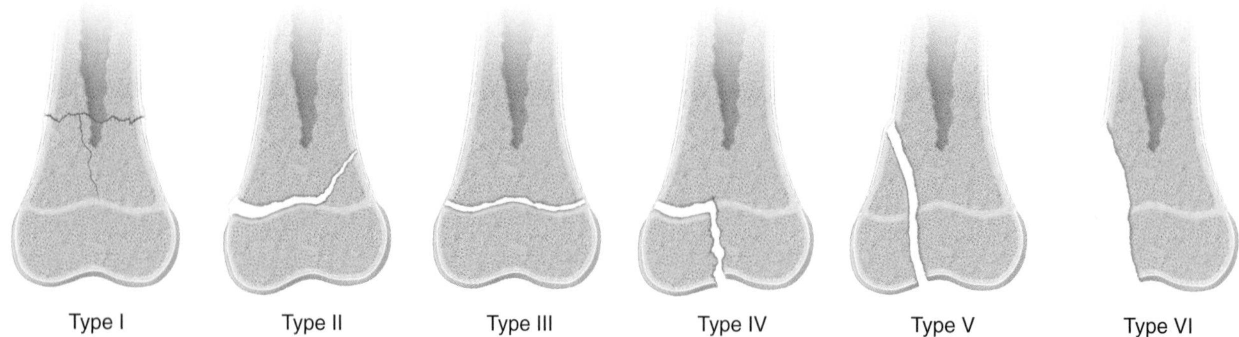

FIGURE 40–11 Peterson's classification of physeal fractures. Type I injuries are frequently seen in the distal radius. Type VI injuries are open and associated with loss of a portion of the physis.

physis with a traumatic reduction of a physeal fracture that has begun to heal. Interestingly, this recommendation has been accepted and repeated with little clinical or experimental evidence to prove its validity. Recently, Egol and colleagues studied the effect of a delay in reduction of Salter-Harris I fractures in rats. There was no evidence that a delay in reduction produced a growth disturbance.[94] Despite this recent animal study, we believe it is still prudent to avoid reduction in late-presenting type I or II physeal fractures. Because of the intra-articular component, displaced type III and IV injuries must be reduced regardless of the time that has elapsed since the injury.

Once a physeal fracture has been reduced, the reduction can be maintained with a cast, pins, internal fixation, or some combination of these three. Specific recommendations regarding the method and duration of immobilization are discussed in specific chapters pertaining to each injury.

COMPLICATIONS OF PHYSEAL INJURIES

Like all fractures, physeal injuries may be complicated by malunion, infection, neurovascular problems, or osteonecrosis. The best treatment of these complications is avoidance, but even under the best of circumstances these problems can arise. The treatment of these complications is discussed in other chapters in the context of specific injuries.

A complication unique to physeal fractures is growth disturbance. Although trauma is the most common cause of growth disturbance, growth disturbance is also seen as a sequela of Blount's disease, infection, irradiation, thermal injury, and laser beam exposure.[32,188,190,262] Although physeal injuries represent 15% to 30% of all fractures, growth arrest occurs after only 1% to 10% of physeal fractures. A number of factors affect the likelihood of development of a growth arrest. Most important is the severity of the injury to the physis. Comminuted fractures from high-energy injury are more likely to result in physeal arrest. Physeal injuries that cross the germinal layer (i.e., Salter-Harris types III and IV injuries) are also more likely to be associated with subsequent growth disturbance. Fortunately, not all patients in whom a physeal arrest develops will require treatment. This is because physeal injuries are most common in adolescents, who often have limited growth remaining.[228,259,282]

Assessment of Growth Disturbance

Growth disturbance from a physeal fracture is usually evident 2 to 6 months after the injury, but it may not become evident for up to a year.[282] Thus, it is important not only to warn parents about this potential problem but to follow patients with physeal fractures long enough to identify growth arrest. Early identification of a traumatic growth disturbance can make its management considerably easier because the treatment can be directed solely toward resolving the arrest, rather than addressing both the arrest and an acquired growth deformity. Growth disturbance is usually the result of the development of a bony bridge, or bar, across the physeal cartilage. However, growth disturbance may occur after traumatic injury without the development of a bony bridge. Presumably, this occurs because the injury slows growth of a portion of the physis rather than stopping it completely. The resulting asymmetric growth can produce clinically significant angular deformity (Fig. 40–12).

The development of a bony bar may create either a complete or partial growth disturbance. If the area of the bar is large, it may stop the growth of the entire physis (Fig. 40–13). More often, a bar forms in a portion of the physis and stops growth at that point, while the rest of the physis continues to grow. This produces a tethering effect, which may result in shortening or progressive angular deformity, or both (Figs. 40–14 and 40–15).

To treat a physeal bar appropriately, both the extent and location of the bar and the amount of growth remaining from the physis must be determined. The anatomy of a physeal bar may be delineated using plain radiography, tomography, computed tomography (CT), or MRI.[32,55,167,208,248] MRI is increasingly used to assess physeal anatomy and has replaced CT as our preferred modality.[63,75,93,281] In particular, fat-suppressed, three-dimensional, spoiled gradient-recalled echo sequences can be obtained and

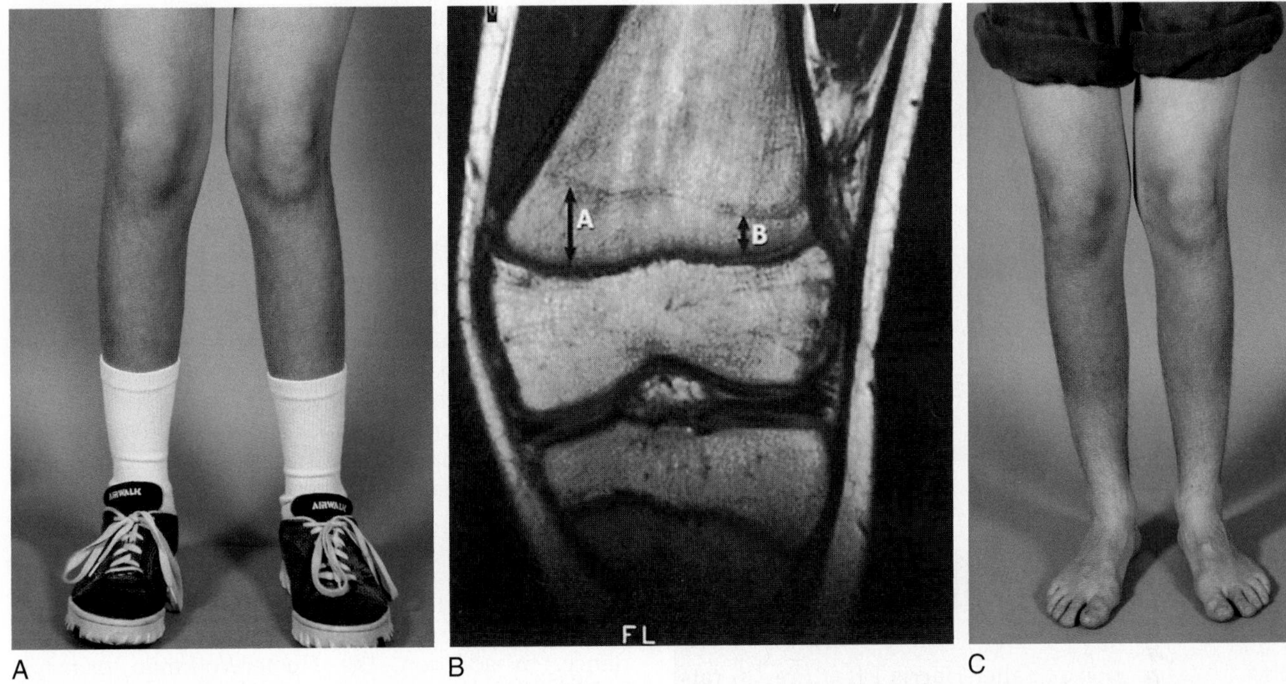

FIGURE 40–12 Asymmetric growth following a Salter-Harris type II distal femoral fracture. **A,** Valgus deformity 15 months after fracture. **B,** Magnetic resonance image demonstrating asymmetric growth of the distal femoral physis. The distance from the physis to the Harris growth arrest line is greater medially (A) than laterally (B). The fact that the growth arrest line has migrated proximally on the lateral aspect reflects a "slowing" of growth rather than a complete "arrest." **C,** Clinical appearance 8 months after a medial distal femoral epiphysiodesis was performed. Lateral growth continued until the deformity was corrected. At this point, a lateral hemiepiphysiodesis and a contralateral epiphysiodesis were performed.

reconstructed to create an accurate three-dimensional model of the physis, including calculation of the percentage of physeal arrest[281] (Fig. 40–16). Partial physeal arrests are usually classified as peripheral (type A) or central (type B or C), depending on their location within the physis (Fig. 40–17). There are two types of central bars. The first, type B, is surrounded by a perimeter of healthy physis. This type of bar may produce a tethering effect that "tents" the epiphysis and produces a joint deformity. In the second type of central bar, type C, the bar traverses the entire physis from front to back (or side to side). The physis on both sides of the bar is normal. This pattern is commonly seen with injuries to the medial malleolus.[32,251]

Once the extent and location of the bar have been defined, the amount of growth remaining from the physis must be determined. This can be accomplished by determining the skeletal age of the patient and using information on growth patterns assembled by Green and Anderson.[11-13,111,112] Skeletal age can be determined by comparing a radiograph of the left hand and wrist with standards in an atlas of skeletal age.[115] It is generally assumed that girls grow until a bone age of 14 years and boys until a bone age of 16 years.[25,225,265,340] Future growth for the distal femur and proximal tibia can be estimated using the graphs initially published by Anderson and colleagues (Fig. 40–18) or by using approximations of yearly physeal growth[12,13,111,112,167,225] (Table 40–2).

Table 40–2 Yearly Growth of Various Long Bone Physes

Location	Yearly Growth (mm)
Proximal femur	2
Distal femur	9
Proximal tibia	6
Distal tibia	4
Proximal humerus	12
Distal radius	8

Treatment of Physeal Arrest

Treatment options for physeal arrests include observation, completion of a partial arrest, or physeal bar resection.

Observation. If the bar appears to involve the entire physis and there is an acceptable existing limb length inequality or angular deformity and little contralateral growth remaining, observation may be the best option.

Completion. Completion of a physeal bar may be indicated if there is an acceptable existing angular deformity that might become clinically unacceptable

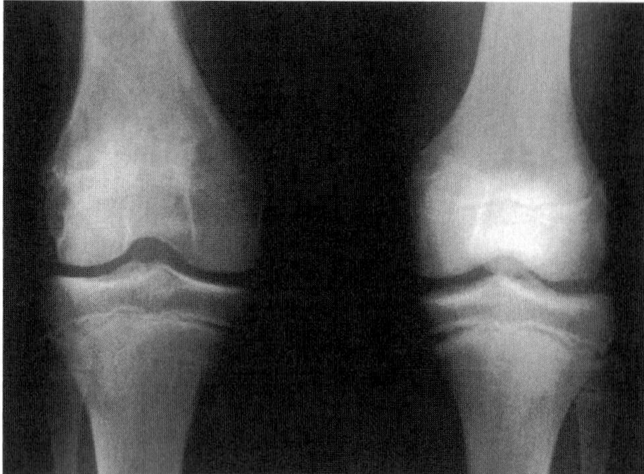

A

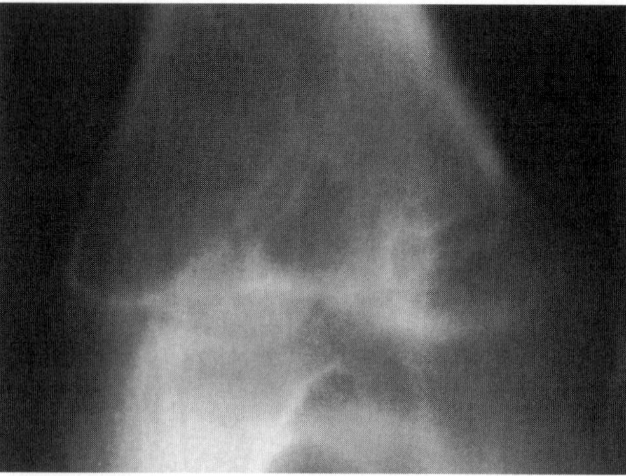

B

FIGURE 40–13 Salter-Harris type II fracture of the right distal femur complicated by pin tract sepsis and complete physeal arrest. **A,** Anteroposterior radiographs of the right and left knee. The uninvolved left knee has a healthy-appearing distal femoral physis. On the right side there is no radiolucency corresponding to the physis. **B,** Tomograph revealing a small amount of physis on the far medial aspect of the right distal femur. Most of the physis has been replaced by radiodense scar. (Radiographic evidence of the cross-pins is present on both the plain radiograph and the tomograph.)

if untreated. With completion of an arrest, the surgeon must evaluate the likelihood of a subsequent limb length inequality. If the likelihood of significant limb length inequality (more than 20 to 25 mm) is high, a contralateral epiphysiodesis should be performed at the time of completion of the partial arrest.

Resection. Resection of a physeal bar is indicated for partial arrests with substantial growth remaining. Physeal bar resection was first introduced by Langenskiöld and has been studied in both human and animal models.[32,44,167,186-189,208] The technique of bar excision involves removing the bone bridging the metaphysis and epiphysis and filling the void created with an interposition material that will prevent reformation of the bony bar. The remaining physis must be undamaged and must be large enough that growth is likely to continue. In addition, there should be a significant amount of growth remaining before skeletal maturity and physiologic physeal closure. Numerous studies have documented that bars involving more than 50% of the physis are unlikely to respond to bar resection.[31,167,186,187,190,249,258] Recommendations regarding requirements of amount of growth remaining are less uniform. Langenskiöld[186] has recommended at least 1 year of growth remaining, whereas Kasser[167] has stated that successful bar resection requires at least 2.5 cm of growth, and Birch[31] has recommended at least 2 years of growth. Clearly, the younger the patient and the more the potential growth from the physis, the greater the benefit of a successful resection.

The surgeon must decide whether an osteotomy is necessary to correct existing angular deformity. Although angular deformities of less than 20 degrees have been reported to correct spontaneously after bar resection, this has not been our universal clinical experience. In addition, the Hueter-Volkman principle indicates that improved alignment may help facilitate more normal growth. We believe that corrective osteotomy should be considered for any angular deformity that is judged to be "clinically unacceptable."[31,167,251,258]

When a peripheral (type A) bar is resected, the bar should be approached directly and removed under direct vision with a wide margin of periosteum (Fig. 40–19). The bar should be resected until the cavity is rimmed completely with normal physis. Types B and C bars are approached through a window in the metaphysis or through an osteotomy. Although some have advocated magnification with loupes or a microscope, we have not routinely used these aids. However, resection of central bars can be facilitated by the use of fluoroscopy, fiberoptic lighting, and dental mirrors (Fig. 40–20).

Once the bar has been completely resected, the cavity created can be filled with fat or Cranioplast. Silicone (Silastic) has been used experimentally in both humans and animals but is currently unavailable for use.[44] Each of these interposition materials has advantages and advocates.[31,167,249,258] Fat is commonly used because it is readily available and autogenous. Its only drawback is that a separate incision in the gluteal area is often required to harvest a graft of adequate size. Methylmethacrylate, available commercially as Cranioplast, is radiolucent and thermally nonconductive. Its solid structure may help support an epiphysis if a large metaphyseal defect has been created. It may, however, be difficult to remove if further reconstructive procedures are required. Some recent animal studies have investigated biologic interposition materials, although none is currently available for clinical use.[195,199,317] Regardless of which interposition material is selected, the goal is to bridge the physis with the material so that bar formation is prevented. Peterson has advocated contouring the epiphyseal defect or creating drill holes or "pods" in the epiphysis to anchor the interposition material in the epiphysis so that the

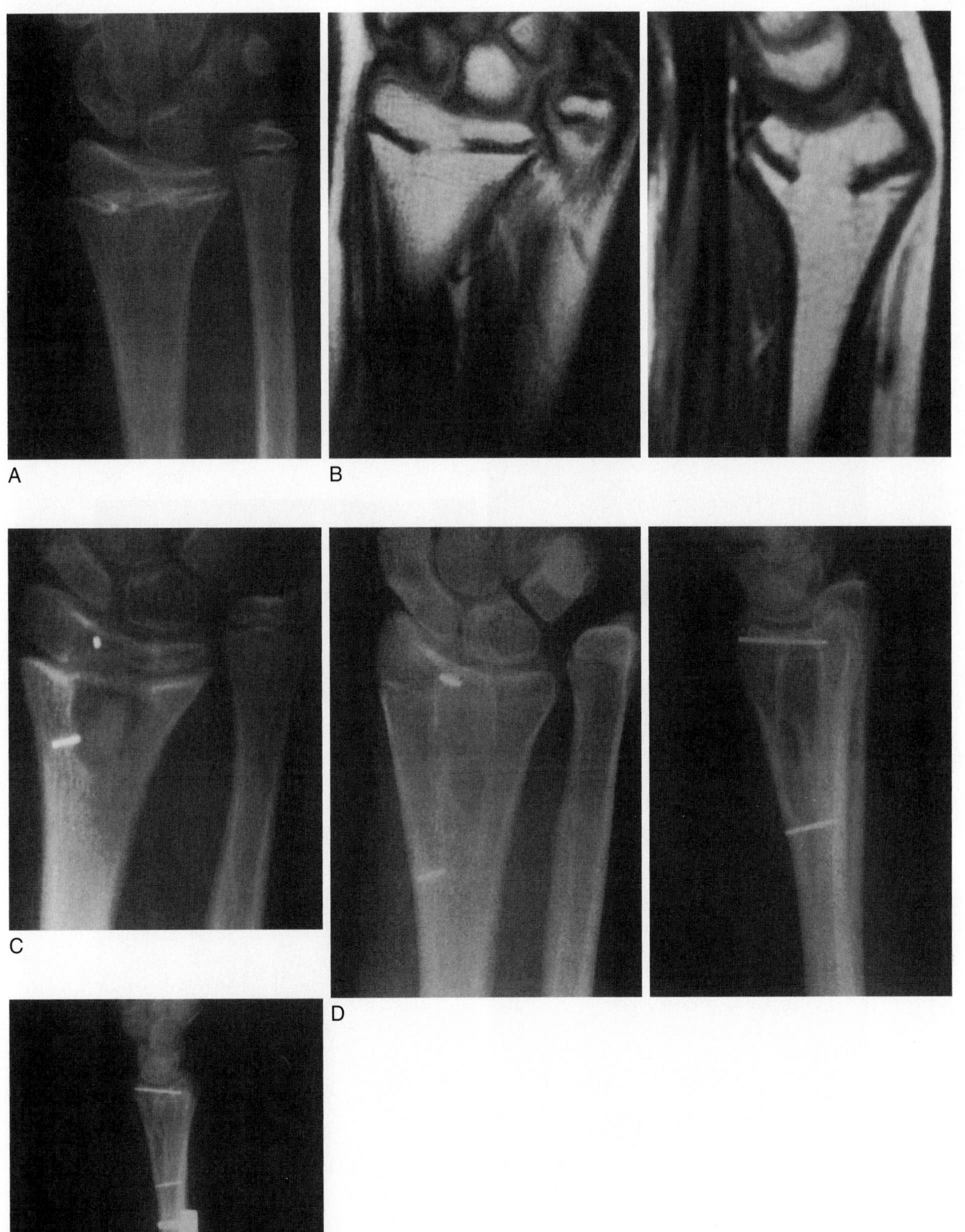

FIGURE 40–14 Partial physeal arrest (type B) producing primarily shortening. **A,** Anteroposterior (AP) radiograph of the wrist of a 12-year-old girl who had sustained a Salter-Harris type II fracture of the distal radius 6 years earlier. Note the ulnar-positive variance as well as the physeal bar in the center of the distal radius. **B,** Coronal and sagittal magnetic resonance images show the extent of the bar. **C,** The bar has been resected and metallic markers placed in the epiphysis and metaphysis. **D,** AP and lateral radiographs showing resumption of growth, as evidenced by an increased distance between metallic markers. The ulnar-positive variance persists. **E,** Lateral radiograph after ulnar shortening to treat symptomatic ulnar-positive variance.

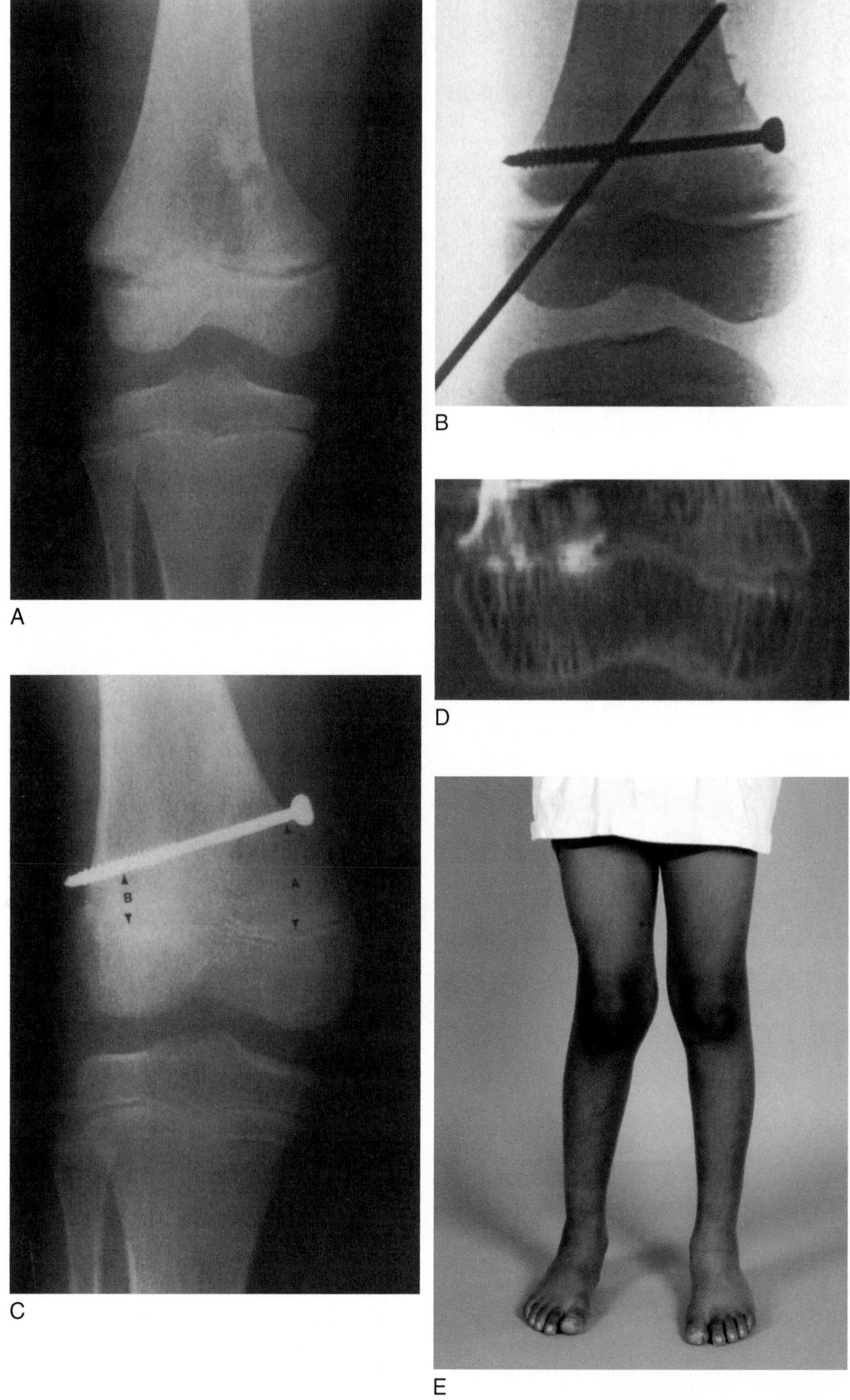

FIGURE 40–15 Physeal arrest producing angular deformity. **A,** Salter-Harris type II fracture of the distal femur. **B,** Immediate postreduction film. **C,** Anteroposterior radiograph 9 months after injury. The distance between the physis and the screw medially (A) is substantially greater than it was immediately before surgery. However, the distance laterally (B) is relatively unchanged. Note the radiodense appearance of the physis laterally. **D,** Computed tomography scan demonstrating lateral bar formation. **E,** The asymmetric growth has produced a valgus clinical appearance.

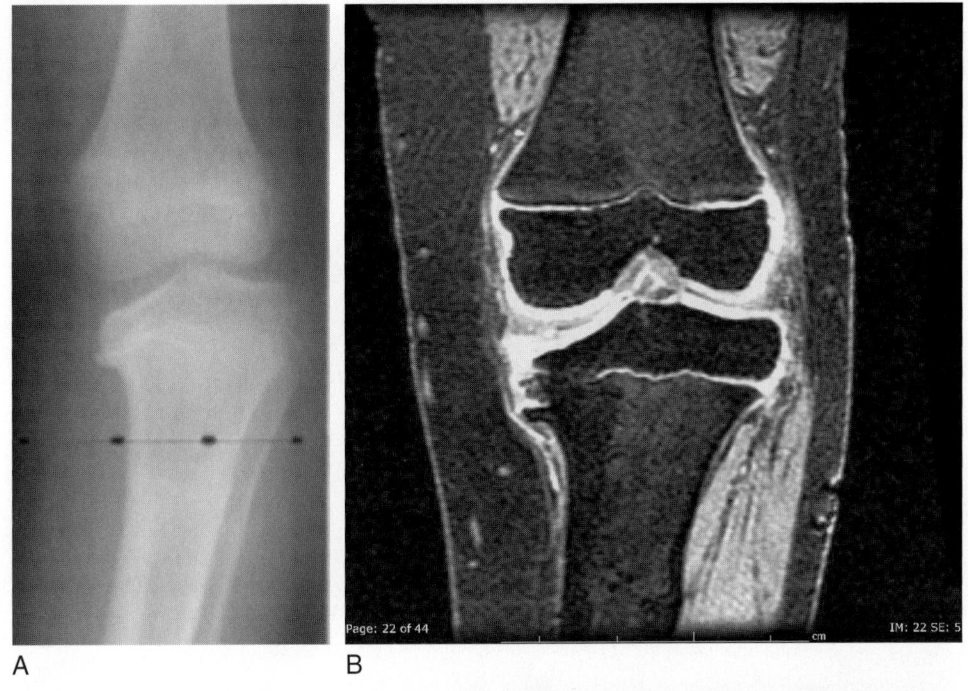

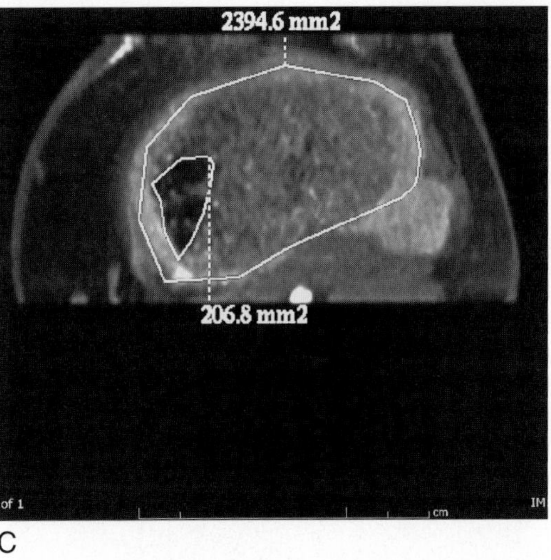

FIGURE 40–16 **A,** Anteroposterior radiograph of a patient with infantile Blount's disease with recurrent and progressive genu varum after a proximal tibial osteotomy. There was clinical and radiographic suspicion of a medial physeal arrest. **B,** Coronal plane magnetic resonance image of a patient with a physeal bar associated with infantile Blount's disease. The fat-suppressed, spoiled gradient-recalled echo sequences can be reconstructed to create an accurate three-dimensional model of the physis. **C,** Three-dimensional axial physeal model reconstructed from fat-suppressed, three-dimensional, spoiled gradient-recalled echo sequences. The workstation allows calculation of the area of the bony bar (*dark area*) as well as the total area (*light area*) to obtain an accurate assessment of physeal involvement.

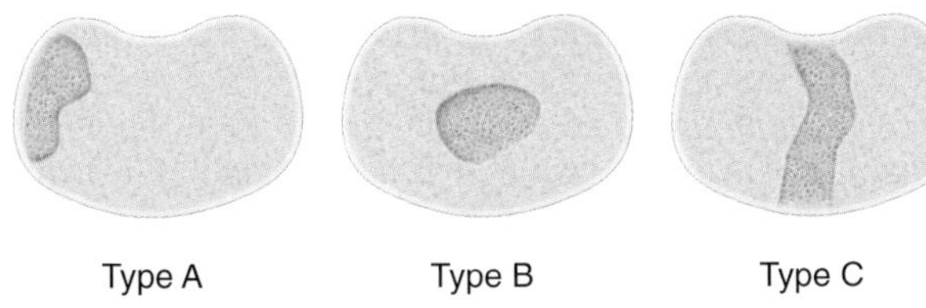

FIGURE 40–17 Classification of partial physeal arrest. Type A, peripheral; type B, central, surrounded by normal physis; type C, central, traversing the physis completely.

interposition material will migrate distally with the epiphysis as growth resumes[258] (Fig. 40–21). Once the bar has been resected and the interposition material has been placed, radiographic markers should be placed on each side of the physis to aid in evaluating resumption of growth (see Fig. 40–14).

Results after bar resection are variable. Nearly all authors report poor results with bars involving more than 50% of the physis.[31,167,249,258] Peterson reported results as a percentage of growth of the normal

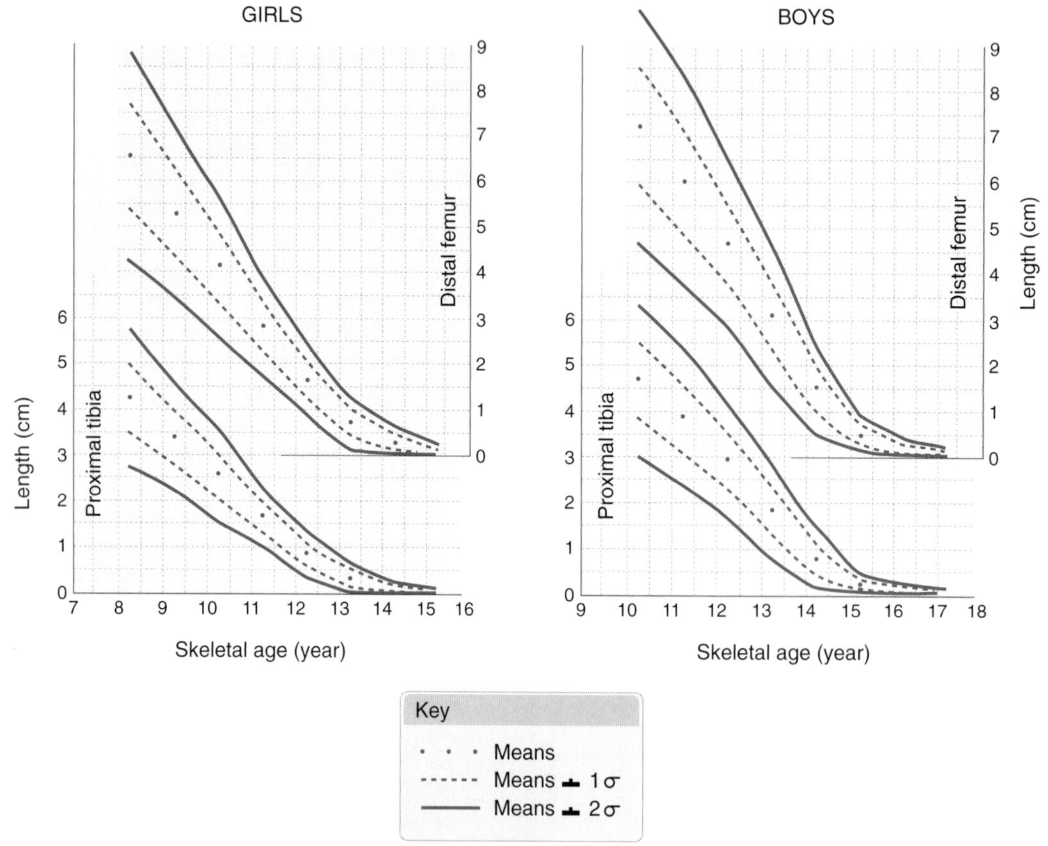

FIGURE 40–18 The Green-Anderson growth-remaining chart. This chart can be used to estimate the growth remaining at the normal distal femur and proximal tibia at the skeletal ages indicated. The means and standard deviations were derived from longitudinal series of 50 girls and 50 boys. (Redrawn from Anderson M, Green WT, Messner MB: Growth and predictions of growth in the lower extremities. J Bone Joint Surg Am 1963;45:10.)

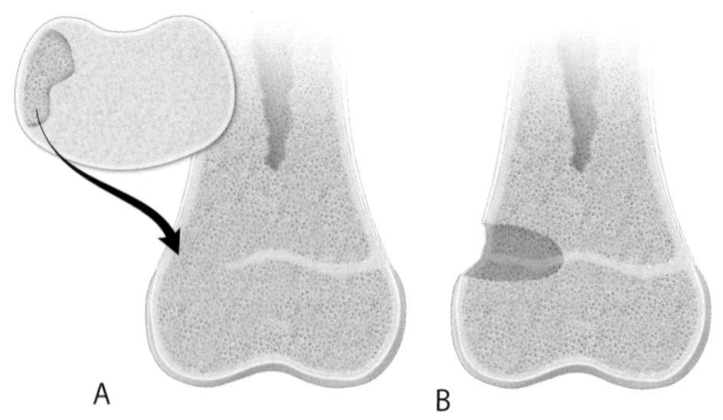

FIGURE 40–19 Schematic representation of peripheral bar resection. **A,** Peripheral physeal bar of the distal femur. **B,** The bar can be approached directly and excised (with a small amount of the metaphysis and epiphysis) using a high-speed burr.

(contralateral) physis ranging from 0% to 200%, with a mean of 84%.[258] In reviewing our results, we found that only 27 of 42 (63%) of our physeal bar resections had at least 50% of "predicted growth" after the resection, and that 32 of the patients required additional procedures.[271] Similarly, Hasler and Foster recently reported "fair" or "poor" results in 14 of 24 patients.[134]

It is important to remember that even if growth resumes, premature closure of the physis is to be expected.[31,167,251,258]

Although physeal bar resection clearly has a role in the management of patients with physeal arrest, the surgeon should be cognizant of the relatively modest results and weigh the potential benefits in the context of the actual amount of growth remaining and the etiology, location, and extent of the physeal arrest. Close clinical follow-up to maturity is imperative.

Care of the Multiply Injured Child

Blunt trauma is the leading cause of death in children older than 1 year of age. Although a number of these deaths are from such massive injuries that there is no chance of resuscitation, there are deaths that could be prevented with proper trauma care.[59,88,90,114] Although most preventable deaths are the result of pulmonary, intracranial, or intra-abdominal lesions, it is important for all physicians, including orthopaedists, caring for victims of acute trauma to be thoroughly familiar with the systematic, multidisciplinary approach to the assessment and resuscitation of the polytraumatized child. The principles of assessment and resuscitation

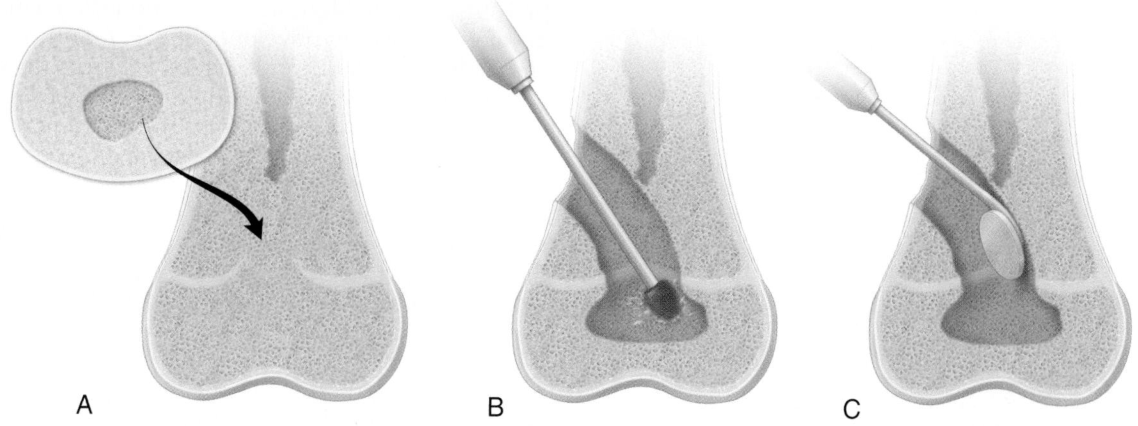

FIGURE 40–20 **A,** Central physeal bar of the distal femur. **B,** A high-speed burr is used to approach the bar through a tunnel in the metaphysis. **C,** A dental mirror (as well as fluoroscopic guidance, fiberoptic suction lighting, and small curved curets) can be helpful in assessing the resection. (Redrawn from Peterson HA: Partial growth plate arrest and its treatment. J Pediatr Orthop 1984;4:246.)

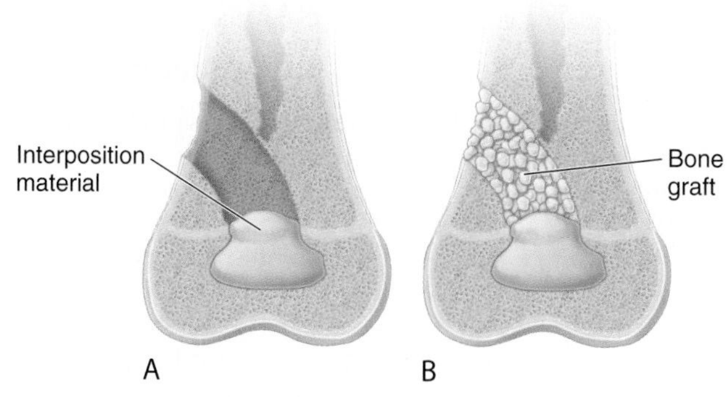

FIGURE 40–21 Once a bar has been successfully resected, the void in the epiphysis and metaphysis should be filled with fat or Cranioplast **(A).** It is helpful to contour and anchor the material into the epiphysis so that it will migrate distally with the physis with growth. The metaphyseal defect can be backed with local bone graft **(B).** (Redrawn from Peterson HA: Partial growth plate arrest and its treatment. J Pediatr Orthop 1984;4:246.)

are outlined and well presented in the Advanced Trauma Life Support course provided by the American College of Surgeons. This comprehensive course provides specific training for the management of the pediatric trauma patient.[313]

Anatomic and Physiologic Characteristics Specific to Children

Children possess a number of anatomic and physiologic characteristics that make their injuries and their injury response different from adults'. Head and visceral injuries are more common in children, whereas chest and thorax injuries are less frequent. Several factors contribute to the fact that head injuries occur in over 80% of polytraumatized children. First, because a child's head is relatively large compared with the trunk, the head is usually the point of first contact during high-energy injuries. Second, the cortical bone of the cranial vault is thinner in children. Finally, a child's brain is less myelinated than an adult's and more easily injured. Fortunately, there are also several characteristics that make recovery from head injury more favorable in children. These include a larger subarachnoid space, greater extracellular space, and open cranial sutures.* Visceral injuries are also more common in children than in adults, in part because there is less abdominal musculature and less subcutaneous fat. Conversely, the elasticity of the thoracic cage makes fractures of the ribs and sternum uncommon in children.[126,174,194,196,202,223,239,313]

A child's response to injury is also different from an adult's. It is unusual for children to have preexisting disease, and they usually have large cardiopulmonary reserves. Consequently they can often maintain a normal systolic blood pressure in the presence of significant hypovolemia, although they will develop tachycardia. Children also become hypothermic rapidly because their surface area is large relative to their body mass. This hypothermia can compound the lactic acidosis associated with hypovolemic shock.

Management of Airway, Breathing, and Circulation

Evaluation and resuscitation of the polytraumatized child begin with the ABCs (airway, breathing, circulation) of trauma. Management of the airway should begin with the assumption that a cervical spinal lesion exists, and cervical spine precautions should be used until the cervical spine is cleared clinically and radiographically. The relatively large head of a child forces the cervical spine into flexion. Thus, appropriate immobilization includes a collar or sand bags as well

*See references 45, 126, 169, 174, 194, 202, 289, 313, 314, 334.

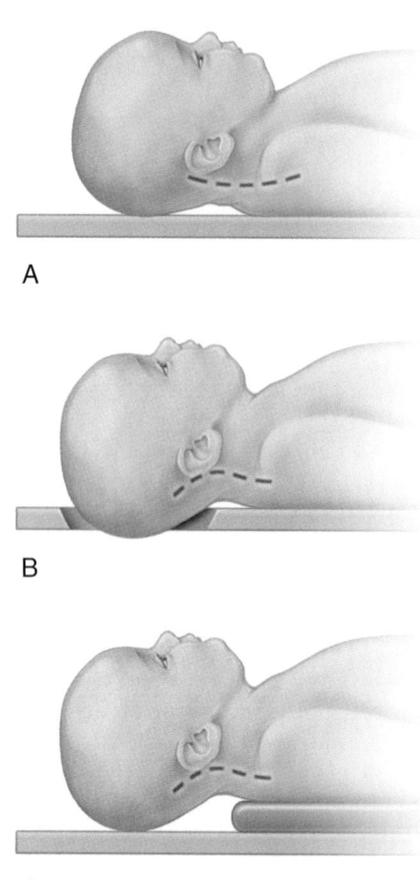

FIGURE 40–22 When placed on an adult backboard, the relatively large head of a child forces the cervical spine into flexion **(A)**. Cervical flexion may be avoided either by using a backboard with a cutout for the head **(B)** or by elevating the torso **(C)**.

as a backboard that has a cutout for the head. If these special backboards are unavailable, children may be safely transported by placing a roll under the shoulders to elevate the torso relative to the head* (Fig. 40–22). With these cervical spine precautions, an adequate airway must be maintained. The jaw thrust or lift will often open the airway. It is also important to remember that the nostrils must be kept clear in infants. All obvious foreign materials (food, mucus, blood, vomit) must be removed from the mouth and oropharynx. Placement of a nasogastric tube will decompress the stomach and help prevent aspiration. In the unconscious or obtunded child, endotracheal intubation ensures a secure airway.[238]

Once an adequate airway has been obtained, breathing and circulation should be assessed. Ventilation should be confirmed by auscultating breath sounds in both lung fields. Absent or decreased breath sounds should alert the surgeon to the possibility of an improperly placed airway or a potential pneumothorax. Assessment of blood volume status in children can be deceptive owing to their large physiologic reserves. Although children often maintain a normal blood pressure despite significant volume loss, tachycardia develops early in hypovolemic shock. Life-threatening hemorrhage in children is usually the result of solid visceral injury because children are less likely than adults to sustain massive blood loss from pelvic or extremity trauma.[65,86,156,324] As assessment and management of the airway, breathing, and circulation is being undertaken, attempts should be made to obtain venous access. Once venous access has been established, fluid resuscitation can begin. A child's circulating blood volume can be estimated as 80 mL/kg. A child's weight in kilograms can be estimated as weight (kg) = (age [yr] × 2) + 8.

As in adults, fluid resuscitation begins with a crystalloid bolus equal to one fourth of the circulating blood volume (20 mL/kg). If tachycardia or other signs of hypovolemia persist after two crystalloid boluses, consideration should be given to transfusion of packed red blood cells. Once fluid resuscitation has begun, the bladder should be decompressed with a Foley catheter. Urine output can then be monitored. Normal urine output in an infant is 1 to 2 mL/kg/hour and in a child or adolescent 0.5 mL/kg/hour.[202,313]

Primary and Secondary Assessments

The primary survey is completed with a quick history, which should include assessment for medical allergies, current medications, significant past medical history, and the details of the accident and management to date. As the primary survey is completed, the secondary survey begins. The secondary survey includes calculation of the Glasgow Coma Scale (GCS) score (Table 40–3) and radiographs of the chest (anteroposterior [AP]), cervical spine (lateral), and pelvis (AP).[246,247] Additional studies (CT of the head and abdomen, radiography of the extremities and thoracolumbar spine) should be performed as indicated. We obtain AP and lateral radiographs of any extremity that is painful, swollen, ecchymotic, or abraded. Routine blood work should include a complete blood cell count as well as a typing and crossmatching. It is prudent to draw ample extra blood at the time venous access is established so that appropriate tests may be added as indicated. The secondary assessment also provides an opportunity to gather information that will allow the computation of an injury score that can be used to classify injury severity and predict morbidity and mortality. A number of scoring systems are available, including the Injury Severity Scale (ISS), the Abbreviated Injury Scale, the Pediatric Trauma Score, the Trauma Score, and the Revised Trauma Score.[15,20,95,105,168,241,253,280,316] The Revised Trauma Score is not specific for children; however, it has the advantage of being universally applicable and has been shown to correlate with survival and with the ISS score as well as with the more specific Pediatric Trauma Score[95,105] (Table 40–4). The ISS score is used primarily for injury classification and outcomes research but also as a measure of quality assurance. It has not been shown to have a direct correlation with mortality.[10,15,18,20,67,95,168,241,316]

*See references 77, 132, 141, 148, 149, 159, 172, 183, 202, 313, 320.

Table 40-3 Glasgow Coma Scale

Variable	Score
Opening of the Eyes	
Spontaneously	4
To speech	3
To pain	2
None	1
Best Verbal Response	
Oriented	5
Confused	4
Inappropriate words	3
Incomprehensible sounds	2
None	1
Children's Best Verbal Response	
Smiles, orients to sound, follows objects, interacts	5
Consolable when crying, interacts inappropriately	4
Inconsistently consolable	3
Moans inconsolably, irritable, restless	2
No response	1
Best Motor Response	
Spontaneous (obedience to commands)	6
Localization of pain	5
Withdrawal	4
Abnormal flexion to pain	3
Abnormal extension to pain	2
None	1

Modified from Armstrong PF, Smith JT: Initial management of the multiply injured child. In Letts RM (ed): Management of Pediatric Fractures. New York, Churchill Livingstone, 1994, p 32.

Table 40-4 Revised Trauma Score

	Variables		
Revised Trauma Score	Glasgow Coma Scale Score	Systolic Blood Pressure (mm Hg)	Respiratory Rate (breaths/min)
4	13-15	>89	10-29
3	9-12	76-89	>29
2	6-8	50-75	6-9
1	4-5	1-49	1-5
0	3	0	0

Each of the three variables (GCS, BP, RR) is given a Revised Trauma Score, and the Revised Trauma Scores are totaled (range: 0-12). A total score ≤11 indicates potentially important trauma.

From Armstrong PF, Smith JT: Initial management of the multiply injured child. In Letts RM (ed): Management of Pediatric Fractures. New York, Churchill Livingstone, 1994, p 34. Originally from American Hospital and Prehospital Resources for Optimal Care of the Injured Patient and Appendices F and J. Chicago, American College of Surgeons, 1986.

Management of the traumatized child is a multidisciplinary process. As the secondary survey begins, continuous monitoring of airway, breathing, and circulation must continue. Deterioration of vital signs or GCS score may warrant emergency consultation with a neurosurgeon or a trauma surgeon. CT of the head is perhaps the single most important study in the management of intracranial trauma. Often, an abdominal CT may be performed at the same time with little or no delay. In today's increasingly specialized environment, the orthopaedist may become involved in the care of a multiply injured child after the initial assessment has begun. One of the advantages of a multidisciplinary approach is that it has a built-in system of checks and balances. Thus, the prudent orthopaedist will *never assume* that the initial assessment has been completed accurately and thoroughly and will begin the assessment with the ABCs and progress to the assessment of any orthopaedic injuries.

Perhaps the two greatest mistakes an orthopaedic surgeon can make in managing a traumatically injured child are to assume that a long bone fracture is an isolated injury and to assume that a patient has an unsurvivable injury. At our acute care institution, we routinely consult a trauma surgeon for patients with isolated long bone fractures and a high-energy mechanism of injury (such as pedestrians or bicyclists hit by automobiles).[161,324] In addition, we aggressively treat all children with the expectation that they will recover from even the most severe head injuries.[196,286,327,351] It is important to remember that the secondary survey continues 24 and 48 hours after the injury. Continuous reassessment will help identify the "missed injuries" that are noted in 2% to 12% of polytraumatized patients.[42,182,196,227] Unlike in adults, early mobilization is not as important in the management of orthopaedic injuries in a polytraumatized child.[38,104,180,207,224,264,360] Nevertheless, orthopaedic injuries should be managed in a fashion that accommodates the needs of all members of the trauma team.

A number of recent reports have investigated the development of post-traumatic stress in children after traumatic injury.[85,166,284,287,291,297,349,350] These studies clearly demonstrate that symptoms of post-traumatic stress disorder are common after pediatric orthopaedic trauma. Symptoms have been shown to correlate with more severe injury requiring hospitalization, pulse at presentation, and parental reports of post-traumatic stress.[166,284,287,297] Winston and colleagues have validated a brief screening questionnaire for injured children and their parents.[349]

Open Fractures

Although the incidence and mechanism of open fractures differ somewhat between children and adults, their management in these two populations is similar, requiring an aggressive, thorough, and systematic approach[119,121,288] (Box 40–1). The most common open fractures in children involve the hand and upper extremity. The majority of these injuries are the result of falls.[125,288] Open fractures of the lower

Box 40-1

Open Fracture Management

1. Thorough assessment for life-threatening injuries
2. Immediate intravenous antibiotics, continue for 48 hours:
   - Grade I—first-generation cephalosporin
   - Grades II and III—first-generation cephalosporin + aminoglycoside
   - "Barnyard" injuries—add anaerobic coverage (penicillin or metronidazole)
3. Tetanus prophylaxis
4. Thorough operative debridement
5. Adequate fracture stabilization
6. Second operative debridement in 48-72 hours *if indicated*
7. Early definitive soft tissue coverage
8. Early bone grafting *if indicated*

Box 40-2

Open Fracture Classification

Type I
Wound <1 cm long
Moderately clean puncture wound
Usually "inside-out" injury
Little soft tissue damage, no crushing
Little comminution

Type II
Wound >1 cm long
No extensive tissue damage
Slight or moderate crush injury
Moderate comminution or contamination

Type III
Extensive soft tissue damage to muscles, skin, and neurovascular structures and a high degree of contamination
Three subtypes:
A: Adequate soft tissue coverage (includes high-energy segmental, comminuted fractures, regardless of normal size)
B: Local or free flap required for coverage
C: Arterial injury requiring repair

Modified from references 120 through 123.

extremities, particularly the tibia, are usually the result of higher-energy trauma, most commonly trauma sustained in automobile–pedestrian or automobile–bicycle accidents.[48,76,117,155,276,306] Although recent reports have highlighted the problems of interobserver and intraobserver reliability, the classification system of Gustilo and Anderson is still the one most widely used for classifying open fractures in both children and adults[46,119,120,122,123,147] (Box 40–2).

Overview of Treatment

The treatment of open fractures begins in the emergency department with a complete and thorough assessment to identify any life-threatening injuries (see previous discussion under Care of the Multiply Injured Child). Once an open fracture has been identified, intravenous (IV) antibiotics should be administered. In a review of over 1100 open fractures, Patzakis and Wilkins found the timely administration of IV antibiotics to be the single most important factor in reducing the infection rate.[257] Other studies have confirmed that early administration of IV antibiotics is more critical than the time to operative debridement.[60,130,302,303] We currently use a first-generation cephalosporin for all open fractures. For grades II and III open fractures, we usually add gram-negative coverage with the addition of an aminoglycoside. For "barnyard" injuries we add anaerobic coverage with penicillin or metronidazole (Flagyl).[123] In addition, the status of the patient's tetanus immunization should be reviewed. The American College of Surgeons recommends a booster of tetanus toxoid to all patients with wounds unless they have completed immunization or received a booster in the past 5 years. Patients with "tetanus-prone" wounds (severe, neglected, or more than 24 hours old) should be given a booster unless it can be confirmed that they have received one in the past year. The decision to provide passive immunization with human tetanus immune globulin must be made on an individual basis. Passive immunization with human immune globulin should be considered in all patients with tetanus-prone wounds who have not been immunized or whose immunization status cannot be confirmed.[9]

All open fractures are an operative emergency and require operative debridement as soon as the patient can be assessed and stabilized. At the time of debridement, all open wounds should be extended proximally and distally and all loose debris and nonviable tissue, including devascularized bone, should be removed. Both ends of the fracture should be visualized and debrided. After a systematic, circumferential, superficial to deep debridement, the wound should be thoroughly irrigated with 5 to 10 L of saline.[119,120,122,123,256,315,322] Although some recent retrospective studies report good results treating Gustilo type I open fractures nonoperatively, we believe that all open fractures should be managed with operative debridement.[153,356]

Once the wound has been thoroughly debrided, the fracture should be stabilized. Fracture stabilization reduces the rate of infection by protecting the integrity of the soft tissue envelope. In children, fracture stabilization can frequently be accomplished with cast

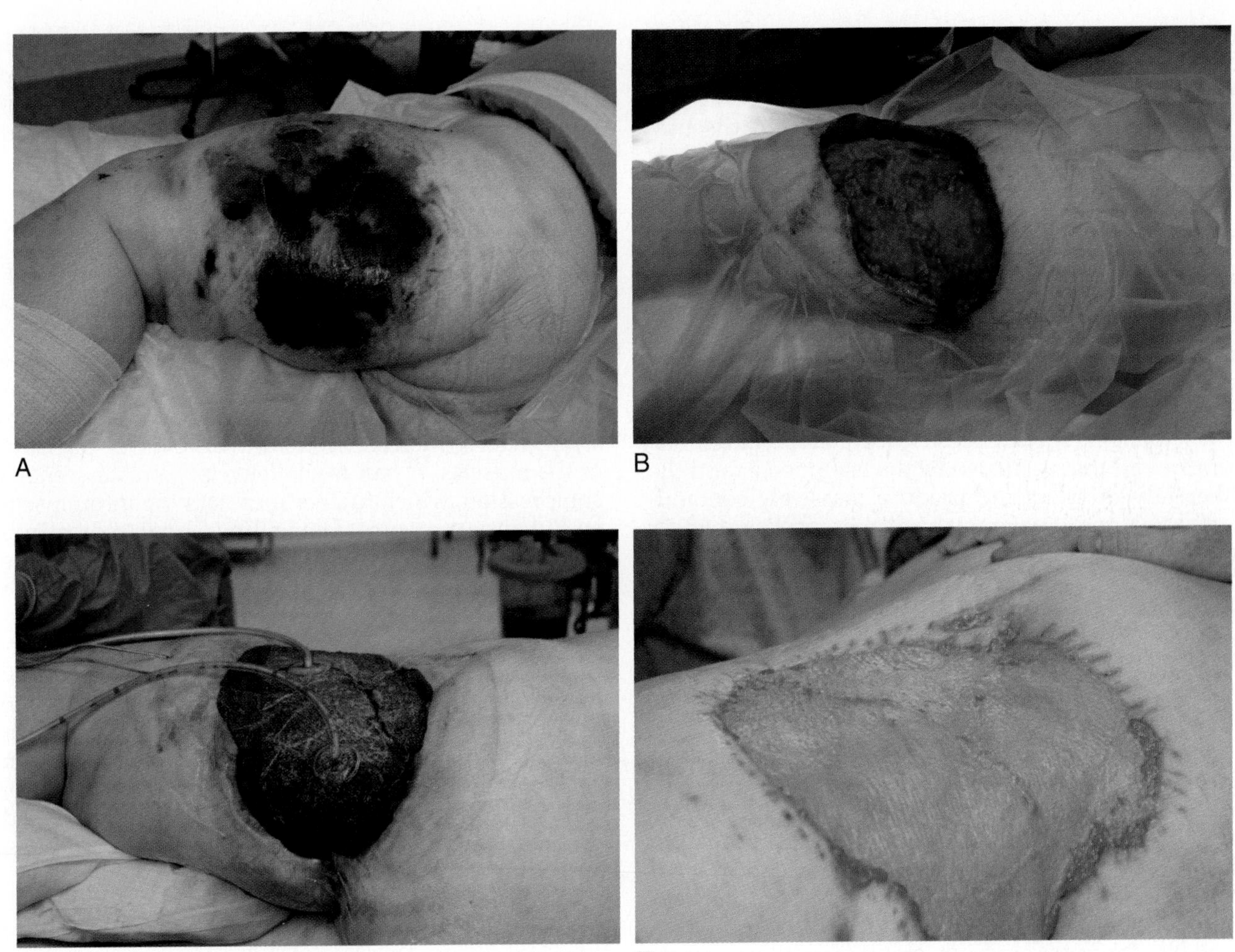

FIGURE 40–23 **A,** Obese 13-year-old with large lateral thigh Morel-Lavallee lesion. **B,** Soft tissue deficit after debridement. **C,** Vacuum-assisted closure dressing in place. **D,** Final appearance after split-thickness skin grafting.

immobilization, often supplemented with percutaneous pin fixation. If there are large soft tissue wounds, however, internal or external fixation may be indicated.[48,125,155,180,276,306,319,354] Recommendations regarding fracture stabilization are discussed with each injury.

The necessity of a second debridement for all open fractures is controversial. Although routine redebridement has been recommended,[119,120,123] there are several large series in which open fractures in children were managed successfully with a single debridement and loose wound closure over a drain.[76,117,155] We make the decision to perform a second debridement on an individual basis, based on the amount of contamination, soft tissue devitalization, and bony comminution present at the initial debridement.

If primary wound closure is not possible either initially or on a delayed basis, wound closure with skin grafts or soft tissue transfer should be accomplished as soon as a clean, stable wound can be achieved, preferably within 5 to 10 days.[49,66,119,123] The development of negative-pressure therapy using the vacuum-assisted closure device has been a significant advance in the management of traumatic soft tissue loss in children as well as adults[52,140,243,298,341] (Fig. 40–23). The use of rotational (gastrocnemius or soleus) flaps or free microvascular tissue transfer in children is well established and based on principles similar to those in adults.[16,64,68,98,255,275,293] Once soft tissue closure has been achieved, attention can be directed at bony reconstruction. Fortunately, open fractures in children rarely go on to delayed union or nonunion; consequently, such procedures are rarely indicated.* The management of bone loss is discussed with specific injuries.

Gunshot Wounds

In large urban settings in the United States, gunshot injuries in children are becoming increasingly common. Gunshot wounds may be classified as either high or low velocity. High-velocity gunshots usually produce extensive soft tissue damage, gross contamination, and comminuted fractures. These injuries should be treated as type III open fractures. Low-velocity gunshot wounds have little soft tissue injury or fracture comminution. Recently, several authors have reported the successful treatment of these

*See references 48, 76, 113, 117, 125, 155, 180, 210, 276, 306.

injuries with local wound debridement and short-term IV or oral antibiotic therapy. It is important to realize that most of these studies have been performed in adults. However, the few reports specifically discussing gunshot wounds in children suggest that, as is often the case, children have a better prognosis than adults.[17,22,87,97,143,150,175,197,231,242,310,312,329,337]

Lawnmower Injury

Lawnmower injuries are another unique subcategory of open fractures. Not surprisingly, most children injured by lawnmowers are bystanders rather than operators or even riders. Most reports note that 30% to 50% of patients require some level of amputation. The vortex of air that is created by the lawnmower and the inherently dirty setting produce massively contaminated wounds. Acute management of lawnmower injuries involves multiple thorough debridements. We routinely debride these wounds multiple times at 48-hour intervals, until there is no evidence of debris and there is a healthy granulation bed. In addition to thorough debridement, initial management should include broad-spectrum antibiotics, including coverage for potential anaerobic infection. If amputation is required, every effort is made to keep the level as distal as possible. Consideration should be given to using the amputated parts to provide cartilaginous caps over any exposed residual bone in the hope of preventing appositional overgrowth of the residual limb. Like most traumatic injuries, many, if not all, lawnmower injuries are easily preventable. There are currently many educational efforts under way to ensure that operators of lawnmowers have adequate knowledge of the potential danger these machines represent not only to operators but to bystanders.[8,14,27,28,89,178,192,203,205,206,209,236,275,298,333]

Compartment Syndrome

Compartment syndrome is a potentially devastating entity that may develop when injury induces increased pressure within a closed space. Because the earliest signs of compartment syndrome are often subtle and the patients are frequently obtunded or difficult to assess for other reasons, the diagnosis may be delayed or altogether missed, resulting in devastating complications that may be avoided with prompt surgical decompression.[129,137,218,219,232-234,318,321,332] The best treatment of a compartment syndrome is avoidance. However, once it has developed it must be promptly recognized and treated.

Incidence

Compartment syndrome has been reported after accidental injury (with or without a fracture), elective surgical procedures (related to the procedure or positioning), infection, snake bites, and IV infiltrations.* A recent report described 24 cases of compartment syndrome in newborn infants—all of whom presented with a sentinel skin lesion.[267] However, in children, compartment syndrome is still most commonly seen after fractures of the supracondylar humerus or tibia.*

Pathophysiology

Eaton and associates have outlined the pathophysiology of compartment syndrome.[92] Initially, ischemia produces anoxia in muscles, which in turn causes release of histamine-like substances, which increases capillary permeability and leads to intramuscular edema. The increasing intramuscular edema produces a progressive increase in the intrinsic tissue pressure of the muscles. A taut fascial envelope creates venous compression, which further increases the intramuscular intrinsic pressure. Unyielding circular dressings on the limb can also contribute to increases in the intramuscular pressure. Pressor receptors within the muscle produce vasospasm, which aggravates the initial vascular compromise, creating a destructive ischemia–edema cycle. The only treatment for this potentially devastating cycle is prompt wide surgical decompression of the fascial compartment.[129,165,213,216,218,219,220,233] Compartment syndrome can be recognized by the so-called six P's: pain out of proportion to physical examination findings, increased pressure, pink skin color, pulse present, paresthesias, and paresis. However, the only early sign may be pain, particularly pain on passive stretching.[174,219,347] In fact, paresis and paresthesias are late findings, often present only after permanent damage has occurred. In a review of 36 children with compartment syndrome, Bae and colleagues found that an increasing analgesia requirement was the most frequent indicator of compartment syndrome.[19]

Diagnosis

Diagnosis of an acute compartment syndrome can be aided by measurement of the pressure within the compartment. Numerous techniques have been described to measure intracompartmental pressure. One of the earliest was the Whitesides needle technique. This technique uses an 18-gauge needle, a syringe, IV tubing, sterile saline, a three-way stopcock, and a mercury manometer (Fig. 40–24A). The needle is placed into the compartment and the plunger is advanced until the fluid column begins to enter the compartment. The pressure reading on the manometer at this point represents the compartment pressure.

Other techniques have been developed to allow continuous monitoring of compartment pressures or to simplify pressure measurement. These include the wick or slit catheter technique, the infusion technique, commercially available gauges, and an IV catheter with an infusion pump or arterial line pressure monitor.[39,232,234,326] Wick and slit catheters were devel-

*See references 57, 146, 193, 235, 244, 267, 290, 294, 309, 358.

*See references 23, 24, 35, 48, 54, 74, 76, 125, 128, 137-139, 155, 160, 217, 218, 233, 276, 277, 296, 308.

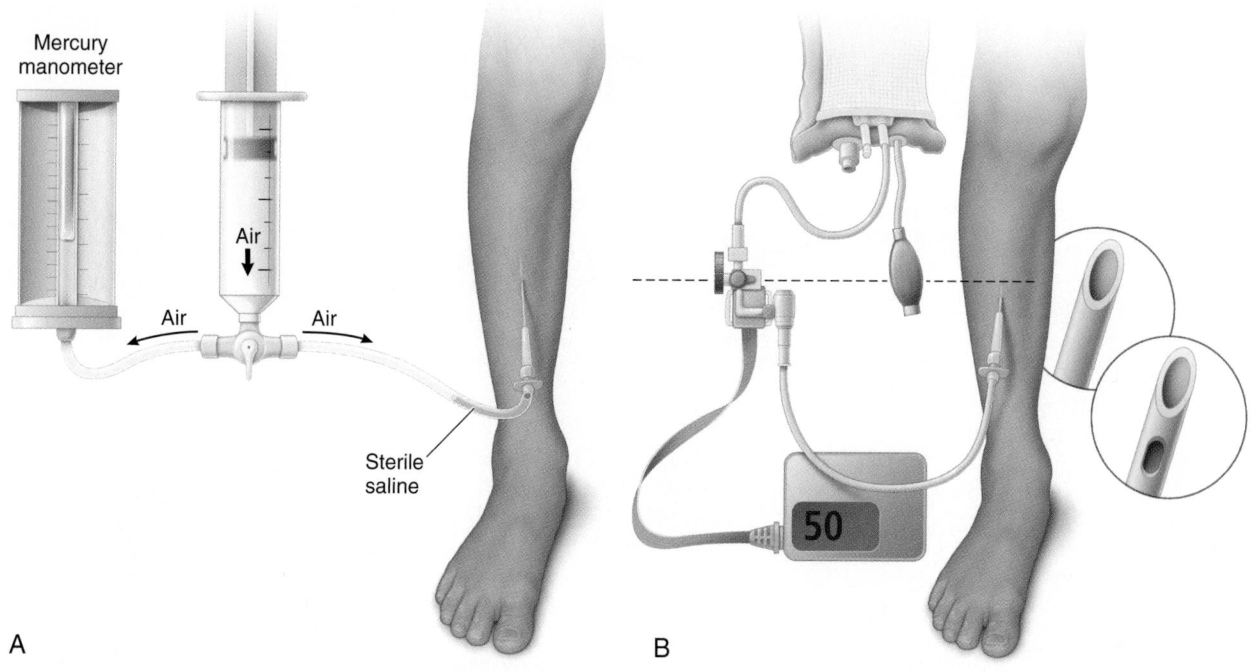

FIGURE 40–24 **A,** Whiteside's needle technique for measuring compartment pressures (see text for technique). **B,** Arterial line technique for compartment pressure measurement (see text for technique).

oped because of theoretical concerns that the injection technique created nonequilibrium conditions at the tip of the catheter and overestimated the compartment pressure.[232,234,279] Wilson and colleagues have shown that slit catheters and 16-gauge IV catheters produce similar compartment pressure measurements.[348] Uppal and colleagues described a technique using an 18-gauge needle and an IV alarm control (IVAC) pump. After zeroing the IVAC pump and adjusting the unit to read in millimeters of mercury rather than millimeters of water, the fluid flow rate is set at 25 mm/hr. An 18-gauge needle is then introduced into the compartment and the "read pressure" button is depressed. The compartmental pressure is displayed on the IVAC pump.[326] Similarly, a needle or Angiocath (with or with out a side port) can be connected to an arterial line monitor. After zeroing the monitor (which requires a small fluid bolus), the pressure is displayed on the arterial line monitor (Fig. 40–24B). This technique can be used with a slit indwelling catheter to provide continuous pressure monitoring.

Boody and Wongworawat compared three commonly used techniques to measure compartment pressure (Whitesides technique, the commercially available Stryker monitor, and an arterial line). They assessed three needle types with each device (straight needles, side-port needles, and slit catheters). They concluded that side-port needles and slit catheters are more accurate than straight needles and that the arterial line manometer is the most accurate device. They found that the Stryker device was also very accurate but thought that the Whitesides manometer apparatus lacked the precision needed for clinical use.[39]

Prevention and Treatment

Appropriate management of "at-risk" extremities may help prevent compartment syndrome. Elevation of affected extremities is recommended immediately after an injury to decrease soft tissue swelling. Although elevation decreases edema, it also decreases arterial blood flow and reduces oxygen perfusion by reducing the arteriovenous gradient.[129,213,216,219,220,355] Thus, if an evolving compartment syndrome is suspected, the limb should be kept at the level of the heart rather than elevated. Circumferential dressings can cause an elevation in compartment pressures, which can accelerate the development of ischemia and the spiraling increase in edema and pressure.[81,137,233,338] Removal of circumferential dressings has been shown to reduce compartment pressure by as much as 85%. Therefore, once a compartment syndrome is suspected, all circumferential dressings should be removed *to the skin*.[30,108] Appropriate management also includes thorough documentation of all physical findings and treatment options. This is particularly important given the frequent medicolegal implications of compartment syndrome.[29,58]

The intracompartmental pressure at which a compartment syndrome exists is unknown, and the pressure may vary with the technique of measurement.[229,292,348] Whitesides and colleagues recommended surgical decompression when compartment pressure rose to within 10 to 30 mm Hg of the diastolic pressure using the needle technique.[342,343] Matsen and coworkers[214,215] have recommended decompression at pressures of 45 mm Hg using the infusion technique,

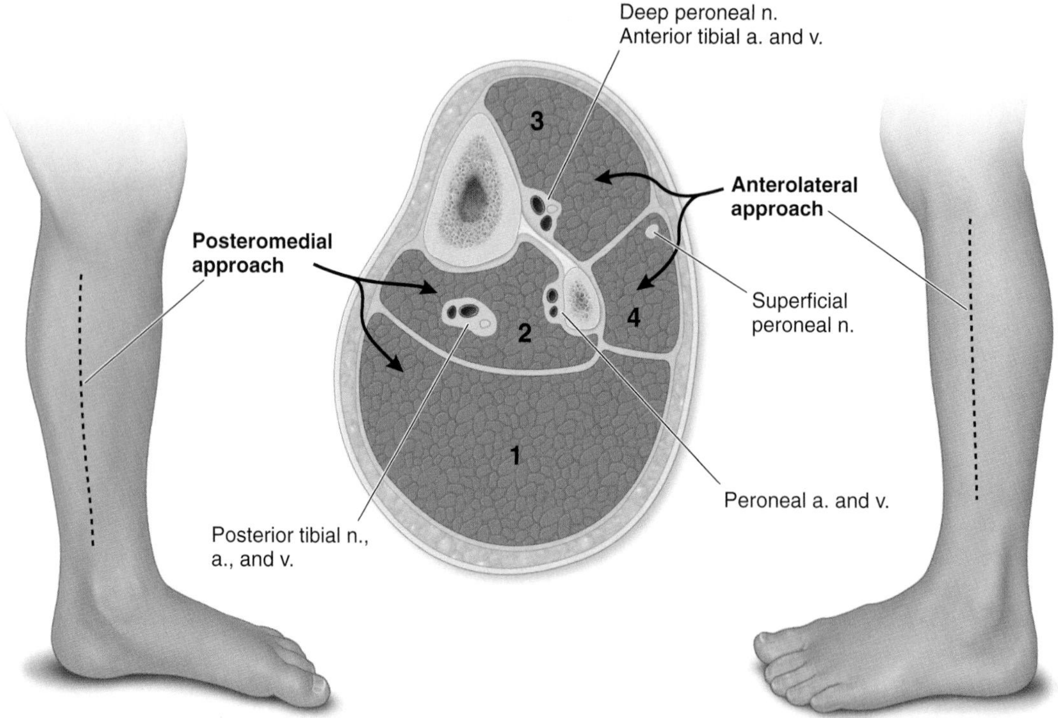

FIGURE 40–25 Two-incision technique for four-compartment fasciotomy of the leg. *Left,* Posteromedial incision for decompression of the superficial and deep posterior compartments. This incision must extend far enough distally to allow complete decompression of the entire deep posterior compartment. *Right,* Anterolateral incision for release of the anterior and lateral compartments. Care should be taken to identify and protect the superficial peroneal nerve. This incision must extend far enough proximally to ensure complete decompression of the muscles near their origin.

whereas Mubarak and colleagues[232] and Rorabeck and associates[43,279] have recommended decompression at 30 to 35 mm Hg using the wick or slit catheter. These thresholds for pressure measurements are guidelines only, and decisions regarding fasciotomy must be made in the context of the entire clinical setting, taking into account the patient's blood pressure, local perfusion, trends of intracompartmental pressures, and symptoms, as well as the patient's ability to cooperate with repeated examinations. It is also important to remember that compartment syndrome is a dynamic entity and that the at-risk extremity must be continuously reassessed.

Although the specific surgical technique for fasciotomy depends on the anatomic location, a few general points merit discussion. When treating compartment syndrome of the leg, it is important that all four compartments be widely released. We prefer to do this with a two-incision technique. The anterior and lateral compartments are released through a lateral incision that extends proximally to the origin of these muscles in the leg. The superficial and deep posterior compartments are addressed through a medial incision that extends distally to allow release of the entire deep posterior compartment (Fig. 40–25). In treating compartment syndrome of the forearm, we use the volar approach of Henry (Fig. 40–26). It is important to remember that there is both a superficial and a deep compartment to the forearm and that the deep compartment, consisting of the flexor profundi, the flexor pollicis longus, and the pronator quadratus, is more susceptible to development of compartment syndrome.[278] Once fasciotomy has been performed, Eaton and Green recommend careful assessment of each individual muscle. If the epimysium is a constricting, compressive structure, they recommend episiotomy.[91] Similarly, Rorabeck recommends external neurolysis if indicated.[278] After decompression, the initial findings may be mild. However, massive swelling is the rule after fascial release; thus, it is wise to use generous incisions that allow full and complete release of the fascia.

Once wide surgical decompression has been achieved, all untreated fractures should be stabilized in a fashion that allows appropriate treatment of the soft tissue wounds. The condition of the underlying muscle is then assessed. Initially ischemic muscle may respond favorably to decompression; thus, all nonviable tissue should be removed but any questionable tissue left alone. A sterile bulky dressing is applied to the extremity and the patient should be returned to the operating room at 48- to 72-hour intervals for continued debridement of nonviable tissue. Once a stable, healthy wound has been achieved, soft tissue closure can be performed either primarily or with split-thickness skin grafting, if necessary. After primary healing has occurred, reconstruction of any permanent deficits can be undertaken. With early

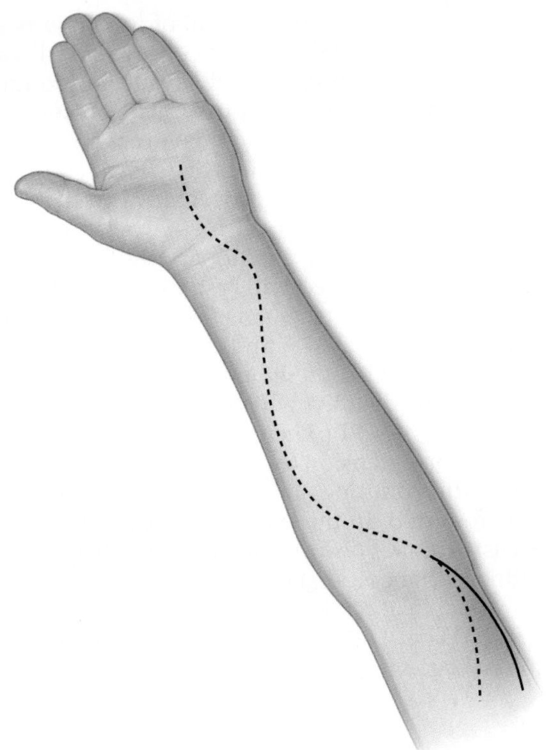

FIGURE 40–26 Skin incision for volar fasciotomy of the forearm. Distally, a skin flap is preserved to cover the median nerve. Proximally, the incision may be extended either medially or anterolaterally.

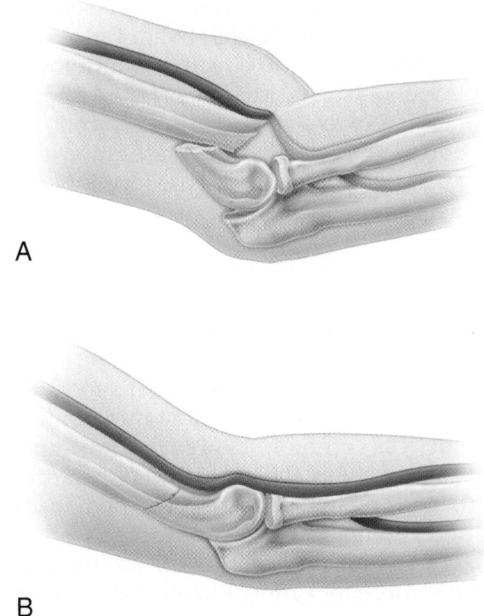

FIGURE 40–27 Emergency realignment of an ischemic extremity **(A)** may reduce the tension on a vessel and restore the circulation **(B)**.

diagnosis and treatment, Bae and colleagues reported full restoration of function in over 90% of 36 children with compartment syndrome.[19]

Although prompt recognition and early appropriate treatment of compartment syndrome can limit or avoid some of the potentially devastating problems, one should remember that as Sir Robert Jones noted, "It cannot be too emphatically stated that despite every precaution ischemic contractures may occur."[26] Littler later echoed these comments, stating, "Occasionally, despite professional awareness and all preventive effort, this distressing complication develops."[26]

Vascular Injuries

Vascular injury may result from severely displaced fractures. This is most commonly seen with extension supracondylar humerus fractures or with fractures of the distal femur or proximal tibia.* Patients who present with an ischemic limb and a fracture should undergo immediate "closed reduction" of the fracture in the emergency department. This closed reduction is actually a simple realignment of the limb, performed with gentle traction to restore the limb to a more anatomic position, thus removing any tension on the neurovascular structures (Fig. 40–27). If, as is frequently the case, realignment of the limb restores circulation to the extremity, fracture management can usually proceed in the normal fashion. However, if a nonviable limb persists after realignment, the patient should be taken immediately to the operating room for fracture stabilization, vascular exploration, and, if indicated, repair. We believe that "preoperative" arteriography in an ischemic/nonviable extremity only prolongs the ischemic time and should not routinely be performed. We proceed immediately to the operating room and stabilize the fracture. Once the fracture has been stabilized, vascular exploration can be accomplished. If necessary, fluoroscopy can be used to obtain an intraoperative arteriogram, although we find that this is seldom necessary because the anatomic location of the vascular injury is usually obvious. Ideally, revascularization should be achieved within 6 to 8 hours. Prolonged ischemia and subsequent revascularization may be associated with the development of compartment syndrome. The surgeon should have a low threshold for performing fasciotomies at the time of revascularization.[48,51,69,72,103,179,254,311,328,336,361]

The management of a viable limb with an absent pulse is controversial. This is often the case with a limb that was initially ischemic but improved with realignment. Some authors have advocated arteriography or exploration with appropriate vascular repair. Others have documented that a viable but pulseless extremity may be safely observed. We manage these patients in consultation with a trauma surgeon, vascular surgeon, or microsurgeon, with decisions made on an individual basis.[72,103] However, we usually recommend a conservative course with close observation.[62,295,345,361] The importance of an adequate period of close observation must be emphasized because

*See references 48, 51, 69, 72, 103, 179, 254, 311, 328, 336, 361.

propagation of a thrombus can turn a pulseless, viable hand to an ischemic, nonviable hand. Pulse oximetry has been reported to be an effective continuous monitoring device in such situations.[110,272] Although the ability of pulse oximetry to accurately reflect tissue oxygenation (a function of oxygen saturation *and* blood flow) has been questioned,[301] we believe it is an effective adjunct in monitoring an extremity for viability.

CASTS

No discussion of the general principles of traumatic injuries in children would be complete without a discussion of the principles involved in good casting. With advances in orthopaedics, cast immobilization is increasingly less common. However, for a number of reasons, casts remain the mainstay of treatment for children's fractures and reconstructive pediatric orthopaedic surgery. Thus, the ability to apply a well-molded cast or splint is an important skill for the pediatric orthopaedic surgeon. Unfortunately, too often the task of reducing and splinting a fracture is delegated to the most junior member of the team, often with little instruction and no supervision. This may result in less-than-desirable outcomes because even an undisplaced buckle fracture can angulate in a poorly applied splint or cast (see Fig. 40–3). It is increasingly common to hear comments regarding the "lost art of casting." Applying a well-molded cast or splint, particularly on a small, moving child with a chubby arm, is indeed an acquired skill.

Principles of Application. A well-applied cast has only two layers of cast padding on all areas except bony prominences, which require a third or fourth. A cast with too much padding will fail to hold a reduction, whereas one with too little may result in pressure sores. Once a cast has been applied it should be molded to provide three-point fixation of the fracture[61] (Fig. 40–28). When applying a cast, one should remember that the length on the convex side of an angle is significantly greater than that on the concave side. Failure to account for this difference will result in too much material on the concave side or insufficient material on the convex side. Technically this problem may be addressed with the use of splints or by fanning the cast material out over the convex side. During cast application, attention must be given to the position of the entire extremity. Moving a joint once the padding and plaster have been applied will result in a crease, which can lead to soft tissue problems (Fig. 40–29). Similarly, applying a short-leg cast with the ankle in equinus or a long-arm cast with the elbow extended may allow the cast to shift distally, which can also lead to pressure sores (Fig. 40–30). There are clinical situations in which a cast in extension (e.g., supracondylar humerus fractures after pinning) or equinus (distal tibia fractures) is required. In these instances, careful molding of the cast around bony prominences will help prevent migration of the cast distally.

Materials. The Dutch military surgeon Antonius Mathijsen began impregnating open meshed bandages

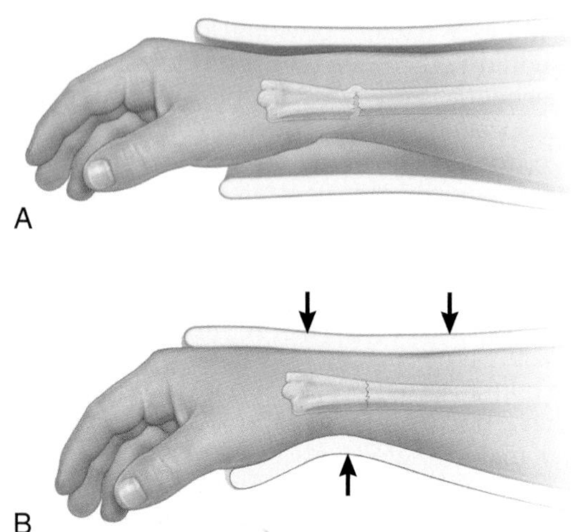

FIGURE 40–28 **A,** A cast with too much padding and an inadequate mold will not maintain a reduction. **B,** Proper casting technique provides three-point fixation of the fracture.

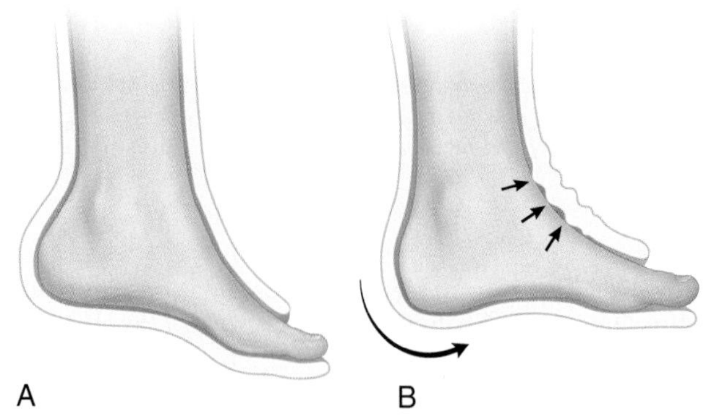

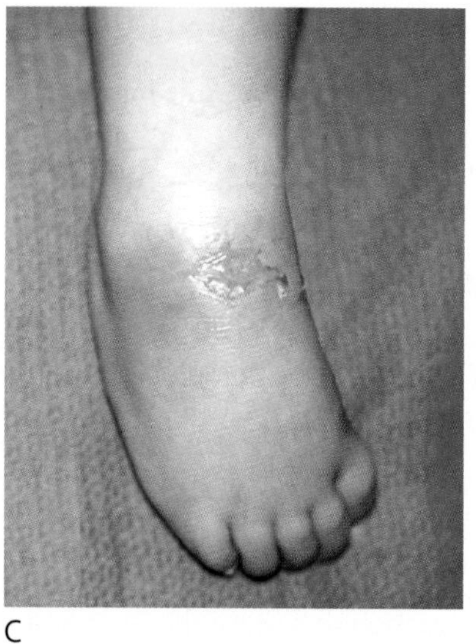

FIGURE 40–29 **A,** Once casting materials have been applied, a joint must not be moved. **B** and **C,** Moving the foot out of equinus creates creases in the cast, which can lead to skin breakdown.

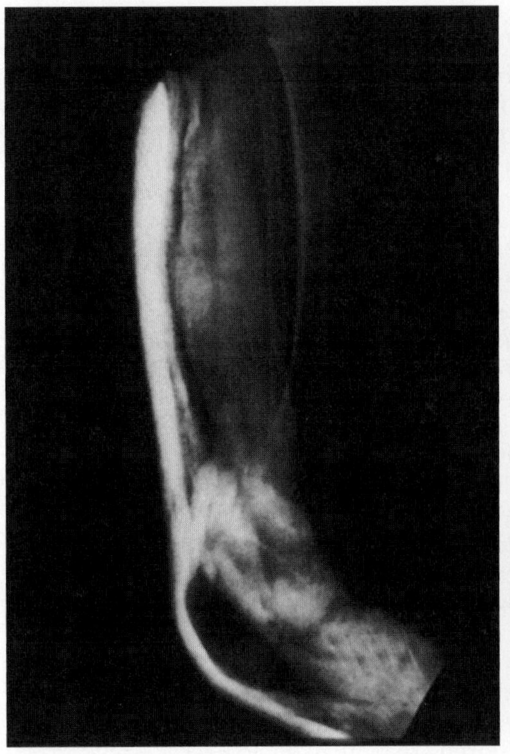

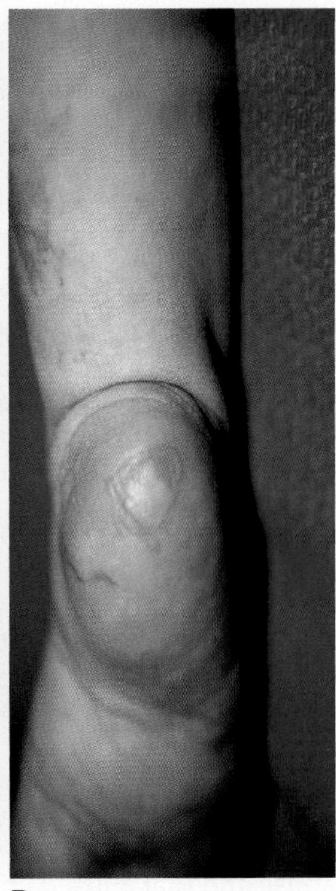

FIGURE 40-30 Pressure sores after distal migration of a splint. **A,** Lateral radiograph of a poorly molded posterior splint. The splint has slid distally and is impinging on the heel. **B,** When the splint is removed, there is blistering on the heel.

with plaster-of-Paris powder in 1852, and for over a century there were few fundamental changes in casting materials.[118] Recently, several new casting materials were introduced. These include fiberglass casting tape and Gore-Tex spica liners. Despite the considerable debate over the efficacy of these new materials, there has been little scientific experimentation with them, and the choice of materials remains primarily a subjective one. Proponents of fiberglass casts note that they are lighter and more durable. Others have argued that fiberglass is more difficult to mold and less forgiving when swelling is expected. In one of the few studies comparing casting material, Davids and coworkers demonstrated that a properly applied fiberglass cast produces less skin pressure than a plaster-of-Paris cast.[81] 3M has developed a fiberglass casting material (Scotchcast) that is removed with simple unrolling. The ease of removal of this material has led to its widespread use in the treatment of clubfeet.[73]

CHILD ABUSE

One of the earliest descriptions of the orthopaedic manifestations of child abuse was by Caffey in 1946. He described six infants with femur fractures and chronic subdural hematomas.[50] In 1953, Silverman[299] implicated the parents and guardians in these traumatic lesions. In 1962, Kempe and colleagues introduced the phrase "battered child syndrome."[170] This paper brought multidisciplinary medical attention to the problem of child abuse and led to mandatory reporting laws, which now exist in all 50 states. Originally, child abuse was defined as physical injury inflicted on children by persons caring for them.[135] Since this early definition in 1968, the definition of abuse has expanded to include physical neglect and endangerment as well as emotional and sexual abuse.

Incidence

The incidence of child abuse is difficult to determine. It has been estimated that 1% to 1.5% of all children are abused each year.[325] In the United States in 1991, there were more than two million reports alleging maltreatment of more than three million children. These reports were substantiated in approximately one million children. Although this represents a nearly 20% increase from 1990, it is difficult to determine whether the increase represents an improvement in reporting or an actual increase in the number of abused children.[325] Statistical analysis of reported cases shows that children are more likely to be abused by caregivers who are young, poor, and of minority status. However, abuse in affluent families may be underreported because of medical practitioners' desire to protect their social peers from the stigma of investigation by public agencies. Abuse is also less likely to be reported if it is emotional rather than physical and if the mother is the perpetrator. There is no doubt that child abuse is a problem that crosses all age, sex, ethnic, and socioeconomic groups.[53,127,185]

Although children of any age can be abused, younger children are more frequently victims.[353] Zimmerman and associates reported that 50% of 243 abused children were younger than 1 year of age and 78% were younger than 3 years.[359] Younger children are also more likely to die from abuse.[53,240] In the United States, in 1996, 76% of the 1077 fatalities from abuse were in children younger than 4 years of age.[326]

Diagnosis

The diagnosis of abuse can be straightforward and obvious or frustratingly difficult. Regardless of the ease with which the diagnosis can be made, a high degree of suspicion is required in order to make the diagnosis. Child abuse has been found in up to half of all children with fractures in the first year of life and in one third of children younger than 3 years of age with a fracture.[21,145,176,177,221,353] A number of the "pathognomonic" signs of abuse are actually rare. The classic finding of "multiple fractures in different stages of healing" has been reported to be present in only 10% to 15% of documented cases of abuse.[106,204] Similarly, corner fractures or bucket-handle metaphyseal fractures are not as frequent as diaphyseal fractures. The importance of soft tissue injuries should not be overlooked. In fact, a number of reports have stressed the fact that fractures rarely exist without other signs of abuse and that abused children are more likely to have soft tissue injuries than fractures.[106,204,222,226] A skeletal survey may be an effective means of clarifying tentative findings in children who were suspected victims of physical child abuse.[37,359] It is important to consider, identify, and report neglect and endangerment. There may be no question of intentional injury when paramedics bring in a toddler who has fallen out of a three-story window; however, such a scenario suggests neglect or endangerment. Allowing a child to return to such an environment may be as dangerous as failing to report physical injury.

As in all areas of orthopaedics, there are few absolutes in child abuse. The best approach to child abuse is to maintain a high degree of vigilance by considering the diagnosis in all children with traumatic injuries. Indeed, nonaccidental trauma has been reported as the cause of nearly every type of musculoskeletal injury, including fractures of the spine and proximal femur as well as compartment syndrome.[163,198,230] Certain factors, such as a changing history or a history not consistent with the injury, a delay in seeking treatment, long-bone fractures in children younger than 1 year of age, multiple fractures in different stages of healing, corner fractures, rib fractures, skull fractures, thermal injuries, and unexplained soft tissue injuries, should raise concern and trigger a report to the appropriate child protective agencies. Perhaps the most frequently overlooked part of the assessment of the abused child is the interview with the child. Children, when time is taken to place them in a comfortable, secure, nonthreatening environment (characteristics that are difficult, if not impossible, to find in most busy emergency departments!), will display remarkable candor. The possibility of nonaccidental trauma should be considered in the fracture clinic as well as the emergency department.[21,252]

Reporting

Despite mandatory reporting laws, physicians are often reluctant to report suspected abuse because of concern over upsetting the parents or caregivers. It has been our experience that when approached in a nonaccusational fashion with a simple explanation of the legal and ethical duty to report suspected abuse, parents are usually understanding of the physician's role. In fact, our suspicions are often heightened when a caregiver so counseled becomes indignant or threatening when informed of the necessity to report.

The consequences of failing to identify and report abuse are high. The reinjury rate of battered children is between 30% and 50% and the risk of death between 5% and 10%.[6,34,106] If a reinjury occurs, it is likely that the caregivers will seek medical attention at a different medical facility. Because the risk of death increases with each subsequent emergency department visit,[5,34] it is of paramount importance to report all cases of *suspected* abuse. However, simply reporting the incident may not ensure adequate safety for the child; hospitalization may be necessary to allow adequate assessment.

Most large urban children's hospitals have developed an interdisciplinary approach to the treatment of abused children. The "child abuse team" includes pediatricians, social workers, chaplains, and, when indicated, specialists such as orthopaedists. This approach streamlines what can be a cumbersome process as the parties involved develop an understanding of the legal issues and a rapport with representatives from the legal system. At our acute care institution, this multidisciplinary approach, which uses mandatory parenting classes and other community resources, allows approximately 80% of abused children to remain safely in their home. Using a similar system, Galleno and Oppenheim demonstrated a decrease in the reinjury rate from 50% to 9%.[106]

SUMMARY

Although managing skeletal injuries in children is usually straightforward, yielding excellent clinical results, there are times when even the simple can become difficult. In his book *Children's Fractures,* Mercer Rang likens fracture management to a game of chess.[269] This classic discussion is full of tips and pearls of wisdom and is well worth the brief time it takes to read. He outlines six principles of fracture care (which apply to all areas of pediatric orthopaedics) that are worth repeating:

1. Use your working knowledge of the various complications to look deliberately for them.
2. Children are uncooperative only when something is wrong.
3. Ensure that your system of follow-up does not permit patients to be lost.
4. Recognize a loose cast.
5. Recognize the earliest signs of a displacing fracture.
6. Talk to the parents ("If parents are a nuisance, it is always your fault").

References

1. Aitken A: The end results of the fractured distal radial epiphysis. J Bone Joint Surg 1935;17:302.
2. Aitken A: End results of fractures of the proximal humeral epiphysis. J Bone Joint Surg 1936;18:1036.
3. Aitken A: The end results of the fractured distal tibial epiphysis. J Bone Joint Surg 1936;18:685.
4. Aitken A, Blackett C, Ciacotti J: Overgrowth of the shaft following fractures in childhood. J Bone Joint Surg Am 1939;21:334.
5. Akbarnia B, Torg JS, Kirkpatrick J, et al: Manifestations of the battered-child syndrome. J Bone Joint Surg Am 1974;56:1159.
6. Akbarnia BA, Akbarnia NO: The role of orthopedist in child abuse and neglect. Orthop Clin North Am 1976; 7:733.
7. Albright J, Brand R: The Scientific Basis of Orthopaedics. New York, Appleton-Century-Crofts, 1979.
8. Alonso JE, Sanchez FL: Lawn mower injuries in children: A preventable impairment. J Pediatr Orthop 1995;15:83.
9. American College of Surgeons: A guide to prophylaxis against tetanus in wound management. Bull Am Coll Surg 1972;57:32.
10. American College of Surgeons: Hospital and Prehospital Resources for Optimal Care of the Injured Patient and Appendices F and J. Chicago, American College of Surgeons, 1986.
11. Anderson M, Green W: Lengths of the femur and tibia: norms derived from orthoroentgenograms of children from five years of age until epiphyseal closure. Am J Dis Child 1948;75:279.
12. Anderson M, Green WT, Messner MB: Growth and predictions of growth in the lower extremities. J Bone Joint Surg Am 1963;45:1.
13. Anderson M, Messner MB, Green WT: Distribution of lengths of the normal femur and tibia in children from one to eighteen years of age. J Bone Joint Surg Am 1964;46:1197.
14. Anger DM, Ledbetter BR, Stasikelis PJ, et al: Injuries of the foot related to the use of lawn mowers. J Bone Joint Surg Am 1995;77:719.
15. Aprahamian C, Cattey RP, Walker AP, et al: Pediatric Trauma Score: Predictor of hospital resource use? Arch Surg 1990;125:1128.
16. Arnez ZM, Hanel DP: Free tissue transfer for reconstruction of traumatic limb injuries in children. Microsurgery 1991;12:207.
17. Arslan H, Subasi M, Kesemenli C, et al: Problem fractures associated with gunshot wounds in children. Injury 2002;33:743.
18. Association for the Advancement of Automobile Medicine: The Abbreviated Injury Scale, 1990 Revision. Des Plaines, Ill, Association for the Advancement of Automotive Medicine, 1990.
19. Bae DS, Kadiyala RK, Waters PM: Acute compartment syndrome in children: Contemporary diagnosis, treatment, and outcome. J Pediatr Orthop 2001;21: 680.
20. Baker SP, O'Neill B, Haddon W Jr, et al: The injury severity score: A method for describing patients with multiple injuries and evaluating emergency care. J Trauma 1974;14:187.
21. Banaszkiewicz PA, Scotland TR, Myerscough EJ: Fractures in children younger than age 1 year: Importance of collaboration with child protection services. J Pediatr Orthop 2002;22:740.
22. Bartonicek J, Havranek P: Gunshot injury of the proximal femoral physis. Arch Orthop Trauma Surg 2004; 124:69.
23. Battaglia TC, Armstrong DG, Schwend RM: Factors affecting forearm compartment pressures in children with supracondylar fractures of the humerus. J Pediatr Orthop 2002;22:431.
24. Baumann E: Mutilation of hand and arm with Volkmann's ischemic contracture following a compound Monteggia fracture treated by circular plaster cast [in German]. Ther Umsch 1973;30:877.
25. Bayley N: Individual patterns of development. Child Dev 1956;27:45.
26. Beasley R, Cooley S, Flatt A, et al: The hand and upper extremity. In Littler J, ed: Reconstructive Plastic Surgery: Principles and Procedures in Corrective Reconstruction and Transplantation, vol 6. Philadelphia, WB Saunders, 1977, p 3131.
27. Benevenia J, Makley JT, Leeson MC, et al: Primary epiphyseal transplants and bone overgrowth in childhood amputations. J Pediatr Orthop 1992;12:746.
28. Bernardo LM, Gardner MJ: Lawn mower injuries to children in Pennsylvania, 1989 to 1993. Int J Trauma Nurs 1996;2:36.
29. Bhattacharyya T, Vrahas MS: The medical-legal aspects of compartment syndrome. J Bone Joint Surg Am 2004;86:864.
30. Bingold AC: On splitting plasters: A useful analogy. J Bone Joint Surg Br 1979;61:294.
31. Birch JG: Surgical technique of physeal bar resection. Instr Course Lect 1992;41:445.
32. Birch JG, Herring JA, Wenger DR: Surgical anatomy of selected physes. J Pediatr Orthop 1984;4:224.
33. Bisgard J, Martenson L: Fractures in children. Surg Gynecol Obstet 1937;65:464.
34. Bittner S, Newberger EH: Pediatric understanding of child abuse and neglect. Pediatr Rev 1981;2: 197.
35. Blakemore LC, Cooperman DR, Thompson GH, et al: Compartment syndrome in ipsilateral humerus and forearm fractures in children. Clin Orthop Relat Res 2000;376:32.
36. Blasier RD, Aronson J, Tursky EA: External fixation of pediatric femur fractures. J Pediatr Orthop 1997;17: 342.
37. Block RW: Follow-up skeletal surveys prove to be valuable in evaluation of child physical abuse. Child Abuse Negl 2005;29:1073.
38. Bone LB, Johnson KD, Weigelt J, et al: Early versus delayed stabilization of femoral fractures: A prospective randomized study. J Bone Joint Surg Am 1989;71: 336.
39. Boody AR, Wongworawat MD: Accuracy in the measurement of compartment pressures: A comparison of three commonly used devices. J Bone Joint Surg Am 2005;87:2415.

40. Borden S 4th: Traumatic bowing of the forearm in children. J Bone Joint Surg Am 1974;56:611.
41. Borden S 4th: Roentgen recognition of acute plastic bowing of the forearm in children. AJR Am J Roentgenol Radium Ther Nucl Med 1975;125:524.
42. Born CT, Ross SE, Iannacone WM, et al: Delayed identification of skeletal injury in multisystem trauma: The "missed" fracture. J Trauma 1989;29:1643.
43. Bourne RB, Rorabeck CH: Compartment syndromes of the lower leg. Clin Orthop Relat Res 1989;240:97.
44. Bright RW: Operative correction of partial epiphyseal plate closure by osseous-bridge resection and silicone-rubber implant: An experimental study in dogs. J Bone Joint Surg Am 1974;56:655.
45. Bruce DA, Schut L, Bruno LA, et al: Outcome following severe head injuries in children. J Neurosurg 1978;48:679.
46. Brumback RJ, Jones AL: Interobserver agreement in the classification of open fractures of the tibia: The results of a survey of two hundred and forty-five orthopaedic surgeons. J Bone Joint Surg Am 1994;76:1162.
47. Buchholz IM, Bolhuis HW, Broker FH, et al: Overgrowth and correction of rotational deformity in 12 femoral shaft fractures in 3-6-year-old children treated with an external fixator. Acta Orthop Scand 2002;73:170.
48. Buckley SL, Smith G, Sponseller PD, et al: Open fractures of the tibia in children. J Bone Joint Surg Am 1990;72:1462.
49. Byrd HS, Cierny G 3rd, Tebbetts JB: The management of open tibial fractures with associated soft-tissue loss: External pin fixation with early flap coverage. Plast Reconstr Surg 1981;68:73.
50. Caffey J: Multiple fractures in the long bones of infants suffering from chronic subdural hematoma. AJR Am J Roentgenol 1946;56:163.
51. Campbell CC, Waters PM, Emans JB, et al: Neurovascular injury and displacement in type III supracondylar humerus fractures. J Pediatr Orthop 1995;15:47.
52. Caniano DA, Ruth B, Teich S: Wound management with vacuum-assisted closure: Experience in 51 pediatric patients. J Pediatr Surg 2005;40:128.
53. Cappelleri JC, Eckenrode J, Powers JL: The epidemiology of child abuse: Findings from the Second National Incidence and Prevalence Study of Child Abuse and Neglect. Am J Public Health 1993;83:1622.
54. Carbonell PG, Prats FL, Fernandez PD, et al: Monitoring antebrachial compartmental pressure in displaced supracondylar elbow fractures in children. J Pediatr Orthop B 2004;13:412.
55. Carlson WO, Wenger DR: A mapping method to prepare for surgical excision of a partial physeal arrest. J Pediatr Orthop 1984;4:232.
56. Carsi B, Abril JC, Epeldegui T: Longitudinal growth after nonphyseal forearm fractures. J Pediatr Orthop 2003;23:203.
57. Cascio BM, Buchowski JM, Frassica FJ: Well-limb compartment syndrome after prolonged lateral decubitus positioning: A report of two cases. J Bone Joint Surg Am 2004;86:2038.
58. Cascio BM, Wilckens JH, Ain MC, et al: Documentation of acute compartment syndrome at an academic health-care center. J Bone Joint Surg Am 2005;87:346.
59. Chan BS, Walker PJ, Cass DT: Urban trauma: An analysis of 1,116 paediatric cases. J Trauma 1989;29:1540.
60. Charalambous CP, Siddique I, Zenios M, et al: Early versus delayed surgical treatment of open tibial fractures: Effect on the rates of infection and need of secondary surgical procedures to promote bone union. Injury 2005;36:656.
61. Charnley J: The Closed Treatment of Common Fractures. Edinburgh, Livingstone, 1980.
62. Cheng JC, Lam TP, Shen WY: Closed reduction and percutaneous pinning for type III displaced supracondylar fractures of the humerus in children. J Orthop Trauma 1995;9:511.
63. Cheon JE, Kim IO, Choi IH, et al: Magnetic resonance imaging of remaining physis in partial physeal resection with graft interposition in a rabbit model: A comparison with physeal resection alone. Invest Radiol 2005;40:235.
64. Chiang YC, Jeng SF, Yeh MC, et al: Free tissue transfer for leg reconstruction in children. Br J Plast Surg 1997;50:335.
65. Ciarallo L, Fleisher G: Femoral fractures: Are children at risk for significant blood loss? Pediatr Emerg Care 1996;12:343.
66. Cierny G 3rd, Byrd HS, Jones RE: Primary versus delayed soft tissue coverage for severe open tibial fractures: A comparison of results. Clin Orthop Relat Res 1983;178:54.
67. Civil ID, Schwab CW: The Abbreviated Injury Scale, 1985 revision: A condensed chart for clinical use. J Trauma 1988;28:87.
68. Clarke HM, Upton J, Zuker RM, et al: Pediatric free tissue transfer: An evaluation of 99 cases. Can J Surg 1993;36:525.
69. Cole WG: Arterial injuries associated with fractures of the lower limbs in childhood. Injury 1981;12:460.
70. Compere E: Growth arrest in long bones as a result of fractures that include the epiphysis. JAMA 1935;105:2140.
71. Compete E, Adams C: Studies of the longitudinal growth of long bones: The influence of trauma to the diaphysis. J Bone Joint Surg 1937;19:922.
72. Copley LA, Dormans JP, Davidson RS: Vascular injuries and their sequelae in pediatric supracondylar humeral fractures: Toward a goal of prevention. J Pediatr Orthop 1996;16:99.
73. Coss HS, Hennrikus WL: Parent satisfaction comparing two bandage materials used during serial casting in infants. Foot Ankle Int 1996;17:483.
74. Costecalde M, Gaubert J, Durand J, et al: Subtotal traumatic amputation of the limb in young children: Analysis of 2 successful repairs [in French]. Chir Pediatr 1988;29:184.
75. Craig JG, Cramer KE, Cody DD, et al: Premature partial closure and other deformities of the growth plate: MR imaging and three-dimensional modeling. Radiology 1999;210:835.

76. Cullen MC, Roy DR, Crawford AH, et al: Open fracture of the tibia in children. J Bone Joint Surg Am 1996; 78:1039.
77. Curran C, Dietrich AM, Bowman MJ, et al: Pediatric cervical-spine immobilization: Achieving neutral position? J Trauma 1995;39:729.
78. Currey JD, Butler G: The mechanical properties of bone tissue in children. J Bone Joint Surg Am 1975;57:810.
79. Dale G, Harris W: Prognosis of epiphyseal separation: an experimental study. J Bone Joint Surg Br 1958; 40:116.
80. Davids JR: Rotational deformity and remodeling after fracture of the femur in children. Clin Orthop Relat Res 1994;302:27.
81. Davids JR, Frick SL, Skewes E, et al: Skin surface pressure beneath an above-the-knee cast: Plaster casts compared with fiberglass casts. J Bone Joint Surg Am 1997;79:565.
82. Davidson JS, Brown DJ, Barnes SN, et al: Simple treatment for torus fractures of the distal radius. J Bone Joint Surg Br 2001;83:1173.
83. de Pablos J, Franzreb M, Barrios C: Longitudinal growth pattern of the radius after forearm fractures conservatively treated in children. J Pediatr Orthop 1994;14: 492.
84. de Sanctis N, Gambardella A, Pempinello C, et al: The use of external fixators in femur fractures in children. J Pediatr Orthop 1996;16:613.
85. de Vries AP, Kassam-Adams N, Cnaan A, et al: Looking beyond the physical injury: Posttraumatic stress disorder in children and parents after pediatric traffic injury. Pediatrics 1999;104:1293.
86. Demetriades D, Karaiskakis M, Velmahos GC, et al: Pelvic fractures in pediatric and adult trauma patients: Are they different injuries? J Trauma 2003;54:1146.
87. Dickey RL, Barnes BC, Kearns RJ, et al: Efficacy of antibiotics in low-velocity gunshot fractures. J Orthop Trauma 1989;3:6.
88. Division of Injury Control, Centers for Disease Control: Childhood injuries in the United States. Am J Dis Child 1990;144:627.
89. Dormans JP, Azzoni M, Davidson RS, et al: Major lower extremity lawn mower injuries in children. J Pediatr Orthop 1995;15:78.
90. Dykes EH, Spence LJ, Bohn DJ, et al: Evaluation of pediatric trauma care in Ontario. J Trauma 1989;29:724.
91. Eaton RG, Green WT: Epimysiotomy and fasciotomy in the treatment of Volkmann's ischemic contracture. Orthop Clin North Am 1972;3:175.
92. Eaton RG, Green WT: Volkmann's ischemia: A volar compartment syndrome of the forearm. Clin Orthop Relat Res 1975;113:58.
93. Ecklund K, Jaramillo D: Patterns of premature physeal arrest: MR imaging of 111 children. AJR Am J Roentgenol 2002;178:967.
94. Egol KA, Karunakar M, Phieffer L, et al: Early versus late reduction of a physeal fracture in an animal model. J Pediatr Orthop 2002;22:208.
95. Eichelberger MR, Gotschall CS, Sacco WJ, et al: A comparison of the Trauma Score, the Revised Trauma Score, and the Pediatric Trauma Score. Ann Emerg Med 1989; 18:1053.
96. Evans EM: Fractures of the radius and ulna. J Bone Joint Surg Br 1951;33:548.
97. Ferraro SP Jr, Zinar DM: Management of gunshot fractures of the tibia. Orthop Clin North Am 1995;26:181.
98. Fleischmann W, Suger G, Kinzl L: Treatment of bone and soft tissue defects in infected nonunion. Acta Orthop Belg 1992;58(Suppl 1):227.
99. Ford L, Gilula L: Plastic bones of the forearm. Orthop Rev 1978;7:101.
100. Foucher M: De la divulsion des epiphyses. Cong Med Fr (Paris) 1863;1:63.
101. Friberg KS: Remodelling after distal forearm fractures in children: I. The effect of residual angulation on the spatial orientation of the epiphyseal plates. Acta Orthop Scand 1979;50:537.
102. Friberg KS: Remodelling after distal forearm fractures in children: III. Correction of residual angulation in fractures of the radius. Acta Orthop Scand 1979;50: 741.
103. Friedman RJ, Jupiter JB: Vascular injuries and closed extremity fractures in children. Clin Orthop Relat Res 1984;188:112.
104. Fry K, Hoffer MM, Brink J: Femoral shaft fractures in brain-injured children. J Trauma 1976;16:371.
105. Furnival RA, Schunk JE: ABCs of scoring systems for pediatric trauma. Pediatr Emerg Care 1999;15:215.
106. Galleno H, Oppenheim WL: The battered child syndrome revisited. Clin Orthop Relat Res 1982;162:11.
107. Garcés GL, Hernández Hermoso JA: Bone growth after periosteal stripping in rats. Int Orthop 1991;15:49.
108. Garfin SR, Mubarak SJ, Evans KL, et al: Quantification of intracompartmental pressure and volume under plaster casts. J Bone Joint Surg Am 1981;63:449.
109. Gascó J, de Pablos J: Bone remodeling in malunited fractures in children: Is it reliable? J Pediatr Orthop B 1997;6:126.
110. Graham B, Paulus DA, Caffee HH: Pulse oximetry for vascular monitoring in upper extremity replantation surgery. J Hand Surg [Am] 1986;11:687.
111. Green WT, Anderson M: Experiences with epiphyseal arrest in correcting discrepancies in length of the lower extremities in infantile paralysis: A method of predicting the effect. J Bone Joint Surg Am 1947;29:659.
112. Green WT, Anderson M: Skeletal age and the control of bone growth. Instr Course Lect 1960;17:199.
113. Greenbaum B, Zionts LE, Ebramzadeh E: Open fractures of the forearm in children. J Orthop Trauma 2001;15:111.
114. Greensher J: Recent advances in injury prevention. Pediatr Rev 1988;10:171.
115. Greulich W, Pyle S: Radiographic Atlas of the Skeletal Development of the Hand and Wrist. Palo Alto, Calif, Stanford University Press, 1959.
116. Griffith JF, Tong MP, Hung HY, et al: Plastic deformation of the femur: Cross-sectional imaging. AJR Am J Roentgenol 2005;184:1495.
117. Grimard G, Naudie D, Laberge LC, et al: Open fractures of the tibia in children. Clin Orthop Relat Res 1996;332:62.
118. Guerra JJ, Bednar JM: Equipment malfunction in common hand surgical procedures: Complications associated with the pneumatic tourniquet and with

the application of casts and splints. Hand Clin 1994; 10:45.
119. Gustilo RB: Current concepts in the management of open fractures. Instr Course Lect 1987;36:359.
120. Gustilo RB, Anderson JT: Prevention of infection in the treatment of one thousand and twenty-five open fractures of long bones: Retrospective and prospective analyses. J Bone Joint Surg Am 1976;58:453.
121. Gustilo RB, Corpuz V, Sherman RE: Epidemiology, mortality and morbidity in multiple trauma patients. Orthopedics 1985;8:1523.
122. Gustilo RB, Mendoza RM, Williams DN: Problems in the management of type III (severe) open fractures: A new classification of type III open fractures. J Trauma 1984;24:742.
123. Gustilo RB, Merkow RL, Templeman D: The management of open fractures. J Bone Joint Surg Am 1990; 72:299.
124. Haas S: The localization of the growing point in the epiphyseal cartilage plate of bone. Am J Orthop Surg 1917;15:563.
125. Haasbeek JF, Cole WG: Open fractures of the arm in children. J Bone Joint Surg Br 1995;77:576.
126. Hahn YS, Chyung C, Barthel MJ, et al: Head injuries in children under 36 months of age: Demography and outcome. Childs Nerv Syst 1988;4:34.
127. Hampton RL, Newberger EH: Child abuse incidence and reporting by hospitals: Significance of severity, class, and race. Am J Public Health 1985;75:56.
128. Hanlon M, Barnes M, Lamb G, et al: Central compartment pressure monitoring following clubfoot release. J Pediatr Orthop 1996;16:63.
129. Hargens AR, Mubarak SJ: Current concepts in the pathophysiology, evaluation, and diagnosis of compartment syndrome. Hand Clin 1998;14:371.
130. Harley BJ, Beaupre LA, Jones CA, et al: The effect of time to definitive treatment on the rate of nonunion and infection in open fractures. J Orthop Trauma 2002;16: 484.
131. Harris H: Lines of arrested growth in the long bones in childhood: The correlation of histological and radiographic appearances in clinical and experimental conditions. Br J Radiol 1931;4:561.
132. Harris MB, Waguespack AM, Kronlage S: "Clearing" cervical spine injuries in polytrauma patients: Is it really safe to remove the collar? Orthopedics 1997; 20:903.
133. Harris W: The endocrine basis for slipping of the upper femoral epiphysis. J Bone Joint Surg Br 1950;32:5.
134. Hasler CC, Foster BK: Secondary tethers after physeal bar resection: A common source of failure? Clin Orthop Relat Res 2002;405:242.
135. Helfer R, Kempe C: The Battered Child. Chicago, University of Chicago Press, 1968.
136. Henderson OL, Morrissy RT, Gerdes MH, et al: Early casting of femoral shaft fractures in children. J Pediatr Orthop 1984;4:16.
137. Henssge J, Linka F: Volkmann's contracture and constricting bandage [in German]. Beitr Orthop Traumatol 1968;15:27.
138. Hernandez J Jr, Peterson HA: Fracture of the distal radial physis complicated by compartment syndrome and premature physeal closure. J Pediatr Orthop 1986; 6:627.
139. Herring JA, Mubarak SJ: Complications of a tibial osteotomy. J Pediatr Orthop 1983;3:625.
140. Herscovici D Jr, Sanders RW, Scaduto JM, et al: Vacuum-assisted wound closure (VAC therapy) for the management of patients with high-energy soft tissue injuries. J Orthop Trauma 2003;17:683.
141. Herzenberg JE, Hensinger RN, Dedrick DK, et al: Emergency transport and positioning of young children who have an injury of the cervical spine: The standard backboard may be hazardous. J Bone Joint Surg Am 1989;71:15.
142. Hirsch C, Evans FG: Studies on some physical properties of infant compact bone. Acta Orthop Scand 1965; 35:300.
143. Hoffer MM, Johnson B: Shrapnel wounds in children. J Bone Joint Surg Am 1992;74:766.
144. Holschneider AM, Vogl D, Dietz HG: Differences in leg length following femoral shaft fractures in childhood [in German]. Z Kinderchir 1985;40:341.
145. Holter JC, Friedman SB: Child abuse: Early case finding in the emergency department. Pediatrics 1968;42:128.
146. Hope MJ, McQueen MM: Acute compartment syndrome in the absence of fracture. J Orthop Trauma 2004;18:220.
147. Horn BD, Rettig ME: Interobserver reliability in the Gustilo and Anderson classification of open fractures. J Orthop Trauma 1993;7:357.
148. Hubbard DD: Injuries of the spine in children and adolescents. Clin Orthop Relat Res 1974;100:56.
149. Huerta C, Griffith R, Joyce SM: Cervical spine stabilization in pediatric patients: Evaluation of current techniques. Ann Emerg Med 1987;16:1121.
150. Hull JB: Management of gunshot fractures of the extremities. J Trauma 1996;40:S193.
151. Hynes D, O'Brien T: Growth disturbance lines after injury of the distal tibial physis: Their significance in prognosis. J Bone Joint Surg Br 1988;70:231.
152. Iannotti J, Goldstein S, Kuhn J, et al: Growth plate and bone development. In Simon S, ed: Orthopaedic Basic Sciences. Rosemont, Ill, American Academy of Orthopaedic Surgeons, 1994, p 191.
153. Iobst CA, Tidwell MA, King WF: Nonoperative management of pediatric type I open fractures. J Pediatr Orthop 2005;25:513.
154. Iqbal QM: Long bone fractures among children in Malaysia. Int Surg 1974;59:410.
155. Irwin A, Gibson P, Ashcroft P: Open fractures of the tibia in children. Injury 1995;26:21.
156. Ismail N, Bellemare JF, Mollitt DL, et al: Death from pelvic fracture: Children are different. J Pediatr Orthop 1996;31:82.
157. Izhar-Ul-Haque, Munkonge L: Femoral fracture in children (a prospective study of two hundred and four fractures). Med J Zambia 1982;16:51.
158. Jacobsen FS: Periosteum: Its relation to pediatric fractures. J Pediatr Orthop B 1997;6:84.
159. Jaffe DM, Binns H, Radkowski MA, et al: Developing a clinical algorithm for early management of cervical spine injury in child trauma victims. Ann Emerg Med 1987;16:270.

160. Janzing H, Broos P, Romnens P: Compartment syndrome as complication of skin traction, in children with femoral fractures. Acta Chir Belg 1996;96:135.
161. Jawadi AH, Letts M: Injuries associated with fracture of the femur secondary to motor vehicle accidents in children. Am J Orthop 2003;32:459.
162. Jenkins DH, Cheng DH, Hodgson AR: Stimulation of bone growth by periosteal stripping: A clinical study. J Bone Joint Surg Br 1975;57:482.
163. Jones JC, Feldman KW, Bruckner JD: Child abuse in infants with proximal physeal injuries of the femur. Pediatr Emerg Care 2004;20:157.
164. Juster M, Moscofian A, Balmain-Oligo N: Formation of the skeleton: VIII. Growth of a long bone: Periostealization of the metaphysial bone [in French]. Bull Assoc Anat (Nancy) 1975;59:437.
165. Kadiyala RK, Waters PM: Upper extremity pediatric compartment syndromes. Hand Clin 1998;14:467.
166. Kassam-Adams N, Garcia-Espana JF, Fein JA, et al: Heart rate and posttraumatic stress in injured children. Arch Gen Psychiatry 2005;62:335.
167. Kasser JR: Physeal bar resections after growth arrest about the knee. Clin Orthop Relat Res 1990;255:68.
168. Kaufmann CR, Maier RV, Rivara FP, et al: Evaluation of the Pediatric Trauma Score. JAMA 1990;263:69.
169. Keen TP: Nursing care of the pediatric multitrauma patient. Nurs Clin North Am 1990;25:131.
170. Kempe CH, Silverman FN, Steele BF, et al: The battered-child syndrome. JAMA 1962;181:17.
171. Kerley ER: The microscopic determination of age in human bone. Am J Phys Anthropol 1965;23:149.
172. Kewalramani LS, Kraus JF, Sterling HM: Acute spinal-cord lesions in a pediatric population: Epidemiological and clinical features. Paraplegia 1980;18:206.
173. Kirschenbaum D, Albert MC, Robertson WW Jr, et al: Complex femur fractures in children: Treatment with external fixation. J Pediatr Orthop 1990;10: 588.
174. Kissoon N, Dreyer J, Walia M: Pediatric trauma: Differences in pathophysiology, injury patterns and treatment compared with adult trauma. CMAJ 1990;142: 27.
175. Knapp TP, Patzakis MJ, Lee J, et al: Comparison of intravenous and oral antibiotic therapy in the treatment of fractures caused by low-velocity gunshots: A prospective, randomized study of infection rates. J Bone Joint Surg Am 1996;78:1167.
176. Kocher MS, Kasser JR: Orthopaedic aspects of child abuse. J Am Acad Orthop Surg 2000;8:10.
177. Kowal-Vern A, Paxton TP, Ros SP, et al: Fractures in the under-3-year-old age cohort. Clin Pediatr (Phila) 1992; 31:653.
178. Krajbich JI: Lower-limb deficiencies and amputations in children. J Am Acad Orthop Surg 1998;6:358.
179. Kreder HJ, Armstrong P: A review of open tibia fractures in children. J Pediatr Orthop 1995;15:482.
180. Kregor PJ, Song KM, Routt ML Jr, et al: Plate fixation of femoral shaft fractures in multiply injured children. J Bone Joint Surg Am 1993;75:1774.
181. Kummer B, Lohscheidt K: Mathematical model of the longitudinal growth of long bones [in German]. Anat Anz 1985;158:377.
182. Laasonen EM, Kivioja A: Delayed diagnosis of extremity injuries in patients with multiple injuries. J Trauma 1991;31:257.
183. Lally KP, Senac M, Hardin WD Jr, et al: Utility of the cervical spine radiograph in pediatric trauma. Am J Surg 1989;158:540.
184. Landin LA: Fracture patterns in children: Analysis of 8,682 fractures with special reference to incidence, etiology and secular changes in a Swedish urban population 1950-1979. Acta Orthop Scand 1983;202:1.
185. Lane WG, Rubin DM, Monteith R, et al: Racial differences in the evaluation of pediatric fractures for physical abuse. JAMA 2002;288:1603.
186. Langenskiöld A: An operation for partial closure of an epiphysial plate in children, and its experimental basis. J Bone Joint Surg Br 1975;57:325.
187. Langenskiöld A: Surgical treatment of partial closure of the growth plate. J Pediatr Orthop 1981;1:3.
188. Langenskiöld A: Growth disturbance after osteomyelitis of femoral condyles in infants. Acta Orthop Scand 1984;55:1.
189. Langenskiöld A: Partial closure of the epiphyseal plate: Principles of treatment. 1978. Clin Orthop Relat Res 1993;297:4.
190. Langenskiöld A, Osterman K: Surgical treatment of partial closure of the epiphysial plate. Reconstr Surg Traumatol 1979;17:48.
191. Larsen E, Vittas D, Torp-Pedersen S: Remodeling of angulated distal forearm fractures in children. Clin Orthop Relat Res 1988;237:190.
192. Lau ST, Lee YH, Hess DJ, et al: Lawnmower injuries in children: A 10-year experience. Pediatr Surg Int 2006:1.
193. Launay F, Paut O, Katchburian M, et al: Leg amputation after intraosseous infusion in a 7-month-old infant: A case report. J Trauma 2003;55:788.
194. Leape L: Progress in pediatric trauma: Anatomy and patterns of injury. In Hearris B, ed: The First National Conference on Pediatric Trauma. Boston, Nob Hill Press, 1985.
195. Lee KM, Cheng AS, Cheung WH, et al: Bioengineering and characterization of physeal transplant with physeal reconstruction potential. Tissue Eng 2003;9:703.
196. Letts M, Davidson D, Lapner P: Multiple trauma in children: Predicting outcome and long-term results. Can J Surg 2002;45:126.
197. Letts RM, Miller D: Gunshot wounds of the extremities in children. J Trauma 1976;16:807.
198. Levin TL, Berdon WE, Cassell I, et al: Thoracolumbar fracture with listhesis: An uncommon manifestation of child abuse. Pediatr Radiol 2003;33:305.
199. Li L, Hui JH, Goh JC, et al: Chitin as a scaffold for mesenchymal stem cells transfers in the treatment of partial growth arrest. J Pediatr Orthop 2004;24:205.
200. Light TR, Ogden DA, Ogden JA: The anatomy of metaphyseal torus fractures. Clin Orthop Relat Res 1984;188:103.
201. Lincoln TL, Mubarak SJ: "Isolated" traumatic radial-head dislocation. J Pediatr Orthop 1994;14:454.
202. Lloyd-Thomas AR, Anderson I: ABC of major trauma. Paediatric trauma: Secondary survey. BMJ 1990;301: 433.

203. Loder RT: Demographics of traumatic amputations in children: Implications for prevention strategies. J Bone Joint Surg Am 2004;86:923.
204. Loder RT, Bookout C: Fracture patterns in battered children. J Orthop Trauma 1991;5:428.
205. Loder RT, Brown KL, Zaleske DJ, et al: Extremity lawnmower injuries in children: Report by the Research Committee of the Pediatric Orthopaedic Society of North America. J Pediatr Orthop 1997;17:360.
206. Loder RT, Dikos GD, Taylor DA: Long-term lower extremity prosthetic costs in children with traumatic lawnmower amputations. Arch Pediatr Adolesc Med 2004;158:1177.
207. Loder RT, Gullahorn LJ, Yian EH, et al: Factors predictive of immobilization complications in pediatric polytrauma. J Orthop Trauma 2001;15:338.
208. Loder RT, Swinford AE, Kuhns LR: The use of helical computed tomographic scan to assess bony physeal bridges. J Pediatr Orthop 1997;17:356.
209. Logar M, Smrkolj V, Veselko M: An unusual lawn mower injury. Unfallchirurg 1996;99:152.
210. Luhmann SJ, Schootman M, Schoenecker PL, et al: Complications and outcomes of open pediatric forearm fractures. J Pediatr Orthop 2004;24:1.
211. Mabrey JD, Fitch RD: Plastic deformation in pediatric fractures: Mechanism and treatment. J Pediatr Orthop 1989;9:310.
212. Mann DC, Rajmaira S: Distribution of physeal and nonphyseal fractures in 2,650 long-bone fractures in children aged 0-16 years. J Pediatr Orthop 1990;10:713.
213. Matsen FA 3rd, Krugmire RB Jr, King RV: Nicolas Andry Award: Increased tissue pressure and its effects on muscle oxygenation in level and elevated human limbs. Clin Orthop Relat Res 1979;144:311.
214. Matsen FA 3rd, Mayo KA, Sheridan GW, et al: Monitoring of intramuscular pressure. Surgery 1976;79:702.
215. Matsen FA 3rd, Mayo KA, Sheridan GW, et al: Continuous monitoring of intramuscular pressure and its application to clinical compartmental syndromes. Bibl Anat 1977;15pt1:112.
216. Matsen FA 3rd, Rorabeck CH: Compartment syndromes. Instr Course Lect 1989;38:463.
217. Matsen FA 3rd, Staheli LT: Neurovascular complications following tibial osteotomy in children: A case report. Clin Orthop Relat Res 1975;110:210.
218. Matsen FA 3rd, Veith RG: Compartmental syndromes in children. J Pediatr Orthop 1981;1:33.
219. Matsen FA 3rd, Winquist RA, Krugmire RB Jr: Diagnosis and management of compartmental syndromes. J Bone Joint Surg Am 1980;62:286.
220. Matsen FA 3rd, Wyss CR, Krugmire RB Jr, et al: The effects of limb elevation and dependency on local arteriovenous gradients in normal human limbs with particular reference to limbs with increased tissue pressure. Clin Orthop Relat Res 1980;150:187.
221. McClelland CQ, Heiple KG: Fractures in the first year of life: A diagnostic dilemma. Am J Dis Child 1982;136:26.
222. McMahon P, Grossman W, Gaffney M, et al: Soft-tissue injury as an indication of child abuse. J Bone Joint Surg Am 1995;77:1179.
223. Meier R, Krettek C, Grimme K, et al: The multiply injured child. Clin Orthop Relat Res 2005;432:127.
224. Mendelson SA, Dominick TS, Tyler-Kabara E, et al: Early versus late femoral fracture stabilization in multiply injured pediatric patients with closed head injury. J Pediatr Orthop 2001;21:594.
225. Menelaus MB: Correction of leg length discrepancy by epiphysial arrest. J Bone Joint Surg Br 1966;48:336.
226. Merten DF, Radkowski MA, Leonidas JC: The abused child: A radiological reappraisal. Radiology 1983;146:377.
227. Metak G, Scherer MA, Dannöhl C: Missed injuries of the musculoskeletal system in multiple trauma: A retrospective study [in German]. Zentralbl Chir 1994;119:88.
228. Mizuta T, Benson WM, Foster BK, et al: Statistical analysis of the incidence of physeal injuries. J Pediatr Orthop 1987;7:518.
229. Moed BR, Thorderson PK: Measurement of intracompartmental pressure: A comparison of the slit catheter, side-ported needle, and simple needle. J Bone Joint Surg Am 1993;75:231.
230. Mooney JF 3rd, Cramer KE: Lower extremity compartment syndrome in infants associated with child abuse: A report of two cases. J Orthop Trauma 2004;18:320.
231. Moyikoua A, Dolama F, Pena-Pitra B, et al: Open fractures caused by gunshot in civilian practice: Apropos of 31 cases [in French]. Ann Chir 1994;48:1020.
232. Mubarak SJ: A practical approach to compartmental syndromes: Part II. Diagnosis. Instr Course Lect 1983;32:92.
233. Mubarak SJ, Carroll NC: Volkmann's contracture in children: Aetiology and prevention. J Bone Joint Surg Br 1979;61:285.
234. Mubarak SJ, Owen CA, Hargens AR, et al: Acute compartment syndromes: Diagnosis and treatment with the aid of the wick catheter. J Bone Joint Surg Am 1978;60:1091.
235. Mueller KL, Farley FA: Superficial and deep posterior compartment syndrome following high tibial osteotomy for tibia vara in a child. Orthopedics 2003;26:513.
236. Munoz-Juárez M, Drugas GT, Hallett JW, et al: Vena caval impalement: An unusual lawn mower injury in a child. Mayo Clin Proc 1998;73:537.
237. Naga AH, Broadrick GL: Traumatic bowing of the radius and ulna in children. N C Med J 1977;38:452.
238. Nakayama DK, Gardner MJ, Rowe MI: Emergency endotracheal intubation in pediatric trauma. Ann Surg 1990;211:218.
239. Nakayama DK, Ramenofsky ML, Rowe MI: Chest injuries in childhood. Ann Surg 1989;210:770.
240. National Child Abuse and Neglect Data Systems: Working Paper 2-1991. Summary Data Component. Washington, DC, Government Printing Office, 1993.
241. Nayduch DA, Moylan J, Rutledge R, et al: Comparison of the ability of adult and pediatric trauma scores to predict pediatric outcome following major trauma. J Trauma 1991;31:452.
242. Nicholas RM, McCoy GF: Immediate intramedullary nailing of femoral shaft fractures due to gunshots. Injury 1995;26:257.

243. Nugent N, Lannon D, O'Donnell M: Vacuum-assisted closure: A management option for the burns patient with exposed bone. Burns 2005;31:390.
244. Obaid L, Byrne PJ, Cheung PY: Compartment syndrome in an ELBW infant receiving low-molecular-weight heparins. J Pediatr 2004;144:549.
245. O'Brien E: Fractures of the hand and wrist region. In Rockwood C, Wilkins K, King R, eds: Fractures in Children, vol 3. Philadelphia, JB Lippincott, 1991.
246. O'Brien T: Growth-disturbance lines in congenital dislocation of the hip. J Bone Joint Surg Am 1985;67:626.
247. O'Brien T, Millis MB, Griffin PP: The early identification and classification of growth disturbances of the proximal end of the femur. J Bone Joint Surg Am 1986;68:970.
248. Oestreich AE: Imaging of the skeleton and soft tissues in children. Curr Opin Radiol 1992;4:55.
249. Ogden J: Skeletal Injury in the Child. Philadelphia, Lea & Febiger, 1981.
250. Ogden JA: Injury to the growth mechanisms of the immature skeleton. Skeletal Radiol 1981;6:237.
251. Ogden JA: The evaluation and treatment of partial physeal arrest. J Bone Joint Surg Am 1987;69:1297.
252. Oral R, Blum KL, Johnson C: Fractures in young children: Are physicians in the emergency department and orthopedic clinics adequately screening for possible abuse? Pediatr Emerg Care 2003;19:148.
253. Ott R, Kramer R, Martus P, et al: Prognostic value of trauma scores in pediatric patients with multiple injuries. J Trauma 2000;49:729.
254. Padovani JP, Rigault P, Mouterde P: Vascular traumatic injuries of the limbs in children [in French]. Chir Pediatr 1978;19:69.
255. Parry SW, Toth BA, Elliott LF: Microvascular free-tissue transfer in children. Plast Reconstr Surg 1988;81:838.
256. Patzakis MJ: Clostridial myonecrosis. Instr Course Lect 1990;39:491.
257. Patzakis MJ, Wilkins J: Factors influencing infection rate in open fracture wounds. Clin Orthop Relat Res 1989;243:36.
258. Peterson HA: Partial growth plate arrest and its treatment. J Pediatr Orthop 1984;4:246.
259. Peterson HA: Physeal fractures: Part 3. Classification. J Pediatr Orthop 1994;14:439.
260. Peterson HA, Burkhart SS: Compression injury of the epiphyseal growth plate: Fact or fiction? J Pediatr Orthop 1981;1:377.
261. Peterson HA, Madhok R, Benson JT, et al: Physeal fractures: Part 1. Epidemiology in Olmsted County, Minnesota, 1979-1988. J Pediatr Orthop 1994;14:423.
262. Peterson HA, Wood MB: Physeal arrest due to laser beam damage in a growing child. J Pediatr Orthop 2001;21:335.
263. Poland J: Traumatic Separation of the Epiphysies. London, Smith, Elder & Co., 1898.
264. Porat S, Milgrom C, Nyska M, et al: Femoral fracture treatment in head-injured children: Use of external fixation. J Trauma 1986;26:81.
265. Prader A: Normal growth and disorders of growth in children and adolescents [in German]. Klin Wochenschr 1981;59:977.
266. Pritchett JW: Growth plate activity in the upper extremity. Clin Orthop Relat Res 1991;268:235.
267. Ragland R 3rd, Moukoko D, Ezaki M, et al: Forearm compartment syndrome in the newborn: Report of 24 cases. J Hand Surg [Am] 2005;30:997.
268. Rang M: Biomechanic differences. In Rang M, ed: Children's Fractures. Philadelphia, JB Lippincott, 1983, p 2.
269. Rang M, ed: Children's Fractures. Philadelphia, JB Lippincott, 1983.
270. Rang M: Injuries of the epiphysis, growth plate and perichondral ring. In Rang M, ed: Children's Fractures. Philadelphia, JB Lippincott, 1983, p 23.
271. Rathjen KE, Hurt JH, Birch JG, et al: Epiphysiolysis for the treatment of partial physeal arrest. Presented at the Pediatric Orthopaedic Society of North America Annual Meeting, Amelia Island, Fla, May 2-4, 2003.
272. Ray SA, Ivory JP, Beavis JP: Use of pulse oximetry during manipulation of supracondylar fractures of the humerus. Injury 1991;22:103.
273. Reed MH: Fractures and dislocations of the extremities in children. J Trauma 1977;17:351.
274. Reisch RB: Traumatic plastic bowing deformity of the radius and ulna in a skeletally mature adult. J Orthop Trauma 1994;8:258.
275. Rinker B, Valerio IL, Stewart DH, et al: Microvascular free flap reconstruction in pediatric lower extremity trauma: A 10-year review. Plast Reconstr Surg 2005;115:1618.
276. Robertson P, Karol LA, Rab GT: Open fractures of the tibia and femur in children. J Pediatr Orthop 1996;16:621.
277. Rodgers WB, Waters PM, Hall JE: Chronic Monteggia lesions in children: Complications and results of reconstruction. J Bone Joint Surg Am 1996;78:1322.
278. Rorabeck CH: A practical approach to compartmental syndrome: Part III. Management. Instr Course Lect 1983;32:102.
279. Rorabeck CH, Castle GS, Hardie R, et al: Compartmental pressure measurements: An experimental investigation using the slit catheter. J Trauma 1981;21:446.
280. Sacco WJ, MacKenzie EJ, Champion HR, et al: Comparison of alternative methods for assessing injury severity based on anatomic descriptors. J Trauma 1999;47:441.
281. Sailhan F, Chotel F, Guibal AL, et al: Three-dimensional MR imaging in the assessment of physeal growth arrest. Eur Radiol 2004;14:1600.
282. Salter R: Epiphyseal plate injuries. In Letts R, ed: Management of Pediatric Fractures. New York, Churchill Livingstone, 1994, p 11.
283. Salter R, Harris W: Injuries involving the epiphyseal plate. J Bone Joint Surg Am 1963;45:587.
284. Sanders MB, Starr AJ, Frawley WH, et al: Posttraumatic stress symptoms in children recovering from minor orthopaedic injury and treatment. J Orthop Trauma 2005;19:623.
285. Sanders WE, Heckman JD: Traumatic plastic deformation of the radius and ulna: A closed method of correction of deformity. Clin Orthop Relat Res 1984;188:58.
286. Schalamon J, von Bismarck S, Schober PH, et al: Multiple trauma in pediatric patients. Pediatr Surg Int 2003;19:417.

287. Schreier H, Ladakakos C, Morabito D, et al: Posttraumatic stress symptoms in children after mild to moderate pediatric trauma: A longitudinal examination of symptom prevalence, correlates, and parent-child symptom reporting. J Trauma 2005;58:353.
288. Schwarz N: Incidence of open fractures in children [in German]. Aktuelle Traumatol 1981;11:133.
289. Seekamp A, Ziegler M, Biank J, et al: The significance of hypothermia in polytrauma patients [in German]. Unfallchirurg 1996;99:100.
290. Seiler JG 3rd: Rattlesnake bite with associated compartment syndrome: What is the best treatment? J Bone Joint Surg Am 2003;85:1163.
291. Sesko AM, Choe JC, Vitale MA, et al: Pediatric orthopaedic injuries: The effect of treatment on school attendance. J Pediatr Orthop 2005;25:661.
292. Shakespeare DT, Henderson NJ, Clough G: The slit catheter: A comparison with the wick catheter in the measurement of compartment pressure. Injury 1982; 13:404.
293. Shapiro J, Akbarnia BA, Hanel DP: Free tissue transfer in children. J Pediatr Orthop 1989;9:590.
294. Shaw BA, Hosalkar HS: Rattlesnake bites in children: Antivenin treatment and surgical indications. J Bone Joint Surg Am 2002;84:1624.
295. Shaw BA, Kasser JR, Emans JB, et al: Management of vascular injuries in displaced supracondylar humerus fractures without arteriography. J Orthop Trauma 1990; 4:25.
296. Shelton WR, Canale ST: Fractures of the tibia through the proximal tibial epiphyseal cartilage. J Bone Joint Surg Am 1979;61:167.
297. Shemesh E, Newcorn JH, Rockmore L, et al: Comparison of parent and child reports of emotional trauma symptoms in pediatric outpatient settings. Pediatrics 2005;115:e582.
298. Shilt JS, Yoder JS, Manuck TA, et al: Role of vacuum-assisted closure in the treatment of pediatric lawnmower injuries. J Pediatr Orthop 2004;24: 482.
299. Silverman FN: The roentgen manifestations of unrecognized skeletal trauma in infants. AJR Am J Roentgenol Radium Ther Nucl Med 1953;69:413.
300. Simonian PT, Hanel DP: Traumatic plastic deformity of an adult forearm: Case report and literature review. J Orthop Trauma 1996;10:213.
301. Singh D: Pulse oximetry and fracture manipulation. Injury 1992;23:70.
302. Skaggs DL, Friend L, Alman B, et al: The effect of surgical delay on acute infection following 554 open fractures in children. J Bone Joint Surg Am 2005; 87:8.
303. Skaggs DL, Kautz SM, Kay RM, et al: Effect of delay of surgical treatment on rate of infection in open fractures in children. J Pediatr Orthop 2000;20:19.
304. Skak SV: A case of partial physeal closure following compression injury. Arch Orthop Trauma Surg 1989; 108:185.
305. Sola CK, Silberman FS, Cabrini RL: Stimulation of the longitudinal growth of long bones by periosteal stripping: An experimental study on dogs and monkeys. J Bone Joint Surg Am 1963;45:1679.
306. Song KM, Sangeorzan B, Benirschke S, et al: Open fractures of the tibia in children. J Pediatr Orthop 1996;16: 635.
307. Stenström R, Gripenberg L, Bergius AR: Traumatic bowing of forearm and lower leg in children. Acta Radiol Diagn 1978;19:243.
308. Stott NS, Zionts LE, Holtom PD, et al: Acute hematogenous osteomyelitis: An unusual cause of compartment syndrome in a child. Clin Orthop Relat Res 1995;317: 219.
309. Stotts AK, Carroll KL, Schafer PG, et al: Medial compartment syndrome of the foot: An unusual complication of spine surgery. Spine 2003;28:E118.
310. Stricker SJ, Volgas DA: Extremity handgun injuries in children and adolescents. Orthopedics 1998;21:1095.
311. Strömqvist B, Lidgren L, Norgren L, et al: Neurovascular injury complicating displaced proximal fractures of the humerus. Injury 1987;18:423.
312. Stucky W, Loder RT: Extremity gunshot wounds in children. J Pediatr Orthop 1991;11:64.
313. Subcommittee of Advanced Trauma Life Support: Advanced Trauma Life Support: Student Manual. Chicago, American College of Surgeons, 1989, p 11.
314. Teasdale G, Jennett B: Assessment of coma and impaired consciousness: A practical scale. Lancet 1974;2:81.
315. Templeman DC, Gulli B, Tsukayama DT, et al: Update on the management of open fractures of the tibial shaft. Clin Orthop Relat Res 1998;350:18.
316. Tepas JJ 3rd, Mollitt DL, Talbert JL, et al: The pediatric trauma score as a predictor of injury severity in the injured child. J Pediatr Surg 1987;22:14.
317. Tobita M, Ochi M, Uchio Y, et al: Treatment of growth plate injury with autogenous chondrocytes: A study in rabbits. Acta Orthop Scand 2002;73:352.
318. Tollens T, Janzing H, Broos P: The pathophysiology of the acute compartment syndrome. Acta Chir Belg 1998;98:171.
319. Tolo VT: External skeletal fixation in children's fractures. J Pediatr Orthop 1983;3:435.
320. Treloar DJ, Nypaver M: Angulation of the pediatric cervical spine with and without cervical collar. Pediatr Emerg Care 1997;13:5.
321. Trice M, Colwell CW: A historical review of compartment syndrome and Volkmann's ischemic contracture. Hand Clin 1998;14:335.
322. Tsukayama DT, Gustilo RB: Antibiotic management of open fractures. Instr Course Lect 1990;39:487.
323. Tupman GS: Treatment of inequality of the lower limbs: The results of operations for stimulation of growth. J Bone Joint Surg Br 1960;42:489.
324. Unal VS, Gulcek M, Unveren Z, et al: Blood loss evaluation in children under the age of 11 with femoral shaft fractures patients with isolated versus multiple injuries. J Trauma 2006;60:224.
325. Uppal GS, Smith RC, Sherk HH, et al: Accurate compartment pressure measurement using the Intravenous Alarm Control (IVAC) pump: Report of a technique. J Orthop Trauma 1992;6:87.
326. U.S. Department of Health and Human Services: Child Maltreatment 1996: Reports from the States to the National Child Abuse and Neglect Data System. Washington, DC, Government Printing Office, 1998.

327. van der Sluis CK, Kingma J, Eisma WH, et al: Pediatric polytrauma: Short-term and long-term outcomes. J Trauma 1997;43:501.
328. Vasli LR: Diagnosis of vascular injury in children with supracondylar fractures of the humerus. Injury 1988; 19:11.
329. Victoroff BN, Robertson WW Jr, Eichelberger MR, et al: Extremity gunshot injuries treated in an urban children's hospital. Pediatr Emerg Care 1994;10:1.
330. Vinz H: Change in the resistance properties of compact bone tissue in the course of aging [in German]. Gegenbaurs Morphol Jahrb 1970;115:257.
331. Vittas D, Larsen E, Torp-Pedersen S: Angular remodeling of midshaft forearm fractures in children. Clin Orthop Relat Res 1991;265:261.
332. von Schroeder HP, Botte MJ: Definitions and terminology of compartment syndrome and Volkmann's ischemic contracture of the upper extremity. Hand Clin 1998;14:331.
333. Vosburgh CL, Gruel CR, Herndon WA, et al: Lawn mower injuries of the pediatric foot and ankle: Observations on prevention and management. J Pediatr Orthop 1995;15:504.
334. Walker M, Storrs B, Mayers T: Head injuries. In Mayers TA, ed: Emergency Management of Pediatric Trauma. Philadelphia, WB Saunders, 1985, p 272.
335. Wallace ME, Hoffman EB: Remodelling of angular deformity after femoral shaft fractures in children. J Bone Joint Surg Br 1992;74:765.
336. Walløe A, Egund N, Eikelund L: Supracondylar fracture of the humerus in children: Review of closed and open reduction leading to a proposal for treatment. Injury 1985;16:296.
337. Washington ER, Lee WA, Ross WA Jr: Gunshot wounds to the extremities in children and adolescents. Orthop Clin North Am 1995;26:19.
338. Weiner G, Styf J, Nakhostine M, et al: Effect of ankle position and a plaster cast on intramuscular pressure in the human leg. J Bone Joint Surg Am 1994;76:1476.
339. West S, Andrews J, Bebbington A, et al: Buckle fractures of the distal radius are safely treated in a soft bandage: A randomized prospective trial of bandage versus plaster cast. J Pediatr Orthop 2005;25:322.
340. Westh RN, Menelaus MB: A simple calculation for the timing of epiphysial arrest: A further report. J Bone Joint Surg Br 1981;63:117.
341. White RA, Miki RA, Kazmier P, et al: Vacuum-assisted closure complicated by erosion and hemorrhage of the anterior tibial artery. J Orthop Trauma 2005;19:56.
342. Whitesides TE, Haney TC, Morimoto K, et al: Tissue pressure measurements as a determinant for the need of fasciotomy. Clin Orthop Relat Res 1975;113:43.
343. Whitesides TE Jr, Haney TC, Harada H, et al: A simple method for tissue pressure determination. Arch Surg 1975;110:1311.
344. Wiley J, McIntyre W: Fracture patterns in children. In Unthoff H, Jaworski ZFG, eds: Current Concepts of Bone Fragility. Berlin, Springer-Verlag, 1986, p 159.
345. Wilkins KE: Supracondylar fractures: What's new? J Pediatr Orthop 1997;6:110.
346. Wilkins KE: Principles of fracture remodeling in children. Injury 2005;36(Suppl 1):A3.
347. Willis RB, Rorabeck CH: Treatment of compartment syndrome in children. Orthop Clin North Am 1990; 21:401.
348. Wilson SC, Vrahas MS, Berson L, et al: A simple method to measure compartment pressures using an intravenous catheter. Orthopedics 1997;20:403.
349. Winston FK, Kassam-Adams N, Garcia-Espana F, et al: Screening for risk of persistent posttraumatic stress in injured children and their parents. JAMA 2003; 290:643.
350. Winston FK, Kassam-Adams N, Vivarelli-O'Neill C, et al: Acute stress disorder symptoms in children and their parents after pediatric traffic injury. Pediatrics 2002;109:e90.
351. Winthrop AL, Brasel KJ, Stahovic L, et al: Quality of life and functional outcome after pediatric trauma. J Trauma 2005;58:468.
352. Worlock P, Stower M: Fracture patterns in Nottingham children. J Pediatr Orthop 1986;6:656.
353. Worlock P, Stower M, Barbor P: Patterns of fractures in accidental and non-accidental injury in children: A comparative study. BMJ 1986;293:100.
354. Wyrsch B, Mencio GA, Green NE: Open reduction and internal fixation of pediatric forearm fractures. J Pediatr Orthop 1996;16:644.
355. Wyss CR, Matsen FA 3rd, King RV, et al: Dependence of transcutaneous oxygen tension on local arteriovenous pressure gradient in normal subjects. Clin Sci 1981;60:499.
356. Yang EC, Eisler J: Treatment of isolated type I open fractures: Is emergent operative debridement necessary? Clin Orthop Relat Res 2003;410:289.
357. Yao L, Seeger LL: Epiphyseal growth arrest lines: MR findings. Clin Imaging 1997;21:237.
358. Yuan PS, Pring ME, Gaynor TP, et al: Compartment syndrome following intramedullary fixation of pediatric forearm fractures. J Pediatr Orthop 2004;24: 370.
359. Zimmerman S, Makoroff K, Care M, et al: Utility of follow-up skeletal surveys in suspected child physical abuse evaluations. Child Abuse Negl 2005;29: 1075.
360. Ziv I, Rang M: Treatment of femoral fracture in the child with head injury. J Bone Joint Surg Am 1983; 65:276.
361. Zonis Z, Weisz G, Ramon Y, et al: Salvage of the severely injured limb in children: A multidisciplinary approach. Pediatr Emerg Care 1995;11:176.

Chapter 41

Spinal Injuries

TRAUMATIC INJURIES OF THE CERVICAL SPINE

Cervical spine injuries are rare in children and are often difficult to diagnose because of an inability to obtain a clear history and the difficulty of imaging an immature spine. Therefore, a high index of suspicion is necessary to avoid missing the diagnosis and incurring associated sequelae. Neurologic injury may be present despite negative imaging studies. The patterns of injury in children older than 10 years are similar to those in adults, with a greater incidence of subaxial injuries than in younger children, in whom injuries more frequently occur between the occiput and C2. The majority of injuries do not result in neurologic injury, and nonoperative treatment is usually effective.

Anatomy

The development of the atlas and axis with their ossification centers was well studied by Bailey.[15] Three ossification centers are present in the immature atlas: one for the anterior ring, which usually appears by 1 year of age, and one each for the posterior neural arches. The connection between the anterior and posterior arches is composed of the neurocentral synchondroses, which fuse at 7 years of age and can be mistaken for fracture before this period. The posterior arch most often closes by the age of 3 years but can remain open or partially closed (Fig. 41–1).

The ossification centers of the axis include one for the body, one for each neural arch, and one for the dens (Fig. 41–2). Fusion of the dens to the neural arches and the anterior body occurs between 3 and 6 years of age. During fetal development, the dens is formed from two ossification centers, which fuse during the seventh month of gestation. An ossification center at the tip of the odontoid appears between 4 and 6 years of age and fuses to the remaining odontoid by 12 years. The lower cervical vertebrae follow a similar pattern of development: the ossification centers at the body and each neural arch close by the third year, and the neurocentral synchondroses fuse between the fourth and sixth years.

The blood supply to the odontoid is derived from the anterior and posterior ascending arteries, which branch from the vertebral arteries at the level of the third cervical vertebra and coalesce in the midline.[232] Anastomoses between the carotid and ascending arteries occur near the apex of the odontoid process.

Epidemiology

Although cervical spine fractures in children account for a small percentage of all cervical spine fractures, cervical spine injuries account for the majority of spine injuries in children, with up to 48% of all spine fractures in children occurring in the cervical spine.[8,41,47] A 20-year review of all cervical spine fractures at the Henry Ford Hospital found that only 12 (1.9%) of 631 patients were younger than 15 years.[118] Others report a similar incidence of fractures in children as in adults.[118]

In contrast to what is seen in adults, most cervical spine injuries in young children occur between the occiput and C2 because of increased ligamentous laxity and hypermobility together with a relatively larger head size, which results in the fulcrum of injury being above C3.* Atlas and axis injuries accounted for 16% of cervical spine injuries in a large series of adults, as compared with 70% in children.[115] As the child gets older and takes on a more adult body habitus, the incidence of cervical spine injuries is more similar to the adult pattern.[36,68,111,130,172,191]

*See references 20, 33, 37, 68, 111, 118, 205, 207, 208, 244.

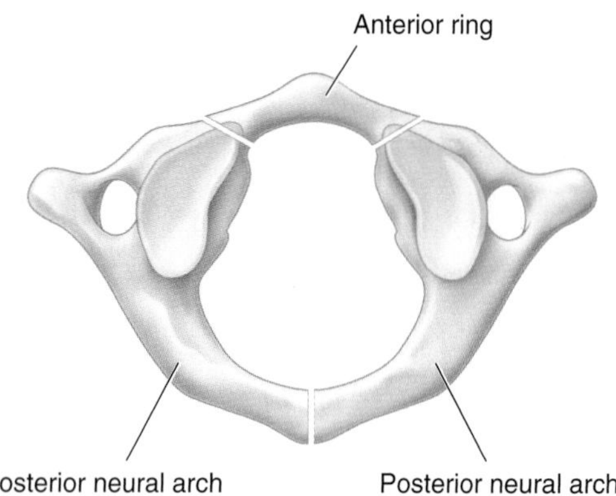

FIGURE 41-1 Ossification centers of the atlas. Note the neurocentral synchondrosis between the anterior ring and the posterior neural arches.

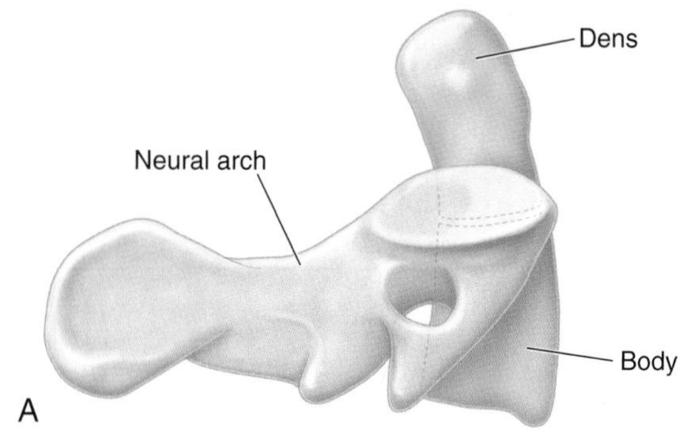

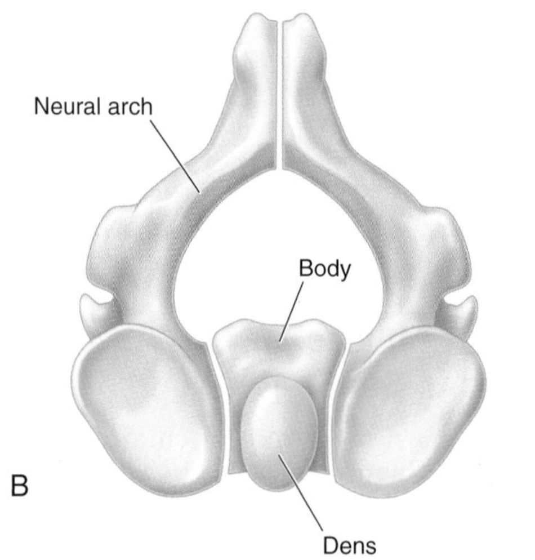

FIGURE 41-2 Schematic sagittal **(A)** and axial **(B)** views of the ossification centers of the axis. The four centers of ossification are depicted. The anterior arch is composed of the body and the dens, whereas two neural arches compose the remaining centers of ossification.

The mechanism of injury depends on the age of the child. Obstetric cervical spine injury can occur, particularly in infants with hyperextension of the head in the breech presentation. Cesarean delivery may prevent this catastrophic complication.[3,6,31,37] Infants with cervical spine injury are most commonly the victims of nonaccidental trauma, usually violent shaking.[53,112,146,262] Careful clinical evaluation is important in this age group because a significant number of these injuries may have normal plain radiographs, or "spinal cord injury without radiographic abnormality" (SCIWORA), which is discussed later under Spinal Cord Injury without Radiographic Abnormality.[33,41,108,196,200,254,262,265,273] In older children, cervical spine injuries are more often due to motor vehicle accidents, pedestrian–motor vehicle encounters, falls from heights, and athletic injuries.[12,20,33,41,47,69,111,112,118,172,204,205]

Diagnosis

Every child evaluated after a traumatic event should be questioned about the mechanism of injury and assessed for injury to the cervical spine. Risk factors for cervical spine injury include facial abrasions or lacerations,[165] head trauma,[17] clavicle fractures, high-speed motor vehicle accidents, and falls from a height. Painful torticollis may be present in an alert child with a cervical spine injury.

Physical examination should include a head-to-toe assessment by the complete trauma team. The head and face should be carefully inspected for lacerations and abrasions. The neck should be palpated to elicit tenderness, muscle guarding, or the presence of a gap in the spinous processes that would indicate a posterior ligamentous injury. A complete orthopaedic assessment of all four extremities and of the remainder of the spine and pelvis should be performed. A thorough neurologic examination must be performed and should include a rectal examination when a neurologic injury is suspected. The importance of a thorough and careful examination cannot be overstated inasmuch as additional orthopaedic injuries have been reported to occur in up to 40% of children with cervical spine injuries, and closed head injuries have been reported in 58% of cases.[65,71]

A child who arrives in the emergency department unconscious is always considered to have a cervical spine injury. The child should wear a cervical collar to stabilize the cervical spine until the patient is awake and can cooperate with the physical examination. A cervical spine injury should be strongly suspected when clonus is present in the extremities without decerebrate rigidity.[249] Surgeons should remember the importance of distracting injuries—particularly other fractures. Chang and coauthors reported that 7% of patients who had a distracting injury as the *only* indication for imaging the spine were found to have vertebral column injuries.[44]

Radiographic Findings

Radiographic evaluation should be performed when a cervical spine injury is suspected. A review of 2133 radiographs obtained in children younger than 18 years over a 7-year period disclosed cervical spine injury in only 1.2% of patients.[216] The two best predictors of cervical spine injury were involvement in a motor vehicle accident and complaints of neck pain.[93] However, we usually obtain radiographs in any patient with cervical tenderness, distracting injuries, altered mental status, alcohol or drug intoxication, or a neurologic deficit.

CERVICAL SPINE RADIOGRAPHS

Although plain radiographic assessment of the child may be difficult, up to 98% of injuries can be diagnosed on lateral cervical spine radiographs, so careful assessment of good-quality radiographs is the critical first step in the evaluation of children with cervical spine injury.[65] In an unstable patient, a screening lateral radiograph of the cervical spine obtained in the emergency department should be viewed as an initial screening test and additional views obtained when the condition of the patient allows (Fig. 41–3).[242] A complete radiographic examination should include anteroposterior (AP), lateral, open-mouth, and oblique views. When injury is suspected despite normal-appearing radiographs, flexion-extension lateral radiographs should be obtained to help identify pathology (Fig. 41–4). When one injury is identified, it is important to obtain and carefully examine radiographs of the entire spine because multiple sites of injury may be present. In one study of 42 children with spine injuries seen over a 16-year period, 50% of injuries were in the cervical spine, and 35% of patients had more than one level of injury, usually contiguous segments.[179] McGrory and colleagues reported injuries in nonadjacent motion segments in 6 (4.2%) of 143 patients.[177]

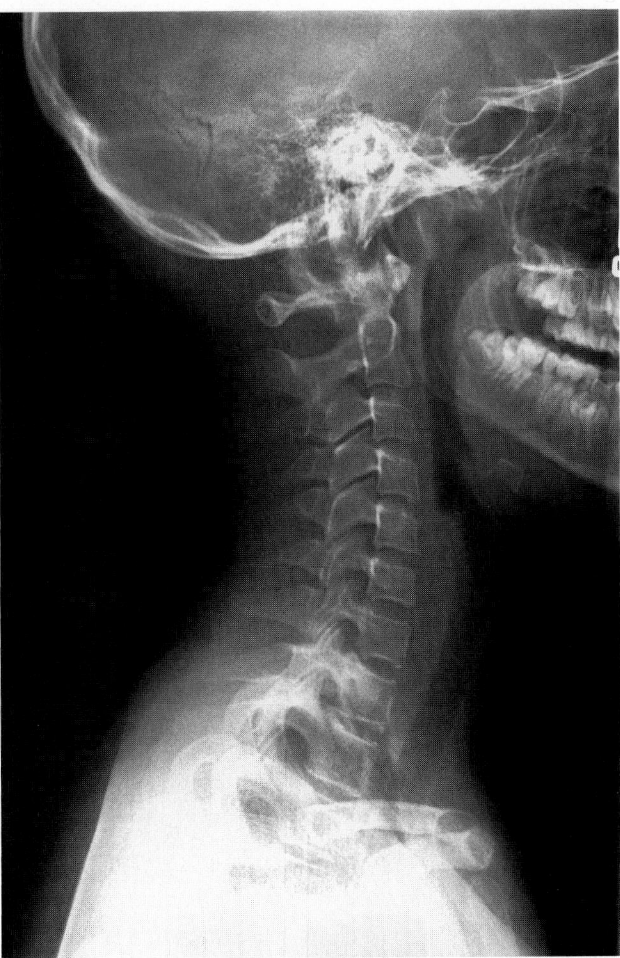

FIGURE 41–3 Screening lateral radiograph of the cervical spine. The radiograph should show all seven cervical vertebrae and should also include the C7-T1 level.

The lateral radiograph should be examined systematically, with the examiner looking first for alignment. Alignment is checked by following the anterior and posterior lines of the vertebral bodies or the spinolaminar line described by Swischuk (Fig. 41–5).[262,263] This line is more important diagnostically than the line connecting the anterior and posterior lines of the vertebral bodies, which may exhibit a step-off, especially at the C2-4 levels. Second, the posterior interspinous process distance should be assessed. Posterior ligamentous instability is manifested on the lateral radiograph by an increase in the interspinous distance, loss of parallelism between the articular processes, and posterior widening of the disk space (Fig. 41–6).[208] Third, the prevertebral soft tissue width should be measured. Normally, it is less than 5 to 6 mm anterior to the body of C2.[48] Apple and colleagues reported that 10 of 11 patients younger than 12 years had injuries involving C1, C2, or the occipitoatlantal articulation, all of whom had retropharyngeal swelling of more than 7 mm anterior to C2.[12] Fourth, cervical lordosis should be examined. Although loss of cervical lordosis does not denote the presence of cervical spine injury, it may indicate muscle guarding and spasm. Fifth, because children have a higher incidence of injuries between the occiput and C3, it is important to carefully evaluate this area and obtain a good open-mouth view.

Accepted criteria for instability of the upper cervical spine in children include more than 10 degrees of forward flexion of C1 on C2 and an atlanto–dens interval (ADI) greater than 4 mm.[168] Pennecot and colleagues reported the upper limit of the ADI in children to be 3 ± 0.7 mm in flexion, with less than 0.5 mm of difference in ADI occurring between flexion and extension radiographs.[207] In a classic article, Fielding and colleagues reported that in adults, the transverse ligament is ruptured when the ADI is between 3 and 5 mm, and the transverse and alar ligaments are ruptured when the ADI is 10 to 12 mm.[79] In the lower cervical spine no accepted criteria have been developed for children; however, White and colleagues reported that in adults, the accepted amount of angulation between the affected vertebra and the adjacent segment is 11 degrees.[191,276,281]

Pseudosubluxation refers to forward translation of the anterior aspect of the vertebral body relative to the inferior level despite normal alignment of the posterior spinolaminar line (Swischuk's line, see Fig. 41–5) This well-described radiographic variant is a result of normal physiologic development of the cervical spine. In the upper cervical spine of young patients, the facet

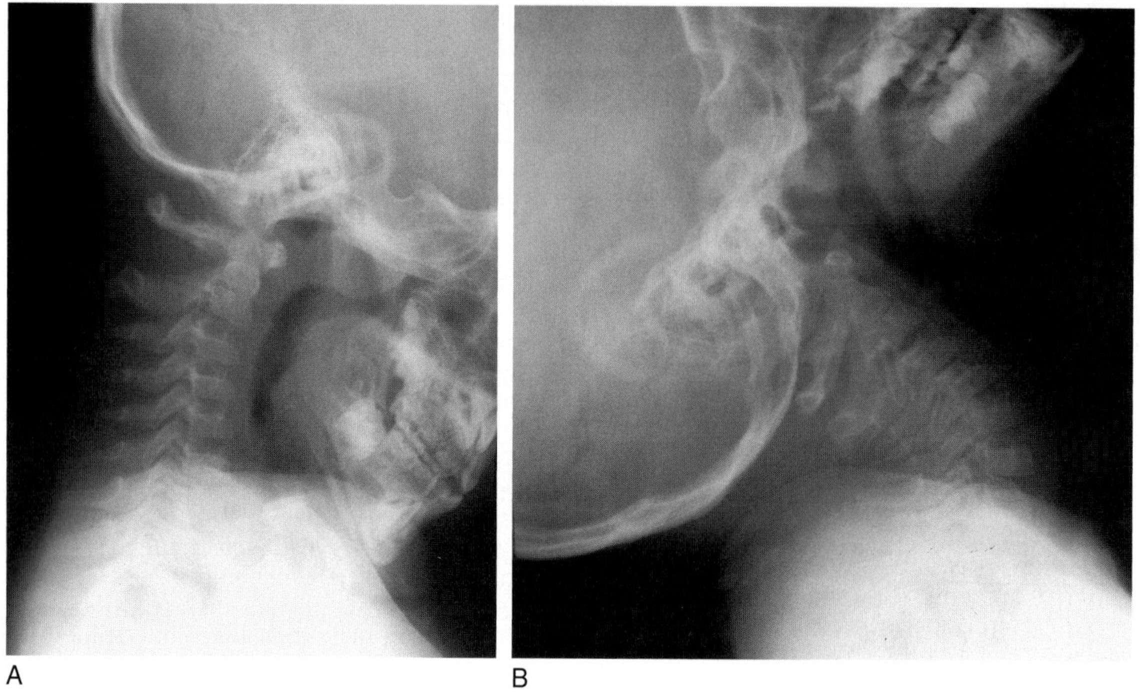

FIGURE 41-4 **A** and **B**, Flexion-extension lateral radiographs.

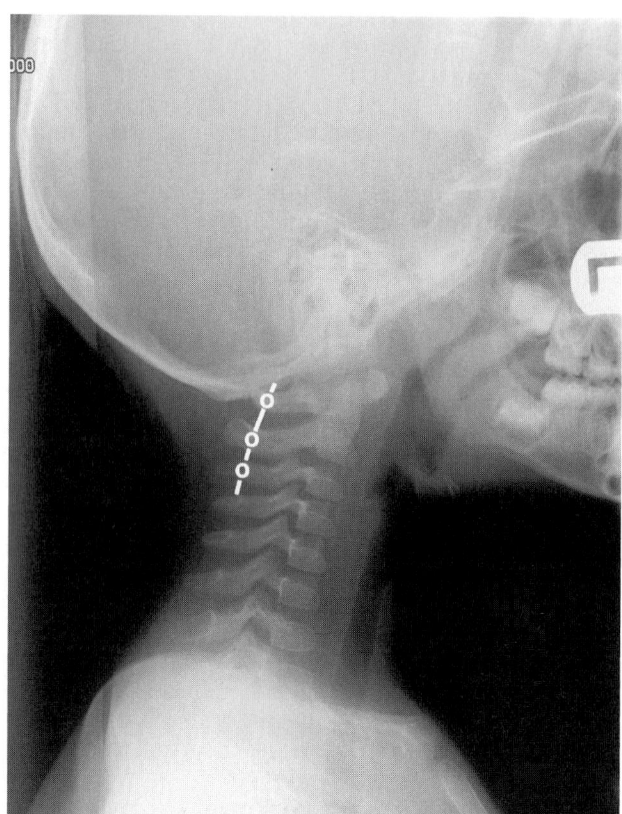

FIGURE 41-5 Lateral radiograph demonstrating the spinal laminar line of Swischuk. This line is drawn by connecting the anterior edge of the spinous processes of C1, C2, and C3.

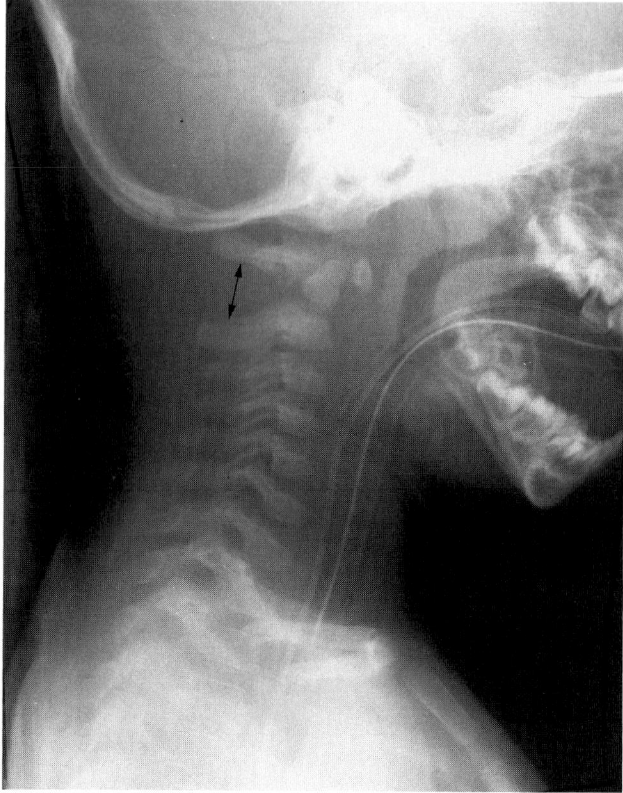

FIGURE 41-6 Posterior ligamentous instability. A lateral radiograph of a 2-year-old child demonstrates widening of the posterior elements between C1 and C2 (*arrow*), indicating a posterior ligamentous injury.

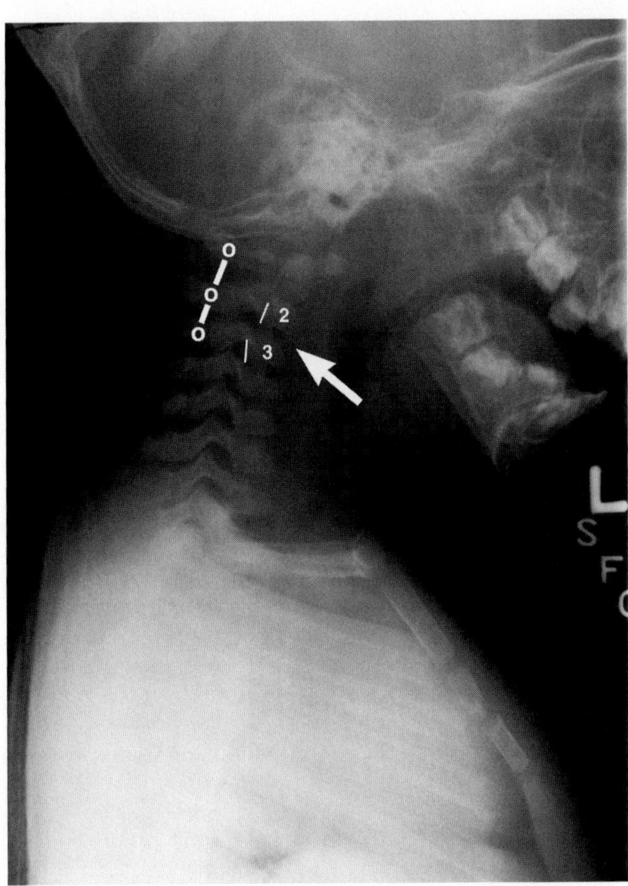

FIGURE 41–7 Pseudosubluxation of the cervical spine in children. On the lateral radiograph there is apparent subluxation of the vertebral bodies of C2 and C3. It appears that C2 is anteriorly subluxed on C3 (*arrow*). However, when the spinal laminar line of Swischuk is drawn, there is no true subluxation.

joints are more horizontal. With growth, the facets become more vertical. Forward displacement of up to 4 mm at C2-3 is normal in children and is most commonly seen in those younger than 8 years (Fig. 41–7).[42,134,170,243,260]

OTHER STUDIES

Further imaging studies, including computed tomography (CT) or magnetic resonance imaging (MRI), are indicated when abnormalities are seen on the initial plain radiographs and when cervical spine injury is suspected despite normal radiographs. CT is best used in children suspected of having osseous fractures, facet dislocations, or vertebral end-plate fractures.[54,70] MRI is best used to evaluate soft tissue injuries, including posterior ligamentous injury, a herniated disk, encroachment of the neuroforamina, spinal cord lesions and edema, or a post-traumatic spinal cord cyst.[85] MRI may have some prognostic value in distinguishing patients with spinal cord edema, who generally recover neurologically, from patients with intraspinal hemorrhage, who often do not recover.[49] MRI may also be useful in demonstrating injuries to the spinal cord that are remote from the bony injury.[18]

A number of studies have assessed the role of CT and MRI scans to clear the cervical spine in adults and children with altered mental status or a distracting injury. Both of these modalities have been shown to be highly sensitive and specific in identifying occult injury. These screening protocols have been shown to decrease length of hospital stay and may be more effective than dynamic radiographs. Although many protocols have been proposed, there is to date no universally accepted standard.* Frank and coauthors reported the results of a protocol to use MRI for clearing the cervical spine in obtunded and intubated pediatric trauma patients who could not be cleared within 72 hours. They reported decreased time to clearance of the cervical spine and decreased length of stay and believed that the MRI protocol was effective and cost-efficient.[82]

Treatment

Because a child's head is proportionally larger than the body, positioning the patient to prevent acute flexion of the neck is important during transport and evaluation. Adult proportions begin to emerge in children at 8 years of age. In 1989, Herzenberg and colleagues reported on 10 children younger than 7 years with unstable cervical spine injuries who were found to have anterior angulation or translation on the lateral radiograph when the patient was positioned on the traditional backboard (Fig. 41–8A).[121] They recommended using a bed or backboard with a posterior recess to allow posterior positioning of the head and thus prevent flexion of the cervical spine (Fig. 41–81B). Initially, the child should be examined with a cervical collar in place. Although a rigid collar provides some stability to the neck, residual motion can occur. This motion can be limited with the use of tape and sandbags.[132] These devices should be gently removed while a second examiner applies a stabilizing force with mild in-line traction as the posterior elements are palpated. The hard collar is then replaced and the appropriate imaging studies performed. When ventilatory support is required, the best method of intubation is controversial.[21,125,138,171,259] It appears that gentle in-line traction with orotracheal or nasotracheal intubation is safe and does not lead to further neurologic injury. Pharmacologic treatment of patients with neurologic injuries is discussed later (under Pharmacologic Treatment of Spinal Cord Injury).

ATLANTO-OCCIPITAL DISLOCATION

This relatively rare injury usually occurs in motor vehicle accidents and is associated with high mortality (Fig. 41–9). Bucholz and Burkhead reported findings in 112 postmortem specimens from victims of multiple trauma, 9 (8%) of which showed atlanto-occipital dislocation.[35] Their series included 20 children younger than 18 years, 3 (15%) of whom had this injury. Although atlanto-occipital dislocation is often fatal,

*See references 34, 82, 88, 114, 120, 124, 160, 218, 219, 236, 271.

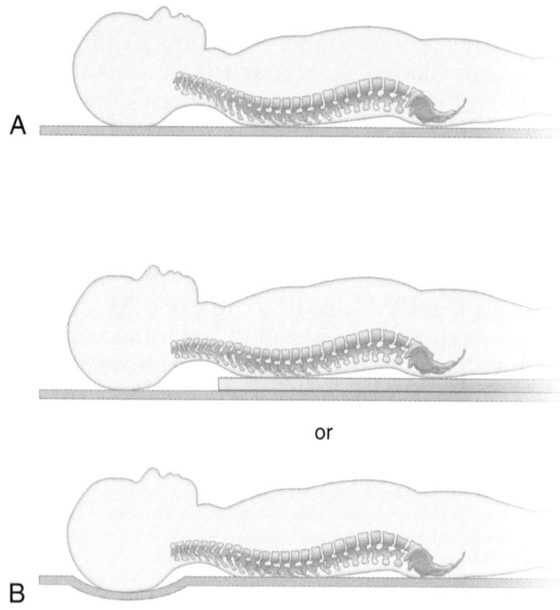

FIGURE 41-8 Proper transport of a child with a suspected cervical injury. **A,** Because of the proportionally large head of a child, a standard backboard will result in cervical spine flexion. **B,** A more appropriate transport backboard is one that includes a double mattress pad or a sunken headrest so that the head can fall back and provide a more normal lordotic position of the cervical spine.

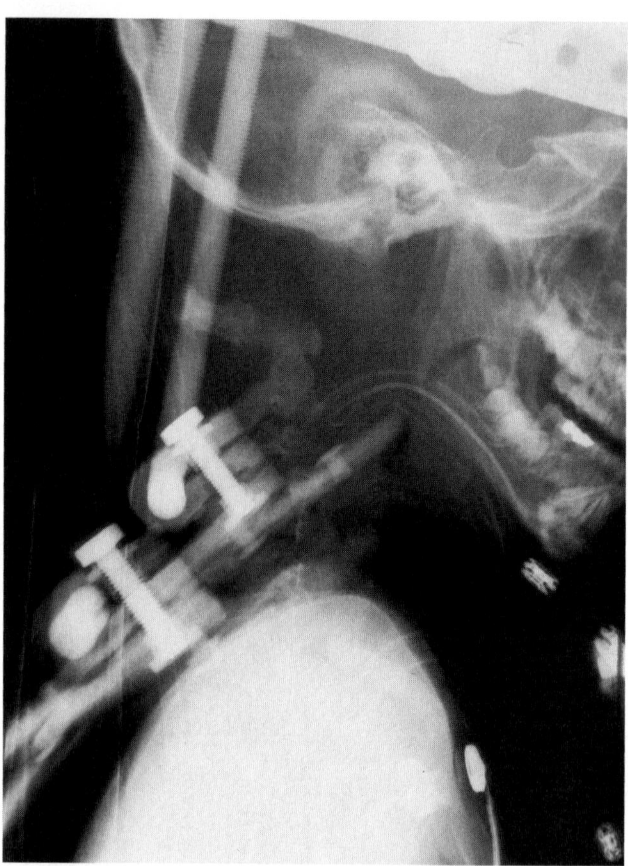

FIGURE 41-9 Atlanto-occipital dislocation shown on a lateral radiograph of a 4-year-old child involved in a motor vehicle accident.

some children will survive this injury. Hosalkar and associates recently reported a 17-year experience with traumatic atlanto-occipital dislocation. Eight of the 16 patients they treated were declared dead on arrival in the emergency department. Three of the patients who survived the initial injury subsequently died from massive head trauma. Of the remaining five survivors, one was neurologically normal, three had mild hemiparesis, and one was a ventilator-dependent quadriplegic.[128] There are numerous case reports of other children who have survived traumatic atlanto-occipital dislocation with a variety of neurologic deficits.[12,20,22,72,75,93,141,154,188,250,261,270,284]

Radiographic assessment of atlanto-occipital dislocation can be difficult because radiographs obtained in the emergency department may appear normal. These injuries may be suspected from subtle plain film findings such as an increased interspinous process distance. Although a number of radiographic measurements have been described, we prefer to use the Powers ratio when evaluating this injury (Fig. 41–10).[215] Historically, when atlanto-occipital injury was strongly suspected in the absence of good radiographic evidence, the diagnosis was made with a lateral radiograph taken with mild traction carefully applied to the head. Currently, however, MRI is increasingly being used to identify this injury, as well as other more subtle injuries to the tectorial membrane.[75,261]

Treatment consists of halo application and stabilization and posterior fusion from the occiput to C1 or C2.[75,93,103,128,138,154,250] Postoperatively, the patient is immobilized in a halo vest or halo cast (Fig. 41–11). Although internal fixation in a young child is difficult, we have placed sutures or metal wire around the posterior elements of C1 and C2 and through the base of the skull. The duration of immobilization should be 3 to

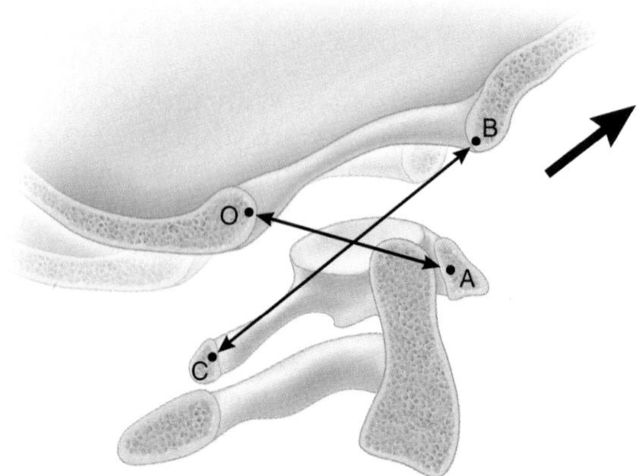

FIGURE 41-10 The Powers ratio. This ratio is determined by drawing a line from the posterior arch of the atlas (C) to the basion (B) and dividing this by the distance from the anterior arch of the atlas (A) to the opisthion (O). A normal Powers ratio is less than 0.9. A ratio greater than 1.0 is diagnostic of atlanto-occipital dislocation.

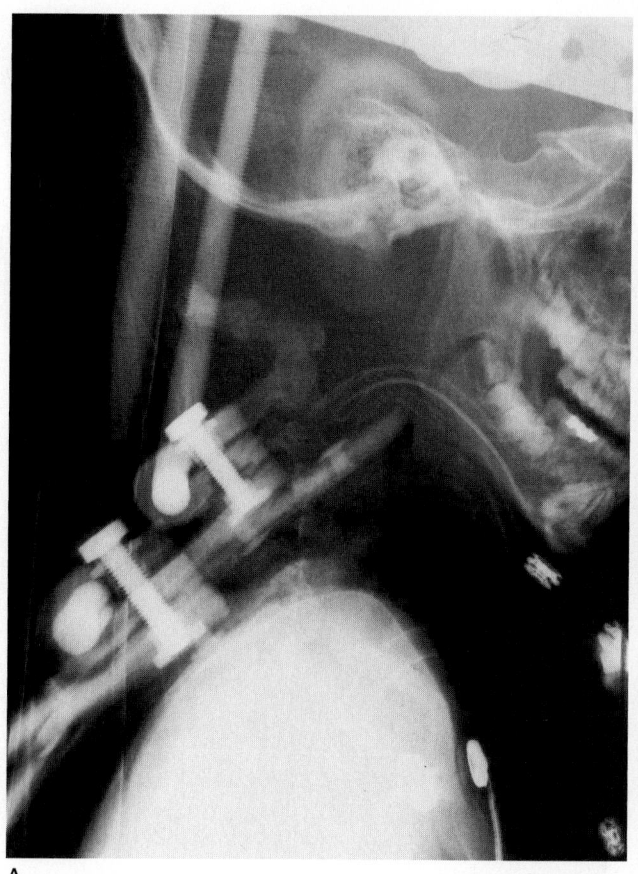

A

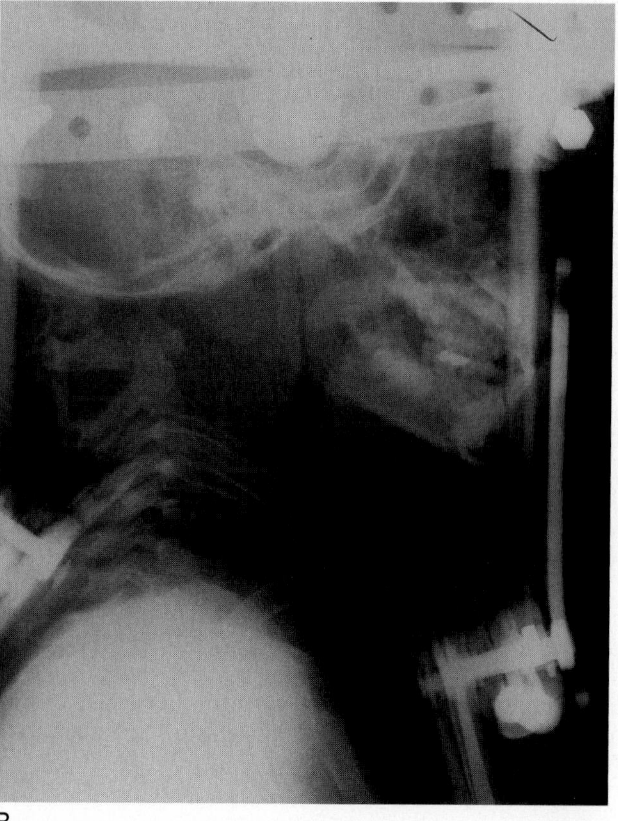

B

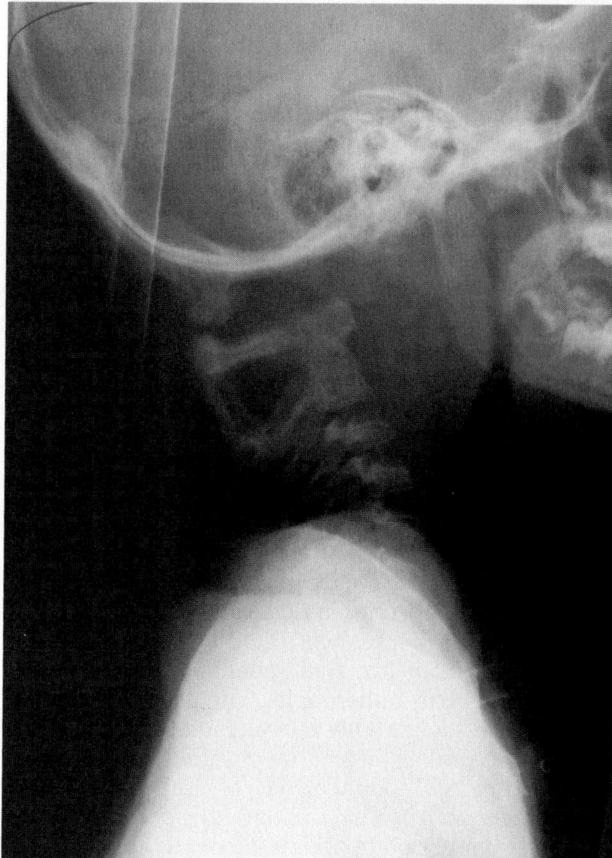

C

FIGURE 41–11 Treatment of atlanto-occipital dislocation. **A,** Lateral radiograph demonstrating atlanto-occipital dislocation. **B,** Lateral radiograph obtained after halo application with reduction. **C,** Lateral radiograph demonstrating fusion 4 months after injury and fusion from the occiput to C2.

4 months. Patients with more stable injuries, such as tectorial membrane abnormalities noted on MRI, may be managed with immobilization without fusion.[75,261]

ATLAS FRACTURES

Fracture of the ring of C1, the so-called Jefferson fracture, is caused by an axial compressive force applied to the head that results in direct compression of the ring of C1 by the occipital condyles. This very rare injury accounts for less than 5% of all cervical spine fractures in children.[12,20,86,173,184,266] The fracture may be at multiple sites within the ring of the atlas or it may be at the neurocentral synchondrosis. Jefferson fractures may be seen on plain radiographs but can usually be detected by displacement of the lateral masses. CT scans will more completely identify one if significant displacement of the fracture occurs. The transverse ligament may become stretched and incompetent and result in C1-2 instability, which should be evaluated with lateral flexion-extension radiographs.

Atlas fractures should be treated by external immobilization for 3 to 4 months. We prefer immobilization with a halo vest or halo cast, although a Minerva cast or noninvasive halo has been used. When C1-2 is unstable, treatment requires fusion and stabilization of this joint, as outlined in the discussion of Traumatic Atlantoaxial Instability.

TRAUMATIC ATLANTOAXIAL INSTABILITY

In adults, instability of the atlantoaxial junction is most often a result of injury to the transverse ligament and the alar ligaments, and it results in an increased ADI. In the pediatric population, traumatic atlantoaxial instability is most commonly seen in older children (Fig. 41–12). In a younger child, traumatic instability may result from injury to the synchondrosis at the base of the dens. Apple and colleagues described three patients who had sustained injuries to this area, which they described as epiphysiolysis dentis. All patients were younger than 5 years.[12] Nontraumatic atlantoaxial instability is also seen in younger children with underlying conditions such as Down syndrome, Morquio's syndrome or other skeletal dysplasias, and juvenile rheumatoid arthritis.

The rule of thirds, first described by Steel, is helpful in assessing atlantoaxial instability. Steel divided the distance between the anterior and posterior arches of C1 into three equal areas (Fig. 41–13).[255] The anterior third is filled with the odontoid, followed by the spinal cord, and finally an unoccupied area, which provides a "cushion" for the spinal cord.

The diagnosis of traumatic atlantoaxial instability is made with plain radiographs. The ADI should initially be assessed on true lateral radiographs of the cervical spine taken in neutral position. If injury is suspected, the ADI should also be assessed on flexion-extension views. Absolute radiographic parameters to guide treatment of traumatic atlantoaxial instability in children do not exist. However, we perform surgical stabilization when anterior translation is greater than 8 to 10 mm or neurologic deficits are present.

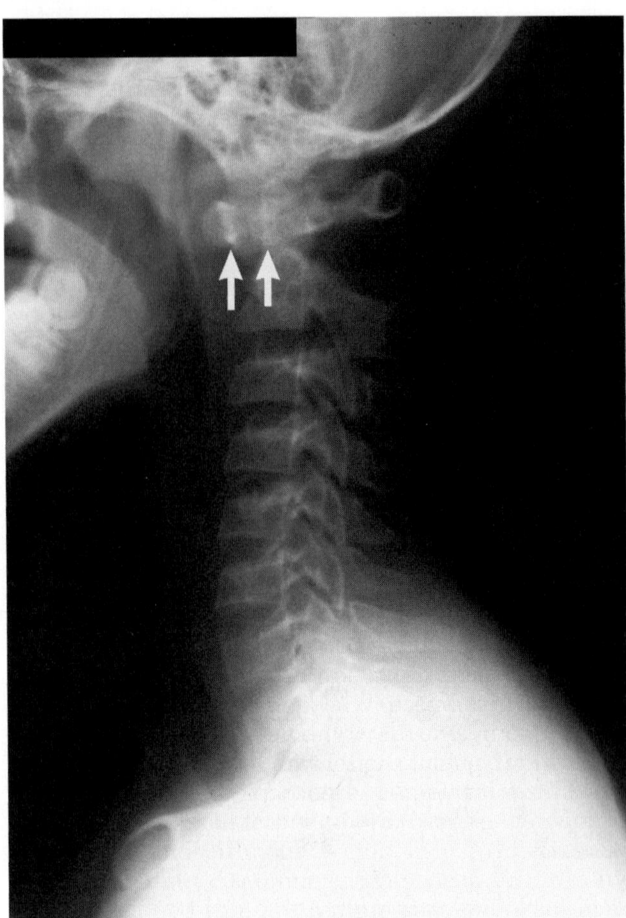

FIGURE 41–12 Lateral radiograph demonstrating atlantoaxial instability. The atlas is displaced anteriorly on the axis. The *arrows* indicate an atlanto–dens interval of 11 mm.

In adults, when the odontoid is displaced posteriorly by a distance equal to its diameter, the spinal cord is endangered, and surgical stabilization of C1-2 is recommended to prevent neurologic injury. Surgical treatment includes the application of a halo ring to facilitate positioning of the head and neck with C1 and C2 in a reduced position, followed by posterior spinal fusion between C1 and C2. Internal fixation in a young child is often difficult; however, a Gallie or Brooks fusion provides additional stability to the C1-2 segment (Fig. 41–14). Halo immobilization should be maintained for approximately 2 to 4 months, depending on radiographic healing and the age of the child.[203,217] In an older child (>11 years), more stable fixation using transarticular screws between C1 and C2 may require less external immobilization. Some authors have used only a soft cervical collar for 8 weeks after transarticular fixation.[38,87,109,135,169,244] We use 3.5-mm cortical screws placed under direct visualization to obtain solid purchase in the anterior cortex of the anterior ring of the atlas. This technique can be supplemented with a Gallie or Brooks fusion (Fig. 41–15). If evaluation is delayed from the time of injury, it may be necessary to

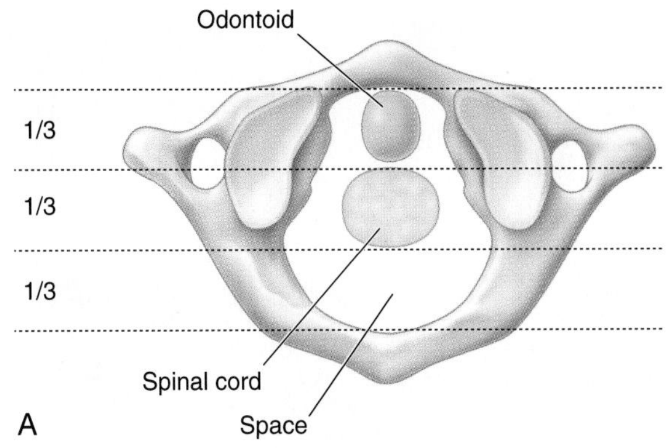

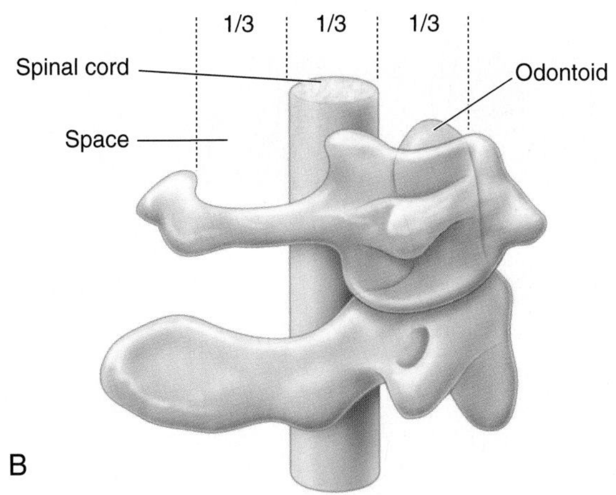

FIGURE 41–13 Schematic axial **(A)** and sagittal **(B)** representation of Steel's rule of thirds. One third of the space is occupied by the odontoid, one third is occupied by the spinal cord, and one third is space.

use halo traction to reduce the anterior translation before surgical stabilization is undertaken.

ODONTOID FRACTURES

Odontoid fractures account for approximately 10% of all cervical spine fractures and dislocations in children.* However, only about 10% of all odontoid fractures occur in children; the vast majority occur in adults.[9] In a child the injury occurs at the synchondrosis at the base of the dens. The mechanism of injury is usually relatively severe, with falls from a significant height and motor vehicle accidents accounting for the majority of injuries.[245] However, in children younger than 4 years, the mechanism of injury may be minor, such as a fall from a bed or a fence[237,240] or a fall from a crib.[78] Consideration should be given to possible associated injuries, most commonly facial fractures, but pulmonary and visceral injuries have been described.[192]

Traditionally, it has been reported that neurologic injury is rare; however, Odent and colleagues reported neurologic injury in 8 of 15 children, all of whom had complete lesions at the level of the cervicothoracic junction.[192] These injuries are often missed because of the innocuous nature of the original injury and the absence of impressive signs and symptoms.[7,192,240] The patient may complain of neck pain, and there may be tenderness on palpation over the upper cervical spine. In the study by Odent and colleagues, the diagnosis was delayed up to 4 months from the time of injury in 5 of 15 children.[192] Persistent pain and neck irritability should alert the physician to injury. Seimon described a clinical sign that he believed correlated well with an odontoid fracture[240]: the patient strongly resists the examiner's attempts to extend the neck. The child will also resist attempts to be brought to either an erect or recumbent position unless the head is supported by the examiner.[240]

The dens is usually displaced anteriorly, often more than 50% of its width on a lateral radiograph. In approximately 10% to 15% of cases the displacement is posterior or there is no displacement. In such cases the injury is difficult to see on plain radiographs, and further imaging studies, such as CT with sagittal images or tomograms, may be necessary. In patients with neurologic injury, MRI may demonstrate spinal cord injury (SCI) distal to C2, which is thought to be due to significant anterior displacement of the upper spine leading to stretch of the spinal cord over the cervicothoracic junction.[117,192]

Children with odontoid fractures can generally be treated successfully by nonoperative means.[19,20,73,118,192,233,240,244] Odent and colleagues reported successfully treating 11 patients with external immobilization, either a Minerva jacket or a halo cast; 7 required reduction and 4 did not. The three patients in this series treated operatively had at least one complication.[192] We prefer closed reduction with the patient sedated to allow constant neurologic assessment. We usually immobilize in a halo vest or cast for 2 to 3 months until solid union is achieved. Before complete removal of the halo, flexion-extension radiographs should be obtained to identify any motion at the fracture site. Nonunion is extremely rare when this fracture is identified and treated early. Nonunion requires operative intervention with either anterior screw fixation or posterior fusion of C1-2. The latter is preferred in a small child, whereas the former may be a reasonable option in an adolescent.[137]

Os odontoideum is a cervical spine anomaly in which the dens is separated from the body of the axis. The dens becomes an ossis with smooth cortical margins (Fig. 41–16). The etiology of os odontoideum has been debated. Some have hypothesized that it is essentially a nonunion from unrecognized remote trauma.[80] Others believe that it represents a congenital anomaly. Sankar and coworkers described 16 patients with symptomatic os odontoideum. Three patients had a history of remote trauma, whereas nine had other congenital abnormalities of the cervical spine or a genetic diagnosis. They concluded that os odontoideum may be the result of trauma or a congenital abnormality.[228] Os odontoideum may be an asymptomatic normal variant or may produce neck pain or

*See references 7, 12, 19, 20, 64, 73, 100, 104, 192, 240, 245.

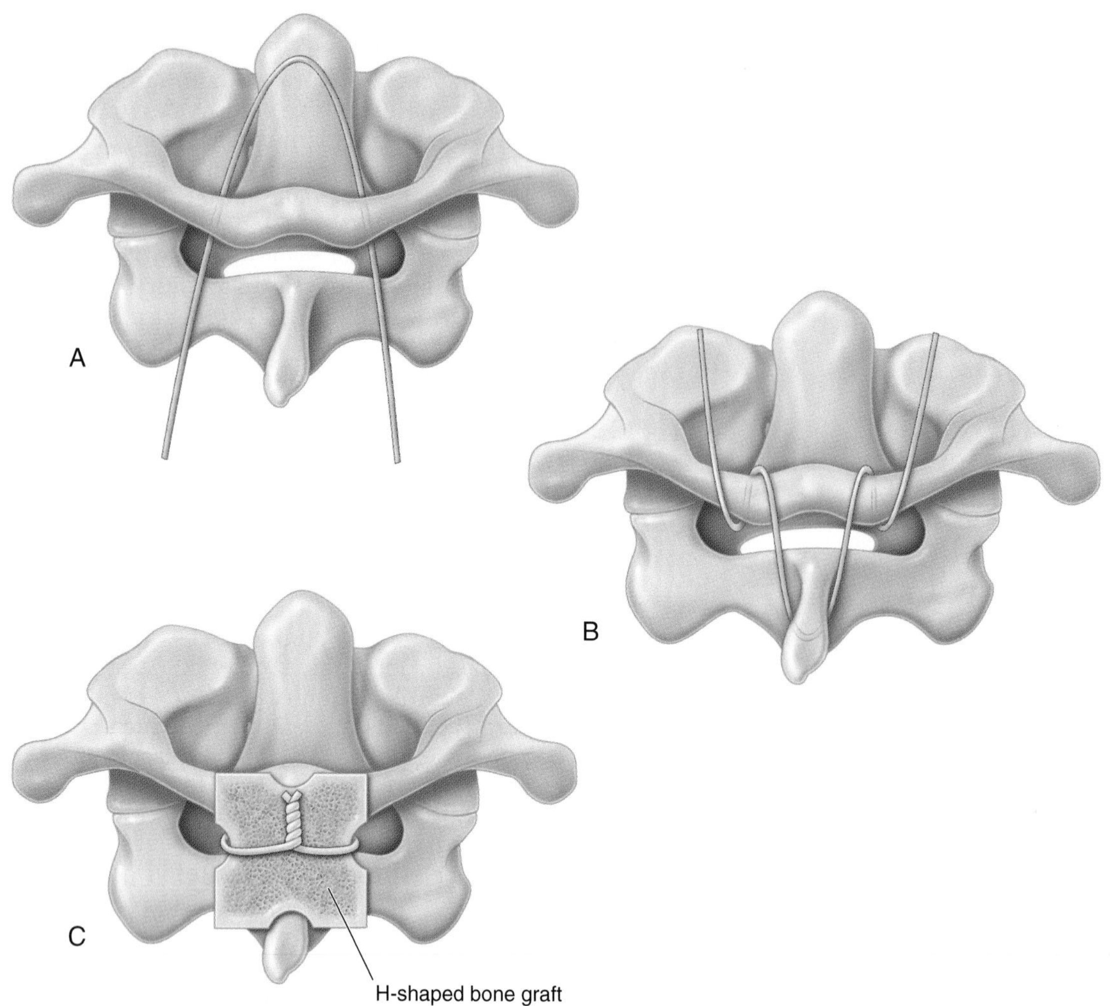

FIGURE 41–14 Posterior C1-2 fusion by the Gallie technique. **A,** A loop of wire is passed below the posterior arch of C1. **B,** The loop is turned back on the posterior arch of C1 and looped around the inferior aspect of the spinous process of C2. **C,** An H-shaped iliac crest bone graft is placed over the posterior arches of C1 and C2. The wire is twist-tied down to provide stable fixation.

neurologic symptoms. Symptomatic patients should be treated by posterior C1-2 fusion.

TRAUMATIC SPONDYLOLISTHESIS OF C2 (HANGMAN'S FRACTURE)

Traumatic spondylolisthesis of C2 is rare in children, with few cases reported in the literature.[12,184,215,232,263,275,284] The mechanism of injury is generally extension and axial loading, with a high incidence of injuries to the face and head. The injury is usually incurred in motor vehicle accidents or a fall from a height. It has also been reported in infants as a result of nonaccidental trauma. Injury in this age group may be difficult to distinguish from a congenital abnormality. Neurologic injury is rare in these injuries, although some have reported neurologic deficits that appeared to resolve over the following year.[12,211,274] We usually obtain a CT scan in all suspected cases of hangman's fracture to fully define the extent of the fracture and the amount of displacement (Fig. 41–17).

In a reliable patient an undisplaced fracture, or a fracture with less than 3 mm of anterior displacement of C2 on C3, can be treated by external immobilization in a hard collar. However, we have a low threshold for using a halo vest. When there is more than 3 mm of displacement, gentle reduction should be performed and the patient immobilized in a halo vest for 2 to 3 months.[268] Pizzutillo and colleagues reported successful treatment in four of five children with a Minerva cast or a halo vest. The fifth child required operative fusion after the fracture failed to unite with conservative treatment.[211]

FRACTURES AND DISLOCATIONS OF THE SUBAXIAL SPINE

Fractures and dislocations of the subaxial spine are relatively rare in young children; however, the incidence in children older than 8 years is similar to that in adults. Of 43 bony injuries in children, 24 (56%) involved the occiput to C2 (average patient age of 6.2

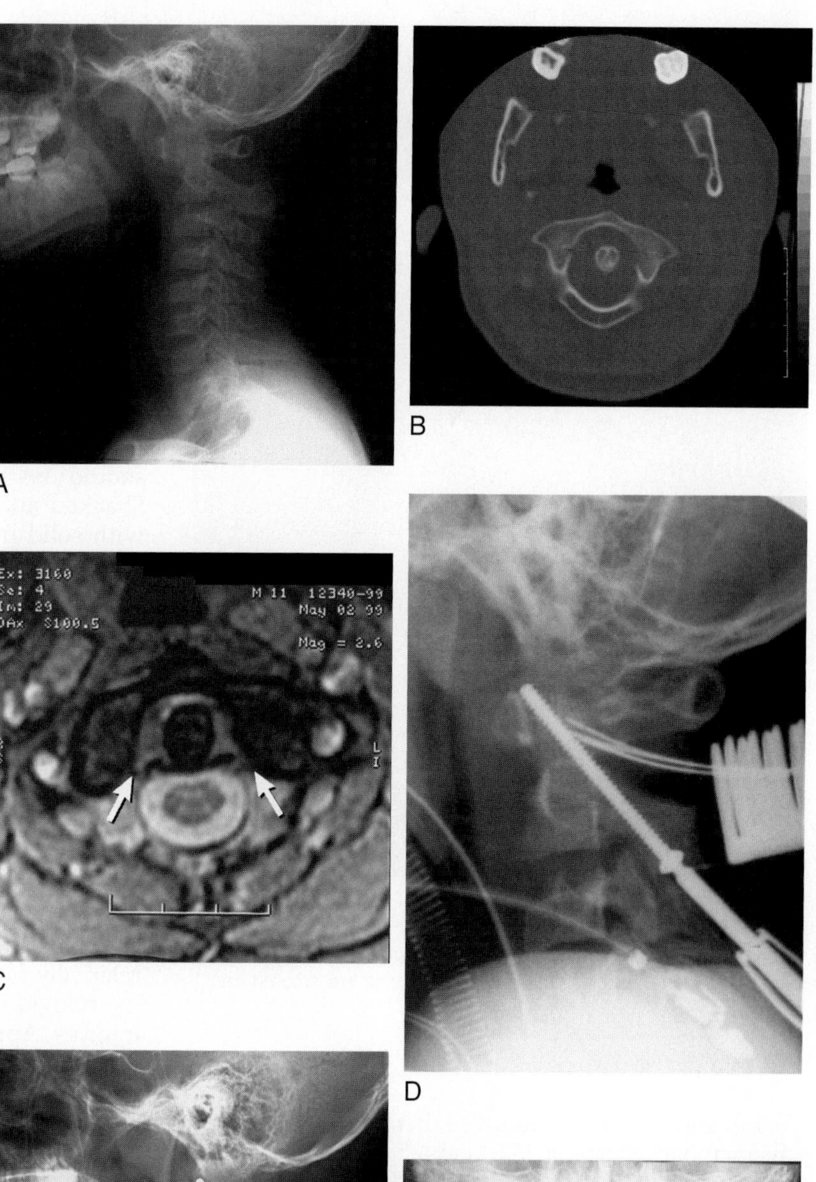

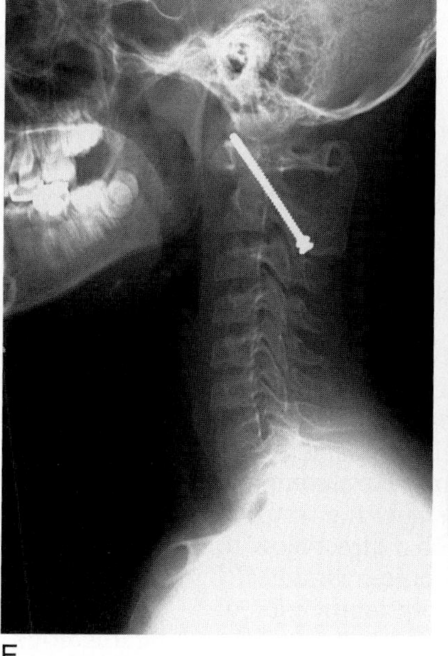

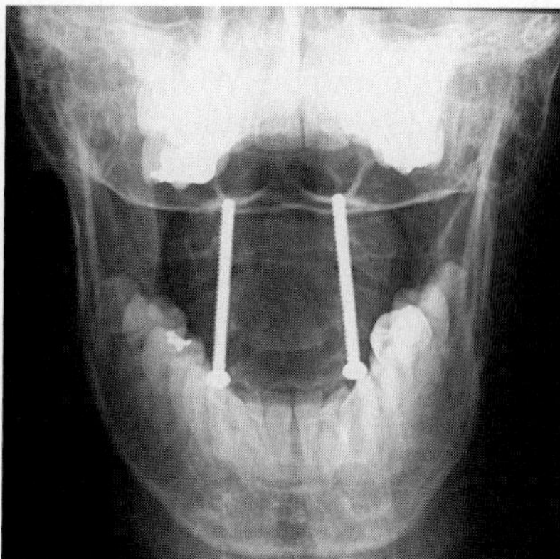

FIGURE 41-15 Transarticular screw fixation between C1 and C2. **A,** Lateral radiograph demonstrating atlantoaxial instability in a 12-year-old boy after a trampoline accident. **B,** Computed tomography scan demonstrating anterior subluxation of the atlas on the axis. **C,** Magnetic resonance image demonstrating avulsion of the transverse ligament (*arrows*), as well as fluid between the anterior aspect of the dens and the posterior arch of C1. **D,** Intraoperative fluoroscopic images demonstrating reduction of C1 on C2. Screws are placed after bone grafting of the articular surfaces. A modified Gallie fusion was also done posteriorly to supplement fixation. **E** and **F,** Six months after surgery there is solid healing of the anterior and posterior fusion. Note the screws traversing the articular facets of C1-2 on the anteroposterior radiograph.

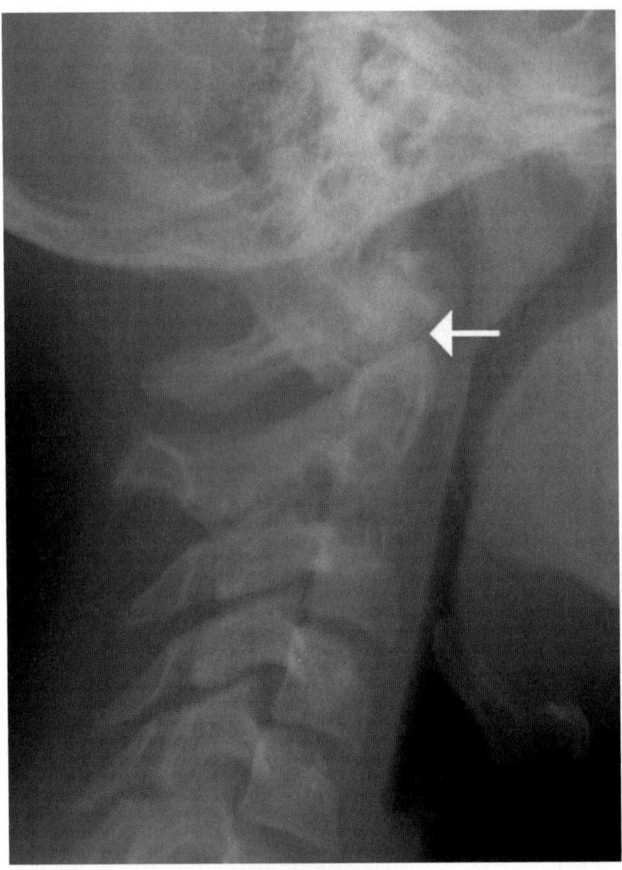

FIGURE 41-16 Lateral radiograph of a patient with an os odontoideum (*arrow*). Note that the dens appears to be separated from the body of C2 but the margins are smooth and regular.

years) and 19 (44%) occurred between C3 and C7 (average patient age of 13.6 years).[20] When all cervical spine injuries are included (including C1-2 rotatory subluxation and SCIWORA), subaxial injuries account for only 23% of injuries.[20] These injuries can be subdivided into fracture-dislocations, burst fractures, compression fractures, posterior ligamentous injuries, unilateral or bilateral facet dislocations, and bilateral facet fractures.[66,148]

A fracture-dislocation injury was the most common subaxial injury reported by Birney and Hanley (Fig. 41–18), with four patients sustaining this injury. Two patients were without neurologic injury, one had a transient incomplete injury, and one had a complete neurologic injury.[20] This injury is usually the result of a motor vehicle accident or a fall with a direct blow to the head. The diagnostic workup should include MRI followed by a reduction maneuver and stabilization of the spine.

A burst fracture is due to axially applied loads to the head, generally with the head slightly flexed. The characteristic fracture pattern includes anterior displacement of the anteroinferior aspect of the body—a "teardrop" fracture. The danger occurs with the posterior aspect of the vertebral body, which fractures in the sagittal plane and can travel posteriorly into the canal. These injuries are most often associated with neurologic injury and are frequently the injury sustained by football players. Birney and Hanley reported six children with a burst fracture; two had a transient incomplete neurologic injury and one had a permanent complete injury.[20] Both CT and MRI are helpful in defining the anatomy of the canal, posterior ligamentous structures, and intervertebral disk. In a patient with a neurologic injury, gentle closed reduction with a halo should be performed, followed by immobilization in a halo cast for 2 to 3 months. If neurologic injury is present and persists despite fracture reduction with in-line traction, anterior decompression with removal of the retropulsed fragments should be performed, followed by strut grafting. Shacked and colleagues[241a] reported excellent results with solid union in six children 3 to 14 years of age who underwent anterior decompression and strut grafting for cervical spine fractures. The anterior approach should be used with caution in very young children because continued posterior growth with a solid anterior fusion may produce excess kyphosis. When a burst fracture is associated with significant posterior ligamentous instability, posterior fusion may decrease the likelihood of postoperative deformity.[253]

Compression fractures are due to a pure flexion moment without significant rotatory or axial loading. This leaves the posterior ligamentous structures intact and does not injure the posterior aspect of the vertebral body; therefore, it does not result in protrusion of bone or disk into the spinal canal. These injuries are relatively rare in children and do not usually result in neurologic injury. In 11 patients with cervical spine injuries, Apple and colleagues noted that only 1, a 9-year-old girl, had compression fractures of the C4-6 bodies; she had been involved in a motor vehicle accident and had no neurologic injury.[12] McGrory and colleagues reported that 10 (7%) of 143 pediatric patients had sustained a compression fracture; 9 of the 10 were older than 10 years.[177] Neurologic injury is rare in these patients because of the lack of posterior body injury and thus less risk of retropulsion into the canal.

Compression fractures are often difficult to diagnose because of the mild radiographic findings and the normal, anteriorly wedged shape of the vertebral body in children. Treatment consists of cervical spine immobilization in a cervical collar for 2 to 4 months, depending on the age of the child and the extent of injury. Surgical treatment is reserved for patients with unacceptable kyphosis, which may not remodel.[238]

Posterior ligamentous injuries result from flexion and flexion-rotation mechanisms with tearing of the posterior ligaments and the facet joint capsule. When the flexion-rotation force is relatively mild, a posterior ligamentous injury occurs. With higher-energy injury, unilateral or bilateral perched or dislocated facets may occur. In children, the cartilaginous portion of the facet may produce the appearance of a perched facet when in fact there is complete dislocation. Pure ligamentous injury is rare in children and is not generally associated with neurologic injury.

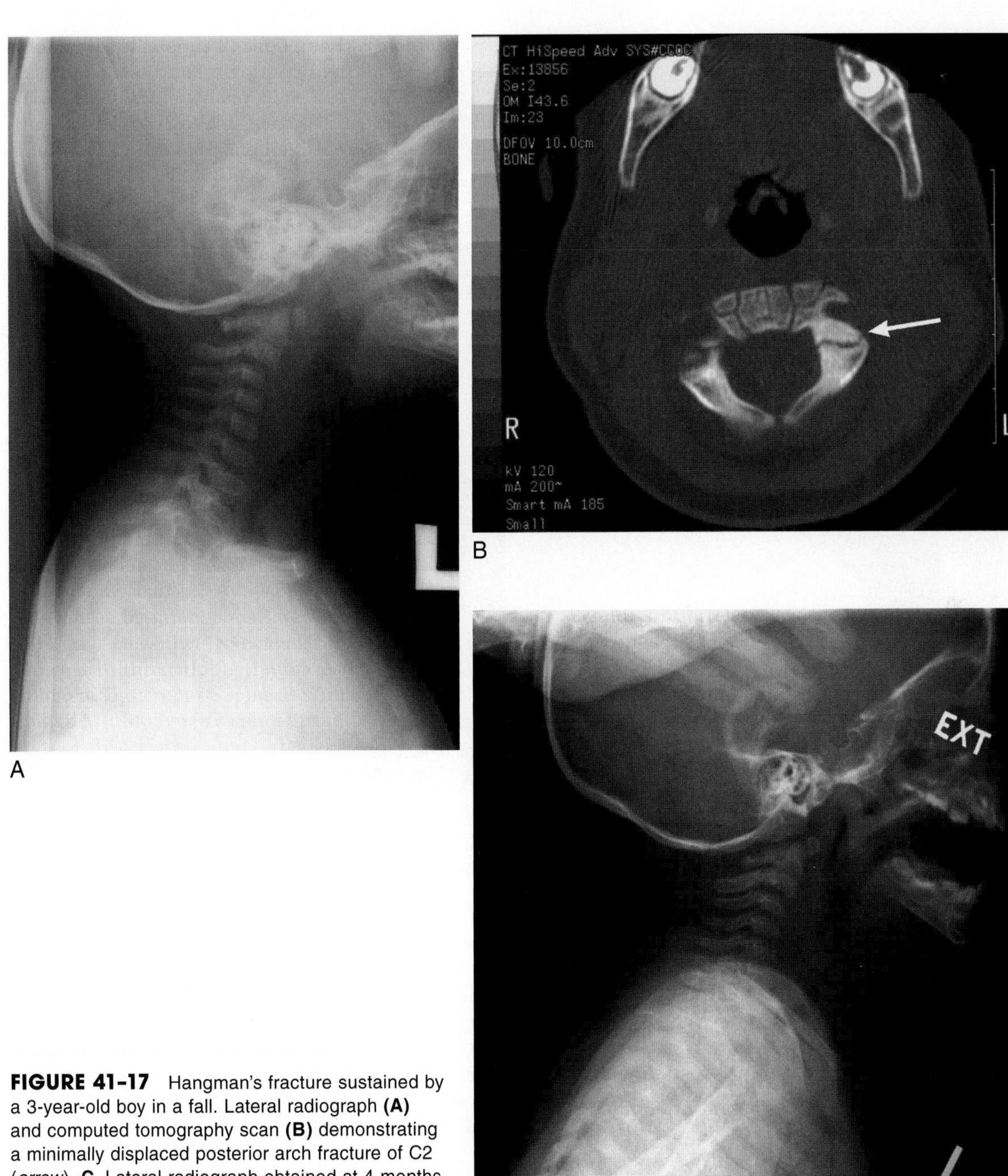

FIGURE 41–17 Hangman's fracture sustained by a 3-year-old boy in a fall. Lateral radiograph **(A)** and computed tomography scan **(B)** demonstrating a minimally displaced posterior arch fracture of C2 (*arrow*). **C,** Lateral radiograph obtained at 4 months showing good bone healing.

Treatment is based on the degree of instability, which has not been fully defined in children. In adults, instability can be defined as angulation between adjacent vertebrae in the sagittal plane of 11 degrees more than the adjacent normal segment or translation in the sagittal plane of 3.5 mm or greater.[201,202,275,276] Because the majority of these injuries occur in patients older than 10 years, similar criteria can be used in children. Significant posterior ligamentous injury requires posterior fusion with autologous bone graft and internal fixation with spinous process wires. Minor ligamentous injuries may be managed conservatively, particularly in a very young (<3 years of age) child.[175] With a unilateral facet dislocation, there is anterior translation between vertebral bodies of 25% to 50% of the sagittal diameter, which may result in unilateral nerve root or spinal cord compression. Bilateral facet dislocations are very unstable injuries with a high risk of causing neurologic injury.[20] Unilateral or bilateral facet dislocation is treated by acute reduction with halo traction and conscious sedation. Reduction is achieved by skeletal traction. Serial lateral radiographs should be obtained after each incremental increase in traction to determine whether reduction has occurred. The head should be in a slightly flexed position and then extended as radiographs demonstrate that the facets

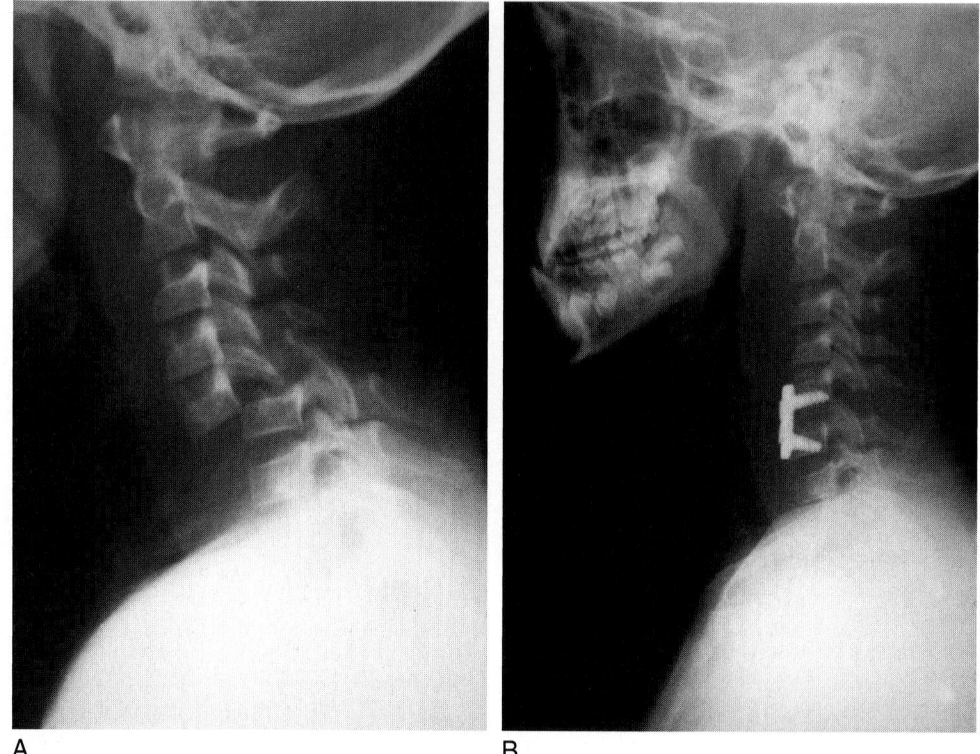

FIGURE 41-18 Fracture-dislocation of the subaxial spine. **A,** Lateral radiograph demonstrating complete dislocation of C5 on C6. **B,** Lateral radiograph obtained after halo reduction and anterior plate fixation with an anterior strut graft.

are aligned and nearly reduced. After closed reduction of a unilateral facet dislocation, most children can be successfully treated with 2 to 3 months of immobilization in a halo cast. Bilateral facet dislocations are usually treated with a posterior arthrodesis, although closed treatment can be successful in a child younger than 3 years. Failure to reduce a unilateral or bilateral facet dislocation requires open reduction and fusion with posterior wiring and halo immobilization for 2 to 4 months.

Traumatic Injuries of the Thoracic and Lumbar Spine

Injuries of the thoracic and lumbar spine are less common in children than are cervical spine injuries. Patients in the first decade of life are more likely to sustain upper thoracic (T4 to T10) injuries and are more likely to be injured from falls or motor vehicle–pedestrian collisions. They may also be injured from abuse.[4,39,61,97,116,126,164,179,231] Patients in the second decade of life are more likely to sustain injuries at the thoracolumbar junction and are commonly injured in motor vehicle collisions or during recreational events.[16,116,119,143,193,206,229,246,277] Neurologic injury occurs in approximately half the patients, with a slight predominance of incomplete lesions.[62,108,142,159,225] These high-energy injuries are frequently associated with other visceral or orthopaedic injuries, including multiple injuries of the spinal column.*

The nomenclature for thoracic and lumbar spine fractures is somewhat confusing because both thoracic and lumbar injuries, as well as injuries at the thoracolumbar junction, are frequently referred to as "thoracolumbar" injuries. We reserve the phrase "thoracolumbar injuries" for injuries occurring between T12 and L1.

Anatomy

An understanding of the anatomy of the immature spine is important in evaluating and treating children with spinal injuries. The pediatric spine is more flexible than the adult spine, which may contribute to the frequency of neurologic injury, as well as the finding of SCIWORA. Several factors contribute to the flexibility of a child's spine. First, the soft tissues are more forgiving, the ligaments are more elastic, the muscles are smaller, and the intervertebral disks are healthy and well hydrated. Second, there is a higher ratio of cartilage to bone. Finally, the facets are more horizontal, thereby allowing greater motion.[5,131,151,163,223,227] Vertebral growth occurs equally from the superior

*See references 4, 10, 13, 27, 41, 47, 50, 98, 99, 113, 116, 123, 161, 167, 182, 220-222, 227, 229, 239, 257, 258, 267, 270, 278.

and inferior apophyses, which develop within the cartilaginous end-plate. These apophyses are wider peripherally than centrally, which gives them a ring appearance, the origin of the term *ring apophysis*. They are similar to the epiphysis of a long bone. Ring apophyses appear radiographically between 8 and 12 years of age and fuse with the body between 21 and 25 years of age.

Management of children with thoracic and lumbar spinal injuries requires an understanding of the "three-column spine," a concept introduced by Denis in 1983.[60] This anatomic description provides the basis for the most efficient means of classification, as well as a foundation for a rational approach to treatment. Denis realized that complete rupture of the posterior ligamentous structures did not produce instability. Rather, instability in flexion required not only rupture of the posterior ligaments but also disruption of what he termed the "middle column"—the posterior longitudinal ligament, the posterior annulus fibrosus, and the posterior wall of the vertebral body (Fig. 41–19). The anterior column consists of the anterior longitudinal ligament, the anterior annulus fibrosus, and the anterior vertebral body. The posterior arch and the posterior ligamentous complex (the supraspinous and interspinous ligaments, facet joint capsules, and ligamentum flavum) make up the posterior column.

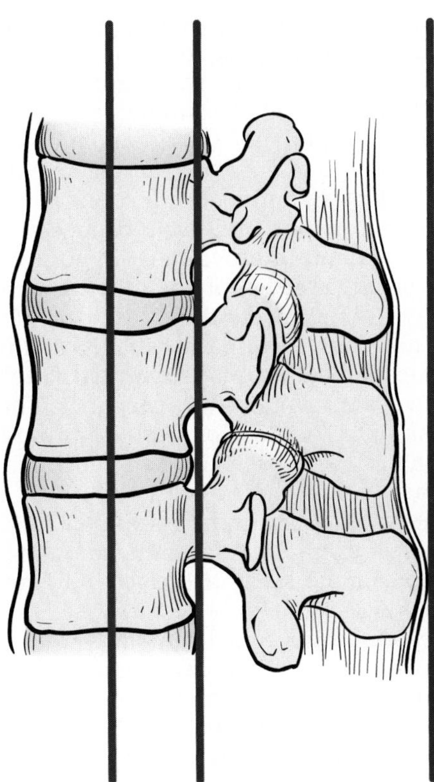

FIGURE 41–19 The three-column spine. The anterior column consists of the anterior longitudinal ligament, the anterior annulus fibrosus, and the anterior vertebral body. The middle column consists of the posterior wall of the vertebral body, the posterior longitudinal ligament, and the posterior annulus fibrosus. The posterior column consists of the posterior arch and the posterior ligamentous complex (supraspinous and interspinous ligaments, facet joint capsules, and ligamentum flavum).

Mechanism of Injury

Thoracic and lumbar spine injuries are most frequently the result of high-energy forces. Motor vehicle–related injuries are the most common, although falls, recreational activities, child abuse, obstetric injury, and gunshots have all been reported as mechanisms.* The force that produces the injury is most commonly flexion, which may be combined with compression, distraction, or shear forces.† Extension injuries have been described but are extremely uncommon.[186]

Roaf in 1960 reported on the events that lead to spinal fracture. As a vertical load is applied, the end-plate bulges toward the vertebral body; there is little change in either the annulus or the nucleus of the disk. As the load increases, deformation of the end-plate forces blood out of the cancellous bone of the vertebral body, thereby decreasing its energy-absorbing ability. Eventually, the elastic limit of vertebral body is exceeded and fracture occurs.[223] The elasticity of the pediatric spine allows these forces to be distributed over multiple levels, which explains why multiple compression fractures are seen more commonly in children. If a distraction or shear force exists concurrently, it may also produce deformity, usually through the end-plate rather than the disk.[45,126,130,143,223,246]

Neurologic injury is classified as primary or secondary. Primary injuries are the result of direct injury to the neural elements and may be due to contusion, stretch, compression, or laceration. Contusion injuries are most common and have a poor prognosis for recovery. Compression produces injury both primarily, through direct neuronal damage, and secondarily, by altering vascular perfusion. Secondary injuries are the result of ischemia and are most common in the "watershed" area of the thoracic spine (T7 to T10). Ischemic injury is a mechanical and biochemical cycle. The initial injury produces a mechanical ischemia, which results in cell death and the release of vasoactive substances. These substances produce both vasoconstriction and edema. The edema leads to further mechanical compression, and the cycle continues.[279] Because of their cyclic nature, ischemic injuries may evolve over time, and a delayed manifestation of neurologic injury is not uncommon.[46,129,183,195] Ischemic SCIs may be exacerbated by systemic hypotension associated with shock from other traumatic injuries. In fact, paraplegia has been reported in both children and adults with hypotensive episodes and no injury to the spinal cord.[1,55,129,147,234,269]

Classification

We use Denis' five-part classification of spinal column injuries (Box 41–1).[60] He classified spinal injuries as

*See references 41, 47, 51,61, 116, 152, 162, 186, 220, 221, 226, 229, 267, 270.

†See references 2, 14, 43, 77, 89, 126, 131, 221, 227, 248.

Box 41-1

Denis' Classification of Thoracic and Lumbar Spine Injuries

Minor Injuries
Articular process fracture
Transverse process fracture
Spinous process fracture
Pars interarticularis fracture

Major Injuries
Compression fractures
Burst fractures
Seat belt injuries
Fracture-dislocation

minor or major and then subdivided major injuries into four classes. Minor injuries include fractures of the spinous and transverse processes, facets, and pars interarticularis. Major injuries include compression fractures, burst fractures, seat belt injuries, and fracture-dislocations. Compression fractures represent failure of only the anterior column. There is no loss of posterior vertebral body height. The intact middle column is pathognomonic for compression fractures. Burst fractures result from failure of the anterior and middle columns in flexion; the posterior column remains intact. A lateral radiograph will reveal fracture of the posterior wall, loss of posterior vertebral body height, and tilting of one or both end-plates. Retropulsion of fragments into the canal may be difficult to appreciate on the lateral radiograph and is best seen on CT scans. The AP radiograph will show loss of vertebral body height and a widened interpedicular distance. Seat belt injuries are the result of a flexion-distraction force. Both the posterior and middle columns fail in tension; the anterior column may remain intact or may fail in compression. Seat belt injuries are further subdivided according to the location (through bone or ligament) of the posterior and middle column injury and whether both columns are injured at the same level or at adjacent levels (Fig. 41–20). Fracture-dislocations are the last and most unstable class of thoracic and lumbar injuries. These injuries represent failure of all three columns in compression, tension, rotation, or shear.

Diagnosis

Thoracic and lumbar spine injuries may be difficult to diagnose. These patients frequently have multiple injuries and an altered state of consciousness. Occasionally, the elasticity of the pediatric spine allows it to "recoil" into a more normal position. If this occurs, the displacement at the time of injury and subsequently the amount of instability may not be appreciated on initial radiographs (Fig. 41–21). Thus, all patients with significant traumatic injuries should be assumed to have spinal column instability until such an injury is excluded.[44,50,182,196] All trauma patients should be logrolled during the initial assessment, and the entire spine should be inspected and palpated for ecchymosis, soft tissue swelling, step-offs, and tenderness. Obviously, the patient's inability to move the extremities heightens the suspicion of spinal column injury, as should significant abdominal injuries and the seat belt sign—a large ecchymosis over the abdomen.

Once one spinal injury has been identified, the entire spine must be imaged because injuries may have occurred at multiple levels.[27,50,98,113,182,222,270] Every patient with a spinal injury requires a careful and thorough neurologic examination. If a neurologic deficit is present, it is important to determine whether the lesion is complete or incomplete. A complete lesion is defined as the absence of both motor and sensory function below the SCI. Spinal shock must have resolved before an injury can be classified as complete. Return of the bulbocavernosus reflex indicates that the S3-4 region of the conus medullaris of the spinal cord is both physiologically and anatomically functional and spinal shock has resolved. In 99% of patients the bulbocavernosus reflex returns within 24 hours.[251] The presence of some neurologic function below the level of injury defines the injury as incomplete. Incomplete lesions have a better prognosis for recovery. Sacral sparing may be the only evidence of an incomplete lesion at the time of initial examination. Sacral sparing is evidenced by perianal sensation, voluntary rectal motor function, and great toe flexor activity. These findings indicate continued function of the lower sacral motor neurons and their connections to the cerebral cortex and improve the prognosis for recovery. Conversely, absence of these sacral nerve functions may be the only finding in a patient with an injury to the conus medullaris or cauda equina. Thus, complete examination of a patient with an SCI must include an assessment of these functions. The American Spinal Injury Association (ASIA) has produced an evaluation form to help ensure complete initial assessment of a patient with an SCI (Fig. 41–22). Another important evaluation at initial assessment is the degree of functional deficit. ASIA recommends using a modified version of the scale, described by Frankel and colleagues (Fig. 41–23).[83]

Thoracic or lumbar spinal injury after minor trauma should raise suspicion of a pathologic fracture. These injuries are most typically compression fractures, and the bone is usually obviously pathologic. Gaucher's disease, all of the mucopolysaccharidoses, osteogenesis imperfecta, idiopathic osteoporosis, metastatic neuroblastoma, Ewing's sarcoma, and leukemia may all be accompanied by back pain and multiple compression fractures (Fig. 41–24).[194,247]

Radiographic Findings

Radiographic imaging begins with a careful assessment of AP radiographs for clues to spinal column

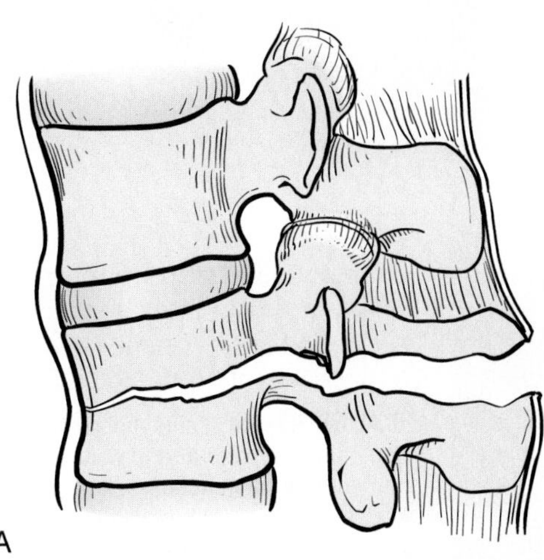

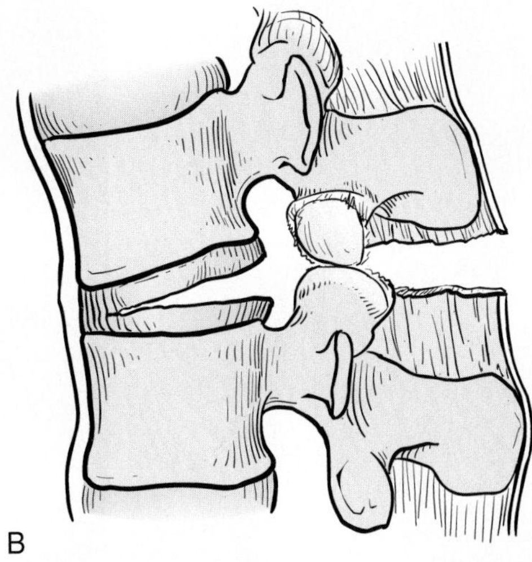

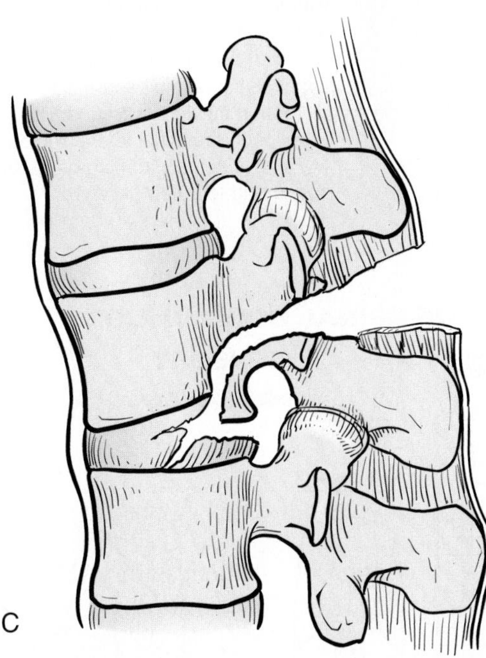

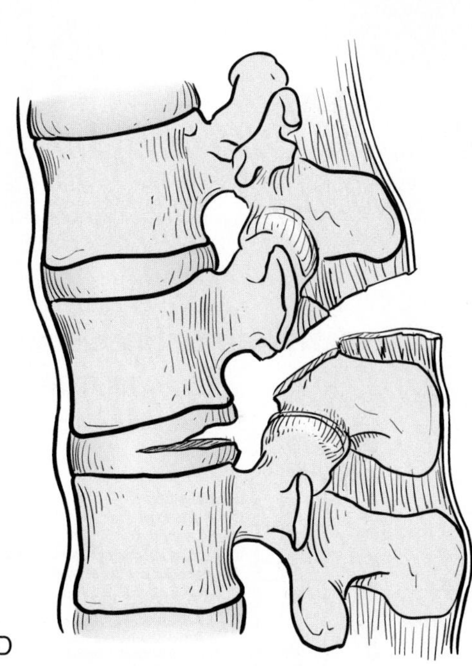

FIGURE 41–20 Flexion-distraction injuries commonly associated with seat belts. **A,** Single-level injury entirely through bone. **B,** Single-level injury entirely through soft tissue. **C,** Two-level injury primarily through bone. Although the supraspinous and interspinous ligaments are disrupted, there is a bony component of the injury in both the posterior and middle columns. This fracture will heal with cast immobilization. **D,** Two-level soft tissue injury. Again, the supraspinous and interspinous ligaments are disrupted. Although there is a fracture through the pars interarticularis, this injury is unlikely to heal with cast immobilization because of the soft tissue nature of the medial column injury.

injury, such as shortening of vertebral height, interpedicular widening, or asymmetry of the spinous process. Lateral radiographs often reveal the nature of the injury. They are particularly helpful for identifying injuries sustained from extension forces. CT defines the three-dimensional anatomy, including the extent of canal involvement. CT with sagittal reconstructions can be helpful in assessing areas that are difficult to see on plain radiographs, such as the cervicothoracic junction and upper thoracic spine (Fig. 41–25). However, CT without sagittal reconstructions may be of limited value in many injuries, including seat belt injuries, because the injury is in the axial plane and can be difficult to appreciate on axial CT scans.[98] MRI is the single best imaging tool for a traumatically injured spine. It provides direct information regarding the cord, canal, intervertebral disk, and posterior ligamentous structures. It is important to realize, however, that false-positive and false-negative MRI studies do occur. Recently, MRI findings at the time of injury have been correlated with functional neurologic outcome.[24,107,174]

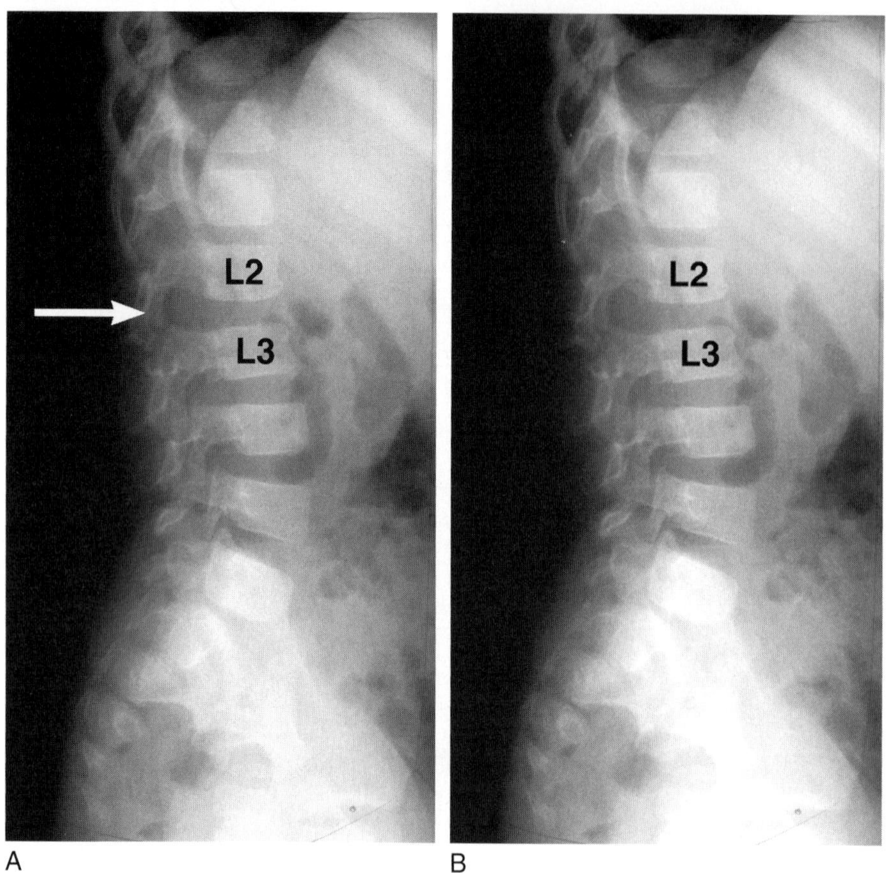

FIGURE 41-21 Initial imaging studies for thoracic and lumbar spine injuries may be nondiagnostic. **A,** Lateral radiograph of a 4-year-old girl involved in a high-speed motor vehicle accident. The films were initially interpreted as normal. **B,** Because of persistent back pain with localized tenderness in the lumbar spine, a flexion stress view was obtained and revealed an acute kyphosis caused by soft tissue disruption between L2 and L3. In retrospect, the initial lateral radiograph **(A)** shows some widening of the disk space and foramen (*arrow*).

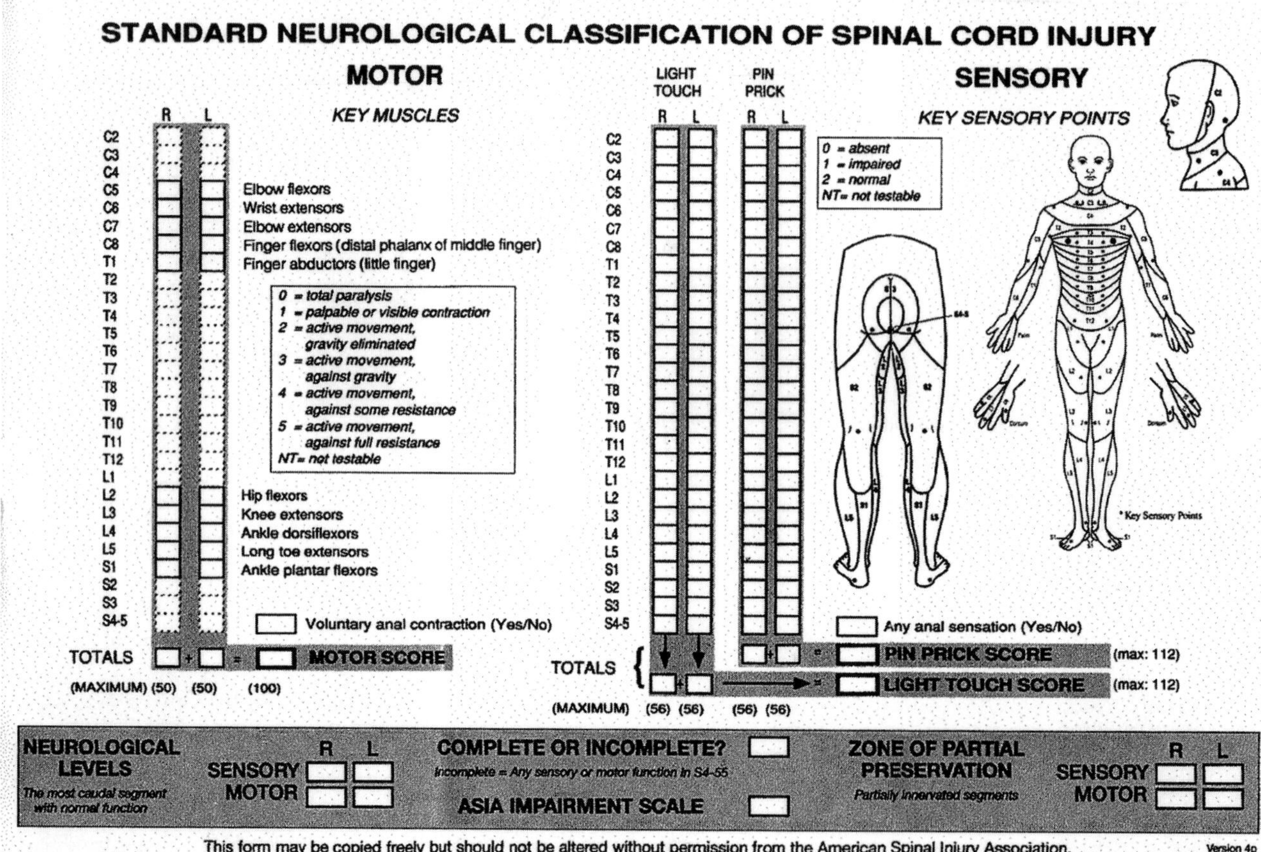

STANDARD NEUROLOGICAL CLASSIFICATION OF SPINAL CORD INJURY

MOTOR

KEY MUSCLES

R L

C2
C3
C4
C5 Elbow flexors
C6 Wrist extensors
C7 Elbow extensors
C8 Finger flexors (distal phalanx of middle finger)
T1 Finger abductors (little finger)
T2
T3
T4
T5
T6
T7
T8
T9
T10
T11
T12
L1
L2 Hip flexors
L3 Knee extensors
L4 Ankle dorsiflexors
L5 Long toe extensors
S1 Ankle plantar flexors
S2
S3
S4-5

0 = total paralysis
1 = palpable or visible contraction
2 = active movement, gravity eliminated
3 = active movement, against gravity
4 = active movement, against some resistance
5 = active movement, against full resistance
NT = not testable

Voluntary anal contraction (Yes/No)

TOTALS + = MOTOR SCORE

(MAXIMUM) (50) (50) (100)

LIGHT TOUCH
PIN PRICK

R L R L

C2 C3 C4 C5 C6 C7 C8 T1 T2 T3 T4 T5 T6 T7 T8 T9 T10 T11 T12 L1 L2 L3 L4 L5 S1 S2 S3 S4-5

SENSORY

KEY SENSORY POINTS

0 = absent
1 = impaired
2 = normal
NT = not testable

Any anal sensation (Yes/No)

TOTALS + = PIN PRICK SCORE (max: 112)

\+ = LIGHT TOUCH SCORE (max: 112)

(MAXIMUM) (56) (56) (56) (56)

* Key Sensory Points

NEUROLOGICAL LEVELS
The most caudal segment with normal function

R L
SENSORY
MOTOR

COMPLETE OR INCOMPLETE?
Incomplete = Any sensory or motor function in S4-S5

ASIA IMPAIRMENT SCALE

ZONE OF PARTIAL PRESERVATION
Partially innervated segments

R L
SENSORY
MOTOR

This form may be copied freely but should not be altered without permission from the American Spinal Injury Association.

Version 4p
GHC 1996

FIGURE 41-22 American Spinal Injury Association form for documentation of acute spinal cord injury. (From Standard Neurological Classification of Spinal Cord Injury, Version 4p, GHC 1996, published by the American Spinal Injury Association.)

Functional Independence Measure (FIM)

LEVELS		
	7 Complete Independence (Timely, Safely) 6 Modified Independence (Device)	No Helper
	Modified Dependence 5 Supervision 4 Minimal Assist (Subject = 75%+) 3 Moderate Assist (Subject = 50%+) **Complete Dependence** 2 Maximal Assist (Subject = 25%+) 1 Total Assist (Subject = 0%+)	Helper

	ADMIT	DISCH
Self Care		
A. Eating	☐	☐
B. Grooming	☐	☐
C. Bathing	☐	☐
D. Dressing-Upper Body	☐	☐
E. Dressing-Lower Body	☐	☐
F. Toileting	☐	☐
Sphincter Control		
G. Bladder Management	☐	☐
H. Bowel Management	☐	☐
Mobility		
Transfer:		
I. Bed, Chair, Wheelchair	☐	☐
J. Toilet	☐	☐
K. Tub, Shower	☐	☐
Locomotion		
L. Walk/wheelChair	W☐ C☐ ☐	W☐ C☐ ☐
M. Stairs	☐	☐
Communication		
N. Comprehension	A☐ V☐ ☐	A☐ V☐ ☐
O. Expression	V☐ N☐ ☐	V☐ N☐ ☐
Social Cognition		
P. Social Interaction	☐	☐
Q. Problem Solving	☐	☐
R. Memory	☐	☐
Total FIM	☐	☐

NOTE: Leave no blanks; enter 1 if patient not testable due to risk.

FIGURE 41-23 The Frankel scale of neurologic injury. (From Frankel HL, Hancock DO, Hyslop G, et al: The value of postural reduction in the initial management of closed injuries of the spine with paraplegia and tetraplegia. I. Paraplegia. 1969;7:179.)

Treatment

Treatment options for thoracic and lumbar spine injuries include symptomatic treatment with reassurance, brace or cast immobilization, and spinal fusion with or without decompression.

NONSURGICAL TREATMENT

Nonoperative treatment is appropriate for all minor injuries (fractures of the spinous and transverse processes, facets, and pars interarticularis), all compression fractures, "bony" seat belt injuries, and many burst fractures. Minor fractures usually require nothing more than symptomatic treatment. The most important aspect of these injuries is to realize that they are frequently the result of high-energy trauma and consequently may be associated with other, often intra-abdominal injuries.[267] Patients with minor fractures may be treated with a few days of bed rest, followed by a gradual return to normal activities. Bracing is not required, although a simple lumbar corset may afford significant pain relief (Fig. 41–26). The retroperitoneal hematoma associated with these injuries in the lumbar spine may produce a significant ileus, and patients being treated on an outpatient basis should be advised accordingly.[96,116]

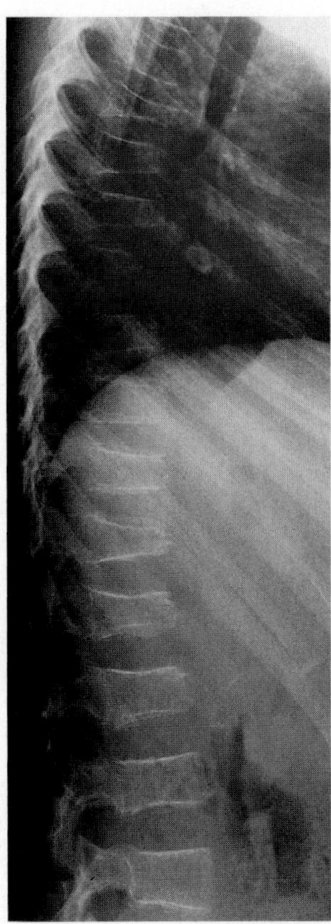

FIGURE 41-24 Lateral radiograph of a patient with back pain. Note the multiple compression fractures. A complete blood cell count revealed acute lymphoblastic leukemia.

Compression fractures can also be treated with simple conservative measures. Most patients with compression fractures are more comfortable with an extension brace.[98,116,140] Studies have shown no difference between bed rest and casting. Regardless of treatment, most patients are symptom-free within a few weeks.[126,130,179] Anterior vertebral height may be restored through remodeling, particularly in younger children.[5,127,139,194] Chance fractures that are entirely through bone (see Fig. 41–25A and C) will heal with immobilization in a hyperextension cast.[162,195,221,270,272]

Burst fractures in children occur most commonly in adolescents, and their management is similar to that for adults. However, management of burst fractures in adults continues to be debated.[40,52,95,122,144,189] We treat the majority of burst fractures in neurologically intact

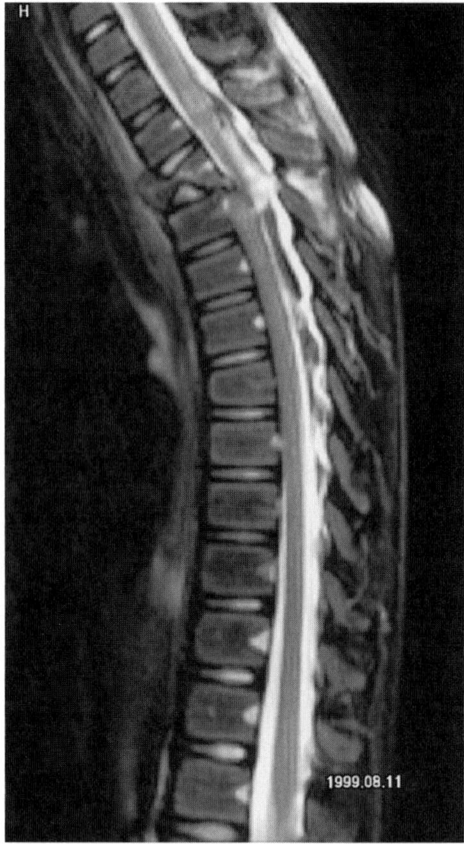

A

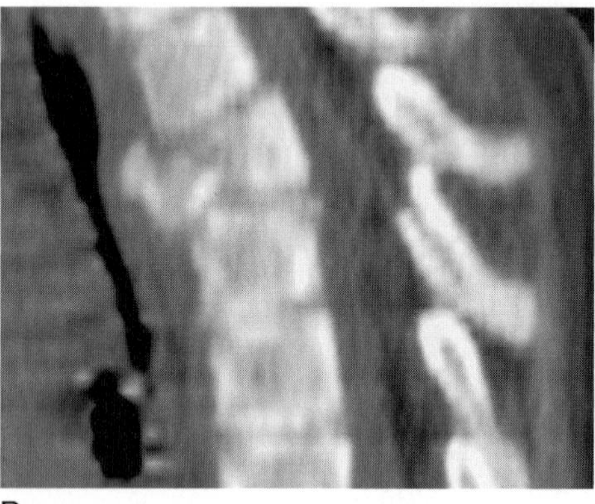

B

FIGURE 41–25 **A,** Sagittal magnetic resonance image of a patient with T3-4 fracture-dislocation. Plain lateral radiographs of this area are often difficult to interpret. **B,** A computed tomography scan with sagittal reconstruction demonstrates the bony deformity.

patients with a period of bed rest, followed by 6 to 12 weeks in a cast or thoracolumbosacral orthosis. Each fracture must be treated on an individual basis by taking into consideration the patient's age and associated injuries, as well as the amount of kyphosis, anterior collapse, and canal compromise. In general, more than 25 degrees of kyphosis (15 degrees if there is greater than 50% collapse of the anterior vertebral body) or 50% canal compromise is thought to preclude conservative treatment.[156,252] If canal compromise is the only surgical indication, it is important to bear in mind that several studies have documented reconstitution of the spinal canal with conservative treatment of burst fractures.[57,58,106,136,139,153,230,280]

SURGICAL TREATMENT

Indications for surgical treatment include the presence of neurologic deficits, seat belt injuries with posterior ligamentous injuries, burst fractures not amenable to conservative treatment, and fracture-dislocations. Surgical treatment consists of spinal fusion with or without decompression. We recommend decompression for all patients with incomplete neurologic injury. We rarely perform decompression in neurologically intact patients (aside from the decompression provided during reduction and stabilization). The decision to perform decompression in patients with complete lesions is made on an individual basis, with the knowledge that these patients have little potential for neurologic recovery. The optimal timing of surgical decompression is unknown. Ideally, decompression should be performed in the first 8 hours after injury. However, such timing is rarely possible. Advocates of early surgery stress the importance of prompt decompression, whereas others express concern that the surgical trauma can contribute to the edema-ischemia cycle.[67,156,187,197,264] The surgical approach is determined by the nature of the fracture and the necessity to decompress the canal. The technique for the surgical approach and instrumentation is the same as that described previously for anterior or posterior fusion for scoliosis (see Chapter 12, Scoliosis).

Most ligamentous seat belt injuries can be treated by simple posterior fusion. If the patient is large enough, we prefer to perform an instrumented fusion. If the patient is too small for even pediatric-size hook-and-rod systems, we perform a spinous process wiring and place the patient in a cast. (We also routinely immobilize patients treated with pediatric-size instrumentation with a cast. Older patients can frequently be managed with no immobilization or with a removable brace.) The length of the fusion is determined by the age of the patient and the extent of the injury. Young patients with a single-level injury may be treated with a two-level posterior fusion. Older patients with two-level injuries may require extension of the fusion two levels above and below (Fig. 41–27).

Burst fractures not amenable to conservative treatment and fracture-dislocations may be managed with either anterior or posterior fusion. In general, we prefer a posterior approach for reduction, decompression, and stabilization, although when circumstances dictate, we will perform decompression and fusion through an anterior approach. Again, the fusion levels are determined by the age of the patient and the magnitude and location of the injury. Advocates of short-segment fusion argue that this technique alters less of the "normal" spine. The trade-off is increased stress within the fused segment and increased risk for loss of correction and pseudarthrosis. Thus, the benefits of

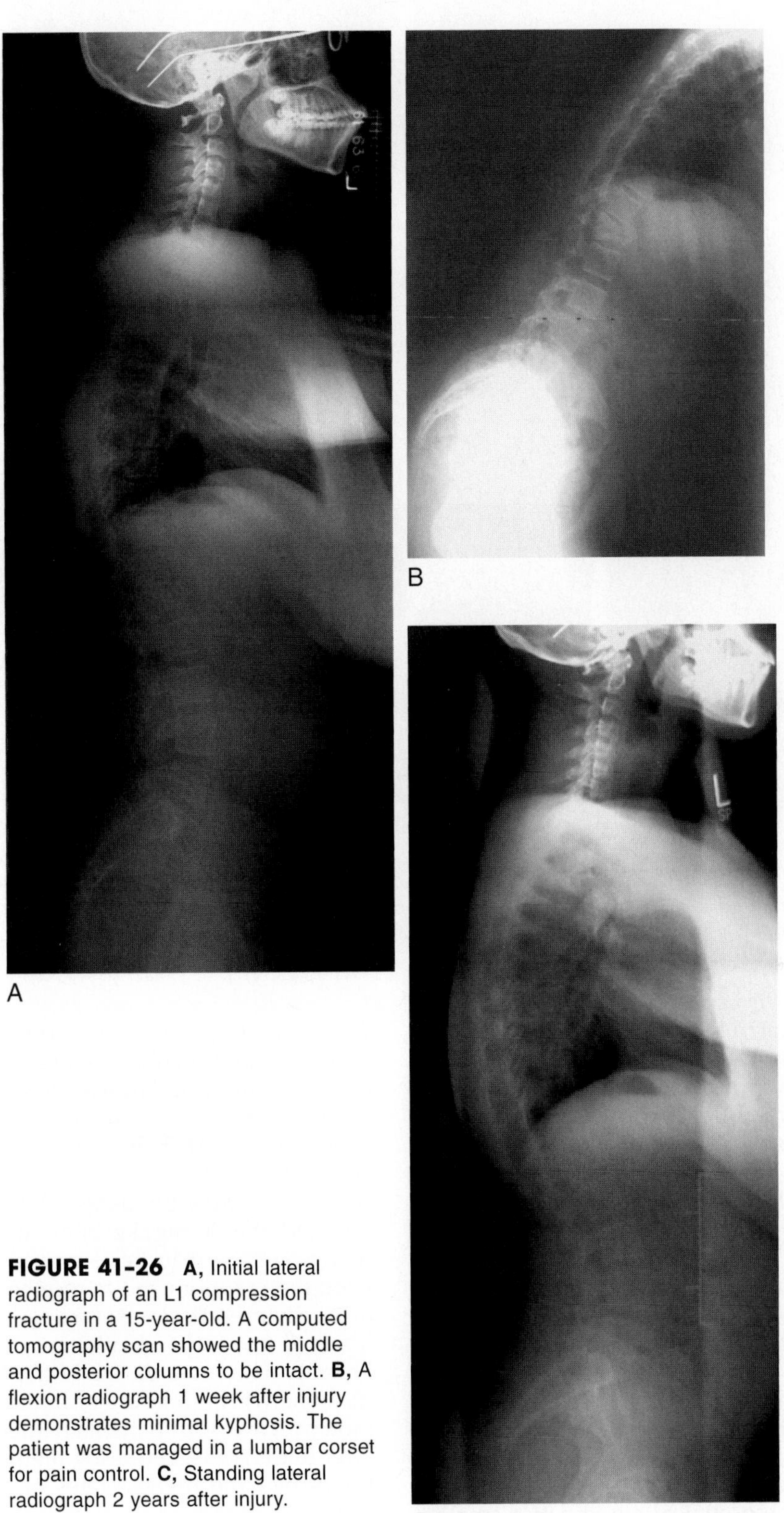

FIGURE 41–26 **A,** Initial lateral radiograph of an L1 compression fracture in a 15-year-old. A computed tomography scan showed the middle and posterior columns to be intact. **B,** A flexion radiograph 1 week after injury demonstrates minimal kyphosis. The patient was managed in a lumbar corset for pain control. **C,** Standing lateral radiograph 2 years after injury.

a shorter fusion segment must be weighed against the increased risk for nonunion or malunion. We believe that restitution of appropriate sagittal balance is a more important factor in the long-term prognosis than the length of the fusion.[23,26,74,155] Thus, we will extend the fusion to whatever level is required to provide a stable construct that can maintain sagittal balance (Fig. 41–28).

Regardless of the surgical plan, it is important to realize that pathology that was not appreciated preoperatively is occasionally uncovered intraoperatively. Subtle laminar, transverse process, or facet fractures

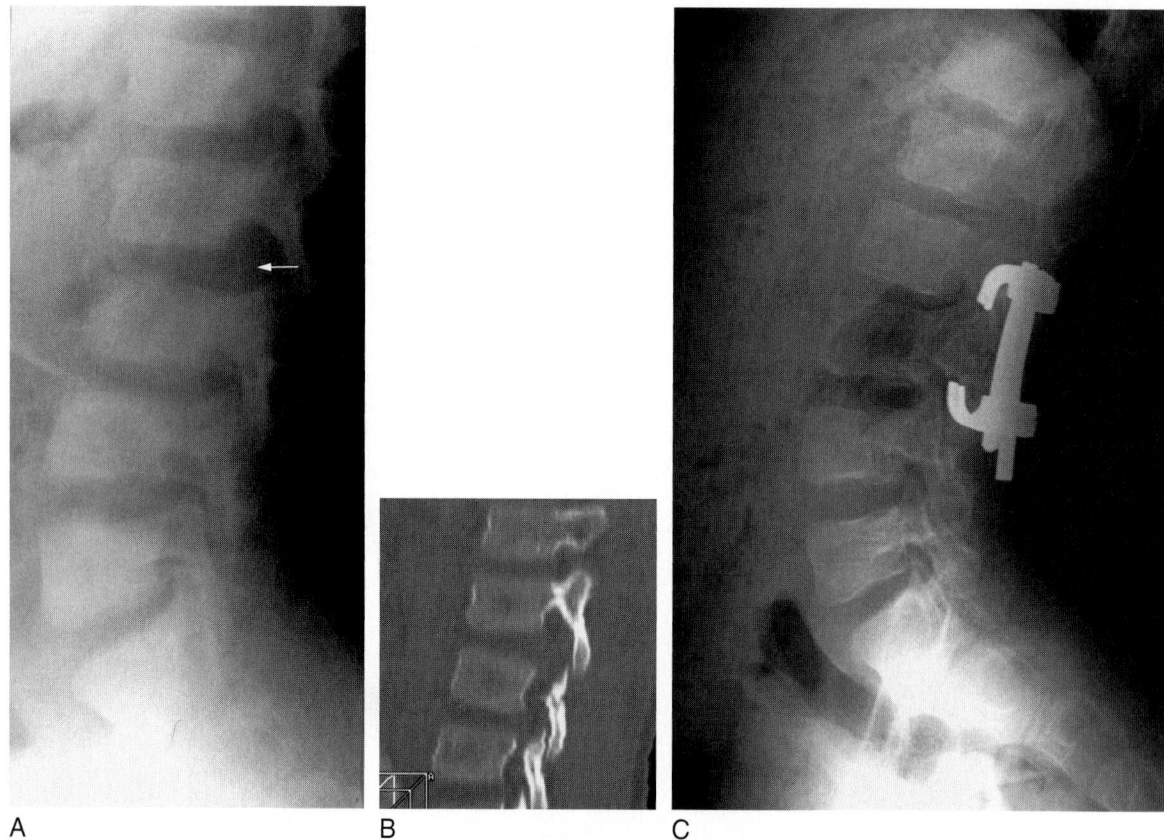

FIGURE 41–27 Soft tissue Chance fracture. **A,** Lateral radiograph showing acute kyphosis at L2-3 with a widened disk space and foramen (*arrow*). **B,** Computed tomography scan confirming the absence of bony involvement. **C,** Appearance 3 years after posterior L2-3 fusion.

discovered intraoperatively will force the surgeon to be flexible with the preoperative plan. Additionally, a traumatically injured spine should be approached cautiously because these subtle injuries may put undamaged neural elements at risk during exposure.

Pharmacologic Treatment of Spinal Cord Injury

A number of pharmacologic agents have been used in an attempt to improve neurologic recovery after SCI. The goal of these agents is to interrupt the cycle of edema and ischemic injury. Several drugs have shown promise in animal studies, including methylprednisolone, thyrotropin-releasing hormone, naloxone, and GM_1 ganglioside. However, only methylprednisolone has received widespread clinical attention. (GM_1 ganglioside has also shown clinical success in a smaller study.*) In 1990, the Second National Acute Spinal Cord Injury Study (NASCIS-II) was the first multicenter study to report improved recovery in patients treated with a pharmacologic agent. Patients who received methylprednisolone within 8 hours of either complete or incomplete SCI had a better neurologic outcome than did patients given placebo or naloxone. This study has been criticized for flaws in experimental design and incomplete data. Perhaps the most significant criticism of NASCIS-II is the lack of a functional outcome measure, which makes it impossible to determine whether the measured improvements were clinically relevant.[59,84,92,94,190,283] In 1997, the results of NASCIS-III were published. All patients in this study received the 30-mg/kg bolus of methylprednisolone that was shown to be useful in NASCIS-II. Patients were then randomized to receive either 24 or 48 hours of methylprednisolone at 5.4 mg/kg/hr or tirilazad, a lazaroid (an antioxidant), every 6 hours for 48 hours. Patients who received the initial bolus of methylprednisolone within 3 hours of injury had similar rates of motor recovery. In patients treated within 3 to 8 hours after injury, those receiving methylprednisolone for 48 hours had the highest rates of recovery, statistically greater than those who received only 24 hours of methylprednisolone. Patients given tirilazad recovered at a rate between the 48- and 24-hour methylprednisolone groups.

Although the NASCIS-II investigators reported no difference in morbidity or mortality between groups, several authors have expressed concern about the potentially adverse effects of massive steroid doses in polytraumatized patients.[59,94,190] Despite concerns, most studies assessing the NASCIS-II protocol are

*See references 29, 59, 84, 89-91, 110, 178, 190, 282, 283.

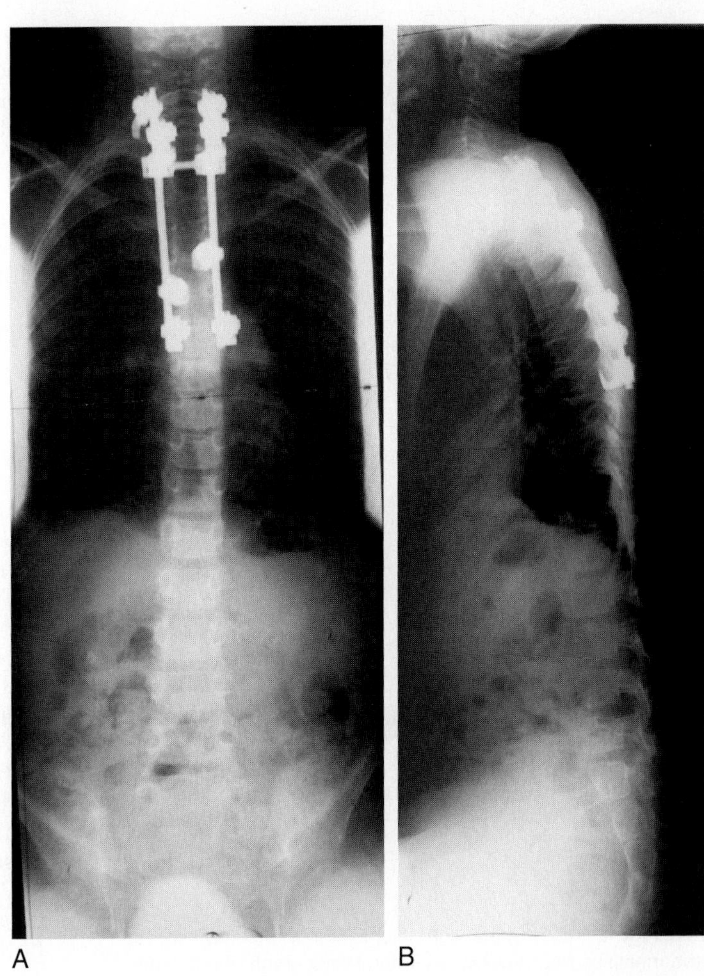

FIGURE 41–28 Postoperative sitting anteroposterior (**A**) and lateral (**B**) radiographs of the patient with T3-4 fracture dislocation shown in Figure 41–24.

similar to the report of Gerndt and colleagues, who noted an increased incidence of pneumonia and a longer intensive care unit stay, but no change in mortality and a decrease in the rehabilitation period.[94] The findings of NASCIS-III were similar: patients receiving 48 hours of methylprednisolone had higher rates of severe sepsis and pneumonia but no difference in mortality.[30]

We follow the recommendations of NASCIS-III. Patients with SCI who receive methylprednisolone within 3 hours of injury are maintained on the treatment regimen (5.4 mg/kg/hr) for 24 hours. When methylprednisolone therapy is initiated 3 to 8 hours after injury, we continue it for 48 hours.[30,59]

Spinal Cord Injury without Radiographic Abnormality

This lesion is overwhelmingly found in children. (Adults may sustain cord injury without fracture but usually have a ligamentous injury noted on MRI.[105]) The term SCIWORA as applied to children was coined by Pang and Wilberger in 1982.[200] In the era of MRI this acronym my be outdated because most, if not all, patients with SCIWORA will have abnormal findings on MRI.[158,166,198] The pathogenesis of SCIWORA lies in the fact that the spinal column is more elastic than the spinal cord. Thus, the spinal column can stretch beyond the elastic limit of the neural elements.[151,196,199,200] When the deforming force is removed, the spinal column returns to its normal state, but the cord is left permanently damaged (Fig. 41–29A). SCIWORA has been reported to account for 15% to 35% of SCIs in children.[63,108,151,196,225] SCIWORA may occur at any age and at any location, but it is most common in the cervical spine. In Pang and Wilberger's original series, half the children had a delay in onset of paralysis of up to 4 days.[200]

The characteristics of SCIWORA vary with age. SCIWORA is more common in young children, who frequently have complete lesions of the cervical spine, with a poor prognosis for neurologic recovery. The disproportionately large head of young children probably serves as the force that deforms the cervical spine beyond the physiologic limit of the cervical cord. Adolescents are more likely to have incomplete lesions, with a better prognosis for recovery.[63,105,196,199,200]

SCIWORA is a diagnosis of exclusion. Therefore, the initial evaluation and management are the same as for any child with an SCI. After initial assessment and resuscitation, plain radiographs and, if indicated, CT scans are obtained. If the preliminary studies fail to reveal pathology, MRI is usually performed. MRI is

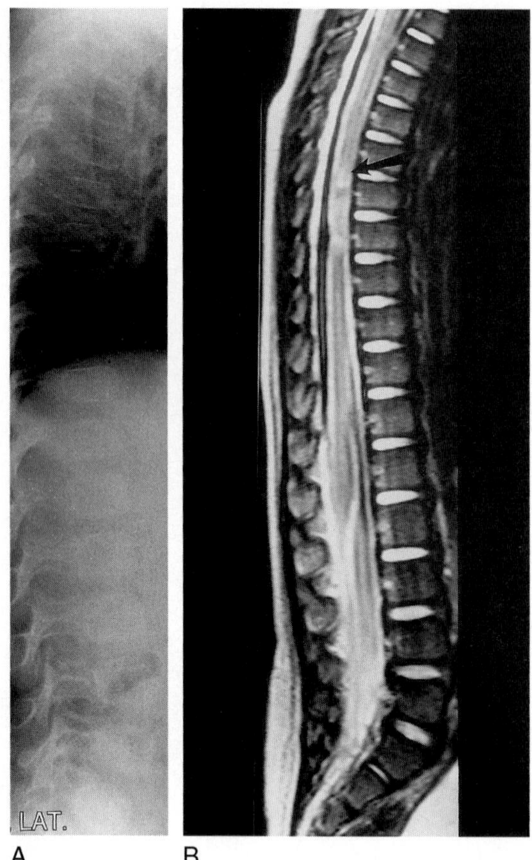

FIGURE 41–29 Spinal cord injury without radiographic abnormalities (SCIWORA). **A,** Lateral radiograph of a patient involved in a high-speed motor vehicle accident who sustained bilateral lower extremity paralysis. There is no abnormality. **B,** Mid-sagittal magnetic resonance image. Note the increased signal within the spinal cord (*arrow*).

diagnostic and reveals abnormal signal in the cord in the absence of changes in the spinal column (Fig. 41–29B).[102] Once the diagnosis has been established, the entire spine should be imaged and the patient treated with spine precautions until awake and alert. Patients seen within 8 hours of injury should be treated with methylprednisolone per the NASCIS-III guidelines. Once the child is awake, alert, and cooperative, dynamic flexion-extension radiographs should be obtained to ensure that there is no subtle ligamentous pathology.

Immobilization of patients with SCIWORA may seem unnecessary because there is, by definition, no abnormality of the spinal column. However, Pang and Pollack noted that 8 (15%) of 55 children with SCIWORA suffered a second SCIWORA 3 days to 10 weeks after their initial injury.[199] They hypothesized that the initial injury made the spine "incipiently unstable" and susceptible to additional, often more severe, neurologic trauma. More recently, Bosch and colleagues published a review that included this same cohort of patients from Children's Hospital of Pittsburgh. Interestingly, they could not identify any patient with permanent neurologic deficit from recurrent SCIWORA and could not identify any benefit from bracing.[28] These conflicting data from one institution make treatment recommendations difficult. It appears that the neurologic risk from secondary SCIWORA is low; thus, the decision to immobilize a patient must be made on an individual basis. Although we still brace patients with "significant" neurologic injury, we believe that bracing for "low-energy" SCIWORA is probably not warranted.[196,199,200,212]

Complications after Spinal Cord Injury

Complications after spine injuries without neurologic deficit are uncommon. Growth arrest or deformity is unusual in children younger than 10 years because of their great remodeling capacity.[5,116,126,130,131,133,214] This ability may be compromised if the end-plate is damaged because it contains the physis. As Roaf has shown, end-plate damage is most likely to occur from the nucleus pulposus during axial loading.[223] Any of the complications associated with spinal fusion, including infection (early or delayed), instrumentation failure, loss of correction, and pseudarthrosis, may develop in patients treated operatively.

Patients with spinal injuries producing a neurologic deficit frequently experience complications. Acute complications include pneumonia, sepsis, autonomic dysreflexia, and pulmonary embolism.[150] In a review of 28,692 pediatric trauma patients, deep vein thrombosis developed in 6 and pulmonary embolism in 2. Both patients with pulmonary embolism had an SCI. The overall incidence of pulmonary embolism was 0.000069%. However, in patients with SCI the incidence was 1.85%.[176] Although deep vein thrombosis and pulmonary embolism are rarely seen in children, prophylaxis would seem prudent in children with SCI.[181]

The long-term complications of patients with SCI are severe. All the complications associated with myelomeningocele can potentially develop in these children; in fact, we routinely refer all patients with SCI to our multidisciplinary spina bifida clinic. In addition to pulmonary and urologic problems, pressure sores, syringomyelia, and scoliosis may develop. Since the advent of MRI, syringomyelia has been noted frequently after SCI. Syringomyelia may develop in the first few months after SCI or decades later. It is more common in patients with complete lesions. The most common initial symptoms include pain, dysesthesias, increased tone, and weakness.[69,81,101,149,209,210,224,241]

Scoliosis is the most common complication of SCI in children. Its incidence has been reported to be between 85% and 100% in patients injured before the adolescent growth spurt, and it does not appear to be related to the level of injury. Mehta and associates found brace treatment effective in delaying surgical treatment of scoliosis after SCI if bracing is initiated when the curves were small, less than 20 degrees. They suggested that bracing may prevent the need for surgery if initiated early (<10 degrees). They did not find an effect of bracing curves greater than 20

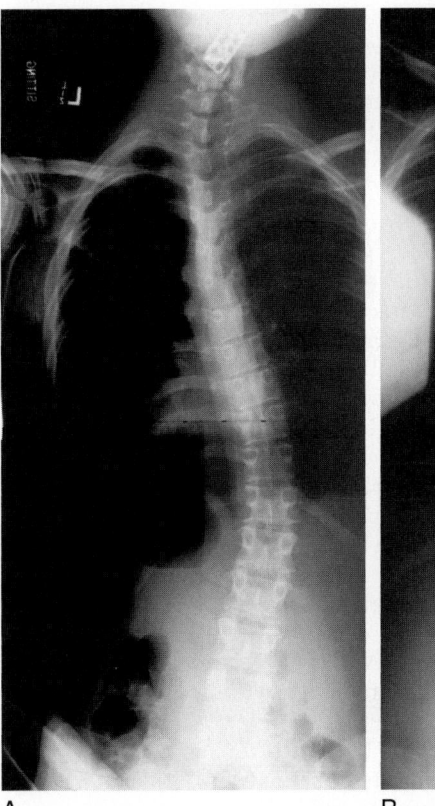

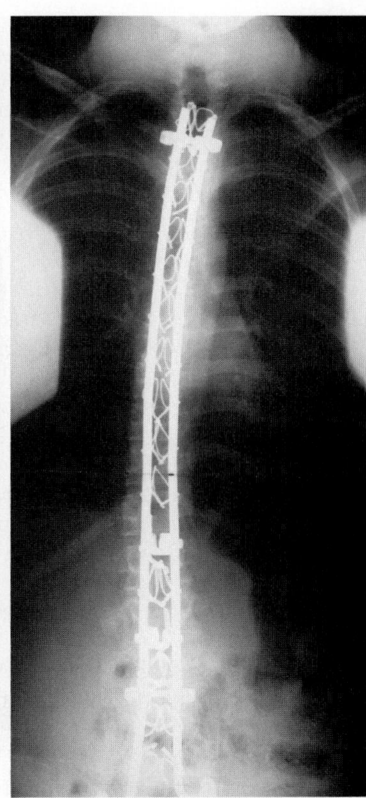

A B

FIGURE 41–30 **A,** Sitting anteroposterior (AP) radiograph of a patient several years after C3-4 fracture-dislocation. Note the long neuromuscular scoliosis and the anterior cervical plate. **B,** AP radiograph after posterior spinal fusion from T2 to the sacrum.

degrees.[180] If untreated, paralytic scoliosis can lead to sitting imbalance and pulmonary problems. It is best treated by posterior spinal fusion from the high thoracic spine to the sacrum. Younger patients in whom the crankshaft phenomenon is a concern and patients with large, stiff curves may benefit from anterior spinal release and fusion (Fig. 41–30).[11,25,32,56,76,145,157,185,213,235,256]

References

1. Abad C, Marti M, Marrero L, et al: [Paraplegia following surgical repair of a ductus and of a coarctation of the aorta in childhood.] Cir Pediatr 1993;6:84.
2. Abel MS: Transverse posterior element fractures associated with torsion. Skeletal Radiol 1989;17:556.
3. Abroms IF, Bresnan MJ, Zuckerman JE, et al: Cervical cord injuries secondary to hyperextension of the head in breech presentations. Obstet Gynecol 1973;41:369.
4. Agran PF, Dunkle DE, Winn DG: Injuries to a sample of seat-belted children evaluated and treated in a hospital emergency room. J Trauma 1987;27:58.
5. Akbarnia BA: Pediatric spine fractures. Orthop Clin North Am 1999;30:521.
6. Allen JP: Birth injury to the spinal cord. Northwest Med 1970;69:323.
7. Alp MS, Crockard HA: Late complication of undetected odontoid fracture in children. BMJ 1990;300:319.
8. Anderson JM, Schutt AH: Spinal injury in children: A review of 156 cases seen from 1950 through 1978. Mayo Clin Proc 1980;55:499.
9. Anderson LD, D'Alonzo RT: Fractures of the odontoid process of the axis. J Bone Joint Surg Am 1974;56:1663.
10. Anderson PA, Henley MB, Rivara FP, et al: Flexion distraction and chance injuries to the thoracolumbar spine. J Orthop Trauma 1991;5:153.
11. Apple DF Jr, Anson CA, Hunter JD, et al: Spinal cord injury in youth. Clin Pediatr (Phila) 1995;34:90.
12. Apple JS, Kirks DR, Merten DF, et al: Cervical spine fractures and dislocations in children. Pediatr Radiol 1987;17:45.
13. Athey AM: A 3-year-old with spinal cord injury without radiographic abnormality (SCIWORA). J Emerg Nurs 1991;17:380.
14. Aufdermaur M: Spinal injuries in juveniles. Necropsy findings in twelve cases. J Bone Joint Surg Br 1974;56:513.
15. Bailey DK: The normal cervical spine in infants and children. Radiology 1952;59:712.
16. Banniza von Bazan UK, Paeslack V: Scoliotic growth in children with acquired paraplegia [proceedings]. Paraplegia 1977;15:65.
17. Bertolami CN, Kaban LB: Chin trauma: A clue to associated mandibular and cervical spine injury. Oral Surg Oral Med Oral Pathol 1982;53:122.
18. Betz RR, Gelman AJ, DeFilipp GJ, et al: Magnetic resonance imaging (MRI) in the evaluation of spinal cord injured children and adolescents. Paraplegia 1987;25:92.
19. Bhattacharyya SK: Fracture and displacement of the odontoid process in a child. J Bone Joint Surg Am 1974;56:1071.

20. Birney TJ, Hanley EN Jr: Traumatic cervical spine injuries in childhood and adolescence. Spine 1989;14:1277.
21. Bivins HG, Ford S, Bezmalinovic Z, et al: The effect of axial traction during orotracheal intubation of the trauma victim with an unstable cervical spine. Ann Emerg Med 1988;17:25.
22. Blauth M, Schmidt U, Lange U: [Injuries of the cervical spine in children.] Unfallchirurg 1998;101:590.
23. Boachie-Adjei O, Dendrinos GK, Ogilvie JW, et al: Management of adult spinal deformity with combined anterior-posterior arthrodesis and Luque-Galveston instrumentation. J Spinal Disord 1991;4:131.
24. Bondurant FJ, Cotler HB, Kulkarni MV, et al: Acute spinal cord injury. A study using physical examination and magnetic resonance imaging. Spine 1990;15:161.
25. Bonnett C, Brown JC, Perry J, et al: Evolution of treatment of paralytic scoliosis at Rancho Los Amigos Hospital. J Bone Joint Surg Am 1975;57:206.
26. Booth KC, Bridwell KH, Lenke LG, et al: Complications and predictive factors for the successful treatment of flatback deformity (fixed sagittal imbalance). Spine 1999;24:1712.
27. Born CT, Ross SE, Iannacone WM, et al: Delayed identification of skeletal injury in multisystem trauma: The "missed" fracture. J Trauma 1989;29:1643.
28. Bosch PP, Vogt MT, Ward WT: Pediatric spinal cord injury without radiographic abnormality (SCIWORA): The absence of occult instability and lack of indication for bracing. Spine 2002;27:2788.
29. Bracken MB: Pharmacological treatment of acute spinal cord injury: Current status and future projects. J Emerg Med 1993;11(Suppl 1):43.
30. Bracken MB, Shepard MJ, Holford TR, et al: Administration of methylprednisolone for 24 or 48 hours or tirilazad mesylate for 48 hours in the treatment of acute spinal cord injury. Results of the Third National Acute Spinal Cord Injury Randomized Controlled Trial. National Acute Spinal Cord Injury Study. JAMA 1997;277:1597.
31. Bresnan MJ, Abroms IF: Neonatal spinal cord transection secondary to intrauterine hyperextension of the neck in breech presentation. J Pediatr 1974;84:734.
32. Bridwell KH, O'Brien MF, Lenke LG, et al: Posterior spinal fusion supplemented with only allograft bone in paralytic scoliosis. Does it work? Spine 1994;19:2658.
33. Brown RL, Brunn MA, Garcia VF: Cervical spine injuries in children: A review of 103 patients treated consecutively at a level 1 pediatric trauma center. J Pediatr Surg 2001;36:1107.
34. Browne GJ, Lam LT, Barker RA: The usefulness of a modified adult protocol for the clearance of paediatric cervical spine injury in the emergency department. Emerg Med (Fremantle) 2003;15:133.
35. Bucholz RW, Burkhead WZ: The pathological anatomy of fatal atlanto-occipital dislocations. J Bone Joint Surg Am 1979;61:248.
36. Burke DC: Traumatic spinal paralysis in children. Paraplegia 1974;11:268.
37. Caird MS, Reddy S, Ganley TJ, et al: Cervical spine fracture-dislocation birth injury: Prevention, recognition, and implications for the orthopaedic surgeon. J Pediatr Orthop 2005;25:484.
38. Campanelli M, Kattner KA, Stroink A, et al: Posterior C1-C2 transarticular screw fixation in the treatment of displaced type II odontoid fractures in the geriatric population—review of seven cases. Surg Neurol 1999;51:596.
39. Campbell J, Bonnett C: Spinal cord injury in children. Clin Orthop Relat Res 1975;112:114.
40. Carl AL, Tranmer BI, Sachs BL: Anterolateral dynamized instrumentation and fusion for unstable thoracolumbar and lumbar burst fractures. Spine 1997;22:686.
41. Carreon LY, Glassman SD, Campbell MJ: Pediatric spine fractures: A review of 137 hospital admissions. J Spinal Disord Tech 2004;17:477.
42. Cattell HS, Filtzer DL: Pseudosubluxation and other normal variations in the cervical spine in children. A study of one hundred and sixty children. J Bone Joint Surg Am 1965;47:1295.
43. Chance GQ: Note on a type of flexion fracture of the spine. Br J Radiol 1948;21:432.
44. Chang CH, Holmes JF, Mower WR, et al: Distracting injuries in patients with vertebral injuries. J Emerg Med 2005;28:147.
45. Cheng JC, Aguilar J, Leung PC: Hip reconstruction for femoral head loss from septic arthritis in children. A preliminary report. Clin Orthop Relat Res 1995;314:214.
46. Choi JU, Hoffman HJ, Hendrick EB, et al: Traumatic infarction of the spinal cord in children. J Neurosurg 1986;65:608.
47. Cirak B, Ziegfeld S, Knight VM, et al: Spinal injuries in children. J Pediatr Surg 2004;39:607.
48. Clark W, Gehweiler JA, Laib R: Twelve significant signs of cervical spine trauma. Skeletal Radiol 1979;3:201.
49. Cotler HB, Kulkarni MV, Bondurant FJ: Magnetic resonance imaging of acute spinal cord trauma: Preliminary report. J Orthop Trauma 1988;2:1.
50. Cramer KE: The pediatric polytrauma patient. Clin Orthop Relat Res 1995;318:125.
51. Crawford AH: Operative treatment of spine fractures in children. Orthop Clin North Am 1990;21:325.
52. Cresswell TR, Marshall PD, Smith RB: Mechanical stability of the AO internal spinal fixation system compared with that of the Hartshill rectangle and sublaminar wiring in the management of unstable burst fractures of the thoracic and lumbar spine. Spine 1998;23:111.
53. Cullen JC: Spinal lesions in battered babies. J Bone Joint Surg Br 1975;57:364.
54. Dake MD, Jacobs RP, Margolin FR: Computed tomography of posterior lumbar apophyseal ring fractures. J Comput Assist Tomogr 1985;9:730.
55. Darwish H, Archer C, Modin J: The anterior spinal artery collateral in coarctation of the aorta. A clinical angiographic correlation. Arch Neurol 1979;36:240.
56. Dearolf WW 3rd, Betz RR, Vogel LC, et al: Scoliosis in pediatric spinal cord–injured patients. J Pediatr Orthop 1990;10:214.
57. Deburge A, Blamoutier A: [Remodeling of the spinal canal after comminuted fracture of the spine. Apropos of a case.] Rev Chir Orthop Reparatrice Appar Mot 1992;78:124.

58. de Klerk LW, Fontijne WP, Stijnen T, et al: Spontaneous remodeling of the spinal canal after conservative management of thoracolumbar burst fractures. Spine 1998; 23:1057.
59. Delamarter RB, Coyle J: Acute management of spinal cord injury. J Am Acad Orthop Surg 1999;7:166.
60. Denis F: The three column spine and its significance in the classification of acute thoracolumbar spinal injuries. Spine 1983;8:817.
61. Diamond P, Hansen CM, Christofersen MR: Child abuse presenting as a thoracolumbar spinal fracture dislocation: A case report. Pediatr Emerg Care 1994; 10:83.
62. Dickman CA, Rekate HL, Sonntag VK, et al: Pediatric spinal trauma: Vertebral column and spinal cord injuries in children. Pediatr Neurosci 1989;15:237.
63. Dickman CA, Zabramski JM, Hadley MN, et al: Pediatric spinal cord injury without radiographic abnormalities: Report of 26 cases and review of the literature. J Spinal Disord 1991;4:296.
64. Diekema DS, Allen DB: Odontoid fracture in a child occupying a child restraint seat. Pediatrics 1988;82:117.
65. Dietrich AM, Ginn-Pease ME, Bartkowski HM, et al: Pediatric cervical spine fractures: Predominantly subtle presentation. J Pediatr Surg 1991;26:995.
66. Dogan S, Safavi-Abbasi S, Theodore N, et al: Pediatric subaxial cervical spine injuries: Origins, management, and outcome in 51 patients. Neurosurg Focus 2006;20: E1.
67. Duh MS, Shepard MJ, Wilberger JE, et al: The effectiveness of surgery on the treatment of acute spinal cord injury and its relation to pharmacological treatment. Neurosurgery 1994;35:240.
68. Eleraky MA, Theodore N, Adams M, et al: Pediatric cervical spine injuries: Report of 102 cases and review of the literature. J Neurosurg 2000;92:12.
69. el Masry WS, Biyani A: Incidence, management, and outcome of post-traumatic syringomyelia. In memory of Mr Bernard Williams. J Neurol Neurosurg Psychiatry 1996;60:141.
70. Epstein NE, Epstein JA: Limbus lumbar vertebral fractures in 27 adolescents and adults. Spine 1991;16: 962.
71. Evans DL, Bethem D: Cervical spine injuries in children. J Pediatr Orthop 1989;9:563.
72. Evarts CM: Traumatic occipito-atlantal dislocation. J Bone Joint Surg Am 1970;52:1653.
73. Ewald FC: Fracture of the odontoid process in a seventeen-month-old infant treated with a halo. A case report and discussion of the injury under the age of three. J Bone Joint Surg Am 1971;53:1636.
74. Farcy JP, Schwab FJ: Management of flatback and related kyphotic decompensation syndromes. Spine 1997;22:2452.
75. Farley FA, Gebarski SS, Garton HL: Tectorial membrane injuries in children. J Spinal Disord Tech 2005;18:136.
76. Farley FA, Hensinger RN, Herzenberg JE: Cervical spinal cord injury in children. J Spinal Disord 1992; 5:410.
77. Ferrandez L, Usabiaga J, Curto JM, et al: Atypical multivertebral fracture due to hyperextension in an adolescent girl. A case report. Spine 1989;14:645.
78. Fielding JW: Disappearance of the central portion of the odontoid process: A case report. J Bone Joint Surg Am 1965;47:1228.
79. Fielding JW, Cochran GB, Lawsing JF 3rd, et al: Tears of the transverse ligament of the atlas. A clinical and biomechanical study. J Bone Joint Surg Am 1974;56: 1683.
80. Fielding JW, Hensinger RN, Hawkins RJ: Os Odontoideum. J Bone Joint Surg Am 1980;62:376.
81. Foo D, Bignami A, Rossier AB: A case of post-traumatic syringomyelia. Neuropathological findings after 1 year of cystic drainage. Paraplegia 1989;27:63.
82. Frank JB, Lim CK, Flynn JM, et al: The efficacy of magnetic resonance imaging in pediatric cervical spine clearance. Spine 2002;27:1176.
83. Frankel HL, Hancock DO, Hyslop G, et al: The value of postural reduction in the initial management of closed injuries of the spine with paraplegia and tetraplegia. I. Paraplegia 1969;7:179.
84. Gabler C, Maier R: [Clinical experiences and results of high-dosage methylprednisolone therapy in spinal cord trauma 1991 to 1993.] Unfallchirurgie 1995;21: 20.
85. Gabriel KR, Crawford AH: Identification of acute posttraumatic spinal cord cyst by magnetic resonance imaging: A case report and review of the literature. J Pediatr Orthop 1988;8:710.
86. Galindo MJ Jr, Francis WR: Atlantal fracture in a child through congenital anterior and posterior arch defects. A case report. Clin Orthop Relat Res 1983;178:220.
87. Gebhard JS, Schimmer RC, Jeanneret B: Safety and accuracy of transarticular screw fixation C1-C2 using an aiming device. An anatomic study. Spine 1998;23: 2185.
88. Geck MJ, Yoo S, Wang JC: Assessment of cervical ligamentous injury in trauma patients using MRI. J Spinal Disord 2001;14:371.
89. Geisler FH: GM-1 ganglioside and motor recovery following human spinal cord injury. J Emerg Med 1993; 11(Suppl 1):49.
90. Geisler FH: Clinical trials of pharmacotherapy for spinal cord injury. Ann N Y Acad Sci 1998;845:374.
91. Geisler FH, Dorsey FC, Coleman WP: Recovery of motor function after spinal-cord injury—a randomized, placebo-controlled trial with GM-1 ganglioside. N Engl J Med 1991;324:1829.
92. George ER, Scholten DJ, Buechler CM, et al: Failure of methylprednisolone to improve the outcome of spinal cord injuries. Am Surg 1995;61:659.
93. Georgopoulos G, Pizzutillo PD, Lee MS: Occipito-atlantal instability in children. A report of five cases and review of the literature. J Bone Joint Surg Am 1987;69:429.
94. Gerndt SJ, Rodriguez JL, Pawlik JW, et al: Consequences of high-dose steroid therapy for acute spinal cord injury. J Trauma 1997;42:279.
95. Ghanayem AJ, Zdeblick TA: Anterior instrumentation in the management of thoracolumbar burst fractures. Clin Orthop Relat Res 1997;335:89.
96. Gilsanz V, Miranda J, Cleveland R, et al: Scoliosis secondary to fractures of the transverse processes of lumbar vertebrae. Radiology 1980;134:627.

97. Glasauer FE, Cares HL: Traumatic paraplegia in infancy. JAMA 1972;219:38.
98. Glass RB, Sivit CJ, Sturm PF, et al: Lumbar spine injury in a pediatric population: Difficulties with computed tomographic diagnosis. J Trauma 1994;37:815.
99. Glassman SD, Johnson JR, Holt RT: Seat belt injuries in children. J Trauma 1992;33:882.
100. Godard J, Hadji M, Raul JS: Odontoid fractures in the child with neurological injury. Direct anterior osteosynthesis with a cortico-spongious screw and literature review. Childs Nerv Syst 1997;13:105.
101. Goldstein B, Hammond MC, Stiens SA, et al: Posttraumatic syringomyelia: Profound neuronal loss, yet preserved function. Arch Phys Med Rehabil 1998;79:107.
102. Grabb PA, Pang D: Magnetic resonance imaging in the evaluation of spinal cord injury without radiographic abnormality in children. Neurosurgery 1994;35:406.
103. Grantham SA, Dick HM, Thompson RC Jr, et al: Occipitocervical arthrodesis. Indications, technic and results. Clin Orthop Relat Res 1969;65:118.
104. Griffiths SC: Fracture of odontoid process in children. J Pediatr Surg 1972;7:680.
105. Gupta SK, Rajeev K, Khosla VK, et al: Spinal cord injury without radiographic abnormality in adults. Spinal Cord 1999;37:726.
106. Ha KI, Han SH, Chung M, et al: A clinical study of the natural remodeling of burst fractures of the lumbar spine. Clin Orthop Relat Res 1996;323:210.
107. Hackney DB, Finkelstein SD, Hand CM, et al: Postmortem magnetic resonance imaging of experimental spinal cord injury: Magnetic resonance findings versus in vivo functional deficit. Neurosurgery 1994;35:1104.
108. Hadley MN, Zabramski JM, Browner CM, et al: Pediatric spinal trauma. Review of 122 cases of spinal cord and vertebral column injuries. J Neurosurg 1988;68:18.
109. Haid RW Jr, Subach BR, McLaughlin MR, et al: C1-C2 transarticular screw fixation for atlantoaxial instability: A 6-year experience. Neurosurgery 2001;49:65.
110. Hamilton AJ, Black PM, Carr DB: Contrasting actions of naloxone in experimental spinal cord trauma and cerebral ischemia: A review. Neurosurgery 1985;17:845.
111. Hamilton MG, Myles ST: Pediatric spinal injury: Review of 174 hospital admissions. J Neurosurg 1992;77:700.
112. Hamilton MG, Myles ST: Pediatric spinal injury: Review of 61 deaths. J Neurosurg 1992;77:705.
113. Harrington T, Barker B: Multiple trauma associated with vertebral injury. Surg Neurol 1986;26:149.
114. Harris MB, Kronlage SC, Carboni PA, et al: Evaluation of the cervical spine in the polytrauma patient. Spine 2000;25:2884.
115. Hasue M, Hoshino R, Omata S, et al: Cervical spine injuries in children. Fukushima J Med Sci 1974;20:115.
116. Hegenbarth R, Ebel KD: Roentgen findings in fractures of the vertebral column in childhood examination of 35 patients and its results. Pediatr Radiol 1976;5:34.
117. Heilman CB, Riesenburger RI: Simultaneous noncontiguous cervical spine injuries in a pediatric patient: Case report. Neurosurgery 2001;49:1017.
118. Henrys P, Lyne ED, Lifton C, et al: Clinical review of cervical spine injuries in children. Clin Orthop Relat Res 1977;129:172.
119. Herkowitz HN, Samberg LC: Vertebral column injuries associated with tobogganing. J Trauma 1978;18:806.
120. Hernandez JA, Chupik C, Swischuk LE: Cervical spine trauma in children under 5 years: Productivity of CT. Emerg Radiol 2004;10:176.
121. Herzenberg JE, Hensinger RN, Dedrick DK, et al: Emergency transport and positioning of young children who have an injury of the cervical spine. The standard backboard may be hazardous. J Bone Joint Surg Am 1989;71:15.
122. Hitchon PW, Torner JC, Haddad SF, et al: Management options in thoracolumbar burst fractures. Surg Neurol 1998;49:619.
123. Hoffman MA, Spence LJ, Wesson DE, et al: The pediatric passenger: Trends in seat belt use and injury patterns. J Trauma 1987;27:974.
124. Hogan GJ, Mirvis SE, Shanmuganathan K, et al: Exclusion of unstable cervical spine injury in obtunded patients with blunt trauma: Is MR imaging needed when multi-detector row CT findings are normal? Radiology 2005;237:106.
125. Holley J, Jorden R: Airway management in patients with unstable cervical spine fractures. Ann Emerg Med 1989;18:1237.
126. Horal J, Nachemson A, Scheller S: Clinical and radiological long term follow-up of vertebral fractures in children. Acta Orthop Scand 1972;43:491.
127. Horsley MW, Taylor TK: Spontaneous correction of a traumatic kyphosis after posterior spinal fusion in an infant. J Spinal Disord 1997;10:256.
128. Hosalkar HS, Cain EL, Horn D, et al: Traumatic atlanto-occipital dislocation in children. J Bone Joint Surg Am 2005;87:2480.
129. Howell JM, McFarling DA, Chisholm CD: Ischemic injury to the spinal cord as a cause of transient paraplegia. Am J Emerg Med 1987;5:217.
130. Hubbard DD: Injuries of the spine in children and adolescents. Clin Orthop Relat Res 1974;100:56.
131. Hubbard DD: Fractures of the dorsal and lumbar spine. Orthop Clin North Am 1976;7:605.
132. Huerta C, Griffith R, Joyce SM: Cervical spine stabilization in pediatric patients: Evaluation of current techniques. Ann Emerg Med 1987;16:1121.
133. Jackson RW: Surgical stabilization of the spine. Paraplegia 1975;13:71.
134. Jacobsen G, Bleeker H: Examination of the atlanto axial joint following injury with particular emphasis on rotational subluxation. AJR Am J Roentgenol 1959;76:1081.
135. Jeanneret B, Magerl F: Primary posterior fusion C1/2 in odontoid fractures: Indications, technique, and results of transarticular screw fixation. J Spinal Disord 1992;5:464.
136. Johnsson R, Herrlin K, Hagglund G, et al: Spinal canal remodeling after thoracolumbar fractures with intraspinal bone fragments. 17 cases followed 1-4 years. Acta Orthop Scand 1991;62:125.
137. Jones A, Mehta J, Fagan D, et al: Anterior screw fixation for a pediatric odontoid nonunion: A case report. Spine 2005;30:E28.
138. Joyce SM: Cervical immobilization during orotracheal intubation in trauma victims. Ann Emerg Med 1988;17:88.

139. Karlsson MK, Hasserius R, Sundgren P, et al: Remodeling of the spinal canal deformed by trauma. J Spinal Disord 1997;10:157.
140. Kathrein A, Huber B, Waldegger M, et al: [Management of injuries of the thoracic and lumbar vertebrae in children.] Orthopade 1999;28:441.
141. Kenter K, Worley G, Griffin T, et al: Pediatric traumatic atlanto-occipital dislocation: Five cases and a review. J Pediatr Orthop 2001;21:585.
142. Kewalramani LS, Kraus JF, Sterling HM: Acute spinal-cord lesions in a pediatric population: Epidemiological and clinical features. Paraplegia 1980;18:206.
143. Kewalramani LS, Tori JA: Spinal cord trauma in children. Neurologic patterns, radiologic features, and pathomechanics of injury. Spine 1980;5:11.
144. Kifune M, Panjabi MM, Liu W, et al: Functional morphology of the spinal canal after endplate, wedge, and burst fractures. J Spinal Disord 1997;10:457.
145. Kilfoyle RM, Foley JJ, Norton PL: Spine and pelvic deformity in childhood and adolescent paraplegia: A study of 104 cases. J Bone Joint Surg Am 1965;47:659.
146. Kleinman PK, Zito JL: Avulsion of the spinous processes caused by infant abuse. Radiology 1984;151:389.
147. Knight RQ, Devanny JR: Spinal cord ischemia and paraplegia in the multiple-trauma patient with aortic arch injury. Case report. Spine 1987;12:624.
148. Koivikko MP, Myllynen P, Santavirta S: Fracture dislocations of the cervical spine: A review of 106 conservatively and operatively treated patients. Eur Spine J 2004;13:610.
149. Kramer KM, Levine AM: Posttraumatic syringomyelia: A review of 21 cases. Clin Orthop Relat Res 1997;334: 190.
150. Krassioukov AV, Furlan JC, Fehlings MG: Autonomic dysreflexia in acute spinal cord injury: An under-recognized clinical entity. J Neurotrauma 2003;20:707.
151. Kriss VM, Kriss TC: SCIWORA (spinal cord injury without radiographic abnormality) in infants and children. Clin Pediatr (Phila) 1996;35:119.
152. Kumar A, Wood GW 2nd, Whittle AP: Low-velocity gunshot injuries of the spine with abdominal viscus trauma. J Orthop Trauma 1998;12:514.
153. Kuner EH, Schlickewei W, Hauser U, et al: [Reconstruction of open width of the spinal canal by internal fixator instrumentation and remodeling.] Chirurg 1996;67: 531.
154. Labbe JL, Leclair O, Duparc B: Traumatic atlanto-occipital dislocation with survival in children. J Pediatr Orthop B 2001;10:319.
155. Lagrone MO, Bradford DS, Moe JH, et al: Treatment of symptomatic flatback after spinal fusion. J Bone Joint Surg Am 1988;70:569.
156. Lalonde F, Letts M, Yang JP, et al: An analysis of burst fractures of the spine in adolescents. Am J Orthop 2001;30:115.
157. Lancourt JE, Dickson JH, Carter RE: Paralytic spinal deformity following traumatic spinal-cord injury in children and adolescents. J Bone Joint Surg Am 1981; 63:47.
158. Launay F, Leet AI, Sponseller PD: Pediatric spinal cord injury without radiographic abnormality: A meta-analysis. Clin Orthop Relat Res 2005;433:166.
159. LeBlanc HJ, Nadell J: Spinal cord injuries in children. Surg Neurol 1974;2:411.
160. Lee SL, Sena M, Greenholz SK, et al: A multidisciplinary approach to the development of a cervical spine clearance protocol: Process, rationale, and initial results. J Pediatr Surg 2003;38:358.
161. LeGay DA, Petrie DP, Alexander DI: Flexion-distraction injuries of the lumbar spine and associated abdominal trauma. J Trauma 1990;30:436.
162. Letts M, Davidson D, Fleuriau-Chateau P, et al: Seat belt fracture with late development of an enterocolic fistula in a child. A case report. Spine 1999;24:1151.
163. Leventhal HR: Birth injuries of the spinal cord. J Pediatr 1960;56:447.
164. Levin TL, Berdon WE, Cassell I, et al: Thoracolumbar fracture with listhesis—an uncommon manifestation of child abuse. Pediatr Radiol 2003;33:305.
165. Lewis VL Jr, Manson PN, Morgan RF, et al: Facial injuries associated with cervical fractures: Recognition, patterns, and management. J Trauma 1985;25:90.
166. Liao CC, Lui TN, Chen LR, et al: Spinal cord injury without radiological abnormality in preschool-aged children: Correlation of magnetic resonance imaging findings with neurological outcomes. J Neurosurg 2005;103:17.
167. Lim LH, Lam LK, Moore MH, et al: Associated injuries in facial fractures: Review of 839 patients. Br J Plast Surg 1993;46:635.
168. Locke GR, Gardner JI, Van Epps EF: Atlas-dens interval (ADI) in children: A survey based on 200 normal cervical spines. Am J Roentgenol Radium Ther Nucl Med 1966;97:135.
169. Lu J, Ebraheim NA, Yang H, et al: Anatomic considerations of anterior transarticular screw fixation for atlantoaxial instability. Spine 1998;23:1229.
170. Lustrin ES, Karakas SP, Ortiz AO, et al: Pediatric cervical spine: Normal anatomy, variants, and trauma. Radiographics 2003;23:539.
171. Majernick TG, Bieniek R, Houston JB, et al: Cervical spine movement during orotracheal intubation. Ann Emerg Med 1986;15:417.
172. Mann DC, Dodds JA: Spinal injuries in 57 patients 17 years or younger. Orthopedics 1993;16:159.
173. Marlin AE, Williams GR, Lee JF: Jefferson fractures in children. Case report. J Neurosurg 1983;58:277.
174. Mascalchi M, Dal Pozzo G, Dini C, et al: Acute spinal trauma: Prognostic value of MRI appearances at 0.5 T. Clin Radiol 1993;48:100.
175. Matsumoto M, Toyama Y, Chiba K, et al: Traumatic subluxation of the axis after hyperflexion injury of the cervical spine in children. J Spinal Disord 2001;14: 172.
176. McBride WJ, Gadowski GR, Keller MS, et al: Pulmonary embolism in pediatric trauma patients. J Trauma 1994;37:913.
177. McGrory BJ, Klassen RA, Chao EY, et al: Acute fractures and dislocations of the cervical spine in children and adolescents. J Bone Joint Surg Am 1993;75:988.
178. McIntosh TK, Faden AI: Opiate antagonist in traumatic shock. Ann Emerg Med 1986;15:1462.
179. McPhee IB: Spinal fractures and dislocations in children and adolescents. Spine 1981;6:533.

180. Mehta S, Betz RR, Mulcahey MJ, et al: Effect of bracing on paralytic scoliosis secondary to spinal cord injury. J Spinal Cord Med 2004;27(Suppl 1):S88.
181. Merli GJ, Crabbe S, Paluzzi RG, et al: Etiology, incidence, and prevention of deep vein thrombosis in acute spinal cord injury. Arch Phys Med Rehabil 1993;74:1199.
182. Metak G, Scherer MA, Dannohl C: [Missed injuries of the musculoskeletal system in multiple trauma—a retrospective study.] Zentralbl Chir 1994;119:88.
183. Meuli M, Sacher P, Lasser U, et al: Traumatic spinal cord injury: Unusual recovery in 3 children. Eur J Pediatr Surg 1991;1:240.
184. Mikawa Y, Watanabe R, Yamano Y, et al: Fracture through a synchondrosis of the anterior arch of the atlas. J Bone Joint Surg Br 1987;69:483.
185. Miladi LT, Ghanem IB, Draoui MM, et al: Iliosacral screw fixation for pelvic obliquity in neuromuscular scoliosis. A long-term follow-up study. Spine 1997;22:1722.
186. Miller JA, Smith TH: Seat belt induced chance fracture in an infant. Case report and literature review. Pediatr Radiol 1991;21:575.
187. Mirza SK, Krengel WF 3rd, Chapman JR, et al: Early versus delayed surgery for acute cervical spinal cord injury. Clin Orthop Relat Res 1999;359:104.
188. Montane I, Eismont FJ, Green BA: Traumatic occipitoatlantal dislocation. Spine 1991;16:112.
189. Muller U, Berlemann U, Sledge J, et al: Treatment of thoracolumbar burst fractures without neurologic deficit by indirect reduction and posterior instrumentation: bisegmental stabilization with monosegmental fusion. Eur Spine J 1999;8:284.
190. Nesathurai S: Steroids and spinal cord injury: Revisiting the NASCIS 2 and NASCIS 3 trials. J Trauma 1998;45:1088.
191. Nitecki S, Moir CR: Predictive factors of the outcome of traumatic cervical spine fracture in children. J Pediatr Surg 1994;29:1409.
192. Odent T, Langlais J, Glorion C, et al: Fractures of the odontoid process: A report of 15 cases in children younger than 6 years. J Pediatr Orthop 1999;19:51.
193. Odom JA, Brown CW, Messner DG: Tubing injuries. J Bone Joint Surg Am 1976;58:733.
194. Oliveri MB, Mautalen CA, Rodriguez Fuchs CA, et al: Vertebral compression fractures at the onset of acute lymphoblastic leukemia in a child. Henry Ford Hosp Med J 1991;39:45.
195. O'Neill MJ: Delayed-onset paraplegia from improper seat belt use. Ann Emerg Med 1994;23:1123.
196. Osenbach RK, Menezes AH: Spinal cord injury without radiographic abnormality in children. Pediatr Neurosci 1989;15:168.
197. Owen JH, Naito M, Bridwell KH, et al: Relationship between duration of spinal cord ischemia and postoperative neurologic deficits in animals. Spine 1990;15:846.
198. Pang D: Spinal cord injury without radiographic abnormality in children, 2 decades later. Neurosurgery 2004;55:1325.
199. Pang D, Pollack IF: Spinal cord injury without radiographic abnormality in children—the SCIWORA syndrome. J Trauma 1989;29:654.
200. Pang D, Wilberger JE Jr: Spinal cord injury without radiographic abnormalities in children. J Neurosurg 1982;57:114.
201. Panjabi MM, White AA 3rd, Johnson RM: Cervical spine mechanics as a function of transection of components. J Biomech 1975;8:327.
202. Panjabi MM, White AA 3rd, Keller D, et al: Stability of the cervical spine under tension. J Biomech 1978;11:189.
203. Parisini P, Di Silvestre M, Greggi T, et al: C1-C2 posterior fusion in growing patients: Long-term follow-up. Spine 2003;28:566.
204. Partrick DA, Bensard DD, Moore EE, et al: Cervical spine trauma in the injured child: A tragic injury with potential for salvageable functional outcome. J Pediatr Surg 2000;35:1571.
205. Patel JC, Tepas JJ 3rd, Mollitt DL, et al: Pediatric cervical spine injuries: Defining the disease. J Pediatr Surg 2001;36:373.
206. Paulson JA: The epidemiology of injuries in adolescents. Pediatr Ann 1988;17:84.
207. Pennecot GF, Gouraud D, Hardy JR, et al: Roentgenographical study of the stability of the cervical spine in children. J Pediatr Orthop 1984;4:346.
208. Pennecot GF, Leonard P, Peyrot Des Gachons S, et al: Traumatic ligamentous instability of the cervical spine in children. J Pediatr Orthop 1984;4:339.
209. Perrouin-Verbe B, Lenne-Aurier K, Robert R, et al: Post-traumatic syringomyelia and post-traumatic spinal canal stenosis: A direct relationship: Rreview of 75 patients with a spinal cord injury. Spinal Cord 1998;36:137.
210. Perrouin-Verbe B, Robert R, Lefort M, et al: [Post-traumatic syringomyelia.] Neurochirurgie 1999;45(Suppl 1):58.
211. Pizzutillo PD, Rocha EF, D'Astous J, et al: Bilateral fracture of the pedicle of the second cervical vertebra in the young child. J Bone Joint Surg Am 1986;68:892.
212. Pollina J, Li V: Tandem spinal cord injuries without radiographic abnormalities in a young child. Pediatr Neurosurg 1999;30:263.
213. Pouliquen JC, Beneux J, Pennecot GF: [The incidence of progressive scoliosis and kyphosis after fractures and dislocations of the spine in children (author's transl).] Rev Chir Orthop Reparatrice Appar Mot 1978;64:487.
214. Povaz F: Behandlungsergebnisse und Prognose von Wirbelbruchen bei Kindern. Chirurg 1969;40:30.
215. Powers B, Miller MD, Kramer RS, et al: Traumatic anterior atlanto-occipital dislocation. Neurosurgery 1979;4:12.
216. Rachesky I, Boyce WT, Duncan B, et al: Clinical prediction of cervical spine injuries in children. Radiographic abnormalities. Am J Dis Child 1987;141:199.
217. Rahimi SY, Stevens EA, Yeh DJ, et al: Treatment of atlantoaxial instability in pediatric patients. Neurosurg Focus 2003;15:ECP1.
218. Ralston ME, Chung K, Barnes PD, et al: Role of flexion-extension radiographs in blunt pediatric cervical spine injury. Acad Emerg Med 2001;8:237.
219. Ralston ME, Ecklund K, Emans JB, et al: Role of oblique radiographs in blunt pediatric cervical spine injury. Pediatr Emerg Care 2003;19:68.

220. Reddy SP, Junewick JJ, Backstrom JW: Distribution of spinal fractures in children: Does age, mechanism of injury, or gender play a significant role? Pediatr Radiol 2003;33:776.
221. Reid AB, Letts RM, Black GB: Pediatric Chance fractures: Association with intra-abdominal injuries and seat belt use. J Trauma 1990;30:384.
222. Rinaldi I, Mullins WJ, Kretz WK, et al: Missed spinal fractures. A serious problem in the patient with multiple injuries. Va Med Mon (1918) 1975;102:305.
223. Roaf R: A study of the mechanics of spinal injuries. J Bone Joint Surg Br 1960;42:810.
224. Robinson LR, Little JW: Motor-evoked potentials reflect spinal cord function in post-traumatic syringomyelia. Am J Phys Med Rehabil 1990;69:307.
225. Ruge JR, Sinson GP, McLone DG, et al: Pediatric spinal injury: The very young. J Neurosurg 1988;68:25.
226. Ruggieri M, Smarason AK, Pike M: Spinal cord insults in the prenatal, perinatal, and neonatal periods. Dev Med Child Neurol 1999;41:311.
227. Rumball K, Jarvis J: Seat-belt injuries of the spine in young children. J Bone Joint Surg Br 1992;74:571.
228. Sankar WN, Wills BP, Dormans JP, et al: Os odontoideum revisited: The case for a multifactorial etiology. Spine 2006;31:979.
229. Santiago R, Guenther E, Carroll K, et al: The clinical presentation of pediatric thoracolumbar fractures. J Trauma 2006;60:187.
230. Scapinelli R, Candiotto S: Spontaneous remodeling of the spinal canal after burst fractures of the low thoracic and lumbar region. J Spinal Disord 1995;8:486.
231. Scher AT: Trauma of the spinal cord in children. S Afr Med J 1976;50:2023.
232. Schiff DC, Parke WW: The arterial supply of the odontoid process. J Bone Joint Surg Am 1973;55:1450.
233. Schippers N, Konings P, Hassler W, et al: Typical and atypical fractures of the odontoid process in young children. Report of two cases and a review of the literature. Acta Neurochir (Wien) 1996;138:524.
234. Schossberger P: Vasculature of the spinal cord: A review. II. Clinical considerations. Bull Los Angeles Neurol Soc 1974;39:86.
235. Schuler TC, Kurz L, Thompson DE, et al: Natural history of os odontoideum. J Pediatr Orthop 1991;11:222.
236. Schuster R, Waxman K, Sanchez B, et al: Magnetic resonance imaging is not needed to clear cervical spines in blunt trauma patients with normal computed tomographic results and no motor deficits. Arch Surg 2005; 140:762.
237. Schwartz GR, Wright SW, Fein JA, et al: Pediatric cervical spine injury sustained in falls from low heights. Ann Emerg Med 1997;30:249.
238. Schwarz N, Genelin F, Schwarz AF: Post-traumatic cervical kyphosis in children cannot be prevented by non-operative methods. Injury 1994;25:173.
239. Sclafani SJ, Florence LO, Phillips TF, et al: Lumbar arterial injury: Radiologic diagnosis and management. Radiology 1987;165:709.
240. Seimon LP: Fracture of the odontoid process in young children. J Bone Joint Surg Am 1977;59:943.
241. Sgouros S, Williams B: Management and outcome of posttraumatic syringomyelia. J Neurosurg 1996;85:197.
241a. Shacked I, Ram Z, Hadani M: The anterior cervical approach for traumatic injuries to the cervical spine in children. Clin Orthop 1993;292:144.
242. Shaffer MA, Doris PE: Limitation of the cross table lateral view in detecting cervical spine injuries: A retrospective analysis. Ann Emerg Med 1981;10:508.
243. Shaw M, Burnett H, Wilson A, et al: Pseudosubluxation of C2 on C3 in polytraumatized children—prevalence and significance. Clin Radiol 1999;54:377.
244. Sherk HH: Fractures of the atlas and odontoid process. Orthop Clin North Am 1978;9:973.
245. Sherk HH, Nicholson JT, Chung SM: Fractures of the odontoid process in young children. J Bone Joint Surg Am 1978;60:921.
246. Shrosbree RD: Spinal cord injuries as a result of motorcycle accidents. Paraplegia 1978;16:102.
247. Sinha AK, Seki JT, Moreau G, et al: The management of spinal metastasis in children. Can J Surg 1997;40:218.
248. Smith WS, Kaufer H: Patterns and mechanisms of lumbar injuries associated with lap seat belts. J Bone Joint Surg Am 1969;51:239.
249. Sneed RC, Stover SL: Undiagnosed spinal cord injuries in brain-injured children. Am J Dis Child 1988;142: 965.
250. Sponseller PD, Cass JR: Atlanto-occipital fusion for dislocation in children with neurologic preservation. A case report. Spine 1997;22:344.
251. Stauffer ES: Diagnosis and prognosis of acute cervical spinal cord injury. Clin Orthop Relat Res 1975;112:9.
252. Stauffer ES: The management of thoracolumbar junction fractures. In Stauffer ES (ed): Thoracolumbar Spine Fractures without Neurologic Deficit. Rosemont, IL, American Academy of Orthopaedic Surgeons, 1993, p 60.
253. Stauffer ES, Kelly EG: Fracture-dislocations of the cervical spine. Instability and recurrent deformity following treatment by anterior interbody fusion. J Bone Joint Surg Am 1977;59:45.
254. Stauffer ES, Mazur JM: Cervical spine injuries in children. Pediatr Ann 1982;11:502.
255. Steel HH: Anatomical and mechanical consideration of the atlanto-axial articulation. J Bone Joint Surg Am 1968;50:1481.
256. Stricker U, Moser H, Aebi M: Predominantly posterior instrumentation and fusion in neuromuscular and neurogenic scoliosis in children and adolescents. Eur Spine J 1996;5:101.
257. Sturm JT, Hynes JT, Perry JF Jr: Thoracic spinal fractures and aortic rupture: A significant and fatal association. Ann Thorac Surg 1990;50:931.
258. Sturm JT, Perry JF Jr: Injuries associated with fractures of the transverse processes of the thoracic and lumbar vertebrae. J Trauma 1984;24:597.
259. Suderman VS, Crosby ET, Lui A: Elective oral tracheal intubation in cervical spine–injured adults. Can J Anaesth 1991;38:785.
260. Sullivan CR, Bruwer AJ, Harris LE: Hypermobility of the cervical spine in children; a pitfall in the diagnosis of cervical dislocation. Am J Surg 1958;95:636.
261. Sun PP, Poffenbarger GJ, Durham S, et al: Spectrum of occipito-atlantoaxial injury in young children. J Neurosurg 2000;93:28.

262. Swischuk LE: Spine and spinal cord trauma in the battered child syndrome. Radiology 1969;92:733.
263. Swischuk LE, Rowe M: The upper cervical spine in health and disease. Pediatrics 1952;10:567.
264. Tator CH, Fehlings MG, Thorpe K, et al: Current use and timing of spinal surgery for management of acute spinal surgery for management of acute spinal cord injury in North America: Results of a retrospective multicenter study. J Neurosurg 1999;91: 12.
265. Taylor AR: The mechanism of injury to the spinal cord in the neck without damage to vertebral column. J Bone Joint Surg Br 1951;33:543.
266. Tolo VT, Weiland AJ: Unsuspected atlas fracture and instability associated with oropharyngeal injury: Case report. J Trauma 1979;19:278.
267. Tyroch AH, McGuire EL, McLean SF, et al: The association between Chance fractures and intra-abdominal injuries revisited: A multicenter review. Am Surg 2005; 71:434.
268. Vaccaro AR, Madigan L, Bauerle WB, et al: Early halo immobilization of displaced traumatic spondylolisthesis of the axis. Spine 2002;27:2229.
269. Vanhulle C, Durand I, Tron P: [Paraplegia due to medullary ischemia after repair of coarctation of the aorta in an infant.] Arch Pediatr 1998;5:633.
270. Vedantam R, Crawford AH: Multiple noncontiguous injuries of the spine in a child: Atlantooccipital dislocation and seat-belt injury of the lumbar spine. Acta Orthop Belg 1997;63:23.
271. Viccellio P, Simon H, Pressman BD, et al: A prospective multicenter study of cervical spine injury in children. Pediatrics 2001;108:E20.
272. Voss L, Cole PA, D'Amato C: Pediatric chance fractures from lapbelts: Unique case report of three in one accident. J Orthop Trauma 1996;10:421.
273. Walsh JW, Stevens DB, Young AB: Traumatic paraplegia in children without contiguous spinal fracture or dislocation. Neurosurgery 1983;12:439.
274. Weiss MH, Kaufman B: Hangman's fracture in an infant. Am J Dis Child 1973;126:268.
275. White AA 3rd, Johnson RM, Panjabi MM, et al: Biomechanical analysis of clinical stability in the cervical spine. Clin Orthop Relat Res 1975;109:85.
276. White AA 3rd, Panjabi MM: The basic kinematics of the human spine. A review of past and current knowledge. Spine 1978;3:12.
277. Wholey MH, Bruwer AJ, Baker HL Jr: The lateral roentgenogram of the neck; with comments on the atlanto-odontoid-basion relationship. Radiology 1958;71:350.
278. Woelfel GF, Moore EE, Cogbill TH, et al: Severe thoracic and abdominal injuries associated with lap-harness seat belts. J Trauma 1984;24:166.
279. Yashon D: Pathogenesis of spinal cord injury. Orthop Clin North Am 1978;9:247.
280. Yazici M, Atilla B, Tepe S, et al: Spinal canal remodeling in burst fractures of the thoracolumbar spine: A computerized tomographic comparison between operative and nonoperative treatment. J Spinal Disord 1996;9: 409.
281. Yngve DA, Harris WP, Herndon WA, et al: Spinal cord injury without osseous spine fracture. J Pediatr Orthop 1988;8:153.
282. Yoon DH, Kim YS, Young W: Therapeutic time window for methylprednisolone in spinal cord injured rat. Yonsei Med J 1999;40:313.
283. Young W, Bracken MB: The Second National Acute Spinal Cord Injury Study. J Neurotrauma 1992;9(Suppl 1):S397.
284. Zigler JE, Waters RL, Nelson RW, et al: Occipito-cervico-thoracic spine fusion in a patient with occipito-cervical dislocation and survival. Spine 1986;11:645.

Chapter 42

Upper Extremity Injuries

INJURIES TO THE CLAVICLE

The clavicle is one of the most frequently broken bones in children,[143,225,295,303] which is not surprising given that it is the only connection between the arm and trunk and consequently is subjected to all the forces exerted on the upper limb.[11,14,93,184] Fortunately, nearly all clavicle fractures in children heal uneventfully with minimal or no treatment.*

Anatomy

The clavicle is the first bone in the body to ossify and has the last physis in the body to close. Initially, the clavicle ossifies via intramembranous bone formation. Later, secondary ossification centers develop at both its medial and lateral ends. The medial epiphysis is the last physis in the body to close, often not until the third decade of life.[14,83,204,217,272,290] The abundant and mobile soft tissue overlying the clavicle makes open fractures unusual.[12,61,307]

In the horizontal plane the clavicle has a double curve, convex forward in its medial two thirds and concave forward in its lateral third. Biomechanically, the point of juncture of the two curves is the weakest point. The superior surface of the clavicle is subcutaneous throughout its length. Along its inferior surface, the costoclavicular ligaments insert medially, the coracoclavicular ligaments (the conoid and trapezoid ligaments) insert laterally, and the subclavius muscle arises along the middle two thirds.[26,98,184] The subclavian vessels and brachial plexus travel beneath the clavicle. In the middle third of the clavicle, the thin subclavius muscle and clavipectoral fascia are the only structures interposed between the clavicle and the medial and lateral cords of the brachial plexus. Fortunately, when fractures of the mid-portion of the clavicle occur, the brachial plexus and subclavian vessels are protected by the thick periosteum, the clavipectoral fascia, and the subclavius muscle.[119,181,216,306]

The physes present at both the medial and lateral ends of the clavicle make true dislocation of the sternoclavicular or acromioclavicular joint a rare occurrence in children. Rather, injuries to either end of the clavicle are usually physeal separations.* The physis at the medial end of the clavicle does not begin to ossify until the 18th year and does not close until between the 22nd and 25th years.[14,83,152,206,208,218,274,292] Thus, most injuries to the medial clavicle in children and young adults are physeal separations, with the lateral metaphyseal fragment displaced either anteriorly or posteriorly and the physeal sleeve left intact. The strong costoclavicular and sternoclavicular ligaments generally remain in continuity with the periosteal sleeve (Fig. 42–1).[26,39,152,191,193] It is important to remember the vital structures immediately posterior to the sternoclavicular joint. The innominate artery and vein, the internal jugular vein, the phrenic and vagus nerves,

*See references 11, 31, 59, 68, 77, 81, 100, 111, 118, 124, 127, 189, 193, 229, 238, 265, 283, 284.

*See references 11, 14, 39, 98, 111, 118, 152, 191, 193, 204, 228, 274, 283, 284, 292.

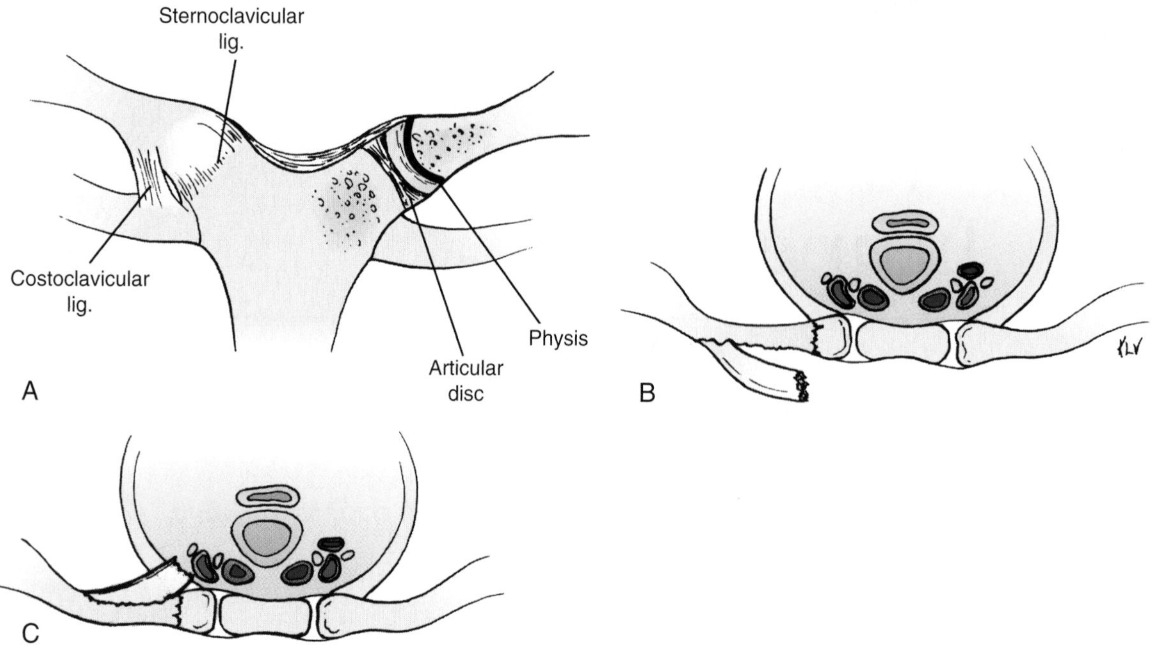

FIGURE 42–1 Anatomy of the medial sternoclavicular joint. **A,** The strong sternoclavicular and costoclavicular ligaments make medial clavicular physeal fractures more common than true dislocation. **B,** Anterior displacement. **C,** Posterior displacement places the great vessels, esophagus, and trachea at risk.

the trachea, and the esophagus all lie immediately posterior to the sternoclavicular joint and can be injured with posterior displacement of the clavicle (see Fig. 42–1).*

Injuries to the lateral clavicle are also more likely to be physeal fractures than true acromioclavicular separations. Laterally, the coracoclavicular ligaments (the conoid and trapezoid ligaments) generally remain in continuity with the periosteal sleeve and the small lateral epiphyseal fragment.[11,93,111,189,193,204,229,232] The medial metaphyseal fragment may be dramatically displaced, similar to a severe acromioclavicular separation (Fig. 42–2). As these fractures heal, the intact periosteal sleeve may form a "new" metaphysis that results in a "duplicated" lateral clavicle (Fig. 42–3). Rockwood has modified the adult classification of acromioclavicular joint injuries to reflect the more common physeal fractures that occur in children (Fig. 42–4).[229] Though uncommon, true dislocations of both the sternoclavicular and acromioclavicular joints can and do occur in children.[14,123,167,193,283,284,292]

Mechanism of Injury

In the newborn, clavicle fractures generally occur from compression of the shoulders during delivery. In children and adolescents, clavicle fractures are usually the result of a fall onto either an outstretched extremity or the side of the shoulder. Fractures may also result from a direct blow. This mechanism accounts for most of the injuries to the lateral end of the clavicle (Fig. 42–5).

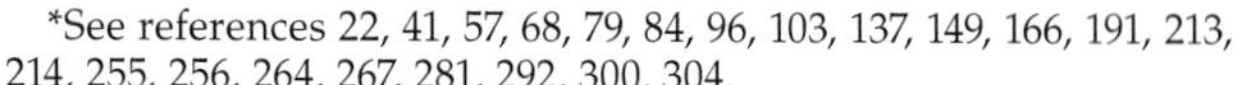

*See references 22, 41, 57, 68, 79, 84, 96, 103, 137, 149, 166, 191, 213, 214, 255, 256, 264, 267, 281, 292, 300, 304.

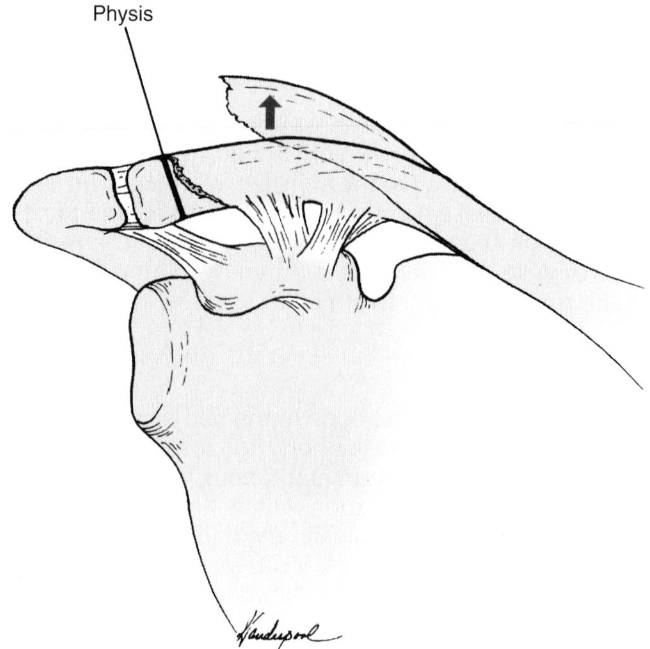

FIGURE 42–2 In a skeletally immature patient, injury around the acromioclavicular joint is more likely to be a physeal fracture than a true separation. *Arrow* indicates upward displacement.

Diagnosis

BIRTH FRACTURES

A fractured clavicle in a newborn may be difficult to diagnose because the infant is often asymptomatic.[54,82,251] In a radiographic survey of 300 newborns, five unsus-

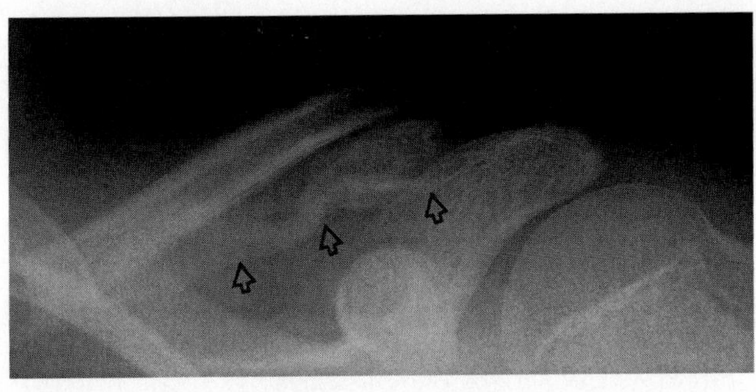

FIGURE 42-3 Anteroposterior radiograph of the left clavicle after lateral physeal separation. The intact periosteal sleeve has formed a "new" lateral clavicle inferior to the superiorly displaced medial fragment (*arrows*).

pected clavicle fractures were discovered.[82] Fractures during delivery usually involve the clavicle, which is most anterior in the birth canal.[54,82] The diagnosis is often made when the child has "pseudoparalysis," or lack of active spontaneous movement of the limb.

The differential diagnosis includes brachial plexus palsy and acute osteoarticular infection. It is important to remember that brachial plexus palsy and clavicle fractures may coexist. Although the clinical diagnosis of a fractured clavicle may be straightforward, assessing the status of the brachial plexus is frequently difficult. Neonatal reflexes such as the Moro and "fencing" reflexes may be helpful in demonstrating active upper extremity muscle function.[251] The diagnosis of osteoarticular infection in a newborn may

Type I

Type II

Type III

Type IV

Type V

Type VI

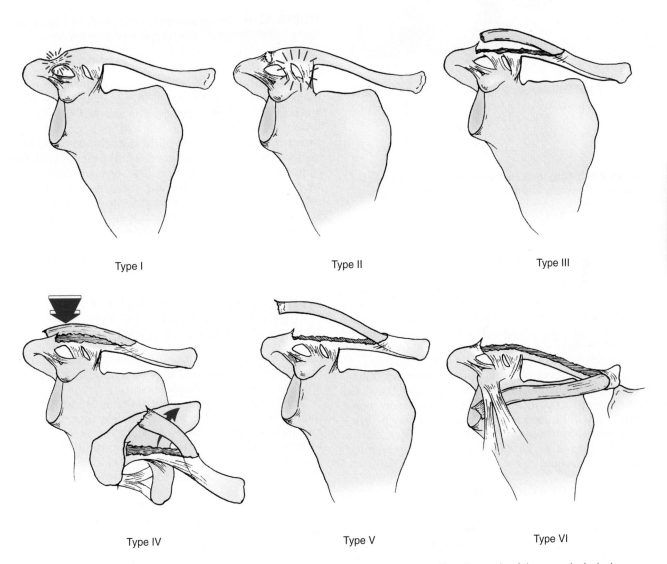

FIGURE 42-4 Rockwood's classification of acromioclavicular joint injuries in children. Type I—sprain of the acromioclavicular ligaments without disruption of the periosteal tube. Type II—partial disruption of the periosteal tube. This may produce some acromioclavicular instability. Type III—large split in the periosteal tube allowing superior displacement of the lateral clavicle. Type IV—large split in the periosteal tube (*large arrow*) with posterior displacement of the lateral clavicle through the trapezius muscle (*curved arrow*). Type V—complete disruption of the periosteal tube with displacement of the clavicle through the deltoid and trapezius muscles into the subcutaneous tissues. Type VI—inferior dislocation of the distal clavicle below the coracoid process. (Redrawn from Sanders JO, Rockwood CA, Curtis RJ: Fractures and dislocations of the humeral shaft and shoulder. In Rockwood CA, Wilkins KE, Beaty JH [eds]: Fractures in Children, vol 3. Philadelphia, Lippincott-Raven, 1996, p 974.)

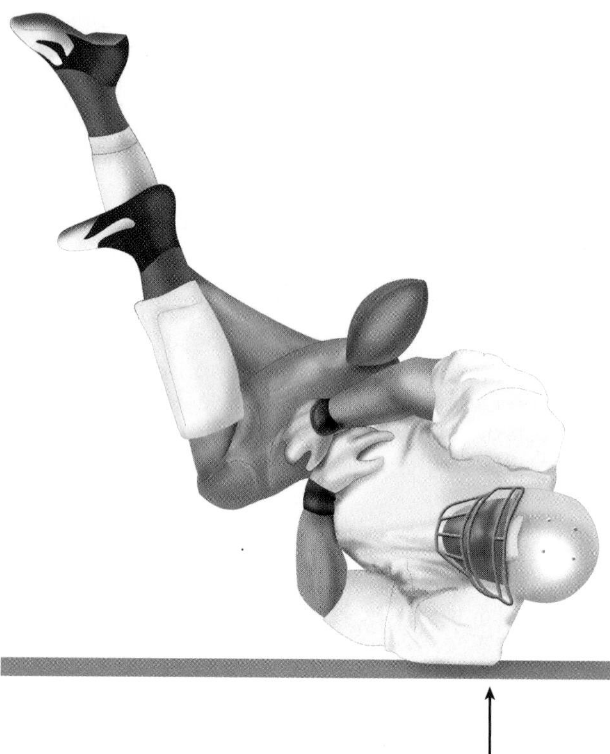

FIGURE 42–5 The most common mechanism of injury to the lateral end of the clavicle is a direct blow sustained during a fall onto the shoulder.

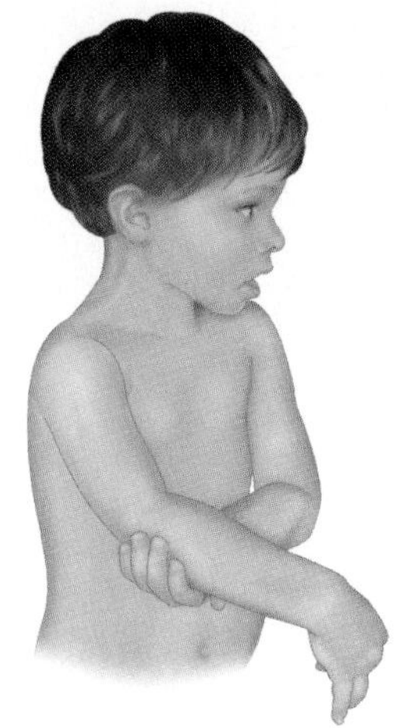

FIGURE 42–6 Clinical appearance of a child with a clavicular fracture. The affected shoulder is displaced anteriorly and inferiorly.

also be difficult to make. Often there are few systemic signs, and bone scans are notoriously unreliable. Infection should be suspected in at-risk patients (i.e., those with indwelling catheters) or in the setting of radiographic lucencies in the metaphysis, diffuse swelling, or increasing pain. Frequently, needle aspiration is required to make the diagnosis.[75,86,125,207,217,299] Occasionally, a birth fracture of the clavicle is accompanied by fracture of the upper humeral physis. Often this injury is not appreciated on the initial radiographs; however, on follow-up films, massive subperiosteal new bone formation will be seen and the condition may be mistaken for osteomyelitis. Fracture of the clavicle in a newborn may also be misdiagnosed as congenital muscular torticollis.[133]

MIDSHAFT CLAVICLE FRACTURES

In an infant or young child, clavicle fractures are often incomplete (greenstick) fractures. These greenstick fractures of the clavicle may escape notice until appearance of the developing callus. In such instances the fracture should not be mistaken for congenital pseudarthrosis of the clavicle, which is also painless. Radiographically, the distinction between congenital pseudarthrosis and acute fracture is straightforward. In congenital pseudarthrosis there is a wide zone of radiolucency with smooth margins at the site of the defect and no evidence of callus formation.[114,246,257,288]

Older children and adolescents usually have completely displaced fractures of the clavicle, which have a classic clinical appearance. The affected shoulder is lower than the opposite normal one and droops forward and inward. The child rests the involved arm against the body and supports it at the elbow with the opposite hand. The tension on the sternocleidomastoid muscle tilts the head toward the affected side and rotates the chin toward the opposite side (Fig. 42–6). Any change in position of the upper limb or the cervical spine is painful. There is local swelling, tenderness, and crepitation over the fracture site. In rare cases the spasm has been severe enough to result in atlantoaxial rotatory instability after a clavicle fracture.[37]

MEDIAL PHYSEAL SEPARATION (PSEUDODISLOCATION) OF THE STERNOCLAVICULAR JOINT

Medial physeal separation, or pseudosubluxation, of the sternoclavicular joint may be manifested as either anterior or posterior displacement.

With anterior displacement of the metaphyseal fragment, the sternal end of the clavicle may be sharp and palpable immediately beneath the skin. The clavicular head of the sternocleidomastoid muscle is pulled anteriorly with the bone and is in spasm, which causes the patient's head to tilt toward the affected side.[14,22,39,68,152,191,193]

Posteromedial displacement is accompanied by local swelling, tenderness, and depression of the medial end of the clavicle. Severe posterior displacement can cause compression of the trachea and result in dyspnea or hoarseness. Posteriorly displaced fractures may also compress the subclavian vessels or brachial plexus and produce vascular insufficiency with diminution or absence of distal pulses or paresthesias and paresis, or both.*

*See references 41, 57, 79, 84, 96, 103, 137, 149, 166, 193, 213, 214, 255, 261, 264, 267, 281, 304.

LATERAL PHYSEAL SEPARATION/ ACROMIOCLAVICULAR JOINT DISLOCATION

When there is separation of the lateral physis of the clavicle, the clinical findings will depend on the type of injury. Rockwood has classified injuries to the distal clavicle in children according to the direction and degree of displacement (see Fig. 42–4).[229] Type I and type II injuries represent the classic mild acromioclavicular joint sprain. Patients complain of pain on all motions of the shoulder, and point tenderness and swelling are present over the acromioclavicular joint. Patients with types III and V injuries have complete disruption of the acromioclavicular joint. The clinical findings are similar to those in patients with types I and II injuries, but with more obvious deformity over the lateral clavicle. With type V injuries the skin may be "tented." The posterior displacement of type IV injuries may be difficult to appreciate unless the patient is examined from above. Patients who sustain the rare inferiorly displaced type VI injury have a prominent acromion and severe limitation of motion.[11,77,81,111,118,138,183,189,193,204,248,262]

Radiographic Findings

Fractures of the middle third of the clavicle will be easily identified on routine anteroposterior (AP) radiographs; however, injuries to the medial end of the clavicle may be difficult to discern with simple AP radiographs. Rockwood has described the serendipity view to assess the medial end of the clavicle. This view is a 40-degree cephalic tilt with both clavicles projected on a chest x-ray cassette.[228] Computed tomography (CT) can also be helpful in assessing the anatomy of the sternoclavicular region.[69,109,158] Laterally, the anatomy of the acromioclavicular joint is often overpenetrated on a routine AP radiograph. A radiograph obtained with soft tissue technique and centered on the acromioclavicular joint will demonstrate pathology of the lateral clavicle. An AP radiograph obtained with a 20-degree cephalic tilt is also helpful in assessing the lateral clavicle. A stress view (an AP radiograph of both clavicles obtained with the patient holding weights in each hand) can help distinguish between type I and type II acromioclavicular joint injuries (Fig. 42–7).[39,111,228] An axillary lateral view may be required to demonstrate a type IV lateral physeal injury.[188,228]

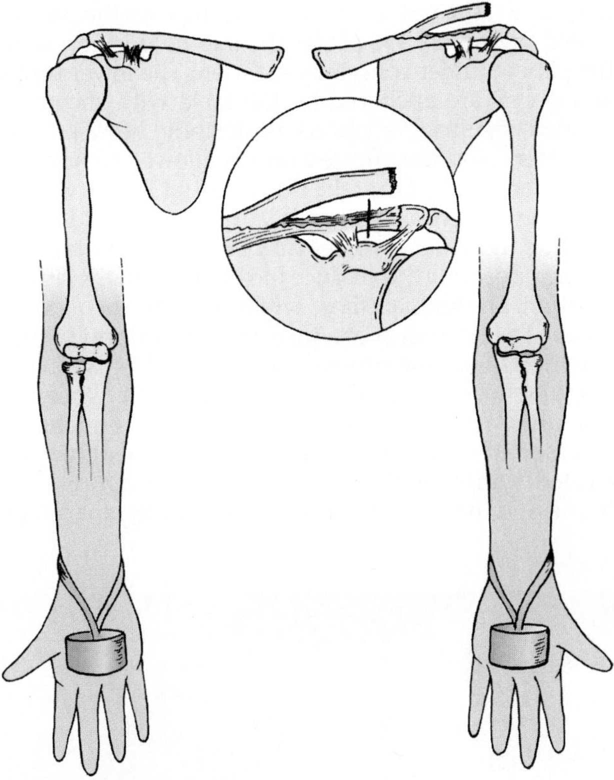

FIGURE 42–7 An anteroposterior radiograph of both clavicles taken with the patient holding weights will distinguish a type I acromioclavicular joint injury from a type II or III injury.

Treatment

BIRTH FRACTURES

An asymptomatic clavicle fracture in a neonate or young infant may be treated with benign neglect. It will unite without external immobilization, and any malalignment will gradually correct with growth. Nurses and parents should be instructed to handle the infant gently and avoid direct pressure over the broken clavicle.[54,82,251]

When the fracture is painful and accompanied by pseudoparalysis, it may be necessary to splint the arm for 1 or 2 weeks. A soft cotton pad is placed in the axilla, and the upper limb is loosely swathed across the chest with two or three turns of an elastic bandage. The parents are instructed in skin care and bathing. Within 7 to 14 days, the pain will subside, the fracture will be united clinically, and the splint is removed. Parents should be warned about the palpable subcutaneous callus that will develop and later resolve.[54,82,251]

MIDSHAFT CLAVICLE FRACTURES

In children and adolescents, displaced fractures of the clavicle rarely, if ever, require reduction. Malalignment and the bump of the callus will remodel and disappear within 6 to 9 months. Treatment consists of keeping the child comfortable with a figure-eight bandage or sling.[265] Well-padded, premade figure-eight clavicular supports are available commercially. The clavicular splints do not immobilize the fracture; their purpose is to provide patient comfort by holding the shoulders back. The fracture sling or harness is worn for 1 to 4 weeks until the pain subsides and the patient can resume normal use of the extremity. Some authors have suggested that clavicle fractures may not even require review by an orthopaedist.[45]

In general, we attempt reduction of a clavicle fracture only when the fragments are displaced so significantly that the integrity of the skin is in jeopardy

(Fig. 42–8). The reduction may be done with the patient seated or supine. We prefer the supine position with the patient under conscious sedation. The lower limbs and pelvis are anchored on the table with sheets. A padded sandbag is placed posteriorly between the shoulders, and the affected arm is allowed to hang in an extended position at the side of the table. The weight of the arm alone is generally sufficient to reduce the fracture; however, if necessary, the shoulders may be pushed posteriorly to reduce the fracture. In the sitting position, anesthesia is best achieved with a hematoma block. The shoulders are then pulled posteriorly and superiorly with the surgeon's knee placed between the scapulae to serve as a fulcrum (Fig. 42–9). Once the fracture is reduced, the stability of the fragments is assessed. If the reduction is stable, the patient may be treated symptomatically with a sling or figure-eight harness. If the reduction is unstable, an attempt can be made to immobilize the patient with a figure-eight harness or cast. We usually find external immobilization to be of little benefit. However, the combination of a reduction maneuver and external immobilization, albeit imperfect, is often adequate to remove the pressure on the overlying skin. If the fracture remains displaced to the point that the skin is still compromised, open reduction may be indicated.

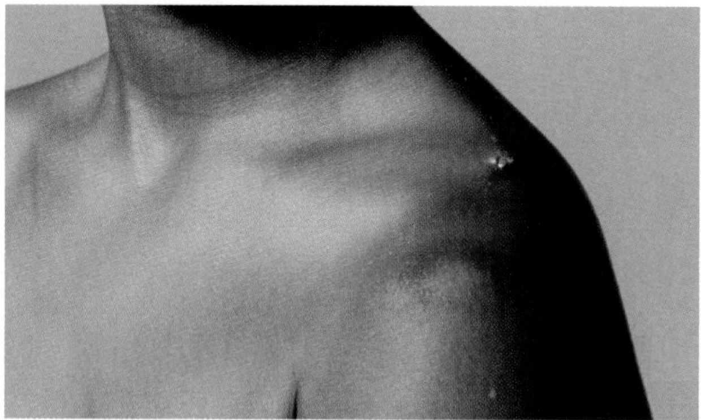

FIGURE 42–8 Clinical photograph of a type V acromioclavicular joint injury that was not reduced. The superiorly displaced fragment eventually eroded through the skin.

Open reduction of clavicle fractures in children is very rarely indicated.[10,61,194,296,311] Even in adolescents, it is far better to accept angulation and deformity than to attempt open reduction. The operative scar is often more displeasing than the bony prominence of the malunited fracture. Generally, we consider open reduction of the clavicle only if there is a neurovascular injury or an open injury that is unstable after irrigation and debridement. Other occasional indications are posterior displacement with impingement of the underlying structures and impending skin penetration by the fracture fragment.[101,141] Usually, a one-third tubular plate provides adequate fixation. We have also been successful in stabilizing some clavicle fractures with a no. 1 or 2 absorbable polydioxanone suture used as a cerclage wire. This technique has the advantage of avoiding permanent hardware without the disadvantages of pin fixation in the shoulder region. We do not use percutaneous pin fixation about the clavicle because of visceral problems associated with pin migration.[53,94,119,128,154,160,181,199,216,221]

MEDIAL PHYSEAL SEPARATION (PSEUDODISLOCATION) OF THE STERNOCLAVICULAR JOINT

Because the physeal sleeve remains intact, a significant amount of remodeling can be expected with medial physeal injuries, and consequently conservative treat-

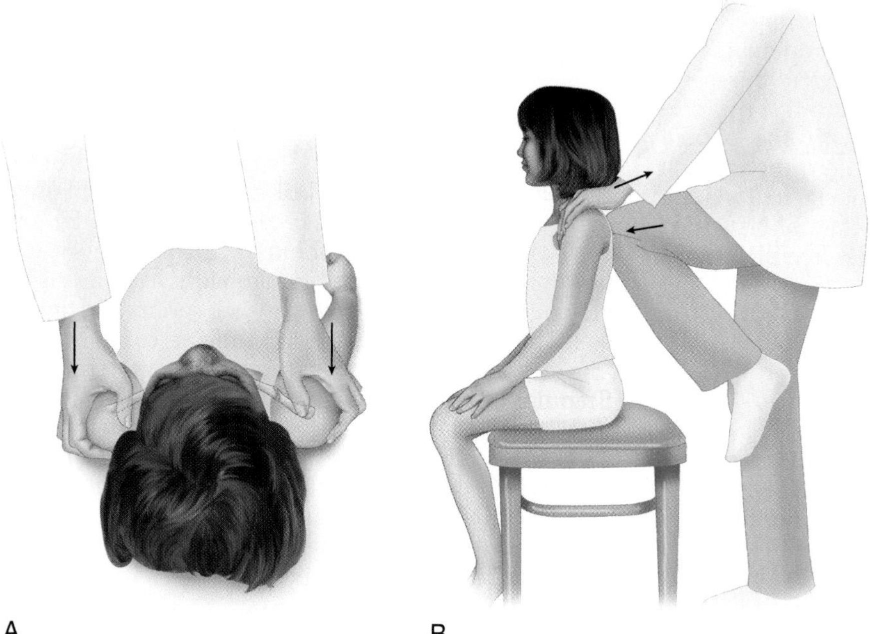

FIGURE 42–9 **A** and **B,** Technique for closed reduction of displaced clavicle fractures. A fulcrum is placed between the shoulders and a posteriorly directed force is applied to the lateral end of the clavicle.

ment is the rule. Patients with anterior displacement and those with posterior displacement without evidence of visceral injury to the mediastinal structures can be managed symptomatically with a sling or figure-eight harness.

If there is a significant cosmetic deformity, we may attempt closed reduction, which frequently achieves stability. If the reduction is lost, we generally accept the deformity and anticipate significant remodeling. If there is posterior displacement with evidence of airway, esophageal, or neurovascular impingement, we will attempt closed reduction on an emergency basis in the operating room. If closed reduction fails, we proceed immediately to open reduction, preferably with the assistance of a general trauma or thoracic surgeon.[22,39,68,101,151,152,191] Suture is preferred for fixation because evaluation of the underlying structures by magnetic resonance imaging (MRI) may be impeded by metallic implants.[151] Long-term outcome after reduction is excellent.[291]

Reduction of Anterior Displacement

Anesthesia is achieved with conscious sedation techniques or a hematoma block. The patient is placed supine with a bolster between the scapulae.[1] An assistant applies longitudinal traction to both upper extremities, and gentle posterior pressure is applied to the displaced medial metaphyseal fragment to obtain reduction. The displaced medial fragment may be grasped with a towel clip to help facilitate reduction. As previously mentioned, if reduction cannot be achieved or if the reduction is unstable, we generally accept the deformity, with the knowledge that significant remodeling nearly always occurs.[22,39,68,152,191]

Reduction of Posterior Displacement

If the metaphyseal fragment is displaced posteriorly with evidence of compression of the mediastinal structures, we first attempt closed reduction under general anesthesia. The patient is placed supine with a bolster between the shoulder blades. Longitudinal traction is applied to the arm with the shoulder adducted. A posteriorly directed force is applied to the shoulder while the medial end of the clavicle is grasped with a towel clip in an effort to bring the metaphyseal fragment anteriorly. If closed reduction fails, we proceed to open reduction, which is best accomplished through an incision superior to the clavicle. Patients with minimal posterior displacement can be managed symptomatically with a sling or harness.*

LATERAL PHYSEAL SEPARATION/ ACROMIOCLAVICULAR JOINT DISLOCATION

Treatment depends on the degree of injury to the joint. All type I and II injuries and type III injuries in patients younger than 15 or 16 years can be managed symptomatically with a sling or harness until the patient can comfortably use the extremity.* Type IV, V, and VI injuries usually require open reduction.[229,248,262] Frequently, fixation can be achieved by repairing the periosteal sleeve. Again, we avoid the use of percutaneous pins in the clavicle because of well-documented problems with migration.[53,94,119,128,154,160,181,199,216]

Complications

Neurovascular complications are extremely rare. They are usually the result of direct force or a comminuted fracture. Laceration of the subclavian artery or vein can occur, although the thick periosteum generally protects the vessels from damage. The presence of a subclavian vessel laceration is suggested by the development of a large, rapidly increasing hematoma. Surgical intervention for repair of the torn vessel should take place immediately because the patient may die of extravasation.[70,119,181,216] Subclavian vein compression after a greenstick fracture of the clavicle with inferior bowing has been reported in a child.[181] Venous congestion and swelling of the involved extremity suggest such a complication.

Nonunion of clavicular fractures is also rare; it is seen most commonly after attempts at open reduction. If nonunion develops, open reduction plus internal fixation with iliac crest bone grafting has been shown to yield excellent results.[99,105,188,198,270,275,297]

The use of pins around the clavicle and shoulder joint should be avoided because of the complication of pin migration, often into vital structures within the mediastinum.[85,94,119,128,160,181,199,216]

Acute atlantoaxial rotary displacement has been reported as a complication of clavicular fractures. The diagnosis may be missed if the orthopaedist inappropriately relates the torticollis to a clavicular fracture.[155]

FRACTURES OF THE SCAPULA

The scapula is a thin triangular bone that is attached to the clavicle by the acromioclavicular joint, the coracoclavicular ligaments, and multiple muscular attachments. The flexibility of the attachment of the scapula to the torso and the thick muscular envelope on both its anterior and posterior surface make it resistant to fracture. When scapular injuries do occur, they are generally the result of high-energy trauma.[1,13,24,108,122,123,150,177,178,192,237,273,294]

Anatomy

Scapular fractures may occur in the body, spine, neck, glenoid, acromion, or coracoid (Fig. 42–10). The scapula contains at least eight secondary ossification centers: one at the inferior margin of the body, one along the vertebral border, one at the inferior glenoid, two for the acromion, two for the coracoid process, and a

*See references 22, 41, 57, 79, 84, 96, 103, 137, 149, 166, 213, 214, 255, 261, 264, 267, 281, 304.

*See references 11, 14, 31, 77, 81, 88, 111, 118, 124, 127, 134, 138, 146, 183, 189, 204, 222, 229.

bipolar physis between the coracoid and body.[111,206] As in all physes, the zone of provisional calcification is a weak link, and avulsion fractures are likely to occur at these growth centers, particularly in adolescents. It is also important to be aware of these ossification centers so that they are not mistaken for injuries.

Fractures of the scapular body are often comminuted, with fracture lines running in multiple directions. The spine of the scapula may also be fractured with the body. (The infraspinous portion is more frequently fractured than the supraspinous portion.) The abundant muscular envelope generally prevents significant displacement of scapular body fractures.[1,24,108,122,123,294]

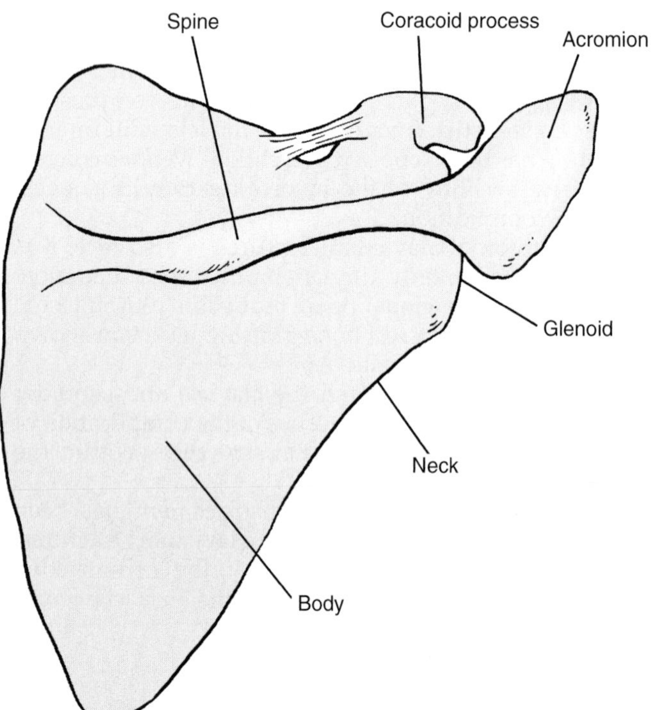

FIGURE 42-10 Scapular anatomy, posterior view.

Fractures of the neck of the scapula usually begin in the suprascapular notch and run inferior laterally to the axillary border of the scapula. The capsular attachments of the glenohumeral joint and the articular surface of the glenoid remain intact. Depending on the force of injury, the fracture may be undisplaced, minimally displaced, markedly displaced, or comminuted. If the coracoclavicular and acromioclavicular ligaments are intact, there is little, if any, displacement of the articular fragment; however, if these ligaments are torn or if the fracture line is lateral to the coracoid process, the articular fragment is displaced downward and inward by the weight of the limb (Fig. 42–11).[1,24,108,123,156,293]

Mechanism of Injury

Scapular fractures are most commonly the result of direct trauma, such as a crush injury in an automobile accident or a fall from a height. Fractures of the glenoid or acromion may result from either direct trauma or force transmitted through the humeral head. Fractures of the inferior rim of the glenoid may also result from eccentric contraction of the long head of the biceps. Similarly, fractures of the coracoid may be caused by either direct injury or an eccentric contraction of the short head of the biceps and the coracobrachialis muscles.[1,24,97,108,112,119,122,123,126,192,204,293]

The high energy required to produce scapular injuries may also result in significant injury to adjacent structures. Thus, scapular fractures are frequently associated with rib or clavicle fractures, pneumothorax, thoracic vertebral fractures, or fractures involving the humerus.[1,24,108,119,122,123,192,204,273,293] Adult studies have shown that patients with scapular fractures have more injuries to the chest and higher injury severity scores, although this may not be clinically significant.[287]

Diagnosis

The diagnosis of scapular fractures is frequently delayed or missed because of the significance of associated injuries. This difficulty is compounded by the

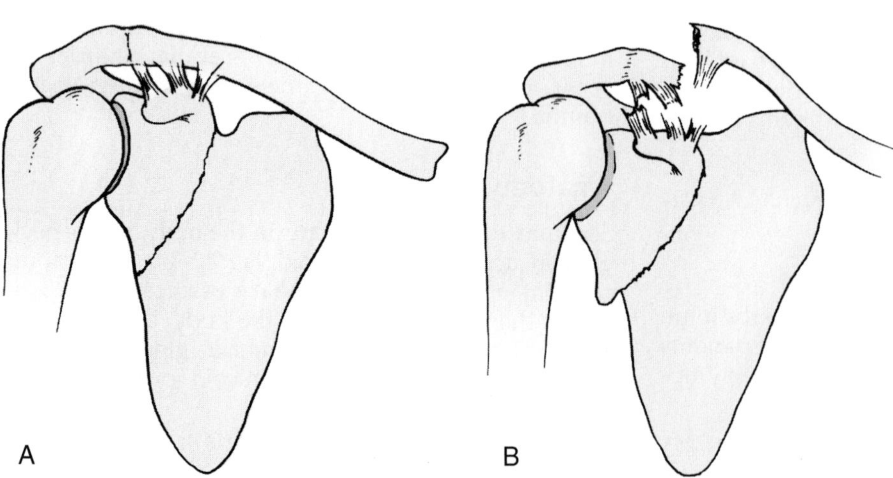

FIGURE 42-11 Fracture of the scapular neck. **A,** If the coracoclavicular and acromioclavicular ligaments are intact, there is little displacement of the glenoid. **B,** Fracture of the scapular neck with disruption of the coracoclavicular and acromioclavicular ligaments creates a floating shoulder.

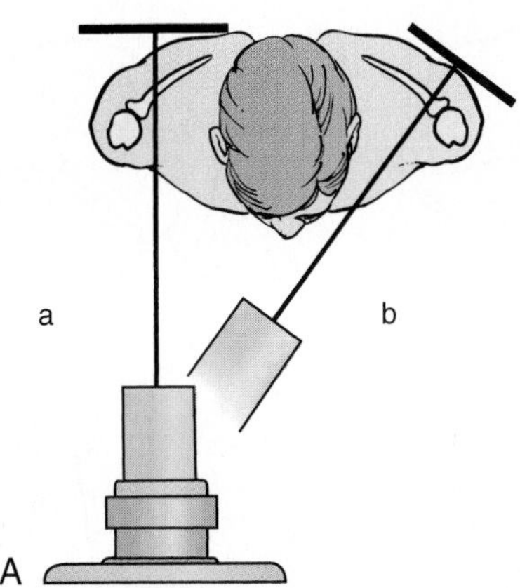

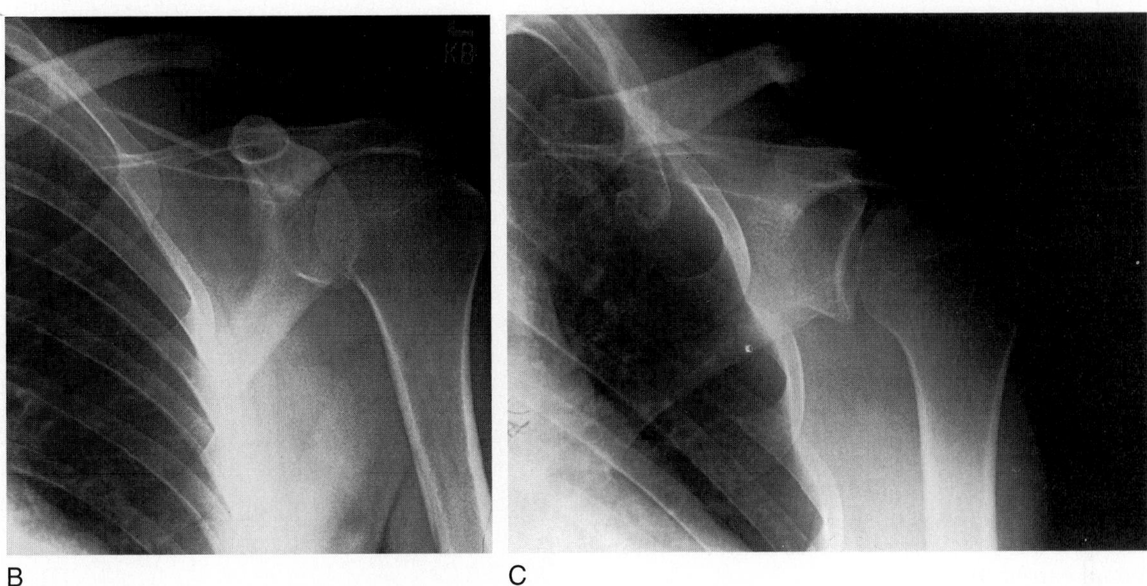

FIGURE 42–12 **A**, The standard chest x-ray technique produces an oblique view of the scapula (a). Orientation of the beam to obtain a true anteroposterior (AP) radiograph of the scapula (b). **B**, The scapula as seen on a chest film. **C**, AP radiograph of the scapula. Compare with the oblique view in **B**. Fractures are more likely to be missed on the oblique projection.

fact that the scapula is projected obliquely on an AP chest radiograph, often the only radiograph of the scapula obtained in a polytraumatized patient. Thus, to make a timely and accurate diagnosis, scapular fractures must be considered in any patient who sustains significant direct trauma to the upper thorax or proximal part of the upper extremity.[1,9,24,108,119,122,123,204,244,273,293] To see the fracture, it is often necessary to obtain a true AP radiograph of the scapula (Fig. 42–12). CT scans will also clearly demonstrate the injury.[150,189,195,209]

Treatment

Fortunately, the vast majority of scapular fractures can be managed conservatively. In general, management is directed toward patient comfort. Most patients do well with minimal immobilization in a sling or a sling and swath or shoulder immobilizer. Gentle range-of-motion exercises can usually be started in the second week after injury, with progression to full use of the upper extremity as tolerated.[1,9,112,119,122,123,204,293]

Although few of the studies of surgical management of scapular fractures deal with injuries in children[1,10,24,108,122,150,156] and little can be definitively stated regarding operative indications, we believe that significantly displaced intra-articular fractures, as well as glenoid rim fractures associated with subluxation of the humeral head, require open reduction and internal fixation.[10,16,24,108,142,150] Additionally, consideration should be given to operative stabilization of unstable fractures through the scapular neck, including ipsilateral fractures of the neck and clavicle and displaced fractures involving both the scapular spine and neck.[1,108,156,293] However, not all floating shoulder injuries require operative treatment, and recent studies in adults confirm that most do well with nonoperative treatment.[76,286]

Complications

Complications from scapular fractures are rare. The most frequent problems encountered with scapular fractures are often related to associated injuries or a delay in diagnosis.[2,24,108,112,122,123,293] Problems related to malunion or nonunion are uncommon.[131,180,216,309] Untreated fractures of the glenoid can result in glenohumeral instability.[10,16,142] Malunion of acromion fractures can result in symptomatic impingement.[180,293] Coracoid fractures, however, have been reported to do well even if they result in fibrous nonunion.[59,97,112,147,174,223,234,251,269,312,313]

Ada and Miller reported no complications in patients with fractures of the body.[1] However, they noted a high incidence of pain, both at rest (50% to 100%) and with exertion (20% to 66%), and weakness (40% to 66%) in patients with displaced fractures of the scapular neck, comminuted fractures of the spine, or intra-articular fractures of the glenoid. They attributed most of these symptoms to rotator cuff impingement and dysfunction and recommended consideration of operative treatment of these fractures.[1]

Associated Conditions

SCAPULOTHORACIC DISSOCIATION

Scapulothoracic dissociation is a rare injury that is usually the result of a massive traction injury to the upper extremity. It represents a traumatic forequarter amputation and is nearly universally associated with major neurovascular injury. Radiographically, lateral displacement of the scapula is noted on an AP chest radiograph. Patients frequently have other life- or limb-threatening injuries, and recognition of the extent of damage to the upper extremity may be delayed, with devastating consequences.[12,64,73,100,210,244] Death has been reported in 10% to 20% of patients.[64,73] Patients nearly universally have a poor result, with a functionless extremity.[1,12,64,74,210,245,250] Sampson and colleagues have noted that if the extremity is viable, attempts at vascular repair are not warranted and do not result in a functional extremity.[250]

OS ACROMIALE

An os acromiale represents failure of the apophysis of the acromion to close. Though considered a normal variant that is present in nearly 10% of shoulders,[74,249] os acromiale is occasionally symptomatic.[74,102,282,290] It has been shown to be associated with pathology of the rotator cuff in some instances.[282,290] Symptomatic os acromiale has been successfully treated with internal fixation and bone grafting, as well as arthroscopic subacromial decompression of the unstable fragment.[215,290,305]

Fractures Involving the Proximal Humeral Physis

Fractures of the proximal humeral physis make up about 3% of all physeal injuries.[182] They may occur in children of any age but are most common in adolescents. Such fractures are almost exclusively Salter-Harris type I or II injuries and are most notable for their tremendous potential to remodel. This remodeling potential is a result of the universal motion of the glenohumeral joint (Wolfe's law) and the fact that approximately 80% of the growth of the humerus comes from its proximal physis* (Fig. 42–13) (see Chapter 40, General Principles of Managing Orthopaedic Injuries).

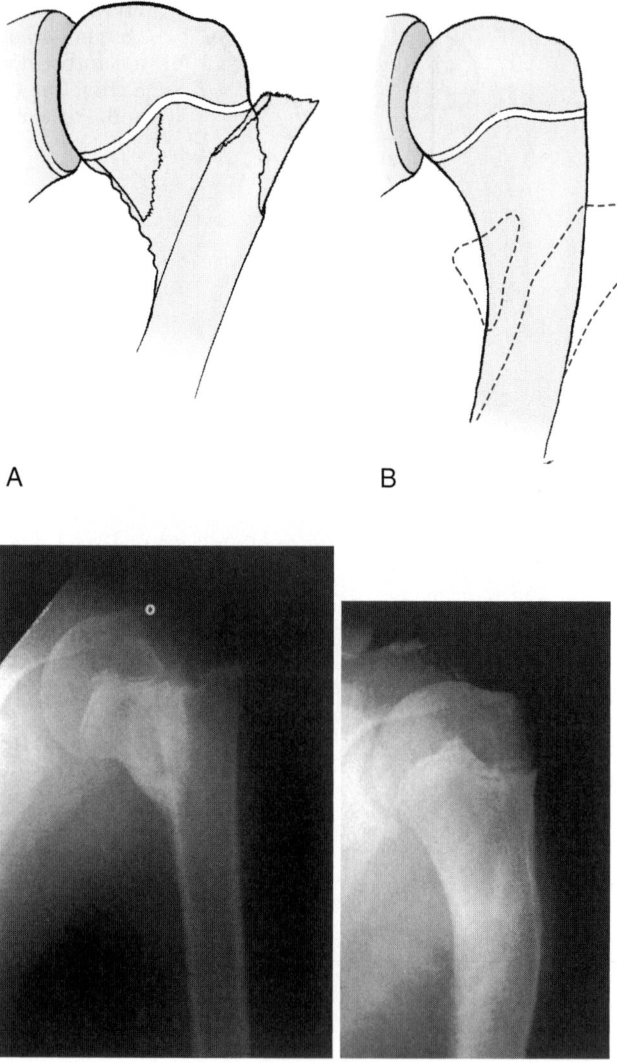

FIGURE 42-13 The remodeling potential of the proximal end of the humerus is great because of the amount of growth (80% of the entire humerus) coming from the proximal physis, as well as the universal motion of the shoulder joint. **A** and **C,** Early remodeling. **B** and **D,** Late remodeling.

Anatomy

The proximal humeral epiphysis develops from three secondary ossification centers: one each for the humeral head, greater tuberosity, and lesser tuberosity. The secondary ossification center for the humeral head usually appears between the ages of 4 and 6 months, although it may be present before birth. The ossification center of the greater tuberosity is generally present by 3 years. The lesser tuberosity ossification center is visible

*See references 6, 7, 25, 27, 36, 42, 46, 47, 58, 63, 115, 140, 145, 176, 190, 197, 259.

radiographically by the age of 5 years. These three ossification centers coalesce into a single large center at around 7 years of age (Fig. 42–14).

The physis of the proximal humerus is concave inferiorly. Medially, it follows the line of the anatomic neck. Laterally, it extends distal to the inferior border of the greater tuberosity. The timing of closure of the proximal humeral physis is variable, with closure occurring as early as 14 years in some girls and as late as 22 years in males.[205]

The supraspinatus, infraspinatus, and teres minor muscles insert onto the greater tuberosity, and the subscapularis inserts on the lesser tuberosity. At the metadiaphyseal junction, the pectoralis major tendon inserts onto the crest of the greater tuberosity, and the teres major attaches to the inferior crest of the lesser tuberosity. The latissimus dorsi arises from the floor of the intertubercular groove.

Dameron and Reibel performed a cadaveric study of the proximal humeri of 12 stillborn infants in an effort to explain the anatomic basis for the displacement of proximal humeral fractures.[63] They found that it was difficult to displace the proximal metaphysis posteriorly but, with the arm extended and adducted, relatively easy to displace it anteriorly. They noted that the periosteum consistently tore just lateral to the biceps tendon and that the stability of the fracture decreased as the periosteal stripping progressed. They attributed the preference for anterior displacement to the asymmetric dome of the proximal humeral physis, with its posteromedial apex, and to the stronger attachment of the periosteum to the posterior surface of the metaphysis. They noted that all 12 humeri fractured through the physis without an attached fragment of metaphyseal bone.[63]

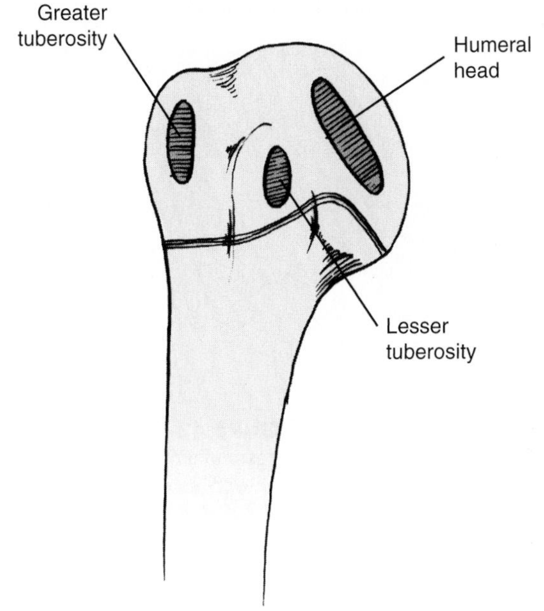

FIGURE 42–14 The three secondary ossification centers of the proximal humerus: the humeral head, greater tuberosity, and lesser tuberosity.

Mechanism of Injury

Fractures involving the proximal humeral physis can result from an indirect force extended through the humeral shaft, such as a fall on an outstretched hand, or from a direct blow to the lateral aspect of the shoulder. Neer and Horwitz attributed 59 of their 89 fractures of the proximal humerus to a direct force, usually applied to the posterolateral aspect of the shoulder.[190] Neonates may sustain proximal humeral fractures as a result of birth trauma. Proximal humeral fractures in infants may be associated with child abuse.[38,87,196]

Classification

Proximal humeral physeal fractures are most commonly classified according to the type of physeal injury or the amount of displacement, or both. Generally, infants and small children with proximal humeral physeal injuries have Salter-Harris type I fractures, whereas older children and adolescents have Salter-Harris type II injuries. The universal motion of the glenohumeral joint makes the proximal fragment resistant to injury. Thus, fractures extending through the proximal segment (i.e., Salter-Harris type III or IV injuries) or physeal fractures combined with dislocation of the glenohumeral joint are rare. However, these injuries have been described, and it is important to carefully assess adequate radiographs to ensure that no unusual occult injuries are present.[196,200,289,302]

Neer and Horwitz used the amount of displacement to classify proximal humeral physeal fractures. In grade I injuries there is less than 5 mm of displacement. Grade II injuries are displaced between 5 mm and a third the diameter of the humeral shaft. Grade III injuries are displaced between one and two thirds the diameter of the shaft, and grade IV fractures are displaced more than two thirds the diameter of the humeral shaft. In grades III and IV displacement there is always a varying degree of angulation.[190]

Diagnosis

Fracture of the proximal humeral physis should be the first diagnosis considered in injuries to the shoulder region in children between ages 9 and 15 years. If the fracture is displaced, the initial findings can be dramatic. The arm is often shortened and held in abduction and extension. The displaced distal fragment causes a prominence in the front of the axilla near the coracoid process. Frequently, the anterior axillary fold is distorted, with a characteristic puckering of the skin caused by the distal fragment. The humeral head may be palpable in its normal position. With minimally displaced fractures, the physical findings may be limited to localized swelling and tenderness.[63,140,190]

In displaced fractures the epiphysis usually remains in the glenoid fossa but is abducted and externally rotated by the pull of the attached rotator cuff. The distal fragment is displaced anteromedially by the combined action of the pectoralis major, latissimus dorsi, and teres major muscles (Fig. 42–15). The intact

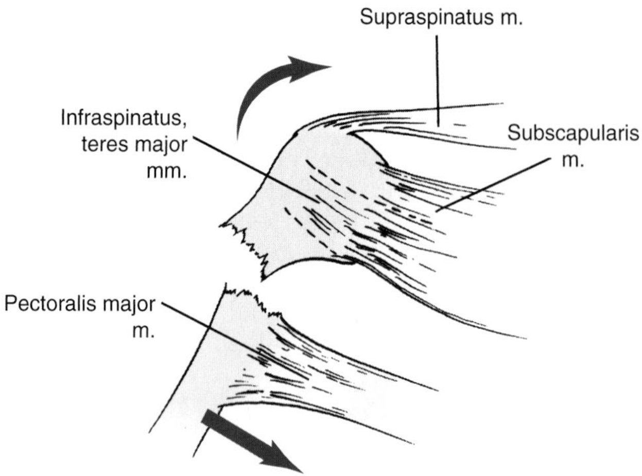

FIGURE 42–15 Displacement of proximal humeral fractures. The muscles of the rotator cuff produce abduction and external rotation of the proximal fragment (*curved arrow*), whereas the pectoralis major, teres major, and latissimus dorsi pull the distal fragment medially (*straight arrow*).

periosteum on the posteromedial aspect of the metaphysis prevents complete displacement and often makes closed reduction difficult. This intact periosteum also serves as a "mold" for the callus and later for the new bone produced by the physis (see Fig. 42–13).[63] Occasionally, the fracture is impacted, with the upper end of the metaphysis driven into the epiphysis.

When assessing trauma about the shoulder it is imperative to obtain two orthogonal radiographs to adequately assess the glenohumeral joint. Often this is difficult because the limb is painful and both the patient and the radiology technician are resistant to moving the extremity. It is incumbent on the treating surgeon to educate the radiology technician on the importance of obtaining a true AP view of the glenohumeral joint (rather than the torso; see Fig. 42–12) and positioning the arm in limited abduction to obtain an axillary lateral view of the proximal humerus. Alternatively, a Y-scapular view can be used to assess the status of the glenohumeral joint, although it is generally more difficult to obtain and interpret this radiograph than to obtain and interpret an axillary lateral view (Fig. 42–16).

The differential diagnosis of a proximal humeral fracture in a neonate or infant includes septic arthritis, osteomyelitis, and brachial plexus palsy. Radiographs of the proximal humerus may be of little help in distinguishing among these entities because much of the anatomy is nonossified cartilage. Ultrasound has proved useful in these instances; it can readily demonstrate proximal humeral fractures and can confirm reduction of the glenohumeral joint and the presence or absence of an intra-articular effusion.[31,87,153,165,253]

Treatment

Nearly all proximal humeral physeal fractures can be treated nonoperatively, regardless of the age of the patient or degree of displacement.[6,7,25,27,36,42,46,47,58,61,63,92,115,132,140,145,176,190,197,259,298]

GRADES I AND II INJURIES

Injuries with grades I and II displacement can be treated symptomatically without an attempt at reduction, regardless of the age of the patient. A simple arm sling or a sling and swath or a hook-and-loop shoulder immobilizer should be worn until the pain subsides. Gentle pendulum exercises can be instituted in the second week, and most patients resume some overhead activities within 4 to 6 weeks.

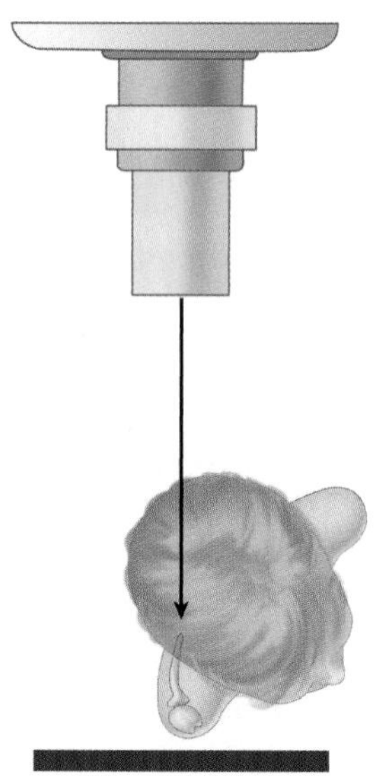

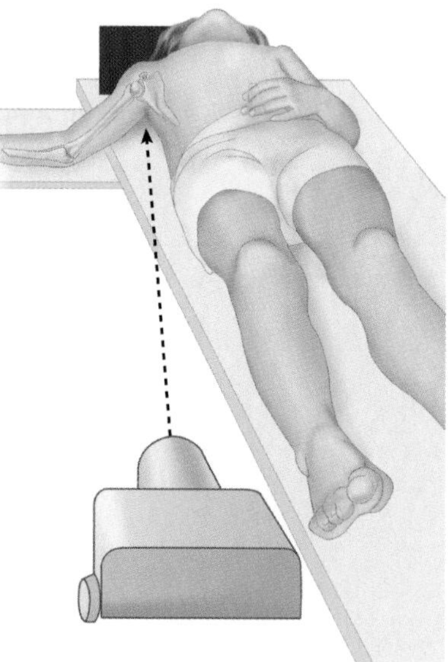

FIGURE 42–16 Sagittal assessment of the glenohumeral joint requires either a Y-scapular view **(A)** or an axillary lateral view **(B).** The Y-scapular view does not require abduction of the arm but is more difficult to obtain and interpret. An axillary lateral view can be obtained with as little as 45 degrees of abduction.

GRADES III AND IV INJURIES

Indications for the treatment of more displaced proximal humeral physeal fractures (i.e., grade III and IV injuries) are controversial. Nearly all authors agree that displaced injuries in younger children (<6 years of age) can be treated symptomatically.* Controversy exists over the management of displaced fractures in older patients. Some authors have advocated open reduction of severely displaced fractures in older children, noting that open reduction is justified on the basis of intraoperative findings, which often include infolded periosteum, interposed biceps tendon, or both.[42,61,140,162,211] However, Lucas and coworkers found that biceps interposition was very unlikely to occur even with completely displaced fractures.[164]

Interestingly, in a review of 48 patients with displaced proximal humeral fractures (all grades III and IV), Beringer and colleagues reported an increased complication rate in patients treated operatively. Complications developed in three of the nine operative patients, whereas none developed in the 39 patients treated by closed reduction. Complications of operative treatment included fracture through a percutaneous pin site, symptomatic impingement requiring hardware removal, and osteomyelitis necessitating four operative debridement procedures. They further explored the functional results by comparing patients who maintained acceptable reduction with those in whom acceptable closed reduction either could not be obtained or could not be maintained. No patient in either group had a functional deficit. To assess the results of closed treatment in patients near skeletal maturity, they examined the results of closed treatment in patients older than 15 years. Again, they found no functional limitations and no significant differences between patients with an "acceptable" reduction and those with persistent malposition. They did note an increased prevalence of "minor abnormalities" in patients with persistent malposition, although these differences were not functionally or cosmetically significant. They concluded that an attempt at maintaining anatomic closed reduction was beneficial, particularly in older adolescents, but that persistent malposition did not warrant open reduction.[27]

Despite these excellent results with conservative treatment, a number of recent reports have advocated surgical treatment. However, it is important to note that these studies do not contain a nonoperative control group.[52,71,254]

Our approach to the treatment of displaced proximal humeral physeal fractures parallels the recommendations of Beringer and colleagues.[27] We attempt closed reduction under conscious sedation in the emergency department in all patients with grades III and IV displacement. Although these fractures generally reduce easily, the reduction is not always stable enough to be maintained (Fig. 42–17).[115] Thus, in younger patients, who have tremendous remodeling potential, we believe that the benefits of a stable closed reduction, primarily less pain and less immediate cosmetic deformity, must be weighed against the risks associated with conscious sedation in patients regardless of age. The technique of closed reduction usually includes traction, abduction, forward flexion, and external rotation of the arm and forearm. Fluoroscopic guidance can be helpful during reduction, particularly if there is atypical displacement of the fracture. Once stable reduction has been achieved, the extremity is placed in a sling and swath or in a shoulder immobilizer for 2 to 3 weeks until the fracture fragments are "sticky." At that point the immobilization can be discontinued and range-of-motion exercises instituted.

*See references 6, 7, 25, 27, 36, 42, 46, 47, 58, 63, 92, 115, 140, 145, 176, 190, 197, 259, 298.

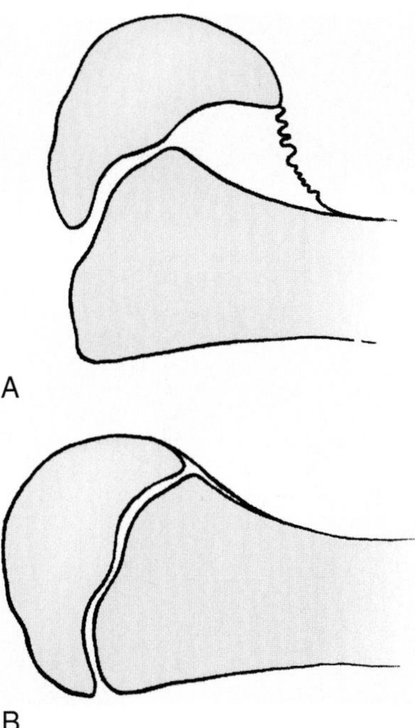

FIGURE 42–17 The intact periosteum on the displaced side of a proximal humeral fracture **(A)** may enhance the stability of the fracture once the fracture has been reduced **(B)**.

In patients in whom reduction can be achieved but is lost once the traction or abduction is removed and in patients in whom we cannot obtain adequate closed reduction, the existing deformity is accepted and patients are managed symptomatically. The parents of these patients usually need a fair amount of reassurance that remodeling will provide an acceptable cosmetic and functional result.

We reserve operative treatment of displaced proximal humeral fractures for patients with intra-articular or open fractures or neurovascular injury. Additionally, we occasionally stabilize a proximal humeral fracture percutaneously in a polytraumatized patient who is undergoing operative treatment of other injuries because we believe that a stabilized extremity is easier to care for in an intensive care unit setting.[196,200,289,302] Though rarer, avulsion fractures of the lesser tuberosity, which may be manifested as chronic shoulder pain without a definite injury, are another injury that may benefit from open reduction and internal fixation.[157]

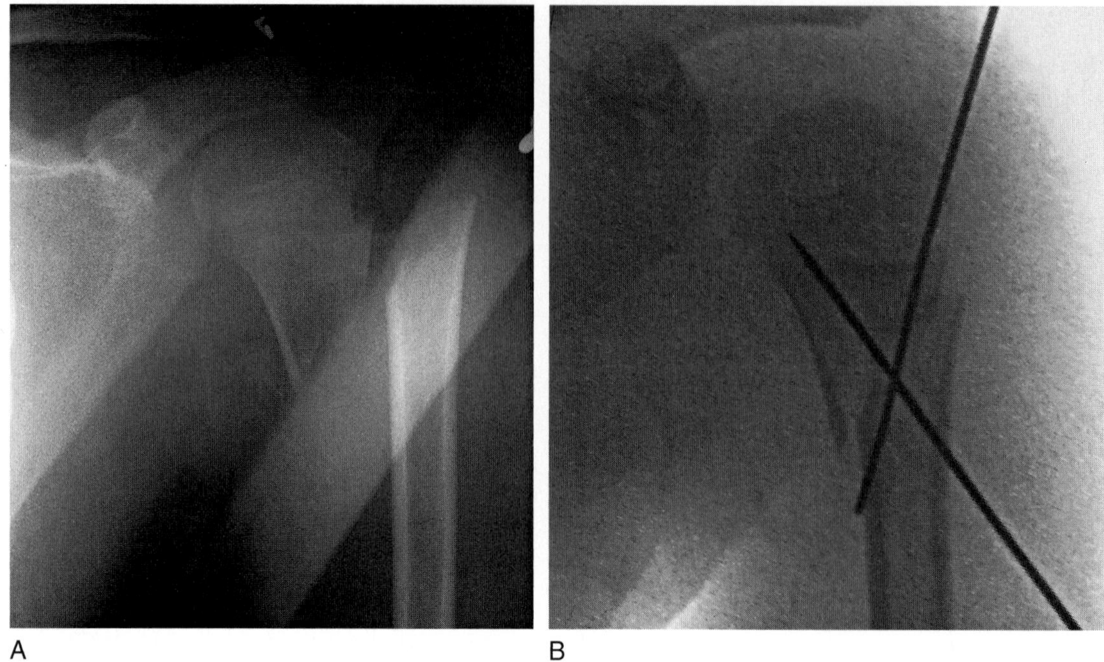

FIGURE 42–18 **A**, Anteroposterior (AP) radiograph of a displaced proximal humeral metaphyseal fracture. **B**, AP radiograph obtained after closed reduction and percutaneous pin fixation. Fracture stabilization eases nursing care in a polytraumatized patient.

Intra-articular fractures require anatomic reduction, which can generally be performed through an anterior arthrotomy via a standard deltopectoral approach. Fixation can be achieved with a combination of screws and percutaneous pins. Every effort should be made to avoid crossing the physis with threaded fixation devices. Our goal in operative treatment of nonarticular fractures is stabilization of the fracture to allow adequate management of concurrent injuries, whether they be neurovascular, soft tissue, or multiorgan injuries. We do not insist on anatomic reduction, and we usually stabilize the fracture with two percutaneous 0.062-inch K-wires (Fig. 42–18).[185,190] We remove the K-wires after 2 to 3 weeks and limit motion of the extremity while they are in place in an attempt to minimize soft tissue complications. As with nonoperative treatment, range-of-motion exercises are begun as soon as all percutaneous pins are removed and the patient is comfortable, generally in 2 to 3 weeks.

Complications

Complications of proximal humeral physeal fractures are rare. The most commonly reported complication is shortening of the humerus. This complication is rarely a functional or cosmetic concern and is noted more frequently in older children with more severely displaced fractures.[6,133] Neer and Horwitz noted inequality of humeral length in 11% of patients with grade I or II displacement and approximately 33% of patients with grade III or IV displacement. No patient had shortening greater than 3 cm, and inequality was seen only in patients older than 11 years at the time of injury.[190] Baxter and Wiley noted shortening greater than 1 cm in 9 of 30 patients.[25] No patient had more than 2 cm of shortening, and none of their patients was clinically aware of the inequality. Unlike Neer and Horwitz, they noted shortening in patients younger than 11 years of age.[25] Beringer and colleagues reported shortening greater than 2 cm in 5 of 18 patients treated conservatively and available for review an average of 4 years after the injury. Again, none of these patients had a functional complaint.[27]

Varus malalignment of the proximal humerus has also been reported as a complication of proximal humeral epiphyseal fractures. Like shortening, this complication is rarely a functional concern and is most commonly noted as an incidental finding at follow-up. There have been cases reported of severe varus combined with shortening that caused significant functional deficits. This complication is rare and probably represents an infantile fracture complicated by growth arrest.[36,78,140,144,165]

Injuries to the brachial plexus and axillary nerve, as well as brachial artery disruption, valgus malalignment, and osteonecrosis of the humeral head, have been reported as rare or unusual complications of proximal humeral fractures.[25,72,173,280]

Associated Conditions

LITTLE LEAGUE SHOULDER

Little League shoulder, also called *proximal humeral epiphysiolysis, osteochondrosis of the proximal humerus,* or

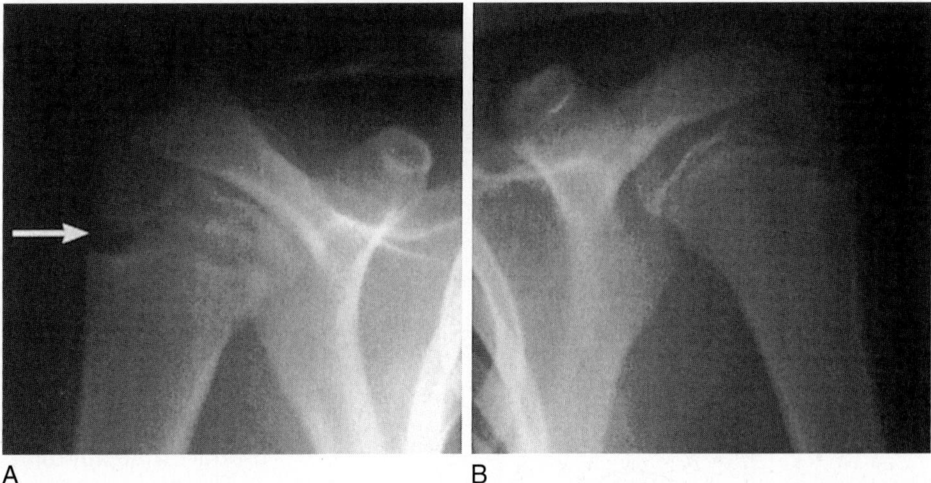

FIGURE 42–19 A and B, Anteroposterior radiographs of both shoulders in an adolescent baseball player. Note the widened right proximal humeral epiphysis (*arrow* in **A**).

traction apophysitis of the proximal humerus, is an overuse injury seen most commonly in pitchers but occasionally in other overhead athletes.[3,4,21,50,62,107,161,277,278] This entity is usually accompanied by nonspecific shoulder pain, often at the beginning of the season or after a significant change in training protocol. There may be point tenderness along the proximal humeral physis and painful or limited range of motion. It is believed to result from rotary torque generated during the cocking and acceleration phases of throwing or from deceleration distraction forces during follow-through.[3,4,107,161,247,278] Meister and associates have shown that shoulder range of motion in adolescent pitchers decreases with age—most dramatically between 13 and 14 years, which corresponds to the age at the peak incidence of Little League shoulder.[179] Radiographs may be normal or may show widening of the proximal humeral physis (Fig. 42–19). Occasionally a stress fracture is present, with metaphyseal lucency and periosteal new bone formation.[277] This condition almost always responds to rest, although displacement through the physis has been reported.[3,4,21,43,62,161,277,278]

Traumatic Dislocation of the Glenohumeral Joint

Traumatic glenohumeral dislocation is an unusual injury in children; it occurs most commonly in older adolescents involved in contact sports.[80,90,110,135,171,200,235] It is important to distinguish traumatic dislocation from atraumatic or voluntary dislocation or subluxation because treatment of these conditions is vastly different.[240,260]

Anatomy

The glenohumeral joint is one of the most mobile joints of the musculoskeletal system. Although its unique anatomic features give it nearly universal motion, they do so at the expense of stability. Conceptually, the shoulder is similar to a ball suspended from a plate. Thus, the glenohumeral joint has little inherent bony stability. Rather, shoulder stability is provided entirely by the muscles and ligaments that suspend the humerus from the glenoid.[28,30,60,175]

The muscles of the rotator cuff—the supraspinatus, infraspinatus, teres minor, and subscapularis—provide dynamic stability to the shoulder, whereas the capsule and ligamentous complex provide static support. The shoulder capsule has about twice the surface area of the humeral head. The capsule extends from the glenoid neck and labrum to the anatomic neck of the humerus. Medially, the capsule extends distally past the physis and inserts on the proximal humeral metaphysis.[60] The inner surface of the capsule is thickened into the anterior glenohumeral ligaments. The most important of these is the anteroinferior glenohumeral ligament, which is the most common site of pathology in anterior shoulder instability.[29,85,201,202,236,242,263,266,272,279]

With traumatic anterior dislocation of the humeral head, the inferior glenohumeral ligament and anterior labrum are usually traumatically disrupted. Although repair of this "essential lesion" was first described by Broca and Hartman, as well as Perthes, it was popularized by Bankart and is commonly referred to as a *Bankart lesion* (or *repair*).[18-20] When displaced anteriorly, the posterior aspect of the humeral head lies against the anterior glenoid, potentially producing a defect in the humeral head, the so-called Hill-Sachs lesion.[113] With posterior dislocation, defects can be found on the anterior aspect of the humeral head (Fig. 42–20).[17,32,44,175,226,271,285]

Mechanism of Injury

Traumatic shoulder dislocation most commonly occurs as a result of an indirect force. Anterior dislocations represent more than 90% of glenohumeral dislocations.[235] Anterior dislocation usually occurs when a force is applied to an arm in an abducted, extended, and externally rotated position. Traumatic shoulder dislocations may also occur posteriorly or inferiorly. Posterior dislocations may be the result of a direct

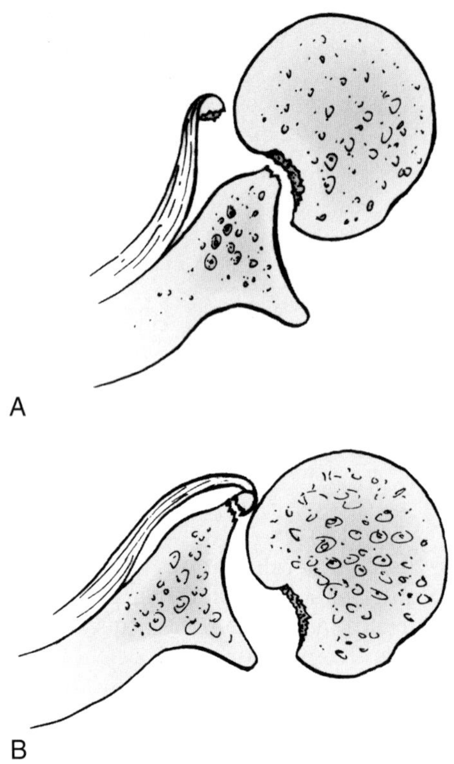

FIGURE 42-20 **A,** Anterior dislocation of the glenohumeral joint produces the characteristic Bankart lesion of the glenoid and a Hill-Sachs lesion of the humeral head. **B,** Anatomy after reduction.

blow to the anterior aspect of the shoulder; an indirect force with the arm in flexion, adduction, and internal rotation; or a massive muscle contraction, as occurs with an electrical shock or seizure.[28,51,90,136,186,187,203,243] Inferior glenohumeral dislocation is also known as *luxatio erecta.* When seen in children or adolescents, luxatio erecta is almost always the result of a high-energy hyperabduction force.[65,66,91,163,169]

Diagnosis

Traumatic dislocation of the glenohumeral joint generally results in a fixed dislocation that is usually acutely painful. With anterior dislocation the arm is typically held in slight abduction and external rotation. Attempts to move the arm are often extremely painful because of the muscle spasm that occurs in an attempt to stabilize the joint. The humeral head is palpable anteriorly, and there is a "defect" inferior to the acromion. Occasionally, patients with recurrent anterior dislocations spontaneously reduce the dislocation, although care must be taken to distinguish these patients from those who "voluntarily" dislocate their shoulders, because the latter have a high incidence of psychological problems.[241,260] It is important to distinguish a psychological voluntary dislocator from a patient who can voluntarily demonstrate the instability but whose primary problem is painful involuntary dislocation.

Historically, posterior dislocation of the glenohumeral joint has been a frequently missed diagnosis. Rowe and Zarins reported that 11 of 14 posterior shoulder dislocations were not recognized by the initial treating physician.[243] However, careful physical examination of a patient with a posterior dislocation will reveal several characteristic findings. The arm is usually held in adduction and internal rotation and has limited and painful external rotation and abduction. Additionally, the shoulder will be flattened anteriorly and have a prominent coracoid process and posterior appearance.[51,90,136,186,187,203,243] Patients with luxatio erecta hold the arm maximally abducted adjacent to the head. The force of the injury may drive the humeral head through the soft tissues of the axilla and produce an open injury.[65,66,91,163,169,252]

The diagnosis of glenohumeral dislocation is often obvious on the basis of the physical examination alone and is simply confirmed radiographically. The high rate of missed diagnoses of posterior dislocations may be due to the nearly normal appearance of a posterior dislocation of the shoulder on an AP radiograph of the torso. This emphasizes the importance of high-quality orthogonal radiographs, as discussed earlier for fractures of the proximal humeral physis (see Figs. 42–12 and 42–16).

Every patient with a traumatic glenohumeral dislocation should undergo a complete neurovascular examination, including assessment of the radial, median, ulnar, musculoskeletal, and axillary nerves. The axillary nerve is the most commonly injured nerve with anterior dislocation. Often the pain associated with an acute shoulder dislocation makes assessment of deltoid muscle function difficult. Thus, it is important to assess the sensory distribution of the axillary nerve in all patients with anterior shoulder dislocations (Fig. 42–21).

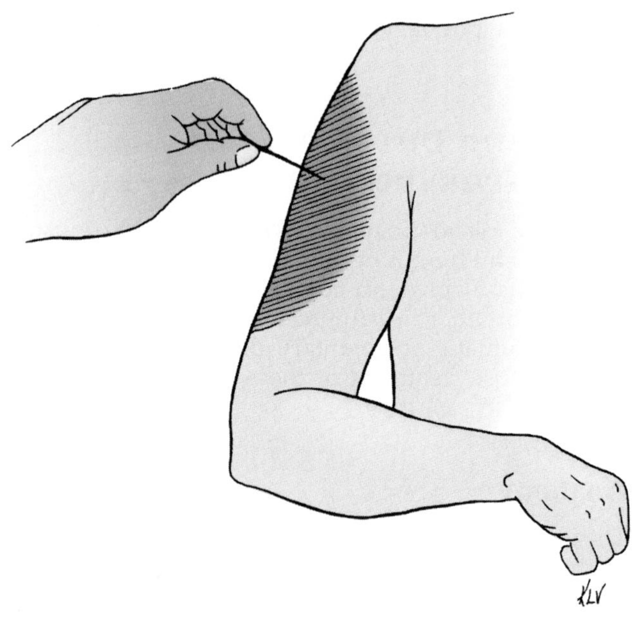

FIGURE 42-21 Sensory distribution of the axillary nerve.

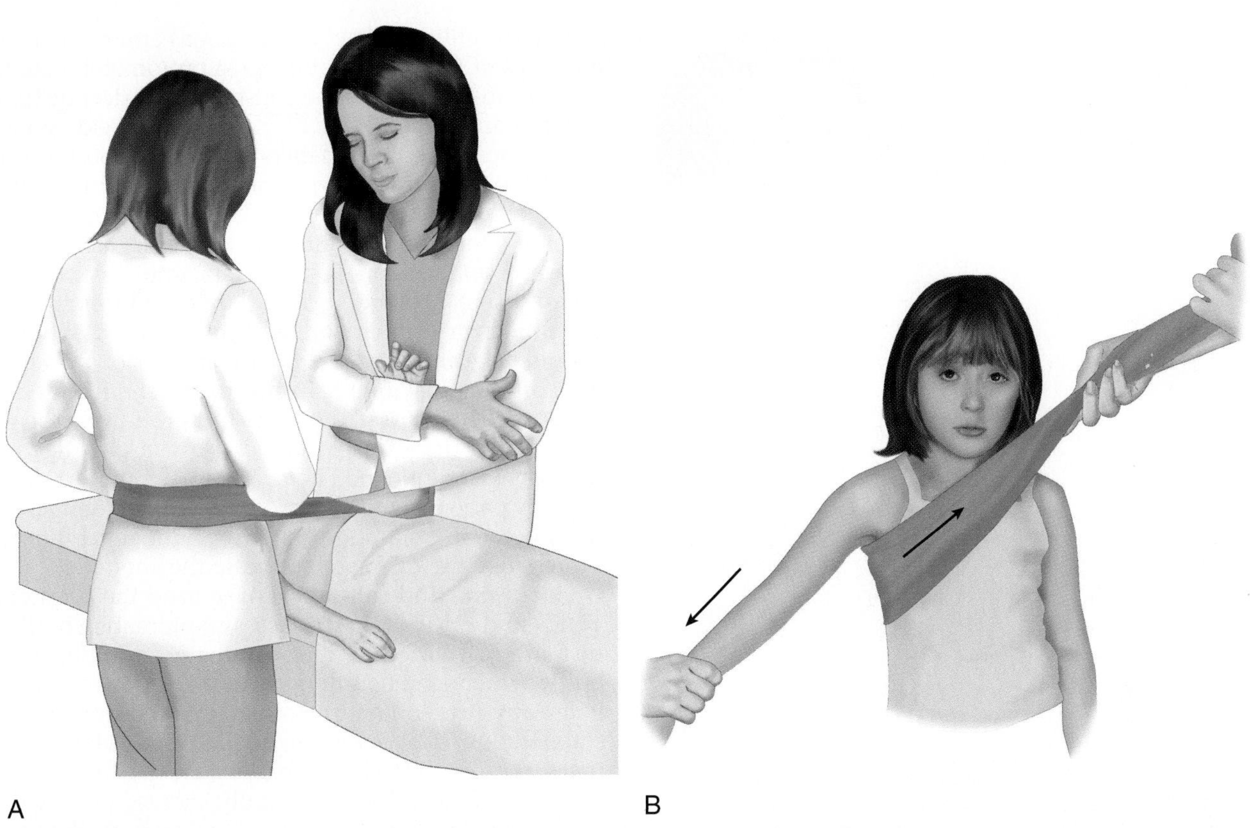

FIGURE 42–22 **A** and **B**, Traction-countertraction technique for reduction of glenohumeral dislocation. Longitudinal traction is applied through the arm and forearm with the arm abducted and the elbow flexed. Gentle internal and external rotation will help reduce the humeral head.

Treatment

Acute traumatic dislocation of the glenohumeral joint should be reduced as quickly and atraumatically as possible. There are numerous techniques for reduction, with descriptions dating to ancient times.[2,268,308] We prefer closed reduction with the traction-countertraction technique performed under conscious sedation. A sheet is placed around the affected axilla to allow an assistant to apply countertraction. Once adequate sedation has been achieved, longitudinal traction is applied through the arm and forearm with the arm abducted and the elbow flexed. Gentle internal and external rotation will help disengage the humeral head. Eventually, the spastic muscles will be fatigued and reduction can be achieved. This technique is effective for both anterior and posterior dislocations (Fig. 42–22). If an assistant is not available, countertraction can be achieved by the surgeon's placing a foot across the anterior and posterior axillary folds and against the chest wall (Fig. 42–23) (This is the technique described by Hippocrates.[2]) Another useful technique that requires no assistant is a modification of the technique described by Stimson. The patient is placed prone with the affected extremity dangling over the edge of the table. With adequate sedation and time, the shoulder will reduce. Reduction can be facilitated by adding weights to the wrist. The amount of weight depends on the size of the patient. We generally start with approximately 5 lb in an athletic adolescent (Fig. 42–24).[268]

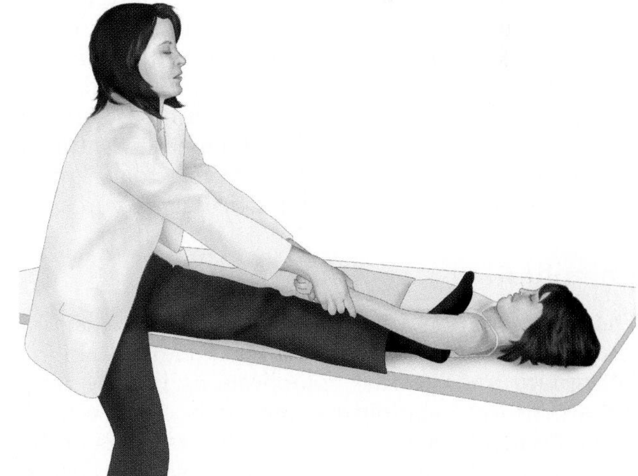

FIGURE 42–23 Hippocrates' technique for reducing a glenohumeral dislocation. This technique is useful when no assistant is available. The surgeon's foot should be placed against the chest wall, not in the axilla.

Postreduction management consists of a careful repeat neurovascular examination, orthogonal radiographs, and sling immobilization. We generally manage patients symptomatically after reduction,

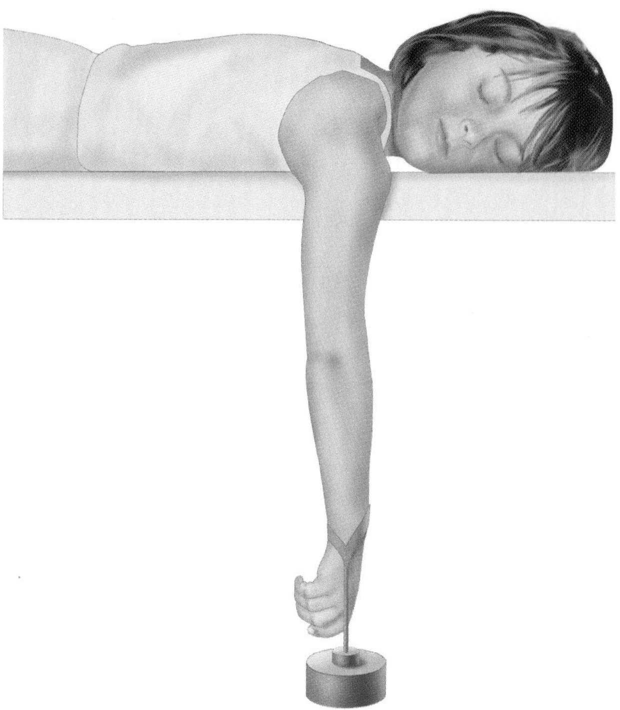

FIGURE 42-24 Modified Stimson technique for reducing a glenohumeral dislocation. The patient is placed prone with the shoulder over the edge of a table and weights suspended from the wrist.

with a sling used for immobilization until upper extremity function can resume, usually in 2 to 3 weeks. Although children and adolescents with traumatic dislocation of the glenohumeral joint are at high risk for recurrence, there is little evidence that prolonged post-reduction immobilization alters the natural history of post-traumatic instability.[80,110,135,171] Operative treatment is reserved for patients with open dislocations, "unreducible" dislocations, and intra-articular fractures.

Complications

The most common complication of traumatic dislocation of the shoulder is recurrent shoulder instability. Other rare but reported complications include fractures, neurovascular injuries, and rarely, osteonecrosis of the humeral head.[16,91,142,163,169,187,200,233] Fractures of the glenoid or humeral head were discussed earlier. In general, intra-articular fractures require open reduction and internal fixation.[16,51,55,142,196,200,203] This is usually best performed through an anterior deltopectoral approach. Effort should be made to avoid threaded fixation across the physis, which may produce growth arrest. Percutaneous pins around the shoulder should be avoided because of the potentially devastating complication of pin migration.[94,128] Open injuries and neurovascular injuries are extremely rare and should be managed individually, with care taken to adhere to the general principles discussed in Chapter 40, General Principles of Managing Orthopaedic Injuries.[66,163]

Recurrent instability can be seen as either repetitive episodes of fixed dislocation or symptomatic instability manifested as a vague sense of shoulder dysfunction or pain.[17,171,233,236,239,242,271,285] Although the diagnosis of recurrent fixed dislocation is relatively straightforward, the diagnosis of symptomatic recurrent instability is often difficult to make. Patients suspected of having symptomatic anterior instability should be assessed for evidence of generalized ligamentous laxity. The contralateral shoulder should be carefully examined for comparison, and the involved shoulder should be examined for evidence of anterior, posterior, and inferior instability. Examination should include the apprehension test, the load-shift or drawer test, the sulcus test, the jerk test, and the push-pull test. As previously mentioned, it is extremely important to identify patients who voluntarily dislocate their shoulders, because no amount of surgery or rehabilitation can change the desire to dislocate the shoulder.

Rockwood and colleagues have used the acronyms TUBS and AMBRI to discuss symptomatic shoulder instability. TUBS describes *t*raumatic shoulder instability, which is generally *u*nilateral. A *B*ankart lesion is usually present, and most patients require *s*urgical stabilization. The acronym AMBRI represents *a*traumatic shoulder instability that is generally *m*ultidirectional and *b*ilateral and is usually successfully treated with a *r*ehabilitation program. If surgery is required, an *i*nferior capsule shift is generally indicated.[56,230]

The incidence of recurrent dislocation in children and adolescents who sustain a traumatic glenohumeral dislocation has been reported to be as high as 70% to 100%.[17,67,80,110,148,171,220,233,236,239,240,242] Although most patients who develop symptomatic post-traumatic recurrent instability—whether they are recurrent dislocators or patients with pain but no dislocation—eventually require surgical stabilization, the first line of treatment is an appropriate rehabilitation program that emphasizes strengthening of the rotator cuff muscles. Although such a program may not alleviate all symptoms, it frequently improves both function and stability and provides an elevated preoperative baseline with regard to strength, range of motion, pain, and an understanding of the postoperative rehabilitative effort required. Surgical treatment of symptomatic anterior instability is most commonly accomplished with a modification of the Bankart repair. It may be performed either in open fashion or arthroscopically. Recently, Deitch and colleagues found no functional difference between patients treated surgically and those treated nonsurgically, although they questioned the ability of available functional instruments to discriminate between patients who do and do not choose surgery.[67] Lawton and coworkers noted similar findings in a review of 70 pediatric patients and adolescents with shoulder instability. Forty-two shoulders received physical therapy, and 28 required surgery. At follow-up, 54 of 70 described their shoulders as "better" or "much better," and 90% were performing at the same or higher levels of sports and work.[148] It is important to realize that some patients have traumatic instability that is compounded by preexisting multidirectional instability.[32,239] Operative repair in these patients should include efforts to "tighten" the redundant inferior capsule. There are numerous references in the adult literature that describe both the open and arthroscopic surgical techniques.[8,17,32,85,171,233,239,271,272,285]

Fractures of the Proximal Metaphysis and Shaft of the Humerus

Fractures of the proximal metaphysis and shaft of the humerus are usually straightforward.[33,48,104,116,121,139] Fractures of the proximal humeral metaphysis are more common in children than adolescents because adolescents are more likely to sustain physeal injuries. Humeral shaft fractures are the second most frequent birth fracture.[87,258] Fractures of the humeral shaft are less common in children than in adults but, as in adults, are frequently associated with radial nerve injury.

Anatomy

The humerus is cylindrical proximally and becomes broad and flat in its distal metaphysis. The deltoid, biceps brachii, and brachialis muscles cover it anteriorly. The coracobrachialis muscle inserts beneath the upper half of the biceps brachii muscle. The pectoralis major inserts into the lateral lip of the bicipital groove. The posterior surface is covered by the deltoid and triceps muscles (Fig. 42–25). On the lateral and medial aspects of the humerus, intermuscular septa divide the arm into anterior and posterior compartments. Anteriorly, the neurovascular bundle, which consists of the brachial vessels and the median, musculocutaneous, and ulnar nerves, courses along the medial aspect of the humerus. The radial nerve lies in the posterior compartment in a shallow groove between the origins of the medial and lateral heads of the triceps. The radial nerve runs obliquely downward and laterally as it passes from the axilla to the anterolateral epicondylar region.[33-35,48,104,116,117,121,139,212,219,256]

Fracture angulation depends on whether the fracture is proximal or distal to the insertion of the deltoid. When the fracture is distal to the deltoid insertion, the action of the supraspinatus, deltoid, and coracobrachialis muscles displaces the proximal fragment laterally and anteriorly, whereas the distal fragment is drawn upward by the biceps and brachialis muscles. If the fracture occurs proximal to the insertion of the deltoid but distal to that of the pectoralis major, the pull of the deltoid will displace the distal fragment laterally and upward, whereas the pectoralis major, latissimus dorsi, and teres major muscles will adduct and medially rotate the proximal fragment. Displace-

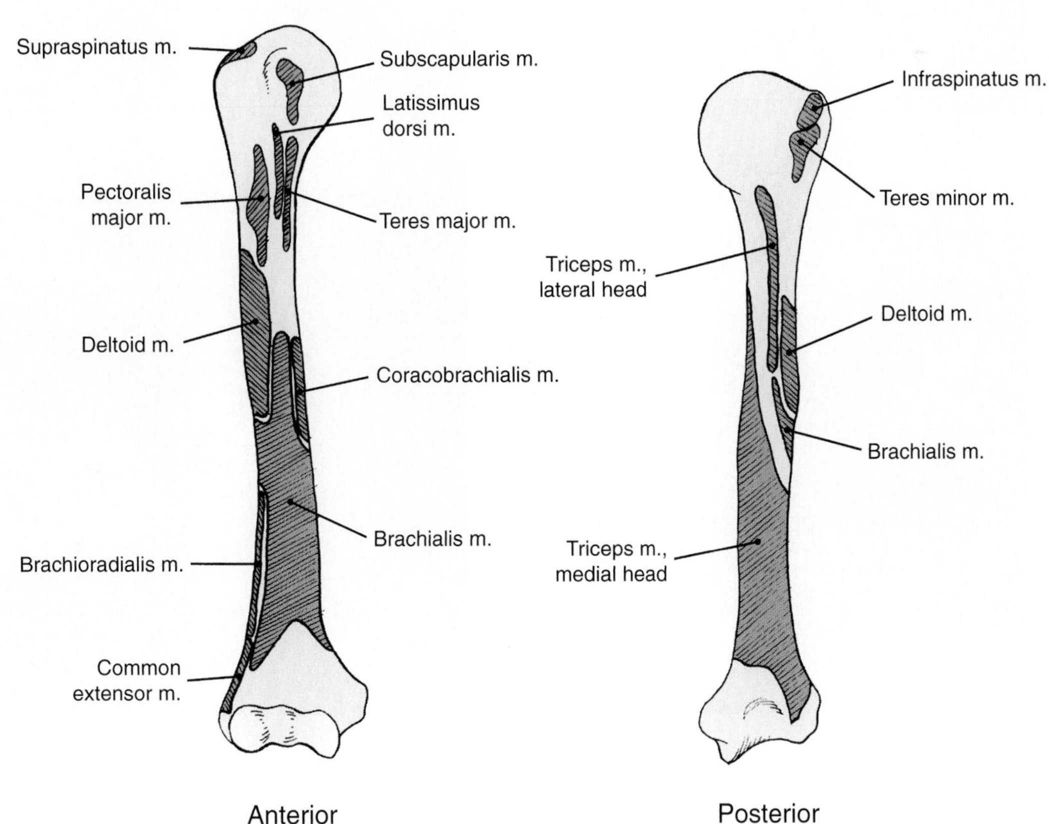

FIGURE 42–25 Anterior and posterior muscular insertions of the humerus.

ment of the fracture fragments is also influenced by gravity, the position in which the upper limb is held, and the forces causing the fracture. The distal fragment is usually internally rotated because the arm is held across the chest while the proximal fragment remains in mid-position.[33,48,104,116,121,139]

Mechanism of Injury

Fractures of the proximal humeral metaphysis are generally a result of a high-energy direct force.[33,48,104,116,121,139] As such, they are frequently associated with multiple trauma. Fractures in this area that occur after minimal trauma should raise suspicion of a pathologic fracture because this is a common location for unicameral bone cysts and other benign lesions (Fig. 42–26). Most fractures of the shaft of the humerus are also caused by a direct force, such as a fall on the side of the arm. Consequently, they are usually transverse or comminuted fractures and are frequently open injuries. An indirect force, such as a fall on an outstretched hand, can produce an oblique or spiral fracture of the humeral shaft. Forceful muscle contraction, such as in throwing a baseball, has also been reported to cause humeral shaft fractures, although such a history should raise the possibility of a pathologic fracture through a lesion such as a unicameral bone cyst or fibrous dysplasia (Fig. 42–27).[5,33,48,89,104,116,121,129,139,172,227]

Diagnosis

The obvious deformity, localized swelling, and pain caused by fractures of the proximal humeral metaphysis or humeral shaft make the clinical diagnosis straightforward. However, due diligence is required to detect associated neurovascular injury. The intimate relationship of the radial nerve to the humerus makes it especially vulnerable to injury. Radial nerve injury results in anesthesia over the dorsum of the hand between the first and second metacarpals and loss of motor strength of the wrist, finger, and thumb extensors, as well as the forearm supinators. The median and ulnar nerves are rarely injured. Vascular injury is also extremely rare.[33-35,48,95,104,116,117,121,139,168,212,219,256,301]

Treatment

In infants with obstetric fractures, the fracture is immobilized for a period of 1 to 3 weeks by bandaging the arm to the side of the thorax in a modified Velpeau bandage or a sling and swath. Parents should be instructed in skin care for the immobilized

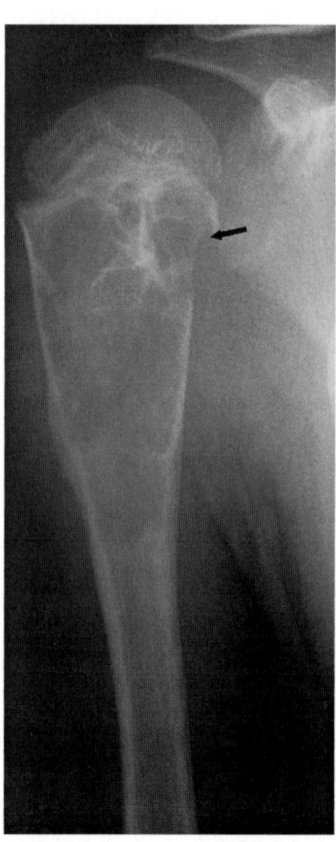

FIGURE 42–26 Anteroposterior radiograph of the proximal end of the humerus showing a fracture of the medial metaphysis (*arrow*) after minimal trauma. Note the large, expansile unicameral bone cyst.

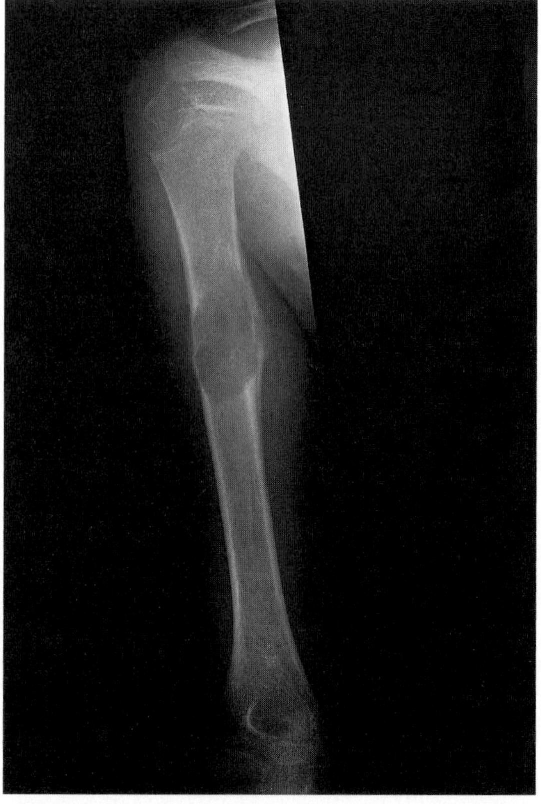

FIGURE 42–27 Anteroposterior radiograph showing a healing pathologic fracture of the humeral shaft. The diaphyseal lesion has the characteristic ground-glass appearance of fibrous dysplasia.

extremity and forewarned of the large palpable callus that will develop in 6 to 8 weeks. Efforts to control alignment are not necessary because the remodeling potential is great. Follow-up examination is required only for assessment of brachial plexus function to ensure that a concomitant nerve palsy does not exist. Primitive reflexes such as the Moro reflex can be valuable in assessing upper extremity function in an infant.[15,38,87,260]

As with fractures involving the proximal humeral physis, the remodeling potential of proximal humeral metaphyseal fractures is great. Consequently, these fractures rarely require more than symptomatic treatment with sling immobilization. Occasionally, we manage polytraumatized patients or open fractures with percutaneous fixation (see Fig. 42–18).[130,245]

Fractures of the humeral shaft are generally best managed with closed techniques.[49] Most commonly, we initially place these patients in a coaptation splint. After 2 to 3 weeks patients can be managed in a sling or hanging arm cast. It is not essential to obtain end-to-end anatomic alignment because overgrowth is common in humeral shaft fractures. Overriding of 1 to 1.5 cm can easily be accepted; however, angulation of more than 15 to 20 degrees in either plane is not desirable, and as with any fracture, rotational remodeling potential is minimal. Consequently, rotational alignment should be maintained. Circumduction and pendulum exercises for the shoulder are demonstrated and begun as soon as pain allows, usually after 2 to 3 weeks. Again, we occasionally treat open injuries or polytraumatized patients with operative techniques.[40,231] External fixation may be indicated for extensive soft tissue injuries, although internal fixation allows easier nursing care.[130] We have found flexible nails to be an easy and effective means of managing humeral shaft fractures in polytraumatized patients (Fig. 42–28).[23,120,245,310]

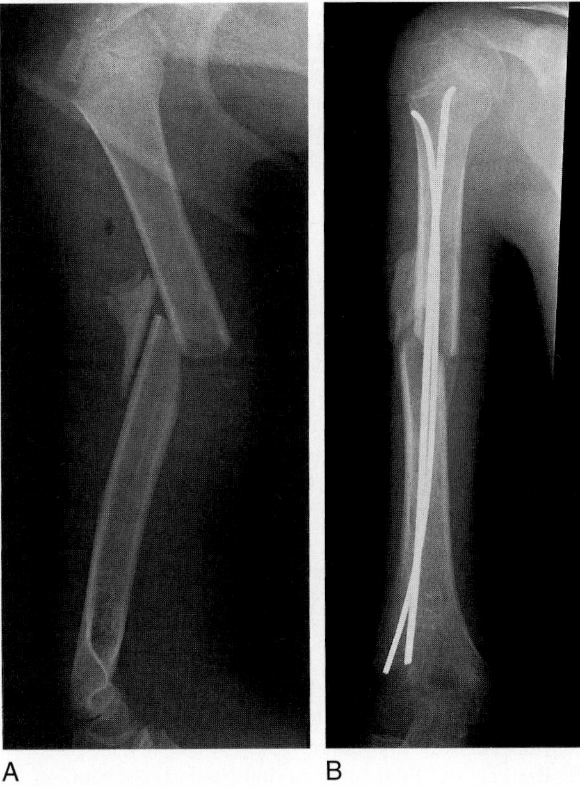

FIGURE 42–28 Comminuted humeral shaft fracture **(A)** treated with flexible intramedullary fixation **(B)**.

Complications

Complications after fractures of the proximal metaphysis or shaft of the humerus are unusual. As with any fracture, open or vascular injuries can occur. These injuries should be managed individually with attention to the guidelines discussed in Chapter 40, General Principles of Managing Orthopaedic Injuries.[95,106]

Radial nerve injury, which is not uncommon in adults, is rare in children. Complete severance of the nerve in closed fractures is very unlikely, and nerve function generally recovers if the fracture is managed conservatively. Thus, these patients should be managed with cast immobilization, with careful splinting of the wrist and hand in a functional position; passive exercises should be performed to maintain full range of motion. If there is no evidence of functional recovery after 3 to 4 months, electromyographic studies or exploration of the nerve may be indicated.[34,35,117,121,212,219,256]

Nonunion of humeral shaft fractures is much less common in children and adolescents than in adults but it does occasionally occur. In general, we prefer to treat nonunion by open reduction and plate fixation.[61,106,159,276]

References

Injuries to the Clavicle, Fractures of the Scapula, Fractures Involving the Proximal Humeral Physis, Traumatic Dislocation of the Glenohumeral Joint, Fractures of the Proximal Metaphysis and Shaft of the Humerus

1. Ada JR, Miller ME: Scapular fractures. Analysis of 113 cases. Clin Orthop Relat Res 1991;269:174.
2. Adams F: The Genuine Works of Hippocrates, vols 1 and 2. New York, William Wood, 1981.
3. Adams JE: Little league shoulder: Osteochondrosis of the proximal humeral epiphysis in boy baseball pitchers. Calif Med 1966;105:22.
4. Adams JE: Bone injuries in very young athletes. Clin Orthop Relat Res 1968;58:129.
5. Ahn JI, Park JS: Pathological fractures secondary to unicameral bone cysts. Int Orthop 1994;18:20.
6. Aitken A: End results of fractures of the proximal humeral epiphysis. J Bone Joint Surg 1936;18:1036.
7. Aitken AP: Fractures of the proximal humeral epiphysis. Surg Clin North Am 1963;43:1573.
8. Aldridge JM 3rd, Perry JJ, Osbahr DC, et al: Thermal capsulorrhaphy of bilateral glenohumeral joints in

a pediatric patient with Ehlers-Danlos syndrome. Arthroscopy 2003;19:E41.
9. Ali Khan MA, Lucas HK: Plating of fractures of the middle third of the clavicle. Injury 1978;9:263.
10. Alkalaj I: Internal fixation of a severe clavicular fracture in a child. Isr Med J 1960;19:306.
11. Allmann F: Fractures and ligamentous injuries of the clavicle and its articulation. J Bone Joint Surg Am 1967;49:774.
12. An HS, Vonderbrink JP, Ebraheim NA, et al: Open scapulothoracic dissociation with intact neurovascular status in a child. J Orthop Trauma 1988;2:36.
13. Armstrong CP, Van der Spuy J: The fractured scapula: Importance and management based on a series of 62 patients. Injury 1984;15:324.
14. Asher MA: Dislocations of the upper extremity in children. Orthop Clin North Am 1976;7:583.
15. Astedt B: A method for the treatment of humerus fractures in the newborn using the S. von Rosen splint. Acta Orthop Scand 1969;40:234.
16. Aston JW Jr, Gregory CF: Dislocation of the shoulder with significant fracture of the glenoid. J Bone Joint Surg Am 1973;55:1531.
17. Baker CL, Uribe JW, Whitman C: Arthroscopic evaluation of acute initial anterior shoulder dislocations. Am J Sports Med 1990;18:25.
18. Bankart A: Recurrent or habitual dislocation of the shoulder joint. BMJ 1923;2:1132.
19. Bankart A: Dislocation of the Shoulder Joints. Robert Jones' Birthday Volume: A Collection of Surgical Essays. London, Oxford University Press, 1928, p 307.
20. Bankart A: The pathology and treatment of recurrent dislocation of the shoulder joint. Br J Surg 1938;26:23.
21. Barnett LS: Little League shoulder syndrome: Proximal humeral epiphyseolysis in adolescent baseball pitchers. A case report. J Bone Joint Surg Am 1985;67:495.
22. Barth E, Hagen R: Surgical treatment of dislocations of the sternoclavicular joint. Acta Orthop Scand 1983; 54:746.
23. Bartl V, Melichar I, Gal P: [Personal experience with elastic stable intramedullary osteosynthesis in children.] Rozhl Chir 1996;75:486.
24. Bauer G, Fleischmann W, Dussler E: Displaced scapular fractures: Indication and long-term results of open reduction and internal fixation. Arch Orthop Trauma Surg 1995;114:215.
25. Baxter MP, Wiley JJ: Fractures of the proximal humeral epiphysis. Their influence on humeral growth. J Bone Joint Surg Br 1986;68:570.
26. Bearn JG: Direct observations on the function of the capsule of the sternoclavicular joint in clavicular support. J Anat 1967;101:159.
27. Beringer DC, Weiner DS, Noble JS, et al: Severely displaced proximal humeral epiphyseal fractures: A follow-up study. J Pediatr Orthop 1998;18:31.
28. Bianchi S, Zwass A, Abdelwahab I: Sonographic evaluation of posterior instability and dislocation of the shoulder: Prospective study. J Ultrasound Med 1994; 13:389.
29. Bigliani LU, Pollock RG, Soslowsky LJ, et al: Tensile properties of the inferior glenohumeral ligament. J Orthop Res 1992;10:187.
30. Birnbaum K, Prescher A, Heller KD: Anatomic and functional aspects of the kinetics of the shoulder joint capsule and the subacromial bursa. Surg Radiol Anat 1998;20:41.
31. Bjerneld H, Hovelius L, Thorling J: Acromio-clavicular separations treated conservatively. A 5-year follow-up study. Acta Orthop Scand 1983;54:743.
32. Blasier RB, Bruckner JD, Janda DH, et al: The Bankart repair illustrated in cross-section. Some anatomical considerations. Am J Sports Med 1989;17:630.
33. Bohler L: Conservative treatment of fresh closed fractures of the shaft of the humerus. J Truama 1965; 5:464.
34. Bostman O, Bakalim G, Vainionpaa S, et al: Immediate radial nerve palsy complicating fracture of the shaft of the humerus: When is early exploration justified? Injury 1985;16:499.
35. Bostman O, Bakalim G, Vainionpaa S, et al: Radial palsy in shaft fracture of the humerus. Acta Orthop Scand 1986;57:316.
36. Bourdillon J: Fracture separation of the proximal epiphysis of the humerus. J Bone Joint Surg Br 1950; 32:35.
37. Bowen RE, Mah JY, Otsuka NY: Midshaft clavicle fractures associated with atlantoaxial rotatory displacement: A report of two cases. J Orthop Trauma 2003; 17:444.
38. Broker FH, Burbach T: Ultrasonic diagnosis of separation of the proximal humeral epiphysis in the newborn. J Bone Joint Surg Am 1990;72:187.
39. Brooks A, Henning G: Injury to the proximal clavicular epiphysis. J Bone Joint Surg Am 1972;54:1347.
40. Brumback RJ, Bosse MJ, Poka A, et al: Intramedullary stabilization of humeral shaft fractures in patients with multiple trauma. J Bone Joint Surg Am 1986;68:960.
41. Buckerfield CT, Castle ME: Acute traumatic retrosternal dislocation of the clavicle. J Bone Joint Surg Am 1984;66:379.
42. Burgos-Flores J, Gonzalez-Herranz P, Lopez-Mondejar JA, et al: Fractures of the proximal humeral epiphysis. Int Orthop 1993;17:16.
43. Cahill BR, Tullos HS, Fain RH: Little league shoulder: Lesions of the proximal humeral epiphyseal plate. J Sports Med 1974;2:150.
44. Calandra JJ, Baker CL, Uribe J: The incidence of Hill-Sachs lesions in initial anterior shoulder dislocations. Arthroscopy 1989;5:254.
45. Calder JD, Solan M, Gidwani S, et al: Management of paediatric clavicle fractures—is follow-up necessary? An audit of 346 cases. Ann R Coll Surg Engl 2002; 84:331.
46. Callahan J: Anatomic considerations: Closed reduction of proximal humeral fractures. Orthop Rev 1984;13: 79.
47. Campbell J, Almond HG: Fracture-separation of the proximal humeral epiphysis. A case report. J Bone Joint Surg Am 1977;59:262.
48. Cartner MJ: Immobilization of fractures of the shaft of the humerus. Injury 1973;5:175.
49. Caviglia H, Garrido CP, Palazzi FF, et al: Pediatric fractures of the humerus. Clin Orthop Relat Res 2005; 432:49.

50. Chapman MW: The role of intramedullary fixation in open fractures. Clin Orthop Relat Res 1986;212:26.
51. Checchia SL, Santos PD, Miyazaki AN: Surgical treatment of acute and chronic posterior fracture-dislocation of the shoulder. J Shoulder Elbow Surg 1998;7:53.
52. Chee Y, Agorastides I, Garg N, et al: Treatment of severely displaced proximal humeral fractures in children with elastic stable intramedullary nailing. J Pediatr Orthop B 2006;15:45.
53. Clark RL, Milgram JW, Yawn DH: Fatal aortic perforation and cardiac tamponade due to a Kirschner wire migrating from the right sternoclavicular joint. South Med J 1974;67:316.
54. Cohen AW, Otto SR: Obstetric clavicular fractures. A three-year analysis. J Reprod Med 1980;25:119.
55. Cohn BT, Froimson AI: Salter 3 fracture dislocation of glenohumeral joint in a 10-year-old. Orthop Rev 1986; 15:403.
56. Collins HR, Wilde AH: Shoulder instability in athletics. Orthop Clin North Am 1973;4:759.
57. Collins J: Retrosternal dislocation of the clavicle. J Bone Joint Surg Br 1972;54:203.
58. Conwell H: Fractures of the surgical neck and epiphyseal separations of the upper end of the humerus. J Bone Joint Surg 1928;8:508.
59. Conwell HE: Fractures of the clavicle: Simple fixation dressing with summary of the treatment and results attained in 92 cases. JAMA 1928;90:838.
60. Cooper D, O'Brien J, Warren R: Supporting layers of the glenohumeral joint: An anatomic study. Clin Orthop Relat Res 1993;289:144.
61. Curtis RJ Jr: Operative management of children's fractures of the shoulder region. Orthop Clin North Am 1990;21:315.
62. Dalldorf PG, Bryan WJ: Displaced Salter-Harris type I injury in a gymnast. A slipped capital humeral epiphysis? Orthop Rev 1994;23:538.
63. Dameron TB Jr, Reibel DB: Fractures involving the proximal humeral epiphyseal plate. J Bone Joint Surg Am 1969;51:289.
64. Damschen DD, Cogbill TH, Siegel MJ: Scapulothoracic dissociation caused by blunt trauma. J Trauma 1997; 42:537.
65. Davids JR, Talbott RD: Luxatio erecta humeri. A case report. Clin Orthop Relat Res 1990;252:144.
66. Davison BL, Orwin JF: Open inferior glenohumeral dislocation. J Orthop Trauma 1996;10:504.
67. Deitch J, Mehlman CT, Foad SL, et al: Traumatic anterior shoulder dislocation in adolescents. Am J Sports Med 2003;31:758.
68. Denham R, Dingley A: Epiphyseal separation of the medical end of the clavicle. J Bone Joint Surg Am 1967;49:1179.
69. Deutsch AL, Resnick D, Mink JH: Computed tomography of the glenohumeral and sternoclavicular joints. Orthop Clin North Am 1985;16:497.
70. Dickson J: Death following fractured clavicle. Lancet 1952;2:666.
71. Dobbs MB, Luhmann SL, Gordon JE, et al: Severely displaced proximal humeral epiphyseal fractures. J Pediatr Orthop 2003;23:208.
72. Drew SJ, Giddins GE, Birch R: A slowly evolving brachial plexus injury following a proximal humeral fracture in a child. J Hand Surg [Br] 1995;20:24.
73. Ebraheim NA, An HS, Jackson WT, et al: Scapulothoracic dissociation. J Bone Joint Surg Am 1988;70:428.
74. Edelson JG, Zuckerman J, Hershkovitz I: Os acromiale: Anatomy and surgical implications. J Bone Joint Surg Br 1993;75:551.
75. Edwards MS, Baker CJ, Wagner ML, et al: An etiologic shift in infantile osteomyelitis: The emergence of the group B streptococcus. J Pediatr 1978;93:578.
76. Edwards SG, Whittle AP, Wood GW 2nd: Nonoperative treatment of ipsilateral fractures of the scapula and clavicle. J Bone Joint Surg Am 2000;82:774.
77. Eidman DK, Siff SJ, Tullos HS: Acromioclavicular lesions in children. Am J Sports Med 1981;9:150.
78. Ellefsen BK, Frierson MA, Raney EM, et al: Humerus varus: A complication of neonatal, infantile, and childhood injury and infection. J Pediatr Orthop 1994;14: 479.
79. Elting JJ: Retrosternal dislocation of the clavicle. Arch Surg 1972;104:35.
80. Endo S, Kasai T, Fujii N, et al: Traumatic anterior dislocation of the shoulder in a child. Arch Orthop Trauma Surg 1993;112:201.
81. Falstie-Jensen S, Mikkelsen P: Pseudodislocation of the acromioclavicular joint. J Bone Joint Surg Br 1982; 64:368.
82. Farkas R, Levine S: X-ray incidence of fractured clavicle in vertex presentation. Am J Obstet Gynecol 1950;59: 204.
83. Fawcett J: The development and ossification of the human clavicle. J Anat Physiol 1913;47:225.
84. Ferry AM, Rook FW, Masterson JH: Retrosternal dislocation of the clavicle. J Bone Joint Surg Am 1957;39: 905.
85. Field LD, Bokor DJ, Savoie FH 3rd: Humeral and glenoid detachment of the anterior inferior glenohumeral ligament: A cause of anterior shoulder instability. J Shoulder Elbow Surg 1997;6:6.
86. Fink CW, Nelson JD: Septic arthritis and osteomyelitis in children. Clin Rheum Dis 1986;12:423.
87. Fisher NA, Newman B, Lloyd J, et al: Ultrasonographic evaluation of birth injury to the shoulder. J Perinatol 1995;15:398.
88. Fleming RE, Tornberg DN, Kiernan H: An operative repair of acromioclavicular separation. J Trauma 1978; 18:709.
89. Flemming JE, Beals RK: Pathologic fracture of the humerus. Clin Orthop Relat Res 1986;203:258.
90. Foster WS, Ford TB, Drez D Jr: Isolated posterior shoulder dislocation in a child. A case report. Am J Sports Med 1985;13:198.
91. Freundlich BD: Luxatio erecta. J Trauma 1983;23:434.
92. Friedlander HL: Separation of the proximal humeral epiphysis: A case report. Clin Orthop Relat Res 1964;35: 163.
93. Fukuda K, Craig EV, An KN, et al: Biomechanical study of the ligamentous system of the acromioclavicular joint. J Bone Joint Surg Am 1986;68:434.
94. Fuster S, Palliso F, Combalia A, et al: Intrathoracic migration of a Kirschner wire. Injury 1990;21:124.

95. Gainor BJ, Metzler M: Humeral shaft fracture with brachial artery injury. Clin Orthop Relat Res 1986;204:154.
96. Gangahar DM, Flogaites T: Retrosternal dislocation of the clavicle producing thoracic outlet syndrome. J Trauma 1978;18:369.
97. Garcia-Elias M, Salo JM: Non-union of a fractured coracoid process after dislocation of the shoulder. A case report. J Bone Joint Surg Br 1985;67:722.
98. Gardner E, Gray DJ: Prenatal development of the human shoulder and acromioclavicular joints. Am J Anat 1953;92:219.
99. Ghormley R, Black J, Cherry J: Ununited fractures of the clavicle. Am J Surg 1941;51:343.
100. Gilchrist DK: A stockinette-Velpeau for immobilization of the shoulder-girdle. J Bone Joint Surg Am 1967;49:750.
101. Goldfarb CA, Bassett GS, Sullivan S, et al: Retrosternal displacement after physeal fracture of the medial clavicle in children treatment by open reduction and internal fixation. J Bone Joint Surg Br 2001;83:1168.
102. Granieri GF, Bacarini L: A little-known cause of painful shoulder: Os acromiale. Eur Radiol 1998;8:130.
103. Greenlee D: Posterior dislocation of the sternal end of the clavicle. JAMA 1944;125:426.
104. Griswold R, Goldberg H, Robertson J: Fractures of the humerus. Am J Surg 1939;43:31.
105. Grogan DP, Love SM, Guidera KJ, et al: Operative treatment of congenital pseudarthrosis of the clavicle. J Pediatr Orthop 1991;11:176.
106. Haasbeek JF, Cole WG: Open fractures of the arm in children. J Bone Joint Surg Br 1995;77:576.
107. Hansen PE, Barnes DA, Tullos HS: Arthrographic diagnosis of an injury pattern in the distal humerus of an infant. J Pediatr Orthop 1982;2:569.
108. Hardegger FH, Simpson LA, Weber BG: The operative treatment of scapular fractures. J Bone Joint Surg Br 1984;66:725.
109. Hatfield MK, Gross BH, Glazer GM, et al: Computed tomography of the sternum and its articulations. Skeletal Radiol 1984;11:197.
110. Heck CC: Anterior dislocation of the glenohumeral joint in a child. J Trauma 1981;21:174.
111. Heppenstall RB: Fractures and dislocations of the distal clavicle. Orthop Clin North Am 1975;6:477.
112. Heyse-Moore GH, Stoker DJ: Avulsion fractures of the scapula. Skeletal Radiol 1982;9:27.
113. Hill H, Sachs M: The grooved defect of the humeral head: A frequently unrecognized complication of dislocations of the shoulder joint. Radiology 1940;35:690.
114. Hirata S, Miya H, Mizuno K: Congenital pseudarthrosis of the clavicle. Histologic examination for the etiology of the disease. Clin Orthop Relat Res 1995;315:242.
115. Hohl JC: Fractures of the humerus in children. Orthop Clin North Am 1976;7:557.
116. Holm CL: Management of humeral shaft fractures. Fundamental nonoperative technics. Clin Orthop Relat Res 1970;71:132.
117. Holstein A, Lewis GM: Fractures of the humerus with radial-nerve paralysis. J Bone Joint Surg Am 1963;45:1382.
118. Horn JS: The traumatic anatomy and treatment of acute acromio-clavicular dislocation. J Bone Joint Surg Br 1954;36:194.
119. Howard FM, Shafer SJ: Injuries to the clavicle with neurovascular complications. A study of fourteen cases. J Bone Joint Surg Am 1965;47:1335.
120. Huber RI, Keller HW, Huber PM, et al: Flexible intramedullary nailing as fracture treatment in children. J Pediatr Orthop 1996;16:602.
121. Hunter SG: The closed treatment of fractures of the humeral shaft. Clin Orthop Relat Res 1982;164:192.
122. Ideberg R, Grevsten S, Larsson S: Epidemiology of scapular fractures. Incidence and classification of 338 fractures. Acta Orthop Scand 1995;66:395.
123. Imatani RJ: Fractures of the scapula: A review of 53 fractures. J Trauma 1975;15:473.
124. Imatani RJ, Hanlon JJ, Cady GW: Acute, complete acromioclavicular separation. J Bone Joint Surg Am 1975;57:328.
125. Ish-Horowicz MR, McIntyre P, Nade S: Bone and joint infections caused by multiply resistant *Staphylococcus aureus* in a neonatal intensive care unit. Pediatr Infect Dis J 1992;11:82.
126. Ishizuki M, Yamaura I, Isobe Y, et al: Avulsion fracture of the superior border of the scapula. Report of five cases. J Bone Joint Surg Am 1981;63:820.
127. Jacobs B, Wade PA: Acromioclavicular-joint injury. An end-result study. J Bone Joint Surg Am 1966;48:475.
128. Janssens de Varebeke B, Van Osselaer G: Migration of Kirschner's pin from the right sternoclavicular joint resulting in perforation of the pulmonary artery main trunk. Acta Chir Belg 1993;93:287.
129. Kaelin AJ, MacEwen GD: Unicameral bone cysts. Natural history and the risk of fracture. Int Orthop 1989;13:275.
130. Kamhin M, Michaelson M, Waisbrod H: The use of external skeletal fixation in the treatment of fractures of the humeral shaft. Injury 1978;9:245.
131. Kaminsky SB, Pierce VD: Nonunion of a scapula body fracture in a high school football player. Am J Orthop 2002;31:456.
132. Karatosun V, Unver B, Alici E, et al: Treatment of displaced, proximal, humeral, epiphyseal fractures with a two-prong splint. J Orthop Trauma 2003;17:578.
133. Kato T, Kanbara H, Sato S, et al: [Five cases of clavicular fractures misdiagnosed as congenital myogenic torticollis]. Seikei Geka 1968;19:729.
134. Kawabe N, Watanabe R, Sato M: Treatment of complete acromioclavicular separation by coracoacromial ligament transfer. Clin Orthop Relat Res 1984;185:222.
135. Kawaguchi AT, Jackson DL, Otsuka NY: Delayed diagnosis of a glenohumeral joint dislocation in a child with developmental delay. Am J Orthop 1998;27:137.
136. Kawam M, Sinclair J, Letts M: Recurrent posterior shoulder dislocation in children: The results of surgical management. J Pediatr Orthop 1997;17:533.
137. Kennedy J: Retrosternal dislocation of the clavicle. J Bone Joint Surg Br 1949;31:74.
138. Kennedy JC, Cameron H: Complete dislocation of the acromio-clavicular joint. J Bone Joint Surg Br 1954;36:202.

139. Klenerman L: Fractures of the shaft of the humerus. J Bone Joint Surg Br 1966;48:105.
140. Kohler R, Trillaud JM: Fracture and fracture separation of the proximal humerus in children: Report of 136 cases. J Pediatr Orthop 1983;3:326.
141. Kubiak R, Slongo T: Operative treatment of clavicle fractures in children: A review of 21 years. J Pediatr Orthop 2002;22:736.
142. Kummel BM: Fractures of the glenoid causing chronic dislocation of the shoulder. Clin Orthop Relat Res 1970;69:189.
143. Landin LA: Fracture patterns in children. Analysis of 8,682 fractures with special reference to incidence, etiology and secular changes in a Swedish urban population 1950-1979. Acta Orthop Scand Suppl 1983;202:1.
144. Langenskiold A: Adolescent humerus varus. Acta Chir Scand 1953;105:353.
145. Larsen CF, Kiaer T, Lindequist S: Fractures of the proximal humerus in children. Nine-year follow-up of 64 unoperated on cases. Acta Chir Scand 1990;61:255.
146. Larsen E, Bjerg-Nielsen A, Christensen P: Conservative or surgical treatment of acromioclavicular dislocation. A prospective, controlled, randomized study. J Bone Joint Surg Am 1986;68:552.
147. Lasda NA, Murray DG: Fracture separation of the coracoid process associated with acromioclavicular dislocation: Conservative treatment—a case report and review of the literature. Clin Orthop Relat Res 1978;134: 222.
148. Lawton RL, Choudhury S, Mansat P, et al: Pediatric shoulder instability: Presentation, findings, treatment, and outcomes. J Pediatr Orthop 2002;22:52.
149. Lee FA, Gwinn JL: Retrosternal dislocation of the clavicle. Radiology 1974;110:631.
150. Lee SJ, Meinhard BP, Schultz E, et al: Open reduction and internal fixation of a glenoid fossa fracture in a child: A case report and review of the literature. J Orthop Trauma 1997;11:452.
151. Lehnert M, Maier B, Jakob H, et al: Fracture and retrosternal dislocation of the medial clavicle in a 12-year-old child—case report, options for diagnosis, and treatment in children. J Pediatr Surg 2005;40:e1.
152. Lemire L, Rosman M: Sternoclavicular epiphyseal separation with adjacent clavicular fracture. J Pediatr Orthop 1984;4:118.
153. Lemperg R, Liliequist B: Dislocation of the proximal epiphysis of the humerus in newborns. Acta Paediatr Scand 1970;59:377.
154. Leonard JW, Gifford RW Jr: Migration of a Kirschner wire from the clavicle into the pulmonary artery. Am J Cardiol 1965;16:598.
155. L-Etani H, D'Astous J, Letts M, et al: Masked rotatory subluxation of the atlas associated with fracture of the clavicle: A clinical and biomechanical analysis. Am J Orthop 1998;27:375.
156. Leung KS, Lam TP: Open reduction and internal fixation of ipsilateral fractures of the scapular neck and clavicle. J Bone Joint Surg Am 1993;75:1015.
157. Levine B, Pereira D, Rosen J: Avulsion fractures of the lesser tuberosity of the humerus in adolescents: Review of the literature and case report. J Orthop Trauma 2005; 19:349.
158. Levinsohn EM, Bunnell WP, Yuan HA: Computed tomography in the diagnosis of dislocations of the sternoclavicular joint. Clin Orthop Relat Res 1979; 140:12.
159. Lewallen RP, Peterson HA: Nonunion of long bone fractures in children: A review of 30 cases. J Pediatr Orthop 1985;5:135.
160. Lindsey RW, Gutowski WT: The migration of a broken pin following fixation of the acromioclavicular joint. A case report and review of the literature. Orthopedics 1986;9:413.
161. Lipscomb AB: Baseball pitching injuries in growing athletes. J Sports Med 1975;3:25.
162. Lorenzo FT: Osteosynthesis with Blount's staples in fractures of the proximal end of the humerus; a preliminary report. J Bone Joint Surg Am 1955;37:45.
163. Lucas GL, Peterson MD: Open anterior dislocation of the shoulder. J Trauma 1977;17:883.
164. Lucas JC, Mehlman CT, Laor T: The location of the biceps tendon in completely displaced proximal humerus fractures in children: A report of four cases with magnetic resonance imaging and cadaveric correlation. J Pediatr Orthop 2004;24:249.
165. Lucas L, Gill J: Humerus varus following birth injury to the proximal humerus. J Bone Joint Surg 1947;29: 367.
166. Lucus GL: Retrosternal dislocation of the clavicle. JAMA 1965;193:850.
167. Lunseth PA, Chapman KW, Frankel VH: Surgical treatment of chronic dislocation of the sterno-clavicular joint. J Bone Joint Surg Br 1975;57:193.
168. Macnicol MF: Roentgenographic evidence of median-nerve entrapment in a greenstick humeral fracture. J Bone Joint Surg Am 1978;60:998.
169. Mallon WJ, Bassett FH 3rd, Goldner RD: Luxatio erecta: The inferior glenohumeral dislocation. J Orthop Trauma 1990;4:19.
170. Manske DJ, Szabo RM: The operative treatment of mid-shaft clavicular non-unions. J Bone Joint Surg Am 1985;67:1367.
171. Marans HJ, Angel KR, Schemitsch EH, et al: The fate of traumatic anterior dislocation of the shoulder in children. J Bone Joint Surg Am 1992;74:1242.
172. Marcove RC, Sheth DS, Takemoto S, et al: The treatment of aneurysmal bone cyst. Clin Orthop Relat Res 1995; 311:157.
173. Martin RP, Parsons DL: Avascular necrosis of the proximal humeral epiphysis after physeal fracture. A case report. J Bone Joint Surg Am 1997;79:760.
174. Martín-Herrero T, Rodríguez-Merchán C, Munuera-Martínez L: Fractures of the coracoid process: Presentation of seven cases and review of the literature. J Trauma 1990;30:1597.
175. Massengill AD, Seeger LL, Yao L, et al: Labrocapsular ligamentous complex of the shoulder: Normal anatomy, anatomic variation, and pitfalls of MR imaging and MR arthrography. Radiographics 1994;14:1211.
176. McBride ED, Sisler J: Fractures of the proximal humeral epiphysis and the juxta-epiphysial humeral shaft. Clin Orthop Relat Res 1965;38:143.
177. McGahan JP, Rab GT, Dublin A: Fractures of the scapula. J Trauma 1980;20:880.

178. McLennan JG, Ungersma J: Pneumothorax complicating fracture of the scapula. J Bone Joint Surg Am 1982; 64:598.
179. Meister K, Day T, Horodyski M, et al: Rotational motion changes in the glenohumeral joint of the adolescent/ Little League baseball player. Am J Sports Med 2005; 33:693.
180. Mick CA, Weiland AJ: Pseudoarthrosis of a fracture of the acromion. J Trauma 1983;23:248.
181. Mital MA, Aufranc OE: Venous occlusion following greenstick fracture of clavicle. JAMA 1968;206:1301.
182. Mizuta T, Benson WM, Foster BK, et al: Statistical analysis of the incidence of physeal injuries. J Pediatr Orthop 1987;7:518.
183. Montgomery SP, Loyd RD: Avulsion fracture of the coracoid epiphysis with acromioclavicular separation. Report of two cases in adolescents and review of the literature. J Bone Joint Surg Am 1977;59:963.
184. Mosely H: The clavicle: Its anatomy and function. Clin Orthop Relat Res 1968;58:17.
185. Naidu SH, Bixler B, Capo JT, et al: Percutaneous pinning of proximal humerus fractures: A biomechanical study. Orthopedics 1997;20:1073.
186. Nakae H, Endo S: Traumatic posterior dislocation of the shoulder with fracture of the acromion in a child. Arch Orthop Trauma Surg 1996;115:238.
187. Naresh S, Chapman JA, Muralidharan T: Posterior dislocation of the shoulder with ipsilateral humeral shaft fracture: A very rare injury. Injury 1997;28:150.
188. Neer CS 2nd: Nonunion of the clavicle. JAMA 1960; 172:1006.
189. Neer CS 2nd: Fractures of the distal third of the clavicle. Clin Orthop Relat Res 1968;58:43.
190. Neer CS 2nd, Horwitz BS: Fractures of the proximal humeral epiphysial plate. Clin Orthop Relat Res 1965;41:24.
191. Nettles JL, Linscheid RL: Sternoclavicular dislocations. J Trauma 1968;8:158.
192. Nettrour LF, Krufky EL, Mueller RE, et al: Locked scapula: Intrathoracic dislocation of the inferior angle. A case report. J Bone Joint Surg Am 1972;54:413.
193. Neviaser JS: Injuries of the clavicle and its articulations. Orthop Clin North Am 1980;11:233.
194. Neviaser RJ, Neviaser JS, Neviaser TJ: A simple technique for internal fixation of the clavicle. A long term evaluation. Clin Orthop Relat Res 1975;109:103.
195. Ng GP, Cole WG: Three-dimensional CT reconstruction of the scapula in the management of a child with a displaced intra-articular fracture of the glenoid. Injury 1994;25:679.
196. Nicastro JF, Adair DM: Fracture-dislocation of the shoulder in a 32-month-old child. J Pediatr Orthop 1982;2:427.
197. Nilsson S, Svartholm F: Fracture of the upper end of the humerus in children. A follow-up of 44 cases. Acta Chir Scand 1965;130:433.
198. Nogi J, Heckman JD, Hakala M, et al: Non-union of the clavicle in a child. A case report. Clin Orthop Relat Res 1975;110:19.
199. Nordback I, Markkula H: Migration of Kirschner pin from clavicle into ascending aorta. Acta Chir Scand 1985;151:177.
200. Obremskey W, Routt ML Jr: Fracture-dislocation of the shoulder in a child: Case report. J Trauma 1994;36:137.
201. O'Brien SJ, Neves MC, Arnoczky SP, et al: The anatomy and histology of the inferior glenohumeral ligament complex of the shoulder. Am J Sports Med 1990;18: 449.
202. O'Connell PW, Nuber GW, Mileski RA, et al: The contribution of the glenohumeral ligaments to anterior stability of the shoulder joint. Am J Sports Med 1990;18:579.
203. Ogawa K, Ogawa Y, Yoshida A: Posterior fracture-dislocation of the shoulder with infraspinatus interposition: The buttonhole phenomenon. J Trauma 1997; 43:688.
204. Ogden JA: Distal clavicular physeal injury. Clin Orthop Relat Res 1984;188:68.
205. Ogden JA: Humerus. In Skeletal Injury in the Child. New York, Springer-Verlag, 1990, p 465.
206. Ogden JA, Conlogue GJ, Bronson ML: Radiology of postnatal skeletal development. III. The clavicle. Skeletal Radiol 1979;4:196.
207. Ogden JA, Lister G: The pathology of neonatal osteomyelitis. Pediatrics 1975;55:474.
208. Ogden JA, Phillips SB: Radiology of postnatal skeletal development. VII. The scapula. Skeletal Radiol 1983;9: 157.
209. Oppenheim WL, Dawson EG, Quinlan C, et al: The cephaloscapular projection. A special diagnostic aid. Clin Orthop Relat Res 1985;195:191.
210. Oreck SL, Burgess A, Levine AM: Traumatic lateral displacement of the scapula: A radiographic sign of neurovascular disruption. J Bone Joint Surg Am 1984; 66:758.
211. Paavolainen P, Björkenheim JM, Slätis P, et al: Operative treatment of severe proximal humeral fractures. Acta Orthop Scand 1983;54:374.
212. Packer JW, Foster RR, Garcia A, et al: The humeral fracture with radial nerve palsy: Is exploration warranted? Clin Orthop Relat Res 1972;88:34.
213. Paterson D: Retrosternal dislocation of the clavicle. J Bone Joint Surg Br 1961;43:90.
214. Peacock HK, Brandon JR, Jones OL Jr: Retrosternal dislocation of the clavicle. South Med J 1970;63:1324.
215. Peckett WR, Gunther SB, Harper GD, et al: Internal fixation of symptomatic os acromiale: A series of twenty-six cases. J Shoulder Elbow Surg 2004;13:381.
216. Penn I: The vascular complications of fractures of the clavicle. J Trauma 1964;27:819.
217. Peters W, Irving J, Letts M: Long-term effects of neonatal bone and joint infection on adjacent growth plates. J Pediatr Orthop 1992;12:806.
218. Poland T: Traumatic Separation of the Epiphysis. London, Smith, Elder, 1898.
219. Pollock FH, Drake D, Bovill EG, et al: Treatment of radial neuropathy associated with fractures of the humerus. J Bone Joint Surg Am 1981;63:239.
220. Postacchini F, Gumina S, Cinotti G: Anterior shoulder dislocation in adolescents. J Shoulder Elbow Surg 2000;9:470.
221. Potter FA, Fiorini AJ, Knox J, et al: The migration of a Kirschner wire from shoulder to spleen: Brief report. J Bone Joint Surg Br 1988;70:326.

222. Powers JA, Bach PJ: Acromioclavicular separations. Closed or open treatment? Clin Orthop Relat Res 1974;104:213.
223. Protass JJ, Stampfli FV, Osmer JC: Coracoid process fracture diagnosis in acromioclavicular separation. Radiology 1975;116:61.
224. Pyper JB: Non-union of fractures of the clavicle. Injury 1978;9:268.
225. Reed MH: Fractures and dislocations of the extremities in children. J Trauma 1977;17:351.
226. Richards RD, Sartoris DJ, Pathria MN, et al: Hill-Sachs lesion and normal humeral groove: MR imaging features allowing their differentiation. Radiology 1994; 190:665.
227. Robins PR, Peterson HA: Management of pathologic fractures through unicameral bone cysts. JAMA 1972; 222:80.
228. Rockwood C: Dislocation of the sternoclavicular joint. Instr Course Lect 1975;24:144.
229. Rockwood C: Fractures of the outer clavicle in children and adults. J Bone Joint Surg kBr 1982;64:642.
230. Rockwood C, Wirth M: Subluxations and dislocations about the glenohumeral joint. In Rockwood C, Green DP: Fractures in Adults, vol 2. Philadelphia, Lippincott-Raven, 1996, p 1193.
231. Rogers JF, Bennett JB, Tullos HS: Management of concomitant ipsilateral fractures of the humerus and forearm. J Bone Joint Surg Am 1984;66:552.
232. Rosenorn M, Pedersen EB: The significance of the coracoclavicular ligament in experimental dislocation of the acromioclavicular joint. Acta Orthop Scand 1974; 45:346.
233. Rothman RH, Marvel JP Jr, Heppenstall RB: Recurrent anterior dislocation of the shoulder. Orthop Clin North Am 1975;6:415.
234. Rounds R: Isolated fracture of the coracoid process. J Bone Joint Surg Am 1949;44:662.
235. Rowe CR: Prognosis in dislocations of the shoulder. J Bone Joint Surg Am 1956;38:957.
236. Rowe CR: Acute and recurrent dislocations of the shoulder. J Bone Joint Surg Am 1962;44:998.
237. Rowe CR: Fractures of the scapula. Surg Clin North Am 1963;43:1565.
238. Rowe CR: An atlas of anatomy and treatment of midclavicular fractures. Clin Orthop Relat Res 1968;58:29.
239. Rowe CR: Recurrent transient anterior subluxation of the shoulder. The "dead arm" syndrome. Clin Orthop Relat Res 1987;223:11.
240. Rowe CR, Patel D, Southmayd WW: The Bankart procedure: A long-term end-result study. J Bone Joint Surg Am 1978;60:1.
241. Rowe CR, Pierce DS, Clark JG: Voluntary dislocation of the shoulder. A preliminary report on a clinical, electromyographic, and psychiatric study of twenty-six patients. J Bone Joint Surg Am 1973;55:445.
242. Rowe CR, Sakellarides HT: Factors related to recurrences of anterior dislocations of the shoulder. Clin Orthop Relat Res 1961;20:40.
243. Rowe CR, Zarins B: Chronic unreduced dislocations of the shoulder. J Bone Joint Surg Am 1982;64:494.
244. Rubenstein JD, Ebraheim NA, Kellam JF: Traumatic scapulothoracic dissociation. Radiology 1985;157:297.
245. Rush L, Rush H: Intramedullary fixation of fractures of the humerus by longitudinal pin. Surgery 1950;27:268.
246. Russo MT, Maffulli N: Bilateral congenital pseudarthrosis of the clavicle. Arch Orthop Trauma Surg 1990;109:177.
247. Sabick MB, Kim YK, Torry MR, et al: Biomechanics of the shoulder in youth baseball pitchers: Implications for the development of proximal humeral epiphysiolysis and humeral retrotorsion. Am J Sports Med 2005;33:1716.
248. Sage J: Recurrent inferior dislocation of the clavicle at the acromioclavicular joint. A case report. Am J Sports Med 1982;10:145.
249. Sammarco VJ: Os acromiale: Frequency, anatomy, and clinical implications. J Bone Joint Surg Am 2000;82: 394.
250. Sampson LN, Britton JC, Eldrup-Jorgensen J, et al: The neurovascular outcome of scapulothoracic dissociation. J Vasc Surg 1993;17:1083.
251. Sanford H: The Moro reflex as a diagnostic aid in fracture of the clavicle in the newborn infant. J Dis Child 1931;41:1304.
252. Sankarankutty M: Traumatic inferior dislocation of the hip (luxatio erecta) in a child. J Bone Joint Surg Br 1967;49:145.
253. Scaglietti O: The obstetrical shoulder trauma. Gynecol Obstet 1938;66:868.
254. Schwendenwein E, Hajdu S, Gaebler C, et al: Displaced fractures of the proximal humerus in children require open/closed reduction and internal fixation. Eur J Pediatr Surg 2004;14:51.
255. Selesnick FH, Jablon M, Frank C, et al: Retrosternal dislocation of the clavicle. Report of four cases. J Bone Joint Surg Am 1984;66:287.
256. Shah JJ, Bhatti NA: Radial nerve paralysis associated with fractures of the humerus. A review of 62 cases. Clin Orthop Relat Res 1983;172:171.
257. Shalom A, Khermosh O, Wientroub S: The natural history of congenital pseudarthrosis of the clavicle. J Bone Joint Surg Br 1994;76:846.
258. Shaw BA, Murphy KM, Shaw A, et al: Humerus shaft fractures in young children: Accident or abuse? J Pediatr Orthop 1997;17:293.
259. Sherk HH, Probst C: Fractures of the proximal humeral epiphysis. Orthop Clin North Am 1975;6:401.
260. Shvartzman P, Guy N: Voluntary dislocation of shoulder. Postgrad Med 1988;84:265.
261. Simurda MA: Retrosternal dislocation of the clavicle: A report of four cases and a method of repair. Can J Surg 1968;11:487.
262. Søndergård-Petersen P, Mikkelsen P: Posterior acromioclavicular dislocation. J Bone Joint Surg Br 1982; 64:52.
263. Speer KP, Deng X, Borrero S, et al: Biomechanical evaluation of a simulated Bankart lesion. J Bone Joint Surg Am 1994;76:1819.
264. Stankler L: Posterior dislocation of the clavicle. A report of 2 cases. Br J Surg 1962;50:164.
265. Stanley D, Norris SH: Recovery following fractures of the clavicle treated conservatively. Injury 1988;19:162.
266. Stefko JM, Tibone JE, Cawley PW, et al: Strain of the anterior band of the inferior glenohumeral ligament

during capsule failure. J Shoulder Elbow Surg 1997;6: 473.
267. Stein AH Jr: Retrosternal dislocation of the clavicle. J Bone Joint Surg Am 1957;39:656.
268. Stimson L: An easy method of reducing dislocations of the shoulder and hip. Med Rec 1900;57:356.
269. Taga I, Yoneda M, Ono K: Epiphyseal separation of the coracoid process associated with acromioclavicular sprain. A case report and review of the literature. Clin Orthop Relat Res 1986;207:138.
270. Taylor AR: Non-union of fractures of the clavicle: A review of thirty-one cases. J Bone Joint Surg Br 1969; 51:568.
271. Taylor DC, Arciero RA: Pathologic changes associated with shoulder dislocations. Arthroscopic and physical examination findings in first-time, traumatic anterior dislocations. Am J Sports Med 1997;25:306.
272. Thomas SC, Matsen FA 3rd: An approach to the repair of avulsion of the glenohumeral ligaments in the management of traumatic anterior glenohumeral instability. J Bone Joint Surg Am 1989;71:506.
273. Thompson DA, Flynn TC, Miller PW, et al: The significance of scapular fractures. J Trauma 1985;25:974.
274. Todd T, DiErrico J: The clavicular epiphyses. Am J Anat 1928;41:25.
275. Tregonning G, MacNab I: Post-traumatic pseudoarthrosis of the clavicle. J Bone Joint Surg Br 1976;58: 264.
276. Trotter DH, Dobozi W: Nonunion of the humerus: Rigid fixation, bone grafting, and adjunctive bone cement. Clin Orthop Relat Res 1986;204:162.
277. Tullos HS, Fain RH: Little league shoulder: Rotational stress fracture of proximal epiphysis. J Sports Med 1974;2:152.
278. Tullos HS, King JW: Lesions of the pitching arm in adolescents. JAMA 1972;220:264.
279. Turkel SJ, Panio MW, Marshall JL, et al: Stabilizing mechanisms preventing anterior dislocation of the glenohumeral joint. J Bone Joint Surg Am 1981;63:1208.
280. Tyagi A, Drake J, Midha R, et al: Axillary nerve injuries in children. Pediatr Neurosurg 2000;32:226.
281. Tyer H, Sturrock W, Callow F: Retrosternal dislocation of the clavicle. J Bone Joint Surg Br 1963;45:132.
282. Uri DS, Kneeland JB, Herzog R: Os acromiale: Evaluation of markers for identification on sagittal and coronal oblique MR images. Skeletal Radiol 1997;26:31.
283. Urist MR: Complete dislocation of the acromioclavicular joint. J Bone Joint Surg 1946;28:813.
284. Urist MR: Follow-up notes to articles previously published in The Journal: Complete dislocation of the acromioclavicular joint. J Bone Joint Surg Am 1963;45: 1750.
285. Valentin A, Winge S, Engstrom B: Early arthroscopic treatment of primary traumatic anterior shoulder dislocation. A follow-up study. Scand J Med Sci Sports 1998;8:405.
286. van Noort A, te Slaa RL, Marti RK, et al: The floating shoulder. A multicentre study. J Bone Joint Surg Br 2001;83:795.
287. Veysi VT, Mittal R, Agarwal S, et al: Multiple trauma and scapula fractures: So what? J Trauma 2003;55: 1145.
288. Wall JJ: Congenital pseudarthrosis of the clavicle. J Bone Joint Surg Am 1970;52:1003.
289. Wang P Jr, Koval KJ, Lehman W, et al: Salter-Harris type III fracture-dislocation of the proximal humerus. J Pediatr Orthop B 1997;6:219.
290. Warner JJ, Beim GM, Higgins L: The treatment of symptomatic os acromiale. J Bone Joint Surg Am 1998; 80:1320.
291. Waters PM, Bae DS, Kadiyala RK: Short-term outcomes after surgical treatment of traumatic posterior sternoclavicular fracture-dislocations in children and adolescents. J Pediatr Orthop 2003;23:464.
292. Wheeler ME, Laaveg SJ, Sprague BL: S-C joint disruption in an infant. Clin Orthop Relat Res 1979;139:68.
293. Wilber MC, Evans EB: Fractures of the scapula. An analysis of forty cases and a review of the literature. J Bone Joint Surg Am 1977;59:358.
294. Wilder RT, Berde CB, Wolohan M, et al: Reflex sympathetic dystrophy in children. Clinical characteristics and follow-up of seventy patients. J Bone Joint Surg Am 1992;74:910.
295. Wiley JJ, McIntyre WM: Fracture patterns in children. In Uhthoff H, Jaworski ZFG: Current Concepts of Bone Fragility. Berlin, Springer-Verlag, 1986, p 159.
296. Wilkes JA, Hoffer MM: Clavicle fractures in head-injured children. J Orthop Trauma 1987;1:55.
297. Wilkins RM, Johnston RM: Ununited fractures of the clavicle. J Bone Joint Surg Am 1983;65:773.
298. Williams DJ: The mechanisms producing fracture-separation of the proximal humeral epiphysis. J Bone Joint Surg Br 1981;63:102.
299. Williamson JB, Galasko CS, Robinson MJ: Outcome after acute osteomyelitis in preterm infants. Arch Dis Child 1990;65:1060.
300. Winter J, Sterner S, Maurer D, et al: Retrosternal epiphyseal disruption of medial clavicle: Case and review in children. J Emerg Med 1989;7:9.
301. Wolfe JS, Eyring EJ: Median-nerve entrapment within a greenstick fracture; a case report. J Bone Joint Surg Am 1974;56:1270.
302. Wong-Chung J, O'Brien T: Salter-Harris type III fracture of the proximal humeral physis. Injury 1988;19: 453.
303. Worlock P, Stower M: Fracture patterns in Nottingham children. J Pediatr Orthop 1986;6:656.
304. Worman LW, Leagus C: Intrathoracic injury following retrosternal dislocation of the clavicle. J Trauma 1967; 7:416.
305. Wright RW, Heller MA, Quick DC, et al: Arthroscopic decompression for impingement syndrome secondary to an unstable os acromiale. Arthroscopy 2000;16:595.
306. Yates DW: Complications of fractures of the clavicle. Injury 1976;7:189.
307. Yokoyama K, Shindo M, Itoman M, et al: Immediate internal fixation for open fractures of the long bones of the upper and lower extremities. J Trauma 1994;37: 230.
308. Zahiri CA, Zahiri H, Tehrany F: Anterior shoulder dislocation reduction technique—revisited. Orthopedics 1997;20:515.
309. Zaricznyj B: Reconstruction for chronic scapuloclavicular instability. Am J Sports Med 1983;11:17.

310. Zatti G, Teli M, Ferrario A, et al: Treatment of closed humeral shaft fractures with intramedullary elastic nails. J Trauma 1998;45:1046.
311. Zenni EJ Jr, Krieg JK, Rosen MJ: Open reduction and internal fixation of clavicular fractures. J Bone Joint Surg Am 1981;63:147.
312. Zettas JP, Muchnic PD: Fractures of the coracoid process based in acute acromioclavicular separation. Orthop Rev 1976;5:77.
313. Zilberman Z, Rejovitzky R: Fracture of the coracoid process of the scapula. Injury 1981;13:203.

FRACTURES ABOUT THE ELBOW

Mercer Rang uses the old saying, "Pity the young surgeon whose first case is a fracture around the elbow," as an introduction to his chapter on elbow fractures, for good reason.[453] Though common—fractures about the elbow account for 5% to 10% of all fractures in children[261,311,458,599,614]—the unique anatomy of the elbow and the high potential for complications associated with elbow fractures make their treatment anxiety producing for many orthopaedic surgeons. Fortunately, with an understanding of the anatomy and adherence to a few basic principles, treatment of such fractures can be straightforward.

It is best to address elbow fractures from an anatomic perspective because each specific fracture has its own challenges in diagnosis and treatment. One frequent source of problems in the management of pediatric elbow injuries is distinguishing fractures from the six normal secondary ossification centers. The six ossification centers develop in a systematic, predictable fashion. The mnemonic CRITOE is helpful in remembering the progression of radiographic appearance of the ossification centers about the elbow in children: *c*apitellum, *r*adius, *i*nternal (or medial) epicondyle, *t*rochlea, *o*lecranon, and *e*xternal (or lateral) epicondyle. In general, the capitellum appears radiographically at around 2 years of age, and the remaining ossification centers appear sequentially every 2 years.[530] It is important to remember that girls mature early and boys late, so the age at which these landmarks appear may vary—earlier for girls, later for boys; however, the sequence remains constant (Fig. 42–29).

The most common fractures about the elbow include fractures of the supracondylar humerus, fractures of the transphyseal distal humerus, fractures of the lateral humeral condyle, fractures of the medial humeral epicondyle (often associated with elbow dislocation), fractures of the radial head and neck, and fractures of the olecranon. Fractures involving the capitellum, coronoid, medial condyle, and lateral epicondyle, as well as intracondylar or T-condylar fractures, occur but are rare. Each of these injuries will be discussed in the context of their unique characteristics, which can assist in diagnosis and treatment.

Supracondylar Fractures of the Humerus

Supracondylar fractures of the humerus are the most common type of elbow fracture in children and adolescents. They account for 50% to 70% of all elbow fractures and are seen most frequently in children between the ages of 3 and 10 years.[153,220] The high incidence of residual deformity and the potential for neurovascular complications make supracondylar humeral fractures a serious injury.[22,345,380,384,484,554,601,604]

ANATOMY

The elbow joint is a complex articulation of three bones that allows motion in all three planes. The distal humerus has unique articulations with the radius and the ulna that make this mobility possible. The radial-humeral articulation allows pronation and supination

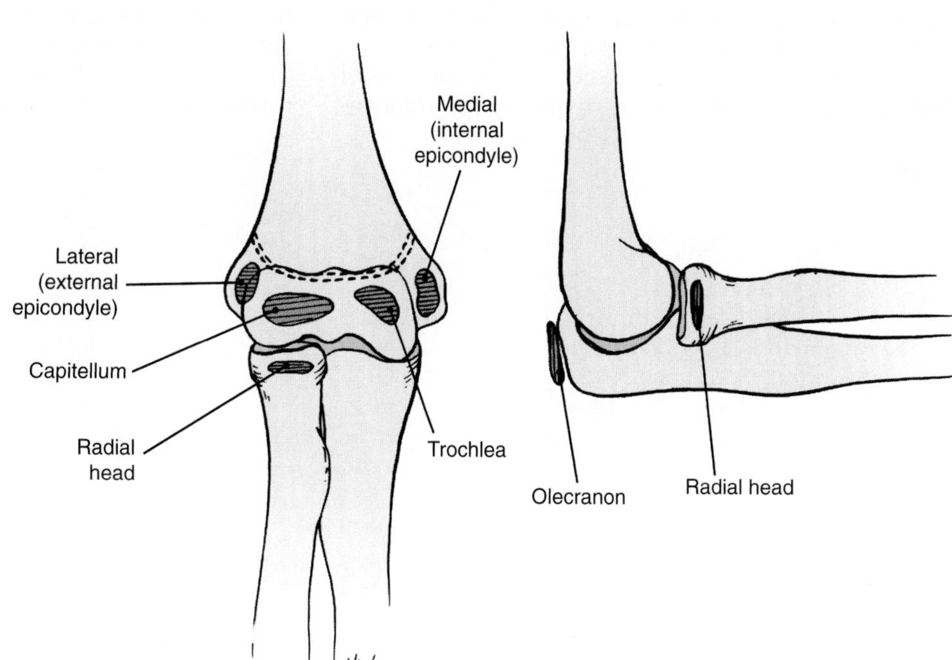

FIGURE 42–29 Secondary ossification centers about the elbow. These landmarks may appear at a younger age in girls and an older age in boys; however, the sequence remains constant.

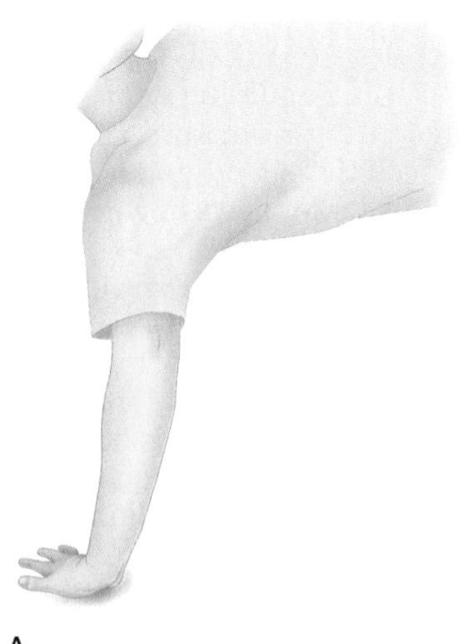
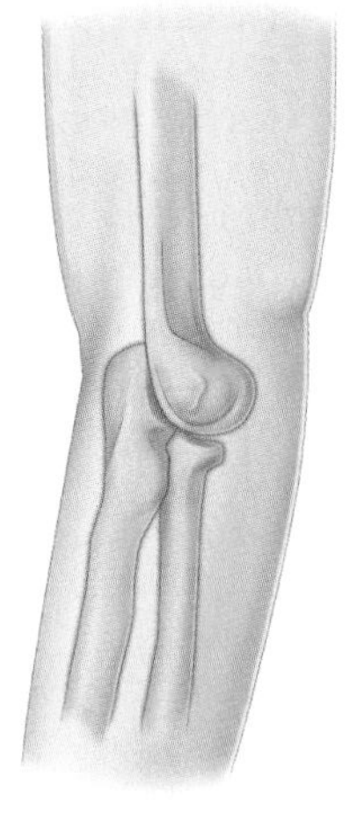
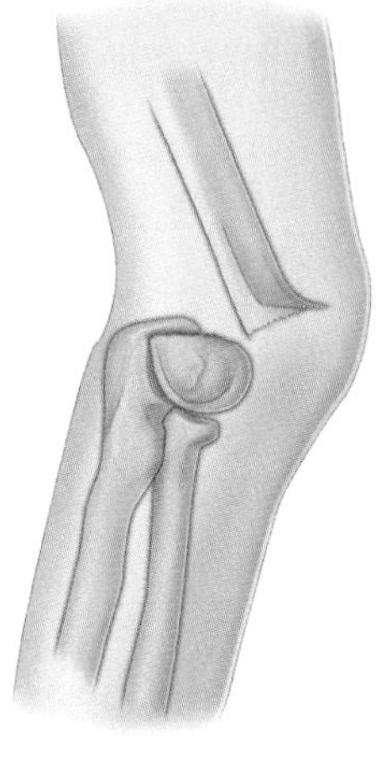

A B C

FIGURE 42-30 **A,** Supracondylar humeral fractures are most commonly the result of a fall onto an outstretched extremity, producing hyperextension of the elbow. **B** and **C,** As the elbow hyperextends, the olecranon serves as a fulcrum to produce the fracture. Thus, supracondylar fractures are most commonly located at the level of the olecranon fossa.

of the forearm, whereas the ulnohumeral articulation allows flexion and extension of the elbow. The separate articulating surfaces of the distal humerus are attached to the humeral shaft via medial and lateral columns. These two columns are separated by a thin area of bone that consists of the coronoid fossa anteriorly and the olecranon fossa posteriorly. This thin area is the weak link in the distal humerus and is where supracondylar humeral fractures originate. When forced into hyperextension, the olecranon can act as a fulcrum through which an extension force can propagate a fracture across the medial and lateral columns (Fig. 42–30). Similarly, a force applied posteriorly with the elbow in flexion can create a fracture originating at the level of the olecranon fossa (Fig. 42–31). Thus, whether the result of an extension or a flexion force, fractures of the supracondylar humerus are usually transverse and at the level of the olecranon fossa. For reasons that are unclear, older patients often have fractures that are oblique rather than transverse. Oblique fractures are less stable than transverse fractures because rotation produces additional angulation (Fig. 42–32).

Although the bony architecture of the distal humerus is responsible for the frequency of supracondylar humeral fractures, it is the soft tissue anatomy that has the potential to produce devastating long-term complications. Anteriorly, the brachial artery and median nerve traverse the antecubital fossa. Laterally, the radial nerve crosses from posterior to anterior just above the olecranon fossa. The ulnar nerve passes behind the medial epicondyle (Fig. 42–33). In extension supracondylar fractures, the brachialis muscle usually shields the anterior neurovascular structures from injury. However, in severely displaced fractures, the proximal fragment may perforate the brachialis muscle and contuse, occlude, or lacerate the vessel or nerve. The vessels or median nerve may also become trapped and compressed between the fracture fragments.[1,543] Even without direct injury, a severely displaced fracture can cause neurovascular injury simply from the stretch or traction that is associated with displacement. Similarly, the radial nerve may be injured by severe anterolateral displacement of the proximal fragment. With flexion-type injuries (anterior displacement of the distal fragment), the ulnar nerve is at risk because it may become "tented" over the posterior margin of the proximal fragment. Neurovascular problems can also develop in minimally

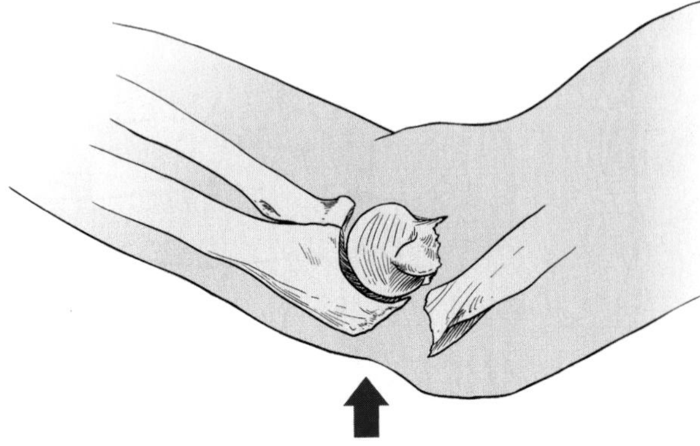

FIGURE 42-31 A posteriorly applied force with the elbow in flexion creates a flexion-type supracondylar humeral fracture (*arrow*). This mechanism accounts for only 2% to 5% of all supracondylar humeral fractures.

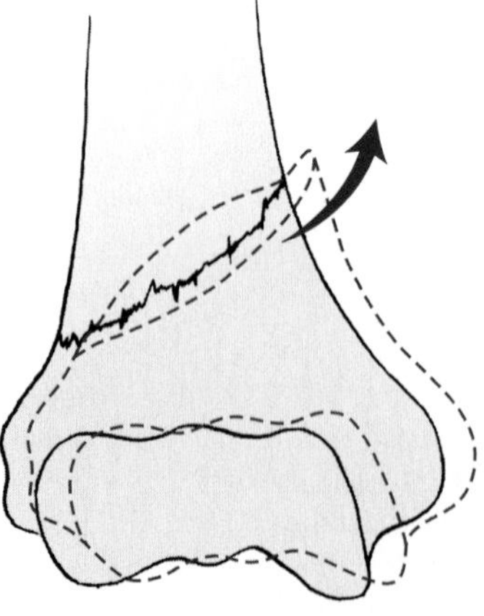

FIGURE 42-32 Oblique fractures, which are more common in older patients, are less stable than transverse fractures.

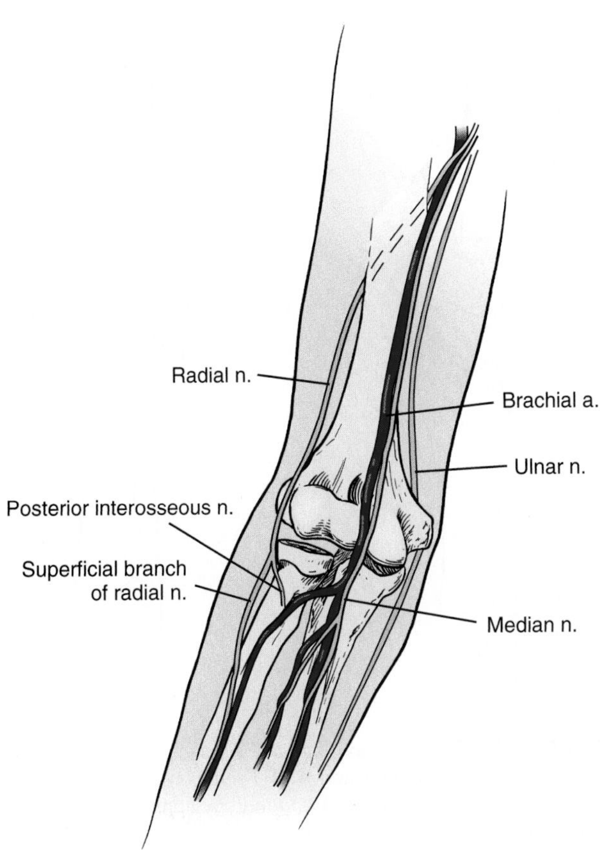

FIGURE 42-33 Neurovascular anatomy around the elbow. The brachial artery and median nerve lie anteromedially. The radial nerve crosses from posterior to anterior, laterally proximal to the lateral condyle. The ulnar nerve lies posteromedially.

displaced fractures as a result of hematoma formation or swelling. Hematomas generally spread anteriorly across the antecubital fossa deep to the fascia and can potentially compress the neurovascular structures.

MECHANISM OF INJURY

Supracondylar humeral fractures may be the result of either an extension or a flexion force on the distal humerus. Most commonly they are the result of a fall on an outstretched hand that causes hyperextension of the elbow.[4,22,345] These *extension-type* supracondylar humeral fractures account for 95% to 98% of all supracondylar fractures. With hyperextension injuries the distal fragment will be displaced posteriorly. *Flexion-type* supracondylar fractures are rare and occur in only 2% to 5% of cases. The mechanism of flexion supracondylar fractures is usually a direct blow on the posterior aspect of a flexed elbow that results in anterior displacement of the distal fragment.[153,380,602]

CLASSIFICATION

Supracondylar humeral fractures are usually initially classified as either extension or flexion injuries. They are then most commonly classified according to the amount of radiographic displacement. This three-part classification system was first described by Gartland in 1959.[182] Recently, it has been shown to be more reliable than most fracture classification systems.[32] Type I fractures are nondisplaced or minimally displaced. Type II fractures have angulation of the distal fragment (posteriorly in extension injuries and anteriorly in flexion injuries), with one cortex remaining intact (the posterior in extension and the anterior in flexion). Type III injuries are completely displaced, with both cortices fractured (Fig. 42–34).

There have been several modifications of this scheme. Wilkins subdivided type III injuries according to the coronal plane displacement of the distal fragment (Fig. 42–35).[602] This modification is clinically helpful in identifying complications from the injury and problems with treatment. Posterolaterally displaced type III fractures, though less frequent and accounting for only 25% of extension supracondylar fractures, are more commonly associated with neurovascular injuries. Undoubtedly, this is because the proximal fragment is displaced anteromedially in the direction of the neurovascular bundle (Fig. 42–36). In extension supracondylar fractures, the coronal plane displacement of the distal fragment also helps predict the stability of the fracture at the time of reduction. In a classic study in monkeys, Abraham and colleagues demonstrated that the periosteal sleeve remains intact on the side to which the distal fragment is displaced.[4] This periosteal sleeve helps stabilize the fracture when it is reduced. Pronation of the forearm tightens the medial sleeve to a greater extent than supination

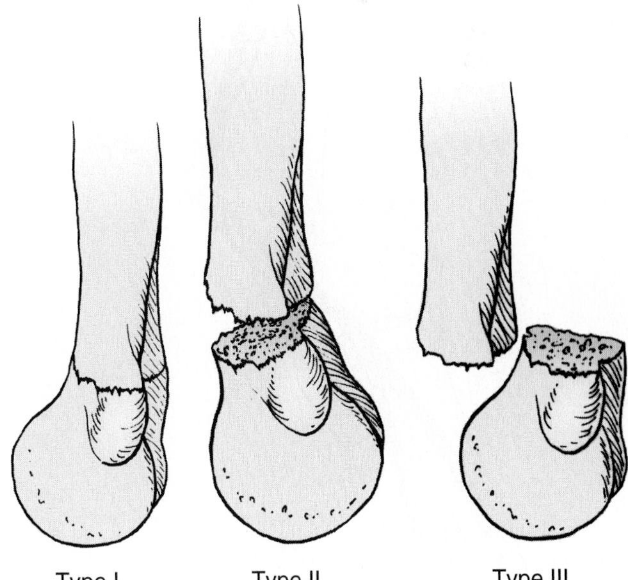

FIGURE 42-34 Classification of extension supracondylar humeral fractures. Type I—the anterior cortex is broken. The posterior cortex remains intact, and there is no or minimal angulation of the distal fragment. Type II—the anterior cortex is fractured and the posterior cortex remains intact. However, plastic deformation of the posterior cortex, or "greensticking," allows angulation of the distal fragment. Type III—the distal fragment is completely displaced posteriorly.

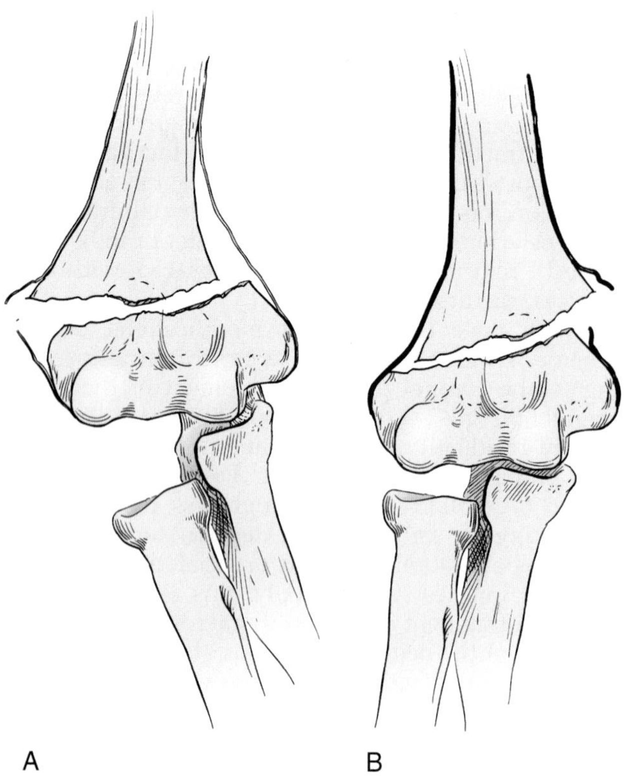

FIGURE 42–35 **A,** Posteromedially displaced fracture. **B,** Posterolaterally displaced fracture.

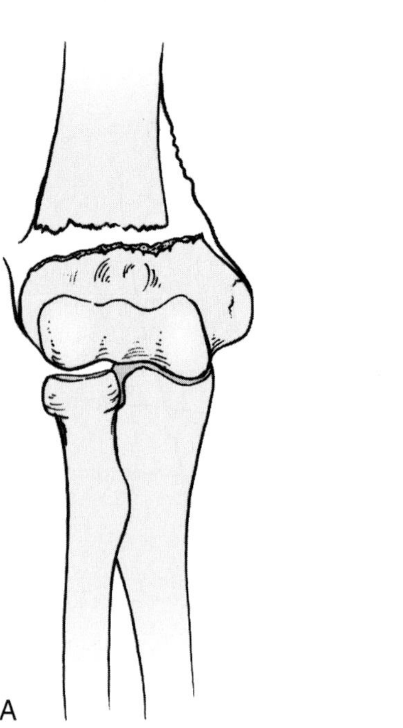

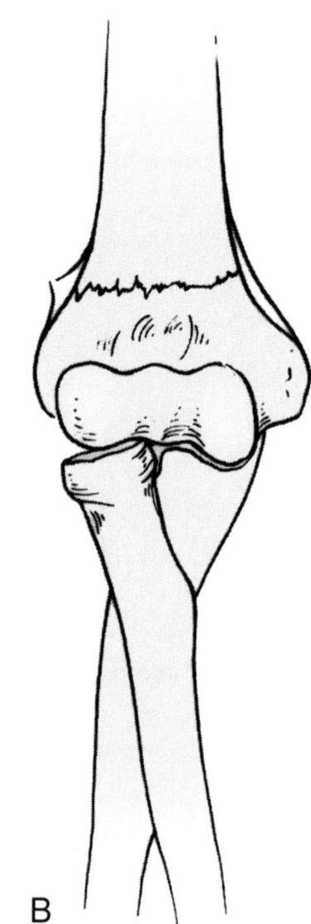

FIGURE 42–37 **A,** Posteromedially displaced fractures have an intact medial periosteal sleeve. **B,** Pronation of the forearm tightens the medial soft tissues and thereby stabilizes the reduction.

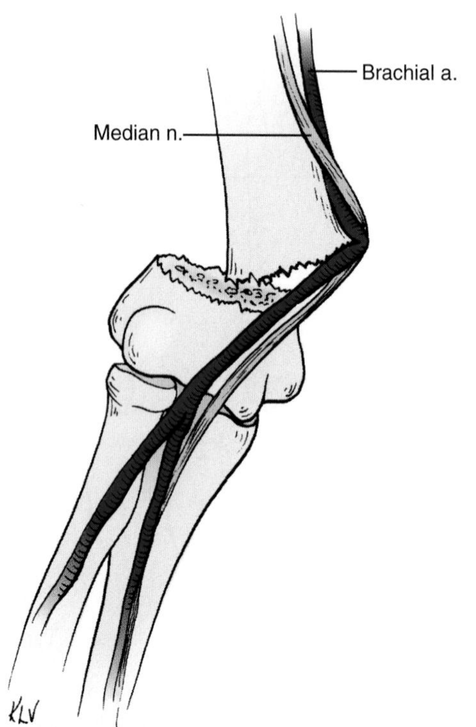

FIGURE 42–36 Posterolaterally displaced type III (extension-type) supracondylar humeral fracture. The proximal fragment displaces anteromedially, thus placing the brachial artery and median nerve at risk.

tightens the lateral sleeve; thus, posterior medial fractures are usually more stable once reduced (Fig. 42–37).

Mubarak and Davids subdivided type I fractures into IA and IB. Type IA injuries are truly nondisplaced fractures, with no comminution, collapse, or angulation. Type IB fractures are characterized by comminution or collapse of the medial column in the coronal plane and may have mild hyperextension in the sagittal plane (Fig. 42–38). They expressed concern that if unreduced, these minimally displaced type IB fractures could lead to a cosmetically unacceptable result, particularly in children with a neutral or varus preinjury carrying angle.[396]

DIAGNOSIS

Supracondylar fractures may be inherently obvious or nearly impossible to diagnose. The clinical findings in severely displaced fractures are generally so obvious that the most difficult part of the diagnosis is remembering to perform a thorough examination to assess for other injuries, as well as possible neurologic injury. This is particularly important given that neurologic injury is present in 10% to 15% of cases and ipsilateral fractures occur in 5% (usually the distal radius).* A complete and thorough assessment of the neurologic

*See references 28, 48, 50, 72, 86, 87, 105, 132, 260, 272, 286, 335, 380, 396, 462, 483, 538, 602.

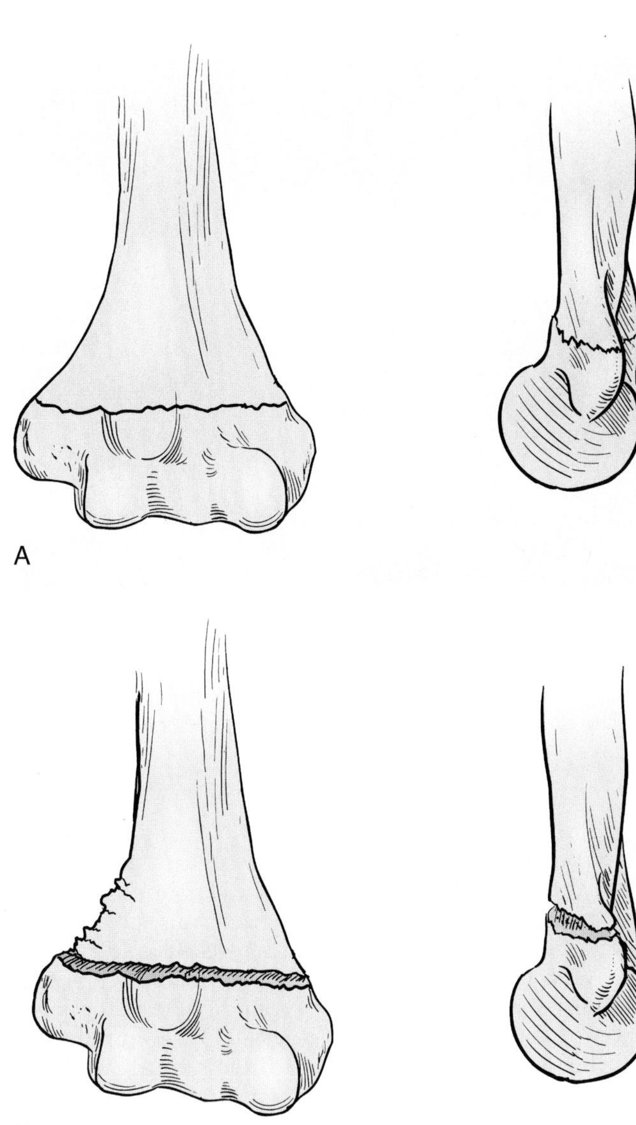

FIGURE 42–38 Type IA and IB supracondylar humeral fractures. **A,** Type IA. There is no angulation in either plane. **B,** Type IB. There is medial column collapse, and there may be slight hyperextension in the sagittal plane.

function of the hand is often difficult in a very young child with an acute elbow fracture. However, if a gentle and deliberate effort is made, most children by the age of 3 or 4 years will cooperate with a two-point sensory and directed motor examination. For uncooperative children, it is important to forewarn the parents that when a thorough examination is possible, there is a 10% to 15% chance that a neurologic injury will be discovered. Fortunately, these injuries nearly always do well.[28,72,87,104,105,132,259,260,272,286,335,483,602]

Although a complete neurologic examination is not always possible, it is always possible to assess the vascular status of patients with displaced supracondylar humeral fractures. It is also of paramount importance to be vigilant for clinical signs of a developing compartment syndrome. The earliest sign of compartment syndrome is pain out of proportion to the physical findings. Obviously, in the emergency department all patients with severely displaced supracondylar fractures have significant pain. However, the pain associated with compartment syndrome is usually of greater intensity and more persistent than that associated with routine injury. Additionally, patients in whom compartment syndrome is developing may experience pain on passive extension of the fingers. Other than pain, the most reliable early sign of compartment syndrome is a full or tense compartment. Unfortunately, by the time that the classic symptoms of pallor, paresthesia, and paralysis develop, there has typically been irreversible damage to the neuromuscular tissue.

The differential diagnosis of severely displaced supracondylar humeral fractures includes elbow dislocations and all conditions that mimic them, such as transphyseal distal humeral fractures and unstable lateral condylar fractures (Milch type II). True elbow dislocations are relatively uncommon. When elbow dislocations do occur, they are generally seen in older children and may be associated with medial epicondylar fractures.[40,128,172,239,518] Transphyseal distal humeral fractures are more common than supracondylar fractures in children younger than 2 years but are uncommon in children older than 2 years. Transphyseal fractures have been reported to be associated with child abuse in as many as 50% of cases.[31,121,361,602,604] Unstable lateral condylar fractures can be differentiated from supracondylar fractures most readily on the lateral radiograph. Supracondylar fractures usually originate at the olecranon fossa and are transverse or, less commonly, short oblique. Lateral condylar fractures originate more distally, often with only a small metaphyseal fragment visible on the lateral radiograph (Thurston-Holland sign) (Fig. 42–39). On the AP view, an unstable lateral condyle fracture (Milch type II) may have a normal-appearing radial-capitellar joint but will demonstrate subluxation of the ulnar-trochlear joint. Conversely, a Milch type I lateral condyle fracture will have a disrupted radial-capitellar joint (Fig. 42–40).

The diagnosis of a minimally displaced supracondylar humeral fracture may be difficult to make.[55,58,62,470] If seen soon after the injury, nondisplaced supracondylar fractures may have minimal swelling and can be difficult to differentiate from minimally displaced lateral condylar, medial epicondylar, or radial neck fractures. The most notable findings may be mild swelling and tenderness over the supracondylar region of the humerus. Careful clinical examination will reveal tenderness both medially and laterally over the supracondylar ridges, whereas with lateral condylar fractures the tenderness is lateral and with medial epicondylar fractures it is medial. In radial neck fractures the tenderness is over the radial neck posterolaterally. However, a small child with a painful elbow does not always cooperate with such a careful examination. In such cases the definitive diagnosis may not be evident until the cast is removed several weeks later (Fig. 42–41).

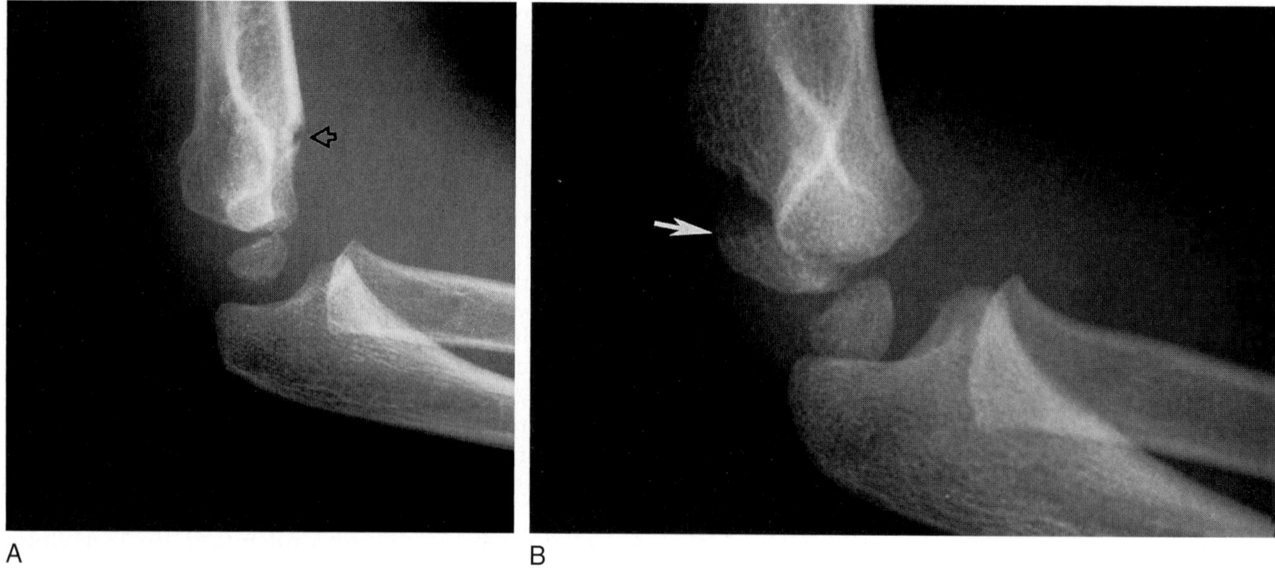

FIGURE 42–39 **A,** Lateral radiograph of a type II extension, supracondylar humeral fracture. The fracture originates just proximal to the "hourglass" of the olecranon fossa (*arrowhead*). **B,** Lateral radiograph of a displaced lateral condylar fracture. The Thurston-Holland, or metaphyseal, fragment is at the posterior aspect of the metaphysis (*arrow*). The fracture originates distal to the "hourglass" of the olecranon fossa.

When the fracture cannot be seen clearly on radiographs, it is important to obtain a thorough history to ensure that there was indeed a witnessed fall and that the symptoms began immediately after the injury because patients with osteoarticular sepsis often have a swollen, painful elbow and a history of trauma. If the elbow pain did not begin immediately after a witnessed traumatic event, consideration should be given to assessment of laboratory indices (complete blood cell count differential, erythrocyte sedimentation rate, and C-reactive protein) to ensure that the symptoms are not a result of occult infection.

RADIOGRAPHIC FINDINGS

The diagnosis of a supracondylar humeral fracture is confirmed radiographically. Obtaining good-quality radiographs is complicated by the fact that the elbow is painful and difficult to move. Because of rotational displacement, it may be impossible to obtain true orthogonal views of severely displaced fractures. However, with proper instruction to the radiographer, true AP and lateral radiographs of fractures with moderate or minimal displacement can be obtained. Obtaining a true AP view of the elbow requires full elbow extension and is therefore seldom possible. Consequently, we obtain an AP view of the distal humerus, which can be achieved with any degree of elbow extension (Fig. 42–42). The importance of obtaining a true lateral radiograph of the distal humerus cannot be overstated because the majority of treatment decisions are made from assessment of the lateral radiograph. Although repeating radiographs is slow, tedious, and frustrating, it is worth the effort because too often "bad x-rays lead to bad decisions."

Several radiographic parameters are helpful in managing patients with supracondylar humeral fractures. One is Baumann's angle, determined from an AP radiograph of the distal humerus. It is the angle between the physeal line of the lateral condyle of the humerus and a line drawn perpendicular to the long axis of the humeral shaft (Fig. 42–43). A number of studies have assessed the use of Baumann's angle in the management of supracondylar humeral fractures.* These studies have shown that although the "normal angle" varies from 8 to 28 degrees, depending on the patient, there is little side-to-side variance in any one individual. It has also been shown that relatively small changes in elbow position, either rotation or flexion, may alter Baumann's angle significantly.[71,290,605,613] Because of the wide range of "normal" values and the potential for positional differences, we find Baumann's angle to be of limited role in the management of supracondylar humeral fractures. Clearly, the presence of a small angle should alert the physician to the possibility of significant varus. Additionally, obtaining a comparison view to calculate Baumann's angle on the uninjured extremity may be a useful adjuvant in the decision-making process for minimally displaced fractures.[20] The AP radiograph should also be assessed for comminution of the medial or lateral columns, as well as for translation. Occasionally a completely displaced fracture will look relatively well aligned on the lateral radiograph but will show translation on the AP film. This translation cannot occur without complete disruption of both the anterior and posterior cortices.

*See references 20, 36, 44, 71, 87, 158, 290, 304, 369, 387, 564, 571, 594, 605, 613.

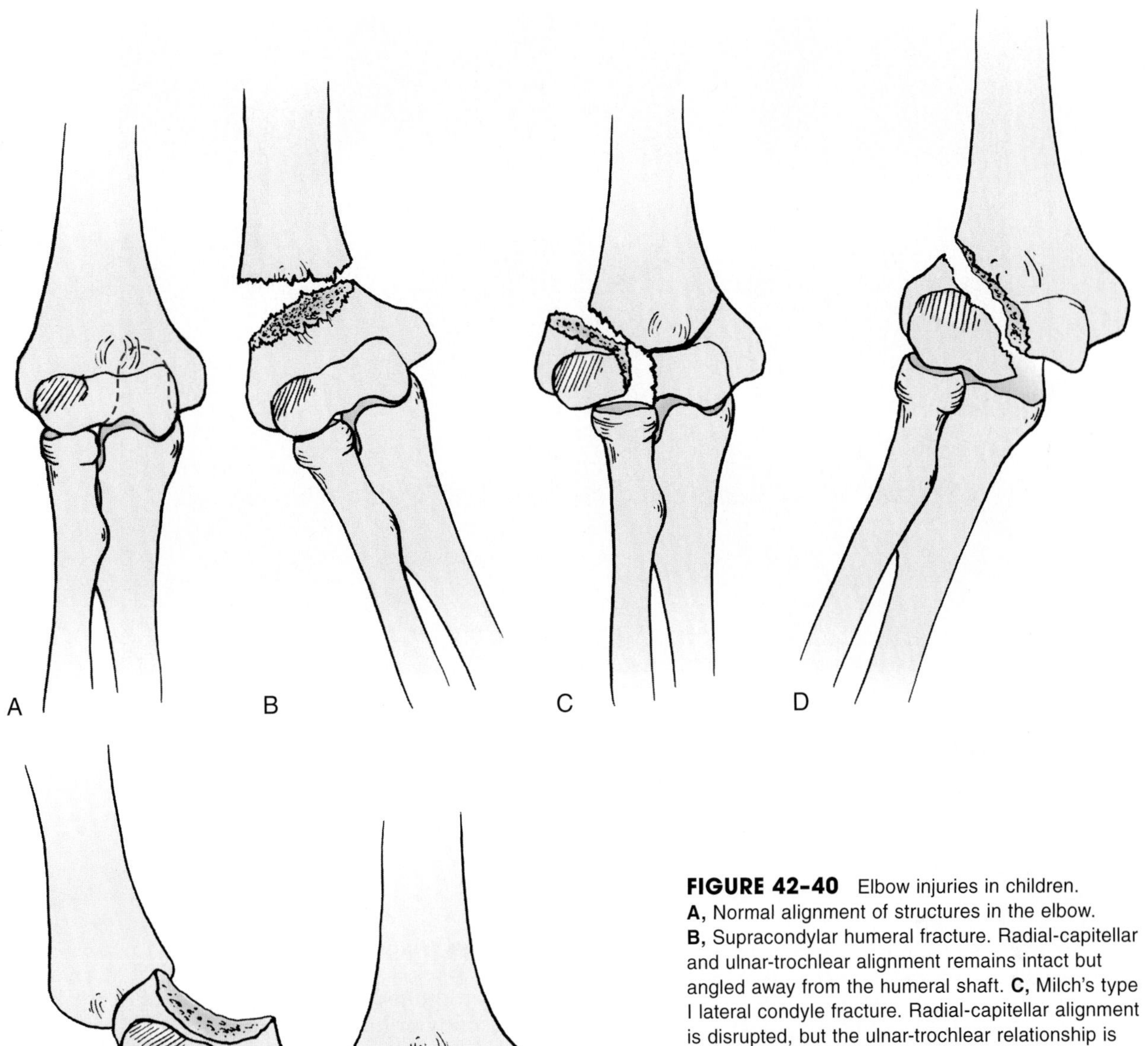

FIGURE 42–40 Elbow injuries in children. **A,** Normal alignment of structures in the elbow. **B,** Supracondylar humeral fracture. Radial-capitellar and ulnar-trochlear alignment remains intact but angled away from the humeral shaft. **C,** Milch's type I lateral condyle fracture. Radial-capitellar alignment is disrupted, but the ulnar-trochlear relationship is normal. **D,** Milch's type II lateral condyle fracture. The fracture extends medial to the trochlear groove, thus making the ulnohumeral joint unstable. However, the radius and capitellum maintain their relationship. **E,** Transphyseal fracture. The radius and capitellum maintain their alignment. If the secondary ossification center of the capitellum has not yet ossified, this injury may be difficult to distinguish from an elbow dislocation. **F,** Elbow dislocation. Both the radial-capitellar and ulnar-trochlear articulations are disrupted. (Redrawn from DeLee JC, Wilkin KE, Rogers LF, et al: Fracture-separation of the distal humeral epiphysis. J Bone Joint Surg Am 1980;62:48.)

Therefore, if present, it always represents an unstable fracture (Fig. 42–44).

There are also several important radiographic parameters on the lateral radiograph. A *fat pad sign* may alert the physician to the presence of an effusion within the elbow. The anterior fat pad is a triangular radiolucency anterior to the distal humeral diaphysis; it is seen clearly, and in the presence of elbow effusion, it is displaced anteriorly. The posterior fat pad is not normally visible when the elbow is flexed at right angles; however, if an effusion is present, it will also be visible posteriorly (Fig. 42–45).

There are several additional radiographic parameters to assess on the lateral radiograph (Fig. 42–46). First, the distal humerus should project as a teardrop or hourglass. The distal part of the teardrop or hourglass is formed by the ossific center of the capitellum (see Fig. 42–46A). It should appear as a nearly perfect

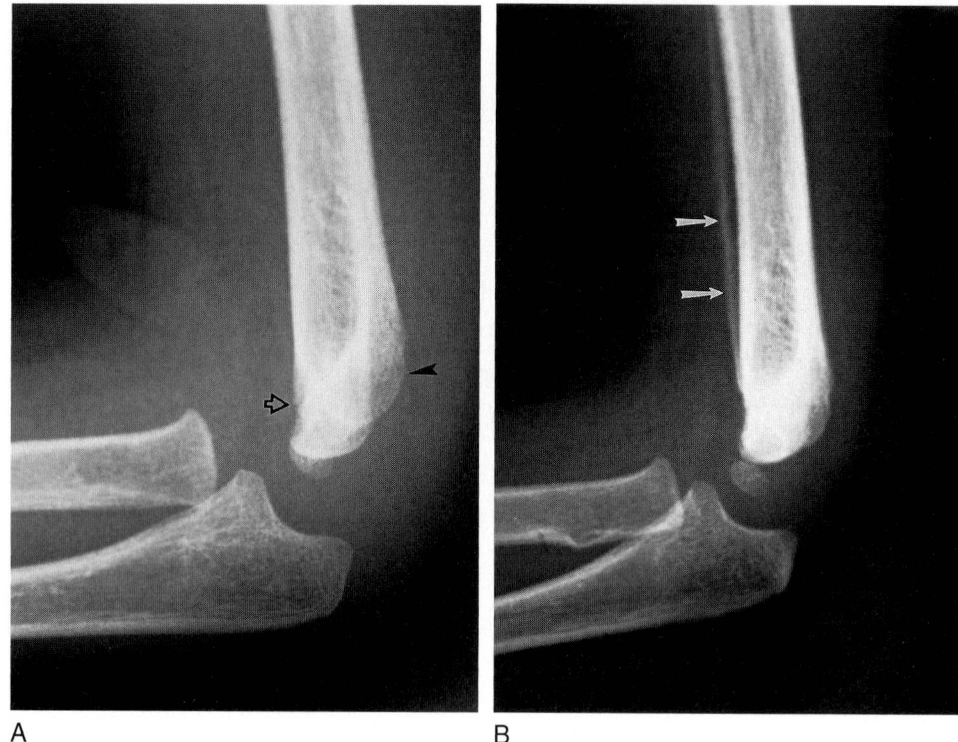

FIGURE 42–41 **A,** Lateral radiograph obtained after a hyperextension elbow injury in a child. Although there is no obvious fracture, there is a suggestion of a break in the anterior cortex (*arrow*), as well as some buckling posteriorly (*arrowhead*). **B,** Two weeks later, abundant periosteal reaction is evident (*arrows*).

circle. An imperfect circle or obscured teardrop or hourglass implies an oblique orientation of the distal portion of the humerus, either from inadequate x-ray technique or from fracture displacement. Second, the angle formed by the long axis of the humerus and the long axis of the capitellum should be approximately 40 degrees (see Fig. 42–46B). In supracondylar fractures with posterior tilting of the distal fragment (seen with extension fractures), the humerocapitellar angle will diminish, whereas with anterior tilting of the distal fragment (seen with less common flexion injuries) it will increase. Third, the anterior humeral line—a line drawn through the anterior cortex of the distal humerus—should pass through the middle third of the ossific nucleus of the capitellum (see Fig. 42–46C). With extension supracondylar fractures the anterior humeral line will pass anterior to the middle of the capitellum. Finally, the coronoid line—a line projected superiorly along the anterior border of the coronoid process—should just touch the anterior border of the lateral condyle of the humerus (see Fig. 42–46D). However, with extension supracondylar fractures, the coronoid line will pass anterior to the anterior border of the lateral condyle.[404]

If a nondisplaced or minimally displaced fracture is suspected but the AP and lateral views do not show a fracture, oblique views may be helpful.

TREATMENT

To again quote Mercer Rang, the goal of treatment of supracondylar humeral fractures is to "avoid catastrophes" (vascular compromise, compartment syndrome) and "minimize embarrassments" (cubitus varus, iatrogenic nerve palsies).[453] With this goal in mind, treatment of supracondylar humeral fractures can be divided into a discussion of their management in the emergency department, the care of nondisplaced fractures, and the treatment of displaced fractures.

Emergency Treatment

It is important that the child and limb receive proper care while awaiting definitive treatment. Unless the patient has an ischemic hand or tented skin, the limb should be immobilized as it lies with a simple splint. If possible, radiographs should be obtained before splinting, or radiolucent splint material should be used. If the distal extremity is initially ischemic, an attempt to better align the fracture fragments should be made immediately in the emergency department. This can be accomplished by extending the elbow, correcting any coronal plane deformity, and reducing the fracture by bringing the proximal fragment posteriorly and the distal fragment anteriorly (Fig. 42–47). Often this simple maneuver immediately restores cir-

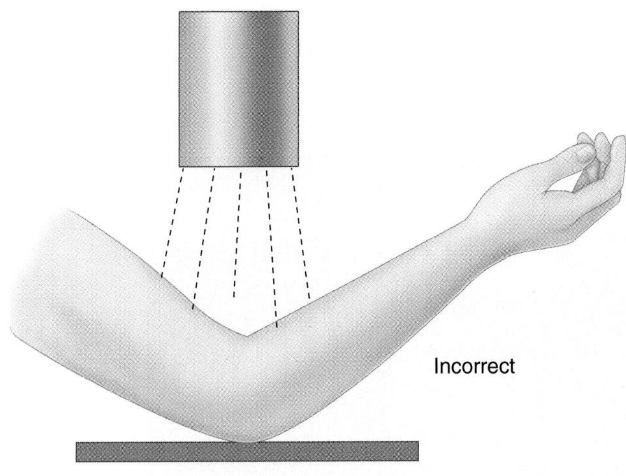

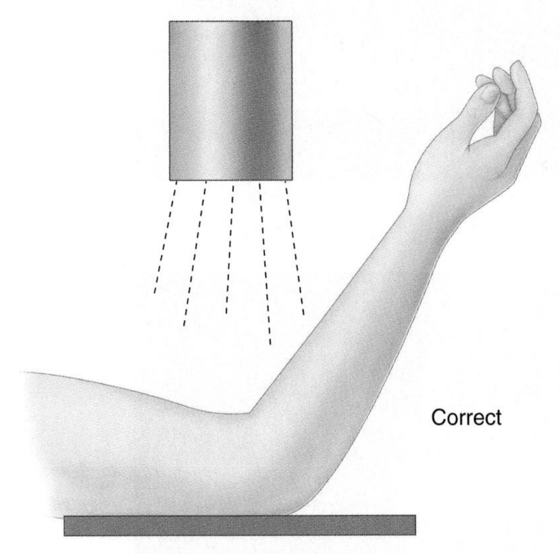

FIGURE 42-42 Radiographic technique to obtain a true anteroposterior (AP) view of the distal humerus. **A,** If the elbow does not fully extend, an attempt to obtain an AP view of the entire elbow will produce an oblique view of both the distal humerus and the proximal radius and ulna. **B,** The distal humerus is placed on the cassette without extending the elbow, and a true AP view of the distal humerus is obtained. An AP view of the proximal radius and forearm can be obtained by placing the forearm on the cassette.

culation to the hand. In extension-type fractures, flexion of the elbow should be avoided because it may cause further damage to the neurovascular structures. The distal circulation should always be checked before and after the splint is applied. Sensation, motor function, and skin integrity should also be carefully checked and recorded.[23] Patients with open fractures should receive intravenous antibiotics and appropriate tetanus prophylaxis (see discussion of open fractures in Chapter 40, General Principles of Managing Orthopaedic Injuries). All patients should be kept from having any food or drink by mouth (NPO) until a definitive treatment plan has been outlined.

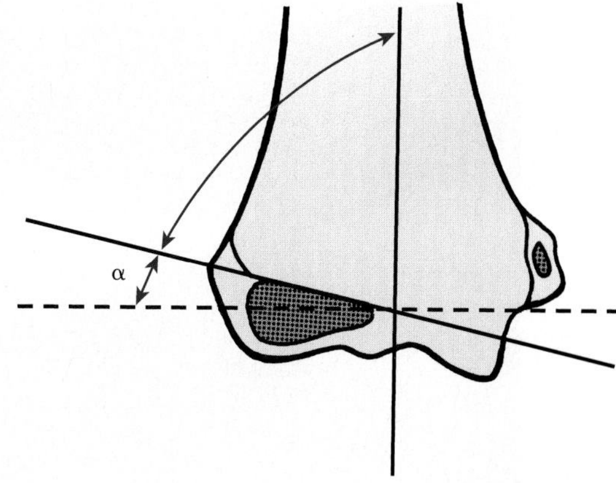

FIGURE 42-43 Baumann's angle is the angle created by the intersection of a line drawn down the proximal margin of the capitellar ossification center and a line drawn perpendicular to the long axis of the humeral shaft.

Treatment of Nondisplaced Fractures

Treatment of nondisplaced fractures is straightforward and noncontroversial. It consists of long-arm cast immobilization for 3 weeks. We often initially treat the patient in the emergency department with a posterior splint with figure-eight reinforcement. The position of the forearm in the long-arm cast has been the subject of a great deal of speculation. For truly nondisplaced fractures there is no theoretical advantage to either pronation or supination. We generally immobilize nondisplaced fractures with the forearm in neutral position. The patient returns 5 to 10 days after injury for removal of the splint. Radiographs are repeated to ensure that no displacement has occurred, and the patient is placed in a long-arm cast for an additional 2 to 3 weeks, at which time immobilization is discontinued. After cast removal the parents are forewarned that normal use of the arm may not resume for 1 to 2 weeks and that some pain and stiffness should be expected for the first 2 months. Children return 6 to 8 weeks after cast removal for review of their range of motion. We have found that patients returning for a range-of-motion check at 3 to 4 weeks may have mild residual deficits in extension or flexion, or both. This can be disconcerting to the parents, who expect everything to be normal at this visit. This parental anxiety (and the long discourse of reassurance) can be avoided by allowing the child to be out of the cast for a longer period before returning for the final checkup.

There are a few potential pitfalls in the management of nondisplaced supracondylar humeral fractures that merit further discussion. The first concerns the diagnosis. Sometimes the only visible radiographic abnormality is the presence of a fat

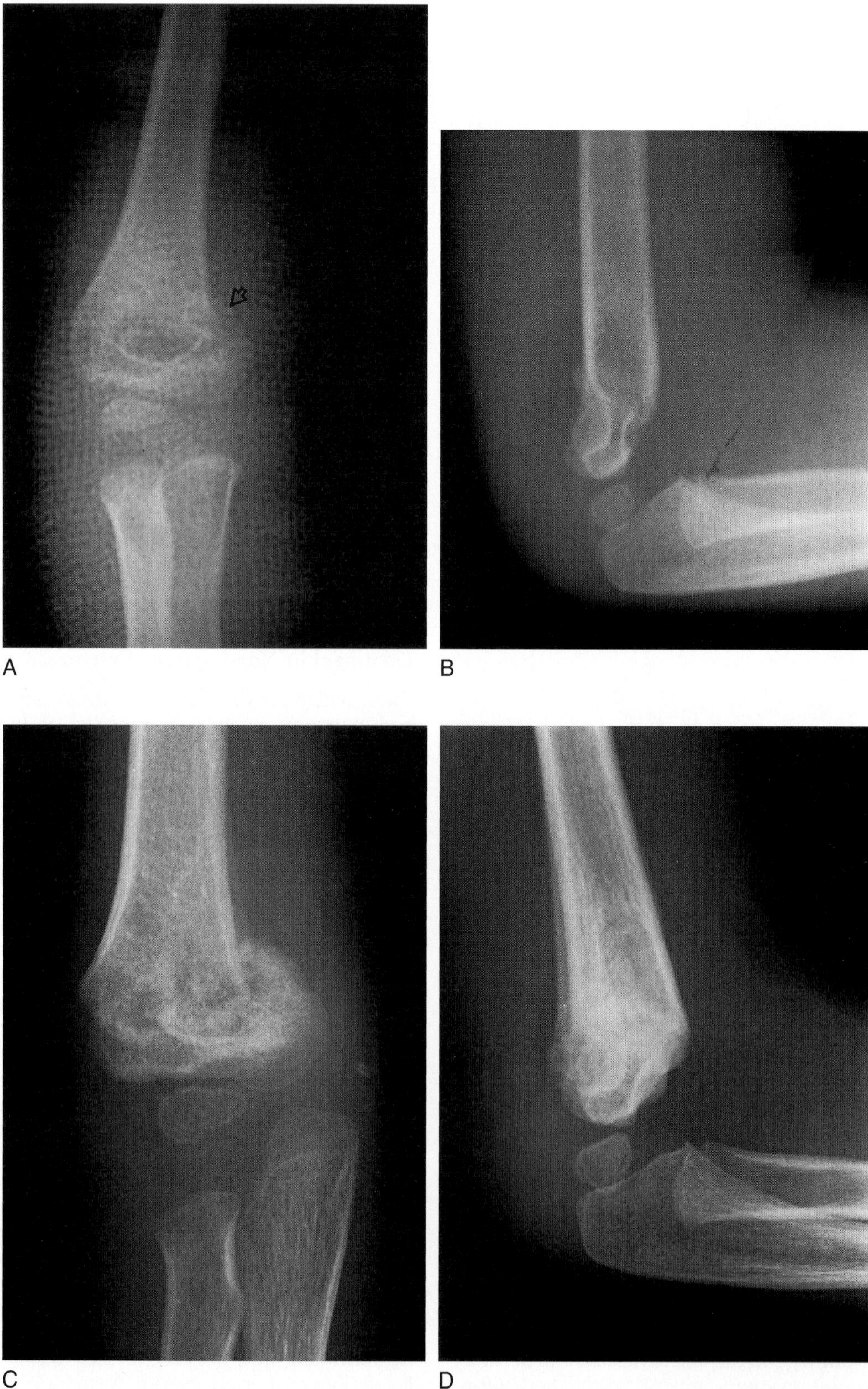

FIGURE 42–44 Anteroposterior (AP) **(A)** and lateral **(B)** radiographs of a minimally displaced supracondylar humeral fracture. The importance of medial translation of the distal fragment on the AP view was not appreciated (*arrow* in part **A**), and the patient was managed in a long-arm cast. **C** and **D,** At the time of cast removal, the fracture had angulated further into varus and hyperextension.

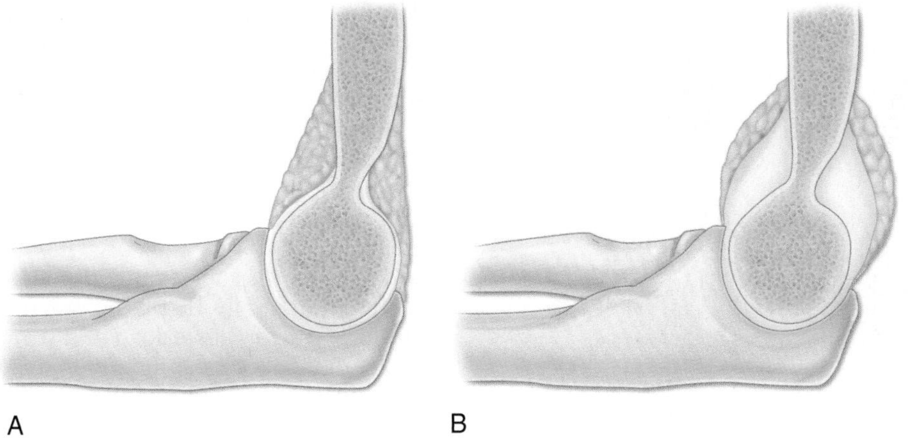

FIGURE 42–45 Fat pad sign. **A,** There is normally both an anterior and a posterior fat pad. These structures may be seen as radiolucencies adjacent to their respective cortices. **B,** In the presence of an effusion, the fat pad will be elevated, thereby creating a radiolucent "sail."

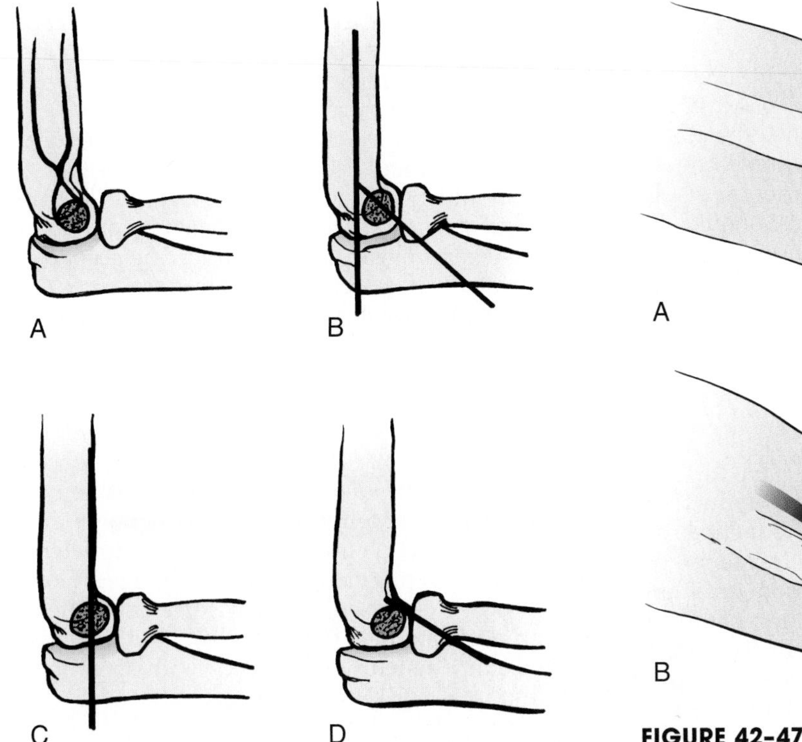

FIGURE 42–46 **A** through **D,** Normal radiographic parameters of a lateral view of the elbow. See text for description.

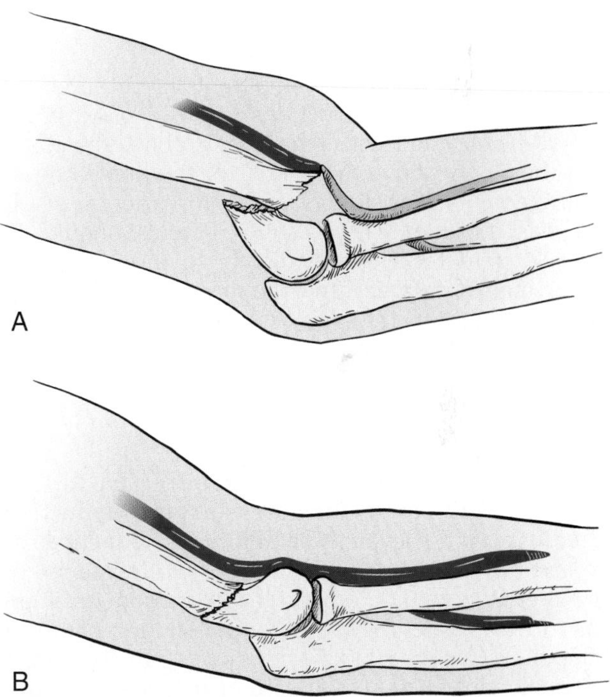

FIGURE 42–47 **A,** Ischemic limb. **B,** Simple realignment may reduce the tension on a vessel and restore the circulation.

pad sign. Frequently after 1 to 3 weeks, the fracture, as well as the periosteal reaction associated with its healing, will be obvious (see Fig. 42–41). Failure to make this diagnosis at the outset is of little concern because the fracture is stable. Of more concern is the possibility of misdiagnosing an occult infection or nursemaid's elbow as a nondisplaced supracondylar humeral fracture. A thorough history will suggest the correct diagnosis. At times, undisplaced fractures cause soft tissue swelling and may even result in compartment syndrome. Thus, we are careful to not immobilize the arm in more than 90 degrees of flexion, and we often use a posterior splint rather than a cast. If a cast is applied, it is generously split. The parents must be educated on the importance of edema control and watching for signs of increased swelling and pressure. Too often patients are discharged from the emergency department with instructions to elevate the arm and use a sling. It should not be surprising that a number of these patients return for follow-up with swollen extremities. Parents, in an effort to follow directions, are dogmatic about use of the sling. Unfortunately, this keeps the extremity in a dependent position and incites swelling. Time should be taken in the emergency

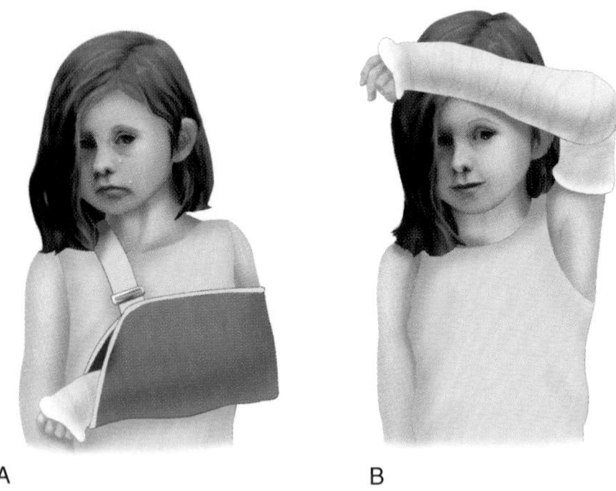

FIGURE 42-48 **A,** A sling holds the hand and elbow in a dependent position, thereby creating edema and pain. **B,** Parents (and patients) should be instructed in true elevation of the extremity, with the fingers above the elbow and the elbow above the heart.

department to explain to the parents (and the nurses giving discharge instructions) that the extremity should be elevated with "the fingers above the elbow and the elbow above the heart" for the first 48 hours after the injury. The sling is for comfort after the swelling has subsided (Fig. 42–48). Parents should be instructed to return immediately to the emergency department if it appears that the splint or cast is becoming too tight or the pain seems to be increasing inappropriately.

Treatment of Displaced Fractures

Several treatment options are available for the management of displaced fractures (types II and III). By definition, all these fractures require reduction. Usually, even for severe type III injuries, reduction can be accomplished in closed fashion. Options exist on the method of maintaining the reduction until the fracture has healed. These methods include cast immobilization, traction, and percutaneous pin fixation. If adequate closed reduction cannot be achieved, open reduction should be performed; this is almost universally followed by pin fixation.

Closed Reduction

Reduction of Extension-Type Fracture. Under general anesthesia, the child is positioned at the edge of the operating table with the arm over a radiolucent table to allow assessment of the reduction with an image intensifier (Fig. 42–49). Some surgeons elect to use the image intensifier itself as the table. An assistant grasps the proximal humerus firmly to allow traction to be placed on the distal fragment. Traction should be applied in a steady continuous force with the elbow in full extension. Once adequate traction has been applied, the coronal plane (varus/valgus) deformity is corrected while traction is maintained (see Fig. 42–49B). Continuing to maintain traction with the nondominant hand, the surgeon uses the fingers of the dominant hand to apply a posterior force to the proximal fragment. The thumb of the dominant hand is advanced along the posterior humeral shaft in an attempt to "milk" the distal fragment further distally. Once the thumb reaches the olecranon, it applies an anterior force to the distal fragment while the fingers continue to pull the proximal fragment posteriorly (see Fig. 42–49C). Concurrently, the nondominant hand flexes the elbow and pronates the forearm for posterior medially displaced fractures and supinates the forearm for posterior lateral fractures. (With the elbow in a flexed position, the patient's thumb should point in the direction of the distal fragment's initial displacement.) While the elbow is being flexed, the surgeon's nondominant hand can continue to exert a distracting force on the distal fragment. With the elbow hyperflexed, the reduction is then assessed on AP and lateral views. The lateral image can be obtained by either externally rotating the shoulder or rotating the image intensifier. With very unstable fractures the surgeon may need to rotate the image intensifier to avoid displacing the fracture. Once the reduction has been confirmed, the fracture can be immobilized with a cast, traction, or percutaneous pin fixation.

Several caveats to achieving successful closed reduction merit further discussion. The first is that every effort should be made to avoid vigorous manipulations and remanipulations because they only damage soft tissue and elicit more swelling. The second is the management of extremely unstable fractures, which are often posterolaterally displaced. Maintenance of reduction is difficult because supination is not as effective at tightening the intact lateral soft tissue hinge as pronation is at stabilizing posteromedially displaced fractures (see Fig. 42–37). During reduction, as the elbow is placed into hyperflexion, these fractures occasionally displace into valgus. When valgus displacement is noted, a different reduction maneuver is required. Traction and the posteriorly directed force to the proximal fragment remain unchanged. However, as the elbow is flexed, a varus force is applied, and flexion is stopped at 90 degrees. The reduction is confirmed and usually stabilized with percutaneous pinning (see Fig. 42–49D and E).

Reduction of Flexion-Type Fractures. Closed reduction is obtained with longitudinal traction and the elbow in extension; the distal fragment is reduced with a posteriorly directed force (Fig. 42–50). Any coronal plane deformity is then corrected. Once adequate reduction has been confirmed, it is most commonly maintained with percutaneous pinning. Severely displaced flexion-type injuries are more likely to require open reduction than the more common extension-type fractures are.[115]

Percutaneous Pinning. The development of image intensifiers and power pin drivers has made percutaneous pin fixation of supracondylar humeral fractures a relatively simple procedure. Because percutaneous pin fixation yields the most predictable results with the

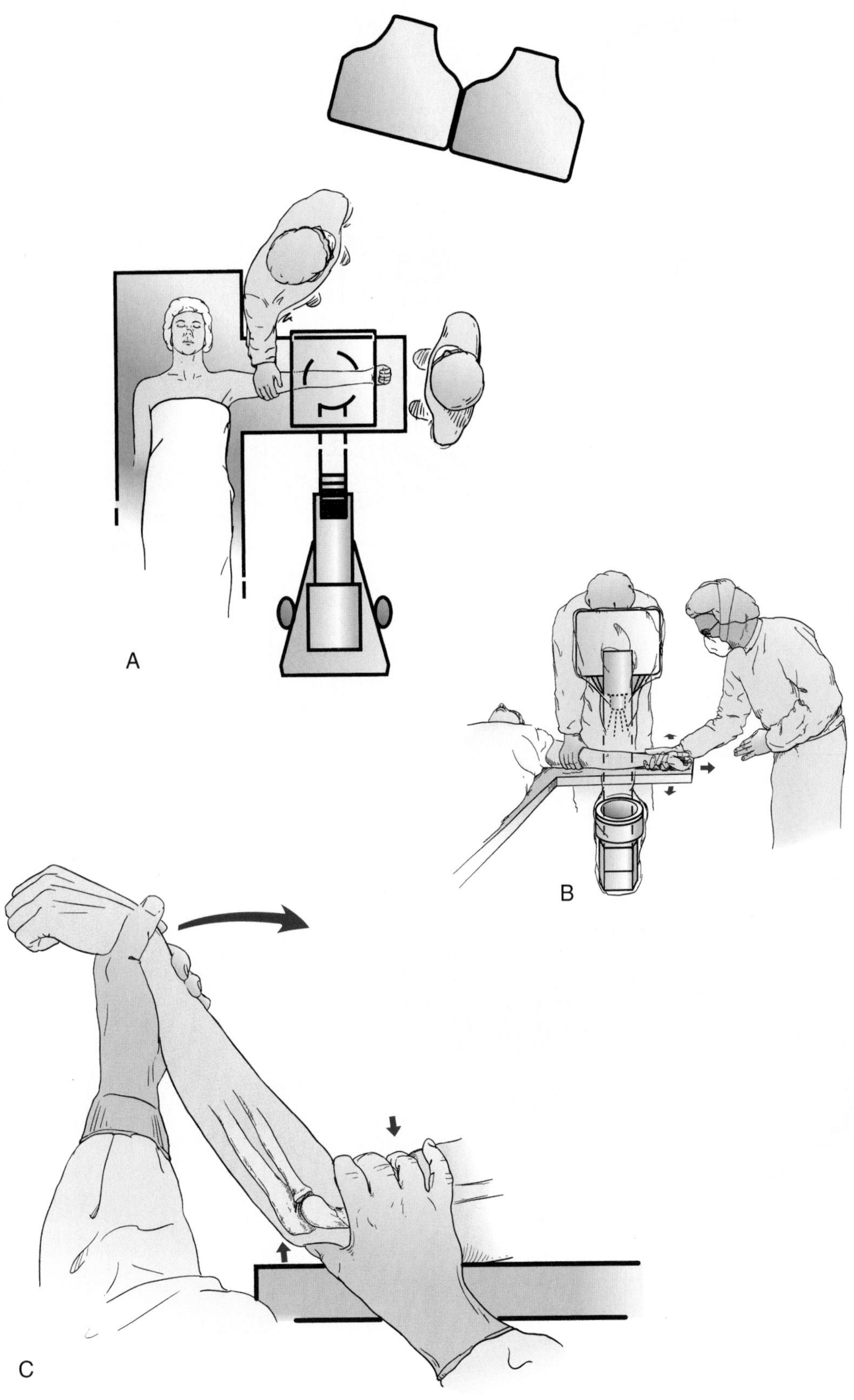

FIGURE 42–49 Technique for closed reduction and percutaneous pinning of supracondylar humeral fracture. **A,** Diagram of patient and C-arm positioning. **B,** Initially, traction is applied and the coronal plane (varus/valgus) deformity is corrected. **C,** The surgeon's dominant hand is used to reduce the fracture in the sagittal plane while the nondominant hand flexes the elbow and pronates (posteromedially displaced fractures) or supinates (posterolaterally displaced fractures) the forearm. The fingers of the dominant hand are used to apply a posteriorly directed force to the proximal fragment while the thumb is slid posteriorly in a proximal-to-distal direction to "milk" the distal fragment anteriorly.

Continued

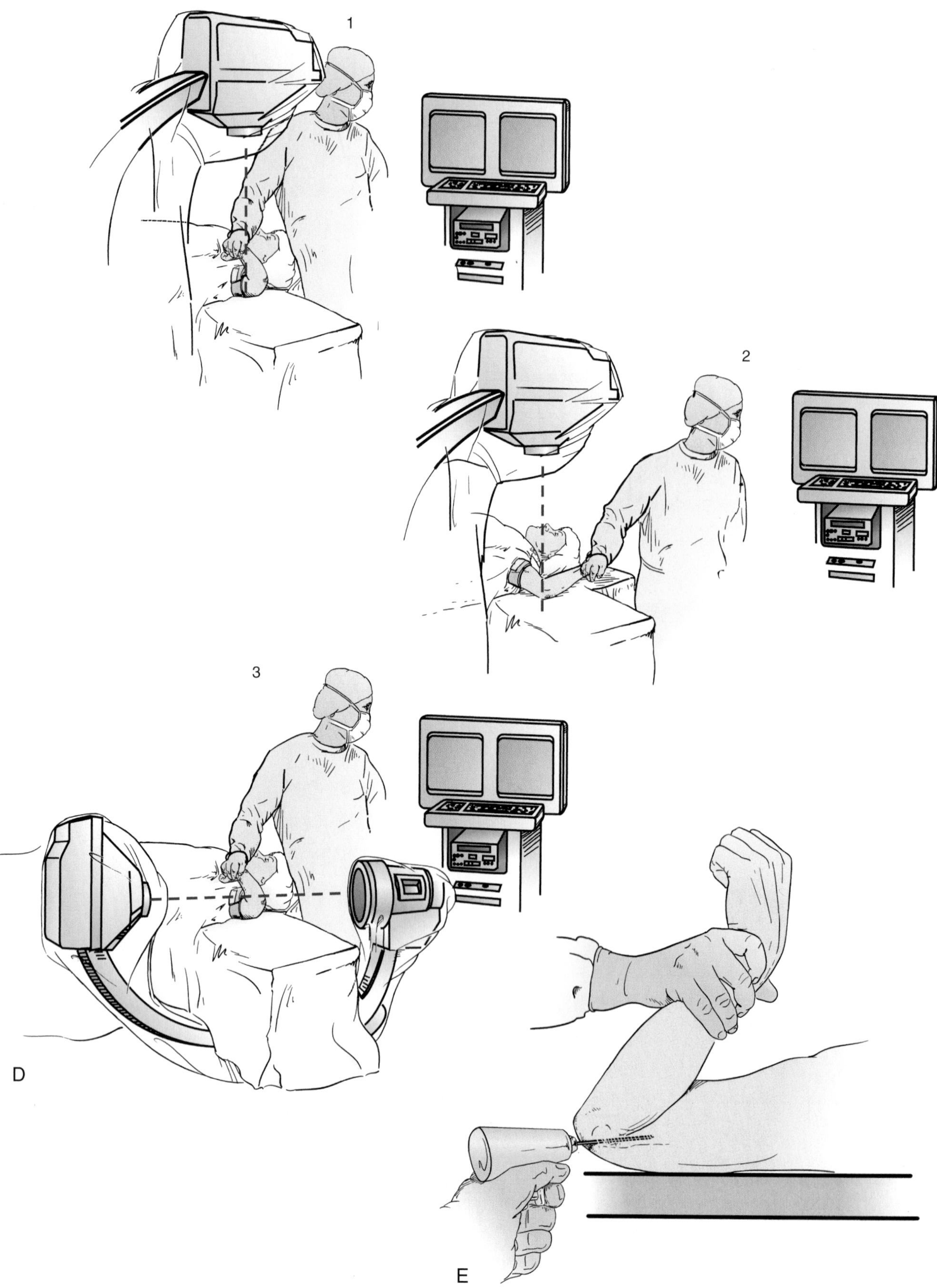

FIGURE 42-49 cont'd **D,** Reduction is confirmed with the arm in a hyperflexed position. The Jones view is used to obtain an anteroposterior (AP) view **(D1).** The lateral view may be obtained by either externally rotating the shoulder **(D2)** or rotating the image intensifier **(D3). E,** The fracture is pinned with the arm in a hyperflexed position, and the reduction and pin placement are confirmed in the AP and lateral planes.

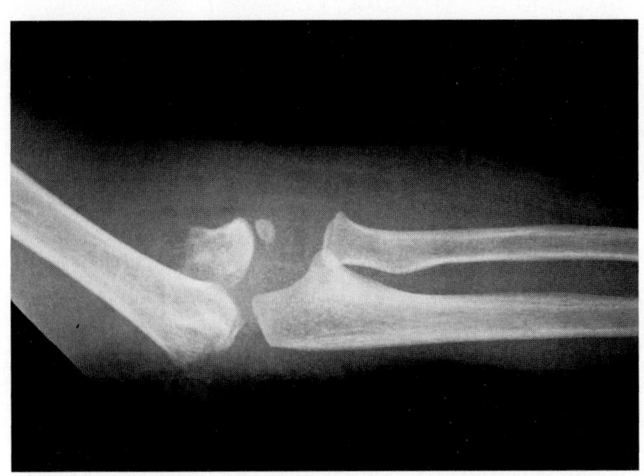

FIGURE 42–50 Lateral radiograph of a type III flexion supracondylar humeral fracture. Note the anterior displacement of the distal fragment.

fewest complications, it is our preferred technique for immobilization of displaced supracondylar humeral fractures.* The technique for percutaneous pinning involves the placement of two or three 0.62-inch smooth K-wires (smaller K-wires may be used in patients younger than 2 years) distally to proximally in a crossed or parallel fashion. (Whether a crossed pin or a parallel pin technique should be used is the subject of considerable debate and is discussed later under Controversies in Treatment.) Once closed reduction has been achieved, the extremity is held in the reduced position by either the surgeon's nondominant hand or an assistant. We usually place the lateral pin first, although occasionally with an unstable posterolaterally displaced fracture, the initial pin may have to be placed medially. If two lateral pins are to be used, the first pin should be placed as close to the midline as possible (just lateral to the olecranon). If only one lateral pin is to be placed, the starting point is the center of the lateral condyle. After the first pin is placed, the second pin is inserted either laterally (in the center of the lateral column) or medially. The relationship of the second pin to the first pin and the fracture is an important aspect of percutaneous pin fixation. The rotational stability of the fixation is enhanced if the second pin crosses the fracture line at a significant distance from the first pin. Careful attention must be given to ensure that the pins do *not* cross the fracture at the same point. This potential error can be made with either crossed or parallel pins. We avoid this problem by attempting to divide the fracture into thirds with the pins (Fig. 42–51).

If a medial pin is used, care must be taken to ensure that the ulnar nerve is not injured. The starting position for a medial pin is the inferiormost aspect of the medial epicondyle (see Fig. 42–51). The pin should be started as far anterior as possible. It is often helpful for the surgeon holding the reduction to "milk" the soft tissue posteriorly, with the thumb left immediately posterior to the medial epicondyle to protect the ulnar nerve (Fig. 42–52). If the elbow is extremely swollen, a small incision can be made to identify and protect the ulnar nerve. It is important to remember that flexion of the elbow displaces the ulnar nerve anteriorly. Thus, it is safer to place a medial pin with the elbow in extension.[418,505,517] Similarly, if the arm is immobilized in flexion, the nerve may be "tented" around the pin, thereby leading to ulnar nerve symptoms without direct penetration of the nerve by the pin (Fig. 42–53).

Placement of K-wires percutaneously through the narrow distal humerus requires some finesse. As in all percutaneous procedures in orthopaedics, it is facilitated by knowing the anatomy and by reducing the task into two separate, two-dimensional problems. Appropriate pin placement is made easier by first lining up the pin driver in the AP plane, locking this angle in, and then lining up the pin driver in the lateral plane without changing the angle in the AP plane. Positioning the pin driver and subsequently the pin *sequentially* in *only* these two orthogonal planes simplifies a conceptually difficult task. The use of a pin driver rather than a drill (which requires a chuck key) also facilitates pin placement because the pin can more readily be advanced in the power driver.

Once the fracture has been stabilized with at least two pins, the elbow is extended and the reduction and pin placement are confirmed on orthogonal x-ray views. If the reduction and pin placement are acceptable, the pins are bent, cut (it is best to leave a few centimeters of pin out of the skin to facilitate removal), and covered with sterile felt to decrease skin motion around the pin. The arm is immobilized in 30 to 60 degrees of flexion in either a posterior splint or a widely split or bivalved cast. The child is observed overnight and discharged with instructions on cast care and elevation. The child usually returns in a week to 10 days for examination, and radiographs are generally taken to check for maintenance of reduction. At 3 weeks the radiographs are repeated, the pins are removed, and the immobilization is discontinued. The parents are instructed to expect gradual return of motion and to avoid forced manipulation. Final follow-up is at 6 to 8 weeks to evaluate alignment and range of motion.

As with all treatment methods, there are potential complications with percutaneous pinning, including pin tract inflammation or infection, iatrogenic ulnar nerve injury, and loss of reduction. Pin tract inflammation or infection occurs in 2% to 3% of patients in most large series of supracondylar humeral fractures treated by pin fixation.[87] Fortunately, these infections usually respond to removal of the pin and a short course of oral antibiotics, although osteomyelitis can develop. Ulnar nerve injury from a medially placed percutaneous pin is another potential complication. The true incidence of this problem is difficult to determine because not all ulnar nerve injuries are iatrogenic. However, the ulnar nerve is the least commonly injured nerve in supracondylar fractures; such injury

*See references 20, 73, 87, 104, 160, 167, 193, 214, 215, 273, 278, 369, 379, 400, 436, 446, 454, 550, 596, 602.

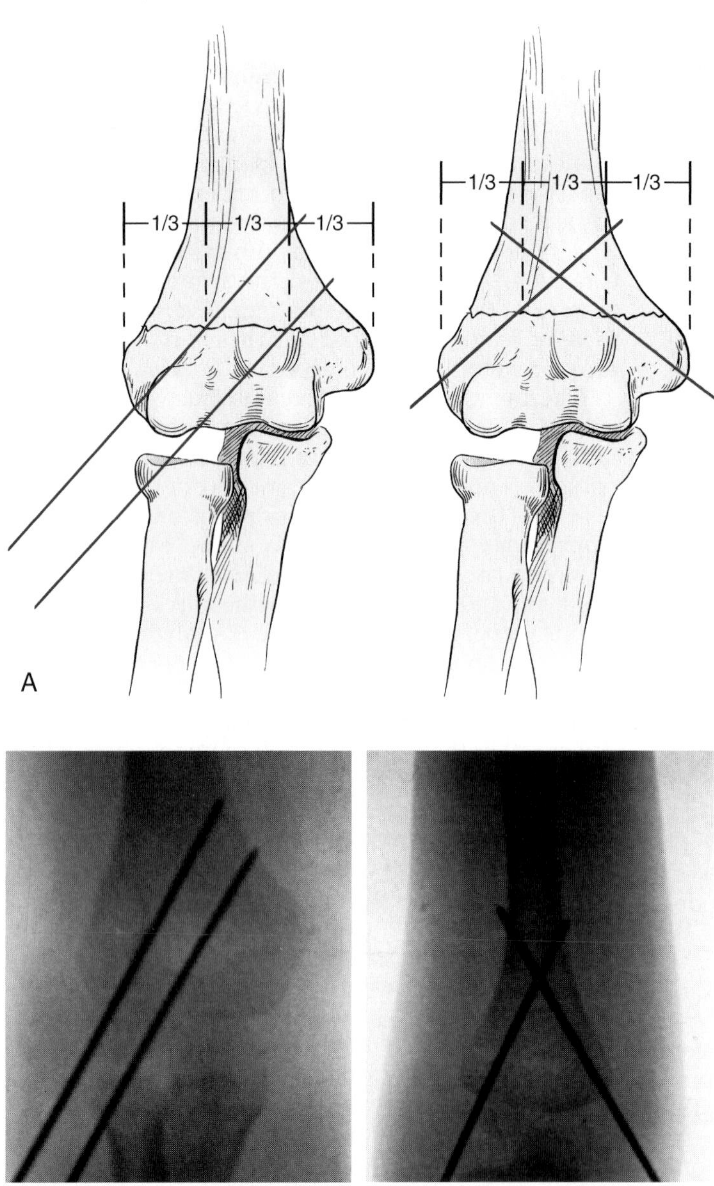

FIGURE 42–51 Pin placement for optimal rotational stability. **A,** Schematic diagram of parallel lateral pins *(left)* and crossed medial and lateral pins *(right)*. Ideally, the pins should be the greatest possible distance from each other at the fracture site. This can be accomplished with either technique. **B,** Anteroposterior radiographs demonstrating fractures fixed with parallel lateral pins *(left)* and crossed medial and lateral pins *(right)*.

occurs most frequently in the rare flexion injuries. If an ulnar nerve deficit is noted postoperatively and a medial pin is present, we recommend removal of the medial pin and observation. Fortunately, in most cases the ulnar nerve makes a complete recovery.* Loss of reduction can occur after closed reduction and percutaneous pinning of supracondylar humeral fractures (Fig. 42–54). This complication is generally the result of inadequate surgical technique and can be minimized by close attention to detail to ensure that the pins are maximally separated at the fracture and have adequate purchase in the proximal fragment.

Cast Immobilization. The advantages of cast immobilization are that a cast is easy to apply, readily available, and familiar to most orthopaedists. Casting does not require sophisticated equipment, there is little chance of iatrogenic infection or growth arrest, and it can yield good results. For these reasons, some surgeons advocate closed reduction and cast immobilization as the initial treatment option for all displaced supracondylar humeral fractures and reserve percutaneous pinning for patients in whom cast management fails.

After closed reduction is obtained, treatment of displaced fractures with a cast is similar to treatment of a nondisplaced fracture.[60] There are, however, a few differences. First, the cast should be carefully applied to avoid compression in the antecubital fossa. Second, patients requiring reduction are admitted to the hospital overnight for observation. Again, it is imperative that the nursing staff and parents understand the importance and the technique of edema control. The final and perhaps most significant difference in the management of displaced fractures with a cast is that the cast is not removed at the initial follow-up visit

*See references 87, 132, 193, 255, 259, 278, 339, 374, 454, 502, 564, 594.

7 to 10 days after the reduction; rather, radiographs are obtained with the arm in the cast. Again, the cast is maintained for 3 to 4 weeks after the reduction, and the parents are warned to expect a period of pain and stiffness after cast removal.

Cast immobilization is not without potential problems. Most displaced supracondylar fractures are stable only if immobilized in more than 90 degrees of flexion. Casting an injured elbow in hyperflexion may lead to further swelling, increased compartment pressure, and possibly the development of Volkmann's ischemic contracture (compartment syndrome). Although Volkmann's ischemic contracture can develop in any patient with a supracondylar humeral fracture regardless of the treatment method, cast immobilization requires flexion of the elbow and a rigid circumferential dressing, both of which may exacerbate the condition.

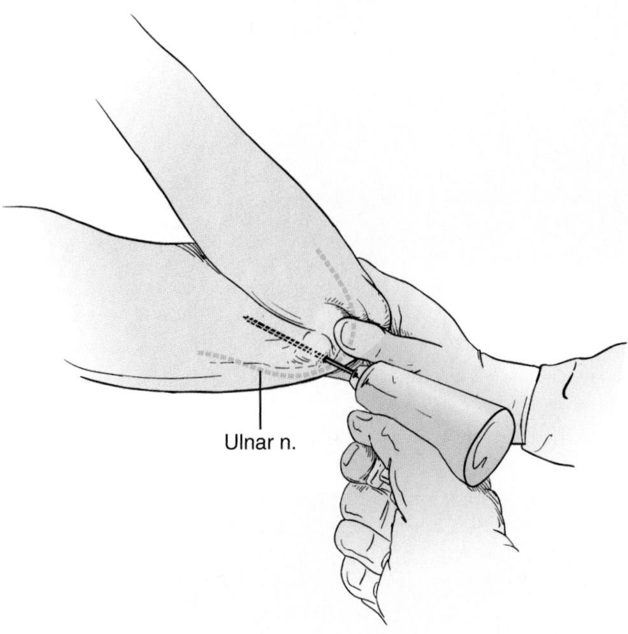

FIGURE 42–52 The assistant holding the reduction protects the ulnar nerve by sweeping the soft tissues posteriorly away from the medial epicondyle.

Loss of reduction is the other potential problem with cast immobilization. As the swelling subsides, a cast inevitably loosens and allows the elbow to extend, which may result in loss of reduction. Often this will occur after the first follow-up radiograph shows maintenance of the reduction. In this scenario, it is not until the cast is removed a few weeks later that the varus hyperextension malunion is discovered. Although good results can be obtained with cast immobilization, particularly with type II fractures, the necessity to immobilize the elbow in flexion and the unpredictable problem of loss of reduction have led us away from cast immobilization of supracondylar fractures that require reduction.

Traction. Traction also yields good results in the management of displaced supracondylar humeral fractures.[13,130,438,615] Numerous traction techniques have been described, including overhead or lateral traction with either skin or skeletal traction applied with an olecranon pin or screw (Fig. 42–55). Traction has been advocated to maintain a closed reduction as well as to achieve reduction of irreducible fractures. A period of traction preceding an attempt at closed reduction in a massively swollen arm has also been described. However, the most effective way to prevent local swelling (or to decrease it if the elbow is already swollen) is to achieve immediate reduction and stabilize the fracture and soft tissue.

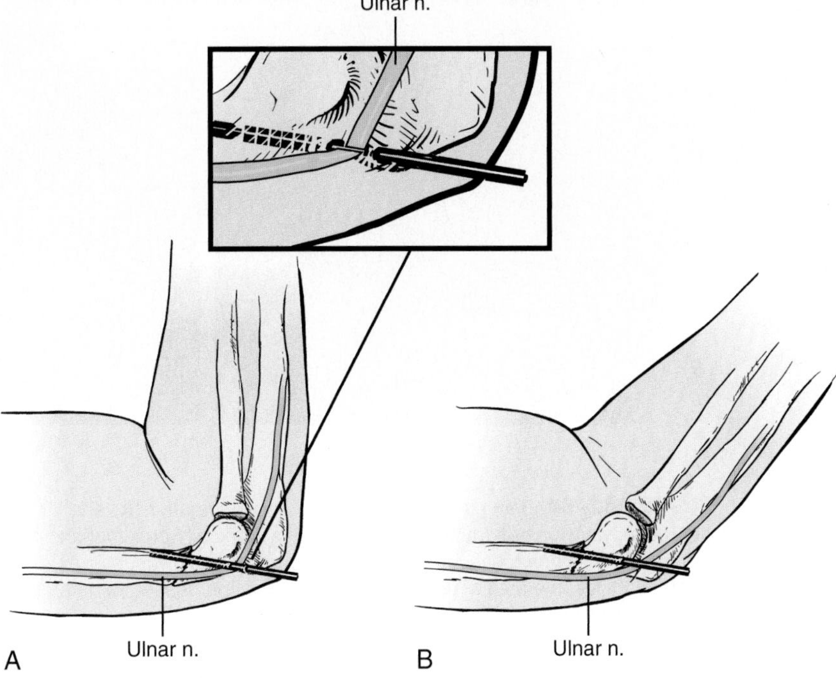

FIGURE 42–53 **A,** Elbow flexion brings the ulnar nerve anteriorly, closer to the medial epicondyle, thereby placing it at greater risk during medial pin placement. Additionally, immobilization of the elbow in flexion may tent the nerve around the pin and produce ulnar nerve symptoms despite a properly placed pin. **B,** With the elbow in extension, the ulnar nerve lies in a safer position, posterior to the medial epicondyle.

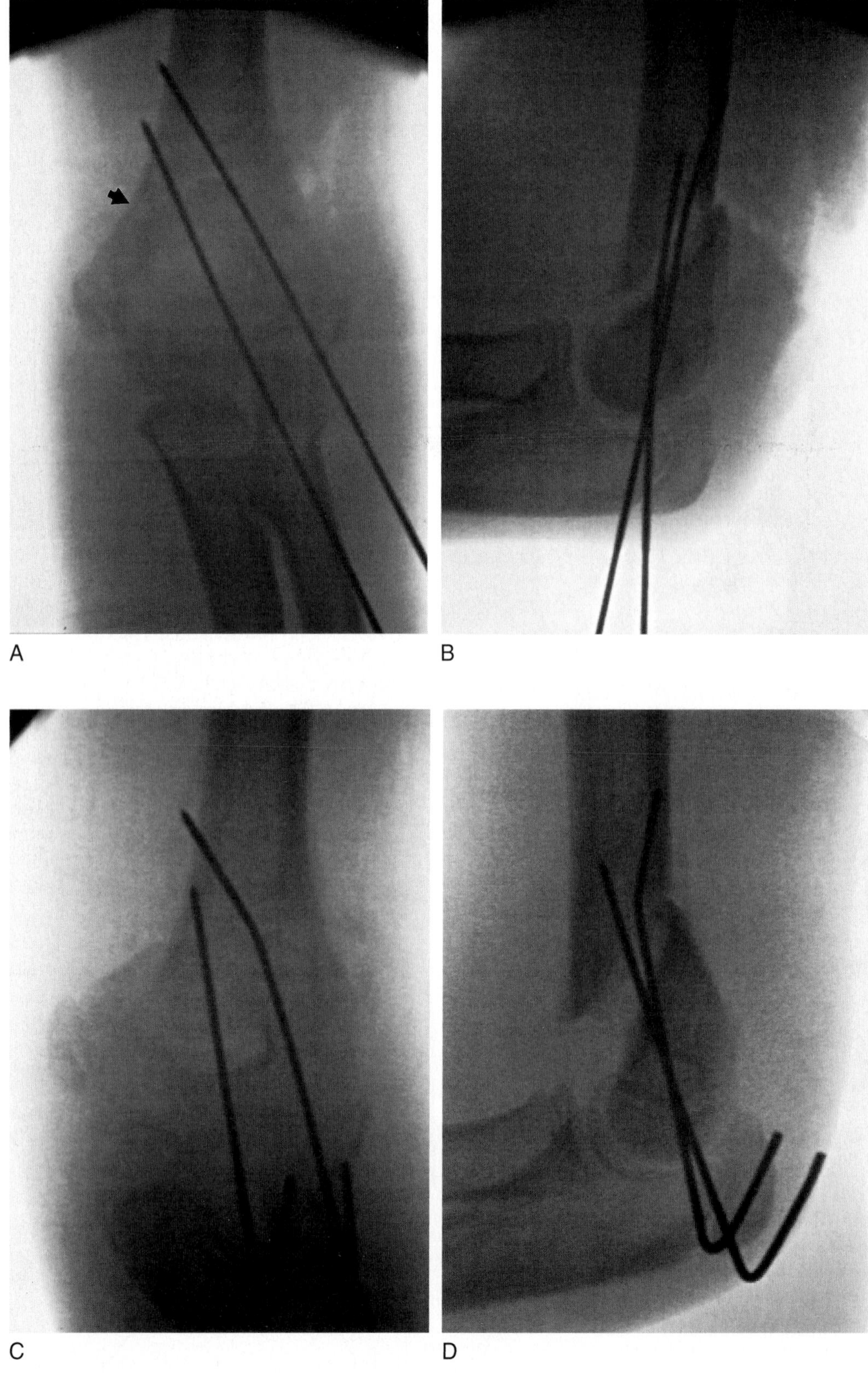

FIGURE 42–54 Immediate postoperative anteroposterior **(A)** and lateral **(B)** radiographs of a type III supracondylar humeral fracture. The fracture is atypically proximal and oblique. Note that the most medial pin has very little purchase in the proximal fragment (*arrowhead* in **A**). **C** and **D,** Eighteen days postoperatively the medial pin has lost its marginal purchase, the lateral pin has bent, and the fracture has migrated into hyperextension and varus.

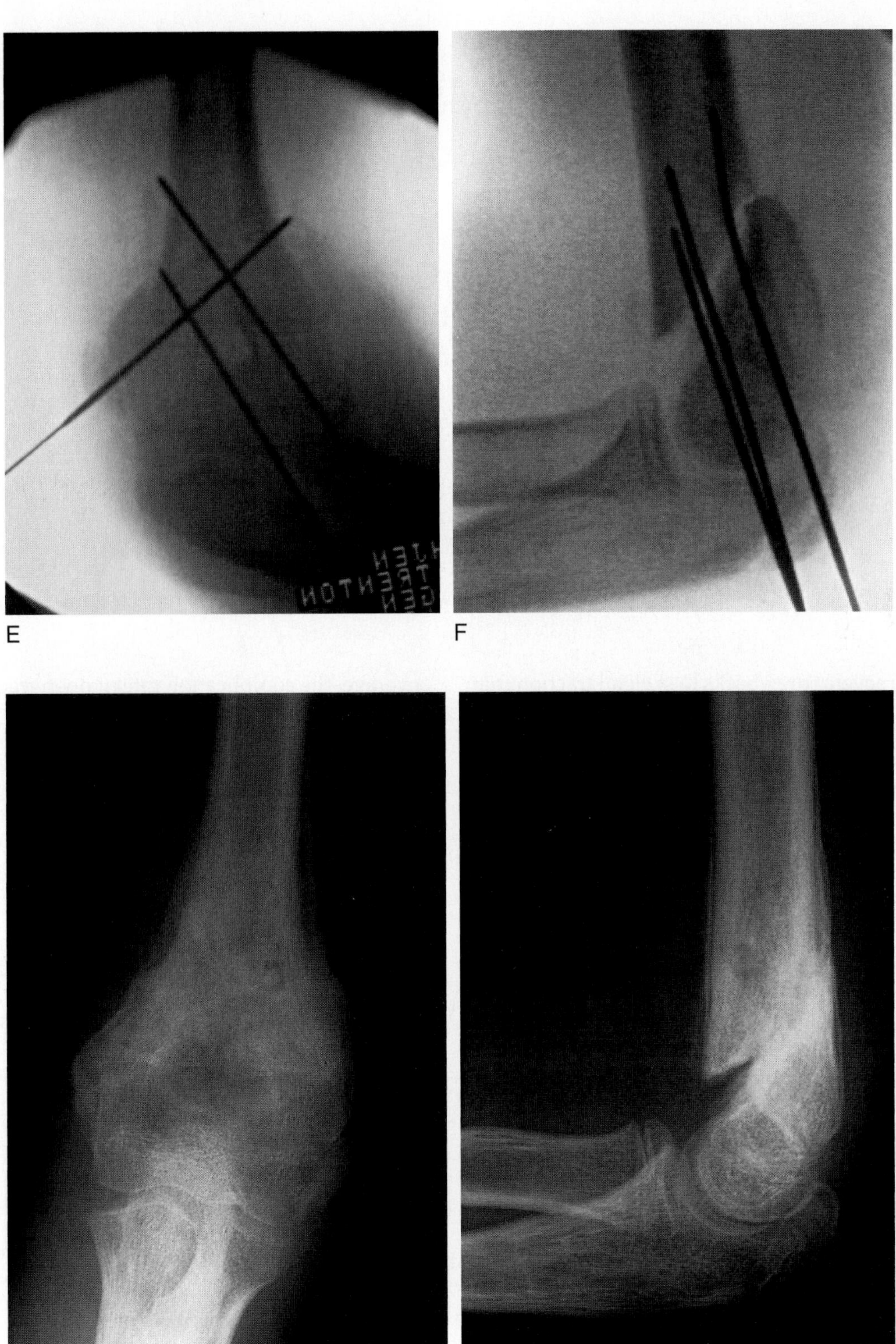

E F G H

FIGURE 42-54 cont'd **E** and **F,** Despite early callus formation, an attempt at closed osteoclasis was made. Note the improved alignment and addition of a medial pin. **G** and **H,** The fracture healed uneventfully.

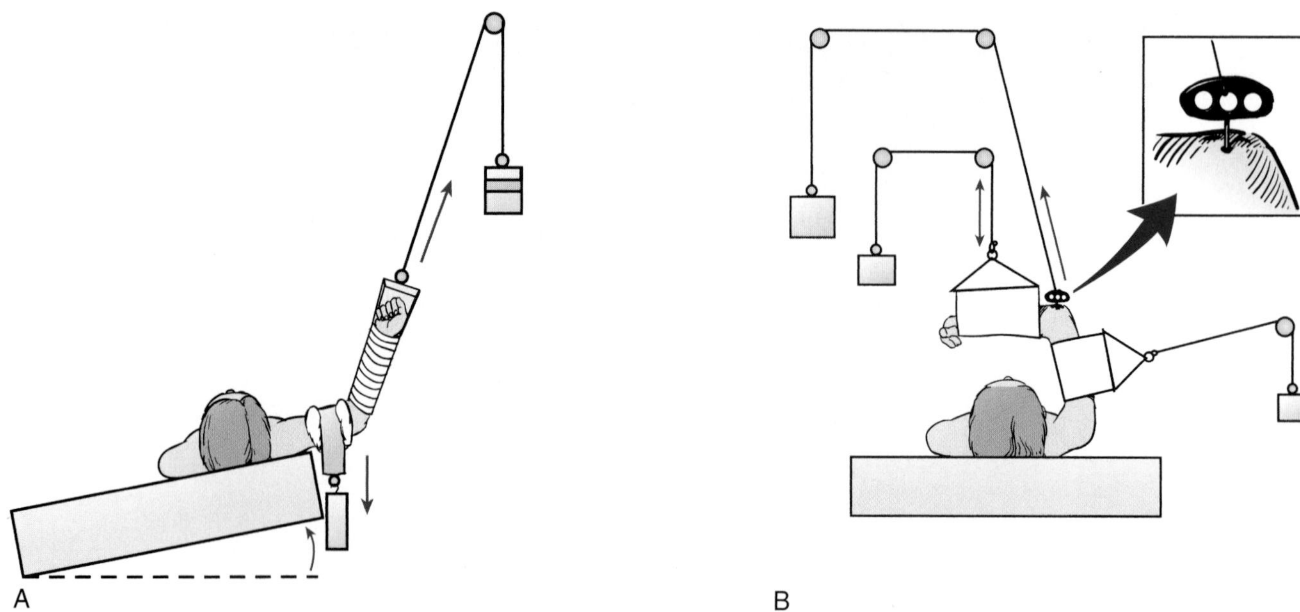

FIGURE 42-55 **A** and **B**, Historically, supracondylar fractures were treated by traction. Traction techniques are rarely used now.

There are several drawbacks to skeletal traction that have led to a steady decline in its use, including the need for prolonged hospitalization, relative discomfort for the child until the fracture becomes "sticky," pin inflammation and infection, the potential for loss of reduction, and the possible development of neurovascular complications, such as ulnar nerve injury from olecranon pins, compartment syndrome from excessive traction or circumferential bandages, and circulatory embarrassment from acute hyperflexion of the elbow while in traction.* We do not use traction in the management of supracondylar humeral fractures. Its use is described for historical completeness. It may have a role in the rare fracture that cannot be managed routinely because of extenuating circumstances.

Open Reduction. Indications for open reduction of a supracondylar humeral fracture include an ischemic, pale hand that does not revascularize with reduction of the fracture, an open fracture, an irreducible fracture, and inability to obtain a satisfactory closed reduction. If the hand remains ischemic after reduction of the fracture, the brachial artery should be immediately explored through an anterior approach. Once the arterial pathology (entrapment, laceration, or compression) has been identified, the fracture should be reduced and percutaneously pinned. If necessary, the arterial pathology can then be addressed.† Open fractures require emergency operative debridement. After debridement, the fracture can be reduced with an open technique and percutaneously pinned. With appropriate debridement, fracture stabilization, and antibiotic coverage, the complication rate of open fractures is not significantly different from that of severely displaced closed fractures.[23,213,227,602]

Supracondylar fractures may be irreducible if the distal aspect of the proximal fragment buttonholes through the brachialis muscle. This buttonholing often produces a characteristic puckering of the skin over the displaced proximal fragment. The presence of this pucker sign is not in itself an indication for open reduction because closed reduction may be successful. However, this sign should alert the surgeon to a potentially refractory fracture that may require open reduction.[122,145,158,436]

The decision that a closed reduction is unacceptable and an open reduction is indicated must be made on an individual basis. We accept mild angulation in the sagittal plane and translation in the coronal plane. A mild amount of valgus angulation in the coronal plane is also acceptable. However, varus angulation in the coronal plane, particularly if associated with either a small amount of hyperextension in the sagittal plane or a contralateral carrying angle that is neutral or varus, is likely to yield a cosmetically poor result that will not remodel (Fig. 42–56). If significant varus deformity exists after the best attempt at closed reduction, we proceed to open reduction. We usually approach the elbow from the side opposite the displaced distal fragment. This allows any interposed soft tissue to be removed from the fracture site. Once reduced with an open technique, the fracture is stabilized with percutaneous pins.

CONTROVERSIES IN TREATMENT

Management of Minimally Displaced Fractures

There is debate regarding the necessity of closed reduction and pinning for all displaced supracondylar

*See references 26, 44, 110, 141, 206, 215, 218, 307, 379, 395, 421, 446, 521, 525, 526, 540, 541, 587.

†See references 19, 72, 99, 132, 158, 310, 324, 394, 503, 576, 579, 587, 596, 602.

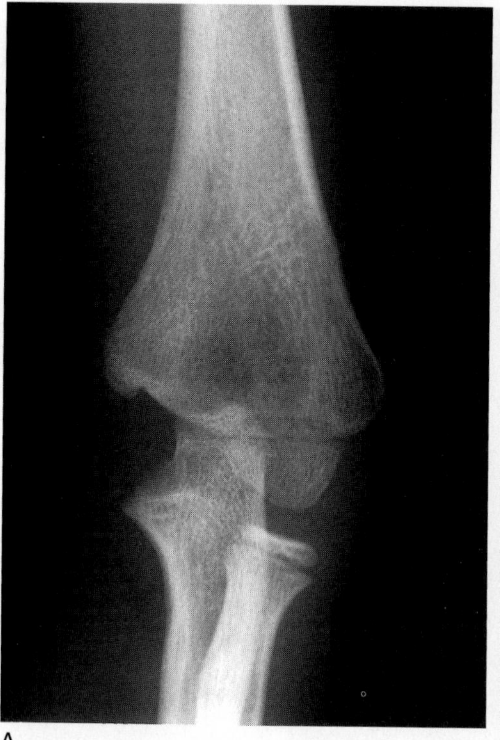
A

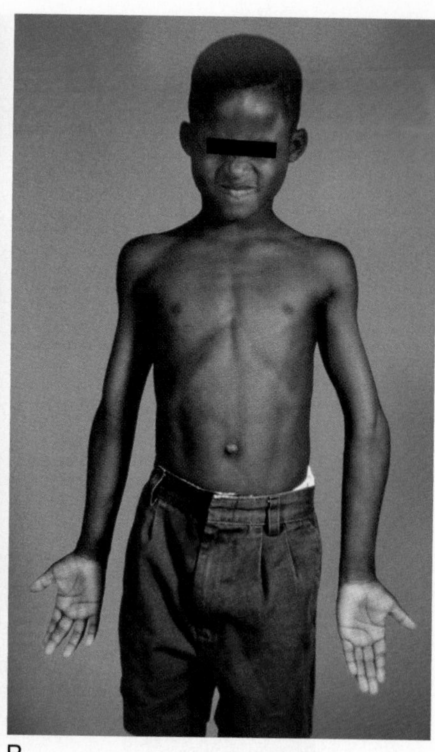
B

FIGURE 42–56
A, Anteroposterior radiograph of varus malunion. **B,** Clinical appearance.

fractures, particularly minimally displaced type IB or II fractures. A number of studies report good results with closed reduction and casting of displaced fractures.[26,215,227,421] However, other studies note superior results with closed reduction and pinning.[1,18,87,369,379,436,587] Although we recognize that some minimally displaced fractures may be managed successfully without pin fixation, we believe that there are several potential hazards with cast management of minimally displaced supracondylar fractures. Type IB fractures with medial column collapse or comminution are difficult, for two reasons. First, they may be more unstable than appreciated on initial radiographs (Fig. 42–57). If treated by simple immobilization, these occultly unstable fractures are likely to displace into varus and hyperextension and lead to malunion and a cosmetically unacceptable result. Second, even if the fracture is stable, collapse of the medial column may produce enough varus and hyperextension to produce a poor result if the fracture is not reduced.[117,396]

There are also two potential problems with closed reduction and cast management of type II fractures. The first is loss of reduction, and the second is increased swelling and the potential development of compartment syndrome secondary to immobilization with the elbow in flexion. The difficulty with cast management of minimally displaced fractures is demonstrated in the study of Hadlow and colleagues.[215] They reported good results in 37 of 48 type II fractures managed by closed reduction and casting without pin fixation. They concluded that pin fixation of *all* type II fractures would result in "unnecessary" pinning 77% of the time. However, they failed to acknowledge that cast treatment produces an unacceptable result in the remaining 23% of cases. Obviously, the problem is correctly identifying which fractures are at risk for malunion. To our knowledge there are no reliable predictors of malunion, and many studies have reported superior results with percutaneous pinning of displaced supracondylar fractures.[117,396,446] Therefore, we prefer closed reduction and pinning for all type IB and type II supracondylar humeral fractures. Although this aggressive management may lead to a few "unnecessary" pinnings, we believe that it also results in the fewest complications.

Timing of Reduction for Type III Fractures

Although there is growing agreement that pin fixation yields the best results for type III fractures, there is some controversy regarding the timing of treatment. Traditionally, type III fractures were regarded as an orthopaedic emergency that had to be treated immediately. Recently, however, good results have been reported when type III fractures were treated on an urgent rather than emergency basis.[210,262,322,367] Those who advocate delayed treatment cite the advantages of an adequate NPO status and a more efficient operative setting.

Provided that the skin is intact and not tented, the swelling is minimal, and the neurovascular examination is normal, we will allow an 8- to 10-hour delay to avoid operating on these fractures in the middle of the night. Type III injuries that are treated in delayed fashion are splinted in extension, with care taken to ensure that the proximal fragment is not displacing the skin, and they are admitted for elevation and observation until definitive treatment. Patients in whom the skin is compromised, the swelling is severe,

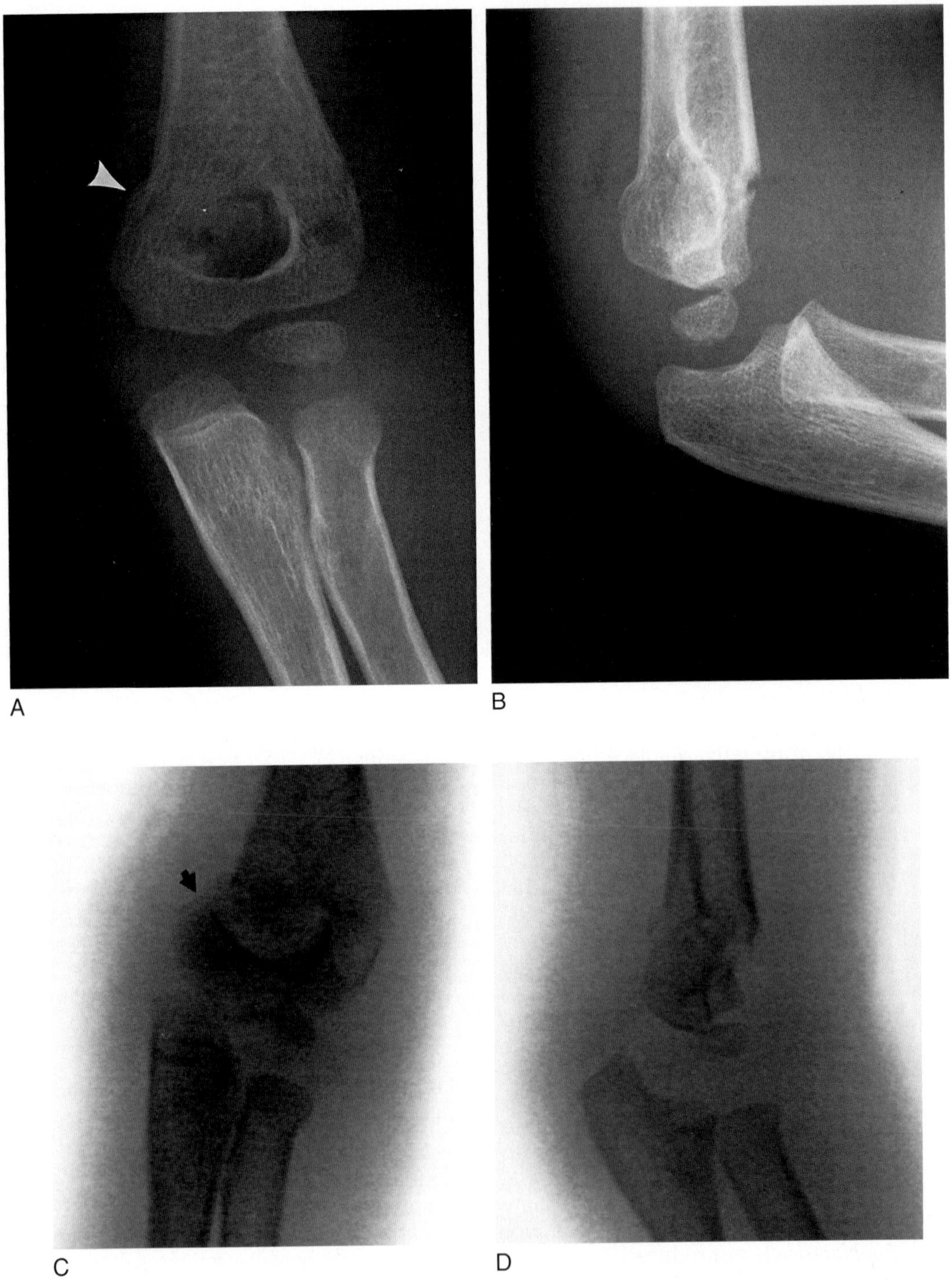

A

B

C

D

FIGURE 42–57 Unstable type IB supracondylar humeral fracture. Initial anteroposterior **(A)** and lateral **(B)** radiographs showing minimal medial comminution (*arrowhead*) and slight hyperextension. **C** and **D,** Intraoperative stress radiographs showing significant varus and hyperextension instability (*arrow*).

or the neurovascular examination is abnormal are treated by closed reduction and pinning on an emergency basis.

Pinning Technique and Iatrogenic Ulnar Nerve Injury

The technique of pin placement and management of iatrogenic ulnar nerve injury are also controversial topics. Although several biomechanical studies have shown that crossed pins are the most stable configuration, recent reports have shown good clinical results with parallel lateral pin fixation.* Though more stable, the crossed pin technique requires placement of a

*See references 20, 87, 119, 163, 193, 196, 278, 339, 396, 454, 501, 505, 517, 564, 602, 622.

medial pin, which may injure the ulnar nerve.* Skaggs and colleagues, in a review of 369 supracondylar fractures, reported that the incidence of ulnar nerve injury could be decreased from 15% to 2% by placing two lateral pins, followed by the selective use of medial pins only for fractures that remain unstable after placement of the lateral pins.[517] In this technique the lateral pins are placed in a parallel or divergent fashion to provide maximal rotational control. The arm is then extended and examined under fluoroscopy. If the fracture remains unstable, a third pin can be placed medially with the arm in extension (Fig. 42–58). This technique not only allows placement of the medial pin with the elbow in the safer extended position (see Fig. 42–53) but also provides a safety net of two lateral pins. If an iatrogenic ulnar nerve injury is noted postoperatively, the medial pin can be removed and two pins will still be present, usually providing adequate stability.

We use both the crossed pin and the double lateral–selective medial pin techniques. We believe that the most important factor in the pinning technique is not where the pins are inserted but where they cross the fracture site. Stability is increased by maximizing the distance between the pins at the fracture sites. This can be accomplished by dividing the fracture into thirds with the pins, regardless of whether pin placement is lateral or medial (see Fig. 42–51).

Treatment of iatrogenic ulnar nerve injury is also controversial. Although iatrogenic ulnar nerve injury almost always recovers, there are case reports of permanent injury.[87,255,278,454,476] Thus, we believe that an ulnar nerve palsy associated with a medial pin requires immediate treatment. Initially, we ensure that the elbow is immobilized in an extended position. Often the ulnar nerve is not directly injured by the K-wire but is stretched around the medial pin when the elbow is in a flexed position (see Fig. 42–53). If the elbow is adequately extended or if extension does not alleviate the ulnar nerve symptoms, we remove the medial pin immediately.

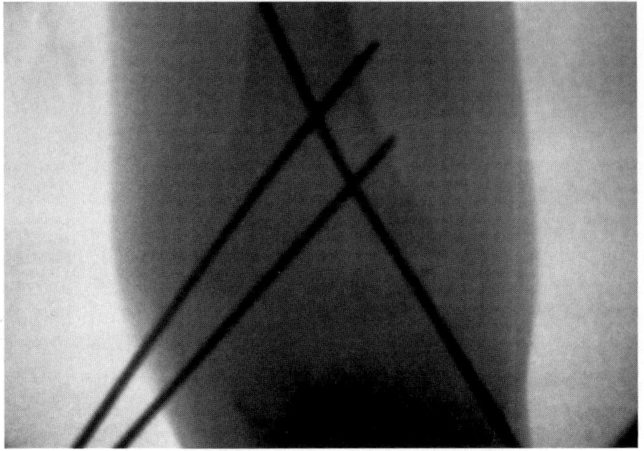

FIGURE 42–58 Anteroposterior radiograph showing a fracture pinned with two lateral pins, the selective medial pin technique.

*See references 196, 204, 255, 278, 339, 374, 454, 476, 505, 564.

Management of a Viable, Pulseless Hand

Controversy exists regarding the best management of a pulseless pink hand. The elbow's abundant collateral circulation allows the distal extremity to remain viable despite complete disruption of the brachial artery (Fig. 42–59). Recommendations for management of a viable but pulseless hand range from observation to arteriography to immediate surgical exploration.* Several groups have shown that the hand can remain viable and a radial pulse can even return after ligation of the brachial artery.[92,579] Nevertheless, some authors recommend aggressive surgical attempts to restore a normal pulse because of concern that conservative management of a pulseless, viable extremity could lead to progressive ischemia as a result of thrombus formation or future problems with cold intolerance, exercise claudication, or growth discrepancy.[64,173,350,441,500,503,507,602] Interestingly, although a number of papers discuss cold intolerance and exercise claudication, only Marck and colleagues actually described a patient with either of these symptoms.[350] They reported a patient who had normal function but cold intolerance 4 years after a supracondylar fracture associated with complete transection of the median nerve and brachial artery. The median nerve had been repaired but the artery was ligated because of good distal perfusion from collateral circulation. It is unclear whether the patient's symptoms (cold intolerance) were due to the vascular or the neurologic injury.

The study by Sabharwal and associates is unique in that the investigators attempted to determine the fate of vascular interventions with noninvasive vascular studies, including magnetic resonance angiography.[482] A normal pulse was restored in 13 patients with pulseless but viable extremities. Eleven of these patients underwent follow-up that included noninvasive vascular studies. Of these 11 patients, a normal pulse was restored by open reduction in 4, by urokinase therapy in 3, and by surgical reconstruction in 4. At follow-up, all patients were asymptomatic and had a normal radial pulse. Five had hypertrophic antecubital scars. Noninvasive vascular studies were normal in three of the four patients treated by open reduction and mobilization of an entrapped brachial artery and in two of the three patients treated with urokinase but in only one of the four patients treated by surgical reconstruction.[482]

Our approach to a viable hand with abnormal pulses is close observation. We believe that the lack of clinical studies documenting late problems, as well as the uncertain fate of aggressive surgical interventions, supports a conservative approach to these injuries. It is important to realize that unidentified vascular pathology can lead to thrombus formation and subsequently to an ischemic limb.[64,99,500,507] Thus, continued

*See references 64, 72, 99, 106, 132, 173, 227, 260, 324, 350, 394, 441, 474, 482, 500, 503, 507, 576, 579, 597, 602.

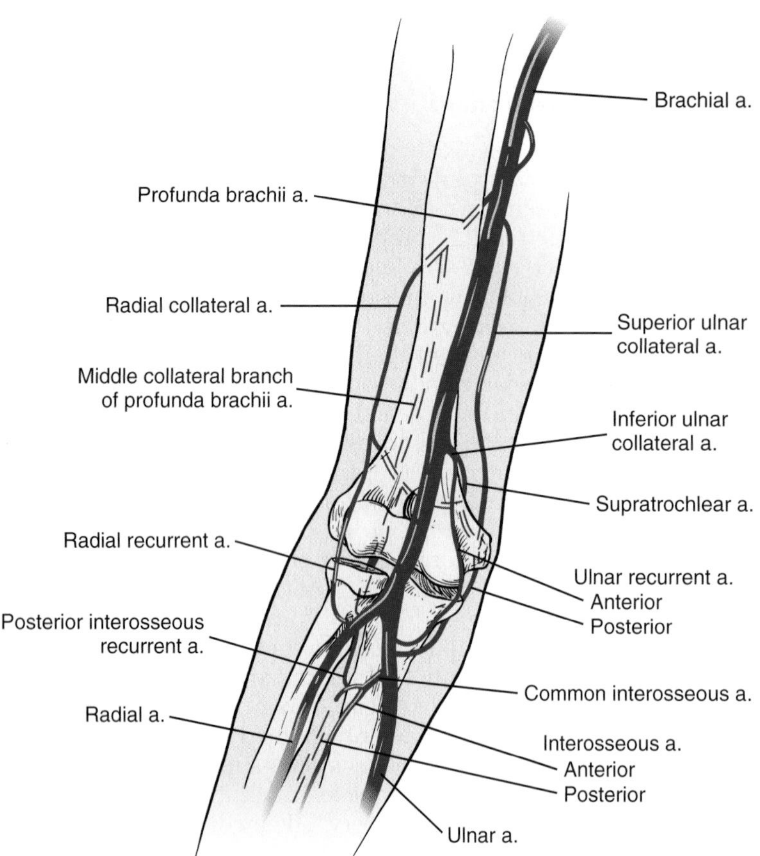

FIGURE 42–59 The collateral circulation around the elbow may provide adequate circulation to the forearm and hand despite complete disruption of the brachial artery.

close observation of these patients is of paramount importance. Though pulse oximetry is controversial, we have found it to be a valuable tool in monitoring these patients after closed reduction and pinning.[198,456,515] If a pulseless, viable limb becomes ischemic, arteriography and thrombolytic therapy may be useful adjuvants.[99,482]

Management of Late-Presenting or Malreduced Fractures

Appropriate management of a patient who is initially evaluated 1 to 2 weeks after injury and found to have a nonreduced or unacceptably reduced fracture is often difficult to determine. Obviously, the condition of the skin and neurovascular structures is an important factor to consider in determining treatment. Other factors include the age of the patient and the time since injury. Some surgeons advocate a "wait and see" approach to these fractures for the reason that attempts at manipulation once early callus begins to form may not improve the reduction and could risk increasing stiffness. This argument is strengthened by the knowledge that functional limitations are rare after nonunion. Others favor a more aggressive approach and attempt closed or even open reduction of these fractures. Unfortunately, there is little in the literature to guide the decision-making progress. Alburger and associates have shown that a 3- to 5-day delay before closed reduction and pinning is not deleterious.[12] Lal and Bhan reported good results in 20 children treated by open reduction 11 to 17 days after injury.[310] Vahvaven and Aalto performed routine remanipulation at 2 weeks for all redisplaced fractures, without adverse sequelae.[571] Devnani recommends gradual reduction with skin traction.[126]

We have had success with remanipulation of supracondylar fractures after delays of 2 to 3 weeks (Fig. 42–60). Management of these injuries must be determined on an individual basis and must take into account such factors as the patient's age, the condition of the soft tissue, the amount of residual deformity, and the degree of radiographic healing. It is important that treatment decisions regarding these malreductions be made with good information. Unfortunately, obtaining an adequate examination and radiographs in a young patient a few weeks after a displaced supracondylar fracture can be extremely difficult and may require examination under anesthesia. Although functional limitations are uncommon with malunion of supracondylar humeral fractures, these injuries have little potential to remodel. Even a small improvement in alignment may represent the difference between a cosmetically acceptable result and one that is unacceptable. If an attempt is made to improve the alignment of a supracondylar fracture in delayed fashion, an anatomic reduction may not be an achievable goal. In such a case we usually accept an adequate

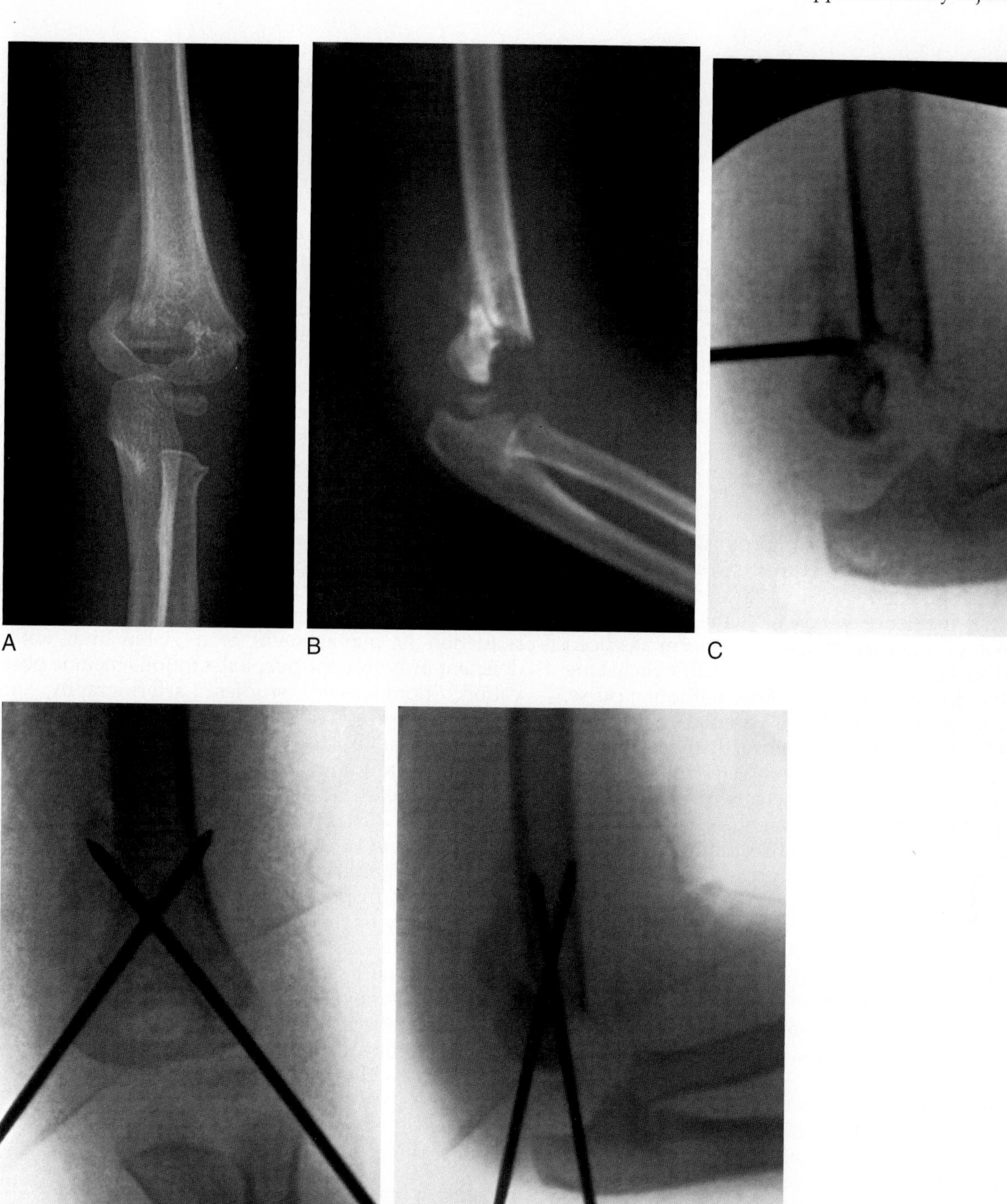

FIGURE 42-60 Anteroposterior (AP) **(A)** and lateral **(B)** radiographs of a type III supracondylar humeral fracture first seen 10 days after the injury. Despite radiographic evidence of early callus formation, closed reduction was attempted. **C,** Intraoperative radiograph showing percutaneous osteoclasis, which was necessary to improve the sagittal alignment. AP **(D)** and lateral **(E)** radiographs obtained after reduction and pinning.

nonanatomic reduction rather than proceed to open reduction.

COMPLICATIONS

The complications of supracondylar humeral fractures can be categorized as either early or late. Early complications include vascular injury, peripheral nerve palsies, and Volkmann's ischemia (compartment syndrome). Late complications include malunion, stiffness, and myositis ossificans. Although attention to detail at the time of initial treatment may limit the long-term sequelae of early complications and minimize late complications, the severity of the injury and the nature of the anatomy make problems from supracondylar fractures unavoidable.

Vascular Injury

The incidence of vascular compromise in type III extension supracondylar fractures has been reported to be between 2% and 38%.[72,86,99,106,132,250,335,336,394,417,474] The reported incidence varies with the definition of vascular compromise inasmuch as this term has been used to describe a wide variety of patients, including those with a diminished pulse, those without a pulse, or those with an ischemic limb. Vascular injury may be induced either directly or indirectly. Direct injury by the fracture may result in complete transection of the brachial artery, an intimal tear, or compression either between the fracture fragments or over the anteriorly displaced fragment.[528] Indirect injury is usually the result of compression. Compression can produce temporary ischemia that is reversible with reduction, reversible spasm, or permanent sequelae such as intimal tears, aneurysms, or thrombosis.[106] If the level of vascular injury, whether produced directly or indirectly, is distal to the inferior ulnar collateral artery, the rich collateral circulation about the elbow will generally provide adequate blood supply to the forearm and hand (see Fig. 42–59).

Management of acute vascular injury associated with supracondylar fractures of the humerus is controversial and must be individualized. The initial treatment consists of a thorough assessment of the skin and neurologic status, as well as evaluation for other injuries. If the hand is obviously ischemic, the arm should be immediately manipulated into an extended position. Often this instantly restores circulation to the hand (see Fig. 42–47). If improving the alignment fails to provide distal circulation, the child should be immediately taken to the operating room for closed reduction and pinning.

We do not believe that arteriography is warranted before an operative attempt at closed reduction, for two reasons. First, reduction of the fracture frequently restores the circulation. Second, even if the limb remains ischemic after reduction, the location of the arterial pathology is known. Thus, an arteriogram provides little information that will alter the clinical management but can significantly prolong the ischemic time. Similarly, we do not generally obtain preoperative vascular or microsurgical consultation because the ischemia frequently resolves with reduction. If the limb remains ischemic, exposure of the brachial vessels can be performed while awaiting the arrival of a vascular surgeon or microsurgeon. If on exploration the artery is found to be trapped within the fracture fragments, the pins can be removed, the artery liberated, the fracture repinned, and circulation of the limb reassessed. Spasm and intimal lesions of the brachial artery may require arteriography for complete assessment, which can usually be performed with little difficulty intraoperatively with the use of standard fluoroscopy. Spasm may be relieved with a stellate ganglion block or local application of papaverine, or resection and reverse interpositional vein grafting may be required. These decisions are generally made in conjunction with a vascular surgeon or microsurgeon. It is important to remember to perform fasciotomies if there has been significant ischemic time or there is any concern regarding elevated compartment pressure.

As previously discussed, management of a limb that is initially ischemic but becomes viable with reduction or management of a viable limb with a deficient pulse is controversial. Options include observation, noninvasive studies, arteriography, and exploration.* We favor a conservative approach with close observation. Although a pulse difference is relatively common and frequently inconsequential, it may be the earliest sign of a potentially devastating complication. Arterial spasm or compression initially producing only a diminished pulse can progress to complete thrombosis, ischemia, and potentially, compartment syndrome. Although we do not routinely use arteriography in the initial management of supracondylar fractures with a vascular injury, the review by Sabharwal and associates points out the potential benefit of arteriography in a patient with a deteriorating examination; such interventional radiographic techniques may allow effective treatment of spasm or thrombosis without surgical exploration.[482]

Peripheral Nerve Injury

Peripheral nerve injury occurs in approximately 10% to 15% of supracondylar humeral fractures.† There is a growing consensus that the anterior interosseous nerve is the most commonly injured nerve with extension-type supracondylar fractures, although the median, radial, and ulnar nerves all may be damaged.[105,132,191,535,602] Anterior interosseous nerve palsy is probably under-reported because it is not associated with sensory loss. Median nerve injury has been reported more commonly with posterolaterally displaced fractures, and radial nerve injury with posteromedial displacement. Although ulnar nerve injury

*See references 12, 72, 92, 99, 132, 324, 347, 482, 503, 528, 569, 576, 579, 587, 602.

†See references 28, 86, 105, 132, 197, 272, 284, 286, 335, 336, 528, 536, 551, 602.

may occur as a consequence of the fracture, the ulnar nerve is more frequently injured iatrogenically from a medial pin.[65,87,132,255,360,374,454,476,564]

Perhaps the single most important and often the most difficult aspect of managing peripheral nerve injuries associated with supracondylar humeral fractures is the challenge of reaching an accurate and timely diagnosis. Unfortunately, it is often impossible to perform an adequate neurologic examination in a young child with a supracondylar humeral fracture in the emergency department. Thus, it is imperative to counsel the parents that as time progresses, there is a chance that a nerve injury will be discovered. Fortunately, the parents can be reassured that nearly all such injuries will spontaneously improve. Because peripheral nerve palsies can be expected to recover spontaneously, little treatment is required other than close monitoring for recovery and perhaps splinting or range-of-motion exercises, or both, to ensure that a fixed contracture does not develop. Although most peripheral nerve injuries recover fully, there are numerous reports of those that do not.* Thus, if within 8 to 12 weeks function is not returning, consideration should be given to performing nerve conduction and electromyographic studies to ensure that the nerve has not been transected. If a peripheral nerve is found to be transected, appropriate reanastomosis with grafting or tendon transfers should be undertaken.

Volkmann's Ischemic Contracture (Compartment Syndrome)

In 1881, Richard von Volkmann described ischemic paralysis and contracture of the muscles of the forearm and hand and, less frequently, the leg after the application of taut bandages in the treatment of injuries occurring in the region of the elbow and knee. He suggested that the pathologic changes primarily resulted from obstruction of arterial blood flow, which if unrelieved would result in death of the muscles.[583] Fortunately, with improved management of elbow fractures in children, the incidence of Volkmann's ischemic contracture after supracondylar humeral fractures is decreasing.[34,51,99,142,372] Patients with floating elbows may be at increased risk for compartment syndrome and should be monitored appropriately.[462] This potentially devastating "complication" may be better described as a "consequence" of a high-energy injury and may develop despite appropriate care.[39]

The pathophysiology, diagnosis, and management of compartment syndrome are discussed in Chapter 40, General Principles of Managing Orthopaedic Injuries. A supracondylar fracture associated with a compartment syndrome is generally best managed by closed reduction and pinning. After decompression of a compartment syndrome, proper splinting and active and passive range-of-motion exercises for the extremity are essential to maintain joint mobility until function returns.

*See references 65, 72, 87, 105, 132, 255, 259, 260, 360, 442, 454, 476, 483, 602.

Malunion: Cubitus Varus and Cubitus Valgus

Cubitus varus and cubitus valgus are the most common complications of supracondylar humeral fractures. The reported incidence ranges from 0% to 50%.* In general, posteromedially displaced fractures tend to develop varus angulation, and posterolaterally displaced fractures tend to develop valgus deviation. Cubitus varus deformity is more commonly noted to be a problem than cubitus valgus, probably because posteromedial fractures are more common. However, varus deformity may be more frequently reported simply because it is more cosmetically noticeable. Although some authors have suggested that angular deformity is a result of growth imbalance,[259] the consensus opinion is that cubitus varus and valgus are the result of malunion (Fig. 42–61).†

Cubitus varus or valgus is assessed by measuring the carrying angle of the arm. The carrying angle is the angle created by the medial border of the fully supinated forearm and the medial border of the humerus with the elbow extended (Fig. 42–62). The carrying angle exhibits considerable individual variation.[38,524] Thus, comparison should be made with the contralateral side rather than with any "normal standard." As the elbow extends, the carrying angle decreases (more varus); thus, hyperextension tends to accentuate a cubitus varus deformity, whereas a flexion contracture can create the appearance of cubitus valgus. Smith has demonstrated that changes in the carrying angle are a result of angular displacement or tilting of the distal fragment, not translation or rotation.[524] However, rotation of the distal fragment can contribute to the cosmetic deformity of a malunion.[460] In fact, a residual rotational deformity is nearly always present after corrective osteotomies for cubitus varus (Fig. 42–63).

Problems arising from cubitus varus or valgus include functional limitation, recurrent elbow fracture, and cosmetic deformity. Fortunately, functional problems are uncommon with either deformity. In cubitus valgus, functional problems may be related either to a coexisting flexion contracture or, in extreme cases, to tardy ulnar nerve symptoms.[116,235,243,315,600] With cubitus varus, functional problems are almost always related to limitation of flexion, although tardy ulnar nerve palsy and elbow instability have also been reported as functional complications of varus deformity.[176,327,389] The limitation in flexion is a result of the hyperextension associated with varus malunion. Usually the arc of elbow motion remains constant. Thus, varus/hyperextension malunion creates a flexion deficit. If significant, this flexion deficit can interfere with activities of daily living.[570,616] Lateral condyle fractures, distal humeral epiphyseal separation, and shoulder instability have also been described as potential complications of varus malunion.[113,211,554] Davids and colleagues have shown that the torsional moment and

*See references 8, 20, 26, 29, 43, 61, 87, 235, 243, 251, 259, 342, 400, 446, 460, 516, 524, 564, 571, 596, 600, 602, 616.
†See references 20, 26, 87, 400, 446, 516, 524, 572, 596, 600, 602.

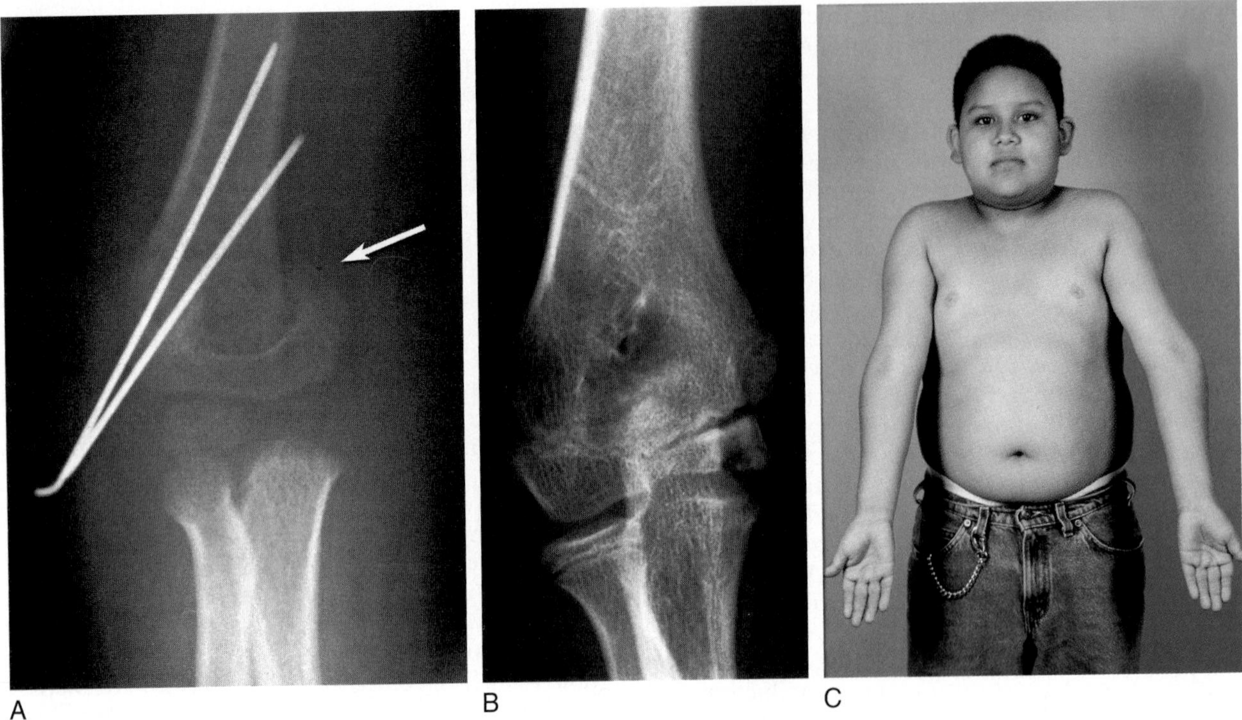

FIGURE 42–61 Malunion producing cubitus varus. **A,** The fracture has been reduced and pinned in varus. Note the shortening of the medial column (*arrow*). **B,** Varus malalignment persists 6 years after injury. **C,** Clinical appearance.

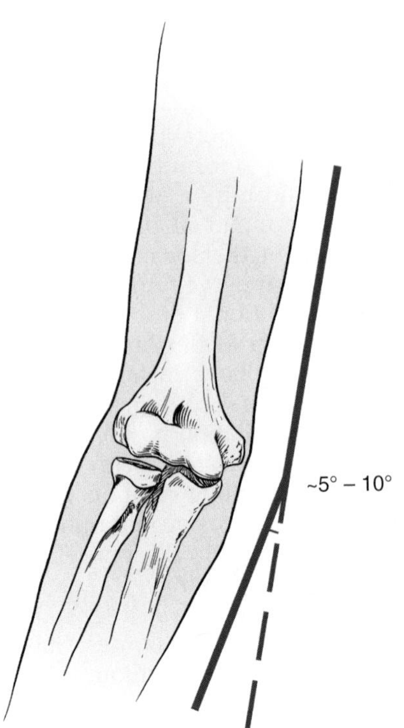

FIGURE 42–62 The carrying angle is the angle defined by the border of the fully supinated forearm and the long axis of the humerus when the elbow is fully extended.

shear force generated across the capitellar physis by a routine fall are increased by varus malalignment.[113] However, cosmetic deformity is by far the most common problem associated with malunion of supracondylar fractures.

Unfortunately, because of the limited growth and the fact that deformity is most commonly perpendicular to the plane of motion, there is little potential for angular malunion of the distal humerus to remodel; therefore, the best treatment of malunion of a supracondylar humeral fracture is avoidance.[306] Awareness of the pitfalls associated with obtaining and maintaining adequate reduction will aid the orthopaedist in minimizing both the occurrence of malunion and the degree of deformity when it does occur. Because both cubitus valgus and varus are primarily cosmetic deformities, mild degrees of malunion can be treated by simple reassurance. However, if the deformity is severe, cosmetic concerns or, less commonly, functional limitations may warrant surgical reconstruction. The reported complication rate with corrective osteotomy is between 30% and 50%; thus, it is important to explain to the parents that surgical reconstruction is a technically demanding procedure with no well-defined indications other than unacceptable cosmesis.[2,26,30,57,123,177,237,328,354,385,389,415,570,584,600]

Loss of fixation and persistent deformity are the most common complications after corrective supracon-

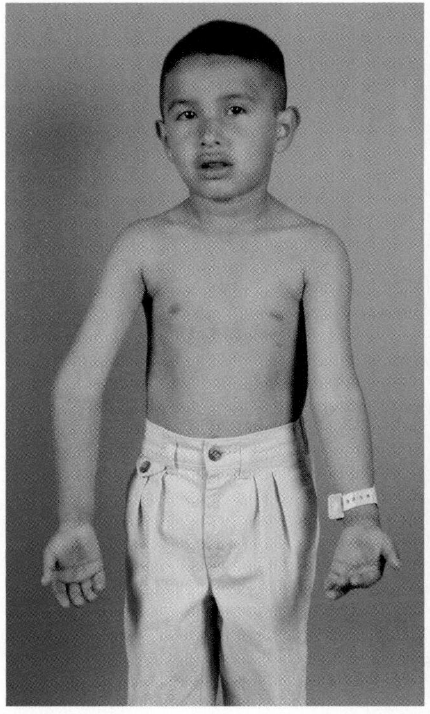
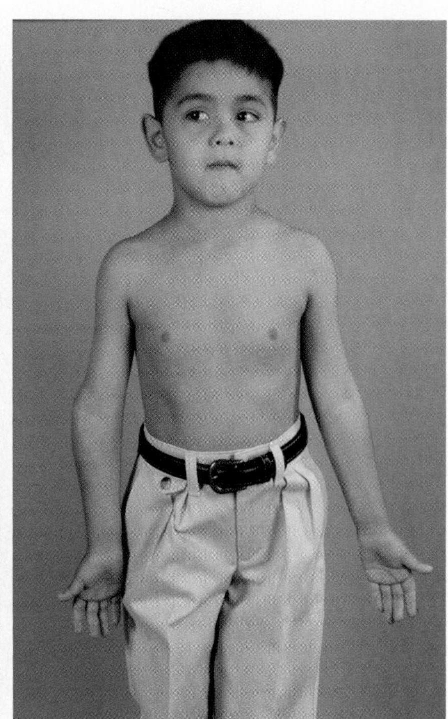

FIGURE 42-63 Persistent rotational deformity. **A,** Preoperative clinical appearance. Note the significant cubitus varus. **B,** Postoperatively, the carrying angle is improved. However, there is still a significant rotational deformity on the lateral aspect of the distal end of the humerus.

dylar osteotomy.* In an effort to limit these complications, a wide variety of osteotomy and fixation techniques have been described. Osteotomy techniques include medial or lateral closing wedge, step-cut, and dome osteotomies. Fixation has been described with crossed pins, staples, screws, screws and tension wires, plates and pins, and external fixation.† In selecting which of these techniques to use, it is important to consider the patient and the individual deformity. Most patients have a complex three-dimensional deformity that includes a significant component of rotational malunion of the distal fragment. Hyperextension in the sagittal plane is also frequently present. In our experience, the distal rotational deformity is not correctable with any of the described techniques. The sagittal plane deformity may be corrected; however, flexion of the distal fragment makes the osteotomy significantly less stable and increases demands on the fixation. We most commonly use a lateral closing wedge osteotomy with single-plane correction and crossed pin fixation (Fig. 42–64). This technique is usually performed through a lateral incision and has the advantage of being stable and technically simple. It is important to note, as well as forewarn the parents, that this technique may actually increase the prominence of the lateral condyle, which may create the appearance of persistent cubitus varus (Fig. 42–65). We have also used a medial opening wedge osteotomy with external fixation and no bone graft (Fig. 42–66).[300,588] This technique affords a more cosmetic medial incision and fixation that is stable enough to allow sagittal plane correction. Another advantage of this technique is that the alignment can be manipulated after the wound is closed. We have found this technique particularly helpful in patients with significant hyperextension deformity (Fig. 42–67).

*See references 2, 26, 30, 57, 123, 177, 237, 328, 354, 385, 389, 415, 570, 584, 600.

†See references 30, 42, 55, 57, 90, 123, 125, 177, 211, 237, 238, 249, 253, 280, 285, 297-300, 305, 308, 328, 354, 385, 389, 399,409, 415, 460, 489, 559, 570, 584, 588, 600.

Elbow Stiffness and Myositis Ossificans

These complications of supracondylar humeral fractures occur rarely.[8,104,110,227,259,310,596] We usually assess elbow range of motion 6 to 8 weeks after the cast has been removed. It is extremely unusual to identify more than a 10- to 15-degree difference in flexion or extension at this point. However, if significant stiffness is present, we begin a supervised home program of gentle range-of-motion exercises and continue to monitor the patient's progress on a monthly basis. Mild stiffness generally resolves with a few months of gentle therapy, although some patients need more intensive therapy, including a splinting program. Persistent stiffness requiring surgical release is extremely uncommon. Mih and associates reported an average 53-degree increase in range of motion in nine pediatric patients who underwent capsular release through a lateral and, if necessary, medial approach.[375,424]

Myositis ossificans is an extremely unusual complication that has been noted to resolve spontaneously over a period of 1 to 2 years (Fig. 42–68).

Transphyseal Fractures

Transphyseal fractures are most common in children younger than 2 years. They have been reported to

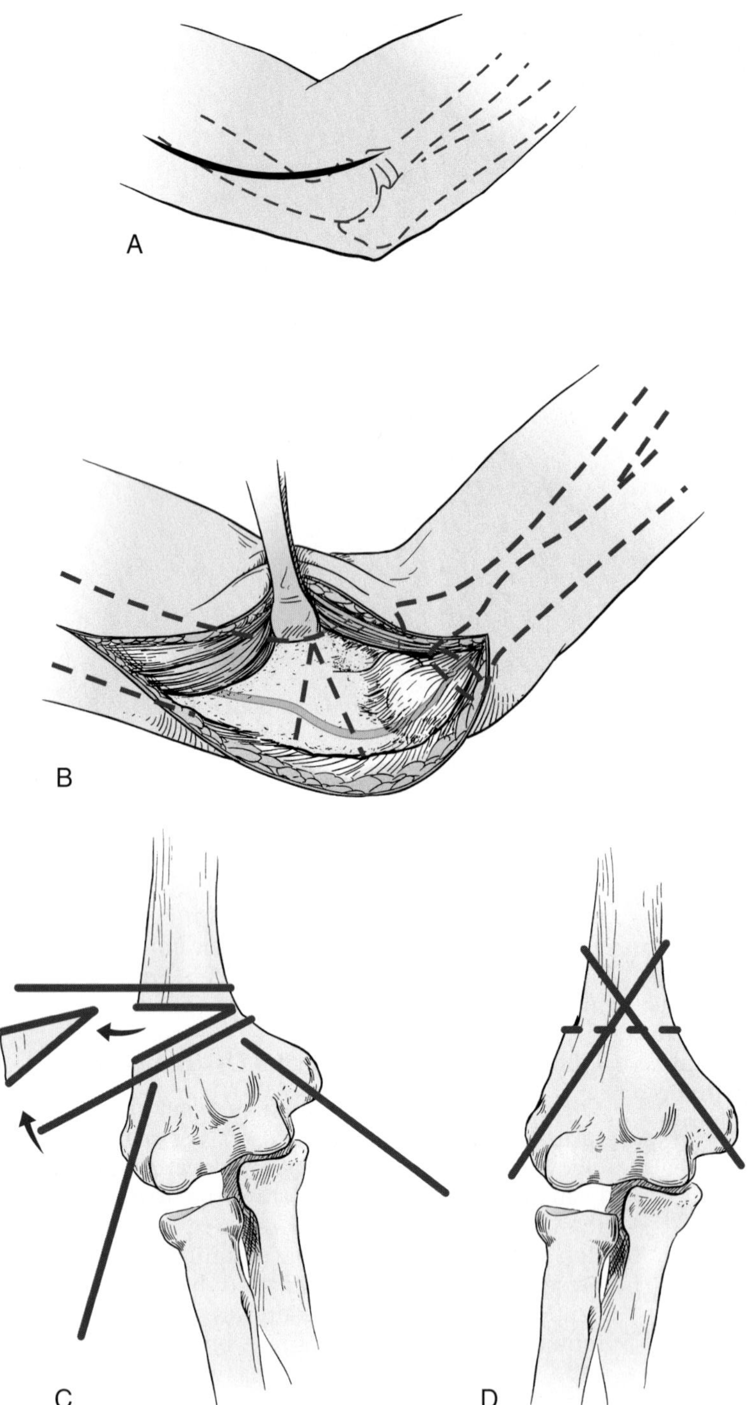

FIGURE 42-64 Technique for lateral closing wedge osteotomy for correction of post-traumatic cubitus varus. **A,** Skin incision. It is helpful to have the uninjured arm exposed in the anatomic position for intraoperative comparison. **B,** The lateral distal aspect of the humerus is approached between the triceps and the common extensor origin. Care must be taken to avoid injury to the radial nerve with proximal exposure. Osteotomy sites are planned parallel to the joint and perpendicular to the humeral shaft. **C,** Medial and lateral pins are introduced before performing the osteotomies. A lateral wedge of bone is then removed. An attempt is made to preserve the medial cortex. **D,** The osteotomy site is closed and the pins are advanced into the proximal fragment.

result from abuse in up to 50% of children younger than 2 years of age.[10,121,370,403] In children of this age, the distal humerus is either entirely cartilaginous or nearly so, thus making interpretation of radiographs difficult and making diagnosis the most difficult aspect of this fracture.

ANATOMY

The anatomic considerations for distal humeral transphyseal fractures are the same as those for supracondylar fractures of the distal humerus. The young age and consequently small anatomy of the children who typically sustain these injuries may make diagnosis and treatment difficult. Interestingly, although transphyseal fractures share the same important anatomic considerations as supracondylar fractures, neurovascular complications are rarely reported with this injury.[2,118,121,244,361]

MECHANISM OF INJURY

The mechanism of injury depends on the age of the patient. In newborns and infants, there is usually a

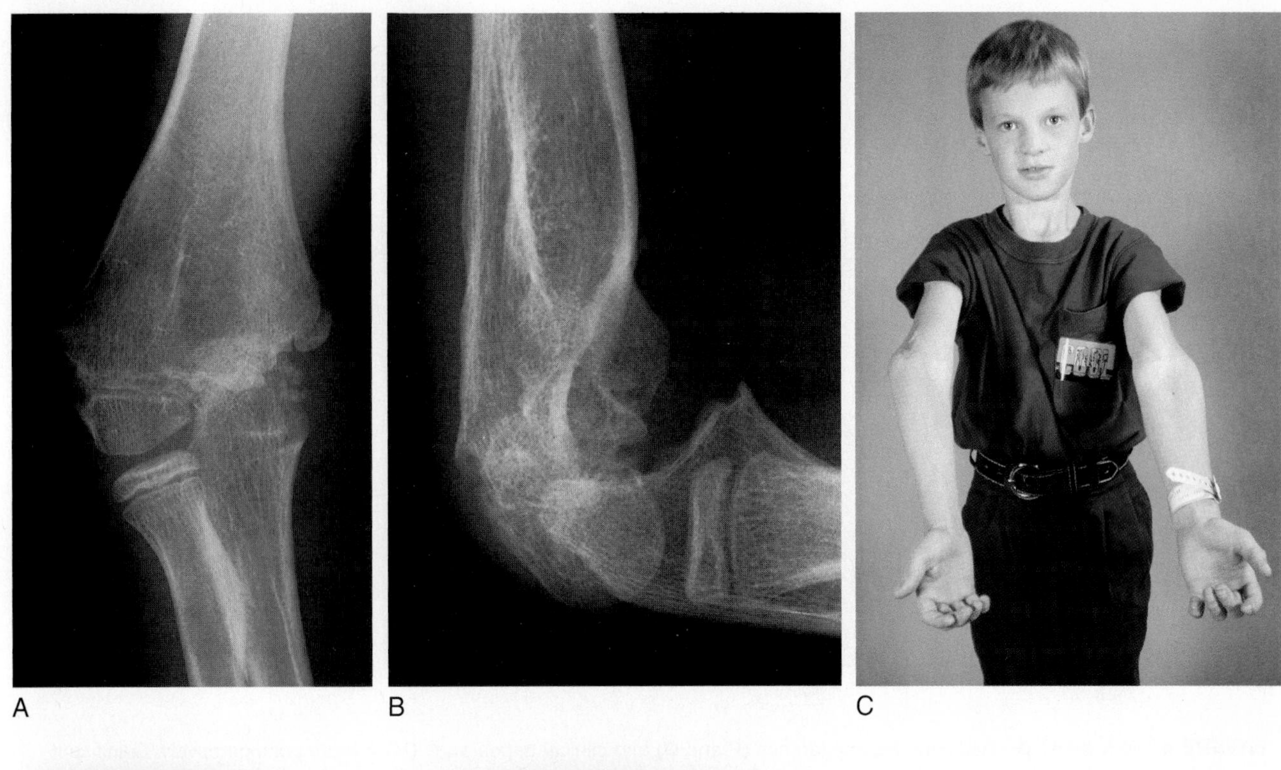

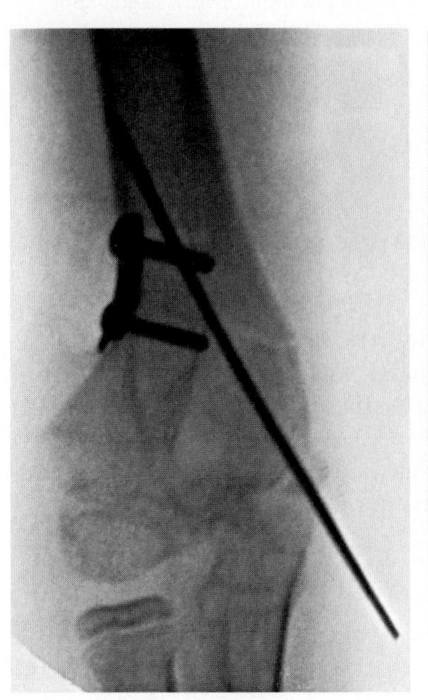

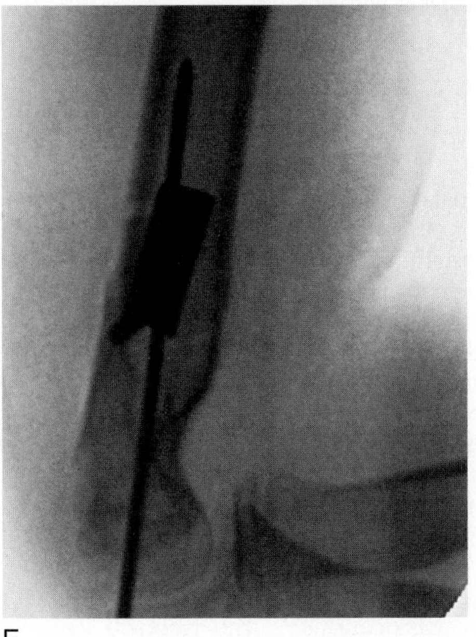

FIGURE 42-65 Example of lateral closing wedge osteotomy for cubitus varus. Varus malunion: anteroposterior **(A)** and lateral **(B)** radiographs and clinical appearance **(C)**. **D** and **E**, Intraoperative radiographs obtained after lateral closing wedge osteotomy. (A medial pin and lateral plate were used rather than crossed pins.) Note the prominence of the lateral condyle.

rotary or shear force associated with birth trauma or child abuse.[10,31,53,78,84,121,356,420,497,508] In older children the mechanism is most commonly a hyperextension force from a fall on an outstretched hand.

CLASSIFICATION

Although classification schemes for transphyseal separations exist, they are not clinically necessary. DeLee and colleagues separated transphyseal fractures into three groups based on their radiographic appearance.[121] Their criteria included the presence or absence of the secondary ossification center of the radial head and the presence and size of the metaphyseal fragment (Thurston-Holland sign). These radiographic parameters correspond to the age of the patient but add little to clinical management.[361] These fractures may also be classified according to the Salter-Harris classification of physeal injuries.[486] In infants these injuries are most commonly Salter-Harris type I fractures. In older children they are usually type II injuries.

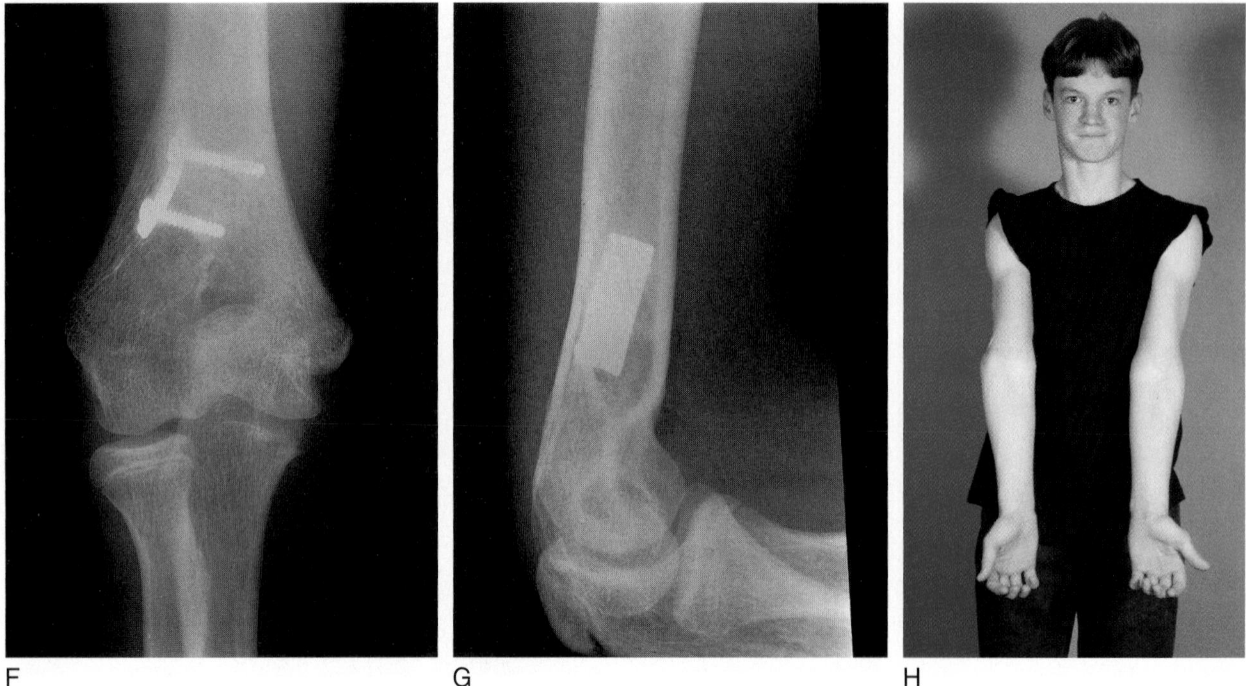

FIGURE 42-65 cont'd Radiographic appearance (**F** and **G**) and clinical appearance (**H**) 4 years postoperatively. Significant remodeling has occurred, and the clinical appearance has improved.

DIAGNOSIS

The most difficult aspect of the diagnosis is distinguishing a transphyseal fracture from an elbow dislocation. Other injuries in the differential include lateral condylar and supracondylar fractures. The key to distinguishing transphyseal separation from true elbow dislocation is the radial head–capitellum relationship.[479] In an elbow dislocation, the radial head does not articulate with the capitellum; however, in a transphyseal fracture, the radial head and capitellum remain congruous (Fig. 42–69A). In a very young patient the capitellum may not be ossified, which makes such distinction difficult if not impossible.[10,53,469,530] In such cases the correct diagnosis can be made with a high degree of suspicion and the knowledge that physeal separations are more common than elbow dislocations in this age group.[121] It may also be difficult to distinguish transphyseal separations from lateral condyle fractures that extend medial to the trochlear notch and consequently produce subluxation of the ulnohumeral joint (Milch type II fractures) (see Fig. 42–40). In both these injuries the radial head–capitellum relationship remains normal. Although oblique radiographs may assist in delineating these details, the distinction may require evaluation with arthrography or MRI in a small child with little ossification of the distal humeral epiphysis.[10,207,221,386,450,479] Supracondylar fractures usually occur at the level of the olecranon fossa, whereas transphyseal separations are more distal (see Fig. 42–40).

RADIOGRAPHIC FINDINGS

As with supracondylar fractures, obtaining good-quality radiographs of transphyseal separations is imperative, but often difficult. Even under the best of circumstances, further evaluation may be required. Ultrasound, MRI, and arthrography have all been used in the evaluation of transphyseal separations.[10,53,129,386,403,420,479,618] Of these modalities, we have the most experience with arthrography because it can be performed at the time of definitive therapy.

TREATMENT

The goal of treatment of transphyseal fractures is to achieve acceptable reduction and maintain it until the fracture unites, usually in 2 to 3 weeks. Some authors have advocated simple splint immobilization for transphyseal separations.[31,121,361,420] However, a number of investigators, including some of those who advocate cast treatment, have reported cubitus varus after simple immobilization of transphyseal fractures.[2,118,121,244] DeLee and associates noted that 3 of 12 patients, all younger than 2 years, had significant varus after closed treatment. Abe and colleagues noted varus in 15 of 21 patients,[2] and Holda and colleagues in 5 of 7.[244] Our experience has paralleled that of authors who have reported significant cubitus varus after cast immobilization, particularly in patients younger than 2 years (see Fig. 42–69). Consequently, we favor closed reduction and pin fixation for most patients with

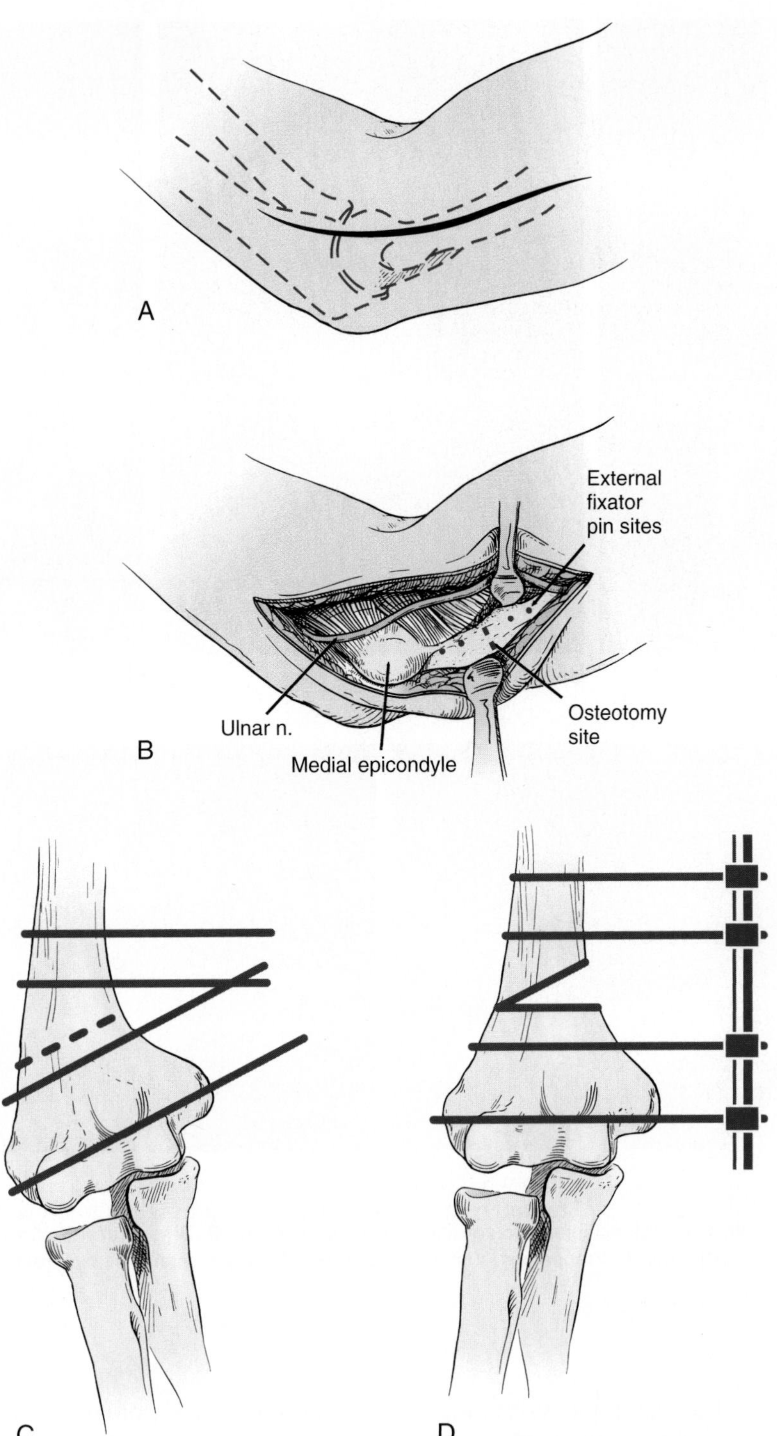

FIGURE 42–66 Technique for medial opening wedge osteotomy with external fixation. **A,** Skin incision. It is helpful to have the uninjured arm exposed in the anatomic position for intraoperative comparison. **B,** The ulnar nerve is dissected and transposed anteriorly. The medial humerus is exposed along the intramuscular septum. **C,** Pins are introduced proximally perpendicular to the humeral shaft. Distally, the pins are placed parallel to the joint and extend to the level of the medial epicondyle. The osteotomy can be made parallel to either group of pins. **D,** After completion of the osteotomy, the deformity is corrected in both planes and the correction is secured with the external fixator. The pins are brought out through the wound. The ulnar nerve is transposed into the flexor origin. Care should be taken to ensure that the ulnar nerve does not contact the proximal pins.

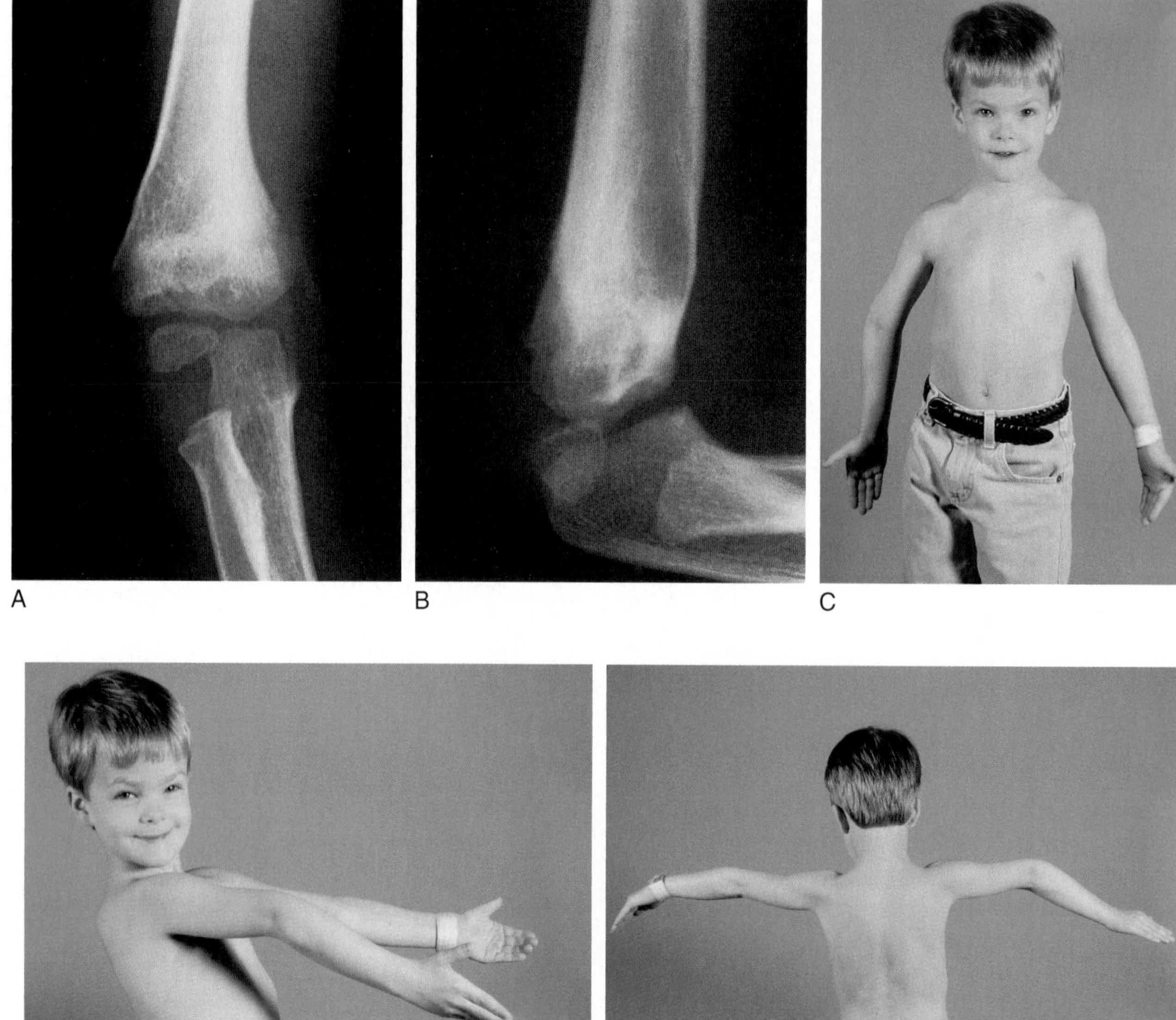

FIGURE 42–67 Medial opening wedge osteotomy to correct cubitus varus. **A** and **B**, Preoperative radiographs showing varus malunion with hyperextension. **C** through **E**, Preoperative clinical appearance. Note the significant hyperextension component of the deformity.

transphyseal separations. The technique for reduction and pinning is identical to that for supracondylar fractures (see Fig. 42–49). We have found arthrography helpful in delineating the pathology, and we do not hesitate to perform arthrography after pin fixation or, if necessary for diagnostic purposes, before reduction and pinning (Fig. 42–70). After reduction and pinning the arm is immobilized in relative extension for 2 to 3 weeks, at which time the cast and pins are discontinued.

COMPLICATIONS

In older children the mechanism of transphyseal separation is the same as for supracondylar fractures. Not surprisingly, the potential complications are similar, although neurovascular injuries are less common. In infants, this injury is most frequently the result of a rotary or shear force applied by an adult. Thus, the most devastating potential complication of transphyseal separation is failure to recognize the possibility of child abuse and to return a child to a dangerous environment. The reinjury rate of abused children is between 30% and 50%, and the risk of death is 5% to 10%.[9,49,181]

The most significant and frequent orthopaedic complication of transphyseal separation is cubitus varus.[2,118,121,244,600] Management of varus deformity after a transphyseal fracture is similar to that after supracondylar fractures (see earlier discussion under

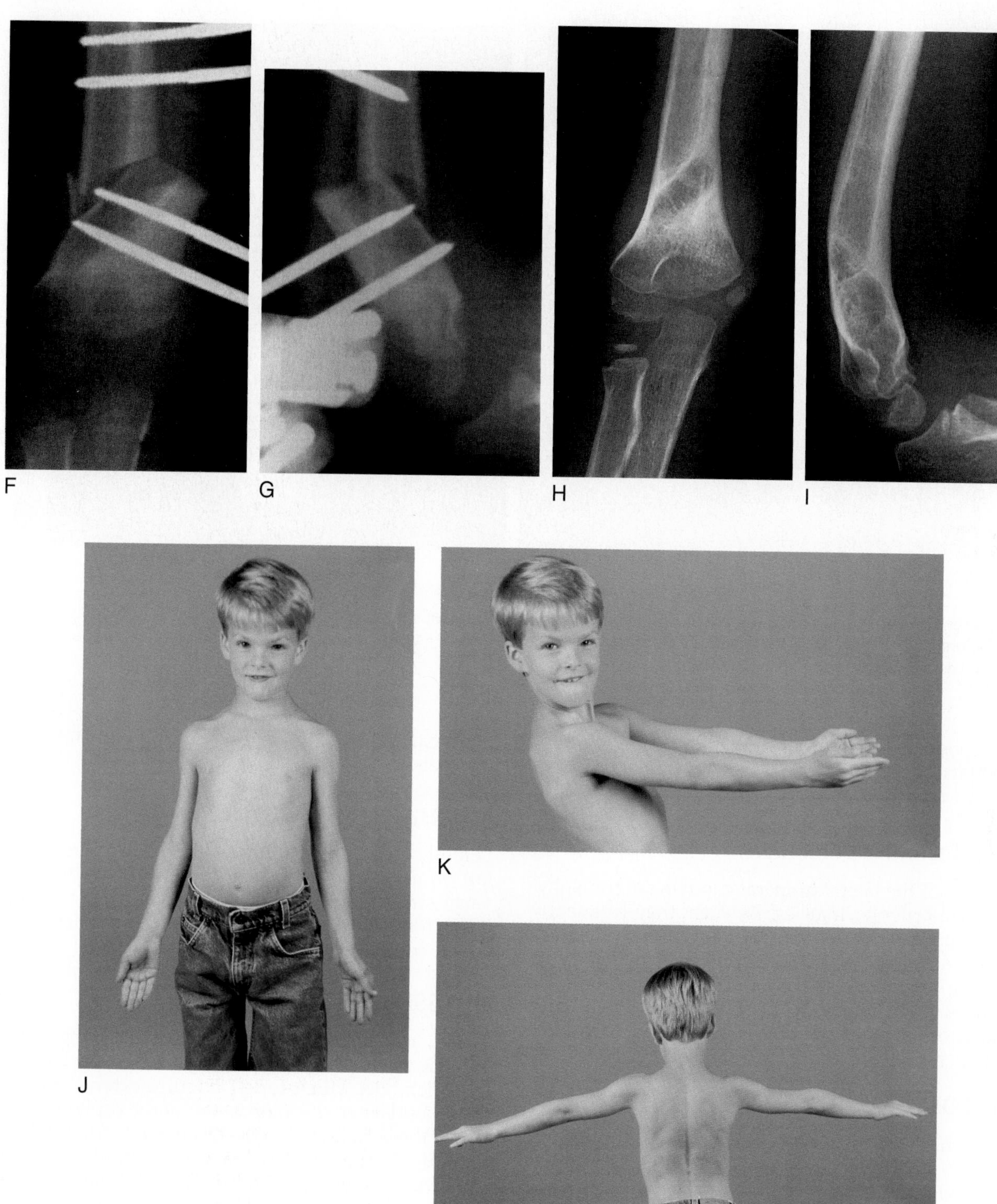

FIGURE 42-67 cont'd **F** and **G,** Immediate postoperative films showing the opening wedge osteotomy without a bone graft. The external fixator allows sagittal plane correction. Anteroposterior **(H)** and lateral **(I)** radiographs obtained 1 year postoperatively. Significant remodeling has occurred. **J** through **L,** Clinical appearance 1 year postoperatively.

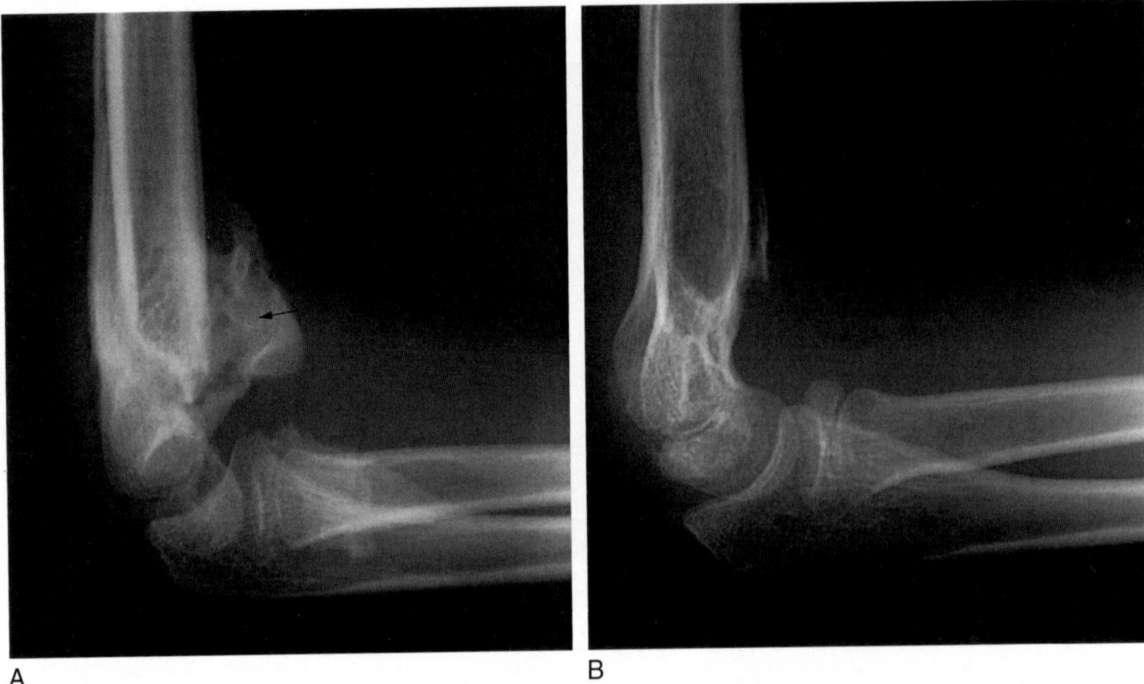

FIGURE 42–68 Myositis ossificans after a type III supracondylar humeral fracture. **A,** Lateral radiograph obtained 3 months after injury. Note the significant calcification in the anterior soft tissues (*arrow*). **B,** Three years after injury, the myositis has resolved without treatment.

Supracondylar Fractures of the Humerus). Deformity secondary to avascular necrosis (AVN) has also been reported after transphyseal separation.[393,617,619]

Lateral Condyle Fractures

Fractures of the lateral humeral condyle are transphyseal, intra-articular injuries. As such, they frequently require open reduction and fixation. In fact, they are the second most common operative elbow injury in children, second in frequency only to supracondylar fractures.[312] Lateral condyle fractures may be difficult to diagnose and have a propensity for late displacement, factors that make their treatment perilous.

ANATOMY

The pertinent anatomic considerations in lateral condyle fractures include the capitellum, the lateral epicondyle, and the soft tissues attached to it, namely, the extensors and supinator. The capitellum is the first secondary ossification center of the elbow to appear, usually around 2 years of age. The lateral epicondyle is the last, often not appearing until 12 or 13 years of age (see Fig. 42–29). The two ossification centers fuse at skeletal maturity.[530] Fractures of the lateral humeral condyle originate proximally at the posterior aspect of the distal humeral metaphysis and extend distally and anteriorly across the physis and epiphysis into the elbow joint. The fracture line may extend through the ossification center of the capitellum or may continue more medially and enter the joint medial to the trochlear groove. If the fracture extends medially to the trochlear groove, the elbow may be unstable and dislocate.

MECHANISM OF INJURY

Lateral condylar fractures are generally the result of a fall on an outstretched arm. The fall may produce a varus stress that avulses the lateral condyle or a valgus force in which the radial head directly pushes off the lateral condyle.[265]

CLASSIFICATION

There are several schemes for classifying lateral condyle fractures. The best known is the one described by Milch.[376] A Milch type I fracture extends through the secondary ossification center of the capitellum and enters the joint lateral to the trochlear groove. A Milch type II fracture extends farther medially, with the trochlea remaining with the lateral fragment, thus making the ulnohumeral joint unstable (Fig. 42–71). Unfortunately, though widely known and frequently used, the Milch classification provides little prognostic information regarding treatment and potential complications.[382]

Lateral condyle fractures involve the physis of the distal humerus and therefore can also be classified according to the Salter-Harris classification. Some controversy exists regarding the appropriate Salter-Harris classification of lateral condyle fractures. We believe, with Salter, that all these fractures begin in the metaphysis, cross the physis, and exit through the epiphysis and should be classified as type IV injuries.[485,486]

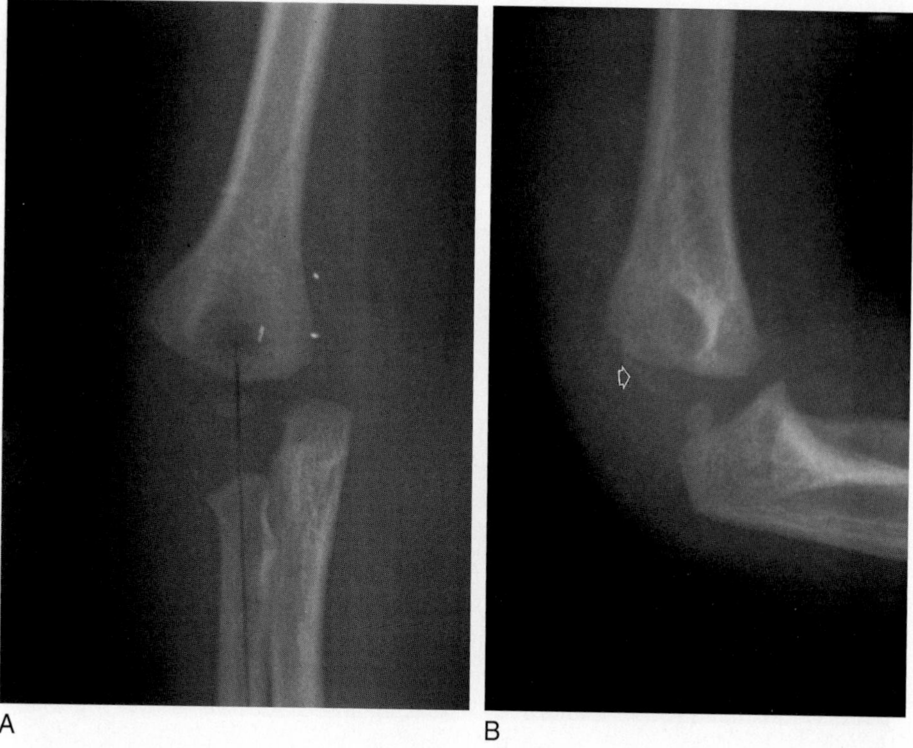

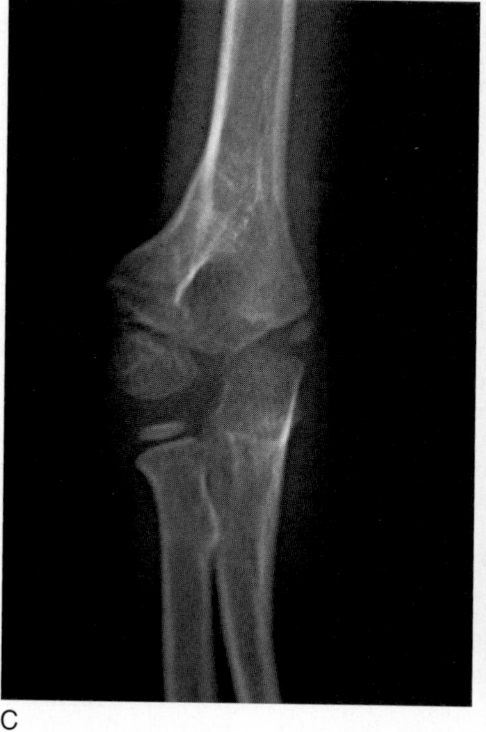

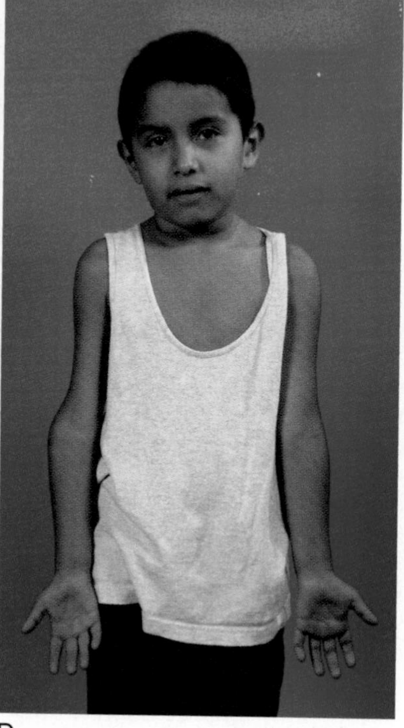

FIGURE 42-69
A, Anteroposterior (AP) radiograph of transphyseal separation of the distal end of the humerus. The medial translation of the forearm gives the appearance of an elbow dislocation; however, the radius and capitellum remain congruent. **B,** Lateral radiograph of transphyseal separation. Note the small posteriorly based metaphyseal (Thurston-Holland) fragment (*arrowhead*). The patient was treated by closed reduction and cast immobilization. **C,** An AP radiograph 3 years after injury shows varus malunion. **D,** Clinical appearance 3 years after the injury.

However, other authors have classified the Milch type II fracture as a Salter-Harris II injury, arguing that the secondary ossification center of the epiphysis is not involved. We believe that the intra-articular, transphyseal nature of these fractures mandates that they be treated as Salter-Harris type IV injuries, with restoration of the articular surface. Regardless, because growth arrest is relatively uncommon after this injury,[480,577] the Salter-Harris classification also adds little useful clinical information.

Unfortunately, the classification that provides the most useful information is not clinically viable. In a cadaver study, Jakob and colleagues reproduced lateral condyle fractures and discovered that the lateral fragment was occasionally hinged on intact medial cartilage.[265] This explains the clinical behavior of lateral

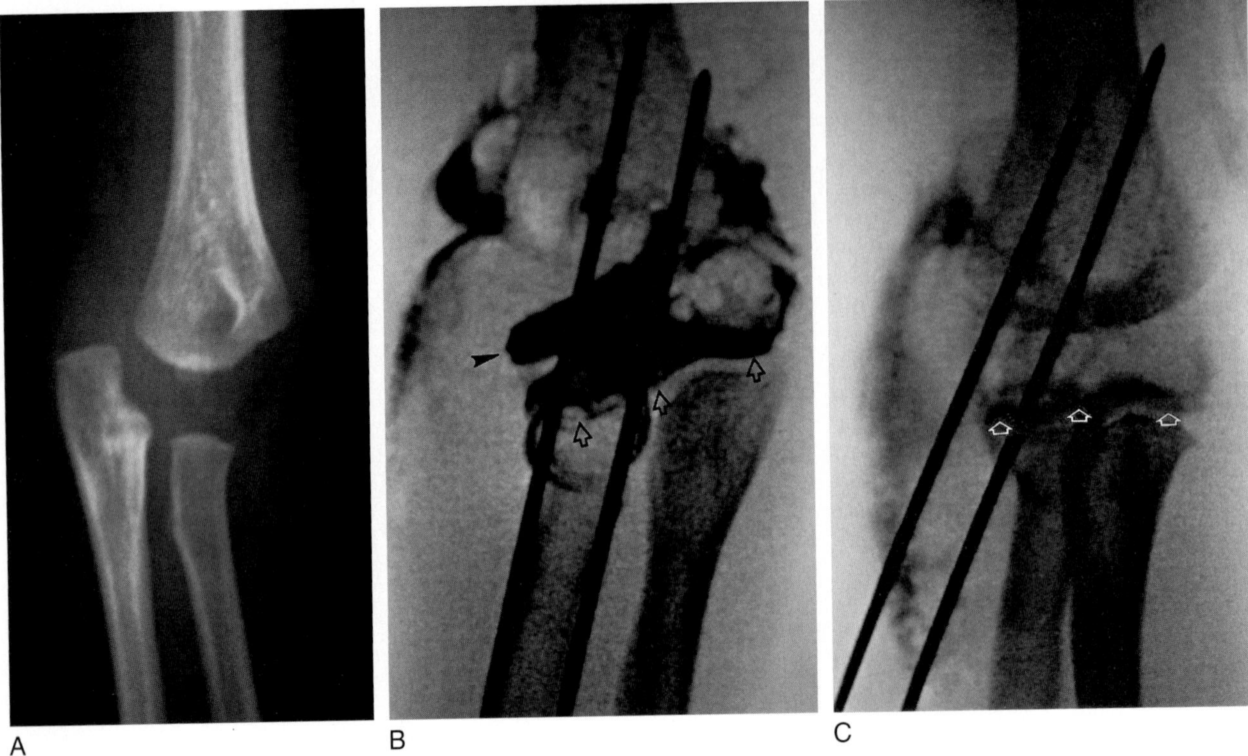

FIGURE 42–70 **A,** Anteroposterior radiograph of transphyseal separation of the distal end of the humerus. The radius and capitellum remain congruent despite medial translation of the forearm. **B,** Arthrogram obtained after an initial attempt at closed reduction and pinning. Note the varus alignment of the joint surface (*open arrows*) and the dye spreading laterally between the metaphysis and the distal fragment (*arrowhead*). **C,** Arthrogram obtained after remanipulation. The joint surface is now anatomically reduced (*arrows*).

condyle fractures. Minimally displaced fractures with an intact medial hinge do not displace further and heal with simple immobilization. However, if the fracture extends completely into the joint, the fracture is at risk for late displacement and potentially nonunion (Fig. 42–72). Thus, the presence or absence of the medial hinge is the key diagnostic factor in lateral condyle fractures. Although a few studies have attempted to identify this hinge and classify lateral condyle fractures accordingly, to date there is no accepted, reproducible, clinically viable method to obtain this information.[33,156,162,247,248,265,279,351,382,557] CT, MRI, and ultrasound have been used to identify the intra-articular fracture in small series.[85,207,450,581]

Finally, lateral condyle fractures may be classified as nondisplaced (traditionally less than 2 mm), minimally displaced (traditionally 2 to 4 mm), or displaced (traditionally greater than 4 mm).[25,33,96,156,165,381,382,425,557] We believe that this classification provides the most clinically useful information because it represents the current best attempt to identify fractures with an intact medial hinge.

DIAGNOSIS

As with all elbow injuries, the diagnosis of lateral condyle fracture may be obvious or frustratingly subtle. A child with a minimally displaced fracture may have complaints of pain and decreased range of motion. The differential diagnosis in these patients includes transphyseal fractures, minimally displaced supracondylar or radial neck fractures, nursemaid's elbow, and infection. Close examination (often not possible in a child with a grossly displaced fracture) may reveal isolated lateral tenderness. A careful history should be elicited to ensure a clear, immediate, traumatic onset of the pain because a history of minor trauma is frequently associated with a delay in the diagnosis of an infectious process. Radiographically, it is often difficult to distinguish between transphyseal fractures and lateral condyle fractures. Both may have a posteriorly based Thurston-Holland fragment on the lateral radiograph (Fig. 42–73; also see Fig. 42–69). The distinction is made by examining the AP radiograph (see Fig. 42–40). In transphyseal fractures the radial head–capitellum relationship remains intact. In displaced lateral condyle fractures the capitellum is laterally displaced in relation to the radial head. Additionally, transphyseal fractures are more likely to exhibit posteromedial displacement, and lateral condyle fractures are more likely to exhibit posterolateral displacement.

RADIOGRAPHIC FINDINGS

The hallmark radiographic finding is a posteriorly based Thurston-Holland fragment in the lateral view

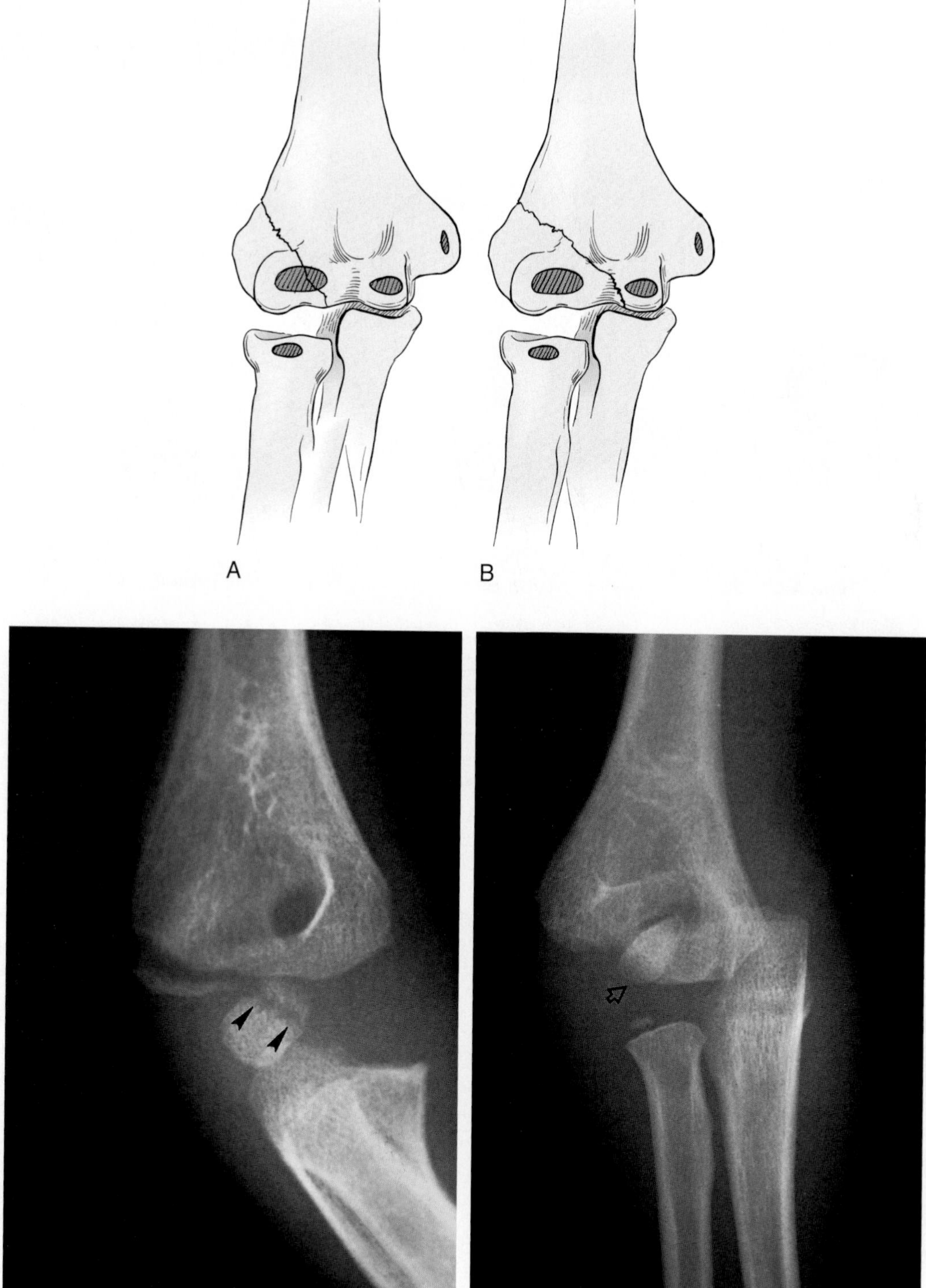

FIGURE 42–71 Milch's classification of lateral condyle fractures. **A,** Type I—the fracture extends through the secondary ossification center of the capitellum. **B,** Type II—the fracture crosses the epiphysis and enters the joint medial to the trochlear groove. Thus, the ulnohumeral joint is potentially unstable. **C,** Anteroposterior (AP) radiograph of a Milch type I fracture. Note that the fracture extends through the secondary ossification center of the capitellum (*arrowheads*). **D,** AP radiograph of a Milch type II fracture of the lateral condyle. The medial displacement of the forearm gives the appearance of an elbow dislocation or a transphyseal fracture. Close examination reveals the radius to be grossly in line with the capitellum. However, the capitular articular surface is subtly rotated (*arrow*).

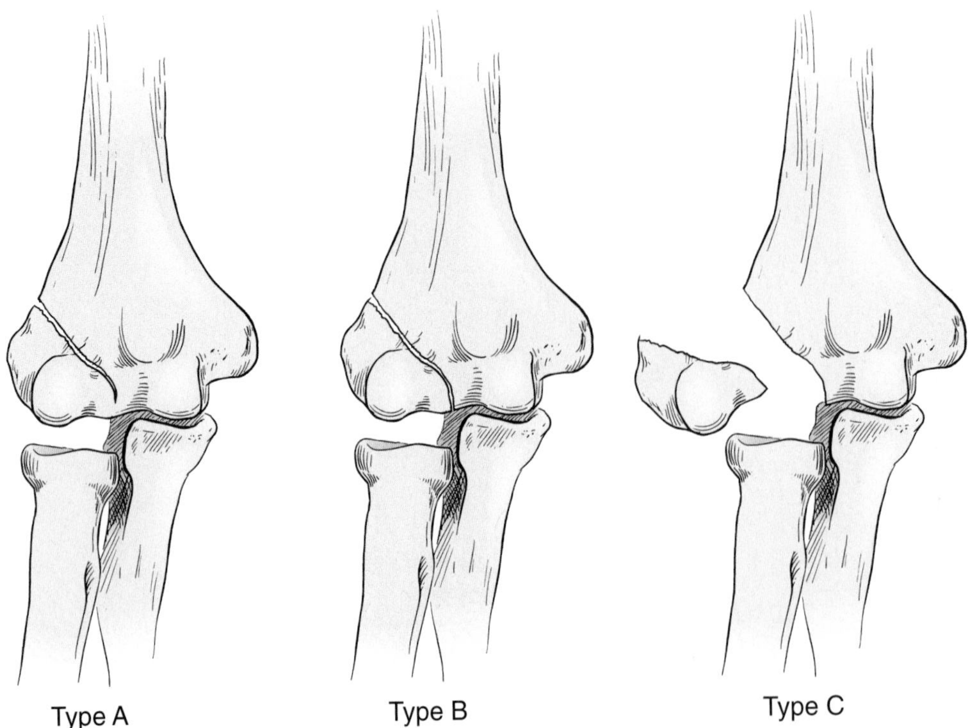

FIGURE 42–72 Classification of lateral condyle fractures based on the presence of an intact articular hinge. Type A—the fracture extends through the metaphysis and physis, but a portion of the articular cartilage remains intact. These fractures are stable, will not displace, and heal with immobilization. Type B—the fracture extends completely through the articular surface. Radiographically, this fracture may be impossible to distinguish from the type A fracture. However, it is potentially unstable and at risk for late displacement and delayed union or nonunion. Type C—grossly displaced lateral condylar fragment (may be significantly rotated).

(see Fig. 42–73A). In minimally displaced fractures, the AP radiograph may show little abnormality, although the fracture line may be seen running parallel to the physis (see Fig. 42–73B). Oblique radiographs or arthrograms are often helpful in identifying minimally displaced fractures.[351,381,574] Recently, sonography, CT, and MRI have been used to help identify which fractures are at risk for late displacement. However, these techniques have not reached widespread clinical acceptance.[85,207,247,279,450,581]

TREATMENT

Treatment of lateral condyle fractures depends on the amount of fracture displacement. The difficulty lies in differentiating stable nondisplaced fractures from potentially unstable, minimally displaced fractures. Unfortunately, there are currently no clinically applicable means of assessing the stability of the medial cartilaginous hinge. However, careful clinical and radiographic examination may offer important information regarding the stability of fractures that appear to be minimally displaced radiographically. Oblique views are often helpful in assessing and monitoring nondisplaced or minimally displaced fractures. Fracture displacement often appears greater on oblique radiographs. We believe that classification as a nondisplaced fracture requires an oblique radiograph with less than 2 mm of displacement. Significant lateral soft tissue swelling identified radiographically or clinically should alert the surgeon to a potentially unstable fracture. The presence of lateral ecchymosis implies a tear in the aponeurosis of the brachioradialis and signals an unstable fracture, regardless of the radiographic appearance (Fig. 42–74). Similarly, palpable crepitus between fragments signals an unstable fracture, irrespective of the radiographic appearance.

Displaced Fractures

Although there is controversy regarding the treatment of nondisplaced and minimally displaced fractures, there is a consensus that displaced lateral condyle fractures require open reduction and fixation (Fig. 42–75).[25,165,241,265,318,382,556] Even though open reduction is most commonly performed through an anterolateral approach, a posterolateral approach has also been described.[388] Because the blood supply of the lateral humeral condyle arises from the posterior soft tissues of the distal fragment, it is important that there be minimal dissection of the posterior soft tissues, and for this reason we prefer the anterolateral approach. Occasionally, there is plastic deformation of the distal fragment, and thus it is important to judge the reduction at the apex of the articular surface rather than by the lateral metaphyseal fragment. Fixation is generally

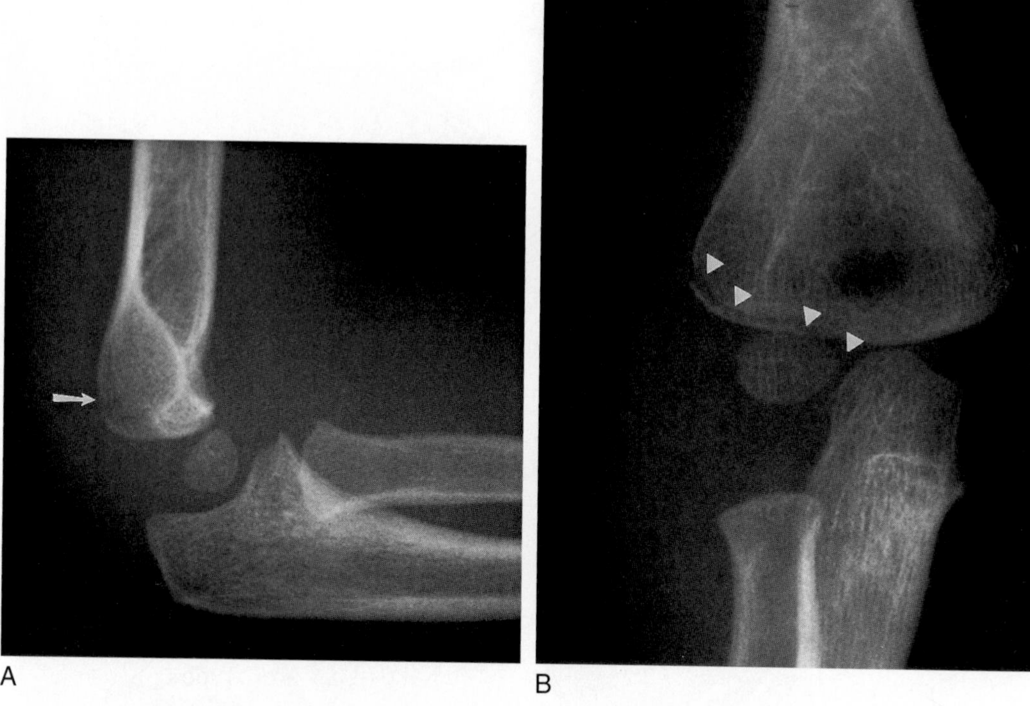

FIGURE 42–73 **A,** Lateral radiograph of a minimally displaced lateral condyle fracture. The small, posteriorly displaced metaphyseal fragment (*arrow*) is often difficult to see. **B,** Anteroposterior radiograph demonstrating the fracture line (*arrowheads*) running parallel to the physis. The fracture extends across the physis into the joint.

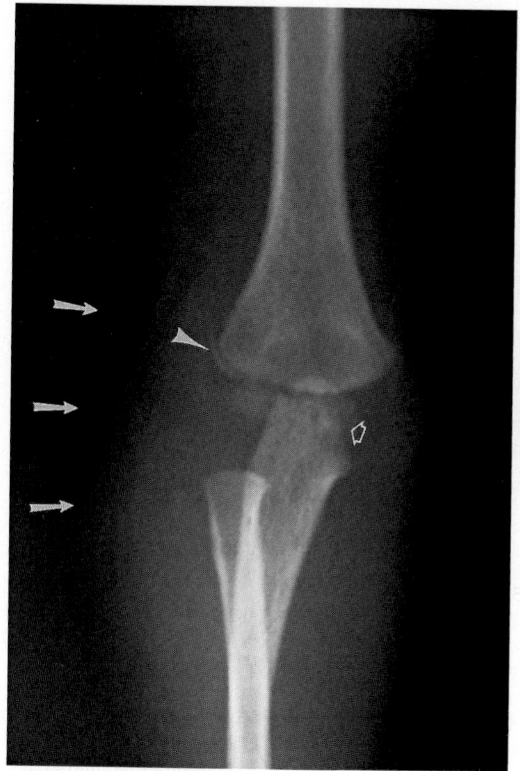

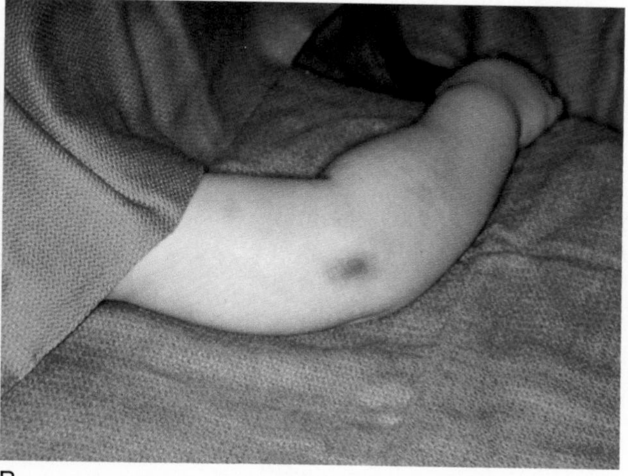

FIGURE 42–74 **A,** Anteroposterior radiograph of a minimally displaced lateral condyle fracture (*arrowhead*). However, there is significant soft tissue swelling laterally (*arrows*), as well as an olecranon fracture (*open arrow*). Despite the minimally displaced radiographic appearance, this is an unstable lateral condyle fracture. **B,** Clinical photograph showing a large lateral ecchymosis associated with this unstable fracture.

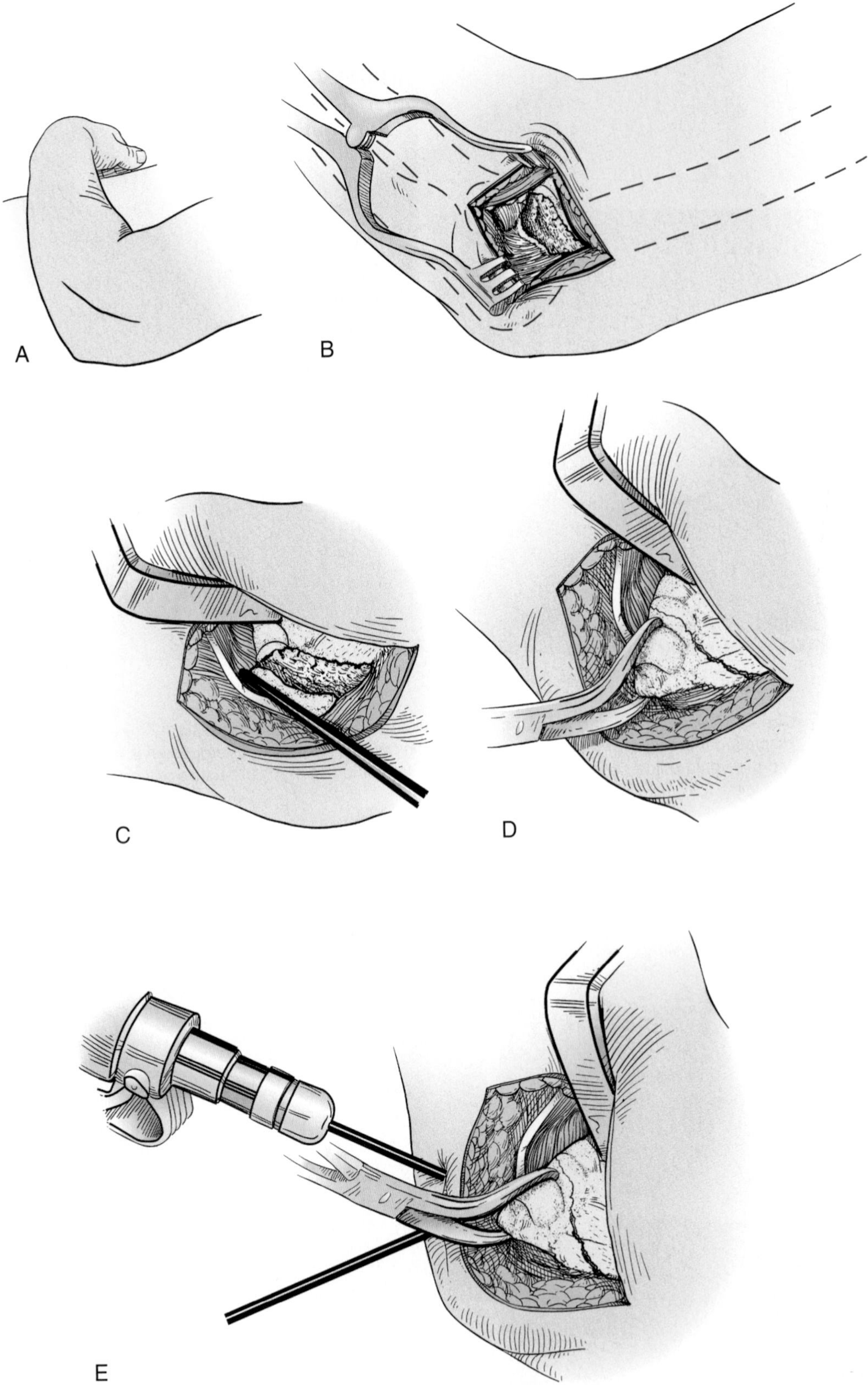

FIGURE 42-75 Technique for open reduction and fixation of a lateral condyle fracture. **A,** A sterile tourniquet is applied and an oblique posterior lateral skin incision is made. **B,** Superficial dissection is carried out in the plane of the fracture hematoma until the distal lateral corner of the proximal fragment is identified. **C,** Once the metaphyseal side of the fracture has been identified, the dissection is carried across the joint to expose the medial articular surface. After exposure of the proximal fragment, the orientation of the distal fragment is defined and the soft tissues are sharply released off the *anterior* aspect of the distal fragment, with extension carried distally to the radial head. **D,** After irrigation and debridement of the fracture hematoma, the distal fragment is reduced with a towel clip. It is important to judge the reduction at the level of the articular surface rather than the metaphysis because plastic deformation or comminution of the metaphyseal fragment may be present. **E,** Pins (usually 0.062 inch) are placed percutaneously to secure the fracture.

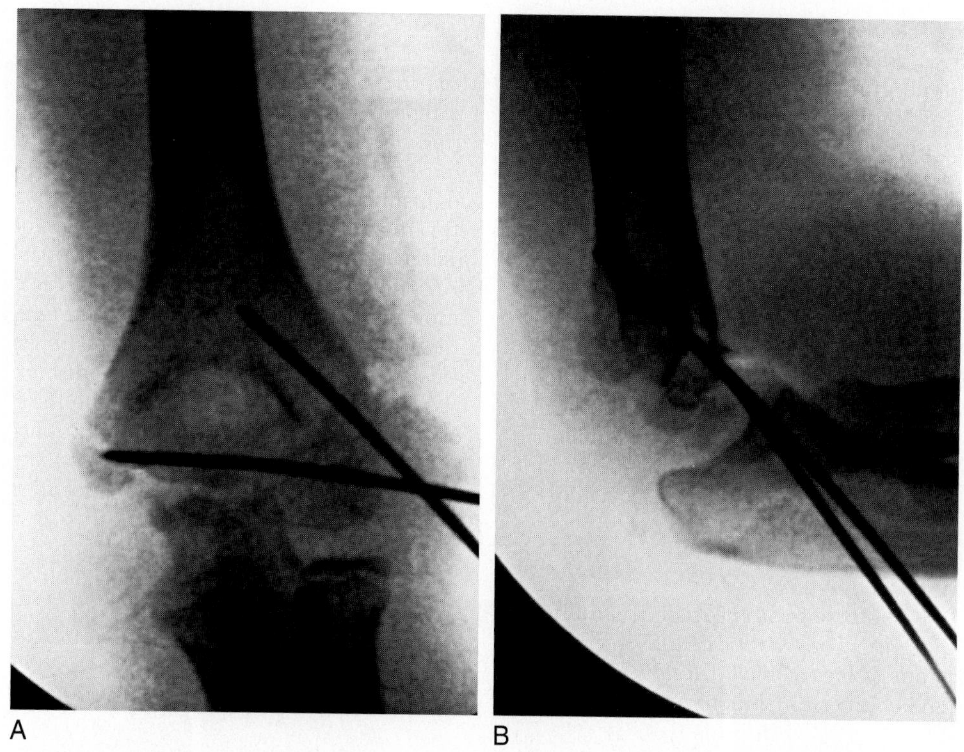

FIGURE 42–76 Anteroposterior **(A)** and lateral **(B)** radiographs demonstrating the technique of percutaneous pin fixation of lateral condyle fractures. The pins are widely divergent at the fracture line to provide maximum rotational stability.

achieved with smooth percutaneous pins, although screws and bioabsorbable pins have been used (Fig. 42–76).[96,229,246,344,502,556] Patients are usually immobilized with the elbow at 90 degrees for 4 weeks postoperatively.

Nondisplaced Fractures

If the fracture is nondisplaced or if there is other radiographic evidence that the medial articular hinge is intact, we treat the fracture by immobilization in 90 degrees of flexion and neutral rotation. Parents must be forewarned that the fracture can displace in the cast and that close follow-up is mandatory and surgery a possibility. Patients usually return 1, 2, and 4 weeks after the injury for radiographic assessment, which may require removal of the cast or splint. The cast is continued until radiographic healing is evident, typically in 4 to 6 weeks. Patients are seen 6 weeks after cast removal to ensure that range of motion has returned. If there was any question regarding union at the time of cast removal, radiographs should be repeated at this time, although they are not routinely necessary.

Minimally Displaced Fractures

Management of minimally displaced lateral condyle fractures is more controversial.* A number of authors have reported good results with conservative treatment. However, these reports all stress the possibility of late displacement and, consequently, potential delayed union or nonunion (Fig. 42–77).[33,124,165] A recent report by Devito and colleagues stressed the feasibility of cast immobilization. Eighty-two of 125 fractures had a fracture gap of 4 mm or less and were initially treated with a closed technique. Nine of the 82 fractures demonstrated late displacement, but only 2 required surgical treatment.[124] Others have advocated percutaneous fixation of minimally displaced lateral condyle fractures.[165,279,381] Mintzer and colleagues reported good results in 12 patients who had more than 2 mm of displacement and were treated by closed reduction and percutaneous pinning. They recommended arthrography to confirm a reduced articular surface.[381] We believe that treatment decisions for minimally displaced lateral condyle fractures must be made on an individual basis, and we use all three treatment techniques (casting, percutaneous fixation, and open reduction). Parents must thoroughly understand the importance of close follow-up if these fractures are to be treated conservatively. We have a low threshold for examination of these fractures under anesthesia with arthrography if necessary.

*See references 25, 33, 96, 156, 159, 161, 162, 165, 223, 265, 351, 381, 382, 426, 440, 557, 576.

COMPLICATIONS

The most common complications after lateral condyle fractures include cubitus varus, lateral spur formation, delayed union, and nonunion with or without cubitus

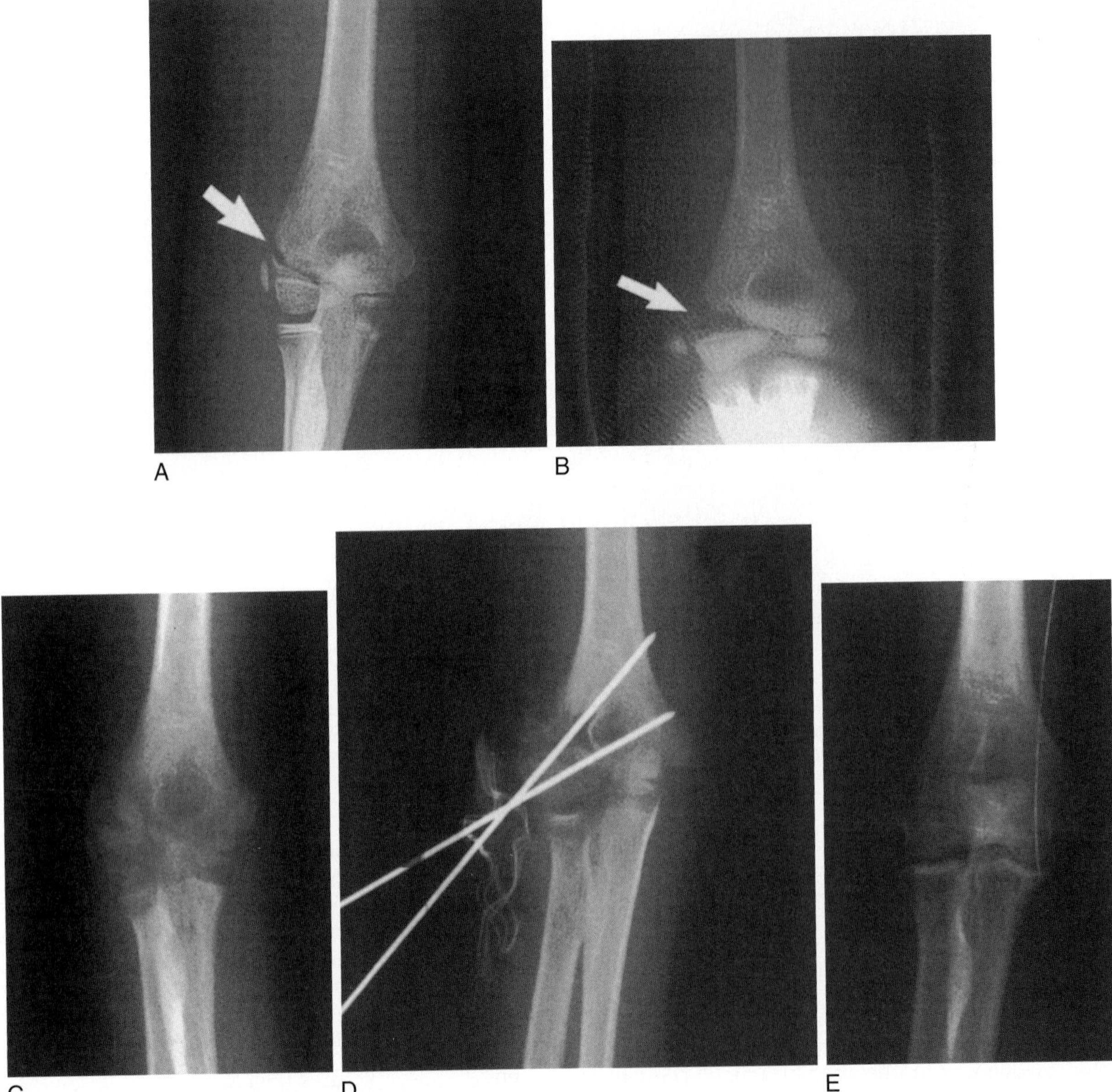

FIGURE 42–77 Radiographic example of a minimally displaced fracture that is displacing with cast immobilization. **A,** Anteroposterior radiograph at the time of injury showing a minimally displaced lateral condyle fracture (*arrow*). **B,** One week after injury, significant displacement of the fracture (*arrow*) had occurred. Cast immobilization was continued. **C,** Two months after the injury, delayed union had developed. **D,** The delayed union was treated by open reduction and stabilization. Note that the fracture was not reduced anatomically but was pinned in a position to provide maximal metaphyseal contact. **E,** Six years postoperatively the fracture has healed with minimal fishtail deformity of the distal humerus.

valgus. Growth arrest and fishtail deformity of the distal humerus can also occur but are rarely clinical problems.[89,299,406,519,582]

Cubitus Varus and Lateral Spur Formation

Cubitus varus is the most commonly reported complication after lateral condyle fractures and occurred in 40% of patients in one series.[165,529] The high incidence of cubitus varus is probably due to the fact that both true cubitus varus and lateral spur formation, which gives the appearance of varus deformity, are often reported as "cubitus varus." Cubitus varus and lateral spur formation are multifactorial in origin. True cubitus varus may be the result of malunion, growth arrest, or growth stimulation of the lateral condylar physis, or a combination of factors. Lateral spur formation occurs in lateral condyle fractures treated with operative as well as nonoperative techniques (Fig. 42–78). It is probably a result of slight displacement of the metaphyseal fragment in addition to disruption of the periosteal envelope.[529,600]

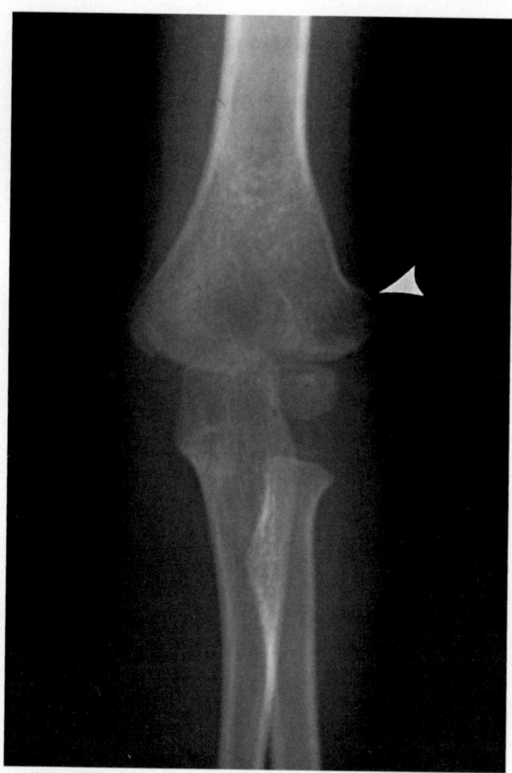

FIGURE 42–78 Anteroposterior radiograph demonstrating lateral spur formation (*arrowhead*) after operative treatment of a displaced lateral condyle fracture. The prominent lateral spur creates the clinical appearance of mild cubitus varus.

Cubitus varus after lateral condylar fractures is rarely as severe as that after supracondylar fractures; it is usually only a coronal plane deformity and does not have the hyperextension and rotary deformity present with supracondylar malunion. Because it is commonly mild and asymptomatic, cubitus varus after lateral condylar fracture rarely requires treatment. Occasionally, a progressive deformity, particularly if involving growth arrest, requires treatment. However, most often this common but mild complication can be treated by simply forewarning the parents at the time of initial treatment that their child may have a prominence on the lateral aspect of the elbow after the fracture has healed.

Delayed Union and Nonunion

Without question, the most frequent problematic complication of lateral condyle fractures is delayed union or nonunion. Several factors contribute to the difficulty in achieving union of lateral condyle fractures.[162,223] First, the fracture is intra-articular and consequently is constantly exposed to synovial fluid. Second, the lateral condyle has a poor blood supply. Finally, if not immobilized, there is constant motion at the fracture site from the pull of the wrist extensors on the distal fragment.

Fractures with Delayed Union. We use the term "delayed union" to refer to either a minimally displaced fracture that does not heal with 6 weeks of immobilization or an untreated fracture that is initially seen more than 2 weeks (but by convention less than 3 months) after the injury. If a conservatively treated fracture appears stable (no progressive displacement), healing usually occurs without further intervention; however, persistent nonunion occasionally develops.[223] Thus, it is important to observe these fractures until radiographic union is achieved. If healing does not occur or if progressive displacement develops (see Fig. 42–77), we recommend surgical treatment. Generally, union can be achieved simply by stabilizing the distal fragment with a screw through the metaphyseal fragment. We do not attempt to anatomically restore the articular surface, and bone grafting is not typically required. The surgical approach to delayed union or nonunion is the same as the surgical approach to an acute fracture (see Fig. 42–75). Care must be taken to ensure that all soft tissue dissection occurs anteriorly to avoid the blood supply of the distal fragment.

Late-Presenting Fractures. Management of late-presenting fractures is controversial. Some authors have reported better results in patients treated with observation rather than delayed open reduction.[127,265] However, a number of authors have recently reported good results with the surgical treatment of late-presenting (2 to 12 weeks) fractures, as well as established nonunion.[114,159,162,164,185,352,506,593,600] Although Flynn initially recommended surgical treatment for late-presenting fractures that were "in good position" and had an open growth plate,[159] other authors have described good results in skeletally mature patients with more displaced fractures. All authors warn of the potential for stiffness, osteonecrosis, and fishtail deformity if surgical treatment is undertaken.[114,159,162,164,185,223,352,506,600] We favor surgical treatment of these fractures (Fig. 42–79).

Nonunited Fractures. We use the term "nonunion" to refer to a fracture that has not healed within 3 months. Clinically, nonunion can be manifested as one of three scenarios.* The first is as a painful nonunion, which is the least common. The pain is usually related to activity. Older patients may have a feeling of lateral instability and apprehension. We manage these patients with an attempt at osteosynthesis. The goal of surgical treatment is to obtain union of the metaphyseal fragment, not to restore the joint surface. Bone grafting may be required, and the posterior soft tissues must be avoided (Fig. 42–80). The second manifestation of delayed union is as a cosmetically unacceptable valgus deformity. These patients generally have an associated flexion contracture and can be managed with a corrective osteotomy, with or without

*See references 114, 159, 185, 268, 277, 352, 391, 392, 500, 523, 561, 562, 600.

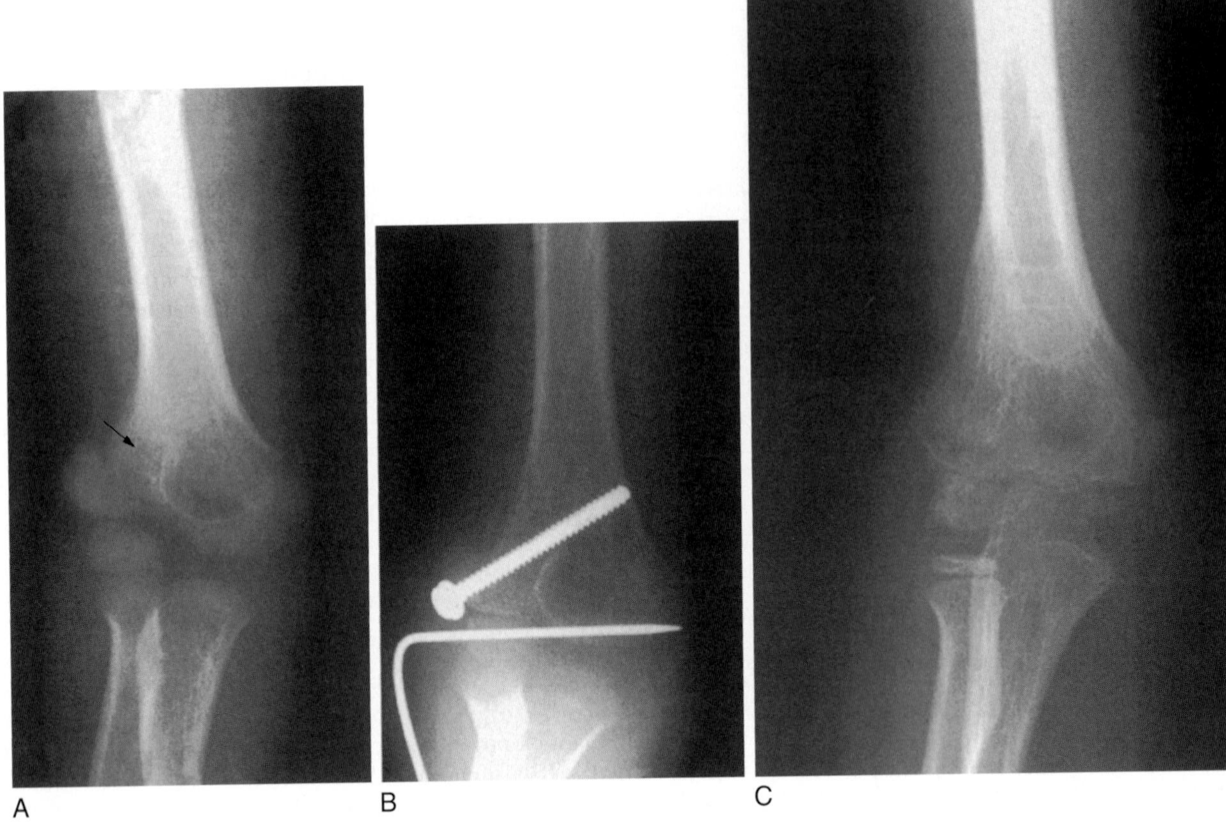

FIGURE 42-79 Treatment of a lateral condyle fracture initially seen 5 weeks after injury. **A,** An anteroposterior (AP) radiograph obtained at initial evaluation showed a displaced lateral condyle fracture (*arrow*). **B,** Open reduction with internal fixation was performed. Note that the fracture was not reduced anatomically but was placed in a position to maximize metaphyseal contact. A screw was used through the metaphyseal fragment because delayed healing was anticipated. A percutaneous pin provided initial rotational stability. **C,** AP radiograph obtained 18 months after treatment.

attempts to achieve healing of the nonunion. Finally, delayed union may be manifested as cubitus valgus and a tardy ulnar nerve palsy.[186,359,378,504] These patients should be managed by ulnar nerve transposition (Fig. 42–81).[523]

Growth Arrest

Although lateral condyle fractures cross the germinal layer of the physis and are classified as Salter-Harris type IV injuries, growth arrest is a rare complication.[25,162,223,381,382,480,523,600] In a review of 39 fractures, Rutherford reported only one case of growth arrest.[480] If growth arrest does occur, a progressive valgus or varus deformity may develop. In young patients this may be treated by bar resection or osteotomy, or both. Because of the limited growth of the distal humerus (20% of the entire humerus, or approximately 3 mm/yr), older patients are probably best treated with completion of the epiphysiodesis and osteotomy.

Fishtail Deformity and Avascular Necrosis

The cause of fishtail deformity of the distal humerus is uncertain. Rutherford noted this deformity in 9 of 10 patients who had unreduced lateral condyle fractures. He hypothesized that malunion at the medial extent of the fracture resulted in growth arrest of the lateral trochlea.[480] However, Morrissey and Wilkins noted it after a variety of fractures of the distal humerus and attributed it to AVN.[393] In all likelihood, both causes occur. Mild deformity after lateral condyle fractures may occur more frequently than reported and is probably related to growth arrest.[393,406,480] More severe deformities are most likely the result of vascular changes, often associated with surgical approaches to the elbow (Fig. 42–82).[617]

Medial Epicondyle Fractures

Fifty percent of medial epicondyle fractures are associated with elbow dislocations. Fractures of the medial epicondyle usually occur between 7 and 15 years of age. They account for approximately 10% of all children's elbow fractures.[40,136,312,313,357,522,606]

ANATOMY

The ossification center of the medial epicondyle of the humerus appears between 5 and 7 years of age and

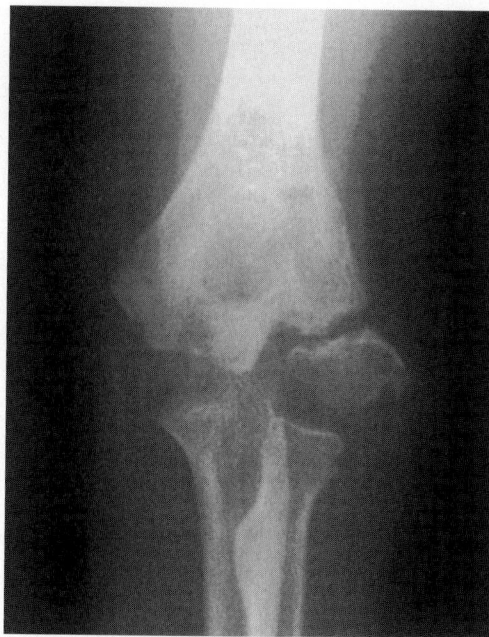

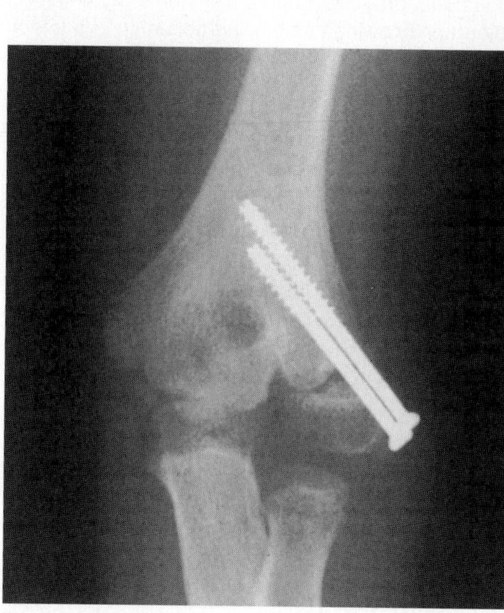

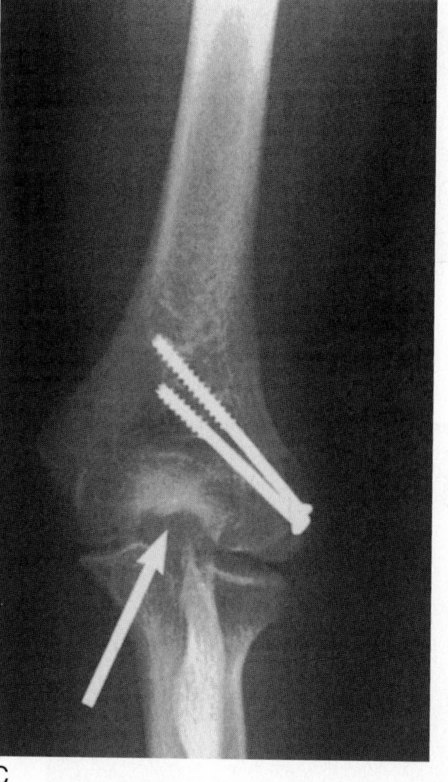

FIGURE 42-80 Symptomatic lateral condyle nonunion. **A,** Anteroposterior radiograph showing established nonunion of the lateral condyle. The patient had elbow pain with vigorous use of the extremity. **B,** Surgical treatment was directed toward achieving union of the distal fragment to the metaphysis. Articular congruity was not restored. **C,** Six years postoperatively the fracture has united. A fishtail deformity is present (*arrow*).

unites with the humeral diaphysis between 18 and 20 years of age.[511,530] The common tendon of the flexor muscles of the forearm and the ulnar collateral ligament of the elbow insert on the medial epicondyle. The ulnar nerve runs in a groove in the posterior aspect of this epicondyle. The medial epicondyle is an apophysis and does not contribute to longitudinal growth of the humerus.

MECHANISM OF INJURY

The mechanism of injury is a valgus stress producing traction on the medial epicondyle through the flexor muscles. The epicondyle may be minimally or severely displaced. If associated with an elbow dislocation, the fragment may become incarcerated in the joint at the time of dislocation or reduction.[152,171,172,430,431,466,472,520,555,586]

CLASSIFICATION

Unfortunately, there is no widely accepted classification of medial epicondyle fractures, and most authors have described unique systems based on what they consider critical information.[611] All of the established classification systems consider whether the fracture is displaced or nondisplaced. However, there is no agreement on what constitutes a displaced fracture.

We believe that the important factors in prognosis and treatment include the amount of displacement

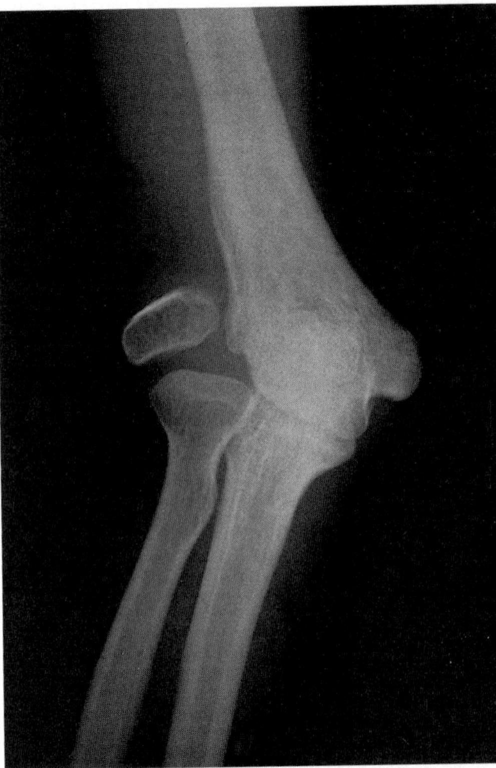

A

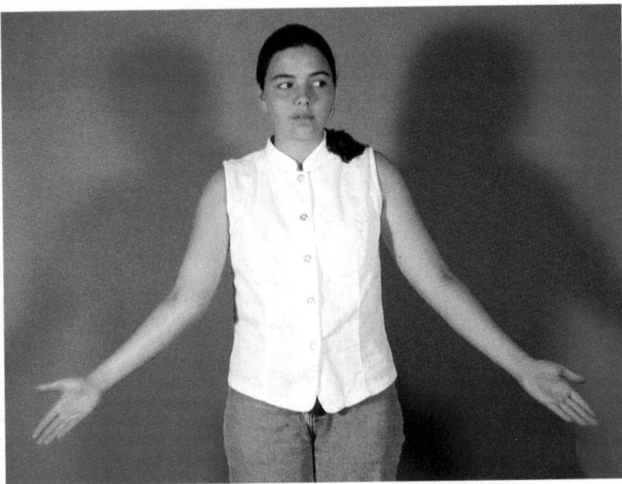

B

FIGURE 42–81 Lateral condyle nonunion producing cubitus valgus and tardy ulnar nerve symptoms. **A,** Anteroposterior radiograph showing established nonunion of a lateral condyle fracture. **B,** Clinical appearance of cubitus valgus. The patient was treated by ulnar nerve transposition.

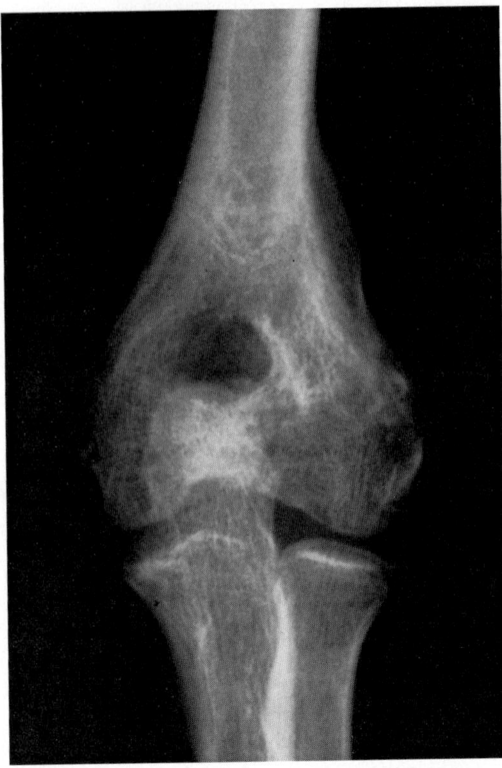

FIGURE 42–82 Anteroposterior radiograph showing a mild fishtail deformity in the distal end of the humerus after uncomplicated treatment of a lateral condyle fracture (also see the fishtail deformities in Fig. 42–80).

(we use a threshold of 5 mm of displacement), the presence of associated elbow injuries or fragment incarceration, and the desired athletic endeavors of the patient.[16,128,239,603]

DIAGNOSIS

The physical findings depend on the degree of displacement of the medial epicondyle. Generally the elbow is held in flexion and any motion is painful. There is tenderness over the medial epicondyle that is exacerbated with valgus stress. Ulnar nerve paresis or dysesthesias may be present.

RADIOGRAPHIC FINDINGS

In older patients (>6 or 7 years of age), the medial epicondylar fragment is usually easily identified radiographically. However, radiographic interpretation in younger patients may be difficult if the secondary ossification center is not yet ossified. In either case, assessment of minimally displaced fractures may be facilitated by comparison views to establish the "normal" width of the cartilaginous space between the metaphysis and medial epicondyle. Fragments trapped in the joint may be difficult to identify, particularly in younger patients with minimal ossification.[430,511] Although medial joint space widening may be present on the AP radiograph, a nonconcentrically reduced

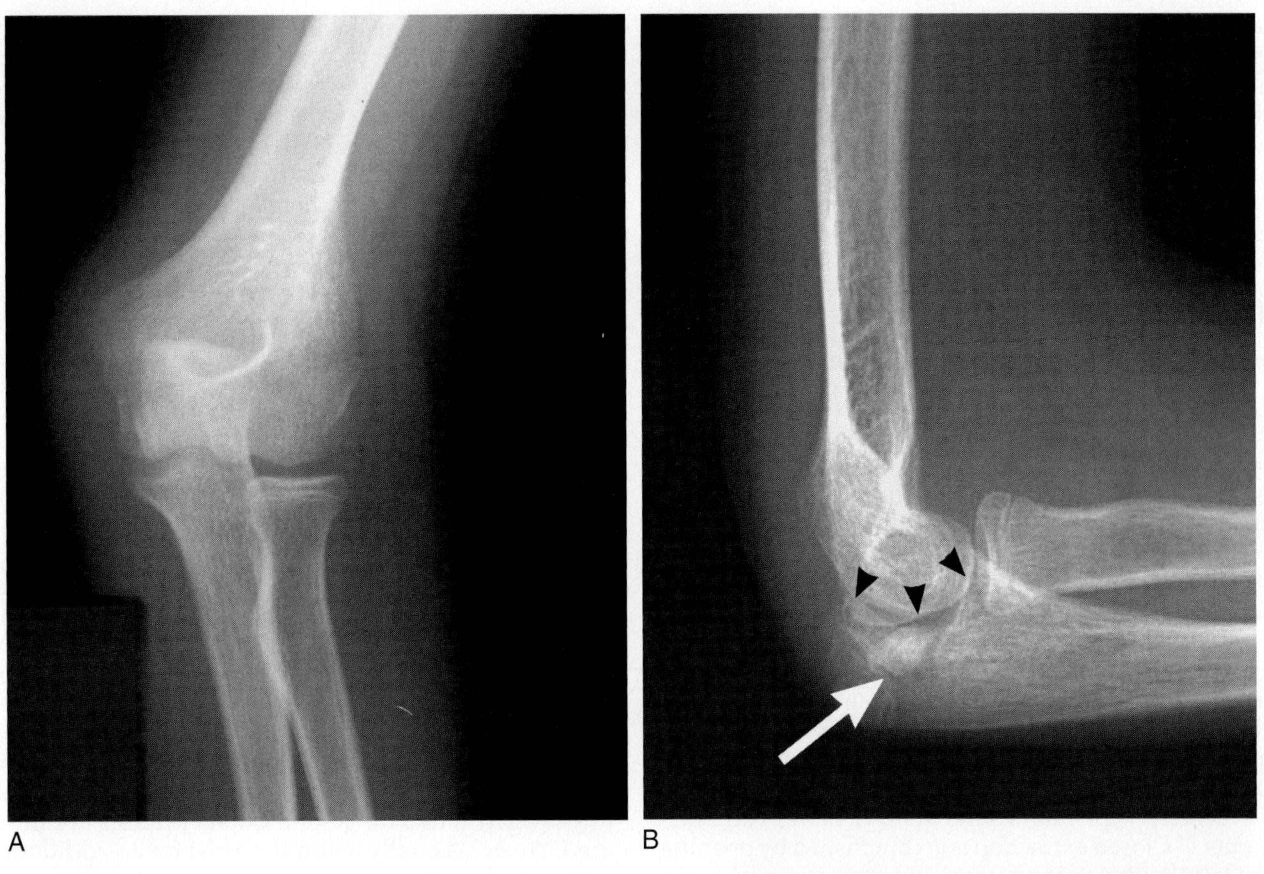

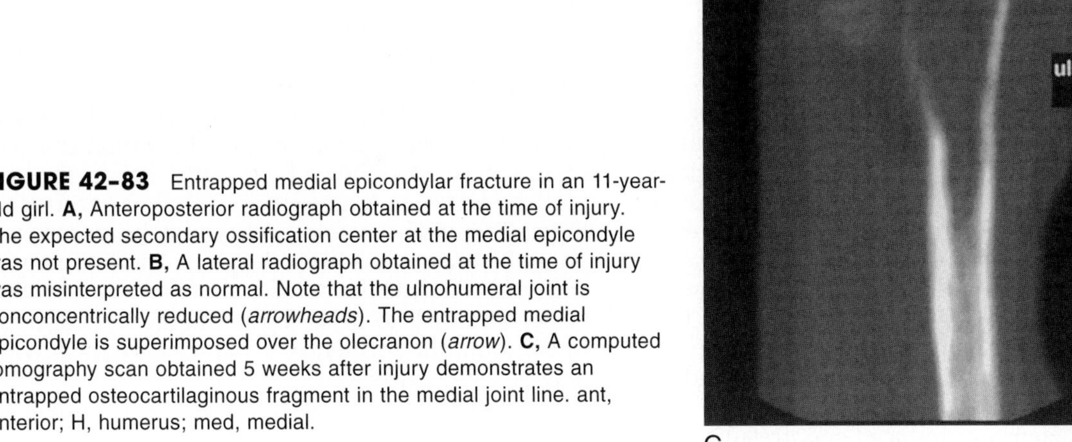

FIGURE 42–83 Entrapped medial epicondylar fracture in an 11-year-old girl. **A,** Anteroposterior radiograph obtained at the time of injury. The expected secondary ossification center at the medial epicondyle was not present. **B,** A lateral radiograph obtained at the time of injury was misinterpreted as normal. Note that the ulnohumeral joint is nonconcentrically reduced (*arrowheads*). The entrapped medial epicondyle is superimposed over the olecranon (*arrow*). **C,** A computed tomography scan obtained 5 weeks after injury demonstrates an entrapped osteocartilaginous fragment in the medial joint line. ant, anterior; H, humerus; med, medial.

ulnohumeral joint on the lateral radiograph is often the only radiographic finding. Thus, whenever a medial epicondyle fracture is suspected, it is imperative that a true lateral radiograph of the elbow be obtained. An inability to obtain a true lateral radiograph should raise suspicion of an entrapped medial epicondyle fragment (Fig. 42–83).

Several authors have advocated an AP valgus stress radiograph for assessment of stability after medial epicondyle fracture.[495,611] This radiograph is obtained with the patient supine, the arm abducted 90 degrees, the shoulder externally rotated 90 degrees, and the elbow flexed at least 15 degrees to eliminate the stabilizing force of the olecranon. In this position gravity will create widening on the medial side of an unstable elbow. Because sedation is generally required, we have found this radiograph to be of little clinical use.

TREATMENT

Nondisplaced and Minimally Displaced Fractures

There is a consensus that nondisplaced and minimally displaced fractures (<5 mm) are best managed by symptomatic treatment, which usually consists of immobilization in a posterior splint, long-arm cast, or sling for 1 to 2 weeks, followed by early active range-of-motion exercises. It is important to warn the parents that radiographic union may not occur but that the functional results are usually excellent.[128,274,607]

It is also agreed that intra-articular fragments should be removed acutely.[439] Although some authors have cautioned against performing such removal with closed techniques because of concern that the ulnar nerve could be damaged, we agree with authors who favor a single attempt at gentle manipulative reduction for acutely (<24 hours after injury) entrapped fragments.[466] Closed extraction is accomplished by opening the joint with a valgus stress and then supinating the forearm and dorsiflexing the wrist and fingers to stretch the flexors and extract the medial epicondylar apophysis from the joint.[56,493] Other authors have suggested that electrical stimulation of the flexor mass or joint distention with saline may help facilitate extraction.[172,430] We do not have experience with these techniques.If we are unable to release an entrapped fragment with closed techniques, we proceed to open reduction.

Displaced Fractures

Treatment of displaced (>5 mm) medial epicondyle fractures is more controversial. Although a number of studies have reported superior results with closed treatment, these series all included a few patients in whom symptomatic nonunion developed. Recently, there have been reports of excellent results with open reduction and internal fixation of medial epicondyle fractures.[76,239,321,429] However, there have also been reports of stiffness and nonunion after operative treatment.[139,518,607] Farsetti and coworkers reviewed 42 patients at an average follow-up of 45 years and found that closed management produced good results in all patients despite failure of the epicondyle to unite. Those treated by open reduction had mostly good results, whereas those who underwent excision of the epicondyle did poorly. Their work strongly supports closed management of this injury.[154] Woods and Tullos have expressed concern that symptomatic treatment of displaced fractures in a high-demand overhead athlete may lead to symptomatic valgus instability because of functional lengthening of the ulnar collateral ligament.[611] Because such late instability can be difficult to treat, they advocate open reduction and internal fixation of medial epicondyle fractures in serious overhead athletes. Unfortunately, it is often difficult to predict whether a young patient with a displaced medial epicondyle fracture will develop into an overhead athlete.

We have had good results with both operative and conservative treatment of displaced medial epicondyle fractures. We treat these injuries on an individual basis after a thorough discussion with the parents. Although some authors have described closed reduction and percutaneous pinning for displaced fractures, we favor open reduction to ensure that the ulnar nerve is not damaged. Open reduction is performed through a medial longitudinal skin incision. The ulnar nerve is identified, dissected free, and retracted posteriorly. The fractured medial epicondyle is identified and is anatomically repositioned with a towel clip. We favor fixation with a partially threaded screw, often using a cannulated system to achieve temporary fixation (Fig. 42–84). Care must be taken in young patients to prevent comminution of the predominantly cartilaginous distal fragment during fixation. After open reduction we immobilize the elbow in flexion for 1 to 3 weeks, after which active range-of-motion exercises are initiated. We occasionally splint the wrist for an additional 3 to 4 weeks after cast removal to prevent active contraction of the flexor muscle mass, which might displace the distal fragment.

COMPLICATIONS

Complications from medial epicondyle fractures include stiffness, ulnar neuritis, missed incarceration, and symptomatic nonunion.[40,239,410,439] Stiffness is the most common complication and is best prevented by avoiding prolonged immobilization. It is important to remember that the soft tissue injury is usually much more significant than the radiographic abnormality. We favor a brief period of immobilization (no more than 3 weeks), followed by early active range-of-motion exercises. Aggressive physical or occupational therapy should be avoided in the early (initial 6 weeks) phase because it has been shown to lead to increased stiffness. The incidence of ulnar nerve dysfunction varies from 10% to 16%.[40] If the fragment is entrapped in the joint, the incidence of ulnar nerve dysfunction may be as high as 50%.[7]

Traditionally, surgical treatment of late-identified entrapped fragments has been avoided.[171,472] However, recent studies have shown good results with late extraction of incarcerated fragments. Fowles and associates reported improved range of motion (80% normal), decreased pain, and improved ulnar nerve symptoms in six patients treated by surgical extraction an average of 14 weeks after injury.[171] Somewhat surprisingly, there are also long-term follow-up reports

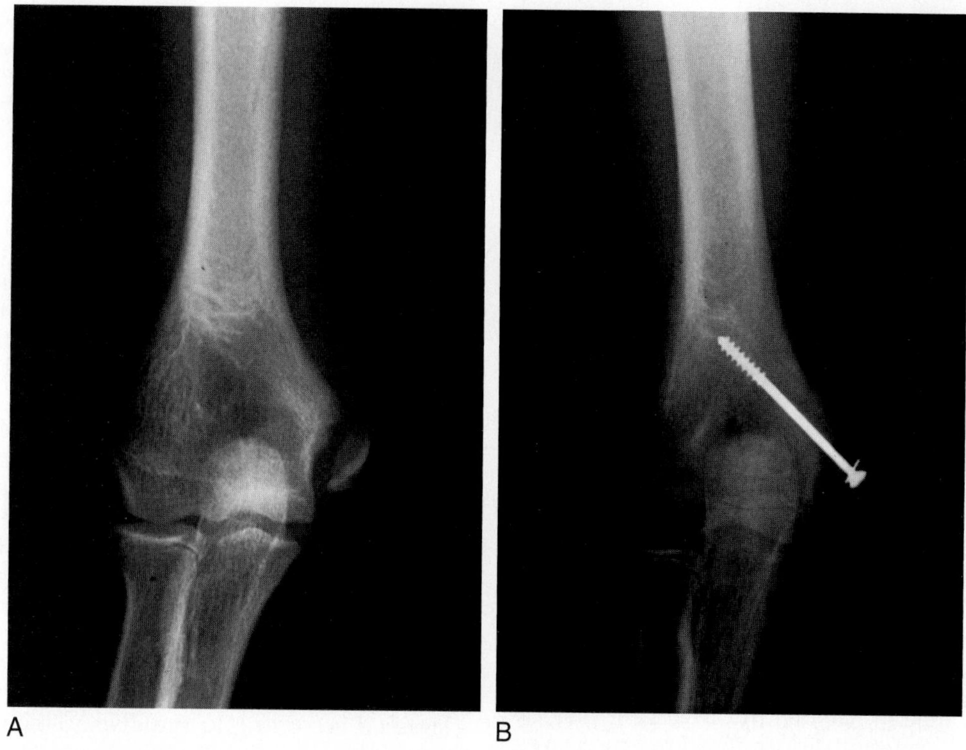

FIGURE 42-84 **A,** Displaced medial epicondyle fracture in a 14-year-old Little League pitcher. The injury was sustained during pitching. **B,** Anteroposterior radiograph obtained after open reduction and fixation of the medial epicondyle fragment.

showing good results with persistently retained fragments.[472]

Symptomatic nonunion in a high-performance athlete is difficult to treat. Wilkins and associates reported the case of a high-performance adolescent baseball pitcher who had to stop pitching after nonoperative management of a medial epicondyle fracture. We have had some success in establishing union in symptomatic patients. Our approach is to stabilize the fragment with in situ fixation and a local bone graft. We do not attempt to mobilize the fragment and reduce it anatomically. Others have advocated simple excision of the symptomatic nonunion with reattachment of the ulnar collateral ligament. We do not have experience with this technique and prefer an initial attempt at establishing union.

Elbow Dislocations

Dislocation of the elbow is a relatively uncommon injury in children. It is frequently associated with fractures, particularly of the medial epicondyle, proximal radius, olecranon, and coronoid process. Elbow dislocations are most common in adolescents and unusual in young children.[200,258,312,473,490,574] An apparent elbow dislocation in a young child should alert the orthopaedist to a potential transphyseal or other fracture. Although most elbow dislocations can be treated by simple closed reduction, it is important to carefully assess the patient and the radiographs to ensure that associated injuries are not missed.

ANATOMY

The anatomic constraints to posterior dislocation include the anterior capsule, the coronoid process (which resists posterior displacement of the ulna), and the collateral ligaments. During posterior elbow dislocation the momentum of the body applied to the lower end of the humerus tears the joint capsule anteriorly. The relatively small coronoid is unable to prevent proximal and posterior displacement of the ulna. The collateral ligaments are stretched or ruptured. The radius and ulna, being firmly bound by the annular ligament and interosseous membrane, are displaced together. The coronoid becomes locked in the olecranon fossa by contraction of the biceps and triceps. In posterolateral dislocations, the biceps tendon serves as a fulcrum about which the distal fragment (the forearm) rotates laterally. The normal cubitus valgus of the elbow also promotes lateral displacement. If only one collateral ligament is torn, one of the forearm bones will dislocate while the other undergoes rotary subluxation.

With posterior and posterior lateral dislocations, the ulnar collateral ligament and medial epicondyle may be avulsed. After reduction, the medial epicondyle may remain incarcerated within the joint (see discussion under Medial Epicondyle Fractures). With posteromedial dislocation, fracture of the lateral condyle may occur. Injury to the radial head or neck is another frequent finding with posterior elbow dislocations.

The neurovascular anatomy of the arm plays an important role in the potential complications that may develop after elbow dislocations (see Fig. 42–33). As with supracondylar fractures, the brachial artery and median nerve lie anterior to the humerus and may be injured when stretched over the displaced proximal fragment. The ulnar nerve lies immediately posterior to the medial epicondyle and is particularly at risk with dislocations associated with medial epicondyle fractures.[47,112,205,233,242,346,353,447,448]

MECHANISM OF INJURY

Elbow dislocations are most commonly the result of a fall on an outstretched arm. The direction of displacement varies according to the direction of the force. The most frequent elbow dislocation is posterior or posterolateral and is usually the result of a fall with the forearm supinated and the elbow either extended or partially flexed (Fig. 42–85).[75,172,316] Though less common, anterior, medial, lateral, and divergent dislocations can occur. Anterior dislocations are caused by a direct blow to or fall on the olecranon process. Medial or lateral dislocations usually result from direct trauma, violent twisting of the forearm, or falls on the hand. In divergent dislocations, which are extremely rare, the radius and ulna are dissociated from each other proximally and dislocated from the humerus.[15,17,54,74,120,192,228,264,341,532,537,543,608]

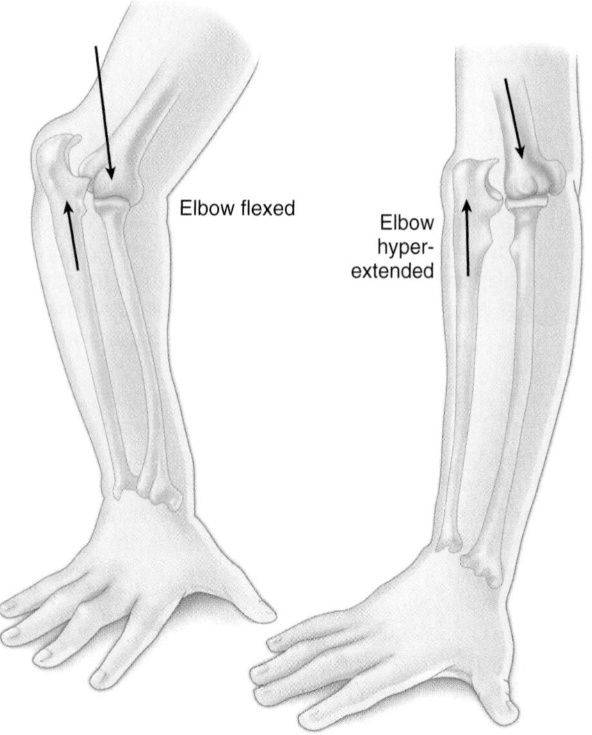

FIGURE 42–85 Elbow dislocations are generally the result of a fall onto a supinated forearm with the elbow in either flexion or extension.

DIAGNOSIS

Immediately after the injury, the patient has a painful and swollen elbow that is held in flexion. Attempts at motion are painful and restricted. From the anterior view the forearm appears to be shortened, whereas from the posterior view the upper part of the arm appears to be decreased in length. The distal humerus creates a fullness within the antecubital fossa.

The differential diagnosis includes transphyseal fractures, supracondylar fractures, Milch type II lateral condylar fractures, and Monteggia fractures (see Fig. 42–40). An accurate diagnosis can be made by assessing good-quality AP and lateral radiographs. The relationship of the radius to the ulna should be analyzed to rule out a divergent dislocation.[15] Radiographs should also be scrutinized to identify any associated fractures, with particular attention to the medial epicondyle, coronoid process, proximal radius, and lateral condyle.[444,531] Elbow dislocations are classified according to the displacement of the distal fragment.[532]

TREATMENT

Thorough examination of the skin and assessment of the vascular and neurologic status of the extremity are imperative because neurovascular injuries are not uncommon.[47,112,205,233,242,346,353,447,448] Reduction of acute posterior dislocations is generally easily accomplished without a general anesthetic.[103,545] We prefer to reduce posterior dislocations with hyperextension and traction followed by flexion (Fig. 42–86).[21,107,219,320] The upper part of the arm is held with one hand and the forearm with the other. The elbow is hyperextended and traction is applied to disengage the tip of the coronoid process from the olecranon fossa. Marked hyperextension of the elbow should be avoided to prevent unnecessary strain on the anterior soft tissues. Traction is continued to restore length. While traction is maintained the elbow is gently flexed. As the olecranon engages the articular surface of the humerus, there is often a palpable and audible click. A second technique places the patient prone with the injured limb hanging over the edge of the table. The weight of the arm provides distal traction while the surgeon pushes the olecranon downward and forward with his or her thumbs.[373]

Anterior dislocation is a very rare injury.[54,93,264,537,543,608] Linscheid and Wheeler reported two cases of anterior dislocation out of 110 elbow dislocations.[333] Anterior dislocations are associated with extensive soft tissue damage and often fracture of the olecranon or the proximal ulna. Reduction is accomplished by longitudinal traction with the elbow in flexion and firm pressure applied distally and posteriorly on the forearm as the elbow is gradually extended. Reduction of the rare medial or lateral dislocation of

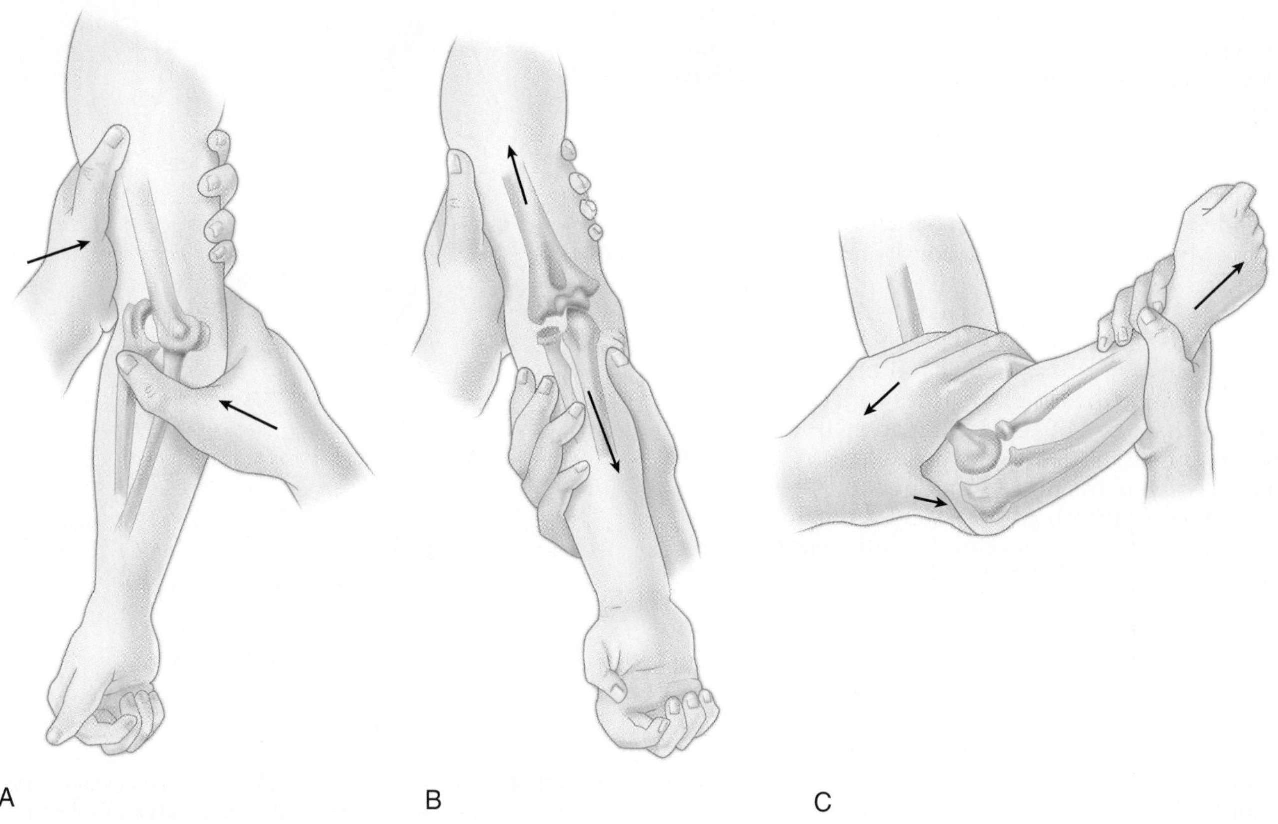

FIGURE 42–86 Technique for closed reduction of posterior elbow dislocation. **A,** The elbow is hyperextended to disengage the coronoid from the olecranon fascia. **B,** Traction is applied to restore length and correct the carrying angle. **C,** The elbow is then reduced with posterior displacement of the distal end of the humerus and flexion of the elbow.

the elbow follows the principles outlined for the treatment of posterior dislocation, that is, traction, correction of coronal plane deformity, and flexion.[532]

After successful closed reduction, good-quality radiographs must be obtained, including a perfect lateral view to ensure that there are no entrapped intra-articular fragments. We immobilize the extremity in a posterior splint. Because compartment syndrome has been reported after elbow dislocation, we recommend admission to the hospital for overnight observation after reduction.[140] The splint is continued for 1 to 2 weeks. Once the splint is removed, active range of motion is encouraged. We reassess the range of motion 6 to 8 weeks after injury. If there is significant stiffness at this time, formal physical or occupational therapy can be initiated. We avoid earlier (<6 weeks after injury) passive range of motion because it has been associated with increased stiffness. Aggressive range-of-motion exercises are never indicated.

When associated with a fracture, the dislocation should be reduced and the fracture reassessed and managed appropriately according to findings on the postreduction radiographs. Late-identified dislocations generally require open reduction.[14,170,316,512,513,534]

COMPLICATIONS

Stiffness is the most common complication after elbow dislocation.[87,172,316,333,452] Other complications include vascular injury, peripheral nerve injury, myositis ossificans, and recurrent dislocation.* Nearly all reports of elbow dislocations, including those in children, list loss of motion as the most common complication. Fortunately, loss of motion in children is rarely significant from a functional or cosmetic standpoint. Stiffness is to some extent a function of the soft tissue damage at the time of injury. However, there are some variables in the management of elbow dislocations that will affect range of motion. Stiffness is more likely after prolonged immobilization and early aggressive passive range-of-motion exercises. Thus, we rarely immobilize elbow dislocations for more than 1 to 2 weeks. After removal of the cast, we immediately begin gentle active motion but do not begin a formal therapy program until 6 to 8 weeks after injury, if necessary. Recently, Stans and coworkers noted that surgical treatment of post-traumatic elbow stiffness was less predictable in children than in adults, although patients with stiffness from dislocation or extra-articular fracture did better than those with stiffness from other causes.[539]

Both heterotopic bone formation and myositis ossificans have been reported after elbow dislocation. Limited amounts of heterotopic bone commonly form along the course of the collateral ligaments.[333] Myositis

*See references 47, 91, 112, 180, 205, 208, 233, 242, 337, 346, 353, 447, 448.

ossificans may occur within the brachialis muscle.[467] A delay in the initial reduction and vigorous passive stretching exercises after cast removal have been reported to lead to myositis ossificans.[337] Rest, gentle active range-of-motion exercises, and anti-inflammatory medications such as indomethacin (Indocin) or naproxen (Naprosyn) are recommended during the active phase of myositis ossificans. Myositis may spontaneously resolve over time (see Fig. 42–68).

Vascular injury is uncommon with elbow dislocation. It is most commonly seen with open injuries.[21,144,208,233,234,242,295,337] Perhaps the most important fact in relation to vascular injuries with elbow dislocation is that the collateral circulation is much more likely to be damaged at the time of injury than with supracondylar fractures. Consequently, most authors have a lower threshold for vascular repair than they do with injuries associated with supracondylar fracture.[24,140,144,208,233,234,242,264,295,333,337,533]

Peripheral nerve injury is more common than vascular injury.[455] The ulnar nerve is most frequently injured, usually in dislocations associated with avulsion of the medial epicondyle. Ulnar nerve symptoms most often arise when displacement of the medial epicondyle results in compression of the nerve by the fibrous band that binds the nerve to the posterior aspect of the epicondyle.[103,171,172,180] With greater awareness of displaced medial epicondylar fractures, the incidence of ulnar nerve symptoms appears to be decreasing, and the ones that are noted are often transient and improve once the incarcerated medial epicondylar fragment is released form the joint.[180,333,591]

Median nerve injury may occur in one of three ways (Fig. 42–87).[47,112,205,346,353,447,448] First, the nerve may be displaced posteriorly behind the medial condylar ridge and trapped between the distal humerus and olecranon (see Fig. 42–87A). Second, the median nerve may be trapped between the fractured surface of the medial epicondyle and the humerus. If the medial epicondyle is allowed to heal in this position, the median nerve will be encased in bone (see Fig. 42–87B).[464] Third, the median nerve can become caught between the trochlea and olecranon during reduction (see Fig. 42–87C).[217,419,544] The diagnosis of median nerve entrapment is made difficult by the lack of pain and the delayed appearance of motor and sensory symptoms. Matev described the radiographic appearance of a chronically displaced median nerve, namely, a sclerotic depression over the posteromedial epicondyle, a finding now referred to as *Matev's sign*.[353] Treatment of median nerve entrapment entails immediate surgical release. Chronic entrapment may require reanastomosis or nerve grafting, or both, and carries a poor prognosis.

Recurrent dislocation is a rare but disabling complication that is difficult to treat. The first case was reported by Albert in 1881.[11] It is most common in young adults who sustained an initial posterior or posterolateral dislocation in late adolescence.[91,363,567] Osborne and Cotterill proposed that the pathologic defect causing recurrent dislocation was laxity of the ligamentous complex of the posterolateral capsule.[416] Initial treatment should be conservative, particularly in a young patient. We have had some success treating these patients with a prolonged period of bracing. If conservative measures fail, we favor the posterolateral capsular reefing technique described by Osborne and Cotterill (Fig. 42–88).[282,416]

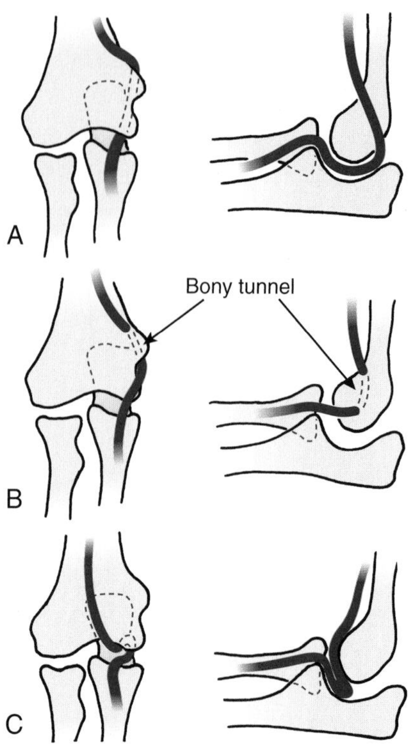

FIGURE 42–87 **A** through **C,** Median nerve entrapment after posterior elbow dislocation. See text for description. (Redrawn from Hallett J: Entrapment of the median nerve after dislocation of the elbow. J Bone Joint Surg Br 1981;63:408.)

Radial Head and Neck Fractures

In children, the cartilaginous radial head is resistant to fracture, and children are more likely to sustain fractures of the radial neck than fractures of the head. About half of radial neck fractures are associated with other injuries to the elbow.[137,331,358,390,589] It is important to warn parents that displaced fractures, particularly those in children older than 10 years, may be associated with loss of forearm rotation.[131,451,459,499]

ANATOMY

The radial head is disk shaped and of greater diameter than the neck, which rotates within the annular ligament. It has a shallow cuplike surface that articulates with the capitellum proximally and the radial notch of the ulna medially. The biceps inserts on its tuberosity immediately distal to the neck. The secondary ossification center of the proximal radius appears as a small sphere between the third and the fifth year of life and

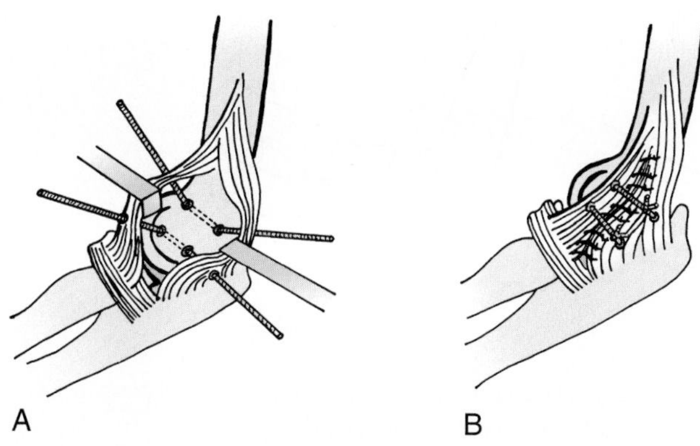

FIGURE 42–88 A and B, Posterolateral capsular reefing technique of Osborne and Cotterill for recurrent elbow dislocation. (Redrawn from Osborne G, Cotterill P: Recurrent dislocation of the elbow. J Bone Joint Surg Br 1966;48:344.)

fuses with the shaft between the ages of 16 and 18 years. Occasionally, the ossification centers are bipartite, which should not be mistaken for a fracture.[530] Because the entire radial head is covered with articular cartilage, the blood supply to the epiphysis is supplied through the more distal metaphysis and may be injured with complete separation through the neck (see Fig. 40–7).[109]

MECHANISM OF INJURY

Fractures of the radial head or neck may occur as a result of two different mechanisms.[269,401] Most commonly they result from a fall onto an outstretched hand with the elbow in extension and valgus. This valgus extension force may also produce other injuries, including avulsion of the medial epicondyle, rupture of the medial collateral ligament, or fracture of the olecranon, proximal ulna, or lateral condyle (Fig. 42–89).[137,184,289,331,499]

Fracture of the radial neck may also occur as a result of dislocation of the elbow. The radial neck may be fractured by impact against the inferior aspect of the capitellum either at the time of posterior dislocation or at the time of spontaneous reduction (Fig. 42–90).[267,407,459,610] Radial head fracture may also occur with anterior dislocation of the elbow and produce anterior displacement of the head.[401,572]

CLASSIFICATION

Fractures of the radial head and neck may be classified according to the magnitude of displacement or the mechanism of injury; fractures involving the physis may be classified according to the type of physeal involvement. O'Brien subdivided radial head and neck fractures into three categories based on the degree of angular displacement of the superior articular surface from the horizontal (Fig. 42–91).[407] This classification has proved to be most effective as a guide in both treatment and prognosis.[407,459] In type I fractures the displacement is 30 degrees or less. Type II fractures have between 31 and 60 degrees of angulation. Type III fractures have more than 60 degrees of displacement.

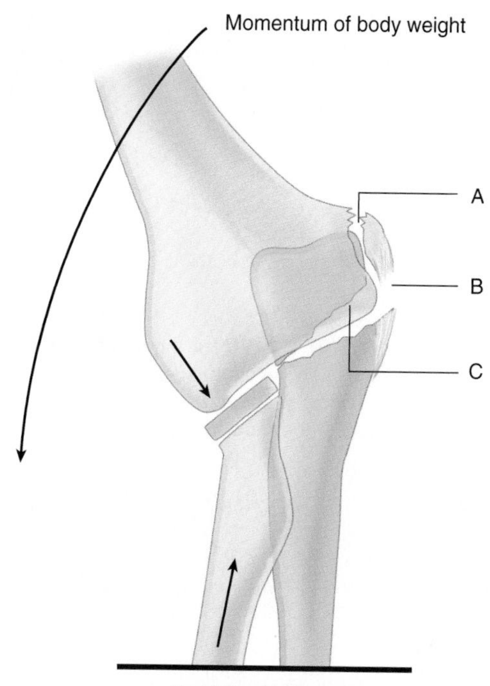

FIGURE 42–89 A valgus hyperextension force to the elbow may produce a radial neck fracture associated with fracture of the olecranon (C) or medial epicondyle (A) or, less commonly, with rupture of the medial collateral ligament (B).

Jeffrey initially recognized two different mechanisms of radial head fracture.[269] Newman later developed a classification system based on the direction of radial head displacement.[402] Wilkins combined and modified these systems to classify radial head and neck fractures according to the mechanism of injury and the location of the fracture line.[80]

Approximately half of fractures of the proximal radius involve the physis and half are completely within the metaphysis.[271] Fractures that involve the physis may also be classified according to the Salter-Harris classification of physeal injuries.[486] Proximal radial physeal fractures are most frequently Salter-Harris type II injuries. Younger children may sustain Salter-Harris type I injuries. Salter-Harris type III or IV fractures involving the radial head and articular surface also occasionally occur. The surgeon should be wary of the rare radial head fracture in which the radial head is flipped 180 degrees with the articular surface facing the radial metaphysis. These injuries most commonly occur in association with a posterior elbow dislocation, generally require open reduction, and are prone to the development of AVN.[89]

DIAGNOSIS

Radial head and neck fractures rarely produce obvious clinical deformity. In fact, the fracture may not be evident on initial radiographs and may be noticed only

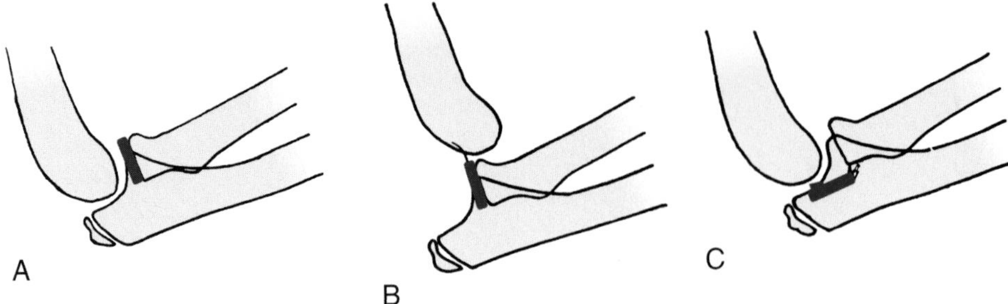

FIGURE 42-90 **A** through **C**, Fracture of the radial neck associated with dislocation of the elbow. The inferior aspect of the capitellum acts as a fulcrum in producing a radial neck fracture. This may occur at the time of dislocation or reduction. (Redrawn from Jeffrey CC: Fractures of the head of the radius in children. J Bone Joint Surg Br 1950;32:3.)

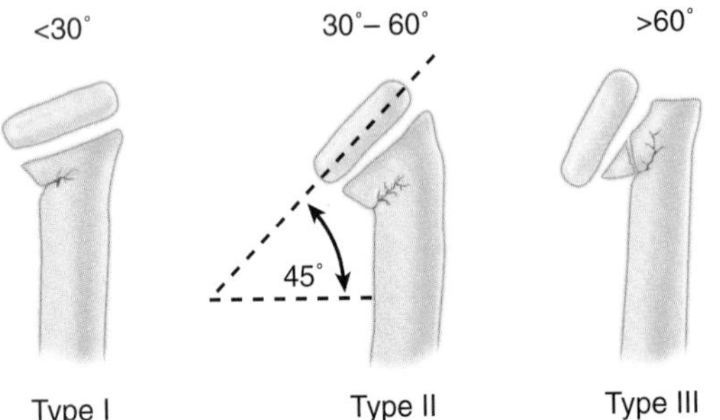

FIGURE 42-91 Classification of radial neck fractures. (The angle measured is the displacement of the superior articular surface of the radial head relative to a perpendicular to the radial shaft.) Type I fractures are angled less than 30 degrees. Type II fractures are angled between 30 and 60 degrees. Type III fractures are angled more than 60 degrees. (Redrawn from O'Brien PI: Injuries involving the proximal radial epiphysis. Clin Orthop Relat Res 1965;41:52.)

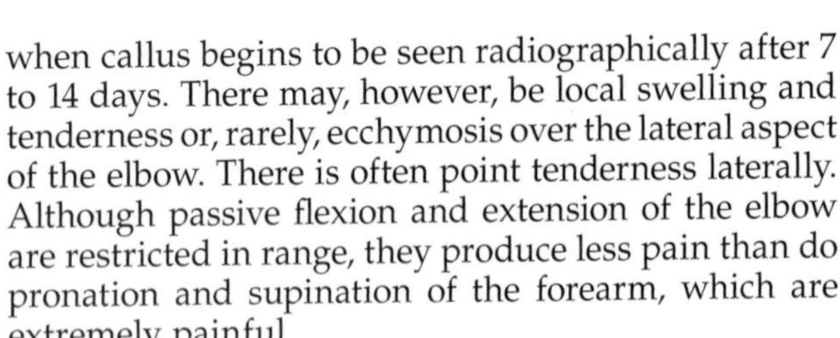

when callus begins to be seen radiographically after 7 to 14 days. There may, however, be local swelling and tenderness or, rarely, ecchymosis over the lateral aspect of the elbow. There is often point tenderness laterally. Although passive flexion and extension of the elbow are restricted in range, they produce less pain than do pronation and supination of the forearm, which are extremely painful.

RADIOGRAPHIC FINDINGS

Fractures of the radial head and neck are often subtle and require close examination of good-quality radiographs. When evaluating and treating fractures of the radial neck and head it is important that AP and lateral radiographs of the *proximal radius* be obtained. The child's inability to fully extend the elbow makes it difficult to obtain a true AP view of an acutely swollen elbow. Thus, if pathology of the proximal radius is suspected, the x-ray technicians should be instructed to obtain an AP radiograph of the proximal radius rather than the elbow (Fig. 42–92). It may be helpful to obtain radiographs with the forearm in different positions of rotation.[405] Careful assessment should be made for associated fractures, particularly of the medial epicondyle and olecranon or proximal ulna.

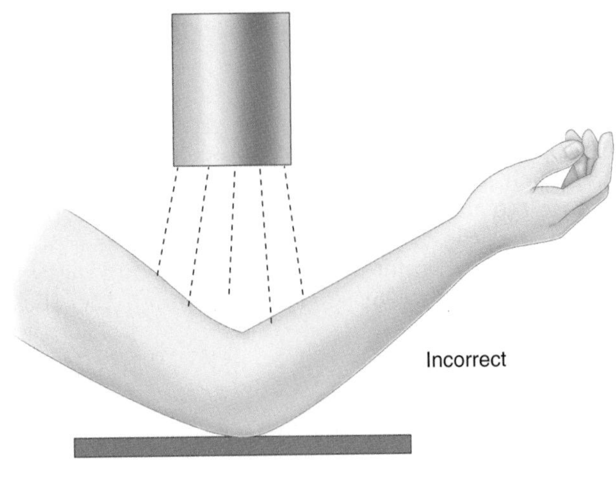

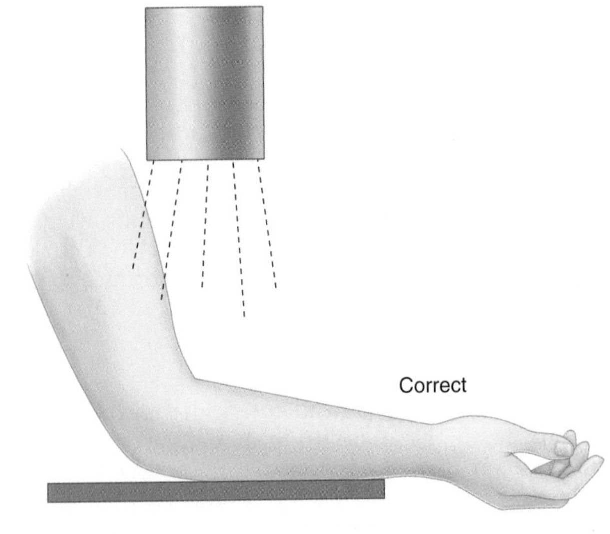

FIGURE 42-92 Technique for obtaining an anteroposterior (AP) radiograph of the proximal radius. **A,** Because an acutely injured elbow is unable to fully extend, placing the apex of the elbow on the cassette produces an oblique view of both the proximal forearm and distal humerus. **B,** A true AP view of the proximal radius and ulna is obtained by placing the proximal part of the forearm directly on the cassette.

TREATMENT

The greatest difficulty in treating radial neck fractures lies in determining which fractures require reduction and which can be treated by simple immobilization. Reduction may be achieved with closed, percutaneous, intramedullary, or open techniques.[194,293,398] The second dilemma that arises with radial neck fractures is determining whether a reduction is acceptable or requires more aggressive treatment. Although O'Brien's classification system, based on the degree of initial angulation, provides vital information and is the most widely accepted, it does not assess all factors that must be considered when making treatment decisions regarding radial neck fractures. Other factors that must be considered include the amount of translation, the age of the patient, and the time elapsed since injury. Perhaps the most important aspect of treating fractures of the radial head and neck in children is for the surgeon to be aware and to educate the parents at the time of injury that significant loss of motion occurs in 30% to 50% of patients.[499,546]

Immobilization

Nondisplaced or minimally displaced fractures (<30 degrees of angulation, minimal translation) may be managed by simple immobilization of the elbow in a sling, posterior splint, or above-elbow cast for 1 to 2 weeks.[499] Because of the limited remodeling potential in children older than 10 years, we attempt closed reduction if more than 15 degrees of angulation is present.

Reduction

What constitutes an acceptable closed, percutaneous, or intramedullary reduction is unclear. A number of authors have reported poor results after open reduction of proximal radius fractures,[402,453,499,558,595] whereas others have shown that results correlate with the quality of reduction.[267,271,434,459,546,558] Not surprisingly, younger children (<10 years) have had better results after open reduction than have older children.[236,271,459] These retrospective studies have a selection bias in that fractures treated by an open technique are generally the most severely displaced and highest-energy injuries. Nevertheless, in reporting better results with closed treatment, Rang and associates believed that the results had more to do with the method of treatment than with the severity of injury.[453] To our knowledge, there are no good studies that have compared closed, percutaneous, intramedullary, and open techniques for similar injuries. We believe that it is probably wiser to leave some residual angulation (up to 45 degrees) than to introduce further soft tissue trauma with an open reduction.[134,402,580]

After successful closed, percutaneous, intramedullary, or open reduction, we usually immobilize the arm in a long-arm cast in neutral position or slight pronation for 2 to 3 weeks. Once the cast is removed, we encourage immediate active range of motion.

Closed Reduction. There are several techniques of closed reduction. Patterson is credited with describing a technique advocated by several subsequent authors.[431] The elbow is fully extended, which usually requires conscious sedation or general anesthesia. An assistant grasps the patient's arm proximal to the elbow joint and places his or her other hand medially over the patient's distal humerus to provide a medial fulcrum for applying a varus stress across the elbow. The surgeon applies distal traction with the forearm supinated to relax the supinators and biceps. Although forearm supination may facilitate relaxation of the supinator muscle, it may not be the best position for manipulation of the head fragment. Jeffrey realized that the tilt of the radial head can be anterior or posterior. He believed that the forearm should be rotated until the maximal tilt of the proximal fragment is felt laterally.[267] A varus force is then applied across the elbow to open up the lateral side of the joint, and the radial head is digitally manipulated back into position (Fig. 42–93). Neher and Torch described a variation of this technique in which an assistant applies a laterally directed force to the distal fragment while the surgeon applies varus force and digitally manipulates the radial head.[267]

Kaufman and colleagues have proposed another technique in which the elbow is manipulated in the flexed position. The thumb is pressed against the anterior surface of the radial head and the forearm is forced into pronation (Fig. 42–94).[289] Reduction has been reported after wrapping the extremity tightly, distally to proximally, with an elastic or Esmarch bandage (Fig. 42–95).[80,294]

Percutaneous and Intramedullary Reduction. In type II (30 to 60 degrees of angulation) and type III (>60 degrees of angulation) radial neck fractures we first attempt closed reduction under conscious sedation or general anesthesia. If we are unable to reduce the angulation to less than 30 degrees, we usually attempt percutaneous or intramedullary reduction. A number of authors have described using a K-wire to percutaneously "joystick" the proximal fragment into position.[46,131,183,451,468] When attempting a percutaneous joystick reduction it is important to avoid injury to the posterior interosseous nerve. The proximal fragment can often be manipulated directly from its subcutaneous position. If the distal fragment requires lateralization, we insert a "joker" as close as possible to the lateral aspect of the olecranon to avoid the posterior interosseous nerve (Fig. 42–96). Métaizeau and colleagues described reducing the radial neck by passing an intramedullary pin in a distal-to-proximal direction (Fig. 42–97).[195,349,371,499,547] This method has been successful when other manipulative techniques have failed. However, our experience is that percutaneous pin manipulation is technically easier than intramedullary reduction and generally produces equivalent results.

Open Reduction. Salter-Harris type III and IV injuries, as well as fractures that remain significantly angled after attempts at closed reduction and minimally invasive techniques, require open reduction. We perform an open reduction through a posterolateral

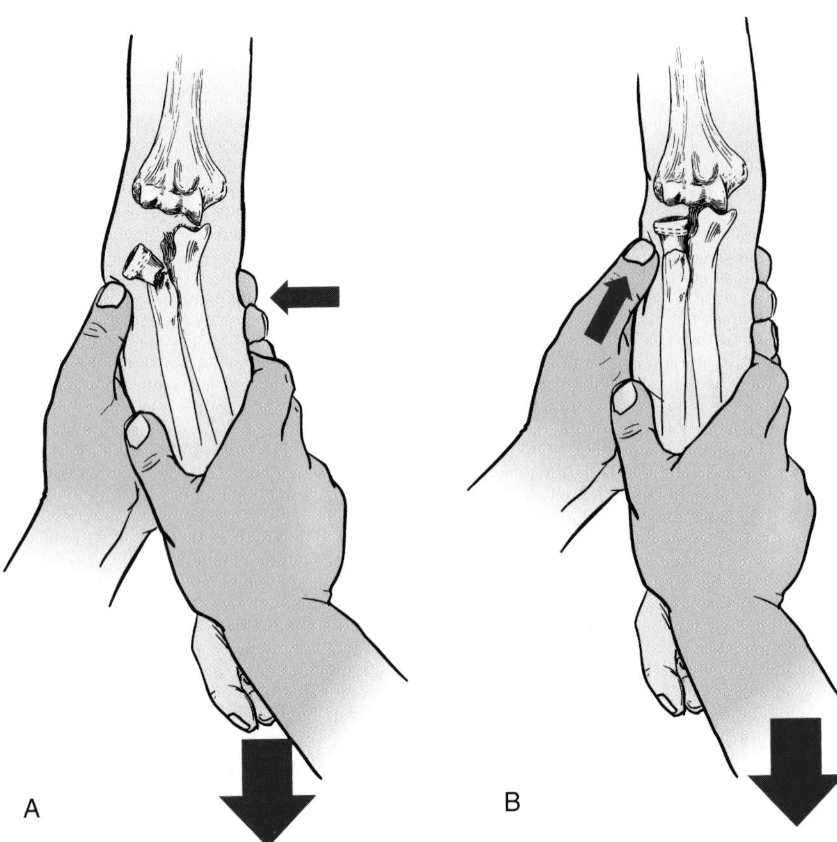

FIGURE 42–93 Technique for closed reduction of the radial head with the elbow in extension. **A,** With the elbow extended, traction and a varus force are applied. The forearm is pronated and supinated to maximize the lateral prominence. **B,** The radial head is digitally manipulated into position. Supination or pronation of the forearm may assist in the reduction.

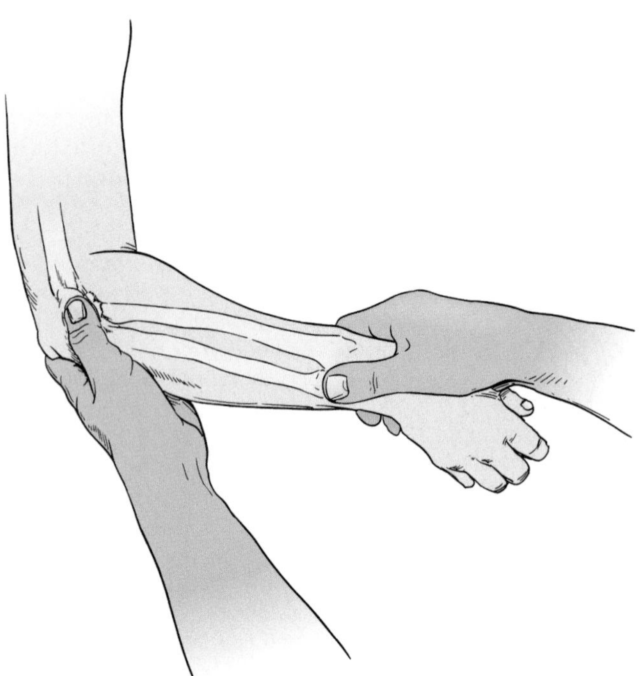

FIGURE 42–94 Technique for closed reduction of the radial head with the elbow in flexion. The forearm is forced into pronation, and the operator's thumb is used to digitally reduce the proximal fragment.

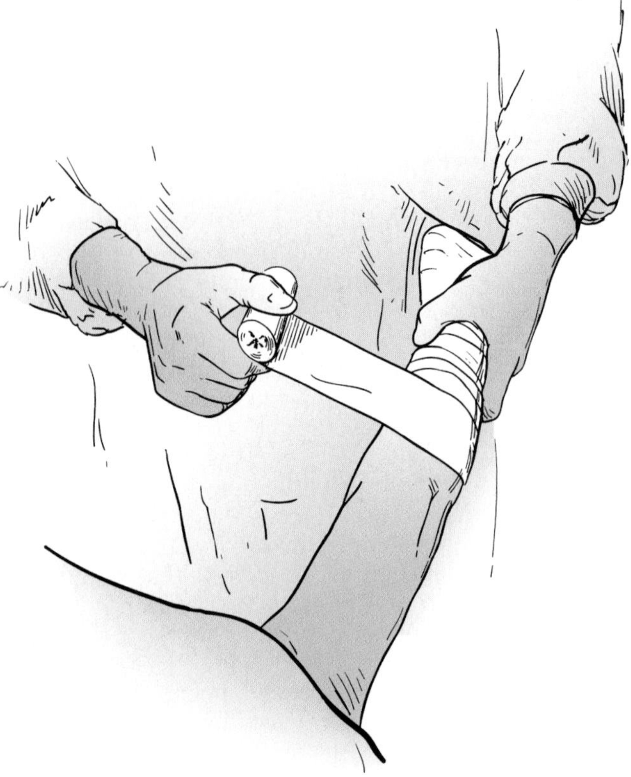

FIGURE 42–95 Reduction of a radial neck fracture has been reported after exsanguination of the extremity with an Esmarch bandage and the elbow in extension.

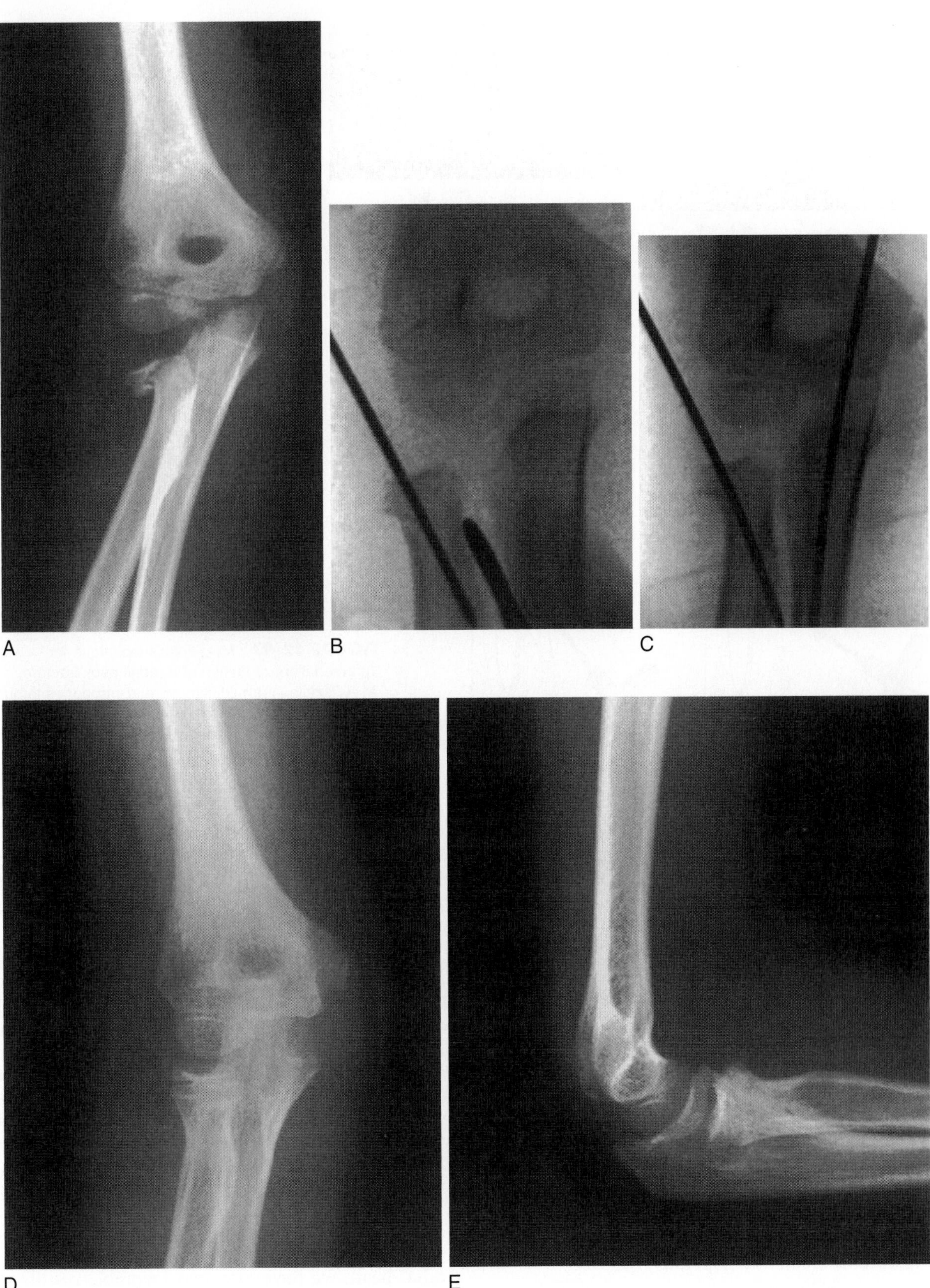

FIGURE 42–96 Percutaneous technique for reduction of radial neck fractures. **A,** Anteroposterior (AP) radiograph obtained at the time of injury showing a displaced radial neck fracture and an associated olecranon fracture. **B,** Intraoperative radiograph showing a percutaneous K-wire used to "joystick" the proximal radial fragment into position. Note that a "joker" has been placed along the lateral border of the ulna to help lateralize the distal fragment and reduce the radial neck. **C,** Both the radial and ulnar fractures are percutaneously fixed. AP **(D)** and lateral **(E)** radiographs obtained 18 months after injury. There is slight hypertrophy of the radial head.

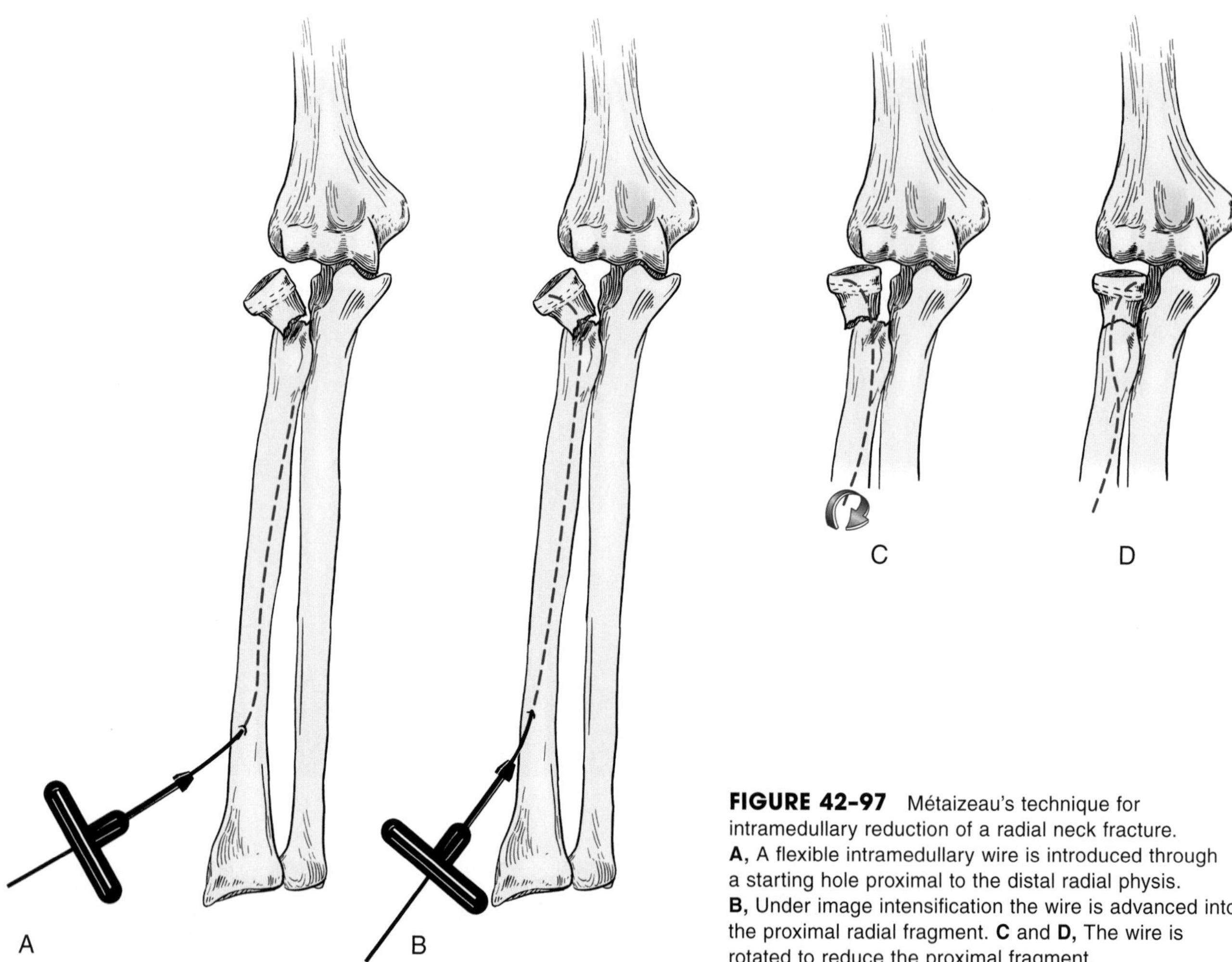

FIGURE 42–97 Métaizeau's technique for intramedullary reduction of a radial neck fracture. **A,** A flexible intramedullary wire is introduced through a starting hole proximal to the distal radial physis. **B,** Under image intensification the wire is advanced into the proximal radial fragment. **C** and **D,** The wire is rotated to reduce the proximal fragment.

approach with as little dissection as possible. A plane is developed between the anconeus and extensor carpi ulnaris muscles. Injury to the posterior interosseous nerve is avoided by staying posterior and positioning the forearm in full pronation. The capsule is divided and the elbow joint is entered. The orbicularis ligament is spared. Occasionally, the head will be subluxated inferior to the ligament. If so, it can usually be reduced with the ligament intact. Fixation is achieved with a K-wire placed percutaneously in a proximal-to-distal direction across the fracture site. Although there is controversy regarding the need for and technique of fixation after percutaneous or open reduction,[271,292,407,459] it is agreed that transcapitellar pins should be avoided.[157,402,595] Although Salter-Harris types III and IV fractures are uncommon (occurring in only 7 of 116 radial neck fractures),[326] Leung and Peterson noted that the prognosis is poor, particularly when the fracture is initially treated nonoperatively.[326]

Treatment of Late-Presenting Displaced Fractures

Management of late-presenting displaced fractures is difficult. Blount advised against attempting reduction after 5 days.[56] Others have reported poor results after longer delays.[371,402,471] Obviously, treatment decisions for late-identified fractures must be made on an individual basis. However, we generally favor a conservative course while remembering that the remodeling potential, particularly in patients younger than 10 years, is great (Fig. 42–98).

Radial Head Excision

The role of radial head excision is poorly defined. Classically, radial head excision has not been advocated in children because of concern regarding growth disturbance and wrist and elbow deformity.[27] Recently, however, Hresko and associates reported good or excellent results in 8 of 12 patients between 12 and 18 years of age who underwent radial head excision for post-traumatic radiocapitellar pain or stiffness. In no patients did cubitus valgus or wrist pain develop.[252] Generally, we favor an initially conservative approach to severe injuries of the radial head. Although we have been impressed by the remodeling potential of the radial head, we have also had favorable results with radial head excision in the rare patient with late pain or stiffness after radial head fracture.

COMPLICATIONS

Loss of joint motion is the most common and problematic complication after radial head and neck fractures.

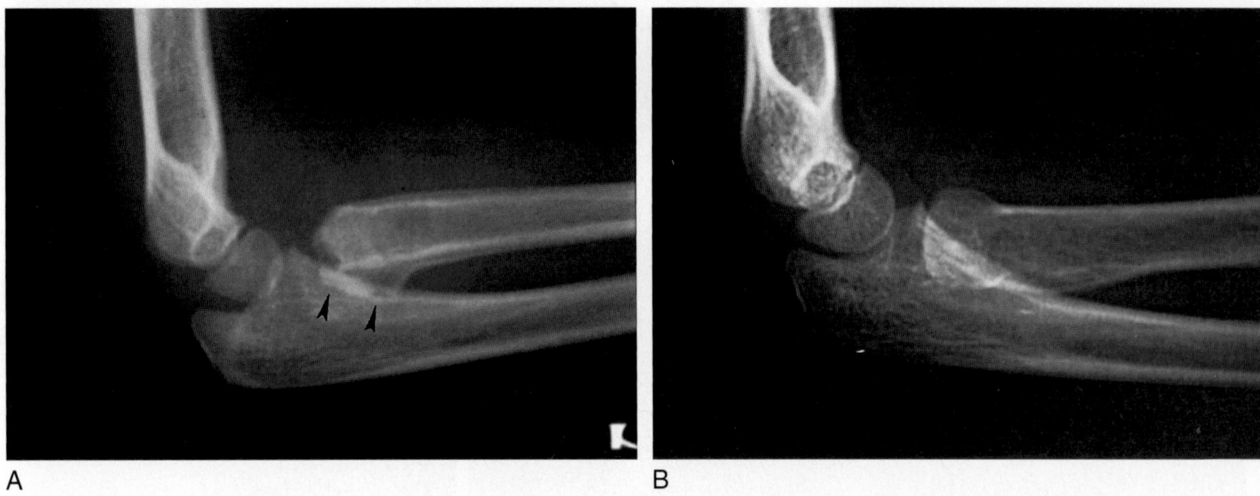

FIGURE 42–98 **A,** Lateral radiograph of the elbow of a 7-year-old girl 4 weeks after injury. The proximal radius is angled 80 degrees (*arrowheads*). There is significant healing, as evidenced by calcification within the intact periosteal sleeve. The patient was treated by observation. **B,** Lateral radiographs obtained 1 year after injury show significant remodeling of the radial head and neck.

Rotation of the forearm is primarily affected, with loss of pronation greater than loss of supination. Loss of motion may be caused by joint incongruity (malunion), enlargement of the radial head (overgrowth), AVN, fibrous adhesions, or proximal radioulnar synostosis. Loss of motion is more likely with (1) severely displaced fractures; (2) fractures associated with other injuries to the elbow, such as dislocation, avulsion of the medial epicondyle, rupture of the medial collateral ligament, or olecranon fracture; (3) patients older than 10 years; (4) a delay in effective treatment; and (5) the quality of reduction achieved.[499] A prudent surgeon should be aware of these risk factors and should forewarn the parents of children at greatest risk for the possibility of loss of forearm rotation.

As with all fractures, malunion results from failure either to achieve adequate reduction or to maintain reduction. Malunion of radial head and neck fractures is most commonly associated with loss of rotation of the forearm. AVN of the radial head develops after radial neck fractures because of its unique blood supply (see Fig. 40–7). AVN has been reported to occur after 10% to 20% of radial neck fractures and is almost always associated with significant loss of motion.[271,402,620] Both synostosis between the proximal radius and ulna[155,407,475] and myositis ossificans within the supinator muscle[572] have been reported to restrict range of motion after radial neck fractures.[109] Although nonunion of the radial neck has been reported, symptoms are generally mild or nonexistent,[536] and healing usually occurs when treated by prolonged immobilization.[80,496] When nonunion occurs, it is most commonly related to initial fracture displacement or inadequate reduction or fixation, or both. Surgical treatment of nonunion is unlikely to improve function.[590] Compartment syndrome has also been reported with fractures of the radial neck.[435]

Overgrowth of the radial head is presumably due to hypervascularity and stimulation of epiphyseal growth and occurs after up to 40% of radial neck fractures. Fortunately, there is rarely any functional deficit.[572] Premature fusion of the upper radial physis has been reported after up to 40% of radial neck fractures.[407,459] Theoretically, physeal arrest may produce shortening and valgus; however, clinical problems are infrequent.[402,407,459]

Olecranon Fractures

Fractures of the olecranon are relatively uncommon and account for only about 5% of elbow fractures.[312] They are associated with other elbow injuries (most commonly the medial epicondyle) in 20% to 50% of cases (Fig. 42–99; see also Fig. 42–96).[108,131,150,201,203,254,312,355] Surgical treatment is required in 10% to 20% of olecranon fractures.[148,178,203,355,401,428]

ANATOMY

Several anatomic factors make olecranon fractures less common and less severe in children than in adults. First, because the olecranon is predominantly cartilage, particularly in younger children, there is a smaller chance of a fracture's occurring with a direct blow to the olecranon. Second, the thick periosteum and relatively thin metaphyseal cortex of the olecranon predispose it to minimally displaced greenstick fractures (Fig. 42–100).

MECHANISM OF INJURY

Olecranon fractures are most often the result of a hyperextension injury. However, they may also be caused by a direct blow to the flexed elbow, a hyperflexion injury, or a shear force.[81] Hyperextension injuries are frequently associated with other elbow injuries. The direction of the associated coronal plane force will determine the corresponding injuries. A valgus hyperextension force may produce an associated radial neck or medial epicondyle fracture (see Figs. 42–96 and 42–99). A varus hyperextension injury

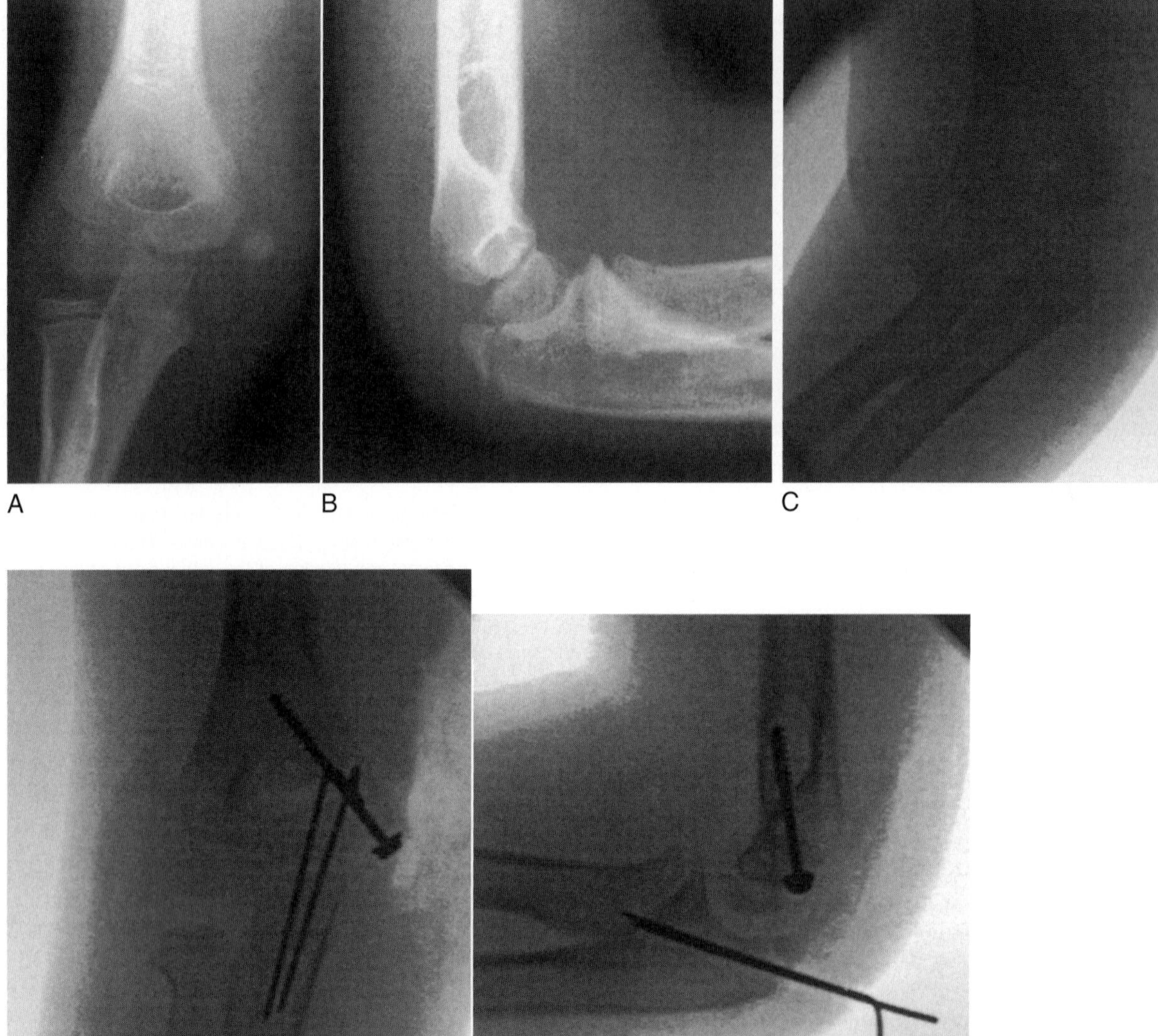

FIGURE 42-99 Anteroposterior **(A)** and lateral **(B)** radiographs of an olecranon fracture with an associated medial epicondyle fracture, the result of a valgus hyperextension injury (which may have been an elbow dislocation) that spontaneously reduced. **C,** Intraoperative stress radiograph showing significant valgus instability. **D** and **E,** The patient was treated by open reduction and internal fixation of the medial epicondyle fragment. Alignment of the olecranon was inspected through the medial incision, and the olecranon fracture was percutaneously pinned before fixation of the medial epicondyle.

may be associated with lateral dislocation of the radial head, a Bado type III Monteggia lesion.

Flexion injuries are usually caused by a fall on an outstretched hand with the elbow flexed. The fracture is the result of a strong eccentric contracture of the triceps in which the olecranon is pulled over the fulcrum of the distal humerus. These fractures are generally transverse (perpendicular to the axis of the ulna), are displaced posteriorly rather than anteriorly, and are rarely associated with other injuries.

Shear injuries are the least common and result from a force to the proximal ulna just anterior to the humeral condyles. The olecranon fractures through metaphyseal bone. The distal fragment is displaced anteriorly, and the radioulnar joint remains intact.

CLASSIFICATION

Unfortunately, nearly every series of olecranon fractures uses a unique classification scheme,[81,148,178,203,355,401,428] and none of these systems provides all the pertinent clinical information. We classify olecranon fractures similar to Graves and Canale[203] and Gaddy and colleagues.[178] Both of these systems describe fractures as either displaced or nondisplaced, although they use different thresholds (Graves and Canale, 5 mm; Gaddy and colleagues, 3 mm). Graves and Canale also have a third classification for open fractures. We believe that the pertinent information required to make sound clinical decisions includes whether the fracture is intra- or extra-articular, whether it is displaced or nondisplaced

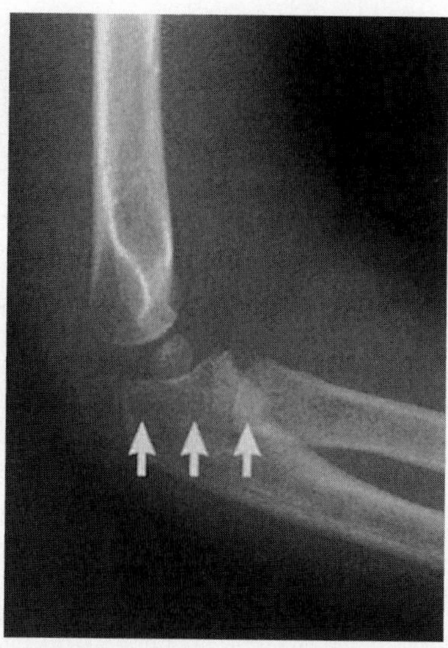

FIGURE 42–100 Lateral radiograph of a buckle fracture (*arrows*) through the metaphyseal bone of the olecranon.

(we favor Gaddy's threshold of 3 mm), and the presence and significance of associated elbow injuries.

DIAGNOSIS

Clinically, an olecranon fracture is most commonly manifested as a swollen elbow. An abrasion or contusion on the posterior aspect of the elbow may provide a clue to the nature of the injury. There may be a palpable defect posteriorly, as well as an inability to extend the elbow. When the olecranon apophysis is not ossified, the examiner may miss a fracture through the olecranon, especially if he or she is unaware of the ossification patterns of an immature elbow.[149] Once the diagnosis has been made, the patient and radiographs should be closely examined for associated injuries, including injuries to the radial head or neck, which have been noted to occur in a third of olecranon fractures.[190]

TREATMENT

Nondisplaced or minimally (3 mm or less) displaced fractures can generally be managed by simple cast immobilization for 3 to 4 weeks. If the fractures are displaced (>3 mm), extra-articular, and stable, they can usually be managed by closed reduction and cast immobilization.[77] This is typically the case for the rare shear-type fractures, which are generally quite stable in flexion. Flexion injuries may require immobilization in extension, which is often awkward and uncomfortable. Intra-articular fractures with more than 3 mm of displacement usually require open reduction and internal fixation. We generally use a standard pin and tension band technique for displaced olecranon fractures (Fig. 42–101).[190,287] Patients with osteogenesis imperfecta and displaced fractures usually require internal fixation and are prone to refracture after implant removal.[212,623] Recently, some authors have described fixation with absorbable implants as an alternative to pins and wires. They note fewer symptoms from hardware with this technique.[81,246] Gicquel has developed a threaded locking pin device that may prove useful for fixation of this fracture.[188,189] Occasionally, hyperextension injuries associated with other elbow fractures will remain unstable after treatment of the associated fracture. In these instances we frequently stabilize the olecranon with simple percutaneous pinning (see Figs. 42–96 and 42–99). In such cases, arthrography may help ensure adequate reduction.

COMPLICATIONS

Complications after olecranon fractures are uncommon. The most common complication of an olecranon fracture is failure to appreciate a concomitant injury. The other common complication after an olecranon fracture is stiffness. Fortunately, this is an unusual finding. Irreducible fractures, loss of reduction, delayed union and nonunion, peripheral nerve injury, and compartment syndrome have all been reported with olecranon fractures.[101,355,621]

Uncommon Elbow Fractures

T-CONDYLAR FRACTURES

Anatomy and Mechanism of Injury

Fractures that involve separation of the medial and lateral columns of the distal humerus from each other and from the humeral shaft are referred to as *T-condylar fractures.* These injuries almost universally result in disruption of the articular surface of the distal humerus and represent a complex reconstructive challenge. These fractures are rare in children. When they do occur, they are usually in adolescents or the result of high-energy trauma (or both).[3,288,427,457] Epright and Wilkins believe that this injury is the result of the olecranon's functioning as a wedge to split the distal humerus at the apex of the trochlea.[147] In adults, the force of the olecranon on the trochlea is greatest when the elbow is flexed 90 degrees or more.[368]

Classification

A number of classifications exist for these fractures in adults.[266,397,463,621] Toniolo and Wilkins have classified these injuries in children into three types.[563] Type I fractures have minimal displacement, type II fractures have displacement but no metaphyseal comminution, and type III fractures have displacement with comminution of the metaphysis.

Treatment

Treatment is directed toward restoring anatomic articular alignment and reestablishing the distal articular surface with the humeral shaft.

Closed Reduction and Percutaneous Pinning. In most type I fractures and in some younger patients with type II and type III fractures, this is possible with closed reduction and percutaneous pinning

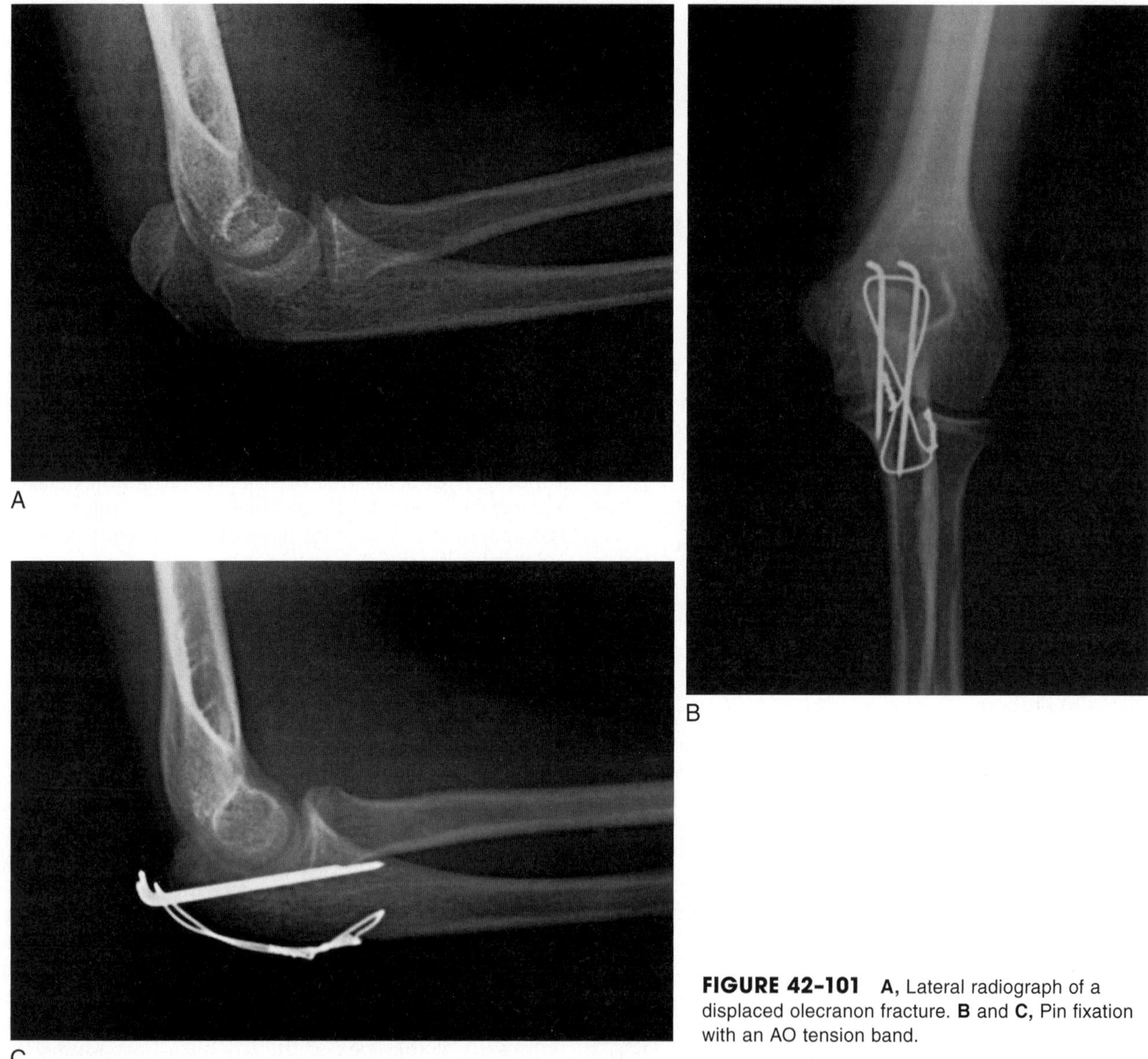

FIGURE 42–101 **A,** Lateral radiograph of a displaced olecranon fracture. **B** and **C,** Pin fixation with an AO tension band.

(Fig. 42–102).[3,281,478] In type I injuries with an intact soft tissue envelope, simple traction may produce adequate reduction through ligamentotaxis. If this is the case, we percutaneously secure the condyles one to another with a transverse pin or screw. The distal fragment can then be secured to the proximal fragment by the same technique as for supracondylar humeral fractures. If traction alone does not reduce the articular surfaces, they may be manipulated percutaneously with large bone reduction forceps; however, if this fails to anatomically reduce the articular surface, open reduction will be required. In younger patients, the largely cartilaginous distal humeral epiphysis may make assessment of the articular surface difficult. In such cases, stress radiography or arthrography may be helpful in assessing the joint surface.[41]

Open Reduction and Internal Fixation. Most patients with types II and III injuries and patients with type I injuries in whom anatomic reduction of the articular surface cannot be achieved with closed or percutaneous techniques require open reduction with rigid internal fixation. A number of different surgical approaches have been described.[41] Although the triceps-splitting approach is the most widely discussed in the literature and the triceps-sparing posterior medial approach has gained recent popularity, we favor a posterior approach with an olecranon osteotomy.[68,275,276,288,291,362,427,457,585] We have found that this approach gives wide surgical exposure, allows rigid fixation, and permits early mobilization. Because most of our experience with these injuries has been in older adolescents, we have not had problems or concerns with the proximal ulnar apophysis. Re and colleagues recently reported improved range of motion (particularly extension) in children and adolescents treated with the posteromedial or olecranon osteotomy approaches.[457]

Once anatomic restoration of the distal humeral articular surface has been achieved, rigid fixation of the articular surface to the humeral shaft must be

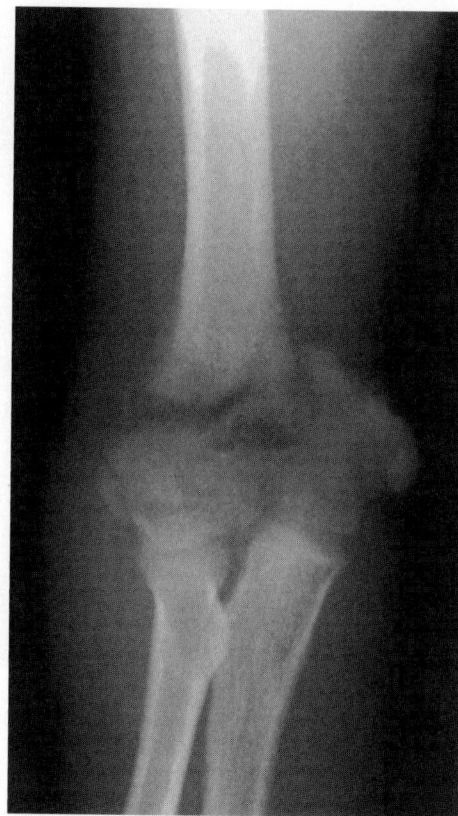

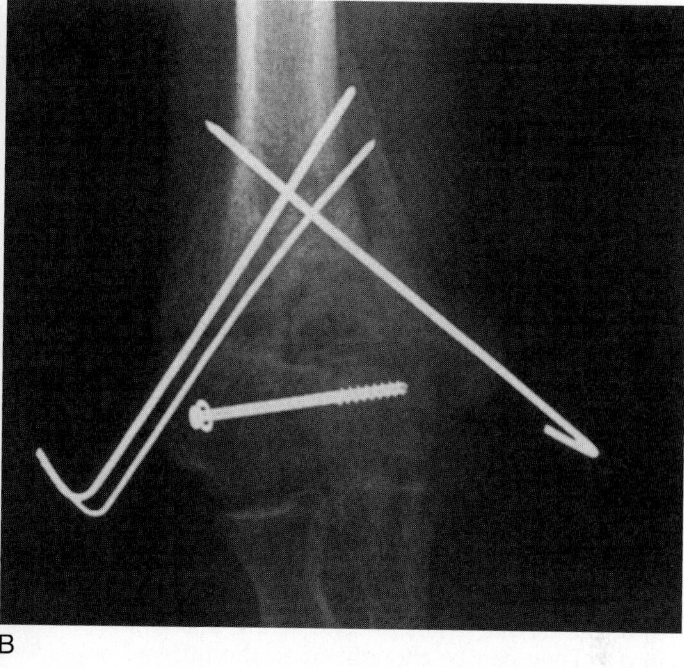

FIGURE 42–102 **A**, Anteroposterior (AP) radiograph of a displaced T-condylar distal humeral fracture **B**, AP radiograph obtained after reduction. The distal fragments were reduced and fixed with a cannulated screw. The distal fragments were then pinned to the proximal fragment.

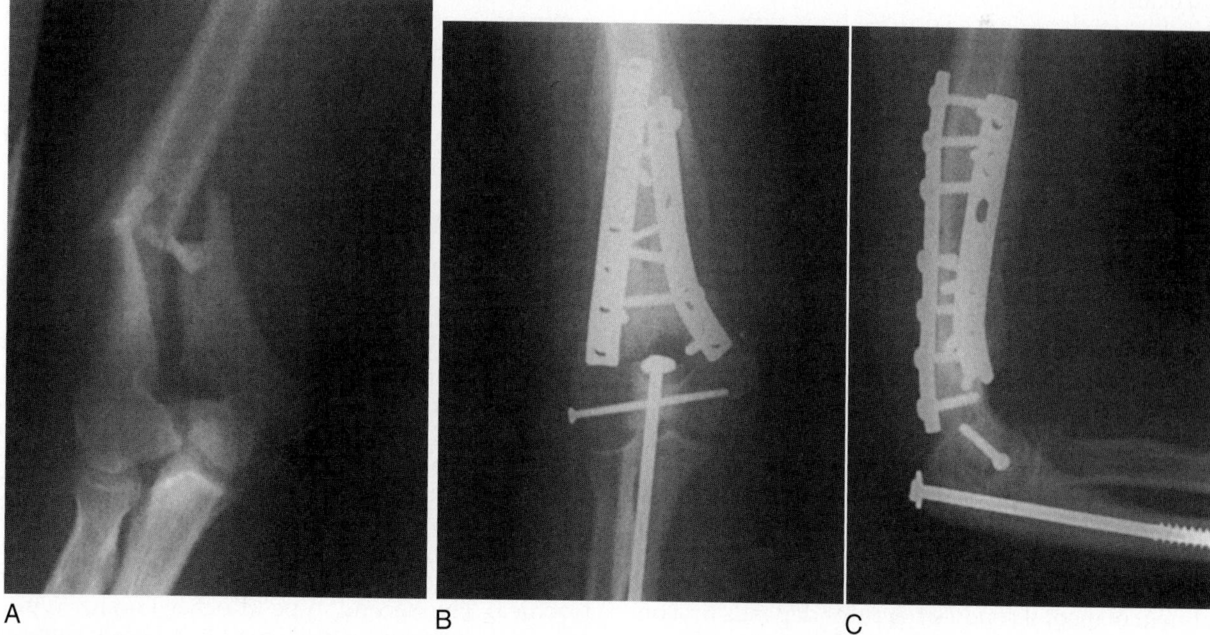

FIGURE 42–103 **A**, Displaced T-condylar distal humeral fracture. Anteroposterior **(B)** and lateral **(C)** radiographs after open reduction and internal fixation through a posterior approach with an olecranon osteotomy and medial and posterior plates.

ensured. Numerous reports in the adult literature have analyzed the problems associated with fixation of these fractures. Current recommendations are for double-plate fixation of the distal fragment to the shaft. One plate should be placed posterior on the lateral column and one medial. Positioning the plates at right angles to each other provides maximum strength (Fig. 42–103). Compression or pelvic reconstruction plates should be used, but thin one-third tubular plates have been found to be inadequate.[231,275,301,362,488,491,498,598]

Complications

The most common complication of T-condylar fractures is stiffness.[275,288,291,362,427,457,498] The likelihood of some permanent loss of motion with these injuries is so high that we counsel the parents preoperatively that the goal of treatment is to *minimize* the stiffness. This can best be accomplished by using rigid internal fixation and minimizing immobilization. Recent reports have shown continuous passive motion in the immediate postoperative period to be beneficial by improving range of motion.[457] As with elbow dislocations, however, it is important that early motion be active rather than passive because overaggressive therapy may exacerbate the stiffness. Failure of internal fixation, nonunion, and AVN of the trochlea have also been reported as complications.[288,427]

MEDIAL CONDYLE FRACTURES

Anatomy and Mechanism of Injury

Fractures of the medial humeral condyle are uncommon injuries. They can be thought of as the mirror image of the more common lateral condyle fracture, not only radiographically but also with respect to classification, treatment, and potential complications. They are thought to be the result of either a direct posterior blow to a flexed elbow[45,79,95,97,100,225,443] or avulsion from a valgus hyperextension injury.[45,143,169]

Classification

There are several ways to classify medial condyle fractures. Milch classified them according to the location of the fracture line. In type I injuries the fracture exits at the trochlear notch. In type II injuries the fracture extends more laterally through the capitellar ossification center.[377] Medial condyle fractures can also be classified as physeal fractures according to the system of Salter and Harris.[486] Like lateral condyle fractures, medial condyle fractures originate in the metaphysis, cross the physis, and exit through the epiphysis into the joint, thus making them Salter-Harris type IV injuries. Finally, medial condyle fractures can be classified according to the amount of displacement.[45,143,296,425] We use a modification of Kilfoyle's classification to describe these fractures as nondisplaced (traditionally <2 mm), minimally displaced (traditionally 2 to 4 mm), or displaced (traditionally >4 mm).[296]

Treatment and Complications

Treatment of medial condyle fractures depends first on making an accurate diagnosis, which may be difficult with this uncommon fracture.[45,111,143,151,169,225,230,490,578] Once an accurate diagnosis has been made, treatment is determined by the amount of displacement (Fig. 42–104). Nondisplaced and minimally displaced fractures can be treated by simple cast immobilization. There is insufficient experience with this injury to know how frequently late displacement of minimally displaced fractures occurs. It is known that this fracture, like lateral condyle fractures, may not unite. Thus,

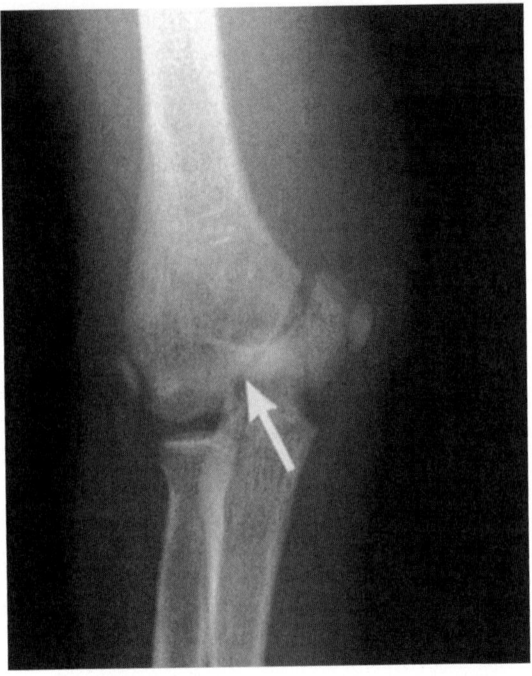

FIGURE 42–104 Displaced medial condyle fracture. Note the intra-articular displacement (*arrow*).

it is important to monitor minimally displaced fractures closely to ensure that further displacement and delayed union or nonunion do not develop. Displaced fractures require open reduction and percutaneous fixation.[45,143,150,169,256,296,425,443]

Complications after medial condyle fracture occur in up to 33% of cases and include stiffness, ulnar neuropathy, delayed union, and nonunion with cubitus varus deformity.[60,80,100,199,222,296,323,578]

CAPITELLAR FRACTURES

Anatomy and Mechanism of Injury

Fractures of the capitellum are rare in children and occur most commonly in adolescents.* Because the capitellum is nearly all cartilaginous, it is resistant to stress and difficult to fracture; therefore, a fall on an outstretched hand is more likely to produce a supracondylar or lateral condyle fracture.[6,16,168,202,270,317,329,589]

Two fracture patterns have been described. The more common type (Hahn-Steinthal type[216]) contains a significant portion of metaphyseal bone from the lateral condyle and, often, the lateral crista of the trochlea. The second type (Kocher-Lorenz type) is even less common in children.[6] It is nearly pure articular cartilage with little or no subchondral or metaphyseal bone. It may be associated with underlying osteochondritis dissecans. Recently, anterior sleeve fractures of the capitellum or trochlea, or both, have been described. Even though a sleeve fracture involves more humerus than capitellum, in principle it func-

*See references 98, 102, 135, 138, 168, 202, 270, 325, 340, 408, 445.

tions as a type II capitellar fracture.[6,133,549] Some authors have described the occasional comminuted fracture as a type III injury.[202]

Treatment

Although most reports of capitellar fractures have been in adults, a few studies have addressed the injury in children.[94,135,138,325,461,479,494] Treatment guidelines can be gained from both the adult and pediatric literature. Frequently, the most difficult aspect of managing capitellar fractures is making the diagnosis.[509] This is particularly true for type II fractures, which have little bone attached to the articular surface. Although some groups have described closed treatment of capitellar fractures,[340,408] we believe that these intra-articular injuries require open reduction and fixation if displaced. Open reduction is usually best accomplished through a posterior or Kocher approach. A variety of implants have been used for fracture fixation, including percutaneous pins, AO screws, Herbert screws, and bioabsorbable pins.* If the fragment is particularly small or if the articular surface is extremely comminuted, excision is a better option than attempts at fixation.[16,138,168,187,365] In general, the results after capitellar fractures are good, although significant stiffness occasionally develops.[135,349,592]

CORONOID FRACTURES

Coronoid fractures are most commonly associated with elbow dislocations and are therefore frequently associated with fractures of the medial epicondyle, olecranon, proximal radius, and lateral condyle. They may also occur in isolation as a result of avulsion from the brachialis. These fractures are rarely displaced and usually require no treatment other than what is appropriate for the associated injuries. Occasionally, a larger fragment is displaced, thus rendering the elbow unstable and requiring open reduction.[179]

TROCHLEAR FRACTURES

True isolated fractures of the trochlea are uncommon. In one report of which we are aware, the fracture is associated with dislocation.[200] There have been a few reports of a concomitant fracture of the anterior trochlea and capitellum.[258,414,549] Treatment of these injuries must be individualized, but open reduction with fixation is usually required because of the intra-articular nature of the injury.

LATERAL EPICONDYLE FRACTURES

In a literature review encompassing 5228 fractures of the distal humerus, Chambers and Wilkins could find only one case of fracture of the lateral epicondylar apophysis.[82] Thus, lateral epicondyle fracture may be the least common children's elbow fracture. The irregular ossification of the secondary ossification center makes the diagnosis of lateral epicondyle fractures difficult. The lateral condylar apophysis ossifies laterally to medially, which creates a space between the secondary ossification center and the metaphysis that can be misinterpreted as a displaced fracture.[510] To correctly diagnose lateral epicondylar pathology, the physician must carefully evaluate the soft tissues, both clinically and radiographically, because trauma generally is associated with noticeable swelling.[82] Comparison views of the opposite elbow may also be helpful. The few reports that deal with lateral epicondyle fractures describe good results with symptomatic treatment despite the development of a fibrous union.[364,411] Entrapment of the fragment has been noted and is the only indication for surgery.[364,592]

*See references 16, 133, 138, 168, 202, 240, 246, 325, 338, 344, 349, 433, 445.

Associated Conditions

NURSEMAID'S ELBOW (PULLED ELBOW, TRAUMATIC SUBLUXATION OF THE RADIAL HEAD)

Pulled elbow or *nursemaid's elbow* refers to traumatic subluxation of the radial head produced by sudden traction on the hand with the elbow extended and the forearm pronated (Fig. 42–105). Hippocrates is said to have recognized the condition, although the first written description did not appear until 1671.[166,573]

Pulled elbow is one of the most common musculoskeletal injuries in children younger than 4 years and is rarely, if ever, found in children older than 5 years. The peak incidence is between the ages of 1 and 3 years.[59,70,175,226,254,330,343,366,481,487,548]

Subluxation of the radial head is possible because of the anatomy of the proximal radius.[343,366,481,487,548] The radial head is actually oval rather than circular. When the forearm is supinated, the anterior aspect of the radial head is elevated sharply from the neck; thus, if traction is applied with the forearm in supination, the annular ligament is pulled against this sharp bony elevation. However, laterally and posteriorly, the radial head rises rather gradually, so when traction is applied with the forearm in pronation, the radial head escapes from under the anterior portion of the annular ligament, which in turn becomes interposed between the radial head and the capitellum when traction is removed. In children 5 years or older, subluxation of the radial head is prevented by a thicker and stronger distal attachment of the annular ligament to the periosteum of the radial neck.[366,487,548]

The diagnosis is made from the history and clinical examination. Immediately after the injury, the child cries with pain and refuses to use the affected limb. A click may have been heard or felt in the child's elbow by the person who pulled it. The child holds the elbow by the side in slight flexion with the forearm pronated and may complain of wrist or elbow pain. If the child is calm and cooperative, passive flexion and extension of the elbow may be possible, but supination of the forearm is limited and voluntarily resisted. Radiographs of the elbow are normal. There is no

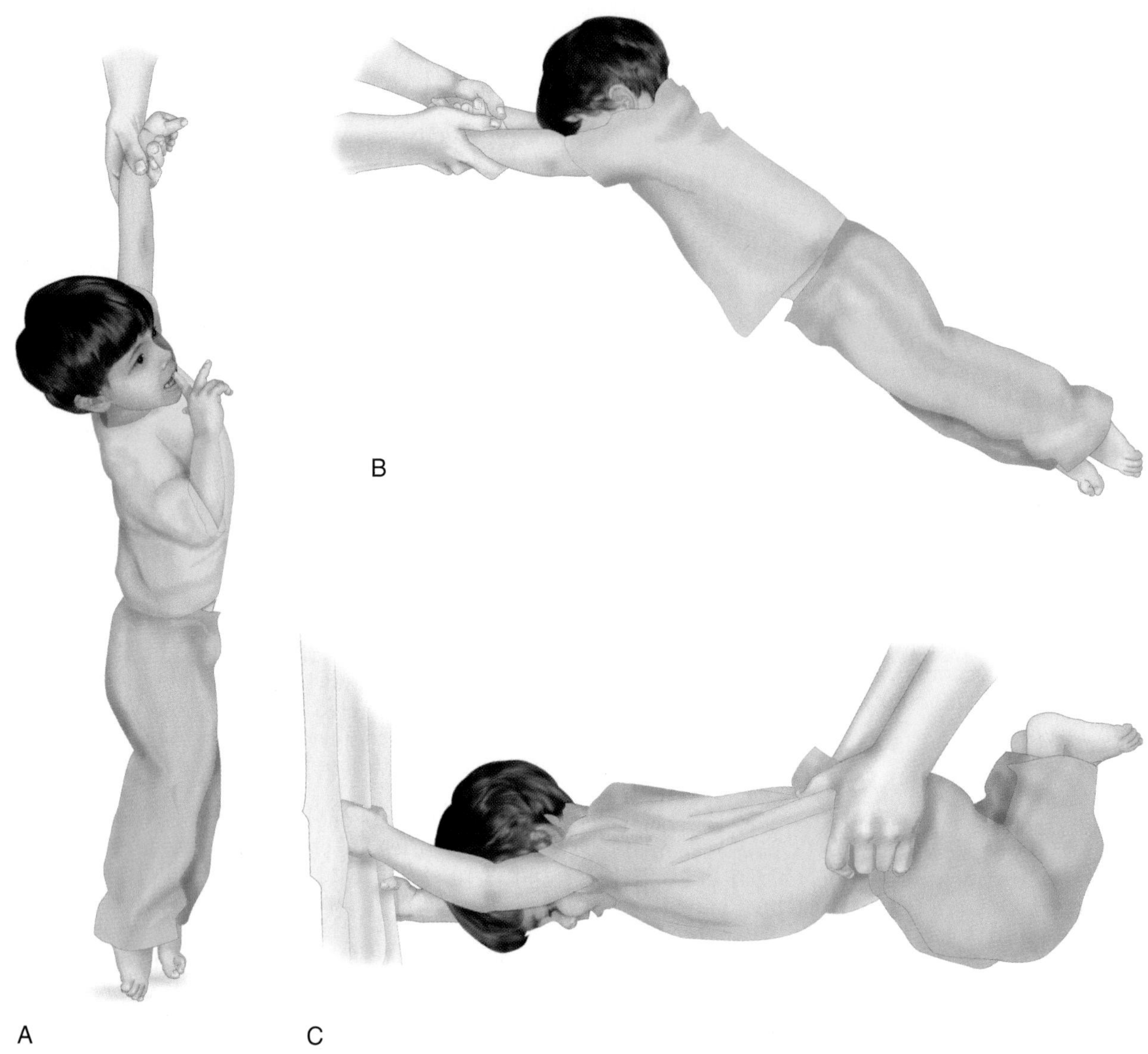

FIGURE 42-105 **A** to **C**, Common mechanisms resulting in nursemaid's (pulled) elbow.

displacement of the proximal radius from the capitellum and no evidence of intra-articular effusion.[343,366,481,487] The history is so classic that the condition can be diagnosed and treated remotely.[283]

Reduction is often unknowingly performed by the x-ray technician, who passively forces the forearm into full supination in an attempt to obtain a true AP projection of the elbow. If the child escapes such treatment, the radial head is reduced by flexing the elbow to 90 degrees and rapidly and firmly rotating the forearm into full supination. As reduction is achieved, a palpable and sometimes audible click can be felt in the region of the radial head. The child should begin to use the arm in a normal manner within minutes. Immobilization is not necessary after reduction. However, the parents should be educated that recurrence, which is seen in about 5% of cases, is preventable by avoiding pulling on the child's hand.

Occasionally, a child has a neglected subluxation that has been present for more than 24 hours. These patients may not have immediate relief with reduction and may benefit from a long-arm cast in supination for 1 to 2 weeks. It is important to be certain of the diagnosis before immobilizing the arm because occult elbow sepsis may also have a history of injury and a flexed, pronated arm. Rarely, a child has multiple chronic recurrences. In addition to thorough education of the caretakers, these children may benefit from 3 to 6 weeks in a long-arm cast with the forearm supinated.

Osteochondroses of the Elbow

Panner first described a lesion in the epiphysis of the capitellum similar to Legg-Calvé-Perthes disease in 1927.[422] In 1964 Smith reviewed the literature and proposed that Panner's disease was a self-limiting condition that was nontraumatic in origin.[527] Since that time, a number of different osteochondroses about the elbow have been described, most of which seem to be related to repetitive stress.* For discussion purposes we will consider three different entities: Panner's disease, osteochondritis dissecans of the capitellum, and other overuse injuries of the elbow.

Panner's Disease

The entity described by Panner and subsequently referred to as *Panner's disease* affects children younger than 10 years and is associated with pain and stiffness in the elbow. These patients do not have constitutional symptoms and rarely have a history of trauma. There may be a flexion contracture and diffuse synovitis. Radiographically, the capitellum will show irregular areas of radiolucency with areas of sclerosis. The radial head may be enlarged and appear skeletally advanced, and an effusion may be noted. Histologic studies of Panner's disease have documented focal areas of AVN with repair and revascularization. The articular cartilage has been noted to be normal.†

Treatment usually consists of reassurance, activity restrictions, and nonsteroidal anti-inflammatory drugs (NSAIDs). Occasionally, extremely symptomatic patients benefit from a period of immobilization in a splint or cast if the symptoms fail to resolve with conservative measures. We recommend arthroscopy to assess the articular cartilage. If the articular surface is intact, antegrade or retrograde drilling of the epiphyseal subchondral bone may stimulate healing. If there is a full-thickness articular cartilage defect with intra-articular loose bodies, we remove the loose bodies and drill the subchondral bone either arthroscopically or through an arthrotomy. It should be stressed that surgical treatment of patients with Panner's disease is extremely uncommon.[69,88,224,232,302,314,319,348,413,422,423,449,527]

Osteochondritis Dissecans of the Capitellum

Osteochondritis dissecans of the capitellum is distinguished from Panner's disease in that it occurs in older children, is usually associated with overhead athletes (most commonly baseball players and gymnasts), and is more likely to require surgical treatment. As with Panner's disease, the initial symptoms are typically pain, stiffness, and occasionally mechanical symptoms.‡ Radiographically, osteochondritis dissecans of the capitellum cannot be distinguished from Panner's disease (Fig. 42–106) other than by the skeletal age of the patient. Although CT, MRI, and ultrasound have all been used in the management of osteochondritis dissecans, we have not found that these imaging studies influence our clinically based decision process.[67,174,245]

Schenck and colleagues have proposed a repetitive microtrauma mechanism for the development of osteochondritis dissecans of the capitellum.[492] In a cadaver study, they noted that the central section of the radial head was significantly stiffer than the lateral capitellum. Presumably, the disparity in the mechanical properties of the central radial head and lateral capitellum would increase strain in the lateral capitellum. During activities associated with high valgus stress, such as throwing, this increased strain may be a factor in the development of osteochondritis dissecans of the elbow.[492]

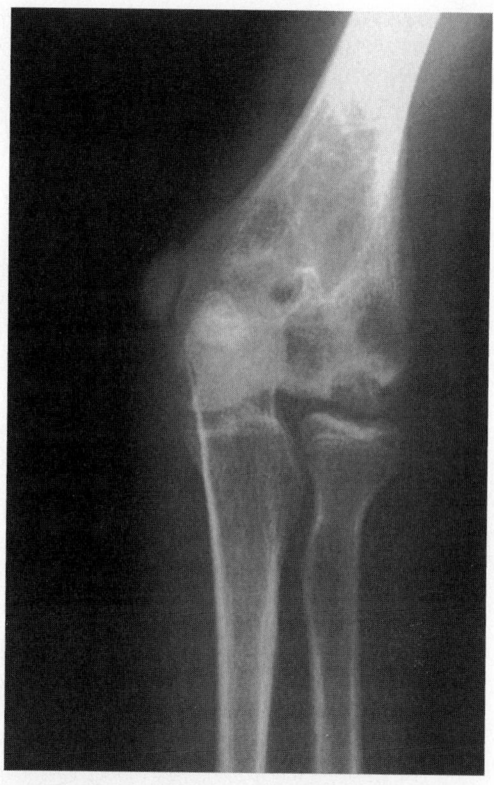

FIGURE 42-106 Anteroposterior radiograph demonstrating osteonecrosis of the capitellum in a 13-year-old.

Initial treatment of osteochondritis dissecans is similar to that for Panner's disease, with an emphasis on activity modification. Patients in whom conservative treatment fails can be treated with arthroscopy for assessment of articular cartilage, followed by drilling and loose body fixation or excision. Reports of fixation of loose osteochondral fragments with Herbert screws or bone pegs are encouraging.[257,309,412] Results after surgical treatment are generally good,[365,437,477,514,560,609] although some authors report an inability to return to high-level competition.[37,83,263] Despite good short-term results, permanent deformity and disability can develop. A number of studies have documented permanent changes in the radial head, presumably the result of growth stimulation because of hypervascularity. The radial head has also been noted to dislocate over time.[35,83,303,477,577] Two long-term studies (17- and 23-year follow-up) reported pain and decreased motion in half the patients with osteochondritis dissecans as adolescents.[35,553]

*See references 5, 35, 37, 63, 66, 146, 263, 309, 332, 334, 338, 365, 383, 412, 437, 465, 477, 514, 552, 553, 560, 566, 568, 575, 612.

†See references 69, 88, 224, 232, 302, 314, 319, 348, 413, 422, 423, 449, 527.

‡See references 5, 63, 146, 332, 334, 383, 465, 566, 568, 612.

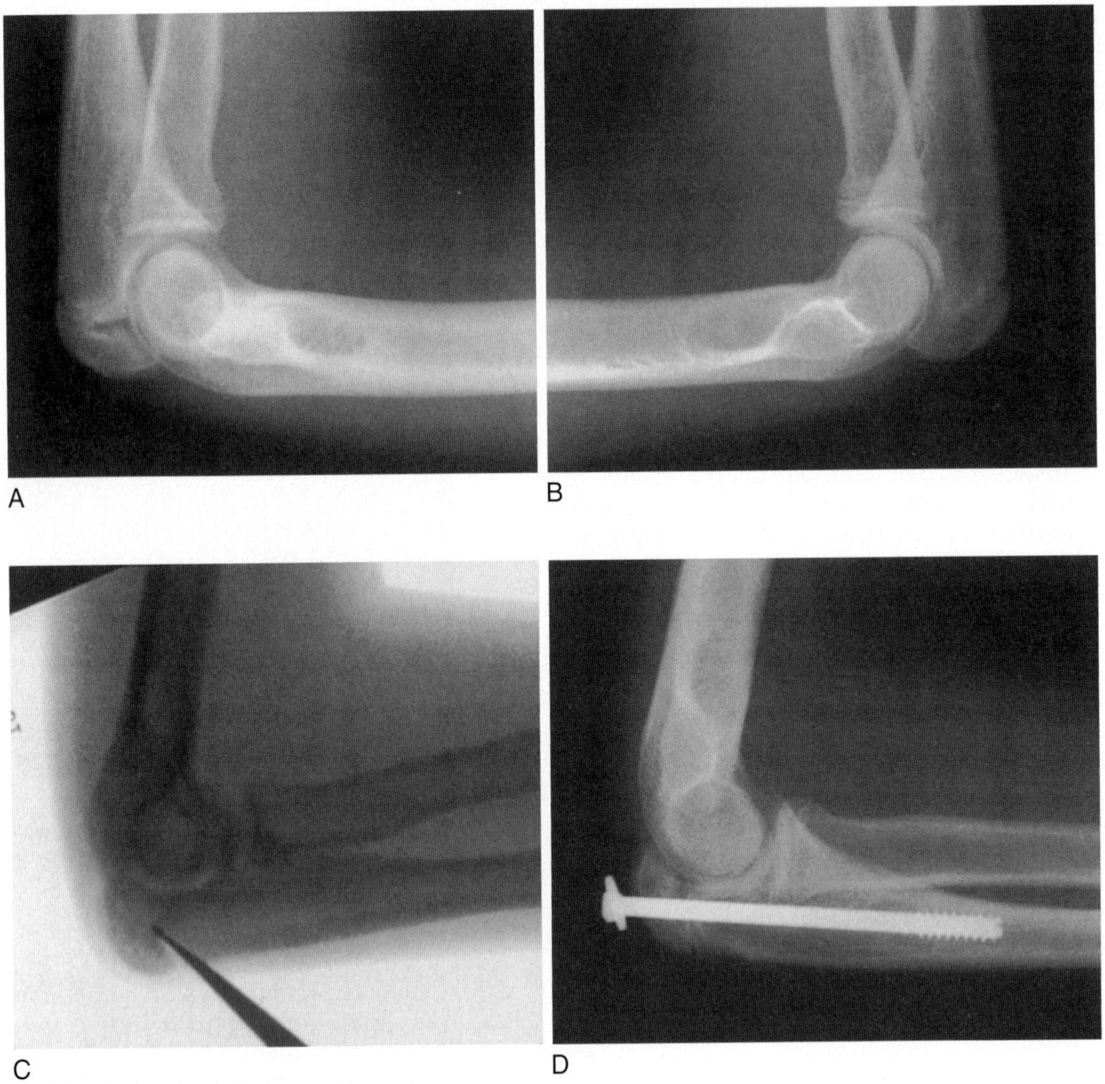

A

B

C

D

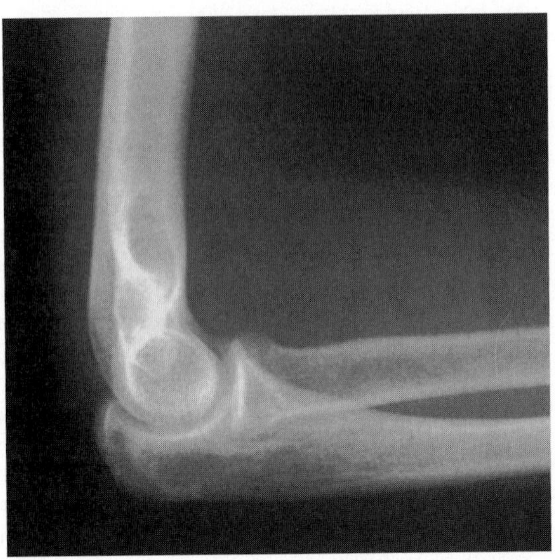

E

FIGURE 42–107 Little League elbow resulting from olecranon apophysitis. **A,** Lateral radiograph of a symptomatic right elbow in a 13-year-old pitcher. Note that the right elbow has an open apophysis and sclerosis on both sides of the apophysis. **B,** Lateral radiograph of an asymptomatic left elbow in the same patient. Note that only the symptomatic right elbow **(A)** has an open apophysis and sclerosis. **C** and **D,** The patient was treated by apophysiodesis and screw fixation. **E,** The symptoms resolved and the patient returned to pitching after screw removal.

Other Osteochondroses about the Elbow

The term *Little League elbow* has been used to describe a multitude of lesions about the elbow, most commonly osteochondritis dissecans of the capitellum, but also Panner's disease, osteochondritis of the trochlea and radial head, and epiphysiolysis of the medial epicondyle and olecranon (Fig. 42–107).[83,209,338,365,432,565] The casual application of this term is unfortunate in that it accurately describes neither the pathology nor the mechanism. These overuse syndromes can be seen in any overhead athlete. Patients usually have localized pain that is activity related. Radiographs may be normal or may reveal characteristic changes consistent with osteonecrosis or epiphysiolysis. Treatment consists of NSAIDs and activity modification. Young athletes may require immobilization to ensure compliance with rigid activity restrictions. Once symptoms have abated, a carefully designed, well-controlled return to athletics should be implemented.

References

Fractures about the Elbow

1. Ababneh M, Shannak A, Agabi S, et al: The treatment of displaced supracondylar fractures of the humerus in children. A comparison of three methods. Int Orthop 1998;22:263.
2. Abe M, Ishizu T, Nagaoka T, et al: Epiphyseal separation of the distal end of the humeral epiphysis: A follow-up note. J Pediatr Orthop 1995;15:426.
3. Abraham E, Gordon A, Abdul-Hadi O: Management of supracondylar fractures of humerus with condylar involvement in children. J Pediatr Orthop 2005;25:709.
4. Abraham E, Powers T, Witt P, et al: Experimental hyperextension supracondylar fractures in monkeys. Clin Orthop Relat Res 1982;171:309.
5. Adams JE: Injury to the throwing arm. A study of traumatic changes in the elbow joints of boy baseball players. Calif Med 1965;102:127.
6. Agins HJ, Marcus NW: Articular cartilage sleeve fracture of the lateral humeral condyle capitellum: A previously undescribed entity. J Pediatr Orthop 1984;4:620.
7. Aitken AP, Childress HM: Intra-articular displacement of the internal epicondyle following dislocation. J Bone Joint Surg 1938;20:161.
8. Aitken AP, Smith L, Blackett CW: Supracondylar fractures in children. Am J Surg 1943;59:161.
9. Akbarnia BA, Akbarnia NO: The role of orthopedist in child abuse and neglect. Orthop Clin North Am 1976;7:733.
10. Akbarnia BA, Silberstein MJ, Rende RJ, et al: Arthrography in the diagnosis of fractures of the distal end of the humerus in infants. J Bone Joint Surg Am 1986;68:599.
11. Albert E: Lehrbuch der Chirurgie and Operationslehre, zweite Auflage, vol II. Wien, Urban & Schwarzenberg, 1881.
12. Alburger PD, Weidner PL, Betz RR: Supracondylar fractures of the humerus in children. J Pediatr Orthop 1992;12:16.
13. Allen PD, Gramse AE: Transcondylar fractures of the humerus treated by Dunlop traction. Am J Surg 1945;67:217.
14. Allende G, Freytes M: Old dislocation of the elbow. J Bone Joint Surg 1944;26:691.
15. Altuntas AO, Balakumar J, Howells RJ, et al: Posterior divergent dislocation of the elbow in children and adolescents: A report of three cases and review of the literature. J Pediatr Orthop 2005;25:317.
16. Alvarez E, Patel MR, Nimberg G, et al: Fracture of the capitulum humeri. J Bone Joint Surg Am 1975;57:1093.
17. Andersen K, Mortensen AC, Gron P: Transverse divergent dislocation of the elbow. A report of two cases. Acta Orthop Scand 1985;56:442.
18. Arino VL, Lluch EE, Ramirez AM, et al: Percutaneous fixation of supracondylar fractures of the humerus in children. J Bone Joint Surg Am 1977;59:914.
19. Aronson DC, Meeuwis JD: Anterior exposure for open reduction of supracondylar humeral fractures in children: A forgotten approach? Eur J Surg 1994;160:263.
20. Aronson DD, Prager BI: Supracondylar fractures of the humerus in children. A modified technique for closed pinning. Clin Orthop Relat Res 1987;219:174.
21. Asher MA: Dislocations of the upper extremity in children. Orthop Clin North Am 1976;7:583.
22. Ashhurst AP: An Anatomical and Surgical Study of Fractures of the Lower End of the Humerus. Philadelphia, Lea & Febiger, 1910.
23. Aufranc OE, Jones WN, Bierbaum BE: Open supracondylar fracture of the humerus. JAMA 1969;208:682.
24. Aufranc OE, Jones WN, Turner RH: Dislocation of the elbow with brachial artery injury. JAMA 1966;197:719.
25. Badelon O, Bensahel H, Mazda K, et al: Lateral humeral condylar fractures in children: A report of 47 cases. J Pediatr Orthop 1988;8:31.
26. Badhe NP, Howard PW: Olecranon screw traction for displaced supracondylar fractures of the humerus in children. Injury 1998;29:457.
27. Baehr FH: Removal of the separated upper epiphysis of the radius. N Engl J Med 1932;24:1263.
28. Bailey GGJ: Nerve injuries in supracondylar fractures of the humerus in children. N Engl J Med 1939;221:260.
29. Bakalim G, Wilppula E: Supracondylar humeral fractures in children. Causes of changes in the carrying angle of the elbow. Acta Orthop Scand 1972;43:366.
30. Barrett IR, Bellemore MC, Kwon YM: Cosmetic results of supracondylar osteotomy for correction of cubitus varus. J Pediatr Orthop 1998;18:445.
31. Barrett WP, Almquist EA, Staheli LT: Fracture separation of the distal humeral physis in the newborn. J Pediatr Orthop 1984;4:617.
32. Barton KL, Kaminsky CK, Green DW, et al: Reliability of a modified Gartland classification of supracondylar humerus fractures. J Pediatr Orthop 2001;21:27.
33. Bast SC, Hoffer MM, Aval S: Nonoperative treatment for minimally and nondisplaced lateral humeral condyle fractures in children. J Pediatr Orthop 1998;18:448.
34. Battaglia TC, Armstrong DG, Schwend RM: Factors affecting forearm compartment pressures in children

with supracondylar fractures of the humerus. J Pediatr Orthop 2002;22:431.
35. Bauer M, Jonsson K, Josefsson PO, et al: Osteochondritis dissecans of the elbow. A long-term follow-up study. Clin Orthop Relat Res 1992;284:156.
36. Baumann E: [Mutilation of hand and arm with Volkmann's ischemic contracture following a compound Monteggia fracture treated by circular plaster cast (author's transl).] Ther Umsch 1973;30:877.
37. Baumgarten TE, Andrews JR, Satterwhite YE: The arthroscopic classification and treatment of osteochondritis dissecans of the capitellum. Am J Sports Med 1998;26:520.
38. Beals RK: The normal carrying angle of the elbow. A radiographic study of 422 patients. Clin Orthop Relat Res 1976;119:194.
39. Beasley RW, Cooley SGE, Flatt AE: The hand and upper extremity. In Littler JW (ed): Reconstructive Plastic Surgery: Principles and Procedures in Correction, Reconstruction, and Transplantation, vol 6. Philadelphia, WB Saunders, 1977, p 3131.
40. Bede WB, Lefebure AR, Rosmon MA: Fractures of the medial humeral epicondyle in children. Can J Surg 1975;18:137.
41. Beghin JL, Bucholz RW, Wenger DR: Intercondylar fractures of the humerus in young children. A report of two cases. J Bone Joint Surg Am 1982;64:1083.
42. Bellemore MC, Barrett IR, Middleton RW, et al: Supracondylar osteotomy of the humerus for correction of cubitus varus. J Bone Joint Surg Br 1984;66:566.
43. Bender J: Cubitus varus after supracondylar fracture of the humerus in children: Can this deformity be prevented? Reconstr Surg Traumatol 1979;17:100.
44. Bender J, Busch CA: Results of treatment of supracondylar fractures of the humerus in children with special reference to the cause and prevention of cubitus varus. Arch Chir Neerl 1978;30:29.
45. Bensahel H, Csukonyi Z, Badelon O, et al: Fractures of the medial condyle of the humerus in children. J Pediatr Orthop 1986;6:430.
46. Bernstein SM, McKeever P, Bernstein L: Percutaneous reduction of displaced radial neck fractures in children. J Pediatr Orthop 1993;13:85.
47. Beverly MC, Fearn CB: Anterior interosseous nerve palsy and dislocation of the elbow. Injury 1984;16:126.
48. Bhuller GS, Connolly JF: Ipsilateral supracondylar fractured humerus and fractured radius. Nebr Med J 1982;67:85.
49. Bittner S, Newberger EH: Pediatric understanding of child abuse and neglect. Pediatr Rev 1981;2:197.
50. Biyani A, Gupta SP, Sharma JC: Ipsilateral supracondylar fracture of humerus and forearm bones in children. Injury 1989;20:203.
51. Blakemore LC, Cooperman DR, Thompson GH, et al: Compartment syndrome in ipsilateral humerus and forearm fractures in children. Clin Orthop Relat Res 2000;376:32.
52. Blanco JS: Ulnar nerve palsies after percutaneous cross-pinning of supracondylar fractures in children's elbows. J Pediatr Orthop 1998;18:824.
53. Blanquart D, Hoeffel JC, Galloy MA, et al: [Separation of the distal humeral epiphysis in young children. Radiologic features.] Ann Pediatr (Paris) 1990;37:470.
54. Blatz DJ: Anterior dislocation of the elbow. Orthop Rev 1981;10:129.
55. Blount WP: Unusual fractures in children. Instr Course Lect 1954;7:57.
56. Blount WP: Fractures in Children. Baltimore, Williams & Wilkins, 1955.
57. Boccanera L, Mohovich F: [Treatment of post-traumatic cubitus varus and cubitus valgus.] Minerva Ortop 1967;18:114.
58. Boyd HB, Altenberg AR: Fractures about the elbow in children. Arch Surg 1944;49:213.
59. Boyette BP, Ahoskie NC, London AHJ: Subluxation of the head of the radius, "nursemaid's elbow." J Pediatr 1939;32:278.
60. Brandberg R: Treatment of supracondylar fractures by reduction followed by fixation in plaster splint. Acta Chir Belg 1939;82:400.
61. Brewster AH, Karp M: Fractures in the region of the elbow in children. Surg Gynecol Obstet 1940;71:643.
62. Brodeur AE, Silberstein MJ, Graviss ER, et al: Three-tier rare-earth imaging system. AJR Am J Roentgenol 1981;136:755.
63. Brogdon BG, Crow NE: Little Leaguer's elbow. AJR Am J Roentgenol 1960;93:671.
64. Broudy AS, Jupiter J, May JWJ: Management of supracondylar fracture with brachial artery thrombosis in a child: Case report and literature review. J Trauma 1979;19:540.
65. Brown IC, Zinar DM: Traumatic and iatrogenic neurological complications after supracondylar humerus fractures in children. J Pediatr Orthop 1995;15:440.
66. Brown R, Blazina ME, Kerlan RK, et al: Osteochondritis of the capitellum. J Sports Med 1974;2:27.
67. Bruns J, Lussenhop S: [Ultrasound imaging of the elbow joint. Loose joint bodies and osteochondrosis dissecans.] Ultraschall Med 1993;14:58.
68. Bryan RS, Morrey BF: Extensive posterior exposure of the elbow. A triceps-sparing approach. Clin Orthop Relat Res 1982;166:188.
69. Busch E: Et tilfaelde af Panners Sygdom. Ugeskr Laeger 1930;92:720.
70. Caldwell CE: Subluxation of the radial head by elongation. Cincinnati Lancet Clin 1891;66:496.
71. Camp J, Ishizue K, Gomez M, et al: Alteration of Baumann's angle by humeral position: Implications for treatment of supracondylar humerus fractures. J Pediatr Orthop 1993;13:521.
72. Campbell CC, Waters PM, Emans JB, et al: Neurovascular injury and displacement in type III supracondylar humerus fractures. J Pediatr Orthop 1995;15:47.
73. Carcassonne M, Bergoin M, Hornung H: Results of operative treatment of severe supracondylar fractures of the elbow in children. J Pediatr Surg 1972;7:676.
74. Carey RP: Simultaneous dislocation of the elbow and the proximal radio-ulnar joint. J Bone Joint Surg Br 1984;66:254.
75. Carlioz H, Abols Y: Posterior dislocation of the elbow in children. J Pediatr Orthop 1984;4:8.

76. Case SL, Hennrikus WL: Surgical treatment of displaced medial epicondyle fractures in adolescent athletes. Am J Sports Med 1997;25:682.
77. Caterini R, Farsetti P, D'Arrigo C, et al: Fractures of the olecranon in children. Long-term follow-up of 39 cases. J Pediatr Orthop B 2002;11:320.
78. Caviglia H, Garrido CP, Palazzi FF, et al: Pediatric fractures of the humerus. Clin Orthop Relat Res 2005; 432:49.
79. Chacha PB: Fracture of the medical condyle of the humerus with rotational displacement. Report of two cases. J Bone Joint Surg Am 1970;52:1453.
80. Chambers HG, Wilkins K: Fractures of the neck and head of the radius. In Rockwood CA Jr, Wilkins K, Beaty J (eds): Fractures in Children, vol 3. Philadelphia, Lippincott-Raven, 1996, p 586.
81. Chambers HG, Wilkins K: Fractures of the olecranon. In Rockwood CA Jr, Wilkins K, Beaty J (eds): Fractures in Children, vol 3. Philadelphia, Lippincott-Raven, 1996, p 613.
82. Chambers HG, Wilkins K: Apophyseal injuries of the distal humerus. In Rockwood CA Jr, Wilkins K, Beaty J (eds): Fractures in Children, vol 3. Philadelphia, Lippincott-Raven, 1996, p 819.
83. Chan D, Aldridge MJ, Maffulli N, et al: Chronic stress injuries of the elbow in young gymnasts. Br J Radiol 1991;64:1113.
84. Chand K: Epiphyseal separation of distal humeral epiphysis in an infant. A case report and review of literature. J Trauma 1974;14:521.
85. Chapman VM, Grottkau BE, Albright M, et al: Multidetector computed tomography of pediatric lateral condylar fractures. J Comput Assist Tomogr 2005;29:842.
86. Cheng JC, Lam TP, Maffulli N: Epidemiological features of supracondylar fractures of the humerus in Chinese children. J Pediatr Orthop B 2001;10:63.
87. Cheng JC, Lam TP, Shen WY: Closed reduction and percutaneous pinning for type III displaced supracondylar fractures of the humerus in children. J Orthop Trauma 1995;9:511.
88. Chiroff RT, Cooke CP 3rd: Osteochondritis dissecans: A histologic and microradiographic analysis of surgically excised lesions. J Trauma 1975;15:689.
89. Chotel F, Vallese P, Parot R, et al: Complete dislocation of the radial head following fracture of the radial neck in children: The Jeffery type II lesion. J Pediatr Orthop B 2004;13:268.
90. Chung MS, Baek GH: Three-dimensional corrective osteotomy for cubitus varus in adults. J Shoulder Elbow Surg 2003;12:472.
91. Ciaudo O, Huguenin P, Bensahel H: [Recurrent dislocation of the elbow (author's transl).] Rev Chir Orthop Reparatrice Appar Mot 1982;68:207.
92. Clement DA: Assessment of a treatment plan for managing acute vascular complications associated with supracondylar fractures of the humerus in children. J Pediatr Orthop 1990;10:97.
93. Cohn I: Forward dislocation of both bones of the forearm at the elbow. Surg Gynecol Obstet 1922;35: 776.
94. Collert S: Surgical management of fracture of the capitulum humeri. Acta Orthop Scand 1977;48:603.
95. Conn J, Wade PA: Injuries of the elbow: A ten-year review. J Trauma 1961;1:248.
96. Conner AN, Smith MG: Displaced fractures of the lateral humeral condyle in children. J Bone Joint Surg Br 1970;52:460.
97. Cooper AP: A Treatise on Dislocations and Fractures of the Joints. Boston, Lilly, Wait, Carter & Hendee, 1832.
98. Cooper SA: Fracture of the external condyle of the humerus. In Lee AC (ed): A Treatise on Dislocations and Fractures of the Joints. London, Joseph Butler, 1841.
99. Copley LA, Dormans JP, Davidson RS: Vascular injuries and their sequelae in pediatric supracondylar humeral fractures: Toward a goal of prevention. J Pediatr Orthop 1996;16:99.
100. Cothay DM: Injury to the lower medial epiphysis of the humerus before development of the ossific centre. Report of a case. J Bone Joint Surg Br 1967;49:766.
101. Cotton FJ: Separation of the epiphysis of the olecranon. Boston Med Surg J 1900:692.
102. Cotton FJ: Elbow fractures in children. Ann Surg 1902;35:262.
103. Cotton FJ: Elbow dislocation and ulnar nerve injury. J Bone Joint Surg 1929;11:348.
104. Cramer KE, Devito DP, Green NE: Comparison of closed reduction and percutaneous pinning versus open reduction and percutaneous pinning in displaced supracondylar fractures of the humerus in children. J Orthop Trauma 1992;6:407.
105. Cramer KE, Green NE, Devito DP: Incidence of anterior interosseous nerve palsy in supracondylar humerus fractures in children. J Pediatr Orthop 1993;13:502.
106. Cregan JC: Prolonged traumatic arterial spasm after supracondylar fracture of the humerus. J Bone Joint Surg Br 1951;33:363.
107. Crosby EH: Elbow dislocations reduced by traction in four different directions. J Bone Joint Surg 1936;18: 1077.
108. Daland EM: Fractures of the olecranon. J Bone Joint Surg 1933;15:601.
109. Dale GG, Harris WR: Prognosis of epiphysial separation: An experimental study. J Bone Joint Surg Br 1958; 40:116.
110. D'Ambrosia RD: Supracondylar fractures of humerus—prevention of cubitus varus. J Bone Joint Surg Am 1972;54:60.
111. Dangles C, Tylkowski C, Pankovich AM: Epicondylotrochlear fracture of the humerus before appearance of the ossification center. A case report. Clin Orthop Relat Res 1982;171:161.
112. Danielsson LG: Median nerve entrapment in elbow dislocation. A case report. Acta Orthop Scand 1986;57: 450.
113. Davids JR, Maguire MF, Mubarak SJ, et al: Lateral condylar fracture of the humerus following posttraumatic cubitus varus. J Pediatr Orthop 1994;14:466.
114. De Boeck H: Surgery for nonunion of the lateral humeral condyle in children. 6 cases followed for 1-9 years. Acta Orthop Scand 1995;66:401.
115. De Boeck H: Flexion-type supracondylar elbow fractures in children. J Pediatr Orthop 2001;21:460.

116. De Boeck H, De Smet P: Valgus deformity following supracondylar elbow fractures in children. Acta Orthop Belg 1997;63:240.
117. De Boeck H, De Smet P, Penders W, et al: Supracondylar elbow fractures with impaction of the medial condyle in children. J Pediatr Orthop 1995;15:444.
118. de Jager LT, Hoffman EB: Fracture-separation of the distal humeral epiphysis. J Bone Joint Surg Br 1991; 73:143.
119. de las Heras J, Duran D, de la Cerda J, et al: Supracondylar fractures of the humerus in children. Clin Orthop Relat Res 2005;432:57.
120. DeLee JC: Transverse divergent dislocation of the elbow in a child. Case report. J Bone Joint Surg Am 1981;63: 322.
121. DeLee JC, Wilkins KE, Rogers LF, et al: Fracture-separation of the distal humeral epiphysis. J Bone Joint Surg Am 1980;62:46.
122. Denis R, Guilleret F: Supracondyloid fractures of the elbow irreducible by external maneuvers. Lyon Chir 1940;36:620.
123. DeRosa GP, Graziano GP: A new osteotomy for cubitus varus. Clin Orthop Relat Res 1988;236:160.
124. Devito DP, Blackstock S, Minkowitz B: Non-operative treatment of lateral condyle elbow fractures in children. Orthop Trans 1995;20:306.
125. Devnani AS: Lateral closing wedge supracondylar osteotomy of humerus for post-traumatic cubitus varus in children. Injury 1997;28:643.
126. Devnani AS: Late presentation of supracondylar fracture of the humerus in children. Clin Orthop Relat Res 2005;431:36.
127. Dhillon KS, Sengupta S, Singh BJ: Delayed management of fracture of the lateral humeral condyle in children. Acta Orthop Scand 1988;59:419.
128. Dias JJ, Johnson GV, Hoskinson J, et al: Management of severely displaced medial epicondyle fractures. J Orthop Trauma 1987;1:59.
129. Dias JJ, Lamont AC, Jones JM: Ultrasonic diagnosis of neonatal separation of the distal humeral epiphysis. J Bone Joint Surg Br 1988;70:825.
130. Dodge HS: Displaced supracondylar fractures of the humerus in children—treatment by Dunlop's traction. J Bone Joint Surg Am 1972;54:1408.
131. Dormans JP, Rang M: Fractures of the olecranon and radial neck in children. Orthop Clin North Am 1990; 21:257.
132. Dormans JP, Squillante R, Sharf H: Acute neurovascular complications with supracondylar humerus fractures in children. J Hand Surg [Am] 1995; 20:1.
133. Drvaric DM, Rooks MD: Anterior sleeve fracture of the capitellum. J Orthop Trauma 1990;4:188.
134. D'Souza S, Vaishya R, Klenerman L: Management of radial neck fractures in children: A retrospective analysis of one hundred patients. J Pediatr Orthop 1993;13:232.
135. Duguet B, Le Saout J: [Capitellum fractures of children (author's transl).] Chir Pediatr 1980;21:331.
136. Dunlop J: Traumatic separation of medial epicondyle of humerus adolescence. J Bone Joint Surg 1935;17: 577.
137. Dunlop J: Separation of medial epicondyle of humerus: Case with displaced upper radial epiphysis. J Bone Joint Surg 1935;17:584.
138. Dushuttle RP, Coyle MP, Zawadsky JP, et al: Fractures of the capitellum. J Trauma 1985;25:317.
139. Duun PS, Ravn P, Hansen LB, et al: Osteosynthesis of medial humeral epicondyle fractures in children. 8-year follow-up of 33 cases. Acta Orthop Scand 1994;65: 439.
140. Ebong WW: Gangrene complicating closed posterior dislocation of the elbow. Int Surg 1978;63:44.
141. Edman P, Lohr G: Supracondylar fractures of the humerus treated with olecranon traction. Acta Chir Scand 1963;126:505.
142. Eichler GR, Lipscomb PR: The changing treatment of Volkmann's ischemic contractures from 1955 to 1965 at the Mayo Clinic. Clin Orthop Relat Res 1967;50:215.
143. El Ghawabi MH: Fracture of the medial condyle of the humerus. J Bone Joint Surg Am 1975;57:677.
144. Eliason EL, Brown RB: Posterior dislocation at the elbow with rupture of the radial and ulnar arteries. Ann Surg 1937;106:1111.
145. Elstrom JA, Pankovich AM, Kassab MT: Irreducible supracondylar fracture of the humerus in children. A report of two cases. J Bone Joint Surg Am 1975;57:680.
146. Elward JF: Epiphysitis of the capitellum of the humerus. JAMA 1939;112:705.
147. Epright RH, Wilkins KE: Fractures and dislocations of the elbow. In Rockwood CA Jr, Green DP (eds): Fractures in Adults. Philadelphia, JB Lippincott, 1975, p 487.
148. Evans MC, Graham HK: Olecranon fractures in children: Part 1: A clinical review; Part 2: A new classification and management algorithm. J Pediatr Orthop 1999;19:559.
149. Fabry J, De Smet L, Fabry G: Consequences of a fracture through a minimally ossified apophysis of the olecranon. J Pediatr Orthop B 2000;9:212.
150. Fahey JJ: Fractures of the elbow in children. Instr Course Lect 1960;17:13.
151. Fahey JJ, O'Brien ET: Fracture-separation of the medial humeral condyle in a child confused with fracture of the medial epicondyle. J Bone Joint Surg Am 1971; 53:1102.
152. Fairbanks HAT, Buxton SJD: Displacement of the internal epicondyle into the elbow joint. Lancet 1934;2:218.
153. Farnsworth CL, Silva PD, Mubarak SJ: Etiology of supracondylar humerus fractures. J Pediatr Orthop 1998;18:38.
154. Farsetti P, Potenza V, Caterini R, et al: Long-term results of treatment of fractures of the medial humeral epicondyle in children. J Bone Joint Surg Am 2001;83:1299.
155. Fielding JW: Radio-ulnar crossed union following displacement of the proximal radial epiphysis. A case report. J Bone Joint Surg Am 1964;46:1277.
156. Finnbogason T, Karlsson G, Lindberg L, et al: Nondisplaced and minimally displaced fractures of the lateral humeral condyle in children: A prospective radiographic investigation of fracture stability. J Pediatr Orthop 1995;15:422.
157. Fischer M, Maroske D: [The broken Kirschner wire as a complication of transarticular fixation of the neck

of the radius in children (author's transl).] Unfallheilkunde 1976;79:277.
158. Fleuriau-Chateau P, McIntyre W, Letts M: An analysis of open reduction of irreducible supracondylar fractures of the humerus in children. Can J Surg 1998; 41:112.
159. Flynn JC: Nonunion of slightly displaced fractures of the lateral humeral condyle in children: An update. J Pediatr Orthop 1989;9:691.
160. Flynn JC, Matthews JG, Benoit RL: Blind pinning of displaced supracondylar fractures of the humerus in children. Sixteen years' experience with long-term follow-up. J Bone Joint Surg Am 1974;56:263.
161. Flynn JC, Richards JF Jr: Non-union of minimally displaced fractures of the lateral condyle of the humerus in children. J Bone Joint Surg Am 1971;53:1096.
162. Flynn JC, Richards JF Jr, Saltzman RI: Prevention and treatment of non-union of slightly displaced fractures of the lateral humeral condyle in children. An end-result study. J Bone Joint Surg Am 1975;57:1087.
163. Foead A, Penafort R, Saw A, et al: Comparison of two methods of percutaneous pin fixation in displaced supracondylar fractures of the humerus in children. J Orthop Surg (Hong Kong) 2004;12:76.
164. Fontanetta P, Mackenzie DA, Rosman M: Missed, maluniting, and malunited fractures of the lateral humeral condyle in children. J Trauma 1978;18:329.
165. Foster DE, Sullivan JA, Gross RH: Lateral humeral condylar fractures in children. J Pediatr Orthop 1985;5:16.
166. Fournier D: L'Oeconomic Chirurgical. Paris, Françoise Clouzier, 1671.
167. Fowles JV, Kassab MT: Displaced supracondylar fractures of the elbow in children. A report on the fixation of extension and flexion fractures by two lateral percutaneous pins. J Bone Joint Surg Br 1974;56:490.
168. Fowles JV, Kassab MT: Fracture of the capitulum humeri. Treatment by excision. J Bone Joint Surg Am 1974;56:794.
169. Fowles JV, Kassab MT: Displaced fractures of the medial humeral condyle in children. J Bone Joint Surg Am 1980;62:1159.
170. Fowles JV, Kassab MT, Douik M: Untreated posterior dislocation of the elbow in children. J Bone Joint Surg Am 1984;66:921.
171. Fowles JV, Kassab MT, Moula T: Untreated intra-articular entrapment of the medial humeral epicondyle. J Bone Joint Surg Br 1984;66:562.
172. Fowles JV, Slimane N, Kassab MT: Elbow dislocation with avulsion of the medial humeral epicondyle. J Bone Joint Surg Br 1990;72:102.
173. Friedman RJ, Jupiter JB: Vascular injuries and closed extremity fractures in children. Clin Orthop Relat Res 1984;188:112.
174. Fritz RC: MR imaging of osteochondral and articular lesions. Magn Reson Imaging Clin N Am 1997;5:579.
175. Frumkin K: Nursemaid's elbow: A radiographic demonstration. Ann Emerg Med 1985;14:690.
176. Fujioka H, Nakabayashi Y, Hirata S, et al: Analysis of tardy ulnar nerve palsy associated with cubitus varus deformity after a supracondylar fracture of the humerus: A report of four cases. J Orthop Trauma 1995;9:435.
177. Gaddy BC, Manske PR, Pruitt DL, et al: Distal humeral osteotomy for correction of posttraumatic cubitus varus. J Pediatr Orthop 1994;14:214.
178. Gaddy BC, Strecker WB, Schoenecker PL: Surgical treatment of displaced olecranon fractures in children. J Pediatr Orthop 1997;17:321.
179. Gadgil A, Roach R, Neal N, et al: Isolated avulsion fracture of the coronoid process requiring open reduction in a paediatric patient: A case report. Acta Orthop Belg 2002;68:396.
180. Galbraith KA, McCullough CJ: Acute nerve injury as a complication of closed fractures or dislocations of the elbow. Injury 1979;11:159.
181. Galleno H, Oppenheim WL: The battered child syndrome revisited. Clin Orthop Relat Res 1982;162:11.
182. Gartland JJ: Management of supracondylar fractures of the humerus in children. Surg Gynecol Obstet 1959; 109:145.
183. Gasperini E, Parmeggiani G: [Separation-fractures of the proximal extremity of the radius in children: Reduction with a percutaneous method.] Arch Ortop 1966; 79:77.
184. Gaston SR, Smith FM, Baab OD: Epiphyseal injuries of the radial head and neck. Am J Surg 1953;85:266.
185. Gaur SC, Varma AN, Swarup A: A new surgical technique for old ununited lateral condyle fractures of the humerus in children. J Trauma 1993;34:68.
186. Gay JR, Love JG: Diagnosis and treatment of tardy paralysis of the ulnar nerve. J Bone Joint Surg 1947;29: 1087.
187. Gejrot W: On intra-articular fractures of the capitellum and trochlea of humerus with special reference to treatment. Acta Chir Scand 1932;71:233.
188. Gicquel P, Giacomelli MC, Karger C, et al: Surgical technique and preliminary results of a new fixation concept for olecranon fractures in children. J Pediatr Orthop 2003;23:398.
189. Gicquel P, Maximin MC, Boutemy P, et al: Biomechanical analysis of olecranon fracture fixation in children. J Pediatr Orthop 2002;22:17.
190. Gicquel PH, De Billy B, Karger CS, et al: Olecranon fractures in 26 children with mean follow-up of 59 months. J Pediatr Orthop 2001;21:141.
191. Gille P, Sava P, Guyot J, et al: [Anterior interosseous nerve syndrome following supracondylar fractures in children (author's transl).] Rev Chir Orthop Reparatrice Appar Mot 1978;64:131.
192. Ginzburg SO, Bukhny AF: [Divergent dislocations and fractures-dislocations of the forearm and elbow joint in children.] Ortop Travmatol Protez 1967;28:33.
193. Gjerloff C, Sojbjerg JO: Percutaneous pinning of supracondylar fractures of the humerus. Acta Orthop Scand 1978;49:597.
194. Goldenberg RR: Closed manipulation for the resolution of fracture of the neck of the radius in children. J Bone Joint Surg 1945;27:267.
195. Gonzalez-Herranz P, Alvarez-Romera A, Burgos J, et al: Displaced radial neck fractures in children treated by closed intramedullary pinning (Métaizeau technique). J Pediatr Orthop 1997;17:325.
196. Gordon JE, Patton CM, Luhmann SJ, et al: Fracture stability after pinning of displaced supracondylar distal

humerus fractures in children. J Pediatr Orthop 2001; 21:313.
197. Gosens T, Bongers KJ: Neurovascular complications and functional outcome in displaced supracondylar fractures of the humerus in children. Injury 2003;34: 267.
198. Graham B, Paulus DA, Caffee HH: Pulse oximetry for vascular monitoring in upper extremity replantation surgery. J Hand Surg [Am] 1986;11:687.
199. Granger B: On a particular fracture of the inner condyle of the humerus. Edinburgh Med Surg J 1818;14:196.
200. Grant IR, Miller JH: Osteochondral fracture of the trochlea associated with fracture-dislocation of the elbow. Injury 1975;6:257.
201. Grantham SA, Kiernan HA Jr: Displaced olecranon fracture in children. J Trauma 1975;15:197.
202. Grantham SA, Norris TR, Bush DC: Isolated fracture of the humeral capitellum. Clin Orthop Relat Res 1981; 161:262.
203. Graves SC, Canale ST: Fractures of the olecranon in children: long-term follow-up. J Pediatr Orthop 1993;13: 239.
204. Green DW, Widmann RF, Frank JS, et al: Low incidence of ulnar nerve injury with crossed pin placement for pediatric supracondylar humerus fractures using a mini-open technique. J Orthop Trauma 2005;19:158.
205. Green NE: Entrapment of the median nerve following elbow dislocation. J Pediatr Orthop 1983;3:384.
206. Griffin PP: Supracondylar fractures of the humerus. Treatment and complications. Pediatr Clin North Am 1975;22:477.
207. Griffith JF, Roebuck DJ, Cheng JC, et al: Acute elbow trauma in children: Spectrum of injury revealed by MR imaging not apparent on radiographs. AJR Am J Roentgenol 2001;176:53.
208. Grimer RJ, Brooks S: Brachial artery damage accompanying closed posterior dislocation of the elbow. J Bone Joint Surg Br 1985;67:378.
209. Gugenheim JJ Jr, Stanley RF, Woods GW, et al: Little League survey: Rhe Houston study. Am J Sports Med 1976;4:189.
210. Gupta N, Kay RM, Leitch K, et al: Effect of surgical delay on perioperative complications and need for open reduction in supracondylar humerus fractures in children. J Pediatr Orthop 2004;24:245.
211. Gurkan I, Bayrakci K, Tasbas B, et al: Posterior instability of the shoulder after supracondylar fractures recovered with cubitus varus deformity. J Pediatr Orthop 2002;22:198.
212. Gwynne-Jones DP: Displaced olecranon apophyseal fractures in children with osteogenesis imperfecta. J Pediatr Orthop 2005;25:154.
213. Haasbeek JF, Cole WG: Open fractures of the arm in children. J Bone Joint Surg Br 1995;77:576.
214. Haddad RJ Jr, Saer JK, Riordan DC: Percutaneous pinning of displaced supracondylar fractures of the elbow in children. Clin Orthop Relat Res 1970;71:112.
215. Hadlow AT, Devane P, Nicol RO: A selective treatment approach to supracondylar fracture of the humerus in children. J Pediatr Orthop 1996;16:104.
216. Hahn NF: Fall von eine besonders Variet der Frakturen des Ellenbogens. Z Wunder Geburt 1953;6:185.
217. Hallett J: Entrapment of the median nerve after dislocation of the elbow. A case report. J Bone Joint Surg Br 1981;63:408.
218. Hamsa RW Sr: A method for aligning supracondylar fractures of the humerus. Clin Orthop Relat Res 1977; 123:104.
219. Hankin FM: Posterior dislocation of the elbow. A simplified method of closed reduction. Clin Orthop Relat Res 1984;190:254.
220. Hanlon CR, Estes WL Jr: Fractures in childhood, a statistical analysis. Am J Surg 1954;87:312.
221. Hansen PE, Barnes DA, Tullos HS: Arthrographic diagnosis of an injury pattern in the distal humerus of an infant. J Pediatr Orthop 1982;2:569.
222. Hanspal RS: Injury to the medial humeral condyle in a child reviewed after 18 years. Report of a case. J Bone Joint Surg Br 1985;67:638.
223. Hardacre JA, Nahigian SH, Froimson AI, et al: Fractures of the lateral condyle of the humerus in children. J Bone Joint Surg Am 1971;53:1083.
224. Haroldsson S: On osteochondrosis deformans juvenilis capituli humeri, including investigation of intraosseous vasculature in distal humerus. Acta Chir Scand Suppl 1959;38:1.
225. Harrison RB, Keats TE, Frankel CJ, et al: Radiographic clues to fractures of the unossified medial humeral condyle in young children. Skeletal Radiol 1984;11:209.
226. Hart GM: Subluxation of the head of the radius in young children. JAMA 1959;169:1734.
227. Hart GM, Wilson DW, Arden GP: The operative management of the difficult supracondylar fracture of the humerus in the child. Injury 1977;9:30.
228. Harvey S, Tchelebi H: Proximal radio-ulnar translocation. A case report. J Bone Joint Surg Am 1979;61: 447.
229. Hasler CC, von Laer L: Prevention of growth disturbances after fractures of the lateral humeral condyle in children. J Pediatr Orthop B 2001;10:123.
230. Hasner E, Husby J: Fracture of epicondyle and condyle of humerus. Acta Chir Scand 1951;101:195.
231. Helfet DL, Hotchkiss RN: Internal fixation of the distal humerus: A biomechanical comparison of methods. J Orthop Trauma 1990;4:260.
232. Heller CJ, Wiltse LL: Avascular necrosis of the capitellum humeri (Panner's disease). A report of a case. J Bone Joint Surg Am 1960;42:513.
233. Henderson RS, Robertson IM: Open dislocation of the elbow with rupture of the brachial artery. J Bone Joint Surg Br 1952;34:636.
234. Hennig K, Franke D: Posterior displacement of brachial artery following closed elbow dislocation. J Trauma 1980;20:96.
235. Henrikson B: Supracondylar fracture of the humerus in children. A late review of end-results with special reference to the cause of deformity, disability and complications. Acta Chir Scand Suppl 1966;369:1.
236. Henrikson B: Isolated fractures of the proximal end of the radius in children epidemiology, treatment and prognosis. Acta Orthop Scand 1969;40:246.
237. Hernandez MA 3rd, Roach JW: Corrective osteotomy for cubitus varus deformity. J Pediatr Orthop 1994; 14:487.

238. Hierholzer G, Horster G, Hax PM: [Supracondylar corrective osteotomies of the humerus in childhood]. Aktuelle Probl Chir Orthop 1981;20:101.
239. Hines RF, Herndon WA, Evans JP: Operative treatment of medial epicondyle fractures in children. Clin Orthop Relat Res 1987;223:170.
240. Hirvensalo E, Bostman O, Partio E, et al: Fracture of the humeral capitellum fixed with absorbable polyglycolide pins. 1-year follow-up of 8 adults. Acta Orthop Scand 1993;64:85.
241. Hoeffel JC, Blanquart D, Galloy MA, et al: [Fractures of the lateral condyle of the elbow in children. Radiologic aspects.] J Radiol 1990;71:407.
242. Hofammann KE 3rd, Moneim MS, Omer GE, et al: Brachial artery disruption following closed posterior elbow dislocation in a child—assessment with intravenous digital angiography. A case report with review of the literature. Clin Orthop Relat Res 1984;184:145.
243. Hofmann V: Causes of functional disorders following supracondylar fractures in childhood. Beitr Orthop Traumatol 1968;15:25.
244. Holda ME, Manoli A 2nd, LaMont RI: Epiphyseal separation of the distal end of the humerus with medial displacement. J Bone Joint Surg Am 1980;62:52.
245. Holland P, Davies AM, Cassar-Pullicino VN: Computed tomographic arthrography in the assessment of osteochondritis dissecans of the elbow. Clin Radiol 1994;49:231.
246. Hope PG, Williamson DM, Coates CJ, et al: Biodegradable pin fixation of elbow fractures in children. A randomised trial. J Bone Joint Surg Br 1991;73:965.
247. Horn BD, Crisci K, MacEwen GD. Fractures of the lateral condyle: The use of magnetic resonance imaging (MRI) to predict fracture displacement. AV Presentation, New Orleans, March 19-23, 1998.
248. Horn BD, Herman MJ, Crisci K, et al: Fractures of the lateral humeral condyle: Role of the cartilage hinge in fracture stability. J Pediatr Orthop 2002;22:8.
249. Horstmann HM, Blyakher AA, Quartararo LG, et al: Treatment of cubitus varus with osteotomy and Ilizarov external fixation. Am J Orthop 2000;29:389.
250. Houshian S, Holst AK, Larsen MS, et al: Remodeling of Salter-Harris type II epiphyseal plate injury of the distal radius. J Pediatr Orthop 2004;24:472.
251. Hoyer A: Treatment of supracondylar fracture of the humerus by skeletal traction in an abduction splint. J Bone Joint Surg Am 1952;24:623.
252. Hresko MT, Rosenberg BN, Pappas AM: Excision of the radial head in patients younger than 18 years. J Pediatr Orthop 1999;19:106.
253. Hui JH, Torode IP, Chatterjee A: Medial approach for corrective osteotomy of cubitus varus: A cosmetic incision. J Pediatr Orthop 2004;24:477.
254. Hume AC: Anterior dislocation of the head of the radius associated with undisplaced fracture of the olecranon in children. J Bone Joint Surg Br 1957;39:508.
255. Ikram MA: Ulnar nerve palsy: A complication following percutaneous fixation of supracondylar fractures of the humerus in children. Injury 1996;27:303.
256. Ingersoll RE: Fractures of the humeral condyles in children. Clin Orthop Relat Res 1965;41:32.
257. Inoue G: Bilateral osteochondritis dissecans of the elbow treated by Herbert screw fixation. Br J Sports Med 1991;25:142.
258. Inoue G, Horii E: Combined shear fractures of the trochlea and capitellum associated with anterior fracture-dislocation of the elbow. J Orthop Trauma 1992;6:373.
259. Ippolito E, Caterini R, Scola E: Supracondylar fractures of the humerus in children. Analysis at maturity of fifty-three patients treated conservatively. J Bone Joint Surg Am 1986;68:333.
260. Iqbal M, Habib-ur-Rehman: Nerve injuries associated with supracondylar fracture of the humerus in children. J Pak Med Assoc 1994;44:148.
261. Iqbal QM: Long bone fractures among children in Malaysia. Int Surg 1974;59:410.
262. Iyengar SR, Hoffinger SA, Townsend DR: Early versus delayed reduction and pinning of type III displaced supracondylar fractures of the humerus in children: A comparative study. J Orthop Trauma 1999;13:51.
263. Jackson DW, Silvino N, Reiman P: Osteochondritis in the female gymnast's elbow. Arthroscopy 1989;5:129.
264. Jackson JA: Simple anterior dislocation of the elbow joint with rupture of the brachial artery. Am J Surg 1940;47:479.
265. Jakob R, Fowles JV, Rang M, et al: Observations concerning fractures of the lateral humeral condyle in children. J Bone Joint Surg Br 1975;57:430.
266. Jarvis JG, D'Astous JL: The pediatric T-supracondylar fracture. J Pediatr Orthop 1984;4:697.
267. Jeffrey CC: Fractures of the head of the radius in children. J Bone Joint Surg Br 1950;32:314.
268. Jeffrey CC: Non-union of the epiphysis of the lateral condyle of the humerus. J Bone Joint Surg Br 1958;40:396.
269. Jeffrey CC: Fractures of the neck of the radius in children: Mechanism of causation. J Bone Joint Surg Br 1972;54:717.
270. Johansson J, Rosman M: Fracture of the capitulum humeri in children: A rare injury, often misdiagnosed. Clin Orthop Relat Res 1980;146:157.
271. Jones ER, Esah M: Displaced fractures of the neck of the radius in children. J Bone Joint Surg Br 1971;53:429.
272. Jones ET, Louis DS: Median nerve injuries associated with supracondylar fractures of the humerus in children. Clin Orthop Relat Res 1980;150:181.
273. Jones KG: Percutaneous pin fixation of fractures of the lower end of the humerus. Clin Orthop Relat Res 1967;50:53.
274. Josefsson PO, Danielsson LG: Epicondylar elbow fracture in children. 35-year follow-up of 56 unreduced cases. Acta Orthop Scand 1986;57:313.
275. Jupiter JB: Complex fractures of the distal part of the humerus and associated complications. Instr Course Lect 1995;44:187.
276. Jupiter JB, Barnes KA, Goodman LJ, et al: Multiplane fracture of the distal humerus. J Orthop Trauma 1993;7:216.
277. Kalenak A: Ununited fracture of the lateral condyle of the humerus. A 50 year follow-up. Clin Orthop Relat Res 1977;124:181.

278. Kallio PE, Foster BK, Paterson DC: Difficult supracondylar elbow fractures in children: Analysis of percutaneous pinning technique. J Pediatr Orthop 1992;12:11.
279. Kamegaya M, Shinohara Y, Kurokawa M, et al: Assessment of stability in children's minimally displaced lateral humeral condyle fracture by magnetic resonance imaging. J Pediatr Orthop 1999;19:570.
280. Kanaujia RR, Ikuta Y, Muneshige H, et al: Dome osteotomy for cubitus varus in children. Acta Orthop Scand 1988;59:314.
281. Kanellopoulos AD, Yiannakopoulos CK: Closed reduction and percutaneous stabilization of pediatric T-condylar fractures of the humerus. J Pediatr Orthop 2004;24:13.
282. Kapel O: Operation for habitual dislocation of the elbow. J Bone Joint Surg Am 1951;33:707.
283. Kaplan RE, Lillis KA: Recurrent nursemaid's elbow (annular ligament displacement) treatment via telephone. Pediatrics 2002;110:171.
284. Karakurt L, Ozdemir H, Yilmaz E, et al: Morphology and dynamics of the ulnar nerve in the cubital tunnel after percutaneous cross-pinning of supracondylar fractures in children's elbows: an ultrasonographic study. J Pediatr Orthop B 2005;14:189.
285. Karatosun V, Alekberov C, Alici E, et al: Treatment of cubitus varus using the Ilizarov technique of distraction osteogenesis. J Bone Joint Surg Br 2000;82:1030.
286. Karlsson J, Thorsteinsson T, Thorleifsson R, et al: Entrapment of the median nerve and brachial artery after supracondylar fractures of the humerus in children. Arch Orthop Trauma Surg 1986;104:389.
287. Karlsson MK, Hasserius R, Karlsson C, et al: Fractures of the olecranon: A 15- to 25-year followup of 73 patients. Clin Orthop Relat Res 2002;403:205.
288. Kasser JR, Richards K, Millis M: The triceps-dividing approach to open reduction of complex distal humeral fractures in adolescents: A Cybex evaluation of triceps function and motion. J Pediatr Orthop 1990;10:93.
289. Kaufman B, Rinott MG, Tanzman M: Closed reduction of fractures of the proximal radius in children. J Bone Joint Surg Br 1989;71:66.
290. Keenan WN, Clegg J: Variation of Baumann's angle with age, sex, and side: Implications for its use in radiological monitoring of supracondylar fracture of the humerus in children. J Pediatr Orthop 1996;16:97.
291. Kelly RP, Griffin TW: Open reduction of T-condylar fractures of the humerus through an anterior approach. J Trauma 1969;9:901.
292. Key JA: Treatment of fractures of the head and neck of the radius. JAMA 1939;96:101.
293. Key JA: Survival of the head of the radius in a child after removal and replacement. J Bone Joint Surg 1946;28:148.
294. Kiefer GN: Fractures of the radial head and neck. In Letts M (ed): Management of Pediatric Fractures. New York, Churchill Livingstone, 1994, p 376.
295. Kilburn P, Sweeney JG, Silk FF: Three cases of compound posterior dislocation of the elbow with rupture of the brachial artery. J Bone Joint Surg Br 1962;44:119.
296. Kilfoyle RM: Fractures of the medial condyle and epicondyle of the elbow in children. Clin Orthop Relat Res 1965;41:43.
297. Kim HS, Jahng JS, Han DY, et al: Modified step-cut osteotomy of the humerus. J Pediatr Orthop B 1998;7:162.
298. Kim HT, Lee JS, Yoo CI: Management of cubitus varus and valgus. J Bone Joint Surg Am 2005;87:771.
299. Kim HT, Song MB, Conjares JN, et al: Trochlear deformity occurring after distal humeral fractures: Magnetic resonance imaging and its natural progression. J Pediatr Orthop 2002;22:188.
300. King D, Secor C: Bow elbow (cubitus varus). J Bone Joint Surg Am 1951;33:572.
301. Kirk P, Goulet JA, Freiberg A: A biomechanical evaluation of fixation methods for fractures of the distal humerus. Orthop Trans 1990;14:674.
302. Klein EW: Osteochondrosis of the capitellum (Panner's disease). Report of a case. Am J Roentgenol Radium Ther Nucl Med 1962;88:466.
303. Klekamp J, Green NE, Mencio GA: Osteochondritis dissecans as a cause of developmental dislocation of the radial head. Clin Orthop Relat Res 1997;338:36.
304. Klinefelter EW: Influence of position on measurement of projected bone angle. AJR Am J Roentgenol 1946;55:722.
305. Koch PP, Exner GU: Supracondylar medial open wedge osteotomy with external fixation for cubitus varus deformity. J Pediatr Orthop B 2003;12:116.
306. Krezel T, Zelaznowski W: [Spontaneous growth correction in supracondylar fractures of the humerus in children.] Chir Narzadow Ruchu Ortop Pol 1967;32:531.
307. Kristensen J, Vibild O: Supracondylar fractures of the humerus in children. Acta Orthop Scand 1976;47:375.
308. Kumar K, Sharma VK, Sharma R, et al: Correction of cubitus varus by French or dome osteotomy: A comparative study. J Trauma 2000;49:717.
309. Kuwahata Y, Inoue G: Osteochondritis dissecans of the elbow managed by Herbert screw fixation. Orthopedics 1998;21:449.
310. Lal GM, Bhan S: Delayed open reduction for supracondylar fractures of the humerus. Int Orthop 1991;15:189.
311. Landin LA: Fracture patterns in children. Analysis of 8,682 fractures with special reference to incidence, etiology and secular changes in a Swedish urban population 1950-1979. Acta Orthop Scand Suppl 1983;202:1.
312. Landin LA, Danielsson LG: Elbow fractures in children. An epidemiological analysis of 589 cases. Acta Orthop Scand 1986;57:309.
313. Lane LC: Fractures of the bones which form the elbow joint and their treatment. Trans Am Surg Assoc 1891;9:431.
314. Lange J: Aseptic necrosis of the capitellum of the humerus; Panner's disease. Acta Chir Scand 1954;108:301.
315. Langenskiold A, Kivilaakso R: Varus and valgus deformity of the elbow following supracondylar fracture of the humerus. Acta Orthop Scand 1967;38:313.
316. Lansinger O, Karlsson J, Korner L, et al: Dislocation of the elbow joint. Arch Orthop Trauma Surg 1984;102:183.
317. Lansinger O, Mare K: Fracture of the capitulum humeri. Acta Orthop Scand 1981;52:39.
318. Launay F, Leet AI, Jacopin S, et al: Lateral humeral condyle fractures in children: A comparison of two

approaches to treatment. J Pediatr Orthop 2004;24:385.
319. Laurent LE, Lindstrom BL: Osteochondrosis of the capitulum humeri: Panner's disease. Acta Orthop Scand 1956;26:111.
320. Lavine LS: A simple method of reducing dislocations of the elbow joint. J Bone Joint Surg Am 1953;35:785.
321. Lee HH, Shen HC, Chang JH, et al: Operative treatment of displaced medial epicondyle fractures in children and adolescents. J Shoulder Elbow Surg 2005;14:178.
322. Leet AI, Frisancho J, Ebramzadeh E: Delayed treatment of type 3 supracondylar humerus fractures in children. J Pediatr Orthop 2002;22:203.
323. Leet AI, Young C, Hoffer MM: Medial condyle fractures of the humerus in children. J Pediatr Orthop 2002;22:2.
324. Lefort G, De Miscault G, Gillier P, et al: [Arterial lesions in supracondylar fractures of the humerus in children. Apropos of 6 cases.] Chir Pediatr 1986;27:100.
325. Letts M, Rumball K, Bauermeister S, et al: Fractures of the capitellum in adolescents. J Pediatr Orthop 1997;17:315.
326. Leung AG, Peterson HA: Fractures of the proximal radial head and neck in children with emphasis on those that involve the articular cartilage. J Pediatr Orthop 2000;20:7.
327. Levai JP, Tanguy A, Collin JP, et al: [Recurrent posterior dislocation of the elbow following malunion of supracondylar fracture of the humerus. Report of a case (author's transl).] Rev Chir Orthop Reparatrice Appar Mot 1979;65:457.
328. Levine MJ, Horn BD, Pizzutillo PD: Treatment of posttraumatic cubitus varus in the pediatric population with humeral osteotomy and external fixation. J Pediatr Orthop 1996;16:597.
329. Liberman N, Katz T, Howard CB, et al: Fixation of capitellar fractures with the Herbert screw. Arch Orthop Trauma Surg 1991;110:155.
330. Lindemann SH: Partial dislocation of the radial head peculiar to children. BMJ 1885;2:1058.
331. Lindham S, Hugosson C: The significance of associated lesions including dislocation in fractures of the neck of the radius in children. Acta Orthop Scand 1979;50:79.
332. Lindholm TS, Osterman K, Vankka E: Osteochondritis dissecans of elbow, ankle and hip: A comparison survey. Clin Orthop Relat Res 1980;148:245.
333. Linscheid RL, Wheeler DK: Elbow dislocations. JAMA 1965;194:1171.
334. Lipscomb AB: Baseball pitching injuries in growing athletes. J Sports Med 1975;3:25.
335. Lipscomb PR: Vascular and neural complications in supracondylar fractures of the humerus in children. J Bone Joint Surg Am 1955;37:487.
336. Louahem DM, Nebunescu A, Canavese F, et al: Neurovascular complications and severe displacement in supracondylar humerus fractures in children: Defensive or offensive strategy? J Pediatr Orthop B 2006;15:51.
337. Louis DS, Ricciardi JE, Spengler DM: Arterial injury: A complication of posterior elbow dislocation. A clinical and anatomical study. J Bone Joint Surg Am 1974;56:1631.
338. Lowery WD Jr, Kurzweil PR, Forman SK, et al: Persistence of the olecranon physis: A cause of "little league elbow." J Shoulder Elbow Surg 1995;4:143.
339. Lyons JP, Ashley E, Hoffer MM: Ulnar nerve palsies after percutaneous cross-pinning of supracondylar fractures in children's elbows. J Pediatr Orthop 1998;18:43.
340. Ma YZ, Zheng CB, Zhou TL, et al: Percutaneous probe reduction of frontal fractures of the humeral capitellum. Clin Orthop Relat Res 1984;183:17.
341. MacSween WA: Transportation of radius and ulna associated with dislocation of the elbow in a child. Injury 1978;10:314.
342. Madsen E: Supracondylar fractures of the humerus in children. J Bone Joint Surg Br 1955;37:241.
343. Magill HK, Aitken AP: Pulled elbow. Surg Gynecol Obstet 1954;98:753.
344. Makela EA, Bostman O, Kekomaki M, et al: Biodegradable fixation of distal humeral physeal fractures. Clin Orthop Relat Res 1992;283:237.
345. Malgaigne JF: Treatise on Fractures. Philadelphia, JB Lippincott, 1859.
346. Mannerfelt L: Median nerve entrapment after dislocation of the elbow. Report of a case. J Bone Joint Surg Br 1968;50:152.
347. Mapes RC, Hennrikus WL: The effect of elbow position on the radial pulse measured by Doppler ultrasonography after surgical treatment of supracondylar elbow fractures in children. J Pediatr Orthop 1998;18:441.
348. March HC: Osteochondritis of the capitellum (Panner's disease). AJR Am J Roentgenol 1944;51:682.
349. Marchiodi L, Mignani G, Stilli S, et al: Retrograde intramedullary osteosynthesis in the surgical treatment of fractures of the radial capitellum during childhood. Chir Organi Mov 1997;82:327.
350. Marck KW, Kooiman AM, Binnendijk B: Brachial artery rupture following supracondylar fracture of the humerus. Neth J Surg 1986;38:81.
351. Marzo JM, d'Amato C, Strong M, et al: Usefulness and accuracy of arthrography in management of lateral humeral condyle fractures in children. J Pediatr Orthop 1990;10:317.
352. Masada K, Kawai H, Kawabata H, et al: Osteosynthesis for old, established non-union of the lateral condyle of the humerus. J Bone Joint Surg Am 1990;72:32.
353. Matev I: A radiological sign of entrapment of the median nerve in the elbow joint after posterior dislocation. A report of two cases. J Bone Joint Surg Br 1976;58:353.
354. Matsushita T, Nagano A: Arc osteotomy of the humerus to correct cubitus varus. Clin Orthop Relat Res 1997;336:111.
355. Matthews JG: Fractures of the olecranon in children. Injury 1980;12:207.
356. Mauer I, Kolovos D, Loscos R: Epiphyseolysis of the distal humerus in a newborn. Bull Hosp Jt Dis 1967;28:109.
357. Maylahn DJ, Fahey JJ: Fractures of the elbow in children; review of three hundred consecutive cases. JAMA 1958;166:220.

358. McBride ED, Monnet JC: Epiphyseal fractures of the head of the radius in children. Clin Orthop Relat Res 1960;16:264.
359. McGowan AJ: The results of transposition of the ulnar nerve for traumatic ulnar neuritis. J Bone Joint Surg Br 1950;32:293.
360. McGraw JJ, Akbarnia BA, Hanel DP, et al: Neurological complications resulting from supracondylar fractures of the humerus in children. J Pediatr Orthop 1986;6: 647.
361. McIntyre WM, Wiley JJ, Charette RJ: Fracture-separation of the distal humeral epiphysis. Clin Orthop Relat Res 1984;188:98.
362. McKee MD, Jupiter JB: A contemporary approach to the management of complex fractures of the distal humerus and their sequelae. Hand Clin 1994;10:479.
363. McKellar Hall R: Recurrent posterior dislocation of the elbow joint in a boy. J Bone Joint Surg Br 1953;35:56.
364. McLeod GG, Gray AJ, Turner MS: Elbow dislocation with intra-articular entrapment of the lateral epicondyle. J R Coll Surg Edinb 1993;38:112.
365. McManama GB Jr, Micheli LJ, Berry MV, et al: The surgical treatment of osteochondritis of the capitellum. Am J Sports Med 1985;13:11.
366. McRae R, Freeman P: The lesion in pulled elbow. J Bone Joint Surg Br 1965;47:808.
367. Mehlman C, Strub W, Crawford A, et al: Displaced supracondylar humeral fractures: Does timing of surgery make a difference? Paper presented at the Annual Meeting of the Pediatric Orthopaedic Society of North America, Lake Buena Vista, Fla, 1999, p 77.
368. Mehne DK, Mata J: Bicolumn fractures of the adult humerus. Paper presented at the 53rd Annual Meeting of the American Academy of Orthopaedic Surgeons, New Orleans, La, 1986.
369. Mehserle WL, Meehan PL: Treatment of the displaced supracondylar fracture of the humerus (type III) with closed reduction and percutaneous cross-pin fixation. J Pediatr Orthop 1991;11:705.
370. Merten DF, Kirks DR, Ruderman RJ: Occult humeral epiphyseal fracture in battered infants. Pediatr Radiol 1981;10:151.
371. Métaizeau JP, Prevot J, Schmitt M: [Reduction and fixation of fractures of the neck of the radious be centromedullary pinning. Original technic.] Rev Chir Orthop Reparatrice Appar Mot 1980;66:47.
372. Meyerding HW: Volkmann's ischemic contracture associated with supracondylar fractures of humerus. JAMA 1936;106:1139.
373. Meyn MA Jr, Quigley TB: Reduction of posterior dislocation of the elbow by traction on the dangling arm. Clin Orthop Relat Res 1974;103:106.
374. Michael SP, Stanislas MJ: Localization of the ulnar nerve during percutaneous wiring of supracondylar fractures in children. Injury 1996;27:301.
375. Mih AD, Cooney WP, Idler RS, et al: Long-term follow-up of forearm bone diaphyseal plating. Clin Orthop Relat Res 1994;299:256.
376. Milch H: Fractures of the external humeral condyle. JAMA 1956;160:641.
377. Milch H: Fractures and fracture dislocations of the humeral condyles. J Trauma 1964;15:592.
378. Miller EM: Late ulnar nerve paralysis. Surg Gynecol Obstet 1924;38:37.
379. Millis MB, Singer IJ, Hall JE: Supracondylar fracture of the humerus in children. Further experience with a study in orthopaedic decision-making. Clin Orthop Relat Res 1984;188:90.
380. Minkowitz B, Busch MT: Supracondylar humerus fractures. Current trends and controversies. Orthop Clin North Am 1994;25:581.
381. Mintzer CM, Waters PM, Brown DJ, et al: Percutaneous pinning in the treatment of displaced lateral condyle fractures. J Pediatr Orthop 1994;14:462.
382. Mirsky EC, Karas EH, Weiner LS: Lateral condyle fractures in children: Evaluation of classification and treatment. J Orthop Trauma 1997;11:117.
383. Mitsunagna MM, Adishian DA, Bianco AJ: Osteochondritis dissecans of the capitellum. J Trauma 1981;22: 1981.
384. Mitsunari A, Muneshige H, Ikuta Y, et al: Internal rotation deformity and tardy ulnar nerve palsy after supracondylar humeral fracture. J Shoulder Elbow Surg 1995;4:23.
385. Miura H, Tsumura H, Kubota H, et al: Interlocking wedge osteotomy for cubitus varus deformity. Fukuoka Igaku Zasshi 1998;89:119.
386. Mizuno K, Hirohata K, Kashiwagi D: Fracture-separation of the distal humeral epiphysis in young children. J Bone Joint Surg Am 1979;61:570.
387. Mohammad S, Rymaszewski LA, Runciman J: The Baumann angle in supracondylar fractures of the distal humerus in children. J Pediatr Orthop 1999;19: 65.
388. Mohan N, Hunter JB, Colton CL: The posterolateral approach to the distal humerus for open reduction and internal fixation of fractures of the lateral condyle in children. J Bone Joint Surg Br 2000;82:643.
389. Mondoloni P, Vandenbussche E, Peraldi P, et al: [Instability of the elbow after supracondylar humeral non-union in cubitus varus rotation. Apropos of 2 cases observed in adults.] Rev Chir Orthop Reparatrice Appar Mot 1996;82:757.
390. Montgomery AH: Separation of the upper epiphysis of the radius. Arch Surg 1925;10:961.
391. Moorhead EL: Old untreated fracture of the external condyle of humerus: Factors in influencing choice of treatment. Surg Clin North Am 1919;3:987.
392. Morgan SJ, Beaver WB: Nonunion of a pediatric lateral condyle fracture without ulnar nerve palsy: Sixty-year follow-up. J Orthop Trauma 1999;13:456.
393. Morrissy RT, Wilkins KE: Deformity following distal humeral fracture in childhood. J Bone Joint Surg Am 1984;66:557.
394. Morwood JB: Supracondylar fracture with absent radial pulse: Report of 2 cases. BMJ 1939;1:163.
395. Mubarak SJ, Carroll NC: Volkmann's contracture in children: Aetiology and prevention. J Bone Joint Surg Br 1979;61:285.
396. Mubarak SJ, Davids JR: Closed reduction and percutaneous pinning of supracondylar fractures of the distal humerus in the child. In Morrey BF (ed): Master Techniques in Orthopaedic Surgery—The Elbow. New York, Raven Press, 1994, p 37.

397. Muller ME, Allgonier M, Schneider R: Manual of Internal Fixation: Technique Recommended by the AO Group. New York, Springer, 1979.
398. Murawski E, Stachow J: [Conservative reduction of radial bone neck fractures in children.] Pol Przegl Chir 1977;49:117.
399. Myint S, Molitor PJ: Dome osteotomy with T-plate fixation for cubitus varus deformity in an adult patient. J R Coll Surg Edinb 1998;43:353.
400. Nacht JL, Ecker ML, Chung SM, et al: Supracondylar fractures of the humerus in children treated by closed reduction and percutaneous pinning. Clin Orthop Relat Res 1983;177:203.
401. Newell RL: Olecranon fractures in children. Injury 1975;7:33.
402. Newman JH: Displaced radial neck fractures in children. Injury 1977;9:114.
403. Nimkin K, Kleinman PK, Teeger S, et al: Distal humeral physeal injuries in child abuse: MR imaging and ultrasonography findings. Pediatr Radiol 1995;25:562.
404. Norell HG: Roentgenologic visualization of the extracapsular fat; its importance in the diagnosis of traumatic injuries to the elbow. Acta Radiol 1954;42:205.
405. Nussbaum AJ: The off-profile proximal radial epiphysis: Another potential pitfall in the X-ray diagnosis of elbow trauma. J Trauma 1983;23:40.
406. Nwakama AC, Peterson HA, Shaughnessy WJ: Fishtail deformity following fracture of the distal humerus in children: Historical review, case presentations, discussion of etiology, and thoughts on treatment. J Pediatr Orthop B 2000;9:309.
407. O'Brien PI: Injuries involving the proximal radial epiphysis. Clin Orthop Relat Res 1965;41:51.
408. Ochner RS, Bloom H, Palumbo RC, et al: Closed reduction of coronal fractures of the capitellum. J Trauma 1996;40:199.
409. O'Driscoll SW, Spinner RJ, McKee MD, et al: Tardy posterolateral rotatory instability of the elbow due to cubitus varus. J Bone Joint Surg Am 2001;83:1358.
410. Ogawa K, Ui M: Fracture-separation of the medial humeral epicondyle caused by arm wrestling. J Trauma 1996;41:494.
411. Ogden JA: Skeletal Injury in the Child. Philadelphia, WB Saunders, 1990.
412. Oka Y, Ohta K, Fukuda H: Bone-peg grafting for osteochondritis dissecans of the elbow. Int Orthop 1999;23:53.
413. Omer GE Jr, Conger CW: Osteochondrosis of the capitulum humeri (Panner's disease). U S Armed Forces Med J 1959;10:1235.
414. Oppenheim W, Davlin LB, Leipzig JM, et al: Concomitant fractures of the capitellum and trochlea. J Orthop Trauma 1989;3:260.
415. Oppenheim WL, Clader TJ, Smith C, et al: Supracondylar humeral osteotomy for traumatic childhood cubitus varus deformity. Clin Orthop Relat Res 1984;188:34.
416. Osborne G, Cotterill P: Recurrent dislocation of the elbow. J Bone Joint Surg Br 1966;48:340.
417. Ottolenghi CE: Acute ischemic syndrome: Its treatment. Prophylaxis of Volkmann's sydrome. Am J Orthop 1960;2:312.
418. Ozcelik A, Tekcan A, Omeroglu H: Correlation between iatrogenic ulnar nerve injury and angular insertion of the medial pin in supracondylar humerus fractures. J Pediatr Orthop B 2006;15:58.
419. Ozkoc G, Akpinar S, Hersekli MA, et al: Type 4 median nerve entrapment in a child after elbow dislocation. Arch Orthop Trauma Surg 2003;123:555.
420. Paige ML, Port RB: Separation of the distal humeral epiphysis in the neonate. A combined clinical and roentgenographic diagnosis. Am J Dis Child 1985;139:1203.
421. Palmer EE, Niemann KM, Vesely D, et al: Supracondylar fracture of the humerus in children. J Bone Joint Surg Am 1978;60:653.
422. Panner HJ: An affection of the capitulum humeri resembling Calvé-Perthes disease of the hip. Acta Radiol 1927;8:617.
423. Panner HJ: A peculiar affection of the capitulum humeri, resembling Calvé-Perthes disease of the hip. Acta Radiol 1929;10:234.
424. Papandrea R, Waters PM: Posttraumatic reconstruction of the elbow in the pediatric patient. Clin Orthop Relat Res 2000;370:115.
425. Papavasiliou V, Nenopoulos S, Venturis T: Fractures of the medial condyle of the humerus in childhood. J Pediatr Orthop 1987;7:421.
426. Papavasiliou VA, Beslikas TA: Fractures of the lateral humeral condyle in children—an analysis of 39 cases. Injury 1985;16:364.
427. Papavasiliou VA, Beslikas TA: T-condylar fractures of the distal humeral condyles during childhood: An analysis of six cases. J Pediatr Orthop 1986;6:302.
428. Papavasiliou VA, Beslikas TA, Nenopoulos S: Isolated fractures of the olecranon in children. Injury 1987;18:100.
429. Partio EK, Hirvensalo E, Bostman O, et al: A prospective controlled trial of the fracture of the humeral medial epicondyle—how to treat? Ann Chir Gynaecol 1996;85:67.
430. Patrick J: Fracture of the medial epicondyle with displacement into the elbow joint. J Bone Joint Surg 1946;28:143.
431. Patterson RF: Treatment of the displaced fracture of the neck of the radius in children. J Bone Joint Surg 1934;16:695.
432. Pavlov H, Torg JS, Jacobs B, et al: Nonunion of olecranon epiphysis: Two cases in adolescent baseball pitchers. AJR Am J Roentgenol 1981;136:819.
433. Pelto-Vasenius K, Hirvensalo E, Rokkanen P: Absorbable implants in the treatment of distal humeral fractures in adolescents and adults. Acta Orthop Belg 1996;62(Suppl 1):93.
434. Pesudo JV, Aracil J, Barcelo M: Leverage method in displaced fractures of the radial neck in children. Clin Orthop Relat Res 1982;169:215.
435. Peters CL, Scott SM: Compartment syndrome in the forearm following fractures of the radial head or neck in children. J Bone Joint Surg Am 1995;77:1070.
436. Peters CL, Scott SM, Stevens PM: Closed reduction and percutaneous pinning of displaced supracondylar humerus fractures in children: Description of a new closed reduction technique for fractures with

brachialis muscle entrapment. J Orthop Trauma 1995; 9:430.
437. Peterson RK, Savoie FH 3rd, Field LD: Osteochondritis dissecans of the elbow. Instr Course Lect 1999;48:393.
438. Piggot J, Graham HK, McCoy GF: Supracondylar fractures of the humerus in children. Treatment by straight lateral traction. J Bone Joint Surg Br 1986;68:577.
439. Pimpalnerkar AL, Balasubramaniam G, Young SK, et al: Type four fracture of the medial epicondyle: A true indication for surgical intervention. Injury 1998;29: 751.
440. Pirker ME, Weinberg AM, Hollwarth ME, et al: Subsequent displacement of initially nondisplaced and minimally displaced fractures of the lateral humeral condyle in children. J Trauma 2005;58:1202.
441. Pirone AM, Graham HK, Krajbich JI: Management of displaced extension-type supracondylar fractures of the humerus in children. J Bone Joint Surg Am 1988; 70:641.
442. Post M, Haskell SS: Reconstruction of the median nerve following entrapment in supracondylar fracture of the humerus: A case report. J Trauma 1974;14:252.
443. Potter CM: Fracture-dislocation of the trochlea. J Bone Joint Surg Br 1954;36:250.
444. Pouliart N, De Boeck H: Posteromedial dislocation of the elbow with associated intraarticular entrapment of the lateral epicondyle. J Orthop Trauma 2002;16:53.
445. Poynton AR, Kelly IP, O'Rourke SK: Fractures of the capitellum—a comparison of two fixation methods. Injury 1998;29:341.
446. Prietto CA: Supracondylar fractures of the humerus. A comparative study of Dunlop's traction versus percutaneous pinning. J Bone Joint Surg Am 1979;61:425.
447. Pritchard DJ, Linscheid RL, Svien HJ: Intra-articular median nerve entrapment with dislocation of the elbow. Clin Orthop Relat Res 1973;90:100.
448. Pritchett JW: Entrapment of the median nerve after dislocation of the elbow. J Pediatr Orthop 1984;4:752.
449. Pritsch M, Engel J, Farin I: [Panner's disease.] Harefuah 1980;99:171.
450. Pudas T, Hurme T, Mattila K, et al: Magnetic resonance imaging in pediatric elbow fractures. Acta Radiol 2005;46:636.
451. Radomisli TE, Rosen AL: Controversies regarding radial neck fractures in children. Clin Orthop Relat Res 1998;353:30.
452. Rana NA, Kenwright J, Taylor RG, et al: Complete lesion of the median nerve associated with dislocation of the elbow joint. Acta Orthop Scand 1974;45:365.
453. Rang M, Barkin M, Hendrick EB: Elbow. Children's Fractures. Philadelphia, JB Lippincott, 1983, p 152.
454. Rasool MN: Ulnar nerve injury after K-wire fixation of supracondylar humerus fractures in children. J Pediatr Orthop 1998;18:686.
455. Rasool MN: Dislocations of the elbow in children. J Bone Joint Surg Br 2004;86:1050.
456. Ray SA, Ivory JP, Beavis JP: Use of pulse oximetry during manipulation of supracondylar fractures of the humerus. Injury 1991;22:103.
457. Re PR, Waters PM, Hresko MT: T-condylar fractures of the distal humerus in children and adolescents. J Pediatr Orthop 1999;19:313.
458. Reed MH: Fractures and dislocations of the extremities in children. J Trauma 1977;17:351.
459. Reidy JA, Vangorder GW: Treatment of displacement of the proximal radial epiphysis. J Bone Joint Surg Am 1963;45:1355.
460. Resch H, Helweg G: [Significance of rotation errors in supracondylar humeral fractures in the child.] Aktuelle Traumatol 1987;17:65.
461. Rhodin R: On the treatment of fracture of the capitellum. Acta Chir Scand 1942;86:475.
462. Ring D, Waters PM, Hotchkiss RN, et al: Pediatric floating elbow. J Pediatr Orthop 2001;21:456.
463. Riseborough EJ, Radin EL: Intercondylar T fractures of the humerus in the adult. A comparison of operative and non-operative treatment in twenty-nine cases. J Bone Joint Surg Am 1969;51:130.
464. Roaf R: Foramen in the humerus caused by the median nerve. J Bone Joint Surg Br 1957;39:748.
465. Roberts N, Hughes R: Osteochondritis dissecans of the elbow joint; a clinical study. J Bone Joint Surg Br 1950;32:348.
466. Roberts NW: Displacement of the internal epicondyle into the elbow joint: Four cases successfully treated with manipulation. Lancet 1934;2:78.
467. Roberts PH: Dislocation of the elbow. Br J Surg 1969; 56:806.
468. Rodriguez Merchan EC: Percutaneous reduction of displaced radial neck fractures in children. J Trauma 1994;37:812.
469. Rogers LF: The radiography of epiphyseal injuries. Radiology 1970;96:289.
470. Rogers LF, Malave S Jr, White H, et al: Plastic bowing, torus and greenstick supracondylar fractures of the humerus: Radiographic clues to obscure fractures of the elbow in children. Radiology 1978;128: 145.
471. Rokito SE, Anticevic D, Strongwater AM, et al: Chronic fracture-separation of the radial head in a child. J Orthop Trauma 1995;9:259.
472. Rosendahl B: Displacement of the medical epicondyle into the elbow joint: The final result in a case where the fragment has not been removed. Acta Orthop Scand 1959;28:212.
473. Rovinsky D, Ferguson C, Younis A, et al: Pediatric elbow dislocation associated with a milch type I lateral condyle fracture of the humerus. J Orthop Trauma 1999;13:458.
474. Rowell PJ: Arterial occlusion in juvenile humeral supracondylar fracture. Injury 1975;6:254.
475. Roy DR: Radioulnar synostosis following proximal radial fracture in child. Orthop Rev 1986;15: 89.
476. Royce RO, Dutkowsky JP, Kasser JR, et al: Neurologic complications after K-wire fixation of supracondylar humerus fractures in children. J Pediatr Orthop 1991; 11:191.
477. Ruch DS, Cory JW, Poehling GG: The arthroscopic management of osteochondritis dissecans of the adolescent elbow. Arthroscopy 1998;14:797.
478. Ruiz AL, Kealey WD, Cowie HG: Percutaneous pin fixation of intercondylar fractures in young children. J Pediatr Orthop B 2001;10:211.

479. Ruo GY: Radiographic diagnosis of fracture-separation of the entire distal humeral epiphysis. Clin Radiol 1987;38:635.
480. Rutherford A: Fractures of the lateral humeral condyle in children. J Bone Joint Surg Am 1985;67:851.
481. Ryan JR: The relationship of the radial head to radial neck diameters in fetuses and adults with reference to radial-head subluxation in children. J Bone Joint Surg Am 1969;51:781.
482. Sabharwal S, Tredwell SJ, Beauchamp RD, et al: Management of pulseless pink hand in pediatric supracondylar fractures of humerus. J Pediatr Orthop 1997;17:303.
483. Sairyo K, Henmi T, Kanematsu Y, et al: Radial nerve palsy associated with slightly angulated pediatric supracondylar humerus fracture. J Orthop Trauma 1997;11:227.
484. Salter RB: Supracondylar fractures in childhood. J Bone Joint Surg Br 1959;41:881.
485. Salter RB: Epiphyseal plate injuries. In Letts M (ed): Management of Pediatric Fractures. New York, Churchill Livingstone, 1994, p 17.
486. Salter RB, Harris WR: Injuries involving the epiphyseal plate. J Bone Joint Surg Am 1963;45:587.
487. Salter RB, Zaltz C: Anatomic investigations of the mechanism of injury and pathologic anatomy of "pulled elbow" in young children. Clin Orthop Relat Res 1971;77:134.
488. Sanders RA, Raney EM, Pipkin S: Operative treatment of bicondylar intraarticular fractures of the distal humerus. Orthopedics 1992;15:159.
489. Sangwan SS, Marya KM, Siwach RC, et al: Cubitus varus—correction by distraction osteogenesis. Indian J Med Sci 2002;56:165.
490. Saraf SK, Tuli SM: Concomitant medial condyle fracture of the humerus in a childhood posterolateral dislocation of the elbow. J Orthop Trauma 1989;3:352.
491. Schemitsch EH, Tencer AF, Henley MB: Biomechanical evaluation of methods of internal fixation of the distal humerus. J Orthop Trauma 1994;8:468.
492. Schenck RC Jr, Athanasiou KA, Constantinides G, et al: A biomechanical analysis of articular cartilage of the human elbow and a potential relationship to osteochondritis dissecans. Clin Orthop Relat Res 1994;299:305.
493. Schmier AA: Internal epicondylar epiphysis and elbow injuries. Surg Gynecol Obstet 1945;80:416.
494. Schneider G, Pouliquen JC: [Old fractures of the lateral humeral condyle (lateralis capitellum humeri) in children.] Rev Chir Orthop Reparatrice Appar Mot 1992;78:456.
495. Schwab GH, Bennett JB, Woods GW, et al: Biomechanics of elbow instability: The role of the medial collateral ligament. Clin Orthop Relat Res 1980;146:42.
496. Scullion JE, Miller JH: Fracture of the neck of the radius in children: Prognostic factors and recommendations for management. J Bone Joint Surg Br 1985;97:491.
497. Segev Z, Tanzman U: [Fracture-separation of the distal humeral epiphyseal complex in a premature newborn.] Harefuah 1985;108:249.
498. Self J, Viegas SF, Buford WL Jr, et al: A comparison of double-plate fixation methods for complex distal humerus fractures. J Shoulder Elbow Surg 1995;4:10.
499. Sessa S, Lascombes P, Prevot J, et al: Fractures of the radial head and associated elbow injuries in children. J Pediatr Orthop B 1996;5:200.
500. Shaker IJ, White JJ, Signer RD, et al: Special problems of vascular injuries in children. J Trauma 1976;16:863.
501. Shannon FJ, Mohan P, Chacko J, et al: "Dorgan's" percutaneous lateral cross-wiring of supracondylar fractures of the humerus in children. J Pediatr Orthop 2004;24:376.
502. Sharma JC, Arora A, Mathur NC, et al: Lateral condylar fractures of the humerus in children: Fixation with partially threaded 4.0-mm AO cancellous screws. J Trauma 1995;39:1129.
503. Shaw BA, Kasser JR, Emans JB, et al: Management of vascular injuries in displaced supracondylar humerus fractures without arteriography. J Orthop Trauma 1990;4:25.
504. Sherren J: Remarks on chronic neuritis of the ulnar nerve due to deformity in the region of the elbow-joint. Edinburgh Med Surg J 1908;23:500.
505. Shim JS, Lee YS: Treatment of completely displaced supracondylar fracture of the humerus in children by cross-fixation with three Kirschner wires. J Pediatr Orthop 2002;22:12.
506. Shimada K, Masada K, Tada K, et al: Osteosynthesis for the treatment of non-union of the lateral humeral condyle in children. J Bone Joint Surg Am 1997;79:234.
507. Shuck JM, Omer GE Jr, Lewis CE Jr: Arterial obstruction due to intimal disruption in extremity fractures. J Trauma 1972;12:481.
508. Siffert RS: Displacement of the distal humeral epiphysis in the newborn infant. J Bone Joint Surg Am 1963;45:165.
509. Silberstein MJ, Brodeur AE, Graviss ER: Some vagaries of the capitellum. J Bone Joint Surg Am 1979;61:244.
510. Silberstein MJ, Brodeur AE, Graviss ER: Some vagaries of the lateral epicondyle. J Bone Joint Surg Am 1982;64:444.
511. Silberstein MJ, Brodeur AE, Graviss ER, et al: Some vagaries of the medial epicondyle. J Bone Joint Surg Am 1981;63:524.
512. Silva JF: Old dislocations of the elbow. Ann R Coll Surg Engl 1958;22:363.
513. Silva JF: The problems relating to old dislocations and the restriction on elbow movement. Acta Orthop Belg 1975;41:399.
514. Singer KM, Roy SP: Osteochondrosis of the humeral capitellum. Am J Sports Med 1984;12:351.
515. Singh D: Pulse oximetry and fracture manipulation. Injury 1992;23:70.
516. Siris IE: Supracondylar fracture of the humerus: An analysis of 330 cases. Surg Gynecol Obstet 1939;68:201.
517. Skaggs DL, Hale JM, Bassett J, et al: Operative treatment of supracondylar fractures of the humerus in children. The consequences of pin placement. J Bone Joint Surg Am 2001;83:735.
518. Skak SV, Grossmann E, Wagn P: Deformity after internal fixation of fracture separation of the medial epicondyle of the humerus. J Bone Joint Surg Br 1994;76:297.
519. Skak SV, Olsen SD, Smaabrekke A: Deformity after fracture of the lateral humeral condyle in children. J Pediatr Orthop B 2001;10:142.

520. Smith FM: Displacement of the medial epicondyle of the humerus into the elbow joint. Ann Surg 1946; 124:425.
521. Smith FM: Kirschner wire traction in elbow and upper arm injuries. Am J Surg 1947;74:770.
522. Smith FM: Medial epicondyle injuries. JAMA 1950;142: 396.
523. Smith FM: An eighty-four year follow-up on a patient with ununited fracture of the lateral condyle of the humerus. A case report. J Bone Joint Surg Am 1973; 55:378.
524. Smith L: Deformity following supracondylar fractures of the humerus. J Bone Joint Surg Am 1960;42: 235.
525. Smith L: Deformity following supracondylar fractures of the humerus. J Bone Joint Surg Am 1965;47: 1668.
526. Smith L: Supracondylar fractures of the humerus treated by direct observation. Clin Orthop Relat Res 1967;50:37.
527. Smith MG: Osteochondritis of the humeral capitulum. J Bone Joint Surg Br 1964;46:50.
528. Smyth EH: Primary rupture of brachial artery and median nerve in supracondylar fracture of the humerus. J Bone Joint Surg Br 1956;38:736.
529. So YC, Fang D, Leong JC, et al: Varus deformity following lateral humeral condylar fractures in children. J Pediatr Orthop 1985;5:569.
530. Sokolowska-Pituchowa J, Goszczynski M: [The age of appearance of centers of ossification in the distal epiphyis of the humerus in the radiologic picture.] Folia Morphol (Warsz) 1968;27:541.
531. Song KS, Jeon SH: Osteochondral flap fracture of the olecranon with dislocation of the elbow in a child: A case report. J Orthop Trauma 2003;17:229.
532. Sovio OM, Tredwell SJ: Divergent dislocation of the elbow in a child. J Pediatr Orthop 1986;6:96.
533. Spear HC, James JM: Rupture of the brachial artery accompanying dislocation of the elbow or supracondylar fracture. J Bone Joint Surg Am 1951;33:889.
534. Speed JS: An operation for reduced posterior dislocation of the elbow. South Med J 1925;18:193.
535. Spinner M, Schreiber SN: Anterior interosseous-nerve paralysis as a complication of supracondylar fractures of the humerus in children. J Bone Joint Surg Am 1969;51:1584.
536. Spitzer AG, Paterson DC: Acute nerve involvement in supracondylar fractures of the humerus in children. J Bone Joint Surg Br 1973;55:227.
537. Srivastava KK, Kochhar VL: Forward dislocation of the elbow joint without fracture of the olecranon. Aust N Z J Surg 1974;44:71.
538. Stanitski CL, Micheli LJ: Simultaneous ipsilateral fractures of the arm and forearm in children. Clin Orthop Relat Res 1980;153:218.
539. Stans AA, Maritz NG, O'Driscoll SW, et al: Operative treatment of elbow contracture in patients twenty-one years of age or younger. J Bone Joint Surg Am 2002;84:382.
540. Staples OS: Supracondylar fractures of the humerus in children: Complications and problems associated with traction treatment. JAMA 1958;168:730.
541. Staples OS: Complications of traction treatment of supracondylar fracture of the humerus in children. J Bone Joint Surg Am 1959;41:369.
542. Staples OS: Dislocation of the brachial artery; a complication of supracondylar fracture of the humerus in childhood. J Bone Joint Surg Am 1965;47:1525.
543. Staunton FW: Dislocation forward of the forearm without fracture of the olecranon. BMJ 1905;2:1570.
544. St Clair Strange FG: Entrapment of the median nerve after dislocation of the elbow. J Bone Joint Surg Br 1982;64:224.
545. Steiger RN, Larrick RB, Meyer TL: Median-nerve entrapment following elbow dislocation in children. A report of two cases. J Bone Joint Surg Am 1969;51:381.
546. Steinberg EL, Golomb D, Salama R, et al: Radial head and neck fractures in children. J Pediatr Orthop 1988;8:35.
547. Stiefel D, Meuli M, Altermatt S: Fractures of the neck of the radius in children. Early experience with intramedullary pinning. J Bone Joint Surg Br 2001;83:536.
548. Stone CA: Subluxation of the head of the radius: Report of a case and anatomical experiments. JAMA 1916;1:28.
549. Stricker SJ, Thomson JD, Kelly RA: Coronal-plane transcondylar fracture of the humerus in a child. Clin Orthop Relat Res 1993;294:308.
550. Swenson AL: Treatment of supracondylar fractures of humerus by Kirschner wire transfixation. J Bone Joint Surg Am 1948;30:993.
551. Symeonides PP, Paschaloglou C, Pagalides T: Radial nerve enclosed in the callus of a supracondylar fracture. J Bone Joint Surg Br 1975;57:523.
552. Takahara M, Ogino T, Fukushima S, et al: Nonoperative treatment of osteochondritis dissecans of the humeral capitellum. Am J Sports Med 1999;27:728.
553. Takahara M, Ogino T, Sasaki I, et al: Long term outcome of osteochondritis dissecans of the humeral capitellum. Clin Orthop Relat Res 1999;363:108.
554. Takahara M, Sasaki I, Kimura T, et al: Second fracture of the distal humerus after varus malunion of a supracondylar fracture in children. J Bone Joint Surg Br 1998;80:791.
555. Tayob AA, Shively RA: Bilateral elbow dislocations with intra-articular displacement of the medial epicondyles. J Trauma 1980;20:332.
556. Thomas DP, Howard AW, Cole WG, et al: Three weeks of Kirschner wire fixation for displaced lateral condylar fractures of the humerus in children. J Pediatr Orthop 2001;21:565.
557. Thonell S, Mortensson W, Thomasson B: Prediction of the stability of minimally displaced fractures of the lateral humeral condyle. Acta Radiol 1988;29:367.
558. Tibone JE, Stoltz M: Fractures of the radial head and neck in children. J Bone Joint Surg Am 1981;63:100.
559. Tien YC, Chih HW, Lin GT, et al: Dome corrective osteotomy for cubitus varus deformity. Clin Orthop Relat Res 2000;380:158.
560. Tivnon MC, Anzel SH, Waugh TR: Surgical management of osteochondritis dissecans of the capitellum. Am J Sports Med 1976;4:121.
561. Toh S, Tsubo K, Nishikawa S, et al: Osteosynthesis for nonunion of the lateral humeral condyle. Clin Orthop Relat Res 2002;405:230.

562. Toh S, Tsubo K, Nishikawa S, et al: Long-standing non-union of fractures of the lateral humeral condyle. J Bone Joint Surg Am 2002;84:593.
563. Toniolo RM, Wilkins KE: T-Condylar fractures. In Rockwood CA Jr, Wilkins KE, Beaty J (eds): Fractures in Children, vol 3. Philadelphia, Lippincott-Raven, 1996, p 833.
564. Topping RE, Blanco JS, Davis TJ: Clinical evaluation of crossed-pin versus lateral-pin fixation in displaced supracondylar humerus fractures. J Pediatr Orthop 1995;15:435.
565. Torg JS, Moyer RA: Non-union of a stress fracture through the olecranon epiphyseal plate observed in an adolescent baseball pitcher. A case report. J Bone Joint Surg Am 1977;59:264.
566. Torg JS, Pollack H, Sweterlitsch P: The effect of competitive pitching on the shoulders and elbows of preadolescent baseball players. Pediatrics 1972;49:267.
567. Trias A, Comeau Y: Recurrent dislocation of the elbow in children. Clin Orthop Relat Res 1974;100:74.
568. Tullos HS, King JW: Lesions of the pitching arm in adolescents. JAMA 1972;220:264.
569. Turra S, Pavanini G, Pasquon PG: [Complications of supracondylar fractures of the humerus in children.] Clin Orthop Relat Res 1974;25:222.
570. Usui M, Ishii S, Miyano S, et al: Three-dimensional corrective osteotomy for treatment of cubitus varus after supracondylar fracture of the humerus in children. J Shoulder Elbow Surg 1995;4:17.
571. Vahvanen V, Aalto K: Supracondylar fracture of the humerus in children. A long-term follow-up study of 107 cases. Acta Orthop Scand 1978;49:225.
572. Vahvanen V, Gripenberg L: Fracture of the radial neck in children. A long-term follow-up study of 43 cases. Acta Orthop Scand 1978;49:32.
573. Van Arsdale WH: On subluxation of the head of the radius in children with a resume of one hundred consecutive cases. Ann Surg 1889;9:401.
574. van Haaren ER, van Vugt AB, Bode PJ: Posterolateral dislocation of the elbow with concomitant fracture of the lateral humeral condyle: Case report. J Trauma 1994;36:288.
575. Vanthournout I, Rudelli A, Valenti P, et al: Osteochondritis dissecans of the trochlea of the humerus. Pediatr Radiol 1991;21:600.
576. van Vugt AB, Severijnen RV, Festen C: Neurovascular complications in supracondylar humeral fractures in children. Arch Orthop Trauma Surg 1988;107:203.
577. van Vugt AB, Severijnen RV, Festen C: Fractures of the lateral humeral condyle in children: Late results. Arch Orthop Trauma Surg 1988;107:206.
578. Varma BP, Srivastava TP: Fracture of the medial condyle of the humerus in children: A report of 4 cases including the late sequelae. Injury 1972;4:171.
579. Vasli LR: Diagnosis of vascular injury in children with supracondylar fractures of the humerus. Injury 1988; 19:11.
580. Vocke AK, Von Laer L: Displaced fractures of the radial neck in children: Long-term results and prognosis of conservative treatment. J Pediatr Orthop B 1998;7:217.
581. Vocke-Hell AK, Schmid A: Sonographic differentiation of stable and unstable lateral condyle fractures of the humerus in children. J Pediatr Orthop B 2001; 10:138.
582. Vocke-Hell AK, von Laer L, Slongo T, et al: Secondary radial head dislocation and dysplasia of the lateral condyle after elbow trauma in children. J Pediatr Orthop 2001;21:319.
583. Volkmann R: Die ischaemischen Muskellahmungen und Kontrakturer. Zentralbl Chir 1881;8:801.
584. Voss FR, Kasser JR, Trepman E, et al: Uniplanar supracondylar humeral osteotomy with preset Kirschner wires for posttraumatic cubitus varus. J Pediatr Orthop 1994;14:471.
585. Wadsworth TG: Screw fixation of the olecranon after fracture or osteotomy. Clin Orthop Relat Res 1976; 119:197.
586. Walker HB: A case of dislocation of the elbow with separation of the internal epicondyle and displacement of the latter into the elbow joint. Br J Surg 1928;15:677.
587. Walloe A, Egund N, Eikelund L: Supracondylar fracture of the humerus in children: Review of closed and open reduction leading to a proposal for treatment. Injury 1985;16:296.
588. Walsh SJ, Lamb GF, Barnes MJ. Medial opening wedge osteotomy with external fixation for correction of cubitus varus. Paper presented at the Annual Meeting of the Pediatric Orthopaedic Society of North America, Miami, 1995.
589. Ward WG, Nunley JA: Concomitant fractures of the capitellum and radial head. J Orthop Trauma 1988;2: 110.
590. Waters PM, Stewart SL: Radial neck fracture nonunion in children. J Pediatr Orthop 2001;21:570.
591. Watson-Jones R: Primary nerve lesions in injuries of the elbow and wrist. J Bone Joint Surg 1930;12:121.
592. Watson-Jones R: Fractures and Joint Injuries. Edinburgh, ES Livingstone, 1956.
593. Wattenbarger JM, Gerardi J, Johnston CE: Late open reduction internal fixation of lateral condyle fractures. J Pediatr Orthop 2002;22:394.
594. Webb AJ, Sherman FC: Supracondylar fractures of the humerus in children. J Pediatr Orthop 1989;9:315.
595. Wedge JH, Robertson DE: Displaced fractures of the neck of the radius. J Bone Joint Surg Br 1982;64:256.
596. Weiland AJ, Meyer S, Tolo VT, et al: Surgical treatment of displaced supracondylar fractures of the humerus in children. Analysis of fifty-two cases followed for five to fifteen years. J Bone Joint Surg Am 1978;60:657.
597. White JJ, Talbert JL, Haller JA Jr: Peripheral artial injuries in infants and children. Ann Surg 1968;167:757.
598. Wildburger R, Mahring M, Hofer HP: Supraintercondylar fractures of the distal humerus: Results of internal fixation. J Orthop Trauma 1991;5:301.
599. Wiley JJ, McIntyre WM: Fracture patterns in children. In Current Concepts of Bone Fragility. Berlin, Springer-Verlag, 1986, p 159.
600. Wilkins KE: Residuals of elbow trauma in children. Orthop Clin North Am 1990;21:291.
601. Wilkins KE: Changing patterns in the management of fractures in children. Clin Orthop Relat Res 1991; 264:136.
602. Wilkins KE: Supracondylar fractures: what's new? J Pediatr Orthop B 1997;6:110.

603. Wilkins KE, Beaty J, Chambers HG: Fractures and dislocations of the elbow region. In Rockwood CA, Wilkins KE, King RE: Fractures in Children. Philadelphia, Lippincott-Raven, 1996.
604. Wilkins KE, Morrey BF, Jobe FW, et al: The elbow. Instr Course Lect 1991;40:1.
605. Williamson DM, Coates CJ, Miller RK, et al: Normal characteristics of the Baumann (humerocapitellar) angle: An aid in assessment of supracondylar fractures. J Pediatr Orthop 1992;12:636.
606. Wilson JN: The treatment of fractures of the medial epicondyle of the humerus. J Bone Joint Surg Br 1960;42:778.
607. Wilson NI, Ingram R, Rymaszewski L, et al: Treatment of fractures of the medial epicondyle of the humerus. Injury 1988;19:342.
608. Winslow R: A case of complete anterior dislocation of both bones of the forearm at the elbow. Surg Gynecol Obstet 1913;16:570.
609. Wood JB, Klassen RA, Peterson HA: Osteochondritis dissecans of the femoral head in children and adolescents: A report of 17 cases. J Pediatr Orthop 1995; 15:313.
610. Wood SK: Reversal of the radial head during reduction of fracture of the neck of the radius in children. J Bone Joint Surg Br 1969;51:707.
611. Woods GW, Tullos HS: Elbow instability and medial epicondyle fractures. Am J Sports Med 1977;5:23.
612. Woodward AH, Bianco AJ Jr: Osteochondritis dissecans of the elbow. Clin Orthop Relat Res 1975;110:35.
613. Worlock P: Supracondylar fractures of the humerus. Assessment of cubitus varus by the Baumann angle. J Bone Joint Surg Br 1986;68:755.
614. Worlock P, Stower M: Fracture patterns in Nottingham children. J Pediatr Orthop 1986;6:656.
615. Worlock PH, Colton CL: Displaced supracondylar fractures of the humerus in children treated by overhead olecranon traction. Injury 1984;15:316.
616. Yamamoto I, Ishii S, Usui M, et al: Cubitus varus deformity following supracondylar fracture of the humerus. A method for measuring rotational deformity. Clin Orthop Relat Res 1985;201:179.
617. Yang Z, Wang Y, Gilula LA, et al: Microcirculation of the distal humeral epiphyseal cartilage: Implications for post-traumatic growth deformities. J Hand Surg [Am] 1998;23:165.
618. Yates C, Sullivan JA: Arthrographic diagnosis of elbow injuries in children. J Pediatr Orthop 1987;7:54.
619. Yoo CI, Suh JT, Suh KT, et al: Avascular necrosis after fracture-separation of the distal end of the humerus in children. Orthopedics 1992;15:959.
620. Young S, Letts M, Jarvis J: Avascular necrosis of the radial head in children. J Pediatr Orthop 2000;20: 15.
621. Zimmerman H: Fractures of the elbow. In Weber BG, Brunner C, Freuler F (eds): Treatment of Fractures in Children and Adolescents. New York, Springer-Verlag, 1980.
622. Zionts LE, McKellop HA, Hathaway R: Torsional strength of pin configurations used to fix supracondylar fractures of the humerus in children. J Bone Joint Surg Am 1994;76:253.
623. Zionts LE, Moon CN: Olecranon apophysis fractures in children with osteogenesis imperfecta revisited. J Pediatr Orthop 2002;22:745.

FRACTURES OF THE FOREARM

Monteggia Fractures

In 1814 Giovanni Monteggia described two cases of fracture of the proximal third of the ulna associated with anterior dislocation of the radial head.[192] In 1844 Cooper described anterior, posterior, and lateral dislocations of the radial head with fracture of the ulnar shaft.[66] Perrin is credited with coining the term *Monteggia fracture* in 1909.[223] The eponym *Monteggia lesion* was used by Bado to describe different types of dislocation of the radial head associated with fracture of the ulnar shaft.[16,17] Although the Monteggia fracture is an uncommon injury, it has been the subject of considerable investigation because of the frequency with which its diagnosis is missed and the serious sequelae that may develop without treatment.

ANATOMY

Pertinent anatomic considerations in Monteggia fractures include the ligamentous structures, which stabilize the radius and ulna; the muscles, which contribute to the deforming forces; and the neurovascular structures, which may be injured with fracture displacement. The radius and ulna are bound together proximally and distally by strong ligaments and throughout their length by the interosseous membrane. The radial head is maintained within the radial notch of the ulna by the annular ligament. The quadrate ligament, radial collateral ligament, and elbow capsule also provide stability to the proximal articulation of the radius and ulna.

The muscular anatomy of the forearm contributes to Monteggia fractures. In hyperextension injuries, the biceps is a major deforming force and acts by pulling the proximal radius away from the capitellum as the elbow extends. The forearm flexors also provide a deforming force in Monteggia fractures by shortening and radially deviating the ulna.[293]

The unique neurovascular anatomy of the elbow predisposes Monteggia fractures to certain complications. The proximity of the displacing radial head to the radial or median nerve makes nerve palsy common. The fascial compartments of the antecubital fossa and forearm can lead to compartment syndrome after Monteggia fractures.[20,89,144,193,195,247,271,276,314]

CLASSIFICATION

The mechanism of injury varies with the type of Monteggia fracture; thus, it is helpful to discuss the classification of Monteggia fractures before discussing the mechanism of injury. Bado's classic classification is still used today.[16,17,71,91,210,239,240,332] This classification is defined by the direction (i.e., anterior, posterior, or lateral) of the radial head dislocation. Radial head displacement is always in the direction of the apex of the ulnar deformity.

In type I fractures, which are most common, the radial head is dislocated anteriorly.

Type II Monteggia fractures have posterior dislocation of the radial head.[16,17,86,219,221]

Type III Monteggia fractures are the second most common. The ulnar fracture is metaphyseal and often greenstick, and the radial head is dislocated laterally.[16,17,141,210,329] If the ulnar fracture extends into the olecranon, there may not be true dissociation between the radial head and the ulna. This fact has led to debate about the proper classification of this injury.[21,43,99,141,210,285,324]

Fracture of both the radius and the ulna with anterior dislocation of the radial head is a type IV Monteggia fracture. Some authors have described the type IV injury as a variant of a type I injury.[16,17,62,71]

Bado described injuries that were "equivalent" to a type I Monteggia fracture based on a similar mechanism of injury, radiographic appearance, or treatment.[16,17] Other authors[27,95,100,210,247,324] have subsequently expanded these equivalent injuries. The most common and recognized equivalents are fracture of the ulnar shaft associated with fracture of the proximal radial epiphysis or radial neck[210] and anterior dislocation of the radial head. Although the latter has been reported as an isolated injury, it is probably always associated with plastic deformation of the ulna.[174] Other uncommon injuries have also been reported as equivalent to Bado type I, II, or III injuries.[27,100,210,221,237,247,274,314,324]

Letts and associates modified Bado's classification for pediatric patients.[171] They described five types, of which the first three—A, B, and C—are subtypes of Bado's type I anterior dislocation. In Letts' type A injuries, anterior dislocation of the radial head occurs as a result of plastic deformation (apex anteriorly) of the ulna.[172] Type B and type C injuries are characterized by anterior dislocation of the radial head, type B by a greenstick fracture of the ulna, and type C by complete fracture of the ulna. Letts' type C injuries include Bado's type IV lesions. Letts' types D and E correspond to Bado's types II and III, respectively.

MECHANISM OF INJURY

Three different theories on the pathogenesis of type I Monteggia fractures have been proposed. The first theory proposes that fracture results from a direct blow to the posterior aspect of the ulna.[38,39,192,266] According to this theory, as the ulna fractures and shortens, it puts stress on the radial head, which either ruptures the annular ligament or dislocates anteriorly from it. A second theory, supported in the original work of Bado, is that of hyperpronation.[17,91,217] According to this hypothesis, the body rotates around a fixed and pronated outstretched hand. Such rotation produces forced hyperpronation, which leads to fracture of the proximal ulna with anterior dislocation of the radial head. The third theory proposes hyperextension as a mechanism. As a child lands on an outstretched hand, the biceps contracts, which dislocates the radial head anteriorly. Thus, the entire body weight is borne by the ulna, which fractures and displaces anteriorly as a result of pull of the intact interosseous membrane and the contracting brachialis.[293] Type II Monteggia fractures occur when the flexed elbow is longitudinally loaded; the forearm may be in pronation, neutral position, or in supination.[210,220,221] Type III Monteggia injuries are most likely the result of a varus-extension force at the elbow.[17,84,197,220,284,332]

DIAGNOSIS

A patient with a Monteggia fracture usually has an obvious deformity of the forearm and elbow. Rotation of the forearm or flexion-extension of the elbow is painful and restricted. The radial head may be palpable and displaced from its normal position in the direction of dislocation—anteriorly, posteriorly, or laterally. Palpation of the ulnar diaphysis will reveal tenderness and deformity. The entire patient must be thoroughly assessed. It is important to be aware of the high incidence of associated ipsilateral extremity fractures in patients with Bado's type II lesions.[162,219]A careful examination of the skin and a careful neurovascular assessment should also be performed, with particular attention to the posterior interosseous nerve.

RADIOGRAPHIC FINDINGS

The most common problem in the management of Monteggia fractures is failure to properly obtain and interpret good-quality radiographs.[42,84,118,244,319] The importance of obtaining radiographs of the elbow in *all* patients with displaced fractures (complete, greenstick, or plastic deformation) of the ulna cannot be overstated.[71,150,151] A recent report highlighted the potential hazards of isolated ulna fractures. Weisman and colleagues described two late-identified Monteggia fractures with initial radiographs documenting a reduced radial head. In these cases the radial head presumably spontaneously reduced and redislocated as the ulna angulated in the cast.[319] The diagnosis cannot be made if the appropriate radiographs are not obtained. The surgeon must carefully assess radial head–capitellar alignment. A line drawn through the longitudinal axis of the radius should pass through the center of the capitellum, regardless of the degree of flexion or extension of the elbow (Fig. 42–108).[266,280]

The only diagnosis in the differential is an ulna fracture associated with congenital dislocation of the radial head. Congenital dislocations of the radial head are usually bilateral and posterior.[7,175] Although anterior congenital dislocation of the radial head has been described, Lloyd-Roberts and others have written that these injuries probably represent chronic, missed traumatic dislocations.[52,175,187] Radiographically, the congenitally dislocated radial head is posterior, enlarged, elliptical, and slightly irregular. The radius appears long relative to the capitellum, which is flattened.[7,45,175]

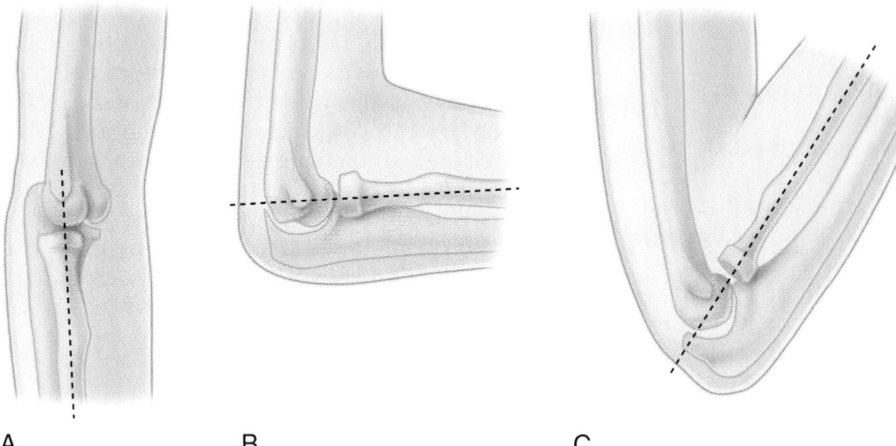

FIGURE 42–108 A through C, Anatomic relationship of the radial head and capitellum. A line through the longitudinal axis of the radius passes through the center of the capitellum, regardless of the degree of elbow flexion.

TREATMENT

Closed Reduction and Cast Immobilization

If seen and diagnosed acutely, Monteggia fractures in children can usually be managed successfully with simple closed reduction and cast immobilization.* The goal of treatment is to obtain and maintain an anatomically reduced radial head. This can often be accomplished with a less than anatomic reduction of the ulna. We routinely accept up to 10 degrees of angulation of the ulna, provided that a concentric radial head reduction is maintained. Satisfactory results have been reported with angulation of up to 25 degrees.[210,229,235] We generally perform closed reduction under conscious sedation in the emergency department.

Type I fractures are reduced with longitudinal traction and reduction of the ulnar fracture. The elbow is then flexed and the radial head is gently reduced with direct pressure. After reduction, the radial head is usually stable as long as the elbow is kept adequately flexed. The arm should be immobilized in 110 to 120 degrees of elbow flexion and neutral or slight supination.[293] This technique is also used for the uncommon type IV Monteggia fracture, although the free-floating proximal radial fragment makes operative treatment more likely, particularly in an adolescent. However, good results have been reported with closed treatment of type IV injuries, provided that radial head reduction is obtained and maintained.[17,210,246]

Type II (posterior) Monteggia fractures are reduced by placing traction on the forearm with the elbow in extension. After the ulnar fracture is anatomically aligned, the radial head is reduced and an above-elbow cast is applied with the elbow in extension and the forearm in neutral rotation.

Type III (lateral) Monteggia fractures are also reduced with the elbow in extension. Reduction is achieved by exerting longitudinal traction on the distal end of the forearm and direct pressure over the radial head and ulna. The arm is immobilized in a long-arm cast with the elbow at 90 degrees and the forearm in supination.[17,84,197,324]

Once adequate closed reduction has been achieved and a long-arm cast applied, postreduction radiographs should be obtained. They must include a true lateral view of the elbow showing the radiocapitellar joint to be reduced. Radiographs in the cast are obtained at weekly intervals for 3 weeks to ensure that the reduction is not lost as the swelling subsides and the cast loosens.[319] If the cast appears loose on the radiographs, it may be wise to replace it before the reduction is lost. It is imperative that radiographic confirmation of the reduced radial head be obtained in the new cast. After 3 weeks the fracture is "sticky" and the reduction is unlikely to be lost. The patient returns at 6 weeks for cast removal and radiographs.

Open Reduction and Fixation

Operative treatment is indicated when anatomic reduction cannot be obtained or maintained by closed methods. If the ulna cannot be maintained in a reduced position, the radial head will often redislocate when the ulnar fracture displaces. In most cases, stabilizing the ulnar fracture will keep the radial head reduced. Ulnar fixation can be accomplished with pins, screws, or plates (Fig. 42–109). We prefer simple pin fixation because it requires a minimal (or no) incision and avoids the problem of retained hardware.* Once the ulnar fracture is stabilized, a long-arm cast is applied with the forearm in the position in which the radial head is most stable (usually supination, although this should be determined intraoperatively under fluoroscopic observation). Radiographs are obtained in the cast 2 weeks later to ensure that the radial head remains reduced. The cast is removed after 6 weeks.

Bado's type IV injuries may require stabilization of both the ulna and radius. The radius may be stabilized by open reduction and plating or by intramedullary reduction and fixation. After fracture stabilization, cast immobilization is continued for 6 weeks with

*See references 11, 27, 39, 44, 84, 99, 171, 210, 220, 239, 240, 244, 264, 266, 324.

*See references 17, 84, 99, 166, 171, 210, 220, 244, 288, 303, 324.

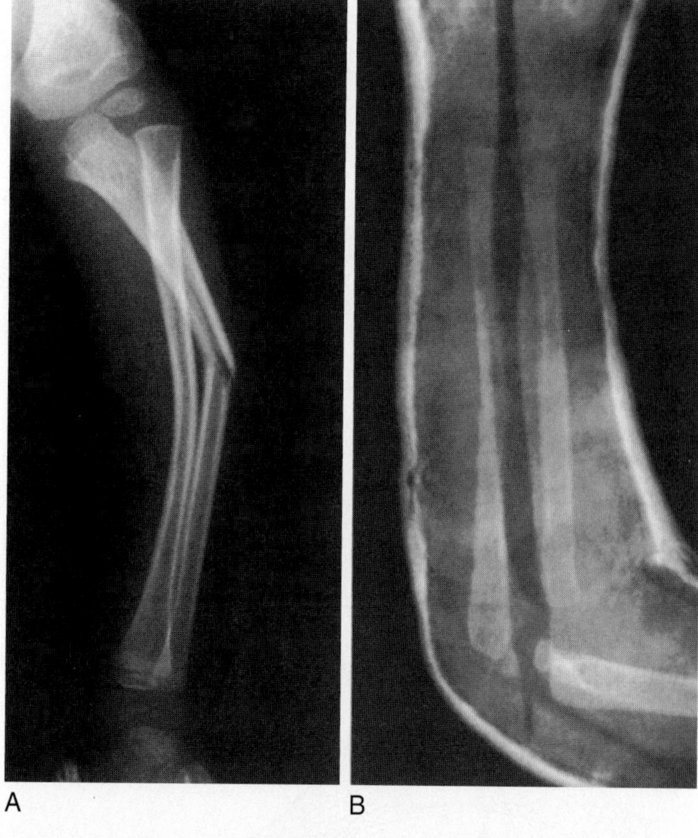

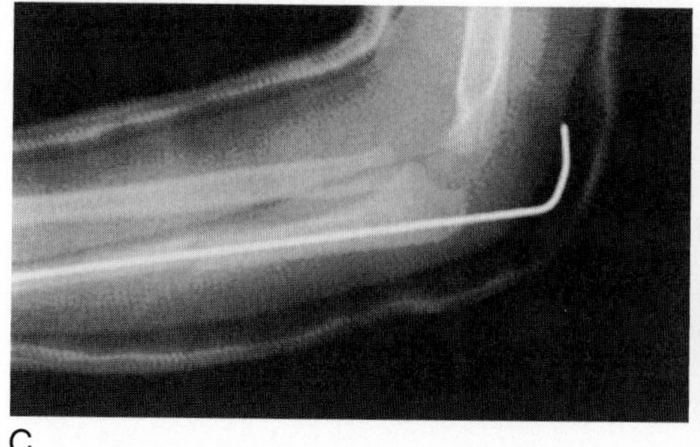

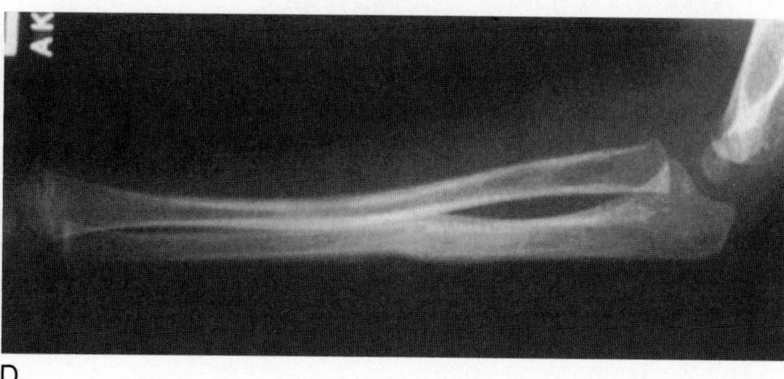

FIGURE 42-109 **A,** Anteroposterior radiograph of the forearm showing a greenstick fracture of the ulna with dislocation of the radial head. **B,** Despite an attempt at closed reduction and casting, the radial head remains anteriorly dislocated. **C,** The radial head is reduced after open reduction and percutaneous pin fixation of the ulna. **D,** The radial head remains reduced after pin removal and fracture union.

close follow-up to ensure that the radial head does not redislocate.

Occasionally, the radial head will not reduce with closed methods because of tissue interposed in the radial notch of the ulna. Possible impediments to closed reduction include either the annular ligament or a cartilaginous or osteochondral fragment. The annular ligament may be intact or ruptured.[208,293,329] In such instances, open reduction of the radial head is required. This can be performed through a simple posterolateral approach or through the more extensile approach described by Boyd. For acute injuries we have found the posterolateral approach between the anconeus and extensor carpi ulnaris to be adequate, although it is important to realize that this approach does not protect the posterior interosseous nerve distal to the annular ligament. Thus, if more extensile exposure is anticipated, the Boyd approach should be used. In this approach, the incision is extended distally and the supinator is elevated off the ulna down to the interosseous membrane to allow exposure of the radiocapitellar joint and visualization of the annular ligament, as well as exposure of both the proximal ulna and radius and the posterior interosseous nerve (Fig. 42–110).[37,39,270] Once the radioulnar joint is exposed, the impediment to reduction can be removed. If the annular ligament remains in continuity, a nerve hook can be used to reduce it over the radial head. If this is unsuccessful, the ligament can be transected and repaired. If the annular ligament is ruptured, primary repair is often possible (Fig. 42–111). If the ligament is not repairable, it may be debrided.

After removal of the impediments to reduction, the ulnar fracture is reduced and stabilized. After fixation

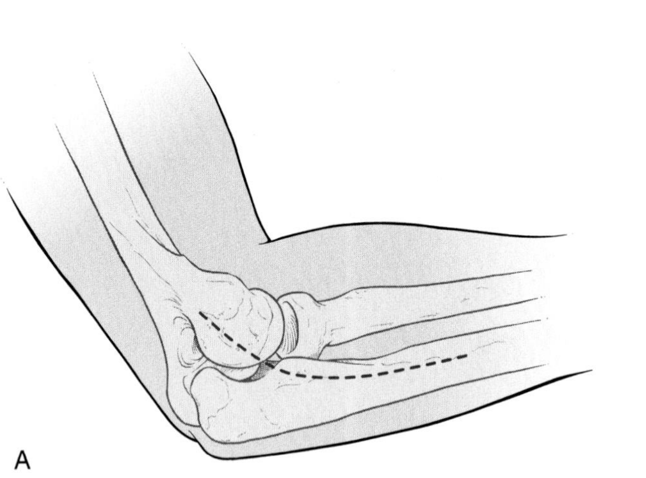

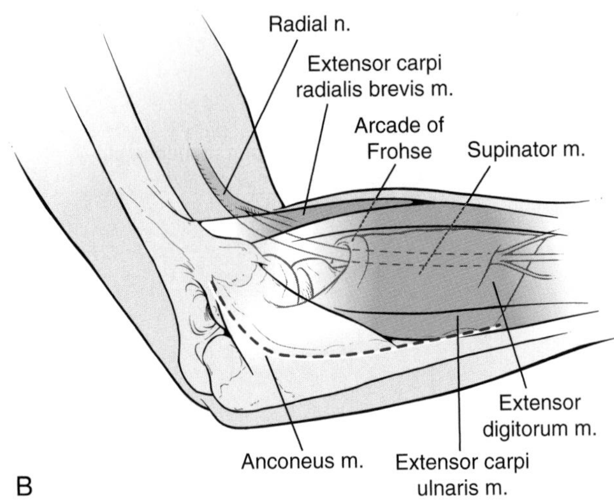

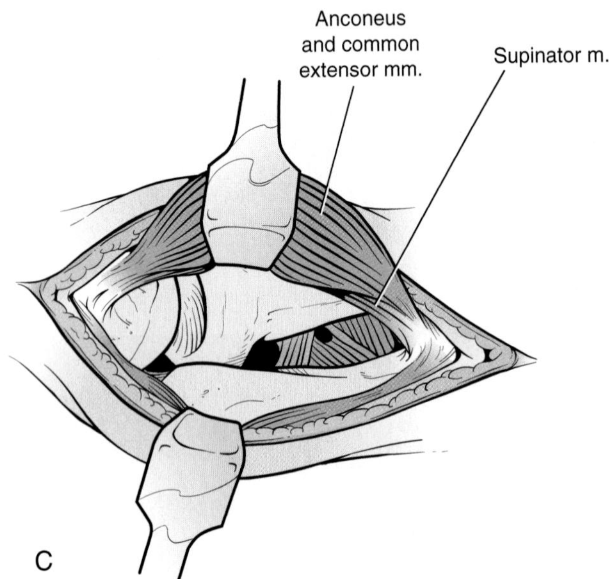

FIGURE 42-110 **A** through **C,** Boyd's approach to the radioulnar joint and proximal radius. The insertion of the anconeus and the common extensor and supinator origin are elevated subperiosteally off the dorsal surface of the ulna. The deep fibers of the supinator arising from below the radial notch must be divided close to the ulna. (Redrawn from Boyd HB: Surgical exposure of the ulna and proximal third of the radius through one incision. Surg Gynecol Obstet 1940;71:86-88, with permission.)

of the ulna, we assess the stability of the radial head and routinely find it to be adequate. Although some authors have advocated routine reconstruction of the annular ligament, we reserve this procedure for unusual cases in which the radial head remains unstable despite removal of the impediments to reduction and stabilization of the ulnar fracture. (The technique of annular ligament reconstruction is discussed under Chronic, Missed, or Neglected Monteggia Fractures.)

After open reduction and ulnar stabilization, the patient is immobilized in a long-arm cast with the arm in the most stable position for 6 weeks. A number of authors have suggested a transcapitellar pin to help hold the radial head reduced. These authors stress that the pin must be of adequate diameter to prevent pin breakage. We have seen AVN of the radial head from a transcapitellar pin that was of "adequate size." We believe that the problems associated with transcapitellar pins (breakage, stiffness, osteonecrosis) outweigh their benefits and we avoid them at all costs.[203,317]

COMPLICATIONS

The most common and serious complication associated with Monteggia fractures is failure to make the appropriate diagnosis, which results in a chronic or neglected Monteggia fracture. Other potential complications include recurrent radial head dislocation, malunion of the ulna, stiffness, posterior interosseous nerve palsy, and Volkmann's ischemic contracture.

Chronic, Missed, or Neglected Monteggia Fracture

Treatment of a child with chronic dislocation of the radial head represents a difficult dilemma. On one hand, numerous reports indicate that most children with persistent dislocation of the radial head have minimal or no symptoms in the short term.[199,226,251,277] However, the long-term prognosis for these elbows is less positive. There are multiple reports of adults with untreated Monteggia lesions who have pain, instability, and restricted motion.[24,45,175,187] Additionally, tardy

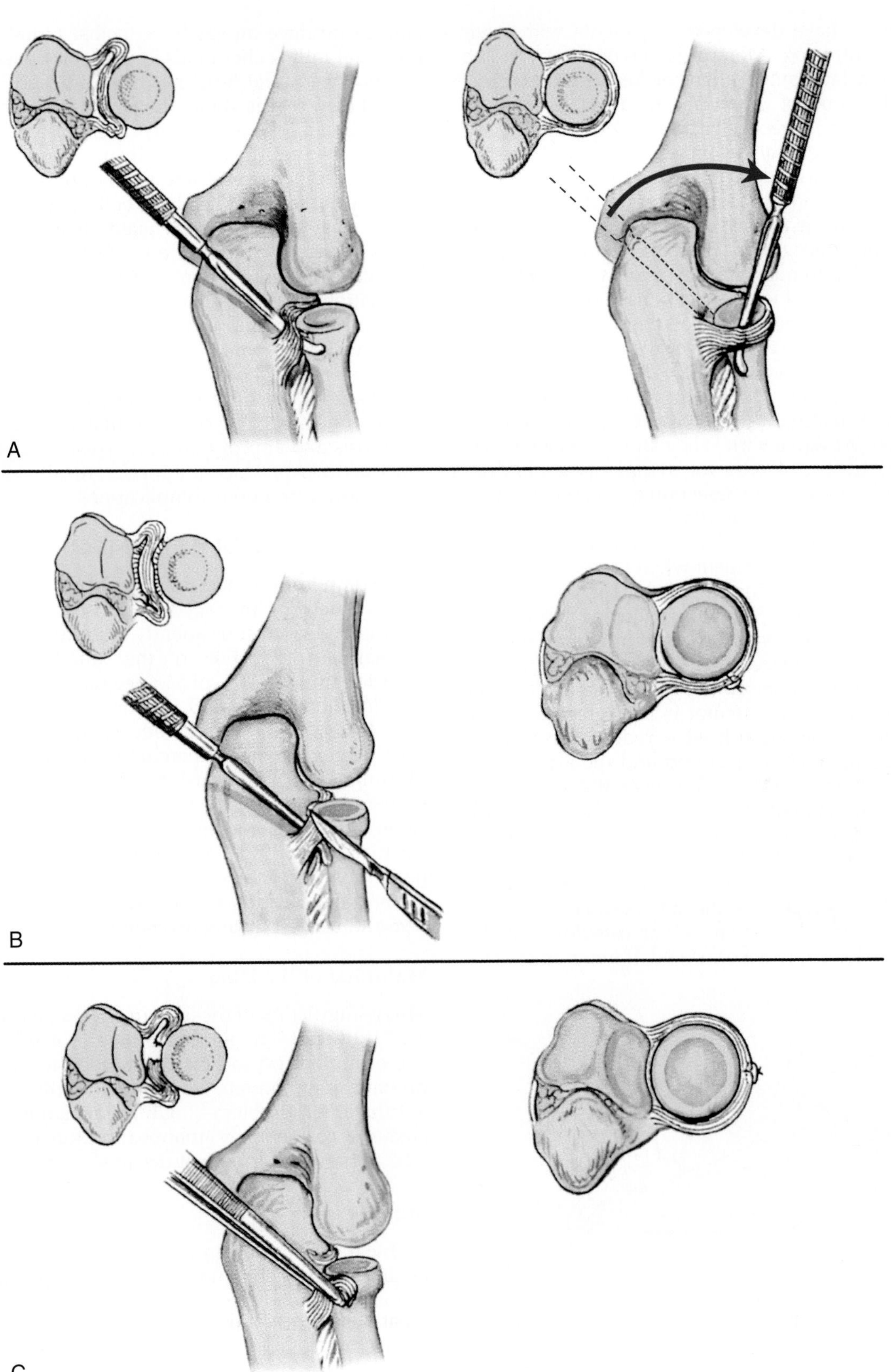

FIGURE 42–111 Techniques for management of the annular ligament after Monteggia fracture-dislocation. **A,** An entrapped annular ligament may be reduced with a nerve hook. **B,** If the annular ligament is irreducible, it may be transected and repaired primarily. **C,** A ruptured annular ligament may be repaired primarily or debrided.

nerve palsies have developed in patients with longstanding untreated Monteggia lesions.[3,15,133,173] The possibility of late complications makes surgical correction at the time of diagnosis an attractive option. However, surgical reconstruction is not simple, and complications are frequent and often severe. Although many studies have described the surgical management of chronic radial head dislocation,* relatively few have described the clinical results.† A recent report by Rodgers and colleagues at Boston Children's Hospital highlights the frequency and severity of complications. They reported 14 complications in seven patients, including 3 ulnar nerve palsies, 1 compartment syndrome, and 2 instances of loss of fixation.[247] Our experience, though limited, parallels that of Rodgers and colleagues and has led us to take a conservative approach to treating a child with chronic radial head dislocation. We agree with Fahey and others who have advocated treatment only for symptomatic children and consider radial head resection a safe, reliable procedure for symptomatic adults.[94]

We will attempt reduction of the radial head and restoration of bone alignment when necessary in children with a symptomatic chronic Monteggia fracture. The most common symptoms during childhood include lack of flexion, restricted pronation/supination, and rarely, unacceptable cosmesis. We favor a Boyd approach to debride the radioulnar joint. After joint debridement, an attempt is made to reduce the radial head. If the radial head is reduced and stable, no further treatment is required and the arm can be immobilized for 6 weeks. If, however, the radial head reduces easily but remains unstable, we proceed with annular ligament reconstruction using the Lloyd-Roberts modification of the Bell Tawse technique (which uses the lateral rather than central triceps tendon) (Fig. 42–112).[25,175] If the radial head is not reducible after joint debridement, ulnar osteotomy at the apex of the deformity is performed. If ulnar osteotomy fails to produce an easily reducible radial head, the proximal radius should also be osteotomized.

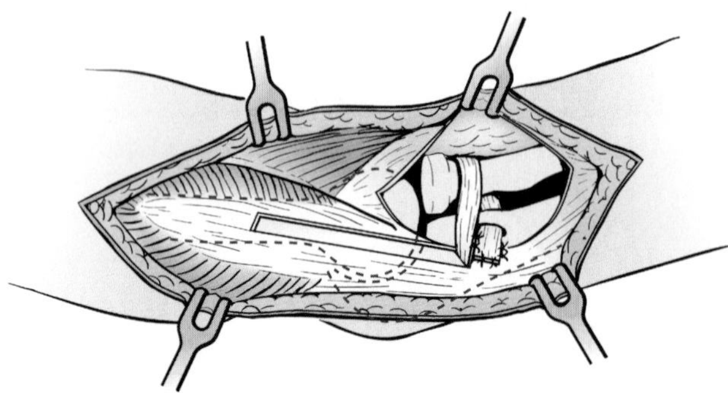

FIGURE 42–112 Bell Tawse technique for reconstruction of the annular ligament. If the radial head remains unstable after reduction of the ulna, the annular ligament can be reconstructed by bringing a lateral strip of triceps tendon around the radial neck and through a drill hole in the proximal ulna.

Once the radial head has been reduced, we assess its stability. If it is stable through a reasonable range of motion and the osteotomies are rigidly fixed, we do not believe that the annular ligament must be reconstructed. If, however, there is any question about the stability of the radial head, we believe that the annular ligament should be reconstructed. Given the frequency and severity of complications after reconstruction of chronic Monteggia lesions, we agree with the recommendations of Rodgers and colleagues for exposure of the entire radial and ulnar nerves, as well as for prophylactic fasciotomies. Although there are descriptions of radial head reduction via ulnar Ilizarov lengthening, we have no experience with this technique.[93,283] There is no question that an accurate initial diagnosis and appropriate early treatment of Monteggia fractures produce a superior result with significantly fewer potential complications.

Recurrence of Radial Head Dislocation

This complication most commonly occurs with Monteggia fractures managed by closed reduction and casting and is most frequently associated with failure to maintain reduction of the ulna.[319] It has been reported in up to 20% of Monteggia fractures.[84] When redislocation occurs and is promptly recognized, we usually repeat the closed reduction and stabilize the ulna, generally with percutaneous intramedullary pinning.[244] If significant healing of the ulna has occurred, management of this problem becomes the same as for a late-identified or neglected Monteggia fracture. Thus, it is of paramount importance that patients with Monteggia fractures be monitored closely so that redislocation of the radial head can be identified and treated in timely fashion.

Malunion of the Ulna

Minor angulation of the ulna in any plane is well tolerated. Although radial displacement is associated with encroachment on the interosseous space and loss of pronation/supination, we have found this to rarely be a functional problem.[229] Ulnar deviation, however, creates a cosmetically unappealing forearm that may lead to parental or patient dissatisfaction.

Stiffness

Stiffness after Monteggia fractures may be the result of simple immobilization, soft tissue (capsular) ossification,[25,141,173,175,277,280] myositis ossificans,[289] or fibrous or bony synostosis between the proximal ulna and radius.[43] Stiffness associated with routine cast immobilization usually improves with active motion in 1 to 2 months. The classic and well-described periarticular ossification is known to resolve over time.[24,141,173,175,277,280] Similarly, myositis ossificans in children generally spontaneously improves in the first year. Myositis is known to be worsened by aggressive passive motion.[202,289] Proximal radioulnar synostosis is a rare

*See references 25, 26, 37, 45, 68, 80, 101, 114, 128, 142, 148, 175, 211, 247, 270, 279, 281, 290, 315.

†See references 26, 77, 80, 120, 140, 144, 156, 215, 247, 279, 311.

complication that is usually seen with fractures associated with significant soft tissue injuries. Resection of the synostosis with interposition material (fat or methyl methacrylate [Cranioplast]) has been described, with variable results.[43,247]

Nerve Palsy

Transient posterior interosseous nerve palsy occurs in about 20% of anterior or lateral Monteggia fracture-dislocations. Fortunately, normal function generally returns within 2 to 3 months of the injury. The anatomic relationships of the proximal part of the forearm help delineate the location and cause of radial nerve palsies associated with Monteggia fractures. The superficial radial nerve (pure sensory) branches from the radial nerve just proximal to the fibrous arch at the proximal extent of the supinator muscle (also known as the arcade of Fröhse). The posterior interosseous nerve (pure motor) passes beneath the arcade. Therefore, a compressive lesion produces a pure motor deficit, whereas a traction or stretch injury produces a combined motor and sensory deficit.[276] If neurologic function does not return within 3 months, electromyography and nerve conduction studies should be performed. If there is no electrophysiologic evidence of reinnervation, consideration should be given to exploration of the nerve. Ulnar and median nerve palsies have been reported with Monteggia fractures, although they are rare.[44,276,315,324]

Compartment Syndrome/Volkmann's Ischemic Contracture

Monteggia fractures are associated with significant disruption of the soft tissues about the elbow. Thus, it is not surprising that compartment syndrome may develop after these injuries.[20,195,247,271,276,314] The possibility of compartment syndrome is increased because closed treatment often requires flexion in a cast past 90 degrees. It is imperative that the surgeon be aware of the potential for compartment syndrome and monitor these patients accordingly, particularly those with altered consciousness.

Fractures of the Shaft of the Radius and Ulna

Fractures of the radial or ulnar shaft, or both, are relatively common and account for 5% to 10% of children's fractures.[182,331] Fractures of the shaft of the radius and ulna may occur in the distal third, middle third, or upper third. Fractures are more common distally than proximally.[33,182,241,294,331] One or both bones may be broken. Fractures may be greenstick or complete in both the radius and ulna, or they may be complete in one and greenstick in the other. Complete fractures may be undisplaced, minimally displaced, or markedly displaced with overriding and angulation. Angulation may be volar, dorsal, or toward or away from the interosseous space. Plastic deformation of one or both bones of the forearm may occur. When only one bone of the forearm is broken, the surgeon should suspect a Monteggia or Galeazzi fracture and obtain radiographs of the wrist and elbow in addition to the forearm. Fractures of the forearm are more easily managed in children than in adults. Closed treatment is usually successful, remodeling is significant, and malunion is uncommon.

ANATOMY

The anatomy of the forearm is responsible for some of the unique features of fractures of the forearm. Fractures are more common distally for several reasons. First, although both bones are thick walled throughout the greater part of their shafts, the cross section of the radius flattens distally. Proximally, it is cylindrical; it becomes triangular in the midshaft and ovoid distally. This geometric change produces a structural weakness in the radius that has been shown to fracture first in both-bone forearm fractures.[294] Second, the muscular envelope of the proximal part of the forearm provides more protection to the underlying bone than distally, where it becomes tendinous.

The soft tissue anatomy is also important in the production of deformities resulting from fractures of both bones of the forearm. The actions of the biceps, supinator, and pronator teres and quadratus all affect the position of the forearm after fracture. In proximal third fractures of the forearm, the proximal fragment of the radius is supinated and flexed because of the unopposed action of the biceps brachii and supinator brevis muscles. The distal fragment is pronated by the action of the pronator teres and pronator quadratus muscles. In middle-third fractures of the forearm (below the insertion of the pronator teres), the proximal fragment of the radius is balanced in neutral rotation because the action of the supinator is counteracted by the pronator teres. It is flexed by the biceps. The distal fragment is pronated and displaced ulnarly by the pronator quadratus. In fractures of the distal third of the forearm, the distal fragment is pronated and ulnarly deviated by the pronator quadratus.

MECHANISM OF INJURY

A fall on an outstretched hand is the most frequent mechanism of fracture of the radial or ulnar shaft (or both). Evans and others have shown that a fall on a supinated, extended arm will produce a volarly angled greenstick fracture, whereas a fall on a pronated, extended arm will produce dorsal angulation of a greenstick fracture.[75,92] Both-bone forearm fractures may also be the result of direct trauma. Frequently these are high-energy, open injuries with significant soft tissue damage. Direct trauma is also involved in fractures sustained when the forearm is raised in self-protection, the so-called nightstick fracture of the ulna.

CLASSIFICATION

There is no established classification system for forearm fractures. Obviously, Monteggia, Galeazzi, and distal metaphyseal or physeal fractures are classified separately. Fractures of the radial and ulnar shaft may be classified according to their completeness—plastic deformation, greenstick, or complete; their location—proximal, middle, or distal third; or the direction of displacement—apex volar, dorsal, radial, or ulnar.

DIAGNOSIS

The diagnosis of forearm fractures is generally straightforward. Fractures of the distal third, which are most common, are often characterized by the classic dinner-fork deformity of the forearm. As with any traumatic injury, a thorough assessment of the entire patient must be completed. Careful attention should be paid to the integrity of the skin because forearm fractures are the most commonly open long-bone fracture in children. It is important to remember that even the smallest inside-to-outside puncture wound represents an operative emergency. These injuries must be treated as open fractures according to the guidelines discussed in Chapter 40, General Principles of Managing Orthopaedic Injuries. Failure to appropriately treat open fractures can have devastating consequences.

Although pain, swelling, crepitus, and deformity make the diagnosis of displaced fractures obvious, plastic deformation injuries and greenstick fractures may be associated with minimal findings. In fact, it is not uncommon for children with mild plastic deformation or minimal buckle or greenstick fractures to initially be seen up to a week after the injury. Often the parents seek care simply because the "sprain" continues to cause minor complaints.

RADIOGRAPHIC FINDINGS

The radiographic diagnosis is usually straightforward. It is important to obtain true AP and lateral views of the forearm because oblique views may not accurately reflect the displacement (Fig. 42–113). The most important aspect of the radiographic diagnosis is to have complete radiographic assessment of the wrist and elbow. This is particularly true when only one bone in the forearm is fractured and the likelihood of a Monteggia or Galeazzi fracture is high.

TREATMENT

Radial and ulnar shaft fractures can almost always be successfully treated by closed reduction and cast immobilization. The indications for operative treatment are few and include fractures associated with an arterial injury requiring repair or a compartment syndrome, open fractures (although after debridement these injuries are often treated by closed techniques), irreducible fractures, failure to maintain adequate reduction, and skeletal maturity. Our approach to an adolescent with minimal growth remaining is to initially treat the individual as skeletally immature. In our experience, if closed reduction can be obtained (generally not problematic) and maintained (frequently problematic), delayed union or nonunion is rare.[229] The difficulty in managing an adolescent with a both-bone forearm fracture lies in determining how much angulation or displacement can be accepted.

Closed Reduction

Position of Immobilization. A great deal of the literature on children's both-bone forearm fractures focuses on the appropriate rotational forearm position to adequately obtain and maintain reduction.[34,53,69,90,92,105,186,227,320] Historically, the classic teaching was that the forearm should be supinated for proximal third fractures, in neutral position for midshaft fractures, and pronated for distal fractures.[34,53,69,92,105,227,320] Evans later challenged this teaching and recommended supination for dorsally angulated greenstick fractures, pronation for volar greenstick fractures, and supination for all complete fractures.[47,90] Evans also advocated using the bicipital tuberosity as a landmark to ensure restoration of appropriate rotational alignment. The bicipital tuberosity should be medial with the forearm in supination, posterior with the forearm in neutral position, and lateral with the forearm in pronation. Evans believed that the fracture could be maximally stabilized by matching the distal forearm position to the position of the bicipital tuberosity on the injury film.[93] In practice, we treat the vast majority of both-bone forearm fractures with the forearm in neutral position.

Reduction is usually performed in the emergency department under conscious sedation. Reduction is obtained by exaggerating the deformity, applying traction, and reducing the fracture. Traction can be applied with the use of finger traps, the aid of an assistant, or the surgeon's lower extremity (Fig. 42–114).

After reduction, a well-molded sugar-tong splint or cast is applied. If a cast is used, it should be widely split or bivalved in the emergency department. The importance of good casting technique cannot be overemphasized. The reduction is sure to be lost if a poorly molded cast is applied. A good cast must fit snugly, which requires a minimal amount of cast padding, as well as a three-point and interosseous mold. Distal slippage of the cast (proximal migration of the forearm) will also lead to loss of reduction and can be minimized by ensuring that the arm is immobilized at a sharp right angle and that the ulnar border of the cast is kept straight (Fig. 42–115). Rang and colleagues have advocated that an eyelet passed proximal to the fracture may help limit migration in the cast.[236]

Immobilization of proximal third fractures and fractures in small, chubby arms (usually any patient younger than 2 years) is difficult because of the large soft tissue envelope that must be molded to control the underlying bone. A number of authors have advocated immobilization of these fractures with the elbow in extension (Fig. 42–116).[107,262,291,309,315] Although this technique is rarely needed—Gainor and Hardy treated only 8 of 130 patients in extension[107]—it can be successful. In an effort to keep the cast from slipping distally, benzoin can be applied to the humeral condyles. One study has shown successful results with fractures at

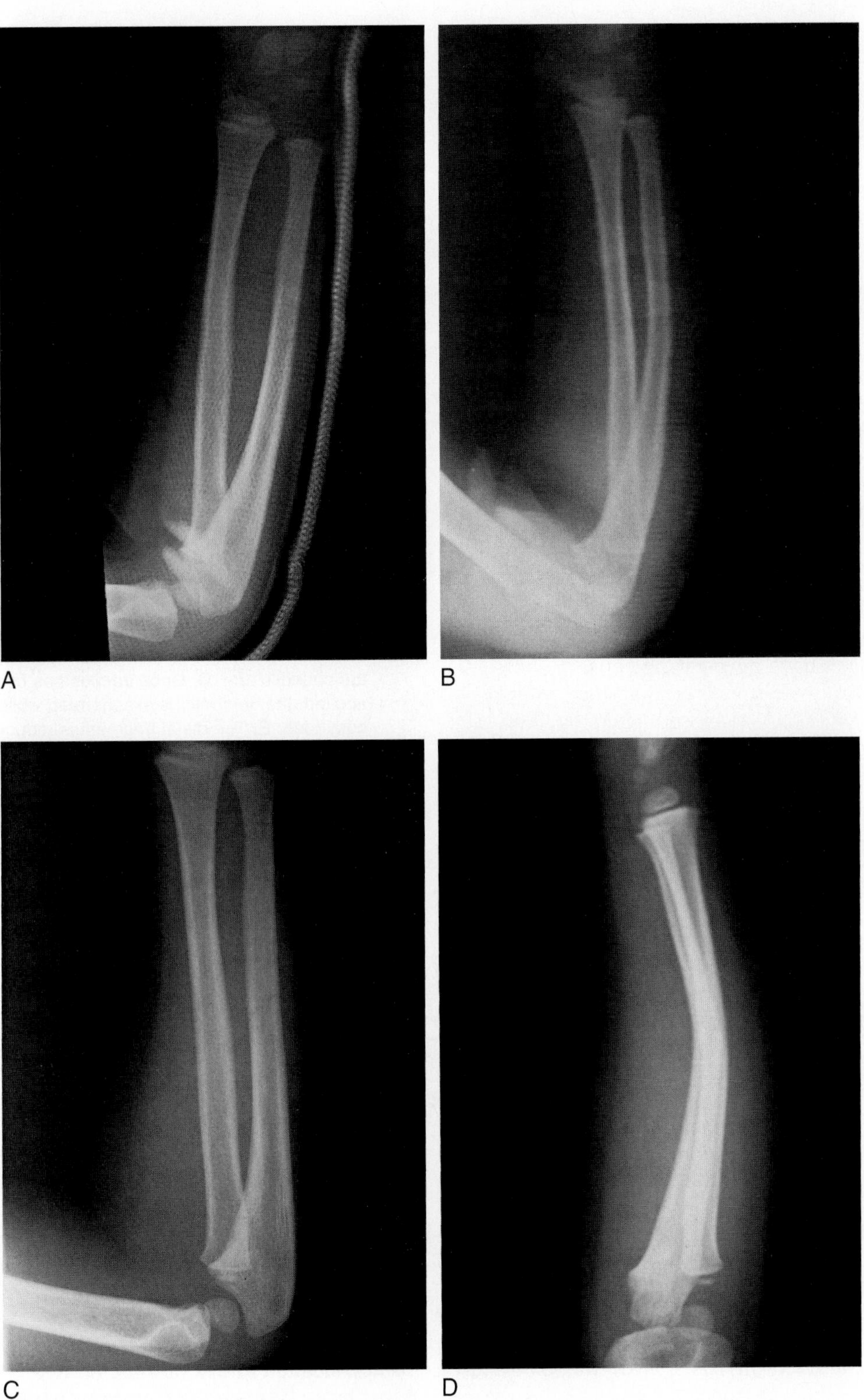

FIGURE 42–113 **A** and **B**, Oblique radiographs show what appears to be a minimally displaced fracture through the ulna. True anteroposterior **(C)** and lateral **(D)** radiographs reveal significant sagittal plane deformity of both bones of the forearm.

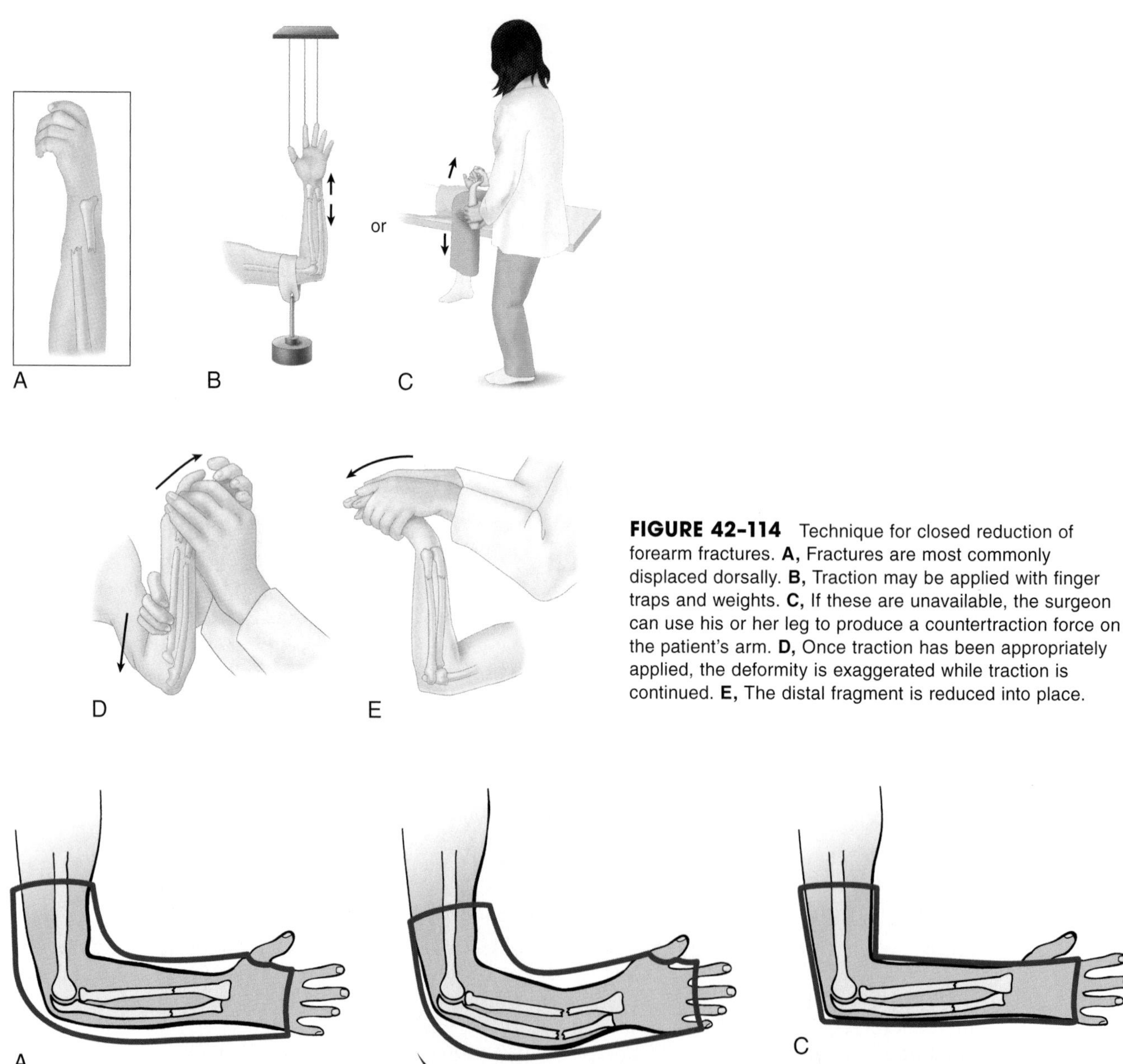

FIGURE 42–114 Technique for closed reduction of forearm fractures. **A,** Fractures are most commonly displaced dorsally. **B,** Traction may be applied with finger traps and weights. **C,** If these are unavailable, the surgeon can use his or her leg to produce a countertraction force on the patient's arm. **D,** Once traction has been appropriately applied, the deformity is exaggerated while traction is continued. **E,** The distal fragment is reduced into place.

FIGURE 42–115 Proper casting technique. **A,** A poorly molded cast is round at the elbow. **B,** Without a proper mold, the cast can migrate distally and produce ulnar deviation of the distal fragment. **C,** A well-molded cast keeps the elbow at 90 degrees, which prevents distal migration and subsequent deformity.

all levels immobilized in casts with the elbow in entension.[35]

Follow-up. After reduction and splinting or casting, the patient is discharged with instructions to elevate the arm "with the fingers above the elbow and the elbow above the heart." It is important to explain to parents that slings are for comfort after the swelling subsides and should be avoided initially because they maintain the extremity in a dependent position. Patients should return 7 to 10 days after reduction for radiographs in the cast. Displacement in the cast must be appreciated and should be treated when first noted. Most large series report, and our experience supports, that remanipulation is required in 5% to 15% of children's both-bone forearm fractures.[56,146,340] Mild displacement may not require formal re-reduction but should alert the surgeon to a loose cast that must be replaced. We have found that cast changes at 10 to 14 days are less painful and less likely to result in displacement than cast changes performed in the first week. If the cast is replaced, it is imperative that the radiographs be repeated to ensure that the reduction was not lost and that the cast fits snugly. In general,

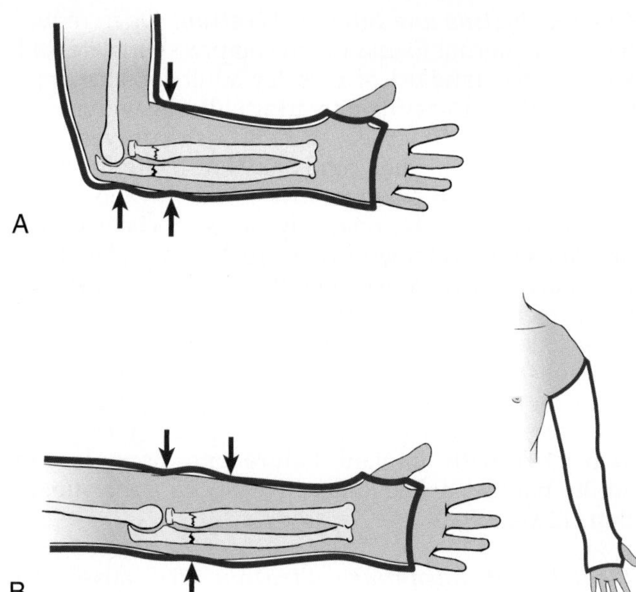

FIGURE 42–116 **A,** Fractures of the proximal third of the forearm may be difficult to maintain in a long-arm cast with the elbow flexed at 90 degrees because it is not possible to obtain three-point fixation. **B,** These fractures can be managed with a long-arm extension cast that allows three-point fixation.

we see patients weekly during the first 3 weeks because this is when loss of reduction is most likely to occur. If after 3 weeks the cast fits snugly and the reduction remains adequate, the patient returns at 6 weeks after injury for cast removal and radiographs.

Parameters of an Acceptable Closed Reduction. Unfortunately, the limits of an acceptable reduction are unknown. The goal of treatment of radial and ulnar shaft fractures is to have a normal-appearing arm with a full or at least functional range of motion. The only sequelae of nonanatomic union that become clinically problematic are the cosmetic appearance of the arm and loss of forearm rotation.[29,229,295] Thus, to establish the limits of an acceptable reduction, it is necessary to know the effect of malunion on appearance and rotation.

A number of studies have shown that malunion does not necessarily correlate with loss of forearm rotation. Daruwalla was unable to correlate residual fracture angulation with limitation of forearm movement,[73] whereas Zionts and colleagues found that the maximal angulation of the radius did correlate with loss of forearm rotation in an older cohort of patients.[340] Other authors have found little correlation between the two factors.[73,130,131,205,227,320,335] In fact, loss of forearm rotation has been shown to occur in patients with "good" radiographic results after pediatric forearm fractures.[205] These studies suggest that factors other than residual angulation may be responsible for the loss of forearm rotation.[131,205,283,335] Complicating the issue further is the observation that a measurable loss of pronation and supination may not produce a *functional* deficit. Carey and associates documented this in five patients older than 10 years who lost 20 to 35 degrees of forearm rotation but had no functional limitations.[53]

The surgeon treating a forearm fracture must analyze a number of factors that contribute to an acceptable result or malunion of a both-bone fracture, including angulation (in both the coronal and sagittal planes), rotation, displacement (translation), radial bowing, and length. Both cadaver and clinical studies have shown that as much as 10 degrees of midshaft angular deformity does not produce clinically significant loss of motion.[186,257,285] Rotational deformity, however, does produce a corresponding loss of motion that does not remodel over time.[69,105,227,320] Price believes that complete bayonet apposition and some loss of radial bowing is acceptable.[206,229] Loss of length is not usually a problem with malunited forearm fractures.[29,78,105,229]

The location of the fracture and the age of the patient also affect the radiographic result. Proximal fractures have been noted in multiple studies to have a worse outcome than distal fractures.* Again, however, the clinical significance of the malunion is unknown. Holdsworth and Sloan noted only three unsatisfactory results in 51 children with malunion of proximal shaft fractures. Consequently, despite the high number of "malunions," they recommended conservative treatment of these fractures.[131] Although children older than 10 years have less capacity for remodeling than younger children do,[105,145,212,227,307] moderate residual angulation may still be well tolerated.[340]

It is apparent from a review of the literature that malunion after pediatric both-bone forearm fractures is not uncommon.† What is surprising, however, is the paucity of reports on the surgical treatment of malunion.[29,31,295] Our review of the literature found only 48 patients younger than 16 years who required surgical treatment for malunion of a radial or ulnar shaft fracture (or both). This supports our clinical bias that "malunion" of these fractures is a radiographic rather than a functional problem. In fact, we more frequently answer questions regarding the unattractive ulnar bowing associated with a malunion than address questions concerning functional limitations (Fig. 42–117). Thus, our experience is that despite a measurable loss of forearm rotation, malunion of forearm fractures, like malunion of supracondylar humeral fractures, is usually a cosmetic rather than a functional problem.

Given the infrequency of functional problems, we favor a generous definition of "acceptable reduction." We consider Price's classic guidelines of 10 degrees of angulation, 45 degrees of malrotation, complete displacement, and loss of radial bowing to be reasonable,[229] and we occasionally accept even more deformity.[286] As in all areas of orthopaedics, each case must be individualized. It is important to know that

*See references 29, 32, 69, 73, 109, 131, 139, 227, 286, 298, 335.

†See references 24, 29, 31, 32, 56, 70, 78, 102, 105, 113, 122, 131, 145, 146, 152, 153, 165, 186, 206, 229, 241, 262, 263, 295, 329, 335.

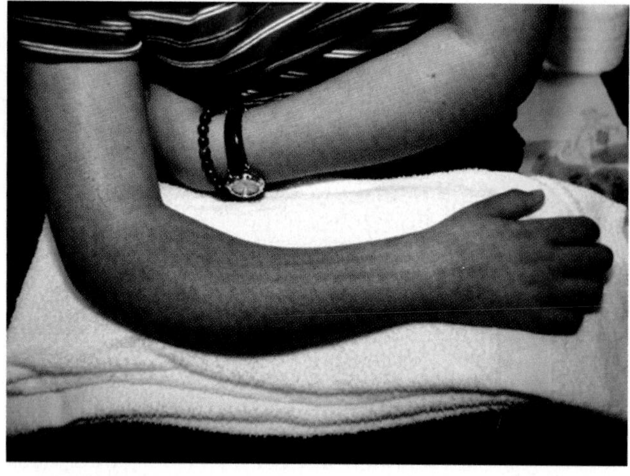

FIGURE 42–117 Unacceptable cosmetic deformity associated with ulnar bowing after a fracture of the proximal third of the radius and ulna.

ulnar bowing, particularly in an adolescent girl, may be poorly tolerated cosmetically. Consequently, we make a diligent effort to keep the ulna from angulating by either appropriate cast application or operative management.

Operative Treatment

Indications for operative management of pediatric radial or ulnar shaft fractures include dysvascular extremities, compartment syndromes, irreducible fractures, entrapped tendons or nerves, open fractures, and failure of closed reduction and casting. In our experience, the most common indications are open fractures and failure to maintain an acceptable closed reduction (usually in an adolescent). Although our definition of an acceptable closed reduction was discussed earlier under Parameters of an Acceptable Reduction, further discussion of operative indications is warranted. Recently there has been a proliferation of reports of operative management of children's both-bone forearm fractures despite good results with conservative management and few reports of functional problems from malunion.* A recent report by Jones and Weiner addressed the proliferation of operative management.[146] In their review of 300 forearm fractures, 22 required remanipulation and 12 required pin fixation.[146] Our experience and that of others[263] agree with their findings, namely, that 90% to 95% of forearm fractures can and should be managed successfully with closed techniques.

Once the decision has been made to treat a fracture surgically, multiple techniques are available, including plates and screws, intramedullary rods, and external fixation, either with fixation devices or with pins and plaster. Oblique crossed pin fixation is generally inadequate for diaphyseal forearm fractures because the bone diameter is small.[326]

Open Reduction and Internal Fixation. Open reduction plus internal fixation with compression plate and screws, the standard of care for adult forearm fractures, is also successful in treating children with radial and ulnar shaft fractures.[8,153,204,214,287,298,333] Advantages of plate fixation include rigid anatomic fixation, which requires minimal postoperative immobilization. Disadvantages include relatively large incisions and problems with retained hardware. We find plate fixation particularly convenient in the management of open fractures because the exposure has been made during debridement. The issue of retained hardware and subsequent stress risers, either with or without removal, can be minimized by using tubular rather than compression plates. Tubular plates have been associated with implant failure and nonunion in adults, but they are adequate in most children younger than 12 years.

Flexible Intramedullary Fixation. The advent of image intensification has made closed reduction and percutaneous intramedullary fixation an attractive alternative in the management of unstable pediatric forearm fractures.[169,198,232,234,268] In adults this technique is problematic because of the high rate of nonunion and the need for immobilization in a cast or splint.[157,183,213,254,267,282] However, in immature patients, nonunion is rare, and external immobilization is not usually a problem. Thus, flexible intramedullary fixation can be used to maintain alignment until union occurs.

Classically, intramedullary devices were started distally in the radius and proximally in the ulna. However, Verstreken and associates have pointed out that starting the ulnar pin distally allows the pin to be advanced proximally up the shaft of the ulna with the elbow in extension and the forearm supinated rather than with the elbow flexed as required with a proximal starting location. This makes obtaining image intensification easier. There may also be fewer problems from symptomatic pin prominence if the pin is started distally.[303]

The technique for intramedullary fixation is shown in Figure 42–118. The starting point for both the radius and ulna is the metaphysis just proximal to the physis. Care must be taken to not damage the superficial radial nerve or the dorsal branch of the ulnar nerve. A small bend placed 5 to 10 mm from the end of the rod may help in reduction. The radius is usually harder to reduce and is generally approached first. In fractures that have failed closed reduction and are subsequently 1 to 3 weeks old there is frequently early callus within the intramedullary canal. Therefore, we have a low threshold for making a small incision to facilitate reduction of the fracture over the rod. We usually immobilize the arm in a long-arm cast (split in the operating room) for 6 weeks, although good results with no or minimal immobilization have been reported.[166,303,318] The pins may be left outside the skin and pulled at 4 to 5 weeks or buried and removed in several months. Shoemaker and colleagues noted loss of reduction and deep infection with percutaneous removal of pins at 4 weeks and recommended leaving

---

*See references 24, 59, 70, 97, 117, 123, 138, 169, 177, 198, 214, 232, 234, 242, 263, 268, 301, 312, 333, 338.

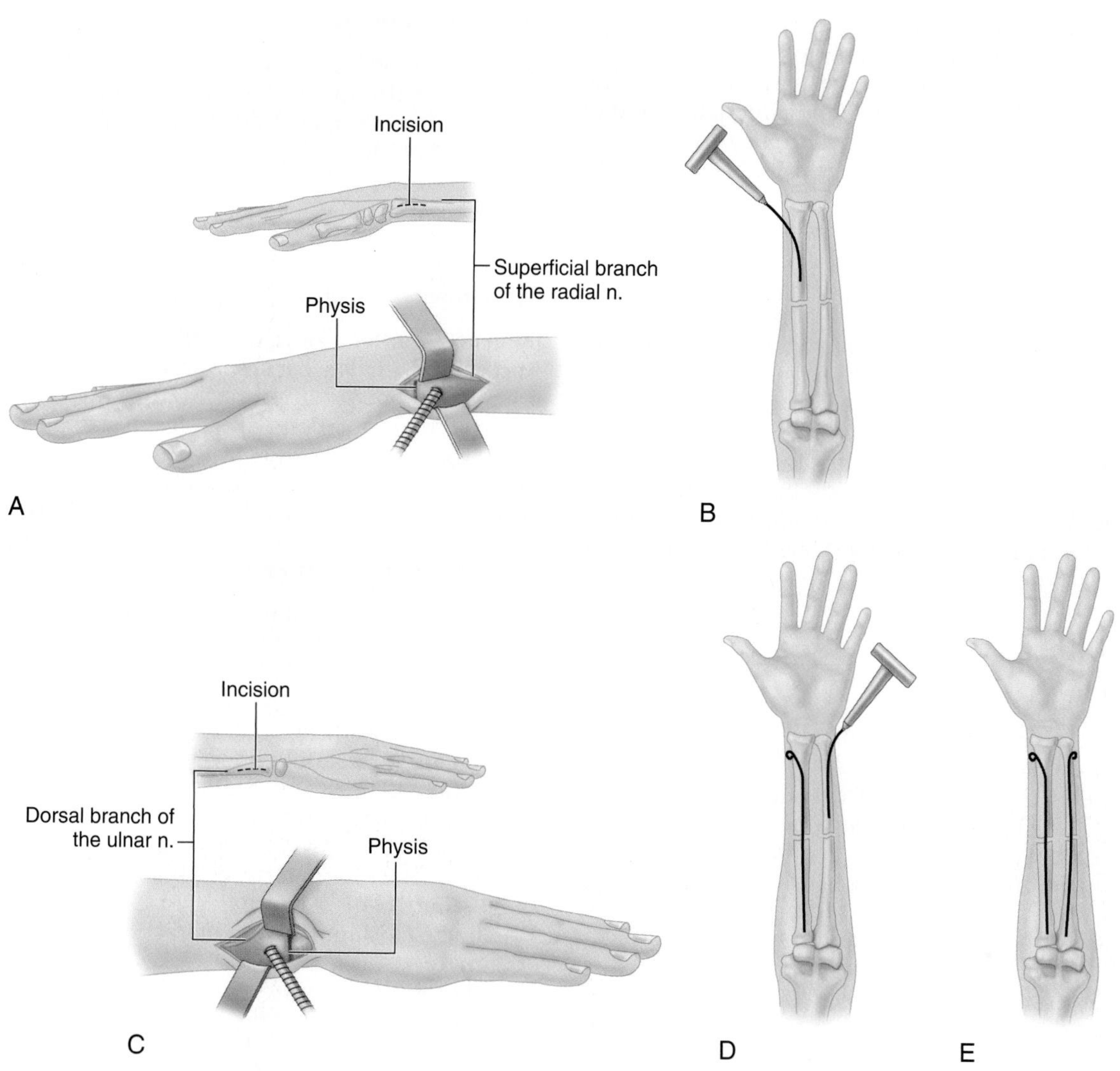

FIGURE 42–118 Technique for intramedullary fixation of forearm fractures. **A,** A distal incision is made over the radius. The superficial branch of the radial nerve is protected and a starting hole is made proximal to the physis. **B,** A flexible intramedullary rod is introduced and advanced to the fracture site. The fracture is then reduced over the rod. The rod is advanced into the proximal fragment to the appropriate length and either buried underneath the skin or left out through the skin. **C,** The dorsal branch of the ulnar nerve is protected for the ulnar starting hole. **D,** A distal starting hole for the ulna makes imaging easier because the fracture can be reduced with the forearm supinated and the elbow extended. **E,** The fracture is reduced over the rod, and final positioning is done under image control.

the pins under the skin, particularly for open fractures, which were slower to heal.[263]

Although there seems to be a recent trend toward intramedullary management of children's forearm fractures, it is important to remember that surgical management is not without risk. Cullen and colleagues reported 18 complications in 10 of 20 patients, including hardware migration, infection, loss of reduction, reoperation, nerve injury, significantly decreased range of motion, synostosis, muscle entrapment, and delayed union.[70]

Single-Bone Fixation. There have been reports of successful management of both-bone forearm fractures with stabilization of only one bone.[97,177,206] The rationale is that the stabilized bone allows the other to be manipulated into a reduced position and maintained with a cast.[169,198,232,234,268] We find this technique attractive because stabilization of the ulna prevents the development of a cosmetically unacceptable bow and provides a fulcrum against which the radius can be maintained in an improved and adequate position. This technique is especially useful in treating a fracture 1 to 2 weeks old in which closed treatment has failed. We often have a difficult time achieving closed intramedullary reduction in these injuries and find that single-bone fixation can be done with a small incision over the ulna, without the need for a second larger incision to reduce and stabilize the radius. This technique is also useful when only one bone has an open fracture (we may use a third tubular plate in such a scenario). Like Shoemaker and colleagues,[263] we have found that as with many fractures treated in a cast, some of the reduction of the nonstabilized bone will be lost over time. However, we have not found this to be a clinical problem, and we believe that the benefits of reduced surgical exposure outweigh the risk of minor loss of reduction (Fig. 42–119).

External Fixation. External fixation of children's forearm fractures can refer to management with traditional external fixation devices or management with pins and plaster. Formal external fixation devices may rarely be indicated for forearm fractures with massive soft tissue loss, although plate fixation and intramedullary techniques usually provide better fixation and consequently better soft tissue stabilization.[233,259] Pins and plaster have yielded good results in unstable forearm fractures.[146]

COMPLICATIONS

Re-fracture

In most large series, re-fracture of the forearm occurs in about 5% of patients.[131,229,304] Re-fracture is more likely to occur after greenstick or open fractures.[121,261,263] The high incidence of re-fracture after plate removal[22,127,154,248,278] has led some authors to abandon routine hardware removal in asymptomatic patients.[22,147,189,258] If displaced, re-fractures can be difficult to reduce and may require surgical stabilization.[13,69,131,229,261] The difficulty in obtaining closed reduction, as well as possible sclerosis of the intramedullary canal, may make open reduction and plate fixation a more attractive option than intramedullary fixation for these injuries.

Malunion

Even with attention to detail and close follow-up, late-identified displacement will occur. If the displacement is appreciated less than a month after the injury, we remanipulate the arm under general anesthesia and usually stabilize at least the ulna. However, if the malunion is identified later, we generally advise the parents that a period of 9 to 18 months of observation is advisable to see how much remodeling will occur. Time must be taken to explain to the parents that remodeling is unpredictable and often surprising. They should be counseled that the atrophy and stiffness associated with immobilization exaggerate the appearance of the deformity and that function frequently returns to normal despite the radiographic malunion.[73,130,131,205,227]

Osteotomy to correct malunion is occasionally necessary. The few reports in the literature describe drill osteoclasis and cast immobilization or osteotomy with compression plate fixation.[29,31,295] We also have little experience in performing osteotomies through limited surgical incisions with intramedullary reduction and cast immobilization (Fig. 42–120).[55]

Delayed Union or Nonunion

Delayed union or nonunion after children's radial or ulnar shaft fractures is uncommon. It is usually associated with open injuries with significant bone or soft tissue loss. If a delayed union does not progress to union with extended observation, compression plate fixation with iliac crest bone graft has been successful.[2,121,333]

Synostosis

Synostosis after forearm fractures in children is uncommon. It has been reported to be more likely after high-energy trauma, surgical intervention, repeated manipulations, and fractures associated with head injury.[70,249,306] Although there are few reports, the results of excision of a radioulnar synostosis do not appear to be as good in children as in adults.[305]

Compartment Syndrome

Compartment syndrome can develop after forearm fractures and may be potentiated by the splint or cast.[126,184,252,337] We believe that it is important to split every cast applied to a freshly injured extremity. If there is clinical suspicion of a compartment syndrome, the cast or splint should be split to the skin or removed altogether. One study found that longer operative times in surgically treated children correlated with the likelihood of development of a compartment syndrome.[337] The diagnosis and management of compartment syndrome are discussed in Chapter 40, General Principles of Managing Orthopaedic Injuries.

Peripheral Nerve Injury

Any of the three nerves of the forearm can be injured with radial and ulnar shaft fractures. Neurologic injury may occur at the time of injury, with closed reduction, or with open reduction. Fortunately, most injuries are related to stretch at the time of injury and recover completely within 2 to 3 months. Entrapment of the median, anterior interosseous, and superficial radial nerves has been reported. Recovery can be expected after release of the entrapped nerves. Although a good neurologic examination can be difficult or impossible to achieve in an anxious child in the emergency department, every effort should be made to assess the child's neurologic status before reduction. A definite loss of neurologic function after reduction should lead to exploration of the fracture, particularly if the reduction is nonanatomic.[70,75,106,110,111,134,200,207,243,263,272,330]

Other Complications

Muscle entrapment, hematogenous osteomyelitis, and gas gangrene have been reported after forearm fractures.[50,70,96,124,158,302]

Fractures of the Distal Forearm

Fractures of the distal part of the forearm are extremely common in children.[18,125,159,164,225,241,325,331] Fractures of the

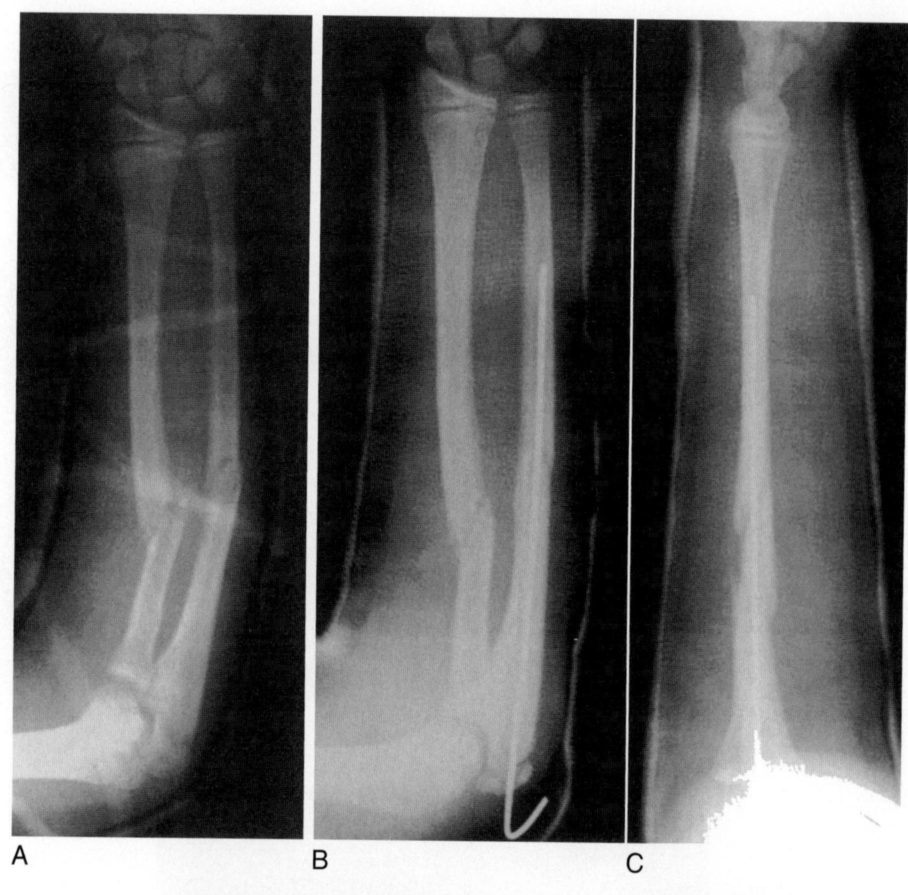

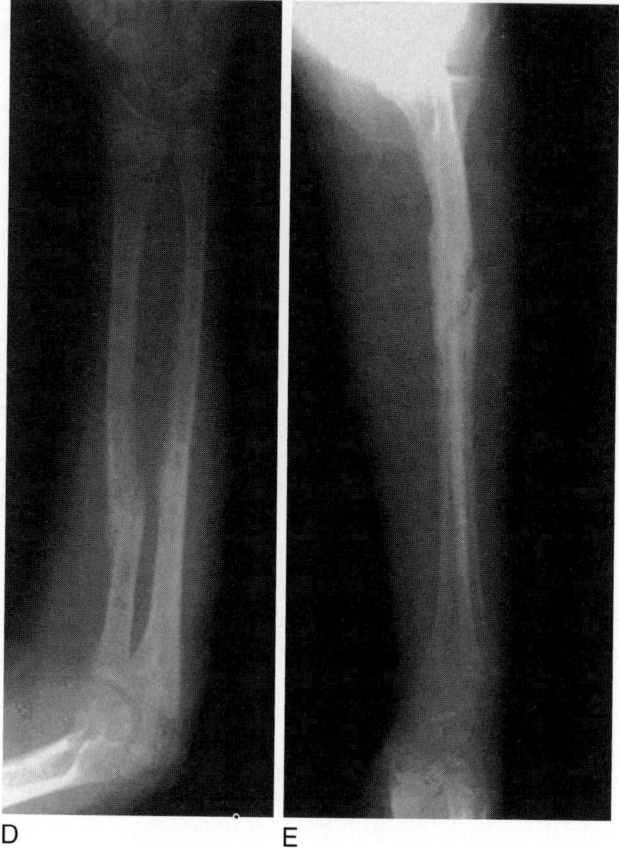

FIGURE 42–119 Single-bone fixation of both-bone forearm fracture. **A,** Anteroposterior (AP) radiograph of a both-bone forearm fracture with the radius fractured proximal to the ulna. Note the ulnar deviation in the cast approximately 2 weeks after injury. AP **(B)** and lateral **(C)** radiographs after open reduction and pin fixation of the ulna. Note that fixation of the ulna has improved alignment of the radius. AP **(D)** and lateral **(E)** radiographs after cast and pin removal.

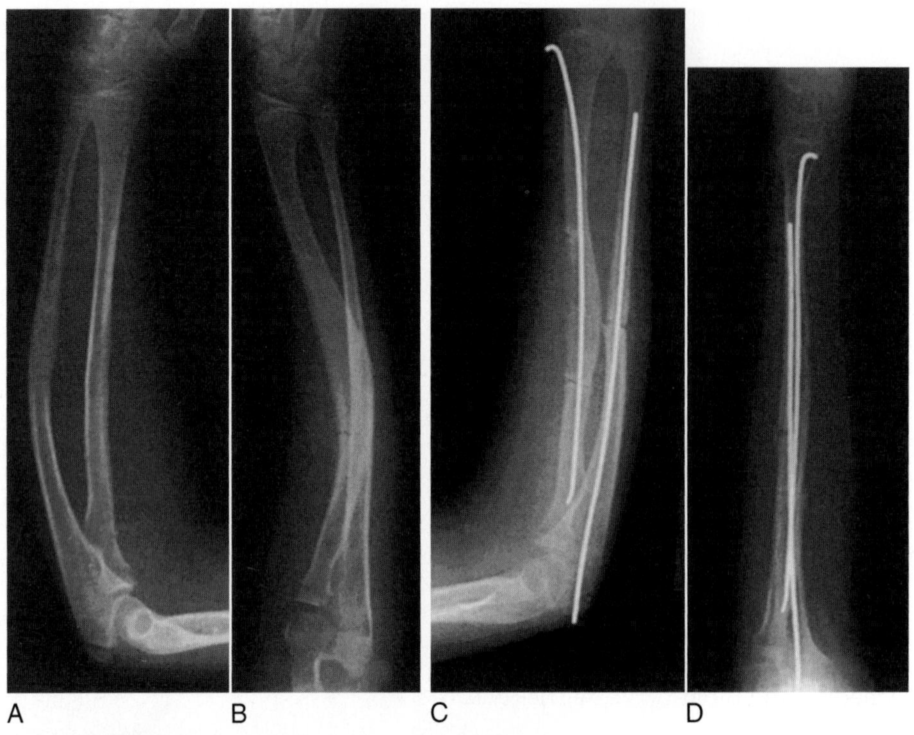

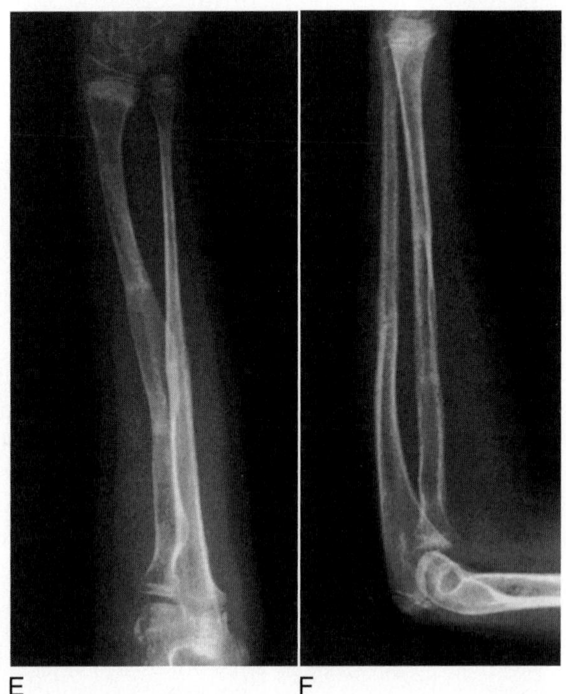

FIGURE 42-120
Anteroposterior **(A)** and lateral **(B)** radiographs showing malunion of a both-bone forearm fracture. Although there were few functional complaints, the patient was unhappy with the appearance of the ulnar bow. **C** and **D,** The ulnar bow was corrected with a closing wedge osteotomy. Correction of the radial deformity required a two-level osteotomy. **E** and **F,** One year postoperatively the patient was pleased with the appearance. She had a 140-degree arc of pronation-supination.

distal forearm include torus or buckle fractures, greenstick fractures, metaphyseal fractures, physeal fractures, and Galeazzi fractures. These fractures can generally be managed by simple closed reduction and casting, with excellent results. However, as with all injuries, complications can develop. Careful attention to detail may allow early identification of these complications and prevent them from becoming disabling long-term problems.

ANATOMY

The pertinent anatomic considerations include the bony anatomy, the distal radioulnar articulation, and the soft tissue envelope of the forearm. The secondary ossification center of the distal radius usually appears before the first birthday, and the distal ulnar ossification center appears between 5 and 7 years of age. The distal radial physis accounts for 75% to 80% of growth of the radius. This rapid growth may predispose the distal radius to fracture because the distal metaphysis is thin from the continuous remodeling.[6,18,125]

The distal radioulnar joint is a pivot that allows the radius to pronate and supinate around the ulna. The distal radioulnar joint has several components, including the triangular fibrocartilage, the ulnar collateral ligament, the volar and dorsal radiocarpal and radioulnar ligaments, and the pronator quadratus muscle. Of these, the triangular fibrocartilage is probably the most important. The triangular fibrocartilage functions to stabilize the distal radioulnar joint against the torsional stress associated with rotation.[264]

The soft tissues of the volar distal forearm include the flexor tendons, the median nerve, and the ulnar neurovascular bundle. With dorsal displacement of the distal fragment these structures may be injured as they are tented over the proximal fragment. In fact, given the frequency of distal forearm fractures and the usual magnitude of displacement, neurovascular injury is surprisingly uncommon, perhaps because the pronator quadratus protects the volar neurovascular structures. Nevertheless, careful examination is required because median and ulnar nerve injuries and open fractures do occur.[61,121,206,300]

MECHANISM OF INJURY

Distal forearm fractures are most commonly the result of a fall onto an outstretched hand. If the wrist is extended or dorsiflexed, as is commonly the case, the distal fragment will be displaced dorsally. Volar displacement of the distal fragment is the result of a fall on a flexed wrist. It is unclear why some falls produce metaphyseal fractures and some produce physeal injuries. Buckle fractures and minimally displaced fractures are thought to be the result of lower energy injury, whereas displaced fractures result from falls from a height or with forward momentum (running, riding a bike, etc.).[265] Forearm fractures have been shown to migrate distally with age, with adolescents more likely to sustain distal fractures and younger children more likely to sustain diaphyseal shaft fractures.[6,18,75,294]

CLASSIFICATION

We classify distal forearm fractures as buckle (or torus), greenstick, metaphyseal, physeal, or Galeazzi fractures. Metaphyseal fractures can be further classified as nondisplaced or displaced. If displaced, they can be classified according to the direction and degree of displacement. Physeal fractures are most commonly classified by the system of Salter and Harris.[255] In his classification of physeal injuries, Peterson identified a fracture seen commonly in the distal part of the forearm.[224] A Peterson I physeal injury is a transverse metaphyseal fracture with longitudinal comminution extending into the physis (Fig. 42–121). It is important to identify these fractures because growth arrest has been reported after such innocuous-appearing injuries.[1,64]

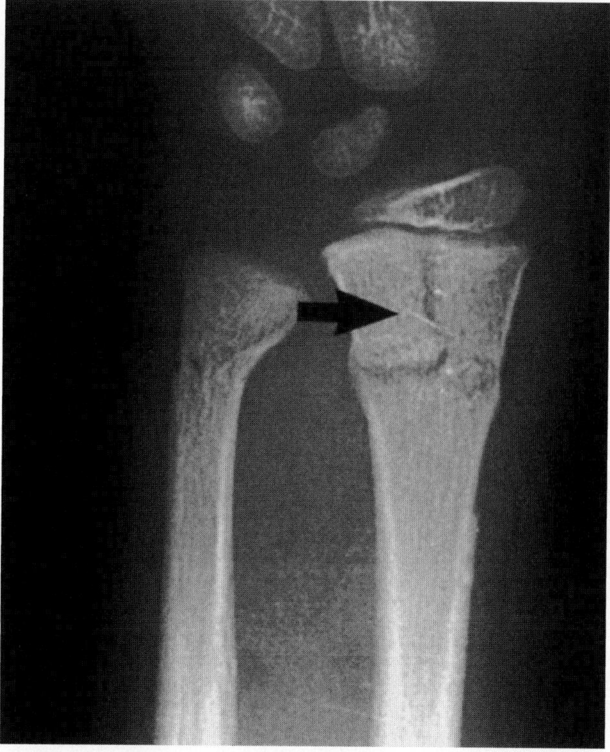

FIGURE 42–121 Anteroposterior radiograph of a Peterson I fracture of the distal end of the radius. Note the metaphyseal fracture of both the radius and the ulna. There is a longitudinal split from the radial metaphysis to the physis (*arrow*).

Though first described by Cooper in 1824,[65] fracture of the distal radius with dislocation of the distal radioulnar joint is known as a *Galeazzi fracture*, after Riccardo Galeazzi, who described 18 cases in 1934.[108] Galeazzi fractures are rare in children. Letts and Rowhani classified Galeazzi fractures in children by the position of the distal ulna (dorsal or volar).[172] They differentiated between complete and greenstick fractures of the distal radius. They included injuries with true ligamentous disruption of the distal radioulnar joint and "equivalents"—fractures of the distal radius with separation of the distal ulnar physis. They classified equivalents according to the position of the distal ulnar metaphysis.

DIAGNOSIS

If the forearm has the classic dinner-fork deformity, the diagnosis is easily made. However, if there is minimal displacement, the findings may be subtle. In fact, patients with buckle fractures are often seen several days or a week after the injury for treatment of a "sprain" that has not resolved. As always, care must be taken to thoroughly assess the patient for associated injuries. The most common concomitant injuries include scaphoid or other carpal fractures distally and supracondylar humeral fractures proximally.[28,63,115,118,137,245,273,296,297,327] Careful assessment of the skin and a neurovascular examination should be performed. In dorsally displaced fractures, median nerve symptoms are common and often transient, with resolution when the deformity is corrected.[129]

RADIOGRAPHIC FINDINGS

As with all injuries, good-quality radiographs of the entire forearm should be obtained. If there is significant displacement or if only one bone is fractured, AP and lateral radiographs of the wrist and elbow should be included in the assessment.

TREATMENT

Buckle Fractures

The goal of treatment of buckle fractures is to keep the child comfortable and to prevent further displacement should the child fall onto the hand again. Most buckle fractures have traditionally been managed in a short-arm cast, which often allows the patient to resume vigorous activities. Several recent randomized prospective studies have shown good results in these stable fractures after minimal immobilization with removable splints or soft bandages.[74,321] Perhaps the most important aspect in managing buckle fractures is to be certain of the diagnosis. Minimally displaced metaphyseal fractures can be mistaken for buckle fractures, and these patients may have significant pain on pronation and supination, suggesting a less stable fracture. These fractures are potentially unstable and will displace further without proper immobilization (Fig. 42–122). Additionally, involvement of the physis (Peterson's type I physeal injury) may lead to growth arrest and should be noted at the time of injury and monitored for 6 to 12 months to ensure that normal growth resumes.[1,10,14,64,81,288]

Greenstick Fractures

Greenstick fractures of the distal part of the forearm can generally be treated by simple closed reduction and long-arm casting. We usually perform closed reduction in the emergency department under conscious sedation. Although a great deal has been written about the position of the forearm after reduction of fractures, we find these fractures very stable once they are reduced and almost always immobilize them with the forearm in neutral position. Patients are generally seen 1 and 2 weeks after reduction to ensure a well-molded cast. Because of an increased risk for re-fracture, we usually immobilize these fractures in a long-arm cast for 6 full weeks and counsel the parents when the cast is removed about the increased risk for re-fracture.[131,229,304]

Metaphyseal Fractures

It is uncommon for metaphyseal fractures of the distal end of the forearm to involve only one bone. The radius is almost always involved as a complete fracture. However, the ulna may have a complete metaphyseal fracture, a metaphyseal greenstick fracture, avulsion of the styloid, a distal physeal fracture, or plastic deformation. In general, treatment is directed at achieving stable reduction of the radius, which usually ensures adequate treatment of the ulna.

Nondisplaced Metaphyseal Fractures. Nondisplaced metaphyseal fractures need only be immobilized in a short- or long-arm cast for 4 weeks. Several recent studies have shown that well-molded short-arm casts are as effective in maintaining reduction as long-arm

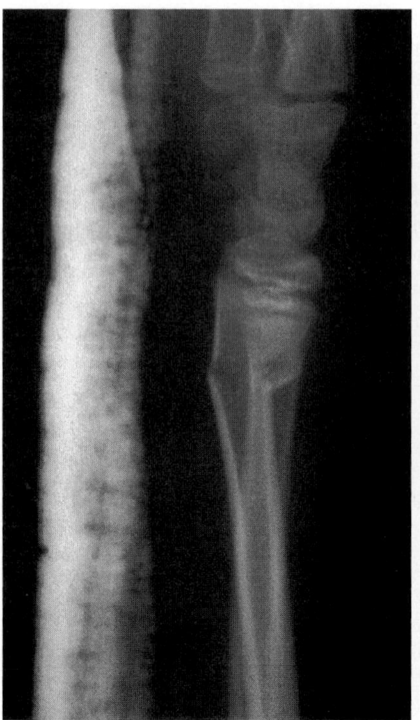
A

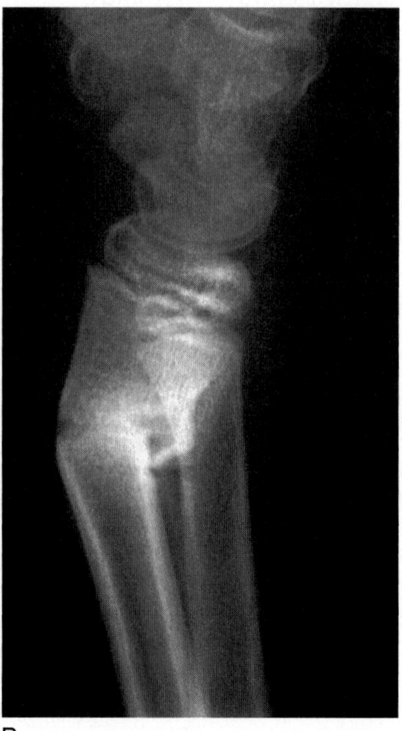
B

FIGURE 42–122 Unstable distal radial buckle fracture. **A,** The distal radius fracture has a buckled appearance. However, both the ulnar and dorsal cortices are fractured. **B,** Angulation of the distal radius after immobilization in a poorly molded splint.

casts.[36,316] We choose a long-arm cast only for patients with significant pain on pronation and supination. Despite the benign nature of these injuries, careful attention to good casting technique will prevent displacement during treatment.

Although mild displacement during treatment usually remodels without functional sequelae, the "worsening" radiographic picture can cause significant parental distress. Recognition of the pattern of a displaced fracture may aid in treatment. Displaced fractures may be "out to length" or may have significant shortening of the distal fragment, so-called bayonet apposition. The reduction is often more difficult if only one bone is shortened. This is frequently the case with metaphyseal radial fractures, which may be completely displaced and shortened while the ulna is minimally displaced. Fractures are most commonly dorsally displaced, with only about 1% of fractures in one large series being volarly displaced.[286] Volar displacement generally requires immobilization with the wrist extended. Supination of the forearm will ease the application of a cast with a three-point volar mold. For dorsally displaced fractures we usually immobilize the forearm in neutral position.

Displaced Distal Metaphyseal Fractures. There is considerable controversy over the treatment of displaced distal fractures of the radius and ulna. The usual treatment is reduction with some form of sedation or block, followed by immobilization until healed. Some authors have shown better maintenance of reduction with K-wire fixation and advocate this approach.[188,191,339] Others note the remarkable ability of a skeletally immature child to remodel displacement and angulation.[83] They recommend immobilization without reduction for fractures in this age group that are angulated 15 degrees or less and shortened up to 1 cm. Others note that stable fractures angulated less than 10 degrees need little radiographic follow-up.[116]

Treatment by Closed Reduction and Casting. Despite recent reports advocating pin fixation for distal forearm metaphyseal fractures,[112,181,188,191,231,322,339] we believe that displaced metaphyseal fractures can generally be treated by closed reduction and casting under conscious sedation in the emergency department. The technique of reduction is the same as that previously described for fractures of the radial or ulnar shaft, namely, traction, exaggeration of the deformity, and restoration of alignment (see Fig. 42–114). One randomized prospective study has shown no difference in the outcome of children treated in short-arm versus long-arm immobilization casts,[35] and we believe that good results can be achieved with both short-arm and long-arm casts. It has been our experience that most patients are more comfortable if initially managed in a long-arm cast.[12,30,33,57,58,151,167,208,209,328]

As with fractures of the diaphysis, we believe that careful attention to the quality of the reduction and the cast is more important than whether a short-arm or a long-arm cast is applied.[56,122] We use both short- and long-arm casts, as well as sugar-tong splints. If a cast is applied, it is usually split to allow for swelling. Patients can generally be sent home from the emergency department unless there is significant swelling or concern over compartment syndrome or neurovascular status, in which case they should be admitted for observation.

The patients and parents are instructed in elevation and seen 1 and 2 weeks after reduction. If the initial cast is still well molded, it is overwrapped. If it is poorly fitting or a splint was applied initially, a new cast is applied and a radiograph is obtained afterward to ensure that the reduction has not been lost and the cast fits snugly. Immobilization is usually continued for a total of 4 to 6 weeks.

Operative Treatment. Indications for operative treatment include open fractures, irreducible fractures, fractures associated with compartment syndrome or carpal tunnel syndrome, fractures with severe swelling (for which a snug-fitting cast is ill-advised), fractures with ipsilateral injuries requiring stabilization (most commonly supracondylar humeral fractures, for which a snug-fitting cast is ill-advised), and fractures requiring remanipulation (acceptable reduction cannot be maintained).[28,112,146,206,273,334]

Most commonly, distal metaphyseal forearm fractures are stabilized with a smooth K-wire placed percutaneously from the radial styloid across the fracture into the proximal metaphysis (Fig. 42–123). We attempt to avoid the physis with the K-wire but find that it is often necessary to cross it. Despite reports of physeal arrest after pin fixation, it is unclear whether the pin or the fracture is responsible for the injury to the physis.[40,135,196,230] We do not believe that a small-diameter smooth pin crossing the physis substantially increases the risk for growth abnormality. Plate fixation and external fixation have also been described.[260,308] We occasionally use single-bone plate fixation to stabilize an open fracture because the debridement often affords adequate exposure for a four-hole tubular plate, which provides more rigid fixation than a single K-wire does. We have limited experience with external fixation. We reserve external fixation for fractures associated with massive soft tissue injury.

It is important that all open fractures, regardless of the size of the wound, be managed with thorough debridement and intravenous antibiotics according to the principles outlined in Chapter 40, General Principles of Managing Orthopaedic Injuries. Fractures may be irreducible because of interposed soft tissue. For dorsally displaced fractures, the soft tissue is usually the pronator quadratus or flexor tendons.[76,98,132] In the rare volarly displaced fracture, the extensor tendons may become entrapped. Patients suspected of having compartment syndrome or carpal tunnel syndrome should undergo immediate stabilization of their fractures because stabilization may help prevent further soft tissue damage and its accompanying swelling. After fracture stabilization, compartment pressures can be measured and managed as discussed in Chapter 40, General Principles of Managing Orthopaedic Injuries, under the heading Compartment Syn-

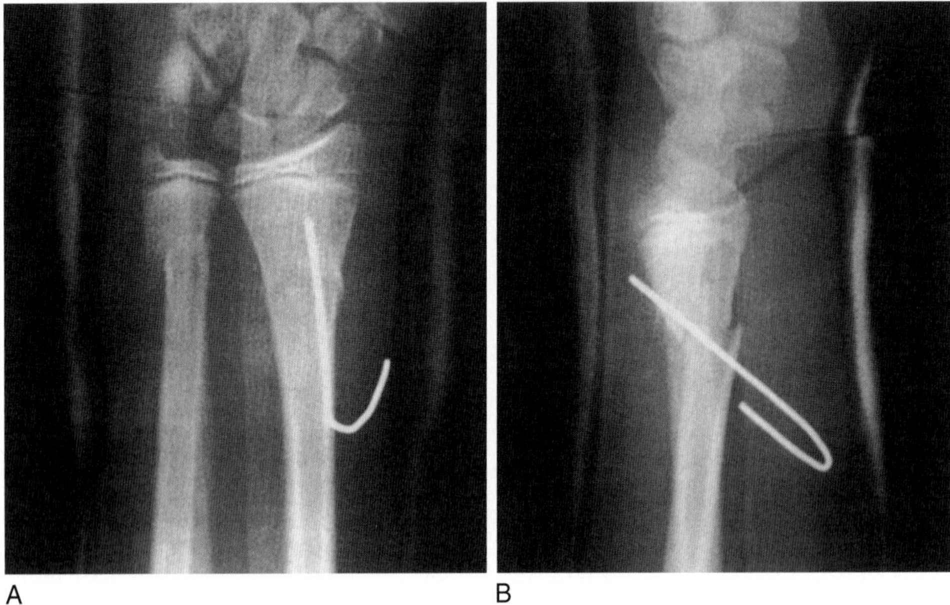

FIGURE 42-123 Anteroposterior **(A)** and lateral **(B)** radiographs of an open distal both-bone forearm metaphyseal fracture that was treated by irrigation, debridement, and percutaneous pinning of the radius. Pin fixation allows the wound to be checked through a window in the cast without concern over loss of reduction.

drome. Patients in whom remanipulation is needed are often older and their fractures are more likely to redisplace; consequently, we have a low threshold for pin fixation of these fractures.[59,112,338]

Parameters of an Acceptable Reduction. The factors that affect remodeling are discussed in detail in Chapter 40, General Principles of Managing Orthopaedic Injuries, and include the amount of growth remaining, the age of the patient, the location of the fracture, and the plane of the deformity, with deformity in the plane of motion having greater remodeling potential.[75,145,165,222,307,335] Because of the significant growth (8 mm/yr) and the proximity to the physis, as well as the plane of motion, distal radial fractures have a large remodeling potential, particularly in the sagittal plane.* As with any fracture, the art of orthopaedics lies in knowing the limits of an acceptable reduction. Obviously, each case must be individualized, although a few generalizations may be made. First, translation, or bayonet apposition, nearly always remodels, although these fractures are less stable and may angle a greater amount. Second, a sagittal plane deformity is more likely to remodel.[75,145,165,222,307] Third, patients younger than 11 years are more likely to remodel distal radial fractures, although older patients may remodel significant deformity (up to 36 degrees in the sagittal plane in a boy aged 12 years 11 months has been reported).[145,165,222,307] In general, in a child younger than 10 years, we will accept at least 30 to 35 degrees of sagittal plane angulation and 20 degrees of coronal plane angulation. The amount of angulation that is acceptable decreases with age. However, we will accept 15 to 20 degrees of sagittal plane angulation in a child with as little as 1 year of growth remaining. As for fractures of the diaphysis, surgical treatment of distal radial metaphyseal malunion is extremely uncommon.[29,105,121,229]

*See references 30, 73, 75, 102-105, 109, 145, 165, 209, 212, 222, 250, 307, 335.

Distal Radial Physeal Fractures

Distal radial physeal fractures are managed similar to displaced metaphyseal fractures, with a few important differences. First, these fractures heal rapidly, with only 3 or 4 weeks of immobilization required. Second, their potential to remodel is even greater than that of distal metaphyseal fractures. Third and most important, attempts at reduction (or re-reduction) after 3 to 7 days may damage the physis and produce growth arrest and consequently less remodeling. Thus, late-identified fractures and fractures in which the reduction has been lost should not be remanipulated but should be managed in a well-molded cast that prevents any further displacement.[4,5,9,34,41,67,81,168] A long-term study with an average follow-up of 25.5 years found only 2 symptomatic patients in 157 studied. Although 10 patients had radial or ulnar shortening of greater than 1 cm, only 2 had severe functional problems.[51] Remodeling of these fractures is especially effective in children up to 10 years of age.[136]

The one absolute indication for operative management is a Salter-Harris type III or IV fracture. By definition, these fractures are intra-articular and should be treated by anatomic reduction (usually open, possibly percutaneous with arthrographic confirmation) and pin fixation. Other operative indications are similar to those for metaphyseal fractures.[162] Distal radial physeal fractures requiring operative fixation can almost always be stabilized with a small, smooth percutaneous K-wire.

Distal Ulnar Physeal Injuries

Although fracture of the distal ulnar physis is uncommon, there are many reports of distal ulnar growth arrest.[4,61,81,88,113,201,218,238] Nelson and colleagues reviewed the literature and found 196 fractures of the distal ulna, 33 of which had sufficient follow-up to assess the growth plate. In 6 of these 33 patients, growth arrest of the distal ulna developed.[201] The reasons for this are unclear. It may be that injuries to the distal ulna are under-recognized and inadequately treated because of concomitant injuries to the ulna. In the series reported by Golz and colleagues, a third of the 18 patients with ulnar physeal injuries had associated fractures of the ulnar metaphysis or styloid.[113] However, open reduction has not been shown to prevent physeal arrest. Golz and colleagues reported growth arrest of the distal ulna in three of the four patients treated by open reduction.[113] Fortunately, symptoms after ulnar physeal arrest are infrequent.[62,81,113,201,218,238]

Fractures of the ulnar styloid (or epiphysis) have been reported in as many as a third of distal radial fractures.[275] These avulsions require no treatment and will usually develop into an asymptomatic nonunion.[51,129] Good results can be achieved with excision of the ulnar styloid nonunion in the unlikely event that it becomes symptomatic.[46,179,212]

Galeazzi Fractures

Galeazzi fractures in children are less common than in adults and rarely require surgical stabilization.[143,161,163,172,178,190,264,310] With disruption of the distal radioulnar joint or separation of the distal ulnar physis, the distal radial fragment may migrate proximally. Although distal radial fracture with separation of the distal ulna has been termed a *Galeazzi equivalent*, Imatani and associates have pointed out that the intact distal radioulnar joint makes proximal migration of the radius without the ulna impossible and suggest that the more accurate term "pseudo–Galeazzi injury" be used.[143] Interestingly, however, Letts and Rowhani noted a poorer prognosis for the equivalents than for the classic Galeazzi lesions.[172] The worse prognosis may be related to the high complication rate associated with distal ulnar physeal separation.[62,81,88,113,201,218,238]

The goal of treatment is to prevent migration of the distal radius and stabilize the distal radioulnar joint. In patients with greenstick fractures of the radius or ulna (or both) and in younger patients with complete fractures, stabilization can usually be accomplished with closed reduction and cast immobilization. Although some authors have recommended supination for dorsally displaced fractures and pronation for volarly displaced fractures, Letts and Rowhani have suggested that all Galeazzi fractures and equivalents be managed with the forearm in supination.[172] Older patients with true Galeazzi fractures that cannot be stabilized by closed reduction and casting may require open reduction. We prefer rigid plate fixation over flexible nail fixation for these injuries. If the distal radioulnar joint remains unstable after reduction and stabilization of the radius, consideration should be given to pinning the distal radioulnar joint in position with a transverse K-wire from the ulna to the radius. Open reduction may also be required for Galeazzi-equivalent lesions with entrapped soft tissue.

COMPLICATIONS

The most common complications after distal forearm fractures include malunion, re-fracture, growth arrest, peripheral nerve injury, and compartment syndrome. Nonunion, cross-union, overgrowth, infection, tendon entrapment, tendon rupture, and reflex sympathetic dystrophy have all also been reported after distal forearm fractures in children.

Malunion. Although radiographic malunion is the most common complication after distal forearm fractures, symptomatic malunion is rare.[29,105,131,229] The most frequent symptom is likely to be displeasure with the cosmetic appearance. This may be more likely with the unusual volarly displaced fracture because there is less soft tissue to cover an apex-dorsal deformity. Symptomatic nonunion, though rare, can be corrected with an osteotomy. Traditionally, this has been performed with drill osteoclasis and casting.[29,31] Some reports, however, have advocated open osteotomy with rigid internal fixation.[295]

Re-fracture. Although re-fracture after distal forearm fractures is less common than with more proximal fractures, it does occur. It has been noted to be more common after greenstick fractures, open fractures, and hardware removal.[121,176,261,263] Even though Price has advocated open reduction and intramedullary fixation of re-fractures because of problems maintaining reduction,[228] Schwarz and colleagues reported good results in 14 of 17 re-fractures treated conservatively. The three patients with poor results were all older than 10 years.[261] We attempt to manage re-fractures conservatively but have a lower threshold for operative treatment, particularly if the original fracture was malunited.

Growth Arrest. Growth arrest is a complication of physeal injury. Although there are reports of arrest after metaphyseal fractures, these injuries probably represent Peterson type I fractures of the physis.[1,64,299] Growth arrest may occur in either the radius or the ulna. Despite the frequency of distal radial physeal fractures, growth arrest is relatively infrequent.[10,14,75,81,299] This may be a function of the high velocity of growth from the distal radial physis (8 mm/yr), as well as the fact that the majority of these injuries result from a relatively low-energy impact. Conversely, ulnar physeal separation is an unusual injury but appears to be associated with a high incidence of growth arrest.[4,62,81,88,113,201,218,238] It is important to explain to the

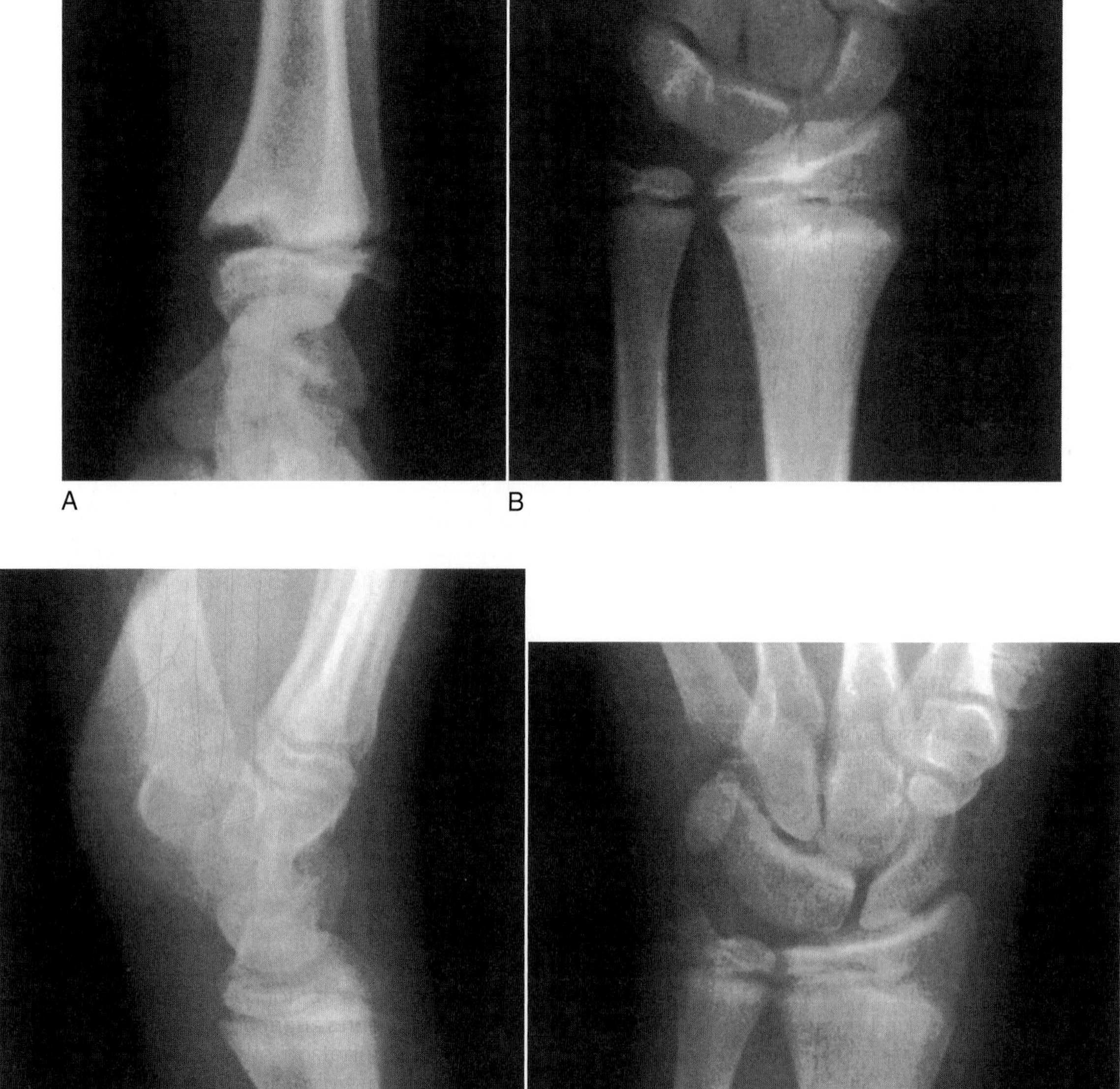

FIGURE 42–124 Chronic overuse injury to the distal radial physis. Anteroposterior **(A)** and lateral **(B)** radiographs of the right wrist in a 13-year-old gymnast. Note the wide and irregular appearance of the physis. **C** and **D,** Radiographic appearance 3 years later, after cessation of gymnastics.

parents of patients with physeal injuries the possibility of growth arrest, as well as the advantage of early identification and consequently the necessity of follow-up for an asymptomatic patient. We recommend follow-up at 4- to 6-month intervals for at least a year.

Treatment of growth arrest is discussed in Chapter 40, General Principles of Managing Orthopaedic Injuries. Generally, options for the treatment of distal radial growth arrest include observation, completion epiphysiodesis (with ulnar epiphysiodesis), or bar resection (Fig. 42–124). Ulnar arrest is not amenable to bar resection and, if identified early, is usually treated by radial epiphysiodesis. Unrecognized growth arrest in either the distal radius or ulna may lead to significant ulnar variance (positive or negative).[10,14,62,81,201,218,238,299] Symptomatic ulnar variance can be treated with either lengthening (acute or gradual) or shortening of the appropriate bone either directly or with epiphyseodesis.[313]

Peripheral Nerve Injury. Peripheral nerve injury is most commonly transient and the result of stretch associated with fracture displacement at the time of injury. It may also be secondary to direct injury, tethering, or entrapment within fracture fragments.[75] The median nerve is most commonly involved, and the symptoms frequently resolve immediately after fracture reduction. Tethering or entrapment can occur at

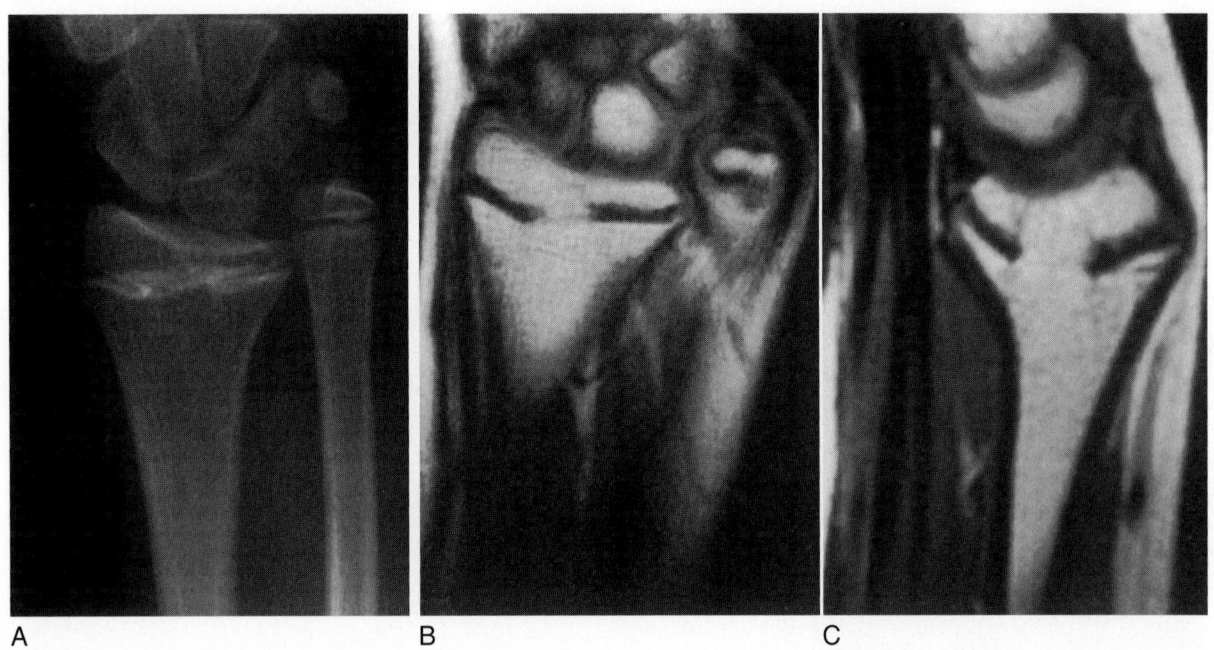

FIGURE 42–125 Physeal arrest (type B) after distal radial fracture. **A,** Anteroposterior (AP) radiograph of the wrist of a 12-year-old girl who had sustained a Salter-Harris type II fracture of the distal radius 6 years earlier. Note the ulnarly positive variance, as well as the physeal bar in the center of the distal radius. Coronal **(B)** and sagittal **(C)** magnetic resonance images show the extent of the bar.

Continued

the time of injury or reduction; thus, it is important to obtain a good pretreatment neurologic examination.[70,81,263] Although this may be difficult in an anxious child, many children will comply with a full examination if placed in a parent's lap and slowly reassured by examining the uninjured limb first. Loss of nerve function after closed reduction is an indication for operative treatment, particularly if the fracture has not been anatomically reduced. If nerve recovery is not evident in 6 to 12 weeks, consideration should be given to electrodiagnostic studies and surgical exploration.

Compartment Syndrome and Acute Carpal Tunnel Syndrome. Both compartment syndrome and acute carpal tunnel syndrome can develop after distal forearm fractures.[70,81,121,128,184,185,200] The hallmark finding in these potentially devastating complications is pain out of proportion to the clinical findings. The key to successful management of these injures is an accurate and timely diagnosis, which requires a high degree of suspicion and vigilant patient management. Diagnosis and treatment are discussed in Chapter 40, General Principles of Managing Orthopaedic Injuries.

Nonunion, Cross-Union, Infection, and Tendon Rupture. Nonunion, cross-union, infection, and tendon rupture are infrequent in children's distal forearm fractures.[306,334] Nonunion of uncomplicated, closed fractures is uncommon enough that its presence should suggest underlying pathology such as congenital pseudarthrosis or osteomyelitis.[23,149] Interestingly, resection of cross-union may be less successful in children than in adults.[306] Overgrowth after distal forearm fractures has not been a clinical problem.[76,336] Although tendon entrapment within the fracture may initially be confused with either nerve injury or compartment syndrome, careful examination usually leads to an accurate diagnosis. Tendon entrapment is not accompanied by sensory changes or pain and is generally associated with some persistent fracture displacement.[55,77,194]

Reflex Sympathetic Dystrophy. Reflex sympathetic dystrophy is a poorly defined entity characterized by pain and vasomotor dysfunction. It frequently develops after trauma and in adults is common in the upper extremity. Although reflex sympathetic dystrophy has been reported after distal forearm fractures in children, it is more common in the lower extremities.* In children, reflex sympathetic dystrophy has been shown to respond to conservative measures, including physical therapy, psychological therapies, transcutaneous electrical stimulation, and tricyclic antidepressant medication. We rarely use sympathetic blocks in managing reflex sympathetic dystrophy in children but have found our child psychology colleagues indispensable.[269,323] Reflex sympathetic dystrophy is discussed in more detail in Chapter 21, Disorders of the Knee.

ASSOCIATED CONDITIONS

Chronic Radial Physeal Injuries

Overuse injuries of the distal radial physis have been increasingly reported, primarily in competitive adolescent gymnasts.[48,49,77,82,180,181,251,253,292,318] A review revealed radiographic changes in the distal radius of 10% of female gymnasts (Fig. 42–125). Additionally, subtle but significant positive ulnar variance has

*See references 19, 54, 60, 72, 85, 87, 160, 216, 269, 323.

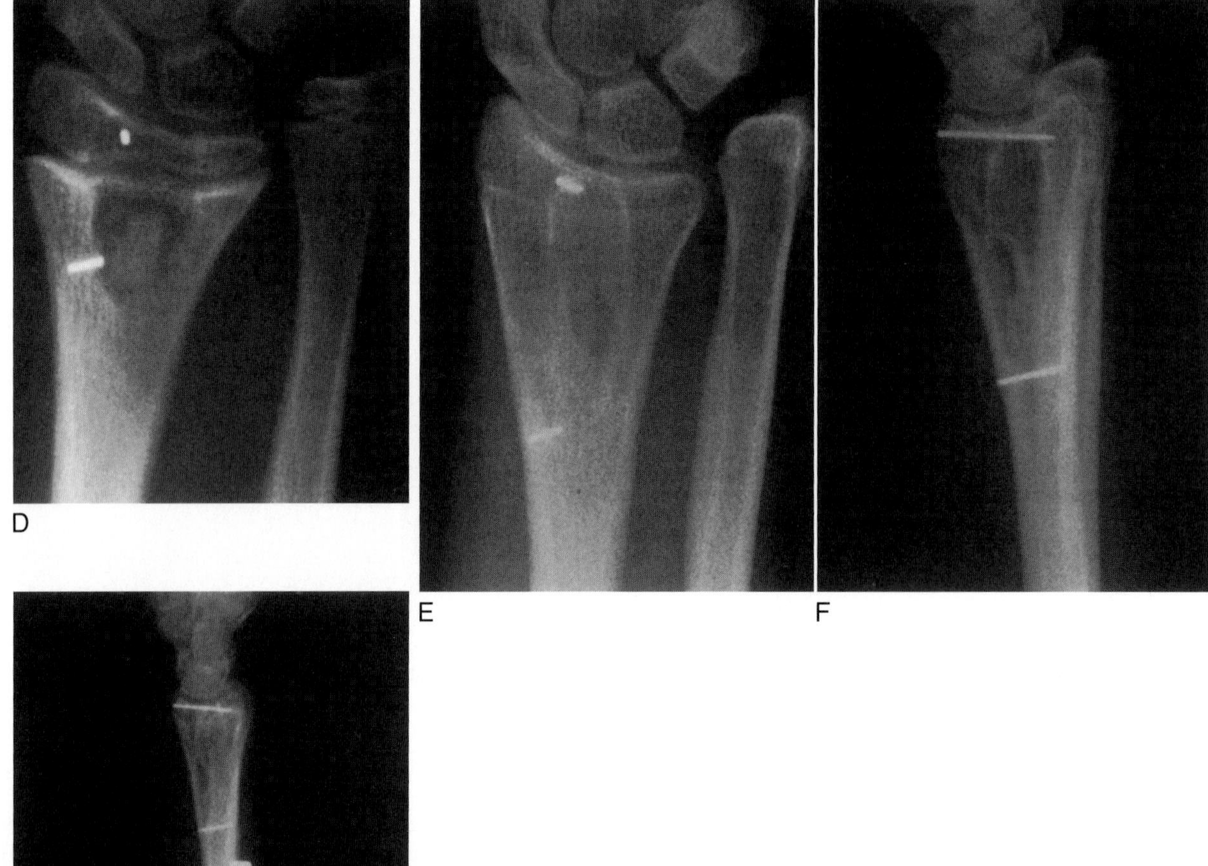

FIGURE 42–125 cont'd **D,** The bar has been resected and metallic markers placed in the epiphysis and metaphysis. AP **(E)** and lateral **(F)** radiographs showing resumption of growth as evidenced by an increased distance between the metallic markers. The ulnarly positive variance persists. **G,** Lateral radiograph after ulnar shortening to treat symptomatic ulnarly positive variance.

been reported in both skeletally mature and immature gymnasts. Like all overuse injuries, "gymnast's wrist " usually resolves with appropriate activity modification.

References

Fractures of the Forearm

1. Abram LJ, Thompson GH: Deformity after premature closure of the distal radial physis following a torus fracture with a physeal compression injury. Report of a case. J Bone Joint Surg Am 1987;69:1450.
2. Adamczyk MJ, Riley PM: Delayed union and nonunion following closed treatment of diaphyseal pediatric forearm fractures. J Pediatr Orthop 2005;25:51.
3. Adams JP, Rizzoli HV: Tardy radial and ulnar nerve palsy: Case report. J Neurosurg 1959;16:342.
4. Aitken AP: The end results of the fractured distal radial epiphysis. J Bone Joint Surg 1935;17:302.
5. Aitken AP: Further observations on fractured distal radial epiphysis. J Bone Joint Surg 1935;17:922.
6. Alexander CG: Effect of growth rate on the strength of the growth plate–shaft junction. Skeletal Radiol 1976; 1:67.
7. Almquist EE, Gordon LH, Blue AI: Congenital dislocation of the head of the radius. J Bone Joint Surg Am 1969;51:1118.
8. Alpar EK, Thompson K, Owen R, et al: Midshaft fractures of forearm bones in children. Injury 1981;13: 153.
9. Altissimi M, Antenucci R, Fiacca C, et al: Long-term results of conservative treatment of fractures of the distal radius. Clin Orthop Relat Res 1986;206:202.
10. Aminian A, Schoenecker PL: Premature closure of the distal radial physis after fracture of the distal radial metaphysis. J Pediatr Orthop 1995;15:495.

11. Anderson HJ: Monteggia fractures. Adv Orthop Surg 1989:201.
12. Armstrong PF, Joughlin VE, Clarke HM: Pediatric fractures of the forearm, wrist, and hand. In Green NE, Swiontkowski MF: Skeletal Trauma in Children. Philadelphia, WB Saunders, 1993, p 127.
13. Arunachalam VS, Griffiths JC: Fracture recurrence in children. Injury 1975;7:37.
14. Aston JW Jr, Henley MB: Physeal growth arrest of the distal radius treated by the Ilizarov technique. Report of a case. Orthop Rev 1989;18:813.
15. Austin R: Tardy palsy of the radial nerve from a Monteggia fracture. Injury 1976;7:202.
16. Bado JL: The Monteggia Lesion. Springfield, IL, Charles C Thomas, 1962.
17. Bado JL: The Monteggia lesion. Clin Orthop Relat Res 1967;50:71.
18. Bailey DA, Wedge JH, McCulloch RG, et al: Epidemiology of fractures of the distal end of the radius in children as associated with growth. J Bone Joint Surg Am 1989;71:1225.
19. Barbier O, Allington N, Rombouts JJ: Reflex sympathetic dystrophy in children: Review of a clinical series and description of the particularities in children. Acta Orthop Belg 1999;65:91.
20. Beaty JH, Kasser JR: Fractures about the elbow. Instr Course Lect 1995;44:199.
21. Beddow FH, Corkery PH: Lateral dislocation of the radio-humeral joint with greenstick fracture of the upper end of the ulna. J Bone Joint Surg Br 1960;42:782.
22. Bednar DA, Grandwilewski W: Complications of forearm-plate removal. Can J Surg 1992;35:428.
23. Bell DF: Congenital forearm pseudarthrosis: Report of six cases and review of the literature. J Pediatr Orthop 1989;9:438.
24. Bellemans M, Lamoureux J: Indications for immediate percutaneous intramedullary nailing of complete diaphyseal forearm shaft fractures in children. Acta Orthop Belg 1995;61(Suppl 1):169.
25. Bell Tawse AJ: The treatment of malunited anterior Monteggia fractures in children. J Bone Joint Surg Br 1965;47:718.
26. Best TN: Management of old unreduced Monteggia fracture dislocations of the elbow in children. J Pediatr Orthop 1994;14:193.
27. Biyani A: Ipsilateral Monteggia equivalent injury and distal radial and ulnar fracture in a child. J Orthop Trauma 1994;8:431.
28. Biyani A, Gupta SP, Sharma JC: Ipsilateral supracondylar fracture of humerus and forearm bones in children. Injury 1989;20:203.
29. Blackburn N, Ziv I, Rang M: Correction of the malunited forearm fracture. Clin Orthop Relat Res 1984;188:54.
30. Blount WP: Fractures in Children. Baltimore, Williams & Wilkins, 1955.
31. Blount WP: Osteoclasis of the upper extremity in children. Acta Orthop Scand 1962;32:374.
32. Blount WP: Forearm fractures in children. Clin Orthop Relat Res 1967;51:93.
33. Blount WP: Fractures in children [reprint]. Huntington, NY, RE Kreiger, 1977.
34. Blount WP, Schaefer AA, Johnson JH: Fractures of the forearm in children. JAMA 1942;120:111.
35. Bochang C, Jie Y, Zhigang W, et al: Immobilisation of forearm fractures in children: Extended versus flexed elbow. J Bone Joint Surg Br 2005;87:994.
36. Bohm ER, Bubbar V, Yong Hing K, et al: Above and below-the-elbow plaster casts for distal forearm fractures in children. A randomized controlled trial. J Bone Joint Surg Am 2006;88:1.
37. Boyd HB: Surgical exposure of the ulna and proximal one-third of the radius through one incision. Surg Gynecol Obstet 1940;71:86.
38. Boyd HB: Treatment of fractures of the ulna with dislocation of the radius. JAMA 1940;115:1699.
39. Boyd HB, Boals JC: The Monteggia lesion. A review of 159 cases. Clin Orthop Relat Res 1969;66:94.
40. Boyden EM, Peterson HA: Partial premature closure of the distal radial physis associated with Kirschner wire fixation. Orthopedics 1991;14:585.
41. Bragdon RA: Fractures of the distal radial epiphysis. Clin Orthop Relat Res 1965;41:59.
42. Brodueur AE, Silberstein MJ, Graviss ER: Radiology of the Pediatric Elbow. Boston, GK Hall, 1981.
43. Bruce HE, Harvey JP, Wilson JC Jr: Monteggia fractures. J Bone Joint Surg Am 1974;56:1563.
44. Bryan RS: Monteggia fracture of the forearm. J Trauma 1971;11:992.
45. Bucknill TM: Anterior dislocation of the radial head in children. Proc R Soc Med 1977;70:620.
46. Burgess RC, Watson HK: Hypertrophic ulnar styloid nonunions. Clin Orthop Relat Res 1988;228:215.
47. Burman M: Primary torsional fracture of the radius or ulna. J Bone Joint Surg Am 1953;35:665.
48. Caine D, Howe W, Ross W, et al: Does repetitive physical loading inhibit radial growth in female gymnasts? Clin J Sport Med 1997;7:302.
49. Caine D, Roy S, Singer KM, et al: Stress changes of the distal radial growth plate. A radiographic survey and review of the literature. Am J Sports Med 1992;20:290.
50. Canale ST, Puhl J, Watson FM, et al: Acute osteomyelitis following closed fractures. Report of three cases. J Bone Joint Surg Am 1975;57:415.
51. Cannata G, De Maio F, Mancini F, et al: Physeal fractures of the distal radius and ulna: Long-term prognosis. J Orthop Trauma 2003;17:172.
52. Caravias DE: Some observations on congenital dislocation of the head of the radius. J Bone Joint Surg Br 1957;39:86.
53. Carey PJ, Alburger PD, Betz RR, et al: Both-bone forearm fractures in children. Orthopedics 1992;15:1015.
54. Cassidy JT: Progress in diagnosing and understanding chronic pain syndromes in children. Curr Opin Rheumatol 1994;6:544.
55. Chambers HG, Wilkins KE: Fractures of the proximal radius and ulna. In Rockwood CA Jr, Wilkins KE, Beaty JH (eds): Fractures in Children, vol 3. Philadelphia, Lippincott-Raven, 1996, p 586.
56. Chan CF, Meads BM, Nicol RO: Remanipulation of forearm fractures in children. N Z Med J 1997;110:249.
57. Chess DG, Hyndman JC, Leahey JL: Short-arm plaster cast for pediatric distal forearm fractures. J Bone Joint Surg Br 1987;69:506.

58. Chess DG, Hyndman JC, Leahey JL, et al: Short-arm plaster cast for distal pediatric forearm fractures. J Pediatr Orthop 1994;14:211.
59. Choi KY, Chan WS, Lam TP, et al: Percutaneous Kirschner-wire pinning for severely displaced distal radial fractures in children. A report of 157 cases. J Bone Joint Surg Br 1995;77:797.
60. Cimaz R, Matucci-Cerinic M, Zulian F, et al: Reflex sympathetic dystrophy in children. J Child Neurol 1999;14:363.
61. Clarke AC, Spencer RF: Ulnar nerve palsy following fractures of the distal radius: Clinical and anatomical studies. J Hand Surg [Br] 1991;16:438.
62. Collado-Torres F, Zamora-Navas P, de la Torre-Solis F: Secondary forearm deformity due to injury to the distal ulnar physis. Acta Orthop Belg 1995;61:242.
63. Compson JP: Trans-carpal injuries associated with distal radial fractures in children: A series of three cases. J Hand Surg Br 1992;17:311.
64. Connolly JF, Eastman T, Huurman WW: Torus fracture of the distal radius producing growth arrest. Nebr Med J 1985;70:204.
65. Cooper AS: A Simple Fracture of the Radius and Dislocation of the Ulna: A Treatise on Dislocation and on Fractures of the Joints. London, Longman & Underwood, 1824.
66. Cooper AS: Dislocations and Fractures of the Joints. Boston, TR Marvin, 1844.
67. Cooper RR: Management of common forearm fractures in children. J Iowa Med Soc 1964;54:689.
68. Corbett CH: Anterior dislocation of the radius and its recurrence. Br J Surg 1931;19:155.
69. Creasman C, Zaleske DJ, Ehrlich MG: Analyzing forearm fractures in children. The more subtle signs of impending problems. Clin Orthop Relat Res 1984;188:40.
70. Cullen MC, Roy DR, Giza E, et al: Complications of intramedullary fixation of pediatric forearm fractures. J Pediatr Orthop 1998;18:14.
71. Curry GJ: Monteggia fracture. Am J Surg 1947;123: 613.
72. Dangel T: Chronic pain management in children. Part II: Reflex sympathetic dystrophy. Paediatr Anaesth 1998;8:105.
73. Daruwalla JS: A study of radioulnar movements following fractures of the forearm in children. Clin Orthop Relat Res 1979;139:114.
74. Davidson JS, Brown DJ, Barnes SN, et al: Simple treatment for torus fractures of the distal radius. J Bone Joint Surg Br 2001;83:1173.
75. Davis DR, Green DP: Forearm fractures in children: Pitfalls and complications. Clin Orthop Relat Res 1976; 120:172.
76. Deeney VF, Kaye JJ, Geary SP, et al: Pseudo–Volkmann's contracture due to tethering of flexor digitorum profundus to fractures of the ulna in children. J Pediatr Orthop 1998;18:437.
77. Degreef I, De Smet L: Missed radial head dislocations in children associated with ulnar deformation: Treatment by open reduction and ulnar osteotomy. J Orthop Trauma 2004;18:375.
78. de Pablos J, Franzreb M, Barrios C: Longitudinal growth pattern of the radius after forearm fractures conservatively treated in children. J Pediatr Orthop 1994;14: 492.
79. De Smet L, Claessens A, Lefevre J, et al: Gymnast wrist: An epidemiologic survey of ulnar variance and stress changes of the radial physis in elite female gymnasts. Am J Sports Med 1994;22:846.
80. Devnani AS: Missed Monteggia fracture dislocation in children. Injury 1997;28:131.
81. Dicke TE, Nunley JA: Distal forearm fractures in children. Complications and surgical indications. Orthop Clin North Am 1993;24:333.
82. DiFiori JP, Puffer JC, Mandelbaum BR, et al: Distal radial growth plate injury and positive ulnar variance in nonelite gymnasts. Am J Sports Med 1997;25:763.
83. Do TT, Strub WM, Foad SL, et al: Reduction versus remodeling in pediatric distal forearm fractures: A preliminary cost analysis. J Pediatr Orthop B 2003;12:109.
84. Dormans JP, Rang M: The problem of Monteggia fracture-dislocations in children. Orthop Clin North Am 1990;21:251.
85. Driessens M, Dijs H, Verheyen G, et al: What is reflex sympathetic dystrophy? Acta Orthop Belg 1999;65: 202.
86. Edwards EG: The posterior Monteggia fracture. Am Surg 1952;18:323.
87. Ehrlich MG, Zaleske DJ: Pediatric orthopedic pain of unknown origin. J Pediatr Orthop 1986;6:460.
88. Eliason EL, Furguson LK: Epiphyseal separation of the long bones. Surg Gynecol Obstet 1934;58:85.
89. Engber WD, Keene JS: Anterior interosseous nerve palsy associated with a Monteggia fracture. A case report. Clin Orthop Relat Res 1983;174:133.
90. Evans EM: Rotational deformity in the treatment of fractures of both bones of the forearm. J Bone Joint Surg 1945;27:373.
91. Evans EM: Pronation injuries of the forearm with special reference to the anterior Monteggia fracture. J Bone Joint Surg Br 1949;31:578.
92. Evans EM: Fractures of the radius and ulna. J Bone Joint Surg Br 1951;33:548.
93. Exner GU: Missed chronic anterior Monteggia lesion. Closed reduction by gradual lengthening and angulation of the ulna. J Bone Joint Surg Br 2001;83:547.
94. Fahey JJ: Fractures of the elbow in children. Instr Course Lect 1960;17:13.
95. Fahmy NR: Unusual Monteggia lesions in children. Injury 1981;12:399.
96. Fee NF, Dobranski A, Bisla RS: Gas gangrene complicating open forearm fractures. Report of five cases. J Bone Joint Surg Am 1977;59:135.
97. Flynn JM, Waters PM: Single-bone fixation of both-bone forearm fractures. J Pediatr Orthop 1996;16:655.
98. Fowles JV, Kassab MT: Displaced fractures of the medial humeral condyle in children. J Bone Joint Surg Am 1980;62:1159.
99. Fowles JV, Sliman N, Kassab MT: The Monteggia lesion in children. Fracture of the ulna and dislocation of the radial head. J Bone Joint Surg Am 1983;65:1276.
100. Frazier JL, Buschmann WR, Insler HP: Monteggia type I equivalent lesion: Diaphyseal ulna and proximal radius fracture with a posterior elbow dislocation in a child. J Orthop Trauma 1991;5:373.

101. Freedman L, Luk K, Leong JC: Radial head reduction after a missed Monteggia fracture: Brief report. J Bone Joint Surg Br 1988;70:846.
102. Friberg KS: Remodelling after distal forearm fractures in children. I. The effect of residual angulation on the spatial orientation of the epiphyseal plates. Acta Orthop Scand 1979;50:537.
103. Friberg KS: Remodelling after distal forearm fractures in children. II. The final orientation of the distal and proximal epiphyseal plates of the radius. Acta Orthop Scand 1979;50:731.
104. Friberg KS: Remodelling after distal forearm fractures in children. III. Correction of residual angulation in fractures of the radius. Acta Orthop Scand 1979;50:741.
105. Fuller DJ, McCullough CJ: Malunited fractures of the forearm in children. J Bone Joint Surg Br 1982;64:364.
106. Gainor BJ, Olson S: Combined entrapment of the median and anterior interosseous nerves in a pediatric both-bone forearm fracture. J Orthop Trauma 1990;4: 197.
107. Gainor JW, Hardy JH 3rd: Forearm fractures treated in extension. Immobilization of fractures of the proximal both bones of the forearm in children. J Trauma 1969; 9:167.
108. Galeazzi R: Di una particulare sindrome, traumatica delle scheletro dell avambraccio. Attie Mem Soc Lombardi Chir 1934;2:12.
109. Gandhi RK, Wilson P, Mason Brown JJ, et al: Spontaneous correction of deformity following fractures of the forearm in children. Br J Surg 1962;50:5.
110. Geissler WB, Fernandez DL, Graca R: Anterior interosseous nerve palsy complicating a forearm fracture in a child. J Hand Surg [Am] 1990;15:44.
111. Genelin F, Karlbauer AF, Gasperschitz F: Greenstick fracture of the forearm with median nerve entrapment. J Emerg Med 1988;6:381.
112. Gibbons CL, Woods DA, Pailthorpe C, et al: The management of isolated distal radius fractures in children. J Pediatr Orthop 1994;14:207.
113. Golz RJ, Grogan DP, Greene TL, et al: Distal ulnar physeal injury. J Pediatr Orthop 1991;11:318.
114. Gordon ML: Monteggia fracture. A combined surgical approach employing a single lateral incision. Clin Orthop Relat Res 1967;50:87.
115. Green WB, Anderson WJ: Simultaneous fracture of the scaphoid and radius in a child. J Pediatr Orthop 1982;2:191.
116. Green JS, Williams SC, Finlay D, et al: Distal forearm fractures in children: The role of radiographs during follow up. Injury 1998;29:309.
117. Griffet J, el Hayek T, Baby M: Intramedullary nailing of forearm fractures in children. J Pediatr Orthop B 1999;8:88.
118. Grundy M: Fractures of the carpal scaphoid in children. A series of eight Cases. Br J Surg 1969:56:523.
119. Guistra P, Killoran PJ, Furman RS: The missed Monteggia fracture. Radiology 1974;110:45.
120. Gyr BM, Stevens PM, Smith JT: Chronic Monteggia fractures in children: Outcome after treatment with the Bell-Tawse procedure. J Pediatr Orthop B 2004;13:402.
121. Haasbeek JF, Cole WG: Open fractures of the arm in children. J Bone Joint Surg Br 1995;77:576.
122. Haddad FS, Williams RL: Forearm fractures in children: Avoiding redisplacement. Injury 1995;26:691.
123. Hahn MP, Richter D, Ostermann PA, et al: [Elastic intramedullary nailing—a concept for treatment of unstable forearm fractures in childhood.] Chirurg 1996;67:409.
124. Hendel D, Aner A: Entrapment of the flexor digitorum profundus of the ring finger at the site of an ulnar fracture. A case report. Ital J Orthop Traumatol 1992;18: 417.
125. Henrikson B: Isolated fractures of the proximal end of the radius in children epidemiology, treatment and prognosis. Acta Orthop Scand 1969;40:246.
126. Hernandez J Jr, Peterson HA: Fracture of the distal radial physis complicated by compartment syndrome and premature physeal closure. J Pediatr Orthop 1986;6:627.
127. Hidaka S, Gustilo RB: Refracture of bones of the forearm after plate removal. J Bone Joint Surg Am 1984;66: 1241.
128. Hirayama T, Takemitsu Y, Yagihara K, et al: Operation for chronic dislocation of the radial head in children. Reduction by osteotomy of the ulna. J Bone Joint Surg Br 1987;69:639.
129. Hoffman BP: Fractures of the distal end of the radius in the adult and in the child. Bull Hosp Jt Dis 1953;14: 114.
130. Hogstrom H, Nilsson BE, Willner S: Correction with growth following diaphyseal forearm fracture. Acta Orthop Scand 1976;47:299.
131. Holdsworth BJ, Sloan JP: Proximal forearm fractures in children: Residual disability. Injury 1983;14:174.
132. Holmes JR, Louis DS: Entrapment of pronator quadratus in pediatric distal-radius fractures: Recognition and treatment. J Pediatr Orthop 1994;14:498.
133. Holst-Nielsen F, Jensen V: Tardy posterior interosseous nerve palsy as a result of an unreduced radial head dislocation in Monteggia fractures: a report of two cases. J Hand Surg [Am] 1984;9:572.
134. Hope PG: Anterior interosseous nerve palsy following internal fixation of the proximal radius. J Bone Joint Surg Br 1988;70:280.
135. Horii E, Tamura Y, Nakamura R, et al: Premature closure of the distal radial physis. J Hand Surg [Br] 1993;18:11.
136. Houshian S, Holst AK, Larsen MS, et al: Remodeling of Salter-Harris type II epiphyseal plate injury of the distal radius. J Pediatr Orthop 2004;24:472.
137. Hove LM: Simultaneous scaphoid and distal radial fractures. J Hand Surg Br 1994;19:384.
138. Huber RI, Keller HW, Huber PM, et al: Flexible intramedullary nailing as fracture treatment in children. J Pediatr Orthop 1996;16:602.
139. Hughston JC: Fractures of the forearm in children. J Bone Joint Surg Am 1962;44:1667.
140. Hui JH, Sulaiman AR, Lee HC, et al: Open reduction and annular ligament reconstruction with fascia of the forearm in chronic monteggia lesions in children. J Pediatr Orthop 2005;25:501.
141. Hume AC: Anterior dislocation of the head of the radius associated with undisplaced fracture of the olecranon in children. J Bone Joint Surg Br 1957;39:508.

142. Hurst LC, Dubrow EN: Surgical treatment of symptomatic chronic radial head dislocation: A neglected Monteggia fracture. J Pediatr Orthop 1983;3:227.
143. Imatani J, Hashizume H, Nishida K, et al: The Galeazzi-equivalent lesion in children revisited. J Hand Surg [Br] 1996;21:455.
144. Jessing P: Monteggia lesions and their complicating nerve damage. Acta Orthop Scand 1975;46:601.
145. Johari AN, Sinha M: Remodeling of forearm fractures in children. J Pediatr Orthop B 1999;8:84.
146. Jones K, Weiner DS: The management of forearm fractures in children: A plea for conservatism. J Pediatr Orthop 1999;19:811.
147. Kahle WK: The case against routine metal removal. J Pediatr Orthop 1994;14:229.
148. Kalamchi A: Monteggia fracture-dislocation in children. Late treatment in two cases. J Bone Joint Surg Am 1986;68:615.
149. Kameyama O, Ogawa R: Pseudarthrosis of the radius associated with neurofibromatosis: Report of a case and review of the literature. J Pediatr Orthop 1990;10:128.
150. Karachalios T, Smith EJ, Pearse MF: Monteggia equivalent injury in a very young patient. Injury 1992;23:419.
151. Kasser JR: Forearm fractures. In MacEwen GD (ed): A Practical Approach to Assessment and Treatment. Baltimore, Williams & Wilkins, 1993, p 165.
152. Kaufman B, Rinott MG, Tanzman M: Closed reduction of fractures of the proximal radius in children. J Bone Joint Surg Br 1989;71:66.
153. Kay S, Smith C, Oppenheim WL: Both-bone midshaft forearm fractures in children. J Pediatr Orthop 1986;6:306.
154. Kessler SB, Deiler S, Schiffl-Deiler M, et al: Refractures: A consequence of impaired local bone viability. Arch Orthop Trauma Surg 1992;111:96.
155. Kim HT, Conjares JN, Suh JT, et al: Chronic radial head dislocation in children, Part 1: Pathologic changes preventing stable reduction and surgical correction. J Pediatr Orthop 2002;22:583.
156. Kim HT, Park BG, Suh JT, et al: Chronic radial head dislocation in children, Part 2: Results of open treatment and factors affecting final outcome. J Pediatr Orthop 2002;22:591.
157. Knight RA, Purvis GD: Fractures of both bones of the forearm in adults. J Bone Joint Surg Am 1949;31:755.
158. Kolkman KA, van Niekerk JL, Rieu PN, et al: A complicated forearm greenstick fracture: Case report. J Trauma 1992;32:116.
159. Kowal-Vern A, Paxton TP, Ros SP, et al: Fractures in the under-3-year-old age cohort. Clin Pediatr (Phila) 1992;31:653.
160. Kozin F, Haughton V, Ryan L: The reflex sympathetic dystrophy syndrome in a child. J Pediatr 1977;90:417.
161. Kraus B, Horne G: Galeazzi fractures. J Trauma 1985;25:1093.
162. Kristiansen B, Eriksen AF: Simultaneous type II Monteggia lesion and fracture-separation of the lower radial epiphysis. Injury 1986;17:51.
163. Landfried MJ, Stenclik M, Susi JG: Variant of Galeazzi fracture-dislocation in children. J Pediatr Orthop 1991;11:332.
164. Landin LA: Fracture patterns in children. Analysis of 8,682 fractures with special reference to incidence, etiology and secular changes in a Swedish urban population 1950-1979. Acta Orthop Scand Suppl 1983;202:1.
165. Larsen E, Vittas D, Torp-Pedersen S: Remodeling of angulated distal forearm fractures in children. Clin Orthop Relat Res 1988;237:190.
166. Lascombes P, Prevot J, Ligier JN, et al: Elastic stable intramedullary nailing in forearm shaft fractures in children: 85 cases. J Pediatr Orthop 1990;10:167.
167. Lawton LJ: Fractures of the distal radius and ulna. In Letts RM: Management of Pediatric Fractures. New York, Churchill Livingstone, 1994, p 345.
168. Lee BS, Esterhai JL Jr, Das M: Fracture of the distal radial epiphysis. Characteristics and surgical treatment of premature, post-traumatic epiphyseal closure. Clin Orthop Relat Res 1984;185:90.
169. Lee S, Nicol RO, Stott NS: Intramedullary fixation for pediatric unstable forearm fractures. Clin Orthop Relat Res 2002;402:245.
170. Lesko PD, Georgis T, Slabaugh P: Irreducible Salter-Harris type II fracture of the distal radial epiphysis. J Pediatr Orthop 1987;7:719.
171. Letts M, Locht R, Wiens J: Monteggia fracture-dislocations in children. J Bone Joint Surg Br 1985;67:724.
172. Letts M, Rowhani N: Galeazzi-equivalent injuries of the wrist in children. J Pediatr Orthop 1993;13:561.
173. Lichter RL, Jacobsen T: Tardy palsy of the posterior interosseous nerve with a Monteggia fracture. J Bone Joint Surg Am 1975;57:124.
174. Lincoln TL, Mubarak SJ: "Isolated" traumatic radial-head dislocation. J Pediatr Orthop 1994;14:454.
175. Lloyd-Roberts GC, Bucknill TM: Anterior dislocation of the radial head in children: Aetiology, natural history and management. J Bone Joint Surg Br 1977;59:402.
176. Lovell ME, Galasko CS, Wright NB: Removal of orthopedic implants in children: Morbidity and postoperative radiologic changes. J Pediatr Orthop B 1999;8:144.
177. Luhmann SJ, Gordon JE, Schoenecker PL: Intramedullary fixation of unstable both-bone forearm fractures in children. J Pediatr Orthop 1998;18:451.
178. Macule Beneyto F, Arandes Renu JM, Ferreres Claramunt A, et al: Treatment of Galeazzi fracture-dislocations. J Trauma 1994;36:352.
179. Maffulli N, Fixsen JA: Painful hypertrophic non-union of the ulnar styloid. J Hand Surg [Br] 1990;15:355.
180. Mandelbaum BR, Bartolozzi AR, Davis CA, et al: Wrist pain syndrome in the gymnast. Pathogenetic, diagnostic, and therapeutic considerations. Am J Sports Med 1989;17:305.
181. Mani GV, Hui PW, Cheng JC: Translation of the radius as a predictor of outcome in distal radial fractures of children. J Bone Joint Surg Br 1993;75:808.
182. Mann DC, Rajmaira S: Distribution of physeal and nonphyseal fractures in 2,650 long-bone fractures in children aged 0-16 years. J Pediatr Orthop 1990;10:713.
183. Marek FM: Axial fixation of forearm fractures. J Bone Joint Surg Am 1961;43:1099.
184. Matsen FA 3rd, Veith RG: Compartmental syndromes in children. J Pediatr Orthop 1981;1:33.

185. Matsen FA 3rd, Winquist RA, Krugmire RB Jr: Diagnosis and management of compartmental syndromes. J Bone Joint Surg Am 1980;62:286.
186. Matthews LS, Kaufer H, Garver DF, et al: The effect on supination-pronation of angular malalignment of fractures of both bones of the forearm. J Bone Joint Surg Am 1982;64:14.
187. McFarland B: Congenital dislocation of the head of the radius. Br J Surg 1936;24:41.
188. McLauchlan GJ, Cowan B, Annan IH, et al: Management of completely displaced metaphyseal fractures of the distal radius in children. A prospective, randomised controlled trial. J Bone Joint Surg Br 2002;84:413.
189. Mih AD, Cooney WP, Idler RS, et al: Long-term follow-up of forearm bone diaphyseal plating. Clin Orthop Relat Res 1994;299:256.
190. Mikic ZD: Galeazzi fracture-dislocations. J Bone Joint Surg Am 1975;57:1071.
191. Miller BS, Taylor B, Widmann RF, et al: Cast immobilization versus percutaneous pin fixation of displaced distal radius fractures in children: A prospective, randomized study. J Pediatr Orthop 2005;25:490.
192. Monteggia GB: Instituzione Chirurgiche. 1814;5:130.
193. Morris AH: Irreducible Monteggia lesion with radial-nerve entrapment. A case report. J Bone Joint Surg Am 1974;56:1744.
194. Morrissy RT, Nalebuff EA: Distal radial fracture with tendon entrapment. A case report. Clin Orthop Relat Res 1977;124:205.
195. Mubarak SJ, Carroll NC: Volkmann's contracture in children: Aetiology and prevention. J Bone Joint Surg Br 1979;61:285.
196. Muller J, Roth B, Willenegger H: Long-term results of physeal fractures to the distal radius treated by percutaneous wire fixation. In Chapchal G (ed): Fractures in Children. New York, Thieme-Stratton, 1981.
197. Mullick S: The lateral Monteggia fracture. J Bone Joint Surg Am 1977;59:543.
198. Myers GJ, Gibbons PJ, Glithero PR: Nancy nailing of diaphyseal forearm fractures. Single bone fixation for fractures of both bones. J Bone Joint Surg Br 2004;86:581.
199. Naylor A: Monteggia fractures. Br J Surg 1942;29:323.
200. Neiman R, Maiocco B, Deeney VF: Ulnar nerve injury after closed forearm fractures in children. J Pediatr Orthop 1998;18:683.
201. Nelson OA, Buchanan JR, Harrison CS: Distal ulnar growth arrest. J Hand Surg [Am] 1984;9:164.
202. Neviaser RJ, LeFevre GW: Irreducible isolated dislocation of the radial head. A case report. Clin Orthop Relat Res 1971;80:72.
203. Newman JH: Displaced radial neck fractures in children. Injury 1977;9:114.
204. Nielsen AB, Simonsen O: Displaced forearm fractures in children treated with AO plates. Injury 1984;15:393.
205. Nilsson BE, Obrant K: The range of motion following fracture of the shaft of the forearm in children. Acta Orthop Scand 1977;48:600.
206. Noonan KJ, Price CT: Forearm and distal radius fractures in children. J Am Acad Orthop Surg 1998;6:146.
207. Nunley JA, Urbaniak JR: Partial bony entrapment of the median nerve in a greenstick fracture of the ulna. J Hand Surg [Am] 1980;5:557.
208. Ogden JA: Skeletal Injury in Children. Baltimore, Lea & Febiger, 1990.
209. Ogden JA: Skeletal Injury in the Child. Philadelphia, WB Saunders, 1990.
210. Olney BW, Menelaus MB: Monteggia and equivalent lesions in childhood. J Pediatr Orthop 1989;9:219.
211. Oner FC, Diepstraten AF: Treatment of chronic post-traumatic dislocation of the radial head in children. J Bone Joint Surg Br 1993;75:577.
212. Onne L, Sandblom PH: Late results in fractures of the forearm in children. Acta Chir Scand 1949;98:549.
213. Ono M, Bechtold JE, Merkow RL, et al: Rotational stability of diaphyseal fractures of the radius and ulna fixed with Rush pins and/or fracture bracing. Clin Orthop Relat Res 1989;240:236.
214. Ortega R, Loder RT, Louis DS: Open reduction and internal fixation of forearm fractures in children. J Pediatr Orthop 1996;16:651.
215. Osamura N, Ikeda K, Hagiwara N, et al: Posterior interosseous nerve injury complicating ulnar osteotomy for a missed Monteggia fracture. Scand J Plast Reconstr Surg Hand Surg 2004;38:376.
216. Oud CF, Legein J, Everaert H, et al: Bone scintigraphy in children with persistent pain in an extremity, suggesting algoneurodystrophy. Acta Orthop Belg 1999; 65:364.
217. Papavasiliou VA, Nenopoulos SP: Monteggia-type elbow fractures in childhood. Clin Orthop Relat Res 1988;223:230.
218. Paul AS, Kay PR, Haines JF: Distal ulnar growth plate arrest following a diaphyseal fracture. J R Coll Surg Edinb 1992;37:347.
219. Pavel A, Pitman JM, Lance EM, et al: The posterior Monteggia fracture: A clinical study. J Trauma 1965;12: 185.
220. Peiro A, Andres F, Fernandez-Esteve F: Acute Monteggia lesions in children. J Bone Joint Surg Am 1977; 59:92.
221. Penrose JH: The Monteggia fracture with posterior dislocation of the radial head. J Bone Joint Surg Br 1951; 33:65.
222. Perona PG, Light TR: Remodeling of the skeletally immature distal radius. J Orthop Trauma 1990;4:356.
223. Perrin J: Les fractures du cubitus accompagnees de luxation de l'extremite superieur du radius. These de Paris. Paris, G Steinheil, 1909.
224. Peterson HA: Physeal fractures: Part 3. Classification. J Pediatr Orthop 1994;14:439.
225. Peterson HA, Madhok R, Benson JT, et al: Physeal fractures: Part 1. Epidemiology in Olmsted County, Minnesota, 1979-1988. J Pediatr Orthop 1994;14:423.
226. Pollen AG: Fractures and Dislocations in Children. Edinburgh, Churchill Livingstone, 1973.
227. Price CT: Fractures of the midshaft radius and ulna. In Letts RM (ed): Management of Pediatric Fractures. New York, Churchill Livingstone, 1994.
228. Price CT: Injuries to the shafts of the radius and ulna. In Rockwood CA Jr, Wilkins KE, Beaty JH (eds): Fractures in Children, vol 3. Philadelphia, Lippincott-Raven, 1996, p 528.
229. Price CT, Scott DS, Kurzner ME, et al: Malunited forearm fractures in children. J Pediatr Orthop 1990;10:705.

230. Pritchett JW: Does pinning cause distal radial growth plate arrest? Orthopedics 1994;17:550.
231. Proctor MT, Moore DJ, Paterson JM: Redisplacement after manipulation of distal radial fractures in children. J Bone Joint Surg Br 1993;75:453.
232. Pugh DM, Galpin RD, Carey TP: Intramedullary Steinmann pin fixation of forearm fractures in children. Long-term results. Clin Orthop Relat Res 2000;376:39.
233. Putnam MD, Walsh TMt: External fixation for open fractures of the upper extremity. Hand Clin 1993;9: 613.
234. Rabinovich A, Adili A, Mah J: Outcomes of intramedullary nail fixation through the olecranon apophysis in skeletally immature forearm fractures. J Pediatr Orthop 2005;25:565.
235. Ramsey RH, Pedersen HE: The Monteggia fracturedislocation in children. Study of 15 cases of ulnar-shaft fracture with radial-head involvement. JAMA 1962;182: 1091.
236. Rang M, Barkin M, Ein SH: Radius and ulna. In Rang M: Children's Fractures. Philadelphia, JB Lippincott, 1983, p 207.
237. Ravessoud FA: Lateral condylar fracture and ipsilateral ulnar shaft fracture: Monteggia equivalent lesions? J Pediatr Orthop 1985;5:364.
238. Ray TD, Tessler RH, Dell PC: Traumatic ulnar physeal arrest after distal forearm fractures in children. J Pediatr Orthop 1996;16:195.
239. Reckling FW: Unstable fracture-dislocations of the forearm (Monteggia and Galeazzi lesions). J Bone Joint Surg Am 1982;64:857.
240. Reckling FW, Cordell LD: Unstable fracture-dislocations of the forearm. The Monteggia and Galeazzi lesions. Arch Surg 1968;96:999.
241. Reed MH: Fractures and dislocations of the extremities in children. J Trauma 1977;17:351.
242. Richter D, Ostermann PA, Ekkernkamp A, et al: Elastic intramedullary nailing: A minimally invasive concept in the treatment of unstable forearm fractures in children. J Pediatr Orthop 1998;18:457.
243. Rijnberg WJ, MacNicol MF: Superficial radial nerve entrapment within a radial fracture in a child. Injury 1993;24:426.
244. Ring D, Waters PM: Operative fixation of Monteggia fractures in children. J Bone Joint Surg Br 1996;78:734.
245. Rogers JF, Bennett JB, Tullos HS: Management of concomitant ipsilateral fractures of the humerus and forearm. J Bone Joint Surg Am 1984:66;552.
246. Rodgers WB, Smith BG: A type IV Monteggia injury with a distal diaphyseal radius fracture in a child. J Orthop Trauma 1993;7:84.
247. Rodgers WB, Waters PM, Hall JE: Chronic Monteggia lesions in children: Complications and results of reconstruction. J Bone Joint Surg Am 1996;78:1322.
248. Rosson JW, Shearer JR: Refracture after the removal of plates from the forearm. An avoidable complication. J Bone Joint Surg Br 1991;73:415.
249. Roy DR: Radioulnar synostosis following proximal radial fracture in child. Orthop Rev 1986;15:89.
250. Roy DR: Completely displaced distal radius fractures with intact ulnas in children. Orthopedics 1989;12: 1089.
251. Roy S, Caine D, Singer KM: Stress changes of the distal radial epiphysis in young gymnasts. A report of twenty-one cases and a review of the literature. Am J Sports Med 1985;13:301.
252. Royle SG: Compartment syndrome following forearm fracture in children. Injury 1990;21:73.
253. Ruggles DL, Peterson HA, Scott SG: Radial growth plate injury in a female gymnast. Med Sci Sports Exerc 1991;23:393.
254. Sage FP: Medullary fixation of fractures of the forearm. A study of the medullary canal of the radius and a report of fifty fractures of the radius treated with a prebent triangular nail. J Bone Joint Surg Am 1959;41: 1489.
255. Salter RB, Harris WR: Injuries involving the epiphyseal plate. J Bone Joint Surg Am 1963;45:587.
256. Salter RB, Zaltz C: Anatomic investigations of the mechanism of injury and pathologic anatomy of "pulled elbow" in young children. Clin Orthop Relat Res 1971; 77:134.
257. Sarmiento A, Ebramzadeh E, Brys D, et al: Angular deformities and forearm function. J Orthop Res 1992; 10:121.
258. Schmalzried TP, Grogan TJ, Neumeier PA, et al: Metal removal in a pediatric population: Benign procedure or necessary evil? J Pediatr Orthop 1991;11:72.
259. Schranz PJ, Gultekin C, Colton CL: External fixation of fractures in children. Injury 1992;23:80.
260. Schuind F, Cooney WP 3rd, Burny F, et al: Small external fixation devices for the hand and wrist. Clin Orthop Relat Res 1993;293:77.
261. Schwarz N, Pienaar S, Schwarz AF, et al: Refracture of the forearm in children. J Bone Joint Surg Br 1996;78: 740.
262. Shaer JA, Smith B, Turco VJ: Mid-third forearm fractures in children: An unorthodox treatment. Am J Orthop 1999;28:60.
263. Shoemaker SD, Comstock CP, Mubarak SJ, et al: Intramedullary Kirschner wire fixation of open or unstable forearm fractures in children. J Pediatr Orthop 1999; 19:329.
264. Shonnard PY, DeCoster TA: Combined Monteggia and Galeazzi fractures in a child's forearm. A case report. Orthop Rev 1994;23:755.
265. Skillern PG: Complete fracture of the lower third of the radius in childhood with greenstick fracture of the ulna. Ann Surg 1915;61:209.
266. Smith FM: Monteggia fractures: An analysis of 25 consecutive fresh injuries. Surg Gynecol Obstet 1947;85: 630.
267. Smith H, Sage F: Medullary fixation of forearm fractures. J Bone Joint Surg Am 1957;39:91.
268. Smith VA, Goodman HJ, Strongwater A, et al: Treatment of pediatric both-bone forearm fractures: A comparison of operative techniques. J Pediatr Orthop 2005;25:309.
269. Song KM, Morton AA, Koch KD, et al: Chronic musculoskeletal pain in childhood. J Pediatr Orthop 1998;18: 576.
270. Speed JS, Boyd HB: Treatment of fractures of ulna with dislocation of head of radius: Monteggia fracture. JAMA 1940;125:1699.

271. Spinner M, Freundlich BD, Teicher J: Posterior interosseous nerve palsy as a complication of Monteggia fractures in children. Clin Orthop Relat Res 1968;58:141.
272. Stahl S, Rozen N, Michaelson M: Ulnar nerve injury following midshaft forearm fractures in children. J Hand Surg [Br] 1997;22:788.
273. Stanitski CL, Micheli LJ: Simultaneous ipsilateral fractures of the arm and forearm in children. Clin Orthop Relat Res 1980;153:218.
274. Stanley E, De La Garza JF: Monteggia fracture-dislocation in children. In Rockwood CA Jr, Wilkins KE, Beaty JH (eds): Fractures in Children, vol 3. Philadelphia, Lippincott-Raven, 1996, p 548.
275. Stansberry SD, Swischuk LE, Swischuk JL, et al: Significance of ulnar styloid fractures in childhood. Pediatr Emerg Care 1990;6:99.
276. Stein F, Grabias SL, Deffer PA: Nerve injuries complicating Monteggia lesions. J Bone Joint Surg Am 1971; 53:1432.
277. Stelling FH, Cote RH: Traumatic dislocation of head of radius in children. JAMA 1956;160:732.
278. Stern PJ, Drury WJ: Complications of plate fixation of forearm fractures. Clin Orthop Relat Res 1983;175: 25.
279. Stoll TM, Willis RB, Paterson DC: Treatment of the missed Monteggia fracture in the child. J Bone Joint Surg Br 1992;74:436.
280. Storen G: Traumatic dislocation of the radial head as an isolated lesion in children; report of one case with special regard to roentgen diagnosis. Acta Chir Scand 1959;116:144.
281. Strachan JC, Ellis BW: Vulnerability of the posterior interosseous nerve during radial head resection. J Bone Joint Surg Br 1971;53:320.
282. Street DM: Intramedullary forearm nailing. Clin Orthop Relat Res 1986;212:219.
283. Tarr RR, Garfinkel AI, Sarmiento A: The effects of angular and rotational deformities of both bones of the forearm. An in vitro study. J Bone Joint Surg Am 1984;66:65.
284. Theodorou SD: Dislocation of the head of the radius associated with fracture of the upper end of the ulna in children. J Bone Joint Surg Br 1969;51:700.
285. Theodorou SD, Ierodiaconou MN, Roussis N: Fracture of the upper end of the ulna associated with dislocation of the head of the radius in children. Clin Orthop Relat Res 1988;228:240.
286. Thomas EM, Tuson KW, Browne PS: Fractures of the radius and ulna in children. Injury 1975;7:120.
287. Thompson GH, Wilber JH, Marcus RE: Internal fixation of fractures in children and adolescents. A comparative analysis. Clin Orthop Relat Res 1984;188:10.
288. Thompson HA, Hamilton AT: Monteggia fracture: Internal fixation of fractured ulna with I. M. Steinmann pin. Am J Surg 1950;79:579.
289. Thompson HC 3rd, Garcia A: Myositis ossificans: Aftermath of elbow injuries. Clin Orthop Relat Res 1967;50:129.
290. Thompson JD, Lipscomb AB: Recurrent radial head subluxation treated with annular ligament reconstruction. A case report and follow-up study. Clin Orthop Relat Res 1989;246:131.
291. Thorndike AJ, Dimmler CJ: Fractures of the forearm and elbow in children: An analysis of 364 consecutive cases. N Engl J Med 1941;225:475.
292. Tolat AR, Sanderson PL, De Smet L, et al: The gymnast's wrist: Acquired positive ulnar variance following chronic epiphyseal injury. J Hand Surg [Br] 1992;17:678.
293. Tompkins DG: The anterior Monteggia fracture: Observations on etiology and treatment. J Bone Joint Surg Am 1971;53:1109.
294. Tredwell SJ, Van Peteghem K, Clough M: Pattern of forearm fractures in children. J Pediatr Orthop 1984; 4:604.
295. Trousdale RT, Linscheid RL: Operative treatment of malunited fractures of the forearm. J Bone Joint Surg Am 1995;77:894.
296. Trumble TE, Benirschke SK, Vedder NB: Ipsilateral fractures of the scaphoid and radius. J Hand Surg Am 1993;18:8.
297. Vahvanen V, Westerlund M: Fracture of the carpal scaphoid in children. A clinical and roentgenological study of 108 cases. Acta Orthop Scand 1980:51: 909.
298. Vainionpaa S, Bostman O, Patiala H, et al: Internal fixation of forearm fractures in children. Acta Orthop Scand 1987;58:121.
299. Valverde JA, Albinana J, Certucha JA: Early posttraumatic physeal arrest in distal radius after a compression injury. J Pediatr Orthop B 1996;5:57.
300. Vance RM, Gelberman RH: Acute ulnar neuropathy with fractures at the wrist. J Bone Joint Surg Am 1978; 60:962.
301. Van der Reis WL, Otsuka NY, Moroz P, et al: Intramedullary nailing versus plate fixation for unstable forearm fractures in children. J Pediatr Orthop 1998;18:9.
302. Veranis N, Laliotis N, Vlachos E: Acute osteomyelitis complicating a closed radial fracture in a child. A case report. Acta Orthop Scand 1992;63:341.
303. Verstreken L, Delronge G, Lamoureux J: Shaft forearm fractures in children: Intramedullary nailing with immediate motion: A preliminary report. J Pediatr Orthop 1988;8:450.
304. Victor J, Mulier T, Fabry G: Refracture of radius and ulna in a female gymnast. A case report. Am J Sports Med 1993;21:753.
305. Vince KG, Miller JE: Cross-union complicating fracture of the forearm. Part I: Adults. J Bone Joint Surg Am 1987;69:640.
306. Vince KG, Miller JE: Cross-union complicating fracture of the forearm. Part II: Children. J Bone Joint Surg Am 1987;69:654.
307. Vittas D, Larsen E, Torp-Pedersen S: Angular remodeling of midshaft forearm fractures in children. Clin Orthop Relat Res 1991;265:261.
308. Voto SJ, Weiner DS, Leighley B: Redisplacement after closed reduction of forearm fractures in children. J Pediatr Orthop 1990;10:79.
309. Walker JL, Rang M: Forearm fractures in children. Cast treatment with the elbow extended. J Bone Joint Surg Br 1991;73:299.
310. Walsh HP, McLaren CA, Owen R: Galeazzi fractures in children. J Bone Joint Surg Br 1987;69:730.

311. Wang MN, Chang WN: Chronic posttraumatic anterior dislocation of the radial head in children: Thirteen cases treated by open reduction, ulnar osteotomy, and annular ligament reconstruction through a Boyd incision. J Orthop Trauma 2006;20:1.
312. Waseem M, Paton RW: Percutaneous intramedullary elastic wiring of displaced diaphyseal forearm fractures in children. A modified technique. Injury 1999;30:21.
313. Waters PM, Bae DS, Montgomery KD: Surgical management of posttraumatic distal radial growth arrest in adolescents. J Pediatr Orthop 2002;22:717.
314. Watson JA, Singer GC: Irreducible Monteggia fracture: Beware nerve entrapment. Injury 1994;25:325.
315. Watson-Jones R: Fractures and Joint Injuries. Edinburgh, ES Livingstone, 1956.
316. Webb GR, Galpin RD, Armstrong DG: Comparison of short and long arm plaster casts for displaced fractures in the distal third of the forearm in children. J Bone Joint Surg Am 2006;88:9.
317. Wedge JH, Robertson DE: Displaced fractures of the neck of the radius. J Bone Joint Surg Br 1982;64: 256.
318. Weiker GG: Hand and wrist problems in the gymnast. Clin Sports Med 1992;11:189.
319. Weisman DS, Rang M, Cole WG: Tardy displacement of traumatic radial head dislocation in childhood. J Pediatr Orthop 1999;19:523.
320. Weiss GA: Forearm fractures in children: A retrospective study. J Pediatr 1986;6:506.
321. West S, Andrews J, Bebbington A, et al: Buckle fractures of the distal radius are safely treated in a soft bandage: A randomized prospective trial of bandage versus plaster cast. J Pediatr Orthop 2005; 25:322.
322. Widmann RF, Waters PM, Reeves S: Complications of closed treatment of distal radius fractures in children. Paper presented at the Annual Meeting of the Pediatric Orthopaedic Society of North America, Miami,1995, p 58.
323. Wilder RT, Berde CB, Wolohan M, et al: Reflex sympathetic dystrophy in children. Clinical characteristics and follow-up of seventy patients. J Bone Joint Surg Am 1992;74:910.
324. Wiley JJ, Galey JP: Monteggia injuries in children. J Bone Joint Surg Br 1985;67:728.
325. Wiley JJ, McIntyre WM: Fracture patterns in children. In Current Concepts of Bone Fragility. Berlin, Springer-Verlag, 1986, p 159.
326. Wilkins K: Fractures of the radius and ulnar shafts. In KE W (ed): Operative Management of Upper Extremity Fractures in Children. Rosemont, IL, Americn Academy of Orthopaedic Surgeons, 1994.
327. Wilkins KE: Supracondylar fractures: What's new? J Pediatr Orthop Br 1997:6:110.
328. Wilkins KE, O'Brien ET: Fractures of the distal radius and ulna. In Rockwood CA Jr, Wilkins KE, Beaty JH: Fractures in Children. Philadelphia, Lippincott-Raven, 1996, p. 451.
329. Wise RA: Lateral dislocation of the head of the radius with fracture of the ulna. J Bone Joint Surg 1941; 23:379.
330. Wolfe JS, Eyring EJ: Median-nerve entrapment within a greenstick fracture; a case report. J Bone Joint Surg Am 1974;56:1270.
331. Worlock P, Stower M: Fracture patterns in Nottingham children. J Pediatr Orthop 1986;6:656.
332. Wright PR: Greenstick fracture of the upper end of the ulna with dislocation of the radio-humeral joint or displacement of the superior radial epiphysis. J Bone Joint Surg Br 1963;45:727.
333. Wyrsch B, Mencio GA, Green NE: Open reduction and internal fixation of pediatric forearm fractures. J Pediatr Orthop 1996;16:644.
334. Young TB: Irreducible displacement of the distal radial epiphysis complicating a fracture of the lower radius and ulna. Injury 1984;16:166.
335. Younger AS, Tredwell SJ, Mackenzie WG, et al: Accurate prediction of outcome after pediatric forearm fracture. J Pediatr Orthop 1994;14:200.
336. Yu Z, Wang Y, Wang C: [The influence on radioulnar joints after single-bone fracture of the forearm in children.] Zhonghua Wai Ke Za Zhi 1996;34:209.
337. Yuan PS, Pring ME, Gaynor TP, et al: Compartment syndrome following intramedullary fixation of pediatric forearm fractures. J Pediatr Orthop 2004;24: 370.
338. Yung SH, Lam CY, Choi KY, et al: Percutaneous intramedullary Kirschner wiring for displaced diaphyseal forearm fractures in children. J Bone Joint Surg Br 1998;80:91.
339. Zamzam MM, Khoshhal KI: Displaced fracture of the distal radius in children: Factors responsible for redisplacement after closed reduction. J Bone Joint Surg Br 2005;87:841.
340. Zionts LE, Zalavras CG, Gerhardt MB: Closed treatment of displaced diaphyseal both-bone forearm fractures in older children and adolescents. J Pediatr Orthop 2005;25:507.

Fractures and Dislocations of the Wrist and Hand

Falling onto an outstretched hand usually causes fractures of the forearm bones in children and, in rare cases, causes carpal fractures until the late teen years. Because the carpus is completely cartilaginous at birth and remains substantially so until late childhood, the cushioning effect of the cartilage protects against carpal fracture in young children. Ossification begins in the capitate between 2 and 3 months of age and proceeds in a clockwise manner to the hamate about a month later. Two years later, ossification is seen in the triquetrum. The lunate appears on the radiographs of older 3-year-olds, the scaphoid at about age 5, and the trapezoid and the trapezium in 6-year-olds. By the time that the child is in first grade, all but the pisiform are beginning to ossify. Ossification of the pisiform begins much later, in the 9th or 10th year of life. Not until adolescence do the carpal bones of the wrist have an adult-like appearance on radiographs.

Fracture of a carpal bone may occur in small children as part of a massive injury and in this case is almost always associated with other fractures of forearm bones, metacarpals, or other carpals. Later in adolescence, more adult-type fracture patterns consisting of isolated carpal fractures may be seen, but they are usually stable. Less common but important, carpal fracture may occur in conjunction with ligamentous injury. In these patients, the injury causes serious instability of the wrist that demands careful treatment. Despite appropriate treatment, these patients generally have residual joint stiffness and weakness.

Fractures of the Scaphoid

Fractures of the scaphoid are the most common carpal fracture in adults, as well as in children. However, unlike in adults and adolescents, the fracture is rare in young children. It tends to occur in the distal pole as an avulsion-type fracture.[1]

A scaphoid fracture is seen most commonly in males between the ages of 15 and 30 years.[1] During adolescence, as in adulthood, the fracture may be the only radiographic evidence of more extensive, severe trauma in which critical ligamentous structures in the wrist may have been injured. Additional ligamentous injuries in these cases may make the associated fracture unstable, might prolong healing, and may eventually lead to nonunion. Any evidence of fracture displacement or instability or a history of wrist dislocation should be treated by internal fixation of the fracture and repair of the torn ligaments. This is a relatively common injury in adolescent athletes.

ANATOMY

The patient is usually an adolescent boy who gives a history of falling onto an outstretched hand in a football game. All too commonly the injury is misinterpreted by the patient, parent, coach, and trainer as "just a sprain." When such an injury is associated with radial-side wrist pain, the orthopaedist must examine the wrist carefully because the physical findings are often subtle and critical.

Mild swelling in the anatomic snuffbox is best appreciated by comparing the injured wrist with the uninjured one (Fig. 42–126). Tenderness in this area should also be compared with the opposite side. When more massive swelling is present, particularly when associated with tenderness over both the scaphoid and the ulnar side of the wrist, the surgeon must consider that a perilunate injury may have occurred. This is important inasmuch as radiologically the wrist may have little or no sign of this injury because the perilunate dislocation may have reduced itself before the x-ray study.

RADIOGRAPHIC FINDINGS

The radiographic findings in scaphoid fracture may be subtle or, in the first few weeks, occasionally absent. It is solid orthopaedic practice to trust the physical examination, and experienced orthopaedists look for well-localized tenderness in the anatomic snuffbox. Nondisplaced scaphoid fractures may not be visible on the initial films. If doubt exists, the wrist should be immobilized in plaster and repeat radiographs obtained in 14 to 21 days. In addition, no imaging technique can accurately evaluate the ligamentous injury that may accompany the deceptively benign appearance of a fractured scaphoid. Here, the surgeon must rely on a high index of suspicion and the presence of widespread tenderness and swelling noted on the physical examination.

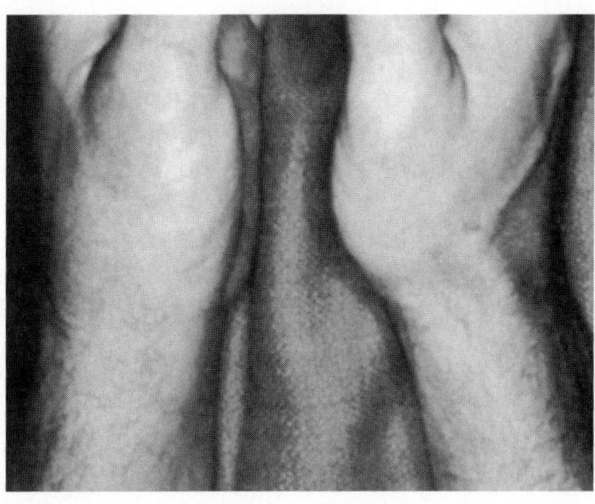

FIGURE 42–126 Subtle swelling in the anatomic snuffbox is more easily demonstrated when the normal side (*right*) and the injured side (*left*) are compared side by side.

Routine Scaphoid X-Ray Series

When properly performed, this series is usually the only imaging study required. Inexpensive and easily carried out, the study requires attention to detail on the part of the x-ray technician. The orthopaedist must insist that at least the following be included:

1. Radial and ulnar deviation posteroanterior views with the wrist in about 30 degrees of extension. (This amount of wrist extension is conveniently realized by asking the patient to make a fist gently during the examination.)
2. A pronated oblique view of the wrist, posteroanterior, with the wrist slightly supinated (about 30 degrees) off the x-ray cassette.
3. A true lateral view of the wrist with the radius and ulna superimposed and in neutral radial and ulnar deviation and neutral extension (this can be verified when the metacarpals are collinear with the long axis of the forearm bones).
4. Comparison views of the opposite wrist in all projections. *The importance of comparison views cannot be overstated.* Subtle changes in the intercalated carpal segment are often normal variants, and without a comparison view of the patient's uninjured wrist, they may be erroneously considered pathologic.

A practical way to obtain the scaphoid series is to use two 10 × 12-inch films as follows:

1. Divide the first film into four quadrants and expose the left wrist on the left two quadrants. In the upper quadrant, obtain the ulnar deviation view to stretch out the scaphoid, and in the lower quadrant, obtain a radial deviation view to check for scaphoid rotation. Repeat the same views of the right wrist in the corresponding two right quadrants. Now the two wrists can readily be compared with minimal shuffling of x-ray films.
2. Divide the second film into thirds. Place the two lateral exposures of the right and left wrists side by side and the oblique film in the remaining third. Figure 42–127 shows an example of the scaphoid x-ray series.

Additional imaging studies are expensive but may be indicated when displacement of the fracture is expected or for complex wrist injuries. They are not routinely indicated.

Computed Axial Tomography Scans

A computed axial tomography (CAT) scan is useful for detecting small or subtle fractures and fracture displacements. It should be undertaken when there is reason to suspect that such findings may exist. Marked swelling, significant ulnar wrist tenderness, comminuted scaphoid fractures, and intercalated segment instability not present in the normal wrist are indications to use this study. It is also helpful in evaluating union of the scaphoid. However, a CAT scan may occasionally underestimate or overestimate the status of osseous union in these fractures.

Bone Scans

Occasionally, the standard scaphoid series just detailed fails to demonstrate a fracture but the patient's clinical findings indicate a scaphoid fracture and persist after 14 to 21 days of a trial of plaster cast immobilization. In this case, a bone scan is a valuable way to assess the presence of a fracture and hence the need for continuing the plaster immobilization. When the bone scan is normal at 4 weeks, the patient can be assured by the surgeon that the scaphoid is not fractured. An abnormal bone scan is an indication for more advanced imaging techniques such as CAT scans.

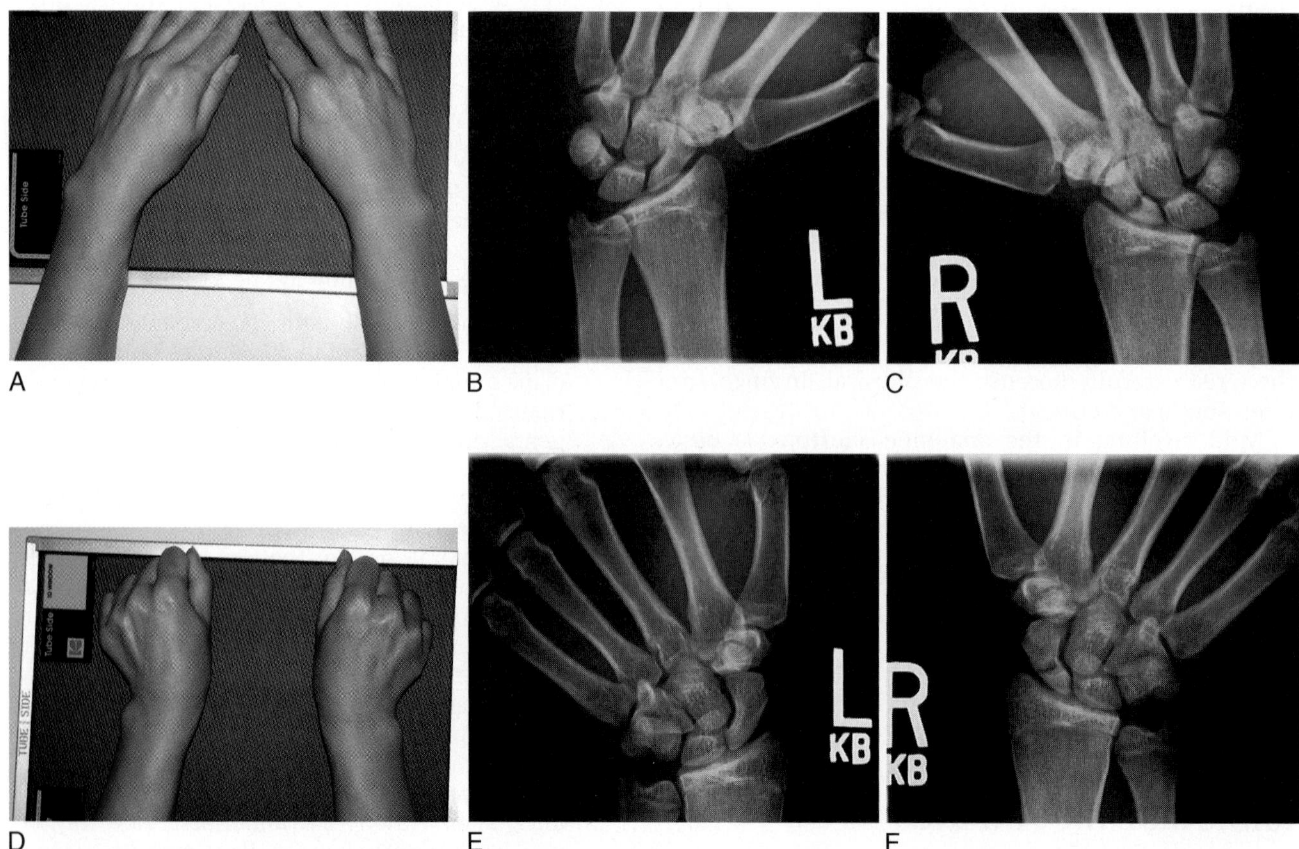

FIGURE 42–127 The scaphoid radiographic series (**B/C, E/F, H/I,** and **K**) provides comparison views side by side, a useful and important aid for locating subtle abnormalities. It is made using two 10 × 12-inch films. Clinical photographs **(A, D, G, J)** show positioning of the wrist on the x-ray cassette. The technique is described in the text.

Magnetic Resonance Imaging

There has been considerable abuse of MRI for evaluating wrist injuries. This expensive study rarely adds information that changes the treatment of such patients. MRI is not a reliable determinant of proximal pole blood supply in this small bone, nor does it accurately reveal concomitant ligamentous injury in patients with a scaphoid fracture. MRI may be useful in imaging the mainly cartilaginous carpus of children, but it is rarely indicated in the treatment of an adolescent with a fracture of the scaphoid.

TREATMENT

Stable or Nondisplaced Scaphoid Fractures

Treatment with a short-thumb spica cast for 4 to 8 weeks is appropriate in younger children. In older adolescents involved in sports, consideration of internal fixation of even nondisplaced fractures may be appropriate in selected cases to allow earlier return to sporting activities. Even with rigid internal fixation, however, it is prudent to protect the patient from overstressing the recently fixed but as yet ununited scaphoid fracture. Usually about 8 weeks is required to obtain adequate osseous union, return of flexibility, and strength before allowing the patient to play vigorous sports without a brace or plaster protection.

Unstable or Displaced Scaphoid Fractures

Displacement of even 1 mm on the radiograph is diagnostic of instability, and open reduction with internal fixation is the appropriate treatment of these scaphoid fractures. Specialized devices such as the Herbert

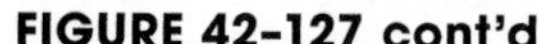
FIGURE 42-127 cont'd

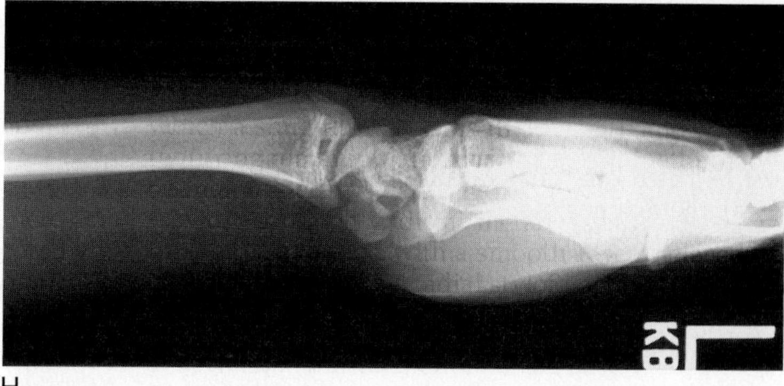

H

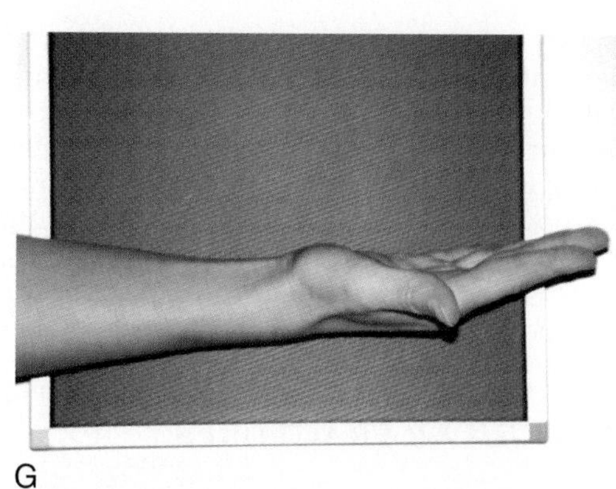
G

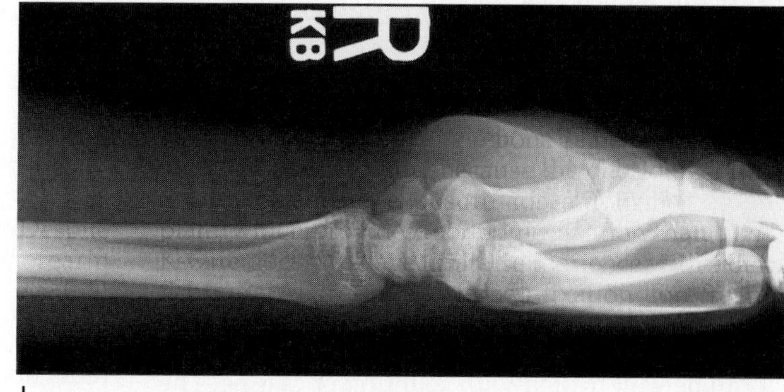

I

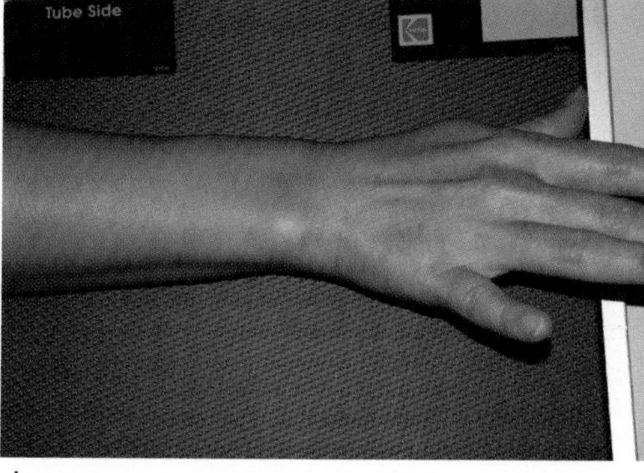

J

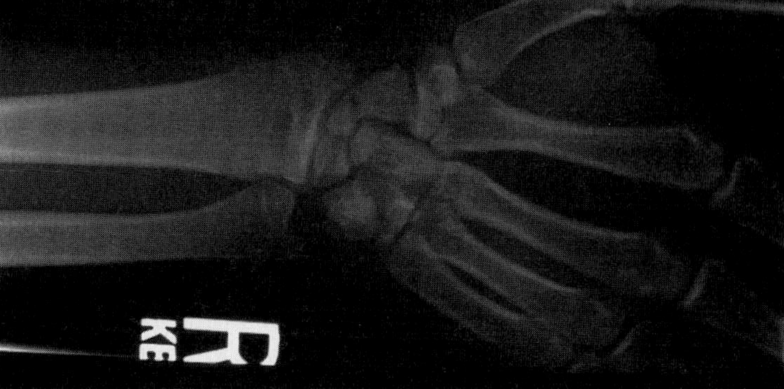

K

scaphoid screw have been used effectively. Considerable skill and experience are required to position the internal fixation device properly in this bone. The target area is small and unforgiving. The patient is wisely referred to a surgeon who performs this technique routinely, especially for more unusual cases in which a perilunate injury accompanies the scaphoid fracture, where the wrist is often very unstable. Open repair of these injuries is one of the most challenging procedures in hand surgery. Wide exposure with incisions on the dorsum as well as anteriorly is needed to achieve adequate ligament repair. These rare injuries are best referred to a hand surgeon for this treatment.

Dislocation and Fracture-Dislocation of the Immature Wrist

Subluxations and dislocations of the wrist can be very difficult to diagnose in an immature carpus because it is unossified. After an injury, if the child's wrist is significantly swollen and unable to flex and extend and if no forearm fracture is evident, this diagnosis must be ruled out. Bilateral films for comparison are critical; the diagnosis is usually made from a carefully positioned lateral radiograph. For lateral views the wrist must be carefully positioned in neutral flexion and extension with the forearm bones superimposed. The orthopaedist must insist that repeat films be done until a proper study is obtained. On the lateral view in a very young patient, often the axial malalignment of the metacarpals and forearm bones is the only tip-off that can be used to identify this injury. If this is noted in a child, MRI and arthrography are necessary for more complete delineation of these rare dislocations, which in a mature carpus would be obvious on a plain radiograph. When no history of trauma is present, juvenile arthritis must be considered.

Other carpal fractures are rare in children and are generally associated with severe trauma.

Fractures and Dislocations of the Hand

Hand fractures in children are usually benign injuries that can be well treated with splinting or casting. The reader is encouraged to review the section on the principles of treatment of acute bony injuries of the hand in Chapter 15, Disorders of the Upper Extremity, for the diagnosis and treatment of these common injuries. Only particularly problematic fractures of the hands of children are covered in this discussion. In general, the need for open reduction of hand fractures is the same as in other areas and is dictated by failure to obtain or maintain reduction of the fracture. The Kirschner wire is the mainstay of stabilization in a hand fracture, and there is essentially never a need for plate fixation of a child's hand bone. A K-wire placed percutaneously under image intensifier control is especially useful. Leaving the wire outside the skin but under a cast until healing is secure facilitates removal at follow-up.

METACARPAL FRACTURES

Although fracture of a single metacarpal tends to be stable and needs protection only while healing, multiple fractures are often unstable. Multiple metacarpal fractures are usually the result of a violent crushing injury and are frequently open. In this case, after appropriate cleansing, temporary K-wire fixation is needed for 4 to 5 weeks.

Occasionally, an isolated but malaligned metacarpal defies closed treatment because of angulatory or rotatory malalignment. Rotatory deformities that cause significant finger overlap do not generally correct with remodeling. K-wire stabilization after reduction is effective.

FRACTURE OF THE PHALANGES

Proximal Phalanx (P1) and Middle Phalanx (P2)

Proximal and middle phalangeal fractures that are markedly angulated and displaced may occasionally be irreducible by closed means because of periosteum, tendon, or sheath interposition. Once released, the reduction is usually easy to obtain but difficult to maintain without supplementary K-wire fixation.

Distal Phalanx (P3)

This bone is so intimately connected to the nail bed, its germinal matrix, and the dorsal skin that a markedly displaced fracture rarely occurs without open injury to the nail bed. The nail plate and any interposed soft tissue must be removed before accurate reduction is possible. Subsequent stabilization of the phalanx with a longitudinal K-wire continued across the distal interphalangeal joint helps provide both soft and hard tissue alignment. Closure of the nail bed should be done with fine (6-0) absorbable suture.

INTRA-ARTICULAR FRACTURES

An intra-articular fracture with marked displacement can be managed by open reduction, which is best done in the acute period. If the fracture is well along in healing, sometimes it is best to let the fracture heal and perform an osteotomy later (see Fig. 15–47). At other times the fracture may be rotated so much that open reduction is the only hope for salvaging any joint function.

Intra-articular fractures that are not displaced rarely need anything other than protection and closed treatment. If the surgeon considers the fracture pattern unstable, such as an oblique fracture of the condyle of a joint, percutaneous pin fixation is usually adequate. Image intensification and a small power drill make fixation easier and less likely to displace the fracture.

Reference

FRACTURES AND DISLOCATIONS OF THE WRIST AND HAND

1. Light TR: Injury to the immature carpus. Hand Clin 1988;4:415.

Chapter 43

Lower Extremity Injuries

PELVIS AND ACETABULUM

Pelvic and Acetabular Fractures

Pelvic and acetabular fractures are much less common in children than in adults and are most often due to high-energy trauma. The person evaluating a child with a pelvic fracture must investigate other organ systems, including the vascular, genitourinary, and neurologic systems, for potentially life-threatening injuries. Treatment is most often nonoperative because of the elastic nature of the child's pelvis and the surrounding soft tissue. Operative treatment usually consists of internal fixation, external fixation, or a combination of both.

ANATOMY

The pelvis is formed from three primary centers of ossification—the ischium, ilium, and pubis—and also includes the sacrum. The three centers of ossification join at the triradiate cartilage, which fuses at the age of 16 to 18 years (Fig. 43–1).[55] At the inferior pubic rami, fusion of the ischium and pubis takes place at 6 to 7 years of age.

The secondary centers of ossification are the iliac crests, which appear at 13 to 15 years of age and fuse at 15 to 17 years, and the ischial apophyses, which appear later, at 15 to 17 years, and fuse at 17 to 19 years.[55] Other secondary centers of ossification include the anterior inferior iliac spine, the pubic tubercle, the angle of the pubis, the ischial spine, and the lateral wing of the sacrum.

The sacroiliac joint owes its stability to its strong anterior and posterior ligamentous structures. The anterior ligamentous structures, weaker than the posterior ones, are composed of a flat ligament running from the ilium to the sacrum. Posteriorly, there are short and long ligaments; the short posterior ligaments travel obliquely from the posterior ridge of the sacrum to the posterior superior and posterior inferior spines of the ilium, whereas the long posterior ligaments are longitudinal fibers running from the lateral sacrum to the posterior superior iliac spines. These ligaments then merge with the sacral tuberous ligament and are the major stabilizing ligaments of the sacroiliac joint.

The development and growth of the acetabulum in children have been described in a classic article by Ponseti.[33] The acetabulum in childhood is composed of growth plate cartilage of the ilium, ischium, and pubis; peripheral articular cartilage; and hyaline cartilage (Fig. 43–2). The acetabulum grows as a result of interstitial growth within the triradiate aspect of the cartilage complex, which causes the hip joint to expand. The presence of the femoral head within the acetabulum promotes the development of the concavity of the acetabulum. Depth increases as a result of interstitial growth in the acetabular cartilage, appositional growth at the periphery, and periosteal new bone formation at the acetabular margin. Secondary centers of ossification appear at puberty and include the os acetabuli (epiphysis of the pubis), which forms the anterior wall; the acetabular epiphysis (epiphysis of the ilium), which forms the superior wall; and the seldom seen epiphysis of the ilium. These secondary centers of ossification appear at approximately 8 to 9 years and unite at around 18 years of age.

Ligamentous structures connect various portions of the pelvic ring to provide stability (Fig. 43–3). The sacrotuberous ligament connects the posterolateral aspect of the sacrum and the dorsal aspect of the posterior iliac spine to the ischial tuberosity. The sacrospinous ligament connects the lateral aspect of the sacrum and coccyx to the sacrotuberous ligament and inserts on the ischial spine. In addition to the ligaments

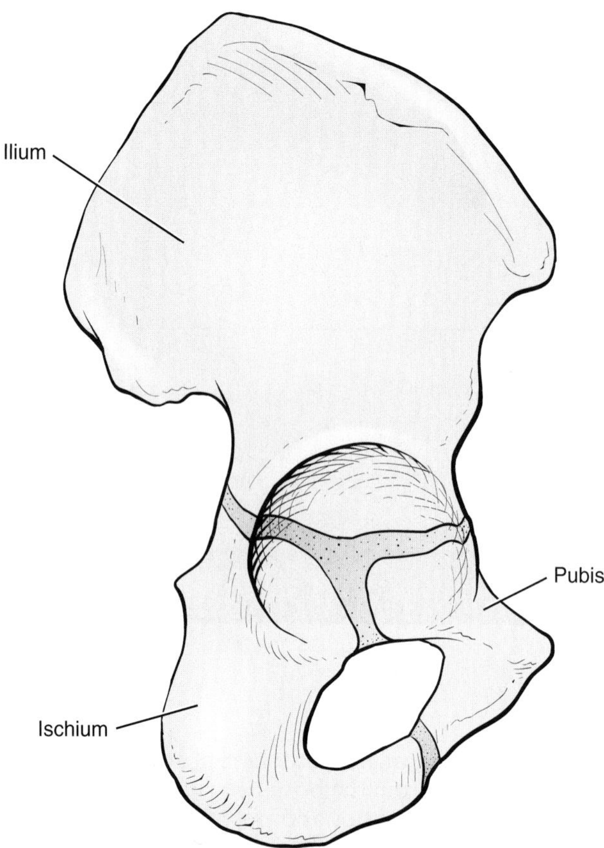

FIGURE 43–1 Lateral view of the pelvis demonstrating the relationship of the ilium, pubis, and ischium and their junction at the triradiate cartilage.

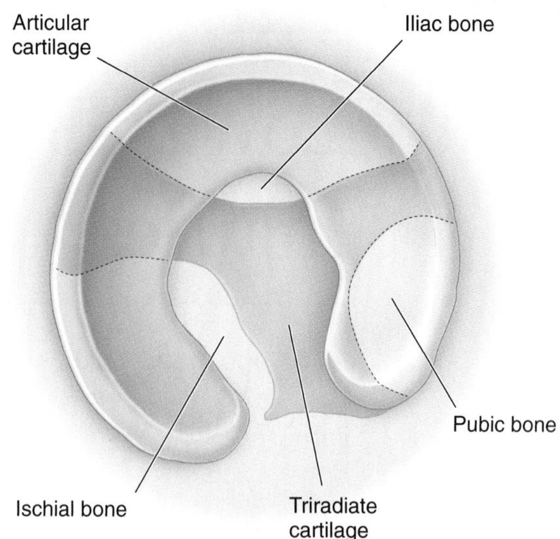

FIGURE 43–2 Diagram of the triradiate cartilage demonstrating the sites occupied by the iliac, ischial, and pubic bones. (Redrawn from Ponseti IV: Growth and development of the acetabulum in the normal child. J Bone Joint Surg Am 1978;60:575.)

connecting various parts of the pelvis, there are numerous connections between the pelvis and spine. The iliolumbar ligaments connect the transverse processes of L4 and L5 to the posterior iliac crest. The lumbosacral ligaments run from the transverse process of L5 to the ala of the sacrum.

The pelvis and acetabulum in children differ from the same structures in adults in several ways. Children are subject to avulsion injuries because of the presence of various apophyses. In addition, growth plate injuries may occur, especially in the acetabulum, and can lead to a dysplastic acetabulum or leg length discrepancy.[5] Moreover, the child's pelvis is more elastic because of the mechanical properties of children's bone and the presence of more cartilaginous structures; consequently, after a significant pelvic injury, radiographs may show only a single innocuous-appearing fracture.

Other organ systems that lie adjacent to or within the pelvis include the nervous, genitourinary, and vascular systems. The lumbosacral coccygeal plexus enters the pelvis and is composed of the anterior rami of T12 through S4. The sciatic nerve exits the pelvis from beneath the piriformis muscle and enters the greater sciatic notch (Fig. 43–4). Major vascular channels lie on the inner wall of the pelvis. The common iliac vessel divides and gives off the internal iliac artery, which lies over the pelvic brim, and the superior gluteal artery, which crosses over the anteroinferior portion of the sacroiliac joint to exit the greater sciatic notch, where it lies directly on bone. The bladder and urethra are the structures of the urinary system that are most often injured after a pelvic fracture. The bladder lies superior to the pelvic floor and the urethra passes through the prostate in males to exit the pelvic floor. The membranous urethra is the initial portion at the upper surface (followed by the bulbous portion, below the pelvic floor) and is the segment most often injured.

MECHANISM OF INJURY

Motor vehicle accidents account for 75% to 90% of all pelvic fractures in children.[35-37,53] Unlike adults who sustain pelvic fractures, who typically were the occupant of the vehicle, children with pelvic fractures are most often pedestrians who have been struck by a motor vehicle; this mechanism of injury accounts for up to 75% of pelvic fractures in children.[53] Many of these children have not only been struck but also directly run over by the vehicle. Quinby described 20 children with pelvic fractures, 19 of whom were pedestrians struck by a vehicle; 8 of them were also directly run over.[35] Other causes of pelvic fractures in children include falls from a height (8% to 10%), bicycle or motorcycle injuries (5% to 8%), and sporting injuries (3% to 5%).[37,53]

Avulsion injuries are produced from milder trauma than pelvic ring fractures are. The majority are sustained during participation in sports and result from an acute powerful muscle contraction. In a review of 198 patients with avulsion fractures, 65% took place during soccer or gymnastics.[38]

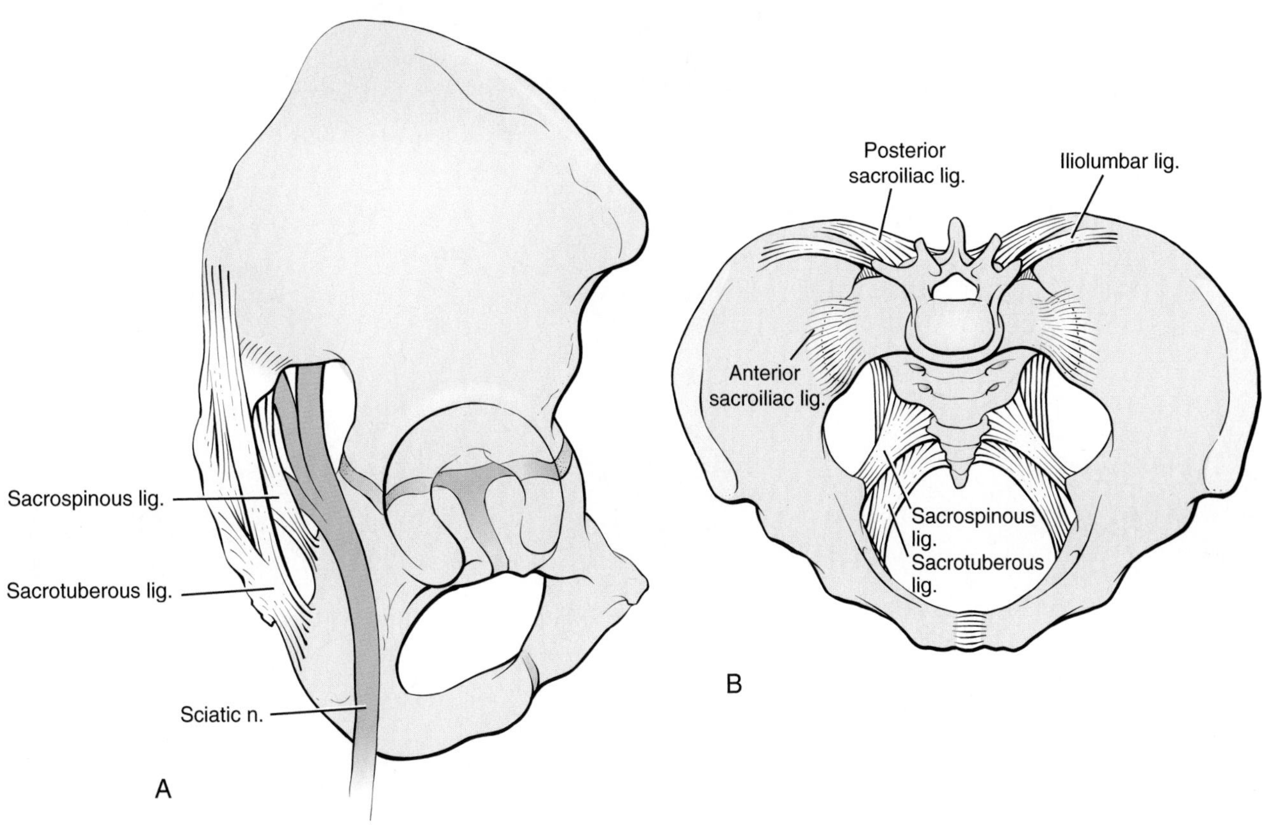

FIGURE 43-3 Ligamentous structures that provide stability to the pelvic ring. **A,** Lateral view of the sacrospinous and sacrotuberous ligaments. **B,** Anteroposterior view of the sacrospinous and sacrotuberous ligaments. Posterior ligamentous structures include the strong posterior sacroiliac and iliolumbar ligaments and the weaker anterior sacroiliac ligaments.

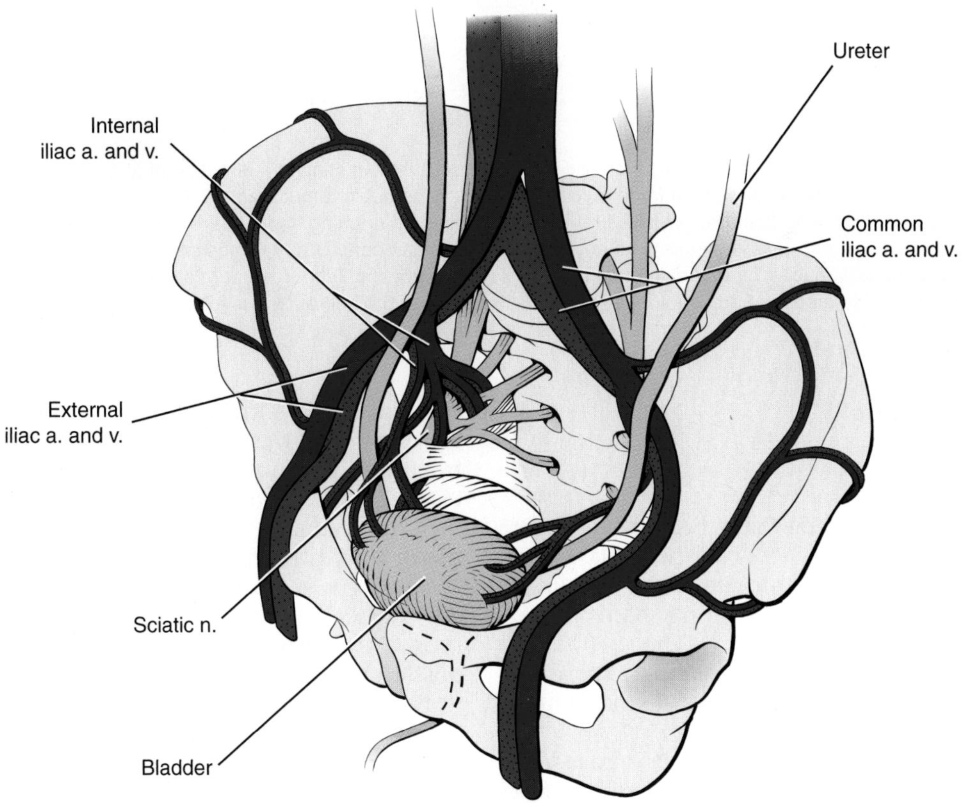

FIGURE 43-4 Internal view of the pelvis showing the relationship of the great vessels, lumbosacral plexus, bladder, and ureters.

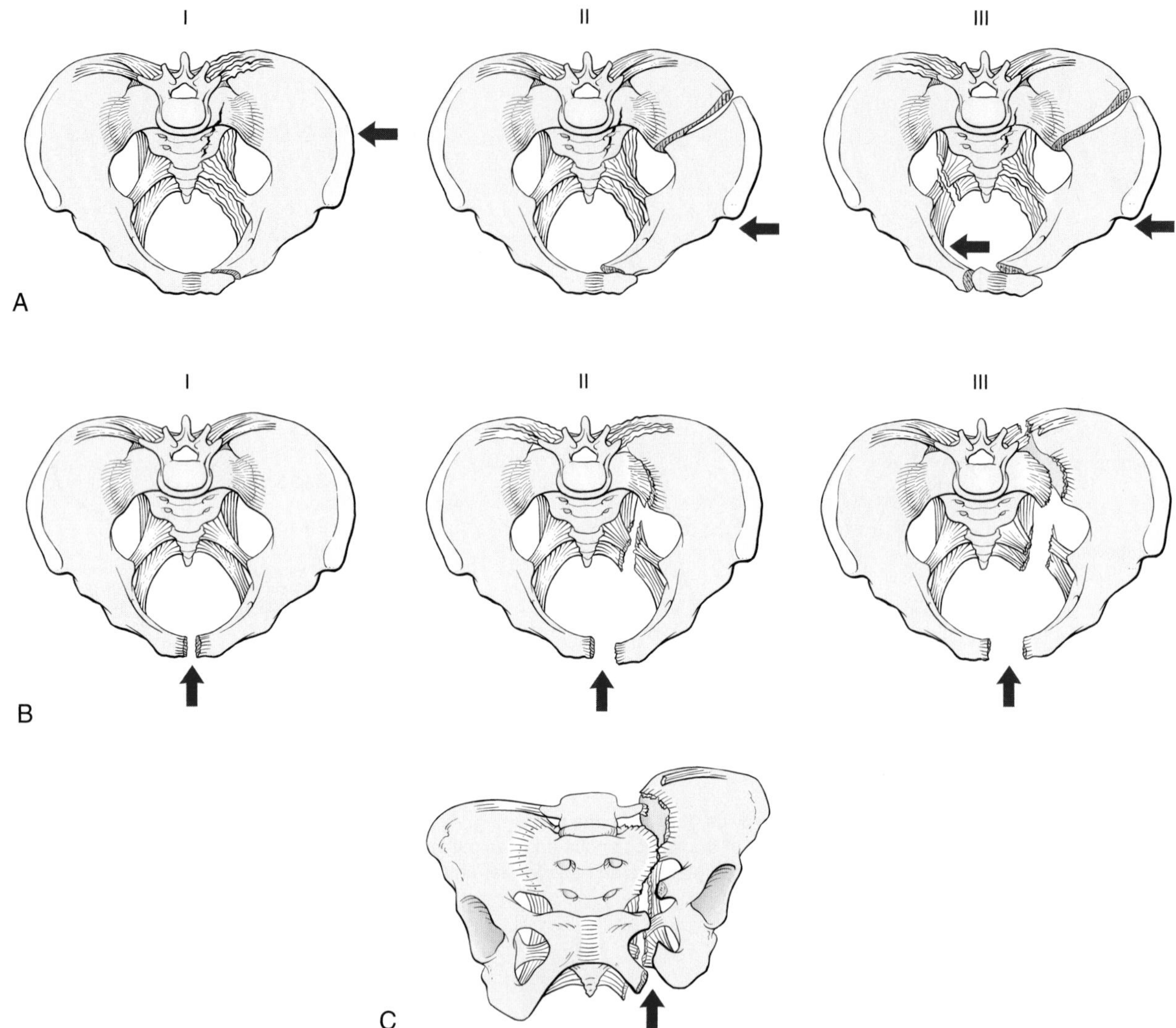

FIGURE 43–5 Young and Burgess' classification of pelvic fractures. *Arrows* show the direction of force. **A,** Lateral compression force. Type I: the posterolateral force results in a sacral and pubic ramus fracture. Type II: the anterolateral force results in an additional iliac wing fracture. Type III: further force creates an opening injury to the contralateral pelvis with disruption of the sacrospinous, sacrotuberous, and anterior sacroiliac ligaments. **B,** Anteroposterior compression force. Type I: disruption of the symphysis pubis. Type II: disruption of the anterior ligaments. Type III: disruption of the posterior ligaments. **C,** Vertically directed force creating fractures in the rami and disruption of the sacrospinous joint.

CLASSIFICATION

Pelvic Fracture

Several classification systems have been devised for pelvic fractures in adults.[4,19,31,51,52,57] These classifications are based on the anatomic site of the fracture,[19] the mechanism of injury,[57] and the mechanism and stability of the pelvic fracture.[51,52] The two most common classification systems used are those of Young and Burgess (Fig. 43–5)[57] and Tile and Pennal (Fig. 43–6).[31,52]

The Young and Burgess classification is based on the direction of the offending force: anteroposterior compression, lateral compression, and a vertically unstable or shear-type injury. The Tile and Pennal classification is similar in determining the mechanism of injury and the stability of the pelvis and aids in treatment planning. Three major categories of fractures are differentiated. A type A fracture is stable and includes avulsion injuries, minimally displaced fractures, and transverse fractures of the sacrum and coccyx; type B fractures include rotationally unstable, but vertically and posteriorly stable fractures; and type C fractures are severe fractures with rotational, posterior, and vertical instability (see Fig. 43–6).

Because of differences in anatomy and fracture patterns in children and adolescents, separate classifications for pediatric pelvic fractures have been developed.[3,35,53,55] In a review of 166 consecutive pediatric pelvic fractures, Silber and Flynn found that skeletal maturity level highly correlated with the need for

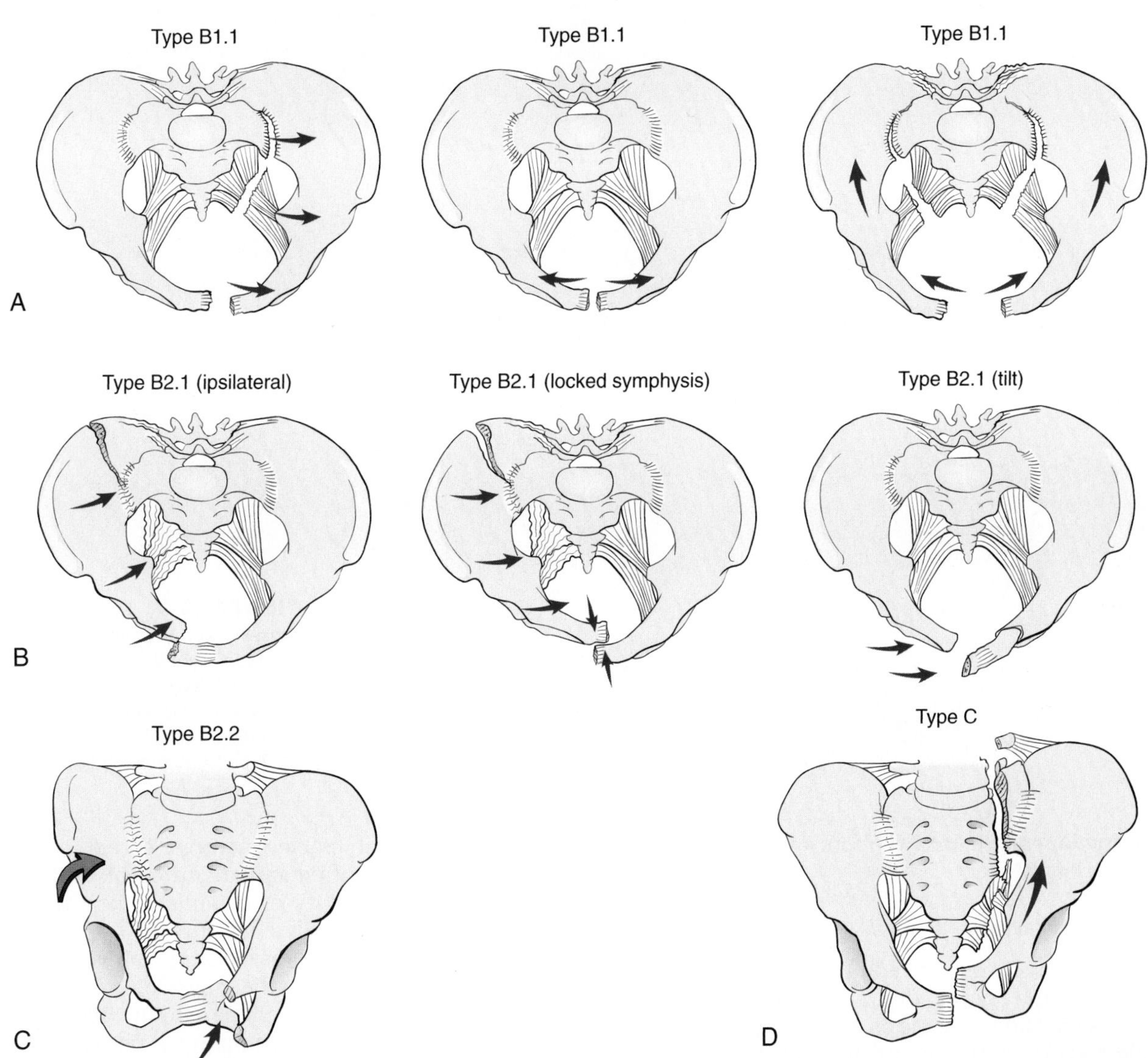

FIGURE 43–6 Tile and Pennal's classification of pelvic fractures. *Arrows* show the direction of force. Stable fractures that do not involve the pelvic ring are not shown. **A** through **C** are rotationally unstable but vertically stable fractures. **A,** External rotation or "open-book" fractures. **B,** Internal rotation or lateral compression injuries with ipsilateral injury only. **C,** Lateral compression injuries with contralateral fracture. **D,** Vertically and rotationally unstable fractures of the pelvis.

operative intervention. No patients with open triradiate cartilage required operative treatment, and fractures of the iliac wing and pubic rami were most common in this group. In patients with closed triradiate cartilage, pubic or sacroiliac diastasis and acetabular fractures were more prevalent.[44]

Quinby divided patients into three categories based on associated injuries: group I, patients needing laparotomy; group II, those not needing laparotomy; and group III, patients with an associated severe vascular injury.[35] This classification has little utility today because of the lower incidence of laparotomy in the pediatric population, but it does illustrate the high prevalence of visceral and vascular injuries in association with pelvic fractures in children.

Watts divided pelvic fractures according to their radiographic findings: group I, avulsion injuries, usually of the anterior superior or inferior iliac spine and the ischial tuberosity; group II, fractures of the pelvic ring, both stable and unstable; and group III, acetabular fractures.[55]

We prefer the more recent pelvic classification scheme described by Torode and Zieg, which is a four-part classification based on the radiographic examination findings: type I, avulsion fractures; type II, iliac wing fractures; type III, simple pelvic ring fractures; and type IV, ring disruption fractures that are unstable (Fig. 43–7).[53] This classification scheme correlates well with fracture outcome and the type of treatment required. Type I injuries were treated symptomatically without admission to the hospital; type II and type III injuries required admission to the hospital, primarily for observation of associated injuries; and type IV injuries required more aggressive management,

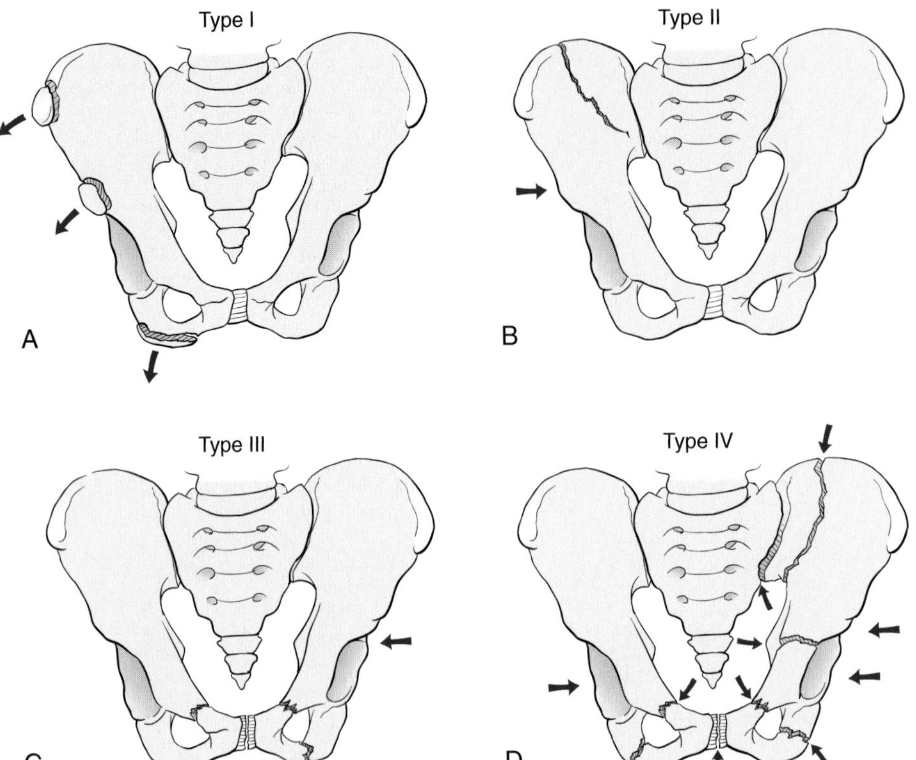

FIGURE 43–7 Torode and Zieg's classification of pelvic fractures. *Arrows* show the direction of force. **A,** Type I: avulsion fractures. **B,** Type II: iliac wing fractures. **C,** Type III: simple ring fractures. **D,** Type IV: ring disruption fractures.

including operative intervention, and had a higher complication rate.

Acetabular Fracture

Acetabular fractures in adults are best classified according to the original descriptions by Letournel.[18-20] This classification scheme is based on five primary simple fracture patterns and five associated fracture types, which in turn are based on the simple fracture patterns. Acetabular fractures in children are best classified into four types:[55]

- Type I Small fragment fractures that occur with dislocation of the hip
- Type II Linear fractures that result in one or more large, stable fragments
- Type III Linear fractures that result in hip instability
- Type IV Fractures that are secondary to central dislocations of the hip

ASSOCIATED INJURIES

The high energy that produces pelvic fractures commonly results in visceral and vascular injuries, which may be fatal. The mortality associated with pelvic fractures in children is reported to be between 2% and 11%.[1,37,53] The probability of associated injuries is highest (60%) when multiple fractures of the pelvic ring are present, followed in frequency by iliac or sacral fractures (15%) and finally by isolated pubic fractures (1%). Similarly, resuscitation requirements are greater in patients with unstable pelvic fractures than in those with stable fractures. Torode and Zieg reported that 27% of patients required blood transfusions, with the majority of patients having the more severe type III or IV pelvic fracture.[53]

The most common associated injuries involve intra-abdominal organs, the neurologic system, the musculoskeletal system, and the genitourinary system. The injuries that may accompany a pediatric pelvic fracture are often more clinically relevant than direct fracture care. Fatalities in children with pelvic fracture result from visceral and head injuries.[46] In a recent review, 91% of pediatric patients requiring transfusion in the setting of a pelvic fracture had hemorrhage attributable to another site.[9] Intra-abdominal injury occurs in up to 15% of pelvic fractures and includes contusions or laceration of the spleen, liver, or kidney and very often mesenteric injuries or injuries to the large or small intestine.[1,3,29,35,37,53] Modern approaches to treating intra-abdominal injuries in children reduced the rate of laparotomies performed for the assessment and management of these injuries.[3,53]

Neurologic injury is the most common associated nonorthopaedic injury in children with a pelvic fracture, with a reported incidence of up to 50%.[53] Concussion is the most common neurologic injury (33%), followed by skull fracture (16%), nerve avulsion (5%), and brain death (4%).[53]

Associated musculoskeletal injuries occur in up to 50% of cases, with a higher incidence in patients with unstable pelvic fractures.[53] The most common fractures involve the femur (25%), skull (15%), upper extremity (15%), and tibia/fibula (15%).[37,53]

Associated injuries related to the vascular system are most often due to venous bleeding and subsequent retroperitoneal hematoma, which occurs in up to 46% of patients.[37] In one series of patients with retroperitoneal hematomas, 10% were in hypovolemic shock at initial evaluation and required the administration of whole blood or packed cells. Major arterial injuries, in contrast, are relatively rare and occur in approximately 3% of patients.

Genitourinary injuries are generally seen in individuals who have sustained more severe pelvic injuries, with a reported incidence of 10% to 20%.[1,3,29,35,37,53] Severe injuries requiring treatment, such as bladder rupture or urethral laceration, occur in association with less than 1% of pelvic fractures in children. Perineal or vaginal laceration may also be seen. In the absence of gross hematuria, genitourinary injury requiring treatment is uncommon.[50]

CLINICAL FEATURES

A history of a child's being struck by a car while walking or running should alert the physician that pelvic trauma has occurred. Because these children often have a head injury and are frequently confused or amnestic, high suspicion for pelvic trauma and associated injury is mandatory. In addition, the initial pelvic radiograph is difficult to interpret and may not indicate the great amount of energy originally imparted to the pelvis. The details of the accident are important, including the speed of the traveling vehicle, the direction in which the child was struck, and whether the child was directly run over by the vehicle. A patient with an avulsion fracture will have less pain and is usually an older child (12 to 16 years) seen after an athletic event.

The physical examination by the orthopaedic surgeon should be thorough and organized and begin with inspection of the entire body, including the perineal area, followed by palpation and assessment of pelvic stability and finally a thorough assessment of the peripheral pulses and a neurologic examination.

The patient should be inspected for lacerations, abrasions, and evidence of tire marks on the skin, with the child "log-rolled" to allow careful inspection of the entire body. A child who sustained a severe crush injury may have a significant soft tissue injury in which subcutaneous fat and skin are sheared off the underlying fascia, the so-called Morel-Lavallee lesion.[11,28] This injury is most often seen in an obese child over the greater trochanteric region in the case of acetabular fractures and in the buttock region in the case of lateral compression–type injuries of the pelvis (Fig. 43–8). Deformity of the pelvis and the extremities should also be evaluated. The child's hips should be rotated to assess for asymmetry, especially in the setting of a lateral compression–type injury. Limb length is also assessed, especially with a vertically unstable pelvic fracture.

Palpation of the pelvis is performed to assess for bony tenderness, sacroiliac joint tenderness, and stability of the pelvis in the anteroposterior, mediolateral, and vertical planes. Any pain on palpation of the bony prominences (as well as pain in the sacroiliac joints or sacrum) should lead to suspicion of a pelvic fracture. Pain with anteriorly directed pressure along the anterior superior iliac spines or with medially directed pressure along the iliac wings should alert

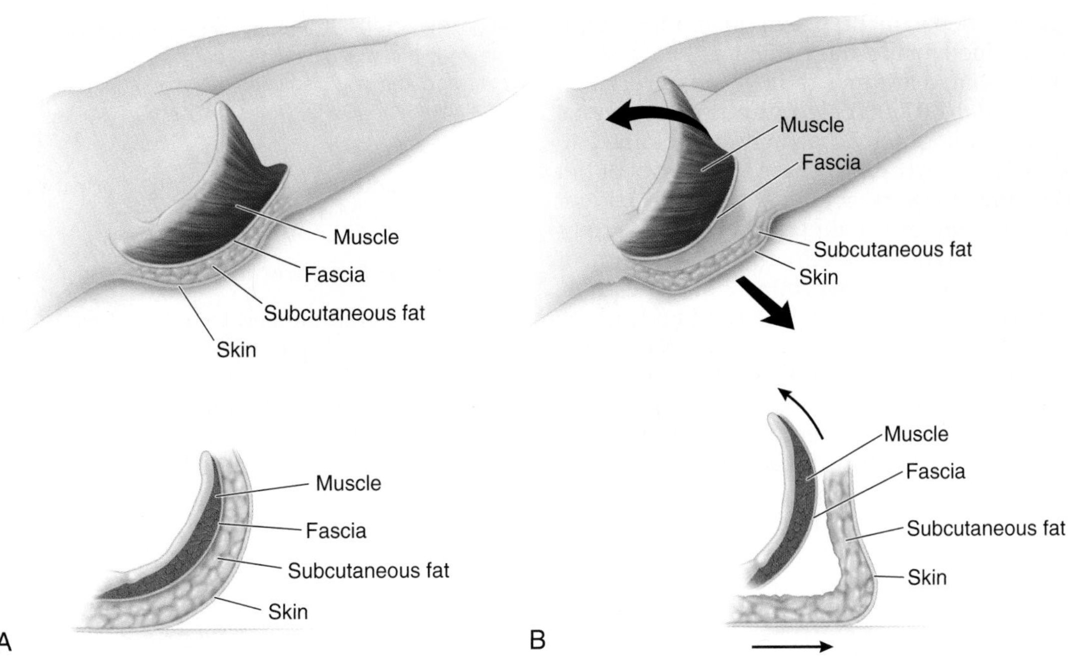

FIGURE 43–8 The Morel-Lavallee lesion, an injury in which subcutaneous fat and skin are sheared off the deep fascia over the buttock. **A,** Relationship between the fascial layer and subcutaneous fat. **B,** Mechanism of shearing of fat and the fascial layers.

the clinician to an open book–type fracture or a lateral compression–type fracture, respectively.

Vertically unstable fractures are difficult to assess by palpation but may be implied by an oblique-appearing pelvis or a limb length discrepancy. Although arterial injuries are rare, the lower extremity pulses should be carefully palpated and further assessed by Doppler examination if a discrepancy between extremities is present. A careful neurologic examination is performed to assess the lumbosacral plexus.

Careful inspection of the perineal area is essential. Blood at the urethral meatus or a scrotal hematoma may indicate a urethral injury. In the setting of significant fracture displacement, the vagina and rectum should be inspected for tears. A rectal examination is performed to assess rectal tone, evaluate the position of the prostate in boys, palpate rectal tears, feel for fractures, and attempt to elicit pain on palpation of the bony pelvis. A digital pelvic examination should be performed in girls. It is best done under sedation, if possible, especially in a young child, and is best performed by a gynecologist.

RADIOGRAPHIC FINDINGS

Pelvic Fracture

Several studies have shown that the majority of clinically significant pelvic fractures can be predicted by physical examination in alert patients without neurologic impairment.[15,43] When young age, neurologic impairment, sedation, or distracting injury might prevent an accurate examination, a screening AP radiograph is recommended. The initial anteroposterior (AP) pelvic radiograph should be obtained as soon as possible in the emergency room suite. A radiology technician should be ready when the patient arrives in the emergency department; the pelvic radiograph should be obtained while the patient is being stabilized, and associated trauma radiographs are taken during the standard trauma algorithmic assessment.

Other plain radiographs that may be obtained to assess for pelvic fractures include inlet and outlet views.[7] The inlet view is obtained with the patient supine and the x-ray beam aimed caudad 60 degrees and therefore at right angles to the pelvic brim; it allows visualization of the iliopectineal line, the pubic rami, the sacroiliac joints, and the alae and body of the sacrum (Fig. 43–9). The inlet view is best used to assess for anterior and posterior displacement of the pelvic ring, especially posterior displacement of the sacroiliac joint, sacrum, or iliac wing; internal rotation deformities of the pelvis; and sacral impaction injuries. The outlet view is obtained by directing the x-ray beam 45 degrees cephalad (Fig. 43–10) and helps define superior-to-inferior displacement of the pelvic ring, superior rotation of the hemipelvis, and the sacral foramina, which are best seen in this view.

Because abdominal computed tomography (CT) is common for the evaluation of visceral injury in pediatric blunt trauma, CT images of the pelvis may be available early in the evaluation of these patients. Recent reviews have confirmed the utility of these CT images for diagnosis and management of pediatric pelvic fractures without the addition of plain radiographs.[10,45]

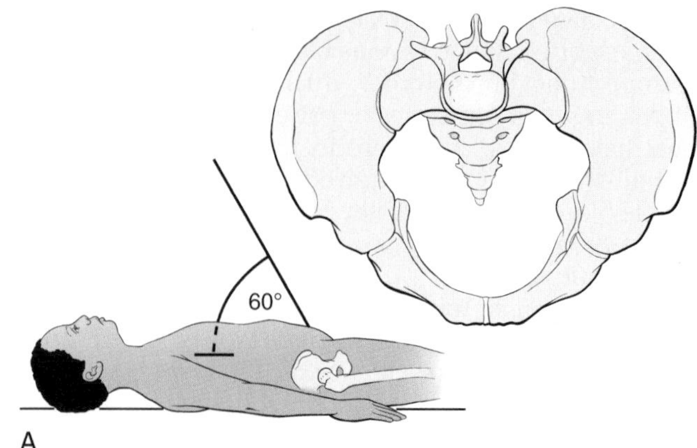

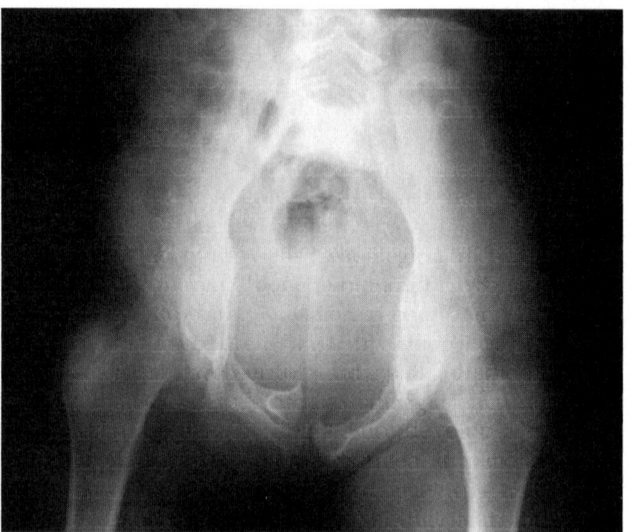

FIGURE 43–9 **A,** For an inlet view, the patient is supine and the x-ray beam is directed 60 degrees caudad. **B,** Radiographic inlet view showing disruption of the anterior ring with fracture displacement.

Acetabular Fracture

Plain radiographs used to assess acetabular fractures include the oblique views described by Judet (Fig. 43–11).[14] The iliac oblique view shows the posterior column, anterior acetabular wall, and iliac wing. The obturator oblique view shows the anterior column, posterior wall, and obturator foramen (Fig. 43–12). Careful inspection of the two oblique views and the AP pelvic view should allow classification of the acetabular wall fracture according to Letournel.[19]

CT is used to assess acetabular fractures only after the fracture has been carefully evaluated and classified on plain radiographs. CT is performed to identify loose fragments and incongruities of the joint and to determine the size and displacement of the wall fracture. Although CT may be useful in older patients with mature pelvic and acetabular fracture patterns, plain radiographs provide information for diagnosis and

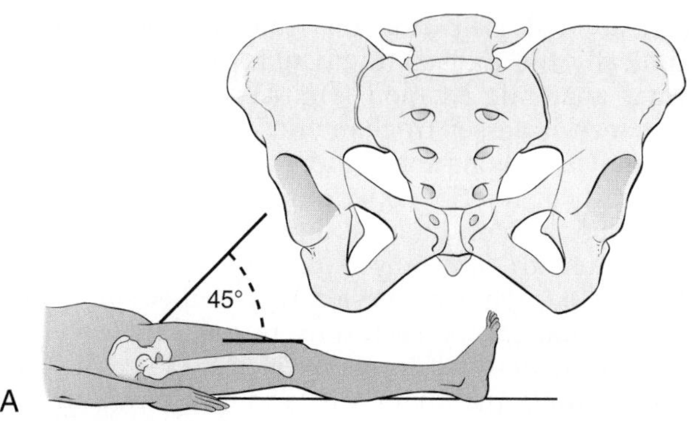

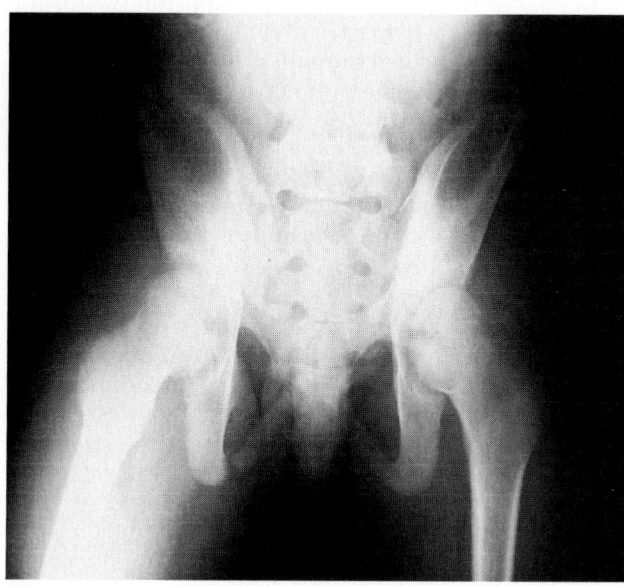

FIGURE 43-10 **A,** For an outlet view, the patient is supine and the x-ray beam is directed 45 degrees craniad. **B,** Radiographic outlet view showing disruption of the anterior ring with fracture displacement.

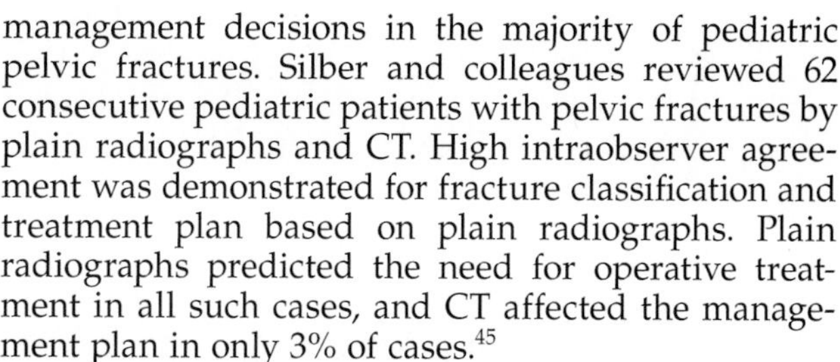

management decisions in the majority of pediatric pelvic fractures. Silber and colleagues reviewed 62 consecutive pediatric patients with pelvic fractures by plain radiographs and CT. High intraobserver agreement was demonstrated for fracture classification and treatment plan based on plain radiographs. Plain radiographs predicted the need for operative treatment in all such cases, and CT affected the management plan in only 3% of cases.[45]

TREATMENT OF PELVIC FRACTURES

Types of Injuries

The classification of Torode and Zieg will serve as the basis for discussion of the treatment of pelvic fractures[53]:

Type I	Avulsion fractures
Type II	Iliac wing fractures
Type III	Simple pelvic ring fractures
Type IV	Pelvic ring disruption fractures

Type I: Avulsion Fractures. The most common avulsion injuries occur in the pelvis at the ischial tuberosity (the attachment of the hamstrings and hip adductors), at the anterior superior iliac spine (the attachment of the sartorius muscle), at the anterior inferior iliac spine (the attachment of the direct head of the rectus), and less often, at the iliac crest and the lesser trochanter of the femur (the attachment of the iliopsoas tendon) (Fig. 43–13).[8,49] Athletic injuries account for the majority of these fractures, boys are affected more often than girls, and the average age at injury is between 12 and 14 years, just before closure of the apophyses.[8] The powerful contraction of the attached muscle results in avulsion of bone. An acute injury is most common; however, chronic repetitive trauma can also result in avulsion injuries.[49,56]

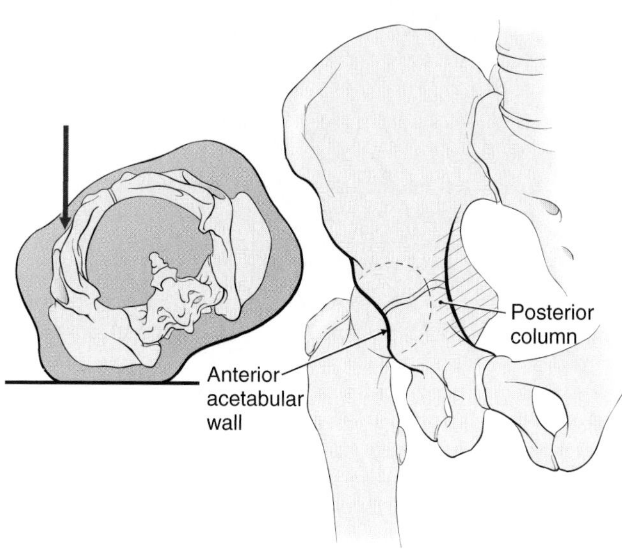

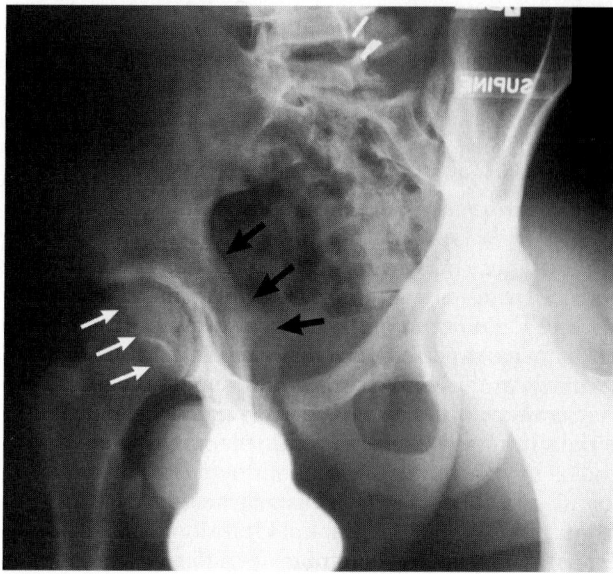

FIGURE 43-11 **A,** The iliac oblique view is imaged with the x-ray beam directed 45 degrees toward the side of the pelvis to be examined. **B,** Radiographic right iliac oblique view showing the anterior wall (*white arrows*) and posterior column (*black arrows*).

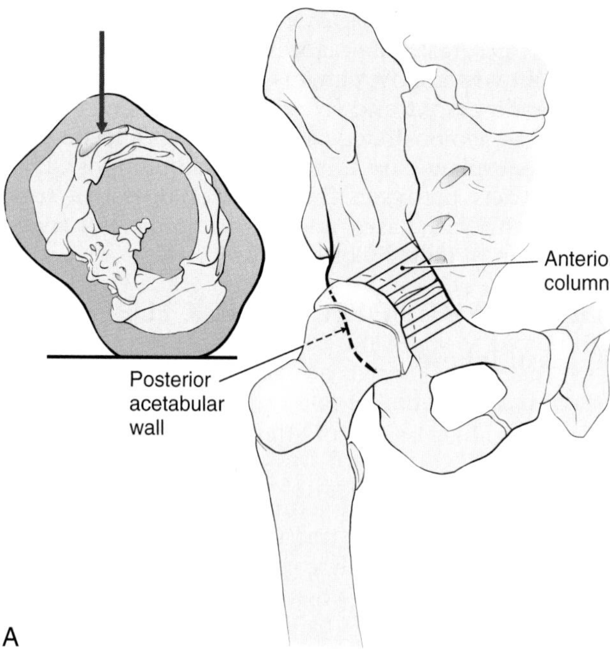

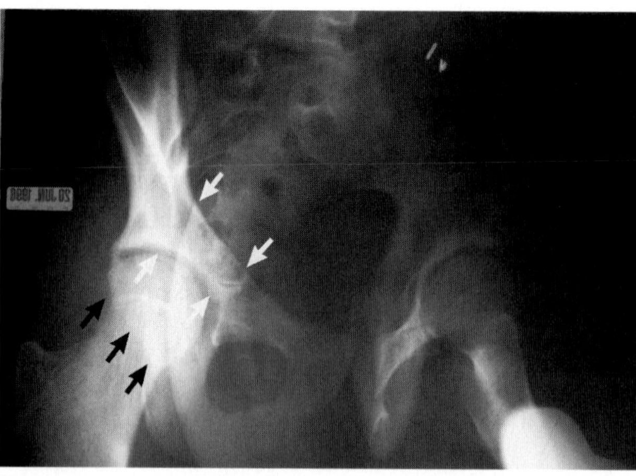

FIGURE 43–12 **A,** The obturator oblique view is imaged with the x-ray beam directed 45 degrees away from the side of the pelvis to be examined. **B,** Radiographic right obturator oblique view showing the anterior column (*white arrows*) and posterior wall (*black arrows*).

The typical history is that of an adolescent athlete who performs a sudden strenuous activity such as kicking a ball or making a quick turn and feels a sudden, sharp pain. The pain is localized to the area of injury and results in limitation of motion, most often motion of the hip joint. The pain is aggravated by passive motion of the hip that places tension on the attached muscle: flexion and abduction of the hip in ischial tuberosity avulsion injuries and extension of the hip in anterior superior and anterior inferior spine injuries and lesser trochanter avulsions. Active contraction of the muscle that produced the avulsion is painful. Localized tenderness of superficial structures such as the anterior superior iliac spine and the ischial tuberosity will help establish the diagnosis. Radiographically, the avulsed fragment is displaced from its normal anatomic location (Fig. 43–14). This is most easily seen in lesser trochanteric injuries and ischial tuberosity avulsions and is more difficult to see radiographically in anterior superior and inferior iliac spine injuries because of the mild displacement that occurs and because the anatomy is difficult to discern on a pelvic radiograph. An anterior inferior iliac spine fracture avulsion can be seen only in an oblique view.[49] Comparison views of the contralateral side are helpful in confirming the diagnosis and avoiding further unnecessary imaging studies.

Conservative treatment of avulsion injuries of the pelvis is usually successful and consists of symptomatic treatment in which the patient is placed on crutches to allow the involved extremity to be rested.[25,49,56] The period of treatment is 2 to 3 weeks, until symptoms resolve and radiographic evidence of healing is present. Avulsion injuries of the ischial tuberosity are most prone to nonunion, with some groups reporting a 68% incidence of nonunion.[55] Such nonunion may result in pain with sitting and excessive physical activity; however, most patients have few symptoms despite the presence of a nonunion. We perform open reduction and internal fixation only for painful nonunion of the ischial tuberosity. Of 14 cases of nonunion of the ischial tuberosity managed by surgical intervention, 10 were treated by excision and 3 by early reattachment, with 1 of the 3 patients continuing to have a nonunion.[55]

Most studies report return to full function after avulsion injuries around the pelvis.[8,25] The 20 patients described by Fernbach and Wilkinson returned to

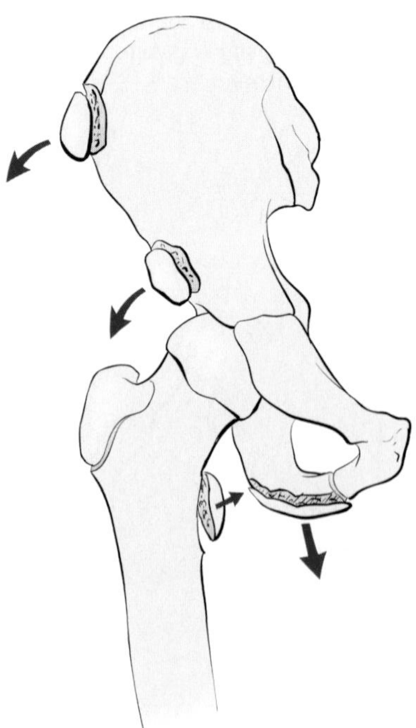

FIGURE 43–13 Torode and Zieg's type I injury—a pelvic avulsion fraction. *Arrows* show the direction of force.

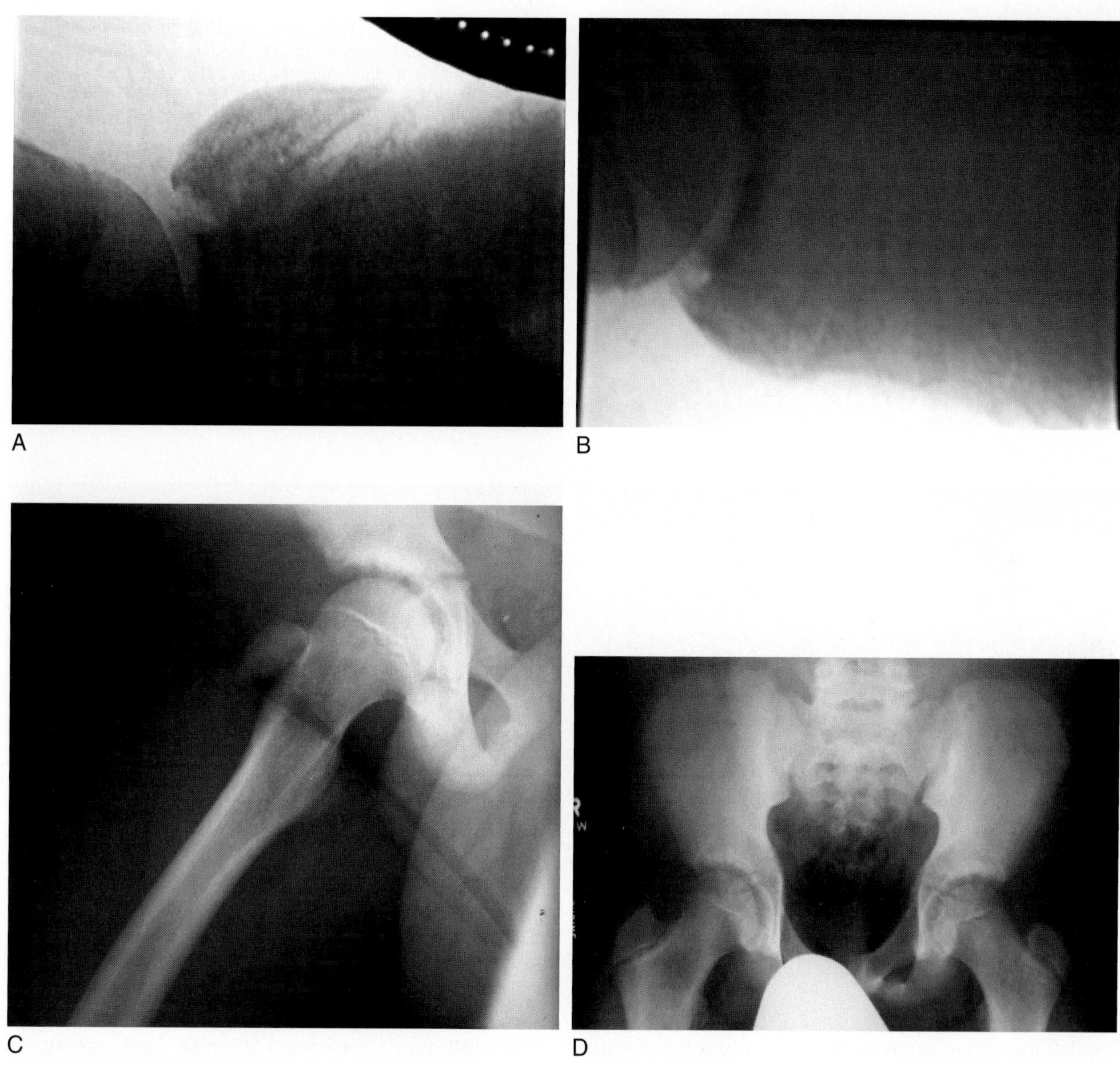

FIGURE 43–14 Avulsion fracture of the pelvis and proximal end of the femur. **A,** Lateral radiograph of avulsion of the anterior inferior iliac spine. **B,** The opposite, normal side. **C,** Greater trochanter avulsion fracture. **D,** Four months after injury, the radiographs appear essentially normal.

their previous level of athletic competition after conservative treatment of an avulsion injury of the pelvis.[8] The worst results occur in patients with avulsion injuries of the ischial tuberosity. Sundar and Carty described three patients with acute avulsion fractures, all of whom had symptoms at follow-up and difficulty resuming sporting activities, whereas five of nine patients with a chronic ischial avulsion injury had reduced sporting ability at follow-up.[49]

To avoid reinjury, the avulsion injury should heal fully before the patient returns to full activities.[25] A conditioning and strengthening program is generally necessary to restore the strength of the affected muscle to normal before the child resumes competitive athletics.

Type II: Iliac Wing Fractures. Type II fractures represent approximately 15% of all pelvic fractures in children, a slightly higher percentage than in adults.[36,53] The mechanism is usually an external force exerted on the iliac wing that results in disruption of the iliac apophysis or a lateral compression–type wing fracture (Fig. 43–15). Patients are most often pedestrians struck by a motor vehicle, although direct trauma from other objects may result in this injury. Associated abdominal injuries are less common than with types III and IV fractures, with the incidence of genitourinary injuries being 6% and laparotomy being needed in 11% of patients.[53] However, these injuries can lead to significant blood loss, and blood transfusions have been necessary in up to 17% of patients.[53] Fracture displacement

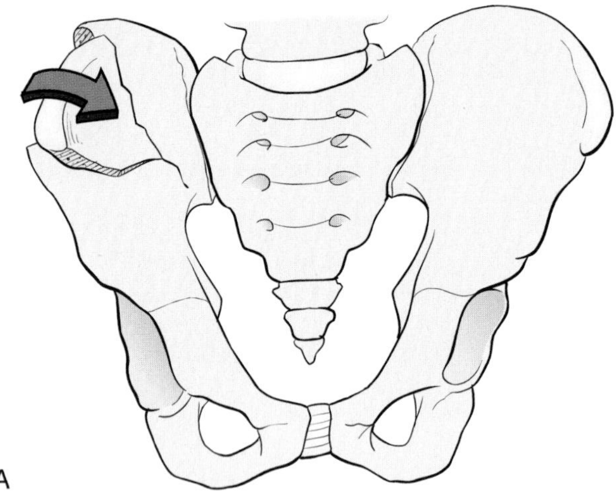

FIGURE 43–15 A, Type II pelvic injury in the Torode and Zieg classification (*arrow*). Radiograph **(B)** and computed tomography scan **(C)** of a type II (iliac wing) fracture.

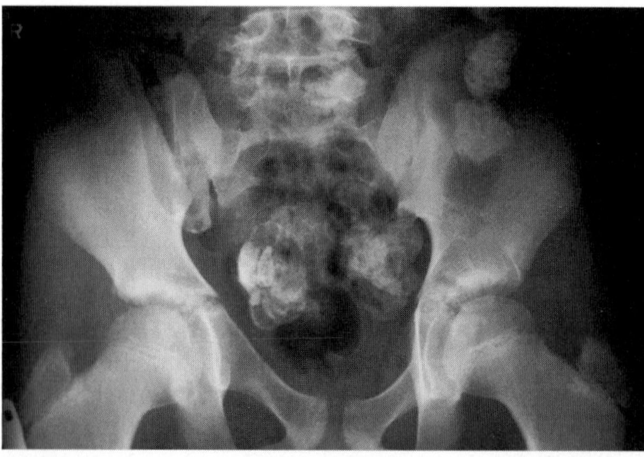

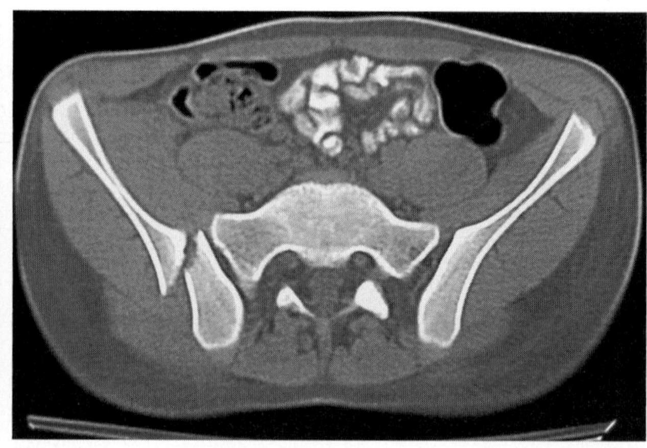

is most often lateral and is usually mild because of the vast muscle attachments.

Treatment generally consists of admission to the hospital for observation of the musculoskeletal injuries, hemodynamic status, and associated intra-abdominal injuries. Ileus may develop after an iliac wing fracture and must be carefully evaluated by a general surgeon, with CT of the abdomen performed if necessary. Treatment of ileus usually consists of placement of a nasogastric tube.

Although pain initially limits the patient's activities after the injury, most patients quickly regain their mobility. Fracture healing is generally rapid, and functional limitations are rare with this type of injury, although some patients may have delayed ossification of the iliac apophysis or a prominent bump from ossification of the injured area.[53]

Type III: Simple Pelvic Ring Fractures. This injury includes fractures of two ipsilateral pubic rami, disruptions of the pubic symphysis, fractures or separations of the sacroiliac joints, or displaced fractures in which no clinical instability can be detected (Fig. 43–16). This is the most common fracture type and accounts for up to 55% of all pelvic fractures in children.[3,35,36,53] Unlike the situation in adults, in whom a pelvic fracture in one part of the ring must be associated with fracture in another part, children can have a fracture or fractures in a single aspect of the pelvic ring without an associated fracture. Presumably, this is due to the elasticity of the sacroiliac joints and pubic symphysis, which allows some strain to occur without radiographic evidence of injury. A single fracture with significant displacement but without posterior ring injury should be classified as a type III fracture because the overall stability of the ring is intact.

Other less common fractures classified as type III include fractures of the sacrum and coccyx. Fractures of the sacrum are relatively rare, with a reported incidence of 1% to 12%.[6,30,36] These fractures are best viewed on an AP or outlet view of the pelvis and are important to recognize because they can result in injury to the sacral nerves. Most sacral fractures are undisplaced transverse fractures through a sacral foramen and rarely require operative intervention. Coccygeal fractures are difficult to diagnose from radiographs because of the considerable normal anatomic variability.[34] The diagnosis is therefore most often made clinically when tenderness is noted over the coccyx. Treatment is conservative with symptomatic pain management, including sitting on a cushioned donut until symptoms resolve.

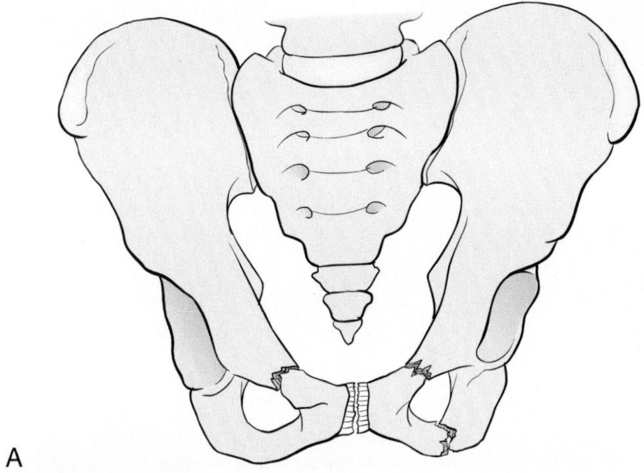

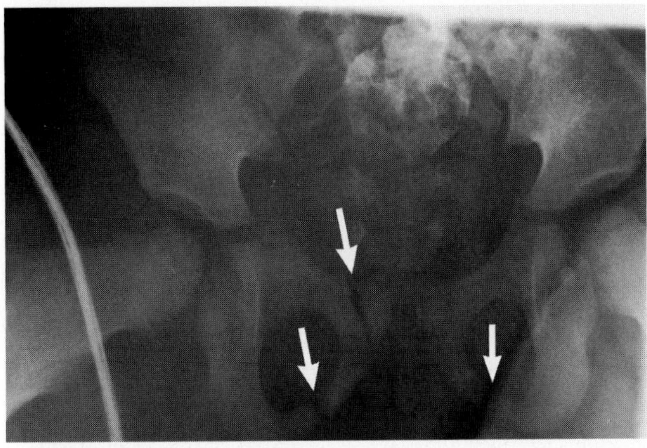

FIGURE 43–16 **A,** Type III pelvic injury in the Torode and Zieg classification. **B,** Radiograph of a type III (simple pelvic ring) fracture (*arrows*).

Type III fractures are associated with a higher incidence of other musculoskeletal injuries than type I or II injuries are, including musculoskeletal (50%), genitourinary (26%), and neurologic (57%) injuries. Careful assessment of these potential associated injuries is important.

Patients with these simple ring fractures do well with conservative treatment consisting of a short period of bed rest followed by progressive weight bearing until the patient is comfortable and independent on crutches. Fracture healing is rapid with an undisplaced fracture; however, it may be delayed with a displaced fracture. Torode and Zieg reported that 2 (3%) of 70 patients with type III fractures had delayed union of displaced pubic rami fractures, which healed approximately 1 year after injury.[53] Disruption of the pubic symphysis may occur as an isolated injury or, more often, with injury to the anterior capsule of the sacroiliac joint or partial separation of the adjacent ilium, or both. However, these injuries are stable because of the posterior structures (joint capsule, periosteum, and ligamentous structures) of the sacroiliac joint. Isolated disruptions of the pubic symphysis without significant injuries to the posterior ring occur at the bone–cartilage level, thus allowing healing to be complete without residual instability.[53] Significant displacement of the pubic symphysis with posterior ring injury may require operative intervention (see subsequent discussion under Treatment Techniques).

Type IV: Pelvic Ring Disruption Fractures. Pelvic ring disruption fractures include bilateral pubic rami fractures, or so-called straddle fractures; double-ring fractures or disruptions (e.g., pubic rami fracture and disruption of the sacroiliac joint); and fractures of the anterior structures and acetabular portion of the pelvic ring (for acetabular fractures, see discussion under Treatment of Acetabular Fractures) (Fig. 43–17).

Type IV fractures have the highest incidence of associated genitourinary (38%), musculoskeletal (56%), and neurologic (56%) injuries and also result in significant intra-abdominal injuries requiring laparotomy (40%). In addition, the mortality rate has been reported to be as high as 13%.[53]

Straddle Fracture. Straddle fractures consist of bilateral fractures of both the superior and inferior rami or separation of the symphysis pubis along with ipsilateral fractures of the superior and inferior rami (Fig. 43–18). A straddle fracture generally occurs after a fall while straddling an object or after a lateral compression–type injury. Associated injuries to the genitourinary system are fairly common; the reported incidence is as high as 20%.[6,30]

Treatment consists of bed rest with the hips slightly flexed to relax the abdominal muscles, which tend to displace the fracture fragments. The hips should also be in mild abduction to prevent adductor muscle tension. The duration of bed rest depends on the amount of displacement and pain present, with most patients needing 2 to 3 weeks.[55] Weight bearing is begun as tolerated by the patient. Fracture union may be delayed up to a few years if fracture displacement is present.[24]

Double-Ring Fracture. The second group of type IV fractures includes vertically or rotationally unstable pelvic fractures (or both), which account for approximately 20% to 30% of all pelvic fractures in children.[36,37] A complete description of the analogous injury in adults has been provided and the injuries classified by Young and Burgess[57] and Pennal and Tile.[31,51] Because these injuries are rare, specific treatment protocols are not as well defined in children. Historically, treatment has consisted of conservative management involving the use of pelvic slings and skeletal traction. However, recent developments in treating adult pelvic fractures have been applied to pediatric fractures, with promising results.[16]

Pelvic asymmetry may predict the need for intervention in pediatric pelvic fractures. Smith and colleagues reviewed 20 patients (average age, 9.5 years) with unstable pelvic fracture patterns at an average of 6.5 years after treatment. In this group, more than 1.1 cm of pelvic asymmetry after operative or nonoperative treatment was associated with lower functional

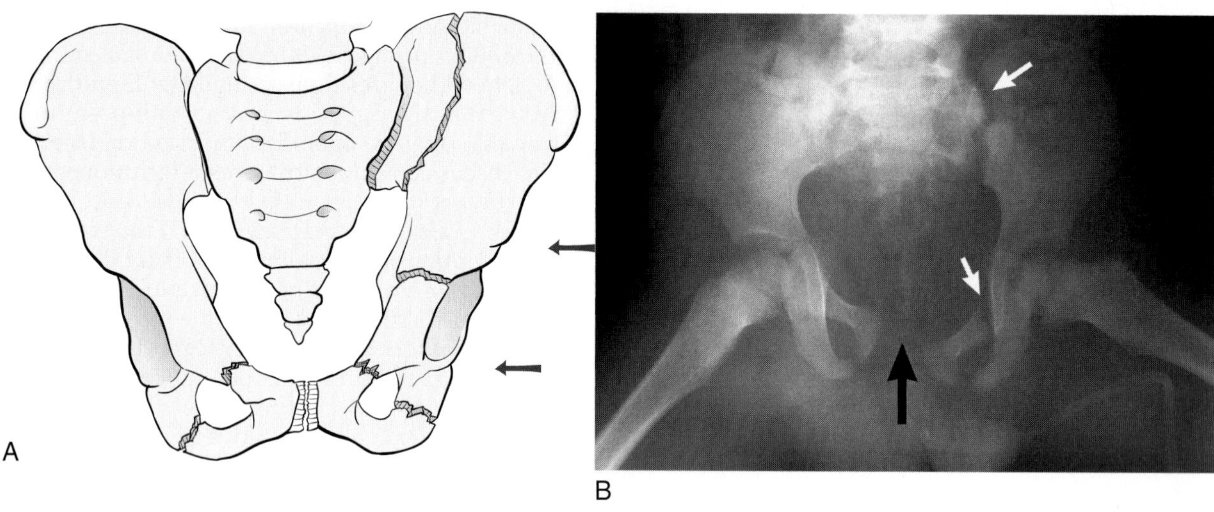

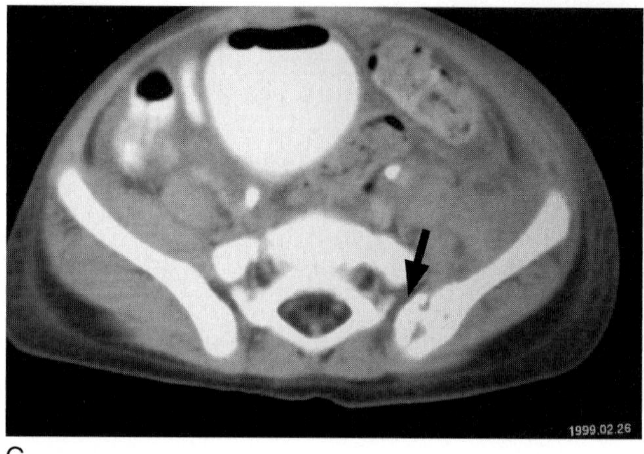

FIGURE 43-17 **A,** Type IV pelvic injury in the Torode and Zieg classification. *Arrows* show the direction of force. **B,** Radiograph demonstrating pubic symphysis diastasis, fracture of the right superior ramus (*lower white arrow*), and right sacroiliac joint widening (*upper white arrow*). *Black arrow* shows the direction of force. **C,** Computed tomography scan demonstrating widening of the sacroiliac joint (*arrow*).

outcome scores. Additionally, no remodeling of pelvic asymmetry was seen in this study group.[48]

The following treatment guidelines are based on the Young and Burgess classification and should be used. In general, children younger than 10 years with minimal pelvic asymmetry do well with nonoperative treatment and need less operative intervention. Lateral compression fractures in which the posterior structures and bone are intact (types A1 to A3) and anterior compression fractures without posterior sacroiliac joint disruption or posterior ring or displaced sacral fractures (types B1 and B2) do not usually need operative intervention. The only exception is when significant hemodynamic instability is present, and in such cases emergency application of a pelvic external fixator is required to decrease pelvic volume and tamponade the venous bleeding. Anterior compression injuries with displaced posterior pelvic fractures or sacroiliac joint disruptions (type B3) and vertically and rotationally unstable fractures (type C) require operative intervention, which generally consists of open reduction and internal fixation.

Anterior and Acetabular Fracture. A lateral compression–type injury (Fig. 43–19) that produces an anterior pelvic ring fracture and partial sacroiliac injury in which the anterior ligaments are injured but the posterior ligaments are intact results in a rotationally unstable but vertically stable pelvis. Therefore, treatment is bed rest, followed by advancement of crutch walking, non–weight bearing on the affected side for 6 to 8 weeks, and then weight bearing as tolerated by the patient. In a patient with a displaced lateral compression fracture of the A2 or A3 type, open reduction and internal fixation can be performed.

Anterior compression–type injuries (Fig. 43–20) in children younger than 10 years usually heal without difficulty and respond to conservative, symptomatic treatment as outlined earlier, which may include immobilization in a hip spica cast. In an older child with a symphysis pubic diastasis of less than 3 cm, conservative treatment is appropriate; however, if the diastasis is greater than 3 cm, open reduction of the diastasis should be considered. In fractures in which there is complete disruption of the posterior structures with complete (vertical and rotational) instability, closed reduction followed by percutaneous screw fixation of the sacroiliac joint, with or without open reduction and internal fixation of the symphysis pubis, should be performed.

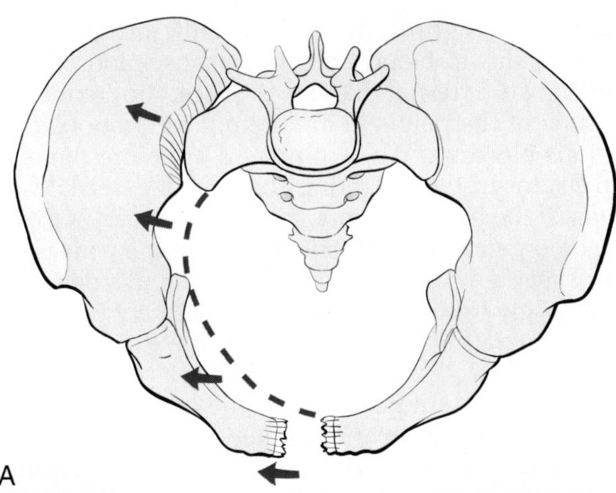

A Malgaigne-type injury (Fig. 43–21) is characterized by complete disruption of the entire hemipelvis with a vertical shear injury and vertical displacement. The patient has a limb length discrepancy with a vertically and rotationally unstable fracture. In a young child this injury can often be treated by skin or skeletal traction to reduce the vertical displacement and stabilize this highly unstable fracture. Traction is generally needed for 2 to 3 weeks, until the fracture has stabilized sufficiently to allow hip spica application or has fully healed.[29] In a child older than 10 years or with remaining pelvic asymmetry, traction to reduce the pelvis is followed by percutaneous fixation of the

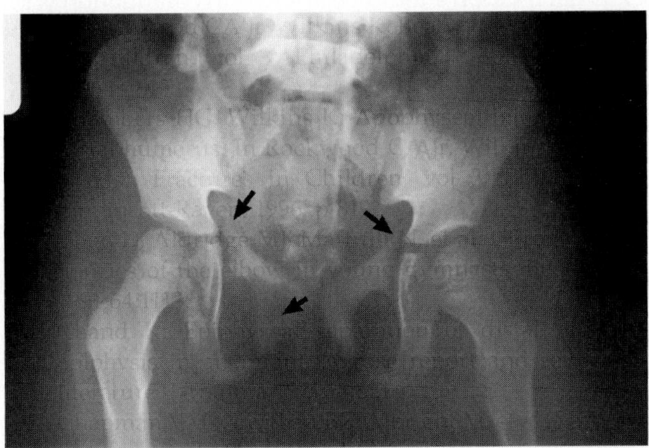

FIGURE 43–18 **A,** Straddle fracture. *Arrows* show the direction of force. Dashed line indicates displacement of the pelvic ring. **B,** Bilateral superior and inferior rami fractures (*arrows*) in a straddle fracture.

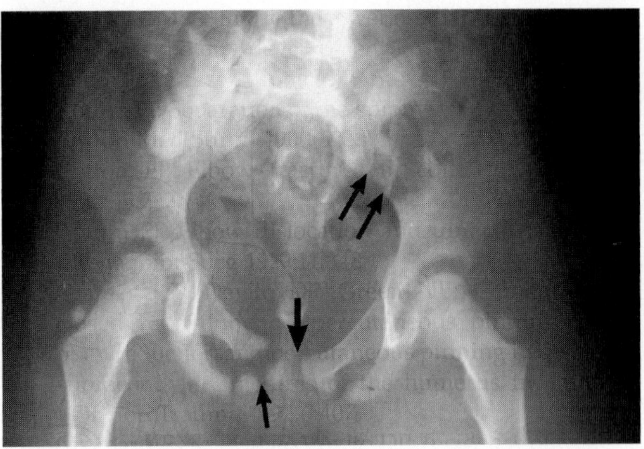

FIGURE 43–19 Radiograph of a lateral compression–type injury causing an anterior pelvic ring fracture and partial sacroiliac joint injury that was unsuccessfully treated conservatively. *Arrows* (from left to right) indicate superior and inferior pubic rami fractures, pubic symphysis diastasis, sacroiliac joint widening, and iliac wing fracture.

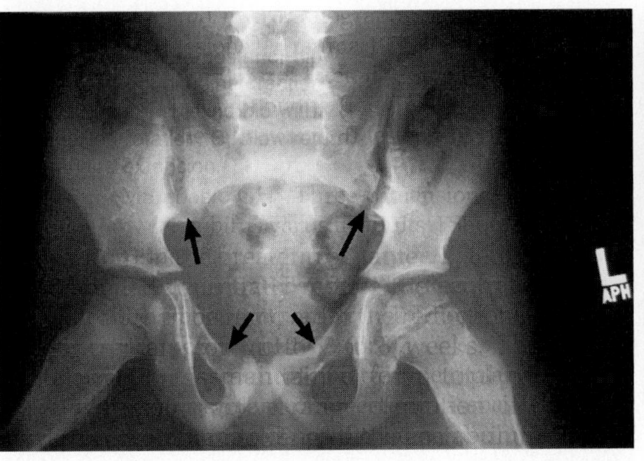

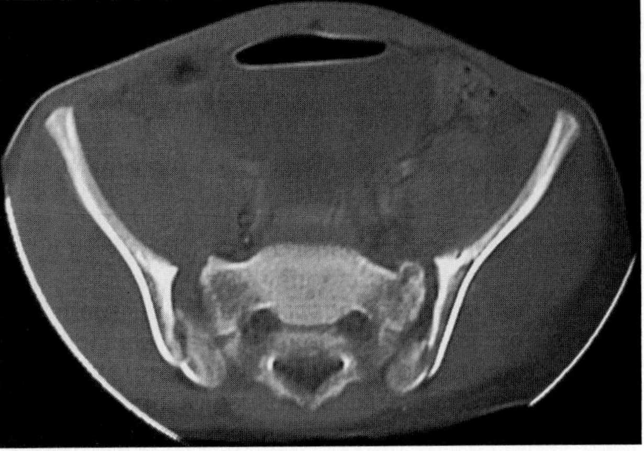

FIGURE 43–20 **A,** Radiograph of an anterior compression injury (*arrows*). **B,** Computed tomography scan of an anterior compression–type injury with disruption of the anterior ring and partial disruption of the posterior ring that was successfully treated conservatively.

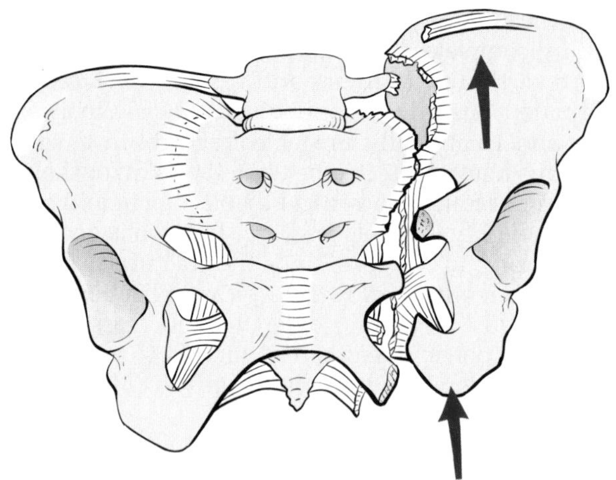

FIGURE 43–21 Malgaigne-type fracture with vertical displacement (*arrows*).

sacroiliac joint. The anterior aspect of the pelvis is stabilized by either external or internal fixation.

Treatment Techniques

External Fixation. There are two main indications for the use of an external fixator. The first is the existence of significant hemodynamic instability that is refractory to blood and fluid resuscitation. In this setting an external fixator is placed to reduce the volume of the pelvis in an attempt to tamponade the venous bleeding. We recommend applying the external fixator in the operating room under sterile conditions. If the hemodynamic instability is very severe in the emergency department, as a temporary measure a bed sheet is wrapped around the patient's pelvis and tied snugly to reduce the pelvis. The sheet is removed in the operating room just before the external fixator is applied.

The second indication for the application of an external fixator is an anterior pelvic ring displacement associated with posterior instability in a rotationally and vertically unstable fracture pattern. In this setting, external fixation should be applied in conjunction with internal fixation of the posterior injury and should not be used alone.

In an emergency situation in which hemodynamic instability is present, an external fixator can usually be applied quickly to the anterior aspect of the pelvis (Fig. 43–22). When emergency application is required, a single pin or screw is placed on each side of the pelvis, and then the external fixator bars are assembled and the pelvic displacement is reduced. The choice of pin size depends on the age and size of the child, with

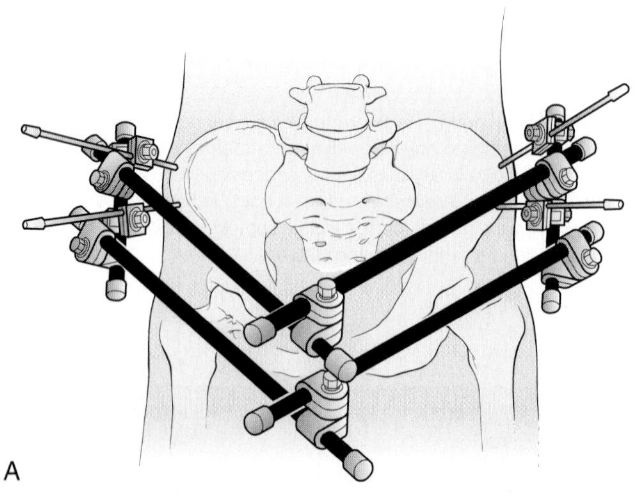

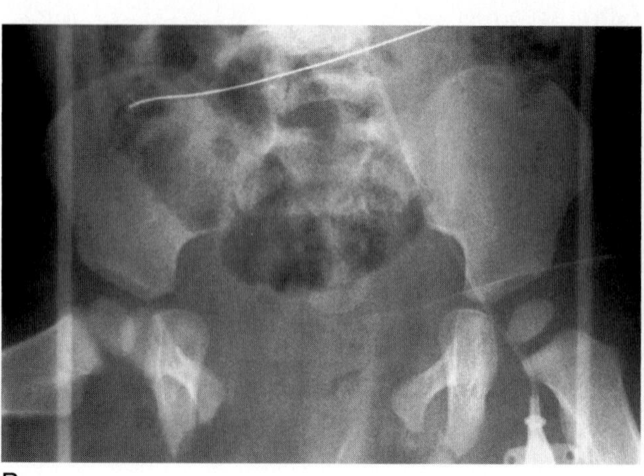

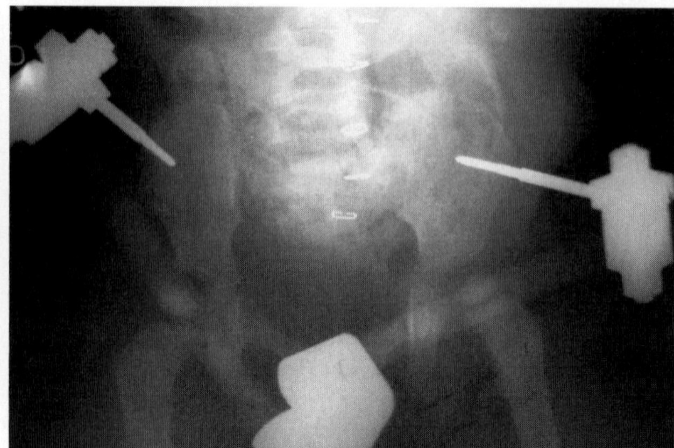

FIGURE 43–22 **A,** Typical arrangement of an external fixator applied to the pelvis for an unstable pelvic ring fracture. **B,** Radiograph of a severely disrupted pelvis with significant pubic diastasis in a 4-year-old child. **C,** Treatment with application of an external fixator.

standard adult-size 5.0-mm Schanz pins used in children older than 8 years and smaller external fixator pins used in younger children.

Because the iliac wing is directed obliquely lateromedially, it is important to direct the drill bit and pins laterally to medially at an approximately 30-degree angle from a vertical line to avoid perforating the medial or lateral cortex. A small incision is made over the anterior superior iliac spine in a transverse direction to allow the pins to slide along the incision during the reduction maneuver. This is followed by predrilling with a 3.2-mm drill bit (if 5.0-mm Schanz pins are used). The pin is then advanced by hand, with a T-handled chuck used to allow the pin to advance between the inner and outer cortical walls of the pelvis. The threaded aspect of the pin should be completely buried in the thickened anterior aspect of the iliac wing. If a second pin is used, it is placed approximately 1 to 2 cm away from the first pin to provide greater stability.

After the pins have been placed, the external fixator bars are loosely attached to the pins just before reduction. The surgeon must understand the nature of the pelvic displacement before undertaking the reduction. With vertical displacement of the pelvis, axial traction on the appropriate extremity is required; with rotational deformity, the pelvis must be rotated to achieve reduction. After reduction, the external fixator frame is tightened to stabilize the pelvis, and radiographs are obtained to confirm the reduction. The frame is inspected to ensure that it allows adequate room for the abdomen, and it should be positioned so that the patient can sit in a reclining chair.

Open Reduction and Internal Fixation of the Symphysis Pubis. The indications for open reduction and internal fixation of the symphysis pubis are similar to those for external fixation of the pelvis: (1) fractures with more than 3 cm of symphyseal displacement and (2) unstable, open book–type fractures with posterior ring disruption. This technique should not be used when the patient is hemodynamically unstable, because soft tissue dissection may aggravate the blood loss and result in hemodynamic instability. External fixation can be done more rapidly and without such tissue disruption.

A Foley catheter should be placed to decompress the bladder. A standard transverse Pfannenstiel incision is made approximately one fingerbreadth above the pubic tubercle and to the point of the external ring (Fig. 43–23). The spermatic cord is identified and retracted out of the operative field. The rectus sheath is divided above the symphysis, and the fatty tissue anterior to the bladder is bluntly dissected off the anterior symphysis. The anterior rectus sheath has usually been avulsed from the pubis at the time of injury; however, if it remains intact, it should be incised transversely, with a small attachment left so that the rectus sheath can be sutured back into place after fixation of the fracture. A sponge should be packed behind the symphysis to protect the bladder. Subperiosteal dissection is then carried out laterally until enough exposure is attained for plate fixation. We prefer dynamic compression or pelvic reconstruction plates (3.5 mm) when the child is large enough and four-hole plates when possible, although two-hole plate fixation appears to be stable enough in children younger than 12 years. In a very young child (<8 years), two-hole semitubular or one-third tubular plates can be used effectively. Hohmann retractors are placed around the symphysis, and reduction is best achieved by placing bone reduction forceps in the obturator foramen. Anatomic reduction should be achieved under direction visualization.

Internal Fixation of the Sacroiliac Joint. Injuries to the sacroiliac joint, including dislocations and fracture-dislocations, can be approached through open exposure of the joint, either anteriorly or posteriorly,[17,23,42,47] or they can be treated by closed reduction followed by percutaneous fixation.[39-41] An open technique is needed to achieve anatomic reduction when the sacroiliac joint has been disrupted. This disruption is rarely seen in children's pelvic injuries and is not generally necessary for appropriate treatment. We prefer to perform closed reduction followed by percutaneous internal fixation under fluoroscopic guidance.[39,40] Posterior open reduction is needed if closed reduction is unsuccessful or there is a significantly displaced sacral fracture.

The posterior approach requires the patient to be placed prone on the operating table. A vertical incision is made 2 cm lateral to the posterior superior iliac crest. The gluteal muscles are subperiosteally reflected off the posterior iliac wing. The origin of the gluteus maximus is reflected off the sacrum, and the greater sciatic notch is exposed to fully visualize the fracture reduction. To identify sacral fractures, the dissection is carried down to the sacral notch by reflecting the gluteus maximus fibers, the erector spinae, and the multifidus muscles. Internal fixation can usually be performed with single- or double-screw fixation, as described later, or with 3.5-mm reconstruction plates.

For percutaneous screw fixation, we prefer to place the patient supine on a radiolucent operating room table with the pelvis positioned on a flat elevated surface (one or two bed sheets). An image intensifier is used to image the sacroiliac joints and the sacrum in three views: a straight AP view, a 40-degree cephalad view (outlet view), and a 40-degree caudad view (inlet view). The inlet view shows the screw placement in the axial projection, and the operator examines the screw to be sure that it is not too anterior or posterior. The outlet view shows the screw in the cephalocaudal orientation, and the operator ensures that the screw is between the neural foramina (Fig. 43–24). In a child older than 10 years, we prefer to use a 6.5- or 7.3-mm cannulated cancellous screw, and in a younger child we use a 5.5-cm cannulated cancellous screw.

Intraoperative stimulus-evoked electromyography can be used to decrease the risk for iatrogenic nerve injury during the placement of percutaneous screws.[26,27] Both legs are prepared and placed in the operative view to allow manipulation for reduction purposes.

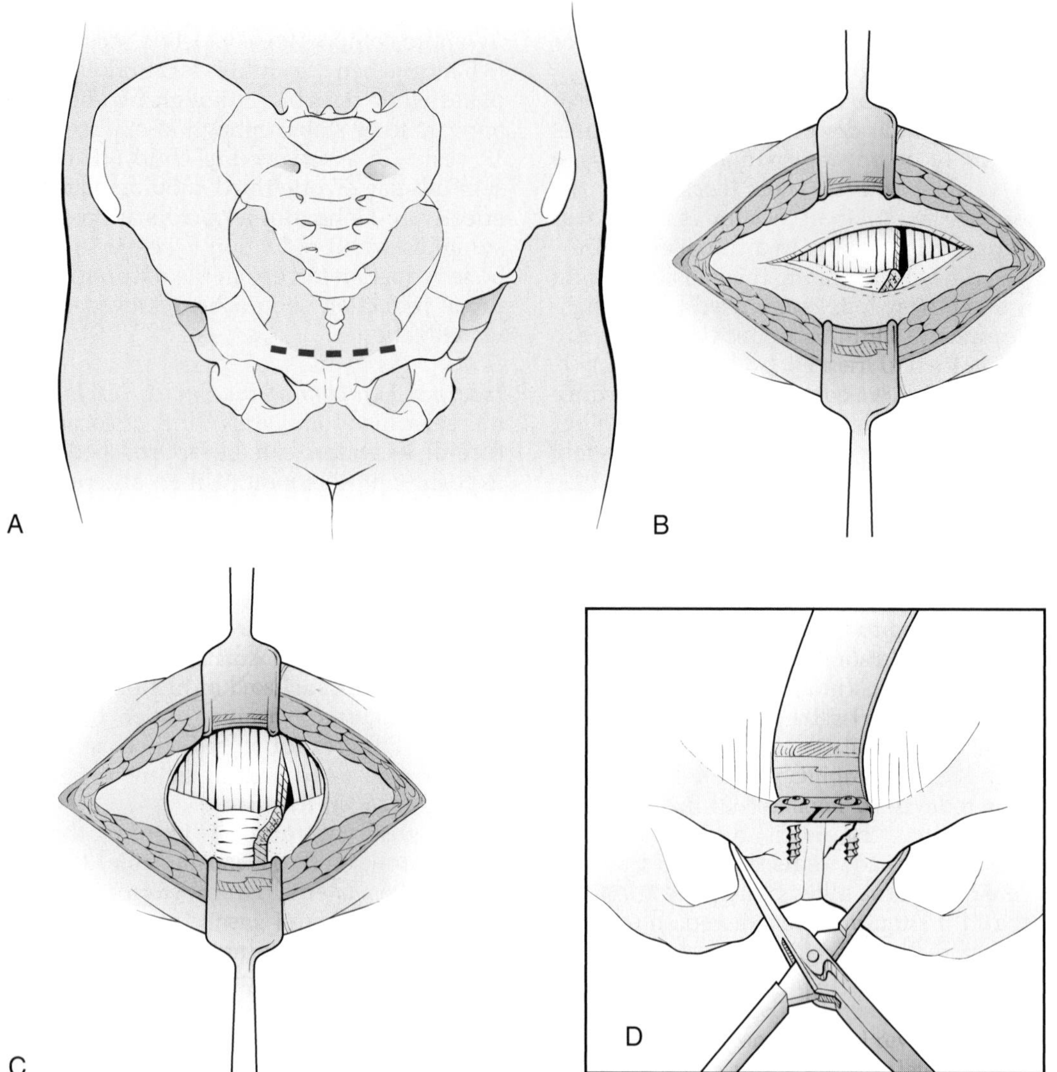

FIGURE 43–23 Surgical exposure for open reduction and internal fixation of pubic symphysis diastasis. **A,** A Pfannenstiel incision is made just superior to the pubic symphysis (*dashed line*). **B** and **C,** A transverse incision is made in the rectus sheath, and subperiosteal dissection is carried out over the pubic tubercle. **D,** Internal fixation with a two-hole dynamic compression plate.

Reduction of the sacroiliac joint requires that traction be placed on the leg and manual compression be applied across the sacroiliac joint. More severely displaced fractures may require the use of skeletal traction, in which case we prefer to use a Schanz pin placed into the anterior superior iliac spine to reduce the disruption. The starting position for the initial screw is approximately 2.5 cm lateral to the posterior superior iliac spine. A small stab incision is made, and under image intensification the initial guidewire is placed superior to the first sacral foramen past the midline. We recommend that a second guide pin be placed between the first and second sacral foramina to help maintain the reduction during screw placement. The initial guide pin is then overdrilled across the sacroiliac joint and the lateral cortex is tapped, after which a partially threaded cancellous screw with a washer is passed over the pin. The screw should travel past the midline and usually has excellent purchase; it should help lag the sacrum to the ilium in a reduced position. We have used single-screw fixation in children's sacroiliac joint disruptions with good success (Fig. 43–25). If good screw purchase is not achieved, screw position should be verified, and if the screw is in the correct position, a second screw should be placed between the first and second sacral foramina. Postoperatively, the patient can be partially weight bearing on the affected side, followed by full weight bearing after 6 weeks.

TREATMENT OF ACETABULAR FRACTURES

Acetabular fractures in children are very rare and account for approximately 5% to 10% of all pelvic fractures. The majority of fractures do not require operative intervention. An isolated injury to the triradiate

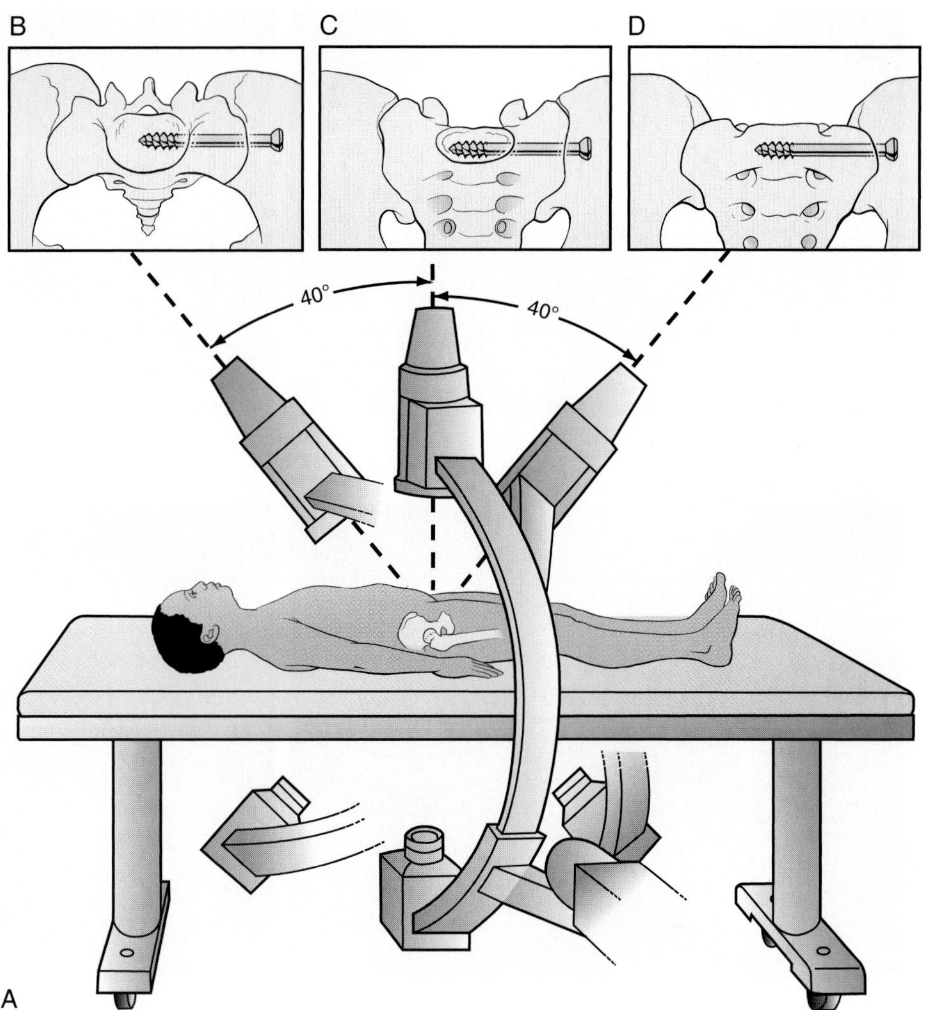

FIGURE 43–24
A, Fluoroscopic imaging for placement of sacroiliac screws. With the patient supine on the operating room table, fluoroscopy is used to image the pelvis in three views. **B,** The inlet view shows the anterior and posterior margins for screw placement. **C,** The anteroposterior view provides a general view of screw placement. **D,** The outlet view shows the superior and inferior margins for screw placement.

cartilage may not be noted at the time of the initial injury but may be manifested later, when premature closure of the triradiate cartilage results in the development of a shallow acetabulum.[53]

Acetabular fractures in children are generally treated nonoperatively, with approximately 25% requiring operative intervention.[12] By contrast, the vast majority of acetabular fractures in adults require operative intervention.[18,19,21-23]

Conservative treatment is indicated for children's acetabular fractures when they are minimally displaced (<2 mm) and for fracture-dislocations in which stable closed reduction of the femoral head results in minimal displacement of the fracture fragments. This includes all type I and most type II fractures in which the fracture fragments are displaced less than 2 mm after hip joint reduction, as well as some type IV fractures in which reduction of the central hip dislocation results in fracture reduction to within 2 mm. All patients with less than 2 mm of displacement have good or excellent functional radiographic results.[12]

Types of Injuries

Type I Fractures. In type I fractures, the patient is placed on bed rest for a short period (3 to 7 days) until comfortable and then begins to ambulate on crutches without bearing weight. Radiographs or CT scans, or both, should be obtained after the patient has been on crutches for a few days to ensure that the fracture fragments have not displaced. Progressive weight bearing is then started after 8 to 10 weeks.

Type II Fractures. Type II fractures are often associated with other pelvic ring fractures, which must be assessed and treated as discussed earlier. The acetabular fracture can generally be treated conservatively, usually with a period of bed rest and skin or skeletal traction. The period of bed rest is typically 4 weeks, followed by progressively increasing weight bearing, with the average time to full weight bearing being 10 weeks.[12] Operative treatment of acetabular fractures of this type is relatively uncommon.

Type III Fractures. Type III fractures are treated similarly to those in adults, with assessment of the fracture pattern, application of skeletal traction to restore articular congruity to within 2 mm, and operative intervention if such congruity is not achieved. In our experience, traction is usually unable to restore or maintain joint congruity within acceptable limits, and

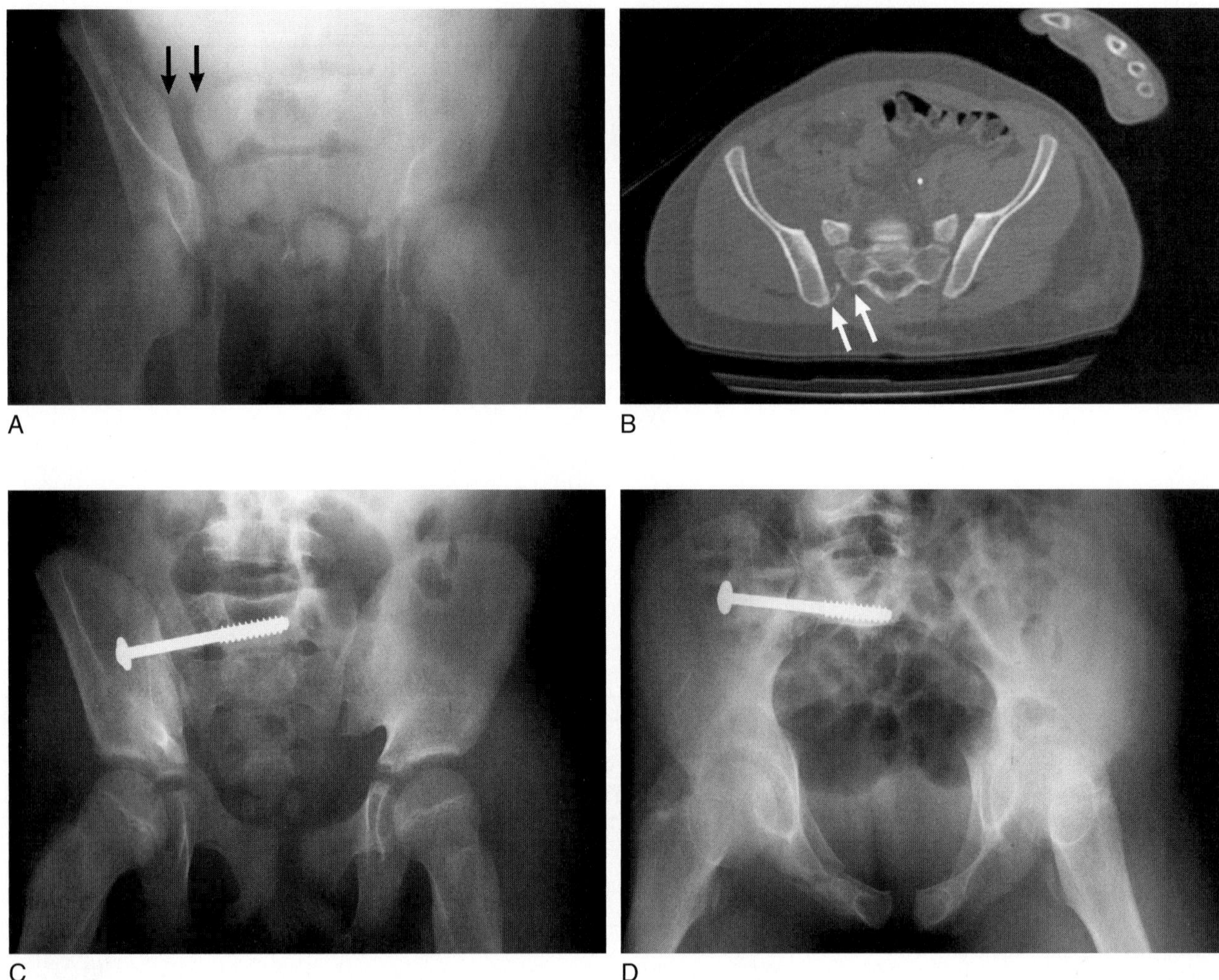

FIGURE 43–25 **A,** Initial outlet radiograph in a 10-year-old boy showing widening of the right sacroiliac joint (*arrows*) along with disruption of the posterior ligaments. **B,** Fracture was confirmed by computed tomography; *arrows* show sacroiliac joint widening with iliac avulsion. Postoperative inlet **(C)** and outlet **(D)** radiographs. The sacroiliac joint disruption has been reduced and fixed with a single percutaneously placed screw.

therefore open reduction with internal fixation is necessary. If traction is successfully used in these fractures, it must be continued for up to 12 weeks to avoid redisplacement of the fracture.

Type IV Fractures. Type IV fractures with a central fracture-dislocation should be treated initially by skeletal traction in an attempt to reduce the dislocation and achieve an acceptable reduction. The few type IV fractures described in the literature have generally required operative intervention.[2,12] Open reduction with stable internal fixation should be performed, although this may not improve the overall result. Heeg and associates described three patients with central fracture-dislocations, all of whom required operative intervention. Anatomic reduction was achieved in two patients, with a fair result in one and an excellent result in the other; the third patient had a poor outcome after anatomic reduction could not be achieved and underwent hip fusion 6 months after injury.[12]

Triradiate Cartilage Injuries. Although isolated triradiate cartilage injuries account for a small percentage of acetabular fractures in children, they must be recognized because these injuries can lead to significant progressive deformity (Fig. 43–26). The acetabulum grows through interstitial growth within the triradiate cartilage, so interruption of this growth secondary to fracture results in a shallow acetabulum, similar to developmental dysplasia of the hip.[33] Heeg and colleagues reported on four patients with triradiate acetabular injuries, all of whom had sustained an injury to the sacroiliac joint.[13] Acetabular deformity with hip subluxation developed in three of the patients, and the authors recommended that any patient who sustains pelvic trauma should be monitored clinically and radiographically for at least 1 year.

Bucholz and coauthors reported on nine patients with triradiate cartilage injuries and classified them into two main patterns of injury based on the Salter-Harris classification.[5] The first type, analogous to

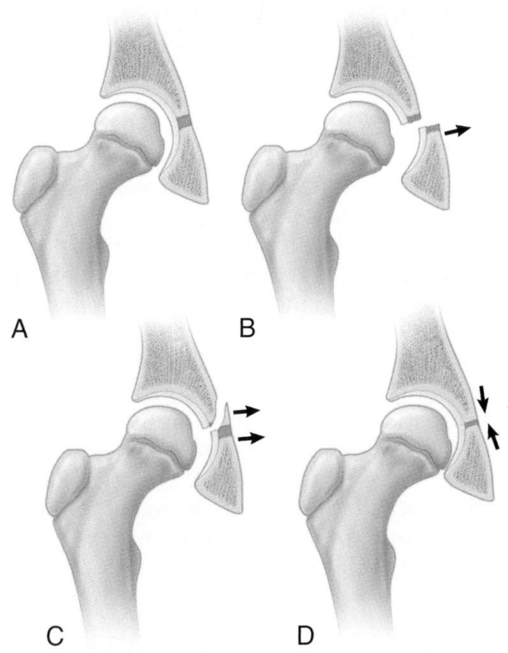

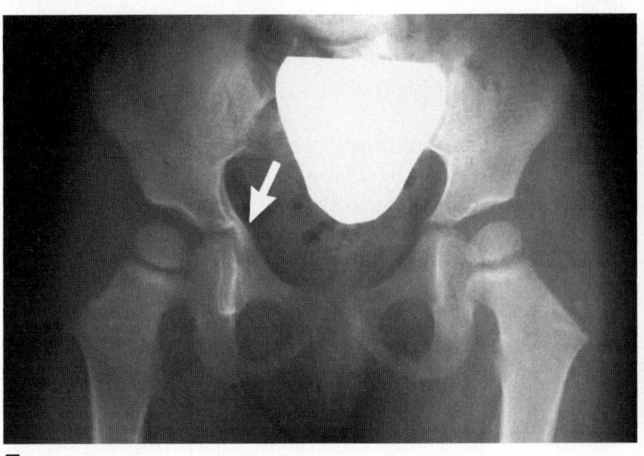

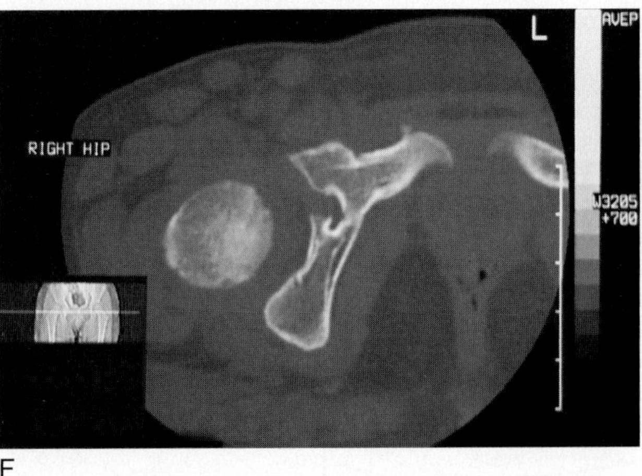

FIGURE 43–26 Triradiate cartilage injuries. **A** through **D**, Classification of injuries. **A**, Normal anatomy. **B** and **C**, The first group of injuries described by Bucholz, in which a Salter-Harris type I **(A)** or II **(B)** fracture occurs; the prognosis for continued growth is good. **D**, The second type of triradiate cartilage injury, in which a Salter-Harris type V injury occurs; the prognosis for continued growth is worse. Radiograph **(E)** and computed tomography scan **(F)** showing premature closure of the triradiate cartilage after injury in a 4-year-old girl who sustained a Salter-Harris type II fracture. *Arrow* in **E** indicates triradiate physeal bar.

Salter-Harris type I or II injury, is a shear injury with central displacement of the distal portion of the acetabulum (see Fig. 43–26B and C); the prognosis for continued normal acetabular growth is favorable. The second type, analogous to a Salter-Harris type V injury, is often difficult to diagnose and generally has a poor prognosis, with premature closure of the triradiate cartilage. The degree of deformity depends on the age of the child at the time of injury; in no patient in their study did significant acetabular dysplasia develop when the injury occurred after 11 years of age.[5] The diagnosis is confirmed by thin-section (2 to 3 mm) CT through the triradiate cartilage (see Fig. 43–26F).

Premature physeal closure of the triradiate cartilage is treated by physeal bar resection and interposition of fat or wax. There are very few reported cases in the literature, and the results have been mixed. Peterson and Robertson reported successful physeal bar resection in a child who had sustained the injury at 5 years of age and in whom over the ensuing 2-year period a shallow acetabulum developed.[32] The second window of the ilioinguinal approach was used to identify the physeal bar, and the exposed bony surfaces were covered with a thin layer of bone wax. Postoperative follow-up was reported to the age of 19 years, at which time the acetabulum had shown increased growth, which was observed by analyzing radiographic markers placed at the time of surgery. We recommend physeal bar resection through an ilioinguinal approach when the patient is younger than 12 years.

Treatment Techniques

The operative approach to the acetabulum depends on the type of fracture present. The posterior column and posterior acetabular wall are best fixed through the Kocher-Langenbeck approach, and the anterior column and inner innominate bone are best approached through an ilioinguinal approach. Both columns can be approached through an extended iliofemoral approach; however, this technique leads to the highest incidence of heterotopic ossification and the longest postoperative recovery period and is rarely used in children's acetabular fractures.

The Kocher-Langenbeck approach requires the patient to be prone on a radiolucent operating table. The incision is begun lateral to the posterior superior iliac spine and extends to the posterior aspect of the greater trochanter and down the lateral aspect of the femoral shaft. The fascia lata is split in line with the femur, the gluteus maximus tendon is taken off its attachment to the femur, and the sciatic nerve is identified superficial to the quadratus femoris. The greater and lesser sciatic notches are then exposed by taking the piriformis and obturator internus tendons off the trochanter. Subperiosteal dissection is then carried out to expose the inferior aspect of the iliac wing, and a capsulotomy is performed to expose the posterior aspect of the acetabulum and femoral head (Fig. 43–27).

The ilioinguinal approach was first described by Letournel, and this classic description should be studied before using this approach.[20] The patient is placed supine on the operating table. The incision begins at the midline approximately 3 to 4 cm above the pubis, continues to the anterior superior iliac spine, and follows the iliac crest. Subperiosteal dissection is then carried out along the iliac crest to expose the anterior sacroiliac joint and the internal iliac fossa. The external oblique aponeurosis is incised to expose the inguinal canal. The spermatic cord is bluntly dissected and isolated, and a Penrose drain is placed around it. The posterior aspect of the inguinal ligament is then incised to allow access to the psoas sheath, the retropubic space of Retzius, and the external aspect of the iliac vessels. A Penrose drain is next placed around the psoas and lateral cutaneous nerve of the thigh, and the iliopectineal fascia is divided. A second Penrose drain is placed around the external iliac vessels and lymphatics. The three windows of the ilioinguinal approach are now present (Fig. 43–28). The first window is between the iliac fossa and the psoas muscle and gives access to the internal iliac fossa, the anterior sacroiliac joint, and the upper portion of the anterior column. The second window is between the psoas muscle and the iliac vessel and provides access to the pelvic brim from the anterior sacroiliac joint to the lateral extremity of the superior pubic ramus. The third window is medial to the iliac vessels and provides access to the symphysis pubis and the retropubic space of Retzius.

The extended iliofemoral approach is rarely necessary and can best be learned by studying Letournel's original description.[18,20]

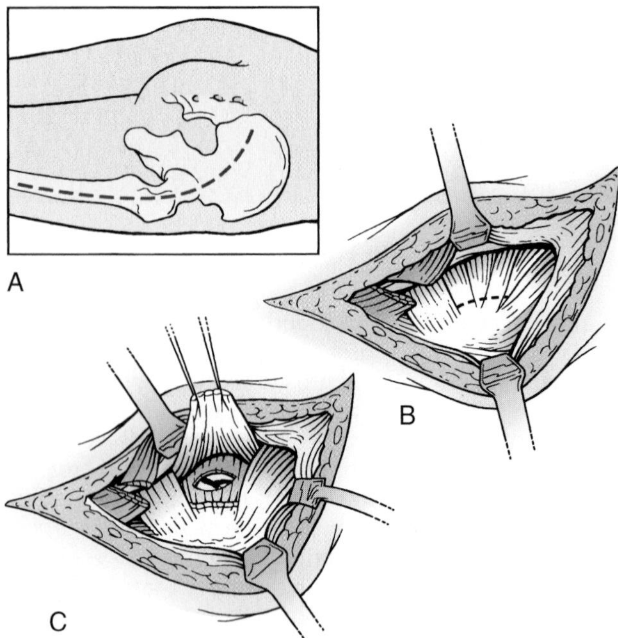

FIGURE 43–27 Kocher-Langenbeck approach to the posterior part of the acetabulum. **A,** The incision is begun lateral to the posterior superior iliac spine and continued to the greater trochanter and laterally down the proximal end of the femur. **B,** The piriformis and obturator internus tendons are then dissected off the greater trochanter. **C,** Subperiosteal dissection followed by capsulotomy is used to expose the posterior aspect of the acetabulum.

COMPLICATIONS

Nonorthopaedic complications are related to the associated injuries as described in the preceding sections and especially include those involving the genitourinary and neurologic systems, hemorrhage, lacerations of the vagina or rectum, and possibly death. Urinary infections have been reported in 10% to 20% of patients, and pulmonary complications, including pneumonia, have occurred in 10% to 30% of patients.[37,54]

Complications related directly to the pelvis and acetabular fractures include delayed union, nonunion, malunion, and sacroiliac joint pain. Nierenberg and coworkers reported no complications related to the pelvic fracture in all 14 patients with stable fractures, but 3 of 6 unstable fractures had malunion.[29] Torode and Zieg reported complications related to the pelvic fracture only in type IV fractures. Of 40 patients, 8 (20%) demonstrated nonunion of the pubic rami and 3 (8%) demonstrated premature closure of the triradiate cartilage. In addition, marked displacement of the pelvic ring was noted in five (13%) patients, although four of these patients were classified as having an excellent result and one (3%) patient demonstrated fusion of the sacroiliac joint, which was partly responsible for the pelvic distortion.[53]

Acetabular fractures are associated with complications early and late. Heeg and colleagues described eight (35%) patients with early complications: four had a urinary or respiratory tract infection, three had pin tract infections, and one had a superficial infection at the operative site. Late complications occurred in three (13%) patients, all of whom underwent operative treatment: two (9%) had premature closure of the triradiate cartilage requiring further operative treatment and one (4%) had a painful hip secondary to extensive

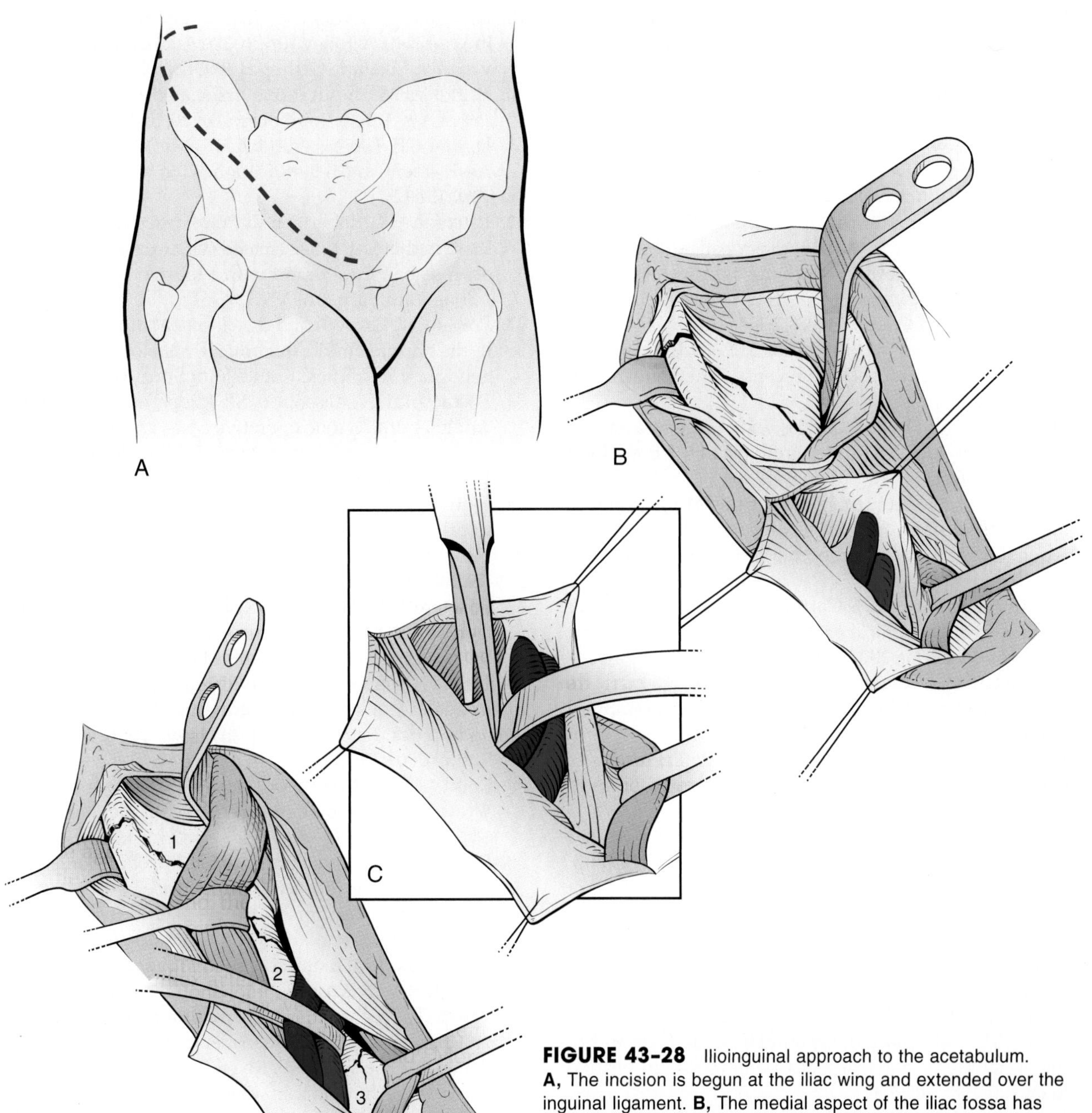

FIGURE 43-28 Ilioinguinal approach to the acetabulum. **A,** The incision is begun at the iliac wing and extended over the inguinal ligament. **B,** The medial aspect of the iliac fossa has been exposed, as have the femoral vessels and the spermatic cord. **C,** The iliopectineal fascia has been incised. **D,** The three windows can now be used to approach the acetabular fracture.

heterotopic ossification and subsequently underwent fusion to treat the painful symptoms.

References

Pelvis and Acetabulum

1. Bond SJ, Gotschall CS, Eichelberger MR: Predictors of abdominal injury in children with pelvic fracture. J Trauma 1991;31:1169.
2. Brooks E, Rosman M: Central fracture-dislocation of the hip in a child. J Trauma 1988;28:1590.
3. Bryan WJ, Tullos HS: Pediatric pelvic fractures: Review of 52 patients. J Trauma 1979;19:799.
4. Bucholz RW: The pathological anatomy of Malgaigne fracture-dislocations of the pelvis. J Bone Joint Surg Am 1981;63:400.
5. Bucholz RW, Ezaki M, Ogden JA: Injury to the acetabular triradiate physeal cartilage. J Bone Joint Surg Am 1982; 64:600.
6. Dunn AW, Morris HD: Fractures and dislocations of the pelvis. J Bone Joint Surg Am 1968;50:1639.
7. Edeiken-Monroe BS, Browner BD, Jackson H: The role of standard roentgenograms in the evaluation of instability of pelvic ring disruption. Clin Orthop Relat Res 1989; 240:63.

8. Fernbach SK, Wilkinson RH: Avulsion injuries of the pelvis and proximal femur. AJR Am J Roentgenol 1981; 137:581.
9. Grisoni N, Connor S, Marsh E, et al: Pelvic fractures in a pediatric level I trauma center. J Orthop Trauma 2002;16:458.
10. Guillamondegui OD, Mahboubi S, Stafford PW, et al: The utility of the pelvic radiograph in the assessment of pediatric pelvic fractures. J Trauma 2003;55:236.
11. Hak DJ, Olson SA, Matta JM: Diagnosis and management of closed internal degloving injuries associated with pelvic and acetabular fractures: The Morel-Lavallee lesion. J Trauma 1997;42:1046.
12. Heeg M, de Ridder VA, Tornetta P 3rd, et al: Acetabular fractures in children and adolescents. Clin Orthop Relat Res 2000;376:80.
13. Heeg M, Visser JD, Oostvogel HJ: Injuries of the acetabular triradiate cartilage and sacroiliac joint. J Bone Joint Surg Br 1988;70:34.
14. Judet R, Judet J, Letournel E: Fractures of the acetabulum: Classification and surgical approaches for open reduction. Preliminary report. J Bone Joint Surg Am 1964;46:1615.
15. Junkins EP Jr, Nelson DS, Carroll KL, et al: A prospective evaluation of the clinical presentation of pediatric pelvic fractures. J Trauma 2001;51:64.
16. Karunakar MA, Goulet JA, Mueller KL, et al: Operative treatment of unstable pediatric pelvis and acetabular fractures. J Pediatr Orthop 2005;25:34.
17. Kellam JF, McMurtry RY, Paley D, et al: The unstable pelvic fracture. Operative treatment. Orthop Clin North Am 1987;18:25.
18. Letournel E: The results of acetabular fractures treated surgically: Twenty-one year's experience. In The Hip: Proceedings of the Seventh Open Scientific Meeting of the Hip Society. St Louis, CV Mosby, 1979, p 42.
19. Letournel E: Acetabulum fractures: Classification and management. Clin Orthop Relat Res 1980;151:81.
20. Letournel E, Judet R: Fractures of the Acetabulum. Berlin, Springer-Verlag, 1981.
21. Matta JM, Anderson LM, Epstein HC, et al: Fractures of the acetabulum. A retrospective analysis. Clin Orthop Relat Res 1986;205:230.
22. Matta JM, Mehne DK, Roffi R: Fractures of the acetabulum. Early results of a prospective study. Clin Orthop Relat Res 1986;205:241.
23. Matta JM, Saucedo T: Internal fixation of pelvic ring fractures. Clin Orthop Relat Res 1989;242:83.
24. McDonald GA: Pelvic disruptions in children. Clin Orthop Relat Res 1980;151:130.
25. Metzmaker J, Pappas AM: Avulsion fractures of the pelvis. Orthop Trans 1980;4:82.
26. Moed BR, Ahmad BK, Craig JG, et al: Intraoperative monitoring with stimulus-evoked electromyography during placement of iliosacral screws. An initial clinical study. J Bone Joint Surg Am 1998;80:537.
27. Moed BR, Anders MJ, Ahmad BK, et al: Intraoperative stimulus-evoked electromyographic monitoring for placement of iliosacral implants: An animal model. J Orthop Trauma 1998;12:85.
28. Morel-Lavallee M: Decollements traumatiques de la peau et des couches sous-jacentes. Arch Gen Med 1863;1:20.
29. Nierenberg G, Volpin G, Bialik V, et al: Pelvic fractures in children: A follow-up in 20 children treated conservatively. J Pediatr Orthop B 1993;1:140.
30. Peltier LF: Complications associated with fractures of the pelvis. J Bone Joint Surg Am 1965;47:1060.
31. Pennal GF, Tile M, Waddell JP, et al: Pelvic disruption: Assessment and classification. Clin Orthop Relat Res 1980;151:12.
32. Peterson HA, Robertson R: Premature partial closure of the triradiate cartilage treated with excision of a physeal osseous bar. Case report with a fourteen-year follow-up. J Bone Joint Surg Am 1997;79:767.
33. Ponseti IV: Growth and development of the acetabulum in the normal child. Anatomical, histological, and roentgenographic studies. J Bone Joint Surg Am 1978;60:575.
34. Postacchini F, Massobrio M: Idiopathic coccygodynia. Analysis of fifty-one operative cases and a radiographic study of the normal coccyx. J Bone Joint Surg Am 1983;65:1116.
35. Quinby WC Jr: Fractures of the pelvis and associated injuries in children. J Pediatr Surg 1966;1:353.
36. Reed MH: Pelvic fractures in children. J Can Assoc Radiol 1976;27:255.
37. Reichard SA, Helikson MA, Shorter N, et al: Pelvic fractures in children—review of 120 patients with a new look at general management. J Pediatr Surg 1980;15:727.
38. Rossi F, Dragoni S: Acute avulsion fractures of the pelvis in adolescent competitive athletes: Prevalence, location and sports distribution of 203 cases collected. Skeletal Radiol 2001;30:127.
39. Routt M, Meir M, Kregor P, et al: Percutaneous iliosacral screws with the patient supine technique. Operat Tech Orthop 1993;3:35.
40. Routt ML Jr, Kregor PJ, Simonian PT, et al: Early results of percutaneous iliosacral screws placed with the patient in the supine position. J Orthop Trauma 1995;9:207.
41. Routt ML Jr, Simonian PT: Closed reduction and percutaneous skeletal fixation of sacral fractures. Clin Orthop Relat Res 1996;329:121.
42. Ruedi T, Hochstetter AVS, Schlumpf R: Surgical Approaches for Internal Fixation. Berlin, Springer-Verlag, 1987.
43. Sauerland S, Bouillon B, Rixen D, et al: The reliability of clinical examination in detecting pelvic fractures in blunt trauma patients: A meta-analysis. Arch Orthop Trauma Surg 2004;124:123.
44. Silber JS, Flynn JM: Changing patterns of pediatric pelvic fractures with skeletal maturation: Implications for classification and management. J Pediatr Orthop 2002;22:22.
45. Silber JS, Flynn JM, Katz MA, et al: Role of computed tomography in the classification and management of pediatric pelvic fractures. J Pediatr Orthop 2001;21:148.
46. Silber JS, Flynn JM, Koffler KM, et al: Analysis of the cause, classification, and associated injuries of 166 consecutive pediatric pelvic fractures. J Pediatr Orthop 2001;21:446.
47. Simpson LA, Waddell JP, Leighton RK, et al: Anterior approach and stabilization of the disrupted sacroiliac joint. J Trauma 1987;27:1332.
48. Smith W, Shurnas P, Morgan S, et al: Clinical outcomes of unstable pelvic fractures in skeletally immature patients. J Bone Joint Surg Am 2005;87:2423.

49. Sundar M, Carty H: Avulsion fractures of the pelvis in children: A report of 32 fractures and their outcome. Skeletal Radiol 1994;23:85.
50. Tarman GJ, Kaplan GW, Lerman SL, et al: Lower genitourinary injury and pelvic fractures in pediatric patients. Urology 2002;59:123.
51. Tile M: Fractures of the Pelvis and Acetabulum. Baltimore, Williams & Wilkins, 1984.
52. Tile M: Pelvic ring fractures: Should they be fixed? J Bone Joint Surg Br 1988;70:1.
53. Torode I, Zieg D: Pelvic fractures in children. J Pediatr Orthop 1985;5:76.
54. Trunkey DD, Chapman MW, Lim RC Jr, et al: Management of pelvic fractures in blunt trauma injury. J Trauma 1974;14:912.
55. Watts HG: Fractures of the pelvis in children. Orthop Clin North Am 1976;7:615.
56. Winkler AR, Barnes JC, Ogden JA: Break dance hip: Chronic avulsion of the anterior superior iliac spine. Pediatr Radiol 1987;17:501.
57. Young J, Burgess A: Radiological Management of Pelvic Ring Fractures. Baltimore, Urban & Schwarzenberg, 1987.

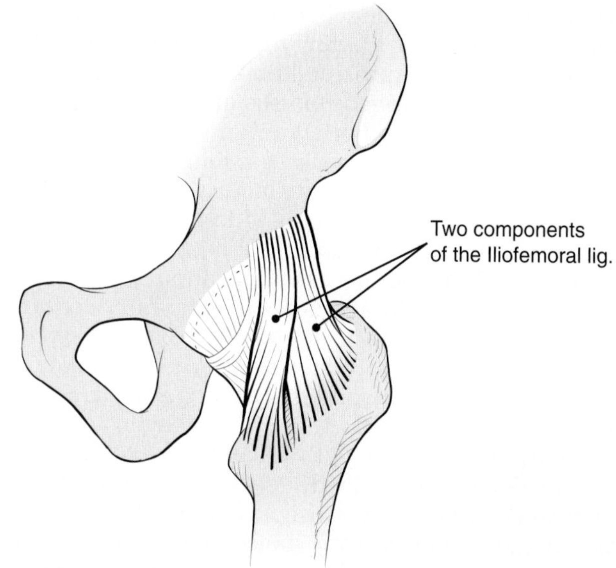

FIGURE 43–29 The iliofemoral ligament is composed of two bands originating on the anterior inferior iliac spine and attaching to the intertrochanteric line anterior to the lesser and greater trochanters.

HIP

Hip Dislocations

Traumatic hip dislocations in children are relatively rare. In a younger child (<5 years), minor trauma such as a slip or a fall from a low height may cause a hip dislocation, whereas in an adolescent a dislocation is usually caused by major trauma such as a motor vehicle accident. Posterior dislocations are approximately eight to nine times more common than anterior dislocations, and treatment generally consists of closed reduction under sedation or general anesthesia, followed by immobilization and a short period of non–weight-bearing activity. Complications are similar to those in adults; however, recurrent hip dislocations are more common in children.

ANATOMY

The iliofemoral ligament, often referred to as the Y ligament of Bigelow, is the major ligamentous structure around the hip joint. It originates on the anterior inferior iliac spine, extends across the anterior aspect of the hip joint, and attaches to the femur at the anterior intertrochanteric line (Fig. 43–29). The iliofemoral ligament limits hyperextension and lateral rotation of the hip joint and is the primary obstacle to reduction in posterior hip dislocations. The ischiofemoral ligament is located posteriorly and lies deep to the short external rotators, which provide additional stability. In a posterior dislocation of the hip, the ligamentum teres is avulsed, the posterior hip capsule is torn, a fragment of the posterior acetabular rim is often fractured, and the labrum may be avulsed or torn. The capsular tear may be at its attachment to the posterior labrum[5,24] or in its midsubstance.[51] The short lateral rotator muscles—obturator internus, piriformis, obturator externus, and quadratus muscles—are either partially or completely torn along with the capsule. The gluteus maximus, medius, and minimus muscles are stretched and translated posteriorly by the femoral head, which lies deep to or within the fibers of these muscles. Structures and conditions that are known to block reduction include the piriformis muscle, which may be displaced across the acetabulum; osteocartilaginous fragments; infolding of the labrum and capsule; and buttonholing of the femoral head through a small tear in the posterior capsule.[5,33,37,48]

Anterior hip dislocations also tear the ligamentum teres and the anterior joint capsule. The muscles anterior to the hip joint may be stretched or partially torn. Rarely, the femoral nerve and artery are also injured during a high-energy injury.[4,12]

MECHANISM OF INJURY

Two main mechanisms of injury result in a hip dislocation. In the younger age group (<5 years), a trivial fall or slip may result in a hip dislocation because of the generalized joint laxity and soft cartilaginous acetabulum in this age group. In older patients (11 to 15 years), the hip dislocation is more often due to higher energy trauma (athletic injury or a motor vehicle accident).[13,23] It is important to obtain a good history because the mechanism of injury has prognostic implications, with high-energy trauma injuries resulting in a worse outcome.[13]

The typical posterior dislocation results from a posteriorly directed axial load applied to the distal end of the femur. It is often seen in motor vehicle accidents in which the patient is in the front seat during a head-on collision and the knee strikes the dashboard and pushes the femoral head posteriorly out of the acetabulum. This mechanism of injury often results in associated injuries, including hip, femoral shaft, distal femoral, patellar, or proximal tibial fractures. A front-seat passenger or driver who sustains these fractures in a motor vehicle accident should always be suspected of having a hip dislocation or subluxation with an associated acetabular injury. Careful physical examination and radiographic examination, often including CT, are necessary to evaluate the hip joint even though the initial AP radiograph may appear normal.

Anterior hip dislocations result from an anteriorly directed force applied to the posterior aspect of the abducted and laterally rotated thigh. The femoral head is displaced forward, commonly lying external to the obturator foramen.

Central dislocations with fractures of the acetabulum are due to a medially directed force on the greater trochanter. A fall from a height is the most common mechanism, followed by a motor vehicle accident in which the knee strikes the dashboard when the hip is extended and abducted.

CLASSIFICATION

There are several classifications of hip dislocation. Because of the rarity of dislocations in children, however, no classification has been widely used. The simplest classification is based on the direction in which the femoral head is dislocated relative to the acetabulum (Fig. 43–30A and B). Most (75% to 90%) hip dislocations are posterior.[6,8,11,34,35] Posterior hip dislocations can be further subdivided according to the resting position of the femoral head: iliac, if the femoral head lies posteriorly and superiorly along the lateral aspect of the ilium; and ischial, if it lies adjacent to the greater sciatic notch. The remaining dislocations are anterior and are subdivided into obturator and pubic dislocations (Fig. 43–30C and D). A central hip dislocation is relatively rare in children and is associated with fracture of the acetabulum.

Hip dislocations in children are associated with acetabular or proximal femoral fractures far less frequently than in adults. The incidence of associated

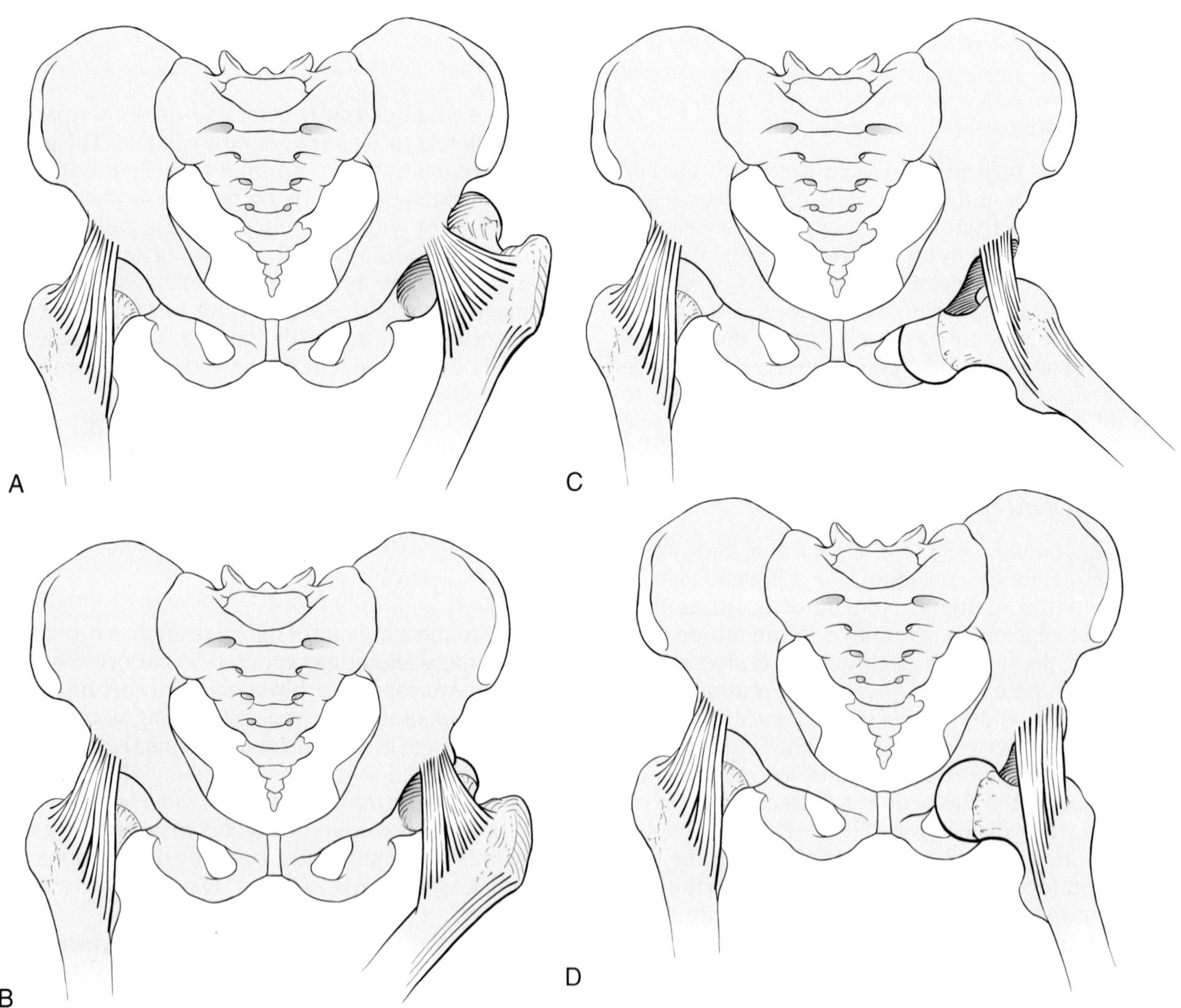

FIGURE 43-30 Classification of hip dislocations. Posterior hip dislocations—iliac **(A)** and ischial **(B)**; anterior hip dislocations—obturator **(C)** and pubic **(D)**.

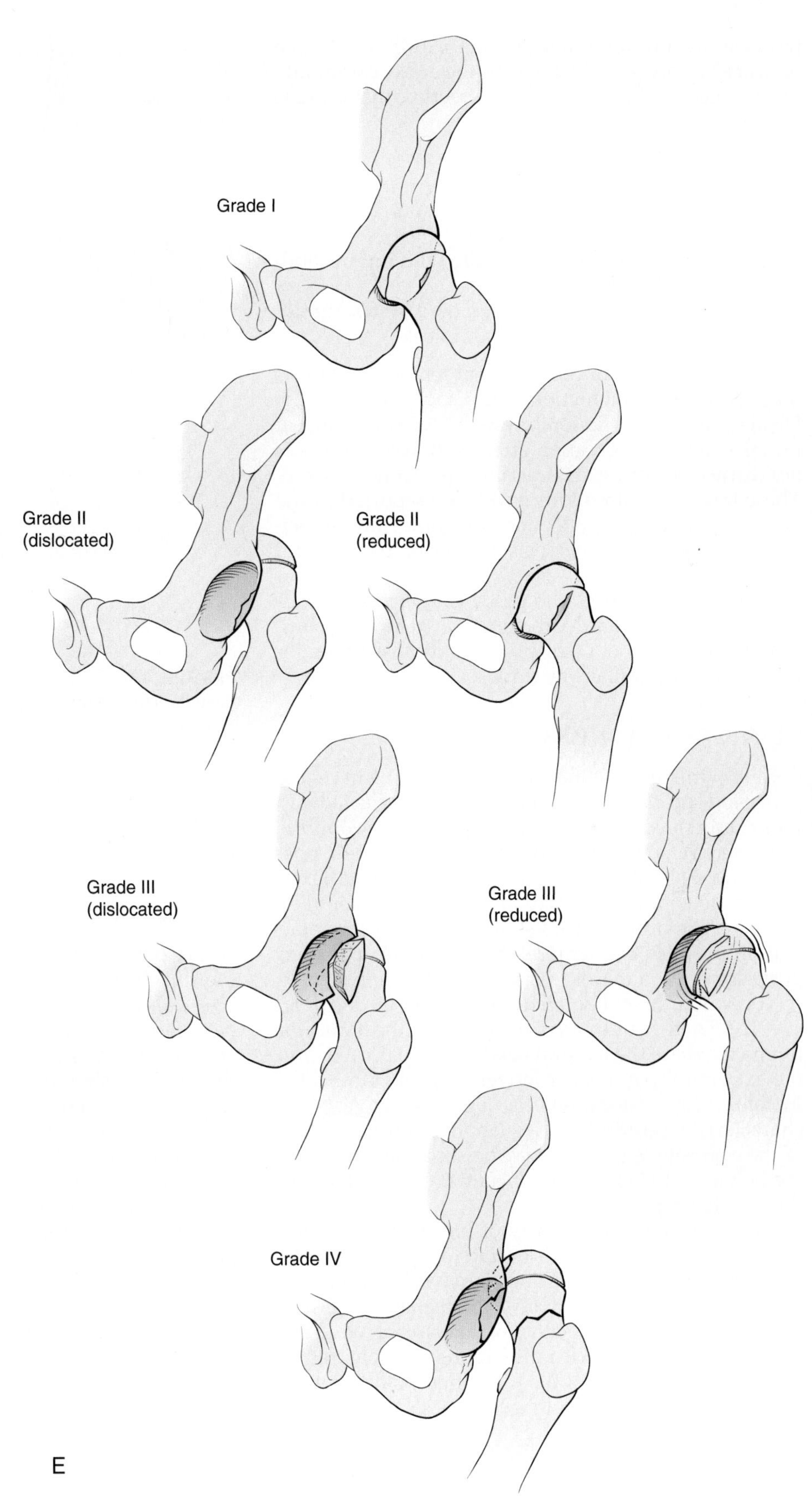

FIGURE 43-30 cont'd
E, Stewart-Milford comprehensive classification.

fractures in children ranges from 4% to 18%.[13,28,34] The Stewart-Milford classification is the most commonly used classification for hip fracture-dislocations (Fig. 43–30E)[44]:

Grade I	No acetabular fracture or only a minor chip fracture
Grade II	Posterior rim fracture, but the hip is stable after reduction
Grade III	Posterior rim fracture with hip instability after reduction
Grade IV	Dislocation accompanied by fracture of the femoral head and neck

Physeal fracture of the proximal femoral epiphysis may occur in conjunction with a hip dislocation. Displacement of the epiphysis may be noted at initial evaluation or after attempted reduction if a nondisplaced physeal fracture is unrecognized. These fracture-dislocations have been reported in the periadolescent age group and are uniformly associated with avascular necrosis (AVN) of the femoral epiphysis.[19,32,50]

Acetabular fractures should be classified individually to allow standard preoperative treatment planning to be carried out (see previous discussion under Pelvic and Acetabular Fractures).

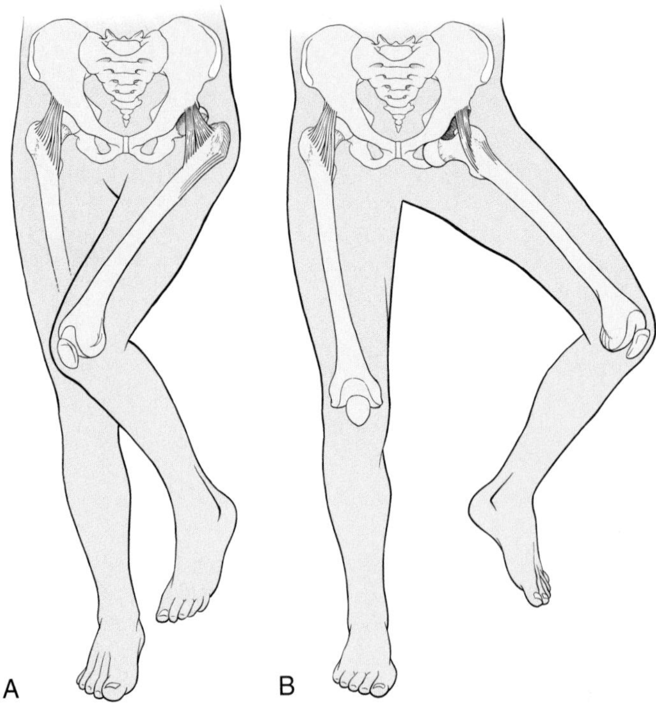

FIGURE 43–31 Clinical position of the lower extremity with posterior **(A)** and anterior **(B)** hip dislocations.

CLINICAL FEATURES

A child with an acute hip dislocation will be in severe pain, and any attempted motion of the affected hip will exacerbate the pain. The position of the limb is characteristic for the type of hip dislocation. In a posterior hip dislocation the involved thigh is held flexed and adducted and in a medially rotated position (Fig. 43–31A). The limb appears shorter than the contralateral limb, and the femoral head can be palpated posteriorly. In anterior dislocations the leg is held in abduction, lateral rotation, and some flexion (Fig. 43–31B). There is fullness in the region of the obturator foramen, where the femoral head can be palpated, and the extremity may appear longer than the other side. In central hip dislocations the leg does not rest in a characteristic position and leg length is similar to that of the opposite leg. There may be some narrowing of the pelvic width as a result of central displacement of the affected hip.

Although the vast majority of hip dislocations are thought to maintain a dislocated position, cases of spontaneously reduced dislocations with subsequent evaluation for pain secondary to interposed tissues have been reported. A child or adolescent with hip pain after injury and radiographs demonstrating asymmetric widening of the hip joints should be evaluated with further imaging techniques such as CT or magnetic resonance imaging (MRI).[36]

A thorough neurologic examination of the affected extremity should be performed, with careful evaluation of sciatic nerve function in posterior dislocations and femoral nerve function in anterior dislocations. The peripheral pulses, including the posterior tibial, dorsalis pedis, and popliteal pulses, should be palpated, and a thorough examination should be performed to assess for other injuries, especially ipsilateral lower extremity fractures and knee injuries.[2,7,21,22,27,41,47]

RADIOGRAPHIC FINDINGS

An AP pelvic radiograph should be obtained to confirm the hip dislocation and rule out other fractures (Fig. 43–32A). Oblique (Judet) views and CT scans should be obtained when an associated acetabular fracture is suspected (Fig. 43–32B and C). Isolated radiographs of the hip joint should be obtained to exclude other fractures before attempts are made to reduce the hip dislocation when a femoral head or femoral neck fracture is seen on the initial AP pelvic film. A fluoroscopic examination before reduction may be considered in the periadolescent age group to evaluate for evidence of epiphyseal motion secondary to unrecognized physeal fracture.[19] After reduction of the hip dislocation, an AP pelvic radiograph should be carefully evaluated to confirm concentric reduction (Fig. 43–33). A postreduction CT study can be performed routinely after an apparently successful closed reduction to ensure that concentric reduction was achieved and to image loose fragments in the joint, which cannot be seen on a plain radiograph. Because associated fractures in children are relatively rare, with a posterior or anterior hip dislocation we prefer to perform a postreduction CT study when concerned that concentric reduction has not been achieved or to assess an acetabular wall or femoral head fracture suspected on the postreduction radiograph. MRI has been reported to

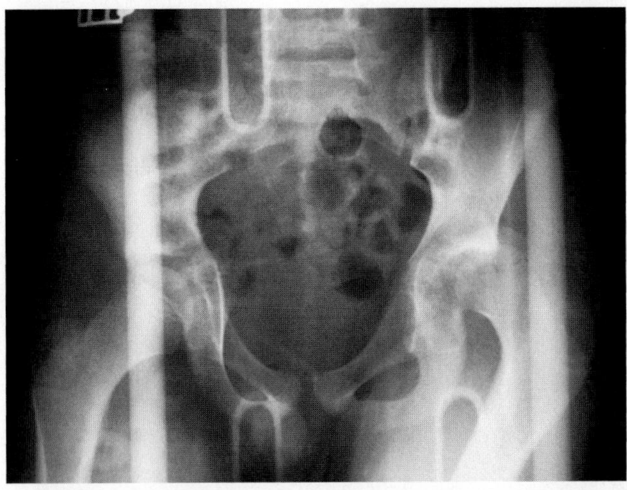

A

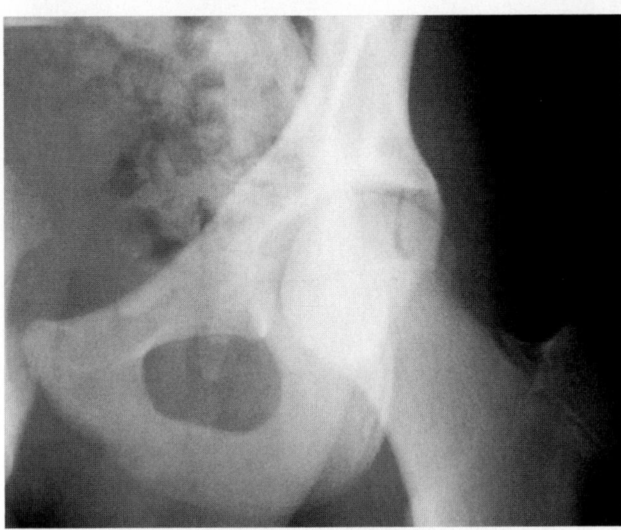

B

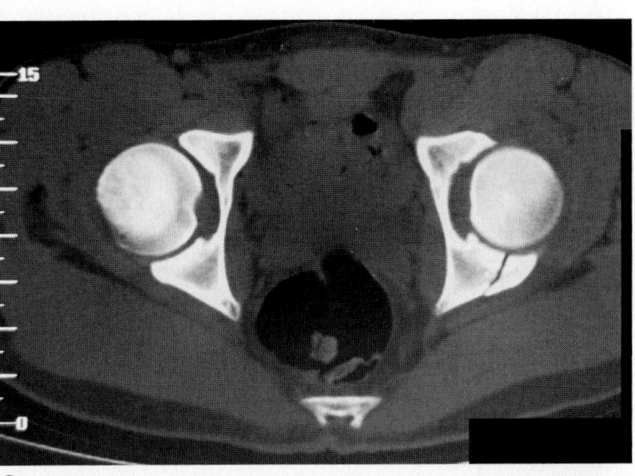

C

FIGURE 43–32 Posterior hip dislocations. **A,** Anteroposterior radiograph of a posterior hip dislocation in a 10-year-old. **B,** Posterior acetabular fracture seen on a postreduction radiograph **(B)** and computed tomography scan **(C)** after a posterior hip dislocation in a 13-year-old boy.

be useful to assess unossified acetabular rim fractures in the uncommon setting of postreduction instability without a visible fracture.[39] An arteriogram should be obtained in any child in whom the clinical findings or Doppler studies indicate a femoral arterial injury.[31]

TREATMENT

Hip dislocations should be treated on an urgent basis with prompt, immediate reduction after a thorough physical examination and evaluation of the plain radiographs. Closed reduction should be attempted under general anesthesia in the operating room if it can be performed without delay or in the emergency room under conscious sedation. The method and duration of immobilization after reduction have not been agreed on, although some form of immobilization should be used.

Closed Reduction

Posterior Dislocation. Closed reduction of a posterior dislocation can be achieved by using the Bigelow,[3] Allis,[1] or Stimson[45] methods, all of which rely on flexion of the hip joint to relax the iliofemoral ligament.

The easiest, most common, and most effective treatment is that described by Allis (Fig. 43–34).[1] The patient is placed supine, and an assistant stabilizes the pelvis by applying direct pressure over the anterior superior iliac spine. The hip and knee are then flexed 90 degrees, with the thigh in slight adduction and medial rotation. The surgeon then places a forearm behind the patient's knee and leg and applies an anteriorly directed force to release the femoral head from behind the posterior lip of the acetabulum. If soft tissue resistance is felt, the medial rotation and hip adduction are increased in an effort to further relax the hip joint capsule, and closed reduction is again attempted. An assistant can apply direct anterior pressure on the femoral head to aid in the reduction.

In the circumduction method of Bigelow, an assistant applies countertraction on the anterior superior iliac spine while the surgeon grasps the affected limb at the ankle with one hand and places the opposite forearm behind the patient's knee (Fig. 43–35). The

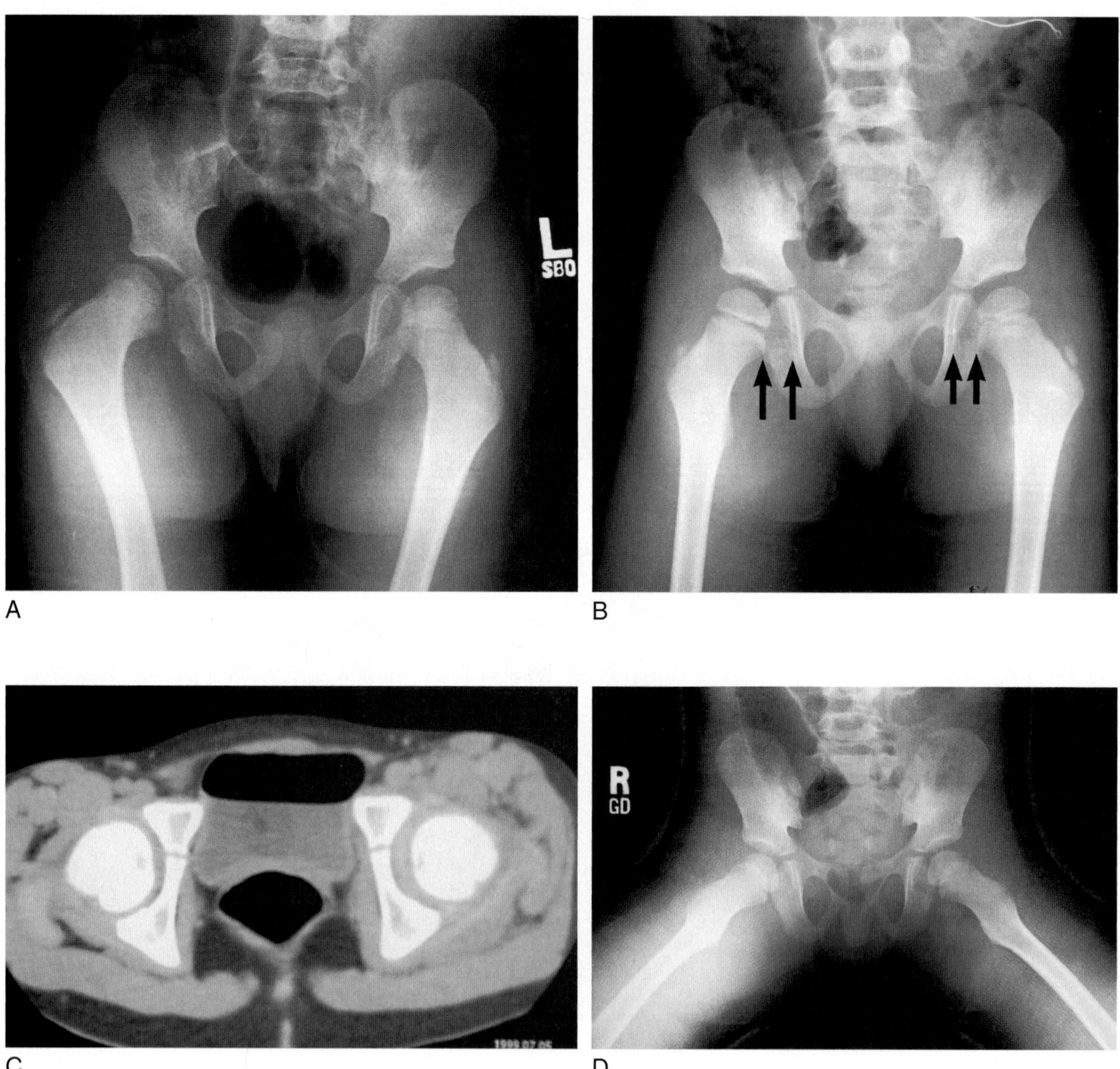

FIGURE 43–33 Nonconcentric reduction of a posterior hip dislocation. **A,** Posterior hip dislocation in a 5-year-old child. **B,** Postreduction anteroposterior radiograph showing increased medial joint space (*arrows*). **C,** Nonconcentric reduction is confirmed with computed tomography. **D,** Open reduction with removal of interposed soft tissue was followed by casting.

initial maneuver is to flex the adducted and medially rotated thigh 90 degrees while longitudinal traction is applied in line with the deformity. This will relax the Y ligament and bring the femoral head near the posterior rim of the acetabulum. The femoral head is then freed from the rotator muscles by gently rotating the thigh back and forth. Finally, the femoral head is levered into the acetabulum by gentle abduction, lateral rotation, and extension of the hip. Manipulation should always be gentle to prevent rupture of the Y ligament or damage to the sciatic nerve. The prone position is required for the Stimson technique, which is difficult to perform in a larger child but can be used in a younger patient (Fig. 43–36).

Anterior Dislocation. To reduce an anterior dislocation of the hip, a modification of the Allis technique entails initially flexing the knee to relax the hamstrings while the hip is fully abducted and flexed to 90 degrees (Fig. 43–37). Traction should be applied directly in line with the longitudinal axis of the femur while an assistant applies posterior pressure on the anteriorly dislocated femoral head. The surgeon then adducts the hip, with the patient's thigh used as the lever, to reduce the femoral head into the acetabulum. The hip can be medially rotated as it is adducted to achieve reduction.

Central Dislocation. Central dislocations require skeletal traction through a distal femoral pin to reduce the femoral head to its anatomic position. Because a central dislocation is associated with an acetabular fracture, which is often comminuted, the medially displaced femoral head must be initially reduced to its anatomic position. This is best accomplished with a skeletal traction pin (Schanz pin placed in a lateromedial direction or a skeletal traction pin placed in the

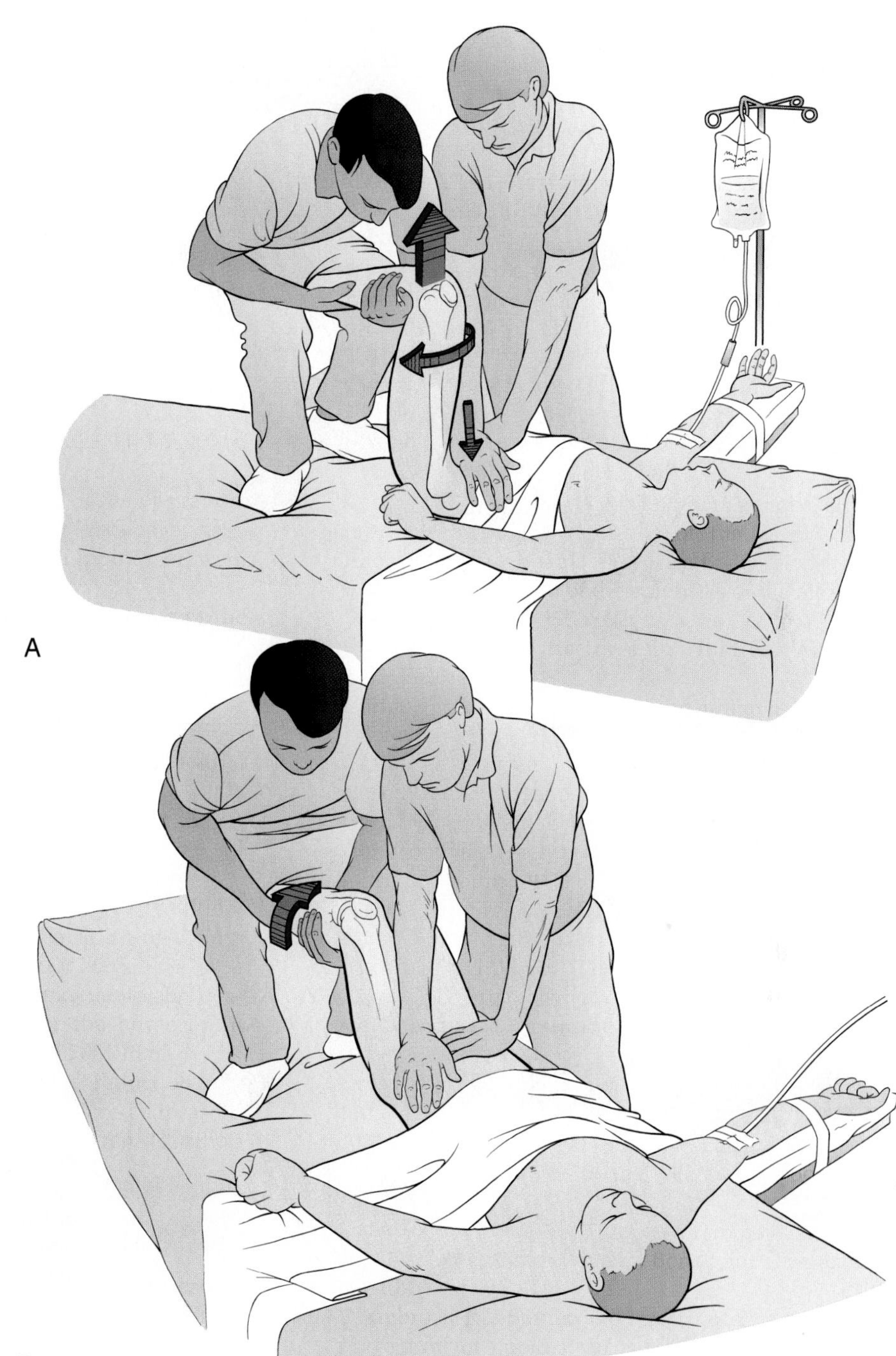

FIGURE 43–34 Allis' direct method for reducing a posterior hip dislocation. **A,** Longitudinal traction through 90 degrees flexed hip with slowly applied rotation. **B,** Slow return to neutral and extension.

AP direction) in the greater trochanter. Lateral traction can be applied to initially reduce the central dislocation and can then be removed if the reduction is stable, or it can remain for up to 2 to 3 weeks. The distal skeletal traction is maintained for a total of 3 to 4 weeks, with some active range of motion of the hip allowed to promote molding of the acetabulum.

Open Reduction

The indications for open reduction of a dislocated hip are failed closed reduction, nonconcentric closed reduction, and a dislocation associated with a displaced femoral head or neck fracture or an acetabular fracture. The surgical approach depends on the direction of the hip dislocation: a posterior approach for posterior dislocations and an anterior approach for anterior dislocations. The goals of surgical intervention are to clear the obstacles preventing reduction of the hip (piriformis tendon, hip capsule), identify objects preventing concentric reduction (inverted limbus, osteocartilaginous loose bodies), anatomically fix any acetabular or femoral head fractures, and repair the soft tissue envelope. Clinical series suggest that as many as 25% of patients may require open reduction.[28,50]

Posterior Approach. A standard posterior approach (Southern or Moore) to the hip is used (Fig. 43–38).[29]

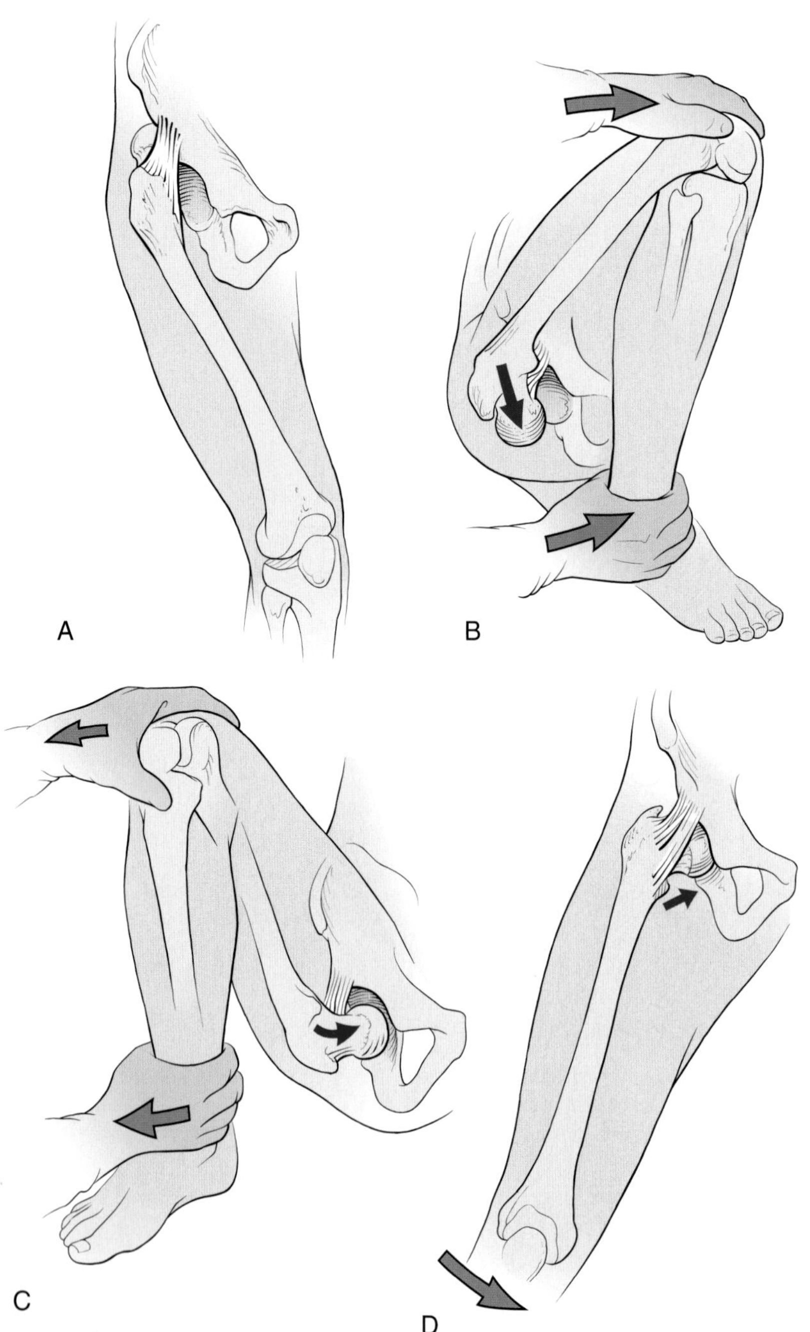

FIGURE 43–35 Bigelow's circumduction method for reducing a traumatic posterior dislocation of the hip. **A,** Posterior hip dislocation. **B,** Hip flexion, thigh adduction, and internal rotation. **C,** Abduction and external rotation. **D,** Return to neutral and extension.

The sciatic nerve should be identified visually and followed both proximally and distally, especially when nerve injury has been identified on the preoperative physical examination. The remaining soft tissue structures should then be inspected and all torn muscles tagged with suture to allow proper closure at completion of the procedure. The short external rotators should be divided 1 cm from their insertion. The femoral head is often protruding through a tear in the posterior capsule, and care should be taken to avoid injuring the articular cartilage at that point. The capsule should be incised to allow complete inspection of the labrum, the posterior wall of the acetabulum, and the articular surfaces of the acetabulum and femoral head. Subluxation or dislocation of the femoral head should be performed to allow good visualization; it is often achieved by means of skeletal traction applied through a Schanz pin placed in the greater trochanter. The joint is irrigated, and any osteocartilaginous debris is removed. Posterior rim fractures should be internally fixed with screws in a young child, and a 3.5-mm pelvic reconstruction plate should be used in an adolescent. Labral avulsions are repaired by fixing the labrum down to the posterior rim of the acetabulum (analogous to a Bankart-type repair in the shoulder), and the posterior capsule should be repaired (see Fig. 43–38C).

Anterior Approach. An anterior approach for an anterior hip dislocation can be either a direct anterior

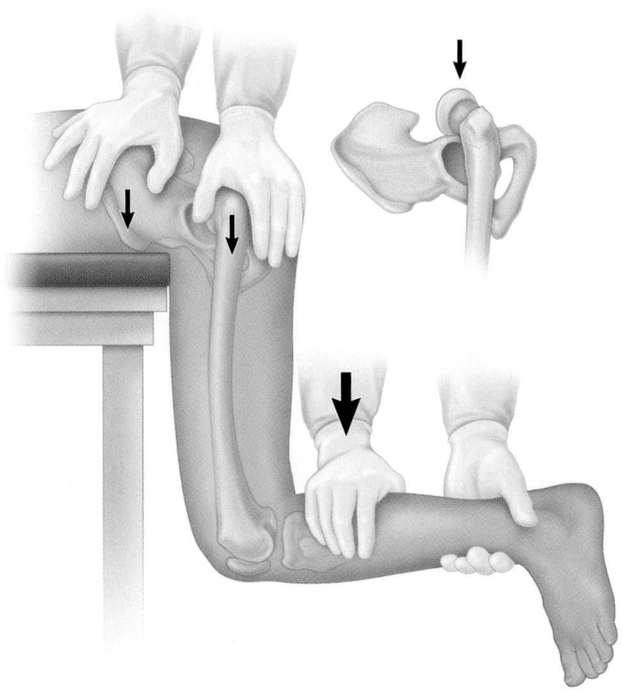

FIGURE 43-36 Stimson's gravity method for reducing a traumatic posterior dislocation of the hip.

(Smith-Peterson) or an anterolateral (Watson-Jones) approach. The literature on surgical intervention for anterior dislocations is sparse because the vast majority are concentrically reduced by closed means.[7,9] However, the goals of surgical treatment remain the same and should be kept in mind when operative intervention is needed.

Postreduction Treatment

Postreduction treatment after concentric reduction depends on the age of the patient and whether associated fractures are present. Children younger than 6 to 7 years should be placed in a hip spica cast with the affected hip in neutral extension and some abduction. An alternative treatment in a young child is a period of skin traction. In an older child, bed rest followed by gradual mobilization on crutches can be used. The period of immobilization or protected motion should be 4 weeks to allow capsular and soft tissue healing. In fracture-dislocations, 6 to 8 weeks of immobilization may be considered to allow fracture healing. After the period of immobilization, partial weight bearing is allowed until there is pain-free full range of motion of the hip, at which time full weight bearing is permitted.[23] Most children will resume full activities and full weight bearing as soon as the immobilization period has ended.[34] Although these guidelines are generally accepted, there is no consensus on the exact duration of immobilization and time to full weight bearing. In addition, there is no correlation between the final result and the period of non–weight bearing after a traumatic hip dislocation.[8,13,14,23,34,40]

COMPLICATIONS

The most common complications after a traumatic hip dislocation in children are AVN of the femoral head, sciatic nerve injury, recurrence of the hip dislocation, late degenerative arthritis, and rarely, femoral arterial injury in anterior dislocations.

Avascular Necrosis. The most frequent complication after a posterior traumatic hip dislocation in children is AVN of the femoral head, with the reported incidence being between 8% and 18%.[13,15,17,23,34] The most important factors predisposing to the development of AVN are older age (>6 years), severe trauma, prereduction or perireduction epiphyseal separation, and a delay of more than 6 hours from the time of injury to the time of reduction (Fig. 43–39).[28] Although radiographic changes can be seen as early as 3 months after injury, AVN can develop up to 2 years later.[13] Therefore, serial radiographs should be obtained for at least 2 years after the original dislocation. Treatment of AVN is difficult and varies with the age of the child. In adolescents, a proximal femoral osteotomy can be performed to position the viable femoral head in the weight-bearing zone.

Sciatic Nerve Palsy. Sciatic nerve palsy is thought to be rare but has been reported in up to 25% of posterior dislocations. It occurs most frequently in older children in the setting of a high-energy injury.[34] In older patients, there is a demonstrated association of delay in reduction of a posterior dislocation with the development of sciatic nerve dysfunction.[20] The sciatic nerve injuries are usually partial, and exploration of the nerve has been recommended in patients who have not demonstrated some recovery by 3 months. Pearson and Mann reported partial return of nerve function in four of five patients (one patient underwent nerve exploration at 3 months), with the fifth patient demonstrating complete recovery.[34]

Recurrent Hip Dislocation. Recurrent hip dislocation is more common in children than in adults, and the reported cases in the literature are all posterior dislocations, usually in children younger than 10 years. No association has been demonstrated between recurrence of a posterior dislocation and the severity of the injury or the type of immobilization used. Some have suggested that a minimum of 2 weeks of immobilization is required to allow the capsule to heal and will lower the incidence of redislocation.[10,18,43] Inadequate healing of the posterior capsule or attenuation of the posterior capsule accounts for the recurrent dislocation and can be treated by open surgical repair[14,25,42,51,52] or by immobilization of the hip in 45 degrees of flexion and 20 degrees of abduction for 4 to 6 weeks.[2,16,52] Evaluation of a recurrent hip dislocation should include CT or MRI to identify loose bodies within the joint and posterior acetabular or femoral head fractures that occurred at the time of redislocation. CT arthrography is useful for identifying a redundant posterior capsule or residual posterior capsular defect, which is seen as

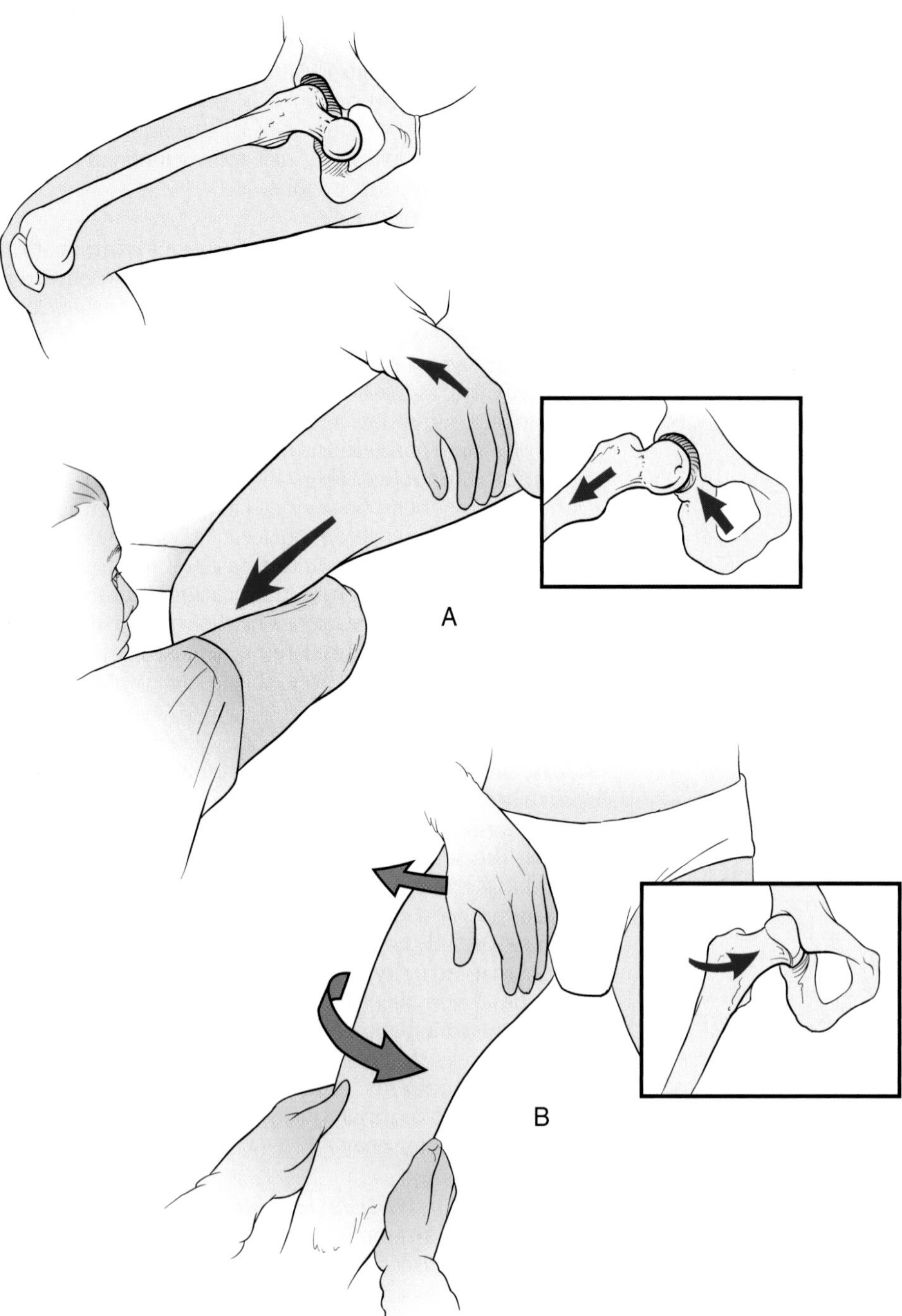

FIGURE 43–37 Allis' method for reducing a traumatic anterior dislocation of the hip. **A,** Longitudinal traction. **B,** Thigh abduction, internal rotation, and return to neutral.

leakage of dye from the capsule.[51] The lesions noted in adults at the time of re-exploration of the hip are labral avulsions,[25,30,38] a tear of the posterior capsule,[24-26,46,49,51] or a markedly attenuated capsule.[16] Operative repair of the torn capsule and a "Bankart-type" repair of the labrum should prevent further dislocation, although supplementation with a posterior bone block has been described.[25,26,38] If a redundant capsule is present, treatment consists of excision of the posterior pouch and repair of the capsular defect.

Degenerative Arthritis. Degenerative arthritis after traumatic hip dislocation is infrequent in the pediatric population and is due to AVN of the femoral head. Predisposing factors may include a delay in reduction, the presence of cartilaginous loose bodies, acetabular labral tears, and nonconcentric reduction secondary to trapped osteocartilaginous fracture fragments or an inverted limbus. When degenerative changes are noted, it is important to look for signs of incomplete reduction. Treatment should be conservative and includes anti-inflammatory medication, modification of activities, and weight control.

Vascular Injury. Vascular injury in anterior dislocations is a surgical emergency that requires prompt

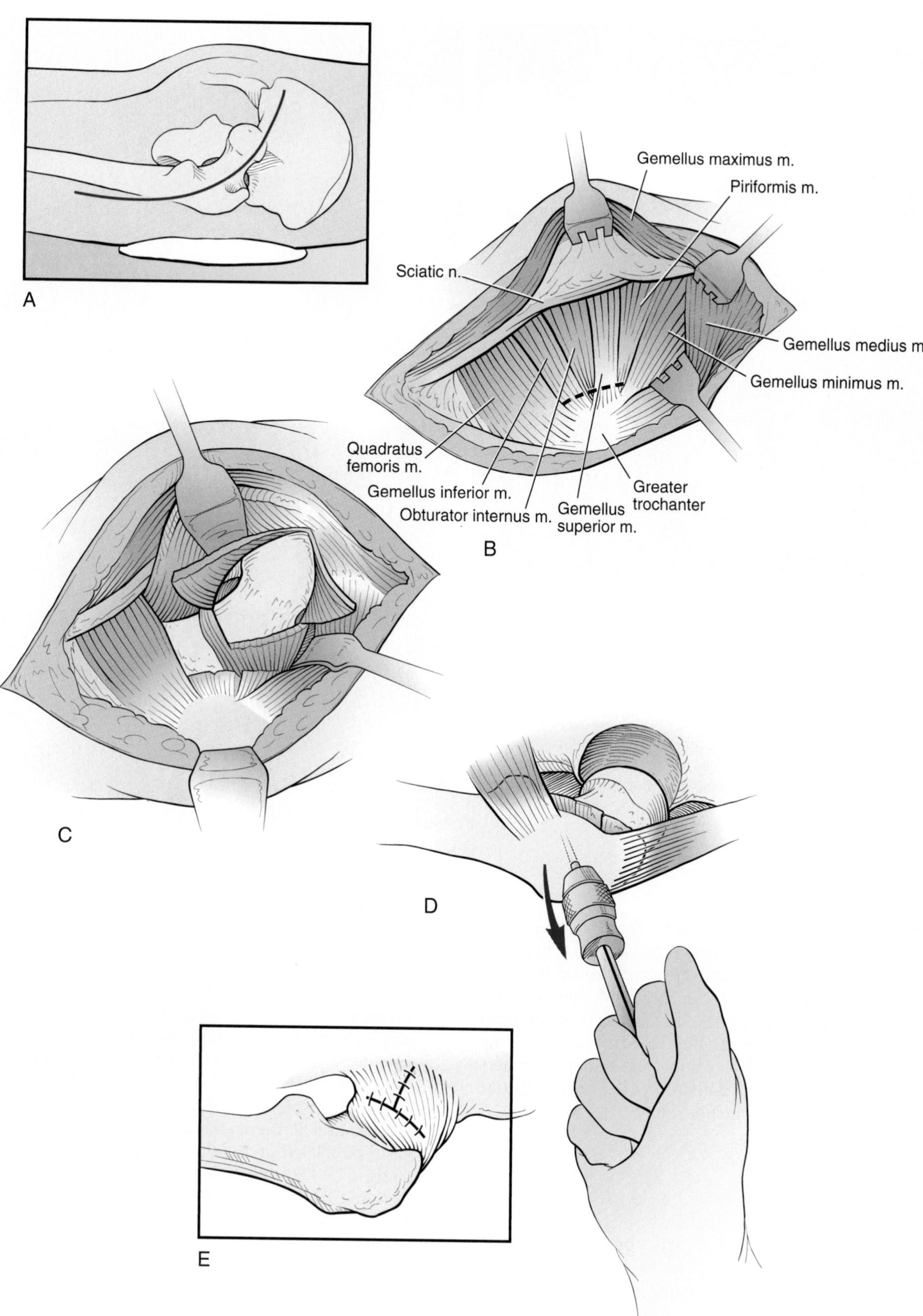

FIGURE 43-38 Posterior approach to the hip. **A,** A skin incision is made from the posterior superior iliac spine over the greater trochanter and down the lateral aspect of the thigh. **B,** The sciatic nerve is identified and retracted. The short rotators are incised at their insertion and retracted. **C,** The posterior capsule, which is partially torn, should be incised to allow visualization of the acetabulum. **D,** A Schanz pin is placed in the greater trochanter to allow the surgeon to distract the femoral head for better observation of the acetabulum. **E,** Repair of labral tears and the capsule.

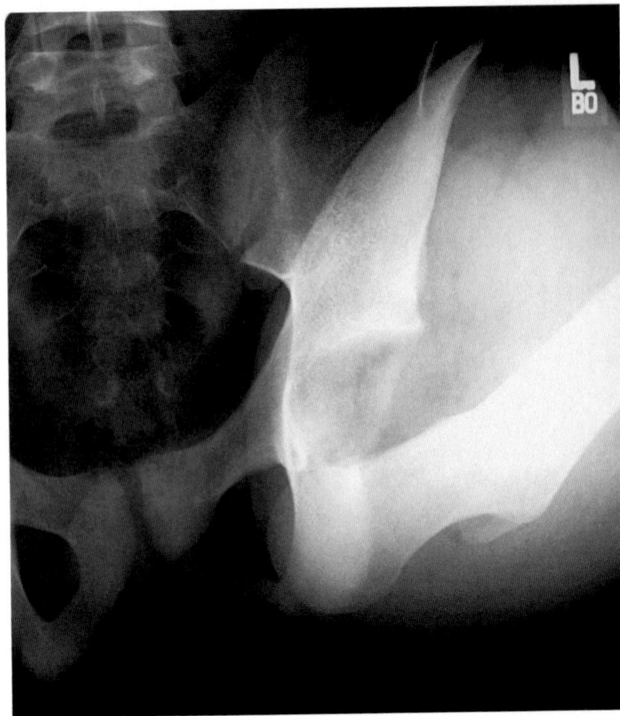

A

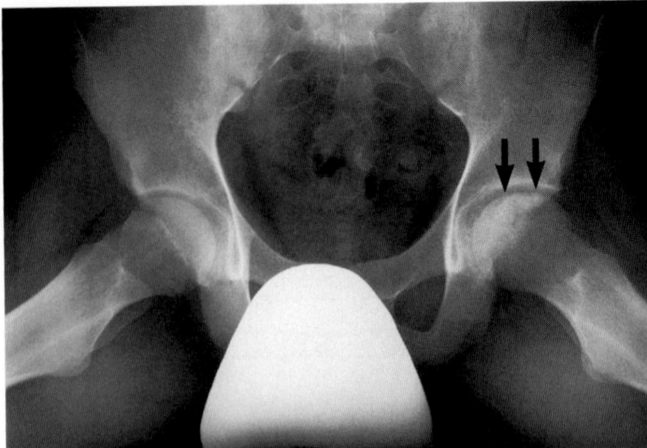

B

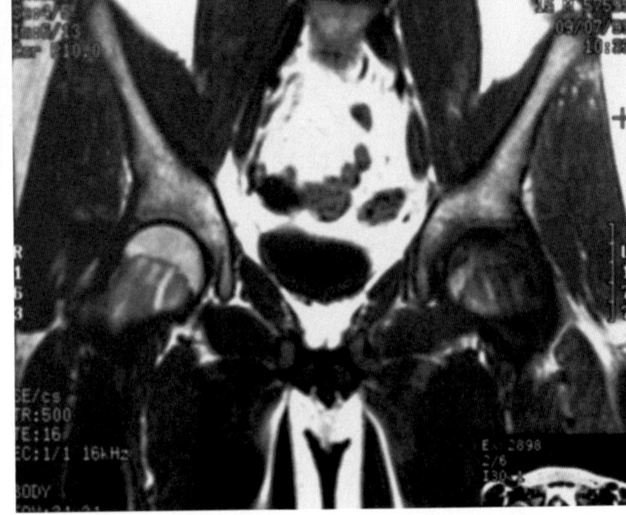

C

FIGURE 43-39 Avascular necrosis (AVN) after hip dislocation in a 15-year-old boy. **A,** Anterior hip dislocation. **B,** Radiographs obtained 6 months after the injury demonstrating AVN (*arrows*). **C,** Magnetic resonance image demonstrating partial femoral head AVN.

reduction of the hip followed by vascular repair.[4,31,42] Examination of the peripheral pulses is extremely important in anterior dislocations and should be done at initial evaluation, after reduction, and then serially over the next 24 to 48 hours. Another rare complication is injury to the triradiate cartilage leading to a shallow acetabulum and hip subluxation.[52] Treatment consists of physeal bar excision if detected early, or acetabular reconstruction when identified late.

References

Hip Dislocations

1. Allis O: An Inquiry into the Difficulties Encountered in the Reduction of Dislocation of the Hip. Philadelphia, 1896.
2. Barquet A: Traumatic hip dislocation with fracture of the ipsilateral femoral shaft in childhood. Report of a case and review of the literature. Arch Orthop Trauma Surg 1981;98:69.
3. Bigelow H: The Mechanics of Dislocation and Fracture of the Hip with the Reduction of the Dislocations by the Flexion Method. Philadelphia, Henry C. Lea, 1869.
4. Bonnemaison MF, Henderson ED: Traumatic anterior dislocation of the hip with acute common femoral occlusion in a child. J Bone Joint Surg Am 1968;50:753.
5. Canale ST, Manugian AH: Irreducible traumatic dislocations of the hip. J Bone Joint Surg Am 1979;61:7.
6. Choyce C: Traumatic dislocation of the hip in childhood and relation of trauma to pseudocoxalgia: Analysis of 59 cases published up to Jan 1924. Br J Surg 1924;12:52.
7. Craig CL: Hip injuries in children and adolescents. Orthop Clin North Am 1980;11:743.
8. Epstein HC: Traumatic dislocations of the hip. Clin Orthop Relat Res 1973;92:116.
9. Epstein HC, Wiss DA: Traumatic anterior dislocation of the hip. Orthopedics 1985;8:130.
10. Freeman GE Jr: Traumatic dislocation of the hip in children: A report of 7 cases and a review of the literature. J Bone Joint Surg Am 1961;43:401.
11. Funk F: Traumatic dislocation of the hip in children: Factors affecting prognosis and treatment. J Bone Joint Surg Am 1962;44:1135.

12. Garcia Mata S, Hidalgo Ovejero A, Martinez Grande M: Open anterior dislocation of the hip in a child. J Pediatr Orthop B 1998;7:232.
13. Gartland JJ, Benner JH: Traumatic dislocations in the lower extremity in children. Orthop Clin North Am 1976;7:687.
14. Gaul RW: Recurrent traumatic dislocation of the hip in children. Clin Orthop Relat Res 1973;90:107.
15. Glass A, Powell H: Traumatic dislocation of the hip in children. J Bone Joint Surg Br 1961;43:29.
16. Graham B, Lapp RA: Recurrent posttraumatic dislocation of the hip. A report of two cases and review of the literature. Clin Orthop Relat Res 1990;256:115.
17. Haliburton RA, Breckenshire F, Barber J: Avascular necrosis of the femoral capital epiphysis after traumatic dislocation of the hip in children. J Bone Joint Surg Br 1961;43:43.
18. Heinzelmann PR, Nelson CL: Recurrent traumatic dislocation of the hip. Report of a case. J Bone Joint Surg Am 1976;58:895.
19. Herrera-Soto JA, Price CT, Reuss BL, et al: Proximal femoral epiphysiolysis during reduction of hip dislocation in adolescents. J Pediatr Orthop 2006;26:371.
20. Hillyard RF, Fox J: Sciatic nerve injuries associated with traumatic posterior hip dislocations. Am J Emerg Med 2003;21:545.
21. Huo MH, Root L, Buly RL, et al: Traumatic fracture-dislocation of the hip in a 2-year-old child. Orthopedics 1992;15:1430.
22. Klasen HJ, Binnendijk B: Fracture of the neck of the femur associated with posterior dislocation of the hip. J Bone Joint Surg Br 1984;66:45.
23. Libri R, Calderon JE, Capelli A, et al: Traumatic dislocation of the hip in children and adolescents. Ital J Orthop Traumatol 1986;12:61.
24. Liebenberg F, Dommisse GF: Recurrent post-traumatic dislocation of the hip. J Bone Joint Surg Br 1969;51:632.
25. Lieberman JR, Altchek DW, Salvati EA: Recurrent dislocation of a hip with a labral lesion: Treatment with a modified Bankart-type repair. Case report. J Bone Joint Surg Am 1993;75:1524.
26. Lutter LD: Post-traumatic hip redislocation. J Bone Joint Surg Am 1973;55:391.
27. Mass DP, Spiegel PG, Laros GS: Dislocation of the hip with traumatic separation of the capital femoral epiphysis: Report of a case with successful outcome. Clin Orthop Relat Res 1980;146:184.
28. Mehlman CT, Hubbard GW, Crawford AH, et al: Traumatic hip dislocation in children. Long-term followup of 42 patients. Clin Orthop Relat Res 2000;376:68.
29. Moore A: The Moore self-locking Vitallium prosthesis in fresh femoral neck fractures: A new low posterior approach (the Southern exposure). In American Academy of Orthopaedic Surgeons Instructional Course Lectures, vol 16. St Louis, CV Mosby, 1959.
30. Nelson CL: Traumatic recurrent dislocation of the hip. Report of a case. J Bone Joint Surg Am 1970;52:128.
31. Nerubay J: Traumatic anterior dislocation of hip joint with vascular damage. Clin Orthop Relat Res 1976;116:129.
32. Odent T, Glorion C, Pannier S, et al: Traumatic dislocation of the hip with separation of the capital epiphysis: 5 adolescent patients with 3-9 years of follow-up. Acta Orthop Scand 2003;74:49.
33. Patterson I: The torn acetabular labrum: A block to reduction of a dislocated hip. J Bone Joint Surg Br 1957;39:306.
34. Pearson DE, Mann RJ: Traumatic hip dislocation in children. Clin Orthop Relat Res 1973;92:189.
35. Pennsylvania Orthopaedic Society: Traumatic dislocation of the hip joint in children: A final report by the Scientific Research Society. J Bone Joint Surg Am 1968;50:79.
36. Price CT, Pyevich MT, Knapp DR, et al: Traumatic hip dislocation with spontaneous incomplete reduction: A diagnostic trap. J Orthop Trauma 2002;16:730.
37. Proctor H: Dislocations of the hip joint (excluding "central" dislocations) and their complications. Injury 1973;5:1.
38. Rashleigh-Belcher HJ, Cannon SR: Recurrent dislocation of the hip with a "Bankart-type" lesion. J Bone Joint Surg Br 1986;68:398.
39. Rubel IF, Kloen P, Potter HG, et al: MRI assessment of the posterior acetabular wall fracture in traumatic dislocation of the hip in children. Pediatr Radiol 2002;32:435.
40. Schlonsky J, Miller PR: Traumatic hip dislocations in children. J Bone Joint Surg Am 1973;55:1057.
41. Schmidt GL, Sciulli R, Altman GT: Knee injury in patients experiencing a high-energy traumatic ipsilateral hip dislocation. J Bone Joint Surg Am 2005;87:1200.
42. Schwartz DL, Haller JA Jr: Open anterior hip dislocation with femoral vessel transection in a child. J Trauma 1974;14:1054.
43. Simmons RL, Elder JD: Recurrent posttraumatic dislocation of the hip in children. South Med J 1972;65:1463.
44. Stewart MJ, Milford LW: Fracture-dislocation of the hip; an end-result study. J Bone Joint Surg Am 1954;36:315.
45. Stimson L: Treatise on Dislocation. Philadelphia, Lea Brothers, 1888.
46. Sullivan CR, Bickel WH, Lipscomb PR: Recurrent dislocation of the hip. J Bone Joint Surg Am 1955;37:1266.
47. Tabuenca J, Truan JR: Knee injuries in traumatic hip dislocation. Clin Orthop Relat Res 2000;377:78.
48. Thompson S: Traumatic dislocation of the hip. In Proceedings of the Sheffield Regional Orthopaedic Club. J Bone Joint Surg Br 1951;42:858.
49. Townsend R, Edwards G, Bazant F, et al: Posttraumatic recurrent dislocation of the hip without fracture. J Bone Joint Surg Br 1969;51:194.
50. Vialle R, Odent T, Pannier S, et al: Traumatic hip dislocation in childhood. J Pediatr Orthop 2005;25:138.
51. Weber M, Ganz R: Recurrent traumatic dislocation of the hip: Report of a case and review of the literature. J Orthop Trauma 1997;11:382.
52. Wilchinsky ME, Pappas AM: Unusual complications in traumatic dislocation of the hip in children. J Pediatr Orthop 1985;5:534.

Hip Fractures

When compared with hip fractures in adults, hip fractures in children are relatively rare and account for less than 1% of all pediatric fractures. The vast majority of hip fractures in children, 80% to 90%, are due to high-energy trauma; the rest are due to moderate trauma or pathologic conditions.

Hip fractures are classified according to their anatomic location, with femoral neck fractures (transcervical or cervicotrochanteric) being the most common. Treatment of most hip fractures in children consists of closed or open reduction and internal fixation, followed by a period of external immobilization. Despite advances in operative technique and more aggressive treatment, the rate of complications from pediatric hip fractures (AVN, coxa vara, premature physeal closure, malunion, nonunion) remains relatively high.

ANATOMY

The proximal femur consists of a single physis at birth that later separates into two distinct centers of ossification—the capital epiphysis and the trochanteric apophysis. Ossification of the femoral epiphysis occurs between 4 and 6 months of age, and the ossific nucleus (Fig. 43–40) of the greater trochanter appears at 4 years. The femoral neck–shaft angle is 135 degrees at birth, increases to approximately 145 degrees by 1 to 3 years of age, and gradually matures to an angle of 130 degrees at skeletal maturity.[18,50,60] Femoral anteversion is approximately 30 degrees at birth and decreases to an average of 10.4 degrees at skeletal maturity.[49,60] The trochanteric physis closes between 16 and 18 years and the proximal femoral physis at approximately 18 years. Growth arrest of the proximal femoral physis before skeletal maturity may result in an abnormal neck–shaft angle, femoral anteversion, and a reduced articulotrochanteric distance (Fig. 43–41). In addition, because the proximal femoral physis contributes approximately 15% of the growth of the entire extremity, mild limb length discrepancy may occur.

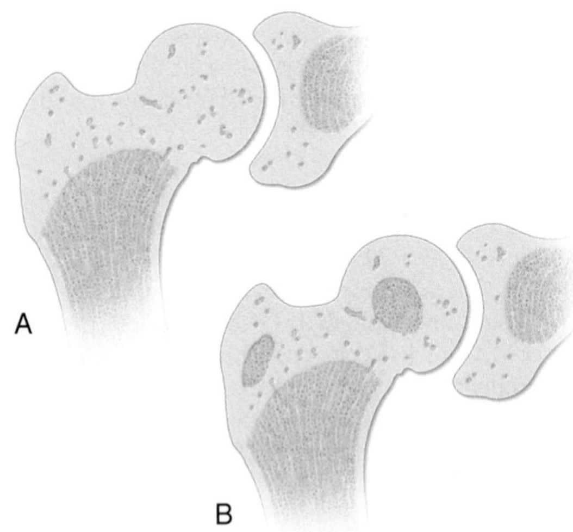

FIGURE 43–40 **A,** The proximal femoral epiphysis is a single physis at birth. **B,** At approximately 4 years of age, the single growth center divides into a separate greater trochanteric and femoral head growth center.

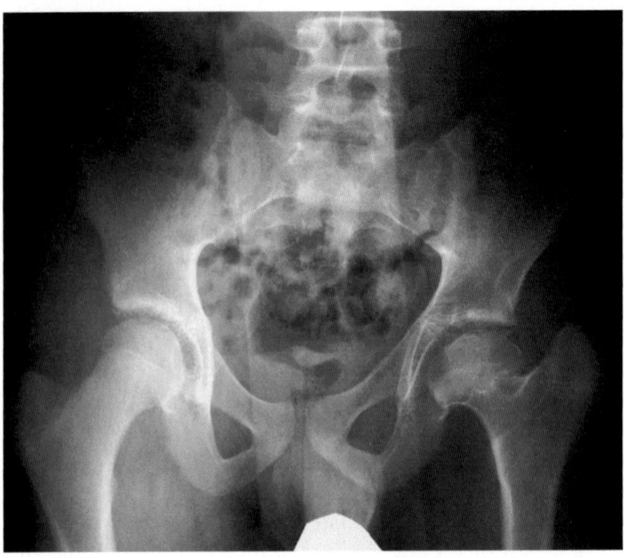

FIGURE 43–41 Proximal physeal growth arrest of the left hip with subsequent coxa breva, coxa magna, and a decreased articulotrochanteric distance after a transcervical hip fracture.

Because of the high incidence of AVN of the femoral head, it is important to understand the vascular anatomy of the proximal femur. It has been extensively studied by Chung,[11] Ogden,[40] and Trueta.[58] The blood supply of the proximal femur comes from two major branches of the profunda femoris artery—the medial and lateral circumflex arteries, which originate at the level of the tendinous portion of the iliopsoas muscle (Fig. 43–42). The lateral circumflex artery travels posterior to the femoral neck, and the medial circumflex artery travels anterior to it. The transverse branch of the lateral circumflex artery divides at the anterolateral border of the intertrochanteric line and gives off branches that penetrate the lateral and anterolateral portions of the greater trochanter. Until the age of 5 to 6 months this branch also supplies much of the anterior portion of the proximal femoral epiphysis and physis.

The major blood supply to the proximal femur comes from the medial circumflex artery, which travels posterior to the iliopsoas tendon and then to the medial side of the proximal femur between the insertion of the inferomedial capsule and the lesser trochanter. Two major branches of the medial circumflex artery are then given off—the posterior inferior branch, which travels along the inferior margin of the posterior neck, and the posterior superior branch, which travels along the superior margin.

At birth the lateral circumflex artery supplies the anterolateral growth plate, the major aspect of the greater trochanter, and the anteromedial aspect of the femoral head. The medial circumflex artery branches to provide blood to the posteromedial proximal epiphysis, the posterior physis, and the posterior aspect of the greater trochanter. The artery of the ligamentum teres supplies a small area of the medial femoral head. Blood vessels, which cross the physis at

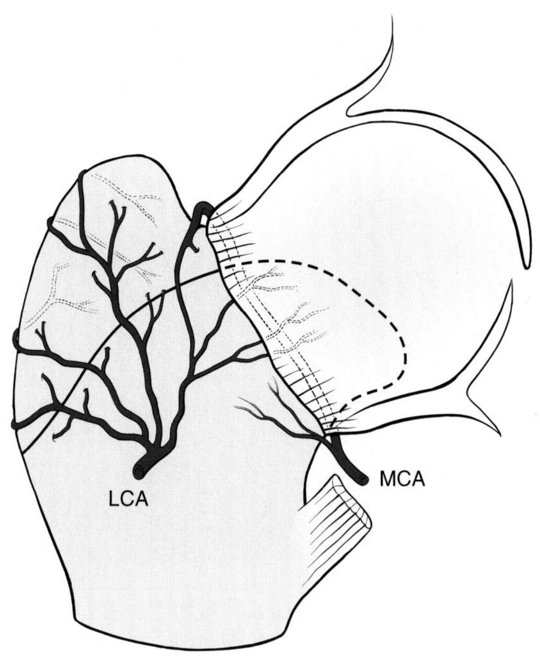

FIGURE 43–42 Blood supply to the femoral head from the medial circumflex artery (MCA) and lateral circumflex artery (LCA), branches of the deep femoral artery at the level of the tendinous portion of the iliopsoas muscle.

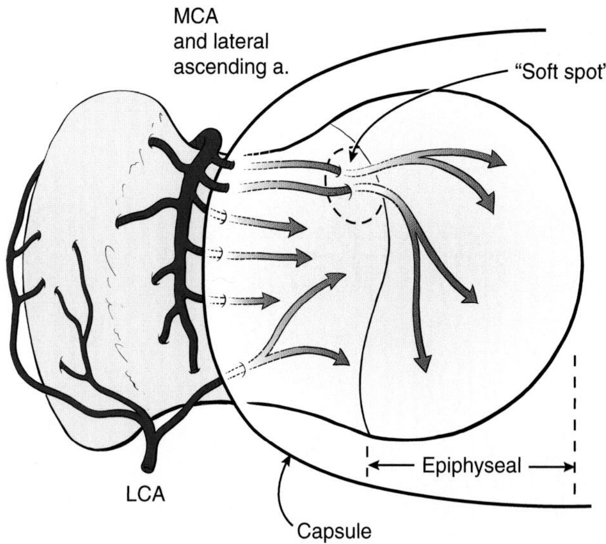

FIGURE 43–43 The medial circumflex artery (MCA) and lateral circumflex artery (LCA) as they enter the femoral head. The major blood supply comes from the lateral cervical ascending artery, a branch of the MCA.

birth, gradually disappear by the age of 15 to 18 months, at which time no vessels are observed crossing the growth plate.

By the age of 3 years the contribution of the lateral circumflex vessel to the blood supply of the proximal femur diminishes and the entire blood supply of the proximal femoral epiphysis and physis comes from the lateral epiphyseal vessels, branches derived from the medial circumflex artery (Fig. 43–43). The posterosuperior and posteroinferior vessels were thought to have prominent roles in the blood supply to the femoral head by Ogden,[40] although Trueta and Morgan[59] thought that the lateral cervical ascending artery (posterosuperior branch) played a more significant role. These vessels lie external to the joint capsule at the level of the intertrochanteric line and then traverse the capsule and travel proximally within the retinacular folds. Very few vessels supplying the femoral head travel within the capsule, and therefore a capsulotomy incision should not compromise the vascularity of the femoral head.[40] This arrangement of the blood supply to the femoral head persists into adulthood. The artery of the ligamentum teres, a branch of the obturator (80%) or the medial circumflex (20%), provides approximately 20% of the blood supply to the femoral head beginning at approximately 8 years of age and is maintained into adulthood.[40,59]

MECHANISM OF INJURY

Hip fractures in children are most frequently the result of severe high-energy trauma (a fall from a height, a motor vehicle accident, or a fall from a bicycle). Such mechanisms account for approximately 85% to 90% of all fractures.[7,15,23,25,27,29,44,47,61] This differs significantly from the situation in the elderly adult population, in which hip fractures are common and result from minimal trauma, most commonly a fall. Because of the significant energy required to produce these fractures in children, associated major injuries are seen in up to 30% of cases.[29,47] Intra-abdominal or intrapelvic visceral injuries and head injuries are the most common associated injuries.[47] Other musculoskeletal injuries seen less often include hip dislocations and pelvic and femoral shaft fractures.[19,26] Because of these associated injuries, any child with a hip fracture must be carefully evaluated.

A small fraction of patients sustain hip fractures from trivial trauma, often associated with a pathologic lesion in the area of the fracture. The most common preexisting conditions include a unicameral bone cyst, osteogenesis imperfecta, fibrous dysplasia, myelomeningocele, and osteopenia from previous polio.[7,27,29,61]

Finally, child abuse may cause hip fractures in children younger than 12 months.[22,61]

CLASSIFICATION

Fractures of the hip in children are classified into four types based on the anatomic location of the fracture as described by Delbet[16] and later popularized by Colonna[13] (Fig. 43–44):

Type I: Transepiphyseal—acute traumatic separation of a previously normal physis (Fig. 43–45). This type of fracture accounts for less than 10% of all children's hip fractures. In 13 reported series, 43 (8%) of 511 hip fractures in children were type I.* Anatomically, these are similar to

*See references 8-10, 15, 23, 25, 27, 29, 42, 44, 47, 56, 61.

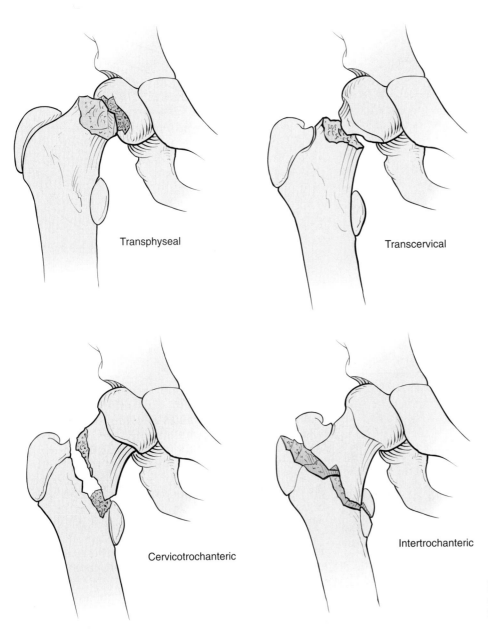

Transphyseal

Transcervical

Cervicotrochanteric

Intertrochanteric

FIGURE 43–44 Delbet's classification of children's hip fractures.

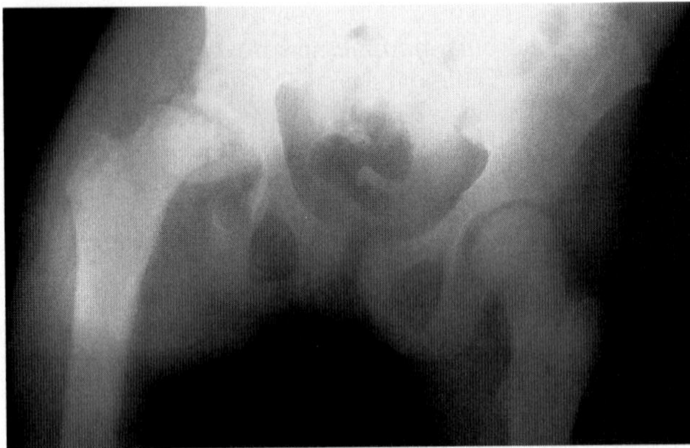

FIGURE 43–45 Transepiphyseal hip fracture in a 10-year-old child with posterior dislocation of the epiphysis.

the type I physeal injury of Salter and Harris and can be distinguished from a slipped capital femoral epiphysis (SCFE) by the younger age of the patient (8 to 9 years), the usually sudden onset of pain secondary to severe trauma, and radiographs showing a more displaced acute separation of the physis. This injury predominantly occurs in two age groups: young infants (<2 years)[20,22,31,41] and children 5 to 10 years of age.[27,47] In a newborn it is known as proximal femoral epiphysiolysis and follows breech delivery; it may be mistaken for congenital dislocation of the hip. The injury is usually recognized late (>2 weeks), after the formation of abundant callus.[41,64] It has also been described in adolescent patients after attempted closed reduction of a posterior hip dislocation.[19,26]

The mechanism of injury is usually severe trauma, often from being struck by a car[45] or a

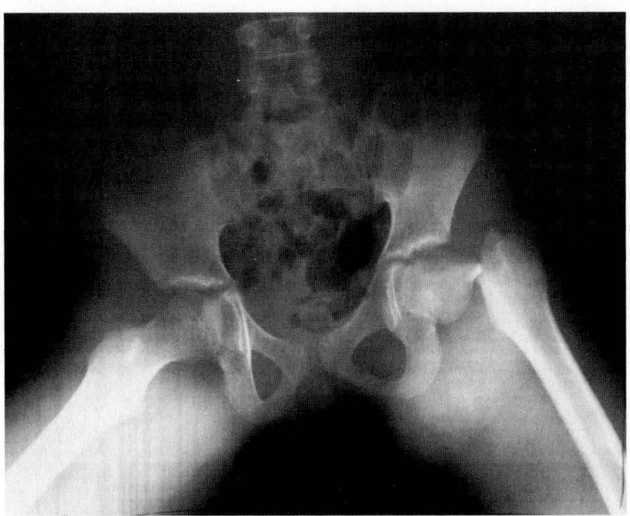

FIGURE 43-46 Transcervical or femoral neck fracture.

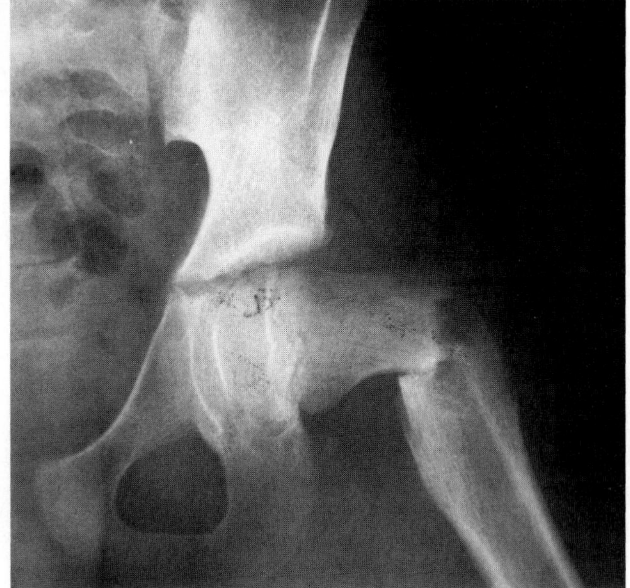

FIGURE 43-47 Left cervicotrochanteric hip fracture in a 9-year-old child.

fall from a height, but it has also been reported in victims of child abuse[20,22] and during difficult labor.[25] It is associated with femoral head dislocation in approximately 50% of cases.[8,20,21,26] Associated injuries occur in up to 60% of cases, with pelvic fractures, often bilateral, being the most common.[45] The results of treatment are relatively poor, with a reported 20% to 100% incidence of AVN of the femoral head.[7,27,29,47]

Type II: Transcervical—fracture through the midportion of the femoral neck (Fig. 43–46). This is the most common fracture type and accounts for 40% to 50% of hip fractures. In the literature, 229 (45%) of 511 hip fractures in children were type II.* These fractures are the result of severe trauma, and the majority (70% to 80%) are displaced when initially seen. The most common complication is AVN, which has historically been reported to occur in up to 50% of patients.[8,27,29,47] However, recent studies that have relied on more aggressive treatment, including evacuation of intracapsular hematoma, have reported a significant reduction in the incidence of AVN.[6,9,56] The best predictor of AVN is displacement of the fracture at the time of injury.[47] Other complications, including loss of reduction, malunion, nonunion, varus deformity, and premature epiphyseal closure, result in relatively poor outcomes when compared with the outcomes of types III and IV fractures.

Type III: Cervicotrochanteric—fracture through the base of the femoral neck (Fig. 43–47). The reported incidence is between 25% and 35%. Of 511 hip fractures, 171 (33%) were type III.* AVN occurs in approximately 20% to 25% of cases and is related to the amount of displacement at the time of injury.

*See references 8-10, 15, 23, 25, 27, 29, 42, 44, 47, 56, 61.

Type IV: Pertrochanteric or intertrochanteric—fracture between the greater and lesser trochanters (Fig. 43–48). The reported incidence is between 6% and 15%. Of 511 hip fractures, 68 (13%) were type IV.* AVN occurs infrequently (<10%), and these fractures have the best overall outcome.

Hip fractures that do not fit into the Delbet classification include fractures of the proximal metaphysis in newborns and stress fractures. Proximal metaphyseal fractures will often be confused with dislocation of the hip because the capital femoral and greater trochanteric epiphyses are not yet ossified (Fig. 43–49). Stress fractures of the femoral neck have been reported in fewer than 20 cases in the literature; the child has a history of a minor injury and vague hip pain.[33,53,55,65] The fracture is often missed on initial evaluation, which may lead to displacement requiring operative intervention (Fig. 43–50).[55,65]

CLINICAL FEATURES

The patient is initially seen after a severe traumatic event with complaints of severe pain in the hip. The history should include the mechanism of injury and a description of other areas of pain. Because of the severity of the hip pain, the patient may not provide a good description of other painful areas, and therefore the examiner must take care to rule out associated injuries. Conversely, other severe injuries can obscure the diagnosis of a hip fracture. Lam reported 75 hip fractures in children, 15 of which were first diagnosed after a period ranging from 1 week to 8 months.[29] One of the principal reasons for a missed diagnosis was the presence of a more serious concomitant injury

*See references 8-10, 15, 23, 25, 27, 29, 42, 44, 47, 56, 61.

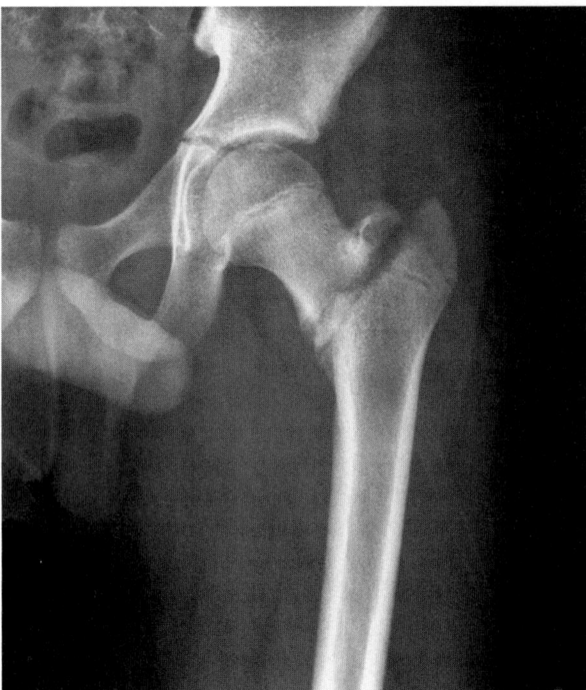
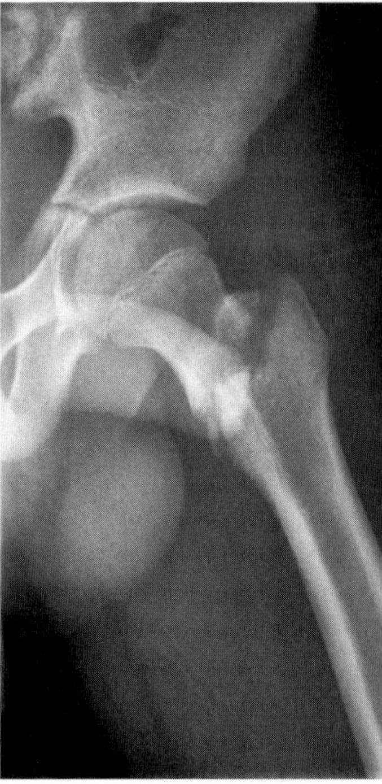

FIGURE 43-48 Left intertrochanteric hip fracture in a 10-year-old child.

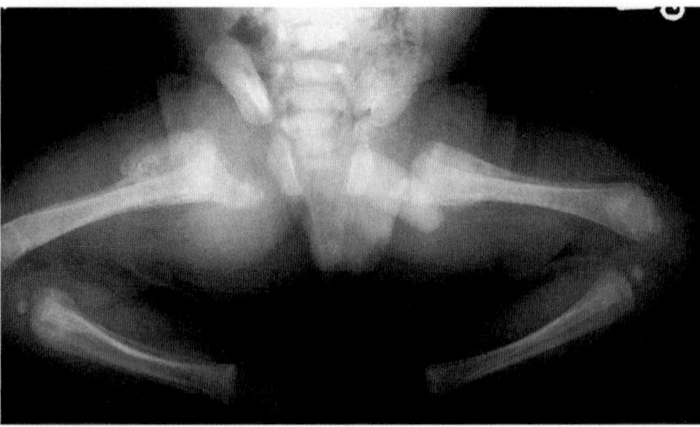

FIGURE 43-49 Proximal femoral metaphyseal fracture in a young infant demonstrating abundant callus formation. Note the multiple fractures in this child abuse case.

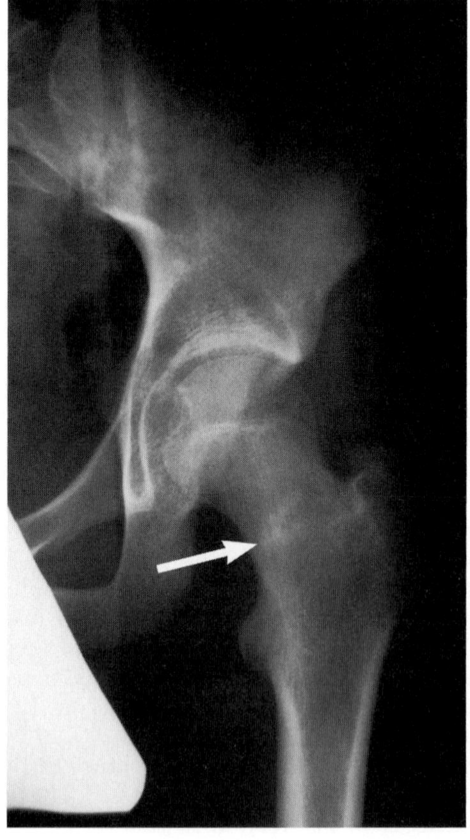

FIGURE 43-50 Stress fracture of the femoral neck (*arrow*).

overshadowing the hip fracture. Undisplaced hip fractures and stress fractures, which occur in approximately 30% of cases,[25,47] may not produce severe pain. The patient may be ambulating at the time of evaluation after a "twisting" or "sprain" of the hip from a slip or athletic mishap.[33,53,55,65]

On physical examination a patient with a displaced hip fracture will hold the injured limb laterally rotated and slightly adducted, and the limb will appear shortened. The patient is in severe pain and unable to actively move the limb. If a dislocation is present, the extremity is held in flexion, adduction, and internal rotation. Local tenderness is elicited on palpation and is most severe posteriorly over the femoral neck. Passive motion of the extremity is markedly restricted, especially with flexion, abduction, and medial rotation. In a nondisplaced fracture the hip examination may not be remarkable, with very mild discomfort elicited during passive range of motion of the extremity. In addition, the patient may be able to ambulate with very little pain. A careful, detailed history, physical examination, and radiographic evaluation are important in these patients to avoid missing the diagnosis.

RADIOGRAPHIC FINDINGS

Radiographic evaluation consists of AP and lateral images of the hip. The radiographs should be analyzed for the type of fracture (Delbet classification), the direction of the fracture line, the amount of displacement, the degree of varus, and the location of the femoral epiphysis. Comparison views of the other hip may assist the surgeon in determining whether a nondisplaced fracture of the femoral neck is present. Such a determination is best done by inspecting the proximal end of the femur for any disruption in the normal trabecular pattern. Nondisplaced or stress fractures can be confirmed by radioisotope bone scanning with pinhole magnification.[14,33,55]

Bone scan imaging must be delayed somewhat from the time of the initial injury to allow increased bone metabolism to occur at the fracture site so that false-negative results are avoided. (In the elderly, the general recommendation is to wait 48 to 72 hours from the time of injury.) Although no data exist on the time delay required in a child or adolescent, we recommend delaying bone scan imaging for 24 to 36 hours after injury.

MRI is the best imaging modality for a nondisplaced or stress fracture of the femoral neck because it provides greater accuracy, earlier diagnosis, and shorter hospital stay, with no exposure to radiation.[4,14,24,51-54] MRI will demonstrate decreased signal on a spin-echo T1 image and a correspondingly increased signal as a result of edema or bleeding on T2-weighted images.[53] An additional advantage of MRI over other imaging modalities is that supplemental information can be obtained, including femoral head viability and the presence of associated bone cysts.

TREATMENT

Improvements in surgical techniques and more aggressive treatment have resulted in improved outcomes in children's hip fractures.[7,8] The most important factors to consider before initiating treatment are the age of the child, the type of hip fracture, the amount of fracture displacement, and the angle of the fracture line. Results in young children (<8 years) with nondisplaced fractures or type III or IV fractures are better than those in older children with a displaced type I or II fracture.

The goals of treatment of children's hip fractures are to achieve anatomic reduction and provide stability to the fracture fragments in order to maintain the reduction and allow complete fracture healing. In general, these goals are best achieved in the operating room, with fracture reduction performed under fluoroscopic guidance and fracture stabilization achieved with rigid internal fixation. Hip spica casting should be used in most children's hip fractures (in addition to internal fixation) to immobilize the extremity and allow complete and solid fracture healing. It is occasionally used as the definitive treatment in small children, in children with minimally displaced cervicotrochanteric and intertrochanteric fractures, and in children with a stress fracture of the femoral neck.

Specific treatment plans for each fracture type are described in the following sections.

Type I: Transepiphyseal Fractures

Historically, transepiphyseal fractures have been associated with a high rate of complications, including loss of reduction and subsequent varus angulation, AVN of the femoral head, and premature epiphyseal closure. The literature reports loss of reduction with resultant varus deformity in approximately 35% of transepiphyseal fractures when treated by cast immobilization.

Although the rate of AVN is most dependent on the amount of displacement at the time of injury, loss of reduction should be limited by stable internal fixation (Fig. 43–51). We recommend anatomic reduction with rigid internal fixation followed by cast immobilization. It is important to determine whether the femoral epiphysis is reduced within the acetabulum on the initial radiographs. If the epiphysis is within the acetabulum, gentle closed reduction similar to that for SCFE is performed because the neck is displaced anterior to the epiphysis. The hip is slowly flexed, slightly abducted, and internally rotated while the surgeon observes the fracture under fluoroscopy. Once anatomic reduction is achieved, internal fixation should be performed through a small lateral incision. We recommend smooth Kirschner wires in a child younger than 4 years, 4.0-mm cannulated screws in a child 4 to 7 years, and 5.0- to 6.5-mm cannulated screws in an older child. To limit the risk of premature physeal closure, threads from wires or screws should not be crossing the physis at completion of the procedure.

If the femoral epiphysis is dislocated from the acetabulum, we recommend a single attempt at closed reduction. However, the likelihood of achieving closed reduction in this situation is low. Multiple attempts may predispose to AVN and are not recommended. Canale reported failure of closed reduction in four of five patients with a type I fracture in which the epiphysis was dislocated from the acetabulum; AVN eventually developed in all five children. Therefore, open reduction should be performed initially in this setting or after a single attempt at gentle closed reduction. The majority of fracture-dislocations occur posteriorly and should be approached with a modified Southern (Moore) technique, whereas an anterior fracture-dislocation requires an anterior (Smith-Peterson) approach. The obstacles to reduction are similar to those for a typical hip dislocation (see discussion in Chapter 16, Developmental Dysplasia of the Hip). A separate lateral incision is then made and the fracture is stabilized by rigid internal fixation.

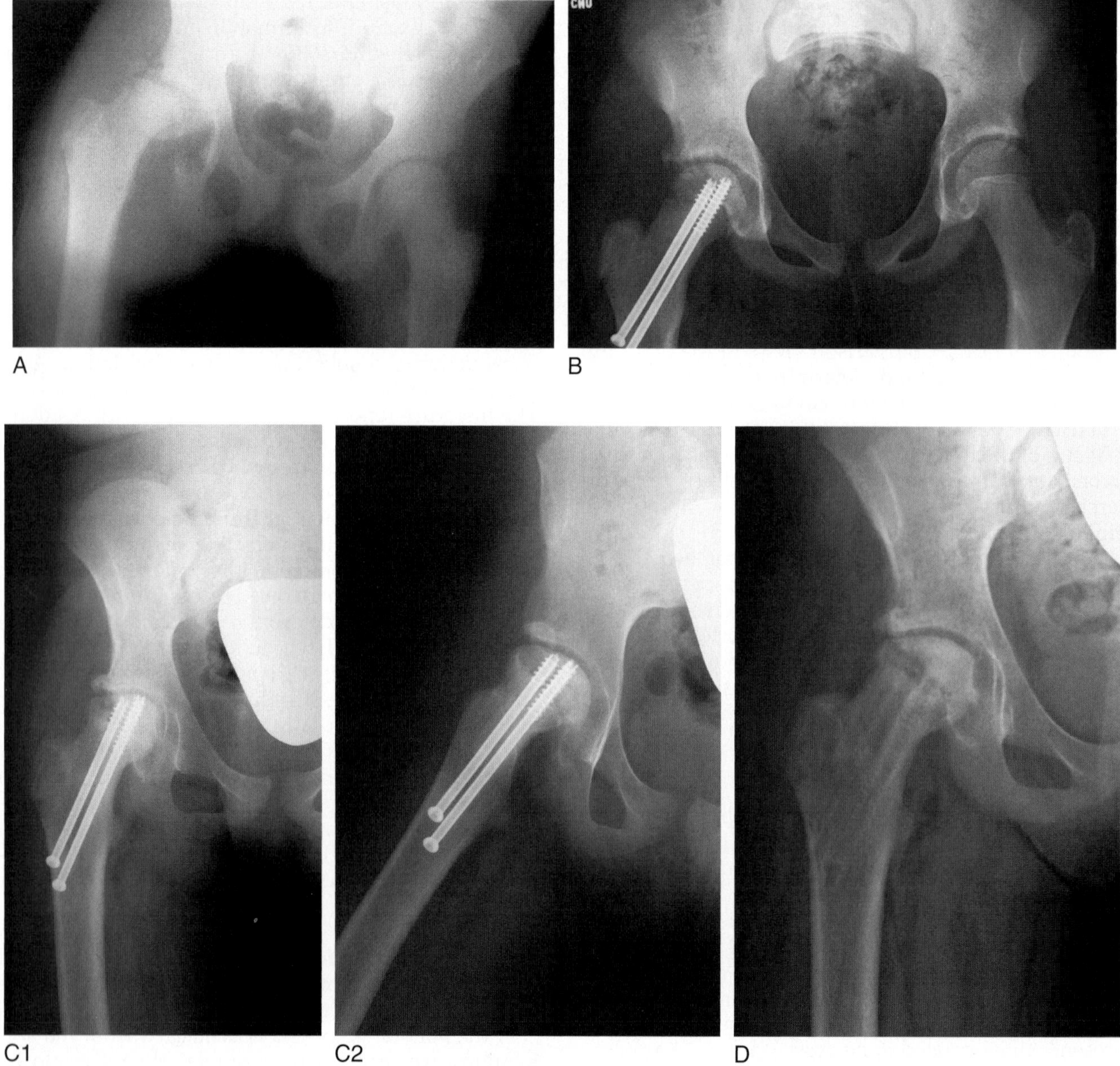

FIGURE 43-51 Transepiphyseal fracture in a 10-year-old that was treated by internal fixation and casting. **A,** Type I fracture-dislocation. **B,** Radiographic appearance after posterior open reduction and internal fixation. Anteroposterior **(C1)** and frog-leg lateral **(C2)** views 4 months later show evidence of avascular necrosis. **D,** Radiographic appearance after screw removal.

We recommend cast immobilization in a one-and-one-half-hip spica cast in all patients after either closed or open reduction and internal fixation. The hip should be positioned in approximately 30 degrees of abduction, neutral extension, and 10 degrees of internal rotation for a minimum of 6 weeks and for up to 12 weeks in an older child if fracture union is delayed. Some surgeons advocate cast immobilization as the principal mode of stabilization in a child younger than 18 months with a transepiphyseal separation because more remodeling potential exists in this age group. However, Forlin and colleagues described five patients with an average age of 15 months who had severely displaced transepiphyseal separations treated by closed reduction and cast immobilization only.[20] Varus angulation developed in all five patients; three required a valgus femoral osteotomy, and in the remaining two patients the varus deformity remodeled. We recommend this treatment in a patient younger than 2 years with minimal or no displacement that does not require manipulation at the time of treatment.

Type II: Transcervical Fractures

We recommend that all transcervical fractures (including nondisplaced fractures) in children of all ages be

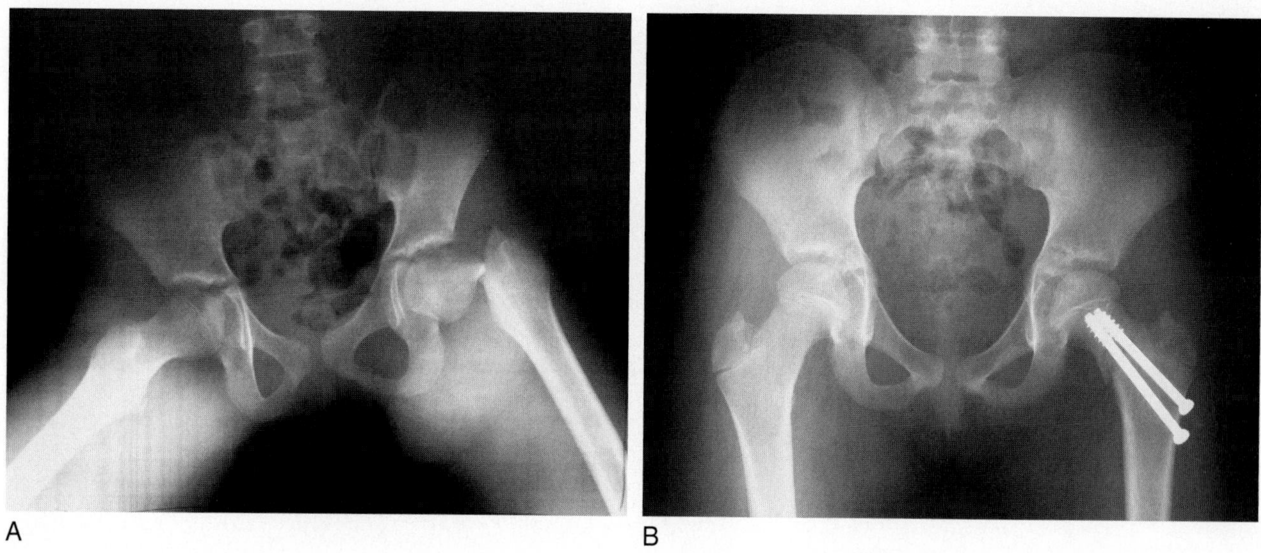

FIGURE 43–52 Transcervical fracture treated by internal fixation and casting. **A,** Injury radiographs of a displaced transcervical hip fracture. **B,** Radiographic appearance after open reduction and internal fixation. Note that the fixation stays distal to the physis.

treated by stable internal fixation to avoid loss of reduction and subsequent malunion, delayed union, or nonunion (Fig. 43–52). These complications are much more common when fractures are stabilized by external immobilization alone.[25,29,47] Anatomic reduction must be achieved to help prevent nonunion, and though not proven, it may diminish the risk for development of AVN. Gentle closed reduction should be attempted under fluoroscopic guidance. The closed reduction maneuver was described in the 1890s by Whitman, who believed that anatomic alignment was mandatory to prevent future deformity.[62,63] The reduction consists of fully abducting the normal hip to stabilize the pelvis, followed by progressive abduction of the extended affected hip. The surgeon then places downward pressure on the greater trochanter and uses the upper border of the acetabular rim as a fulcrum to restore the normal relationship of the proximal femur while the hip is abducted (Fig. 43–53). During abduction of the hip, the extremity is internally rotated to 20 to 30 degrees to complete the reduction maneuver. Once reduction is achieved, the extremity should be slowly adducted to allow placement of internal fixation through a lateral approach.

If closed manipulation fails to achieve anatomic reduction, open reduction through an anterior or anterolateral approach must be performed (Fig. 43–54). Once reduction is achieved, the fracture should be stabilized with threaded Kirschner wires in a young child and cannulated screws in an older child. Internal fixation devices should be kept distal to the physis; however, fracture stability is of prime importance and should not be compromised in an attempt to avoid the growth plate (Fig. 43–55). In an older child a minimum of two screws should be placed parallel to one another and in lag-type fashion, with screw threads in the proximal fracture fragment producing compression across the fracture site. To avoid fracture displacement, we recommend having two guidewires in place while the third guidewire is overdrilled, tapped, and then used as a guide for screw placement.

Cast immobilization in a one-and-one-half-hip spica cast is recommended postoperatively for 6 to 12 weeks until good healing callus is seen. Though still controversial, there is increasing evidence that hip decompression through needle aspiration of the hip joint results in a lower incidence of AVN in type II hip fractures.[9,37,56] Needle aspiration through a subadductor approach has little risk and should be performed after reduction and internal fixation (Fig. 43–56).

Type III: Cervicotrochanteric Fractures

Although type III fractures have a better overall outcome than type II fractures do, a displaced fracture has equally poor results.[8,29]

We recommend that a displaced fracture be treated by closed reduction and internal fixation in all age groups. Nondisplaced fractures in an older child (>6 years) should also be treated by internal fixation (Fig. 43–57). Although some have recommended closed reduction and abduction spica casting without internal fixation, varus deformity develops in 65% to 85% of cases so treated. Undisplaced fractures in a child younger than 6 years may be treated with an abduction cast. In a child younger than 6 years with a displaced fracture, closed reduction and hip spica casting may stabilize the fracture, but maintenance of the reduction relies on the position of the extremity and the molding of the cast. In most cases we prefer the stability of internal fixation. In addition, because of the distal location of this fracture relative to the physis, internal fixation with cannulated screws or Kirschner wires is technically easier than in a type II fracture. However, the distal location of the fracture may not afford good purchase for cannulated screws, which

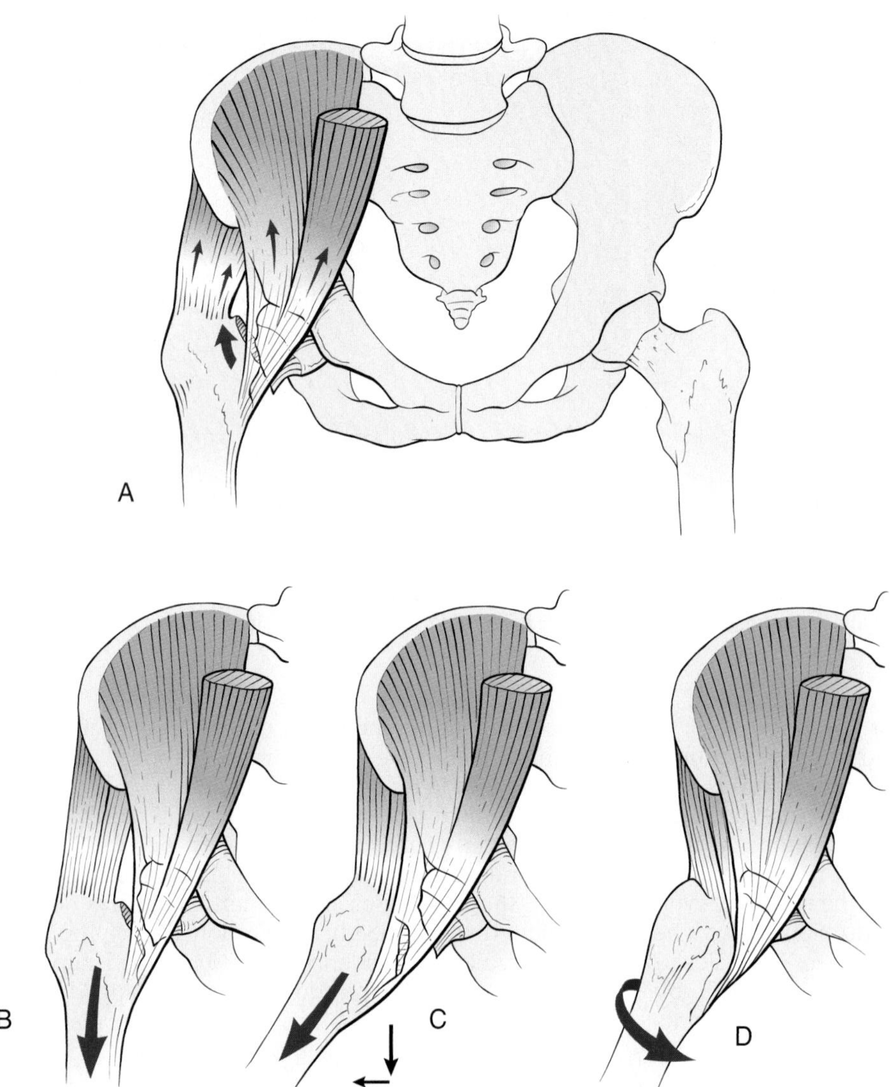

FIGURE 43–53 Closed reduction maneuver to reduce a femoral neck fracture. In-line traction (**A** and **B**) is followed by progressive abduction (**C**) and internal rotation (**D**).

could result in loss of reduction and subsequent varus. We recommend hip spica casting to supplement cannulated screw fixation or the use of a hip screw and side plate construct.

Type IV: Pertrochanteric or Intertrochanteric Fractures

This fracture type results in the best outcome and can often be treated nonoperatively in a child younger than 6 years. As in types II and III fractures, closed reduction with internal fixation is the treatment of choice for a displaced fracture in any age group and for a nondisplaced fracture in an older child (Fig. 43–58).

Stress Fractures

Stress fractures occur predominantly in the adult population as a result of repetitive loading of pathologic bone (rheumatoid arthritis, osteoporosis) or normal bone (military recruits).[5,57] Stress fractures have been subgrouped into the transverse or tension type, which appears as a small radiolucency in the superior part of the femoral neck and requires internal fixation to prevent displacement, and the compression type, which appears as a haze of callus on the inferior aspect of the neck and rarely displaces if treated conservatively.[17]

Only 13 cases have been reported in the literature in children and adolescents.[12,17,33,53,55,65] Stress fractures in children usually occur in the 8- to 14-year-old age group and are accompanied by mild symptoms of pain that can mimic transient synovitis, a pre-SCFE lesion, avulsion injuries of the pelvis, muscle strains, and benign lesions such as osteoid osteoma. The patient complains of mild hip pain, which often does not prevent participation in normal activities such as cross-country running.[55] Physical examination findings are essentially normal, with minimal pain on hip motion. Radiographic evidence of the hip fracture is often not seen for up to 4 to 6 weeks from the time of appearance of the original symptoms or the initial evaluation. Bone scans will generally show a stress fracture; however, MRI is the most helpful method of

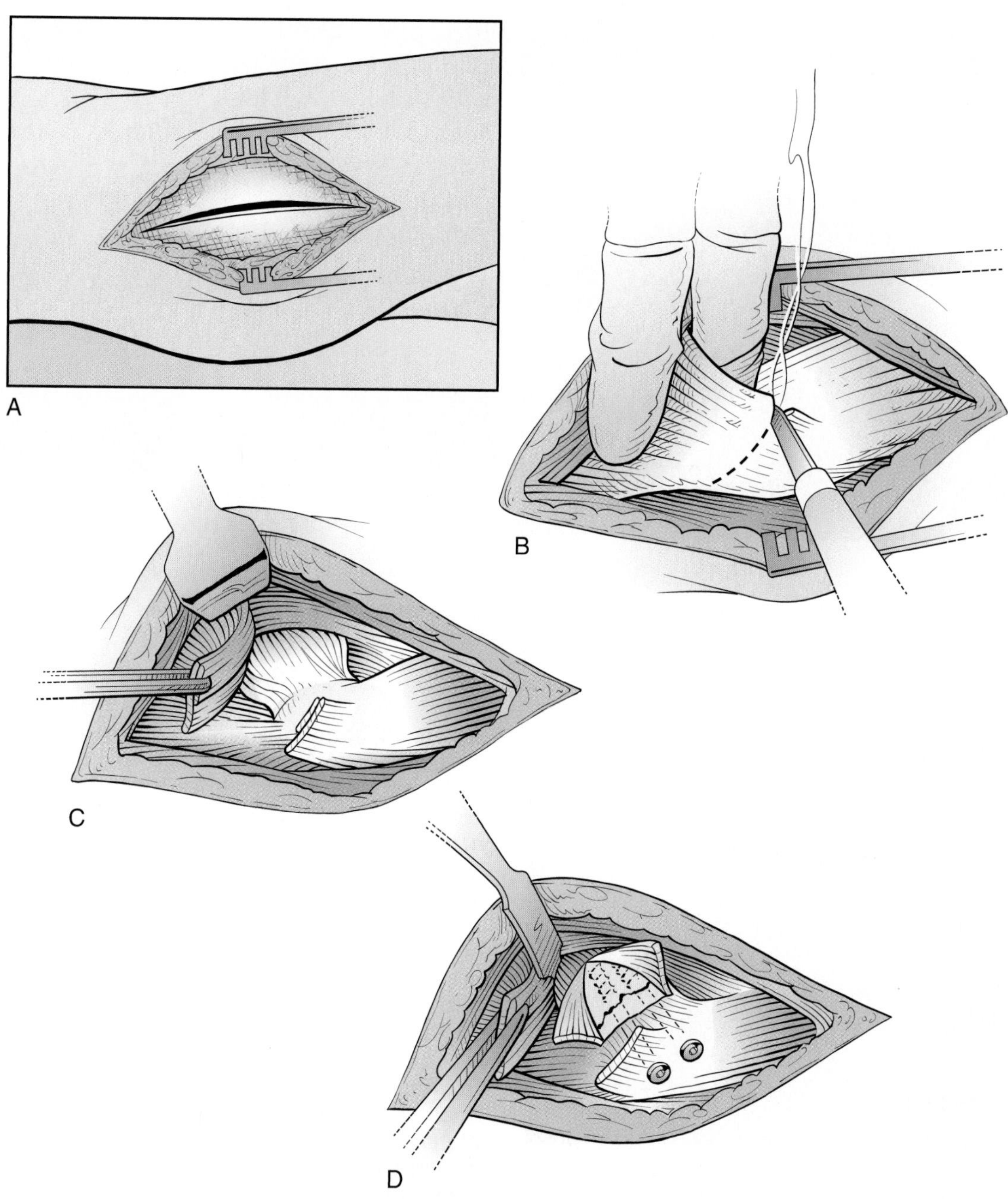

FIGURE 43–54 Open reduction and internal fixation of a femoral neck fracture through an anterolateral approach. **A,** The lateral incision is made and the tensor fasciae latae is incised. **B** and **C,** The gluteus medius and minimus are incised at their tendinous portions and retracted proximally as one layer to allow reapproximation. **D,** The capsule is opened. The fracture is reduced and fixed with two cannulated screws.

making a diagnosis.[28] Displacement of stress fractures in children has been reported when normal activities were continued or after a fall.[55,65]

Algorithms for the treatment of femoral neck stress fractures in children are based on the premise that only compression-type fractures occur in children and conservative treatment yields excellent results.[55] Once the diagnosis is made, treatment should consist of non–weight bearing in a cooperative patient or hip spica casting in a patient whose weight-bearing status cannot be controlled. When painful symptoms have resolved (usually within 4 to 6 weeks), partial weight bearing can be resumed. Full weight bearing is started only after solid radiographic union of the fracture. Internal fixation should be performed on any fracture that is displaced at the time of initial evaluation or begins to show displacement or evidence of delayed union or nonunion.

COMPLICATIONS

Treatment of hip fractures in children is associated with a high incidence of complications, especially with displaced fractures and in older children.[8,27,44,47] The

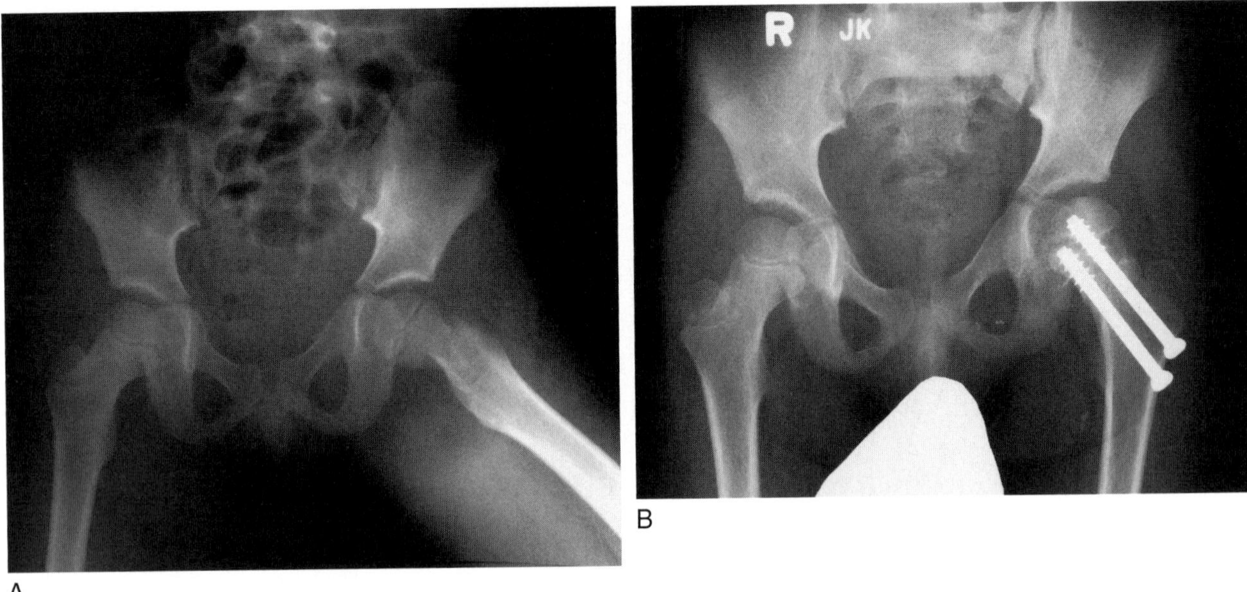

FIGURE 43-55 A and B, Transcervical hip fracture in a 12-year-old adolescent that was treated by screw fixation. The screw threads are proximal to the fracture and provide compression across the fracture site.

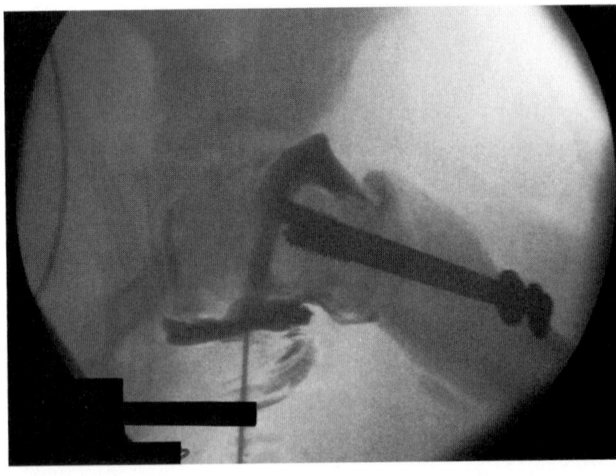

FIGURE 43-56 Arthrogram of the hip to ensure needle presence in the joint followed by aspiration after closed reduction and screw fixation of a basicervical hip fracture in a 10-year-old child.

incidence of each complication has diminished with more aggressive operative management, including prompt closed or open reduction, stable internal fixation that avoids the physis, and external immobilization. Complications in children's hip fractures include AVN, coxa vara, nonunion, premature physeal closure, and infection.

Avascular Necrosis

AVN is the most common and most devastating complication associated with hip fractures in children. Because of the high incidence of AVN and the severity of symptoms, AVN is the principal cause of poor results in children's hip fractures. Historically, the incidence of AVN has been reported to be 100%, 50%, 25%, and 15% for types I, II, III, and IV fractures, respectively, with an overall incidence of 43%.[8] In the most recent literature review, the incidence of AVN is lower: 38%, 28%, 18%, and 5% for types I, II, III, and IV fractures, respectively.[34] AVN of the femoral head is thought to occur as a result of disruption or compromise of the blood supply of the femoral head at the time of the initial trauma (displacement of the fracture) and the tamponade effect of the hip hemarthrosis.

Predisposing Factors. Several studies have found that risk factors predisposing to AVN are fracture displacement, which is the most important factor; the presence of a type I or II fracture; and a fracture in an older child (>12 years).[7,8,25,34,44] Although early reduction (within 24 hours) with fixation improves the overall outcome of hip fractures in adults, few studies have directly compared early and late treatment in children. Pforringer and Rosemeyer reported improved outcomes in children and adolescents with early operative treatment (within 36 hours of injury).[44]

Risk Reduction. Even though the mode of treatment has not been thought to have an effect on the incidence of AVN, there is growing evidence that more aggressive operative management, including decompressive hip arthrotomy, reduces this risk.[7,9,37,56] Cheng and Tang reported on 10 patients (average age, 12.9 years) with displaced hip fractures; seven underwent decompression of the hip joint with needle aspiration followed by closed reduction and internal fixation, and three required open reduction and internal fixation. AVN had not developed in any patient at an average

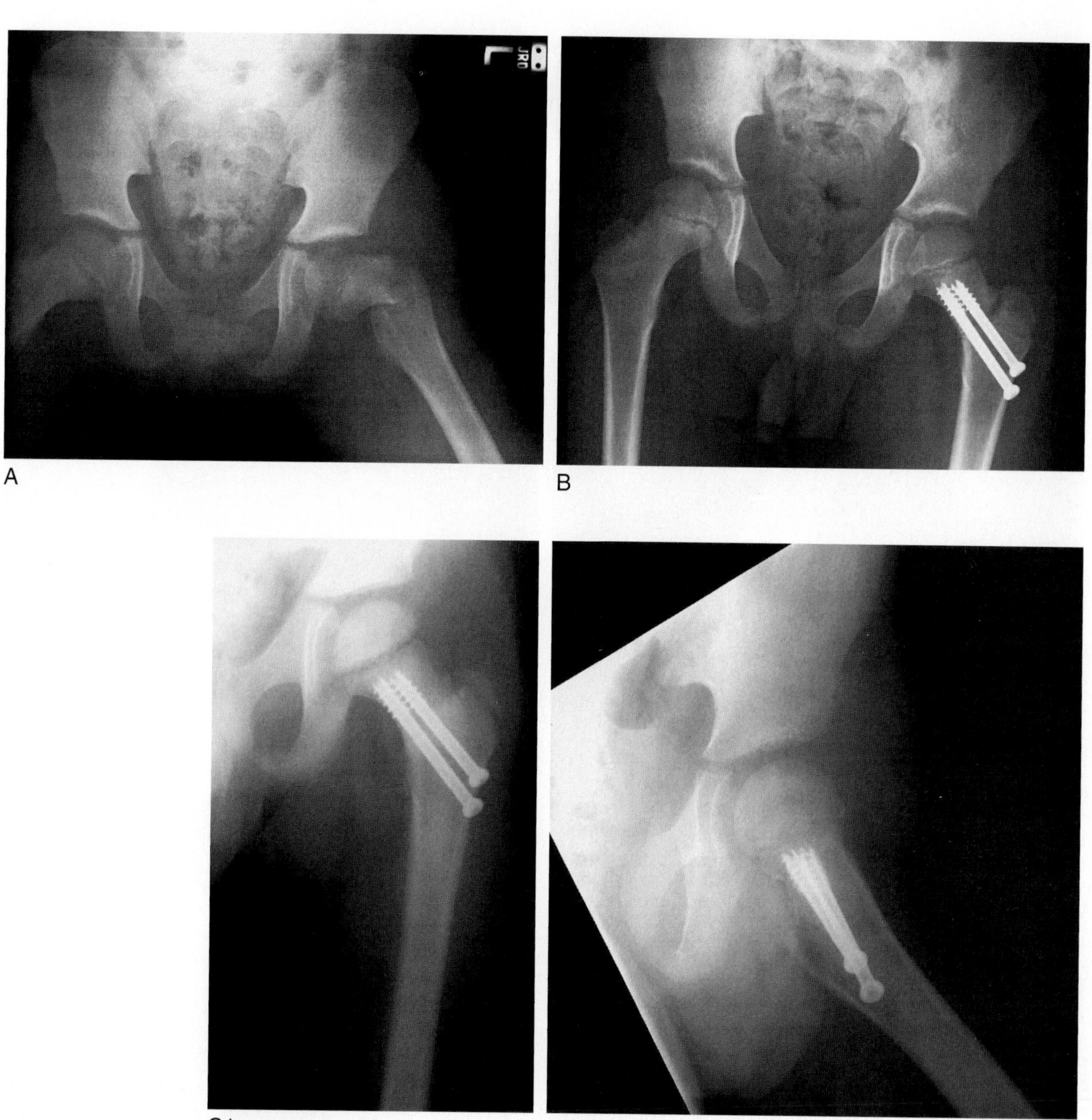

FIGURE 43–57 **A,** Cervicotrochanteric fracture in a 7-year-old child. **B,** Treatment by closed reduction, internal fixation, and casting. Anteroposterior **(C1)** and frog-leg lateral **(C2)** images show final healing at 8 months.

follow-up of 4.6 years.[9] Ng and Cole combined their six cases of displaced hip fractures in children who underwent hip decompression with 39 similar cases reported in the literature and compared them with 48 cases reported by Canale that were treated without hip decompression.[37] They concluded that hip decompression lowers the incidence of AVN, especially in types II and III fractures. However, Gerber and associates reviewed the experience with open reduction and internal fixation of hip fractures in children at seven Swiss hospitals and could not demonstrate an improvement in the incidence of AVN.[23] Although the data are not conclusive, they do suggest that hip decompression helps lower the incidence of AVN, is relatively easy to perform, and is associated with minimal complications. Therefore, we recommend needle aspiration of the hip joint performed with an 18-gauge needle via a subadductor approach at the time of initial treatment. It should be done at the completion of reduction and fixation to minimize the reaccumulation of fracture hematoma.

Clinical Features and Radiographic Findings. Symptoms of AVN may occur early, with complaints of groin pain. Radiographic evidence of AVN can be seen as early as 2 months after injury and is generally present

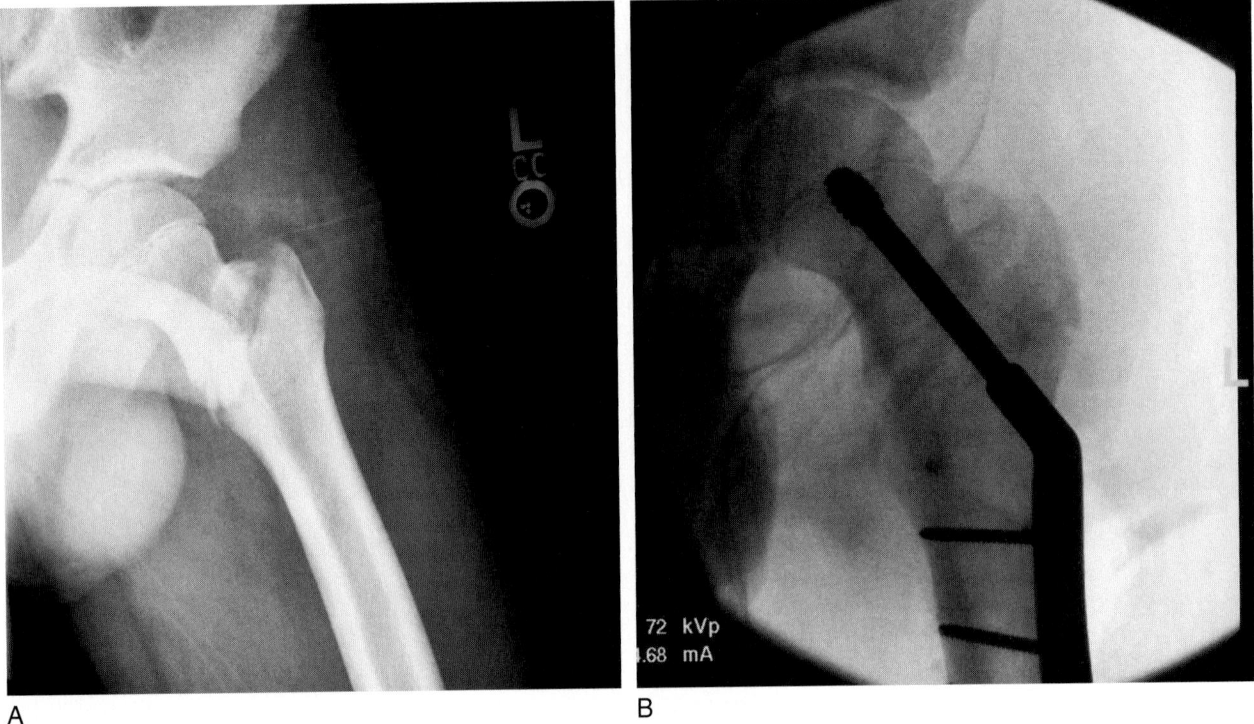

FIGURE 43–58 **A,** Left intertrochanteric hip fracture in a 10-year-old child. **B,** Treatment with a compression screw and side plate.

within 1 year of injury (Fig. 43–59).[8,48] Radiographs may demonstrate osteopenia of the femoral head, followed later by sclerosis, fragmentation, and often collapse and deformity. MRI is the most sensitive test to confirm the diagnosis and also defines the extent of femoral head and neck involvement. Radioisotope scanning shows decreased uptake in the femoral head or neck (or both) and is useful in a hip that has stainless steel internal fixation.[26,39]

Patterns. Three patterns of AVN have been described by Ratliff (Fig. 43–60).[47]

In type I AVN there is severe diffuse necrosis totally involving the femoral head and the proximal fragment of the femoral neck (Fig. 43–61). The femoral head necrosis is accompanied by various degrees of collapse of the femoral head, from segmental necrosis with minimal collapse to diffuse complete collapse with subluxation. Type I AVN results from interruption of the lateral epiphyseal and metaphyseal vessels. This is the most common pattern of AVN; it accounts for more than 50% of cases and has the worst prognosis. In Ratliff's study, type I necrosis occurred in 33 of 55 cases (60%). The patients with partial collapse had fair results, whereas those with complete collapse had poor results.[47] Canale reported that 80% of patients with AVN had the type I pattern.

Type II AVN is characterized by more localized necrotic changes, often in the anterosuperior aspect of the femoral head, with little collapse (Fig. 43–62). It is usually due to interruption of the lateral epiphyseal vessels before entrance into the epiphysis. This type is

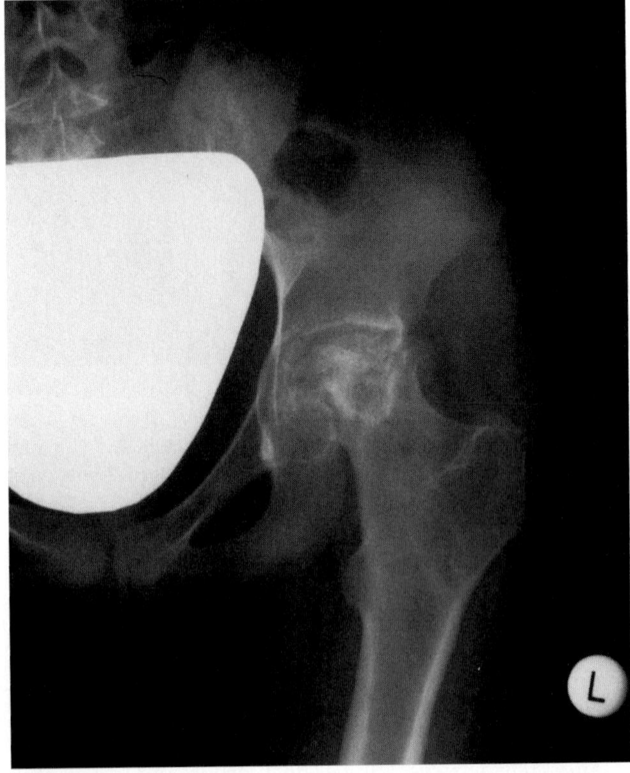

FIGURE 43–59 Severe avascular necrosis of the femoral head after a hip fracture.

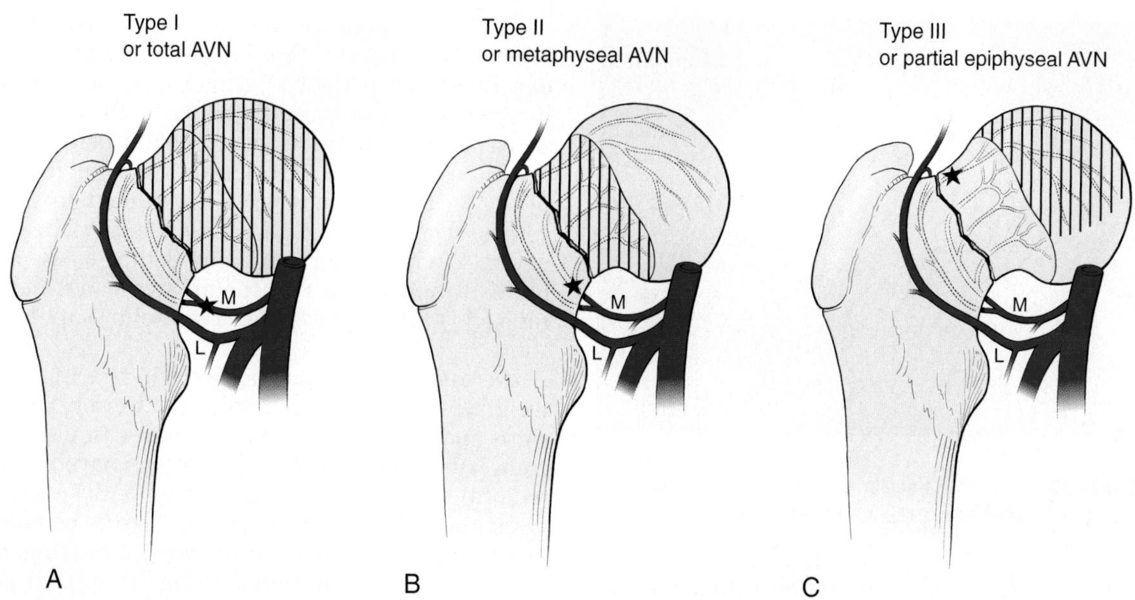

FIGURE 43–60 Patterns of avascular necrosis (AVN) of the femoral head after hip fractures in children, as described by Ratliff. Note the location of the vascular compromise (★) that leads to each pattern. **A,** Type I or total AVN of the entire femoral capital epiphysis and proximal fragment of the femoral neck. **B,** Type II or metaphyseal AVN from the level of the fracture to the physis. **C,** Type III or partial epiphyseal AVN. The AVN is confined to the femoral head. L, lateral femoral circumflex artery; M, medial femoral circumflex artery.

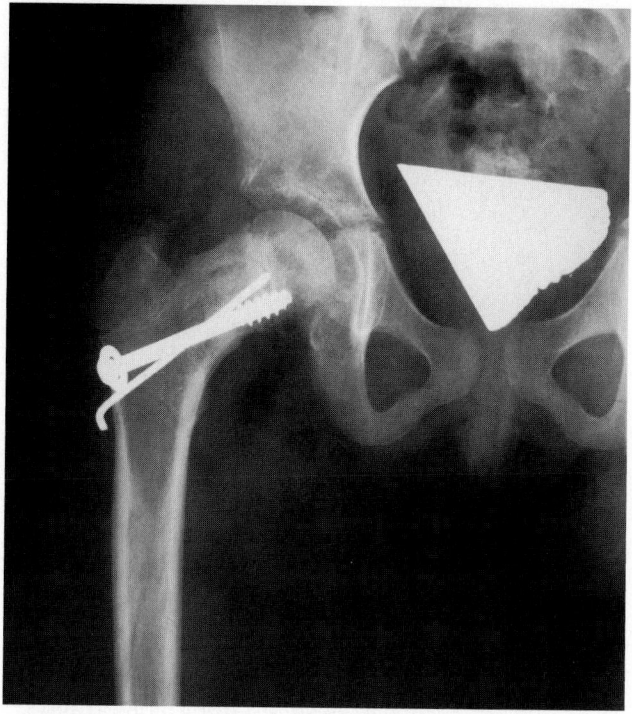

FIGURE 43–61 Type I avascular necrosis in an 8-year-old child, proximal to the femoral neck fracture.

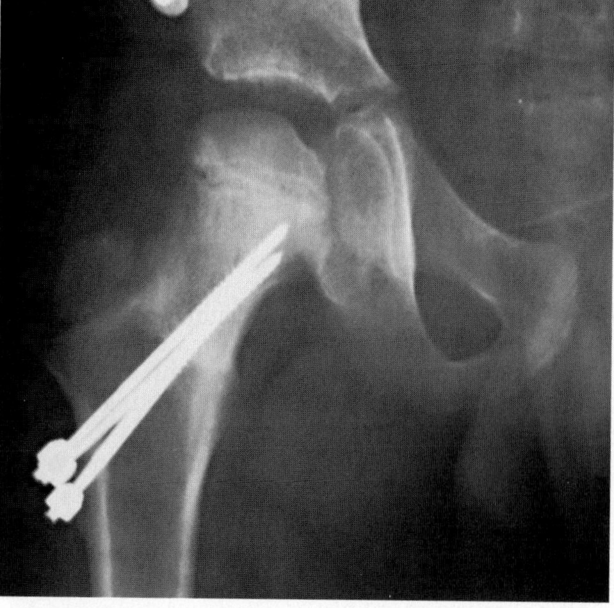

FIGURE 43–62 Type II avascular necrosis (AVN) in a 6-year-old child after closed reduction and internal fixation of a cervicotrochanteric hip fracture. The AVN extends from the fracture site to the physes.

seen in approximately 25% of cases and has a better prognosis than type I AVN does.[48]

Type III AVN is characterized by sclerosis from the fracture line of the femoral neck to the physis, with sparing of the femoral head (Fig. 43–63). It accounts for 25% of cases of AVN and has the best results.

Treatment and Prognosis. In general, AVN after hip fractures in children results in poor outcomes in up to 60% of cases. In a long-term follow-up study, Davison and Weinstein reported that 64% (9 of 14) of patients with AVN had severe pain, limited range of motion, and proximal femoral deformities and that 4 (44%) required arthroplasty an average of 5.6 years after

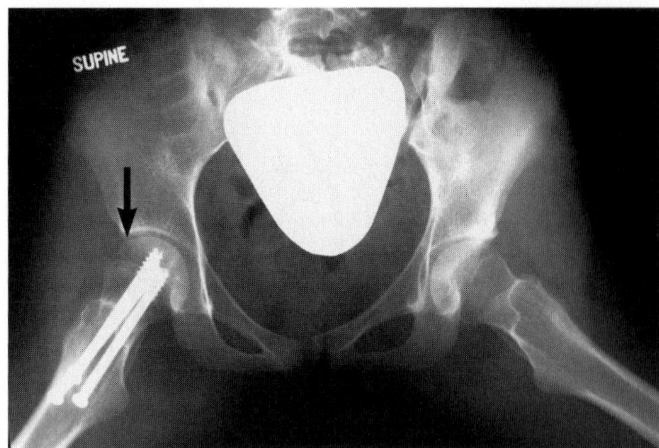

FIGURE 43–63 Type III avascular necrosis (AVN), or partial femoral head AVN, after a femoral head fracture.

injury.[15] Leung and Lam, in a long-term follow-up of hip fractures in children 13 and 23 years after injury, found that 20% of patients had severe collapse and deformity as a result of AVN.[30]

Treatment of AVN has been relatively unsuccessful, and some have suggested that treatment does not affect the natural history.[35] Canale and Bourland reported that 60% of patients with AVN after hip fractures had poor results, regardless of whether treatment was specifically undertaken to treat the AVN.[8] Limited data are available on the treatment of AVN after hip fractures in children, which makes defining the superiority of one treatment modality over others difficult.[8,47]

The goals of treatment are to preserve the functional range of hip motion, maintain containment of the femoral head within the acetabulum, and preserve as much femoral head viability as possible. In general, treatment of AVN should begin at the onset of symptoms and should entail partial weight bearing or non–weight bearing until the painful symptoms resolve. Canale and Bourland treated 22 hips with AVN; 7 were managed by bed rest or non–weight-bearing ambulation started at the time that AVN was first recognized and continued for an average of 8 years. One patient had a good result, three had fair results, and three had poor results.[8] In a study by Ratliff, 20 patients with type I AVN, without subluxation of the femoral head, had fair results at final follow-up after treatment with a weight-relieving caliper.[47]

Operative treatment has resulted in poor outcomes principally because of selection bias; the most severe cases of AVN have undergone operative treatment. When AVN is first recognized, the initial step is removal of internal fixation devices to prevent penetration of the hardware into the joint. Further operative treatment options include intertrochanteric osteotomy (usually valgus) to place viable head in the weight-bearing zone, capsulotomy, and arthrodesis. Ratliff reported seven cases of type I necrosis with subluxation of the femoral head that were treated by subtrochanteric osteotomy in an attempt to allow revascularization of the femoral head. All seven patients had poor results, and this procedure was not recommended.[47] Similarly, Canale and Bourland described one patient who had a cortical bone graft inserted into the avascular area, with a poor result, and a patient who underwent a valgus osteotomy, with a fair result.[8] Cup arthroplasty or total hip arthroplasty in this setting has also resulted in poor outcomes. Davison and Weinstein reported on four patients who underwent cup arthroplasty or total hip arthroplasty. In two the arthroplasties have been revised, and in the other two follow-up has been short.[15]

We recommend partial weight bearing or non–weight bearing on the involved extremity at the first signs and symptoms of AVN until revascularization is complete and the painful symptoms have resolved. If femoral head necrosis is associated with severe symptoms and subluxation, intertrochanteric osteotomy to place more viable head in the weight-bearing zone or arthrodesis is recommended (Fig. 43–64). In general, we do not recommend cup arthroplasty or total hip arthroplasty in an adolescent with AVN because of the relatively short life span of these prostheses in a young, active patient.

Coxa Vara

Coxa vara may have four main causes: malreduction, in which the fracture is left in a varus position; loss of reduction because of inadequate fracture stabilization, usually when external immobilization alone is used; delayed union or nonunion, in which varus eventually develops; and premature closure of the proximal femoral physis with overgrowth of the greater trochanter. Coxa vara occurs in 10% to 32% of cases, depending on the type of treatment.[8,15,25,27,29,47,61]

Closed reduction plus external immobilization with abduction casting results in the highest incidence of coxa vara, most often caused by loss of reduction. Although closed reduction and internal fixation can result in coxa vara, the varus deformity tends to be mild when compared with that in patients treated by closed reduction and casting. Canale and Bourland reported coxa vara in 13 patients (21% of their study group). In seven children treated by closed reduction and internal fixation, the coxa vara resulted in an average neck–shaft angle of 127 degrees, whereas in five children treated by reduction and casting, the varus deformity averaged 94 degrees.[8] McDougall reported a 50% incidence of coxa vara and noted bending of the femoral neck because of bone plasticity at the fracture site, despite radiographic union.[32] Others believe that the obliquity of the fracture line (a Pauwels angle >50 degrees) results in fracture instability and predisposes to varus deformity.[1] Some remodeling occurs with milder deformity, especially in a younger child.[25] However, a neck–shaft angle of less than 100 degrees is associated with a poor outcome, and such a deformity has little ability to remodel, even in a young child.

Coxa vara deformity is best prevented by anatomic reduction and rigid internal fixation followed by

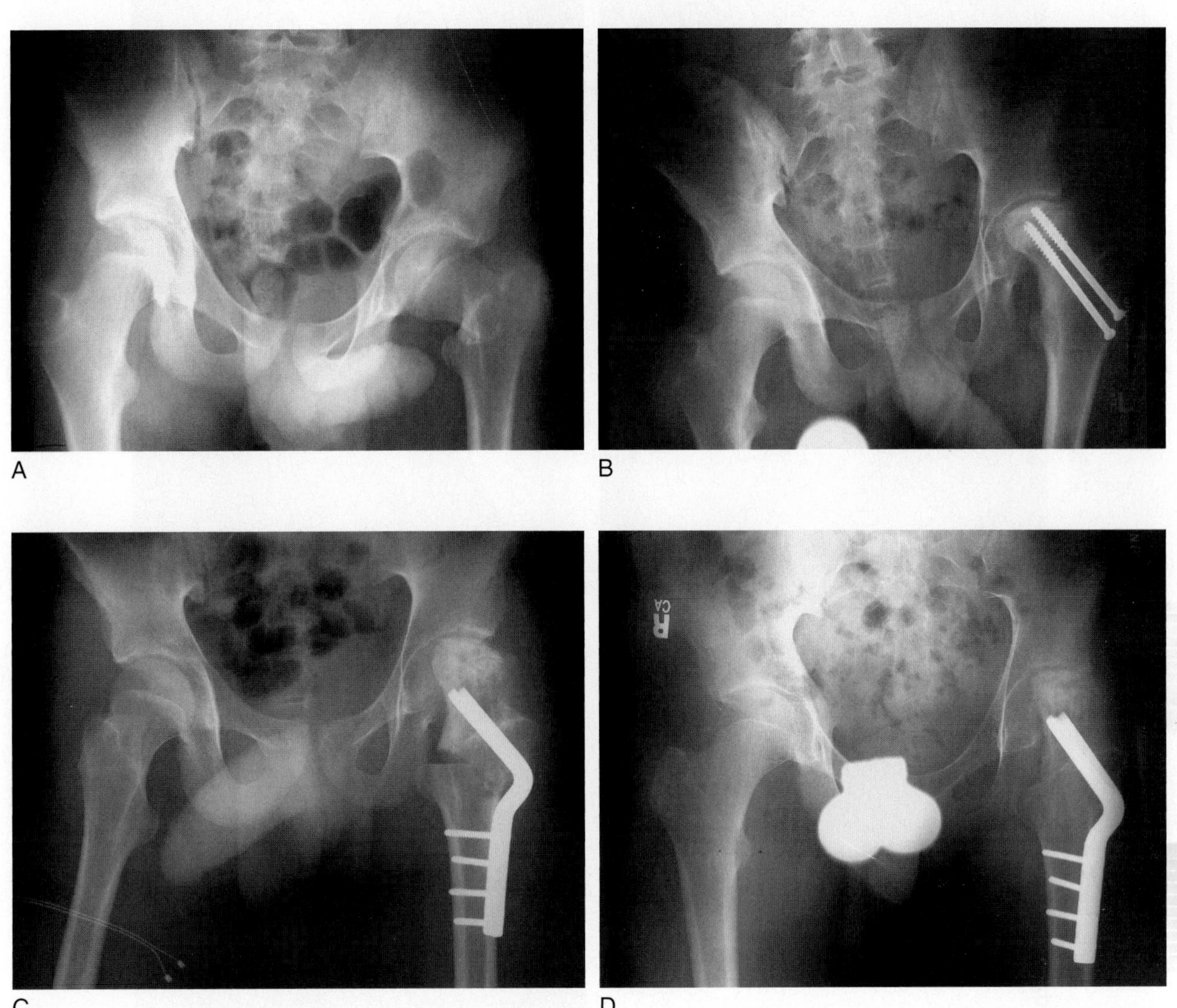

FIGURE 43–64 Intertrochanteric osteotomy to reposition viable femoral head in the weight-bearing zone in a 16-year-old male adolescent with a displaced femoral neck fracture. **A,** Preoperative radiograph. **B,** Radiographs obtained months after operative fixation showing femoral head collapse. **C,** A valgus osteotomy was performed with blade plate fixation to get viable femoral head into the weight-bearing zone. **D,** Appearance at final healing.

external immobilization in most cases. To lessen the risk for premature physeal closure and subsequent coxa vara, internal fixation devices should avoid the growth plate as long as good screw purchase can be achieved. We recommend valgus osteotomy with blade plate fixation in a child with a neck–shaft angle of less than 110 degrees or when reduction is lost (Fig. 43–65).

Nonunion

The incidence of nonunion varies between 6.5% and 12.5% and appears to be related to the method of treatment.[8,25,27,47] Higher rates of nonunion were reported in various series of patients in which the majority were treated by external immobilization[27,47] than in more recent series in which internal fixation was used.[8,25] Additional factors associated with nonunion include poor reduction, distraction of the fracture fragments at the time of internal fixation, and a Pauwels angle greater than 60 degrees. Nonunion can lead to coxa vara and can predispose to other complications such as AVN and premature physeal arrest; the results are ultimately poor when an established nonunion occurs. Therefore, prevention by means of anatomic reduction, rigid internal fixation, and external immobilization is important.

Nonunion should be treated when it is diagnosed to prevent further complications. In a child younger than 10 years, we recommend autogenous bone grafting and rigid internal fixation, with screws placed in lag-type fashion to gain compression across the fracture site. A subtrochanteric valgus osteotomy should be performed as described by Pauwels in an older child or in any child with a Pauwels angle greater than 60 degrees or when unreducible coxa vara is present (Fig. 43–66).[43] The goal of valgus osteotomy is to alter

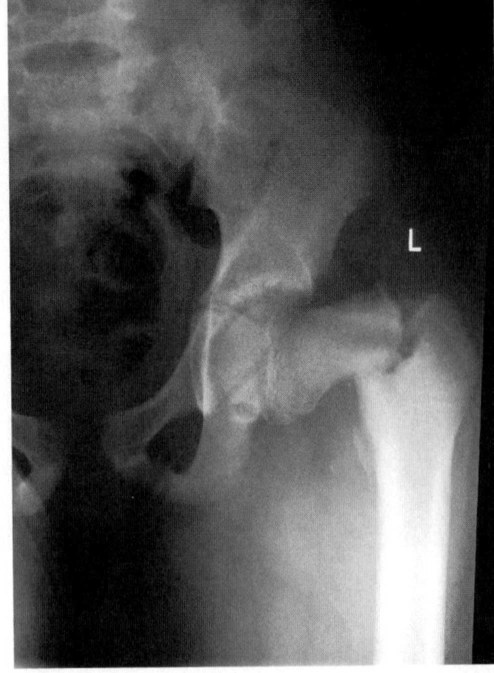

A

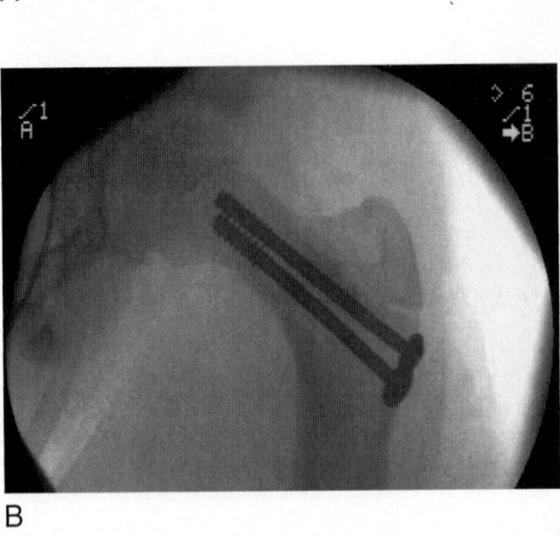

B

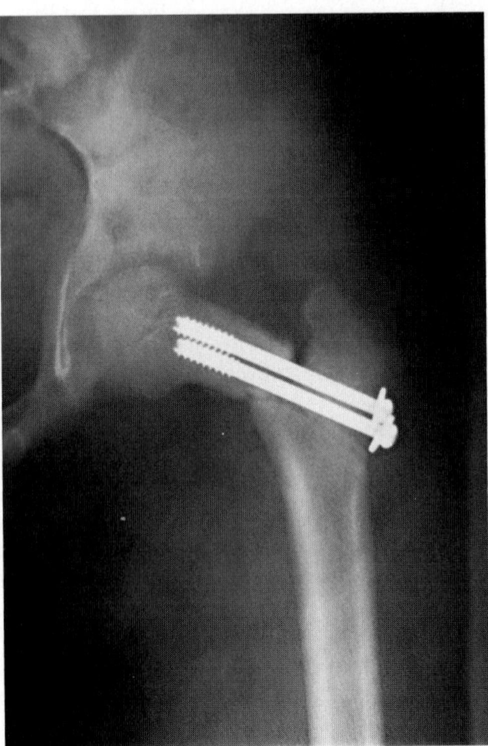

C

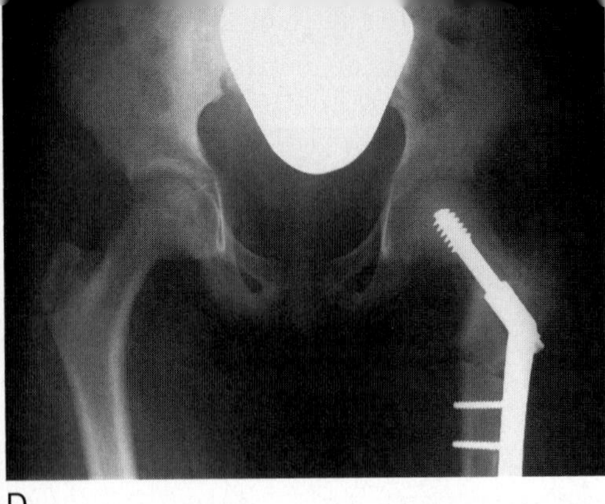

D

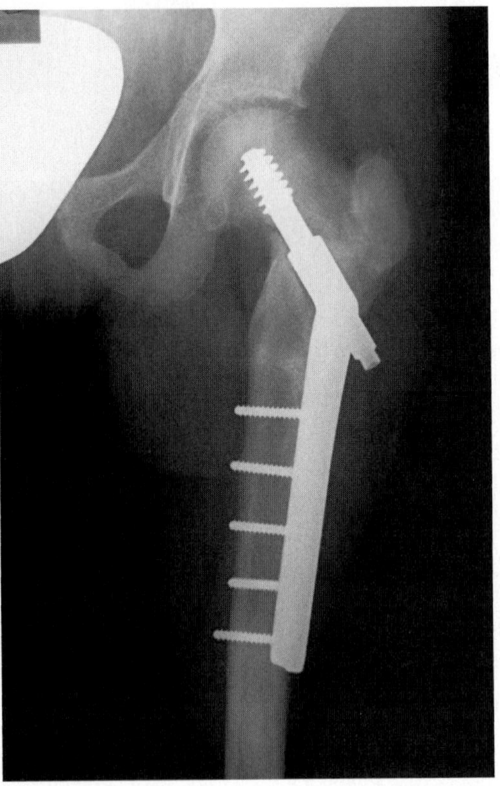

E

FIGURE 43–65 Cervicotrochanteric fracture in a 10-year-old girl. **A,** Initial injury films. **B,** Closed reduction plus percutaneous pinning with two 6.5-mm cannulated screws was performed, followed by immobilization in a hip spica cast. **C,** The fracture line is vertical, and at the 4-week follow-up evaluation the fracture reduction has been lost because of screw cut-out in the metaphysis with resultant varus deformity. **D,** Valgus intertrochanteric osteotomy was then performed. The cannulated screws were removed after the guidewires were placed. The large compression screw was placed over the inferior guidewire, whereas the superior guidewire prevented rotation of the femoral neck. Preoperative planning resulted in using a 20-degree laterally based wedge to produce a valgus correction osteotomy and align the fracture in a more horizontal position. **E,** Appearance at final healing.

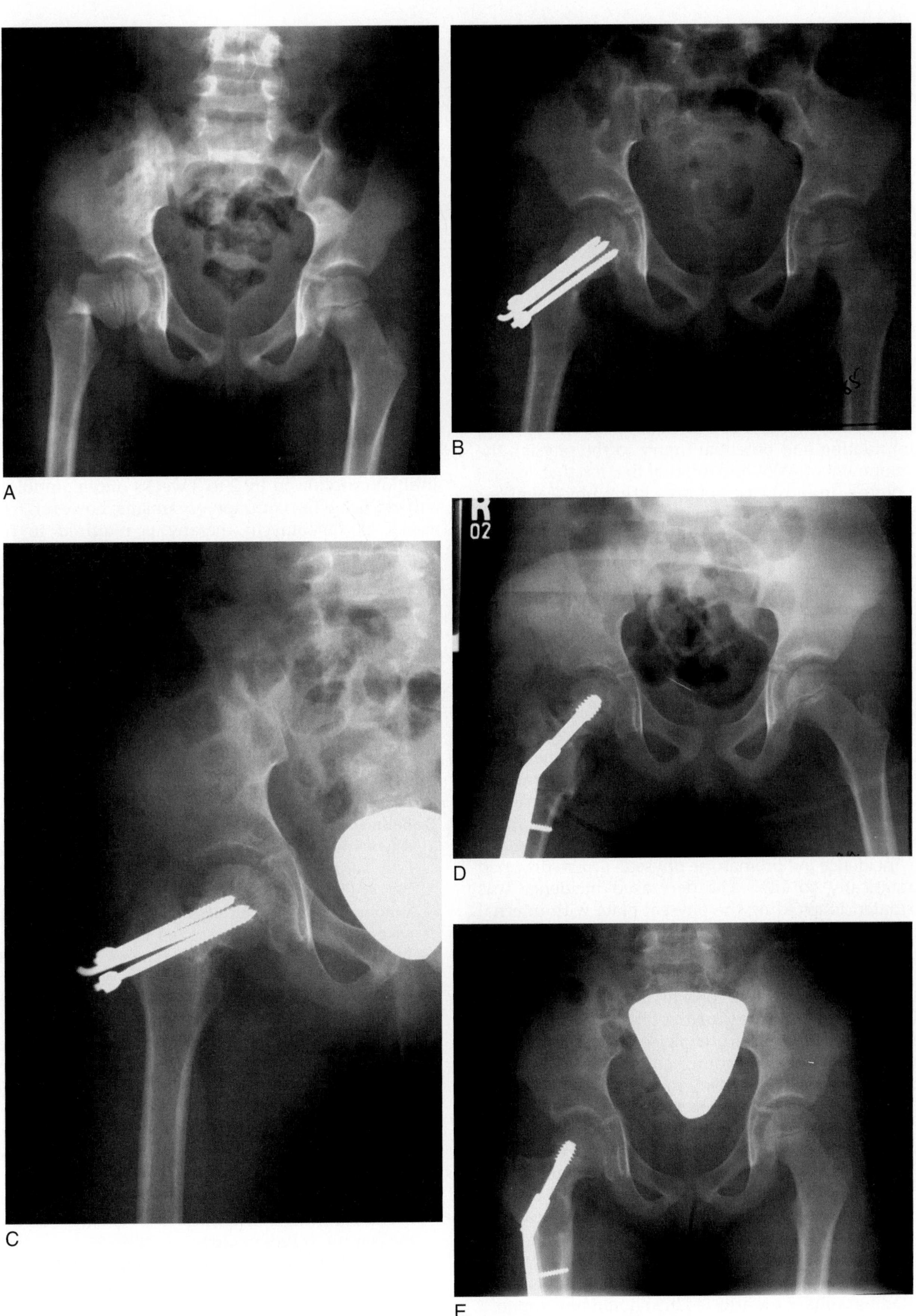

FIGURE 43–66 Radiographs of a femoral neck fracture with a relatively steep Pauwels angle. Because union was delayed, a valgus osteotomy was performed to promote fracture healing. **A,** Initial injury radiographs of a 5-year-old girl who was struck by a car. **B,** Closed reduction followed by three-screw fixation was performed. **C,** At 4 months, delayed union with some varus angulation was noted. **D,** A subtrochanteric valgus osteotomy was performed. **E,** Healing of the fracture and the osteotomy.

the plane of the fracture to produce compressive loads across the fracture site for enhancement of healing. Preoperative planning should be performed to restore a normal neck–shaft angle, which generally requires removing an approximately 25-degree laterally based wedge with the osteotomy placed just superior to the lesser trochanter, followed by blade plate fixation.[36] In adults, excellent results have been reported with this technique, and fracture union was achieved in nearly all cases.[2,3,38] Canale and Bourland reported four children with nonunion treated successfully by subtrochanteric valgus osteotomy without bone grafting.[8]

Premature Physeal Arrest

The reported incidence of premature physeal arrest varies between 10% and 62%.[8,25,29,44,47] Factors that contribute to premature physeal arrest are the amount of displacement at the time of injury (requiring more manipulation and potential injury to the physis), the development of AVN, and internal fixation that crosses the physis. In most cases of premature physeal arrest there is associated AVN of the femoral head. The development of AVN with collapse may lead to premature physeal arrest; however, it is more likely that these fractures are displaced at the time of injury, thereby leading to compromised blood supply to both the epiphysis, which results in AVN, and the physis, which results in physeal arrest. Lam reported that eight of nine patients with premature physeal arrest had associated AVN,[29] whereas Heiser and Oppenheim reported AVN in five of their nine cases.[25]

Internal fixation, when it crosses the physis, may predispose to premature physeal arrest. Canale and Bourland reported a 62% incidence of premature physeal arrest in their initial series. Of the 23 cases in which Knowles pins crossed the physis, 18 closed prematurely and 5 remained open.[8] In their later study, the incidence of premature physeal arrest dropped dramatically, to 12%. The decreased incidence was attributed to avoiding the physeal plate with internal fixation devices and to using as few pins as possible.[7]

Premature physeal closure by itself does not generally result in significant deformity or limb length discrepancy because the proximal growth plate contributes only 15% of the growth of the entire extremity. However, when premature physeal closure is combined with AVN in a young child, significant limb length discrepancies develop in virtually all cases.

To prevent premature physeal arrest, treatment of the displaced hip fracture should consist of gentle closed reduction to avoid further injury to the physis in type I fractures. This is followed in a young child by smooth pin fixation and in an older child by cannulated screws in which the threads do not span the physis. In all other fractures, internal fixation devices should be left short of the physis as long as fracture stability is not compromised.

Radiographs of the affected hip should be compared with those of the contralateral side to determine whether premature physeal arrest and AVN have occurred. Serial scanograms and bone age measurements should be performed to predict the eventual limb length discrepancy, with the Moseley straight-line graph used to accurately predict the appropriate timing of a contralateral epiphysiodesis.

Infection

Infection is relatively rare in children and adolescents after a hip fracture; the reported incidence is approximately 1%.[7,8,46] Infection is usually associated with subsequent AVN, and patients generally have poor outcomes because of pain and deformity. Davison and Weinstein reported that 2 (10.5%) of 19 patients who underwent total cup arthroplasty because of pain and poor hip function had septic arthritis and associated AVN.[15] Treatment consists of debridement of the hip joint until gross infection is cleared, followed by intravenous administration of antibiotics. The duration of intravenous antibiotic therapy depends on the virulence of the offending organism and the clinical course of the patient. In general, 2 to 3 weeks of intravenous antibiotics followed by 2 to 3 weeks of oral antibiotics will eradicate the common organisms; however, 6 to 8 weeks of vancomycin therapy is required to treat methicillin-resistant *Staphylococcus aureus*.

References

Hip Fractures

1. Allende G, Lezama LG: Fractures of the neck of the femur in children; a clinical study. J Bone Joint Surg Am 1951;33:387.
2. Anglen JO: Intertrochanteric osteotomy for failed internal fixation of femoral neck fracture. Clin Orthop Relat Res 1997;341:175.
3. Ballmer FT, Ballmer PM, Baumgaertel F, et al: Pauwels osteotomy for nonunions of the femoral neck. Orthop Clin North Am 1990;21:759.
4. Berger PE, Ofstein RA, Jackson DW, et al: MRI demonstration of radiographically occult fractures: what have we been missing? Radiographics 1989;9:407.
5. Blickenstaff LD, Morris JM: Fatigue fracture of the femoral neck. J Bone Joint Surg Am 1966;48:1031.
6. Boitzy A: Fractures of the proximal femur. In Weber B, Brunner C, Grueler F (eds): Treatment of Fractures in Children and Adolescents. Berlin, Springer-Verlag, 1980.
7. Canale ST: Fractures of the hip in children and adolescents. Orthop Clin North Am 1990;21:341.
8. Canale ST, Bourland WL: Fracture of the neck and intertrochanteric region of the femur in children. J Bone Joint Surg Am 1977;59:431.
9. Cheng JC, Tang N: Decompression and stable internal fixation of femoral neck fractures in children can affect the outcome. J Pediatr Orthop 1999;19:338.
10. Chong KC, Chacha PB, Lee BT: Fractures of the neck of the femur in childhood and adolescence. Injury 1975; 7:111.
11. Chung SM: The arterial supply of the developing proximal end of the human femur. J Bone Joint Surg Am 1976;58:961.

12. Coldwell D, Gross GW, Boal DK: Stress fracture of the femoral neck in a child (stress fracture). Pediatr Radiol 1984;14:174.
13. Colonna P: Fracture of the neck of the femur in childhood: A report of six cases. Ann Surg 1928;88:902.
14. Connolly LP, Treves ST, Connolly SA, et al: Pediatric skeletal scintigraphy: Applications of pinhole magnification. Radiographics 1998;18:341.
15. Davison BL, Weinstein SL: Hip fractures in children: A long-term follow-up study. J Pediatr Orthop 1992;12: 355.
16. Delbet P: Cited in Colonna PC: Fracture of the neck of the femur in childhood: A report of six cases. Ann Surg 1928;88:902.
17. Devas MB: Stress fractures of the femoral neck. J Bone Joint Surg Br 1965;47:728.
18. Fabry G, MacEwen GD, Shands AR Jr: Torsion of the femur. A follow-up study in normal and abnormal conditions. J Bone Joint Surg Am 1973;55:1726.
19. Fiddian NJ, Grace DL: Traumatic dislocation of the hip in adolescence with separation of the capital epiphysis. Two case reports. J Bone Joint Surg Br 1983;65:148.
20. Forlin E, Guille JT, Kumar SJ, et al: Transepiphyseal fractures of the neck of the femur in very young children. J Pediatr Orthop 1992;12:164.
21. Funk F: Traumatic dislocation of the hip in adolescence with separation of the capital epiphysis: Factors affecting prognosis and treatment. J Bone Joint Surg Am 1962;44:1135.
22. Gaudinez RF, Heinrich SD: Transphyseal fracture of the capital femoral epiphysis. Orthopedics 1989;12: 1599.
23. Gerber C, Lehmann A, Ganz R: Femoral neck fractures in children: A multicenter follow-up study. Z Orthop 1985;123:767.
24. Haramati N, Staron RB, Barax C, et al: Magnetic resonance imaging of occult fractures of the proximal femur. Skeletal Radiol 1994;23:19.
25. Heiser JM, Oppenheim WL: Fractures of the hip in children: A review of forty cases. Clin Orthop Relat Res 1980;149:177.
26. Herring JA, McCarthy RE: Fracture dislocation of the capital femoral epiphysis. J Pediatr Orthop 1986;6:112.
27. Ingram AJ, Bachynski B: Fractures of the hip in children; treatment and results. J Bone Joint Surg Am 1953;35: 867.
28. Keene JS, Lash EG: Negative bone scan in a femoral neck stress fracture. A case report. Am J Sports Med 1992;20: 234.
29. Lam SF: Fractures of the neck of the femur in children. J Bone Joint Surg Am 1971;53:1165.
30. Leung PC, Lam SF: Long-term follow-up of children with femoral neck fractures. J Bone Joint Surg Br 1986; 68:537.
31. Lindseth RE, Rosene HA Jr: Traumatic separation of the upper femoral epiphysis in a new born infant. J Bone Joint Surg Am 1971;53:1641.
32. McDougall A: Fractures of the neck of the femur in childhood. J Bone Joint Surg Br 1961;43:16.
33. Miller F, Wenger DR: Femoral neck stress fracture in a hyperactive child. A case report. J Bone Joint Surg Am 1979;61:435.
34. Moon ES, Mehlman CT: Risk factors for avascular necrosis after femoral neck fractures in children: 25 Cincinnati cases and meta-analysis of 360 cases. J Orthop Trauma 2006;20:323.
35. Morrissy R: Hip fractures in children. Clin Orthop Relat Res 1980;152:202.
36. Muller M: Intertrochanteric osteotomy: Indication, preoperative planning, technique. In Schatzker J (ed): The Intertrochanteric Osteotomy. Berlin, Springer-Verlag, 1984, p 25.
37. Ng GP, Cole WG: Effect of early hip decompression on the frequency of avascular necrosis in children with fractures of the neck of the femur. Injury 1996;27:419.
38. Nierenberg G, Volpin G, Bialik V, et al: Pelvic fractures in children: A follow-up in 20 children treated conservatively. J Pediatr Orthop B 1993;1:140.
39. Ogden J: Skeletal Injury in the Child. Philadelphia, WB Saunders, 1990.
40. Ogden JA: Changing patterns of proximal femoral vascularity. J Bone Joint Surg Am 1974;56:941.
41. Ogden JA, Lee KE, Rudicel SA, et al: Proximal femoral epiphysiolysis in the neonate. J Pediatr Orthop 1984;4: 285.
42. Ovesen O, Arreskov J, Bellstrom T: Hip fractures in children. A long-term follow up of 17 cases. Orthopedics 1989;12:361.
43. Pauwels F: Der Schenkelhalsbruch: ein mechanisches Problem. Translated by Hildegard Spital. Beirlageheft zur Zeitschrift fur Orthopaedischechirurgie 1963;63.
44. Pforringer W, Rosemeyer B: Fractures of the hip in children and adolescents. Acta Orthop Scand 1980;51: 91.
45. Ratliff A: Complications after fractures of the femoral neck in children and their treatment. J Bone Joint Surg Br 1970;52:175.
46. Ratliff AH: Fractures of the neck of the femur in children. J Bone Joint Surg Br 1962;44:528.
47. Ratliff AH: Traumatic separation of the upper femoral epiphysis in young children. J Bone Joint Surg Br 1968; 50:757.
48. Ratliff AH: Fractures of the neck of the femur in children. Orthop Clin North Am 1974;5:903.
49. Reikeras O, Bjerkreim I, Kolbenstvedt A: Anteversion of the acetabulum in patients with idiopathic increased anteversion of the femoral neck. Acta Orthop Scand 1982;53:847.
50. Reikeras O, Hoiseth A, Reigstad A, et al: Femoral neck angles: A specimen study with special regard to bilateral differences. Acta Orthop Scand 1982;53:775.
51. Rizzo PF, Gould ES, Lyden JP, et al: Diagnosis of occult fractures about the hip. Magnetic resonance imaging compared with bone-scanning. J Bone Joint Surg Am 1993;75:395.
52. Rubin SJ, Marquardt JD, Gottlieb RH, et al: Magnetic resonance imaging: A cost-effective alternative to bone scintigraphy in the evaluation of patients with suspected hip fractures. Skeletal Radiol 1998;27:199.
53. Scheerlinck T, De Boeck H: Bilateral stress fractures of the femoral neck complicated by unilateral displacement in a child. J Pediatr Orthop B 1998;7:246.
54. Shin AY, Morin WD, Gorman JD, et al: The superiority of magnetic resonance imaging in differentiating the

cause of hip pain in endurance athletes. Am J Sports Med 1996;24:168.
55. St Pierre P, Staheli LT, Smith JB, et al: Femoral neck stress fractures in children and adolescents. J Pediatr Orthop 1995;15:470.
56. Swiontkowski MF, Winquist RA: Displaced hip fractures in children and adolescents. J Trauma 1986;26:384.
57. Tountas AA, Waddell JP: Stress fractures of the femoral neck. A report of seven cases. Clin Orthop Relat Res 1986;210:160.
58. Trueta J: The normal vascular anatomy of the human femoral head during growth. J Bone Joint Surg Br 1957;39:358.
59. Trueta J, Morgan JD: The vascular contribution to osteogenesis. I. Studies by the injection method. J Bone Joint Surg Br 1960;42:97.
60. Vonlanz T, Mayet A: Die Gelenkorper des menschlichen Hufgelenkes in der profredienten Phase ihrer umwegigen Ausformung. Z Anat 1953;117:317.
61. Weiner DS, O'Dell HW: Fractures of the hip in children. J Trauma 1969;9:62.
62. Whitman R: Fracture of the neck of the femur in a child. Med Rec 1891;39:165.
63. Whitman R: Observations on fractures of the neck of the femur in childhood with special reference to treatment and differential diagnosis from separation of the epiphysis. Med Rec 1893;43:22.
64. Wojtowycz M, Starshak RJ, Sty JR: Neonatal proximal femoral epiphysiolysis. Radiology 1980;136:647.
65. Wolfgang GL: Stress fracture of the femoral neck in a patient with open capital femoral epiphyses. J Bone Joint Surg Am 1977;59:680.

FEMUR

Femoral Shaft Fractures

Management of femoral shaft fractures in children continues to be challenging and controversial. Traditional treatment has relied on nonoperative approaches because fracture healing occurs relatively rapidly in children and good results are generally seen. However, with a better understanding of the biology of fracture healing and with advances in fixation methods and operative techniques, there has been a general trend toward operative stabilization of femoral shaft fractures in children.

ANATOMY AND DEVELOPMENT

The femur first appears during the fourth week of gestation as a condensation of mesenchymal tissue. By the eighth week, enchondral ossification has begun and growth is rapid. The primary ossification center is the femoral shaft, with ossification of the secondary centers beginning in the upper epiphysis at 6 months as a single center of ossification that later becomes the femoral head and the greater trochanter. The distal secondary center of ossification develops during the seventh fetal month. The femoral head ossifies at approximately 4 to 5 months of postgestational age, the greater trochanter ossifies at approximately 4 years of age, and the lesser trochanter ossifies at the age of 10 years.

The femoral shaft grows initially by enchondral ossification and production of a medullary cavity with calcification in the periphery and vascularization in the center, a process that results in a large primary ossification center. Woven bone results from this ossification and persists for the first 18 months of life, later becoming more adult-type lamellar bone. This longitudinal and peripheral growth continues until skeletal maturity.

The blood supply of the femoral shaft is from both endosteal and periosteal blood vessels. The endosteal supply is typically derived from two nutrient vessels that enter the femur from a posteromedial direction. The periosteal capillaries supply the outer 25% to 30% of cortical bone and are most prominent in the areas of muscular attachments to the femoral shaft (Fig. 43–67). These two circulatory systems, together with the metaphyseal complex of vessels, are interconnected to provide a strong vascular supply that allows rapid fracture repair.

MECHANISM OF INJURY

The mechanism of injury in femoral shaft fractures is largely correlated with age. Child abuse, the leading cause of femoral fractures before walking age, accounts for 70% to 80% of fractures in this age group.[42] Between 1 and 4 years of age, 30% of femoral shaft fractures are attributed to abuse. A high suspicion of abuse must therefore be entertained, and an appropriate history

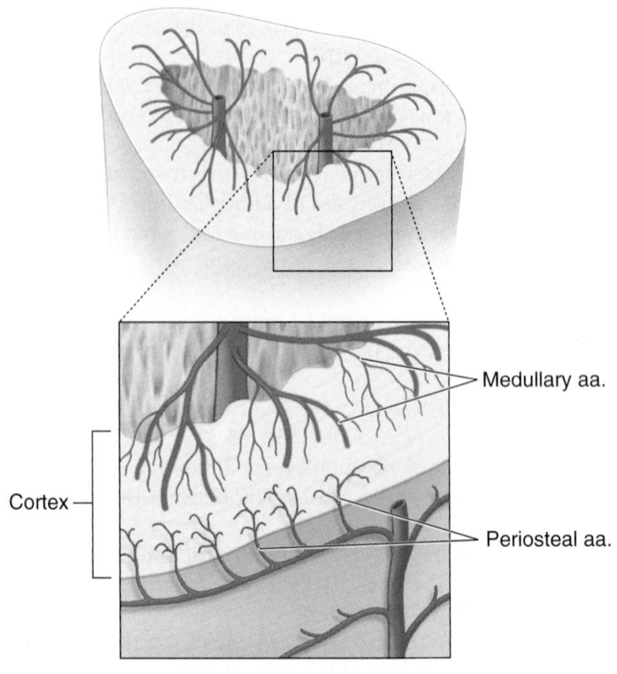

FIGURE 43-67 The blood supply to the femoral diaphysis. The medullary artery supplies the inner two thirds, and the periosteal vessels supply the outer third.

and directed physical examination should be undertaken to look for other injuries. In addition to age, other factors that should raise the suspicion of child abuse include a first-born child, preexisting brain damage of the child, bilateral fractures, subtrochanteric or distal metaphyseal beak fractures, and delay by the family in seeking treatment.[9] Careful analysis is needed because returning a child to a home where abuse has occurred can result in more abuse (approximately 50%) and death in 10% of cases.[40]

In the adolescent age group, high-velocity motor vehicle accidents are more often the mechanism of injury and account for up to 90% of all femoral shaft fractures.[50,70] High-energy trauma results in more significant fracture displacement, which should alert the clinician to the high probability that life-threatening intra-abdominal or intrathoracic injuries (or both) and head injuries are present. Rang has coined the term *Waddel's triad* to include a femoral fracture associated with head and thoracic injury sustained in an automobile-pedestrian accident.[90] In a review of pediatric femoral fractures secondary to motor vehicle–related events, 14% were associated with head injuries.[60] An organized, thorough initial examination and treatment are imperative in this setting and should reflect the current treatment algorithms for a polytraumatized patient.[14,70]

The timing of fixation of femoral shaft fractures in pediatric patients has been studied in a large series of polytraumatized patients. Unlike the case in adults, pulmonary complications rarely develop in children with multiple injuries and an associated femoral shaft fracture, and the timing of fracture stabilization does not appear to affect the prevalence of pneumonia or respiratory distress syndrome.[46]

Minor trauma or repetitive fractures should alert the clinician to the possibility of an underlying pathologic condition, including osteogenesis imperfecta, which is largely a diagnosis based on the typical signs of the disease (dentinogenesis imperfecta, blue sclerae, hearing loss, and multiple fractures). The diagnosis can be confirmed by analysis of collagen produced by cultured dermal fibroblasts. Generalized osteopenia from cerebral palsy, myelomeningocele, and other neuromuscular conditions also predisposes to fracture.[37]

Radiographs should always be carefully evaluated for localized pathologic conditions that can predispose to fracture. The most common benign conditions include aneurysmal bone cyst, unicameral bone cyst, nonossifying fibroma, and eosinophilic granuloma (Fig. 43–68). Malignant conditions are far less common and include osteogenic sarcoma, Ewing's sarcoma, and rarely, metastatic disease.

Another rare entity is a femoral shaft stress fracture, which is often accompanied by a long-standing complaint of pain in the thigh region in an adolescent athlete. No preceding trauma is recalled, and multiple medical opinions are usually sought without a conclusive diagnosis.[19] Timely diagnosis and treatment are essential to prevent a subsequent complete fracture.

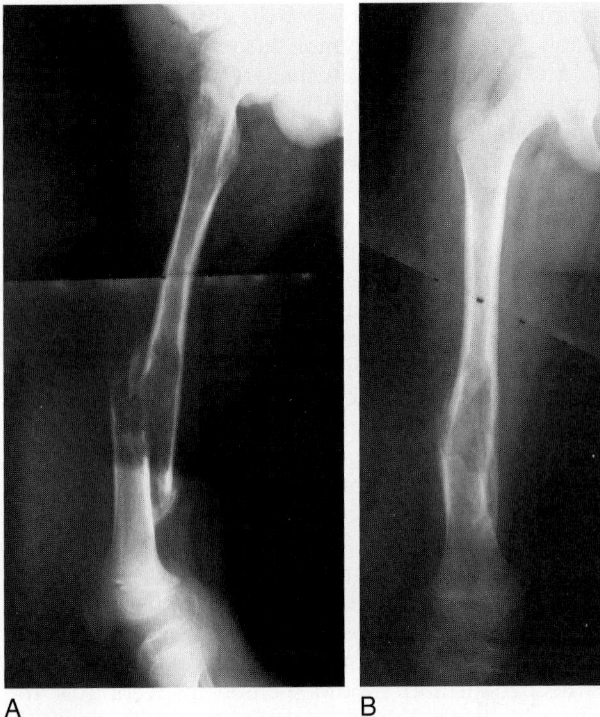

FIGURE 43–68 Pathologic femoral fracture through a unicameral bone cyst in a 10-year-old child. **A,** Preoperative radiograph. **B,** Radiograph obtained 2 months after injury.

CLASSIFICATION

Like most diaphyseal fractures, classification of femoral shaft fractures is based on the radiographic examination and the condition of the soft tissue envelope (closed or open fracture). Radiographs are evaluated for fracture location (proximal, middle, or distal third), configuration (transverse, oblique, or spiral), angulation, the degree of comminution, and the amount of displacement, translation, and shortening. Winquist and colleagues classified the amount of comminution, which is especially useful when rigid intramedullary nailing is used to treat a femoral shaft fracture.[113] Shortening is best classified as more than 3 cm (unacceptable shortening) or less than 3 cm (acceptable shortening) at the time of initial evaluation. The physical examination determines whether an open injury is present, defined as a fracture that communicates with the external environment, usually because of penetration of the fracture fragment in an inside-to-outside fashion. The three-part Gustilo system is used to classify all open fractures and helps determine the specific treatment plan, including the antibiotic regimen.[43]

CLINICAL FEATURES

Examination of an injured child must be individualized according to the age of the child and the circumstances of the injury. A patient with a femoral shaft fracture has localized tenderness and swelling and usually has a deformity with associated shortening and obvious crepitus on palpation. Careful and circumferential evaluation of the soft tissue envelope to look for areas of ecchymosis around the buttock and hip area may suggest an ipsilateral femoral neck or intertrochanteric fracture or hip dislocation. The skin should be thoroughly inspected to identify an open injury, which should be classified according to the Gustilo classification.[43]

A neurologic and vascular examination of the involved extremity should be performed and the findings compared with those on the contralateral side. The findings on repeat neurovascular examination after gentle reduction and immobilization in a splint or in boot traction should remain normal. If the child's neurovascular status declines after manipulation, the splint should be promptly removed and re-manipulation carried out.

Because many patients with femoral shaft fractures have sustained high-energy trauma, a multidisciplinary team approach is necessary. The initial resuscitative treatment is usually carried out by a general surgeon and should follow well-established guidelines.[4] The secondary definitive, injury-specific examination should not be limited to the primary complaint of the patient and should include inspection of the back and spine. Every extremity must be carefully inspected and palpated to avoid missing injuries, which can become extremely difficult to treat if detected late. This is especially important in a head-injured patient who is unable to communicate symptoms. Repeated examinations are a necessary part of the evaluation in this clinical situation.

RADIOGRAPHIC FINDINGS

Standard AP and lateral radiographs of the entire femur, including the hip and knee joint, are necessary. In the proximal femur, femoral neck and intertrochanteric fractures and hip dislocations can be associated with a diaphyseal fracture and are missed in up to a third of cases.[12,31,54,101] In the distal femur, associated physeal injuries and ligamentous and meniscal injuries are often seen.[106] Poor-quality radiographs are unacceptable, and the study must be repeated before the patient leaves the emergency department or radiology suite. In an older child, a Thomas traction splint that has been applied either in the field or on arrival in the emergency department often obscures the proximal femur on the initial radiographs (Fig. 43–69). This splint should be adjusted or removed to allow complete imaging of the proximal femoral bony anatomy.

The radiographs should be evaluated for fracture configuration, degree of comminution, displacement, angulation, and degree of shortening. This information is important in understanding the mechanism of injury and the force imparted to the bone and soft tissue, information ultimately used in planning treatment. The deforming forces of the surrounding musculature result in characteristic displacement patterns (Fig. 43–70). For example, a proximal third fracture will result in flexion (iliopsoas), abduction (abductor muscle group), and lateral rotation (external rotators) of the proximal fragment.

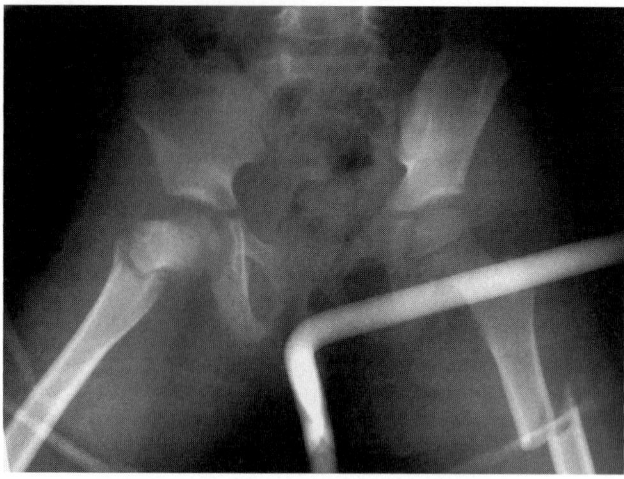

FIGURE 43–69 Femoral fracture. The initial anteroposterior radiograph, shown here, demonstrates a fracture of the diaphysis of the femur; however, the proximal femur cannot be seen because of obstruction by the traction splint. A basicervical neck fracture is seen on the right.

Plain radiographs are usually all that is needed to evaluate femoral shaft fractures. Rarely, stress fractures require CT[19] or MRI to confirm the diagnosis. CT is best used to evaluate intra-articular fractures of the femoral head and distal femur, hip dislocations (to assess for intra-articular loose fragments after reduction), and physeal injuries. Angiography is indicated in the setting of diminished or absent pulses associated with a femoral shaft fracture, all knee dislocations,[105,111] and the presence of an ipsilateral tibial fracture (floating knee).

TREATMENT

Several methods can be used to treat femoral shaft fractures in children. The age and size of the child are the most important factors in deciding which treatment modality is most appropriate. In general, we prefer to treat a younger child nonoperatively in a Pavlik harness or hip spica cast and an older child with some form of skeletal fixation. Additional factors to consider include the mechanism of injury, the presence of multiple injuries, the soft tissue condition, the family support environment, and the economic resources available. Finally, as in any form of orthopaedic treatment, the experience, skill, and preference of the treating physician play a significant role in determining treatment. We use the following guidelines, based on the age of the patient, to determine treatment.

Age Guidelines

0 to 6 Months. In a child 6 months or younger or a small child up to 12 months of age, immediate application of a Pavlik harness results in an excellent outcome, with time to union averaging 5 weeks.[87,99] Advantages of the Pavlik harness include ease of application without requiring a general anesthetic or sedation, minimal hospitalization, ability to adjust the harness

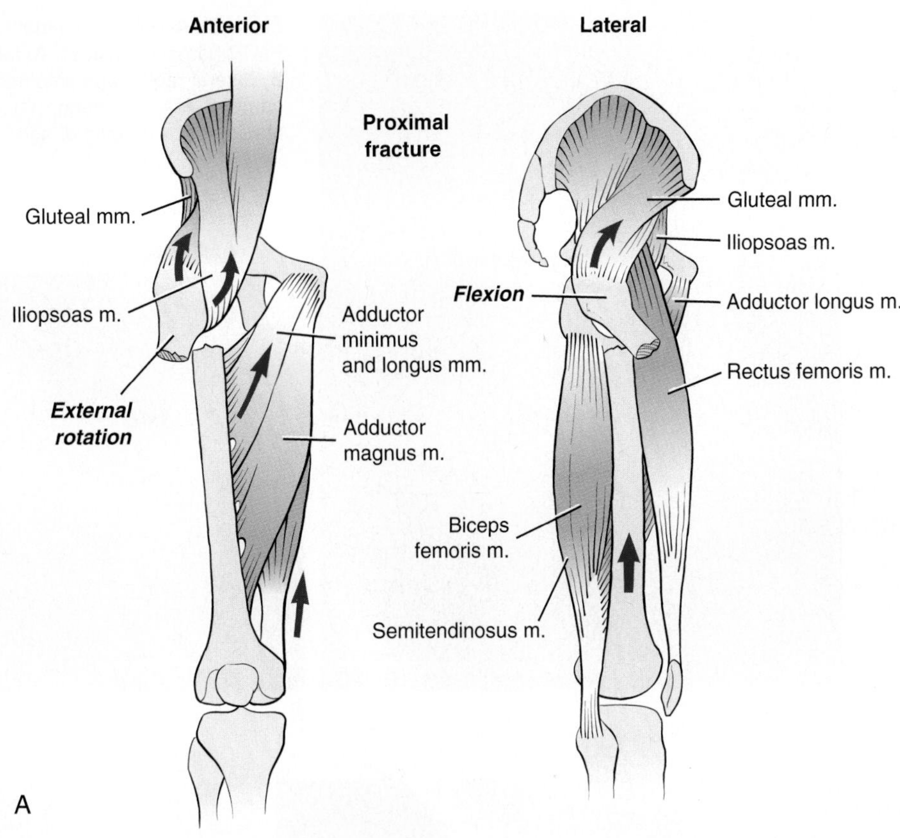

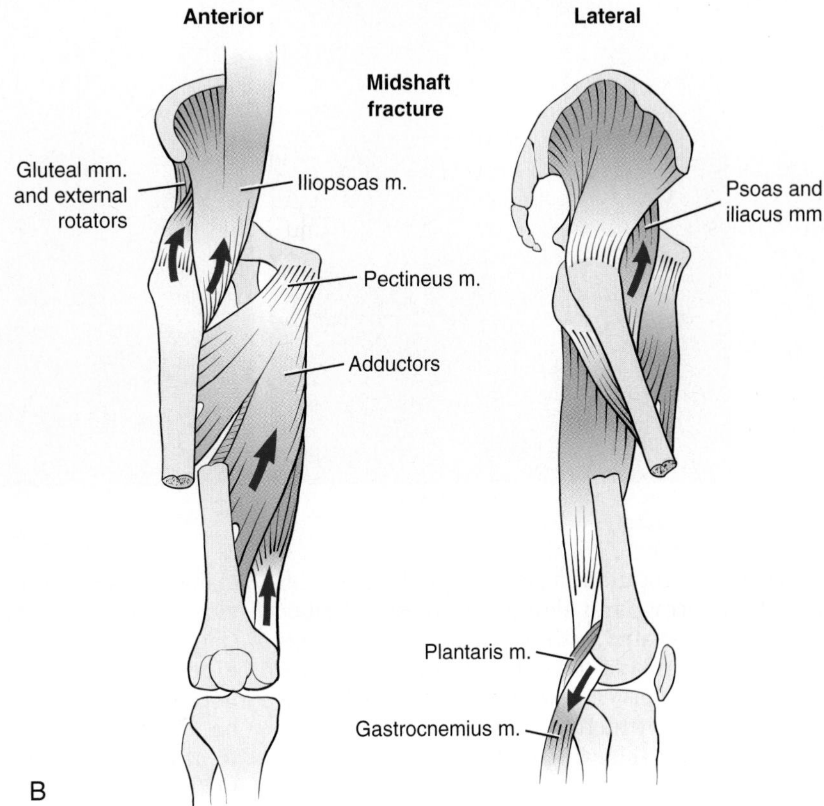

FIGURE 43-70 Characteristic displacement patterns in femoral shaft fractures. **A,** Displacement of fragments in fractures of the upper third of the femoral shaft. **B,** Displacement of fragments in fractures of the middle third of the femoral shaft.

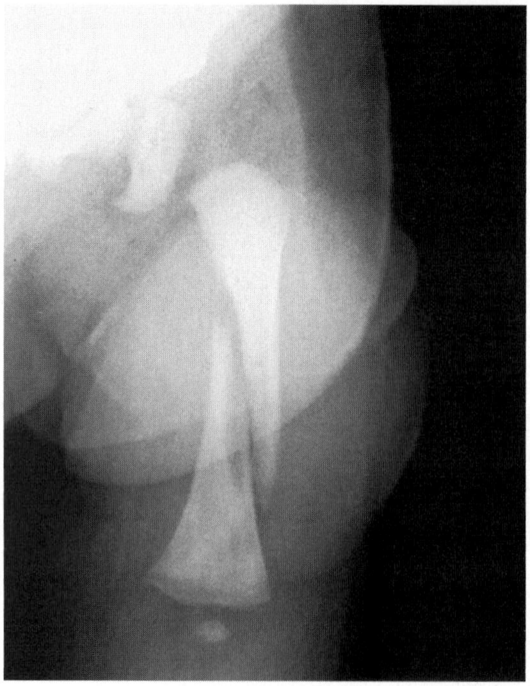

FIGURE 43–71 Treatment of a femoral fracture with a Pavlik harness (infants). **A,** Initial injury in a 3-week-old infant. **B,** Lateral radiograph obtained with the infant in the Pavlik harness. Anteroposterior **(C)** and lateral **(D)** radiographs obtained at 4 months of age.

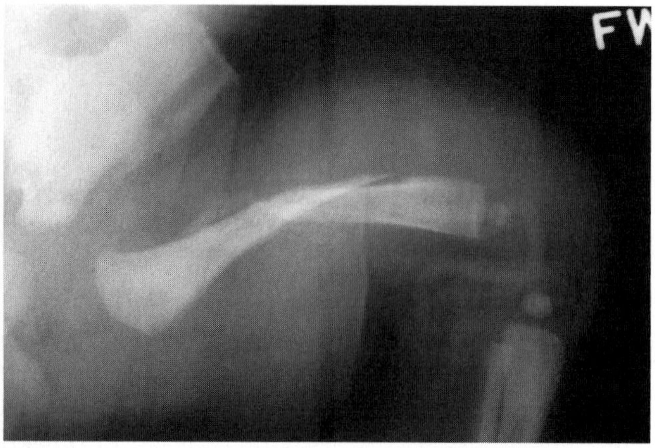

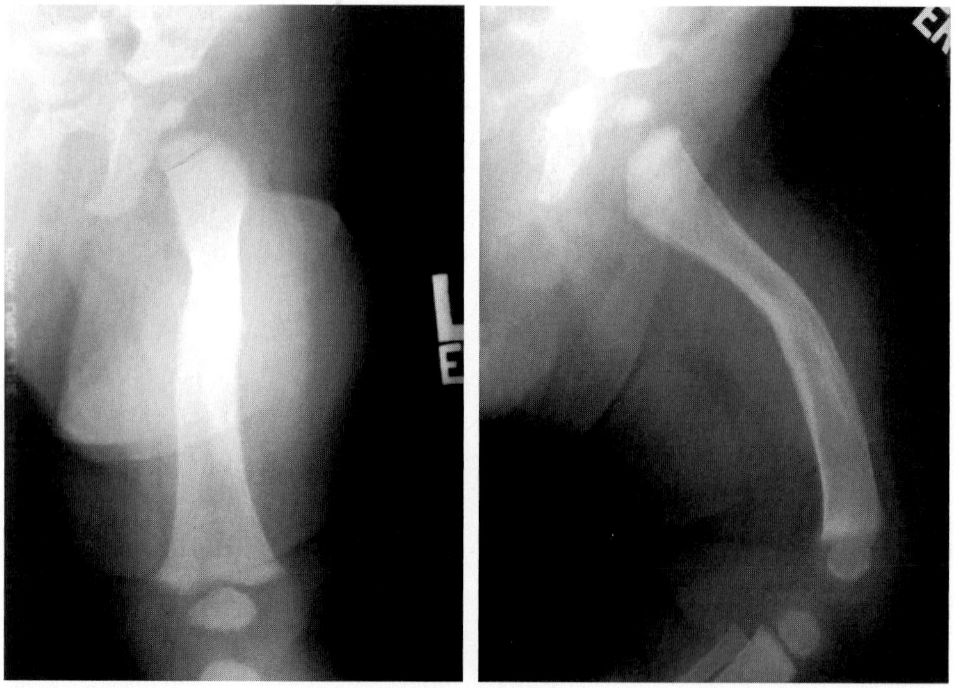

when fracture manipulation is required, ease of nursing and diapering, and absence of the skin irritation commonly associated with casting.[87] Excessive hip flexion in the presence of a swollen thigh may compress the femoral nerve, and the surgeon should monitor quadriceps function during treatment to detect such an injury (Fig. 43–71).

7 Months to 5 Years. When shortening of the fracture is limited to less than 2 to 3 cm and the fracture has a stable, simple pattern, we prefer to treat the child by closed reduction and immediate spica cast application (Fig. 43–72). Skin or skeletal traction is required when excess shortening (>3 cm) or angulation (>30 degrees) is present. In a multiply injured patient, traction may be used until associated injuries permit definitive treatment, without negatively affecting outcomes.[46,76] Definitive treatment may be casting, flexible intramedullary rods, or external fixation, depending on associated injuries. In larger 5-year-old children with a stable

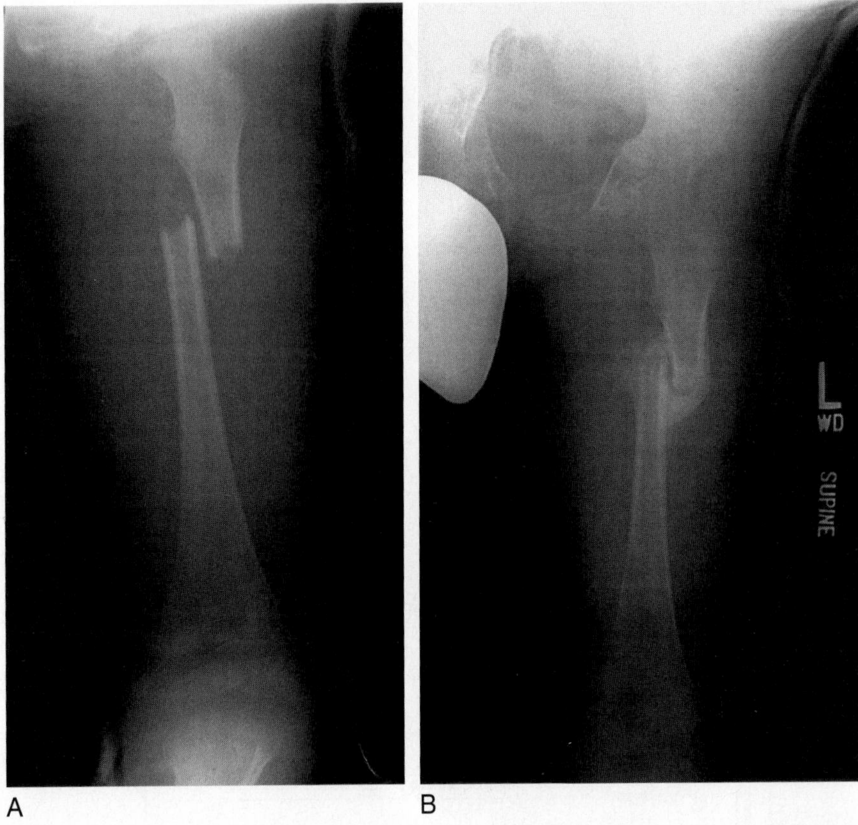

FIGURE 43–72 Treatment of a femoral fracture in a young child (7 months to 5 years). **A,** Initial postreduction radiograph showing 2 cm of shortening in a child 3 years 6 months of age who was treated by immediate closed reduction and spica casting. **B,** Radiographic appearance after 7 weeks in the cast.

fracture pattern, we may use Enders intramedullary rods (Synthes, Paoli, Pa).

6 to 10 Years. Femoral shaft fractures in children between 6 and 10 years of age are treated by closed or open reduction and stabilized with flexible rods (Enders stainless steel or Nancy titanium elastic nails), especially when a stable transverse fracture pattern is present. Additional modes of treatment include initial skeletal traction followed by spica cast treatment, compression plate fixation, submuscular bridge plating, or external fixation (Fig. 43–73).

11 Years to Skeletal Maturity. Flexible intramedullary rodding is an excellent choice with a stable fracture pattern. Submuscular plate fixation may be considered for unstable patterns. A rigid locked intramedullary rod is preferred in some centers, but it must be placed with the proximal starting point in the tip of the greater trochanter to minimize the risk for AVN of the femoral head.

Treatment Techniques

Traction

Skin Traction. Skin traction is a noninvasive technique that is used in the two settings. First, in a small child whose fracture is too shortened (>3 cm) to allow immediate spica casting, traction is used to align the fracture until enough callus formation has occurred to permit spica cast application. Second, in any child who is to undergo definitive skeletal fixation on a delayed

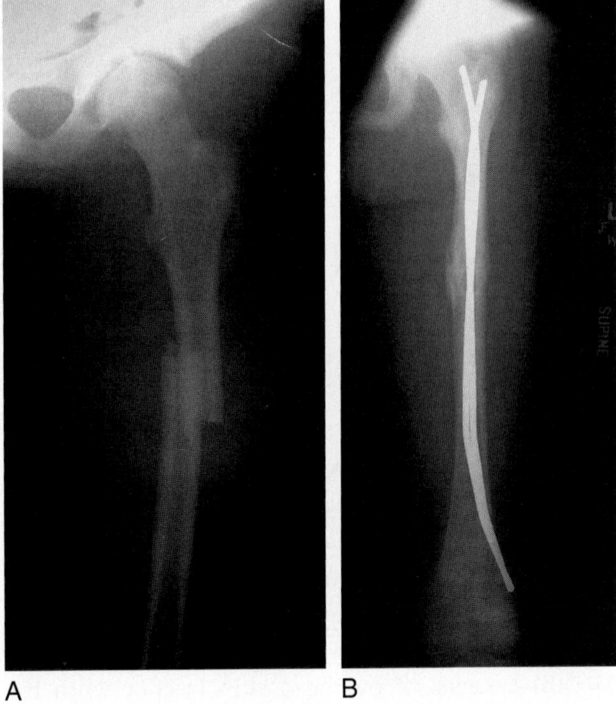

FIGURE 43–73 Stabilization of femoral shaft fractures in children 6 to 10 years of age. **A,** A 7-year-old child with a transverse fracture of the femur treated with two Enders flexible nails placed in retrograde fashion **(B).**

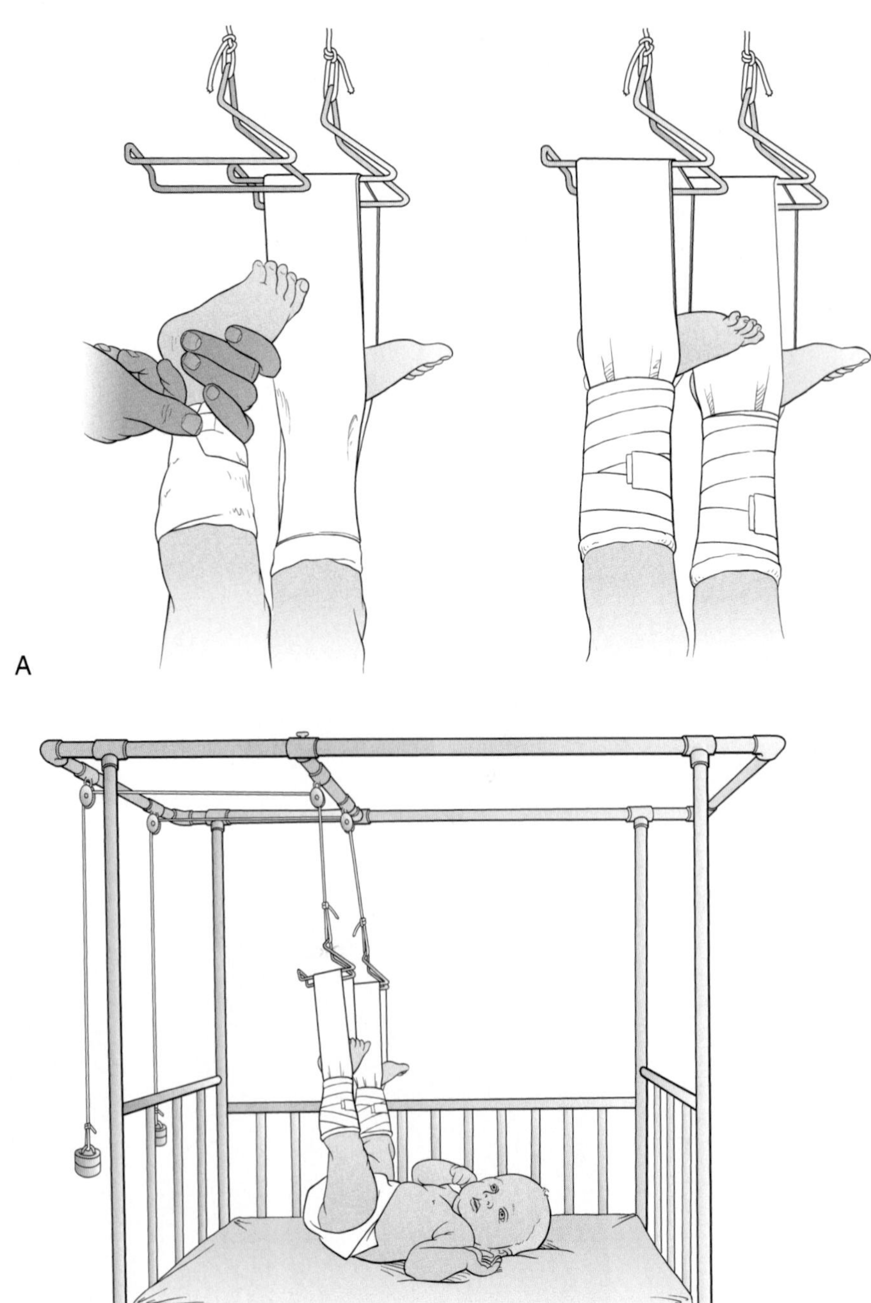

FIGURE 43–74 Traction for the treatment of a femoral shaft fraction. **A,** Application of skin traction initially entails placing cotton cast padding onto the skin and taping it in place in a U shape, which is then overwrapped with an elastic bandage. **B,** Small child placed in Bryant's traction. In this overhead skin traction technique, just enough weight is placed to elevate the buttock off the surface of the bed.

basis, skin traction will temporarily stabilize and align the leg and thereby provide some stability and comfort in the interim period (Fig. 43–74A).

Although skin traction is effective in these settings, there are potential problems and complications. Used in a very young child (<2 years), Bryant's traction (Fig. 43–74B) consists of overhead skin traction with the hips flexed to 90 degrees and the knees fully extended.[16] Because the traction is applied through the skin, patients with abnormal sensation in the lower extremities should not be treated in this fashion. Vascular insufficiency is the most serious complication and results from the vertical position of the legs (increased resistance to distal leg perfusion), extension of the knees (stretching of the popliteal artery) and from compression of the external wrapping on the leg.[83] The complications of overhead Bryant's traction can be avoided by applying traction in a position of 90 degrees of hip flexion and 45 degrees of knee flexion,[34] which is recommended when skin traction is to be used. Skin blistering and sloughing must be avoided with any form of skin traction; these problems are minimized when the amount of weight used is no more than 5 to 10 lb, depending on the size of the child. When more weight is required to control the fracture, we prefer to use skeletal traction.

Skeletal Traction. Skeletal traction is a more powerful technique to apply traction to the femur. It is used in an older child with a diaphyseal fracture, when more than 5 to 10 lb of weight is required, and in any child with a proximal femoral fracture in whom 90-90 traction is needed. The distal end of the femur is the best site for placement of the traction pin, which should be inserted parallel to the knee joint to prevent varus or valgus deformity (Fig. 43–75).[27] Under sedation and sterile conditions, the distal femoral traction pin should be inserted just superior to the adductor tubercle and advanced laterally (Fig. 43–76). When soft tissue injury and contamination prevent femoral traction pin placement, the traction pin can be inserted in the proximal end of the tibia, but only after the knee has been carefully examined to exclude ligamentous injuries. The proximal tibial traction pin should be placed distal to the tibial tubercle physis to avoid anterior growth arrest and the development of a recurvatum deformity.[5,58,80]

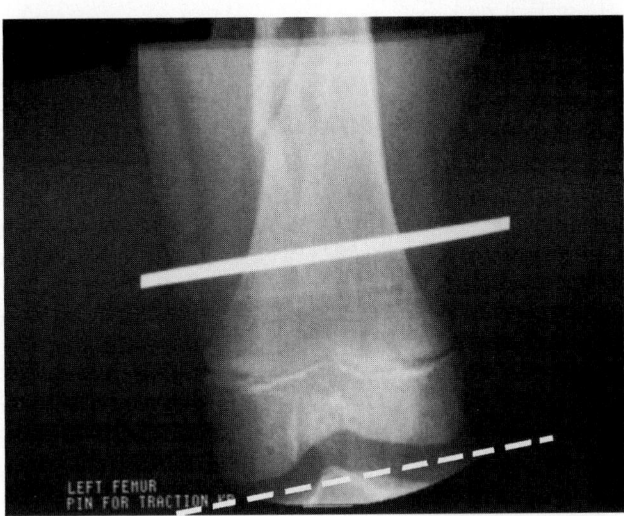

FIGURE 43–75 Distal femoral traction pin placed perpendicular to the femur and parallel to the knee joint line (*dotted line*).

Results and Cautions. Traction should reduce the fracture to within 2 cm in a younger child, and end-to-end apposition should be achieved in a child older than 11 years.[5] Radiographs of the femur should be obtained in both the AP and lateral views to check alignment and callus formation. Traction can be continued for 2 to 3 weeks, until callus forms and the child has no or minimal tenderness on palpation at the fracture site. Traction pins can be incorporated into a hip spica cast at an early period to better control the fracture; however, this is frequently complicated by pin tract infection and pin breakage. **(We do not recommend this technique.)**

Spica Casting. Immediate spica casting has been advocated in a child with an isolated stable femoral shaft fracture and less than 3 mm of shortening, in a child younger than 8 years, and for a fracture without massive swelling of the thigh.[33,59,99] If these conditions are not present, a period of traction should be used. Another important factor is the social situation in which the child is living because the most difficult problems encountered by families have to do with transportation of the child and keeping the child clean in the cast. Preschool children tolerate a spica cast much better than school-aged children do because younger children can be transported more easily and have shorter healing times.[56]

The cast should be placed with the child's hips flexed approximately 60 to 90 degrees (the more proximal the fracture, the more the hip should be flexed) and 30 degrees of abduction; the knees should be flexed to 90 degrees (Fig. 43–77). Some external

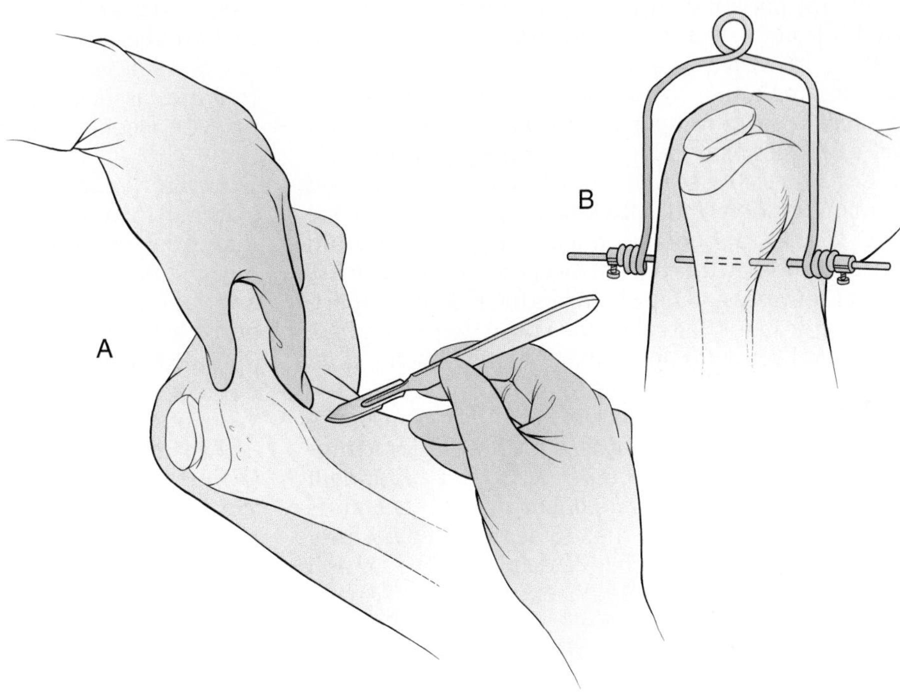

FIGURE 43–76 Placement of a femoral traction pin just superior to the adductor tubercle. **A,** The site is prepared with sterile technique, and a local anesthetic is used. **B,** Traction pin in place with a traction bow.

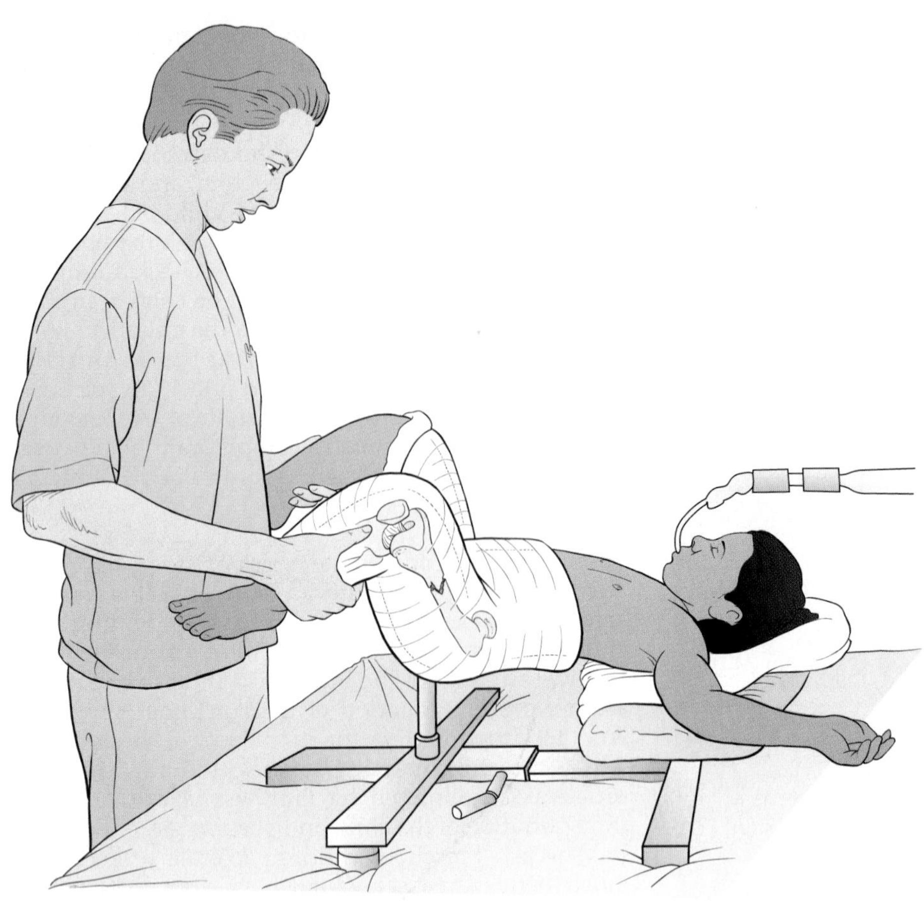

FIGURE 43–77 Hip spica casting for a left femoral shaft fracture in a young child. The hips are flexed to approximately 60 degrees and the knees to 90 degrees.

rotation will correct the rotational deformity of the distal fragment. Several authors have recommended placing a long-leg cast initially and then transferring the patient to the hip spica table and applying the remainder of the cast.[3,59] We and others[98] recommend placing the patient on the spica table and applying the cast while an assistant holds the fracture in a reduced position. However, care must be taken to avoid excessive compression or traction through the region of the popliteal fossa, as compartment syndrome of the lower part of the leg is a recognized complication of early spica casting.[67] If a segmental below-knee cast is used for manipulation and subsequent extension into the spica, special caution and junctional padding should be used; however, this type of cast is not recommended, as focal compression may increase the risk of compartment syndrome. Preferably, the entire cast is applied, and a good condylar and buttock mold is then placed into the cast.

Radiographs in the lateral and AP planes are obtained before the cast hardens to allow mild manipulation as needed in the cast. Acceptable alignment depends on the age of the patient but, in general, is considered to be no more than 15 degrees of deformity in the coronal plane and 25 to 30 degrees in the sagittal plane.[2,59] Shortening should not exceed 2.0 cm. Radiographs should be obtained weekly during the first 2 to 3 weeks to allow correction of any loss of the initial reduction. Excessive shortening within this period is corrected only by removal of the cast and a short time in traction followed by recasting. Wedging of the cast will allow some correction of angular deformity (up to 15 degrees) but must be done with caution because peroneal palsy has been reported during correction of valgus deformities (Fig. 43–78).[112] Femoral fractures that are more susceptible to losing reduction are fractures resulting from a high-energy mechanism and fractures associated with polytrauma. Careful follow-up with weekly radiographs should be performed.

External Fixation. The main indications today for external fixation are (1) an open fracture; (2) severe disruption of the soft tissue envelope, including severe burns; (3) multiple trauma; (4) an extremity with an arterial injury requiring immediate revascularization of the extremity; (5) an unstable fracture pattern; and (6) failed conservative management.[2,6,13,25,28,57,104] External fixation is generally indicated in children 5 to 11 years of age.

The most commonly used fixators today are the Orthofix Dynamic Axial Fixator (EBI)[57] (Orthofix, Winston-Salem, NC) and the AO Fixator (Synthes Ltd., Paoli, PA). These unilateral fixators are relatively easy to apply and allow angular correction during the follow-up period (Fig. 43–79). The fixators are generally left on for 10 to 16 weeks, until solid union has been achieved. Weight bearing is permitted as early as tolerated and depends to some degree on the stability

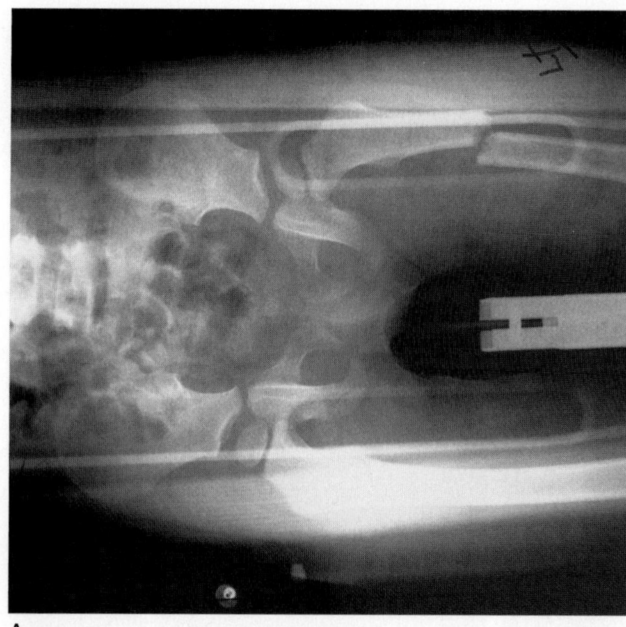

FIGURE 43-78 Manipulation and wedging of a malunited femoral fracture. **A,** Initial radiograph of a left femoral fracture in a 3-year-old. **B,** At 5 weeks there was excess varus angulation. **C,** Percutaneous osteoclasis was performed, followed by casting. The initial casting resulted in residual varus. Wedging of the cast with an opening medial wedge osteotomy corrected the deformity. **D,** Six weeks after osteoclasis and cast wedging, the fracture has healed in good alignment.

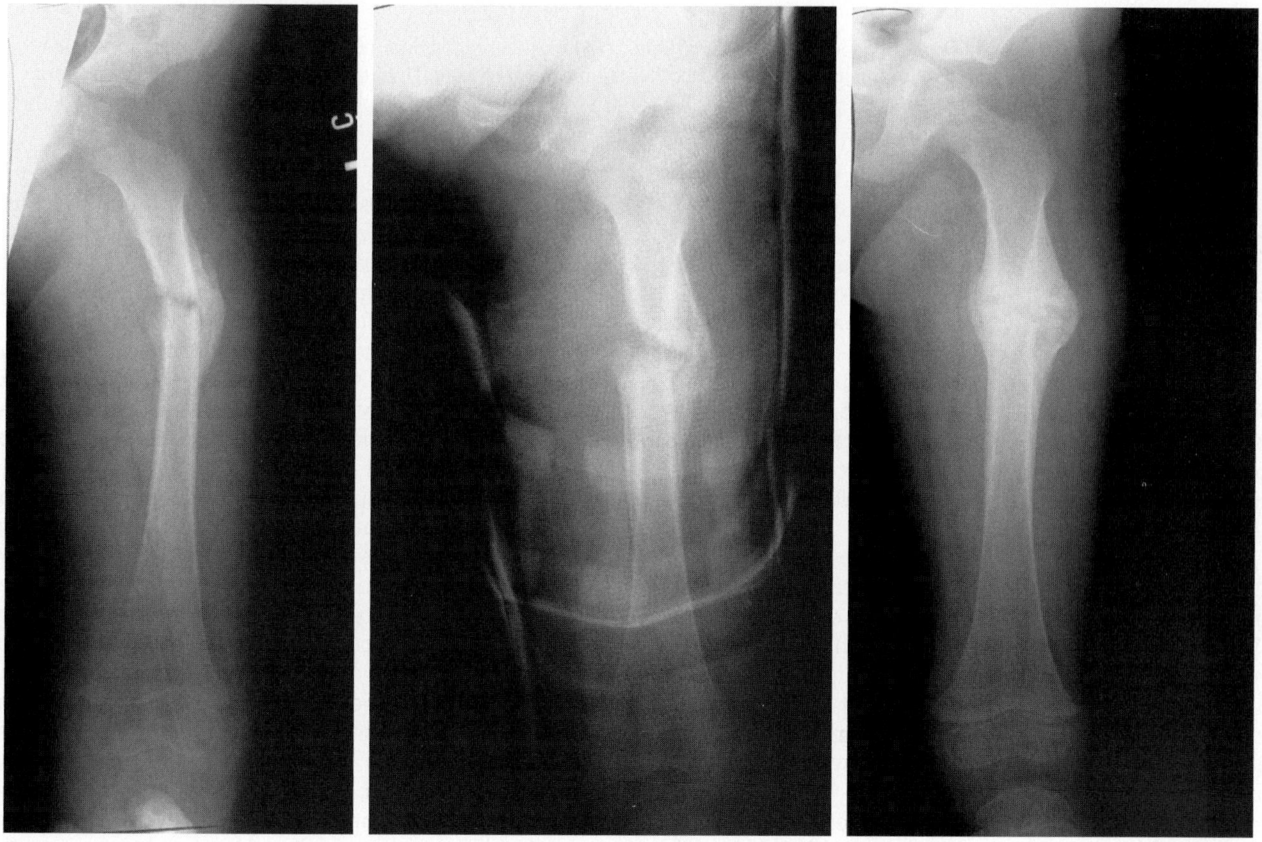

A

B C D

of the fracture and the external fixator. Blasier and colleagues reported a large series of 139 femoral fractures treated with an external fixator in children whose average age was 9 years. Progressive weight bearing was encouraged, and the time in the external fixator averaged 11.4 weeks, with no reported nonunions.[13]

The most common complication of treatment with an external fixator is pin tract infection (approximately 50% of cases), which generally responds to good pin care and antibiotics. Rates of nonunion, delayed union, and angular deformity are generally reported to be slightly higher than when more rigid fixation

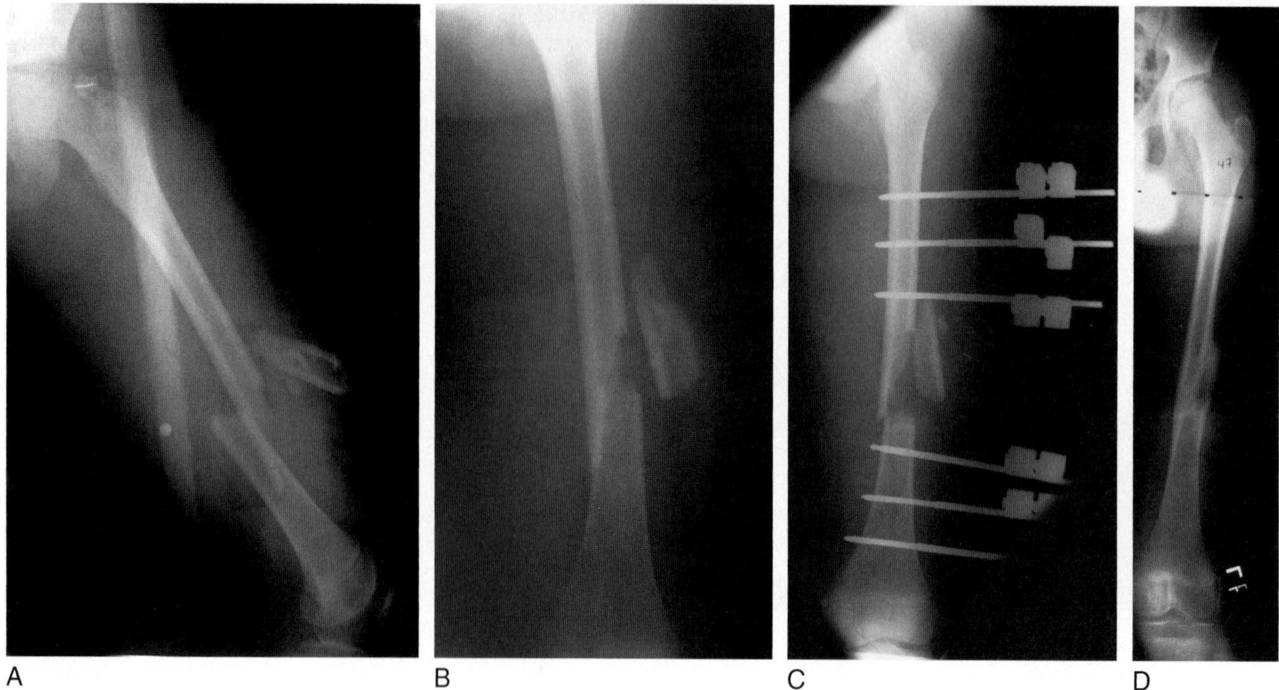

FIGURE 43-79 External fixation of a femoral shaft fracture. Lateral (**A**) and anteroposterior (**B**) initial radiographs in a 12-year-old child with an open femoral fracture. **C**, Appearance after application of an external fixator. **D**, Final healing at 1-year follow-up. Bone grafting had been performed at 4 months.

techniques are used. Refracture is also more common, with a reported incidence of 1.5% to 21% (Fig. 43–80).[6,13,23,49,81,88,103,104] These complications are most common in fractures with a short oblique fracture pattern. Because refracture occurs at the previous fracture site as a consequence of incomplete union, the fixator should be left in place until solid union is seen radiographically. Shortening and overgrowth have not been a major issue, with less than 5 mm of overgrowth commonly reported, and complete apposition of the fracture fragments should be achieved at the time of initial reduction.[17,48]

Open Reduction and Internal Fixation. Proponents of internal fixation with plates and screws recommend this form of treatment for children with multiple trauma or patients with closed head injuries. The main advantages of this technique are that fracture stabilization is performed quickly, anatomic reduction is achieved, and the fracture is rigidly fixed, thereby allowing early mobilization. Open reduction with plate fixation is relatively easy to perform, and this method can be used in any age group (Fig. 43–81). The disadvantages are the large incision and soft tissue stripping, the risk of plate breakage and refracture, and the need for plate removal, with a risk for recurrent fracture. Because anatomic reduction with end-to-end bony apposition is achieved, overgrowth can be seen, although it has not been reported to be a clinical problem.[110]

Most reports of the use of open reduction with internal fixation in a child's femur involve patients with multiple injuries. Ward and colleagues reported on 25 patients, 22 of whom had multiple injuries. Fracture union occurred in 11 weeks in 23 of the 24 patients available for follow-up. They concluded that this technique is acceptable in a child who is younger than 11 years and has a severe head injury or associated polytrauma.[110] Similarly, Kregor and colleagues reported on 15 fractures, 6 of which were open, in patients who had sustained multiple injuries or a head injury. Radiographic union of the fracture occurred at an average of 8 weeks. The compression plates were removed at an average of 10 months postoperatively, with no restriction of activities at an average follow-up of 26 months.[65] In a series of 60 patients with varied clinical findings who were treated with compression plating, the following complications were reported: one case of hardware failure, two refractures, two symptomatic leg length inequalities, and one hypertrophic scar. Average time to union in this series was 8 weeks.[20]

Submuscular Bridge Plating. Submuscular plating through a limited approach with indirect fracture reduction has been shown to be a useful technique for comminuted fractures and other patterns with significant potential for fracture shortening.[1,62,94] In this technique, a 12- to 16-hole, 4.5-mm limited-contact plate is inserted submuscularly and superficial to the periosteum through a 2-cm incision over the proximal or distal metaphyseal flare. The fracture is reduced with manual traction or the assistance of a fracture table, and the plate is used to bridge the unstable portion of the fracture. Fluoroscopic assistance is used to reduce

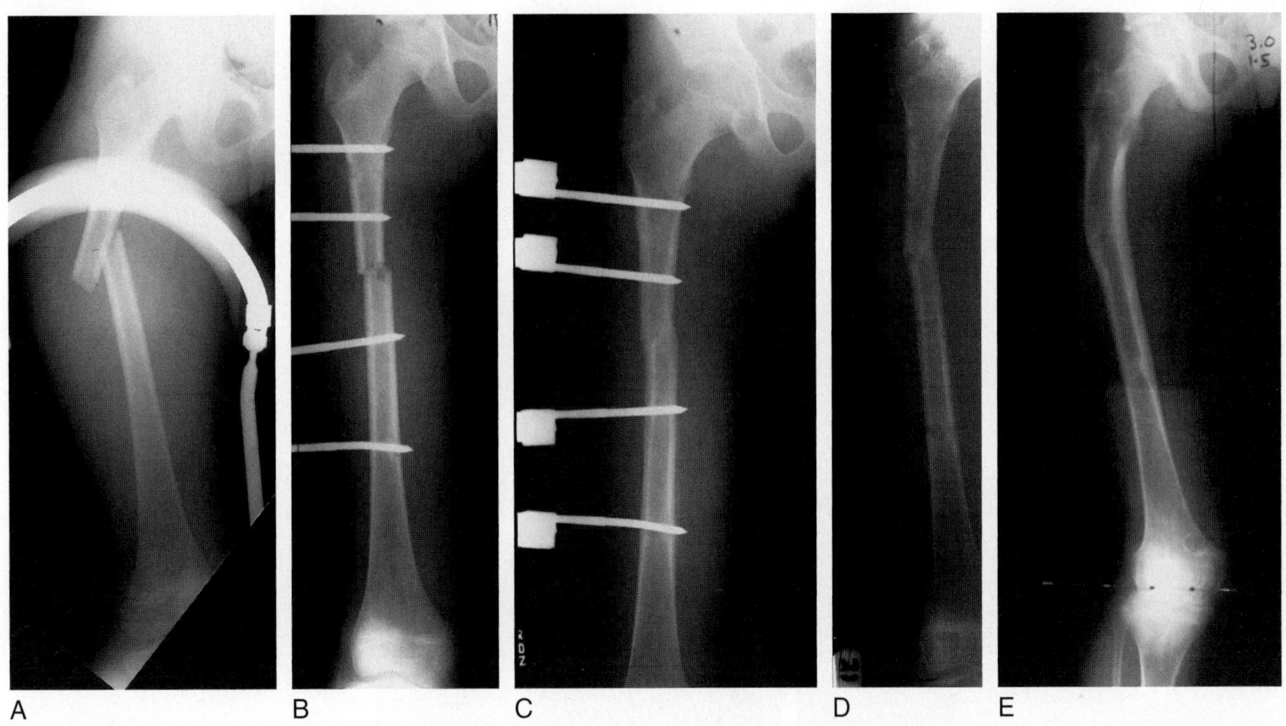

FIGURE 43–80 Femoral shaft refracture after removal of an external fixator. **A,** Initial radiograph obtained in a 12-year-old child with a proximal femoral shaft fracture. **B,** Radiographic appearance after the application of an external fixator. **C,** Radiographic appearance at 9 weeks. Adequate fracture healing allowed removal of the fixation. **D,** Refracture through the original fracture site occurred days after removal of the fixator. A hip spica cast was used to treat the refracture. **E,** Radiograph obtained after complete healing.

fracture and place screws in a percutaneous fashion through small-spaced stab incisions. Initial plate placement may be maintained by the use of Kirschner wires in the proximal and distal holes, and screws may be used to achieve reduction of the femur to the plate. At least three screws, in a spaced fashion, are recommended proximal and distal to the fracture.

The plate is removed 6 to 9 months after insertion.[47] Several series have demonstrated minimal complications with an average time to union of 12 weeks.[1,62,94] The ability to maintain length reduction through a limited approach makes this technique a viable alternative to flexible intramedullary fixation for fracture patterns with the potential for length instability (Fig. 43–82).

Intramedullary Fixation. Intramedullary fixation has assumed a more prominent role in the treatment of femoral shaft fractures in children and adolescents. The main advantages of intramedullary fixation are that external immobilization is not usually required and, because of the load-sharing capability of the rod or rods, immediate or early weight bearing is allowed. The two implants most often used are flexible Enders nails in younger children and rigid locked intramedullary nails in older children and adolescents.

Flexible Intramedullary Fixation

INDICATIONS. Flexible nail fixation has generally been reported to result in excellent fracture union with few complications in the pediatric population (Fig. 43–83).[8,22,32,51,55,63,74,75,95] The additional advantage of a flexible nail over a rigid interlocking rod is that the proximal insertion site avoids the piriformis fossa and the greater trochanter, thus preventing the possibility of AVN of the femoral head and growth arrest, respectively. In addition, the distal insertion site does not require dissection into the knee joint or violation of the distal physis. Enders flexible nails can be used in children 6 to 16 years of age, although they have been reported to be used in children as young as 4 years. Flexible nailing may be done in a child with multiple injuries, concomitant head injury, open fractures, and an extremity with an ipsilateral tibial fracture (floating knee).

PROCEDURE. The fracture pattern most amenable to this treatment is a transverse stable fracture with minimal comminution. Long spiral fractures are a relative contraindication because rotational deformity and shortening are likely to occur. Flexible nails can be used with caution for long oblique and spiral fractures; however, the stability of the fracture site should be evaluated at the time of surgery. Any concern about the stability of the fracture in this setting should prompt the surgeon to apply a single-limb hip spica cast to supplement the fixation for a short period. Carey and Galpin reported on 25 femoral fractures, 8 of which were long oblique or spiral fractures treated by antegrade flexible nailing.[22] No significant problems occurred with regard to angular or rotational

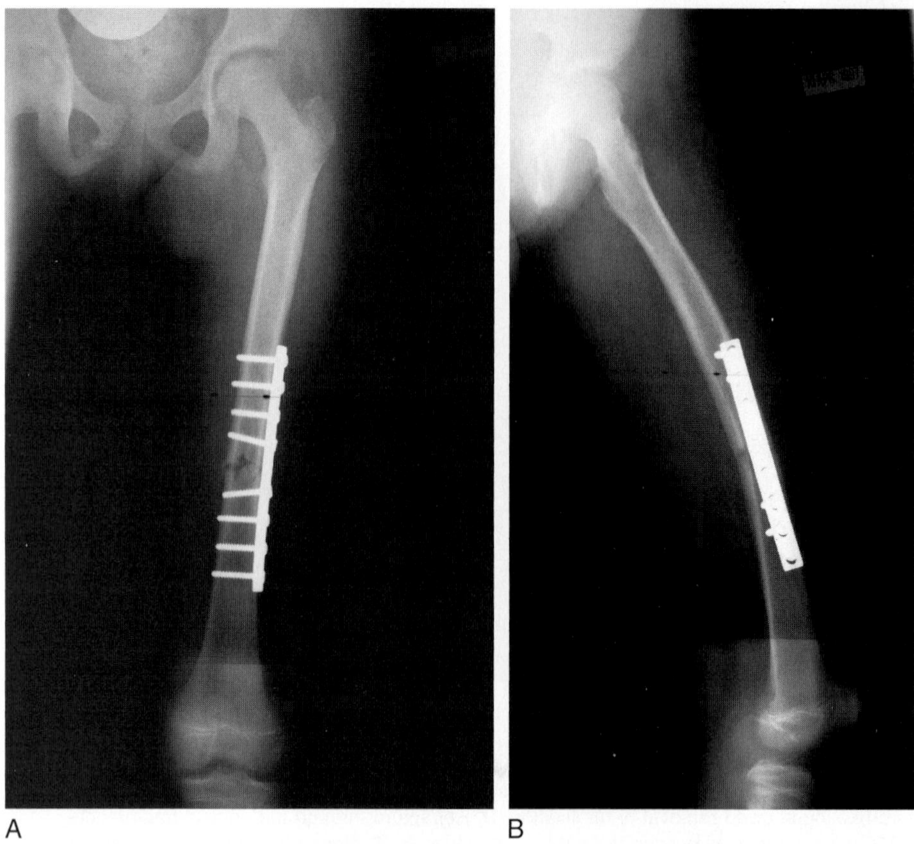

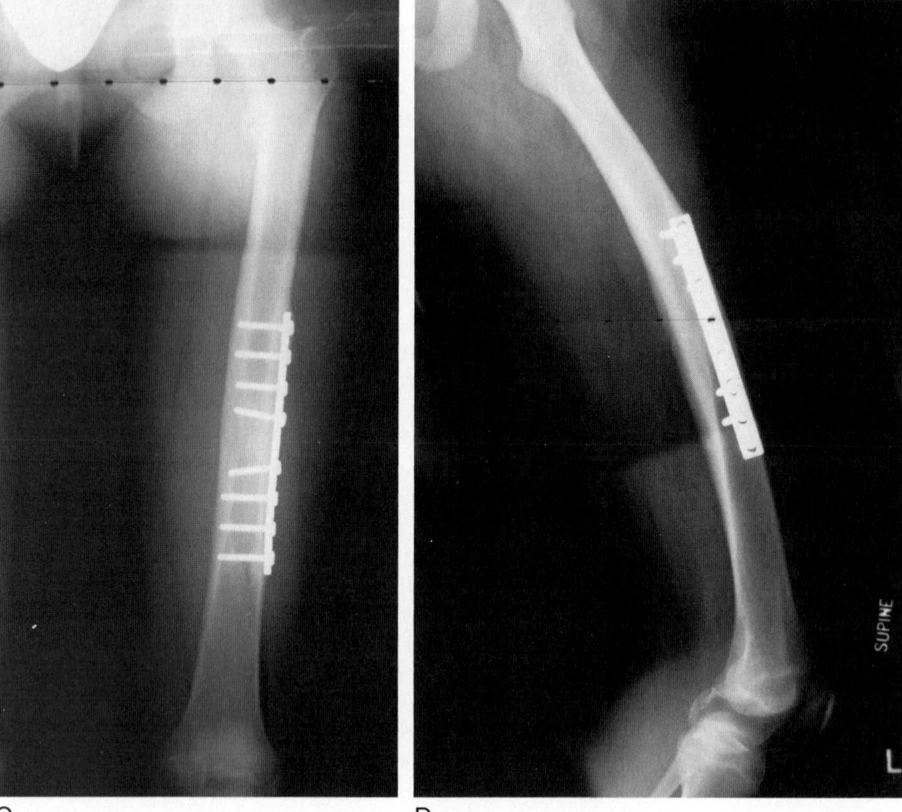

FIGURE 43–81 Plate fixation of a femoral shaft fracture. Anteroposterior **(A)** and lateral **(B)** radiographic appearance in a 12-year-old with a transverse femoral fracture. **C** and **D,** The same views at 8 months after injury, showing abundant callus formation and solid healing. The plate was not removed.

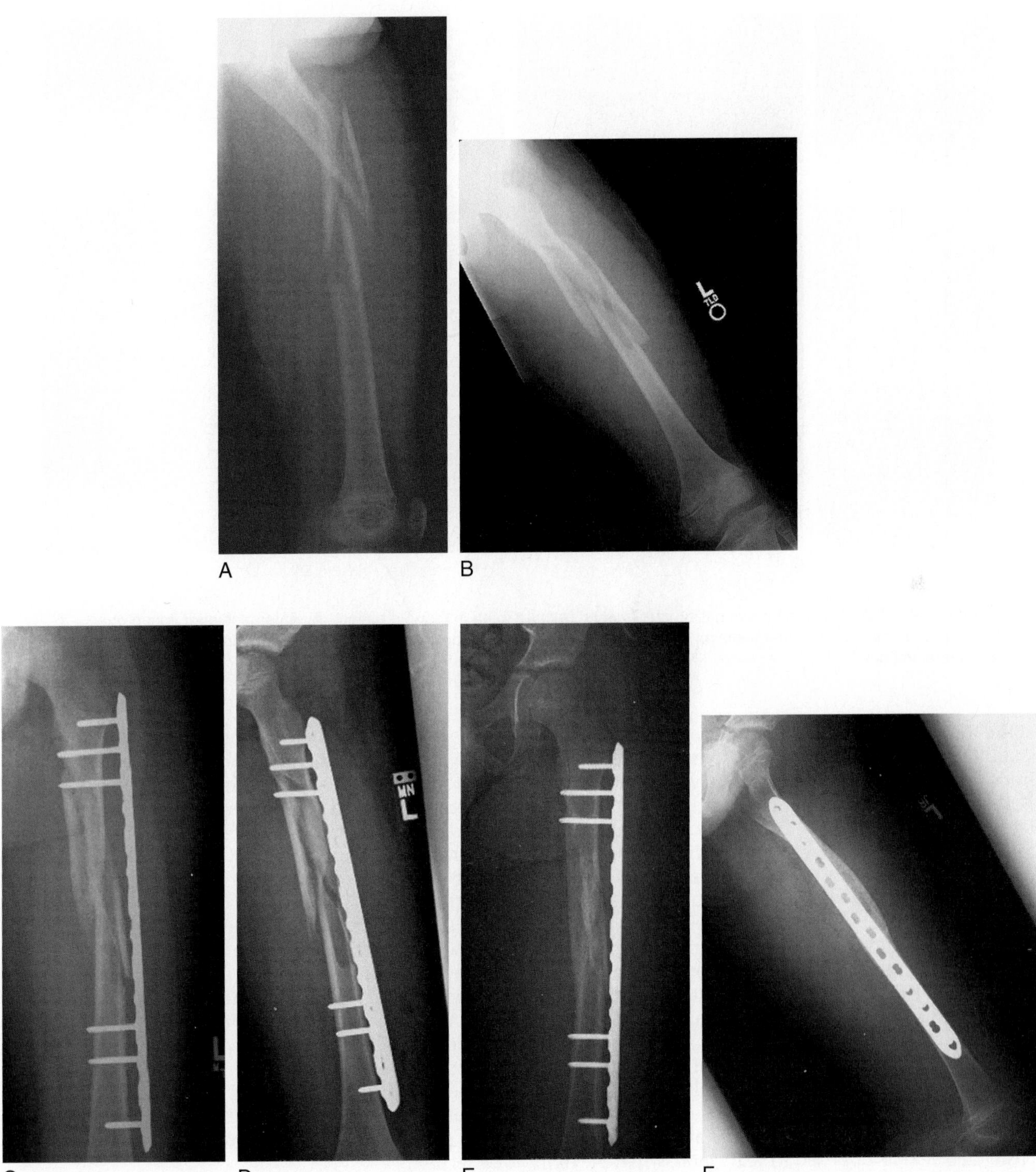

FIGURE 43–82 Plate fixation with a femoral submuscular plate. **A,** Lateral image showing a comminuted diaphyseal fracture. **B,** Anteroposterior (AP) image. **C,** AP image showing submuscular plate fixation. **D,** Lateral image. **E,** Early union with maintenance of reduction. **F,** Lateral image.

deformity or shortening. Postoperatively, weight bearing is generally started immediately, as tolerated by the patient, especially in children with a stable fracture pattern, although some authors wait 4 to 8 weeks before allowing full weight bearing.[32,75] We prefer to have the patient fully bear weight without any external immobilization, but unstable or distal fractures may require a knee immobilizer or walking single-limb hip spica cast (Fig. 43–84).

The flexible nails may be placed antegrade or retrograde, depending on the location of the fracture site and the overall preference and experience of the surgeon. We prefer to use the larger of the two fragments for the insertion site to promote greater stability

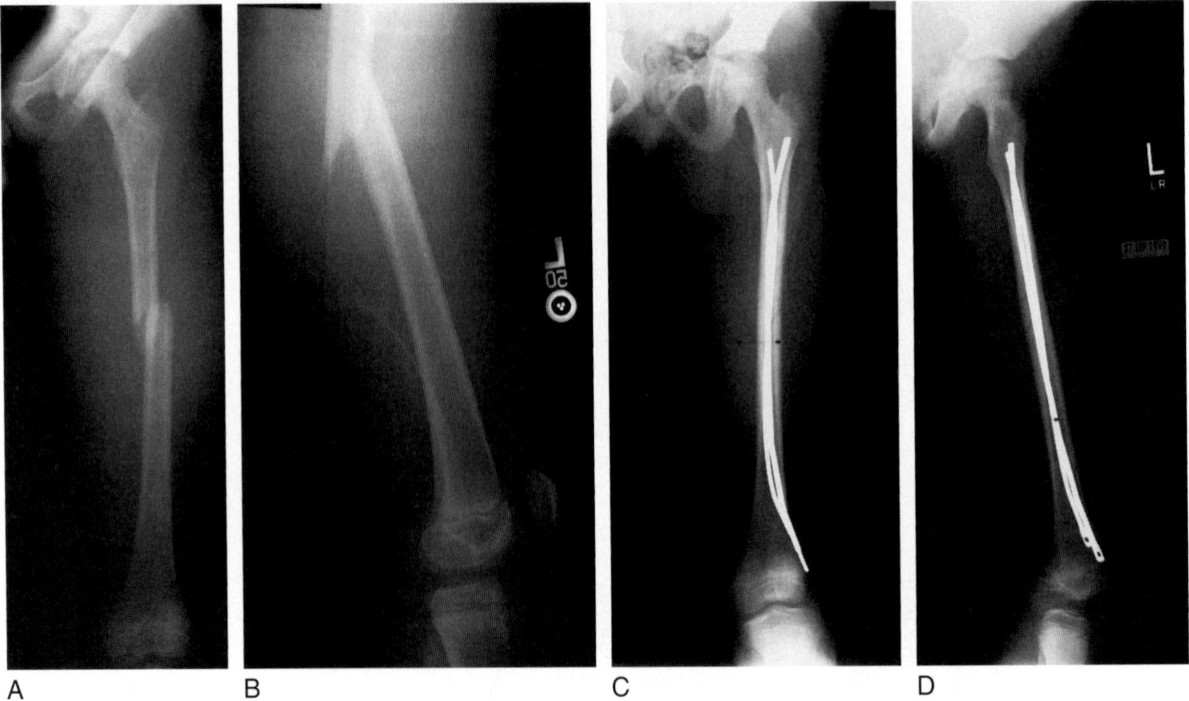

FIGURE 43–83 Flexible Enders nailing of a femoral fracture in an 8-year-old patient. **A,** Anteroposterior image of a short oblique fracture. **B,** Lateral image. **C,** Retrograde Enders intramedullary rods in place, with maintenance of reduction. **D,** Lateral image.

at the fracture site. Two flexible nails of equal diameter should be used to allow three-point fixation of the fracture site. When beginning distally with more rigid Enders rods, we prefer to place a single starting hole laterally and insert two flexible nails through this insertion site, the C-shaped rod ending in the metaphyseal region of the greater trochanter and the S-shaped rod ending at the mid-area or base of the femoral neck (Fig. 43–85). We prefer to use 4.5-mm rods whenever possible, using 3.5-mm rods in a child with a small intramedullary canal or when a second 4.5-mm rod cannot be placed. The nail should be left in place until solid union has occurred; we do not recommend removal until 1 year after placement. Whether to remove an asymptomatic flexible intramedullary nail is controversial. The theoretical advantages of nail removal are that stress risers at the insertion site are eliminated and nail removal is far easier at 1 year as opposed to years later, when the nail end is covered by bone.

COMPLICATIONS. The incidence of complications with flexible nails in appropriate fracture patterns is low. Complications are more frequent in larger children and those older than 10 years.[53] Prominence of the nails after insertion resulting in pain and skin breakdown is reported in 8% to 52% of cases.[35,36,71,82] Although mild angular deformities and refracture can occur, the majority of significant complications are related to length instability. Unstable fracture patterns may exhibit mild shortening with resultant nail migration and prominence. Occasionally, significant shortening may necessitate reoperation.[82,93] Biomechanical models have demonstrated torsional and length stability in flexible intramedullary nail models, but 5 mm of shortening with distal rod migration was observed at the equivalent of 18 kg of weight bearing in a comminuted fracture model.[44,68] Heinrich and associates reported an 11% incidence of varus or valgus malalignment, an 8% incidence of anterior or posterior malalignment, and an 8% incidence of rotational malalignment, with 68% of patients having equal limb lengths at follow-up.[51] Skak and colleagues reported a 16-year follow-up of 52 femoral shaft fractures treated by plate fixation, rigid intramedullary rodding, or flexible nailing. An average shortening of 9 mm occurred in the flexible nail group, and shortening was more likely to occur in older patients than in younger ones.[95] Sink and coworkers reported a 21% reoperation rate after titanium flexible nails as a result of distal nail migration or significant shortening in unstable fracture patterns.[93]

RESULTS. Comparison studies of other techniques generally indicate that flexible nails yield superior results in treating femoral diaphyseal fractures without significant length instability.[8,63,73,95,96] Kissel and Miller compared external fixation with flexible intramedullary nailing and concluded that retrograde nailing provides superior results, with the main advantage being early discharge from the hospital and return to school.[63] Similarly, Bar-On and associates compared external fixation with flexible intramedullary nailing and found less limb length discrepancy, malalignment, and other complications and greater parental satisfaction when flexible nails were used.[8] They

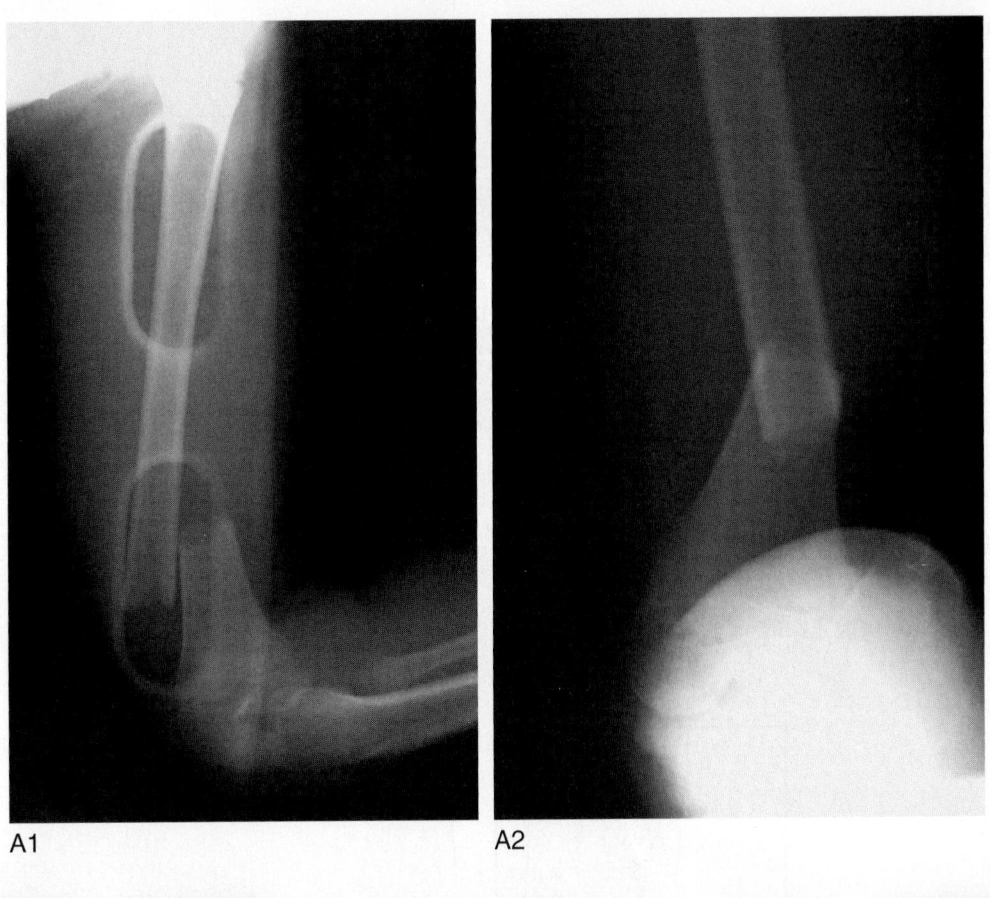

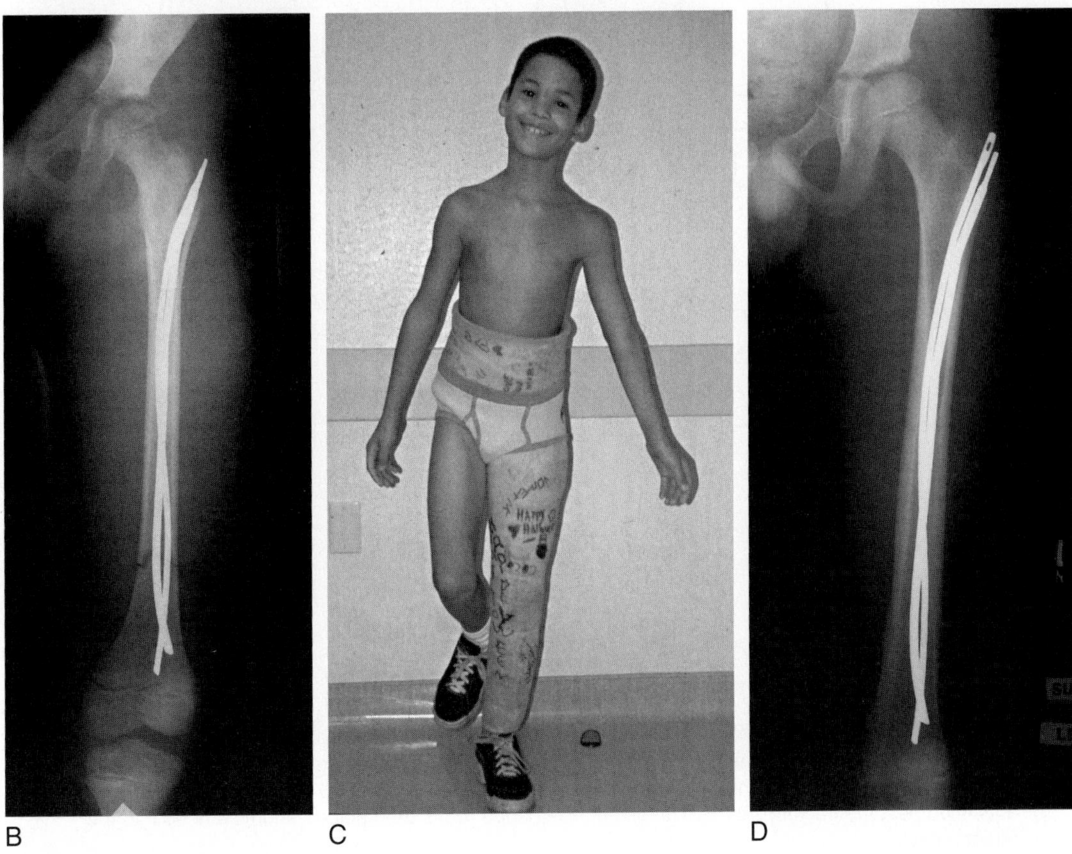

FIGURE 43-84 Radiographic and clinical appearance of a 9-year-old boy who sustained a distal femoral shaft fracture that was treated by Enders nailing, supplemented with a single-limb hip spica walking cast for 4 weeks for rotational control of the fracture. **A,** Initial radiographs demonstrating the distal location and displacement of the fracture. **B,** Postoperative radiograph. **C,** Clinical photograph at 10 days. The boy is fully weight bearing. **D,** Radiograph obtained at 4 months.

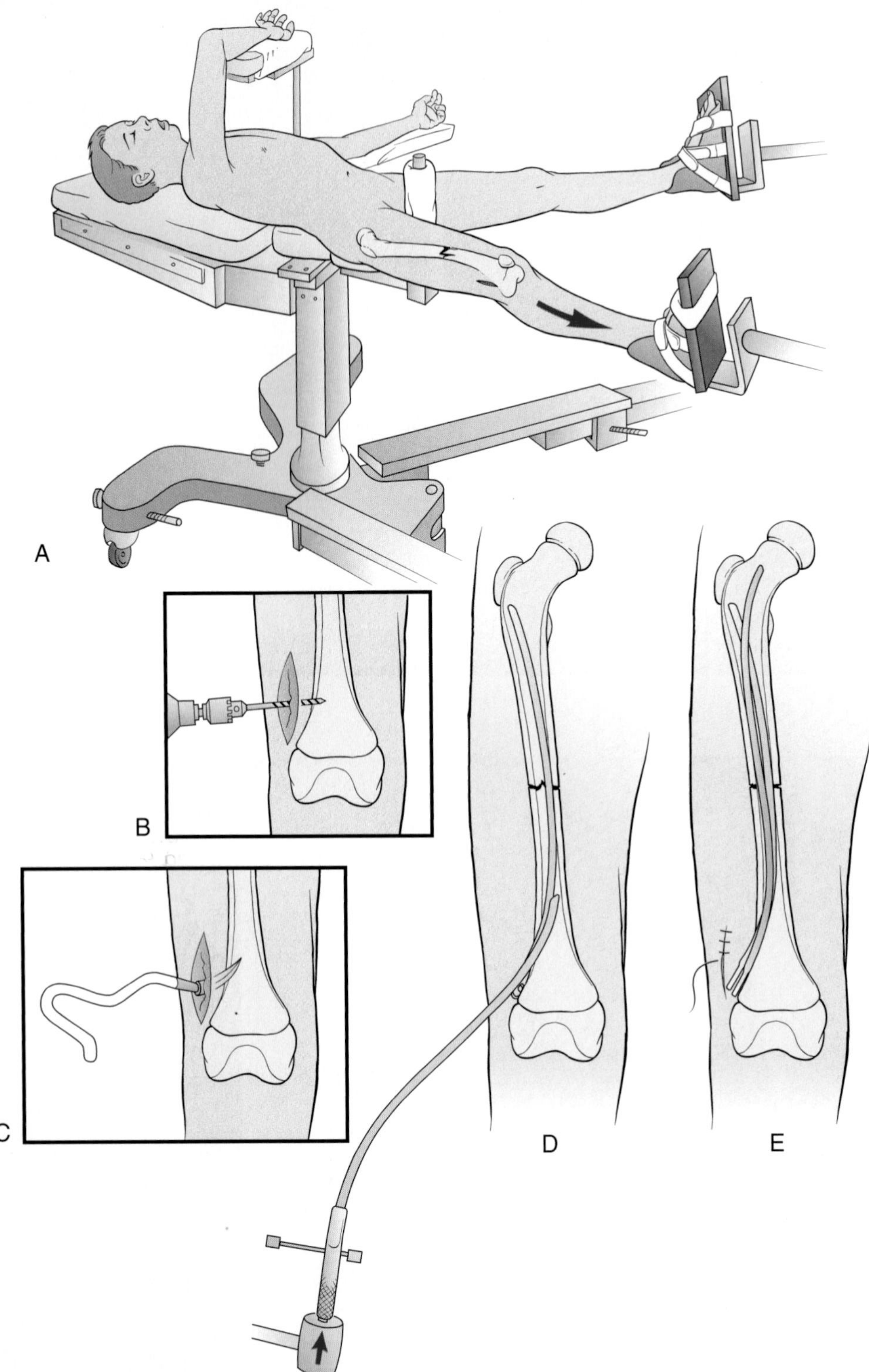

FIGURE 43–85 Enders nailing of a femoral fracture. **A,** Patient positioning on the fracture table. **B,** A lateral skin incision is made just proximal to the physis, and a starting drill hole is made. **C,** The drill hole is enlarged with a sharp awl and rongeurs in an oval pattern. **D,** The initial C-shaped rod is advanced past the fracture site. **E,** The second S-shaped rod is then placed and advanced into the femoral neck.

concluded that flexible intramedullary nailing is the treatment of choice for femoral shaft fractures in children 5 to 13 years of age and that external fixation should be reserved for open and severely comminuted fractures. In 1998 Greene reviewed treatment options for children with a displaced femoral shaft fracture and concluded that flexible intramedullary nails have several advantages over other techniques and are the treatment of choice.[41]

Rigid Intramedullary Nailing

Indications. Rigid interlocking intramedullary nailing has been successfully used in the treatment of femoral shaft fractures in adults. The rigid fixation imparted by the nail, along with the rotational control from the interlocking screws, allows this device to be used in highly unstable fractures, permits weight bearing immediately postoperatively, limits the risk for angular deformity, and can be dynamized to promote fracture healing. These advantages have led some to use rigid intramedullary nails in the adolescent population, with relatively good results (Fig. 43–86).[10,11,38,102,114] A recent series reported 55 femoral shaft fractures treated with an intramedullary rod in children at an average age of 12.8 years.[11] All fractures united without rotational or angular deformity, and the average limb length discrepancy was 0.7 cm.

Complications. Complications occurred in 13 patients: 5 had an articulotrochanteric distance difference of more than 1 cm, 7 had a limb length discrepancy of more than 2 cm, and in 1 patient AVN of the entire femoral head developed. All complications occurred in younger patients (average age, 11.7 years) in whom an adult-type nail with a large diameter (10 and 11 mm) and larger proximal diameter (13 mm) had been placed. The recommendations from this study were to use pediatric-type nails with smaller diameters (8 to 10 mm) and to place the insertion site at the greater trochanter.

Though relatively rare, the most severe complication from intramedullary nailing of a femoral shaft fracture in an adolescent is AVN of the femoral head (Fig. 43–87). It is thought that injury to the medial circumflex artery occurs during insertion of the nail medial to the tip of the greater trochanter, as was recognized by Küntschner during the development of his intramedullary nail.[66] There have been at least 18 reported cases of AVN after intramedullary nailing in children and adolescents; all occurred in children in whom a large, adult-sized nail had been placed through the piriformis fossa.* Because of this complication, newer nails have a smaller diameter throughout the entire length of the nail (8 to 10 mm) and a design that allows insertion through the greater trochanter. However, entrance of the nail through the greater trochanter can lead to premature greater trochanteric epiphysiodesis, coxa valga, and hip subluxation.[39,89] Orler and colleagues suggested that the entry point in a child or adolescent with an open proximal femoral physis should not be in the piriformis fossa (to avoid AVN), but below the greater trochanteric physis (to avoid epiphysiodesis and subsequent deformity).[86]

In a recently reported series, 20 skeletally immature patients underwent nail insertion through the tip of the trochanter without AVN's developing in any case and articular trochanteric distance asymmetry averaging less than 5 mm.[61] In an earlier series, 60 pediatric patients with femoral shaft fractures were treated by intramedullary nailing, with the entry portal placed slightly more lateral and posterior to the piriformis fossa to avoid the retinacular vessels of the femoral neck region. In 33 patients the nail was removed at 10 months, and only 2 patients had subclinical AVN detected on MRI. The AVN was attributed to the soft tissue dissection necessary to remove the implant.[18]

At present, there are no rigid nails specifically designed for entrance below the greater trochanter. We prefer to use flexible nails or submuscular plating wherever possible to avoid the complications associated with the use of rigid intramedullary nails. Strict adherence to greater trochanter insertion technique is recommended when rigid intramedullary nailing is used.

COMPLICATIONS

Limb Length Inequality. Limb length inequality is the most common complication after a femoral shaft fracture in children and may be due to accelerated growth in the involved femur or to shortening at the fracture site. Femoral growth is greatest within the first 3 months after fracture and declines to normal by 18 to 24 months.[91,92] Overgrowth is generally thought to occur more often in younger patients (<10 years),[97] in boys,[24] in those with comminuted or long oblique fractures,[29] and in those with more proximal fractures. The average amount of overgrowth is reported to be between 0.8 and 1.5 cm. In addition, overgrowth of the ipsilateral tibia is seen in the majority of patients, with an average overgrowth of approximately 0.3 cm.[92] Because of the overgrowth phenomenon, an ideal reduction of a femoral shaft fracture in a younger child should allow for up to 1.5 to 2.0 cm of shortening.

Treatment of excessive shortening of the fractured femur depends on the time when it is recognized. If immediate spica casting results in excess shortening, the cast should be removed and the surgeon should repeat a closed reduction with cast application under anesthesia. If this fails to regain length, the child may be placed in traction for a short period, followed by hip spica casting after the fracture begins to consolidate. If excess shortening is seen at a time when callus has already formed, the surgeon should consider osteoclasis followed by external fixation or traction. An alternative is to allow healing to continue and perform an equalization procedure at a later time.

Unacceptable Angulation. Acceptable angular alignment is most dependent on the age of the patient, the proximity of the fracture to the physis, and the plane

*See references 7, 10, 30, 52, 69, 77, 78, 85, 86, 108.

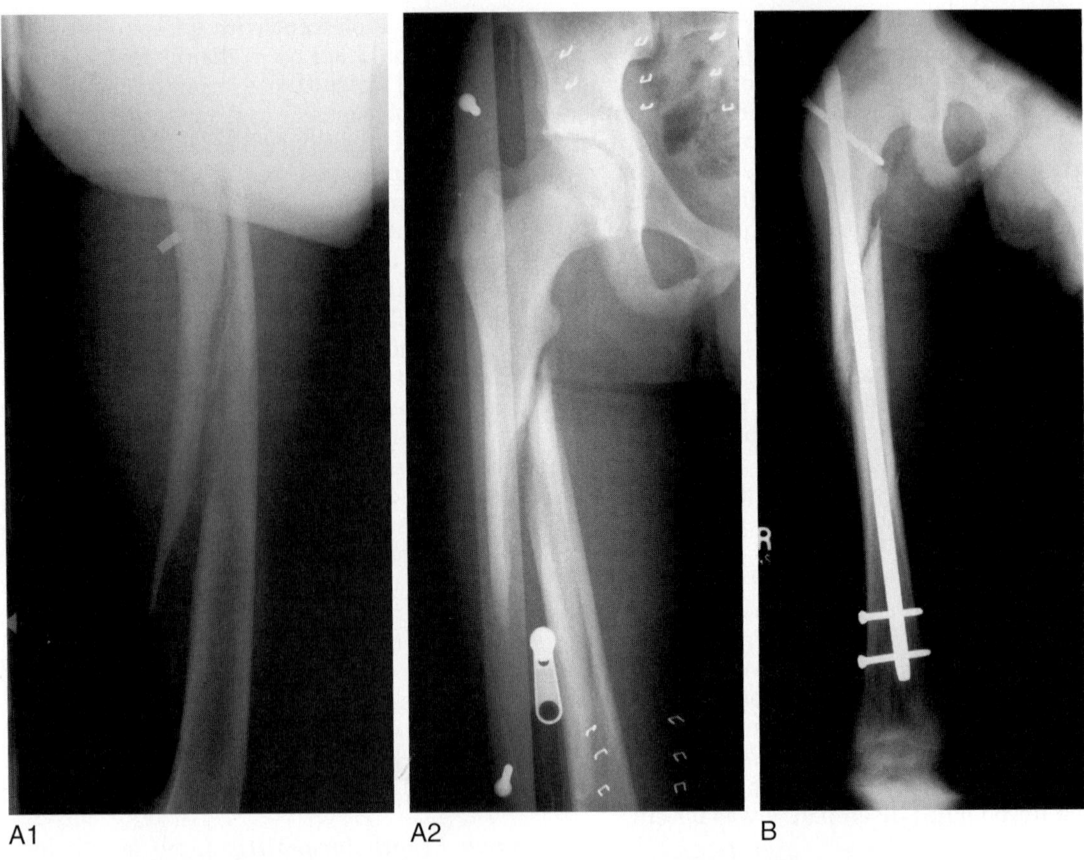

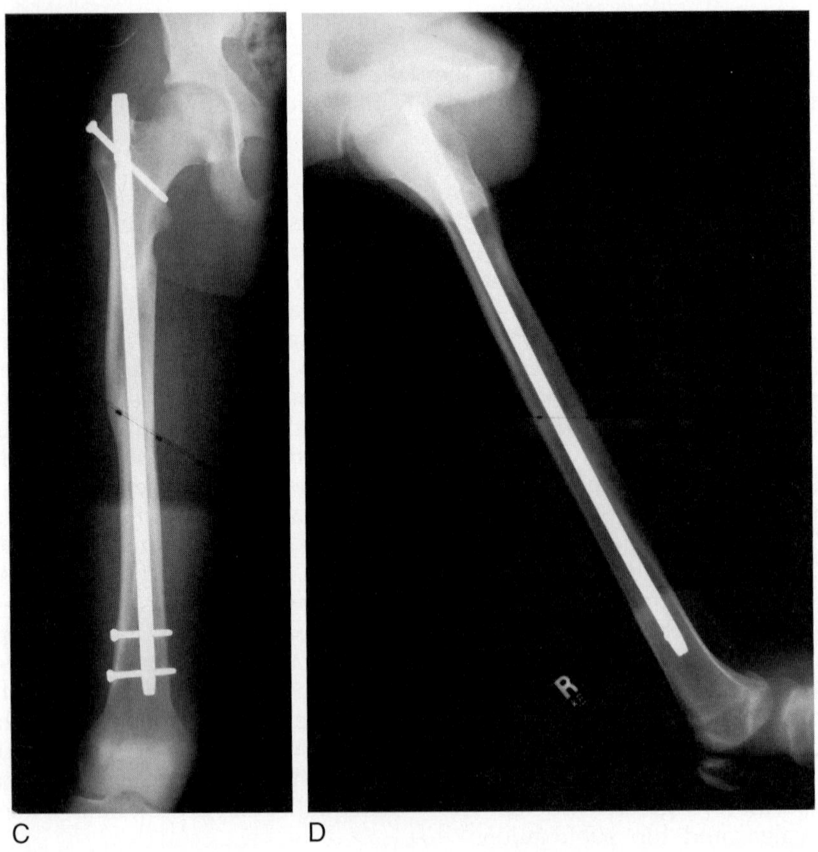

FIGURE 43–86 Locked intramedullary nailing of a femoral fracture in a skeletally mature patient. **A,** Initial injury films in a 14-year-old boy who sustained a twisting injury while playing football. **B,** Initial postoperative film obtained after statically locked intramedullary nailing. Final anteroposterior **(C)** and lateral **(D)** radiographs obtained 8 months postoperatively.

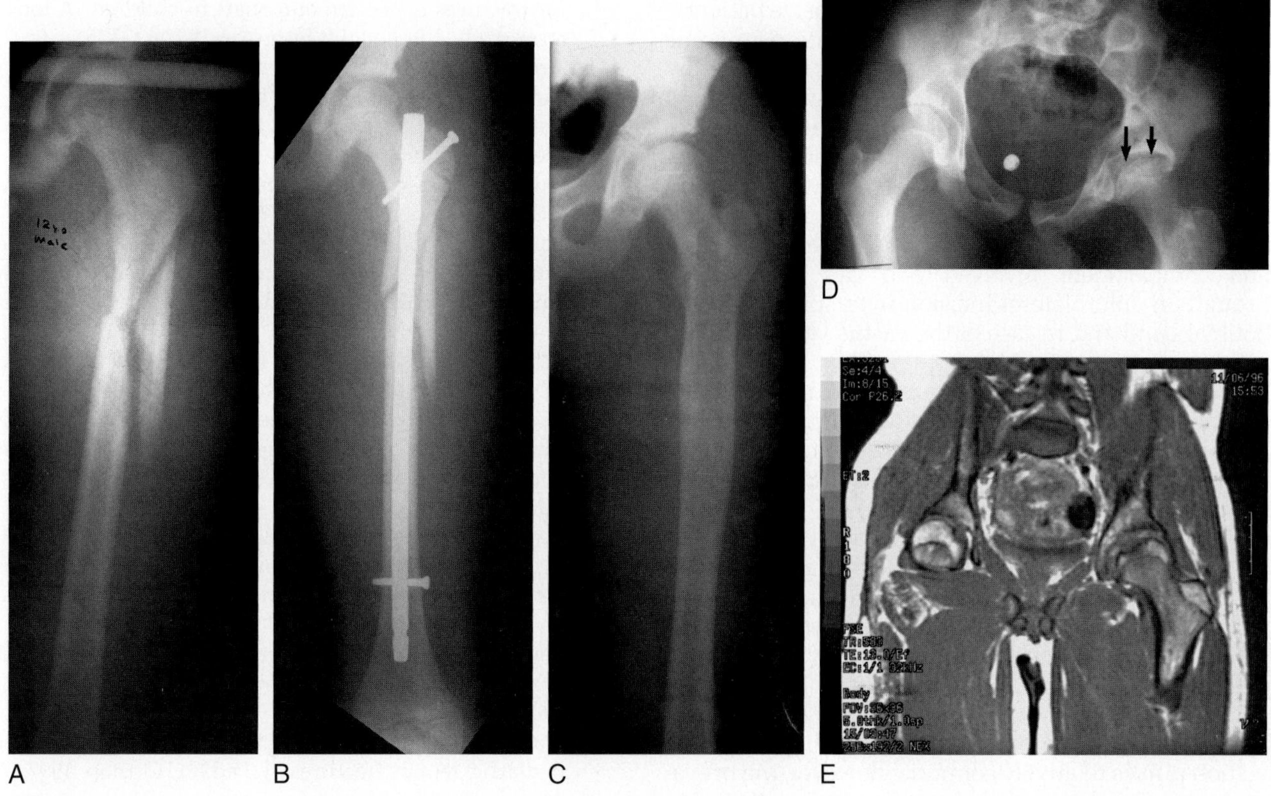

FIGURE 43-87 Avascular necrosis (AVN) as a complication of intramedullary nailing of a femoral shaft fracture in a 12-year-old boy. **A,** Initial radiograph showing a left femoral shaft fracture. **B,** An intramedullary rigid nail was placed beginning at the piriformis fossa. **C,** The rod was removed. **D,** Two years after the injury the patient complained of left hip pain. There was evidence of AVN of the femoral head (*arrows*). **E,** A magnetic resonance image confirmed the presence of AVN.

of the angular deformity. Younger children, fractures near the physis, and angular deformity in the plane of motion of the adjacent joint tend to have greater remodeling potential. General guidelines for acceptance of angular alignment should be followed, although there is some controversy concerning these numbers. (Wallace and Hoffman state that as much as 25 degrees of angular deformity can be accepted in any plane in a child younger than 13 years.[109]) When significant angular deformity persists after fracture healing, corrective osteotomy should be performed. General principles regarding corrective osteotomy are to perform the osteotomy as close to the apex of the deformity as possible; rigidly fix the osteotomy site, preferably with an interlocking rod, to promote healing; and use an Ilizarov frame or similar device in the situation of concomitant shortening.

Rotational Deformities. Rotational deformities of the femur are generally agreed to have less remodeling potential than angular deformities do.[27] However, in animal models an average rotational remodeling potential of 55% has been demonstrated.[100] Others have shown remodeling of rotational deformities in patients with femoral shaft fractures, although the remodeling has been somewhat limited.[15,45,84] Some reports suggest that rotational deformities of 15 or even 25 degrees are well tolerated. These deformities may occur more often than was previously thought; however, they are usually asymptomatic,[72,107] and only the most severe deformities require corrective surgery.

Nonunion and Delayed Union. Nonunion and delayed union of femoral shaft fractures in the pediatric population are relatively rare. We treat established nonunion with rigid fixation and add autogenous bone graft unless the nonunited bone is hypertrophic. In younger children we use plate fixation and in older children, flexible intramedullary rods. Delayed union is most often seen in a child treated with an external fixator and should be treated by dynamization of the fixator. An alternative treatment is removal of the fixator followed by internal fixation with an intramedullary rod in an older child or with plates and screws. However, the risk for infection is increased as a result of the previous treatment with an external fixator, and a 10- to 14-day course of oral antibiotics is recommended before fixation.

Compartment Syndrome. Although compartment syndrome after a femoral fracture is rare because of the large muscle mass of the thigh, the soft tissue envelope should be evaluated in every patient with a femoral fracture. Risk factors are fractures that resulted from high-impact direct trauma, prolonged Bryant's traction,[83] elevation of the leg in a hypotensive patient,[26] and treatment with intramedullary fixation in some patients.[79] The diagnosis should be suspected in any patient with excessive pain and a tense, swollen thigh. When these findings are present, pressure should be measured in all three compartments (adductor, hamstrings, and quadriceps), and fasciotomy of the compartment or compartments should be performed if pressure is elevated. The quadriceps is the most common compartment involved and can be released through an anterolateral incision with splitting of the iliotibial band and release of the vastus lateralis fascia.

Infection. Infection is very rare when nonoperative treatment is used. Canale and colleagues reported three cases of osteomyelitis of closed fractures, two of which were femoral fractures.[21] Symptoms began 1 and 6 weeks after the original injury, respectively, and were characterized as constant pain that was unrelieved by rest. Fever is associated with an uncomplicated femoral fracture but should subside in 2 to 3 days.[97] Treatment of osteomyelitis should consist of open debridement followed by intravenous antibiotics.

Inflammation. Inflammation surrounding external fixation pins is relatively common; however, the prevalence of true infection is reported to be less than 5%, and the infection can be treated with a short course of oral or intravenous antibiotics.[6,13]

Vascular Injury. Vascular injury after a femoral fracture is rare, reported in approximately 1% of cases.[64] If there are clinical signs of arterial insufficiency and an abnormal Doppler examination, angiography may be indicated to look for a complete vascular disruption or intimal tear. If a vascular injury is present, immediate fixation of the bony anatomy with external fixation or plating should precede exploration and repair of the vessel. Careful serial examination of the peripheral pulses is necessary in every patient with a femoral shaft fracture to detect vascular injuries.

References

Femur

1. Agus H, Kalenderer O, Eryanilmaz G, et al: Biological internal fixation of comminuted femur shaft fractures by bridge plating in children. J Pediatr Orthop 2003; 23:184.
2. Allen BL Jr, Kant AP, Emery FE: Displaced fractures of the femoral diaphysis in children. Definitive treatment in a double spica cast. J Trauma 1977;17:8.
3. Alonso JE, Horowitz M: Use of the AO/ASIF external fixator in children. J Pediatr Orthop 1987;7:594.
4. American College of Surgeons: Advanced Trauma Life Support Course. Chicago, American College of Surgeons, 1985.
5. Aronson DD, Singer RM, Higgins RF: Skeletal traction for fractures of the femoral shaft in children. A long-term study. J Bone Joint Surg Am 1987;69:1435.
6. Aronson J, Tursky EA: External fixation of femur fractures in children. J Pediatr Orthop 1992;12:157.
7. Astion DJ, Wilber JH, Scoles PV: Avascular necrosis of the capital femoral epiphysis after intramedullary nailing for a fracture of the femoral shaft. A case report. J Bone Joint Surg Am 1995;77:1092.
8. Bar-On E, Sagiv S, Porat S: External fixation or flexible intramedullary nailing for femoral shaft fractures in children. A prospective, randomised study. J Bone Joint Surg Br 1997;79:975.
9. Beals RK, Tufts E: Fractured femur in infancy: The role of child abuse. J Pediatr Orthop 1983;3:583.
10. Beaty JH, Austin SM, Warner WC, et al: Interlocking intramedullary nailing of femoral-shaft fractures in adolescents: preliminary results and complications. J Pediatr Orthop 1994;14:178.
11. Beaty JH, Herman MJ, Warner WC, et al: Interlocking intramedullary nailing of femoral shaft fracture in adolescents. Banff, Alberta, Canada, Pediatric Orthopaedic Society of North America, 1997.
12. Bennett FS, Zinar DM, Kilgus DJ: Ipsilateral hip and femoral shaft fractures. Clin Orthop Relat Res 1993; 296:168.
13. Blasier RD, Aronson J, Tursky EA: External fixation of pediatric femur fractures. J Pediatr Orthop 1997;17: 342.
14. Bone L: Emergency treatment of the injured patient. In Browner BD, Levine AM, Trafton PG (eds): Skeletal Trauma, vol 1. Philadelphia, WB Saunders, 1992, p 127.
15. Brouwer KJ, Molenaar JC, van Linge B: Rotational deformities after femoral shaft fractures in childhood. A retrospective study 27-32 years after the accident. Acta Orthop Scand 1981;52:81.
16. Bryant T: The Practice of Surgery. Philadelphia: HC Lea, 1873.
17. Buchholz IM, Bolhuis HW, Broker FH, et al: Overgrowth and correction of rotational deformity in 12 femoral shaft fractures in 3-6-year-old children treated with an external fixator. Acta Orthop Scand 2002; 73:170.
18. Buford D Jr, Christensen K, Weatherall P: Intramedullary nailing of femoral fractures in adolescents. Clin Orthop Relat Res 1998;350:85.
19. Burks RT, Sutherland DH: Stress fracture of the femoral shaft in children: Report of two cases and discussion. J Pediatr Orthop 1984;4:614.
20. Caird MS, Mueller KA, Puryear A, et al: Compression plating of pediatric femoral shaft fractures. J Pediatr Orthop 2003;23:448.
21. Canale ST, Puhl J, Watson FM, et al: Acute osteomyelitis following closed fractures. Report of three cases. J Bone Joint Surg Am 1975;57:415.
22. Carey TP, Galpin RD: Flexible intramedullary nail fixation of pediatric femoral fractures. Clin Orthop Relat Res 1996;332:110.
23. Carmichael KD, Bynum J, Goucher N: Rates of refracture associated with external fixation in pediatric femur fractures. Am J Orthop 2005;34:439.

24. Clement DA, Colton CL: Overgrowth of the femur after fracture in childhood. An increased effect in boys. J Bone Joint Surg Br 1986;68:534.
25. Clinkscales CM, Peterson HA: Isolated closed diaphyseal fractures of the femur in children: Comparison of effectiveness and cost of several treatment methods. Orthopedics 1997;20:1131.
26. Dameron TB Jr, Thompson HA: Femoral-shaft fractures in children. Treatment by closed reduction and double spica cast immobilization. J Bone Joint Surg Am 1959; 41:1201.
27. Davids JR: Rotational deformity and remodeling after fracture of the femur in children. Clin Orthop Relat Res 1994;302:27.
28. de Sanctis N, Gambardella A, Pempinello C, et al: The use of external fixators in femur fractures in children. J Pediatr Orthop 1996;16:613.
29. Edvardsen P, Syversen SM: Overgrowth of the femur after fracture of the shaft in childhood. J Bone Joint Surg Br 1976;58:339.
30. Ekelund A, Gretzer H: Intramedullary nailing of femoral fractures in children. Acta Orthop Scand 1989; 60(Suppl):231.
31. Fardon DP: Fracture of neck and shaft of same femur. Report of a case in a child. J Bone Joint Surg Am 1970;52:797.
32. Fein LH, Pankovich AM, Spero CM, et al: Closed flexible intramedullary nailing of adolescent femoral shaft fractures. J Orthop Trauma 1989;3:133.
33. Ferguson J, Nicol RO: Early spica treatment of pediatric femoral shaft fractures. J Pediatr Orthop 2000;20:189.
34. Ferry AM, Edgar MS Jr: Modified Bryant's traction. J Bone Joint Surg Am 1966;48:533.
35. Flynn JM, Hresko T, Reynolds RA, et al: Titanium elastic nails for pediatric femur fractures: A multicenter study of early results with analysis of complications. J Pediatr Orthop 2001;21:4.
36. Flynn JM, Luedtke L, Ganley TJ, et al: Titanium elastic nails for pediatric femur fractures: Lessons from the learning curve. Am J Orthop 2002;31:71.
37. Fry K, Hoffer MM, Brink J: Femoral shaft fractures in brain-injured children. J Trauma 1976;16:371.
38. Galpin RD, Willis RB, Sabano N: Intramedullary nailing of pediatric femoral fractures. J Pediatr Orthop 1994; 14:184.
39. Gonzalez-Herranz P, Burgos-Flores J, Rapariz JM, et al: Intramedullary nailing of the femur in children. Effects on its proximal end. J Bone Joint Surg Br 1995;77:262.
40. Green M, Haggerty R: Ambulatory Pediatrics. Philadelphia, WB Saunders, 1968.
41. Greene WB: Displaced fractures of the femoral shaft in children. Unique features and therapeutic options. Clin Orthop Relat Res 1998;353:86.
42. Gross RH, Stranger M: Causative factors responsible for femoral fractures in infants and young children. J Pediatr Orthop 1983;3:341.
43. Gustilo RB, Anderson JT: Prevention of infection in the treatment of one thousand and twenty-five open fractures of long bones: Retrospective and prospective analyses. J Bone Joint Surg Am 1976;58:453.
44. Gwyn DT, Olney BW, Dart BR, et al: Rotational control of various pediatric femur fractures stabilized with titanium elastic intramedullary nails. J Pediatr Orthop 2004;24:172.
45. Hagglund G, Hansson LI, Norman O: Correction by growth of rotational deformity after femoral fracture in children. Acta Orthop Scand 1983;54:858.
46. Hedequist D, Starr AJ, Wilson P, et al: Early versus delayed stabilization of pediatric femur fractures: Analysis of 387 patients. J Orthop Trauma 1999;13:490.
47. Hedequist DJ, Sink E: Technical aspects of bridge plating for pediatric femur fractures. J Orthop Trauma 2005;19:276.
48. Hedin H, Hjorth K, Larsson S, et al: Radiological outcome after external fixation of 97 femoral shaft fractures in children. Injury 2003;34:287.
49. Hedin H, Hjorth K, Rehnberg L, et al: External fixation of displaced femoral shaft fractures in children: A consecutive study of 98 fractures. J Orthop Trauma 2003; 17:250.
50. Hedlund R, Lindgren U: The incidence of femoral shaft fractures in children and adolescents. J Pediatr Orthop 1986;6:47.
51. Heinrich SD, Drvaric DM, Darr K, et al: The operative stabilization of pediatric diaphyseal femur fractures with flexible intramedullary nails: A prospective analysis. J Pediatr Orthop 1994;14:501.
52. Herzog B, Affolter P, Jani L: Spatbefunde nach Marknagelung kindlicher Femurfracturen. Z Kinderchir 1976;19:74.
53. Ho CA, Skaggs DL, Tang CW, et al: Use of flexible intramedullary nails in pediatric femur fractures. J Pediatr Orthop 2006;26:497.
54. Hoeksema HD, Olsen C, Rudy R: Fracture of femoral neck and shaft and repeat neck fracture in a child. Case report. J Bone Joint Surg Am 1975;57:271.
55. Huber RI, Keller HW, Huber PM, et al: Flexible intramedullary nailing as fracture treatment in children. J Pediatr Orthop 1996;16:602.
56. Hughes BF, Sponseller PD, Thompson JD: Pediatric femur fractures: Effects of spica cast treatment on family and community. J Pediatr Orthop 1995;15:457.
57. Hull JB, Sanderson PL, Rickman M, et al: External fixation of children's fractures: Use of the Orthofix Dynamic Axial Fixator. J Pediatr Orthop B 1997;6:203.
58. Humberger FW, Eyring EJ: Proximal tibial 90-90 traction in treatment of children with femoral-shaft fractures. J Bone Joint Surg Am 1969;51:499.
59. Irani RN, Nicholson JT, Chung SM: Long-term results in the treatment of femoral-shaft fractures in young children by immediate spica immobilization. J Bone Joint Surg Am 1976;58:945.
60. Jawadi AH, Letts M: Injuries associated with fracture of the femur secondary to motor vehicle accidents in children. Am J Orthop 2003;32:459.
61. Kanellopoulos AD, Yiannakopoulos CK, Soucacos PN: Closed, locked intramedullary nailing of pediatric femoral shaft fractures through the tip of the greater trochanter. J Trauma 2006;60:217.
62. Kanlic EM, Anglen JO, Smith DG, et al: Advantages of submuscular bridge plating for complex pediatric femur fractures. Clin Orthop Relat Res 2004;426:244.
63. Kissel EU, Miller ME: Closed Ender nailing of femur fractures in older children. J Trauma 1989;29:1585.

64. Kluger Y, Gonze MD, Paul DB, et al: Blunt vascular injury associated with closed mid-shaft femur fracture: A plea for concern. J Trauma 1994;36:222.
65. Kregor PJ, Song KM, Routt ML Jr, et al: Plate fixation of femoral shaft fractures in multiply injured children. J Bone Joint Surg Am 1993;75:1774.
66. Küntscher G: Intramedullary surgical technique and its place in orthopaedic surgery: My present concept. J Bone Joint Surg Am 1965;47:809.
67. Large TM, Frick SL: Compartment syndrome of the leg after treatment of a femoral fracture with an early sitting spica cast. A report of two cases. J Bone Joint Surg Am 2003;85:2207.
68. Lee SS, Mahar AT, Newton PO: Ender nail fixation of pediatric femur fractures: A biomechanical analysis. J Pediatr Orthop 2001;21:442.
69. Letts M, Jarvis J, Lawton L, et al: Complications of rigid intramedullary rodding of femoral shaft fractures in children. J Trauma 2002;52:504.
70. Loder RT: Pediatric polytrauma: Orthopaedic care and hospital course. J Orthop Trauma 1987;1:48.
71. Luhmann SJ: Acute traumatic knee effusions in children and adolescents. J Pediatr Orthop 2003;23:199.
72. Malkawi H, Shannak A, Hadidi S: Remodeling after femoral shaft fractures in children treated by the modified Blount method. J Pediatr Orthop 1986;6:421.
73. Mani US, Sabatino CT, Sabharwal S, et al: Biomechanical comparison of flexible stainless steel and titanium nails with external fixation using a femur fracture model. J Pediatr Orthop 2006;26:182.
74. Mann DC, Weddington J, Davenport K: Closed Ender nailing of femoral shaft fractures in adolescents. J Pediatr Orthop 1986;6:651.
75. Mazda K, Khairouni A, Pennecot GF, et al: Closed flexible intramedullary nailing of the femoral shaft fractures in children. J Pediatr Orthop B 1997;6:198.
76. Mendelson SA, Dominick TS, Tyler-Kabara E, et al: Early versus late femoral fracture stabilization in multiply injured pediatric patients with closed head injury. J Pediatr Orthop 2001;21:594.
77. Mileski RA, Garvin KL, Crosby LA: Avascular necrosis of the femoral head in an adolescent following intramedullary nailing of the femur. A case report. J Bone Joint Surg Am 1994;76:1706.
78. Mileski RA, Garvin KL, Huurman WW: Avascular necrosis of the femoral head after closed intramedullary shortening in an adolescent. J Pediatr Orthop 1995;15:24.
79. Miller DS, Markin L, Grossman E: Ischemic fibrosis of the lower extremity in children. Am J Surg 1952;84:317.
80. Miller PR, Welch MC: The hazards of tibial pin replacement in 90–90 skeletal traction. Clin Orthop Relat Res 1978;135:97.
81. Miner T, Carroll KL: Outcomes of external fixation of pediatric femoral shaft fractures. J Pediatr Orthop 2000;20:405.
82. Narayanan UG, Hyman JE, Wainwright AM, et al: Complications of elastic stable intramedullary nail fixation of pediatric femoral fractures, and how to avoid them. J Pediatr Orthop 2004;24:363.
83. Nicholson JT, Foster RM, Heath RD: Bryant's traction; a provocative cause of circulatory complications. JAMA 1955;157:415.
84. Oberhammer J: Degree and frequency of rotational deformities after infant femoral fractures and their spontaneous correction. Arch Orthop Trauma Surg 1980;97:249.
85. O'Malley DE, Mazur JM, Cummings RJ: Femoral head avascular necrosis associated with intramedullary nailing in an adolescent. J Pediatr Orthop 1995;15:21.
86. Orler R, Hersche O, Helfet DL, et al: [Avascular femur head necrosis as a severe complication after femoral intramedullary nailing in children and adolescents.] Unfallchirurg 1998;101:495.
87. Podeszwa DA, Mooney JF 3rd, Cramer KE, et al: Comparison of Pavlik harness application and immediate spica casting for femur fractures in infants. J Pediatr Orthop 2004;24:460.
88. Probe R, Lindsey RW, Hadley NA, et al: Refracture of adolescent femoral shaft fractures: A complication of external fixation. A report of two cases. J Pediatr Orthop 1993;13:102.
89. Raney EM, Ogden JA, Grogan DP: Premature greater trochanteric epiphysiodesis secondary to intramedullary femoral rodding. J Pediatr Orthop 1993;13:516.
90. Rang M: Children's Fractures. Philadelphia, JB Lippincott, 1974.
91. Reynolds DA: Growth changes in fractured long-bones: A study of 126 children. J Bone Joint Surg Br 1981;63:83.
92. Shapiro F: Fractures of the femoral shaft in children. The overgrowth phenomenon. Acta Orthop Scand 1981;52:649.
93. Sink EL, Gralla J, Repine M: Complications of pediatric femur fractures treated with titanium elastic nails: A comparison of fracture types. J Pediatr Orthop 2005;25:577.
94. Sink EL, Hedequist D, Morgan SJ, et al: Results and technique of unstable pediatric femoral fractures treated with submuscular bridge plating. J Pediatr Orthop 2006;26:177.
95. Skak SV, Overgaard S, Nielsen JD, et al: Internal fixation of femoral shaft fractures in children and adolescents: A ten- to twenty-one-year follow-up of 52 fractures. J Pediatr Orthop B 1996;5:195.
96. Song HR, Oh CW, Shin HD, et al: Treatment of femoral shaft fractures in young children: Comparison between conservative treatment and retrograde flexible nailing. J Pediatr Orthop B 2004;13:275.
97. Staheli LT: Femoral and tibial growth following femoral shaft fracture in childhood. Clin Orthop Relat Res 1967;55:159.
98. Staheli LT, Sheridan GW: Early spica cast management of femoral shaft fractures in young children. A technique utilizing bilateral fixed skin traction. Clin Orthop Relat Res 1977;126:162.
99. Stannard JP, Christensen KP, Wilkins KE: Femur fractures in infants: A new therapeutic approach. J Pediatr Orthop 1995;15:461.
100. Strong ML, Wong-Chung J, Babikian G, et al: Rotational remodeling of malrotated femoral fractures: A model in the rabbit. J Pediatr Orthop 1992;12:173.

101. Swiontkowski MF, Hansen ST Jr, Kellam J: Ipsilateral fractures of the femoral neck and shaft. A treatment protocol. J Bone Joint Surg Am 1984;66:260.
102. Timmerman LA, Rab GT: Intramedullary nailing of femoral shaft fractures in adolescents. J Orthop Trauma 1993;7:331.
103. Tolo VT: External skeletal fixation in children's fractures. J Pediatr Orthop 1983;3:435.
104. Tolo VT: External fixation in multiply injured children. Orthop Clin North Am 1990;21:393.
105. Treiman GS, Yellin AE, Weaver FA, et al: Examination of the patient with a knee dislocation. The case for selective arteriography. Arch Surg 1992;127:1056.
106. Vangsness CT Jr, DeCampos J, Merritt PO, et al: Meniscal injury associated with femoral shaft fractures. An arthroscopic evaluation of incidence. J Bone Joint Surg Br 1993;75:207.
107. Verbeek HO: Does rotation deformity, following femur shaft fracture, correct during growth? Reconstr Surg Traumatol 1979;17:75.
108. von der Oelsnitz G: Marknagelung kindlicher Oberschenkelfrakturen. Z Kinderchir 1972;11(Suppl):803.
109. Wallace ME, Hoffman EB: Remodelling of angular deformity after femoral shaft fractures in children. J Bone Joint Surg Br 1992;74:765.
110. Ward WT, Levy J, Kaye A: Compression plating for child and adolescent femur fractures. J Pediatr Orthop 1992;12:626.
111. Wascher DC, Dvirnak PC, DeCoster TA: Knee dislocation: Initial assessment and implications for treatment. J Orthop Trauma 1997;11:525.
112. Weiss AP, Schenck RC Jr, Sponseller PD, et al: Peroneal nerve palsy after early cast application for femoral fractures in children. J Pediatr Orthop 1992;12:25.
113. Winquist RA, Hansen ST Jr, Clawson DK: Closed intramedullary nailing of femoral fractures. A report of five hundred and twenty cases. J Bone Joint Surg Am 1984;66:529.
114. Ziv I, Rang M: Treatment of femoral fracture in the child with head injury. J Bone Joint Surg Br 1983;65:276.

KNEE

Distal Femoral Injuries and Fractures

Fractures of the distal femur are relatively rare, are due to high-energy trauma, and are frequently associated with other injuries. Treatment consists of anatomic reduction and usually stable internal fixation. Complications are common and frequently often further operative intervention is needed to take down a physeal bar, correct an angular deformity or limb length discrepancy, or reconstruct an anterior cruciate ligament (ACL) injury.

ANATOMY

The distal femoral epiphysis is formed from a single ossific nucleus that is present at birth and is the first epiphysis in the body to ossify. The distal femoral physis grows at a rate of 8 to 10 mm per year and contributes approximately 40% of growth of the lower extremity. It closes at around 13 years in girls and 15 years in boys.[7,97] The ossific nucleus of the proximal tibial epiphysis appears by 2 months of age, and the secondary center of ossification of the tibial tubercle appears between 10 and 14 years. The proximal tibial physis grows approximately 6 mm per year, and the proximal tibial physis fuses at about 14 to 15 years of age.

The distal femur has a characteristic rhomboid shape and inclination of the joint line at the knee. The anatomic axis of the femur (a line drawn down the femoral shaft) angles medially approximately 9 degrees from vertical, and the mechanical axis of the femur (a line drawn between the center of the femoral head and the center of the knee) deviates 3 degrees from vertical, with the difference between the mechanical and anatomic axes being 6 degrees (Fig. 43–88). The distal femoral articular angle, best measured between the mechanical axis of the femur and the knee joint line, is 3 degrees of valgus, or an angle of 87 degrees between the mechanical axis line and the lateral articular surface.

The muscular attachment of both heads of the gastrocnemius and the plantaris muscles is on the posterior aspect of the distal femoral metaphysis, just proximal to the physis. This will lead to flexion of the distal fracture fragment when the fracture line is proximal to the muscle insertion. The adductor magnus muscle attaches to the medial aspect of the femoral metaphysis, which leads to varus of the distal fracture

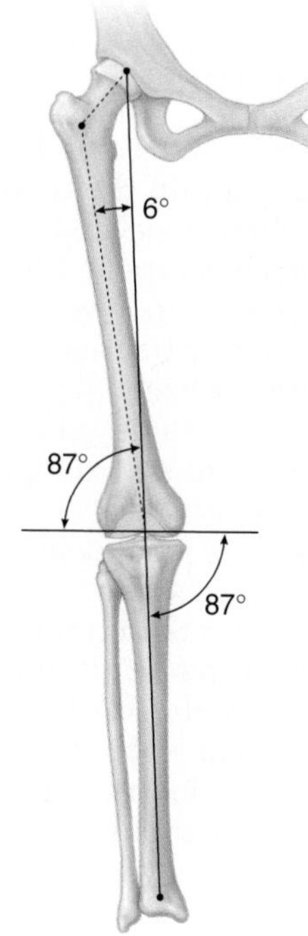

FIGURE 43–88 Relationship between the mechanical axis (*solid line*) and the anatomic axis (*dotted line*) of the lower extremity. The distal, femoral, and proximal tibial articular angles are shown.

fragment when the fracture line is proximal to its insertion. The collateral ligaments, however, attach distal to the physis at the level of the distal femoral epiphysis. Excess varus or valgus stress on the knee in a growing child will place tension on the collateral ligaments, which transfer these forces to the distal femoral physis, thereby frequently resulting in injury to the physis without injury to the collateral ligaments. The ACL and posterior cruciate ligament (PCL) attach to the distal femoral epiphysis at the intercondylar notch and can be injured at the time of distal femoral epiphyseal fracture or physeal injury.[23]

Knowledge of the vascular anatomy is important in managing knee injuries in the pediatric population. The femoral artery travels through the adductor canal medially, just above the distal femoral metaphysis, and then courses posteriorly directly behind the popliteal space. The popliteal artery is directly posterior to the distal femur, from which it is separated by a thin layer of soft tissue. It trifurcates at this level into the anterior interosseous, posterior interosseous, and peroneal arteries. The superior genicular arteries branch from the popliteal artery at the distal femoral metaphyseal area and travel to the distal epiphysis deep to the muscle layer. Because of relatively poor collateral circulation around the knee, popliteal artery injury frequently results in loss of lower limb viability.

The peroneal nerve travels laterally, posterior to the biceps femoris muscle and the lateral head of the gastrocnemius muscle, and descends just distal to the fibular head. At the knee level the peroneal nerve lies superficial and is vulnerable to both direct trauma and stretch injury when a varus stress is applied to the knee.

MECHANISM OF INJURY

The mechanism of injury is varied and partly dependent on the age of the child. In the newborn period, breech presentation is often associated with birth fractures and usually results in a type I Salter-Harris fracture.[156] In the age group from 3 to 10 years, the fractures are more often due to severe trauma, especially falls from a significant height or being struck by an automobile, and only a few fractures result from sports activities.[220] In the adolescent age group the majority of fractures result from sports injuries, with a smaller percentage being caused by automobile accidents in which the patient was a pedestrian.[220] Overall, pedestrian–motor vehicle accidents account for approximately 45% to 50% of fractures, sports injuries for 25%, and falls for approximately 20% of injuries.[58,156,220]

Another component that should be included in defining the mechanism of injury is the direction in which the direct force was applied to the knee. The two most common are a valgus-type force and a hyperextension force. Direct trauma results in epiphyseal separation on the tension side of the knee, with fracture of the metaphysis, epiphysis, or both on the compression side of the knee.

A valgus type of force is caused by a blow to the lateral side of the distal femur, usually occurring on the high-school football field. It generally results in a Salter-Harris type II or III physeal injury with the periosteum ruptured on the medial side and the distal femoral epiphysis displaced laterally with a lateral fragment of the metaphysis (Fig. 43–89). Torg and colleagues reported on six Salter-Harris type III fractures of the medial femoral condyle that occurred while the adolescents were playing football (five fractures) or soccer (one fracture).[269] These six fractures were caused by direct trauma to a fixed leg in which a valgus stress was imparted to the knee and resulted in physeal separation on the medial side and a fracture through the center of the epiphysis.

A hyperextension-type injury results in anterior displacement of the distal femoral epiphysis by the hyperextension force and by the pull of contraction of the quadriceps muscle. The periosteum on the posterior aspect is torn, and the fibers of the gastrocnemius muscle are stretched or partially torn (Fig. 43–90). The triangular metaphyseal fragment and the intact periosteal hinge are anterior in location. The distal end of the femoral shaft is driven posteriorly into the soft tissues of the popliteal fossa, where it may injure the popliteal vessels as well as the common peroneal or posterior tibial nerves. Hyperextension of the knee without direct trauma may result in physeal fracture when the energy is significant. Grogan and Bobechko reported on a triple long-jumper who sustained a Salter-Harris type II fracture of the distal femoral epiphysis while landing.[100]

Distal femoral fractures have been reported in a variety of conditions, including arthrogryposis multiplex congenita (after manipulation of stiff knees)[67] and myelomeningocele. In patients with myelomeningocele, a longer period of external immobilization may be needed for fracture healing.[70,149,256]

CLASSIFICATION

Distal femoral fractures in children can be separated into two groups—isolated fractures of the metaphysis and physeal injuries. Injuries to the distal femoral physis represent approximately 7% of all lower extremity physeal fractures[166,208] and can be grouped according to the Salter-Harris classification.

A Salter-Harris type I injury is rare and accounts for 7.7% of all physeal injuries of the distal femur.[58,156,220,261] It is most often seen in two age groups, newborns and adolescents. In a newborn, these birth fractures are more often associated with breech presentation and are frequently undisplaced and therefore unrecognized at initial evaluation until fracture callus is seen 2 to 3 weeks later (Fig. 43–91).[220] In an adolescent, the injury can also go undetected when undisplaced and should be confirmed with stress radiographs.

Salter-Harris type II fractures are by far the most common distal femoral physeal injury and account for approximately 6%.[58,156,220,261] The majority of these fractures occur in the adolescent age group and are displaced when initially seen (Fig. 43–92).

Salter-Harris types III and IV fractures each account for approximately 10% of physeal injuries and are

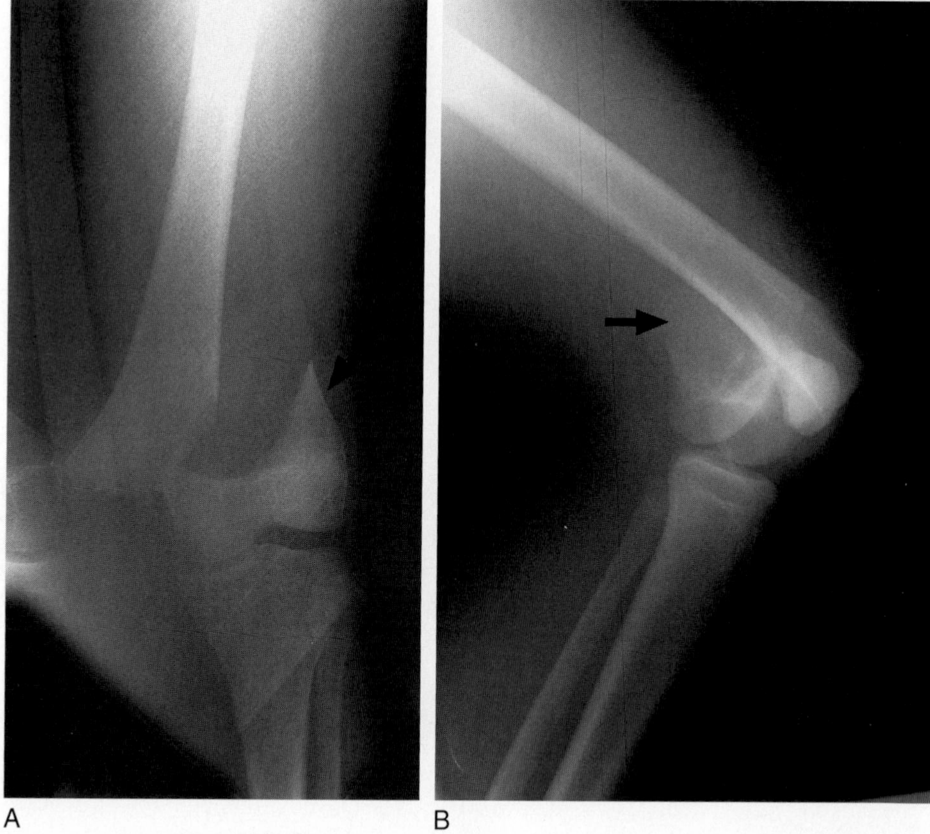

FIGURE 43–89 Anteroposterior **(A)** and lateral **(B)** images of a typical Salter-Harris type II fracture of the distal femur in a 15-year-old boy who sustained a valgus force to the knee while playing football. Note the significant displacement in the lateral Thurston-Holland fragment (*arrow*).

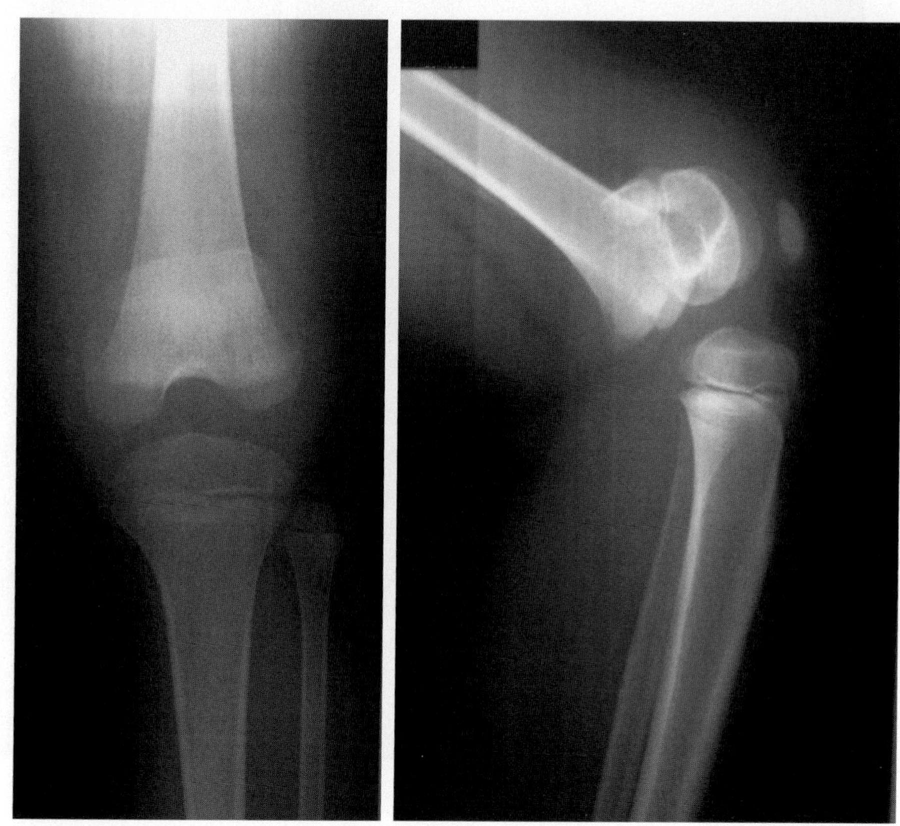

FIGURE 43–90 Anteroposterior **(A)** and lateral **(B)** images of hyperextension-type injury of the distal femoral physis in a 4-year-old patient.

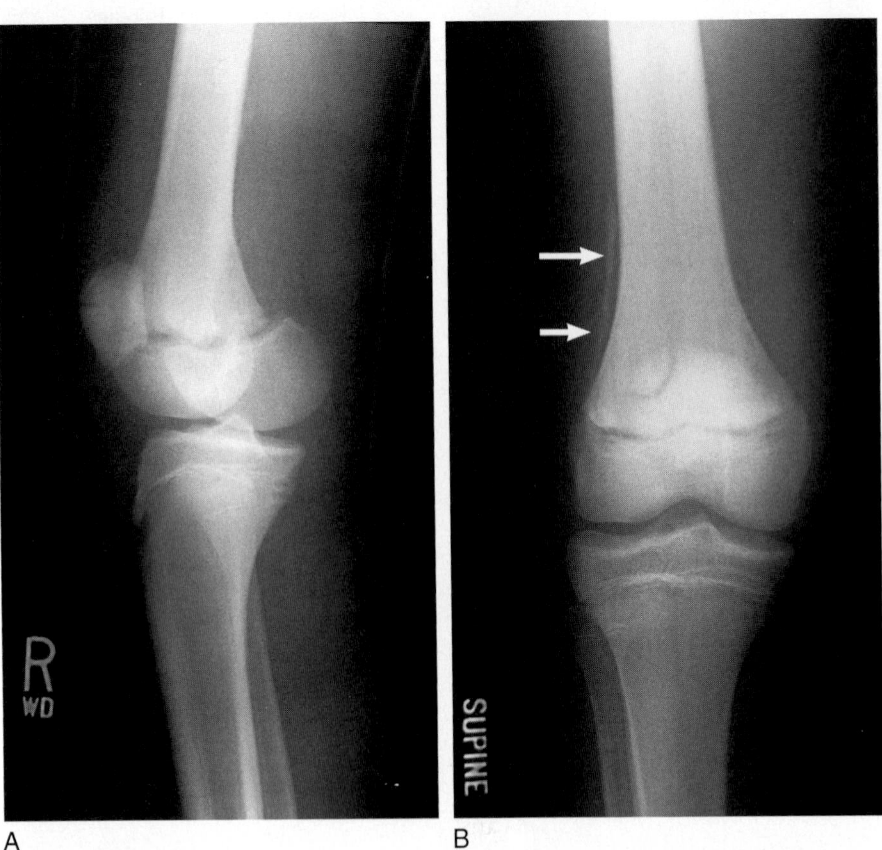

FIGURE 43-91 Salter-Harris type I distal femoral fracture. **A,** Oblique radiograph of the distal femur suggesting physeal injury with minimal rotational displacement of the distal epiphysis and physeal widening. **B,** After 6 weeks of long-leg cast treatment, evidence of healing is present, with periosteal elevation and new bone formation (*arrows*).

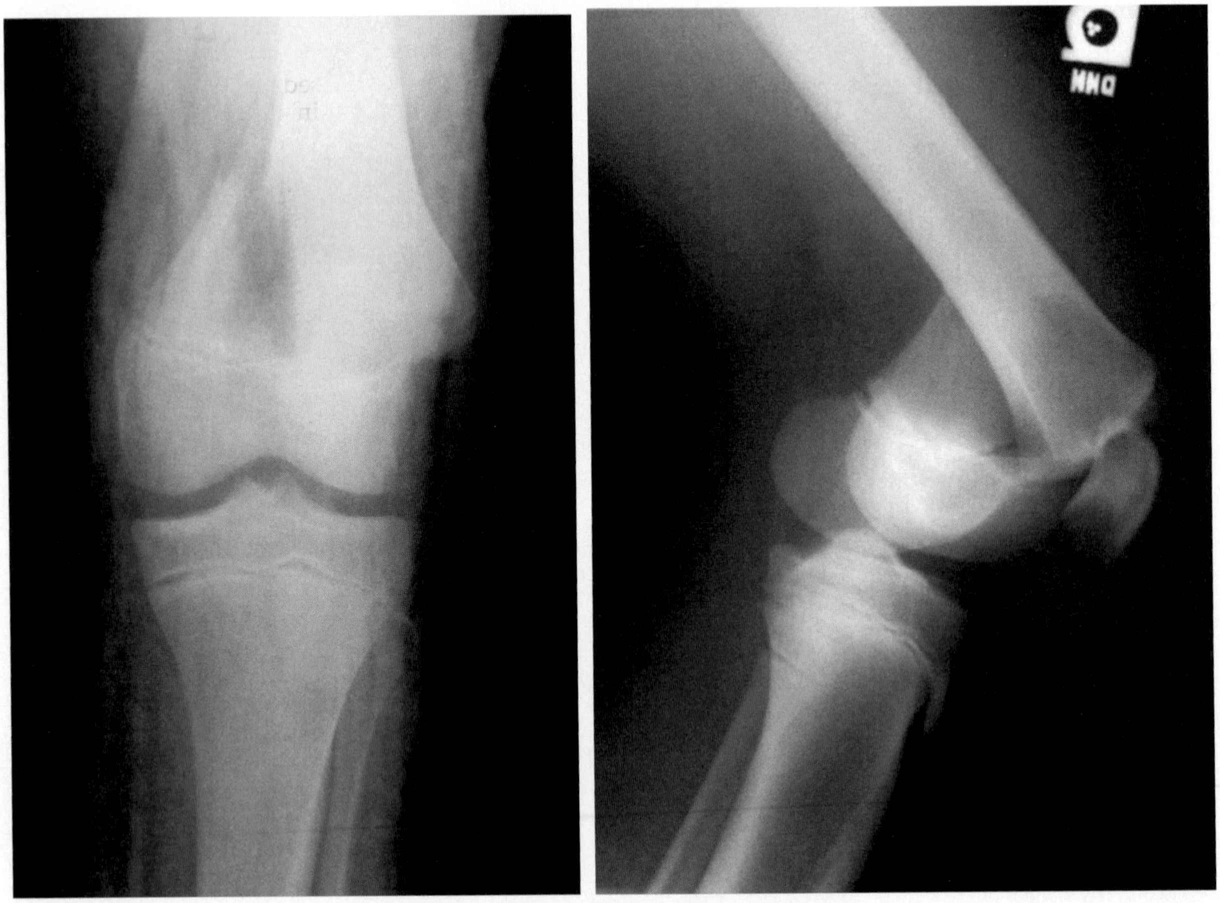

FIGURE 43-92 Anteroposterior **(A)** and lateral **(B)** images of a displaced Salter-Harris type II distal femoral fracture in an 11-year-old boy. The Thurston-Holland fragment is on the medial aspect of the distal femur.

usually displaced; operative intervention is required. A Salter-Harris type V fracture is relatively rare and accounts for approximately 6% of all distal femoral physeal injuries.

Unlike the case with other physeal injuries, the Salter-Harris classification alone has not been as accurate in predicting the overall outcome of distal femoral fractures with respect to future growth arrest, limb length discrepancy, and angular deformity. The mechanism of injury and the degree of initial displacement should be determined at the time of initial evaluation because these factors, in combination with the Salter-Harris classification, have been shown to be accurate predictors of outcome.[156,220]

CLINICAL FEATURES

There is usually a history of significant trauma. More energy is required to produce a distal femoral physeal fracture in patients younger than 11 years (juveniles) than in adolescents. Most often, it involves being struck by a motor vehicle or falling from a significant height. In an adolescent, sports injuries, especially football, account for a large proportion of injuries. The direction of the direct trauma is important to identify because many injuries may appear undisplaced radiographically at initial evaluation but may have been displaced at the time of injury, thereby predisposing to soft tissue, vascular, or neurologic injury.

On physical examination, the patient is in acute distress secondary to pain in the knee region and is unable to walk. With a displaced fracture the knee is swollen and tense, although a patient with a nondisplaced separation will have less pain and may be able to ambulate. The knee is often in a flexed position because of hamstring muscle spasm, and deformity of the knee may be present with extension of the distal extent of the femur or valgus deformity. The skin should be inspected for open skin lesions. Ecchymotic areas will provide information on the deforming forces, such as a valgus stress with ecchymosis on the medial aspect of the knee from displacement of the medial distal femoral metaphysis at the time of injury. Swelling in the popliteal space may alert the surgeon to a vascular injury or disruption.

A careful neurovascular examination should be performed in all patients with a distal femoral fracture or physeal injury. The soft tissue envelope should be palpated to evaluate for compartment syndrome at the time of initial evaluation and during the first 48 hours after injury.

Finally, a thorough orthopaedic evaluation of the remaining extremities, pelvis, and spine is always necessary, especially in patients who have sustained high-energy injuries.

RADIOGRAPHIC FINDINGS

Radiographic examination should include AP and lateral images of the knee and entire femur including the hip joint. When no fracture is present radiographically despite strong suspicion that a fracture exists based on the history and physical examination findings, oblique views should be obtained. They may reveal a fracture when one is not seen on the initial radiographs. Additional radiographs should include stress views of the knee supervised by a physician. The patient should be relaxed with intravenous sedation to alleviate the muscle spasm and allow a good examination.[253]

Additional imaging studies may be required. CT is helpful to define the amount of displacement and step-off in Salter-Harris types III and IV fractures. Though relatively rare in this type of injury, arteriography is indicated in any patient who has diminished peripheral pulses relative to the opposite extremity to identify arterial injury. In a newborn it is often difficult to diagnose a distal femoral physeal separation because of the limited ossification, which can best be visualized with MRI or ultrasound.

A Salter-Harris type V fracture is relatively rare, difficult to diagnose at initial evaluation, and often missed. Lombardo and Harvey reported on 34 fractures of the distal femur, of which there was 1 type V fracture that was not initially recognized.[156] Radiographs of the affected knee and the contralateral knee should be compared, especially with regard to the thickness and configuration of the physis.

TREATMENT

General treatment guidelines include the following: all reduction maneuvers should be performed under general anesthesia or sedation to allow gentle reduction and avoid further injury to the growth plate. Birth fractures heal well with conservative measures, and most deformities in the sagittal plane remodel. Displaced Salter-Harris types III and IV fractures generally require closed or open reduction, followed by internal fixation and external immobilization. Internal fixation should avoid the physis whenever possible and should consist of smooth Kirschner wires if the physis is crossed.

Distal Femoral Metaphyseal Fractures

Distal femoral metaphyseal fractures are treated differently from typical distal femoral physeal injuries. The various treatment options include external fixation, skeletal traction followed by casting, closed or open reduction followed by percutaneous pinning and casting, or open reduction and internal fixation. In general, we recommend closed reduction, percutaneous pinning, and cast immobilization whenever possible and do not often use skeletal traction and casting techniques. Skeletal traction and casting will not be described here but can be found under Skeletal Traction in discussion of Fractures of the Femoral Shaft. Fracture reduction should be as close to anatomic as possible, with acceptable residual angulation in the sagittal plane being less than 20 degrees in a child younger than 10 years and less than 10 degrees in a child nearing skeletal maturity.[28] No rotational malalignment is acceptable. Less than 5 degrees of varus or valgus alignment is acceptable.

External Fixation. We limit the indications for external fixation to significant soft tissue injury associated with an open fracture; a polytrauma patient when urgent stabilization is needed so that the patient can be transported for multiple diagnostic studies; and finally, highly comminuted fractures, which may require stabilization across the knee joint.

The fracture should be reduced before the external fixator is applied. The external fixator should be placed with two pins in the distal metaphyseal fragment and two pins proximal to the fracture site. To avoid injury, the pins should be placed at least 1 cm from the distal physis.[268] Under fluoroscopic guidance, the pins are inserted laterally and placed parallel to the distal femoral articular surface to avoid malalignment and malunion. At completion of the application of the external fixator, the knee should be fully extended and its overall alignment should be checked visually and radiographically. Varus and valgus malalignment should be corrected, as should any rotational deformities. If the configuration of the fracture is stable, the patient can be partially weight bearing at the start of the rehabilitation process and gradually advanced to full weight-bearing status. With an unstable fracture, the patient should be non–weight bearing initially until good fracture callus is seen radiographically and then slowly advanced to full weight bearing. To avoid refracture through the initial fracture site, mature callus should be present and the external fixator should be dynamized for a period of 3 to 4 weeks before the external fixator is removed.[267] An alternative is to remove the external fixator and then apply a long-leg walking cast until solid callus formation is present. In the rare case in which application of the external fixator spans the knee joint in a patient with a highly comminuted fracture, two pins are placed in the proximal end of the tibia, at least 3 cm distal to the tibial tubercle. The external fixation of the tibia should be removed to allow range of motion of the knee in approximately 4 to 6 weeks, when fracture stability has improved.

The most common complication associated with external fixation of distal metaphyseal fractures is pin tract infection, which can usually be treated with oral antibiotics and aggressive pin care. Malunion can occur and is best prevented by careful assessment of alignment at the time of application of the external fixator. Assessment includes extending the knee and clinically evaluating alignment of the lower extremity and fluoroscopic visualization of the knee joint when a mechanical axis line is made with the Bovie cord held over the femoral head and the center of the ankle. Radiographs should be obtained weekly for 2 to 3 weeks after fracture stabilization to ensure that reduction of the fracture has been maintained. Finally, distal femoral physeal injury may occur when pins are placed less than 1 cm from the physis.

Closed Reduction and Internal Fixation. The method of closed reduction of the distal metaphyseal fracture depends on the deformity at the time of treatment. In a hyperextension-type injury the distal fragment is flexed because of the pull of the gastrocnemius muscles, and the proximal fragment is posteriorly displaced. In a hyperflexion type of fracture, again the distal fragment is flexed because of the pull of the gastrocnemius muscle, but the proximal fragment is anterior to the distal fragment. Reducing these fractures is often difficult because the plane of displacement and the plane of knee joint motion are in the same direction and there is an inadequate lever arm of the distal femoral fragment. The technique we prefer for reduction is performed with the patient supine on a radiolucent operating table.

For a hyperextension-type fracture the hip is flexed to relax the quadriceps muscle and the knee is flexed to relax the gastrocnemius and hamstring muscles. Longitudinal traction is applied to the lower part of the leg while knee flexion is increased in an attempt to bring the distal femoral fragment posteriorly. Manual pressure is applied to the distal femoral condyles to push them posteriorly while the proximal femoral segment is pushed anteriorly (Fig. 43–93). The knee should be flexed 60 degrees at this point to help stabilize the fracture, and the reduction is checked on fluoroscopy. For a hyperflexion-type injury, reduction is begun by placing axial traction on the injured leg with the knee in extension. The posteriorly displaced distal fragment is then pushed anteriorly as the proximal fragment is pushed posteriorly.

Once acceptable reduction is achieved, threaded Steinmann pins are placed in crossed fashion, beginning as far from the physis as possible without jeopardizing stability. Because the pins are often close to the knee joint, we prefer to cut the pins just below the skin so that they do not communicate with the external environment or rub the inside of the cast. External immobilization is required after fracture reduction and stabilization and can vary from a hip spica cast with the knee flexed 60 degrees to a long-leg cast with the knee flexed 30 degrees. This depends on the surgeon's assessment of fracture stability at the time of reduction and pin fixation and should err on the side of caution. In fractures stabilized by external immobilization only, the knee should be flexed to 60 degrees for the first 2 to 3 weeks and then gradually brought up into knee extension.[5,99]

Open Reduction and Internal Fixation. Indications for this technique include fractures that are irreducible by closed means and a requirement for stable internal fixation, such as when an associated arterial injury is present. Failure of closed reduction is usually due to the proximal fracture fragment's buttonholing through the quadriceps muscle, which becomes interposed between the fracture fragments and prevents fracture reduction.

The operative approach is generally through a standard lateral approach; however, when an arterial injury is present, a medial approach to both the fracture and the arterial injury is necessary. The lateral approach passes through the tensor fasciae latae and the fascia of the vastus lateralis. The musculature of the vastus lateralis is then gently teased off its fascia posteriorly to the posterolateral aspect of the femur, followed by

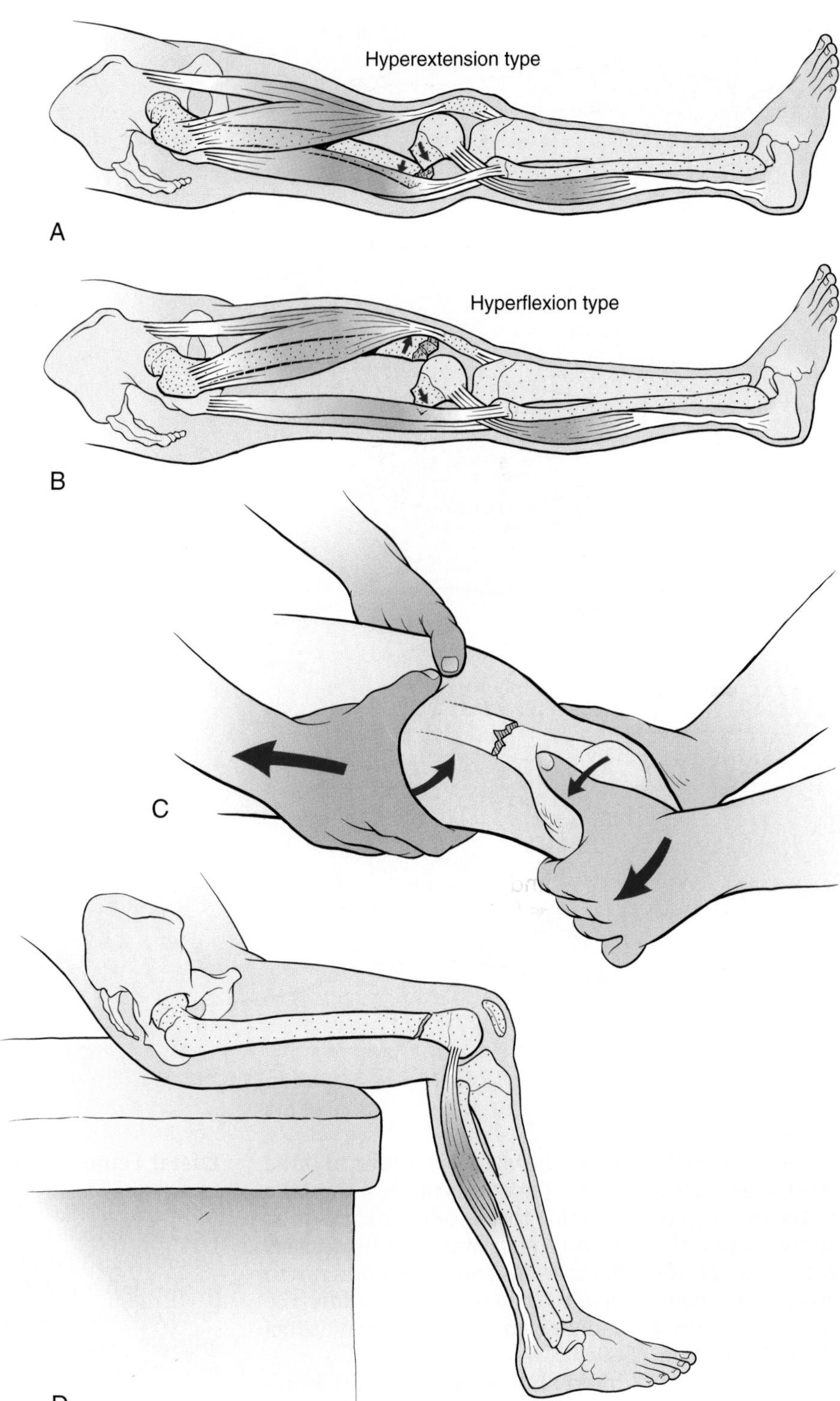

FIGURE 43–93 Reduction of a distal femoral physeal injury. **A,** Hyperextension-type injury. **B,** Hyperflexion-type injury. Note the distal fragment posterior to the proximal fragment. **C,** Reduction maneuver to reduce a hyperextension-type distal femoral physeal injury. Axial traction is initially applied with the knee in extension, followed by gradual flexion of the knee to bring the distal fragment posteriorly. **D,** The knee is flexed to hold the reduction and then placed in a cast in this position.

subperiosteal dissection. Usually, the soft tissue injury created by the fracture will disturb the tissue planes, which may alter the dissection slightly. Once the fracture has been exposed, the interposed muscle must be cleared from the fracture site to allow fracture reduction (Fig. 43–94). The reduction maneuver is similar to that used for closed reduction.

The most common indication for a medial approach to these fractures is a concomitant arterial injury requiring repair. The medial approach facilitates exposure to carry out fracture and arterial repair and saphenous vein harvest for the arterial anastomosis. The medial incision is begun in the mid-coronal plane, just proximal to the knee. An incision is made directly over the adductor tubercle, which lies on the posterior aspect of the medial femoral condyle and defines the interval between the vastus medialis and the medial hamstring muscles. Superficially the interval is

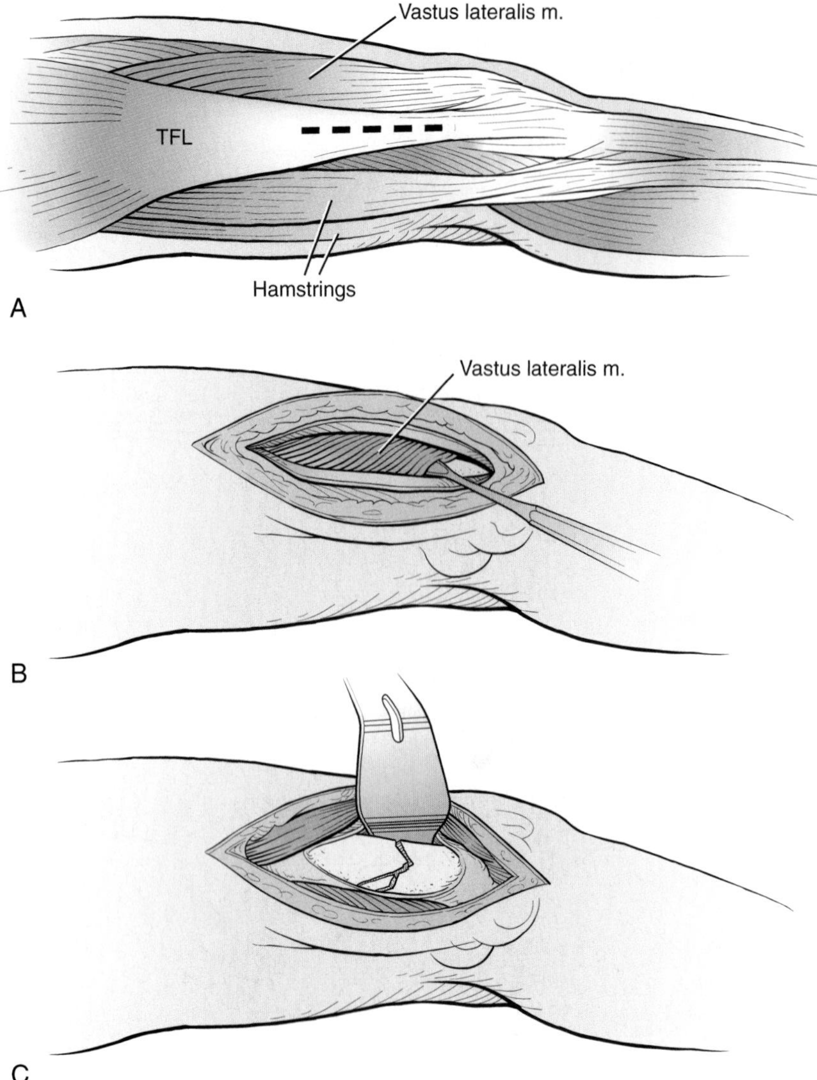

FIGURE 43–94 Lateral approach to the distal femur. **A,** The skin incision is made directly over the lateral aspect of the distal part of the thigh. TFL, tensor fasciae latae. **B,** The TFL is incised and the posterior aspect of the vastus lateralis is dissected off the lateral aspect of the femur. **C,** The vastus lateralis is retracted anteriorly to expose the fracture site.

between the sartorius and the vastus medialis, and the deep dissection is between the vastus medialis and the adductor magnus. Posterior to the adductor magnus lie the popliteal artery and vein and the tibial nerve. Retraction of the adductor magnus posteriorly will protect the neurovascular structures and allow the vastus medialis to be dissected off the medial aspect of the femur (Fig. 43–95).

We prefer rigid internal fixation with a 4.5-mm dynamic compression plate or a clover-type plate in a child older than 12 years or a patient with a severely comminuted fracture (Fig. 43–96). Any internal fixation device should be placed at least 1 cm proximal to the distal physis. In most children, threaded Steinmann pins placed in crossed fashion provide enough stability; this fixation is supplemented with a long-leg cast with the knee in approximately 30 degrees of flexion for a duration of 6 to 8 weeks. The pins should be left deep to the skin and can be removed after good callus formation at 4 weeks, followed by an additional 2 to 4 weeks in a long-leg cast.

Distal Femoral Physeal Fractures

Treatment Principles. The general principles applicable to treating physeal fractures must be followed when treating a distal femoral physeal injury because of the higher risk for development of a physeal osseous bridge with subsequent limb length discrepancy or angular deformity. These principles include the following:

1. All attempts at a closed reduction should be performed under general anesthesia or sedation.
2. The reduction maneuver should consist of predominantly traction, followed by manipulation.
3. The reduction should not be performed more than 10 days after the original injury.
4. Anatomic reduction should be achieved, especially in types III and IV injuries.
5. Internal fixation should avoid the physis and should be nonthreaded if passing across the physis.[229]

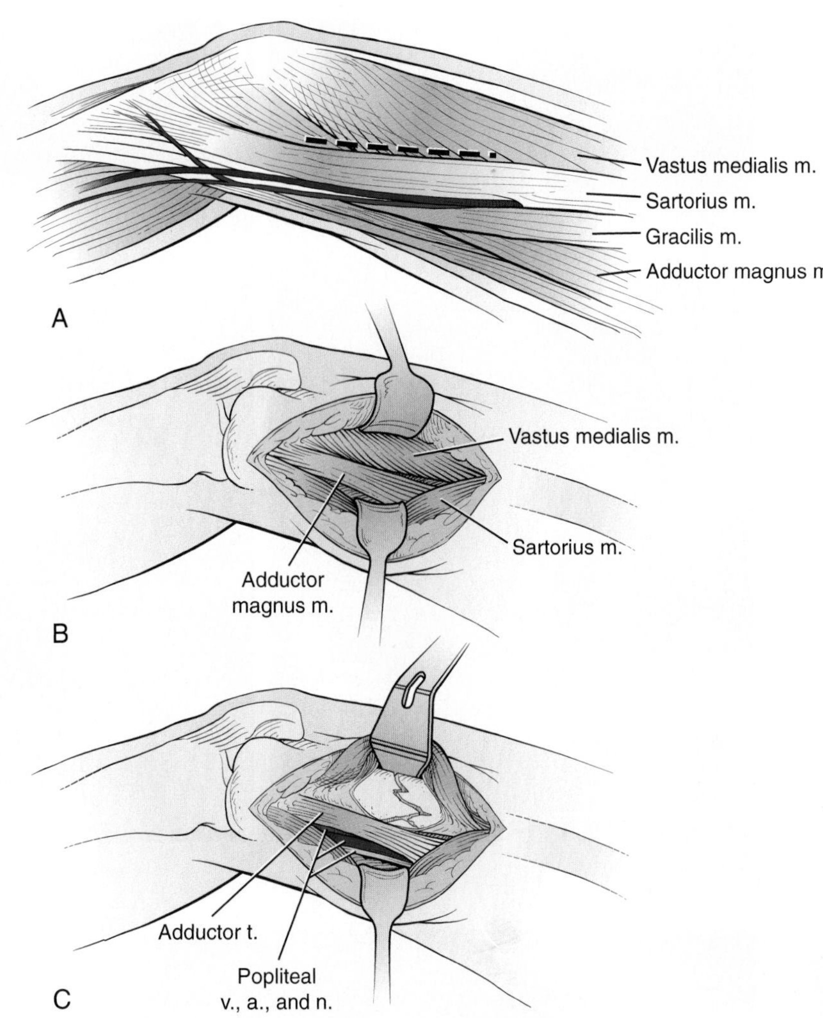

FIGURE 43-95 Medial approach to the distal femur. **A,** A skin incision (*dashed line*) is made parallel and just superior to the sartorius. **B,** Dissection is carried out between the sartorius and vastus medialis. The adductor magnus is seen in this interval. **C,** Subperiosteal dissection is carried out at the distal femur. Access to the neurovascular structure can be achieved below the adductor magnus.

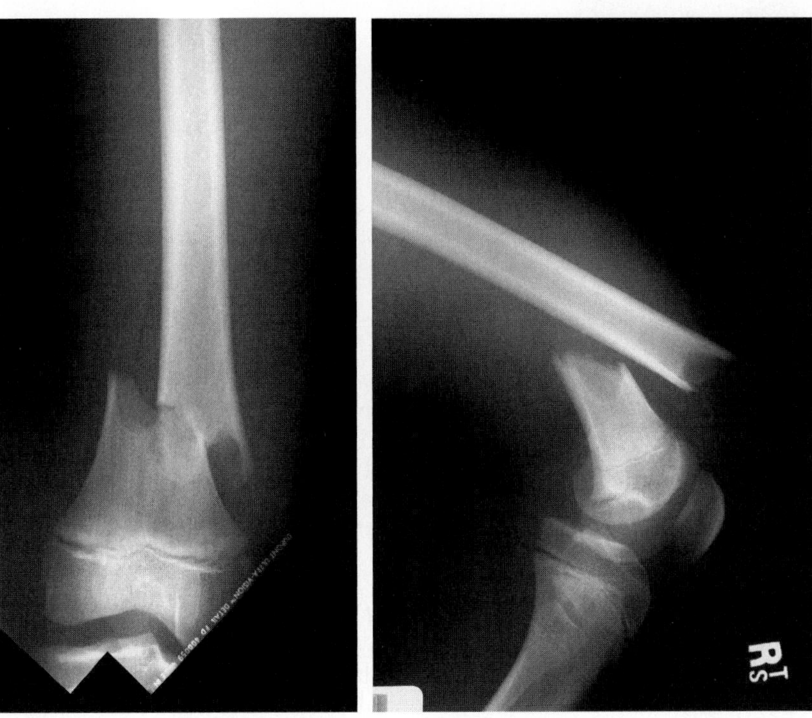

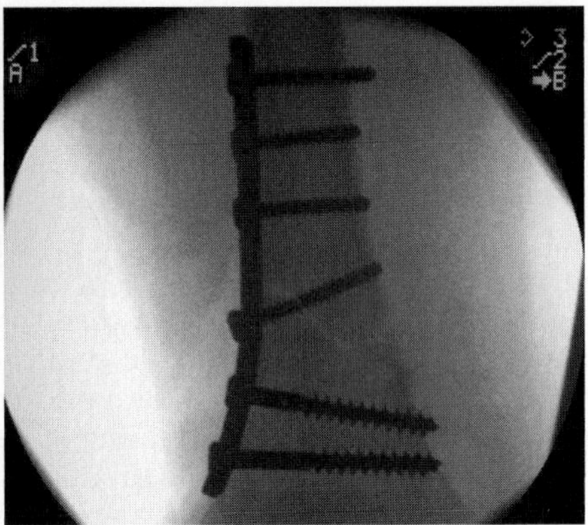

FIGURE 43-96 **A** through **C,** Distal femoral metaphyseal fracture treated by open reduction and internal fixation through a lateral approach.

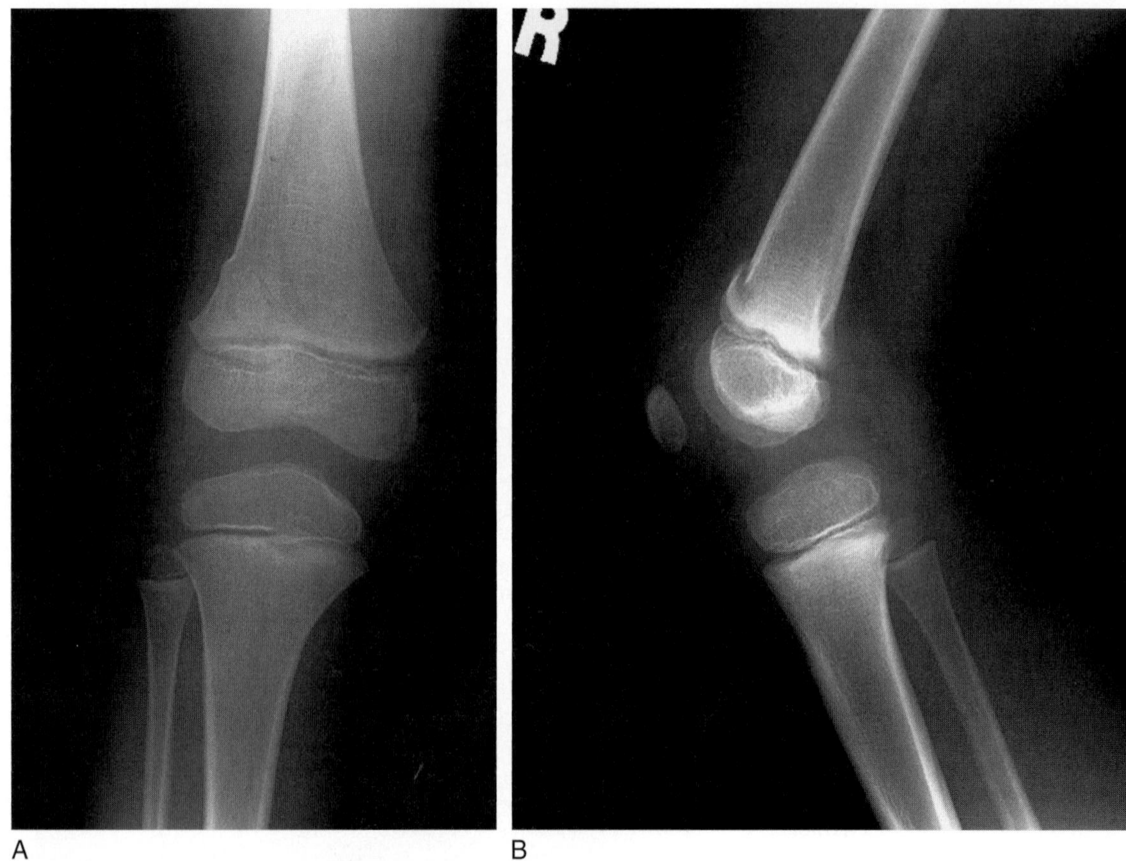

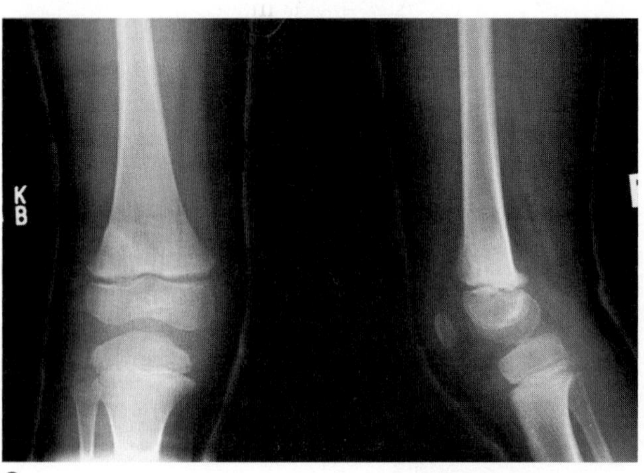

FIGURE 43–97 Undisplaced Salter-Harris type II fracture treated by casting. Anteroposterior **(A)** and lateral **(B)** initial radiographs demonstrating the undisplaced fracture in a 5-year-old child. **C,** At 5 weeks the fracture has healed and the cast has been removed.

Salter and colleagues have stated that when excessive manipulation appears to be necessary to achieve acceptable reduction, it is better to maintain growth potential and perform corrective osteotomy at a later date than to overstress the physis and cause more injury.[228]

The goal of treatment of a distal femoral physeal injury is to gain an anatomic reduction with stable fixation, especially in an older child (>10 years). In a younger child, acceptable alignment includes up to 20 degrees of angulation in the sagittal plane,[28] less than 5 degrees of varus or valgus angulation, and no rotational deformity.

Nondisplaced Physeal Fractures. Nondisplaced physeal injuries can be treated with a long-leg cast for 4 to 6 weeks, depending on the age of the child (Fig. 43–97). Non–weight-bearing crutch walking is continued during this time, followed by weight bearing as tolerated and range-of-motion knee exercises when the cast is discontinued.

Salter-Harris Type I Fractures. A Salter-Harris type I injury in a newborn can be treated by immobilization without attempts at reduction because significant remodeling potential exists.[220] Immobilization in a newborn is difficult but often requires only a bulky soft dressing. An older child with complete physeal separation will need closed reduction performed under general anesthesia. Reduction of a hyperextension injury in which the distal fragment is displaced anteriorly and flexed relative to the tibia is similar to that described for distal femoral metaphyseal fractures. Immobilization is accomplished with a hip spica or long-leg cast with the knee flexed, usually to 60 degrees, followed by gradual extension of the knee over the ensuing 3 to 4 weeks. However, Aitken and Magill pointed out that the distal femoral physeal separation occurs distal to the medial head of the gastrocnemius, with the distal fragment displaced posteriorly, and therefore reduction of these fractures should occur with the knee in extension. Likewise, the knee should be immobilized in extension to allow "the taut medial head of the gastrocnemius to act as a posterior splint and prevent posterior displacement."[5] In an older child or a patient with an unstable physeal separation, smooth pin fixation may be necessary to provide stable fixation. We prefer to place smooth wires or pins in crossed fashion; they are removed at 4 weeks, and the limb is then recasted for an additional 2 weeks in a long-leg cast (Fig. 43–98). To prevent knee contractures, aggressive therapy is then started to regain range of motion of the knee. We prefer a long-leg cast in most children except an obese child, in whom control of the knee in a long-leg cast is difficult, or if there is any concern about compliance with non–weight-bearing status.

Salter-Harris Type II Fractures. Of all type II fractures, 60% to 75% are displaced at the time of initial evaluation.[58,156,220] In the juvenile group, the incidence is closer to 100%[220] because of the high energy required to disrupt the thick periosteal and perichondrial sheaths in children younger than 11 years.[34]

Nondisplaced or minimally displaced type II fractures can be successfully treated by closed reduction and external immobilization. The reduction maneuver should be performed under general anesthesia or sedation, with the principal maneuver being in-line traction followed by an overcorrection maneuver to reduce the angulation of the distal fragment. This should tighten the intact periosteum attached to the metaphyseal fragment. For example, when the metaphyseal fragment is on the lateral side, the distal fragment will be in valgus and can be reduced with a varus-producing maneuver to overcorrect the deformity. A well-molded plaster long-leg cast is applied with the knee in 20 to 30 degrees of flexion and overwrapped in fiberglass. It is important to identify any knee ligamentous injury because such injury will make the reduction maneuver difficult, may cause further damage to the ligament, and will usually require internal fixation to maintain the reduction. Bertin and Goble reported that 6 of 16 patients with distal femoral physeal injuries (three of which were type II fractures) had associated ligamentous injuries; all three had residual coronal and sagittal plane deformity.[23]

In a displaced type II fracture, closed reduction under general anesthesia is performed, followed by percutaneous fixation to fix the metaphyseal fragment. In a young child, Kirschner wires should be used, and in a child older than 10 years, cannulated screws (4.0- or 6.5-mm screws) should be placed percutaneously (Fig. 43–99). Although the literature reports only a 10% to 15% rate of type II fracture stabilization with internal fixation,[156,220] we prefer anatomic reduction under general anesthesia, followed by stable internal fixation of the metaphyseal fragment. The leg should be placed in a cast with the knee in 20 to 30 degrees of flexion until healing occurs, which is generally in 6 weeks. Failed closed reduction of a type II fracture of the distal femur requires open reduction in approximately 5% of cases.[156] This irreducible type II fracture is most often due to interposed periosteum on the tension side of the fracture or, less often, muscle interposition, and it requires open reduction followed by internal fixation.

Salter-Harris Type III Fractures. Type III injuries of the distal femur are relatively less common, are usually displaced, and generally require open reduction and internal fixation. Type III fractures must be anatomically reduced to preserve the articular anatomy and reduce the likelihood of growth arrest. Historically, some of these fractures have been treated successfully by closed reduction and casting[220]; however, reduction can easily be lost because little control of the fracture fragments is achieved in a long-leg cast. We prefer open reduction of all type III fractures to anatomically reduce the joint surface and physis and to provide stable fixation of the fracture. An anteromedial or anterolateral incision is made, depending on the fracture pattern. Anatomic reduction must be achieved under direct visualization, followed by percutaneous fixation of the epiphysis, preferably with cannulated cancellous screws (4.0 or 6.5 mm). If possible, two screws should be placed in the epiphysis, and they should be placed so that the threads are on only one side of the fracture line to gain compression across the fracture (Fig. 43–100). Long-leg cast immobilization for 6 weeks with the knee in 20 to 30 degrees of flexion is required. It is rare to have a type III fracture that is nondisplaced at initial evaluation, and in this setting we continue to prefer internal fixation of these fractures to maintain anatomic reduction.

Salter-Harris Type IV Fractures. Management of type IV fractures is similar to that for type III fractures: anatomic reduction to preserve the joint and prevent growth arrest. This usually means open reduction stabilized with internal fixation. Cannulated screws or Kirschner wires should be placed parallel to the joint line in both the metaphysis and the epiphysis to achieve stable fixation.

For all types of distal femoral physeal injuries, long-leg casting is continued for 6 to 8 weeks, depending on the age of the child and the radiographic appearance of fracture healing. In general, after callus formation becomes evident on radiographs, range-of-motion exercises should be started, with the patient using a removable cast or knee immobilizer until solid fracture healing has occurred. Close follow-up of these

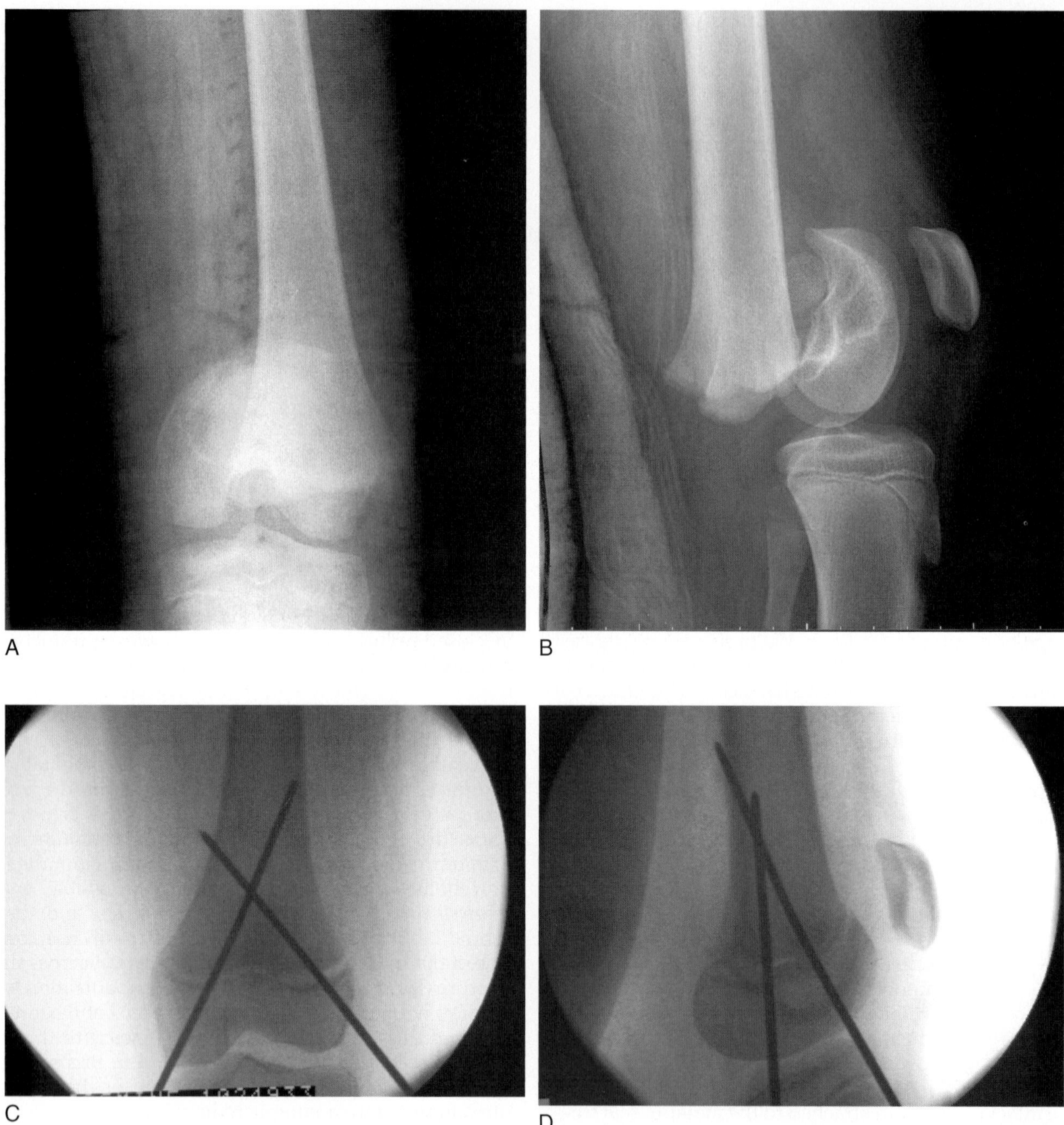

FIGURE 43–98 Closed reduction and percutaneous pinning of a distal femoral physeal injury. Anteroposterior **(A)** and lateral **(B)** initial radiographs in a 5-year-old girl showing a Salter-Harris type II hyperextension distal femoral physeal injury. **C** and **D**, Intraoperative radiographs obtained after closed reduction and percutaneous pinning. The pins were cut below the skin, and a long-leg cast was applied.

patients should continue for at least 18 months to monitor the growth of the distal femoral epiphysis.

The prognosis for these fractures depends on the age of the child at the time of injury, the amount of fracture displacement, the adequacy of the reduction and fracture stabilization, and the type of fracture. Distal femoral physeal injuries in the juvenile age group (<11 years) are the result of a high-energy injury that imparts greater trauma to the physis; such injuries have worse outcomes than do similar fractures in adolescents.[220] Riseborough and colleagues reported that 83% of the juvenile age group who sustained distal femoral physeal fractures had growth problems as compared with 50% of the adolescent age group.[220] This difference is also related to the amount of residual growth remaining in the two age groups, with adolescents having less time than younger patients for limb length discrepancies or angular deformities to develop. Fracture displacement at the time of injury is a strong predictor of outcome.[156] Lombardo and Harvey

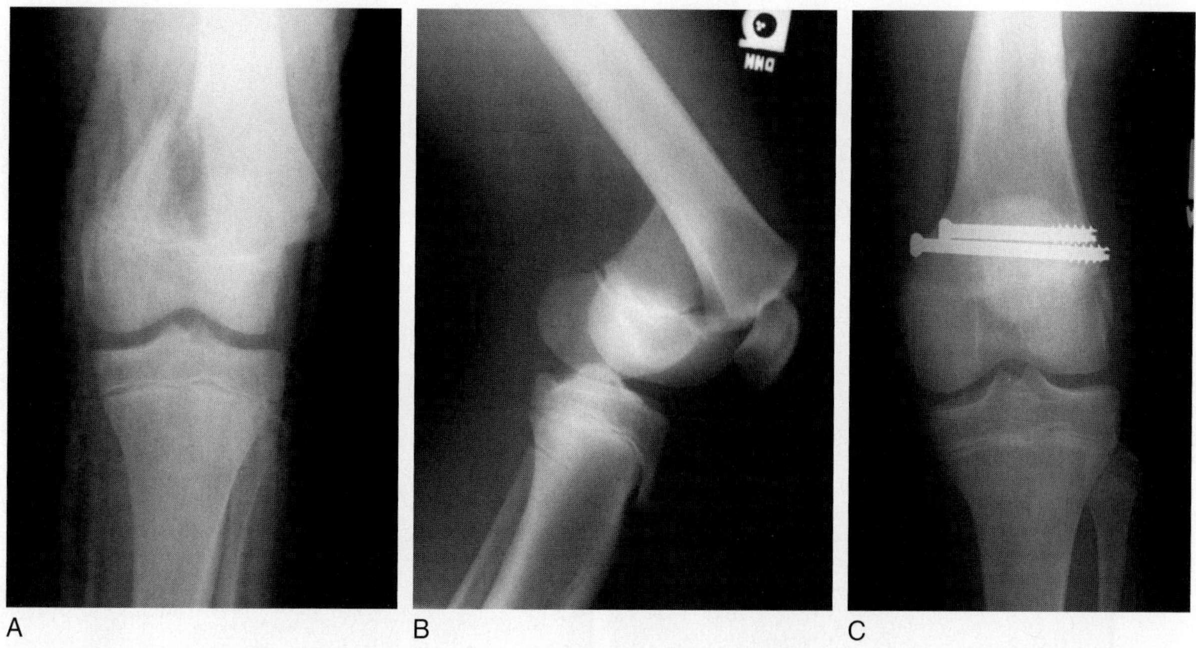

FIGURE 43–99 Closed reduction and screw fixation of Salter-Harris type II fracture. Anteroposterior **(A)** and lateral **(B)** initial radiographs demonstrating displacement in a Salter-Harris type II fracture in a 13-year-old boy. **C,** Closed reduction with percutaneous screw fixation was performed, with healing at 1 year after injury.

reported limb length discrepancies of 5 and 8 mm, respectively, in nondisplaced fractures and displaced fractures that were reduced satisfactorily. Failure to obtain adequate reduction is a poor prognostic indicator, with patients in whom adequate reduction is not achieved having a limb length discrepancy of 25 mm.[156] Finally, types I and II fractures generally have a better outcome than types III, IV, and V fractures do.[58,156,220,261]

COMPLICATIONS

Acute complications are relatively rare and include associated injuries to the popliteal artery, peroneal nerve, or knee ligaments and loss of fracture reduction. Late complications are more common and include limb length discrepancy, angular deformity, knee contracture and stiffness, and residual knee instability secondary to ligamentous injury.

Acute Complications

Arterial Injury. Arterial injury is rare in a distal femoral epiphyseal injury; it is most common with complete separation of the physis in a hyperextension injury in which the posteriorly displaced proximal fragment injures the popliteal artery (Fig. 43–101). To our knowledge, injury to the arterial wall has been reported in only three cases in the literature.[187,220] In another report, a patient with ipsilateral injuries to the distal femur and proximal tibia underwent exploration of the popliteal artery because of a cool, pulseless foot with findings consistent with severe spasm of the popliteal artery; the spasm responded to papaverine injection.[261]

Careful physical examination of the peripheral pulses is necessary at initial evaluation. If a discrepancy between limbs is identified, gentle, closed reduction should be performed and the pulses reexamined. If the examination findings remain unchanged after reduction, the patient undergoes arteriography and arterial exploration. Although some recommend immediate exploration of the artery without arteriography, we prefer to obtain an arteriogram to identify the site and nature of the injury before exploration, especially in light of the fact that arterial injury is so rare. However, excessive delays are unacceptable because warm ischemia times longer than 6 hours have been associated with worse outcomes with respect to limb salvage, neurologic compromise, and muscle death.[151]

Fasciotomy of the leg should be considered in the following situations: prolonged warm ischemia time, significant hypotension in the perioperative period, tense soft tissue compartments, and associated crush injury with significant venous injury in the popliteal or femoral area.[85] When an arterial injury is present, the fracture should be stabilized urgently via a medial approach to the fracture to allow rapid open reduction and internal fixation and subsequent arterial repair. A patient with a warm foot without palpable pulses and a normal arteriogram should be observed in the hospital for 48 hours.

Peroneal Nerve Injury. Peroneal nerve injury may be due to direct trauma on the posterolateral aspect of the leg or to a severe varus-producing injury causing overstretching of the nerve. The incidence is approximately 5% (6 of 111 cases in a compilation of five

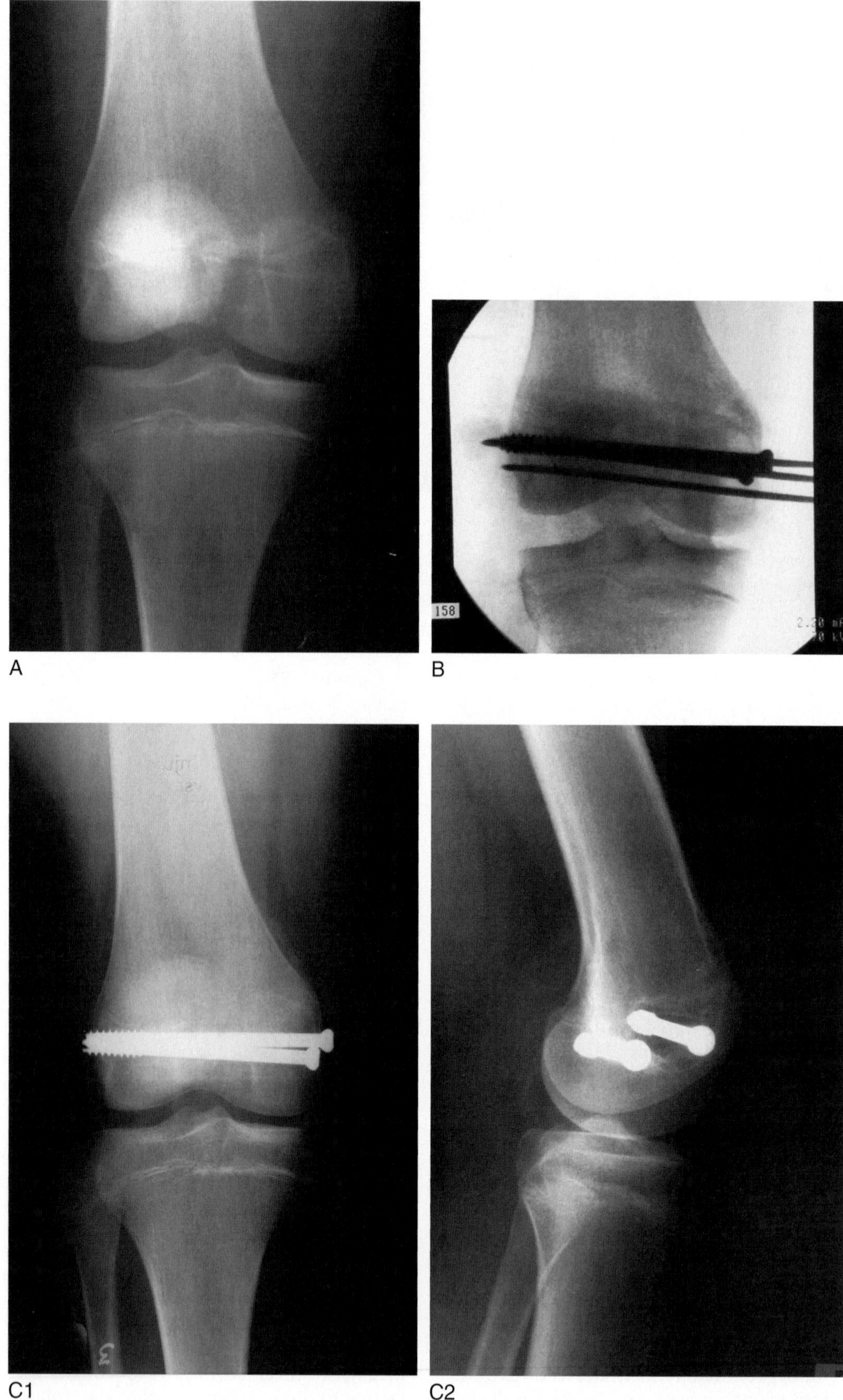

FIGURE 43-100 Salter-Harris type III distal femoral fracture in a 13-year-old boy that was treated by open reduction and internal fixation. **A,** Initial radiograph showing displacement of approximately 4 to 5 mm. **B,** Open reduction plus internal fixation was performed with percutaneously placed screws. Anteroposterior **(C1)** and lateral **(C2)** images 4 months after injury. Healing has occurred, with no loss of reduction.

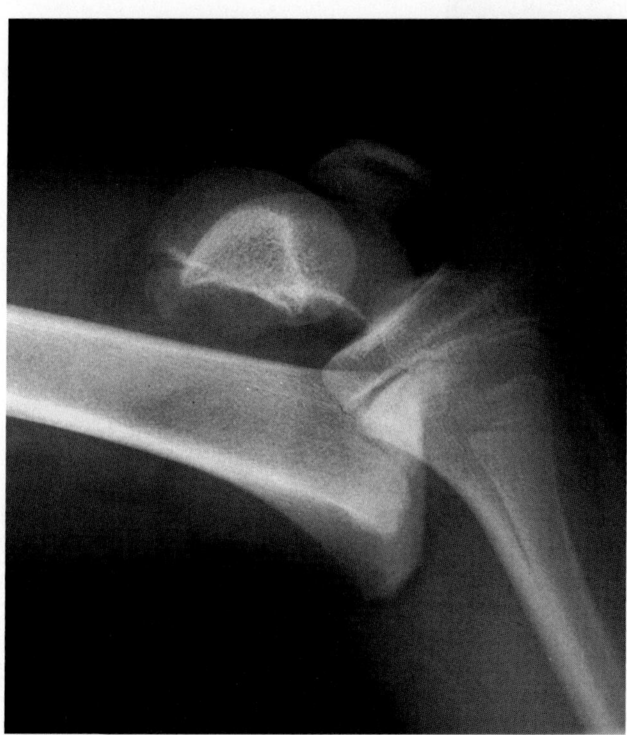

FIGURE 43–101 Severely displaced Salter-Harris type II fracture with hyperextension. Arterial injury was caused by the high-energy force driving the proximal fragment into the posterior compartment of the knee. Arterial reconstruction was performed after closed reduction with pin fixation.

studies).[5,23,58,156,261] All peroneal nerve injuries reported in the literature have resolved completely over a 6-month period. If nerve function has not shown some return of function by 3 months, an electromyographic study should be performed. Exploration of the nerve with direct repair or nerve grafting is indicated if fibrillation or denervation is seen or if there is a delay in nerve conduction velocity. Open fractures with associated peroneal nerve injury should be explored at the time of initial irrigation and should be debrided, with microscopic direct repair if the nerve is divided.

Ligamentous Injuries. Associated ligamentous injuries occur relatively commonly in injuries to the distal femoral physis. Bertin and Goble specifically reported on ligamentous injuries associated with physeal fractures about the knee and noted that 6 (38%) of 16 patients with distal femoral physeal injuries had ACL instability; 1 also had valgus instability.[23] A compilation of 111 patients from five studies showed 26 associated ligamentous injuries (23%),[5,58,156,261,269] with the most commonly injured ligament being the ACL, followed by the lateral collateral ligament (LCL) and then the medial collateral ligament (MCL). It is often difficult to fully assess the integrity of the knee ligaments at the time of initial evaluation. However, they should be carefully assessed as soon as early fracture union is present. It is also important to examine for meniscal pathology, and arthroscopic examination and treatment may be necessary.

Loss of Reduction. Loss of reduction occurs because of suboptimal stabilization of the unstable fracture, usually a result of inadequate external immobilization. Aitken and Magill reported nine fractures treated by closed reduction and cast immobilization, with only two patients maintaining anatomic reduction.[5] They attributed this outcome to not maintaining knee flexion when immobilizing the anteriorly displaced fractures and inadequate knee extension when immobilizing the posteriorly displaced fractures. Others have reported loss of reduction in 40% of fractures after the initial reduction and cast immobilization.[18] With the greater use of internal fixation devices and strict adherence to correct leg immobilization techniques, loss of reduction has become less prevalent in more recent studies.[58,220]

Late Complications

Physeal Arrest. Physeal arrest with residual limb length discrepancy or angular deformity continues to occur relatively frequently despite more exact anatomic reductions and greater use of stable internal fixation (Fig. 43–102). A review of retrospective series showed that limb length inequality of greater than 2 cm has been reported to occur in approximately one third of cases.[58,156,220,261] Risk factors for development of a growth disturbance include high-energy trauma, juvenile age group, severely displaced fractures, and comminuted fractures that produce injury in multiple areas of the physis.[156]

Suspected physeal injury should be thoroughly evaluated with CT. Physeal bar resection is indicated when less than 50% of the physis is involved and the growth remaining is at least 2.5 cm.[132] Limb lengths should be plotted on the Moseley straight-line graph (see Chapter 24, Limb Length Discrepancy) over a 1- to 2-year period to determine the projected discrepancy at skeletal maturity.[184] An alternative method to estimate the discrepancy at initial evaluation of the patient or after identification of the physeal bar is evaluation of growth remaining with the Anderson-Green tables.[97]

General treatment guidelines are the following: no treatment is necessary when the discrepancy is less than 2 cm; between 2 and 6 cm, epiphysiodesis of the contralateral distal femur or proximal tibia is indicated; and larger discrepancies should be treated by a femoral lengthening procedure. In an excessively short femur after injury in a young child, multiple femoral lengthening procedures or a femoral lengthening procedure with contralateral epiphysiodesis is necessary.

Angular Deformity. Angular deformity is less frequently seen than limb length discrepancy, with a reported incidence of 29% (49 of 171 patients in five series).[5,58,156,220,261] The risk factors are similar to those for development of a limb length discrepancy, and the indications for physeal bar resection are the same. No correlation has been found between the direction of fracture displacement and the development of a valgus or varus deformity.[220] Treatment is indicated when more than 5 degrees of abnormal angulation is present

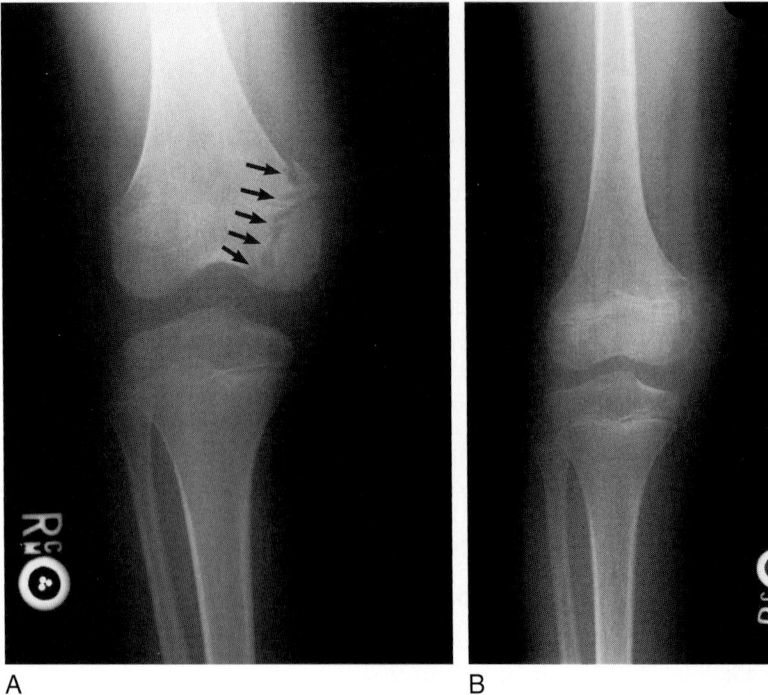

A B

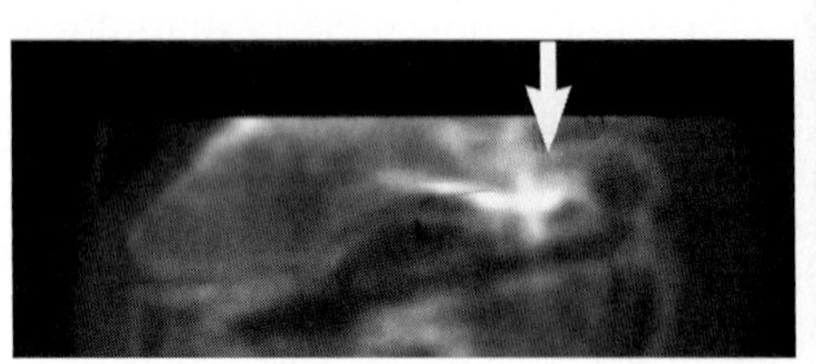

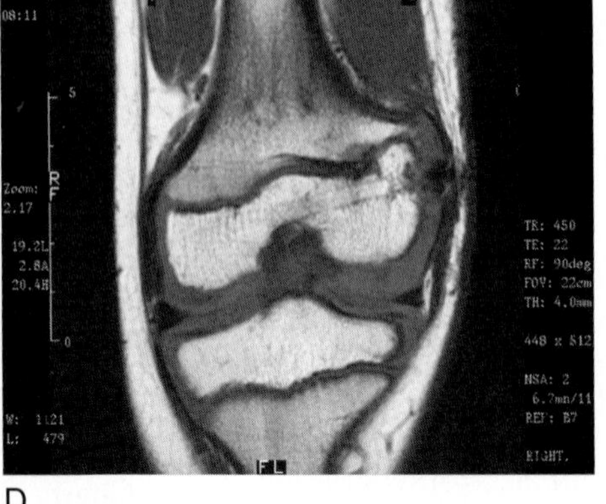

C D

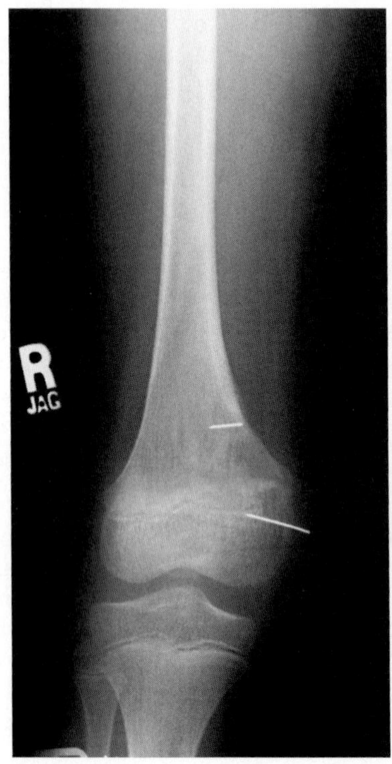

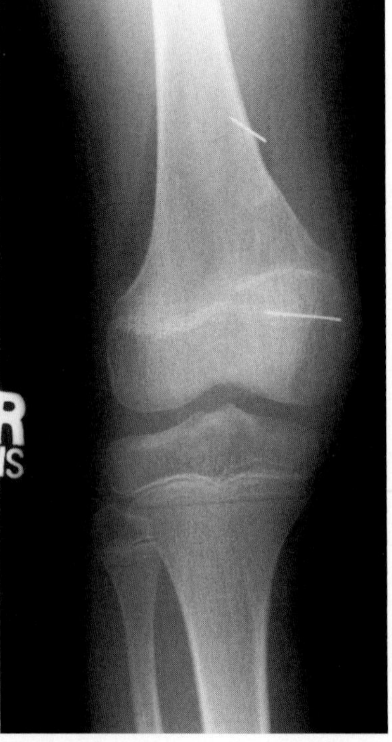

E F

FIGURE 43–102 Physeal arrest after a Salter-Harris type IV fracture of the distal femoral shaft. **A,** Injury radiograph of a 7-year-old boy showing the distal femoral injury (*arrows*). **B,** Radiographic evidence of physeal arrest was apparent after 6 weeks of cast treatment. Physeal arrest was evident on computed tomography **(C)** (*arrow*) and confirmed by magnetic resonance imaging **(D).** **E,** Epiphysiolysis with fat interposition and placement of a metal marker was performed. **F,** Two years later, resumption of growth was confirmed by increasing distance of the markers.

and consists of angular corrective osteotomies or epiphysiolysis.

Loss of Knee Motion. Loss of knee motion occurs in approximately 27% of distal femoral physeal injuries (45 of 167 patients in five series).[5,58,156,220,261] It may be due to excessive duration of immobilization with intra-articular adhesions, capsular contraction, or hamstring or quadriceps contraction. In addition, articular incongruities from Salter-Harris types III and IV injuries may predispose to knee joint contractures. Contractures are best prevented by restricting the duration of external immobilization, removing crossed Kirschner wires as soon as possible, and performing anatomic reduction of intra-articular fractures. Aggressive active and active assisted range-of-motion exercises should be started as soon as 4 to 6 weeks from the time of fracture. A removable posterior splint can be worn at 4 weeks so that the patient can begin range-of-motion exercises twice per day as the fracture heals.

Once fracture healing occurs, knee ligament integrity should be reevaluated and appropriate treatment instituted if necessary (see subsequent discussion of ACL injuries under Ligament Injuries).

Patellar Fractures

Fractures of the patella in children are rare, accounting for less than 5% of all knee injuries.[21,195,216,235] The injury is often caused by direct anterior knee trauma or an eccentric load during extension of the knee while jumping or landing. As in the treatment of adult patellar fractures, the majority of fractures require open reduction and internal fixation. Although the complication rate is low with operative fixation, late reconstruction of missed injuries may result in an extensor lag and an unsatisfactory outcome.

ANATOMY

The patella is a sesamoid bone that lies within the quadriceps tendon and provides added mechanical advantage for knee extension. The patellar ossification center usually appears at 2 to 3 years of age but may be delayed until the sixth year. Although a single ossification center is most common, there can be up to six smaller associated centers of ossification peripheral to the primary. These centers of ossification coalesce, and ossification begins centrally and continues in peripheral fashion. A bipartite patella is thought to occur when the cartilaginous segments fail to coalesce. It is most often seen with a superolateral fragment and is generally thought to occur in less than 5% of the population.[92,98,198,201]

The articular surface is divided into seven facets separated by ridges. A major vertical ridge separates the medial and lateral facets, with a secondary ridge near the medial border that demarcates the odd facet. Two transverse ridges separate the superior, intermediate, and inferior facets. The distal-most pole is nonarticular.[32,217]

The quadriceps mechanism converges onto a single, trilaminar tendon, with the rectus femoris superficial, the vasti in the middle layer, and the intermedius in the deep layer.[156] The fascia lata extends as the deep fascial layer that spreads over the anterior aspect of the knee, and these fibers combine with the vastus medialis and lateralis to form the patellar retinaculum, which inserts into the tibia. The retinaculum is completed by contributions from the patellofemoral ligaments, the lateral aspect of the vastus lateralis, and the iliotibial tract.[156] The infrapatellar ligament is primarily an extension of the rectus femoris and inserts into the tibial tubercle. Expansions of the iliotibial tract and patellar retinaculum converge onto the infrapatellar ligament at its insertion into the tibia.

The blood supply of the patella has been thoroughly studied by Scapinelli[232] and Crock.[55] It is organized into two arterial networks. The first is the extraosseous arterial ring, which lies in the thin layer of connective tissue, with contributions from the supreme genicular, superior medial and lateral genicular, and inferior medial and lateral genicular arteries and the anterior tibial recurrent artery (Fig. 43–103). The inferior genicular arteries branch into the ascending parapatellar, oblique prepatellar, and transverse infrapatellar arteries. These arteries anastomose with branches from the superior genicular arteries. The second network is the intraosseous arterial pattern, which consists of midpatellar vessels that enter in the middle third of the patella and infrapatellar branches that run upward from behind the patellar ligament. AVN of the patella after transverse fractures is most often seen in the superior pole, which is more easily isolated from blood flow than the inferior pole is.

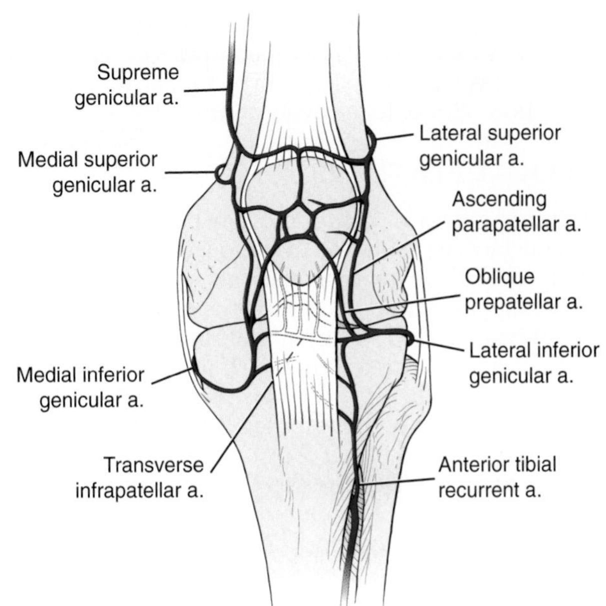

FIGURE 43–103 Arterial blood supply of the patella. The extraosseous arterial ring depicted here demonstrates the rich blood supply of the patella.

MECHANISM OF INJURY

The mechanism of injury is associated with the pattern of the patellar fracture seen radiographically. The majority of transverse mid-patellar fractures are due to direct anterior trauma to a flexed knee or a fall onto the knee.[21,164,195,216] Less frequently, traumatic impact results in a vertical or a stellate-type fracture. Maguire and Canale reported that 22 of 24 patients with patellar fractures sustained the fracture as a result of a direct blow or fall or an impact incurred in a motor vehicle accident; only 2 patients sustained the fracture in a sports activity. There were 20 fractures of the mid-portion of the patella (comminuted, transverse, or vertical fractures) and 4 chip or avulsion fractures.[164] Sleeve fractures are most often associated with forceful contraction of the quadriceps muscle, which usually occurs at the start of a jump during basketball or in the track and field events of high or long jumping.[37,115,289] Wu and colleagues reported on five patients with sleeve fractures, all of whom sustained their injuries at the time of take-off for a long or high jump.[289] However, direct trauma may also result in an inferior sleeve fracture.[216] A superior sleeve or avulsion fracture is often due to a direct blow, and a medial avulsion fracture is associated with lateral dislocation of the knee.

CLASSIFICATION

In children, patellar fractures can be divided into two basic patterns: primary osseous fractures and sleeve or avulsion fractures. The most common bony fracture is a transverse fracture through the mid-portion of the patella; however, vertical fractures and stellate-type fractures also occur.[164] The second major group of patellar fractures is the avulsion-type, or sleeve, fractures.[115] This fracture type most often occurs at the inferior pole of the patella; however, it can also occur at the proximal pole. An avulsion fracture along the medial aspect of the patella may be encountered in association with patellar dislocations.[101,127]

CLINICAL FEATURES

Patellar fractures in children occur between the ages of 8 and 14 years, with the average age being approximately 11 to 12 years. Most patients are boys.[164,216]

The history should elicit the type of injury and the mechanism, as well as any manifestations of patellar dislocation at the time of injury. If a direct injury has resulted in a patellar fracture, the instrument or offending object should be determined, especially when an open injury has occurred.

In a complete fracture or avulsion, the patient's symptoms are more pronounced and the physical examination is diagnostic. The knee is swollen, often with a tense hemarthrosis, and tender. Patients are often unable to bear weight because of pain. Knee extension is frequently difficult, though possible because of residual integrity of the retinacular fibers. However, full active knee extension is not usually possible. Active firing of the quadriceps will further pull the patella superiorly. Palpation reveals a high-riding patella in the inferior sleeve and a transverse type of fracture, and a palpable defect is present and tender.

In an incomplete injury (an undisplaced transverse patellar fracture, a minimally displaced inferior sleeve fracture), symptoms and physical examination findings are less dramatic. Grogan and colleagues reported findings in 8 of 17 patients with inferior sleeve fractures who were initially evaluated 1 week to 4 months after the onset of symptoms. These patients were all involved in competitive sports; however, none could document a specific traumatic episode that triggered the symptoms.[101] Similarly, undisplaced stress fractures of the patella result in minimal symptoms and inability to recognize a specific inciting event.[65]

The orthopaedic examination should always include evaluation of the entire skeleton and the soft tissue envelope to inspect for open fractures. Associated fractures are reported to occur in up to a third of cases, with ipsilateral diaphyseal fractures of the tibia or femur, or both, accounting for the majority of associated injuries.[164] Open fractures account for approximately 30% to 40% of all patellar fractures in children and are generally associated with a motor vehicle accident and direct trauma.[164,216]

RADIOGRAPHIC FINDINGS

Radiographic examination includes AP and lateral radiographs of the knee. The lateral radiograph should be taken with the knee flexed 30 degrees and is usually more informative than the AP radiograph for patellar fractures. The fracture may be undisplaced, mildly displaced with the anterior aspect displaced and the articular surface remaining intact, or completely displaced (Fig. 43–104).[21] Sleeve fractures are often difficult to detect radiographically. It is important to obtain a good lateral radiograph of the knee to discern the typical findings. The radiograph should be inspected for small bony fragments coming from the inferior pole of the patella associated with patella alta. The bony fragment seen radiographically is often small but is associated with a large cartilaginous fragment attached to the patellar tendon. The radiograph must be used in conjunction with clinical assessment to make the diagnosis. A patient with indeterminate radiographs but significant tenderness at the level of the injury or a palpable defect should be treated as though a sleeve fracture were present. Other entities that can resemble a sleeve fracture include accessory centers of ossification, which are more often on the anterior aspect of the distal pole of the patella, and the Sinding-Larsen-Johansson lesion, an overuse condition manifested as small calcifications within the patellar tendon.[249]

The AP radiograph is used to detect a bipartite patella, generally seen on the superolateral aspect of the patella. In addition, the uncommon vertical fracture is best seen in this view, as is a comminuted fracture (Fig. 43–105). Comparison radiographs are helpful in defining the normal anatomy of the particu-

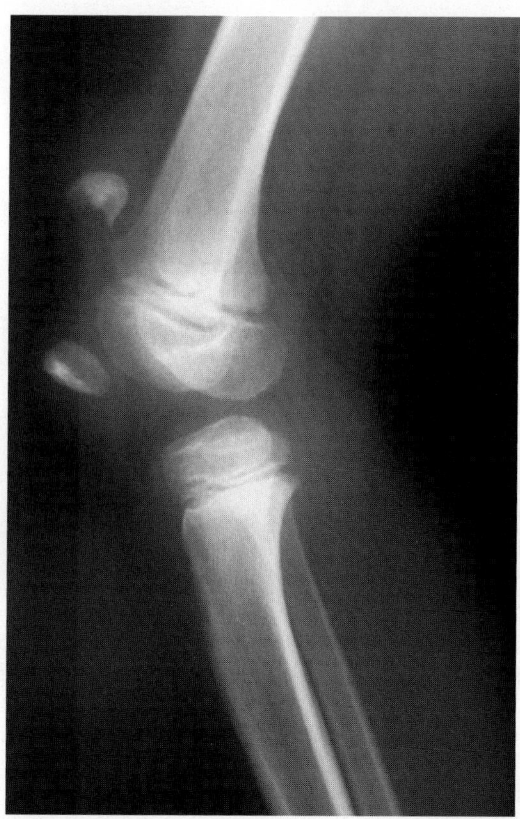

FIGURE 43–104 Displaced transverse fracture of the patella in a 5-year-old.

lar patient, including confirmation of the presence of a bipartite patella.

TREATMENT

The indications for nonoperative and operative treatment are similar to those in adults. Nonoperative treatment is used for an undisplaced fracture,[164,215,216] especially when active knee extension is present, which indicates that the supporting soft tissue structures (retinaculum) are intact. External immobilization in the form of a long-leg cast with near extension is worn for 6 to 8 weeks and is followed by progressive weight bearing. Maguire and Canale report 83% good results in patients with undisplaced patellar fractures treated by external immobilization only.[164]

Operative treatment is indicated for a displaced fracture with more than 4 mm of articular displacement or if the articular step-off is greater than 3 mm.[21,115,164,215,216] The most important aspect of evaluation is to assess the integrity of the articular surface. We prefer operative intervention if displacement or step-off of the articular surface exceeds 2 to 3 mm. In addition, open fractures require operative intervention, which should include irrigation, debridement, and if necessary, reduction and internal fixation.[21,115,164,215,216]

Sleeve Fracture. For a young child (10 years or younger) with a sleeve fracture, we prefer nonabsorbable suture repair followed by immobilization in a long-leg cast for 6 to 8 weeks. Anatomic reduction of the sleeve fracture is followed by suture repair, with the suture placed in the cartilaginous sleeve and the patellar tendon to provide stable fixation (Fig. 43–106). In a child older than 10 years we prefer firm fixation with tension band wiring and Kirschner wire fixation (Fig. 43–107). Patients are allowed to bear weight in the cast and should begin straight-leg-raising exercises 2 weeks after cast application. Grogan and colleagues reported successful treatment with full return to function in nine patients (10 knees) with acute sleeve fractures that were treated operatively.[101]

Sleeve fractures that are seen late are often minimally displaced. These injuries may be treated by cast immobilization in extension, and despite lack of radiographic union, many patients return to full function.[101] If extensor lag is noted at the time of initial evaluation, operative intervention is required to prevent extensor lag.[101]

Displaced Transverse Patellar Fracture. For a displaced transverse patellar fracture we prefer open reduction and internal fixation with tension band wiring and Kirschner wires. A vertical incision is made over the patella, and fracture reduction is performed while ensuring that the articular surface is reduced anatomically. Wires are then placed starting inferiorly and coming out superiorly, followed by AO-type tension band wiring (Fig. 43–108). Weber and coworkers compared several wiring techniques and demonstrated that Magnusson wiring and the modified tension band wiring techniques prevented separation of the fracture fragments better than circumferential or tension band wiring did.[278] Some have advocated the circumferential wiring technique in children to avoid intraosseous penetration and the potential risk for growth disturbance. This, however, has not been seen with internal fixation of patellar fractures in children and may be due, in part, to the older age of the patients.[21,164,216] Ray and Hendrix reported excellent results and radiographic healing in four transverse patellar fractures treated by open reduction and internal fixation—two with suture repair, two with tension band wiring.[216]

Comminuted Fracture. Comminuted fractures are difficult to treat and tend to have worse results.[164] Operative intervention is generally required and should consist of thorough evaluation of the fracture pattern and inspection of the joint. The larger fragments should be anatomically reduced, followed by either excision and removal of small nonarticular fragments or internal fixation of the remaining fragments to the larger fragments, if possible. Although patellectomy was used in the past for the comminuted fracture pattern in children and was not necessarily associated with a poor result,[164,216] we prefer to save the patella at all costs.

Ipsilateral Femoral or Tibial Fracture. Patellar fractures associated with ipsilateral femoral or tibial

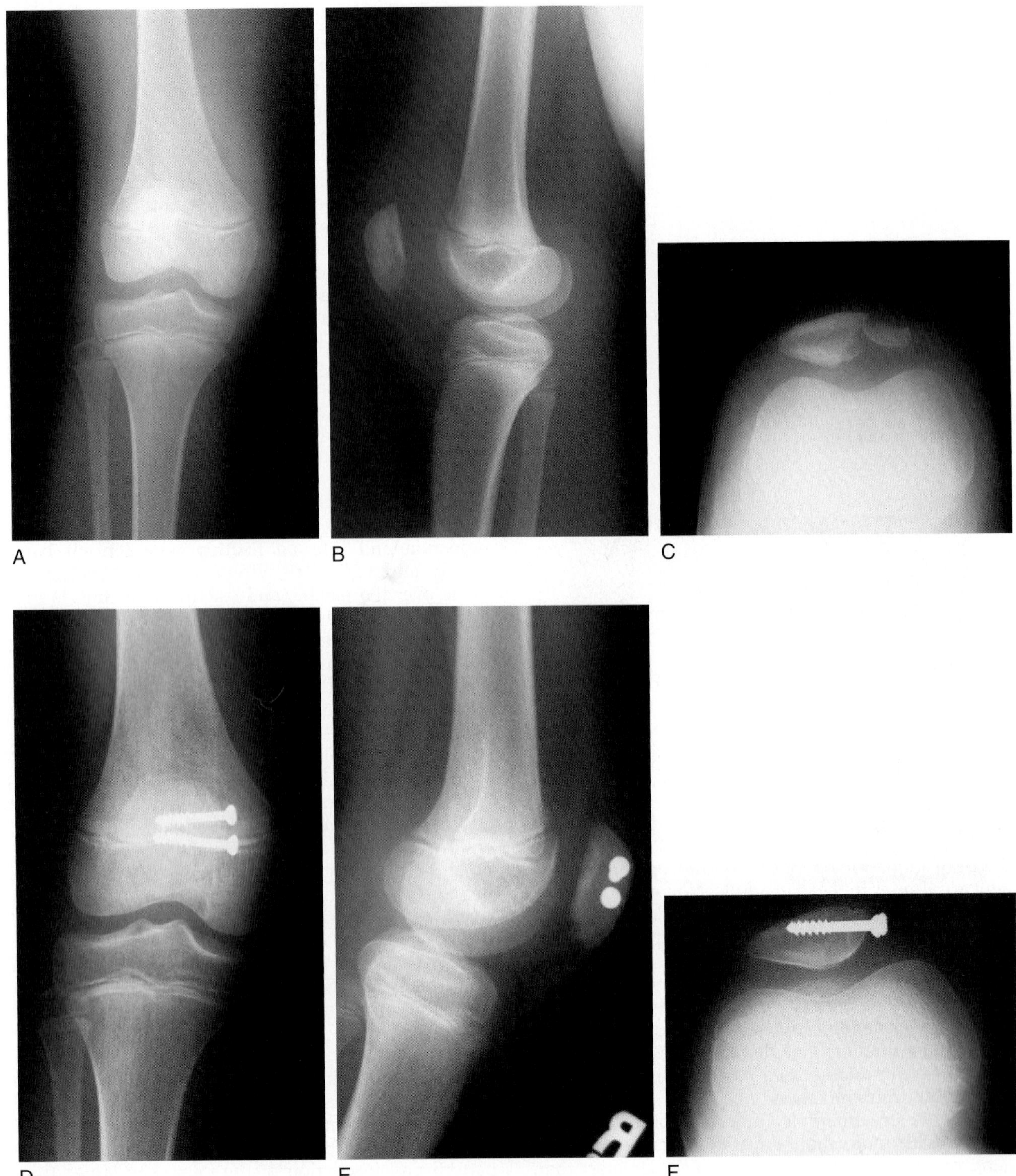

FIGURE 43–105 Vertical patellar fracture in a 10-year-old girl. Anteroposterior **(A)**, lateral **(B)**, and Merchant **(C)** views obtained at the time of injury. Anteroposterior **(D)**, lateral **(E)**, and Merchant **(F)** views obtained after open reduction and screw fixation with anatomic reduction and complete healing.

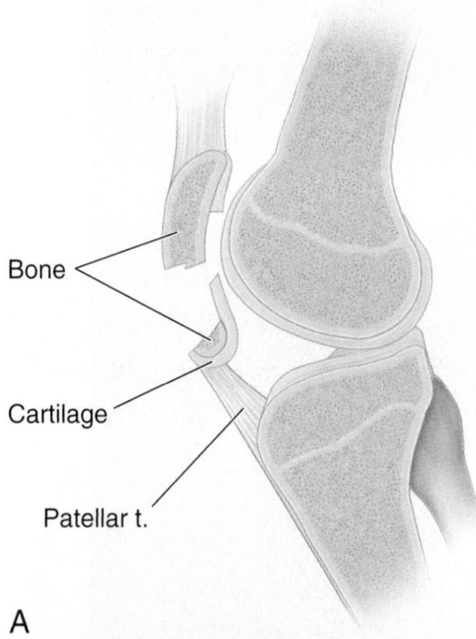

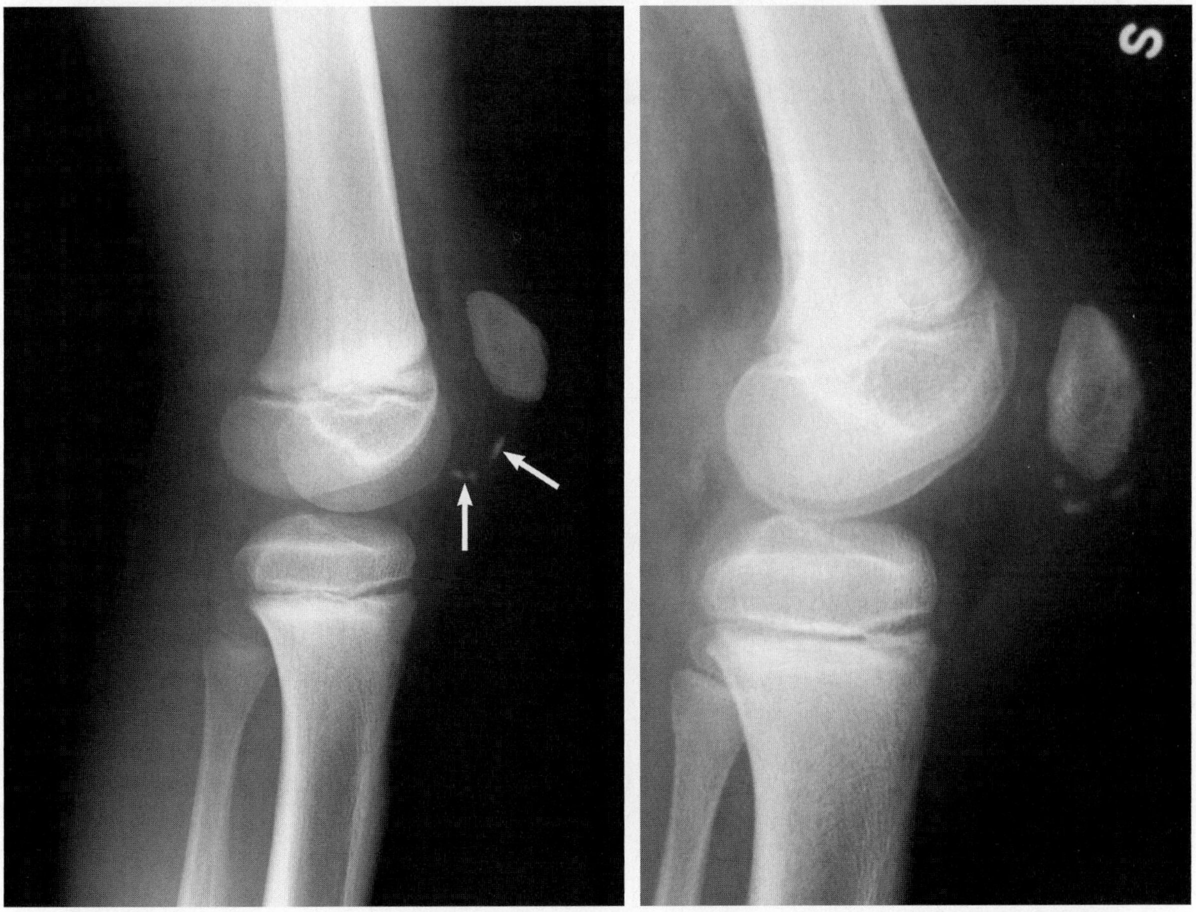

B

C

FIGURE 43–106 Patellar sleeve fracture in an 8-year-old boy. **A,** Diagram of a patellar sleeve fracture. The patellar tendon has avulsed an osteocartilaginous fragment from the distal pole of the patella. **B,** Initial radiograph demonstrating a patellar sleeve fracture with the distal osteocartilaginous fragment seen (*arrows*). **C,** Lateral radiograph obtained 6 weeks after open reduction and suture fixation with No. 2 nonabsorbable suture.

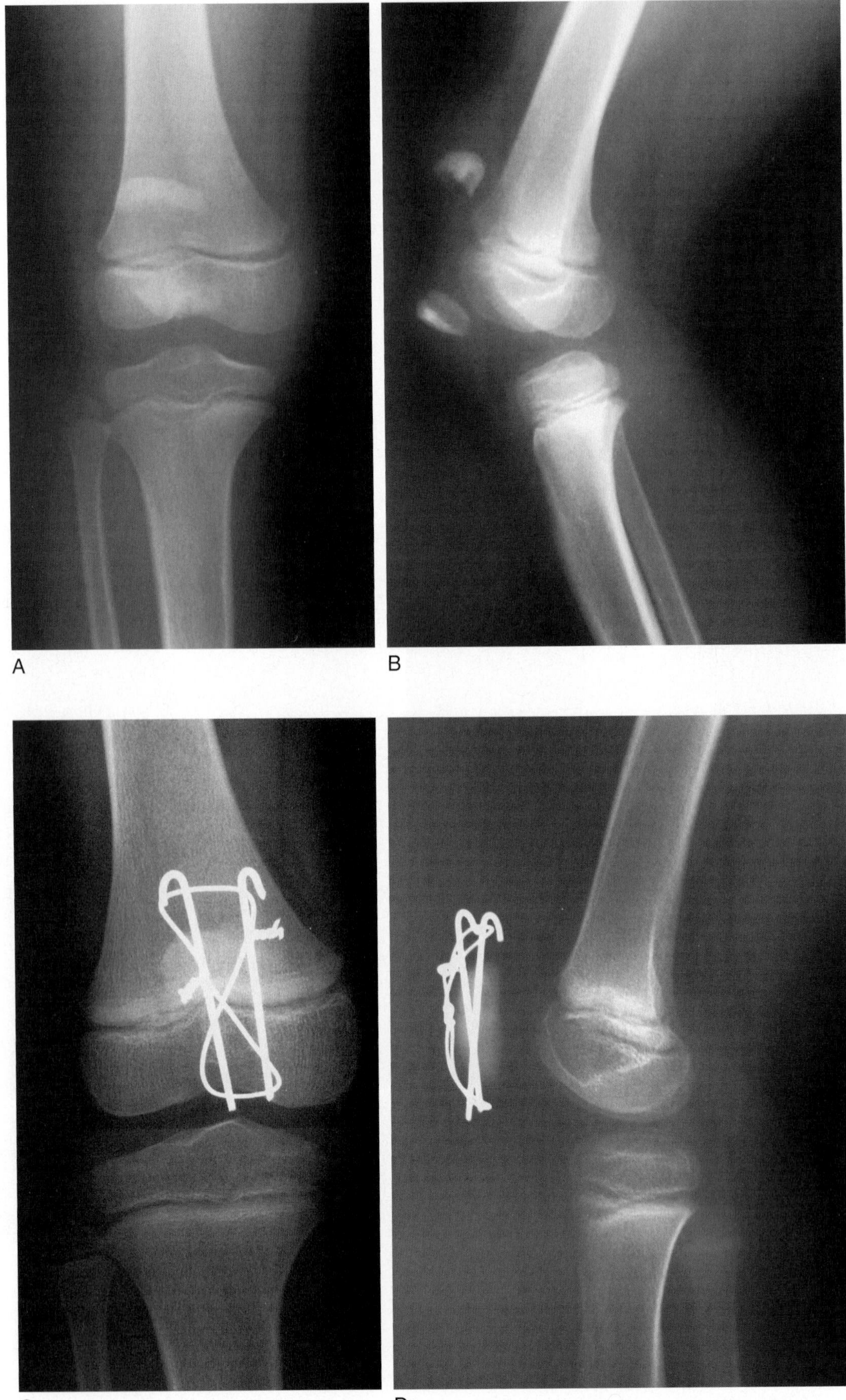

FIGURE 43–107 The tension band technique used to treat a displaced transverse patellar fracture in a 5-year-old girl. Initial anteroposterior (AP) **(A)** and lateral **(B)** radiographs. AP **(C)** and lateral **(D)** radiographic appearance of the same views 4 months after open reduction and internal fixation with a tension band technique.

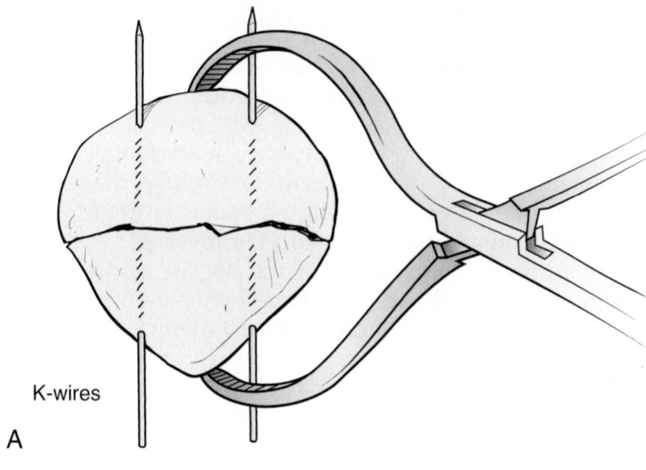

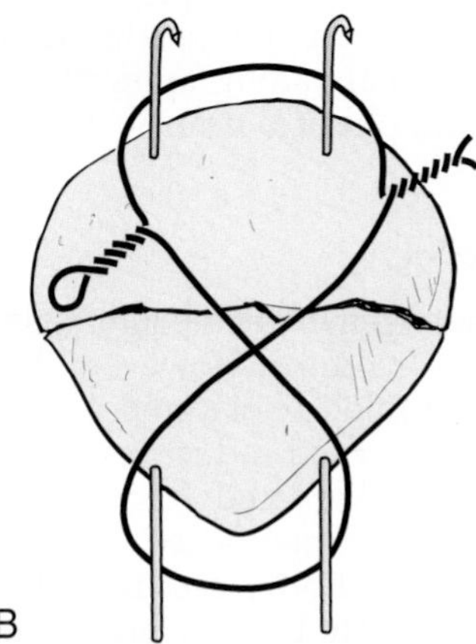

FIGURE 43–108 Tension band technique. **A,** After open reduction, Kirschner wires are placed in parallel fashion in an inferior-to-superior direction. **B,** A loop of wire is next placed in figure-eight fashion. A loop is then placed both medially and laterally to allow compression across the fracture site.

fractures have been reported to have the worst results.[164] However, the authors point out that treatment of these fractures was traction followed by hip spica casting without internal fixation. In the setting of an ipsilateral femoral shaft fracture, we recommend stable fixation of both fractures with flexible intramedullary nailing of the femur and open reduction with internal fixation of the patella. Casting or brace treatment may be indicated, depending on fracture stability. Knee range of motion can generally be initiated 4 weeks after fixation. When an ipsilateral tibial fracture is present, displaced fractures of the patella should be internally fixed and closed reduction of the tibia performed, followed by immobilization in a long-leg cast. Flexible intramedullary nailing of the tibia may be indicated, depending on the fracture pattern or associated injuries.

Marginal Fracture. For marginal fractures of the patella that are not large and do not contain a significant portion of the articular surface, excision of the fragment usually yields good results.

COMPLICATIONS

Sleeve fractures have few complications when they are recognized early and treated by anatomic reduction and internal fixation.[101] Reported complications, however, include nonunion as a result of inadequate fixation and loss of flexion.[289] Inadequate fixation may also lead to an extensor lag, as was reported in two of three patients with sleeve fractures treated inadequately by suture and casting alone, respectively.[115]

Undisplaced transverse patellar fractures have uniformly good results with cast immobilization. Displaced transverse patellar fractures do well with anatomic reduction and stable internal fixation; however, loss of reduction may result in extensor lag, chronic infection, and rarely, AVN of the patella.

Tibial Tuberosity Fractures

Tibial tuberosity fractures are the result of forced extension of the knee or being struck with the leg planted on the ground. Operative treatment is the management of choice for any displaced fracture or a minimally displaced fracture with significant soft tissue swelling. The results of operative treatment are universally good. Compartment syndrome has been reported in displaced fractures that were treated by closed reduction and casting. Patients awaiting operative treatment should be monitored closely for impending compartment syndrome, and all displaced fractures require operative treatment.

ANATOMY

The tibial tubercle is the most anterior aspect of the proximal tibial epiphysis and contributes to growth of the proximal tibia. The cartilaginous aspect of the tibial tubercle is the initial stage of development and persists until the age of 9 or 10 years. The two or three secondary centers of ossification begin to appear at the tibial tubercle at 8 to 12 years in girls and 10 to 14 years in boys. This stage is then followed by the formation of a single tibial tubercle as the secondary centers of ossification begin to fuse, later followed by physeal closure between the epiphysis and metaphysis.[73] Fusion of the physis begins centrally and proceeds centrifugally, with the area beneath the tuberosity fusing last.

In the early stages of development of the tibial tubercle the patellar ligament inserts into fibrous cartilage near the secondary center of ossification. Later, the insertion is through fibrocartilage on the anterior aspect of the proximal tibial epiphysis, with final insertion directly into bone after ossification of the tibial tubercle. Retinacular fibers reinforce the attachment of the patellar ligament to the tibial tubercle; the fibers are distributed from both the medial and lateral margins of the patella and distally. These accessory attachments may allow the patient to continue to demonstrate some knee extension despite a tibial tubercle avulsion.

MECHANISM OF INJURY

Tibial tuberosity fractures are most often incurred during jumping activities, with the most common sports being basketball, football, long jumping, and high jumping.[46,108,202,210,286] This injury occurs as a result of two types of simultaneous mechanisms: active extension of the knee with sudden, strong contraction of the quadriceps, especially during jumping, and acute passive flexion against a contracted quadriceps, which often occurs when a football player is tackled.[277]

Several authors have described an association between Osgood-Schlatter disease and tibial tuberosity fractures.[62,154,202,286] Ogden and colleagues reported that 64% of patients in their series had an associated Osgood-Schlatter lesion,[202] and Levi and Coleman reported a 27% incidence in their series.[154] Ogden and colleagues suggest that this may be due to a change in the secondary center of ossification of the tibial tubercle in which the primarily fibrocartilaginous pattern turns into hypertrophic columnar cartilage, which is structurally weaker.[202]

CLASSIFICATION

Watson-Jones first classified tibial tubercle fractures into three types.[277] This classification was later modified by Ogden to better define the pathomechanics of this injury (Fig. 43–109).[202] In type 1 injuries, the fracture is distal to the normal junction of the ossification centers of the proximal end of the tibia and tuberosity. Type 1A injuries are minimally displaced and type 1B injuries are hinged anteriorly and proximally. Type 2 fractures occur at the junction of the ossification of the proximal end of the tibia and the tuberosity. Type 2A injuries are simple fractures and type 2B injuries are comminuted. Type 3 fractures extend to the joint and are associated with displacement of the anterior fragment and discontinuation of the joint surface; a type 3A injury has a single fragment, and a type 3B injury has a comminuted fragment.

CLINICAL FEATURES

A patient with a tibial tubercle fracture has a history of pain in the knee, most often with onset during basketball or football or at the time of a jump. The patient is unable to fully extend the leg and complains of pain and weakness.

On physical examination, swelling and tenderness are noted over the tibial tubercle area, and the knee is usually held in 20 to 40 degrees of flexion. In many types 2 and 3 injuries a defect can be palpated at the level of the tibial tubercle. In displaced fractures the patella rides abnormally high on the femur. The patient is unable to extend the leg, and extension is painful when attempted. It is important to examine the soft tissue compartments of the leg, especially the anterior compartment, because anterior compartment syndromes have been reported.[205,210,286] In addition, a neurovascular examination should be performed.

RADIOGRAPHIC FINDINGS

A lateral radiograph of the knee will show the fracture, which can then be classified according to the Ogden classification.[202] In a skeletally mature patient the diagnosis is readily apparent; however, in a younger child various stages of development may make diagnosis more difficult. In this situation a lateral radiograph of the contralateral knee is helpful. The level of the patella is an important indication of the degree of displacement of the tibial tubercle. This is best estimated by using either the Blumensaat or the Insall technique.[29,123] The Insall technique compares the longitudinal distance of the patella with the distance from the inferior pole of the patella to the tibial tubercle. This ratio should be 0.8 or greater, with smaller numbers indicating some disruption of the patellar ligament or tibial tubercle. Associated bony injuries are rare and do not warrant additional radiographs unless indicated by the history and physical examination.

TREATMENT

Operative management is the mainstay of treatment of tibial tubercle fractures. However, Ogden type I fractures with minimal displacement have been successfully treated by closed reduction and casting.[46,108,202,210] In a minimally displaced fracture the knee can be extended fully and then flexed to 30 degrees and held in a long-leg or cylinder cast for 6 to 8 weeks. After cast removal, weight bearing begins as tolerated.

We prefer operative management for all types II and III fractures to allow decompression of the fracture hematoma, anatomic reduction, assessment of intra-articular pathology in type III fractures, and stable internal fixation. A longitudinal incision is made medial to the inferior patellar tendon and tuberosity. Fracture hematoma is thoroughly evacuated and the fracture bed is cleared of any interposed soft tissue. The fracture fragments are anatomically reduced with the knee extended. We prefer two 4.0- or 6.5-mm cancellous screws placed parallel to the joint surface. Washers may be used to prevent the screw head from penetrating the anterior cortex (Fig. 43–110). The fragment can be provisionally fixed with the first drill bit or a smooth Kirschner wire while the second screw is placed. The patellar tendon and its lateral attachments are then sutured securely. Because these fractures are most often seen in patients nearing skeletal maturity and because physeal arrest with angular deformity has not been reported after these fractures, it is not necessary to go to great efforts to avoid the physis. In a comminuted fracture multiple screws may be necessary, or a tension band wiring technique can be used to allow fracture stabilization and provide a buttress for the small fracture fragments.[210]

Postoperatively, a long-leg or cylinder cast should be used for 4 to 6 weeks, followed by active and active assisted range-of-motion and quadriceps strengthening exercises. Full athletic activities are generally restricted for an additional 4 to 6 weeks until full range of motion and quadriceps strength return.

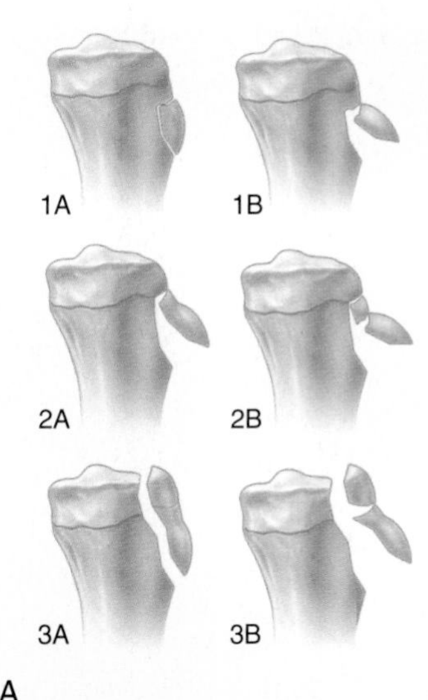

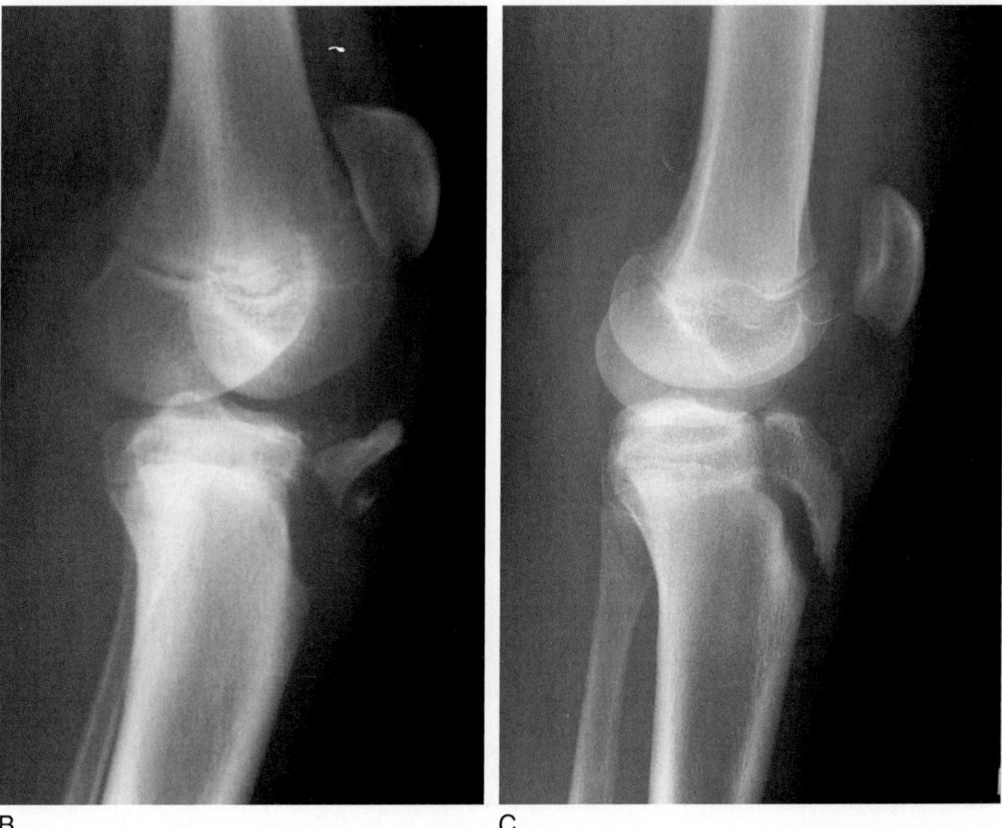

FIGURE 43-109 Ogden modification of the Watson-Jones classification of tibial tubercle fractures. **A,** Ogden classification. **B,** Lateral radiograph of a type II tibial tubercle fracture. **C,** Lateral radiograph of a type III tibial tubercle fracture.

COMPLICATIONS

In general, operative repair of tibial tubercle avulsion injuries produces excellent results with return to full, preinjury activities. Though rare, the most common complications after these injuries are compartment syndrome, loss of knee motion, a prominent tibial tubercle, and reinjury.

Compartment syndrome has been reported in six patients. It occurred in the anterior compartment in all, and all patients had been managed without or were awaiting operative treatment.[205,210,286] Pape and colleagues described two patients who had been treated by external immobilization for types II and III fractures.[205] These authors noted the proximity of the tibial tubercle to the anterior compartment and the anterior tibial recurrent artery. They suggested that tibial tuberosity fractures are associated with significant soft tissue injury, which predisposes to compartment syndrome. The treating physician should be aware of this complication and monitor any patient who initially has a displaced tibial tubercle fracture and is

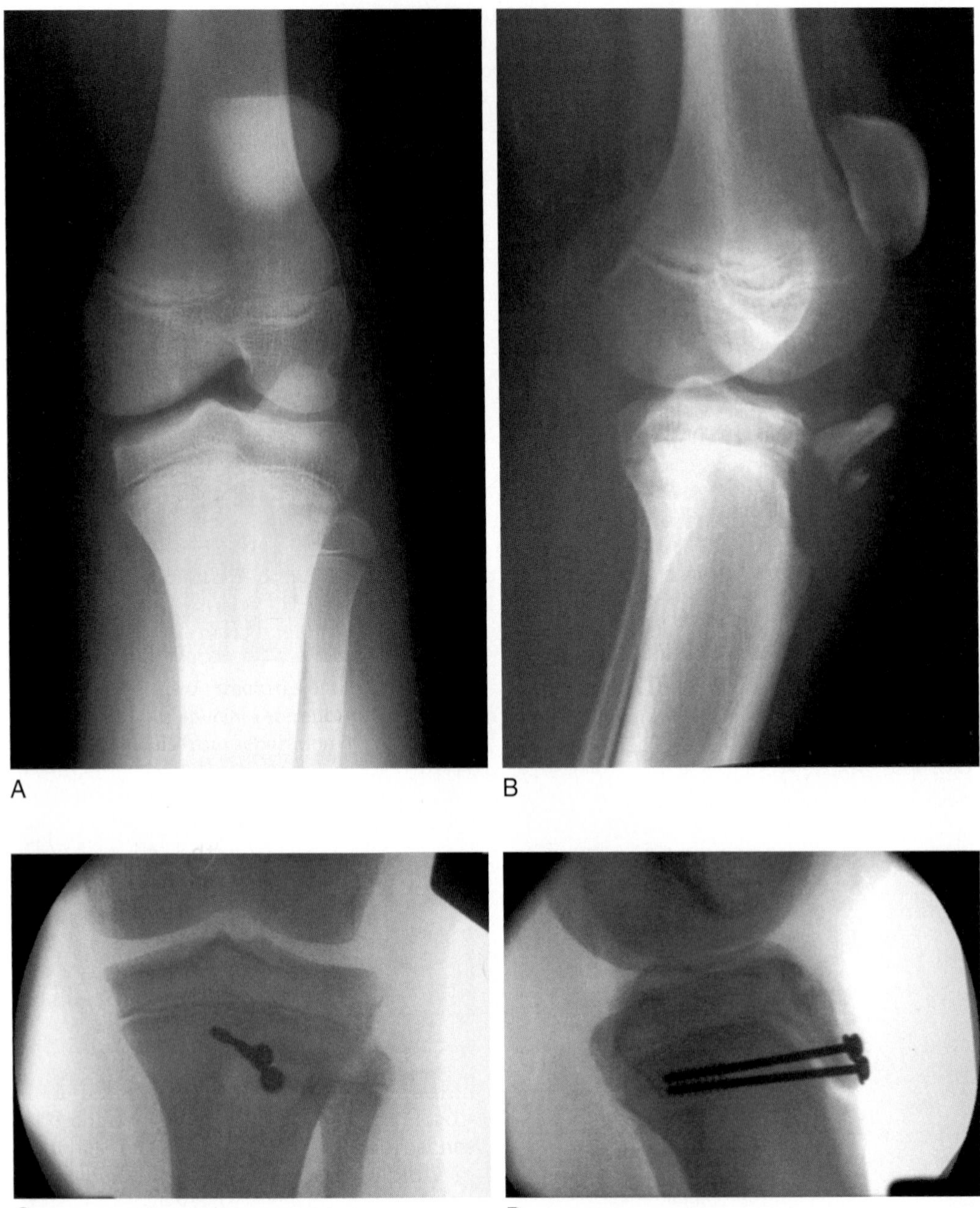

FIGURE 43–110 Internal fixation of a displaced (type II) tibial tubercle fracture in a 14-year-old boy who sustained the fracture while long jumping. **A** and **B,** Initial radiographs. **C** and **D,** Postoperative views showing anatomic reduction with internal fixation achieved by using partially threaded cancellous screws with washers.

awaiting operative treatment or has an undisplaced or minimally displaced fracture treated by nonoperative methods.

In type III fractures, meniscal injury may occur and should therefore be evaluated at the time of surgery through a small knee arthrotomy. The medial or lateral meniscus, or both, may be torn at the time of the initial injury. Wiss and associates reported that 2 of 15 patients with type III avulsions had peripheral detachments of both menisci and that a third had a transverse tear of the anterior horn of the medial meniscus.[286] Loss of motion of the knee has been reported in a single case in which there was lack of extension by 25 degrees after open reduction and internal fixation of a type III injury. Other complications are rare and include infection, nonunion, refracture when activities are begun early, nonunion of the distal fragment in a type III fracture, and in a single reported case, pulmonary embolism, which was treated successfully.[46,202,286] Bursitis over the screw heads has been reported in 5 of 15 patients treated by open reduction and internal fixation for type III fractures; the bursitis resolved after screw removal.[286]

Proximal Tibial Physeal Fractures

Injuries to the proximal tibial physis are rare and account for approximately 0.5% to 3% of all physeal injuries in children.[39,187,208] This rareness is due to the lack of collateral ligamentous attachments to the proximal tibial epiphysis, which allows valgus or varus forces to be transmitted through these ligaments to their attachments on the distal femoral physis, fibular head, and tibial metaphysis. These fractures may be difficult to diagnose when radiographs look normal, and complications, including significant arterial injury, are relatively common.

ANATOMY

The proximal tibial ossific nucleus forms at approximately 2 months of age, with the secondary center of ossification of the tibial tubercle appearing between 10 and 14 years. It unites with the proximal tibial epiphysis at about 15 years. Closure of the proximal tibial physis is thought to begin centrally and proceed to the periphery.[202] Radiographic investigations of patients 12 to 20 years of age have shown that the proximal tibial physis appears to fuse posteriorly, followed by anterior fusion.[27]

The joint capsule incompletely surrounds the knee, allowing the popliteus tendon to travel from the proximal tibia to the posterior aspect of the distal femoral epiphysis. The capsule inserts into the tibial epiphysis, and the LCL and MCL attach distally to the fibular head and the proximal medial tibial metaphysis, respectively.

The vascular anatomy is important in understanding the relatively high incidence of vascular injuries associated with this fracture. The popliteal artery travels close to the proximal tibia and has fibrous attachments to the posterior capsule. At the level of the proximal tibial epiphysis it branches and gives off the lateral and medial inferior genicular arteries, which further tether the popliteal artery. The three major branches (peroneal, anterior tibial, and posterior tibial arteries) divide off the popliteal artery distal to the soleus muscle. Immediately distal to the trifurcation the anterior tibial artery penetrates the interosseous membrane and travels to the anterior compartment of the leg, again tethering the artery. Additional fixation points include the connective tissue septa in the terminal aspect of the adductor canal, in the posterior aspect of the articular capsule, and in the deep portion of the peroneal muscle. These multiple levels of tethering and the proximity of the artery to the proximal tibial epiphysis result in a high incidence of arterial injury.

MECHANISM OF INJURY

Both indirect and direct trauma to the knee can result in fractures of the proximal tibial physis. The most common mechanism is an indirect blow to a hyperextended knee when the lower part of the leg is in a fixed position.[39,212,247,288] Similarly, valgus, varus, and rarely, flexion-type indirect trauma can result in these injuries.[27,39,247,288] Direct trauma can account for these injuries, with the leg fixed and then struck while the individual is playing football or is run over by a motor vehicle or lawnmower.[39,281,287]

Sporting activities and motor vehicle accidents account for most of these fractures reported in the literature. Shelton and Canale reported that 18 (47%) of 38 patients were injured while participating in sports—most commonly football, then basketball—and that 12 (32%) were injured in automobile or motorcycle accidents. Others have reported a higher incidence of proximal tibial physeal injuries' being incurred in motor vehicle accidents.[39,212] Flexion-type injuries are rare and have been reported only in patients who were engaged in jumping activities, which can produce the avulsion, shear, and compression stress that produce this injury.[27] The patients are typically older (16 years), an age when the anterior proximal tibial physis remains open but the posterior physis has closed. Lawnmower accidents are most often reported in younger children (2 to 6 years of age) and accounted for up to 18% of patients in one series.[39]

Associated injuries may occur in up to 42% of patients, with fibular fractures being most common.[247,288] Other associated injuries include ipsilateral tibial and femoral shaft fractures, collateral ligament tears, patellar fractures, quadriceps rupture, and patellar avulsion injuries.[39,207,247]

Finally, miscellaneous causes account for a small percentage of proximal tibial physeal injuries. Among them are a difficult birth, especially with a breech presentation,[254] and myelomeningocele; a patient with myelomeningocele does not have a history of trauma but will have local warmth, redness, swelling, and increased body temperature. Patients with myelomeningocele and proximal tibial physeal fractures are usually initially seen in a later stage, have callus formation on radiographs, and require immobilization for at least 8 weeks.[149]

CLASSIFICATION

Fractures of the proximal tibial physis should be classified according to both the Salter-Harris classification and the mechanism of injury to provide a guideline for patient evaluation and fracture treatment and give the most accurate prognosis. For example, a patient with a displaced, hyperextension Salter-Harris type I injury is at high risk for vascular injury; a type I fracture is also associated with a high incidence of physeal arrest.[39,247,288]

Type I fractures account for 15% of proximal tibial physeal fractures and are usually nondisplaced. These injuries must be carefully evaluated to avoid missing an undisplaced fracture. When a type I injury is suspected because of focal tenderness and soft tissue swelling, cast treatment and should be initiated. If the diagnosis is uncertain or associated injuries are suspected, MRI may be used for diagnosis. Stress radiographs are not recommended; they require sedation or anesthesia and provide no additional information for the plan of care.

Type II injuries are the most common and accounted for approximately 37% in a combined series of patients (41 of 112 in four series).[39,212,247,288] These injuries are generally the result of a valgus stress to the knee with a lateral metaphyseal fragment on a medial physis injury (Fig. 43–111).[39,247,287] The majority of type II fractures are displaced at the time of evaluation, with Shelton and Canale reporting that 71% of fractures were displaced, predominantly in the medial direction.[247] If significant displacement exists, these injuries may not be reducible by closed reduction because of the interposition of soft tissue structures such as the periosteum or pes anserinus.[287] The rare flexion type II fracture is caused by an injury while jumping and results in the metaphyseal fragment being posterior.[27]

Type III injuries are relatively rare and account for 21% of these injuries (24 of 112 in four combined series).[39,212,247,288] Two major types of fractures occur. The first—and the more common—travels through either the lateral or the medial plateau and is best seen on an AP radiograph. The second is an injury involving both the tibial tubercle and the anterior aspect of the proximal tibial epiphysis and is best seen on a lateral radiograph.[247] These fractures are commonly displaced, and the majority require operative intervention.

Type IV fractures are the least common and account for 16% of all proximal tibial physeal injuries (18 of 112).[39,212,247,288] Patients who have sustained indirect trauma usually have injury to the lateral tibial plateau and require operative intervention (Fig. 43–112). Of the five patients with lawnmower injuries in the series

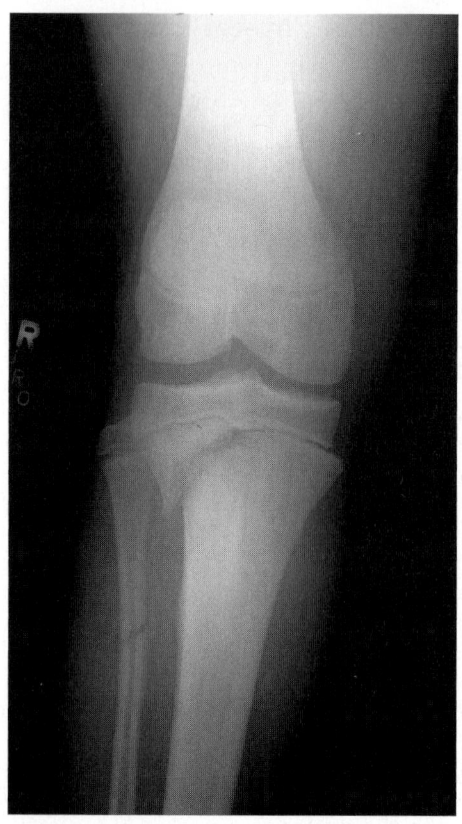

FIGURE 43–111 Salter-Harris type II fracture of the proximal tibia with an associated proximal fibular fracture. It was caused by a valgus force applied to the lateral aspect of the knee while the patient was playing football.

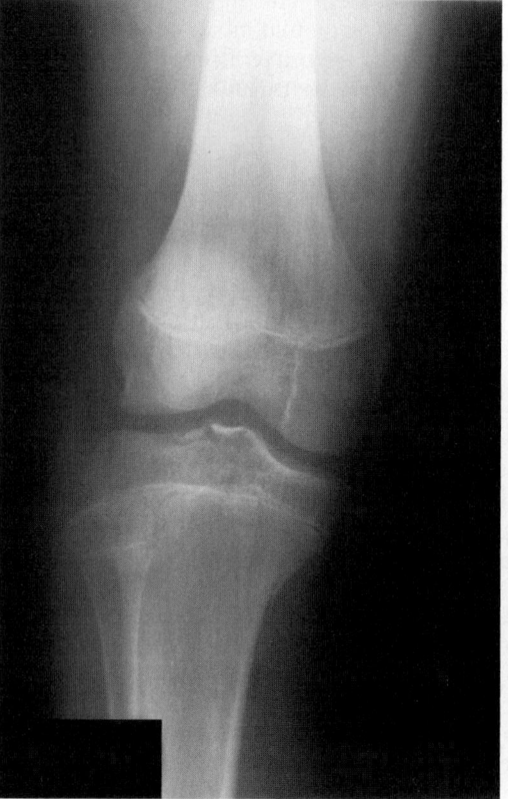

A

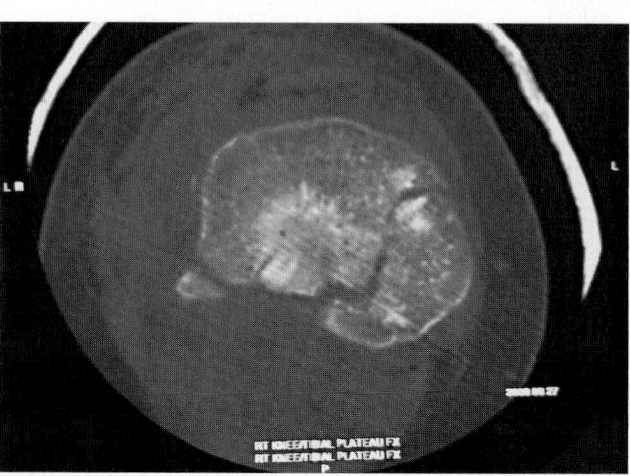

B

FIGURE 43–112 Salter-Harris type IV fracture of the proximal tibia sustained by a 12-year-old boy who was struck on the medial aspect of the knee while playing football. **A,** A radiograph reveals a mildly displaced Salter-Harris type IV fracture. **B,** The intra-articular fracture is seen on computed tomography, with a split in the medial plateau.

reported by Burkhart and Peterson, all had type IV injuries; osteomyelitis developed in four, and physeal arrest developed in the fifth patient.[39]

Type V fractures are rare, often being recognized only after physeal arrest has occurred. Burkhardt and Peterson were the first to report a type V proximal tibial physeal injury in two patients who had an associated distal tibial fracture and unrecognized proximal physeal injuries. Both patients had limb length discrepancies, which were treated by 5-cm shortening of the contralateral femur in the first patient and by lengthening of the tibia (which was complicated by compartment syndrome) in the second patient.[39] A second report in the literature described an associated displaced tibial spine injury in a patient who, at final follow-up, had a varus deformity, a flexion contracture of 30 degrees, and early degenerative joint disease.[212]

CLINICAL FEATURES

The typical patient is a boy between the ages of 13 and 16 years.[27,39,247,288] A careful history is important to determine the mechanism of injury (direct or indirect trauma), the time that the injury occurred, and the location of pain and other symptoms.

On examination, the affected knee usually has an effusion and is held in a flexed position. Knee extension is painful and resisted by hamstring spasm. The alignment of the leg may provide information regarding the mechanism of injury. With a hyperextension injury the knee may be flexed only 10 degrees, whereas in a flexion-type injury the knee is more flexed at the time of initial evaluation. An injury caused by direct impact on the lateral aspect of the leg will produce a valgus-type deformity that is often a Salter-Harris type II injury, with the metaphyseal fragment on the lateral side and an associated fibular fracture and MCL tear.

Because vascular injury is relatively common, palpation of the distal pulses (dorsalis pedis and posterior tibial) is critical in any patient who may have a proximal tibial physeal injury. Serial examination of a leg with normal pulses is mandatory during the initial 24 to 48 hours, no matter what type of treatment has been rendered. In a displaced fracture with absent pulses, fracture reduction should be performed urgently, followed by reexamination of the pulses. The pulses usually return at this point and serial examinations should be performed. Arteriography is indicated if the pulses do not return to normal after fracture reduction.

The leg should be carefully evaluated to make sure that a compartment syndrome is not present or developing. The soft tissue compartments should be palpated to ensure that they are supple and not tense. Passive hyperextension of the toes should not result in excess pain in the anterior compartment of the leg.

RADIOGRAPHIC FINDINGS

Radiographic examination should include a true AP and lateral view of the knee. It is imperative that a true lateral radiograph be obtained so that pure flexion or extension injuries are not missed. The radiograph should be analyzed for separation or displacement of the physis and for metaphyseal or epiphyseal fracture lines.

Further imaging studies are useful for Salter-Harris type III and IV injuries to assess joint incongruity, fracture line orientation, and fracture displacement. MRI is rarely used in assessing these injuries; however, it may be useful in a patient with a suspected ligamentous injury or when soft tissue interposition at the fracture site is thought to be present.

TREATMENT

Only after careful analysis of the distal pulses can treatment of these fractures begin. The goals of treatment are to obtain anatomic reduction without imparting further damage to the proximal tibial physis and to maintain the reduction until healing has occurred. Treatment of a displaced fracture that requires manual reduction should be performed at least under conscious sedation and preferably under general anesthesia to allow a gentle reduction to be performed without stressing the physis unnecessarily.

Closed Reduction

Nonoperative treatment is indicated for a nondisplaced fracture, as well as for a minimally displaced fracture that can be reduced under general anesthesia and is stable with external immobilization without excess flexion of the knee (>60 degrees).

The most common type of fracture is a hyperextension Salter-Harris type I or II fracture. Reduction is performed by anteriorly directed translation of the metaphyseal fragment while manual traction is applied to the leg with the thigh stabilized by an assistant. Flexion of the knee is necessary to obtain and maintain the reduction. Cast immobilization should be used for 4 to 6 weeks, with the knee in no more than 60 degrees of flexion to avoid increasing the risk for arterial compromise and subsequent compartment syndrome. The cast should be removed at 3 weeks to place the knee in 20 to 30 degrees of knee flexion. Aitken described nine patients who had mild displacement after reduction but experienced complete spontaneous correction without deformity or clinical shortening in all cases.[4] Similar results were reported by Burkhart and Peterson, who treated 12 patients with type I or II fractures by casting alone or closed reduction followed by casting. Two patients required operative procedures at a later date to excise a physeal bar.[39] However, Shelton and Canale described two patients with displaced hyperextension-type Salter-Harris type II injuries who initially underwent closed reduction.[247] One patient had a satisfactory result despite some mild recurrence of the posterior displacement, and in the other patient unsuccessful closed reduction necessitated open reduction. Similarly, Wozasek and colleagues reported successful casting or closed reduction and casting in 6 of 11 patients with type II fractures.[288]

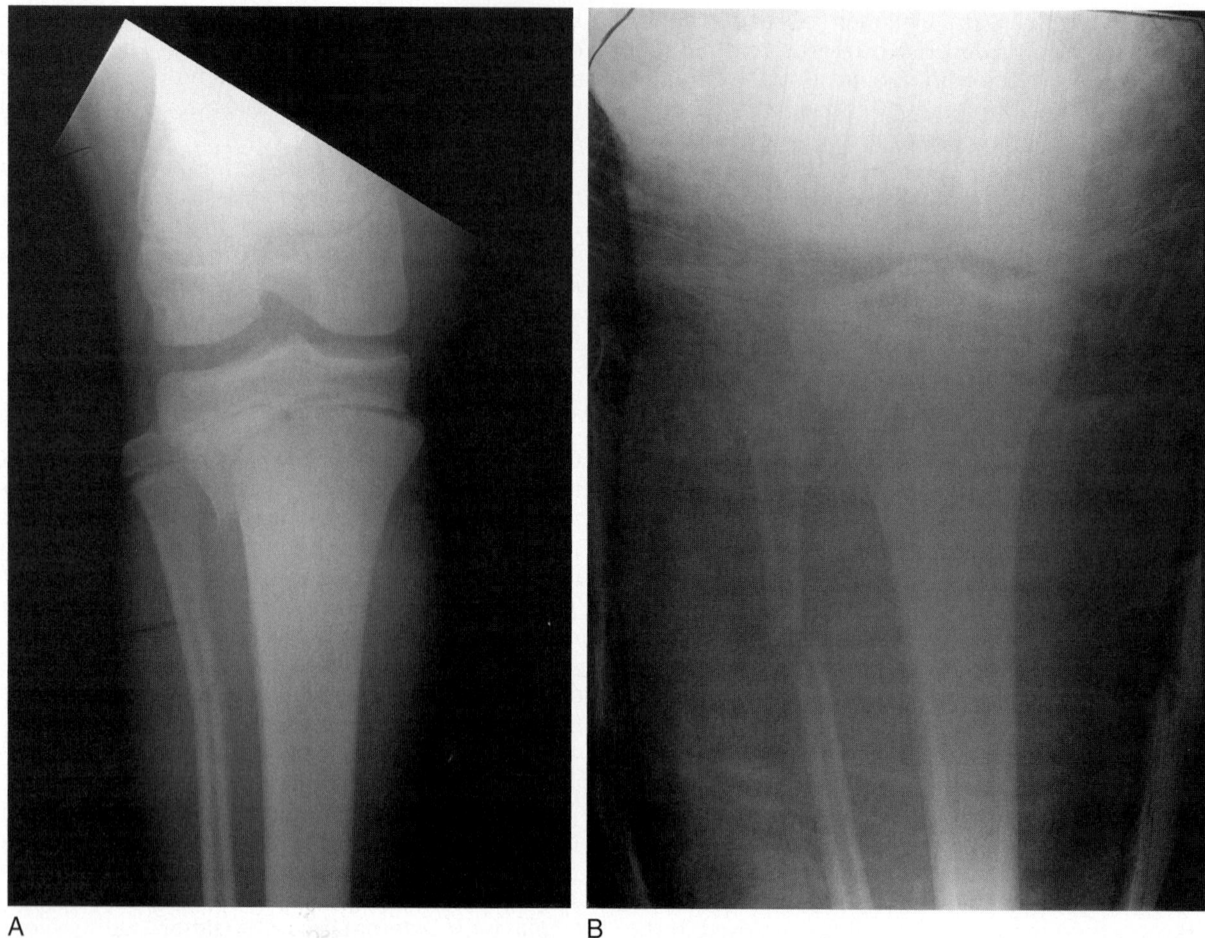

FIGURE 43–113 Closed reduction and casting of a Salter-Harris type II fracture in a 13-year-old boy. **A,** Initial radiograph. **B,** Accurate reduction was achieved by applying axial traction and a varus force to the knee.

A patient with a valgus-type Salter-Harris type II injury may initially be treated by closed reduction and casting. The reduction maneuver entails the use of a varus force applied to the knee while axial traction is applied to the leg with the knee extended, followed by immobilization in a long-leg cast, with mild varus molded into the cast (Fig. 43–113). Successful closed reduction plus casting was reported in seven patients with displaced valgus-type injuries.[247] Anatomic reduction should be achieved without any excess widening of the physis or a springy feeling when a varus reduction maneuver is applied because soft tissue interposition (pes anserinus or periosteum) may be present.[287]

If closed reduction is to be performed, careful assessment of the peripheral pulses is required after reduction and casting. We prefer to apply a well-molded cast followed by leg elevation and close observation of the patient in the hospital for 24 to 48 hours, with serial examination of peripheral pulses and passive motion of the toes. If significant swelling is present at the time of reduction or there is any concern that a compartment syndrome is impending, the cast should be bivalved at the time of application. Radiographs should be obtained weekly for the initial 2 weeks to ensure that the fracture reduction is maintained. Mild displacement of a few millimeters is acceptable within the first 2 weeks because re-reduction may increase the risk for physeal bar formation.

Open Reduction

In the patient with a Salter-Harris type III or IV fracture that is undisplaced, long-leg casting can be performed.[247,288] In type III fractures that involve the anterior aspect of the epiphysis, displacement is usually present, and the fracture should be treated by open reduction and internal fixation.[247]

Indications for operative treatment of these injuries include the following: (1) failed closed reduction (after a maximum of two attempts) with residual displacement in types I and II fractures, (2) failure to maintain reduction in a long-leg cast with less than 40 degrees of knee flexion, (3) all displaced types III and IV fractures, (4) the presence an associated arterial injury, and (5) the presence of an associated ipsilateral fracture that makes immobilization of the leg difficult or impossible.

In an unstable physeal injury that cannot be maintained with external immobilization, smooth pins should be placed in crossed fashion, crossing distal to the physis. The pins can be left out of the skin to make removal at 4 to 6 weeks easier (Fig. 43–114). Cast immobilization is used for 6 to 8 weeks. In a displaced type II fracture, pin fixation should be used to stabilize the metaphyseal fragment to prevent penetration across the physis.

Open reduction with internal fixation is required for displaced types III and IV fractures. A small arthrotomy is used to visualize the articular surface to allow anatomic reduction. This is then followed by percutaneous screw fixation of the epiphysis for type III injuries or the metaphyseal fragment in type IV injuries. An alternative method is to use arthroscopic visualization of the articular surface to guide fracture reduction and confirm articular congruity after percutaneous fixation of the fracture fragments. We prefer cancellous screw fixation (4.0- or 6.5-mm screws) to gain some compression across the fracture site (Fig. 43–115). Cast immobilization should be performed for 6 to 8 weeks. Early motion can be started at 4 to 6 weeks by allowing the patient to wear a removable splint, which can be taken off to perform these exercises.

Arterial injury in the setting of a hyperextension injury requires stable fixation of the fracture before repair of the arterial injury. Fixation can be achieved with percutaneous smooth pin fixation.

COMPLICATIONS

The results of treatment of proximal tibial physeal injuries are good (when lawnmower injuries are excluded), with satisfactory outcomes reported in 74% to 86% of cases.[39,247,288] All patients with lawnmower injuries had unsatisfactory results.[39]

The most devastating complication is injury to the popliteal artery, which is reported to occur in 3% to 7% of cases.[39,212,247] The importance of a thorough vascular examination at the time of initial assessment, after fracture reduction, and serially within the first 48 hours cannot be overemphasized. A delay in diagnosis and therefore in treatment significantly decreases the likelihood of a good outcome. Detection of discrepant or absent peripheral pulses should be followed by immediate reduction of the fracture. If peripheral pulses do not return, emergency arterial exploration is required. There is no role for arteriography in the setting of an isolated proximal tibial physeal injury with absent distal pulses because arteriography delays definitive treatment and will confirm only the level of injury posterior to the knee. If the study is required by the vascular surgeon, it can be performed in the operating room. In the setting of a viable foot with diminished or absent distal pulses, arteriography is indicated and should be performed on an emergency basis. Fracture fixation should be performed expeditiously, followed by thrombectomy, repair, or vein grafting.

Compartment syndrome has been associated with these fractures and should be carefully monitored for at the time of initial evaluation and throughout the hospital stay. Clinical examination should evaluate the soft tissue envelope for tense compartments, distal pulses, pain with passive range of motion of the toes, and so forth. The long-leg cast should be split immediately after application if there is any concern for an impending compartment syndrome, if the patient is unreliable, or if the patient has an associated head injury with altered consciousness. Compartment pressures should be measured if there is any concern regarding the use of standard techniques.[185,283] Patients with pressures above 40 mm Hg or less than 30 mm Hg below diastolic pressure should undergo four-compartment fasciotomy.

Physeal arrest and angular deformity or limb length discrepancy is relatively common, with the reported incidence being between 10% and 20%.[39,212,247,288] Patients at risk for physeal arrest and limb length discrepancy include those with displaced type I or II fractures,[247] those with any type IV or V fracture,[39] patients with an associated ipsilateral fracture,[288] and patients with lawnmower injuries.[39] Physeal arrest should be treated in standard fashion.[132,209]

Associated ligamentous injuries should be assessed at the time of initial evaluation. Often this is difficult because of instability, or potential instability, at the fracture site. Assessment of ligamentous instability should therefore be completed after operative stabilization of the fracture or soon after fracture healing has occurred. The incidence of associated ligamentous injury is reported to be as high as 60%, as reported by Bertin and Goble. In their study, 8 of 13 patients with proximal tibial physeal injuries had anterior instability at the time of healing.[23] Similarly, Poulsen and colleagues reported an associated avulsion of the anterior tibial spine with anterior instability in 5 (33%) of 15 patients.[212] These studies are in contrast to larger series in which only one patient in the combined series had a collateral ligament injury and no patient had sagittal plane instability.[39,247]

Patellar Dislocations

Patellar dislocation is most often due to a twisting injury or direct trauma. The majority of injuries occur in the early adolescent age group, and most dislocations are lateral. Historically, the incidence of acute patellar dislocation has been estimated at 43 per 100,000 children younger than 16 years.[169] Fithian and coauthors reported a lower incidence of first-time dislocation of 29 per 100,000 in patients 10 to 17 years of age.[86] Osteochondral fractures of both the patella and the femur are associated with an acute patellar dislocation. The most common complication is recurrence of dislocation or chronic instability. Recurrent subluxation is reported more commonly in girls than in boys.[26,74,86,93,113,135] Younger children (<14 years) are more likely than older children to experience recurrent dislocations.[43] The initial treatment of acute patellar dislocation is nonoperative.

ANATOMY

The extensor mechanism of the knee is formed from the quadriceps, its tendon, the patella, and the patellar

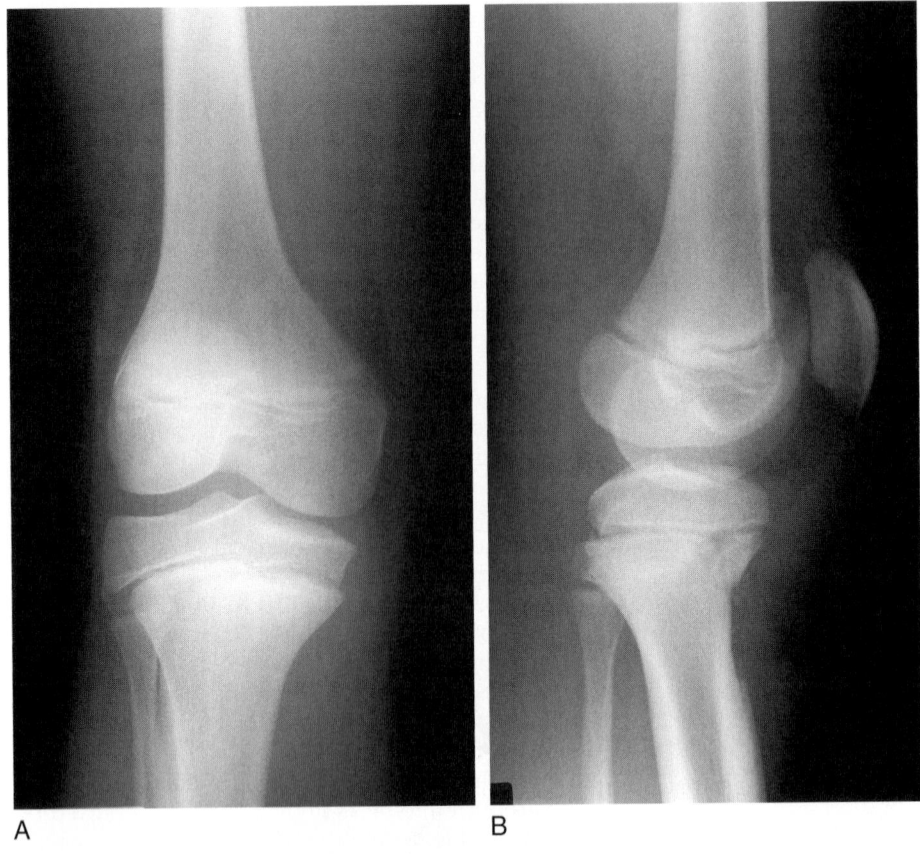

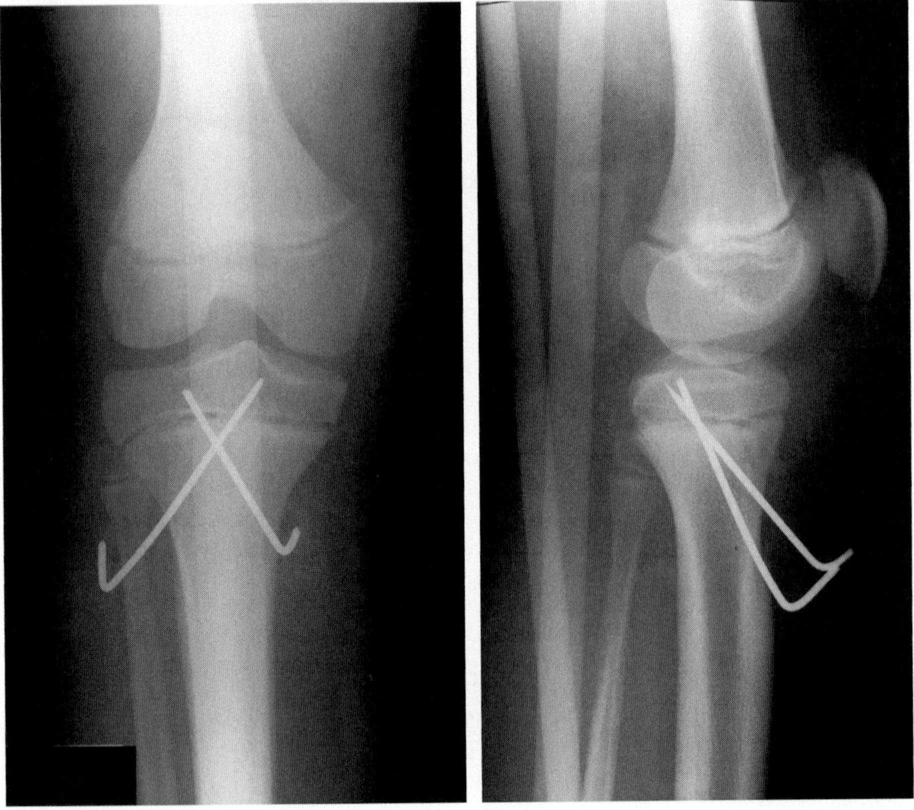

FIGURE 43–114 Salter-Harris type I fracture in a 9-year-old child. Initial anteroposterior **(A)** and lateral **(B)** radiographs demonstrating mild displacement. **C** and **D,** Same views after closed reduction and percutaneous pinning in which the pins were flared in retrograde fashion.

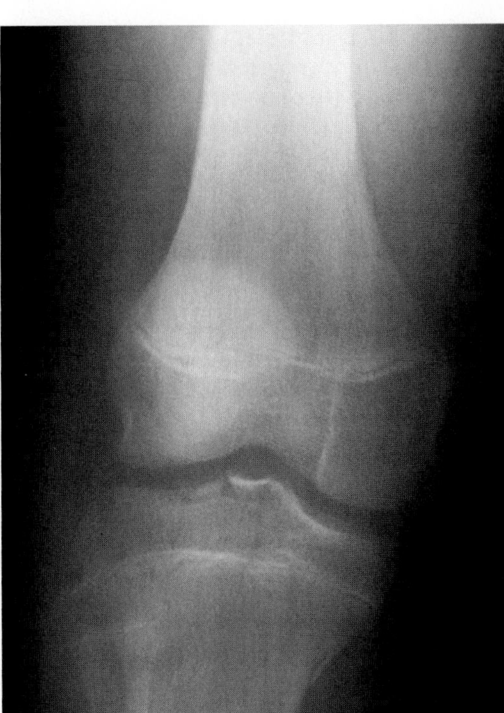

A

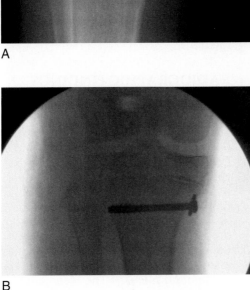

B

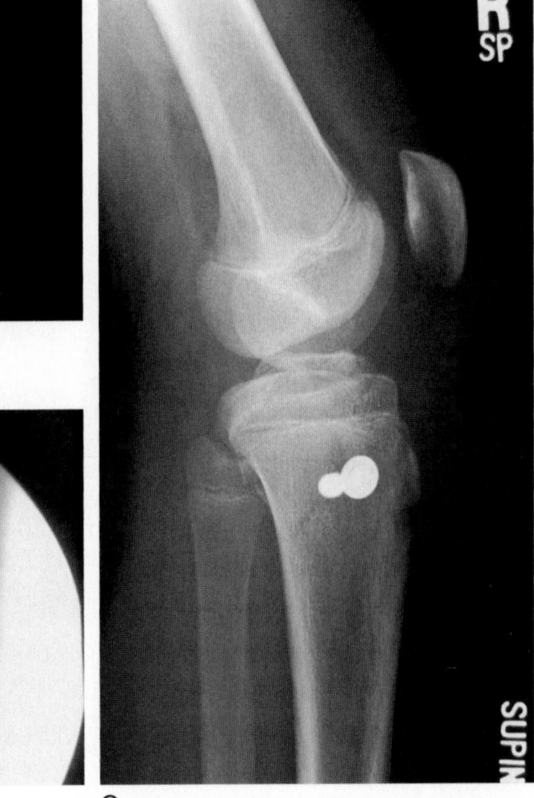

C

FIGURE 43-115 Salter-Harris type IV fracture involving the medial proximal aspect of the tibia in a 13-year-old boy who was playing football when a varus force was directed to his knee. **A,** Initial radiograph showing a minimally displaced Salter-Harris type IV fracture. Anteroposterior **(B)** and lateral **(C)** views showing closed reduction with single-screw fixation.

tendon. The alignment of this mechanism is in slight valgus, with the apex at the center of the knee. The patella articulates with the femoral groove beginning at approximately 20 degrees of knee flexion, and the contact area between the patella and the femoral groove increases with greater degrees of flexion. Medial soft tissue restraints account for resistance to lateral patellar translation in lesser degrees of flexion. At 30 and greater degrees of flexion, bony constraint affords patellofemoral stability.[80]

Many patients sustaining patellar dislocation have anatomic variables that predispose to lateral instability. Patella alta, genu valgum, internal torsion of the femur, trochlear dysplasia, quadriceps force imbalance, and primary or secondary laxity of the medial patellofemoral ligament (MPFL) are recognized factors contributing to patellar instability.[11,54,64,146,218,240] With increasing numbers of these variables present, the balance of vectors across the patellofemoral joint shifts laterally, and the force required to dislocate the patella decreases.[43]

The majority of lateral patellar dislocations occur with the knee in lesser degrees of flexion. In this position, the patella is superior to the osseous constraints of the femoral sulcus, and the MPFL acts as the primary soft tissue restraint to lateral translation. The MPFL was first described by Warren and Marshall as lying superficial to the joint capsule and deep to the vastus medialis obliquus (VMO).[276] In cadaver studies it has been demonstrated that this ligament extends from the

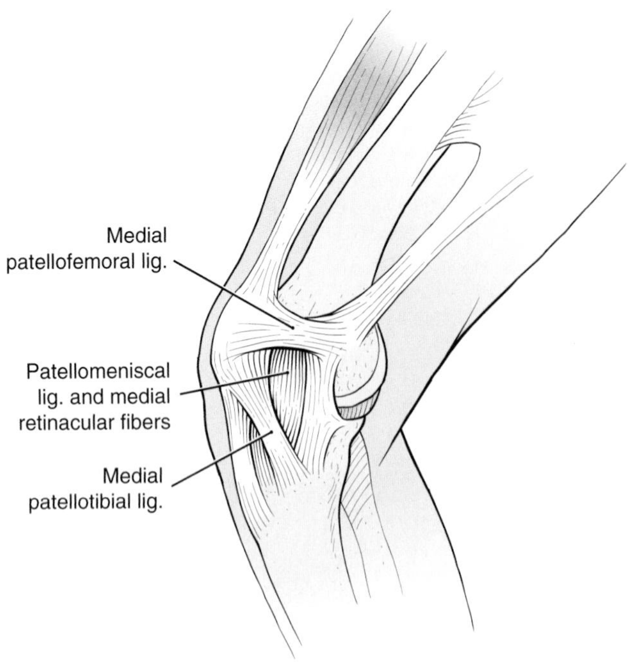

FIGURE 43–116 The medial patellofemoral ligament, which extends from the superomedial margin of the femoral epicondyle to the superomedial margin of the patella.

anterior aspect of the femoral epicondyle to the superomedial margin of the patella (Fig. 43–116).[83] The fibers of the MPFL fan out and insert with the vastus medialis tendon. The function of the MPFL is to act as a static stabilizer of the patella and prevent it from subluxing or dislocating laterally. Cadaveric studies have shown that 41% to 80% of the restraint to lateral translation is provided by the MPFL.[54,64,240]

MECHANISM OF INJURY

Patellar dislocations occur in two ways. The first is indirect trauma in which the femur is internally rotated on a fixed foot. Contraction of the quadriceps muscle during this twisting injury further pulls the patella laterally and results in patellar dislocation.[119] The second type of mechanism is a direct force applied either to the lateral aspect of the knee, which creates a valgus stress that leads to lateral patellar dislocation, or medially, applied to the patella and pushing it directly laterally. After both types of injuries the patella will often reduce spontaneously without requiring formal reduction. The most common activities in which these injuries are incurred are ball sports (football, basketball, baseball), falls, and gymnastics.[43,173]

CLINICAL FEATURES

The clinical history generally includes a twisting injury or direct blow while the individual is engaged in a sports activity. At the time of initial evaluation patients frequently report a "giving way" or "going out of joint" sensation. Although girls are more often thought to have patellar instability, this may not hold true for initial traumatic patellar dislocations. Some studies report a greater proportion of boys having this injury,[43] whereas others report a higher incidence in girls.[188,225] Fithian and colleagues, in a prospective review of all age groups, reported 52% of primary dislocations occurring in females. The female-to-male ratio of first-time dislocation was slightly higher in the pediatric population.[86] The patella most often reduces spontaneously with extension of the knee or with a combination of extension of the knee along with manipulation of the patella at the scene of the injury. On the rare occasion when the patella remains dislocated at the time of initial evaluation, the knee is in the flexed position and the patient has significant pain and swelling. The knee is maintained in the flexed position, and active motion is resisted; however, passive extension of the knee can be performed. The patella can be palpated on the lateral aspect of the knee, the femoral condyles are easily palpated, occasionally a longitudinal tear on the medial aspect of the joint capsule and patellar retinaculum is felt, and there is usually a large knee effusion. In the more common situation the patella has been reduced to an anatomic position. There is a knee effusion, which may be tense, especially when an osteochondral fracture is present,[188,225] and there is tenderness on the medial aspect of patella and the insertion of the vastus medialis.

RADIOGRAPHIC FINDINGS

Radiographic assessment should include AP, lateral, and tangential views of both knees. The radiographs are assessed for osteochondral fractures of the patella, most often on the medial aspect, and fractures of the lateral femoral condyle. It is important to obtain tangential views of both knees for comparison. Although many techniques are available for obtaining a tangential view of the patella, we prefer the Merchant view of the knee in which the knee is supported at 35 to 45 degrees of flexion to allow evaluation of the patellofemoral articulation with a relaxed quadriceps mechanism and before bony constraint of the patella within the femoral sulcus.[176] The Merchant view may be analyzed for the sulcus angle, the lateral patellofemoral angle, and lateral patellar displacement. Although these parameters may be used to assess the relative position of the patella, they have not been found to be independently predictive of *recurrent* dislocations, and therefore they are not a useful guide to treatment.[173]

MRI is not routinely indicated for evaluation after patellar dislocation. It is useful for the evaluation of osteochondral injury in the setting of a persistent effusion or when the diagnosis is in question. Sanders and coworkers reported 70% accuracy in prediction of MPFL disruption and vastus medialis muscle elevation in 12 of 14 patients by MRI.[230] Elias and colleagues reported MRI findings in 82 patients with lateral patellar dislocation. In this series, 35 of 71 visualized MPFLs showed signs of disruption, 45% of patients had significant elevation of the VMO from the plane of the adductor tendon, and concave impaction deformity of the inferior patella (44%) was specific for lateral patellar dislocation when compared with controls.[75]

TREATMENT

Conservative Treatment. Acute treatment of a patellar dislocation rarely requires reduction of the patella because most patients are initially seen with the patella reduced. Even in an occasional patient with an unreduced patella, the diagnosis should be evident, and radiographs are not necessary. (We prefer to obtain radiographs only after reduction.) After sedation, gentle closed reduction should be performed by slowly extending the knee while applying medially directed pressure on the patella. Care must be taken to achieve gentle reduction because some investigators believe that osteochondral injury can occur after the acute dislocation when the medial edge of the patella slides back tangentially over the lateral condyle.[225,251]

In the more common situation in which the patient has a reduced patella, arthrocentesis of the joint can be performed to reduce the patient's discomfort and may be useful for diagnosing an associated osteochondral fracture when fatty marrow is present. This diagnostic aspect of knee aspiration is especially important in a young child, in whom an osteochondral fracture can be difficult to ascertain radiographically.

The majority of patellar dislocations can be treated with a brief period of immobilization in extension and protected weight bearing. After 5 to 10 days of cast or brace treatment, range-of-motion and strengthening exercises should be started. Bracing may be used to prevent lateral displacement of the patella. Rehabilitation, including vastus medialis strengthening and muscular endurance training, should be accomplished before return to sport at 8 to 12 weeks after injury. In a review of patellar dislocations in children by McManus and colleagues, 6 (21%) of 29 patients who were treated by cast immobilization later underwent operative intervention for recurrent dislocation.[173] Of the 21 patients who did not have a recurrent dislocation, 50% had some symptoms but were participating in their preinjury activities. Cash and Hughston reported 52% good results in patients with some evidence of congenital abnormality of the knee as opposed to 75% good results in those without congenital abnormality.[43] In a prospective review of nonoperative treatment, Atkin and colleagues found that 58% of patients had continued limitation in strenuous activities.[11] Fithian and coworkers found that females accounted for 70% of patients with recurrent instability after acute patellar dislocation. This series also demonstrated that a history of recurrent instability (two or more episodes) is most predictive of future instability.[86]

Treatment of Osteochondral Fracture. The primary indication for operative intervention after acute patellar dislocation is the presence of an osteochondral fracture. An osteochondral fracture may occasionally be diagnosed on the initial radiographs. In the setting of persistent effusion or mechanical symptoms, MRI should be performed to screen for chondral and smaller osteochondral injuries. Nietosvaara and colleagues described three patients who had loose osteochondral fragments and two medial marginal patellar avulsions that were not seen radiographically.[188] Osteochondral fractures associated with an acute patellar dislocation have been reported to occur in 5% to 39% of cases.[173,188,225] Nomura and Inoue reported fissuring and higher degrees of chondral injury in 77% of patients. The primary location was the central and medial patellar facet.[190] Nietosvaara and associates reported 26 (39%) patients to have a significant osteochondral fracture, 21 of which were detached, and only 3 of these injuries were fixed intraoperatively. Similarly, Rorabeck and Bobechko reported only 1 of 18 patients undergoing operative repair of an osteochondral fracture; their best results were achieved after excision of the osteochondral fragment combined with repair of soft tissues to prevent recurrent dislocation.[225]

When there is an osteochondral fracture, we recommend arthroscopy and fixation of the fragment. We use headless compression screw or absorbable pin fixation. This is performed arthroscopically or through a small arthrotomy, depending on the remaining continuity of the lesion.[266] At times, the osteochondral fragment is too small for fracture fixation, and excision is performed.[173,188,225] Microfracture of the lesion is most often the treatment of choice in this setting; however, osteochondral grafting or autologous chondrocyte implantation may be considered for larger lesions (generally >15 mm).[258,259] Medial soft tissue injury may be addressed by open repair of the MPFL and VMO. Frequently, the MPFL is avulsed from the femur, and direct repair via suture anchors can be performed. The MPFL may be attenuated and reconstruction with a hamstring graft (as described later) may be performed. Postoperatively, the patient is placed in a brace with protected weight bearing for 4 weeks and started on physical therapy for range-of-motion and strengthening exercises.

MPFL or VMO Repair. The indications for isolated MPFL or VMO repair (or repair of both structures) after acute patellar dislocation are unclear. There is significant evidence of the importance of the MPFL as a stabilizer of lateral patellar translation and that injury to this ligament is a primary component of lateral patellar dislocation.[12,40,54,64,189,227,230,240] Some ability of these structures to heal without operative intervention is presumed by their extra-articular location and by the large number of individuals who have only a single dislocation. Although redislocation is more likely to occur in younger children and those with the anatomic variables previously discussed, there may be other factors not yet identified that predispose to recurrence. The results of acute repair have been varied and no randomized studies are available. Ahmad and coworkers reported patient satisfaction and no recurrent instability after acute MPFL and VMO repair in eight patients at an average follow-up of 3 years.[2] Buchner and colleagues reported no difference in the redislocation rate (26%) or reported outcomes in patients treated nonoperatively or by acute medial repair.[38] In general, we advocate nonoperative management of primary patellar dislocations in the absence of an osteochondral fracture.

COMPLICATIONS

Recurrent dislocation is the most common complication of an acute patellar dislocation and is more often seen in children whose dislocation occurred before 16 years of age, in those with an increased Q angle, in those with evidence of ligamentous laxity, in patients with radiographic evidence of femoral condylar or patellar dysplasia, and in children with a weak VMO.[152] Initial treatment is similar to that for acute patellar dislocation, followed by aggressive rehabilitation of the VMO and quadriceps, with operative intervention indicated in patients in whom this treatment protocol fails.

Operative treatment of recurrent lateral patellar dislocation should be focused on re-establishing the medial soft tissue restraints. In the setting of recurrent dislocation, the MPFL is often attenuated, and reconstruction of the ligament with semitendinosus tendon, quadriceps tendon, or adductor tendon has been described with good results.[12,61,173,265] Ellera Gomes and colleagues reported that 15 of 16 patients treated by semitendinosus graft reconstruction of the MPFL experienced good and excellent results at an average follow up of 5 years.[76] At 2-year follow-up, Drez and coworkers reported 93% good and excellent results with the use of hamstring or fascia lata grafts.[68] This procedure is commonly used for recurrent patellar instability in our practice. The knee is inspected arthroscopically and any chondral injury is addressed. The semitendinosus tendon (or gracilis in larger patients) is harvested and fashioned into a double-stranded 4- to 5-mm graft. The medial retinaculum is inspected and subfascial elevation of the VMO is performed via an incision centered between the patella and adductor tubercle. The remnant MPFL is used to locate the position for graft fixation just distal to the adductor insertion and anterior to the MCL origin. In skeletally immature patients, radiographic confirmation of fixation distal to the physis is mandatory. A tenodesis screw at the femur and a suture anchor at the patella are used for graft fixation. The site of patellar fixation is the superior third and middle third junction on the medial border of the patella. The graft is tensioned with the knee flexed 30 to 40 degrees to allow the patella to engage the femoral sulcus. Manual translation confirms adequate passive stability before final fixation. The VMO is advanced moderately distally and laterally and sutured to the graft and distal retinaculum with the knee held in 60 degrees of flexion to avoid overtightening of the tissue. Postoperatively, partial weight bearing in extension is allowed. Full flexion and accelerated muscle rehabilitation are initiated at 3 to 4 weeks. Return to sports and unrestricted activity is permitted at 4 months.

The Dewar-Galeazzi procedure has also often been used for recurrent dislocation with good results and avoids fixation around the physis in younger patients.[153] In this procedure the semitendinosus is transferred to the patella to act as a checkrein, combined with a medial retinacular and VMO advancement procedure (Fig. 43–117).

Continued translation or malrotation of the patella may be treated with the Roux-Goldthwait procedure, in which the lateral portion of the patellar tendon may be detached and resutured beneath the medial portion of the patellar tendon. Several reports document generally good results with this procedure, but patellar tendon pain or continuing instability may occur.[14,66,106,168]

Tibial Spine Fractures

Tibial spine fractures are uncommon injuries in skeletally immature children. They usually occur after a fall from a bicycle or a motorcycle, and associated injuries are rare. A three-part classification described by Meyers and McKeever is used for treatment decision making.[178,179] Type I injuries are treated in a long-leg cast in extension, type II injuries are generally treated by closed reduction followed by casting, and type III injuries should be treated by open reduction, performed either arthroscopically or through an open arthrotomy, followed by internal fixation and casting. The outcome of treatment is usually good despite some residual anterior laxity.

ANATOMY

The intercondylar eminence is the region between the articular portions of the adjacent plateaus of the tibia. The eminence consists of two bone spines or tuberosities: the medial spine, which is associated with attachments of the ACL, and the lateral spine. Adjacent to these two elevations are the bony attachments of the anterior and posterior horns of the medial and lateral menisci. The ACL fibers fan out at its attachment and its fibers merge with the intermeniscal ligament and attachments of the menisci. The PCL does not attach to either tibial spine but attaches to the tibia just posterior to the tibial eminence, with its fibers extending distally on the posterior aspect of the tibia (Fig. 43–118).

In a skeletally immature child the intercondylar eminence is incompletely ossified and is more prone to fail than the ligamentous structures that attach to it. Failure occurs through the cancellous bone beneath the subchondral plate. Injuries to the anterior condylar eminence have been simulated in cadavers by placing traction on the ACL after osteotomy of the tibial eminence.[222] The fracture line is usually confined to the intercondylar eminence; however, it may propagate into the weight-bearing portion of the tibial plateau, most often the medial plateau.[284]

MECHANISM OF INJURY

Both ACL ruptures and tibial spine fractures may occur in the skeletally immature population. Either injury may occur while twisting on a partially flexed

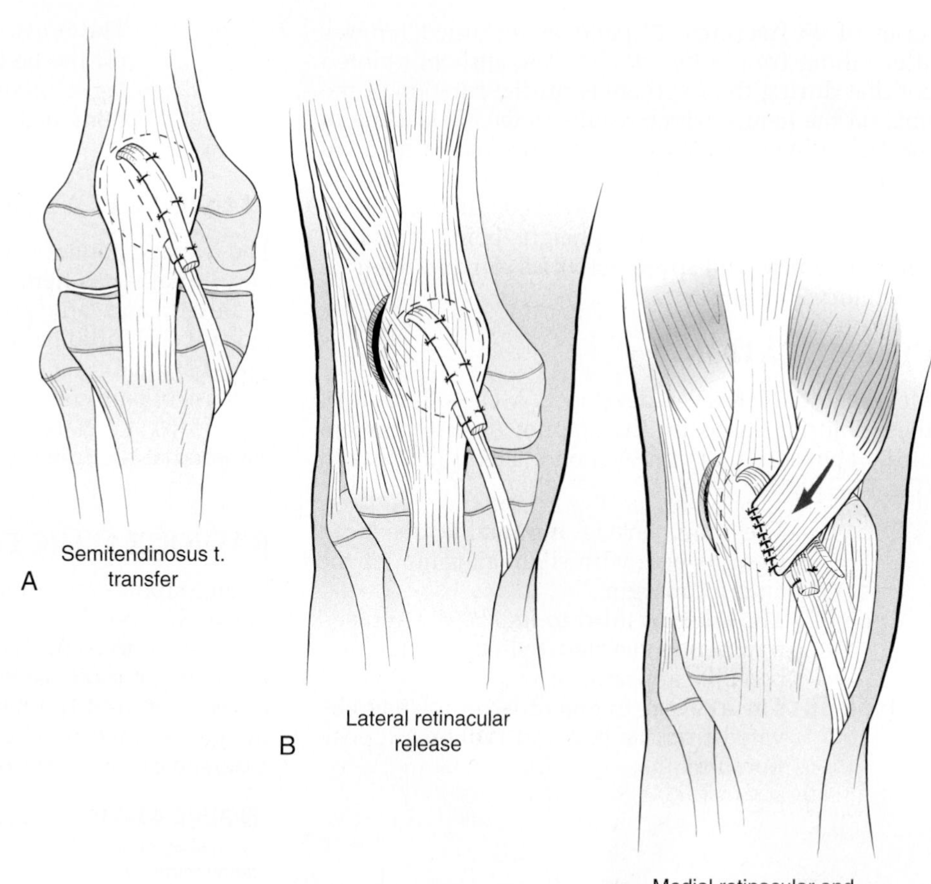

FIGURE 43–117 Galeazzi-type procedure for realignment of the knee extensor mechanism. **A,** Semitendinosus transfer through the patella; the semitendinosus is then sutured back onto itself. **B,** Lateral retinacular release. **C,** Medial retinacular and vastus lateralis advancement.

knee. The factors that predispose to one or the other of these injuries are unclear. In a retrospective radiographic review, Kocher and colleagues found the intercondylar notch to be narrower in patients who had sustained mid-substance ACL injury.[140] Avulsion of the anterior spine may occur when an axially loaded knee undergoes hyperextension and rotation with the femur externally rotated. A blow to the superoanteriorly flexed knee may drive the femur posteriorly on the fixed tibia and result in avulsion of the anterior part of the tibial spine. The most common activity in which tibial avulsion occurs is a fall from a bicycle or motorcycle, which accounts for approximately 50% to 65% of injuries.[179,284,285] In Meyers and McKeever's

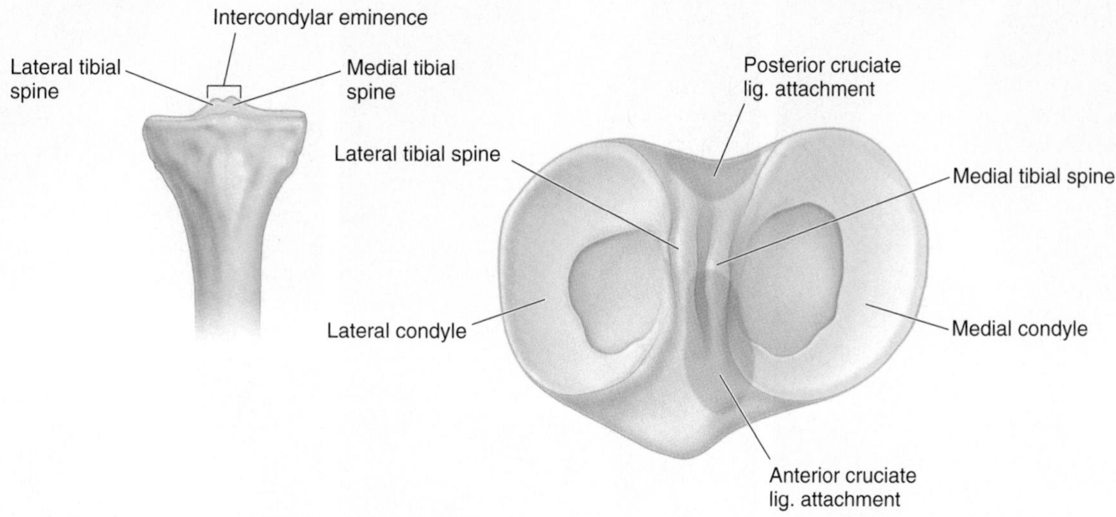

FIGURE 43–118 Diagram of a tibial plateau depicting the relationship of the anterior cruciate ligament, posterior cruciate ligament, and the medial and lateral tibial spine.

series of 35 fractures, 17 patients sustained injuries after falling from a bicycle.[178,179] The authors pointed out that during the fall there is medial rotation of the tibia on the femur, which results in tensile loading of the ACL. When an adolescent has knee pain after a fall from a bicycle, the radiographs should be carefully inspected for a tibial spine avulsion injury. Other activities such as falls from a height, being struck by a motor vehicle, and sports activities can also result in this injury.

CLASSIFICATION

Meyers and McKeever developed a classification of these injuries based on the amount of displacement of the avulsion injury as seen on a lateral radiograph (Fig. 43–119).[178,179]

Type I The fragment is minimally displaced from its bed, with slight elevation of the anterior margin.

Type II The anterior third to half of the avulsed fragment is elevated, thereby producing a beaklike appearance.

Type III The avulsed fragment is completely elevated from its bed and no bony apposition remains.

Type IV The avulsed fragment is completely lifted off the bed and rotated so that the cartilaginous surface of the fragment faces the bony bed.

CLINICAL FEATURES

The average patient is between 10 and 14 years of age and initially has hemarthrosis of the knee. The knee is flexed, and any attempt at passive extension is painful and inhibited by muscle spasm. At the time of initial evaluation it is difficult to assess knee stability because of pain-mediated muscular spasm and guarding. However, varus and valgus instability can be assessed at the initial evaluation.

RADIOGRAPHIC FINDINGS

Radiographic assessment includes AP and lateral views. The notch view or oblique views are occasionally needed to confirm the diagnosis. The lateral radiograph is the most useful for visualizing displacement of the fractured fragment. CT is occasionally used to image the fracture when displacement cannot be fully assessed on plain radiographs.

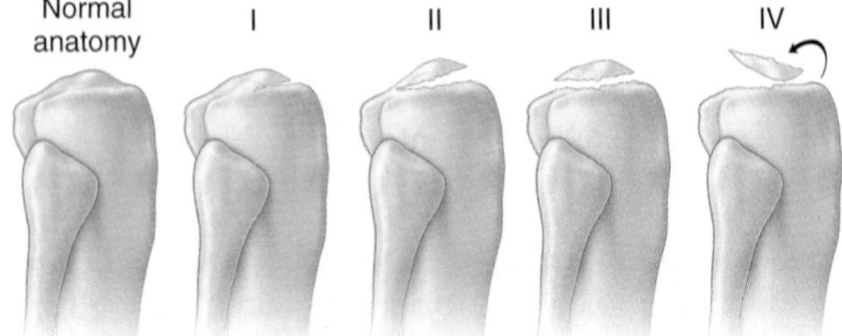

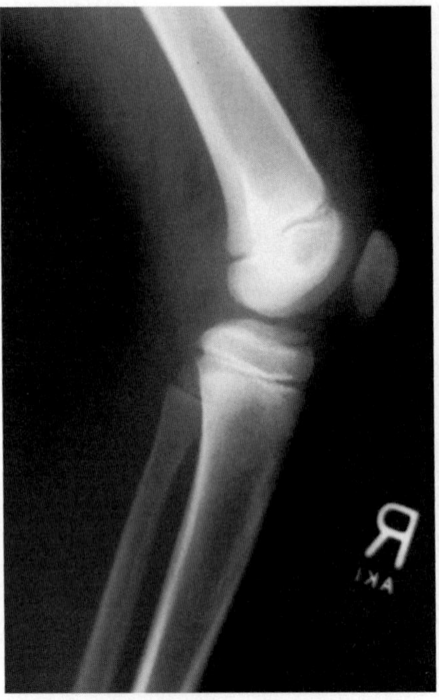

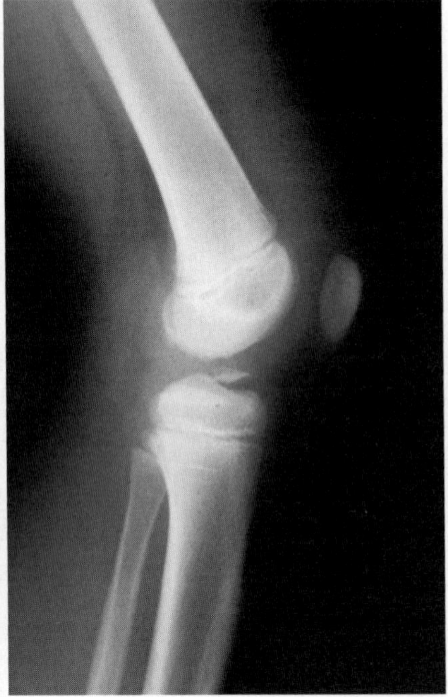

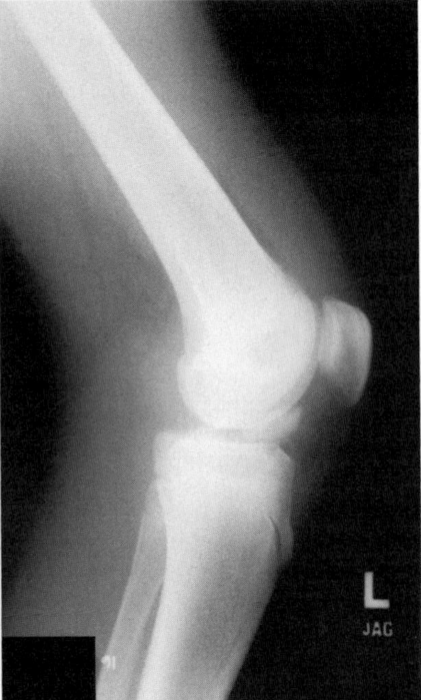

FIGURE 43–119 **A,** Meyers and McKeever classification of tibial spine injuries in children. **B,** Lateral radiograph demonstrating a nondisplaced type I tibial spine injury. **C,** Lateral radiograph demonstrating a type II tibial spine injury. **D,** Lateral radiograph demonstrating a type III tibial spine injury.

TREATMENT

The treatment guidelines that Meyers and McKeever outlined in their initial works are still followed today.[178,179]

Type I Fractures

For all type I injuries, in which the fracture is nondisplaced or minimally displaced, closed treatment is indicated. We prefer treatment in a long-leg cast with the knee in approximately 10 degrees of flexion. Slight flexion may afford benefit over full extension because of positional tension within the ACL. The ACL is taut with the knee in hyperextension, relaxed at the start of flexion, and then becomes tight again in full flexion. When a tense hemarthrosis is present, needle aspiration and intra-articular lidocaine injection will provide additional comfort and help bring the knee out to the extended position.

Type II Fractures

For a type II fracture in which the fracture fragment is anteriorly displaced, we prefer an initial attempt at closed reduction. It is controversial whether closed reduction can reduce the fracture or may, in fact, result in displacement of the fracture. Meyers and McKeever reported a patient who had a type II fracture that was converted to a type III fracture after manipulation and subsequently required open reduction.[179] Others have reported closed reduction and casting in an attempt to reduce the displaced type II fracture, but documented reductions were not discussed.[19,102,129,172,284,285] However, Bakalim and Wilpulla described 10 patients who underwent successful closed reduction without evidence of anterior laxity at final follow-up.[13] Reduction of type II and III fractures may be prevented by anterior intra-articular soft tissues. Kocher and colleagues reviewed the operative records of 80 cases of operatively treated tibial spine fractures. Entrapment of the medial meniscus or intermeniscal ligament was reported in 42 cases, with lateral meniscal entrapment seen in only 1 case. Only six of these cases with soft tissue blocking reduction were type II fractures.[141] Lowe and coworkers, however, found no tissue interposition in a smaller review of irreducible type III fractures and proposed that inability to achieve closed reduction was related to the superolateral pull of the anterior horn of the lateral meniscus, which was attached to the fracture fragment in each of the 12 cases.[160]

Closed reduction is performed after aspiration of hemarthrosis and injection of intra-articular lidocaine. The knee is extended to full extension or hyperextension and then slowly returned to a position of 5 to 10 degrees of flexion, and a long-leg cast is applied (Fig. 43–120). A radiograph is then taken to view the position of the tibial spine and confirm the reduction. If reduction has been achieved, radiographs are taken on a weekly basis for the first 2 weeks to ensure that the reduction has been maintained.

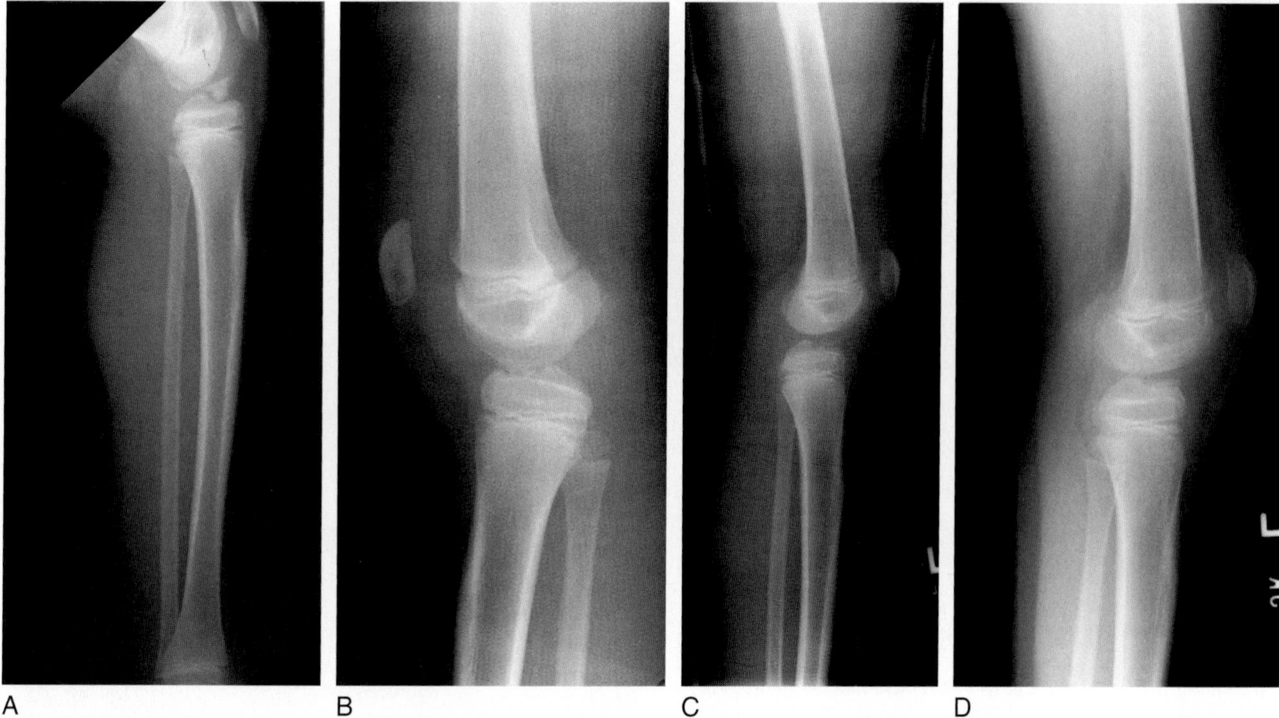

FIGURE 43–120 Closed reduction of a tibial spine fracture in a 9-year-old patient. **A,** Initial injury radiograph demonstrating a displaced tibial spine fracture. **B,** Hyperextension of the leg to reduce the fracture. **C** and **D,** Final radiographic appearance at 6 months. The fracture has healed in a mildly displaced position.

Type III Fractures

Type III fractures are best treated operatively with either an arthroscopic or an open technique. McLennan reviewed 10 type III injuries that had been treated by various techniques and concluded that arthroscopic reduction and internal fixation provided better results than did closed reduction or arthroscopic reduction without internal fixation.[172] Mah and coworkers reported excellent results in 10 type III fractures fixed with an arthroscopic suture technique.[165] Senekovic and Veselko reported less than 2 mm of anterior laxity and excellent Lysholm scores in 32 (pediatric and adult) patients after arthroscopic screw fixation without immobilization.[241] In six skeletally immature patients, Kocher and colleagues reported all excellent functional results after screw fixation despite persistent Lachman (five) and pivot shift (two) signs postoperatively.[138]

We prefer an arthroscopic technique to reduce and repair type III or persistently elevated type II injuries. The knee is inspected for associated osteochondral or meniscal injury. Though less common, meniscal tears have been reported in the setting of tibial spine fractures.[141] The intermeniscal ligament and medial meniscus should be well visualized and removed from below the osteochondral fragment. An 18-gauge needle placed through the anterior soft tissues to maintain retraction of the intermeniscal ligament and anterior soft tissues may aid in visualization of the fracture bed. After debridement of the hematoma, the fragment is reduced with the aide of a probe, a suture through the ACL base, or the single tip of a pointed reduction clamp placed through the anteromedial portal. The fragment may be fixed with sutures through bony tunnels or a cannulated 3.5- or 4.0-mm screw. In a young child the fragment is often large, and fixation through the avulsed fragment will provide stable fixation (Fig. 43–121). In an older child and adolescent the osteochondral fragment is smaller, which requires that fixation begin within the distal aspect of the ACL. This can best be done by inserting a spade-tipped guide-

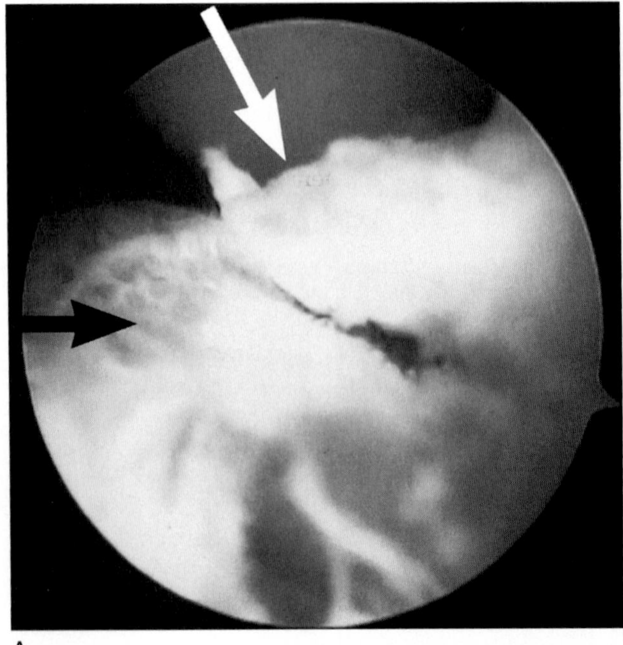

A

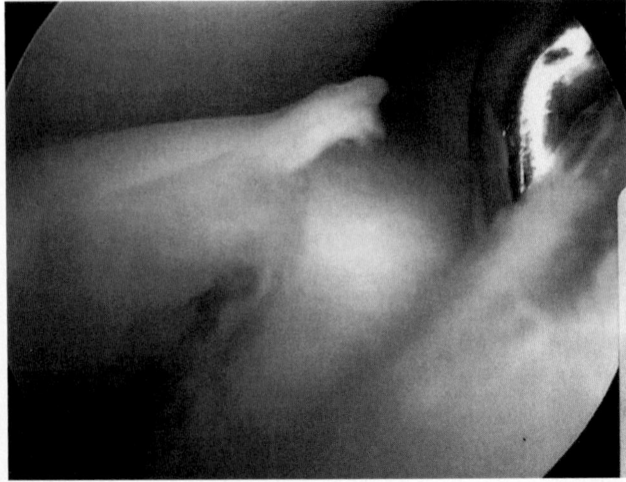

B

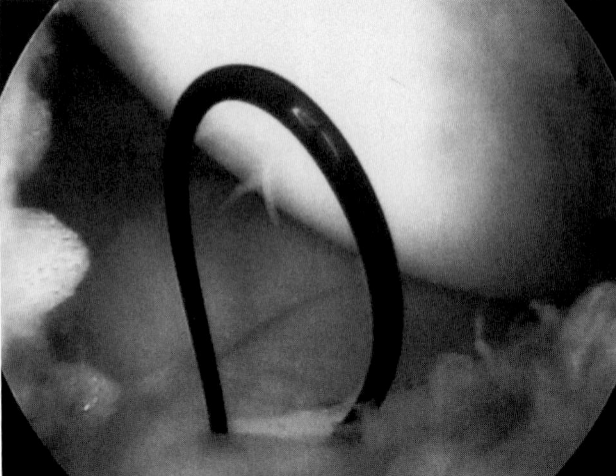

C

FIGURE 43–121 **A,** Intraoperative arthroscopic view of a patient with a tibial spine fracture. The avulsed fragment is displaced (*white arrow*) and lying over the medial meniscus (*black arrow*). **B,** A hook probe is used to pull the meniscus from beneath the fracture fragment to allow reduction of the tibial spine. **C,** The fragment in the reduced position. Sutures travel through the fragment, and a transtibial guide is in place.

wire into the ACL and passing No. 1 nonabsorbable sutures and tying them to allow fixation of the ACL. It is performed so that double-stranded sutures hold the ACL/bony fragment in a reduced position. The sutures can then be pulled down through the proximal tibia with the aid of a suture passer and tied as the fragment is visualized (Fig. 43–122). Use of a cannulated screw requires both an adequate osteochondral fragment for fixation and a significant amount of intact epiphyseal bone below the fracture to allow secure fixation. Insertion of the guidewire and screw from a parapatellar portal and screw length less than 20 mm will routinely allow fixation of the fragment without encroachment on the physis. The screw is positioned within the anterior insertion of the ACL fibers to prevent any impingement in full extension. Transphyseal screw fixation in a skeletally immature child should not be performed because it leads to anterior epiphysiodesis and a recurvatum deformity.[186] In addition, although no cases of physeal arrest have been reported, the physis should be avoided when placing drill holes for suture passage as long as the ability to achieve stable fixation is not compromised.

In the open technique, a small anteromedial incision is made at the joint line and the menisci and avulsed fragment are inspected. The fracture bed is cleared of fracture hematoma and menisci, and the knee is extended to reduce the fracture and allow the passage of sutures. The sutures are passed much as in the arthroscopic technique, by drilling from the proximal epiphysis into the avulsed fragment. Sutures are then placed into the ACL by using a Krackow-type stitch, after which the sutures are passed through the avulsed fragment and out the two drill holes (Fig. 43–123). The knee is extended and the sutures are tied down over the anterior aspect of the proximal tibia.

After the repair, performed by either the open or the arthroscopic technique, radiographs should be taken to be used for later comparison. The knee is then placed in a long-leg cast in nearly full extension. Radiographs are obtained at 1 week postoperatively to ensure that the fragment remains in the reduced position. The cast is left in place for 4 weeks, followed by strengthening and active range-of-motion exercises.

PCL Avulsion Fractures

Treatment of PCL avulsion fractures is somewhat controversial.[59,96,170,177,226,231,270] In patients with an undisplaced fracture, casting for 6 weeks provides excellent results.[177] A minimally displaced fracture has a high propensity to displace while in the cast and should therefore be repaired.[177] A displaced fracture always requires open reduction and internal fixation.[96,177,226,270] We prefer a direct posterior incision in the knee with anatomic reduction. Internal fixation is best accomplished with screw fixation when the fragment is large enough and with suture fixation when a smaller avulsed fragment is present. Postoperatively, the patient should be placed in a long-leg cast for 4 weeks, followed by active range-of-motion and strengthening exercises.

COMPLICATIONS

The overall prognosis for these injuries is good, especially in patients in whom anatomic reduction is achieved and maintained, with 85% of patients in one series returning to preinjury levels of activity.[285] The two most prominent complications from this injury are residual anterior instability and loss of motion, especially knee extension.[19,102,129,172,179,252,284,285]

ACL laxity has been objectively measured and reported in 38% to 100% of cases.[129,252,285] However, only a small proportion of patients have symptomatic instability. The laxity may be due to inadequate reduction of the avulsed fragment or may be a result of the initial injury, in which stretching of the ACL initially occurs before avulsion of the tibial spine.[110] Unrecognized injuries of the MCL have been reported and should be assessed during the initial evaluation.[102,110,252]

One of the most common complications is loss of extension from a displaced fragment impinging on the femoral notch. Wiley and Baxter reported that all 45 patients in their series had some loss of knee extension, with 60% having greater than 10 degrees of loss.[284] Treatment of symptomatic knee extension loss of more than 10 degrees has been successfully reported in 10 patients who had between 10 and 25 degrees of loss of extension.[204] These patients underwent arthroscopic debridement and abrasion of the tibial spine, and five patients had a notchplasty performed at the same time. At final follow-up, eight patients had full extension and two had residual extension deficits between 3 and 5 degrees.

Proximal Tibiofibular Joint Dislocations

These injuries are extremely rare and occur during athletic activities in which the patient's foot is inverted and plantar flexed, with simultaneous flexion of the knee and twisting of the body. Approximately a third of these injuries are missed on initial evaluation. Treatment of tibiofibular dislocation or subluxation is closed reduction followed by long-leg casting. Some injuries become recurrent, with a chronic subluxating proximal fibula. These patients are best treated by soft tissue reconstruction to prevent future subluxation or by resection of the proximal fibular head.

ANATOMY

Ogden has classified the proximal tibiofibular joint into two basic types. The first type is a horizontal joint in which the fibular articular surface is circular and planar and articulates with a similar surface on the tibia. This type of joint is usually under and behind the lateral edge of the tibia and provides some stability (Fig. 43–124). The second type is an oblique tibiofibular joint in which the joint line is angled more than 20 degrees as compared with the tibiofemoral joint; this type generally has less articular surface area than the horizontal type does.[199] More than 70% of subluxations and dislocations occur in patients with an oblique joint pattern.

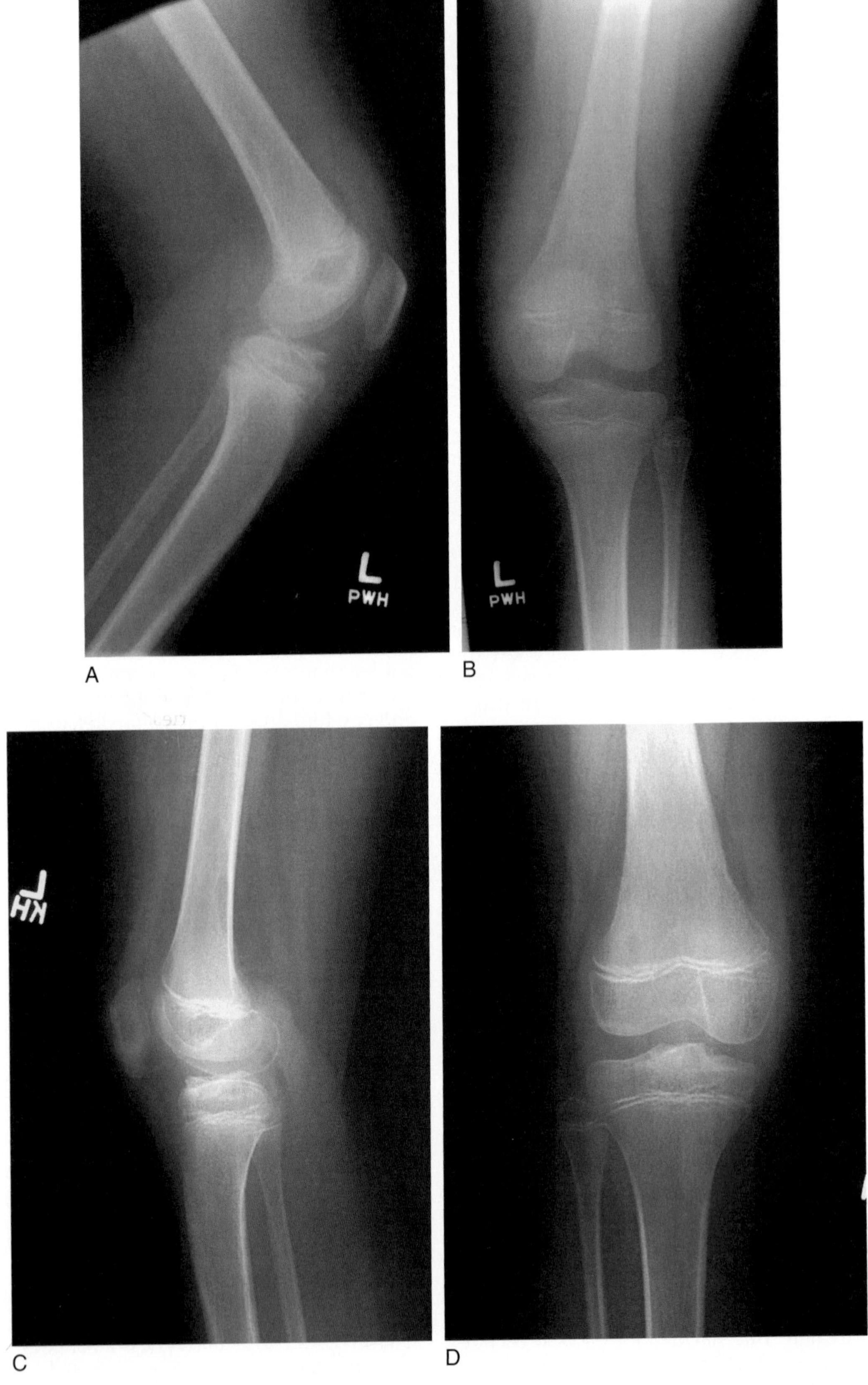

FIGURE 43-122 Mildly displaced tibial spine fracture in a 9-year-old patient treated by arthroscopically assisted reduction. **A** and **B,** Initial radiographic appearance. **C** and **D,** Arthroscopically assisted reduction plus casting was performed. This final radiographic picture shows minimal displacement of the tibial spine fracture.

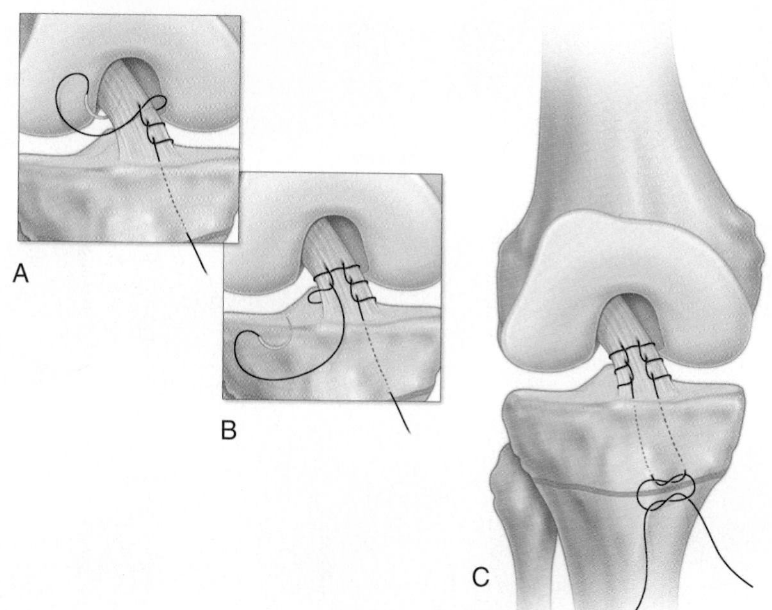

FIGURE 43–123 Open reduction and internal fixation of a tibial spine fracture. **A** and **B,** Krackow-type suture placed in the anterior cruciate ligament. **C,** Sutures are brought out through the proximal tibial epiphysis and tied.

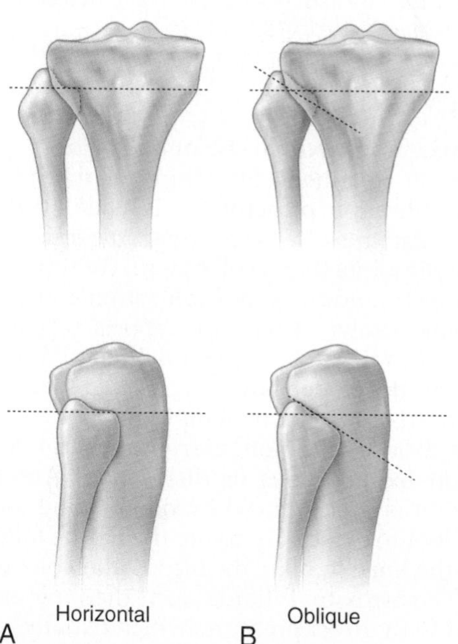

FIGURE 43–124 Anatomy of the proximal tibiofibular joint. **A,** Horizontal-type joint. **B,** Oblique-type joint.

The syndesmosis between the proximal tibia and fibula provides stability to the joint and is supplemented by the fibular collateral ligament and the biceps femoris, which insert into the fibular head.

MECHANISM OF INJURY

Most injuries occur in adolescents engaged in athletic activities, parachute landings, or motor vehicle accidents.[57,79,94,199,200,279] The best understood mechanism results in an anterolateral dislocation. Initially, sudden inversion plus plantar flexion of the foot results in an anteriorly directed pull of the fibular head by the peroneals and long toe extensors. Simultaneously, flexion of the knee relaxes the biceps tendon and fibular collateral ligament while twisting of the body results in external rotation of the tibia. The combined forces pull the fibula out laterally and anteriorly. Associated injuries are relatively rare, but a proximal tibial fracture is seen with these injuries.[244] Other injuries include hip fractures, fracture-dislocations of the ankle, and fracture-dislocations of the distal femoral epiphysis.[199,200] Posterolateral dislocations are more often a result of violent direct trauma as opposed to the twisting athletic injury resulting in anterolateral dislocation.

Conditions such as generalized ligamentous laxity and muscular dystrophy may predispose patients to the development of a subluxating or dislocated joint.[203]

CLASSIFICATION

The classification of proximal tibiofemoral joint dislocations was first described by Lyle in 1925.[162] Ogden later developed the more commonly used classification in 1974, when he described four basic types of injuries to the proximal tibiofibular joint (Fig. 43–125).[199,200]

1. The most common type of dislocation is an anterolateral dislocation, which accounts for 67% of cases; in this type of dislocation the proximal fibula displaces laterally to free itself from the lateral edge of the tibia, followed by anterior displacement.
2. Subluxation of the joint occurs in approximately 25% of cases when the fibula exhibits increased motion laterally, medially, anteriorly, and posteriorly.
3. Posteromedial dislocation is relatively rare (5%) and occurs with posterior displacement of the fibula followed by medial displacement.

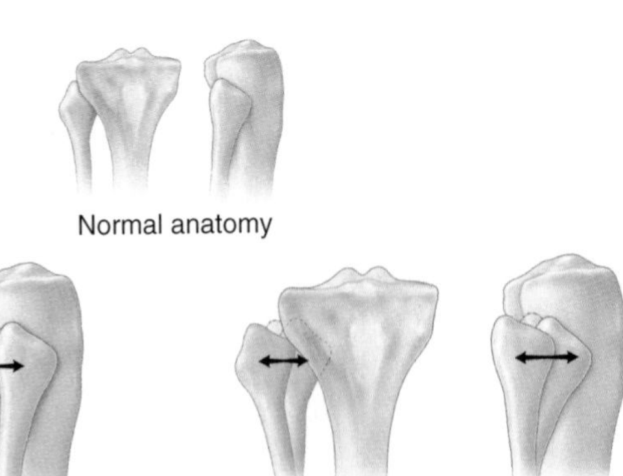
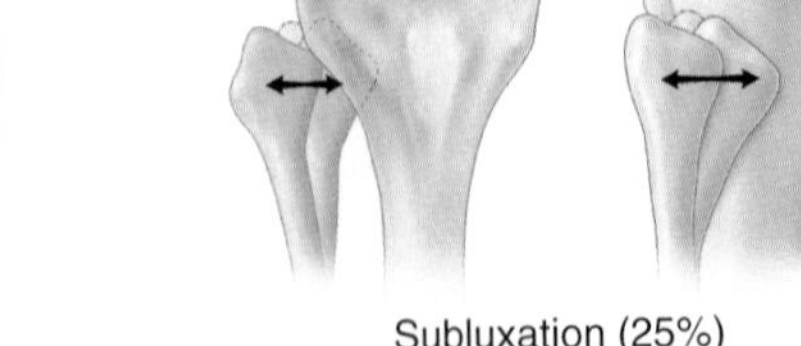
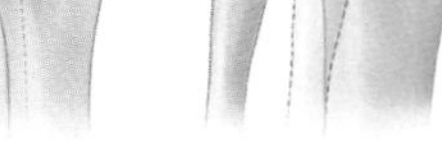 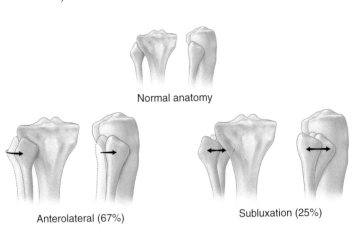
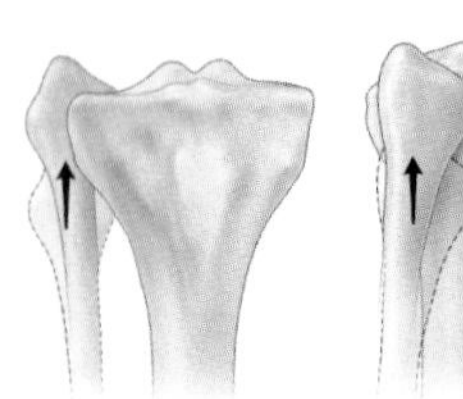

FIGURE 43–125 Classification of proximal tibiofibular dislocations.

4. Superior dislocation is the least common (2%) and occurs when upward displacement occurs along with mild lateralization.

CLINICAL FEATURES

A patient with subluxation of the fibula usually has pain along the lateral aspect of the knee and lower limb. These patients typically have generalized joint hyperlaxity or an underlying condition such as Ehlers-Danlos syndrome. Patients with dislocation of the joint seek care after an injury that usually involved twisting of the extremity during an athletic activity. Patients will often have symptoms in the lateral popliteal fossa in the location of the biceps tendon that has been stretched, and dorsiflexing and everting the foot may accentuate the pain. In addition, the patient may complain of transient paresthesias along the distribution of the peroneal nerve, although footdrop is rare.

The physical examination in patients with chronic subluxation will elicit tenderness on deep palpation over the fibular head. One of the most striking features in a patient with a dislocated tibiofibular joint is a prominent fibular head on visual inspection. It is important to fully image any injured extremity to search for a proximal tibiofibular dislocation. Ogden described 16 of 43 patients with associated fractures, and these were the patients in whom the tibiofibular dislocation was most often missed.[199] The knee can often be put through its range of motion without significant symptoms and may lack only a small amount of full knee extension; a knee joint effusion is rare.

RADIOGRAPHIC FINDINGS

Radiographic examination includes AP and lateral views of the knee and often an oblique radiograph to fully image the dislocation.

TREATMENT

A subluxated proximal tibiofibular joint generally requires no treatment. Stretching of the hamstrings with modification of activities is usually all that is required. Patients often have some generalized hyperlaxity of the joints that resolves with continued growth and maturity, and the joint subluxation and associated symptoms resolve. There are reports of adults with habitual chronic subluxation in whom peroneal nerve symptoms developed and required resection of the fibular heads for relief of symptoms.[63]

For a dislocated tibiofibular joint, we prefer closed reduction for all types of dislocation. Anterolateral dislocation is best reduced by dorsiflexing and everting the foot to externally rotate the fibula, followed by flexing the knee to relax the biceps and collateral ligament. The proximal fibula can then be manually reduced with direct pressure, which usually results in a loud, audible popping sound (Fig. 43–126). A long-leg cast with the knee flexed to 30 degrees is then used for 2 to 3 weeks, after which normal activities are gradually resumed.

Posteromedial dislocation is a more severe injury, with disruption of the LCL and the biceps tendon. This injury requires open reduction and reconstruction of these structures, followed by brace immobilization and protected range of motion.

Superior dislocation is very rare and most often associated with a proximal tibial fracture, which requires open reduction and internal fixation.

COMPLICATIONS

Long-term studies of patients with proximal tibiofemoral joint dislocations are not available. In the short term, patients do very well. The exceptions are those who continue to have a chronically subluxating joint,

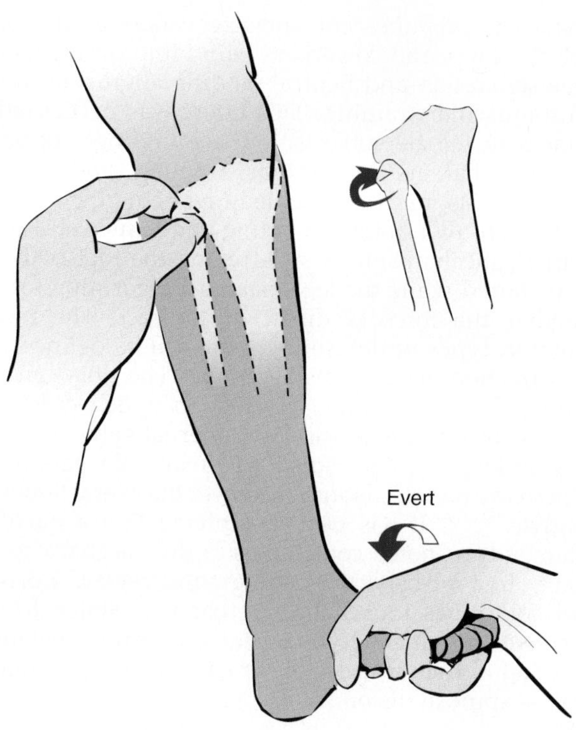

FIGURE 43–126 Reduction maneuver for a proximal tibiofibular dislocation. As the foot is manually everted, the fibular head is palpated and reduced, and a "clunk" is generally heard.

which is best treated by capsuloligamentous reconstruction or proximal fibular head resection.[175,239] We do not recommend fusion of the proximal tibiofibular joint because symptoms at the ankle usually develop as a result of restricted motion of the proximal joint. This ultimately requires proximal fibular head resection or osteotomy below the arthrodesed joint.

Recurrent dislocation of the tibiofibular joint is rare.[94,203,242,279] Treatment of a child with joint hyperlaxity does not usually require any treatment, and the child can be watched until skeletal maturity, when the symptoms resolve.[203] In patients in whom conservative treatment fails, surgical options include resection of the proximal fibular head or reconstruction of the stabilizing structures of the joint. We prefer to attempt to surgically stabilize the joint with a split biceps tendon, an iliotibial band, or a combination of both.[94,242,279]

Ligament Injuries

ANATOMY

The ACL originates on the lateral wall of the intercondylar notch at its posterior margin and inserts just anterior to the tibial spine on the tibia (Fig. 43–127). The orientation of the ACL within the knee results in its fibers being twisted approximately 90 degrees as the knee moves from flexion to extension. Because of this, the fibers can be functionally differentiated into two bundles, the anteromedial bundle and the posterolateral bundle. In flexion, the anteromedial bundle lengthens and the posterolateral bundle shortens, whereas in extension the opposite occurs. The ACL is intracapsular but is surrounded by a synovial fold. Its primary blood supply is derived from the middle genicular artery, which comes off the popliteal artery and penetrates the posterior joint capsule. An indirect blood supply comes from the inferior medial and lateral genicular arteries, which penetrate the fat pad.

The PCL originates on the posteromedial aspect of the intercondylar notch and inserts into the posterior sulcus of the tibia between the medial and lateral joint surfaces. Like the ACL, the PCL has two functionally separate bundles—the anterolateral fibers, which are taut in flexion, and the posteromedial fibers, which are taut in extension.

The capsuloligamentous constraints include the MCL, the lateral ligament complex (fibular collateral ligament, popliteus tendon, and popliteofibular

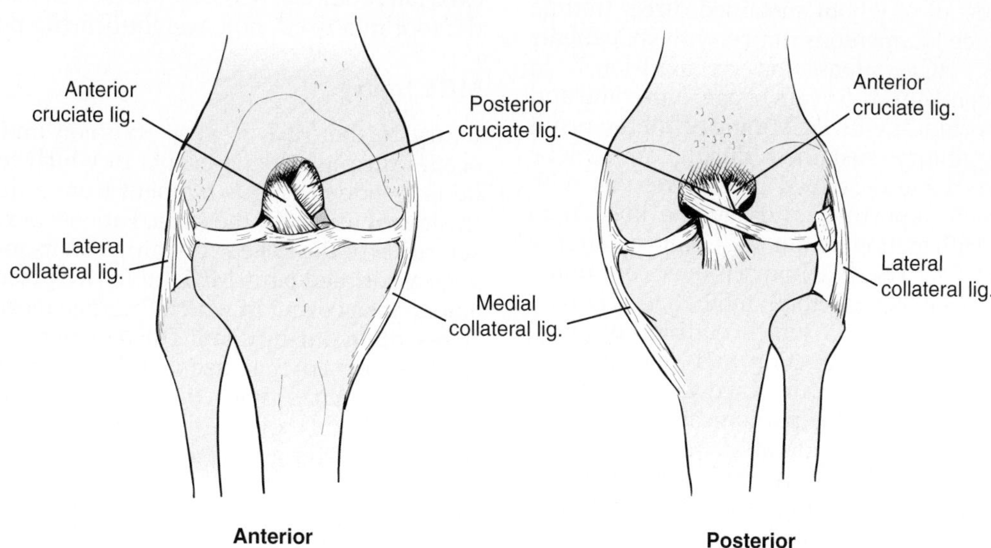

FIGURE 43–127 Anatomic location of the anterior cruciate and posterior cruciate ligaments, along with the lateral and mediolateral ligaments.

ligament), and the joint capsule. On the medial aspect of the knee, three layers of soft tissue structural support can be identified. The first layer is the deep fascia, which overlies the gastrocnemius muscles posteriorly; anteriorly it becomes confluent with the second layer and the medial patellar retinaculum. The second layer contains the superficial MCL, which is the primary stabilizer of the knee to valgus forces; the MCL travels from the medial epicondyle to the medial tibia deep to the gracilis and semitendinosus. The third layer consists of the joint capsule, which is thin anteriorly, becomes the deep MCL medially, and blends with the second layer posteriorly to become the posteromedial capsule.

On the lateral aspect of the knee the three layers include the lateral retinaculum, composed of the superficial oblique and deep transverse components. The second layer is composed of the fibular collateral ligament, which runs from the lateral epicondyle to the proximal fibula, and the arcuate ligament, a triangular ligament that fans out proximally from the fibula and inserts onto the femur. The third layer is the joint capsule, which is thin anteriorly and stronger posteriorly, with support from the arcuate complex and the popliteus tendon.

These ligamentous structures work synchronously to provide stability to the knee joint. The ACL is the primary restraint to anterior translation, whereas the deep MCL is a secondary restraint. The PCL is the primary restraint to posterior translation, and the LCL, posterolateral complex, and superficial MCL are secondary restraints.

MECHANISM OF INJURY

ACL Injury

Two types of injuries result in an ACL tear: a direct traumatic event and a twisting injury of the knee, most often occurring during participation in an athletic event. In a younger child, direct trauma is more often the cause of a tear or avulsion of the ACL. Clanton and colleagues described nine children with an average age of 10 years, all of whom sustained direct trauma resulting in knee ligamentous injury, with six patients demonstrating ACL attenuation or avulsion.[51] In patients between 12 and 15 years of age, Lipscomb and Anderson reported 24 with ACL injuries, all the result of a twisting injury sustained during an athletic event.[155] Others have described similar results, with most adolescents reporting injury to the knee with subsequent confirmation of an ACL injury after a twisting injury.[206,282] The ACL injury is most commonly seen in sports such as basketball, football, soccer, volleyball, and gymnastics, in which cutting, jumping, and sudden changes in direction and velocity (predominantly deceleration) occur. Knee valgus is a recognized component in the pathomechanics of the injury. There is increasing literature to suggest that neuromuscular control and relative knee position during jumping and landing are important biomechanical factors in ACL injury. In an evaluation of jump-landing kinematics, Swartz and colleagues demonstrated increased knee valgus and decreased hip flexion in prepubescent subjects versus adult controls.[262] Noyes and coworkers found improvements in knee separation and neutral landing alignment after neuromuscular training. This effect was particularly evident in female subjects.[193] These findings support theories that neuromuscular training and sport-specific skills may be of value in reducing the significant rate of ACL injury in young and female athletes.

In all mechanisms of ACL injury, the foot is fixed or anchored while the leg sustains a deforming force, whether the force is direct or indirect. The most common types of deforming force can be defined by the direction of tibial displacement. The tibia can be adducted and internally rotated, in which case the ACL is stretched over the PCL; alternatively, the tibia may undergo a valgus stress with external rotation, in which case the ACL is stretched over the lateral femoral condyle.[93,117,194] It has been postulated that a narrow intercondylar notch contributes to this mechanism of injury. In a retrospective radiographic review, Kocher and colleagues found the intercondylar notch to be narrower in patients who sustained a mid-substance ACL injury than in those of similar age who sustained a tibial spine avulsion.[140]

PCL Injury

PCL injury usually occurs either from a motor vehicle accident, in which case there are often other ligamentous or bony injuries, or during athletic activities.[56,120,134,157,271] In athletic injuries the typical mechanism is a fall onto a flexed knee while the foot is in a plantar flexed position, which results in posterior displacement of the tibia on the femur. A direct blow to the anterior aspect of the tibia while the knee is flexed may also result in a tear of the PCL. When a PCL rupture is associated with other ligamentous injuries, more severe trauma is often required to produce this injury. It is usually due to a rotatory force combined with a varus or valgus deforming force. For example, a PCL-MCL injury results from a valgus–external rotation stress sustained by a flexed knee with the foot in a fixed, non–weight-bearing position.[243]

MCL Injury

Injury to the MCL is very common and most often occurs during athletic events in which the knee sustains a sudden valgus moment from a direct blow to the lateral aspect of the knee. Patients often describe a sensation of the knee's "opening" on its medial aspect, with associated pain. MCL injury may also occur from a noncontact event in which the knee receives a valgus stress, often during a fall. The patient feels pain on the medial aspect of the knee that slowly subsides over the first 30 minutes, with the athlete often wishing to resume play. The knee then stiffens, with increasing pain and swelling over the ensuing 12 to 16 hours.

LCL Injury

Isolated injury to the LCL is far less frequent than MCL injury and occurs with a varus displacement of the knee. Because isolated injury of the LCL is rare, careful assessment for other ligamentous and meniscal injuries is necessary.

CLINICAL FEATURES

ACL Injury

A patient with an ACL tear describes a characteristic sudden movement in the knee, often with a "giving way" or "shifting" sensation. Patients report hearing a "pop" at the time of the initial injury in 40% to 60% of cases.[85,194] The patient is unable to resume participating in the event and is generally assisted off the field, with the subsequent development of a large effusion. Although the majority of patients describe significant pain at the time of injury and shortly thereafter, some have mild symptoms and attempt to return to activities before seeking a medical opinion. This most often results in the athlete's realizing that the knee is unstable and prevents performance at the preinjury level.

The physical examination is diagnostic of an injury to the ACL. The knee should be inspected for effusion and ecchymosis because the majority of ACL injuries are associated with a knee effusion.[8,33,51,74] Stanitski and colleagues demonstrated that in the presence of an acute traumatic knee hemarthrosis, 47% of preadolescents (7 to 12 years of age) and 65% of adolescents had an injury to the ACL.[257] Range of motion of the knee should be evaluated, with careful attention to the amount of extension of the knee. In the acute phase, extension may be limited by pain and guarding as a result of bony contusion.

The Lachman test is the most sensitive test for isolating an ACL injury. It is performed by applying an anteriorly directed force to the proximal tibia with the knee in 30 degrees of flexion and the leg slightly externally rotated to relax the hip flexors (Fig. 43–128). The amount of anterior displacement of the tibia should be estimated and categorized into one of the following categories:

Grade 1	1 to 5 mm
Grade 2	6 to 10 mm
Grade 3	11 to 15 mm
Grade 4	16 to 20 mm

The end point should also be characterized as firm (normal), marginal, or soft. In a larger adolescent it is often difficult to stabilize the thigh while performing this test, and therefore it is helpful for the examiner to place his or her flexed knee on the examining table and rest the patient's distal thigh on it (Fig. 43–129). The examiner can then control the distal part of the thigh by applying posteriorly directed pressure to it to perform the examination.

The anterior drawer test is performed with the knee flexed to 90 degrees (Fig. 43–130). The examiner ensures that the hamstrings are relaxed and applies an anteriorly directed force to the proximal end of the tibia.

The final test, the pivot shift test, is the most difficult to perform, especially in a patient with an acutely injured knee, and requires considerable cooperation from the patient. Although there are many variations of this test, they all rely on anterior subluxation of the tibia on the femur when the knee is in extension and reduction of the tibia with knee flexion of 20 to 40 degrees as the iliotibial band directs the anterior lateral tibia posteriorly.[158,159] Relocation of the tibia should be classified as follows:

0	No relocation (normal)
1+	Glide with reduction
2+	Shift of the tibia with reduction
3+	Temporary locking of the tibia before reduction

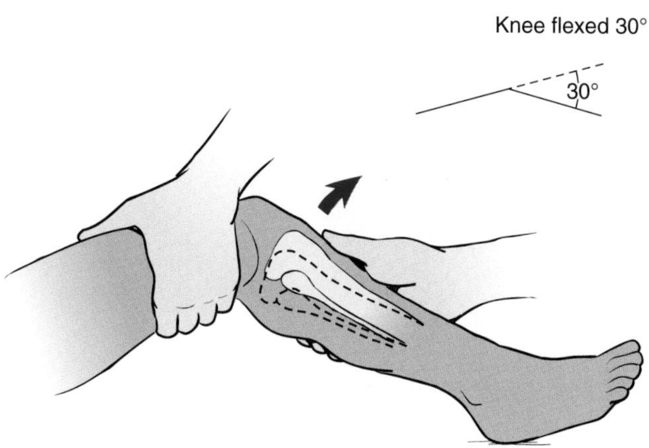

FIGURE 43–128 The Lachman test. The knee is flexed to 30 degrees with slight external rotation of the hip. The examiner holds the distal end of the patient's thigh with one hand while stabilizing the proximal end of the tibia with the other (the thumb is placed on the tibial tubercle to determine the amount of displacement anteriorly). An anteriorly directed force is then applied to the proximal end of the tibia.

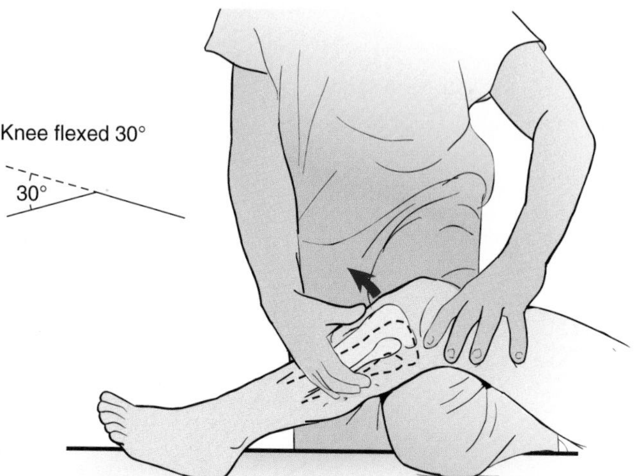

FIGURE 43–129 Modified position for the Lachman test in a larger patient. The examiner stabilizes the patient's thigh by placing it over the examiner's flexed thigh on the examination table. The examiner then fully stabilizes the thigh with one hand while applying an anteriorly directed force with the other hand.

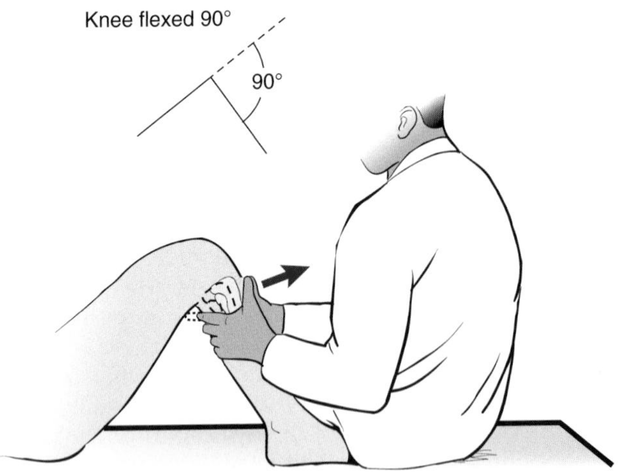

FIGURE 43–130 Anterior drawer test. With the patient's knee flexed to 90 degree, the examiner stabilizes the patient's foot on the bed. The examiner then uses both hands to provide an anterior force while the index fingers ensure that the patient's hamstrings are relaxed.

PCL Injury

The physical examination findings consistent with a PCL injury are similar to those for ACL injuries but opposite in direction. Initially, the position of the tibia can be evaluated with the knee flexed to 90 degrees while the heel is supported. The examiner looks for "posterior sag" of the proximal tibia as compared with the opposite extremity.[95]

The posterior drawer test at 90 degrees is most useful in a suspected PCL-deficient knee.[41,91] With the patient supine on the examining table, the patient's knee is flexed to 90 degrees. The examiner can sit lightly on the distal aspects of both feet. The examiner grasps the proximal aspect of the tibia with both hands and ensures that the hamstrings are relaxed, then applies a direct posterior force to the proximal tibia. The examiner's thumbs are placed on the tibial tubercle during this maneuver and are used to identify the amount of posterior displacement of the tibia, which is graded as in the anterior drawer test. Comparisons can be made with the opposite side when the examination is difficult to perform or when the starting point is obscure, for example, when the proximal tibia is subluxated posteriorly before the posteriorly directed force is applied to the tibia.

Frequently, a PCL tear is associated with injuries of the posterolateral corner (arcuate complex, popliteus, and LCL). The Hughston and Norwood posterolateral drawer test helps define associated posterolateral corner injuries.[121] When a posterolateral corner injury is associated with a PCL injury, there is more posterolateral spin of the tibia on the femur with the knee flexed to 90 degrees than when it is flexed to 30 degrees. This is best assessed with the patient supine and the hip flexed to 90 degrees, followed by external rotation of the tibia on the femur; the amount of external foot progression is then compared at 30 and 90 degrees of knee flexion. An isolated posterolateral corner injury has a greater thigh–foot progression angle at 30 degrees than at 90 degrees (Fig. 43–131).

Another test for PCL instability is the reverse pivot shift test, which relies on the tibia subluxating posteriorly when the knee is flexed to approximately 20 to 30 degrees.[128]

MCL Injury

A patient with a suspected MCL injury should be evaluated by initial palpation of the MCL at its points of insertion on the medial femoral condyle and at its insertion on the anteromedial aspect of the proximal tibia just under the pes anserinus. Tenderness along the ligament or at its insertion points raises suspicion of a ligament tear. Stress tests are performed with the knee in full extension while a valgus stress is applied

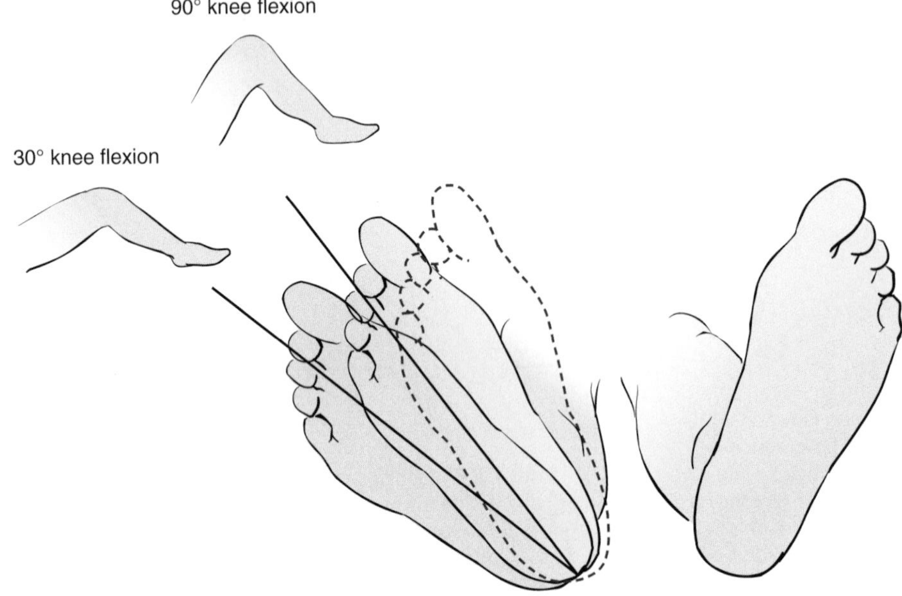

FIGURE 43–131 Asymmetric thigh–foot angles are present in a posterolateral corner tear of the right knee, more prominent in 30 degrees of knee flexion than in 90 degrees of knee flexion.

to the knee. Opening on the medial aspect of the knee in this position indicates a substantial tear of the MCL along with the medial capsule and one or both cruciate ligaments. The knee should be flexed to 10 to 15 degrees and the valgus stress repeated because this position of the knee relaxes the posterior capsule and allows specific testing of the MCL.[84,103] MCL injuries are best classified according to the Marshall grading system, which is easy to use and offers prognostic information:[84]

Grade I	MCL tender without laxity
Grade II	Increased valgus laxity in flexion without instability in full extension
Grade III	Valgus laxity in both flexion and full extension

LCL Injury

The LCL can easily be palpated with the knee in the figure-four position as it travels from the lateral femoral condyle to the head of the fibula. Tenderness or obvious disruption of the ligament indicates injury to the fibular collateral ligament. Stress testing of the knee should be performed with the knee in an extended position because normal varus laxity occurs with knee flexion.

Combination Injuries

Although isolated injuries of the various ligaments occur, there is a high incidence of associated injuries within the knee; these injuries should be carefully evaluated before determining treatment. One of the most common injury patterns is that of a combined ACL-MCL injury, which has a reported incidence of 15% to 40%.[89,196,197,246] Meniscal tears are relatively common in patients with an ACL tear. It is generally agreed that the medial meniscus is more often torn in a normal knee and in an ACL-deficient knee. However, with an acutely torn ACL, the lateral meniscus is more often torn at the time of injury.[20,25,45,47,48,136,238]

RADIOGRAPHIC FINDINGS

Radiographs of the knee should be obtained in any patient with a suspected ligamentous injury to assess for fractures or bony avulsions indicating ligamentous injury. Images should include AP, lateral, tunnel, and patellar views. Skeletal maturity should be assessed on these radiographs, with careful inspection of the physes to determine their degree of closure. Bony abnormalities should be assessed, including tibial spine avulsion fractures, physeal fractures, and collateral ligament avulsions of the MCL or LCL. The clinician should evaluate for associated osteochondral lesions, which are seen in up to 23% of acute ACL injuries.[81,82] In a chronically ACL-deficient knee the incidence is far higher. A capsular avulsion on the lateral aspect of the proximal tibia, the so-called Segond fracture, is seen in approximately 10% of cases and can help make the diagnosis of an ACL tear.

MRI should be used only as an adjunct to a good history and physical examination when the extent and degree of associated injuries are difficult to determine.

TREATMENT

ACL Injury

The initial treatment of an ACL-deficient knee is to restore the normal range of motion of the knee. Although treatment of an ACL-deficient knee depends partly on the activity level of the child and the status of the physes, in most cases the ultimate treatment is surgical reconstruction to reestablish joint stability. Such treatment allows the patient to return to normal physical activity without jeopardizing the remaining intact structures of the knee. A comparison of young patients treated nonoperatively with those treated by reconstruction demonstrated that those who underwent nonoperative treatment experienced instability, with recurrent pain and effusion, and many did not return to sports activities.[171] Several studies have shown that rates of meniscal and osteochondral injury increase with increasing time interval between ACL injury and reconstruction. Injury to the medial meniscus is most significantly associated with a delay in stabilization.[3,88,181]

Surgical Treatment. The goal of ACL reconstruction is restoration of functional knee stability, which is accomplished by replacement of the injured ligament with graft material. A ligament that has sustained significant injury is rarely functional. Kocher and colleagues found that partial ACL tears may occasionally be managed nonoperatively when the tear is anteromedial and less than 50% and when functional examination signs are nearly normal (Lachman and pivot shift tests). Posterolateral tears and those involving more than 50% of the diameter of the ligament had poor functional results.[142] There is no role for direct repair of the ligament because of the rapid inflammatory reaction that occurs soon after injury. In a skeletally mature adolescent, a standard arthroscopically assisted technique is used with either a patellar tendon or a hamstring graft (Fig. 43–132). Proposed advantages of the patellar tendon include greater strength and better fixation to the femur and tibia.[49,69,77,131,150,191] The advantages of a hamstring graft include less donor site morbidity and patellar pain, and material properties similar to the ACL.[35,260] In an evaluation of functional outcome after ACL reconstruction, Kocher and coworkers found that elimination of pivot shift instability was most highly correlated with reported patient satisfaction.[144] This suggests that technical aspects of reconstruction for restoration of rotational control are as important as those for decreasing anterior tibial translation.

Treatment in Skeletally Immature Patients. The most controversial issue surrounding ACL injury in a skeletally immature child is whether to perform surgical intervention shortly after injury or to postpone intra-articular surgical reconstruction until the physes

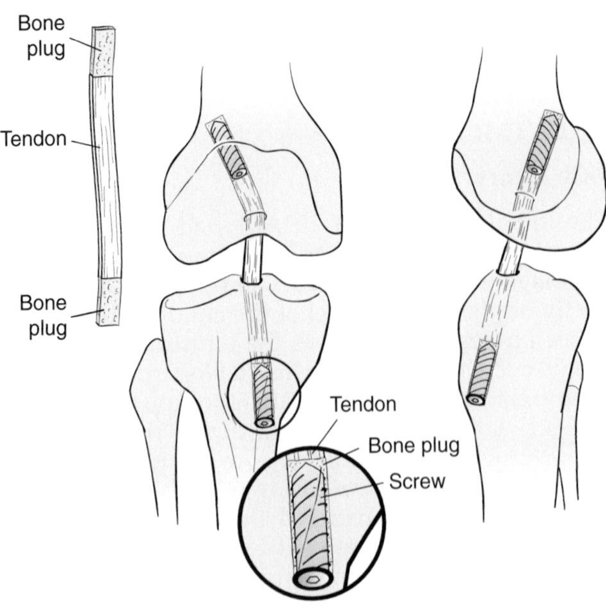

FIGURE 43-132 Surgical reconstruction of the anterior cruciate ligament in a skeletally mature patient.

have closed. Animal studies, in both rabbit and canine models, suggest that tensioned soft tissue grafts across the physis may result in arrest or deformity.[72,116] However, several clinical reviews have reported series of transphyseal reconstructions performed with soft tissue grafts in skeletally immature patients without physeal injury.[71,90,155] In a review of reported complications after ACL reconstruction in the skeletally immature, Kocher and coworkers found that the majority of physeal complications occurred with fixation devices or bone plugs placed directly across the physis or when large (12 mm) tunnels were used.[143] Graft placement through both the tibial and femoral physes, with fixation in the metaphyses, has been reported in series in which the majority of patients had 2 to 4 years of growth remaining (average age, 13 years).[71,90] Hybrid intra-articular reconstruction techniques without physeal complications have been described in children of younger chronologic and Tanner age. In these techniques, transphyseal (femur or tibia) placement is used on one side of the joint, with corresponding intraepiphyseal fixation, or graft passage external to the physis on the other end of the graft.[104,155] Lipscomb and Anderson reported results in 24 adolescent patients with open physes who had undergone open intra-articular reconstruction performed with semitendinosus and gracilis tendons. The tibial tunnel was centered through the tibia and penetrated the physis, whereas the femoral tunnel exited distal to the distal femoral physis. They reported 96% good or excellent results, and only one patient had a limb length discrepancy of 2 cm.[155]

The lower age limit for complete transphyseal reconstruction without growth disturbance remains unclear. Alternative techniques in prepubescent children are intraepiphyseal graft placement and fixation and complete extraphyseal reconstruction. Anderson has reported excellent results with an all-epiphyseal technique; however, the smaller size of the epiphysis in younger age groups may make this technique technically demanding.[6] A well-studied technique of physeal-sparing reconstruction, described by Kocher and colleagues, provides an excellent option in this age group. In this series, 44 patients who were Tanner stage 2 or less (average age, 10.3 years) underwent reconstruction without physeal complications. Eleven of 42 patients had moderately abnormal pivot shift test results, but only 2 patients required revision reconstruction at an average follow-up of 5.3 years.[139]

We prefer to treat a skeletally immature child nonoperatively if the child and parents have limited goals for participation in athletic activities and if there are no symptoms of instability. Nonoperative treatment should consist of initial measures to maintain comfort, followed by directed rehabilitation to regain normal range of motion of the knee. A good home exercise program consists of quadriceps and hamstring strengthening exercises and neuromuscular conditioning to help restore knee stability. A patient is placed in a functional brace to help prevent subluxation. Although the mechanisms by which braces afford stability are unclear, Kocher and coworkers found that functional bracing status was significantly associated with injury-free activity in an athletic population.[145] Within 6 to 8 weeks the patient should have achieved normal motion and strength and can begin to participate in increased activities. These activities should be limited to noncontact sports and restricted participation in sports that require rapid directional changes.

If the patient experiences symptoms of instability, we perform an intra-articular reconstruction with an iliotibial band or a hamstring graft, which is tunneled through the center of the tibial physis but placed extracortically in the over-the-top femoral position to avoid the distal femoral physis (Fig. 43–133). In a periadolescent (2 to 3 years of growth remaining), we prefer a transphyseal hamstring graft with fixation that avoids the physes.

ACL and MCL Injuries

Combined ACL and MCL tears are relatively common and should therefore be carefully sought in any patient with a suspected ACL tear. Patients with a grade I or II MCL injury should be treated with a hinged knee brace for 4 to 6 weeks, followed by rehabilitation to obtain normal range of motion and strength. Surgical reconstruction of the ACL is then managed as previously described. The results of operative treatment of the ACL without surgical repair of the MCL have been uniformly good, without residual valgus instability.[15,16,114,233,245] In a patient with a grade III MCL injury, we recommend operative treatment to directly repair the torn ligament, with simultaneous reconstruction of the ACL in an older child. Aggressive rehabilitation is needed to regain motion of the knee, especially in patients with MCL disruptions at or proximal to the joint line.[223]

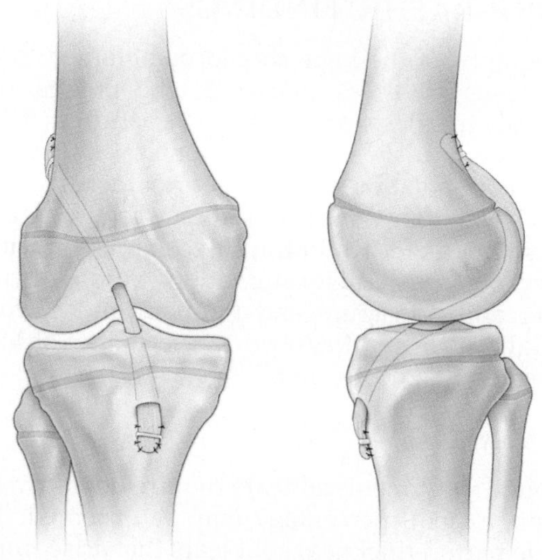

FIGURE 43–133 Surgical reconstruction of the anterior cruciate ligament in a skeletally immature patient.

PCL Injury

Treatment of a patient with a PCL tear is generally nonoperative, with good results reported.[56,248] In an acutely torn PCL, the initial treatment is symptomatic, together with active range-of-motion and strengthening exercises. Grade III instability after a PCL tear may result in continued instability requiring reconstruction, especially in a high-performance athlete.[50]

MCL Injury

Isolated MCL injuries are treated nonoperatively, with excellent results. Grades I and II injuries are treated symptomatically with a hinged brace or crutches until the patient is asymptomatic, which usually occurs between 1 and 3 weeks. Grade III injuries should be treated by immobilization in a hinged knee brace for 4 to 6 weeks. During this period quadriceps and hamstring strengthening exercises should be performed. Athletic activities can be resumed when full range of motion of the knee is achieved and the strength of the leg is similar to that on the opposite side.

LCL Injury

Isolated tears of the LCL are uncommon. Pain in the posterolateral complex without instability is treated by protected range of motion and strengthening as described earlier. Grades II and III injuries are evaluated with MRI to assess for the presence of associated injuries and determine the extent of injury to the posterolateral corner. Acute direct repair of the fibular collateral ligament, popliteofibular ligament, and arcuate complex may then be performed. Grade III injuries are most often associated with tears of the ACL. Treatment of this clinical situation is controversial, with little data available in the pediatric literature. In a skeletally immature child, a grade III LCL tear should be repaired primarily, with reconstruction of the ACL performed at skeletal maturity. In an adolescent, simultaneous reconstruction of the ACL and direct repair of the LCL should be performed.

Meniscal Injuries

ANATOMY

The menisci are composed of fibrocartilage, with circumferentially arranged collagen fibers designed to bear the tensile loads of the weight-bearing surface. In addition to the circumferential arrangement, some collagen fibers are arranged in radial fashion to provide additional support. The blood supply to the menisci comes from the surrounding capsular and synovial perimeniscal capillary plexus, which branches from the medial, lateral, and middle genicular arteries.[10] The peripheral 30% of the meniscus, the so-called red-red zone, has the richest blood supply. Development of the menisci begins during the 10th week of fetal life, at which time they have a semilunar appearance.[52] At birth there is an abundance of cells in comparison to matrix, and this proportion slowly declines until the age of 10, when the adult microscopic appearance of the menisci is present.

The medial meniscus is larger than the lateral meniscus and takes on a more C-shaped structure that is narrower and thinner. The anterior attachment of the medial meniscus is anterior to the intercondylar eminence and the ACL. The posterior horn attaches anterior to the attachment of the PCL and just posterior to the intercondylar eminence. At its periphery, the meniscus is attached to the medial capsule and attaches to the proximal tibia through the coronary ligaments. The lateral meniscus is thicker, smaller, and more mobile than the medial meniscus. The anterior horn attaches to the tibia anterior to the tibial eminence, and the posterior horn attaches to the intercondylar eminence just anterior to the posterior attachment of the medial meniscus. Additional attachments via the meniscofemoral ligaments (ligaments of Humphrey and Wrisberg) help stabilize the posterior horn of the lateral meniscus.

MECHANISM OF INJURY

The majority of meniscal tears occur with a twisting motion of the knee without direct trauma to the knee. This most often occurs when the knee is partially flexed and a rotational force drives the femoral condyle into the meniscus and produces a shearing force that results in meniscal failure. These tears usually occur in older children who are involved in relatively strenuous, highly competitive activities that involve quick cuts and turns. Direct trauma to the knee may also result in meniscal injury when the blow forces the knee to suddenly rotate, and shearing force is exerted on the menisci.

CLASSIFICATION

The four basic types of meniscal tears are longitudinal, horizontal, oblique, and radial (Fig. 43–134). Tears may

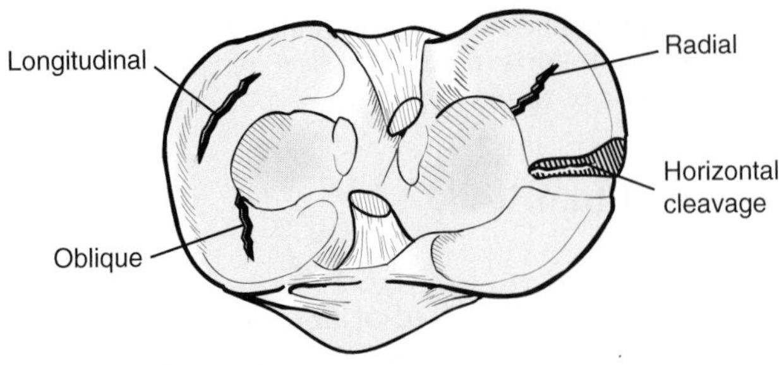

FIGURE 43–134 The four basic types of meniscal tears: longitudinal, oblique, radial, and horizontal cleavage.

occur in one of these basic patterns or in a combination of these patterns. In a longitudinal tear the collagen fibers split in line with the circumferentially directed fibers, which can result in instability of the innermost fragment when the tear is full thickness. The location of the tear with respect to the peripheral aspect of the meniscus should be identified to help determine whether repair can be performed. A partial longitudinal tear may begin on the superior or inferior surface of the meniscus and should be carefully evaluated. A horizontal cleavage tear occurs in a plane parallel to the superior and inferior surfaces of the meniscus and is rare in children. An oblique tear is a full-thickness vertical tear through the inner free margin of the meniscus that extends peripherally. A radial tear begins on the innermost aspect of the free edge of the meniscus and extends peripherally perpendicular to the free edge. In a series of 23 meniscal tears in skeletally immature patients, Vaquero and coworkers reported that 18 were longitudinal and in the peripheral zone.[275]

CLINICAL FEATURES

Patients may remember the traumatic event in which they sustained a twisting injury to the knee and may have heard or felt a "pop." However, up to 40% experience a spontaneous onset of symptoms without a known inciting event.[135] Frequently, the pain diminishes after injury; however, it returns and is associated with a knee effusion 24 to 48 hours later. Other symptoms include locking, giving way, and clicking sensations. King reported pain in 82% of patients, giving way in 63%, locking in 43%, a sensation of clicking in the knee in 45%, but recurrent effusions in only 34%—a lower rate than in adults.[135]

The physical examination should include a thorough assessment of the ligamentous structures of the knee. A focused examination for meniscal pathology includes inspection of the knee for joint effusion and palpation of the medial and joint line in an attempt to elicit tenderness. The provocative maneuvers of McMurray and Apley may help confirm or identify pathology, especially tears of the most posterior horn of the medial meniscus.

RADIOGRAPHIC FINDINGS

Radiographs of the knee should be obtained to identify occult fractures, injuries to the physes, osteochondral injuries, or avulsion fractures. MRI is commonly used to identify a meniscal injury in the pediatric population, with a reported accuracy of up to 95%.[24,122,163,180,214,263,290] This accuracy level depends on interpretation of MRI findings in conjunction with the history and physical examination. Studies by both Kocher and colleagues and Luhman and coworkers highlight the lower diagnostic performance of MRI as an isolated diagnostic tool.[137,161]

TREATMENT

Although most meniscal tears require operative intervention, a small percentage may be observed. These include partial-thickness split tears that arise from the femoral or tibial surfaces and are stable to probing, and short vertical peripheral tears, which often heal sufficiently to resolve symptoms.[280]

It is well established that complete meniscectomy as treatment of a torn or injured meniscus is detrimental to the long-term outcome of the knee.[9,118,174,213,264,273] Today, the preferred options for treatment include partial meniscectomy and meniscal repair.

The primary indications for partial meniscectomy are tears that are not amenable to repair because of location, chronicity of the tear, or configuration. The goal of partial meniscectomy is to remove the torn aspect of the meniscus while preserving as much of the meniscus as possible. The zone between torn and normal meniscus should be tapered to create a smooth transition area, thus decreasing the likelihood of creating a starting point for a new tear. The results of partial meniscectomy are generally very good, with immediate and long-term symptom relief.[1,17,22,30,111-113,130,133,147,148,169,234,255]

Indications for meniscal repair include long (15 to 25 mm) vertical longitudinal tears at the periphery without significant damage to the body of the meniscus.[44,60,107,237] Although the tear should clearly be in the vascular zone of the meniscus, the greater vascular penetration in children than in adults allows greater potential for healing. For example, the best results of meniscal repair in adults are achieved in tears within 3 mm of the periphery; however, in children it is likely that tears extending more than 3 mm from the periphery will heal. In a review of patients 19 years or younger, Noyes and Barber-Westin reported a 75% success rate at 4.3 years for repair of meniscal tears extending into the avascular zone.[192] Various techniques for repair have been described, including inside-out, outside-in, and all-inside procedures (Fig. 43–135).* Fibrin clot sutured into the repair site appears to increase the likelihood of healing.[87,109,124-126,211,221,272,274] Newer techniques for meniscal repair include fixation with meniscal suture anchors, arrows, or darts. Although inside-to-out vertical mattress suture

*See references 36, 42, 53, 78, 167, 182, 183, 219, 224, 236, 250.

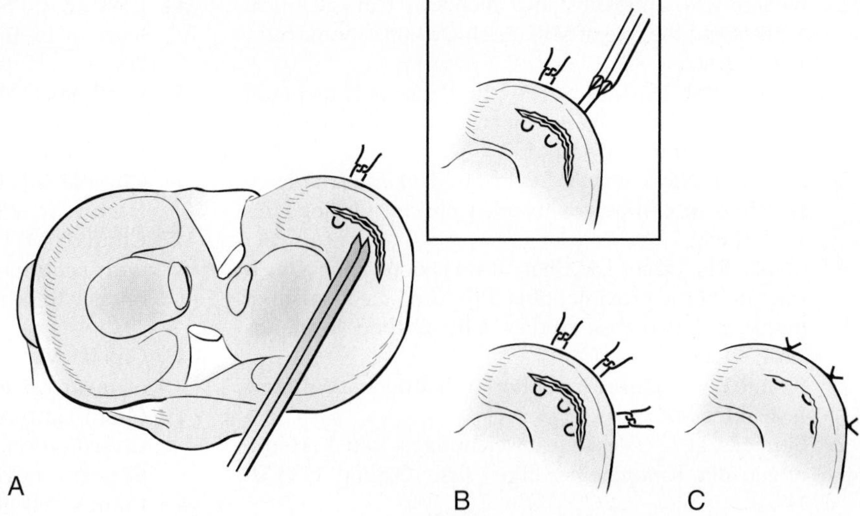

FIGURE 43–135 Meniscal repair techniques. **A,** The inside-out (or outside-in [*inset*]) technique. **B,** Sutures have been placed in horizontal fashion. **C,** The sutures are then tied on the outside.

techniques remain the gold standard, suture anchor constructs have demonstrated similar strength and excellent early outcomes.[31,105,291]

References

Knee

1. Aglietti P, Zaccherotti G, De Biase P, et al: A comparison between medial meniscus repair, partial meniscectomy, and normal meniscus in anterior cruciate ligament reconstructed knees. Clin Orthop Relat Res 1994;307:165.
2. Ahmad CS, Stein BE, Matuz D, et al: Immediate surgical repair of the medial patellar stabilizers for acute patellar dislocation. A review of eight cases. Am J Sports Med 2000;28:804.
3. Aichroth PM, Patel DV, Zorrilla P: The natural history and treatment of rupture of the anterior cruciate ligament in children and adolescents. A prospective review. J Bone Joint Surg Br 2002;84:38.
4. Aitken AP: Fractures of the proximal tibial epiphysial cartilage. Clin Orthop Relat Res 1965;41:92.
5. Aitken AP, Magill HK: Fractures involving the distal femoral epiphyseal cartilage. J Bone Joint Surg Am 1952;34:96.
6. Anderson AF: Transepiphyseal replacement of the anterior cruciate ligament using quadruple hamstring grafts in skeletally immature patients. J Bone Joint Surg Am 2004;86(Suppl 1):201.
7. Anderson M, Green WT, Messner MB: Growth and predictions of growth in the lower extremities. J Bone Joint Surg Am 1963;45:1.
8. Angel KR, Hall DJ: Anterior cruciate ligament injury in children and adolescents. Arthroscopy 1989;5:197.
9. Appel H: Late results after meniscectomy in the knee joint. A clinical and roentgenologic follow-up investigation. Acta Orthop Scand Suppl 1970;133:1.
10. Arnoczky SP, Warren RF: Microvasculature of the human meniscus. Am J Sports Med 1982;10:90.
11. Atkin DM, Fithian DC, Marangi KS, et al: Characteristics of patients with primary acute lateral patellar dislocation and their recovery within the first 6 months of injury. Am J Sports Med 2000;28:472.
12. Avikainen VJ, Nikku RK, Seppanen-Lehmonen TK: Adductor magnus tenodesis for patellar dislocation. Technique and preliminary results. Clin Orthop Relat Res 1993;297:12.
13. Bakalim G, Wilppula E: Closed treatment of fracture of the tibial spines. Injury 1974;5:210.
14. Baker RH, Carroll N, Dewar FP, et al: The semitendinosus tenodesis for recurrent dislocation of the patella. J Bone Joint Surg Br 1972;54:103.
15. Ballmer PM, Ballmer FT, Jakob RP: Reconstruction of the anterior cruciate ligament alone in the treatment of a combined instability with complete rupture of the medial collateral ligament. A prospective study. Arch Orthop Trauma Surg 1991;110:139.
16. Barber FA: Snow skiing combined anterior cruciate ligament/medial collateral ligament disruptions. Arthroscopy 1994;10:85.
17. Barrett GR, Treacy SH, Ruff CG: The effect of partial lateral meniscectomy in patients > or = 60 years. Orthopedics 1998;21:251.
18. Bassett FH 3rd, Goldner JL: Fractures involving the distal femoral epiphyseal growth line. South Med J 1962;55:545.
19. Baxter MP, Wiley JJ: Fractures of the tibial spine in children. An evaluation of knee stability. J Bone Joint Surg Br 1988;70:228.
20. Bellabarba C, Bush-Joseph CA, Bach BR Jr: Patterns of meniscal injury in the anterior cruciate–deficient knee: A review of the literature. Am J Orthop 1997;26:18.
21. Belman DA, Neviaser RJ: Transverse fracture of the patella in a child. J Trauma 1973;13:917.
22. Benedetto KP, Rangger C: Arthroscopic partial meniscectomy: 5-year follow-up. Knee Surg Sports Traumatol Arthrosc 1993;1:235.
23. Bertin KC, Goble EM: Ligament injuries associated with physeal fractures about the knee. Clin Orthop Relat Res 1983;177:188.

24. Biedert RM: Intrasubstance meniscal tears. Clinical aspects and the role of MRI. Arch Orthop Trauma Surg 1993;112:142.
25. Binfield PM, Maffulli N, King JB: Patterns of meniscal tears associated with anterior cruciate ligament lesions in athletes. Injury 1993;24:557.
26. Bisson LJ, Wickiewicz T, Levinson M, et al: ACL reconstruction in children with open physes. Orthopedics 1998;21:659.
27. Blanks RH, Lester DK, Shaw BA: Flexion-type Salter II fracture of the proximal tibia. Proposed mechanism of injury and two case studies. Clin Orthop Relat Res 1994;301:256.
28. Blount W: Fractures in Children. Baltimore, Williams & Wilkins, 1955.
29. Blumensaat C: Die Lageabweichungen und Verrenkungen der Kniescheibe. Ergeb Chir Orthop 1938;31: 149.
30. Bolano LE, Grana WA: Isolated arthroscopic partial meniscectomy. Functional radiographic evaluation at five years. Am J Sports Med 1993;21:432.
31. Borden P, Nyland J, Caborn DN, et al: Biomechanical comparison of the FasT-Fix meniscal repair suture system with vertical mattress sutures and meniscus arrows. Am J Sports Med 2003;31:374.
32. Bostrom A: Fracture of the patella. A study of 422 patellar fractures. Acta Orthop Scand Suppl 1972; 143:1.
33. Bradley GW, Shives TC, Samuelson KM: Ligament injuries in the knees of children. J Bone Joint Surg Am 1979;61:588.
34. Bright RW, Burstein AH, Elmore SM: Epiphyseal-plate cartilage. A biomechanical and histological analysis of failure modes. J Bone Joint Surg Am 1974;56:688.
35. Brown CH Jr, Steiner ME, Carson EW: The use of hamstring tendons for anterior cruciate ligament reconstruction. Technique and results. Clin Sports Med 1993;12:723.
36. Brown GC, Rosenberg TD, Deffner KT: Inside-out meniscal repair using zone-specific instruments. Am J Knee Surg 1996;9:144.
37. Bruijn JD, Sanders RJ, Jansen BR: Ossification in the patellar tendon and patella alta following sports injuries in children. Complications of sleeve fractures after conservative treatment. Arch Orthop Trauma Surg 1993;112:157.
38. Buchner M, Baudendistel B, Sabo D, et al: Acute traumatic primary patellar dislocation: long-term results comparing conservative and surgical treatment. Clin J Sport Med 2005;15:62.
39. Burkhart SS, Peterson HA: Fractures of the proximal tibial epiphysis. J Bone Joint Surg Am 1979;61:996.
40. Burks RT, Desio SM, Bachus KN, et al: Biomechanical evaluation of lateral patellar dislocations. Am J Knee Surg 1998;11:24.
41. Butler DL, Noyes FR, Grood ES: Ligamentous restraints to anterior-posterior drawer in the human knee. A biomechanical study. J Bone Joint Surg Am 1980;62:259.
42. Cannon WD Jr: Arthroscopic meniscal repair. Inside-out technique and results. Am J Knee Surg 1996;9:137.
43. Cash JD, Hughston JC: Treatment of acute patellar dislocation. Am J Sports Med 1988;16:244.
44. Cassidy RE, Shaffer AJ: Repair of peripheral meniscus tears. A preliminary report. Am J Sports Med 1981;9: 209.
45. Cerabona F, Sherman MF, Bonamo JR, et al: Patterns of meniscal injury with acute anterior cruciate ligament tears. Am J Sports Med 1988;16:603.
46. Christie MJ, Dvonch VM: Tibial tuberosity avulsion fracture in adolescents. J Pediatr Orthop 1981;1:391.
47. Cimino PM: The incidence of meniscal tears associated with acute anterior cruciate ligament disruption secondary to snow skiing accidents. Arthroscopy 1994;10: 198.
48. Cipolla M, Scala A, Gianni E, et al: Different patterns of meniscal tears in acute anterior cruciate ligament (ACL) ruptures and in chronic ACL-deficient knees. Classification, staging and timing of treatment. Knee Surg Sports Traumatol Arthrosc 1995;3:130.
49. Clancy WG Jr, Nelson DA, Reider B, et al: Anterior cruciate ligament reconstruction using one-third of the patellar ligament, augmented by extra-articular tendon transfers. J Bone Joint Surg Am 1982;64:352.
50. Clancy WG Jr, Shelbourne KD, Zoellner GB, et al: Treatment of knee joint instability secondary to rupture of the posterior cruciate ligament. Report of a new procedure. J Bone Joint Surg Am 1983;65:310.
51. Clanton TO, DeLee JC, Sanders B, et al: Knee ligament injuries in children. J Bone Joint Surg Am 1979;61: 1195.
52. Clark CR, Ogden JA: Development of the menisci of the human knee joint. Morphological changes and their potential role in childhood meniscal injury. J Bone Joint Surg Am 1983;65:538.
53. Coen MJ, Caborn DN, Urban W, et al: An anatomic evaluation of T-Fix suture device placement for arthroscopic all-inside meniscal repair. Arthroscopy 1999;15:275.
54. Conlan T, Garth WP Jr, Lemons JE: Evaluation of the medial soft-tissue restraints of the extensor mechanism of the knee. J Bone Joint Surg Am 1993;75:682.
55. Crock HV: The arterial supply and venous drainage of the bones of the human knee joint. Anat Rec 1962; 144:199.
56. Cross MJ, Powell JF: Long-term followup of posterior cruciate ligament rupture: A study of 116 cases. Am J Sports Med 1984;12:292.
57. Crothers OD, Johnson JT: Isolated acute dislocation of the proximal tibiofibular joint. Case report. J Bone Joint Surg Am 1973;55:181.
58. Czitrom AA, Salter RB, Willis RB: Fractures Involving the distal epiphyseal plate of the femur. Int Orthop 1981;4:269.
59. Dandy DJ, Pusey RJ: The long-term results of unrepaired tears of the posterior cruciate ligament. J Bone Joint Surg Br 1982;64:92.
60. DeHaven KE, Black KP, Griffiths HJ: Open meniscus repair. Technique and two to nine year results. Am J Sports Med 1989;17:788.
61. Deie M, Ochi M, Sumen Y, et al: A long-term follow-up study after medial patellofemoral ligament reconstruction using the transferred semitendinosus tendon for patellar dislocation. Knee Surg Sports Traumatol Arthrosc 2005;13:522.

62. Deliyannis SN: Avulsion of the tibial tuberosity: report of two cases. Injury 1973;4:341.
63. Dennis JB, Rutledge BA: Bilateral recurrent dislocations of the superior tibiofibular joint with peroneal-nerve palsy. J Bone Joint Surg Am 1958;40:1146.
64. Desio SM, Burks RT, Bachus KN: Soft tissue restraints to lateral patellar translation in the human knee. Am J Sports Med 1998;26:59.
65. Devas MB: Stress fractures of the patella. J Bone Joint Surg Br 1960;42:71.
66. Dewar RP, Hall JE: Recurrent dislocation of the patella. J Bone Joint Surg Br 1957;39:798.
67. Diamond LS, Alegado R: Perinatal fractures in arthrogryposis multiplex congenita. J Pediatr Orthop 1981;1: 189.
68. Drez D Jr, Edwards TB, Williams CS: Results of medial patellofemoral ligament reconstruction in the treatment of patellar dislocation. Arthroscopy 2001;17: 298.
69. Drez DJ Jr, DeLee J, Holden JP, et al: Anterior cruciate ligament reconstruction using bone–patellar tendon–bone allografts. A biological and biomechanical evaluation in goats. Am J Sports Med 1991;19:256.
70. Edvardsen P: Physeo-epiphyseal injuries of lower extremities in myelomeningocele. Acta Orthop Scand 1972;43:550.
71. Edwards PH, Grana WA: Anterior cruciate ligament reconstruction in the immature athlete: Long-term results of intra-articular reconstruction. Am J Knee Surg 2001;14:232.
72. Edwards TB, Greene CC, Baratta RV, et al: The effect of placing a tensioned graft across open growth plates. A gross and histologic analysis. J Bone Joint Surg Am 2001;83:725.
73. Ehrenhorg G: The Osgood-Schlatter lesion: A clinical and experimental study. Acta Chir Scand 1962;288:1.
74. Eiskjaer S, Larsen ST, Schmidt MB: The significance of hemarthrosis of the knee in children. Arch Orthop Trauma Surg 1988;107:96.
75. Elias DA, White LM, Fithian DC: Acute lateral patellar dislocation at MR imaging: Injury patterns of medial patellar soft-tissue restraints and osteochondral injuries of the inferomedial patella. Radiology 2002;225: 736.
76. Ellera Gomes JL, Stigler Marczyk LR, Cesar de Cesar P, et al: Medial patellofemoral ligament reconstruction with semitendinosus autograft for chronic patellar instability: A follow-up study. Arthroscopy 2004;20: 147.
77. Eriksson E: Reconstruction of the anterior cruciate ligament. Orthop Clin North Am 1976;7:167.
78. Esser RD: Arthroscopic meniscus repair: the easy way. Arthroscopy 1993;9:231.
79. Falkenberg P, Nygaard H: Isolated anterior dislocation of the proximal tibiofibular joint. J Bone Joint Surg Br 1983;65:310.
80. Farahmand F, Naghi Tahmasbi M, Amis A: The contribution of the medial retinaculum and quadriceps muscles to patellar lateral stability—an in-vitro study. Knee 2004;11:89.
81. Feagin JA Jr: The syndrome of the torn anterior cruciate ligament. Orthop Clin North Am 1979;10:81.
82. Feagin JA Jr, Lambert KL: Mechanism of injury and pathology of anterior cruciate ligament injuries. Orthop Clin North Am 1985;16:41.
83. Feller JA, Feagin JA Jr, Garrett WE Jr: The medial patellofemoral ligament revisited: An anatomical study. Knee Surg Sports Traumatol Arthrosc 1993;1: 184.
84. Fetto JF, Marshall JL: Medial collateral ligament injuries of the knee: A rationale for treatment. Clin Orthop Relat Res 1978;132:206.
85. Fetto JF, Marshall JL: The natural history and diagnosis of anterior cruciate ligament insufficiency. Clin Orthop Relat Res 1980;147:29.
86. Fithian DC, Paxton EW, Stone ML, et al: Epidemiology and natural history of acute patellar dislocation. Am J Sports Med 2004;32:1114.
87. Forman SK, Oz MC, Lontz JF, et al: Laser-assisted fibrin clot soldering of human menisci. Clin Orthop Relat Res 1995;310:37.
88. Foster A, Butcher C, Turner PG: Changes in arthroscopic findings in the anterior cruciate ligament deficient knee prior to reconstructive surgery. Knee 2005; 12:33.
89. Frolke JP, Oskam J, Vierhout PA: Primary reconstruction of the medial collateral ligament in combined injury of the medial collateral and anterior cruciate ligaments. Short-term results. Knee Surg Sports Traumatol Arthrosc 1998;6:103.
90. Fuchs R, Wheatley W, Uribe JW, et al: Intra-articular anterior cruciate ligament reconstruction using patellar tendon allograft in the skeletally immature patient. Arthroscopy 2002;18:824.
91. Fukubayashi T, Torzilli PA, Sherman MF, et al: An in vitro biomechanical evaluation of anterior-posterior motion of the knee. Tibial displacement, rotation, and torque. J Bone Joint Surg Am 1982;64:258.
92. George R: Bilateral bipartite patellae. Br J Surg 1935;22: 555.
93. Gersoff WK, Clancy WG Jr: Diagnosis of acute and chronic anterior cruciate ligament tears. Clin Sports Med 1988;7:727.
94. Giachino AA: Recurrent dislocations of the proximal tibiofibular joint. Report of two cases. J Bone Joint Surg Am 1986;68:1104.
95. Godfrey J: Ligamentous injuries of the knee. Curr Pract Orthop Surg 1973;5:56.
96. Goodrich A, Ballard A: Posterior cruciate ligament avulsion associated with ipsilateral femur fracture in a 10-year-old child. J Trauma 1988;28:1393.
97. Green WT, Anderson M: Epiphyseal arrest for the correction of discrepancies in length of the lower extremities. J Bone Joint Surg Am 1957;39:853.
98. Green WT Jr: Painful bipartite patellae. A report of three cases. Clin Orthop Relat Res 1975;110:197.
99. Griswold A: Early motion in the treatment of separation of the lower femoral epiphysis: report of a case. J Bone Joint Surg 1928;10:75.
100. Grogan DP, Bobechko WP: Pathogenesis of a fracture of the distal femoral epiphysis. A case report. J Bone Joint Surg Am 1984;66:621.
101. Grogan DP, Carey TP, Leffers D, et al: Avulsion fractures of the patella. J Pediatr Orthop 1990;10:721.

102. Gronkvist H, Hirsch G, Johansson L: Fracture of the anterior tibial spine in children. J Pediatr Orthop 1984; 4:465.
103. Grood ES, Noyes FR, Butler DL, et al: Ligamentous and capsular restraints preventing straight medial and lateral laxity in intact human cadaver knees. J Bone Joint Surg Am 1981;63:1257.
104. Guzzanti V, Falciglia F, Stanitski CL: Preoperative evaluation and anterior cruciate ligament reconstruction technique for skeletally immature patients in Tanner stages 2 and 3. Am J Sports Med 2003;31:941.
105. Haas AL, Schepsis AA, Hornstein J, et al: Meniscal repair using the FasT-Fix all-inside meniscal repair device. Arthroscopy 2005;21:167.
106. Hall JE, Micheli LJ, McManama GB Jr: Semitendinosus tenodesis for recurrent subluxation or dislocation of the patella. Clin Orthop Relat Res 1979;144:31.
107. Hamberg P, Gillquist J, Lysholm J: Suture of new and old peripheral meniscus tears. J Bone Joint Surg Am 1983;65:193.
108. Hand WL, Hand CR, Dunn AW: Avulsion fractures of the tibial tubercle. J Bone Joint Surg Am 1971;53:1579.
109. Hashimoto J, Kurosaka M, Yoshiya S, et al: Meniscal repair using fibrin sealant and endothelial cell growth factor. An experimental study in dogs. Am J Sports Med 1992;20:537.
110. Hayes JM, Masear VR: Avulsion fracture of the tibial eminence associated with severe medial ligamentous injury in an adolescent. A case report and literature review. Am J Sports Med 1984;12:330.
111. Hede A, Larsen E, Sandberg H: The long term outcome of open total and partial meniscectomy related to the quantity and site of the meniscus removed. Int Orthop 1992;16:122.
112. Hede A, Larsen E, Sandberg H: Partial versus total meniscectomy. A prospective, randomised study with long-term follow-up. J Bone Joint Surg Br 1992;74:118.
113. Hede A, Larsen E, Sandberg H: [Partial versus total meniscectomy. A prospective, randomized study.] Ugeskr Laeger 1994;156:48.
114. Hillard-Sembell D, Daniel DM, Stone ML, et al: Combined injuries of the anterior cruciate and medial collateral ligaments of the knee. Effect of treatment on stability and function of the joint. J Bone Joint Surg Am 1996;78:169.
115. Houghton GR, Ackroyd CE: Sleeve fractures of the patella in children: A report of three cases. J Bone Joint Surg Br 1979;61:165.
116. Houle JB, Letts M, Yang J: Effects of a tensioned tendon graft in a bone tunnel across the rabbit physis. Clin Orthop Relat Res 2001;391:275.
117. Howe J, Johnson RJ: Knee injuries in skiing. Clin Sports Med 1982;1:277.
118. Huckell JR: Is meniscectomy a benign procedure? A long term follow-up study. Can J Surg 1965;8:254.
119. Hughston JC: Reconstruction of the extensor mechanism for subluxating patella. J Sports Med 1972;1:6.
120. Hughston JC, Bowden JA, Andrews JR, et al: Acute tears of the posterior cruciate ligament. Results of operative treatment. J Bone Joint Surg Am 1980;62:438.
121. Hughston JC, Norwood LA Jr: The posterolateral drawer test and external rotational recurvatum test for posterolateral rotatory instability of the knee. Clin Orthop Relat Res 1980;147:82.
122. Hutchinson CH, Wojtys EM: MRI versus arthroscopy in evaluating knee meniscal pathology. Am J Knee Surg 1995;8:93.
123. Insall J, Salvati E: Patella position in the normal knee joint. Radiology 1971;101:101.
124. Ishimura M, Ohgushi H, Habata T, et al: Arthroscopic meniscal repair using fibrin glue. Part I: Experimental study. Arthroscopy 1997;13:551.
125. Ishimura M, Ohgushi H, Habata T, et al: Arthroscopic meniscal repair using fibrin glue. Part II: Clinical applications. Arthroscopy 1997;13:558.
126. Ishimura M, Tamai S, Fujisawa Y: Arthroscopic meniscal repair with fibrin glue. Arthroscopy 1991;7:177.
127. Iwaya T, Takatori Y: Lateral longitudinal stress fracture of the patella: report of three cases. J Pediatr Orthop 1985;5:73.
128. Jakob RP, Hassler H, Staeubli HU: Observations on rotatory instability of the lateral compartment of the knee. Experimental studies on the functional anatomy and the pathomechanism of the true and the reversed pivot shift sign. Acta Orthop Scand Suppl 1981;191:1.
129. Janarv PM, Westblad P, Johansson C, et al: Long-term follow-up of anterior tibial spine fractures in children. J Pediatr Orthop 1995;15:63.
130. Jaureguito JW, Elliot JS, Lietner T, et al: The effects of arthroscopic partial lateral meniscectomy in an otherwise normal knee: A retrospective review of functional, clinical, and radiographic results. Arthroscopy 1995;11: 29.
131. Jones KG: Reconstruction of the anterior cruciate ligament. A technique using the central one-third of the patellar ligament. J Bone Joint Surg Am 1963;45:925.
132. Kasser JR: Physeal bar resections after growth arrest about the knee. Clin Orthop Relat Res 1990;255:68.
133. Katz JN, Harris TM, Larson MG, et al: Predictors of functional outcomes after arthroscopic partial meniscectomy. J Rheumatol 1992;19:1938.
134. Kennedy JC, Grainger RW: The posterior cruciate ligament. J Trauma 1967;7:367.
135. King AG: Meniscal lesions in children and adolescents: A review of the pathology and clinical presentation. Injury 1983;15:105.
136. King SJ, Carty HM, Brady O: Magnetic resonance imaging of knee injuries in children. Pediatr Radiol 1996;26:287.
137. Kocher MS, DiCanzio J, Zurakowski D, et al: Diagnostic performance of clinical examination and selective magnetic resonance imaging in the evaluation of intraarticular knee disorders in children and adolescents. Am J Sports Med 2001;29:292.
138. Kocher MS, Foreman ES, Micheli LJ: Laxity and functional outcome after arthroscopic reduction and internal fixation of displaced tibial spine fractures in children. Arthroscopy 2003;19:1085.
139. Kocher MS, Garg S, Micheli LJ: Physeal sparing reconstruction of the anterior cruciate ligament in skeletally immature prepubescent children and adolescents. J Bone Joint Surg Am 2005;87:2371.
140. Kocher MS, Mandiga R, Klingele K, et al: Anterior cruciate ligament injury versus tibial spine fracture in the

skeletally immature knee: A comparison of skeletal maturation and notch width index. J Pediatr Orthop 2004;24:185.
141. Kocher MS, Micheli LJ, Gerbino P, et al: Tibial eminence fractures in children: Prevalence of meniscal entrapment. Am J Sports Med 2003;31:404.
142. Kocher MS, Micheli LJ, Zurakowski D, et al: Partial tears of the anterior cruciate ligament in children and adolescents. Am J Sports Med 2002;30:697.
143. Kocher MS, Saxon HS, Hovis WD, et al: Management and complications of anterior cruciate ligament injuries in skeletally immature patients: Survey of the Herodicus Society and The ACL Study Group. J Pediatr Orthop 2002;22:452.
144. Kocher MS, Steadman JR, Briggs KK, et al: Relationships between objective assessment of ligament stability and subjective assessment of symptoms and function after anterior cruciate ligament reconstruction. Am J Sports Med 2004;32:629.
145. Kocher MS, Sterett WI, Briggs KK, et al: Effect of functional bracing on subsequent knee injury in ACL-deficient professional skiers. J Knee Surg 2003;16:87.
146. Koskinen SK, Kujala UM: Patellofemoral relationships and distal insertion of the vastus medialis muscle: A magnetic resonance imaging study in nonsymptomatic subjects and in patients with patellar dislocation. Arthroscopy 1992;8:465.
147. Kruger-Franke M, Kugler A, Trouillier HH, et al: [Clinical and radiological results after arthroscopic partial medial meniscectomy. Are there risk factors?] Unfallchirurg 1999;102:434.
148. Kruger-Franke M, Siebert CH, Kugler A, et al: Late results after arthroscopic partial medial meniscectomy. Knee Surg Sports Traumatol Arthrosc 1999;7:81.
149. Kumar SJ, Cowell HR, Townsend P: Physeal, metaphyseal, and diaphyseal injuries of the lower extremities in children with myelomeningocele. J Pediatr Orthop 1984;4:25.
150. Lambert KL: Vascularized patellar tendon graft with rigid internal fixation for anterior cruciate ligament insufficiency. Clin Orthop Relat Res 1983;172:85.
151. Lange RH, Bach AW, Hansen ST Jr, et al: Open tibial fractures with associated vascular injuries: Prognosis for limb salvage. J Trauma 1985;25:203.
152. Larsen E, Lauridsen F: Conservative treatment of patellar dislocations. Influence of evident factors on the tendency to redislocation and the therapeutic result. Clin Orthop Relat Res 1982;171:131.
153. Letts RM, Davidson D, Beaule P: Semitendinosus tenodesis for repair of recurrent dislocation of the patella in children. J Pediatr Orthop 1999;19:742.
154. Levi JH, Coleman CR: Fracture of the tibial tubercle. Am J Sports Med 1976;4:254.
155. Lipscomb AB, Anderson AF: Tears of the anterior cruciate ligament in adolescents. J Bone Joint Surg Am 1986;68:19.
156. Lombardo SJ, Harvey JP Jr: Fractures of the distal femoral epiphyses. Factors influencing prognosis: A review of thirty-four cases. J Bone Joint Surg Am 1977;59:742.
157. Loos WC, Fox JM, Blazina ME, et al: Acute posterior cruciate ligament injuries. Am J Sports Med 1981;9:86.
158. Losee RE: Concepts of the pivot shift. Clin Orthop Relat Res 1983;172:45.
159. Losee RE: Diagnosis of chronic injury to the anterior cruciate ligament. Orthop Clin North Am 1985;16:83.
160. Lowe J, Chaimsky G, Freedman A, et al: The anatomy of tibial eminence fractures: Arthroscopic observations following failed closed reduction. J Bone Joint Surg Am 2002;84:1933.
161. Luhmann SJ, Schootman M, Gordon JE, et al: Magnetic resonance imaging of the knee in children and adolescents. Its role in clinical decision-making. J Bone Joint Surg Am 2005;87:497.
162. Lyle H: Traumatic luxation of the head of the fibula. Ann Surg 1925;82:635.
163. Magee TH, Hinson GW: MRI of meniscal bucket-handle tears. Skeletal Radiol 1998;27:495.
164. Maguire JK, Canale ST: Fractures of the patella in children and adolescents. J Pediatr Orthop 1993;13:567.
165. Mah JY, Adili A, Otsuka NY, et al: Follow-up study of arthroscopic reduction and fixation of type III tibial-eminence fractures. J Pediatr Orthop 1998;18:475.
166. Mann DC, Rajmaira S: Distribution of physeal and nonphyseal fractures in 2,650 long-bone fractures in children aged 0-16 years. J Pediatr Orthop 1990;10:713.
167. Maruyama M: The all-inside meniscal suture technique using new instruments. Arthroscopy 1996;12:256.
168. Marziani R: Sulla iussazione della rotula e sul suo trattamento operativo. Arch Orthop 1930;46:797.
169. Matsusue Y, Thomson NL: Arthroscopic partial medial meniscectomy in patients over 40 years old: A 5- to 11-year follow-up study. Arthroscopy 1996;12:39.
170. Mayer PJ, Micheli LJ: Avulsion of the femoral attachment of the posterior cruciate ligament in an eleven-year-old boy. Case report. J Bone Joint Surg Am 1979; 61:431.
171. McCarroll JR, Rettig AC, Shelbourne KD: Anterior cruciate ligament injuries in the young athlete with open physes. Am J Sports Med 1988;16:44.
172. McLennan JG: Lessons learned after second-look arthroscopy in type III fractures of the tibial spine. J Pediatr Orthop 1995;15:59.
173. McManus F, Rang M, Heslin DJ: Acute dislocation of the patella in children. The natural history. Clin Orthop Relat Res 1979;139:88.
174. Medlar RC, Mandiberg JJ, Lyne ED: Meniscectomies in children. Report of long-term results (mean, 8.3 years) of 26 children. Am J Sports Med 1980;8:87.
175. Mena H, Brautigan B, Johnson DL: Split biceps femoris tendon reconstruction for proximal tibiofibular joint instability. Arthroscopy 2001;17:668.
176. Merchant AC, Mercer RL, Jacobsen RH, et al: Roentgenographic analysis of patellofemoral congruence. J Bone Joint Surg Am 1974;56:1391.
177. Meyers MH: Isolated avulsion of the tibial attachment of the posterior cruciate ligament of the knee. J Bone Joint Surg Am 1975;57:669.
178. Meyers MH, McKeever FM: Fracture of the intercondylar eminence of the tibia. J Bone Joint Surg Am 1959;41:209.
179. Meyers MH, McKeever FM: Fracture of the intercondylar eminence of the tibia. J Bone Joint Surg Am 1970; 52:1677.

180. Miller GK: A prospective study comparing the accuracy of the clinical diagnosis of meniscus tear with magnetic resonance imaging and its effect on clinical outcome. Arthroscopy 1996;12:406.
181. Millett PJ, Willis AA, Warren RF: Associated injuries in pediatric and adolescent anterior cruciate ligament tears: Does a delay in treatment increase the risk of meniscal tear? Arthroscopy 2002;18:955.
182. Miura H, Kawamura H, Arima J, et al: A new, all-inside technique for meniscus repair. Arthroscopy 1999;15:453.
183. Morgan CD: The "all-inside" meniscus repair. Arthroscopy 1991;7:120.
184. Moseley CF: A straight-line graph for leg-length discrepancies. J Bone Joint Surg Am 1977;59:174.
185. Mubarak SJ, Hargens AR, Owen CA, et al: The wick catheter technique for measurement of intramuscular pressure. A new research and clinical tool. J Bone Joint Surg Am 1976;58:1016.
186. Mylle J, Reynders P, Broos P: Transepiphysial fixation of anterior cruciate avulsion in a child. Report of a complication and review of the literature. Arch Orthop Trauma Surg 1993;112:101.
187. Neer CS 2nd: Separation of the lower femoral epiphysis. Am J Surg 1960;99:756.
188. Nietosvaara Y, Aalto K, Kallio PE: Acute patellar dislocation in children: Incidence and associated osteochondral fractures. J Pediatr Orthop 1994;14:513.
189. Nomura E: Classification of lesions of the medial patello-femoral ligament in patellar dislocation. Int Orthop 1999;23:260.
190. Nomura E, Inoue M: Cartilage lesions of the patella in recurrent patellar dislocation. Am J Sports Med 2004;32:498.
191. Noyes FR, Barber-Westin SD: The treatment of acute combined ruptures of the anterior cruciate and medial ligaments of the knee. Am J Sports Med 1995;23:380.
192. Noyes FR, Barber-Westin SD: Arthroscopic repair of meniscal tears extending into the avascular zone in patients younger than twenty years of age. Am J Sports Med 2002;30:589.
193. Noyes FR, Barber-Westin SD, Fleckenstein C, et al: The drop-jump screening test: Difference in lower limb control by gender and effect of neuromuscular training in female athletes. Am J Sports Med 2005;33:197.
194. Noyes FR, Matthews DS, Mooar PA, et al: The symptomatic anterior cruciate–deficient knee. Part II: The results of rehabilitation, activity modification, and counseling on functional disability. J Bone Joint Surg Am 1983;65:163.
195. Nummi J: Fracture of the patella. A clinical study of 707 patellar fractures. Ann Chir Gynaecol Fenn Suppl 1971;179:1.
196. Odensten M, Gillquist J: Functional anatomy of the anterior cruciate ligament and a rationale for reconstruction. J Bone Joint Surg Am 1985;67:257.
197. O'Donoghue DH: Treatment of acute ligamentous injuries of the knee. Orthop Clin North Am 1973;4:617.
198. Oetteking B: Anomalous patellae. Anat Rec 1922;23:269.
199. Ogden JA: Subluxation and dislocation of the proximal tibiofibular joint. J Bone Joint Surg Am 1974;56:145.
200. Ogden JA: Subluxation of the proximal tibiofibular joint. Clin Orthop Relat Res 1974;101:192.
201. Ogden JA, McCarthy SM, Jokl P: The painful bipartite patella. J Pediatr Orthop 1982;2:263.
202. Ogden JA, Tross RB, Murphy MJ: Fractures of the tibial tuberosity in adolescents. J Bone Joint Surg Am 1980;62:205.
203. Owen R: Recurrent dislocation of the superior tibiofibular joint. A diagnostic pitfall in knee joint derangement. J Bone Joint Surg Br 1968;50:342.
204. Panni AS, Milano G, Tartarone M, et al: Arthroscopic treatment of malunited and nonunited avulsion fractures of the anterior tibial spine. Arthroscopy 1998;14:233.
205. Pape JM, Goulet JA, Hensinger RN: Compartment syndrome complicating tibial tubercle avulsion. Clin Orthop Relat Res 1993;295:201.
206. Parker AW, Drez D Jr, Cooper JL: Anterior cruciate ligament injuries in patients with open physes. Am J Sports Med 1994;22:44.
207. Perez Carro L: Avulsion of the patellar ligament with combined fracture luxation of the proximal tibial epiphysis: Case report and review of the literature. J Orthop Trauma 1996;10:355.
208. Peterson CA, Peterson HA: Analysis of the incidence of injuries to the epiphyseal growth plate. J Trauma 1972;12:275.
209. Peterson HA: Partial growth plate arrest and its treatment. J Pediatr Orthop 1984;4:246.
210. Polakoff DR, Bucholz RW, Ogden JA: Tension band wiring of displaced tibial tuberosity fractures in adolescents. Clin Orthop Relat Res 1986;209:161.
211. Port J, Jackson DW, Lee TQ, et al: Meniscal repair supplemented with exogenous fibrin clot and autogenous cultured marrow cells in the goat model. Am J Sports Med 1996;24:547.
212. Poulsen TD, Skak SV, Jensen TT: Epiphyseal fractures of the proximal tibia. Injury 1989;20:111.
213. Raber DA, Friederich NF, Hefti F: Discoid lateral meniscus in children. Long-term follow-up after total meniscectomy. J Bone Joint Surg Am 1998;80:1579.
214. Rand T, Imhof H, Breitenseher M, et al: [Comparison of diagnostic sensitivity in meniscus diagnosis of MRI examinations with a 0.2 T low-field and a 1.5 T high field system.] Radiologe 1997;37:802.
215. Rang M: Children's Fractures. Philadelphia, JB Lippincott, 1974.
216. Ray JM, Hendrix J: Incidence, mechanism of injury, and treatment of fractures of the patella in children. J Trauma 1992;32:464.
217. Reider B, Marshall JL, Koslin B, et al: The anterior aspect of the knee joint. J Bone Joint Surg Am 1981;63:351.
218. Reider B, Marshall JL, Warren RF: Clinical characteristics of patellar disorders in young athletes. Am J Sports Med 1981;9:270.
219. Reigel CA, Mulhollan JS, Morgan CD: Arthroscopic all-inside meniscus repair. Clin Sports Med 1996;15:483.
220. Riseborough EJ, Barrett IR, Shapiro F: Growth disturbances following distal femoral physeal fracture-separations. J Bone Joint Surg Am 1983;65:885.

221. Ritchie JR, Miller MD, Bents RT, et al: Meniscal repair in the goat model. The use of healing adjuncts on central tears and the role of magnetic resonance arthrography in repair evaluation. Am J Sports Med 1998;26:278.
222. Roberts JM, Lovell WW: Fractures of the intercondylar eminence of the tibia. J Bone Joint Surg Am 1970;52:827.
223. Robins AJ, Newman AP, Burks RT: Postoperative return of motion in anterior cruciate ligament and medial collateral ligament injuries. The effect of medial collateral ligament rupture location. Am J Sports Med 1993;21:20.
224. Rodeo SA, Warren RF: Meniscal repair using the outside-to-inside technique. Clin Sports Med 1996;15:469.
225. Rorabeck CH, Bobechko WP: Acute dislocation of the patella with osteochondral fracture: A review of eighteen cases. J Bone Joint Surg Br 1976;58:237.
226. Ross AC, Chesterman PJ: Isolated avulsion of the tibial attachment of the posterior cruciate ligament in childhood. J Bone Joint Surg Br 1986;68:747.
227. Sallay PI, Poggi J, Speer KP, et al: Acute dislocation of the patella. A correlative pathoanatomic study. Am J Sports Med 1996;24:52.
228. Salter RB, Czitrom AA, Willis RB: Fractures involving the distal femoral epiphyseal plate. In Kennedy JC (ed): Injury to the Adolescent Knee. Baltimore, Williams & Wilkins, 1979.
229. Salter RB, Harris WR: Injuries involving the epiphyseal plate. J Bone Joint Surg Am 1963;45:587.
230. Sanders TG, Morrison WB, Singleton BA, et al: Medial patellofemoral ligament injury following acute transient dislocation of the patella: MR findings with surgical correlation in 14 patients. J Comput Assist Tomogr 2001;25:957.
231. Sanders WE, Wilkins KE, Neidre A: Acute insufficiency of the posterior cruciate ligament in children. Two case reports. J Bone Joint Surg Am 1980;62:129.
232. Scapinelli R: Blood supply of the human patella. Its relation to ischaemic necrosis after fracture. J Bone Joint Surg Br 1967;49:563.
233. Schierl M, Petermann J, Trus P, et al: Anterior cruciate and medial collateral ligament injury. ACL reconstruction and functional treatment of the MCL. Knee Surg Sports Traumatol Arthrosc 1994;2:203.
234. Schimmer RC, Brulhart KB, Duff C, et al: Arthroscopic partial meniscectomy: A 12-year follow-up and two-step evaluation of the long-term course. Arthroscopy 1998;14:136.
235. Schoenbauer H: Bruche der Kniescheibe. Ergeb Chir Orthop 1959;42:56.
236. Schulte KR, Fu FH: Meniscal repair using the inside-to-outside technique. Clin Sports Med 1996;15:455.
237. Scott GA, Jolly BL, Henning CE: Combined posterior incision and arthroscopic intra-articular repair of the meniscus. An examination of factors affecting healing. J Bone Joint Surg Am 1986;68:847.
238. Seitz H, Marlovits S, Wielke T, et al: [Meniscus lesions after isolated anterior cruciate ligament rupture.] Wien Klin Wochenschr 1996;108:727.
239. Sekiya JK, Kuhn JE: Instability of the proximal tibiofibular joint. J Am Acad Orthop Surg 2003;11:120.
240. Senavongse W, Amis AA: The effects of articular, retinacular, or muscular deficiencies on patellofemoral joint stability. J Bone Joint Surg Br 2005;87:577.
241. Senekovic V, Veselko M: Anterograde arthroscopic fixation of avulsion fractures of the tibial eminence with a cannulated screw: Five-year results. Arthroscopy 2003;19:54.
242. Shapiro GS, Fanton GS, Dillingham MF: Reconstruction for recurrent dislocation of the proximal tibiofibular joint. A new technique. Orthop Rev 1993;22:1229.
243. Shelbourne K, Mesko J: Combined posterior cruciate-medial collateral ligament rupture: Mechanism of injury. J Knee Surg 1990;3:41.
244. Shelbourne KD, Pierce RO, Ritter MA: Superior dislocation of the fibular head associated with a tibia fracture. Clin Orthop Relat Res 1981;160:172.
245. Shelbourne KD, Porter DA: Anterior cruciate ligament–medial collateral ligament injury: Nonoperative management of medial collateral ligament tears with anterior cruciate ligament reconstruction. A preliminary report. Am J Sports Med 1992;20:283.
246. Shelbourne KD, Whitaker HJ, McCarroll JR, et al: Anterior cruciate ligament injury: Evaluation of intraarticular reconstruction of acute tears without repair. Two to seven year followup of 155 athletes. Am J Sports Med 1990;18:484.
247. Shelton WR, Canale ST: Fractures of the tibia through the proximal tibial epiphyseal cartilage. J Bone Joint Surg Am 1979;61:167.
248. Shino K, Horibe S, Nakata K, et al: Conservative treatment of isolated injuries to the posterior cruciate ligament in athletes. J Bone Joint Surg Br 1995;77:895.
249. Sinding-Larsen M: A hitherto unknown affection of the patella in children. Acta Radiol 1922;1:171.
250. Skie MC, Mekhail AO, Deitrich DR, et al: Operative technique for inside-out repair of the triangular fibrocartilage complex. J Hand Surg [Am] 1997;22:814.
251. Smillie IS: Injuries of the Knee. Edinburgh, E & S Livingstone, 1951.
252. Smith JB: Knee instability after fractures of the intercondylar eminence of the tibia. J Pediatr Orthop 1984;4:462.
253. Smith L: A concealed injury to the knee. J Bone Joint Surg Am 1962;44:1659.
254. Snedcor S, Wilson H: Some obstetrical injuries to the long bones. J Bone Joint Surg Am 1949;31:378.
255. Sommerlath KG: Results of meniscal repair and partial meniscectomy in stable knees. Int Orthop 1991;15:347.
256. Soutter FE: Spina bifida and epiphysial displacement. Report of two cases. J Bone Joint Surg Br 1962;44:106.
257. Stanitski CL, Harvell JC, Fu F: Observations on acute knee hemarthrosis in children and adolescents. J Pediatr Orthop 1993;13:506.
258. Steadman JR, Miller BS, Karas SG, et al: The microfracture technique in the treatment of full-thickness chondral lesions of the knee in National Football League players. J Knee Surg 2003;16:83.
259. Steadman JR, Rodkey WG, Briggs KK: Microfracture to treat full-thickness chondral defects: Surgical

technique, rehabilitation, and outcomes. J Knee Surg 2002;15:170.
260. Steiner ME, Hecker AT, Brown CH Jr, et al: Anterior cruciate ligament graft fixation. Comparison of hamstring and patellar tendon grafts. Am J Sports Med 1994;22:240.
261. Stephens DC, Louis E, Louis DS: Traumatic separation of the distal femoral epiphyseal cartilage plate. J Bone Joint Surg Am 1974;56:1383.
262. Swartz EE, Decoster LC, Russell PJ, et al: Effects of developmental stage and sex on lower extremity kinematics and vertical ground reaction forces during landing. J Athl Train 2005;40:9.
263. Takeda Y, Ikata T, Yoshida S, et al: MRI high-signal intensity in the menisci of asymptomatic children. J Bone Joint Surg Br 1998;80:463.
264. Tapper EM, Hoover NW: Late results after meniscectomy. J Bone Joint Surg Am 1969;51:517.
265. Teitge RA: The treatment of complications of patellofemoral joint surgery. Operat Tech Sports Med 1994;2: 317.
266. ten Thije JH, Frima AJ: Patellar dislocation and osteochondral fractures. Neth J Surg 1986;38:150.
267. Tolo VT: External skeletal fixation in children's fractures. J Pediatr Orthop 1983;3:435.
268. Tolo VT: External fixation in multiply injured children. Orthop Clin North Am 1990;21:393.
269. Torg JS, Pavlov H, Morris VB: Salter-Harris type-III fracture of the medial femoral condyle occurring in the adolescent athlete. J Bone Joint Surg Am 1981;63:586.
270. Torisu T: Isolated avulsion fracture of the tibial attachment of the posterior cruciate ligament. J Bone Joint Surg Am 1977;59:68.
271. Trickey EL: Rupture of the posterior cruciate ligament of the knee. J Bone Joint Surg Br 1968;50:334.
272. Tsai CL, Liu TK, Liu CN, et al: [Meniscal repair with autogenous periosteum and fibrin adhesive system.] Zhonghua Yi Xue Za Zhi (Taipei) 1992;49:170.
273. Vahvanen V, Aalto K: Meniscectomy in children. Acta Orthop Scand 1979;50:791.
274. van Trommel MF, Simonian PT, Potter HG, et al: Arthroscopic meniscal repair with fibrin clot of complete radial tears of the lateral meniscus in the avascular zone. Arthroscopy 1998;14:360.
275. Vaquero J, Vidal C, Cubillo A: Intra-articular traumatic disorders of the knee in children and adolescents. Clin Orthop Relat Res 2005;432:97.
276. Warren LF, Marshall JL: The supporting structures and layers on the medial side of the knee: an anatomical analysis. J Bone Joint Surg Am 1979;61:56.
277. Watson-Jones R: Fractures and Joint Injuries. New York, Churchill Livingstone, 1982.
278. Weber MJ, Janecki CJ, McLeod P, et al: Efficacy of various forms of fixation of transverse fractures of the patella. J Bone Joint Surg Am 1980;62:215.
279. Weinert CR Jr, Raczka R: Recurrent dislocation of the superior tibiofibular joint. Surgical stabilization by ligament reconstruction. J Bone Joint Surg Am 1986; 68:126.
280. Weiss CB, Lundberg M, Hamberg P, et al: Nonoperative treatment of meniscal tears. J Bone Joint Surg Am 1989;71:811.
281. Welch PH, Wynne GF Jr: Proximal tibial epiphyseal fracture-separation: Case report. J Bone Joint Surg Am 1963;45:782.
282. Wester W, Canale ST, Dutkowsky JP, et al: Prediction of angular deformity and leg-length discrepancy after anterior cruciate ligament reconstruction in skeletally immature patients. J Pediatr Orthop 1994;14:516.
283. Whitesides TE, Haney TC, Morimoto K, et al: Tissue pressure measurements as a determinant for the need of fasciotomy. Clin Orthop Relat Res 1975;113:43.
284. Wiley JJ, Baxter MP: Tibial spine fractures in children. Clin Orthop Relat Res 1990;255:54.
285. Willis RB, Blokker C, Stoll TM, et al: Long-term follow-up of anterior tibial eminence fractures. J Pediatr Orthop 1993;13:361.
286. Wiss DA, Schilz JL, Zionts L: Type III fractures of the tibial tubercle in adolescents. J Orthop Trauma 1991; 5:475.
287. Wood KB, Bradley JP, Ward WT: Pes anserinus interposition in a proximal tibial physeal fracture. A case report. Clin Orthop Relat Res 1991;264:239.
288. Wozasek GE, Moser KD, Haller H, et al: Trauma involving the proximal tibial epiphysis. Arch Orthop Trauma Surg 1991;110:301.
289. Wu CD, Huang SC, Liu TK: Sleeve fracture of the patella in children. A report of five cases. Am J Sports Med 1991;19:525.
290. Zaman TM, Roberts J, Oni OO, et al: MRI findings in simultaneous bilateral meniscal lesions. Injury 1997;28: 303.
291. Zantop T, Eggers AK, Musahl V, et al: Cyclic testing of flexible all-inside meniscus suture anchors: biomechanical analysis. Am J Sports Med 2005;33:388.

TIBIA AND FIBULA

Anatomy

The tibia has a triangular shape with an anteriorly directed apex that gradually broadens distally. The anteromedial surface of the tibia has no muscular or ligamentous attachments distal to the pes anserinus and has a mildly concave shape in the mid-diaphyseal area. This anteromedial surface is immediately subcutaneous and easily palpable. The anterolateral surface has many muscular attachments and forms the medial wall of the anterior compartment of the leg. The tibialis anterior, extensor hallucis longus, and the neurovascular bundle are adjacent to this surface. Posteriorly, the tibia has a large soft tissue envelope with attachments from the semimembranosus, popliteus, soleus, tibialis posterior, and flexor digitorum longus muscles. The anterolateral and posterior aspects of the tibia are not palpable.

The fibula is subcutaneous proximally and has attachments from the LCL and the biceps femoris to the fibular head. At its proximal end the peroneal nerve travels anteriorly over the distal aspect of the fibular head and then divides into superficial and deep portions. A large soft tissue envelope surrounds the fibula and is composed predominantly of muscular attachments. The lateral malleolus is the distal aspect of the fibula. It articulates with the distal tibia and talus and provides significant stability to the ankle joint. In the midleg area the tibia and fibula are connected through a thick interosseous membrane running between the lateral crest of the tibia and the anteromedial border of the fibula. The anterior tibial artery and vein course over the interosseous membrane and enter the anterior compartment of the leg.

Three ossification centers arise to form the tibia. The tibial diaphysis ossifies at 7 weeks' gestation, the proximal epiphysis appears a few months after birth, and the distal epiphysis develops in the second year of life. The fibular diaphysis ossifies at 8 weeks' gestation, whereas the proximal secondary center of ossification appears at 4 years and the distal epiphysis at 2 years. Closure of the proximal physis occurs between 16 and 18 years, and the distal physis usually closes at 16 years.

The blood supply to the tibia comes from three main areas: the nutrient artery, a branch of the posterior tibial artery that provides the endosteal and medullary supply; the epiphyseal vessels; and the periosteal vessels.[79] The nutrient artery enters the posterior aspect of the proximal portion of the tibia and then courses proximally and distally to anastomose with the metaphyseal endosteal vessels (Fig. 43–136). The inner two thirds of the tibial diaphysis is supplied by this nutrient artery and the outer third by the anastomosing periosteal vessels.[80] After a fracture of the tibia, the peripheral vessels are recruited to supply the majority of blood flow to the tibial cortex for revascularization of necrotic areas.[79,80,102]

There are four compartments in the leg (Fig. 43–137). The anterior compartment contains the dorsiflexors of the ankle and toes (the tibialis anterior, extensor hallucis longus, and extensor digitorum communis) and the neurovascular bundle, which consists of the anterior tibial artery and vein and the deep peroneal nerve. The artery is assessed through palpation of the dorsalis pedis pulse, and the nerve provides sensation between the first and second toes. The lateral compartment contains the peroneus brevis and longus muscles and the superficial peroneal nerve, which provides sensation to the dorsum of the foot. The superficial posterior compartment contains the ankle flexors, the gastrocnemius, the plantaris muscles, and the sural nerve, which provides sensation to the lateral aspect of the heel. The deep posterior compartment contains the posterior tibial vessels, the peroneal artery, the tibial nerve, the flexor digitorum longus, the flexor hallucis longus, the tibialis posterior, and the plantar intrinsic muscles.

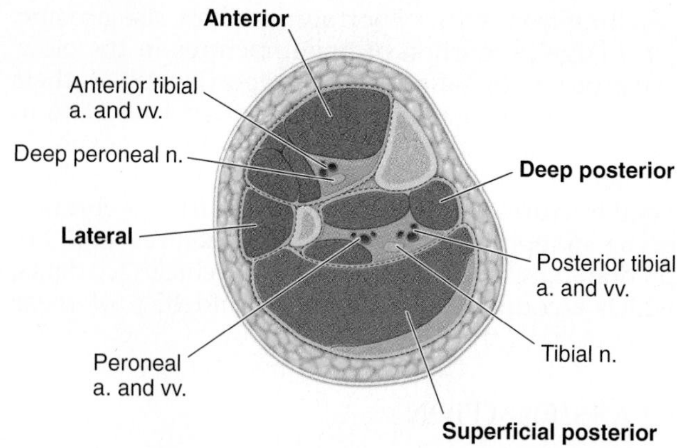

FIGURE 43–137 The four compartments of the leg.

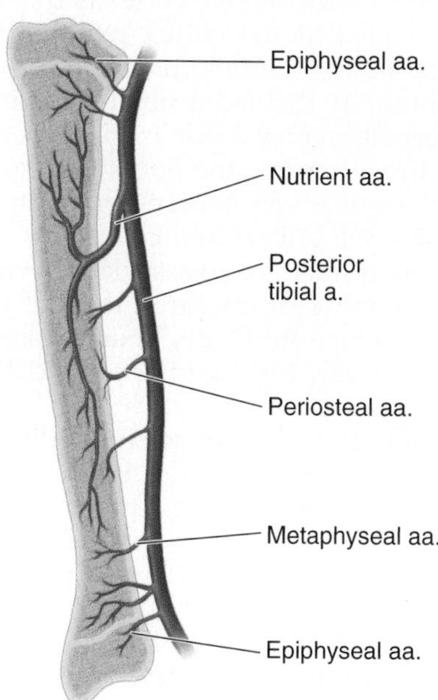

FIGURE 43–136 Blood supply to the tibial diaphysis.

Tibial and Fibular Fractures

Diaphyseal fractures of the tibia and fibula are common in children, being third in frequency, after fractures of the femur and both-bone forearm fractures. They occur most commonly in boys younger than 10 years. The mechanism depends on the age of the child, with more benign fractures occurring in the younger age group. The typical tibial fracture is usually treated by external immobilization, with or without reduction, and outcomes are generally good. Open fracture, which is relatively rare, requires meticulous evaluation and treatment, with generally satisfactory results.

MECHANISM OF INJURY

Tibial fractures in children can be due to indirect or direct trauma, and fractures vary with the age of the child. In an infant and child younger than 4 years, an indirect injury caused by a fall from a height or from a standing position or a bicycle spoke injury results in a spiral or oblique fracture.[20,50,112] In a child older than 4 years, the most common injury is the result of a pedestrian accident in which the child is struck by a car and sustains a complete, often comminuted fracture.[50,93,101,112] Shannak reported 63% of tibial fractures to be due to road traffic accidents, with 18%

resulting from falls.[93] Sporting activities also account for a large proportion of tibial fractures in the older age group, with Yang and Letts reporting 41% of their cases to be due to skiing or skating accidents, 40% to be due to falls, and only 16% to be due to motor vehicle accidents.[112] Child abuse accounts for less than 5% of tibial fractures in children.[50] Open injuries in children occur in up to 8% of all tibial fractures and are predominantly incurred in motor vehicle accidents, which account for between 75% and 85% of these injuries.[11,31,43,51,82,98]

CLASSIFICATION

Tibial and fibular fractures that do not involve the physis are best classified by the anatomic location of the fracture: proximal metaphyseal, diaphyseal, and distal metaphyseal fractures. Diaphyseal fractures are further subdivided into proximal, middle, and distal third fractures. The configuration of the fracture is defined as a torus or compression, greenstick, or complete fracture. Standard nomenclature applicable to all diaphyseal fractures should be used for classification, including the amount of angulation and displacement, the presence and degree of comminution, whether a segmental fracture is present, and whether there is an open injury, which can be defined according to the Gustilo and Anderson classification.[33] All these factors play a role in determining treatment and the prognosis of these fractures.

CLINICAL FEATURES

A good history should be obtained from the patient, parents, or other witnesses. It is important to determine whether the mechanism of injury was a direct or indirect force. Direct trauma to the leg, such as being run over by a motor vehicle, may have grave complications because the soft tissue injury is much greater than may be apparent on the initial examination. Often the mechanism of injury in a young child is uncertain, with the only information being pain over the tibia and an inability to walk.

Physical examination begins with inspection of the leg for soft tissue injury, including evidence of an open injury. Frequently there is no obvious deformity of the leg because the majority of tibial fractures are undisplaced or minimally displaced. In a young child who is unable to ambulate, palpation of the thigh and leg is necessary to help define the location of the injury. In an older child who is able to point to the location of the pain, it is not necessary to deeply palpate the leg in an attempt to identify the fracture. However, it is of paramount importance to assess the condition of the soft tissue envelope surrounding the leg at the time of initial evaluation, especially in a child who has sustained direct trauma to the leg in a pedestrian–motor vehicle accident or a severe twisting injury to the leg. Although compartment syndromes are relatively rare in a child with a tibial fracture, a full assessment should include evaluation of the pain elicited on passive dorsiflexion and plantar flexion of the toes; a complete neurologic examination, including a motor and sensory examination; palpation of the distal pulses; and assessment of capillary refill time. At completion of the physical examination the injured leg should be splinted if transport of the patient is necessary.

RADIOGRAPHIC FINDINGS

Radiographic examination consists of AP and lateral radiographs of the leg to include the knee and ankle joints. Most fractures of the tibia can be seen on at least one view of the tibia; however, in a young child with a nondisplaced fracture, a radiograph of the contralateral leg is occasionally used for comparison.

Rarely are further diagnostic studies required for a patient with a tibial fracture. Instances in which further tests are needed include a suspected occult fracture, in which a technetium-enhanced bone scan can detect the fracture, which appears as mildly increased uptake along the entire length of the tibia,[57,74,77] and a pathologic fracture, in which CT may be helpful to define the extent and nature of the lesion. A skeletal survey or bone scan may be indicated if child abuse is suspected.

Proximal Tibial Metaphyseal Fractures

Fractures of the proximal aspect of the tibia are most common in the 3- to 6-year-old age group and are usually nondisplaced complete fractures or greenstick fractures.[29,36,49,60,81,107,117,118]

MECHANISM OF INJURY

The mechanism of injury is generally a torsional stress applied to the medial aspect of the leg or a direct blow to the lateral aspect of the extended knee.

The most common fracture pattern is a greenstick fracture in which the medial cortex is fractured while the lateral aspect of the cortex remains intact (Fig. 43–138). The fibula is often not fractured in a greenstick or minimally displaced tibial fracture, although plastic deformation may occur. In high-energy injuries involving direct trauma, the fibula is frequently fractured despite a relatively benign-appearing tibial fracture (Fig. 43–139). Robert and colleagues reported 13 proximal fibular fractures in association with 25 proximal tibial metaphyseal fractures, most of which were due to motor vehicle accidents.[81] Neurovascular injury is rare in minimally displaced or greenstick proximal tibial fractures.

The second major type of proximal tibial metaphyseal fracture, a complete fracture, is much less common and involves significant high-energy trauma in an older child. This type of injury was discussed previously under Proximal Tibial Physeal Fractures.

CLINICAL FEATURES AND RADIOGRAPHIC FINDINGS

A patient with the typical proximal metaphyseal fracture usually has pain in the proximal aspect of the

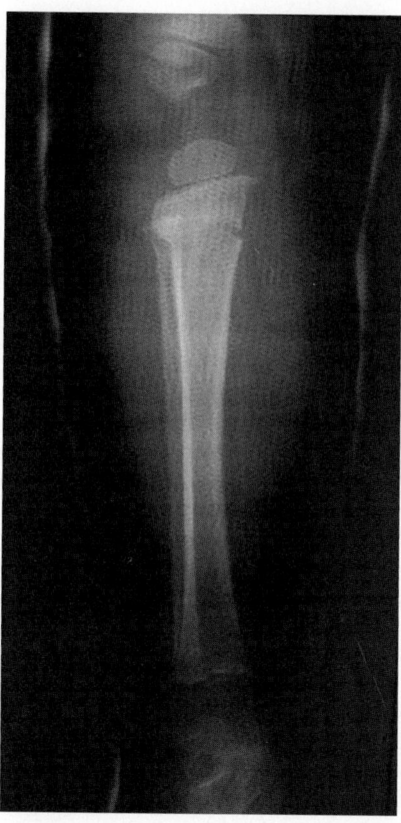

FIGURE 43–138 Proximal tibial fracture demonstrating a greenstick injury to the lateral cortex and a medial cortical fracture.

tibia, minimal soft tissue swelling, and little or no clinical deformity. Radiographic examination reveals three basic fracture patterns: torus, greenstick, and complete fractures, with the majority of fractures being nondisplaced. Robert and colleagues reported 9 torus, 10 greenstick, and 6 complete fractures. All torus fractures were nondisplaced, and approximately 50% of greenstick and complete fractures were displaced at the time of the initial injury.[81]

TREATMENT

Treatment of proximal tibial metaphyseal fractures is nonoperative in the majority of cases. We prefer to have the patient under conscious sedation to obtain a reduction when there is valgus deformity of the tibia after injury. An angled greenstick fracture of the proximal tibia should be broken through by bending the leg toward the angulation and slightly overcorrecting the deformity. The leg is then placed in a long-leg cast with three-point fixation to maintain the reduction. After reduction, a true AP radiograph of the tibia should be taken to document normal alignment, and a radiograph of the contralateral leg can be obtained for comparison. The patient is kept non–weight bearing while in the long-leg cast, and serial radiographs are obtained for the first 2 weeks to ensure maintenance of alignment. The long-leg cast should be worn for approximately 5 to 7 weeks, depending on the age of the child.

After the cast is removed, the patient can be fully weight bearing and should be monitored at regular

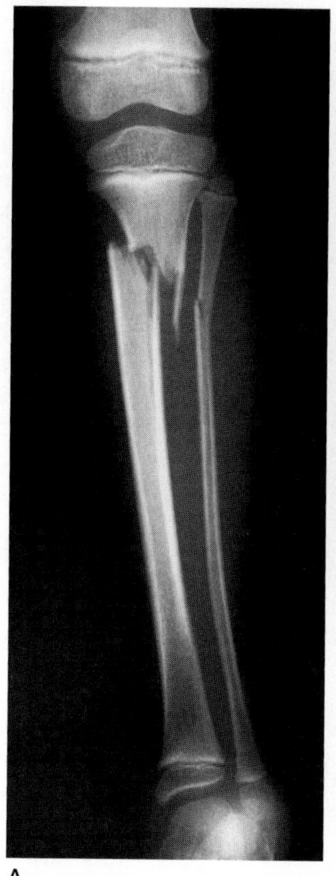

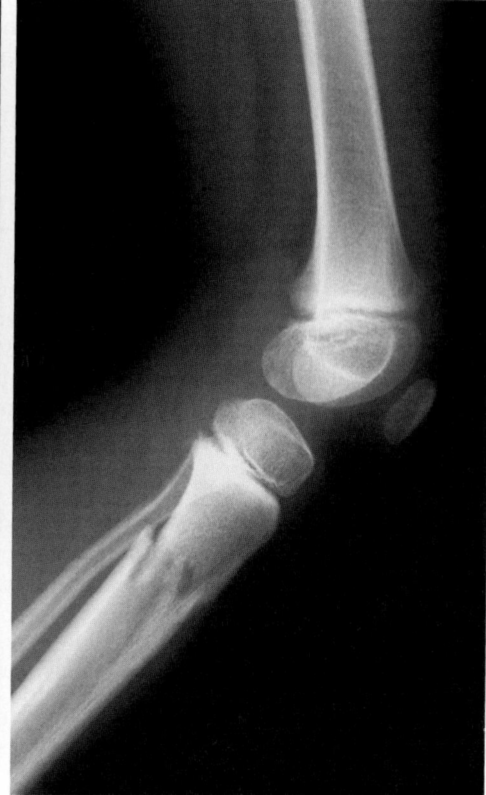

A B

FIGURE 43–139 **A** and **B,** High-energy proximal tibial fracture in which the proximal fibula was also fractured.

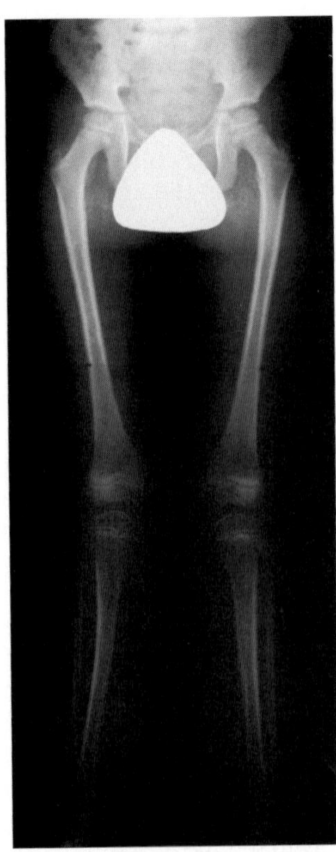

FIGURE 43–140 Spontaneous improvement of a valgus deformity of the proximal tibia in a young child.

intervals of approximately 3 to 6 months. The evolution of a developing valgus deformity has been characterized.* The time at which deformity is greatest is between 12 and 18 months after injury, with an average maximum deformity of 18 degrees.[107] Resolution of the deformity generally takes place within 3 years of the initial injury, with correction occurring through both the proximal and distal physes.[3,97] Residual radiographic deformity averaging 6 degrees persists, with the knee slightly medial to the mechanical axis; however, this is not usually apparent clinically (Fig. 43–140).[107]

Operative treatment is rarely indicated for these fractures. The only exception is when closed reduction fails to reduce the valgus deformity, most often because of soft tissue interposition (pes anserinus, periosteum, or the MCL). A small medial incision is made over the fracture site, the soft tissue interposition is removed, and anatomic reduction is performed under direct vision. We recommend suturing the torn periosteum and applying a long-leg cast. If fracture stability is a concern, Kirschner wires can be placed in crossed fashion, but no internal plate fixation is required for these fractures.

COMPLICATIONS

The most common complication or difficulty encountered with proximal metaphyseal fractures is a valgus deformity, which develops within the first 6 months and continues to progress up to 2 years after injury (Fig. 43–141).* The likelihood of tibial valgus' developing after a proximal tibial metaphyseal fracture must be discussed with the parents at the time of initial treatment and reiterated at each subsequent visit.

Several theories have been proposed to explain the development of post-traumatic tibial valgus deformity: lack of initial accurate reduction, early weight bearing, tethering of the iliotibial tract, tethering by the intact fibula, soft tissue interposition, asymmetric growth of the proximal tibial epiphysis, and injury to the lateral proximal tibial physis.

- The theory of inadequate reduction was proposed early because of the apparently innocuous nature of these fractures and the initial lack of attempted reduction.[2,6,78,89] However, there are reports of post-traumatic valgus' developing after adequate fracture reduction, including over-reduction of the tibia into varus.[49]
- Early weight bearing has been postulated to result in compressive forces on the lateral aspect of the tibia and distractive forces on the medial aspect, thereby leading to increased valgus,[6,76,89] although valgus deformity has occurred in nonambulatory patients after these fractures.[62]
- Soft tissue imbalance with tethering of the iliotibial tract on the lateral aspect of the tibia or disruption of the pes anserinus on the medial aspect has been proposed as a cause of valgus deformity.[109] Similarly, some believe that the fibula tethers the tibia and results in overgrowth on the medial side and inhibition of growth laterally.[104,109]
- Soft tissue interposition has been reported by many authors, with the most common offending tissues being the pes anserinus, periosteum, and MCL.[44,81,108,109] Weber reported two cases of post-traumatic tibia valgus that were explored and interposed pes anserinus removed, followed by uncomplicated fracture healing.[109] However, others have reported valgus deformity after similar treatment.[81]
- Asymmetric growth of the proximal tibial epiphysis caused by premature arrest of the lateral portion has been postulated to cause tibial valgus.[64] One proposed mechanism is that a valgus moment creates a Salter-Harris type V injury of the lateral epiphysis that results in asymmetric growth between the medial and lateral aspects of the proximal tibia.[49,69] Asymmetric growth has also been theorized to develop as a result of an asymmetric vascular response to injury.[16,36,117]

It is often difficult to persuade concerned parents that the marked valgus deformity will improve with time because they have observed a progressive, worsening deformity for up to 18 months after injury. The

*See references 10, 16, 29, 70, 81, 97, 104, 108, 109, 117.

*See references 3-6, 10, 29, 36, 42, 44, 49, 56, 60, 81, 83, 89, 107, 108, 117, 118.

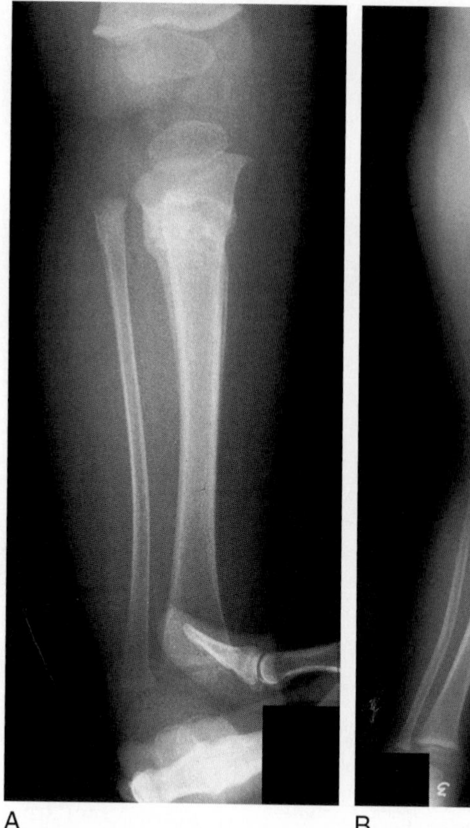

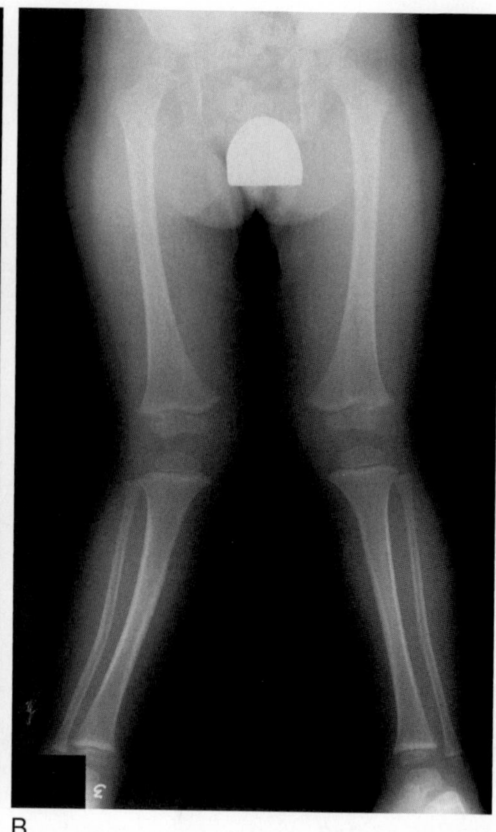

FIGURE 43–141 Valgus deformity after a proximal metaphyseal tibial fracture in a 3-year-old boy. **A,** Radiograph showing the fracture. **B,** One year later there was obvious valgus deformity of the injured leg.

deformity resolves gradually over a period of years. It is important for the surgeon to avoid the temptation to perform a varus tibial osteotomy for two main reasons. The first is that the osteotomy may initiate the same process that the fracture caused and result in recurrence of the deformity. The second is the significant incidence of compartment syndrome. Robert and colleagues reported that after four varus osteotomies performed for post-traumatic valgus deformity, valgus deformity recurred in two patients and compartment syndrome occurred in two.[81] Balthazar and Pappas described nine patients in whom a valgus deformity developed after treatment of a proximal tibial fracture.[3] Six underwent a corrective osteotomy, but all did poorly, with recurrence of the valgus deformity.[3] Others have reported similar results.[10,36]

We prefer to treat residual valgus deformity if it is greater than 15 to 20 degrees. Treatment with a well-timed medial proximal tibial epiphysiodesis is best performed near the end of growth (Fig. 43–142). The indications for a varus osteotomy in a younger child are limited and include severe valgus deformity (>20 degrees) that persists for at least 3 years after injury. A fibular osteotomy and a tibial osteotomy are performed proximally and must be accompanied by fasciotomy of the anterior and lateral compartments of the leg. We prefer to internally fix the fracture with crossed Kirschner wires. The patient wears a long-leg cast until healing occurs, usually around 6 weeks.

In addition to the angular deformity after these injuries, overgrowth of the affected extremity is also seen and averages approximately 1.0 cm, with maximum overgrowth of 1.7 cm.[107,118] The overall outcome in these patients is universally good with respect to daily activities; however, some complain of occasional knee discomfort with strenuous athletic activities.[107]

Tibial and Fibular Diaphyseal Fractures

Fractures of the diaphysis of the tibia are of two major types, displaced and nondisplaced, depending on the age of the child and the mechanism of injury. In a child younger than 11 years, the fracture is typically a nondisplaced or minimally displaced fracture of the tibia, often without an associated fracture of the fibula. The fracture pattern in a child younger than 6 years is generally an oblique or spiral fracture with minimal displacement. The mechanism of injury is usually indirect trauma resulting from a fall or a twisting injury. In children 6 to 11 years of age, the most common fracture is a simple transverse fracture with a fractured fibula; it typically results from direct trauma. In adolescents, fractures of the tibia are usually associated with fibular fractures, are due to higher energy trauma, and behave as adult fractures.

MECHANISM OF INJURY

Shannak reported on 117 children with tibial shaft fractures; their average age was 8 years and the male-to-female ratio was 2.7:1.[93] In a study by Karrsholm and

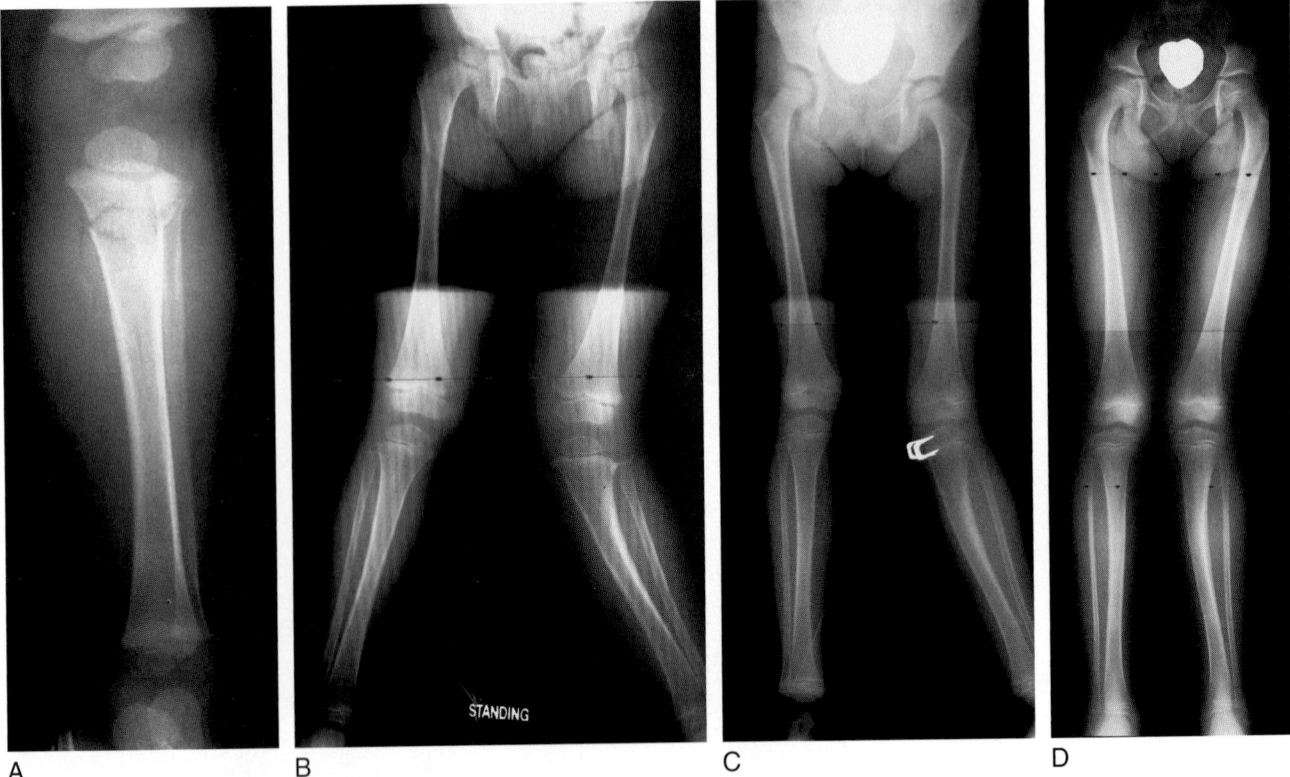

FIGURE 43–142 Epiphysiodesis to correct residual proximal tibial valgus deformity after a fracture in a 12-month-old girl. **A,** Injury radiograph showing the proximal tibial fracture. **B,** Three years later there was progressive valgus deformity. **C,** Medial proximal tibial physeal stapling was performed. **D,** Two years after physeal stapling the valgus deformity has resolved.

colleagues, the peak incidences in boys were undisplaced fractures at 3 to 4 years of age and transverse fractures resulting from athletic and motor vehicle accidents at 15 to 16 years.[50] In girls the incidence was more evenly distributed up to 11 or 12 years of age, with a steady decline thereafter.[50] The mechanism of injury is thought to be predominantly indirect trauma; however, this varies among series, depending on the geographic location. In northern climates, 30% to 40% of tibial fractures occur while skiing or skating, 30% of injuries result from falls, and 15% to 25% of tibial fractures result from motor vehicle accidents.[38,50,112] In more temperate climates, motor vehicle accidents can account for up to 63% of tibial fractures.[93] Child abuse accounts for up to 3% of these injuries[112] and bicycle spoke injuries account for 7% to 10% of injuries.[50]

CLASSIFICATION

Tibial fractures in children are located in the proximal third in 13%, in the middle third in 45%, and in the lower third in 42%.[93] Approximately 70% of all children's tibial fractures have an associated fibular fracture.[9,50,93] Open fractures are rare in children, occurring in less than 5% of all tibial fractures,[50,93] are associated with delayed union, and have a relatively high complication rate when compared with closed fractures.[11,31,43,51,82,98]

CLINICAL FEATURES

In a young child, very little history may be available because of an unwitnessed event or an event that was not thought to cause a fracture. A young patient may refuse to ambulate or may ambulate with a significant limp. No deformity is present, and there is little swelling; however, there is tenderness on palpation at the fracture site. In contrast, an older child with a complete tibial fracture, with or without a fibular fracture, will have sustained fairly significant trauma, will be unable to ambulate, and may have a significant deformity. The mechanism of injury should be elicited, especially the nature of the deforming force and whether a crush-type injury occurred. This information is important to have at the outset so that special precautions can be taken to diagnose and treat compartment syndrome.

The physical examination in any child with a tibial fracture includes assessment of the clinical deformity and a search for evidence of an open soft tissue injury.[33] The soft tissue envelope should be palpated and assessed for the presence of an impending compartment syndrome. This examination includes passive flexion and extension of the toes, assessment of capillary refill time, and a thorough neurologic evaluation. An associated vascular injury is rare in these injuries; however, the posterior tibial and dorsalis pedis pulses should be evaluated.

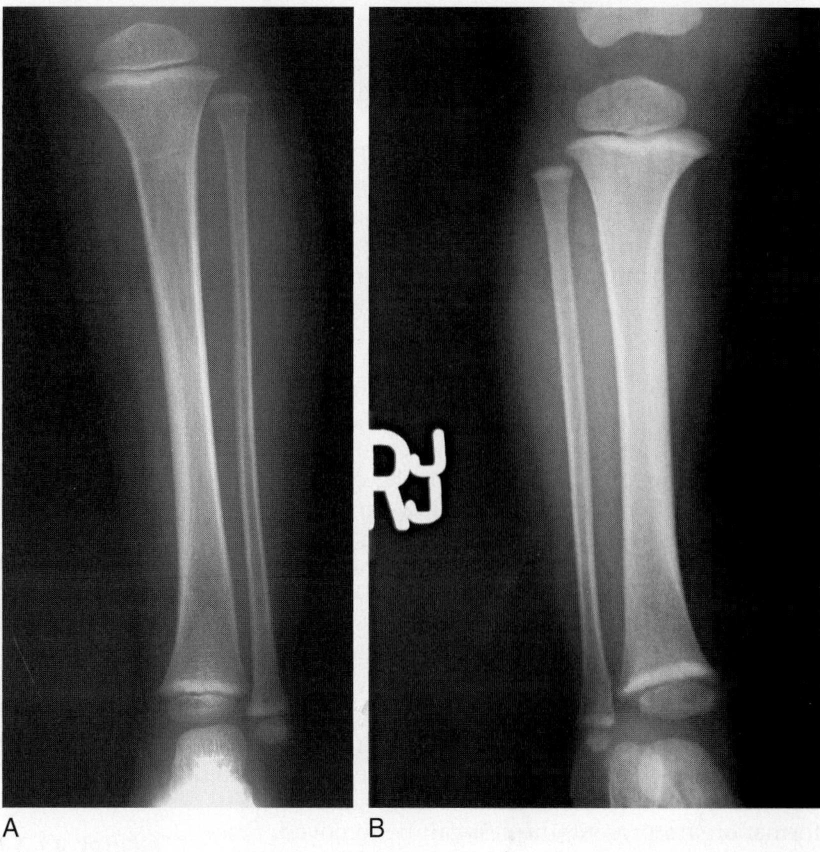

FIGURE 43–143 Diagnosis of an undisplaced tibial fracture in an infant. **A,** Radiographic appearance. The undisplaced distal tibial fracture is difficult to identify. **B,** A contralateral radiograph used for comparison helps the examiner identify the fracture in the injured leg.

RADIOGRAPHIC FINDINGS

Radiographic evaluation should include AP and lateral radiographs of the tibia that include the knee and the ankle joints. Rarely are contralateral views necessary; however, an undisplaced, incomplete fracture is not always easily seen, and comparison views should be taken in this circumstance (Fig. 43–143). Stress fractures are not often seen early and are confirmed by CT, MRI, or bone scan.[25,77]

TREATMENT

In general, open tibial fractures fare worse than closed fractures. The outcome depends on the condition of the soft tissue envelope, on healing without infection, on revascularization of the limb when arterial injury is present, and on prompt assessment and treatment of any compartment syndrome. The incidence of infection in these open injuries is between 5% and 15% and depends most on the severity of the open injury and the time between injury and surgical debridement. Kreder and Armstrong reported a 14% incidence of infection in a series of 56 open tibial fractures in children.[51] However, a delay of more than 6 hours correlated with a 25% infection rate as opposed to a 12% infection rate in children operated on less than 6 hours from the time of injury.[51] Most infections involve *Staphylococcus aureus,* which can be treated with aggressive debridement and administration of intravenous antibiotics. It is important to be aggressive in debriding all areas of necrotic soft tissue to provide the optimal chance for soft tissue healing to occur and to avoid infection. Arterial injury occurs in 2% to 10% of cases.[11,31,43,51,82,98] Approximately 50% of all type IIIC open injuries result in amputation, either at the initial debridement because of the severe nature of the injury or later because of failed vein interposition grafting.[11,82] Although severe soft tissue injury occurs with these fractures, compartment syndromes develop in up to 5% of patients; most of these injuries are grade II open fractures.[11,43]

The average time to union is approximately 5 to 6 months and depends on the extent of the soft tissue injury, the age of the child at the time of injury, the fracture pattern, the amount of segmental bone loss, and the presence of infection.[11,17,31,43,51,82,98] Buckley and colleagues reported an average healing time of 4.8 months; however, comminuted fractures healed at 5.7 months, spiral and transverse fractures healed at approximately 4.2 months, fractures with segmental bone loss healed at 14.7 months, and fractures associated with infection healed in 7.1 months as compared with 4.6 months when infection was not present.[11] Children older than 11 years behave more like adults, with delayed fracture healing when compared with younger children.[31,51,98] Angular deformity occurs in a small proportion of patients and can usually be corrected by manipulation of the external fixator or wedging of the cast. Overgrowth of the affected tibia by up to 3 cm occurs in approximately 8% to 10% of cases, most often in patients who had an initial reduction in which restoration of limb length was achieved.[11]

Nonoperative Treatment

The majority of children's tibial fractures can be treated by cast immobilization after fracture reduction.

Nondisplaced Oblique or Spiral Tibial Fracture with an Intact Fibula ("Toddler's Fracture"). The so-called toddler's fracture was first described by Dunbar and colleagues in 1964.[21] This fracture is seen in children, usually younger than 6 years, who sustained a twisting injury of the foot while walking or running that resulted in a nondisplaced oblique or spiral fracture of the tibia with an intact fibula.[72,106] An oblique radiograph may best show the fracture. Once the diagnosis is made, the limb should be immobilized in a long-leg cast. The cast is left on for approximately 3 to 4 weeks, depending on the age of the child and the amount of callus formation on follow-up radiographs. When the cast is removed the child is allowed full weight-bearing status without further immobilization. It is not necessary to obtain serial weekly radiographs in a child with a toddler's fracture.

Because of the innocuous nature of the injury and the difficulty in making the diagnosis, it is often beneficial to place a child who is thought to have a toddler's fracture in a long-leg cast. Radiographs can be obtained 2 weeks after application of the cast to identify whether a fracture is present. If no signs of callus formation are present, the cast can be removed. Fracture callus confirms the diagnosis, and immobilization should continue for an additional 2 to 3 weeks.

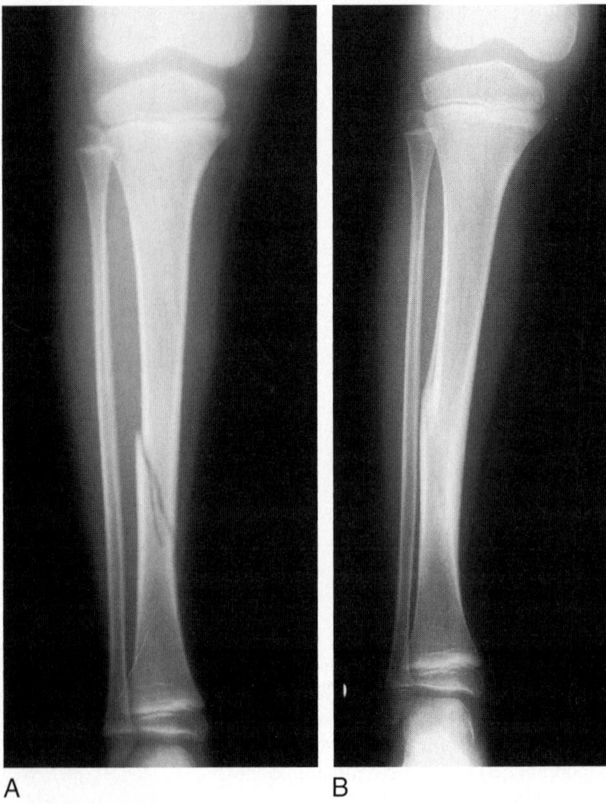

FIGURE 43–144 Isolated tibial fracture in a 5-year-old patient. **A,** Spiral fracture in the mid-portion of the tibia. The fibula is intact. **B,** At the time of healing there was slight varus angulation, which often occurs secondary to the presence of an intact fibula.

Displaced Tibial Fracture with an Intact Fibula in an Older Child. The second category of fracture amenable to nonoperative treatment is a displaced tibial fracture with an intact fibula in an older child. These fractures tend to angle into a varus position secondary to anterolateral muscle forces pulling the distal fragment medially while the fibula stabilizes the lateral aspect of the leg (Fig. 43–144). We prefer to manipulate the fracture with the child under conscious sedation in the emergency room and use a minifluoroscopy unit to check the reduction after the application of an initial roll of plaster cast material. The surgeon should counter the fracture's tendency to reduce into a varus position during the reduction maneuver and during cast application. An initial role of plaster below the knee to create a three-point bending force is essential to obtain adequate reduction. Acceptable fracture reduction is alignment to within 5 to 10 degrees in all planes, with special emphasis on obtaining nearly anatomic alignment in the coronal plane. The remaining cast is then applied after the plaster cast has set and adequate fracture reduction is confirmed. The patient is non–weight bearing in the cast for 4 to 6 weeks, after which the cast may be changed to a short-leg walking cast, depending on the age of the child and the amount of radiographic healing. Radiographs should be obtained weekly during the first 2 to 3 weeks after reduction to assess whether reduction has been maintained and to permit manipulation, if necessary. We recommend manipulation of the fracture when varus angulation of greater than 5 degrees is present on follow-up radiographs.

Yang and Letts reported on 95 children with isolated tibial fractures, most of which were distal third spiral fractures. Angular deformity was present initially in 76 (80%) fractures and recurred after closed reduction in 32 patients, all of which recurrences drifted into varus and were posteriorly angled. Wedging of the cast with manipulation of the fracture was most successful in patients with a single-plane deformity.[112] Yang and Letts recommended close monitoring of isolated tibial fractures on a weekly basis for the first 3 weeks. Teitz and colleagues reported similar difficulties in adults with an isolated tibial fracture: 26% of fractures had a varus malunion, and radiographic changes and pain developed in the affected ankle in 33% of these patients within 2 years of injury.[105]

Displaced Tibial Fracture with a Fibular Fracture in an Older Child. The third major category of tibial diaphyseal fractures in children is a displaced fracture with an associated fibular fracture in an older child. These injuries are generally seen in children older than 10 years and result from direct, high-energy trauma. Because of significant instability from the associated fibular fracture, these injuries may be difficult to reduce adequately, and conscious sedation or general anesthesia is frequently required for reduction. Acceptable reduction must include at least 50% bony apposition of the fracture fragments and less than 5 to 8 degrees of angulation in both the sagittal and coronal planes. These fractures are prone to residual varus in the coronal plane and posterior angulation (apex anterior) in the sagittal plane. To correct this, a three-point mold should be placed to compensate for varus, and the ankle should be placed in 15 to 20 degrees of plantar flexion to prevent posterior angulation. Reduction is facilitated by placing the patient's hip at the edge of the elevated stretcher with the leg dependent to aid in reduction and cast molding. A skilled assistant is valuable for placement of an optimal cast. Once an initial below-knee cast has set, the remaining part of the cast can be applied with the knee in 30 to 45 degrees of knee flexion to provide rotational control of the fracture and restrict the patient from bearing weight on the affected extremity. These patients should be admitted to the hospital for soft tissue monitoring, with the leg elevated, ice packs placed at the level of the fracture, and neurovascular assessment performed every 2 hours by the nursing staff. Requests for excess narcotic medication throughout the night should raise suspicion that a compartment syndrome is impending. Close radiographic monitoring is required at 2 to 3 weeks to ensure that the initial fracture reduction is maintained.

Operative Treatment

Operative treatment is rarely required in a closed tibial fracture in children, (<5% of cases). The main indications are (1) excessive fracture instability that cannot be maintained with external immobilization, (2) loss of reduction that cannot be corrected by cast wedging during the follow-up period, (3) significant comminution and shortening that cannot be corrected with closed treatment, and (4) a displaced fracture in a skeletally mature patient. The primary modes of operative treatment in a pediatric patient include flexible intramedullary rods, percutaneous pin fixation after adequate closed reduction, external fixation, open reduction with internal fixation, and locking rigid intramedullary rods.

For a patient with an unstable fracture pattern or one that has demonstrated recurrent instability in a cast, flexible intramedullary rods have been shown to be a good option. Two recent reviews report excellent outcomes with antegrade flexible intramedullary nails in closed fractures and in a small number of open fractures.[52,68] In a third clinical review, Goodwin and coworkers also reported overall satisfactory results but highlighted technique-related complications that may be seen with flexible nailing of tibial fractures. Excessive coronal plane angulation may occur when the nails are introduced on the same side of the tibia (C and S construct), and we agree with the recommendation for a medial and lateral entry technique (double-C construct). Additionally, a report of physeal injury highlights the requirement for fluoroscopic confirmation of an adequate starting-hole distance from the proximal physis and tubercle apophysis.[28]

External fixation may also be used in a highly unstable closed tibial fracture to provide fracture stability for 4 to 6 weeks, until adequate callus is present (Fig. 43–145). Removal may require a general anesthetic and is followed by the application of a short-leg walking cast for an additional 3 to 4 weeks. Percutaneously placed crossed Kirschner wires are also an option in younger patients with potential for rapid healing. The wires are left outside the skin to allow easy removal in the clinic 4 weeks from the time of injury (Fig. 43–146). Cast immobilization is performed as for a closed fracture, without internal fixation. We do not recommend plate fixation of diaphyseal fractures in children because of the significant soft tissue stripping required, the increased risk for infection and nonunion, and the need to remove the hardware at a later date. Rigid intramedullary fixation has revolutionized the treatment of tibial fractures in adults and can be used in an older adolescent who is skeletally mature (Fig. 43–147).

Open Tibial Diaphyseal Fractures

Although open fractures in children account for less than 5% of all tibial fractures, the topic has taken on considerable interest recently.[11,17,31,43,51,82,98,115]

MECHANISM OF INJURY

Unlike closed tibial fractures, these injuries are due to high-energy trauma that results in significant injury to the surrounding soft tissues, which can lead to delayed union and a high risk for infection. These fractures are often associated with other fractures and with chest and abdominal trauma. The mechanism of injury in more than 80% of open tibial fractures is an automobile striking a pedestrian, bicyclist, or motorcyclist.[11,17,31,43,51,82,98,115] The average age of the children is between 8 and 10 years, boys are injured more frequently than girls by a 3:1 ratio, and the left leg is injured more often than the right.[11,31,43,51,82,98,115]

Because of the high energy required to produce these injuries, associated injuries occur in up to 58% of patients.[11,17] These injuries include other skeletal injuries, closed head injuries, abdominal and thoracic injuries, and maxillofacial injuries.[11,31,51,82,98] In addition, open tibial diaphyseal fractures can be associated with a mortality rate of up to 7% because of the severe head, chest, and abdominal trauma.[31,51]

CLASSIFICATION

Fractures should be classified according to the Gustilo and Anderson classification for open fractures:

Type I Low-energy injury in which the wound is less than 1 cm in length and there is little soft tissue injury or wound contamination

Type II A moderately low-energy injury in which the wound is longer than 1 cm, there is

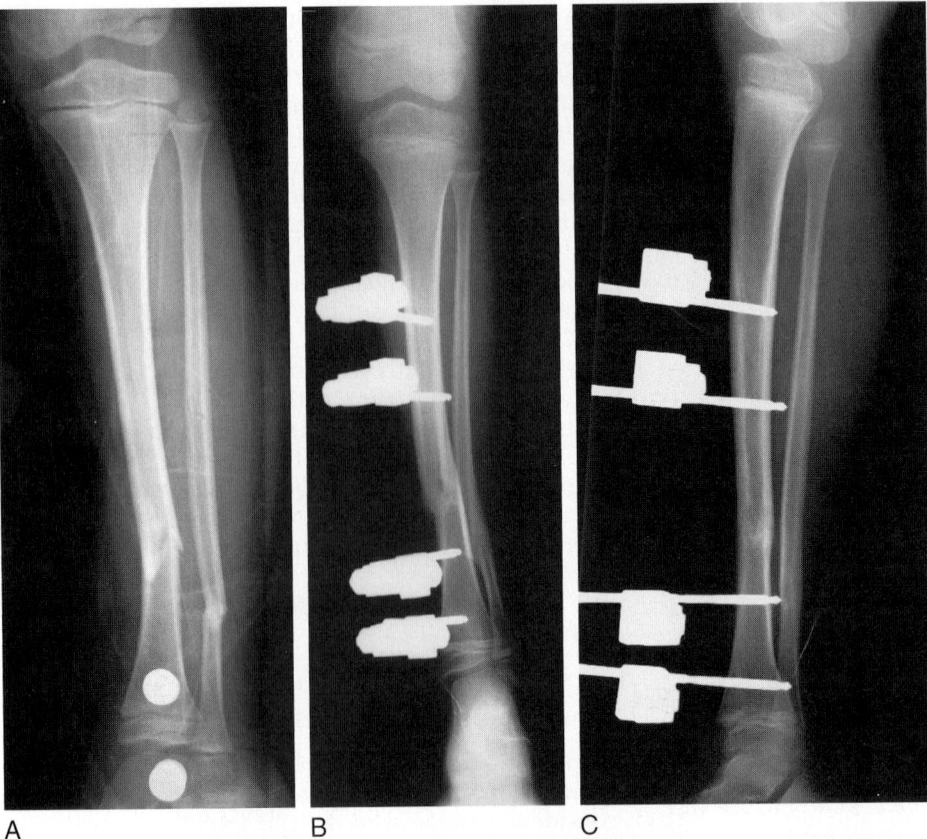

FIGURE 43–145 External fixation of an open tibiofibular fracture. **A,** Injury film demonstrating a distal tibiofibular fracture. **B** and **C,** Following external fixation, adequate alignment and healing occurred after 2 months.

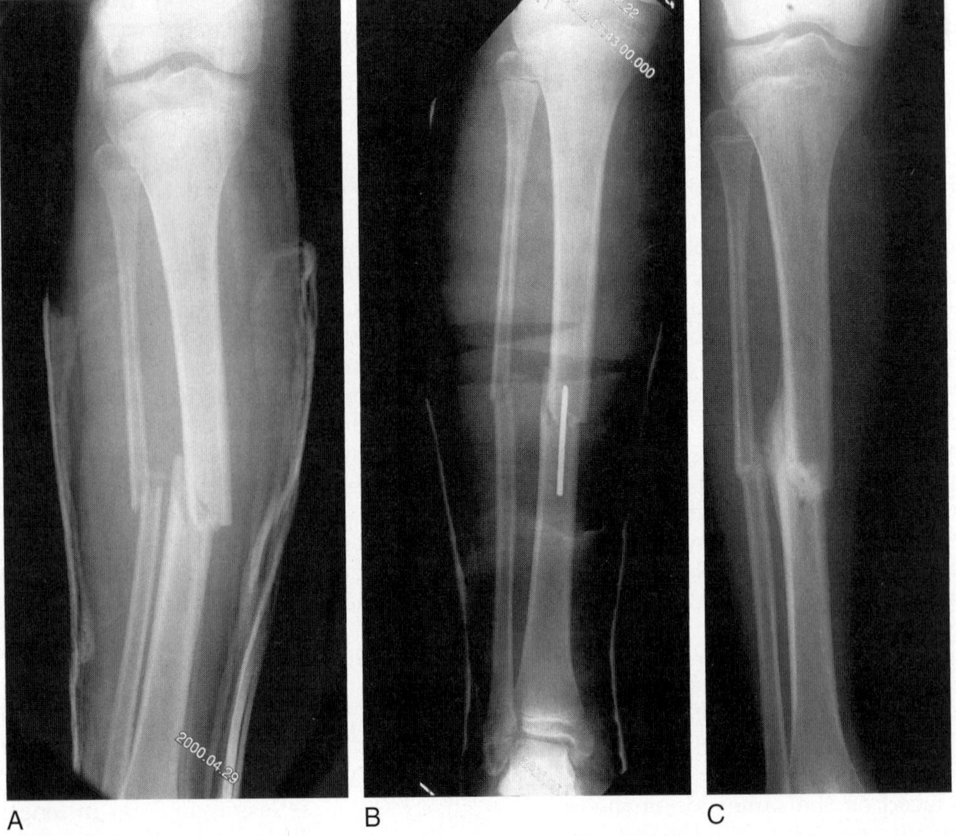

FIGURE 43–146 Percutaneous closed reduction and percutaneous pinning of a tibial fracture. **A,** Radiograph of a 15-year-old boy with a displaced midshaft tibiofibular fracture. Attempts at closed reduction and casting were unsuccessful because of unacceptable alignment. **B,** Closed reduction with percutaneous pinning was performed. **C,** Healing with nearly anatomic alignment was achieved at 4 months.

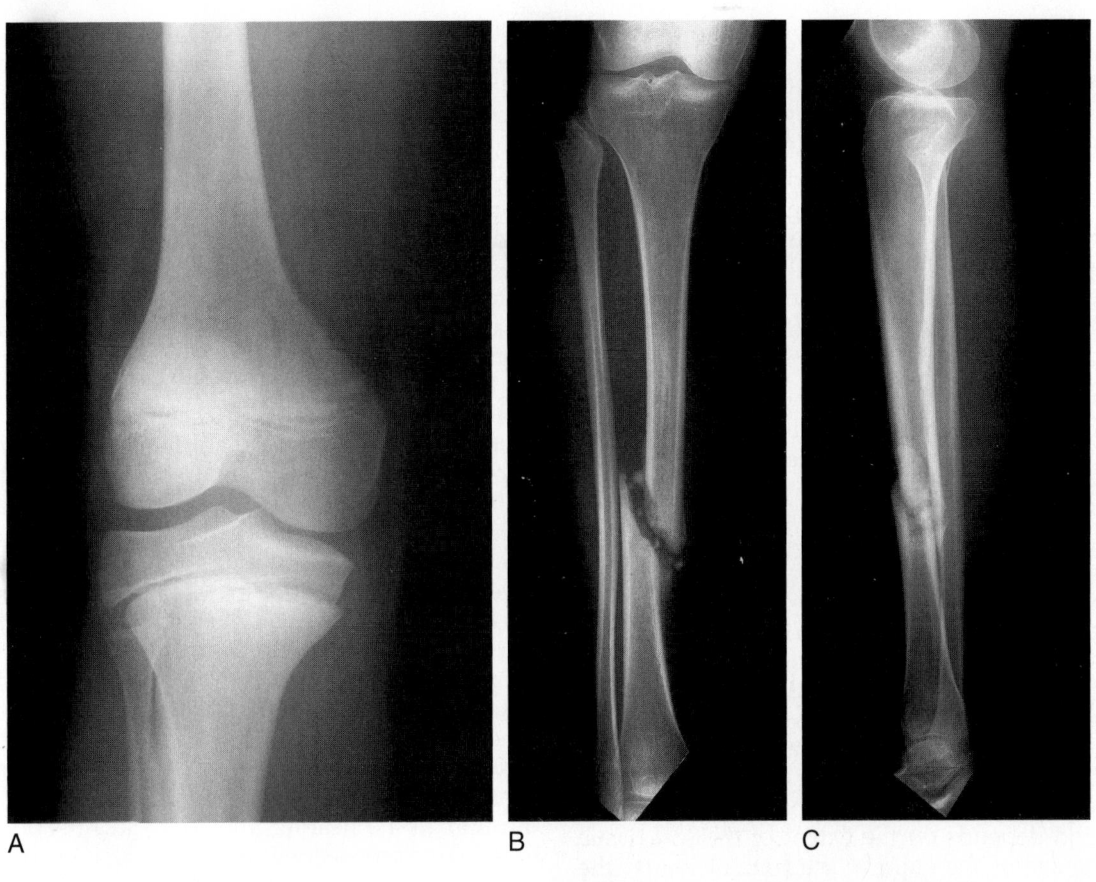

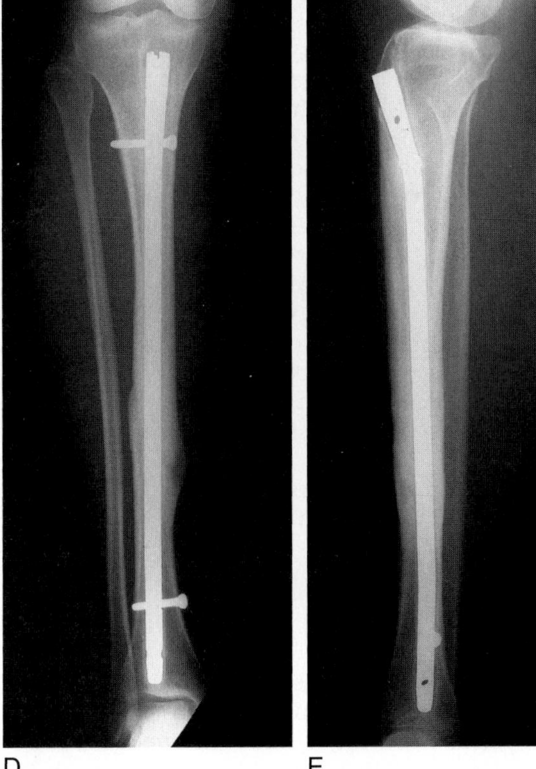

FIGURE 43–147 Rigid intramedullary fixation of an isolated fracture in an adolescent patient. **A** through **C,** Injury radiographs demonstrating an isolated midshaft tibial fracture. **D** and **E,** Three months after surgery the fracture has healed in anatomic alignment.

	little soft tissue injury, and the wound is mildly contaminated
Type III	Significant soft tissue injury with wound contamination
IIIA	Despite significant soft tissue injury the fracture can be adequately covered without using a skin graft or tissue flap.
IIIB	The local soft tissue envelope cannot cover the fracture site and a skin graft or a muscle flap is required
IIIC	An associated arterial injury is present and requires revascularization of the limb

In a compilation of five series, open fractures were evenly distributed among Gustilo and Anderson grades I, II, and III: 32% were grade I, 38% were grade II, and 30% were grade III (17% A, 8% B, and 5% C).[11,31,51,82,98]

TREATMENT

In general, open tibial fractures fare worse than closed fractures. The outcome depends on the condition of the soft tissue envelope, on healing without infection, on revascularization of the limb when arterial injury is present, and on prompt assessment and treatment of any compartment syndrome.

The average time to union is approximately 5 to 6 months and depends on the extent of the soft tissue injury, the age of the child at the time of injury, the fracture pattern, the amount of segmental bone loss, and the presence of infection.[11,17,31,43,51,82,98] Buckley and colleagues reported an average healing time of 4.8 months; however, comminuted fractures healed at 5.7 months, spiral and transverse fractures healed at approximately 4.2 months, fractures with segmental bone loss healed at 14.7 months, and fractures associated with infection healed in 7.1 months as compared with 4.6 months when infection was not present.[11] In children older than 11 years fractures behave more like adult fractures, with delayed fracture healing when compared with younger children.[31,51,98] Angular deformity occurs in a small proportion of patients and can usually be corrected by manipulation of the external fixator or wedging of the cast. Overgrowth of the affected tibia by up to 3 cm occurs in approximately 8% to 10% of cases, most often in patients who had an initial reduction in which restoration of limb length was achieved.[11]

Treatment of open fractures in children is similar to that in adults and should follow an established protocol.

Early Treatment: Antibiotics, Debridement, and Splinting

The first step in management is prompt evaluation and initial classification of the soft tissue injury in the emergency department, followed by the application of a povidone-iodine (Betadine)-soaked dressing and splinting of the fracture. Most infections involve *Staphylococcus aureus,* which can be treated with aggressive debridement and administration of intravenous antibiotics. Intravenous administration of a second-generation cephalosporin (cefazolin) is indicated for all fractures, with the addition of an aminoglycoside for all grade III injuries and severely contaminated wounds and penicillin for all farm-related accidents. Several studies have established early treatment with appropriate intravenous antibiotics as an important independent predictor for prevention of infection in open fractures.[75,95,96] Iobst and coworkers reported one infection (2.5%) in a series of 40 pediatric patients with grade I fractures managed nonoperatively with intravenous antibiotics alone.[41]

In a retrospective multicenter review, Skaggs and colleagues reported no higher infection rates of open fractures debrided after 6 hours when compared with those debrided before 6 hours after injury.[95] Historically, however, the incidence of infection in these open injuries is between 5% and 15% and depends most on the severity of the open injury and the time between injury and surgical debridement. Kreder and Armstrong reported a 14% incidence of infection in a series of 56 open tibial fractures in children.[51] A delay of more than 6 hours correlated with a 25% infection rate as opposed to a 12% infection rate in children operated on less than 6 hours from the time of injury.[51] It is important to be aggressive in debriding all areas of necrotic soft tissue to provide the optimal chance for soft tissue healing and to avoid infection. In the absence of prospective controlled data, we continue to recommend urgent operative irrigation and debridement of the wound, followed by stabilization for all open fractures.

Wound Management

Initial wound management entails extending grade I and smaller grade II wounds to allow thorough debridement of bone and soft tissue. If the wound is on the medial aspect of the leg, with little soft tissue coverage, an anterolateral incision should be used to gain access to the fracture site and injured soft tissue. All incisions made by the surgeon can be closed at the initial surgery, whereas traumatic wounds are left open. We prefer to place nonabsorbable horizontal mattress sutures in the traumatic portions of grade II wounds without tying the sutures (Fig. 43–148). This will allow drainage of the leg to help prevent the accumulation of infectious material. These sutures can be closed at the bedside in 24 to 48 hours. Any bony fragment with little or no soft tissue attachment should be discarded. Any concern regarding the amount of contamination of grade I or II wounds at the initial surgery warrants serial repeat irrigation and debridement every 48 hours until adequate, viable tissue is seen. All grade III injuries require repeat irrigation and debridement. Necrotic muscle or muscle that is thought to be ischemic should be debrided. Signs of muscle viability are muscle contraction when stimulated by pinching with forceps, arterial bleeding when incised, and the presence of a healthy pink color. Repeat irrigation of the soft tissue with 5 to 10 L of normal saline via a pulse lavage system should be performed.

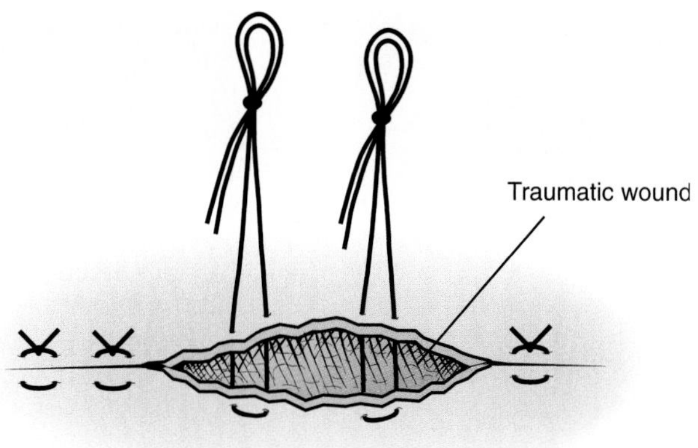

FIGURE 43–148 Suture placement in a traumatic wound at the time of the initial debridement. The sutures are not tied. In areas in which the traumatic wound was extended, suture placement with tying at the time of surgery is appropriate.

Soft Tissue Management

Soft tissue management in a severely injured leg often requires coverage with the use of split- or full-thickness skin grafts, myocutaneous flaps, or free muscle flaps. We prefer to have the plastic surgeon present to assess the wound as soon as possible, certainly by the second debridement, to gain that individual's input regarding the type of soft tissue coverage needed and the timing of this procedure. Coverage procedures should be done as soon as possible, preferably within 5 to 7 days, to prevent seeding of the leg with a secondary infection.[12,13,15,71,75,88] Vacuum-assisted closure (VAC) devices are valuable for managing large soft tissue defects awaiting definitive closure. Recent reviews in adult and pediatric patients have demonstrated trends toward decreasing need for free tissue transfer and revision amputation in higher grade wounds and traumatic amputations.[37,94] Most injuries in children can be treated with a split-thickness skin graft or with a local flap consisting of a gastrocnemius flap in the proximal part of the leg or a soleus flap in the middle aspect of the leg.[39] However, injuries in the lower part of the leg often require a vascularized free flap.[61,113] Free muscle flaps are used for massive soft tissue injuries in any part of the leg. Free flaps are an excellent barrier to secondary infection and have a rich blood supply, which enhances soft tissue and bone healing.[27,61,99,113]

Management of Bony Defects

The surgeon addressing large bony defects must first ensure that the native bony bed is clear of all infection. This is best done with antibiotic-impregnated polymethyl methacrylate beads. Although these beads are commercially available, we prefer to prepare them at the time of surgery by mixing 1 g of powdered cefazolin and 2.4 g of powdered tobramycin with powdered cement. The beads are rolled by hand and strung together on heavy Prolene suture. An alternative is to shape the cement into a solid spacer, which will prevent the ingrowth of soft tissue into the defect site and provide some additional stability to the tibia. When reentering this site for bone grafting, the surgeon often finds surrounding the cement spacer a pseudoperiosteum that provides a confined space for the graft material. Options for treating large segmental bony defects include bone transport, a vascularized fibular transfer, or autologous bone grafting. We prefer to perform autologous bone grafting of the defect 6 to 10 weeks after soft tissue coverage once the flap has completely epithelialized and the edges of the wound are free of all eschar. This time delay eliminates bacterial contamination of the operative site and enhances fracture healing by the autologous bone.[32] Christian and colleagues reported eight adult patients with grade IIIB open tibial fractures and an average segmental bone loss of 10 cm in whom the tibia successfully healed by 9 months with massive autologous bone grafting.[14] The patient is placed prone initially so that bone can be obtained from the posterior iliac crest and is then placed supine. If a free flap was used for soft tissue coverage, the plastic surgeon should be present to elevate the flap without injuring the vascular pedicle.

Patients with deformity, shortening, or chronic osteomyelitis in addition to a large bony defect are best managed with the Ilizarov apparatus[73,99] or other external fixation.

Fracture Stabilization

The primary modes of fracture stabilization for open tibial fractures in children are long-leg cast immobilization with a window over the traumatic wound, flexible intramedullary nails, and external fixation. Approximately 50% of all open tibial fractures are treated by cast immobilization, and the rest are treated with an external fixator or internal fixation and a cast.[11,31,51,82] In 1996 Cullen and colleagues reported that 48% of children with open tibial fractures were treated by percutaneous pin fixation and had a shorter healing time and fewer complications than did patients treated with an external fixator.[17] Kubiak and coworkers reported earlier union and greater satisfaction in patients treated with flexible intramedullary nailing for open tibial fractures than in those treated with external fixation (Fig. 43–149).[52]

We prefer cast immobilization for all grade I and smaller grade II wounds that will not require repeat debridement in the operating room. A window is placed in the cast at the time of application to allow wound access. For larger grade II and all grade III injuries, intramedullary nails or a monolateral external fixator provide stabilization and subsequent soft tissue access. Flexible intramedullary nails have been used in open fractures without the complication of subsequent infection; however, experience in higher grade and grossly contaminated open fractures is limited.[52,68] Therefore, in the setting of gross contamination we most often use an AO external fixator with two sets of half-pins to span the fracture (Fig. 43–150). This provides excellent stability and allows multiple debridement of the soft tissue injury without jeopardizing fracture fixation. An external fixator pin should

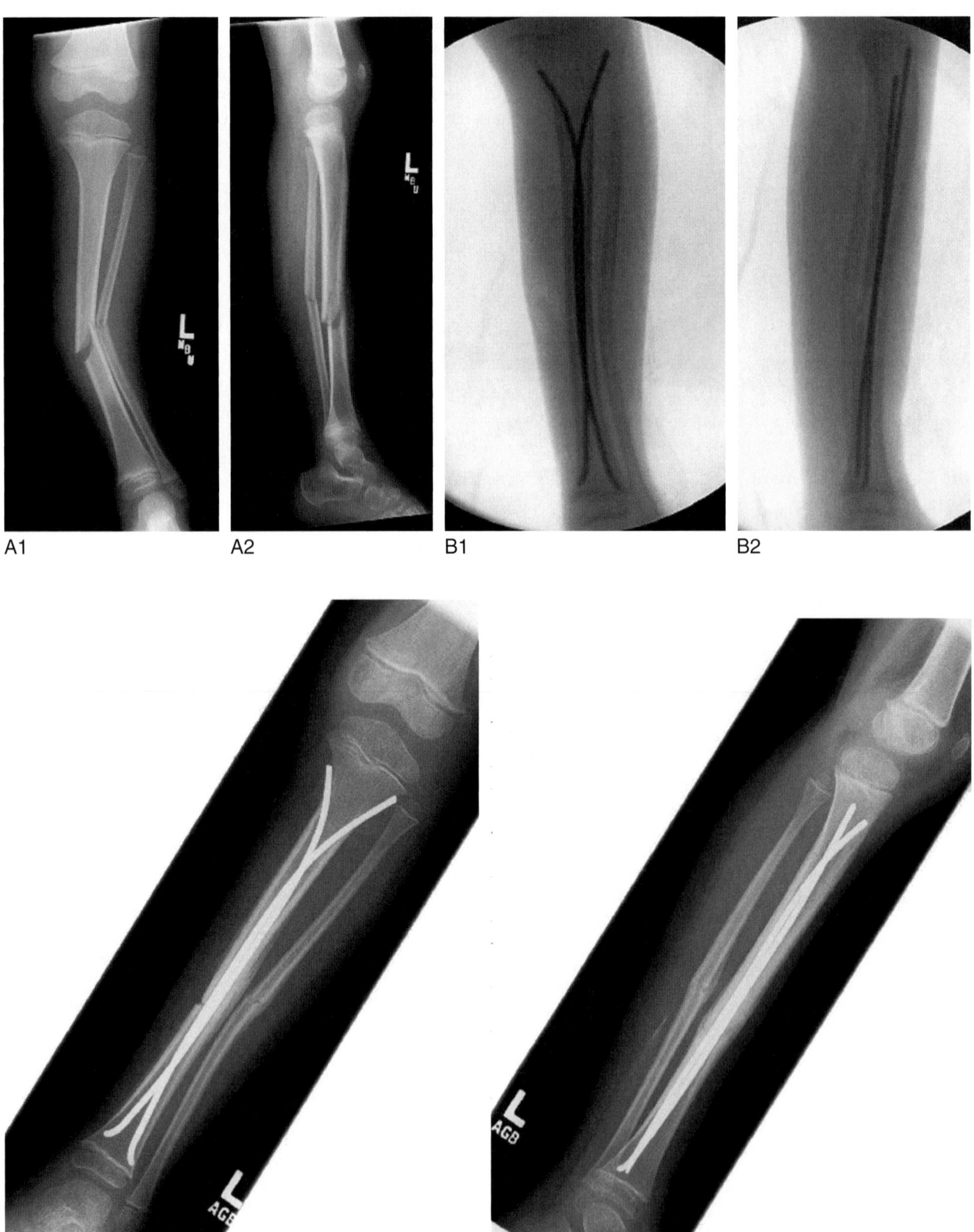

FIGURE 43–149 Flexible intramedullary tibial fixation. **A,** Open fracture with extensive soft tissue injury. **B** and **C,** Titanium elastic nail fixation providing stability for soft tissue management.

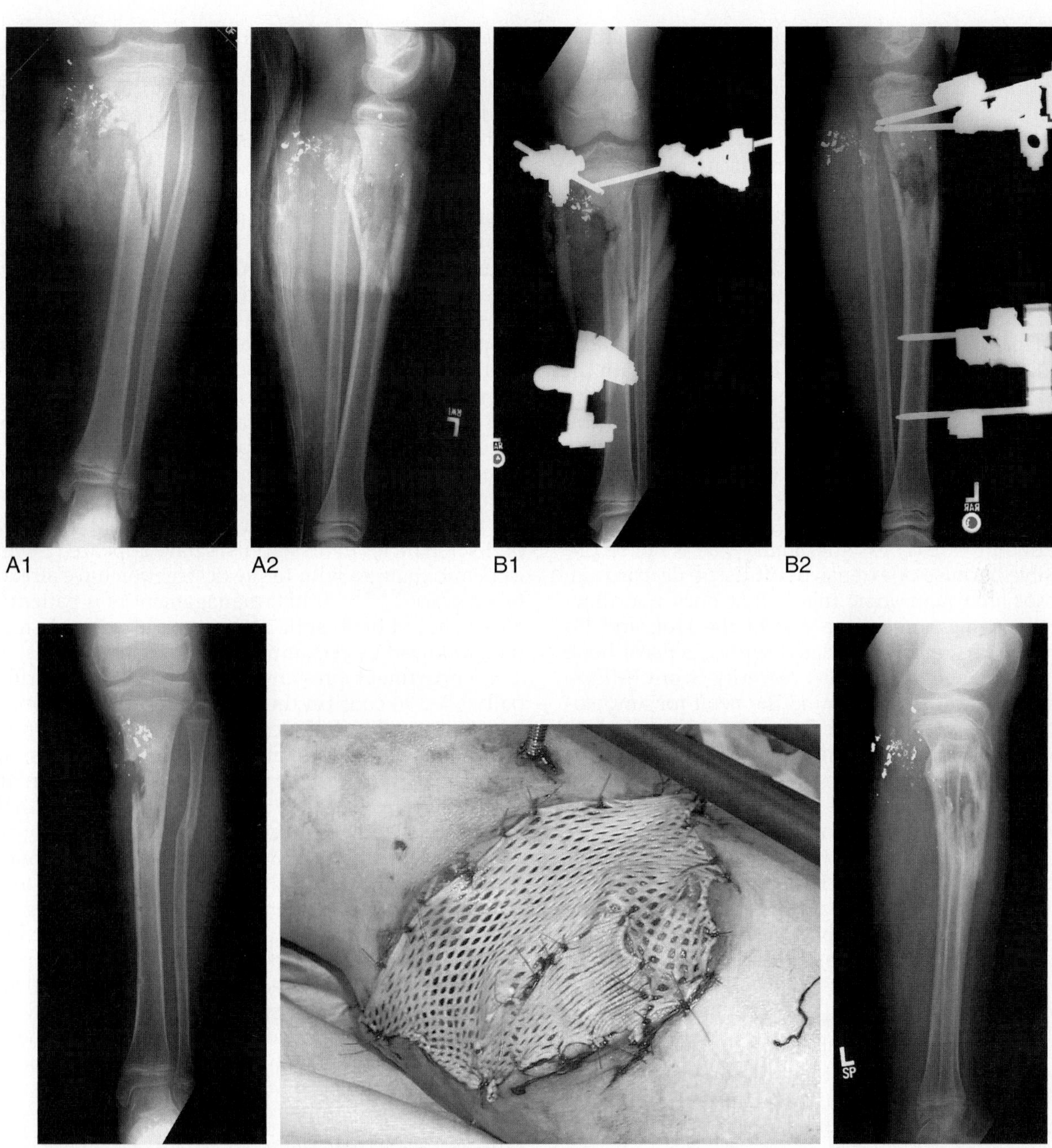

FIGURE 43–150 External fixation in a 10-year-old patient who sustained a gunshot wound to the proximal tibia and subsequently an open tibiofibular fracture. **A,** Injury radiographs. Note the significant bone loss and comminution of the proximal tibia. **B,** The initial treatment was placement of an external fixator, with two proximal half-pins placed parallel to the joint and connected to two distal half-pins in a T fashion. **C,** To allow closure of the soft tissue defect, a shortening fibular osteotomy was performed, followed by skin grafting over the muscle. **D,** Healing was evident 4 months after injury. Bone grafting was not required.

be placed on each side of the fracture no closer than 1 cm to the physis. The bars should then be attached to the pins and a reduction maneuver performed, after which the external fixator is tightened. When good callus is seen, the external fixator frame is removed and a short-leg walking cast is applied.

Treatment of Neurovascular Injury

A severe open tibial fracture with neurovascular injury is rare in children and accounts for approximately 5% of all tibial fractures.[11,43,82] Revascularization of the leg should be done within 4 to 6 hours of injury and should not be delayed by arteriography in the radiology suite. If the ischemia time is approaching the 4-hour limit, an arteriogram obtained with the patient on the operating room table is the best way to determine the exact location of the arterial injury. The timing of bony stabilization and revascularization also depends on the ischemia time. We prefer to stabilize the fracture by applying an external fixator so that definitive revascularization can be performed. However, if the ischemia time is approaching 4 hours, insertion of temporary intraluminal shunts to provide a vascular supply to the distal part of the leg takes precedence over fracture stabilization.[47] Compartment pressures should be measured in any child with an open fracture that requires revascularization, and the surgeon should have a low threshold for performing four-compartment fasciotomies. Prophylactic fasciotomies should be performed in any patient with an ischemia time of 4 hours or longer.[85]

Indications for amputation in a child with a severe tibial fracture are (1) vascular injury that is not reconstructible because of extensive soft tissue destruction, (2) associated neurologic injury that does not allow protective sensation on the sole of the foot, and (3) severe muscle injury associated with extensive bone loss. The Mangled Extremity Severity Score (MESS) can be used to help determine the need for amputation; a score greater than 7 indicates the need to perform an amputation in adults.[48] Fagelman and colleagues have reported retrospective agreement of MESS and clinical decisions for limb salvage in a pediatric series.[24] Although maximal tissue preservation is often advisable, MESS may be a useful adjunct for clinical decision making. It is imperative to avoid sepsis from attempts at salvaging limbs that are on the borderline of survivability because of the potential for multisystem organ failure and death.[8]

COMPLICATIONS

The most common complications associated with tibial diaphyseal fractures are compartment syndrome, delayed union or nonunion, limb length discrepancy, angular deformity, malrotation, and vascular injury. Arterial injury occurs in 2% to 10% of cases.[11,31,43,51,82,98] Approximately 50% of all type IIIC open injuries result in amputation, either at the initial debridement because of the severe nature of the injury or later because of failed vein interposition grafting.[11,82] Although severe soft tissue injury occurs with these fractures, compartment syndromes develop in up to 5% of patients; most of these injuries are grade II open fractures.[11,43]

Compartment Syndrome

Compartment syndrome is due to increased fluid in the compartments of the leg. The increased fluid raises intracompartmental pressure, which inhibits venous return. Compartment syndrome can occur in any or all four compartments of the leg and is seen with tibial fractures in both adults and children.[22,53,66] As the pressure continues to increase, the smaller arterioles and capillaries become occluded and ischemia develops, which results in muscle and nerve injury within 6 hours.[35,92]

The diagnosis is often difficult to make, and the medical team must have a high index of suspicion and act promptly on the basis of serial history taking and physical examination when warning signals are present. Compartment syndrome should be suspected in any patient who has pain out of proportion to the injury, especially a child who has sustained direct trauma to the leg; any child who is unresponsive because of associated head or other injuries; and a young child who is unable to describe symptoms or cooperate with the physical examination.[67] Physical findings that warn of a compartment syndrome are pain on passive range of motion of the toes, and swollen and tense compartments that are tender on palpation. When these signs and symptoms are present, prompt compartment pressure measurements and four-compartment fasciotomies should be performed. By the time sensory and motor neurologic abnormalities or discrepancies in distal pulses have appeared, severe ischemic changes with tissue destruction have already taken place.[35,66,84,85] Initial management of a patient in a cast should be to split the cast, padding, and stockinet, followed by reexamination of the leg.

Compartment pressure measurements are principally used to confirm the diagnosis and can be made by a variety of techniques.[59,65,67,84-86,110] The slit-catheter technique works well at the bedside; however, we prefer to obtain compartment measurements in the operating room with the needle technique. Threshold pressures that have been used to define abnormal compartment pressure have included pressures greater than 45 mm Hg (using the continuous infusion technique), pressures greater than 35 mm Hg (using the slit-catheter technique), and compartment pressures within 15 to 30 mm Hg of diastolic pressure. The pressure in all four compartments should be measured and documented. Although some compartments may not have elevated pressure, all four compartments should be released. We prefer the two-incision technique for the fasciotomies (Fig. 43–151).

Other Complications

Delayed union or nonunion is relatively rare in a child with a closed tibial fracture. Predisposing factors include isolated tibial fracture without a fibular fracture, severe soft tissue injury, treatment in an external fixator, infection, a tibial fracture in an older child, or an open fracture. Delayed union in a young child without a fibular fracture is best treated with a fibular osteotomy distant to the tibial fracture to allow compression across the fracture site. A young patient can then be recasted until healing occurs. Iliac crest bone grafting can be performed through a posterolateral approach to promote healing of an atrophic nonunion (Fig. 43–152). The tibia can be stabilized with plate fixation in a young child and with intramedullary nailing in an older child.

Limb length discrepancy after tibial fractures is due to overgrowth of the affected tibia and is most often

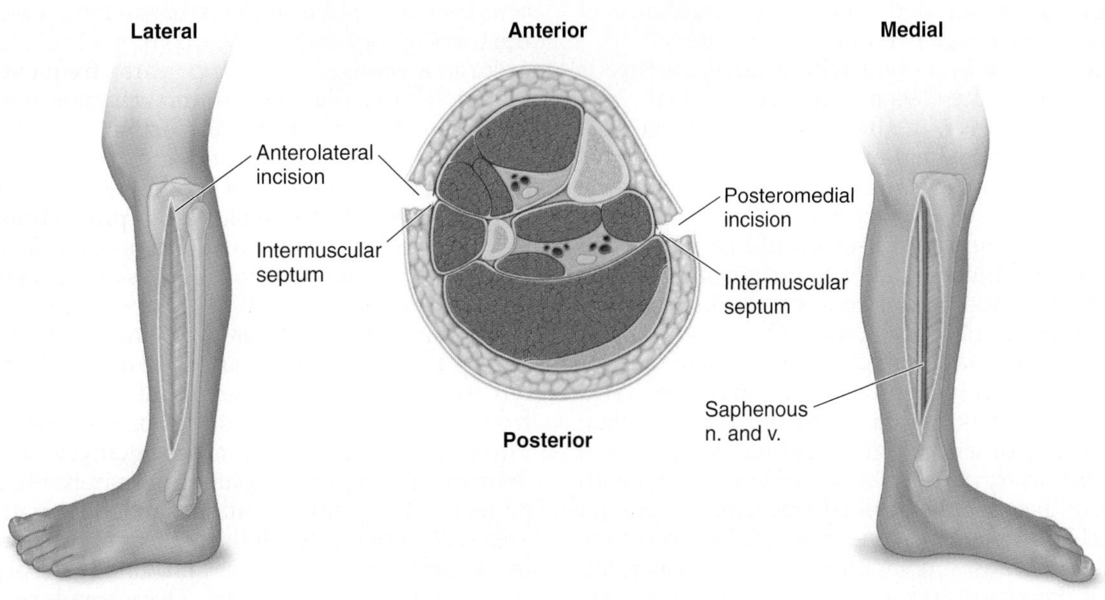

FIGURE 43-151 Four-compartment release for fasciotomy. An anterolateral and a posteromedial incision are made for entrance into all four compartments of the leg.

seen in children younger than 10 years with comminuted fractures, proximal and distal fractures, and open tibial fractures.[11,93] The overgrowth seen in tibial fractures is less than that seen in femoral shaft fractures, with the average overgrowth measuring 4 mm.[93] Although overgrowth after tibial fractures is not usually clinically apparent, discrepancies projected to be more than 2 cm require monitoring with serial scanograms to plan for an appropriately timed epiphysiodesis.

Angular deformity is most often due to inadequate reduction and stabilization or to asymmetric growth. Although remodeling occurs after angular deformity in the tibia, the potential is far less than in the femur. The greatest potential for tibial remodeling occurs in young children (girls younger than 8 years and boys younger than 10 years)[103] who have single-plane deformities, procurvatum, varus deformities, and deformities that are close to the physis.[93] Rotational deformities are rare after tibial diaphyseal fractures in children and generally do not require operative treatment when they do occur. At the time of reduction, rotational malalignment should not be accepted because remodeling of this deformity does not usually occur, especially in an older child.[34,93,100] Shannak reported a 3% incidence of rotational deformities after closed tibial fractures; all occurred in children older than 11 years.[93] We prefer to observe rotational deformities of less than 30 degrees and perform a derotational tibial osteotomy at the supramalleolar level together with a fibular osteotomy when greater than a 30-degree deformity persists 2 years after injury. Proximal osteotomies are performed only if most of the deformity is in the proximal aspect of the tibia because these corrective

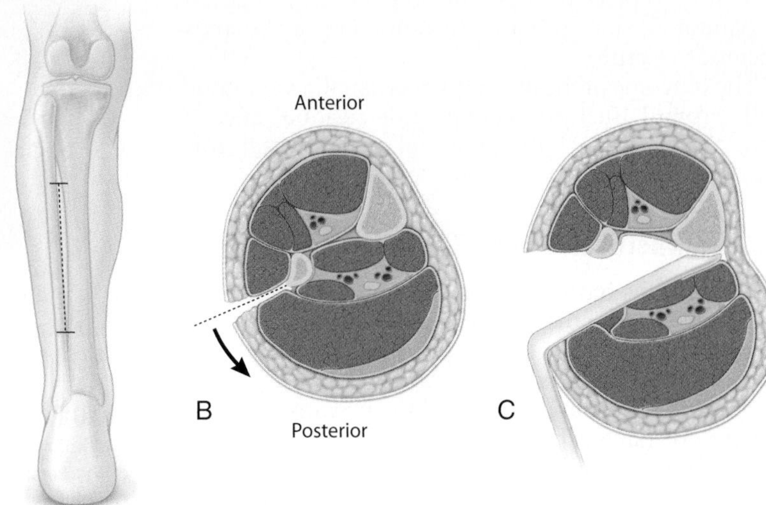

FIGURE 43-152 Approach for posterolateral bone grafting to treat delayed union or nonunion of the tibia. **A,** The skin incision is made over the posterolateral aspect of the leg. **B,** The dissection is carried out between the lateral and posterior compartments down to the fibula. **C,** The dissection is carried further between the deep posterior compartment and the intermuscular septum between the tibia and fibula. A large Hohmann retractor can be placed around the posterior aspect of the tibia to allow direct observation and bone grafting.

procedures are associated with a high incidence of compartment syndrome and neurologic injury.[45,58,91]

Vascular injury in a child with a tibial fracture is rare and most often seen with open tibial fractures.[11,31,82,98] However, it can occur with closed fractures, especially proximal metaphyseal or diaphyseal fractures, and is associated with a high complication rate, particularly when recognized late.[1,26] Careful assessment of the distal pulses should be performed at the initial examination, after reduction, and serially thereafter. Any question or concern about a discrepancy in the peripheral pulses, including Doppler examinations, should prompt an immediate arteriogram.[26,111] Proximal tibial metaphyseal and diaphyseal fractures are at risk for injury to the anterior tibial artery because of its proximity and tethering by soft tissues; this artery can also be injured in patients with posteriorly directed distal tibial fractures. Treatment of arterial injuries should consist of stabilization of the bony anatomy, most often with an external fixator, followed by definitive arterial repair or reconstruction and four-compartment fasciotomies.

Distal Tibial Metaphyseal Fractures

These fractures are similar to proximal metaphyseal fractures in that they occur in younger patients, are generally torus or greenstick fractures, and heal well with closed treatment in a cast. A greenstick fracture is the most common fracture pattern: the posterior cortex is fractured while the anterior cortex undergoes compression, thereby resulting in an impaction type of fracture.

Treatment consists of cast immobilization for a nondisplaced fracture or minimally displaced fracture in a young child or fracture reduction under conscious sedation or general anesthesia followed by cast immobilization. In a young child (<6 years) with a minimally displaced fracture, a short-leg cast may be sufficient to maintain adequate alignment of the fracture for 4 to 6 weeks. In an older child or in any child with a displaced fracture, a long-leg cast with the knee flexed to 40 degrees for 3 to 4 weeks is necessary, followed by 2 to 3 weeks in a short-leg cast. It is often necessary to place the cast with the foot in 20 degrees of plantar flexion to maintain reduction of the apex-posterior fracture.

The outcome of these fractures is usually very good, with prompt fracture healing, little residual angulation, and—unlike with proximal metaphyseal fractures—no subsequent angular deformity.

Stress Fractures of the Tibia

The tibia is the most common site of stress fractures in the pediatric population. Tibial stress fractures are more common in boys than in girls and occur most often in adolescents active in sports.[23,63]

Patients have pain over the mid to proximal leg area but do not have a history of a traumatic injury. The incidence of these injuries peaks between 10 and 15 years, when children are participating in strenuous activities that place undue stress on the tibia. Stress fractures of the fibula are less common in children and occur at a younger age (3 to 8 years), frequently in ice skaters.[30,40] Usually, the children were not prepared or conditioned for the particular activity that they were involved in. The pain is mild and aching, with onset dependent on activity level and relieved by rest.[18] Typically the patient can point to the exact location of the pain, and there is point tenderness at the level of the stress fracture, without soft tissue swelling, erythema, or discoloration.

Radiographic findings are not usually present within the first 2 weeks after the onset of symptoms but are seen later as thickening of the cortical surface from periosteal and endosteal bone formation.[18,19,23,90] Three phases of radiographic changes have been defined, although these phases are rarely seen in each patient.[23] The initial findings include a radiolucent area within the cortex, followed by periosteal and endosteal new bone formation and, finally, resorption of this new bone (Fig. 43–153). Occasionally, a fracture line is seen during the second phase. The most common site for a tibial stress fracture is on the posteromedial or posterolateral aspect.

Tibial stress fractures are often difficult to diagnose from plain radiographs or may need to be confirmed with other tests to rule out infection, osteoid osteoma,

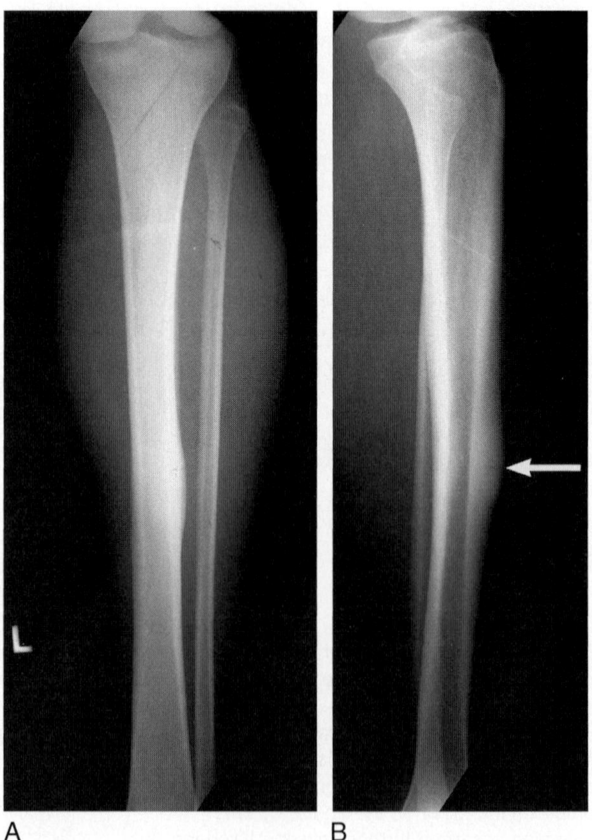

FIGURE 43–153 Tibial stress fracture. Anteroposterior **(A)** and lateral **(B)** radiographs demonstrating periosteal thickening of the cortex consistent with a tibial stress fracture. Note the radiolucent area on the anterior cortex (*arrow*).

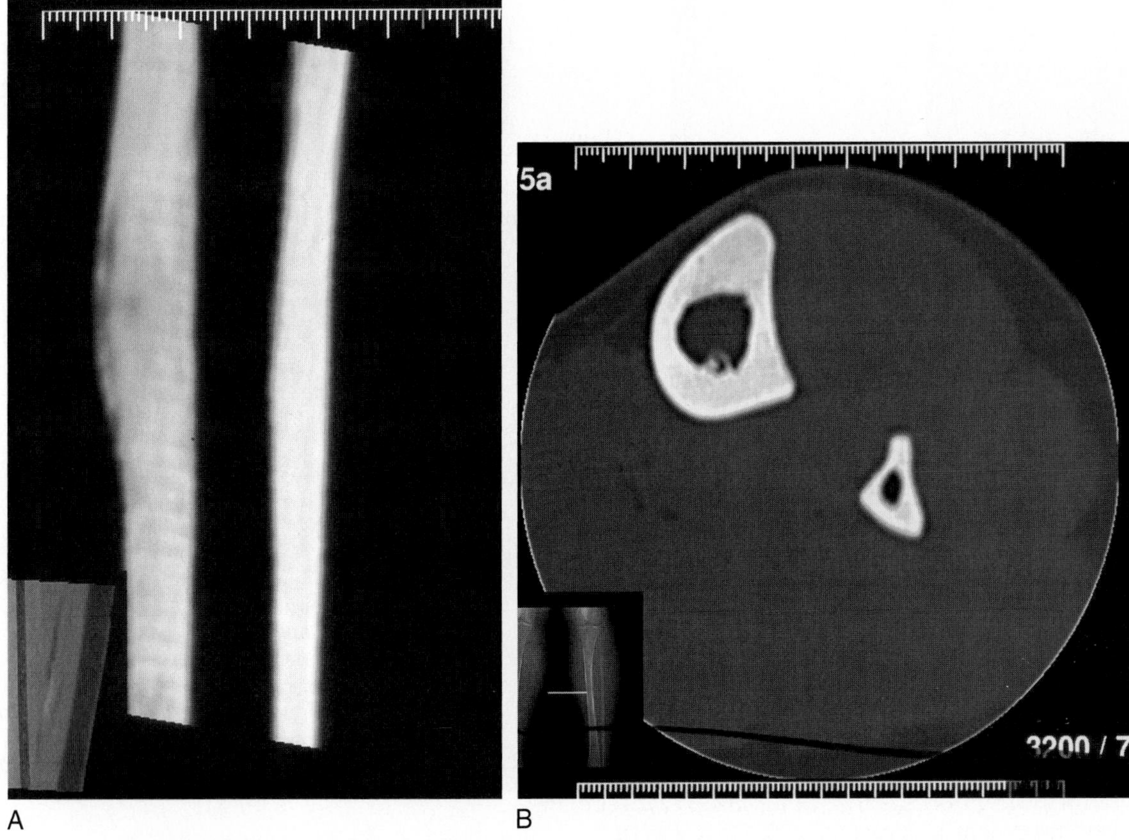

FIGURE 43-154 Computed tomography scans of a stress fracture of the tibia. A, Sagittal image demonstrating the thickened anterior cortex with a radiolucent area in the center. B, Axial image demonstrating thickened cortices and evidence of endosteal bone formation.

or osteogenic sarcoma. A technetium-enhanced bone scan can help the physician make the diagnosis earlier when plain radiographs may not reveal a discernible fracture.[57,77,87] The findings on bone scan consist of increased uptake in a localized area that is sharply demarcated. Other tests to confirm the diagnosis include CT and MRI. CT will demonstrate endosteal and periosteal new bone formation (Fig. 43–154), and MRI will demonstrate intracortical low signal intensity that is continuous with the intramedullary space, as well as surrounding areas of decreased signal intensity on T1-weighted images.[54]

The mainstay of treatment of tibial stress fractures is activity modification to decrease the continuous forces placed on the tibia. The fracture should heal completely before these activities are resumed. Cast immobilization is not required unless the patient is uncooperative with treatment. Restriction of activity should continue for 6 weeks or until symptoms completely resolve, followed by gradual resumption of activities. Stress fractures in children have universally good outcomes when treated appropriately.

Ipsilateral Femoral and Tibial Fracture ("Floating Knee")

Children involved in significant trauma can sustain a fracture of the tibia and the ipsilateral femur, the so-called floating knee. These injuries are relatively uncommon in children, are usually due to pedestrian–motor vehicle accidents, are often open fractures, and are associated with other organ system injuries.[46] The results of treatment are generally satisfactory; however, these injuries are associated with higher complication rates than an isolated tibial or femoral fracture is.

Careful assessment of the soft tissue structures, including the neurovascular system, is very important. These injuries are often associated with a popliteal artery injury, and an arteriogram should be obtained whenever any concern for this injury is present.

Treatment of a floating knee in a child depends on the age and particular injury to the child, including the state of the soft tissue envelope. In general, we prefer to obtain stable fixation whenever possible so that reduction is not lost. This also provides stability for transportation. Letts and colleagues reviewed 15 patients, all of whom had been involved in a motor vehicle accident that resulted in a floating knee and had undergone a variety of treatment modalities. The worst results occurred in patients after nonoperative treatment of both fractures, and they recommended that one or both bones be rigidly fixed.[55] Yue and coworkers also reported improved outcomes after operative stabilization of ipsilateral femoral and tibial fractures in all age groups. Hospital stay and time to weight bearing were also reduced.[116] In children 20 kg

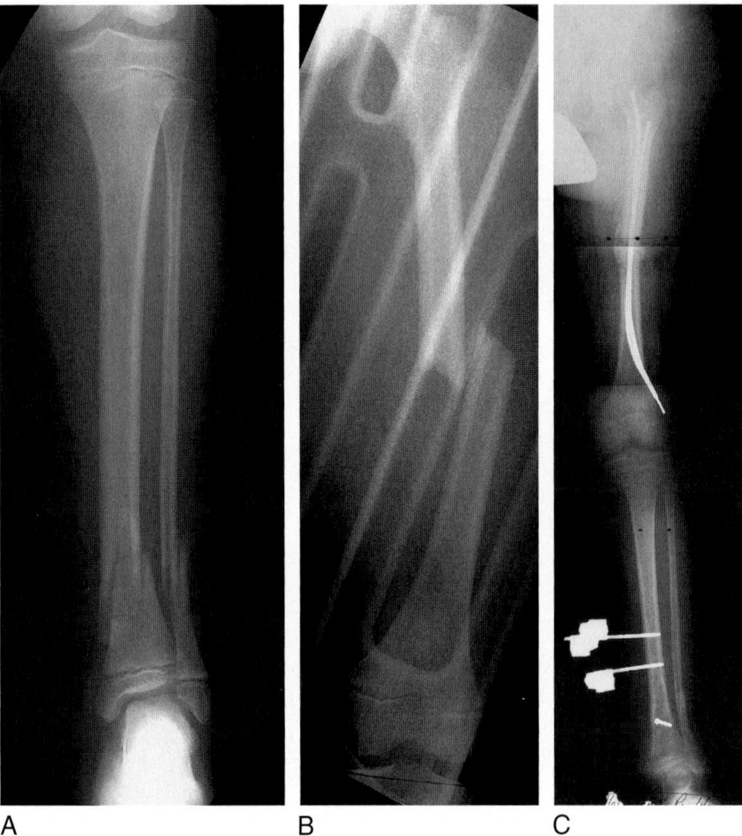

FIGURE 43–155 Treatment of a floating knee in an 11-year-old. Radiographs of a tibial/fibular fracture **(A)** and a transverse diaphyseal femur fracture **(B)** demonstrating ipsilateral femoral and distal tibial fractures. **C,** The femoral fracture was treated with retrograde Enders nailing, whereas the distal tibiofibular fracture was treated with an ankle-bridging external fixator and percutaneous screw fixation.

and larger, surgical stabilization of the femoral fracture with flexible intramedullary rodding will provide stable fixation of the fracture and allow easier manipulation and cast immobilization or fixation of the tibia; it will also prevent angular deformity and shortening (Fig. 43–155). In an adolescent, stable intramedullary fixation of both the femur and the tibia will allow treatment without external immobilization and permit early weight bearing and range-of-motion exercises of the knee and ankle.

The results of treatment of ipsilateral femoral and tibial fractures in children are generally satisfactory; however, complication rates are high. Complications include malunion, premature physeal closure, nonunion, pin tract infection, limb length discrepancy, and knee ligament injuries. Yasko and colleagues reported a 29% complication rate, with four of six patients requiring additional surgical procedures, including bone grafting for tibial nonunion and osteotomy for angular deformity.[114] It is important to evaluate the stability of the knee joint at the time of initial evaluation because many patients return at follow-up with unrecognized ligamentous injuries.[7]

References

Tibia and Fibula

1. Allen MJ, Nash JR, Ioannidies TT, et al: Major vascular injuries associated with orthopaedic injuries to the lower limb. Ann R Coll Surg Engl 1984;66:101.
2. Bahnson D, Lovell W: Genu valgum following fracture of the proximal tibial metaphysis in children. Orthop Trans 1980;4:306.
3. Balthazar DA, Pappas AM: Acquired valgus deformity of the tibia in children. J Pediatr Orthop 1984;4:538.
4. Bassey LO: Valgus deformity following proximal metaphyseal fractures in children: Experiences in the African tropics. J Trauma 1990;30:102.
5. Ben-Itzhak I, Erken EH, Malkin C: Progressive valgus deformity after juxta-epiphyseal fractures of the upper tibia in children. Injury 1987;18:169.
6. Best TN: Valgus deformity after fracture of the upper tibia in children. J Bone Joint Surg Br 1973;55:222.
7. Bohn WW, Durbin RA: Ipsilateral fractures of the femur and tibia in children and adolescents. J Bone Joint Surg Am 1991;73:429.
8. Bondurant FJ, Cotler HB, Buckle R, et al: The medical and economic impact of severely injured lower extremities. J Trauma 1988;28:1270.
9. Briggs TW, Orr MM, Lightowler CD: Isolated tibial fractures in children. Injury 1992;23:308.
10. Brougham DI, Nicol RO: Valgus deformity after proximal tibial fractures in children. J Bone Joint Surg Br 1987;69:482.
11. Buckley SL, Smith G, Sponseller PD, et al: Open fractures of the tibia in children. J Bone Joint Surg Am 1990;72:1462.
12. Byrd HS, Spicer TE, Cierney G 3rd: Management of open tibial fractures. Plast Reconstr Surg 1985;76:719.
13. Caudle RJ, Stern PJ: Severe open fractures of the tibia. J Bone Joint Surg Am 1987;69:801.

14. Christian EP, Bosse MJ, Robb G: Reconstruction of large diaphyseal defects, without free fibular transfer, in grade-IIIB tibial fractures. J Bone Joint Surg Am 1989; 71:994.
15. Cierny G 3rd, Byrd HS, Jones RE: Primary versus delayed soft tissue coverage for severe open tibial fractures. A comparison of results. Clin Orthop Relat Res 1983;178:54.
16. Cozen L: Fracture of the proximal portion of the tibia in children followed by valgus deformity. Surg Gynecol Obstet 1953;97:183.
17. Cullen MC, Roy DR, Crawford AH, et al: Open fracture of the tibia in children. J Bone Joint Surg Am 1996; 78:1039.
18. Devas MB: Stress fractures in children. J Bone Joint Surg Br 1963;45:528.
19. Devas MB, Sweetnam R: Stress fractures of the fibula; a review of fifty cases in athletes. J Bone Joint Surg Br 1956;38:818.
20. Drewes J, Schulte H: Bruche im Beriech des Unterschenkels bei Kindern infolge von Fahrradspeichenverletzungen. Chirurg 1965;36:464.
21. Dunbar JS, Owen HF, Nogrady MB, et al: Obscure tibial fracture of infants—the toddler's fracture. J Can Assoc Radiol 1964;15:136.
22. Ellis H: Disabilities after tibial shaft fractures; with special reference to Volkmann's ischaemic contracture. J Bone Joint Surg Br 1958;40:190.
23. Engh CA, Robinson RA, Milgram J: Stress fractures in children. J Trauma 1970;10:532.
24. Fagelman MF, Epps HR, Rang M: Mangled extremity severity score in children. J Pediatr Orthop 2002;22: 182.
25. Fredericson M, Bergman AG, Hoffman KL, et al: Tibial stress reaction in runners. Correlation of clinical symptoms and scintigraphy with a new magnetic resonance imaging grading system. Am J Sports Med 1995;23: 472.
26. Friedman RJ, Jupiter JB: Vascular injuries and closed extremity fractures in children. Clin Orthop Relat Res 1984;188:112.
27. Georgiadis GM, Behrens FF, Joyce MJ, et al: Open tibial fractures with severe soft-tissue loss. Limb salvage compared with below-the-knee amputation. J Bone Joint Surg Am 1993;75:1431.
28. Goodwin RC, Gaynor T, Mahar A, et al: Intramedullary flexible nail fixation of unstable pediatric tibial diaphyseal fractures. J Pediatr Orthop 2005;25:570.
29. Green NE: Tibia valga caused by asymmetrical overgrowth following a nondisplaced fracture of the proximal tibial metaphysis. J Pediatr Orthop 1983;3:235.
30. Griffiths AL: Fatigue fracture of the fibula in childhood. Arch Dis Child 1952;27:552.
31. Grimard G, Naudie D, Laberge LC, et al: Open fractures of the tibia in children. Clin Orthop Relat Res 1996;332:62.
32. Gustilo RB: Bone grafting in open fractures. J Orthop Trauma 1976;2:54.
33. Gustilo RB, Anderson JT: Prevention of infection in the treatment of one thousand and twenty-five open fractures of long bones: Retrospective and prospective analyses. J Bone Joint Surg Am 1976;58:453.
34. Hansen BA, Greiff J, Bergmann F: Fractures of the tibia in children. Acta Orthop Scand 1976;47:448.
35. Harman J, Guinn R: The recovery of skeletal muscle fibers from acute ischemia as determined by histologic and chemical methods. Am J Pathol 1948;25:751.
36. Herring JA, Moseley C: Posttraumatic valgus deformity of the tibia. J Pediatr Orthop 1981;1:435.
37. Herscovici D Jr, Sanders RW, Scaduto JM, et al: Vacuum-assisted wound closure (VAC therapy) for the management of patients with high-energy soft tissue injuries. J Orthop Trauma 2003;17:683.
38. Hill SA: Incidence of tibial fracture in child skiers. Br J Sports Med 1989;23:169.
39. Horowitz JH, Nichter LS, Kenney JG, et al: Lawnmower injuries in children: Lower extremity reconstruction. J Trauma 1985;25:1138.
40. Ingersoll C: Ice skater's fracture: A form of fatigue fracture. AJR Am J Roentgenol 1943;50:469.
41. Iobst CA, Tidwell MA, King WF: Nonoperative management of pediatric type I open fractures. J Pediatr Orthop 2005;25:513.
42. Ippolito E, Pentimalli G: Post-traumatic valgus deformity of the knee in proximal tibial metaphyseal fractures in children. Ital J Orthop Traumatol 1984;10: 103.
43. Irwin A, Gibson P, Ashcroft P: Open fractures of the tibia in children. Injury 1995;26:21.
44. Jackson DW, Cozen L: Genu valgum as a complication of proximal tibial metaphyseal fractures in children. J Bone Joint Surg Am 1971;53:1571.
45. Jackson JP, Waugh W: The technique and complications of upper tibial osteotomy. A review of 226 operations. J Bone Joint Surg Br 1974;56:236.
46. Jawadi AH, Letts M: Injuries associated with fracture of the femur secondary to motor vehicle accidents in children. Am J Orthop 2003;32:459.
47. Johansen K, Bandyk D, Thiele B, et al: Temporary intraluminal shunts: Resolution of a management dilemma in complex vascular injuries. J Trauma 1982; 22:395.
48. Johansen K, Daines M, Howey T, et al: Objective criteria accurately predict amputation following lower extremity trauma. J Trauma 1990;30:568.
49. Jordan SE, Alonso JE, Cook FF: The etiology of valgus angulation after metaphyseal fractures of the tibia in children. J Pediatr Orthop 1987;7:450.
50. Karrholm J, Hansson LI, Svensson K: Incidence of tibiofibular shaft and ankle fractures in children. J Pediatr Orthop 1982;2:386.
51. Kreder HJ, Armstrong P: A review of open tibia fractures in children. J Pediatr Orthop 1995;15:482.
52. Kubiak EN, Egol KA, Scher D, et al: Operative treatment of tibial fractures in children: Are elastic stable intramedullary nails an improvement over external fixation? J Bone Joint Surg Am 2005;87:1761.
53. Leach RE, Hammond G, Stryker WS: Anterior tibial compartment syndrome. Acute and chronic. J Bone Joint Surg Am 1967;49:451.
54. Lee JK, Yao L: Stress fractures: MR imaging. Radiology 1988;169:217.
55. Letts M, Vincent N, Gouw G: The "floating knee" in children. J Bone Joint Surg Br 1986;68:442.

56. Mahnken RF, Yngve DA: Valgus deformity following fracture of the tibial metaphysis. Orthopedics 1988;11: 1317.
57. Matin P: The appearance of bone scans following fractures, including immediate and long-term studies. J Nucl Med 1979;20:1227.
58. Matsen FA 3rd, Staheli LT: Neurovascular complications following tibial osteotomy in children. A case report. Clin Orthop Relat Res 1975;110:210.
59. Matsen FA 3rd, Winquist RA, Krugmire RB Jr: Diagnosis and management of compartmental syndromes. J Bone Joint Surg Am 1980;62:286.
60. McCarthy JJ, Kim DH, Eilert RE: Posttraumatic genu valgum: Operative versus nonoperative treatment. J Pediatr Orthop 1998;18:518.
61. Meland NB, Fisher J, Irons GB, et al: Experience with 80 rectus abdominis free-tissue transfers. Plast Reconstr Surg 1989;83:481.
62. Mellick LB, Reesor K: Spiral tibial fractures of children: A commonly accidental spiral long bone fracture. Am J Emerg Med 1990;8:234.
63. Micheli LJ, Gerbino P: Etiologic assessment of stress fractures of the lower extremity in young athletes. Orthop Trans 1980;41:51.
64. Morton KS, Starr DE: Closure of the anterior portion of the upper tibial epiphysis as a complication of tibial-shaft fracture. J Bone Joint Surg Am 1964;46:570.
65. Mubarak SJ: A practical approach to compartmental syndromes. Part II. Diagnosis. Instr Course Lect 1983; 32:92.
66. Mubarak SJ, Carroll NC: Volkmann's contracture in children: Aetiology and prevention. J Bone Joint Surg Br 1979;61:285.
67. Mubarak SJ, Owen CA, Hargens AR, et al: Acute compartment syndromes: Diagnosis and treatment with the aid of the wick catheter. J Bone Joint Surg Am 1978;60:1091.
68. O'Brien T, Weisman DS, Ronchetti P, et al: Flexible titanium nailing for the treatment of the unstable pediatric tibial fracture. J Pediatr Orthop 2004;24: 601.
69. Ogden JA: Skeletal Injury in the Child. Philadelphia, Lea & Febiger, 1982.
70. Ogden JA, Ogden DA, Pugh L, et al: Tibia valga after proximal metaphyseal fractures in childhood: A normal biologic response. J Pediatr Orthop 1995;15:489.
71. Ostermann PA, Henry SL, Seligson D: Timing of wound closure in severe compound fractures. Orthopedics 1994;17:397.
72. Oudjhane K, Newman B, Oh KS, et al: Occult fractures in preschool children. J Trauma 1988;28:858.
73. Paley D, Catagni MA, Argnani F, et al: Ilizarov treatment of tibial nonunions with bone loss. Clin Orthop Relat Res 1989;241:146.
74. Park HM, Kernek CB, Robb JA: Early scintigraphic findings of occult femoral and tibial fractures in infants. Clin Nucl Med 1988;13:271.
75. Patzakis MJ, Wilkins J: Factors influencing infection rate in open fracture wounds. Clin Orthop Relat Res 1989;243:36.
76. Pollen A: Fractures and Dislocations. Edinburgh, Churchill Livingstone, 1973.
77. Prather JL, Nusynowitz ML, Snowdy HA, et al: Scintigraphic findings in stress fractures. J Bone Joint Surg Am 1977;59:869.
78. Rang M: Children's Fractures. Philadelphia, JB Lippincott, 1974.
79. Rhinelander FW: Tibial blood supply in relation to fracture healing. Clin Orthop Relat Res 1974;105: 34.
80. Rhinelander FW: Blood supply to developing mature and healing bone. In Sumner-Smith G (ed): Bone in Clinical Orthopaedics. Philadelphia, WB Saunders, 1982, p 81.
81. Robert M, Khouri N, Carlioz H, et al: Fractures of the proximal tibial metaphysis in children: Review of a series of 25 cases. J Pediatr Orthop 1987;7:444.
82. Robertson P, Karol LA, Rab GT: Open fractures of the tibia and femur in children. J Pediatr Orthop 1996;16: 621.
83. Rooker G, Salter R: Prevention of valgus deformity following fracture of the proximal metaphysis of the tibia in children. J Bone Joint Surg Br 1980;62:527.
84. Rorabeck CH: A practical approach to compartmental syndrome. Part III. Management. Instr Course Lect 1983;32:102.
85. Rorabeck CH: The treatment of compartment syndromes of the leg. J Bone Joint Surg Br 1984;66:93.
86. Rorabeck CH, Macnab L: Anterior tibial-compartment syndrome complicating fractures of the shaft of the tibia. J Bone Joint Surg Am 1976;58:549.
87. Roub LW, Gumerman LW, Hanley EN Jr, et al: Bone stress: A radionuclide imaging perspective. Radiology 1979;132:431.
88. Russell GG, Henderson R, Arnett G: Primary or delayed closure for open tibial fractures. J Bone Joint Surg Br 1990;72:125.
89. Salter R, Best TN: The pathogenesis and prevention of valgus deformity following fractures of the proximal metaphyseal region of the tibia in children. J Bone Joint Surg Am 1973;55:1324.
90. Savoca CJ: Stress fractures. A classification of the earliest radiographic signs. Radiology 1971;100:519.
91. Schrock RD Jr: Peroneal nerve palsy following derotation osteotomies for tibial torsion. Clin Orthop Relat Res 1969;62:172.
92. Scully R, Shannon J, Dickerson J: Factors involved in recovery from experimental skeletal ischemia in dogs. Am J. Pathol 1961;39:721.
93. Shannak AO: Tibial fractures in children: Follow-up study. J Pediatr Orthop 1988;8:306.
94. Shilt JS, Yoder JS, Manuck TA, et al: Role of vacuum-assisted closure in the treatment of pediatric lawnmower injuries. J Pediatr Orthop 2004;24:482.
95. Skaggs DL, Friend L, Alman B, et al: The effect of surgical delay on acute infection following 554 open fractures in children. J Bone Joint Surg Am 2005; 87:8.
96. Skaggs DL, Kautz SM, Kay RM, et al: Effect of delay of surgical treatment on rate of infection in open fractures in children. J Pediatr Orthop 2000;20:19.
97. Skak SV, Jensen TT, Poulsen TD: Fracture of the proximal metaphysis of the tibia in children. Injury 1987; 18:149.

98. Song KM, Sangeorzan B, Benirschke S, et al: Open fractures of the tibia in children. J Pediatr Orthop 1996;16:635.
99. Spiro SA, Oppenheim W, Boss WK, et al: Reconstruction of the lower extremity after grade III distal tibial injuries using combined microsurgical free tissue transfer and bone transport by distraction osteosynthesis. Ann Plast Surg 1993;30:97.
100. Stanford TC, Rodriguez RP Jr, Hayes JT: Tibial-shaft fractures in adults and children. JAMA 1966;195:1111.
101. Steinert V, Bennek J: [Tibial fractures in children.] Zentralbl Chir 1966;91:1387.
102. Strachan RK, McCarthy I, Fleming R, et al: The role of the tibial nutrient artery. Microsphere estimation of blood flow in the osteotomised canine tibia. J Bone Joint Surg Br 1990;72:391.
103. Swaan JW, Oppers VM: Crural fractures in children. A study of the incidence of changes of the axial position and of enhanced longitudinal growth of the tibia after the healing of crural fractures. Arch Chir Neerl 1971;23:259.
104. Taylor S: Tibial overgrowth: A cause of genu valgum. J Bone Joint Surg Am 1963;45:659.
105. Teitz CC, Carter DR, Frankel VH: Problems associated with tibial fractures with intact fibulae. J Bone Joint Surg Am 1980;62:770.
106. Tenenbein M, Reed MH, Black GB: The toddler's fracture revisited. Am J Emerg Med 1990;8:208.
107. Tuten HR, Keeler KA, Gabos PG, et al: Posttraumatic tibia valga in children. A long-term follow-up note. J Bone Joint Surg Am 1999;81:799.
108. Visser JD, Veldhuizen AG: Valgus deformity after fracture of the proximal tibial metaphysis in childhood. Acta Orthop Scand 1982;53:663.
109. Weber BG: Fibrous interposition causing valgus deformity after fracture of the upper tibial metaphysis in children. J Bone Joint Surg Br 1977;59:290.
110. Whitesides TE, Haney TC, Morimoto K, et al: Tissue pressure measurements as a determinant for the need of fasciotomy. Clin Orthop Relat Res 1975;113:43.
111. Wolma FJ, Larrieu AJ, Alsop GC: Arterial injuries of the legs associated with fractures and dislocations. Am J Surg 1980;140:806.
112. Yang JP, Letts RM: Isolated fractures of the tibia with intact fibula in children: A review of 95 patients. J Pediatr Orthop 1997;17:347.
113. Yaremchuk MJ: Acute management of severe soft-tissue damage accompanying open fractures of the lower extremity. Clin Plast Surg 1986;13:621.
114. Yasko AW, Thompson GH, Wilber JH: Ipsilateral fractures of the femur and tibia in children. Paper presented at a combined meeting of the Paediatric Orthopaedic Society of North America and the Eruopean Pediatric Orthopaedic Society, 1990, Montreal.
115. Yasko AW, Wilber JH: Open tibial fractures in children. Orthop Trans 1989;13:547.
116. Yue JJ, Churchill RS, Cooperman DR, et al: The floating knee in the pediatric patient. Nonoperative versus operative stabilization. Clin Orthop Relat Res 2000;376:124.
117. Zionts LE, Harcke HT, Brooks KM, et al: Posttraumatic tibia valga: A case demonstrating asymmetric activity at the proximal growth plate on technetium bone scan. J Pediatr Orthop 1987;7:458.
118. Zionts LE, MacEwen GD: Spontaneous improvement of post-traumatic tibia valga. J Bone Joint Surg Am 1986;68:680.

ANKLE

Anatomy

The distal tibial epiphysis ossifies between 6 and 12 months of age, and the medial malleolus appears at 7 years in girls and 8 years in boys. The medial malleolus usually ossifies as a downward extension of the distal tibial ossific nucleus, although it may develop as a separate center of ossification and can be mistaken for a fracture line. The distal aspect of the tibia is completely ossified by 14 to 15 years of age and fuses with the diaphysis at 18 years. Closure of the physis begins centrally, progresses medially, and continues laterally, with the entire process lasting approximately 18 months. This is responsible for the fracture patterns seen in the distal tibia before complete physeal closure, with physeal fractures of the lateral distal tibial physis occurring without injury to the medial side. The distal tibial physis contributes 45% of the growth of the tibia. The distal fibula ossifies during the second year of life, generally between the ages of 18 and 20 months. This physis usually closes 12 to 24 months later than the distal tibial physis.

The ankle joint is composed of the dome of the talus and the distal aspect of the tibia and fibula, which are joined together by a syndesmosis composed of three distinct ligaments: the inferior transverse ligament, the anteroinferior tibiofibular ligament, and the posteroinferior tibiofibular ligament (Fig. 43–156). Ligamentous structures stabilize the distal tibia-fibula complex to the talus and foot. On the medial aspect of the ankle the medial malleolus is attached to the foot by the deltoid ligament, which has a deep component attaching to the talus (the anterior tibiotalar ligament) and a superficial component that is composed of three distinct ligaments and named according to the anatomy that they span—the calcaneotibial, tibionavicular, and posterior talotibial ligaments (Fig. 43–157). The lateral aspect of the ankle is stabilized by three ligaments that originate at the lateral malleolus and insert onto the talus (anterior and posterior talofibular ligaments) and the calcaneus (calcaneofibular ligament). These ligaments are attached to the distal tibia and fibula at the epiphysis, distal to the physis. Because ligamentous structures are stronger than the physis in children, avulsion-type injuries, in which traumatic forces exerted through the ankle ligaments create physeal fractures, are common.

For the purpose of classifying distal tibial injuries, four major headings will be used in the discussion of injuries and their treatment:

Ankle fractures:
- Supination-inversion injury
- Supination–plantar flexion injury
- Supination–external rotation fracture

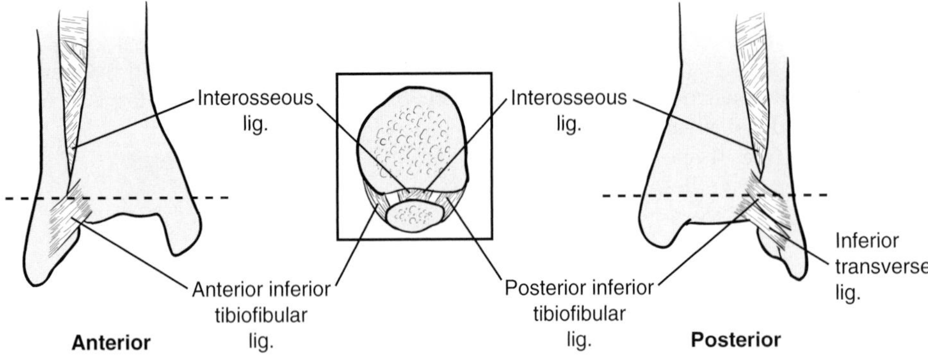

FIGURE 43–156 The ankle syndesmosis, anterior and posterior views. The syndesmosis is composed of the interosseous ligament, the anterior and posterior inferior tibiofibular ligaments, and the inferior transverse ligament posteriorly.

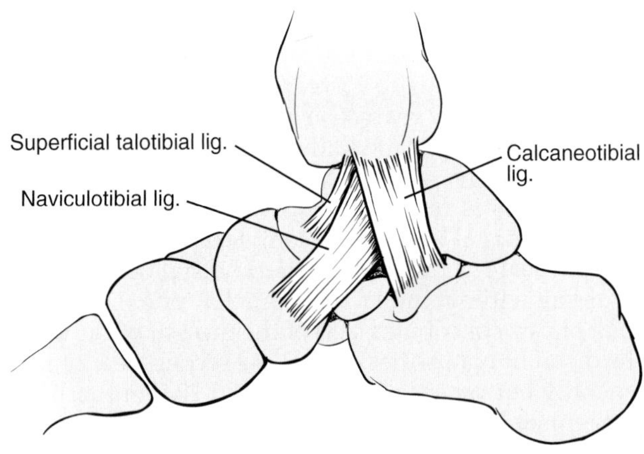

FIGURE 43–157 The medial collateral ligamentous complex of the ankle.

Pronation–eversion–external rotation fracture
Axial compression injuries
Other physeal injuries
 Tillaux fractures
 Triplane fractures
 Isolated distal fibular fractures

Ankle Fractures

Distal tibia and fibula fractures are relatively common, second only to distal radius fractures as the most common physeal fractures in children.[173] The horizontal orientation of the physis and the strong ligamentous attachments distal to the physis make the physis more vulnerable to injury. Fractures of the distal tibia and fibula occur most frequently between 10 and 15 years of age and are more common in boys than in girls. These physeal injuries more often require operative intervention than do fractures of the distal radius and are also more likely to be associated with subsequent premature growth arrest.

CLASSIFICATION

The well-known Salter-Harris classification of physeal fractures describes the anatomic characteristics of distal tibial injuries, provides treatment guidelines, and best prognosticates the status of the growth plate. However, the complexity of the ankle anatomy and its ligamentous attachments, together with various deforming forces at the time of ankle injury, makes it important to use a classification scheme that provides information on the mechanism of injury. This is most important in predicting the likelihood of achieving closed reduction and in determining the type of maneuver necessary to achieve reduction.

The first mechanistic classification of ankle fractures in children was proposed by Bishop, who modified the adult Ashhurst-Bromer classification.[17] Carothers and Crenshaw further modified the classification to include the direction of the injuring force.[37] The most commonly used ankle classification in adults was described by Lauge-Hansen and is based on three characteristics: the position of the foot at the time of injury, the axial load at the time of injury, and the direction of the deforming force.[119-123] However, this classification does not specifically apply to children because it does not take into account the presence of the distal physis of the tibia and fibula. Therefore, Dias and Tachdjian modified the Lauge-Hansen classification to include the Salter-Harris classification so that it applies to injuries in children.[60,61] The original classification defined four types of fractures, each with a two-part name; the first term refers to the position of the foot at the time of injury and the second term to the direction of the deforming force, with grades of injury described in increasing severity (Fig. 43–158). Subsequently, the last four types of fractures were added: juvenile Tillaux, triplane, axial compression, and miscellaneous physeal injuries.[218] To fully use this classification, the following characteristics should be defined: the Salter-Harris type of injury, the direction of the fracture line, the direction of displacement of the epiphyseal-metaphyseal fracture fragment, and the relation of this fracture fragment to localized swelling and tenderness.

Supination-Inversion Injury

This injury occurs with an inversion deforming force applied to the foot in the supinated position.

Grade I injuries occur when traction by the lateral ligaments produces a Salter-Harris type I or II fracture, separation of the distal fibular physis. The fracture may occasionally be at the tip of the lateral malleolus, and rarely, the lateral ligaments are injured. Displace-

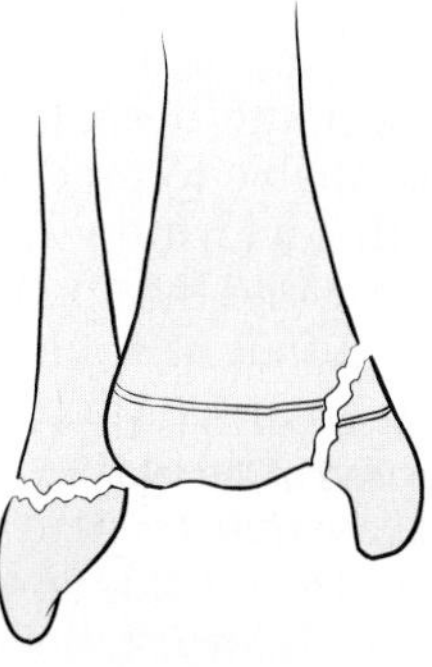

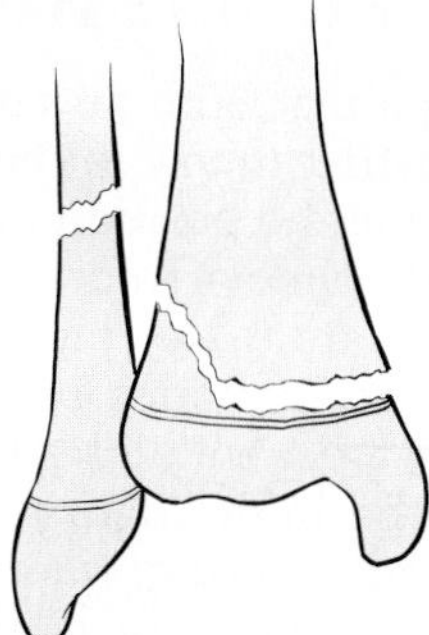

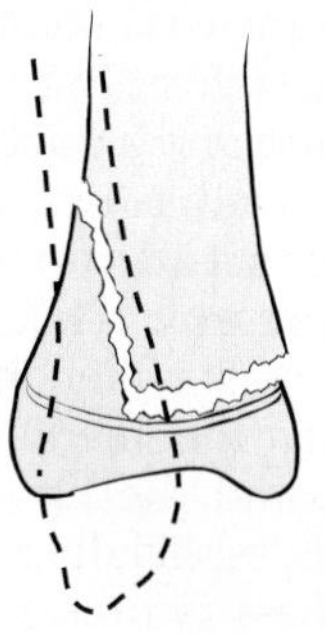

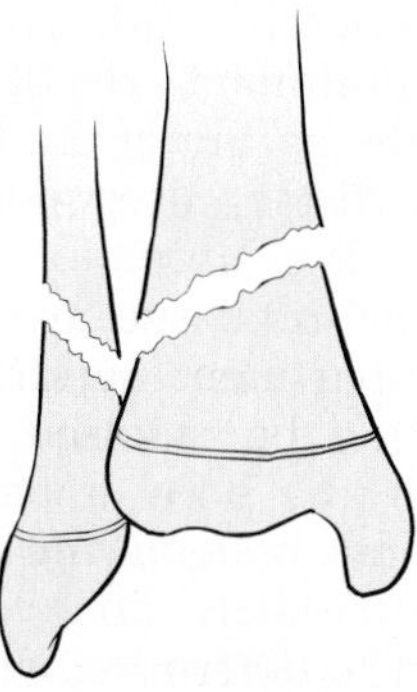

FIGURE 43–158 The Dias-Tachdjian modification of the Lauge-Hansen classification of ankle fractures in children.

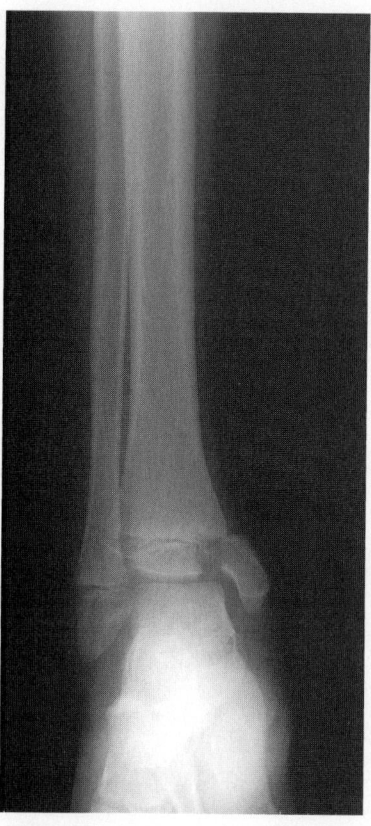

FIGURE 43–159 Grade II supination-inversion injury pattern in a 12-year-old who sustained a distal tibial Salter-Harris type III fracture and a displaced Salter-Harris type I distal fibular fracture as a result of an inversion injury of the ankle.

ment of the distal fibular epiphysis is minimal, and injury to the distal fibular physis may go undiagnosed because of this minimal displacement.

Grade II injuries are a continuation of a grade I injury in which the talus is further pushed medially against the medial malleolus and tilts the talus up into the medial half of the distal end of the tibia (Fig. 43–159). This results in a Salter-Harris type III or IV injury. A type III fracture extends from the articular surface to the zone of the hypertrophic cartilage cells of the physis and exits medially. In a type IV fracture the epiphysis, the physis, and a portion of the metaphysis are completely split, with upward displacement of the medial fragment (Fig. 43–160). Occasionally there is a Salter-Harris type II fracture of the distal tibia in which the distal tibial fracture involves the lateral physis and exits medially through a metaphyseal fracture. Rarely, the fracture extends through the distal tibial physis only, thereby resulting in a Salter-Harris type I injury.

Supination–Plantar Flexion Injury

This injury occurs with the foot fixed in full supination while a plantar flexion force is exerted on the ankle (see Fig. 43–158).

The most common fracture pattern is one in which a Salter-Harris type II physeal injury of the distal tibial physis occurs along with posterior displacement of the epiphyseal-metaphyseal fracture fragment and no fracture of the fibula. The metaphyseal fragment of the tibia is posterior and best seen on a lateral radiograph (Fig. 43–161).

Supination–External Rotation Fracture

This injury occurs with the foot fixed in full supination while a lateral rotation force is exerted on the ankle (see Fig. 43–158).

Grade I injuries result in a Salter-Harris type II fracture of the distal tibial epiphysis with a posterior metaphyseal-diaphyseal fragment and posterior displacement of the fracture. The distal tibial fracture begins on the lateral distal aspect and spirals medially and proximally. The fibula remains intact (Fig. 43–162). This fracture is similar to a supination–plantar flexion injury, especially when seen on the lateral radiograph; the distinction is that the distal tibial fracture line begins on the distal lateral aspect and spirals medially when viewed on the AP projection.

Grade II injuries result from a further lateral rotation force that produces a spiral fracture of the fibula. The fracture begins medially and extends superiorly and posteriorly.

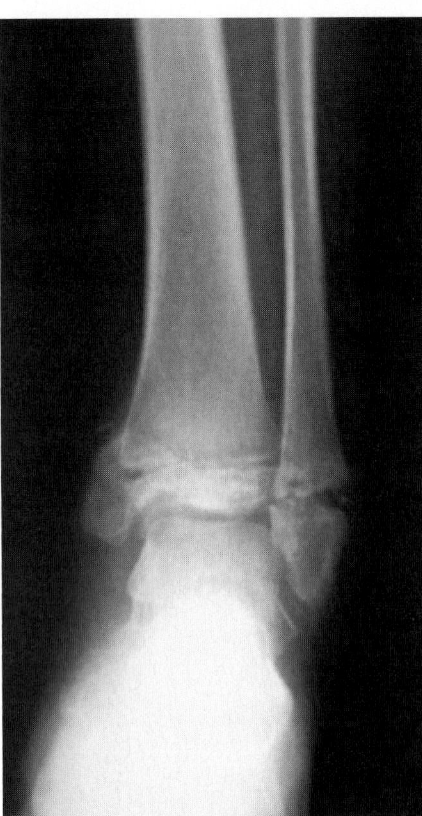

FIGURE 43–160 Grade II supination injury pattern in which treatment was not undertaken. There is a partially healed Salter-Harris type IV injury of the distal tibia and a Salter-Harris type I injury of the distal fibula.

Pronation–Eversion–External Rotation Fracture

This injury results when an eversion and lateral rotation force is applied to a fully pronated foot (see Fig. 43–158). Typically, a Salter-Harris type I or II fracture of the distal tibia occurs, together with a transverse or short oblique fibular fracture located 4 to 7 cm proximal to the tip of the lateral malleolus. When a Salter-Harris type II fracture occurs, the metaphyseal fragment is located laterally or posterolaterally and the distal tibial fragment is displaced laterally and posteriorly (Fig. 43–163).

Axial Compression Injuries and Other Physeal Injuries

These Salter-Harris type V injuries result from an axial load applied to the distal tibia and are often recognized late because of subsequent physeal arrest. They are rare injuries that account for less than 1% of all distal tibial physeal or ankle fractures.[212] When this injury is suspected and it is difficult to ascertain from radiographs whether a Salter-Harris type V fracture has occurred, MRI may be helpful in identifying this injury.[209]

Other physeal injuries are fractures that cannot be classified according to the current ankle fracture classification and include stress fractures and miscellaneous injuries of the distal fibula.

CLINICAL FEATURES

A patient with an ankle fracture usually describes a twisting injury to the ankle but is unable to precisely define the position of the foot or the deforming force at the time of injury. The history provided by a patient with an ankle fracture is slightly different from the history provided by a patient with an ankle sprain in that a patient with a fracture will have pain at the time of the initial injury that persists, as well as pain on weight bearing, whereas a patient with an ankle sprain has initial pain at the time of the injury, followed shortly by some relief of the pain, which slowly returns along with increasing swelling and progressive pain with weight bearing.

The physical examination should include a visual inspection of the skin for lacerations and evidence of an open fracture. The site of any ecchymosis and the predominant area of swelling will provide some clue to the nature of the injury and the deforming forces. The distal pulses should be evaluated and a good neurologic examination performed, as well as evaluation of the soft tissue envelope to ensure that an impending compartment syndrome is not present. The ankle should be assessed for specific areas of tenderness over the bony anatomy, especially the medial and lateral malleoli, the anterior tibia, and the tibial and fibular shafts. In a young child it is especially important to determine whether tenderness is present over the distal fibular physis or the distal medial tibial physis, or both, because radiographs may not show a Salter-Harris type I fracture. Tenderness of the soft tissue structures of the ankle should also be assessed, particularly the lateral ankle ligaments (anterior and posterior talofibular and calcaneofibular ligaments). Examination of the medial ankle ligaments is especially important with an isolated distal fibular fracture. Tenderness medially in this situation requires careful assessment of the stability of the ankle and, in a skeletally mature patient, requires internal fixation of the fibular fracture.[152-154] Though rare, subluxation of the peroneal tendons is often missed and mistaken for an ankle sprain or a distal fibular fracture.[68,151,215] Tenderness posterior to the distal fibula with subluxation of the peroneal tendons elicited on dorsiflexion and eversion of the ankle confirms the diagnosis, and operative treatment usually provides good results.[215]

RADIOGRAPHIC FINDINGS

Radiographic examination of a suspected ankle fracture should include AP, lateral, and mortise views of the ankle (Fig. 43–164). If only two views can be obtained, it is best to obtain the mortise and lateral views and omit the AP view. The radiographs should be closely inspected for fracture, the relationship of the tibia and fibula, and the presence of an intact mortise by comparing the joint space throughout the mortise to confirm that there is symmetry. In injuries in which instability is suspected with an innocuous-appearing fracture, stress radiographs should be obtained to help define the presence of instability (Fig. 43–165).

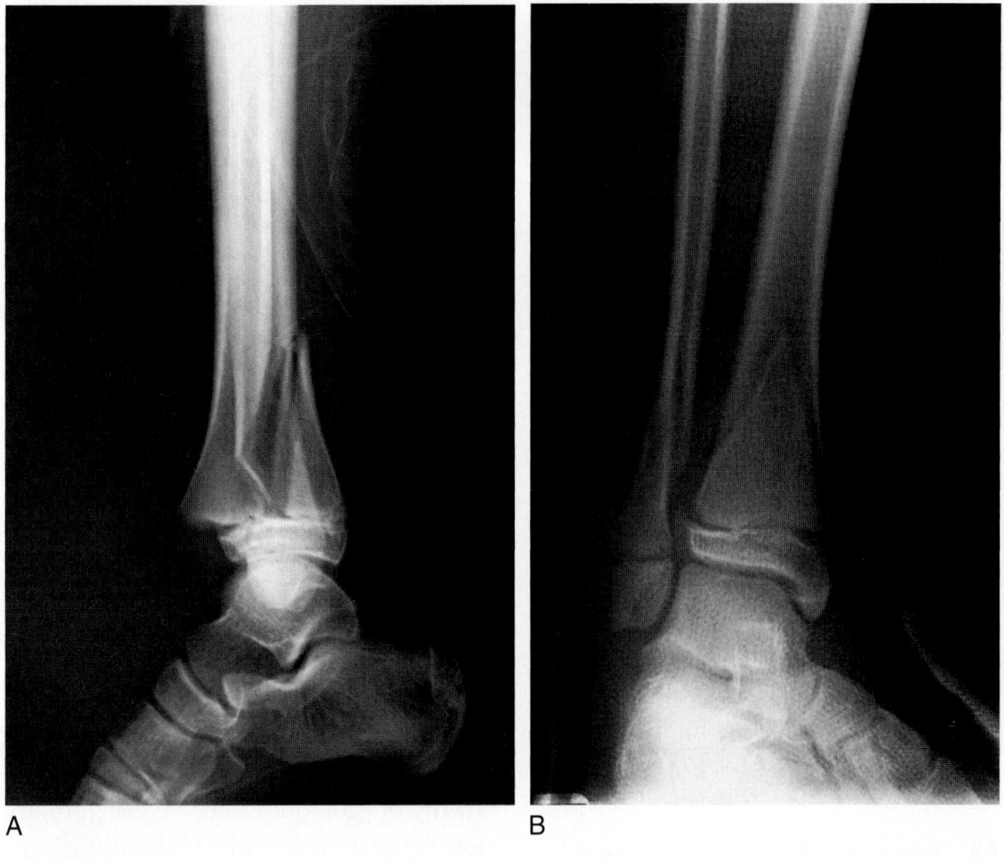

FIGURE 43-161 Radiographic appearance of a supination–plantar flexion injury. **A,** Lateral radiograph showing the posterior metaphyseal fragment on the distal tibia. **B,** Anteroposterior radiograph similarly demonstrating this metaphyseal fragment on the distal tibia, as well as the distal fibular fracture.

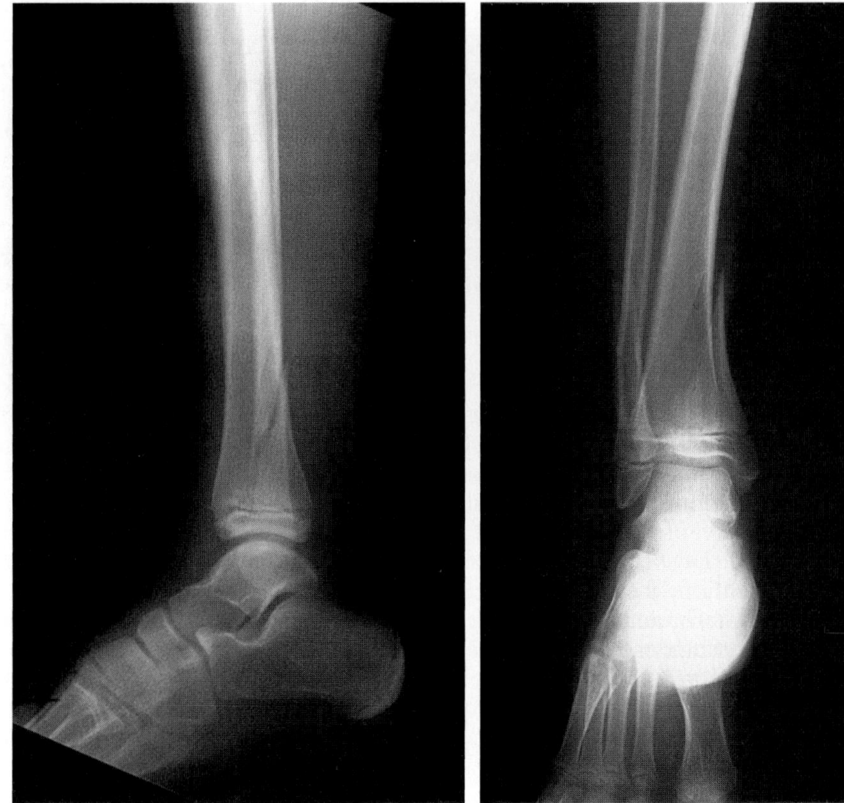

FIGURE 43-162 **A** and **B,** Radiographic appearance of a supination–lateral rotation fracture pattern. The distal tibial fracture begins distolaterally and spirals proximomedially. The distal fibula has sustained a spiral fracture as a result of the external rotation force.

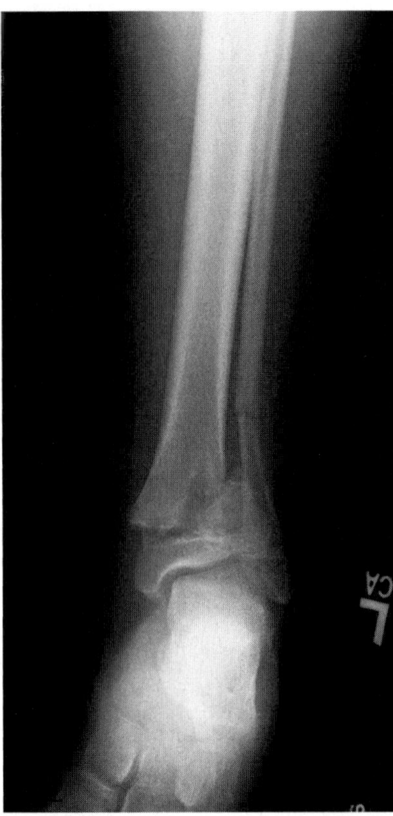

FIGURE 43–163 Radiographic appearance of a pronation–eversion–lateral rotation injury. Note the Salter-Harris type II fracture of the distal tibia with the metaphyseal fragment on the lateral aspect. The distal fibular fracture is a transverse fracture that occurs just proximal to the syndesmosis.

Accessory centers of ossification may be seen on the medial and lateral aspects of the ankle, are commonly bilateral, and can be seen on both the medial and lateral aspects of the foot (Fig. 43–166).[83,118,125,164] On the medial side the os subtibiale can be seen in up to 20%. On the lateral side the os subfibulare is seen less often, in only 1% of cases.[182] This is often mistaken for an avulsion injury and is best evaluated by assessing for the presence of tenderness distal to the medial and lateral malleoli.

TREATMENT

The mechanistic classification described by Dias and Tachdjian is invaluable in understanding the deforming forces of the fracture and therefore the reduction maneuver required to obtain satisfactory reduction. The majority of ankle fractures in children can be treated by closed reduction followed by external immobilization; therefore, a thorough understanding of this classification and the mechanism of injury is important. The type of anesthesia required for closed reduction of ankle fractures in children depends on the age of the child, the type of fracture, and the amount of fracture displacement. A young child with a minimally displaced fracture that can be easily reduced without a great deal of force may require only a hematoma block, whereas a larger child with a significantly displaced fracture may need conscious sedation or a general anesthetic. As in any physeal injury, the reduction should be performed as gently and as soon as possible to avoid having to use considerable force. Each day of delay makes it more difficult to achieve fracture reduction and places the viability of the physis at risk when forceful reduction is required. When the time from injury to treatment is 10 days or longer, we recommend that reduction be avoided because excess force is required for reduction and has a high likelihood of injuring the physis. The initial deformity is accepted, especially when it is in the sagittal plane, and time is allowed for remodeling to occur. If the deformity is in the coronal plane and the fracture is seen late, we prefer to allow fracture consolidation, thereby preserving the growth of the distal tibial physis, followed by corrective osteotomy at a later date.

When operative treatment is required, it is easiest and more useful to use the Salter-Harris classification to guide the surgeon in the treatment plan. In addition, the Salter-Harris classification provides better prognostic information because it correlates with the incidence and type of complications.[212] In a review of 237 distal tibial fractures, three groups of fractures were differentiated according to their risk for the development of complications; these groups were best correlated with the type of fracture (Salter-Harris classification), the severity of displacement or comminution, and the adequacy of reduction.[212]

The primary indications for operative treatment of ankle fractures in children are an inability to achieve or maintain closed reduction, displaced physeal fractures, displaced articular fractures, open fractures, and ankle fractures with significant tissue injury.

The following treatment outline uses the Salter-Harris classification as a framework to guide fracture treatment and the Dias-Tachdjian classification principally to identify the deforming forces and the type of closed reduction maneuvers.

Salter-Harris Types I and II Distal Fibular Fractures

A type I fracture of the fibula is the most common fracture of the ankle in children and is often misdiagnosed as an ankle sprain. Because children are more likely to sustain physeal injuries than ankle sprains, surgeons should have a high index of suspicion that an injury to the distal fibular physis has occurred. The mechanism of injury is usually inversion of a supinated foot and can be associated with a distal tibial physeal fracture. The average age of patients with a type I injury is 12 years, whereas type II injuries are seen in younger patients, with an average age of 10 years.[212]

The physical examination begins with inspection of the lateral aspect of the ankle to identify swelling and ecchymosis, followed by palpation of the distal physis and the lateral ligaments. In addition, the medial aspect of the ankle should be palpated, including the

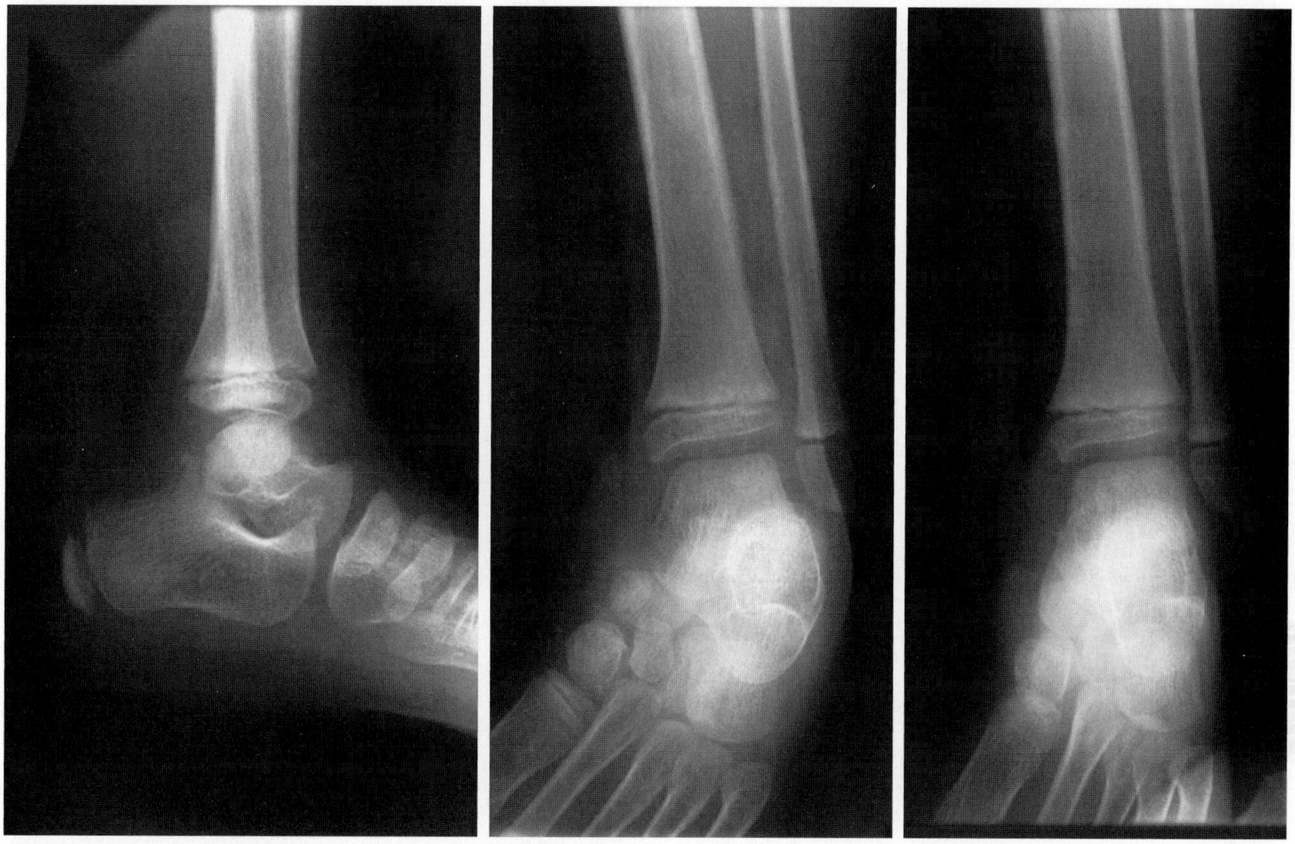

A B C

FIGURE 43-164 A complete radiographic examination for suspected ankle fracture should include lateral **(A)**, mortise **(B)**, and anteroposterior **(C)** views of the ankle.

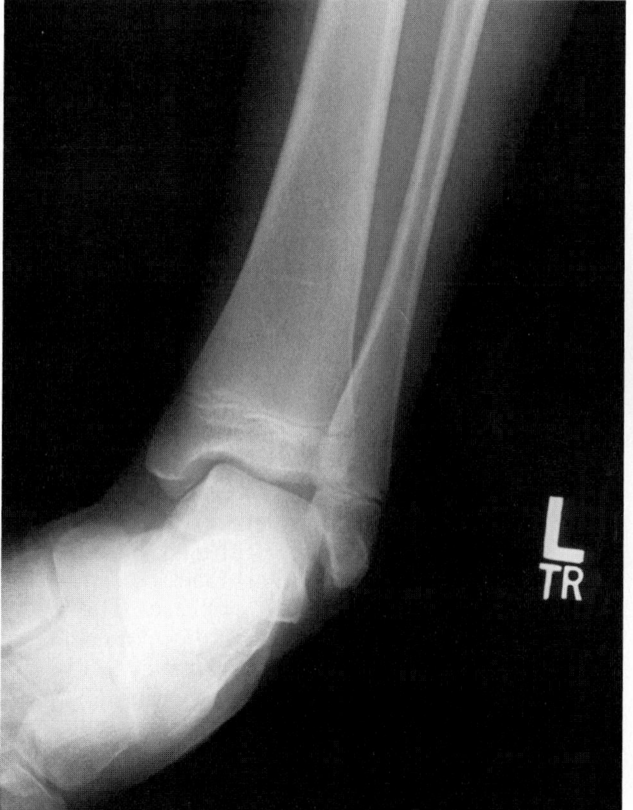

A

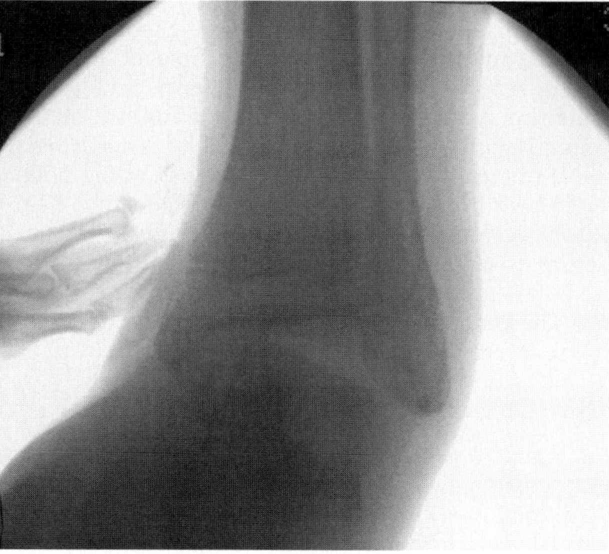

B

FIGURE 43-165 Stress radiographs obtained with the examiner inverting the foot in an attempt to define a ligamentous injury. **A,** Normal stress radiograph with less than 20 degrees of talar tilt. **B,** Abnormal stress radiograph with more than 20 degrees of talar tilt.

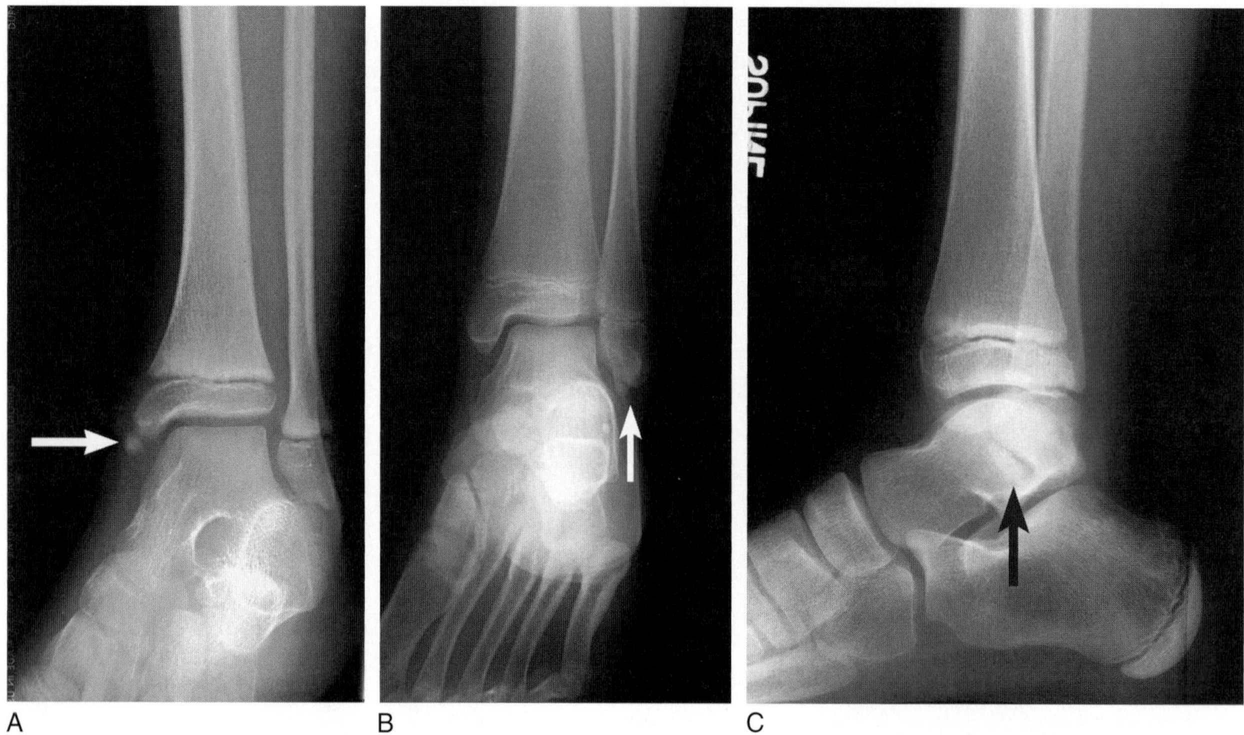

FIGURE 43–166 Accessory centers of ossification. **A,** Accessory center of ossification on the medial malleolus (*arrow*) in a 10-year-old patient. Anteroposterior **(B)** and lateral **(C)** radiographs demonstrating a lateral accessory center of ossification (*arrows*).

ligaments and the medial malleolus. An undisplaced Salter-Harris type I injury is most often not identified on radiographs; however, a soft tissue swelling is seen directly over the distal fibular physis and the diagnosis is confirmed by the presence of tenderness directly over this physis. Salter-Harris type II fractures and displaced Salter-Harris type I fractures are easily identified and are frequently associated with a distal tibial Salter-Harris type III or IV injury.

Treatment of an isolated nondisplaced distal fibular Salter-Harris type I injury consists of a short-leg walking cast or fracture boot for 4 weeks. A displaced fracture requires closed reduction and a short-leg non–weight-bearing cast for 4 to 6 weeks. Complications from this injury are rare, although Spiegel and colleagues reported that 3 of 16 patients underwent premature symmetric physeal closure, with 2 of the patients having subsequent shortening.[212] Salter-Harris type II fractures can be treated with a short-leg non–weight-bearing cast for 4 to 6 weeks and generally heal without complications.[212] A displaced distal fibular fracture associated with a displaced distal tibial fracture will usually reduce on reduction of the tibial fracture. The reduction is generally stable and does not require internal fixation.

Salter-Harris Type I Tibial Fractures

This injury is relatively rare in children and accounts for approximately 15% of all distal tibiofibular fractures in children. It occurs in younger children (average age, 10 years).[212] All four mechanisms of injury described by Dias and Tachdjian can result in this injury,[60,61] and the exact mechanism can be determined by the location of the fracture fragments at the time of the initial radiographic examination. An associated fibular fracture is seen in approximately 25% of tibial fractures and helps determine the mechanism of injury.

Treatment consists of gentle closed reduction with reversal of the original mechanism of injury, followed by cast immobilization. We prefer a long-leg cast for most fractures, especially those that are displaced at the time of the initial injury. A short-leg cast can be applied at 4 weeks and worn for an additional 2 weeks. Complications from these injuries, though rare, include premature physeal arrest with subsequent limb length discrepancy, which has been reported in 3% of cases. Growth stimulation on the affected side has also been reported but does not usually exceed 1.5 cm.[212]

Salter-Harris Type II Distal Tibial Fractures

This injury is the most common distal tibial physeal injury in children and accounts for 40% of all ankle fractures.[212] The average age of these children is 12.5 years, and an associated fibular fracture occurs in the diaphysis in approximately 20% of cases. The mechanism of injury can be any of the four mechanisms described by Dias and Tachdjian; however, the most common are supination–external rotation (57%) and supination–plantar flexion injuries (32%), with pronation-eversion and miscellaneous injuries each accounting for 5%.[212] The location of the metaphyseal fragment is most helpful in determining the mechanism of

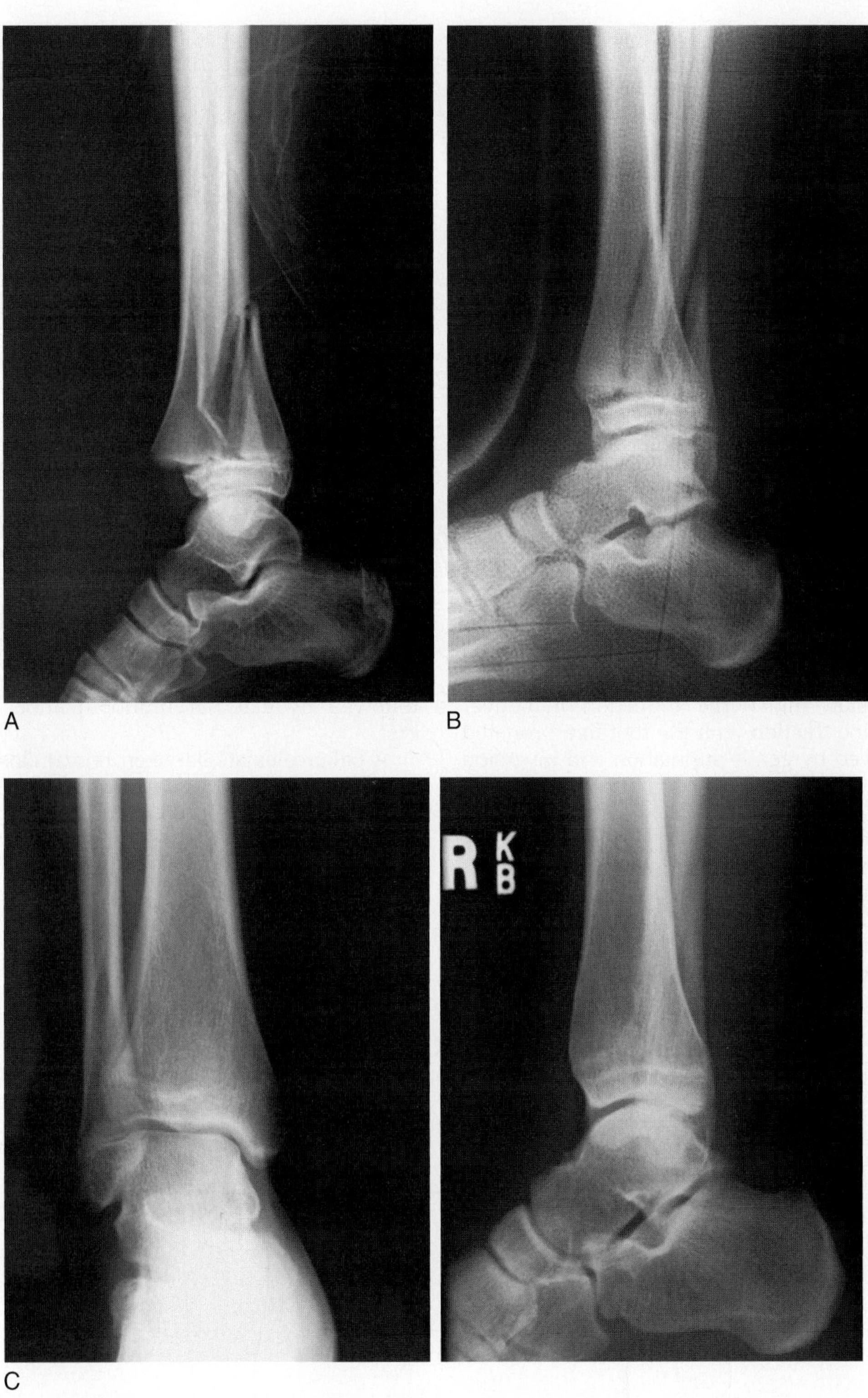

FIGURE 43–167 Supination–plantar flexion injury. **A,** Injury radiographs demonstrating the distal posterior tibial metaphyseal fragment and the fibular fracture. **B,** Postreduction radiographs demonstrating acceptable reduction. **C,** Radiographs demonstrate healing at 1-year follow-up.

injury. A posterior metaphyseal fragment indicates a supination–plantar flexion injury and therefore requires reversal of this mechanism with anterior displacement of the distal fragment to reduce the fracture (Fig. 43–167).

Treatment of nondisplaced fractures require a well-molded long-leg cast for 3 weeks, which can then be modified to a short-leg cast for an additional 2 to 3 weeks. A displaced Salter-Harris type II fracture requires gentle closed reduction, which should be performed under sedation or a general anesthetic to allow muscle relaxation so that further injury to the physis is limited. A long-leg cast should be worn for 4 weeks, followed by a short-leg cast for 2 to 3 weeks. Closed reduction should include initial flexion of the knee 90 degrees and plantar flexion of the foot to relax the triceps surae. An assistant should apply countertraction to the thigh while the surgeon grasps the foot at the heel while steadying the distal tibia with the opposite hand. Axial traction on the distal segment is first applied in line with the deformity, followed by manipulation opposite the initial deforming force (Fig. 43–168). For supination–external rotation injuries, distal traction is initially applied medially, followed by eversion of the foot. A cast is first applied distal to the knee, with the foot slightly internally rotated and in pronation to maintain reduction of the fracture. For a supination–plantar flexion injury the reduction maneuver includes initial axial traction with the foot in the plantar flexed position, followed by gradual dorsiflexion of the foot to approximately 20 degrees. The foot should then be placed in neutral position and a provisional short-leg cast applied. After a radiograph of the ankle confirms that adequate reduction has been achieved, the cast is extended above the knee. For a pronation-eversion injury the reduction maneuver consists of in-line traction with the foot in a pronated position, followed by gentle supination and inversion of the foot past the neutral position and then casting of the leg.

It is imperative that the patient be relaxed during the reduction maneuver to limit the number of attempts needed to achieve adequate reduction. Relaxation can be achieved with adequate conscious sedation in the emergency department or with general anesthesia in the operating room. This is best judged by the treating surgeon and depends on the age of the child, the amount of fracture displacement, the type of fracture, and the quality of conscious sedation provided by the emergency department. Any active guarding by the patient during the initial in-line traction maneuver warrants more medication to sedate the patient or changing the plan to include a general anesthetic so that an unimpeded initial attempt at closed reduction can be performed. This will allow the best attempt at closed reduction and instills confidence in the surgeon that a failed attempt at closed reduction is due to interposition of periosteum or other soft tissue and not to resistance by the patient. If an attempt at closed reduction does not succeed, open reduction should be performed, with removal of interposed soft tissue. This situation most often arises in a patient with a supination–plantar flexion injury in which the anterior periosteum is torn and interposed in the fracture site, thereby preventing reduction. Grace reported three cases of irreducible Salter-Harris type II fractures of the distal tibia that were due to interposition of the anterior neurovascular bundle; the result was a dysvascular foot in two cases after closed reduction.[79] Satisfactory results are achieved when open reduction with removal of the interposed soft tissue is performed, followed by external immobilization in a long-leg cast.

A balance exists between repeat closed reductions and acceptance of the reduction to avoid premature growth arrest. The amount of fracture displacement that is acceptable has not been fully established or agreed upon.[37,111,112,173,195,212] Recently, Barmada and colleagues reported an increased rate of premature physeal closure with a residual physeal gap of greater than 3 mm. The number of reported reduction attempts was not found to be correlated with physeal arrest in

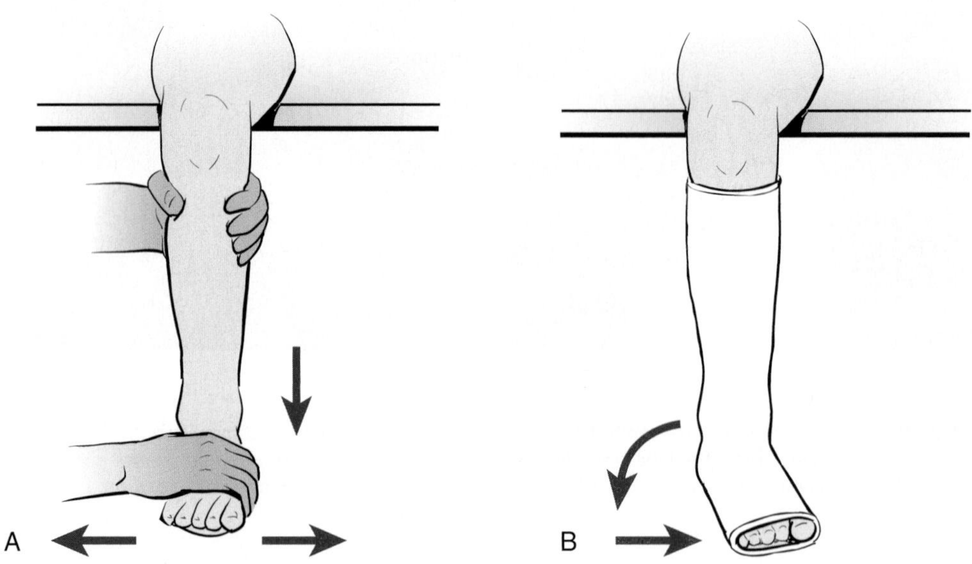

FIGURE 43–168 Reduction of ankle fractures. **A,** After conscious sedation, the leg can be placed over the hospital bed. Axial traction is applied, followed by reversal of the mechanism of injury. **B,** A temporary short-leg cast is then placed and allowed to set in the desired position. The cast is then extended approximately above the knee for optimal control.

this study.[12] We prefer to obtain nearly anatomic reduction of these injuries to prevent residual angular deformity, especially in a child older than 10 years and when the deformity is in the coronal or frontal plane. An initial reduction attempt can be performed under adequate intravenous sedation in the emergency department; however, failure to achieve adequate reduction should be followed by repeat reduction performed under general anesthesia and by open reduction if necessary. Spiegel and colleagues reported that in Salter-Harris type II fractures of the distal tibia, angular deformity does not remodel and thus anatomic reduction is necessary.[212]

Salter-Harris Type III Distal Tibial Fractures

These injuries occur in approximately 20% of all distal tibiofibular fractures in children at an average age of 11 to 12 years.[212] The mechanism is always a supination-inversion injury as described by Dias and Tachdjian and is associated with a distal fibular fracture in 25% of cases. The supinated foot sustains an inversion force that stresses the lateral ligaments of the ankle, with the distal fibula being avulsed while the talus is driven into the medial aspect of the distal tibia. The epiphyseal fracture component of a Salter-Harris type III fracture is always medial to the midline, not to be mistaken for a Tillaux or triplane fracture when the epiphyseal fracture is at the midline or lateral to it (Fig. 43–169).

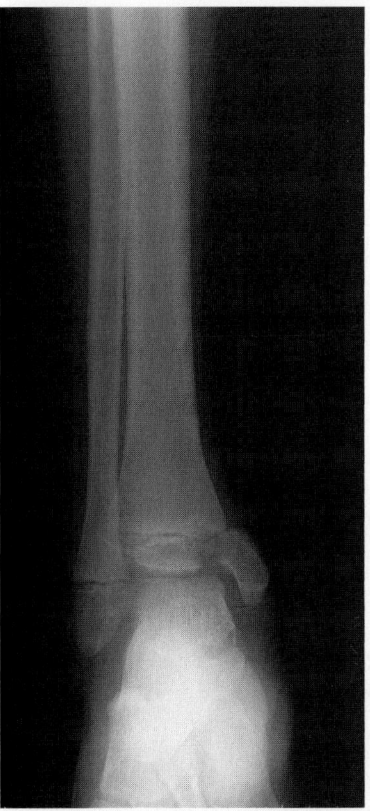

FIGURE 43-169 Radiograph of a Salter-Harris type III fracture caused by a supination-inversion injury in which the talus is driven into the medial malleolus. Note the epiphyseal fracture line medial to the midline, unlike a Tillaux fracture, which is located more laterally in the epiphysis.

Treatment of nondisplaced fractures consists of 4 weeks in a long-leg cast, followed by an additional 4 weeks in a short-leg cast. The initial plaster cast should be applied with the foot in 5 to 10 degrees of eversion and with a good mold on the medial aspect of the ankle. Spiegel and colleagues reported results in 26 patients with mildly displaced or nondisplaced type III fractures treated by closed reduction; premature closure of the medial physis and a resultant 5-degree angular deformity developed in 1 patient.[212] Careful follow-up of these fractures on a weekly basis to ensure maintenance of fracture reduction is essential.

Fractures that are displaced more than 2 mm should be reduced in the operating room by either closed or open reduction followed by screw fixation. In minimally displaced fractures, we attempt closed reduction with a large periarticular reduction clamp followed by percutaneous epiphyseal screw fixation. If anatomic reduction is unable to be achieved in closed fashion, we prefer to view the articular cartilage in the displaced distal tibial fracture through a small, 3- to 4-cm anterior arthrotomy in the interval between the extensor digitorum longus and the extensor hallucis longus (Fig. 43–170). The fracture can then be reduced with Weber bone reduction forceps and rigidly fixed with percutaneously placed screws (Fig. 43–171). Short-leg cast immobilization is required for 6 weeks, followed by progressive weight bearing. The results of operative fixation of these displaced fractures are generally good, with an approximately 15% incidence of premature physeal closure and subsequent angular deformity.[212] When displaced fractures are not reduced anatomically, early degenerative arthritis can occur, and the onset of painful symptoms begins 5 to 8 years after the injury.[40] In addition, patients treated by closed reduction tend to have only a growth disturbance secondary to a bony bridge.[112]

Salter-Harris Type IV Distal Tibial Fractures

These fractures are rare and account for approximately 1% of distal tibial injuries in children.[212] The mechanism of injury is a supination-inversion injury in which the talus is pushed medially into the medial malleolus, and the fracture line travels from the articular surface through the epiphysis and metaphysis.

Open reduction is usually required for these fractures because most are displaced and the fracture line extends into the joint. These fractures are likely to be associated with subsequent early degenerative arthritis and growth arrest if not treated by open reduction and internal fixation.[112] The approach is the traditional one for a medial malleolus fracture, with the skin incision being curvilinear and the convexity anterior to allow direct viewing of the intra-articular component, as well as the metaphyseal fragment (Fig. 43–172). The saphenous vein is dissected free of soft tissue to allow posterior retraction out of the surgical site, and then both the intra-articular and metaphyseal fracture lines

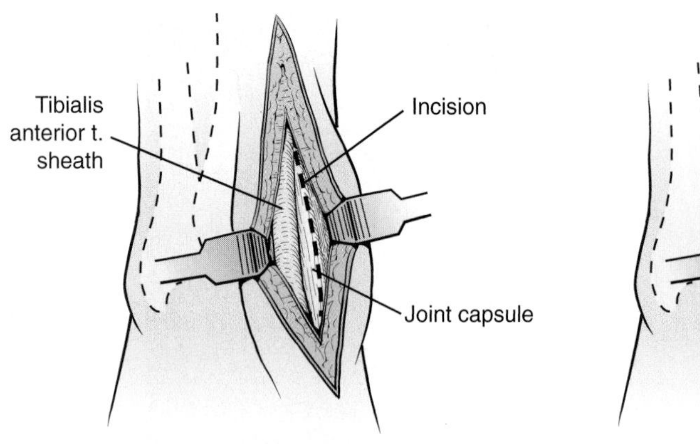

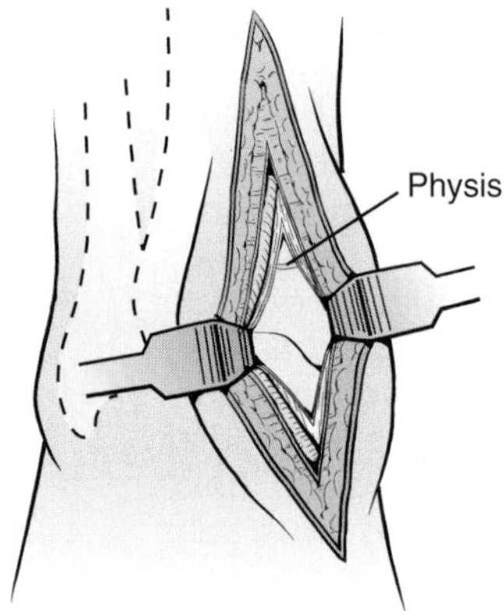

FIGURE 43–170 Anterior approach to the medial ankle joint. An incision is made over the anterior tibialis tendon. The incision is carried just distal to the joint line. The tendon sheath is left intact, and the incision is carried just medial to this. This approach will preserve the tendon and allow access to the medial aspect of the ankle joint for visualization of Salter-Harris type III injuries.

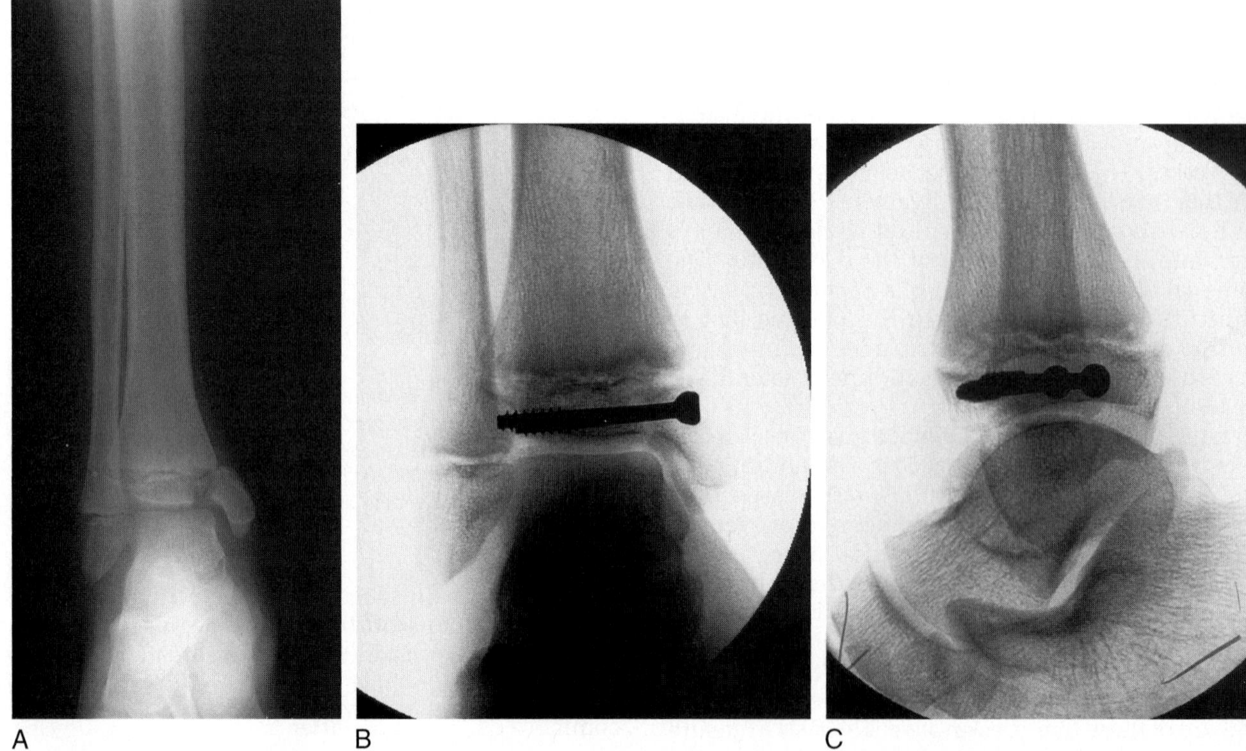

FIGURE 43–171 Open reduction and internal fixation of a Salter-Harris type III distal tibial fracture. **A,** Injury radiograph showing a supination-inversion injury of the ankle with a resultant Salter-Harris type III distal tibial fracture. Anteroposterior **(B)** and lateral **(C)** radiographs obtained after open reduction via the anterior approach to the ankle, as noted in Figure 43–170, followed by percutaneous screw fixation with cannulated screws. Note the reduction and the screw fixation to achieve compression across the fracture site.

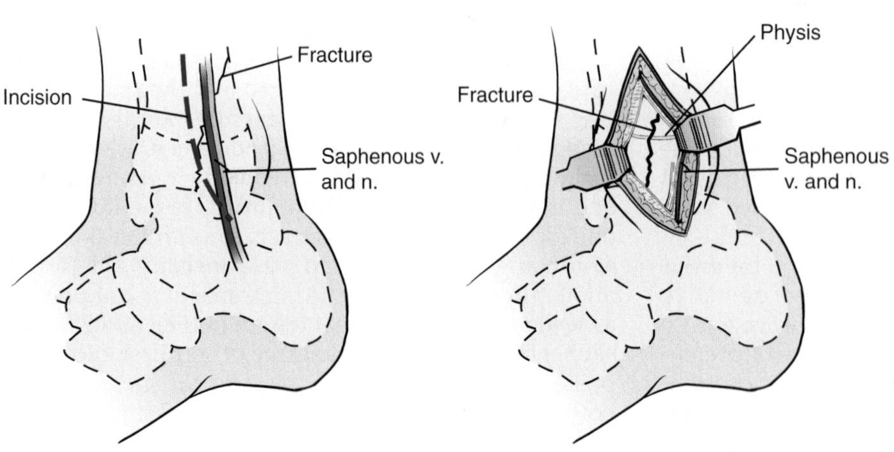

FIGURE 43–172 Approach to the medial aspect of the ankle in the treatment of Salter-Harris type IV fractures of the distal tibia. A curvilinear incision is made over the anterolateral aspect of the distal tibia. This incision affords access to the medial aspect of the joint and allows direct observation of the fracture fragment. The saphenous nerve is carefully retracted posteriorly.

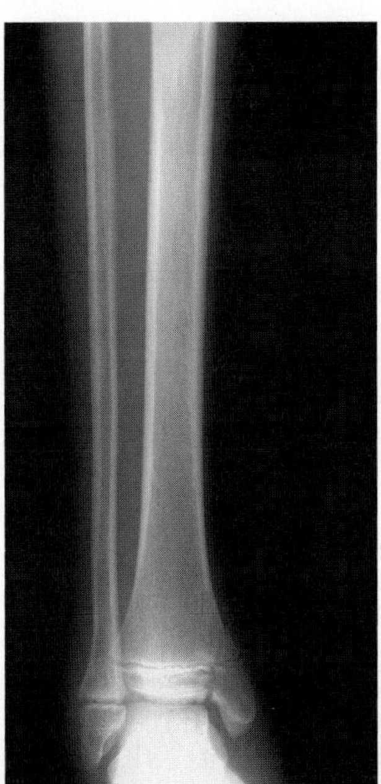

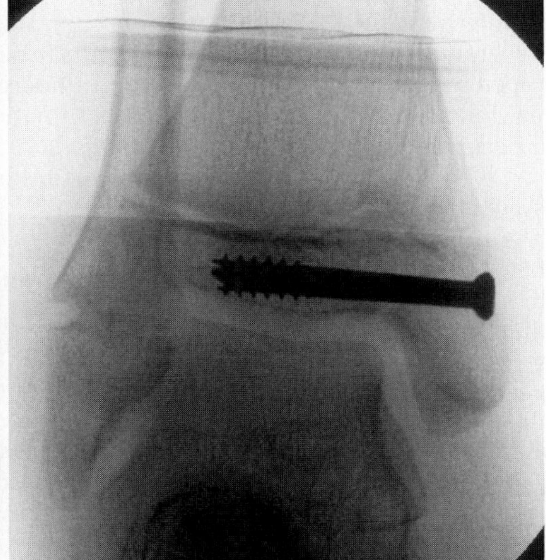

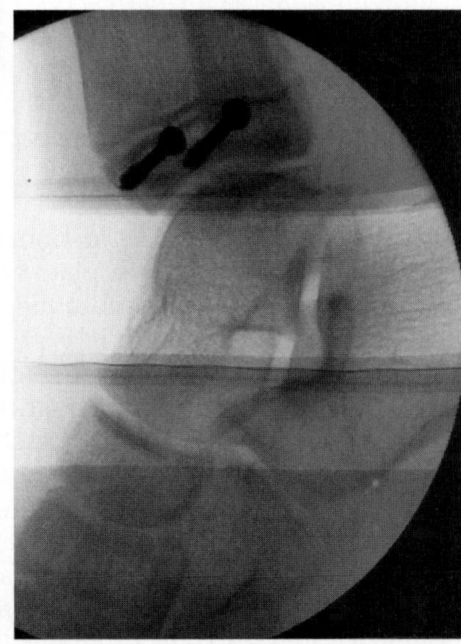

A B1 B2

FIGURE 43–173 Open reduction and internal fixation of a Salter-Harris type IV distal tibial fracture caused by a supination-inversion injury. **A,** Anteroposterior radiograph demonstrating the fracture. Although it is mildly displaced, there is a significant risk for further displacement. **B,** Intraoperative radiographs obtained after open reduction and internal fixation with cannulated screws.

are identified. Reduction is performed with bone reduction forceps and screw fixation parallel to the physis in the epiphysis and the metaphysis (Fig. 43–173). Postoperatively, a long-leg cast should be worn for 3 to 4 weeks, followed by a short-leg cast for an additional 3 weeks.

After treatment of these fractures, monitoring of the distal tibial physis with serial radiographs or scanograms (or both) every 6 months is warranted. If growth arrest is suspected, screw removal followed by CT or MRI is necessary to fully define the presence and extent of a physeal osseous bridge.

The need for routine implant removal after union of distal tibial epiphyseal fractures is unclear. A recent cadaveric biomechanical study suggests that total force transmission and peak contact pressures are significantly increased over baseline with epiphyseal screws in place.[43] Our current practice is to remove these implants after fracture union. The use of bioabsorbable pins and screws has been reported in adult ankle fractures, with mixed results.[14,20,21,29,93] The efficacy and utility of bioabsorbable screws in pediatric distal epiphyseal fractures have not been established.

Salter-Harris Type V Distal Tibial Fractures

These extremely rare injuries are due to an axial compression force and are usually noted after the appearance of physeal arrest of the distal tibia following trauma without radiographic findings. The mechanism of injury to the physis is compression of the germinal layer, vascular insult, or both. These injuries should be analyzed in the same fashion as all physeal arrests and treated appropriately.

COMPLICATIONS

Premature Closure of the Physis

Injury to the germinal layer of the physis may lead to asymmetric or symmetric growth arrest, the most common complication after a distal tibial physeal injury in children. Fractures at highest risk are displaced Salter-Harris types III and IV injuries.* Although it is the most common complication seen with these injuries, it is still relatively rare. Spiegel and colleagues reported findings in 39 patients with a Salter-Harris type III or IV fracture who had adequate follow-up. Premature growth arrest developed in 3 (7.7%) patients.[212]

The adduction force imparted in these fractures leads to injury to the medial aspect of the distal tibial physis and produces asymmetric growth arrest and a subsequent varus deformity. Kling and colleagues reported findings in 16 patients with Salter-Harris type III fractures and 12 patients with Salter-Harris type IV fractures who experienced growth arrest of the distal tibia with subsequent varus and shortening.[112] The average age of the patients was 8 to 9 years, and the time to the development of partial physeal

*See references 12, 37, 51, 60, 61, 77, 117, 150, 173, 212.

growth arrest was 17 months for type III fractures and 20 months for type IV fractures. The average shortening was 1.6 and 1.1 cm for type III and type IV injuries, respectively, and both types of fracture had an average varus deformity of 15 degrees. Most of these fractures had been treated by closed reduction followed by external immobilization in a cast. Kling and colleagues studied a second group of 20 patients at their institution with an acute Salter-Harris type III or IV fracture that was treated by open reduction and internal fixation; 19 healed without evidence of a growth disturbance. It is therefore imperative that open reduction of these physeal fractures be performed, followed by stable internal fixation to prevent the occurrence of this complication.

Even though anatomic reduction is achieved, significant injury to the growth plate at the time of the initial event may lead to subsequent growth arrest (Fig. 43–174).[39] A Salter-Harris type II fracture with significant displacement at the time of injury is also at risk for the development of premature growth arrest and should be treated by open reduction and internal fixation if anatomic reduction cannot be achieved by closed means. Spiegel and colleagues reported that angular deformity of greater than 5 degrees developed in 6 (9%) of 66 patients with Salter-Harris type II fractures after closed treatment.[212] Barmada and coworkers reported a 60% rate of premature physeal closure in these injuries when the residual physeal fracture gap was greater than 3 mm.[12] In younger patients with significant growth remaining, open reduction to decrease this degree of residual physeal displacement may be indicated for prevention of deformity secondary to physeal arrest. It is important to monitor patients with distal tibial physeal injuries closely during the first 2 years after the injury. Physeal arrest can appear more than 2 years after the injury, and therefore follow-up should be extended to near skeletal maturity.

When growth arrest is suspected on plain radiographs, further diagnostic studies should be performed. Plain radiographs should be analyzed for evidence of an osseous bar within the physis. Park-Harris growth arrest lines should be observable and can be helpful in determining the presence of premature asymmetric growth arrest.[95] Internal fixation devices should be removed before further studies, which should include CT or MRI (see Fig. 43–174D). Treatment of growth arrest depends on its location, size, and the amount of growth remaining. In general, when there is more than 2 years of growth remaining and the physeal arrest is less than 50% of the width of the physis, we prefer to resect the osseous bar and replace the area with adipose tissue or Cranioplast (see Fig. 43–174E). Small metal markers should be placed in the epiphysis and metaphysis to allow accurate assessment of future growth and the success of this procedure. When the patient is closer to skeletal maturity (girls older than 11 years and boys older than 13 years), epiphysiodesis of the lateral aspect of the tibial physis and the entire fibular physis is performed. This procedure should be combined with contralateral epiphysiodesis to prevent a large limb length discrepancy. If significant varus deformity is present at the time of epiphysiodesis, an opening wedge osteotomy of the tibia can be performed together with a fibular osteotomy. The opening wedge osteotomy is made 2 cm proximal to the distal physis with the interposition of tricortical iliac crest graft and fixation with crossed Kirschner wires or screws, and the fibula is cut obliquely proximal to the tibial cut (Fig. 43–175). External cast immobilization is used until healing of the osteotomy occurs. Takakura and associates recently reviewed the results in seven adult and two adolescent patients who had undergone an opening wedge osteotomy for post-traumatic varus of the ankle.[219] Both adolescent patients had a significant improvement in their preoperative ankle scores and had resumed athletic activities.

Delayed Union or Nonunion

This complication is very rare in younger children, although it may occur in adolescents with a distal tibial fracture. In the largest series of distal tibial fractures reported in children, nonunion or delayed union did not develop in any patient. If nonunion is present, we prefer an open procedure to debride fibrous tissue at the fracture site, followed by autologous bone grafting and internal fixation, especially if there is motion at the fracture site.

Valgus Deformity Secondary to Malunion

This complication usually results from inadequate reduction of a pronation–eversion–lateral rotation fracture. A valgus tilt of the ankle of more than 15 to 20 degrees will not correct by remodeling with skeletal growth and must be treated surgically. When sufficient growth remains, epiphyseal arrest of the medial distal tibia can be performed to allow the lateral tibial and the distal fibula to continue to grow and correct the deformity. We prefer to perform distal medial epiphysiodesis by placing a single screw across the medial physis so that medial growth will be disturbed; the screw can be removed for resumption of medial growth if overcorrection is anticipated. When growth is complete, the distal tibial osteotomy is best performed by using the Wiltse technique to achieve correction without excess shortening of the limb or the creation of a prominent medial aspect of the ankle (Fig. 43–176).[26]

Tillaux Fractures

Fractures of the lateral portion of the distal end of the tibia in adults were first described by Sir Astley Cooper[47]; however, this fracture is referred to as the fracture of Tillaux.

MECHANISM OF ACTION

Tillaux fracture results from external rotation of the ankle and occurs because of asymmetric closure of the distal tibial physis, which initially begins centrally,

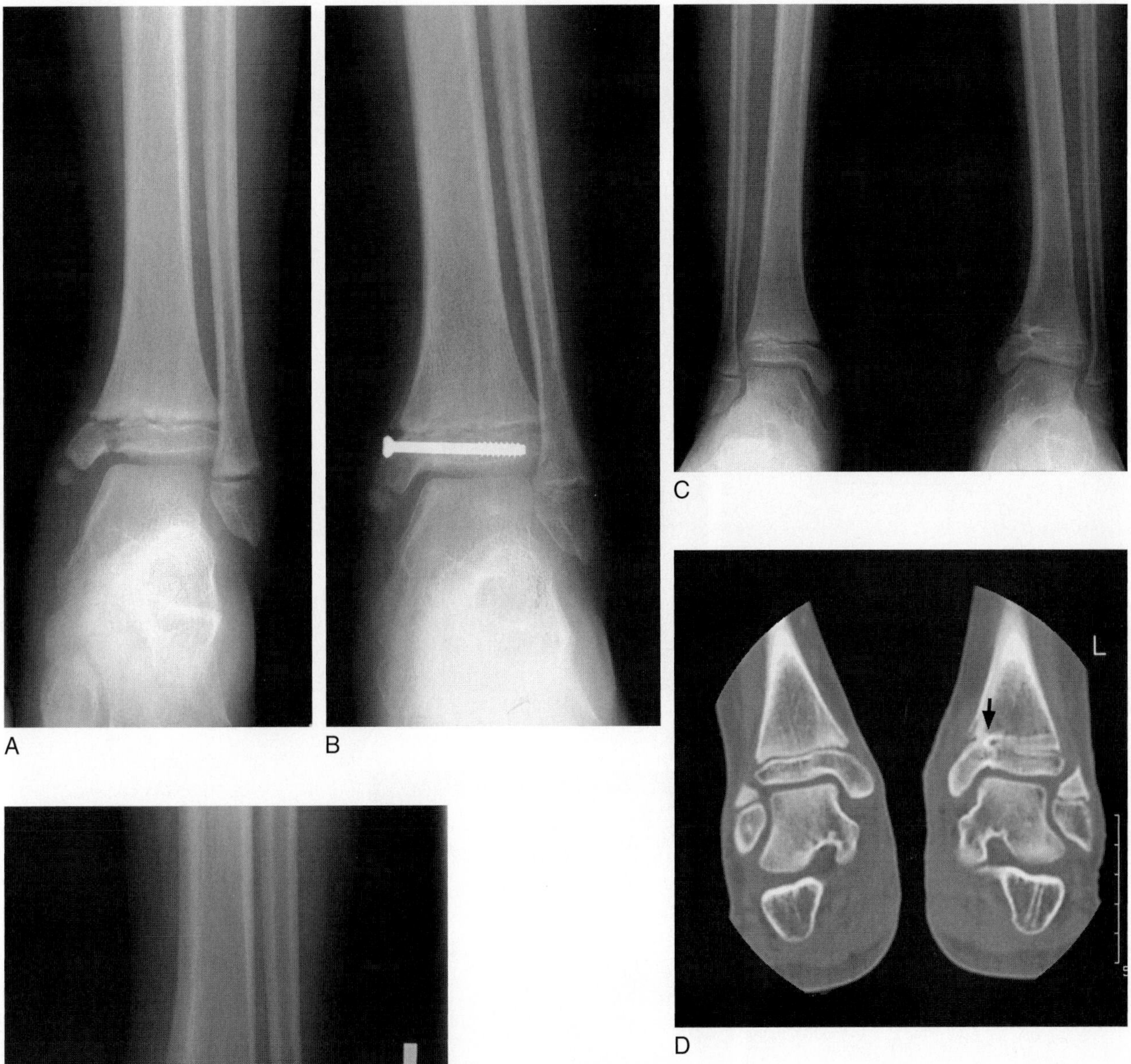

A B C D

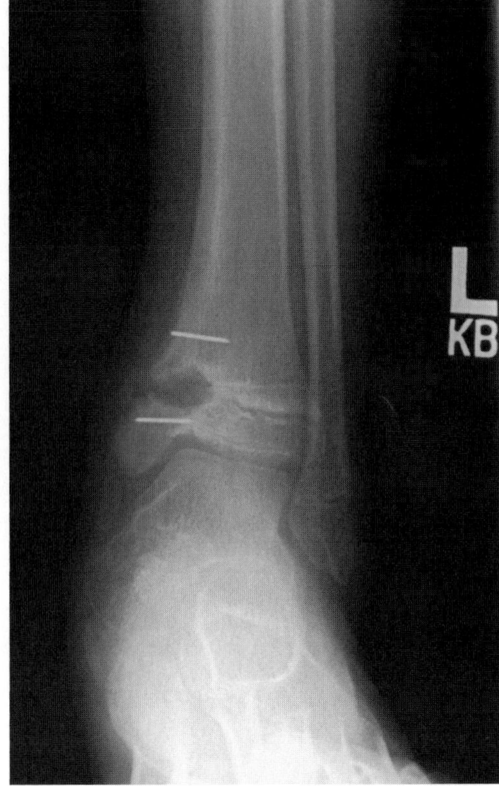

E

FIGURE 43-174 Distal tibial growth arrest after a Salter-Harris type III fracture in a 9-year-old girl. **A,** Injury radiograph. **B,** Open reduction with screw fixation was performed. **C,** Varus deformity of the distal tibia developed secondary to a medial physeal bar. **D,** Computed tomography scan showing distal tibial physeal growth arrest (*arrow*). **E,** Postoperative radiograph obtained after excision of the physeal bar, followed by interposition of fat for distal tibial physeal growth arrest. Small K-wires were placed on both sides of the resection. Their distance should increase if the physis resumes symmetric growth.

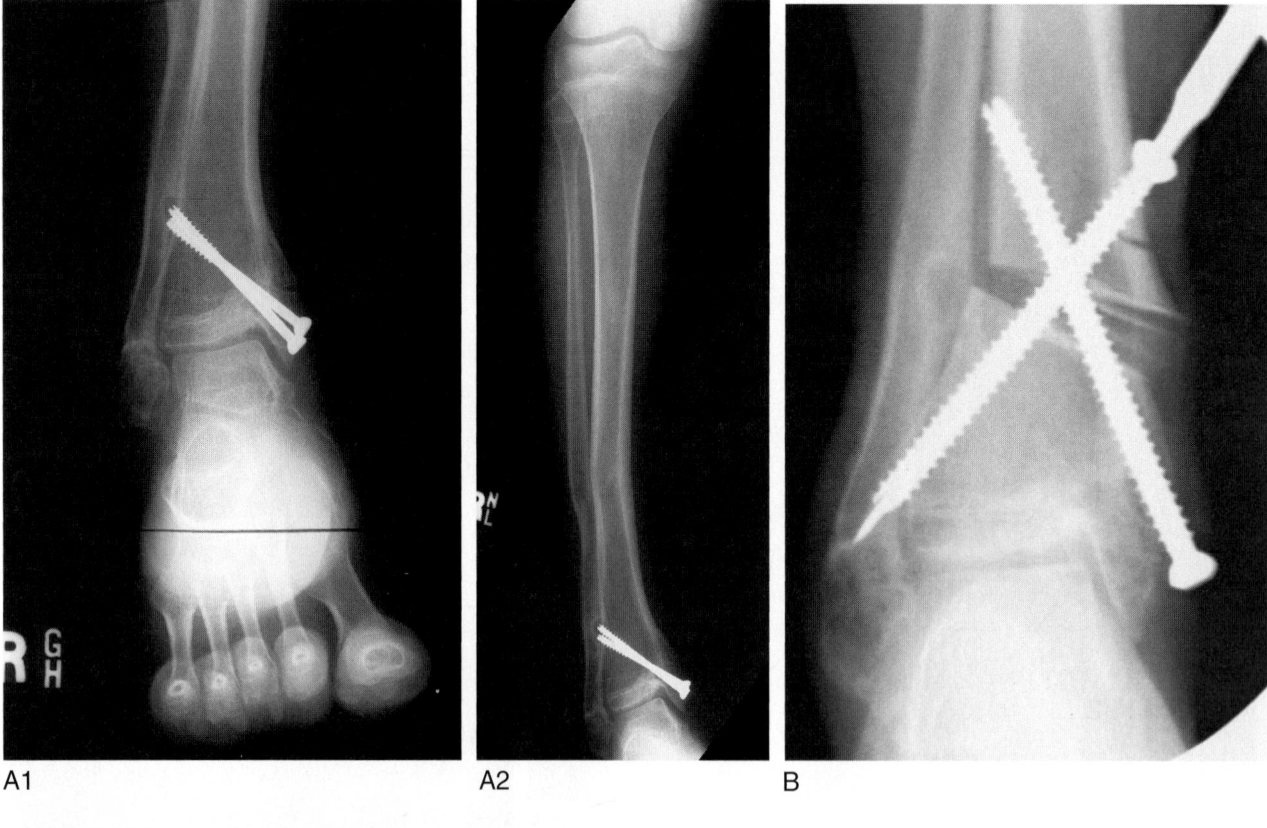

A1 A2 B

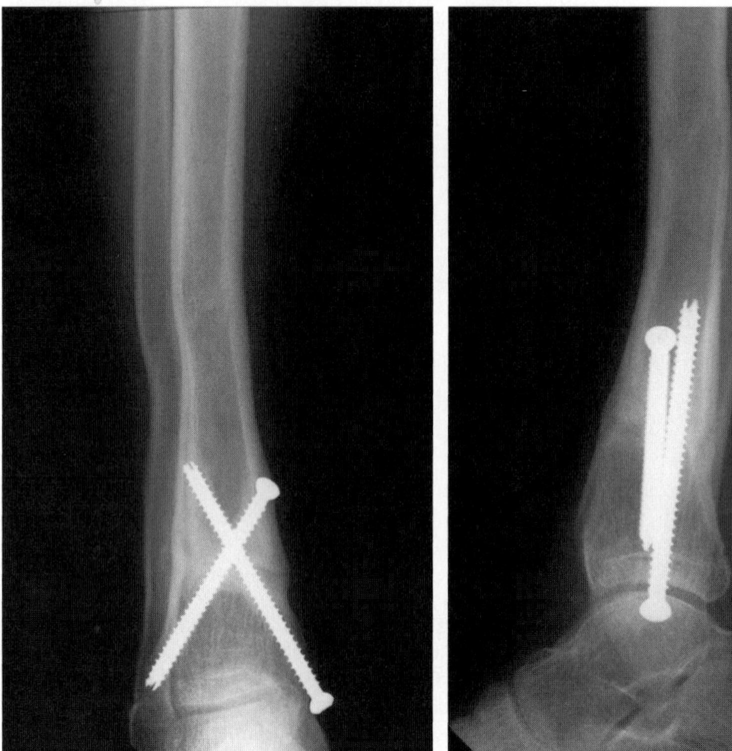

C1 C2

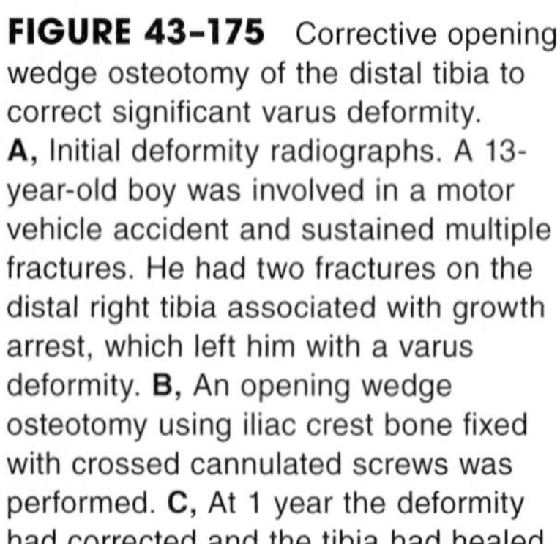

FIGURE 43–175 Corrective opening wedge osteotomy of the distal tibia to correct significant varus deformity. **A,** Initial deformity radiographs. A 13-year-old boy was involved in a motor vehicle accident and sustained multiple fractures. He had two fractures on the distal right tibia associated with growth arrest, which left him with a varus deformity. **B,** An opening wedge osteotomy using iliac crest bone fixed with crossed cannulated screws was performed. **C,** At 1 year the deformity had corrected and the tibia had healed.

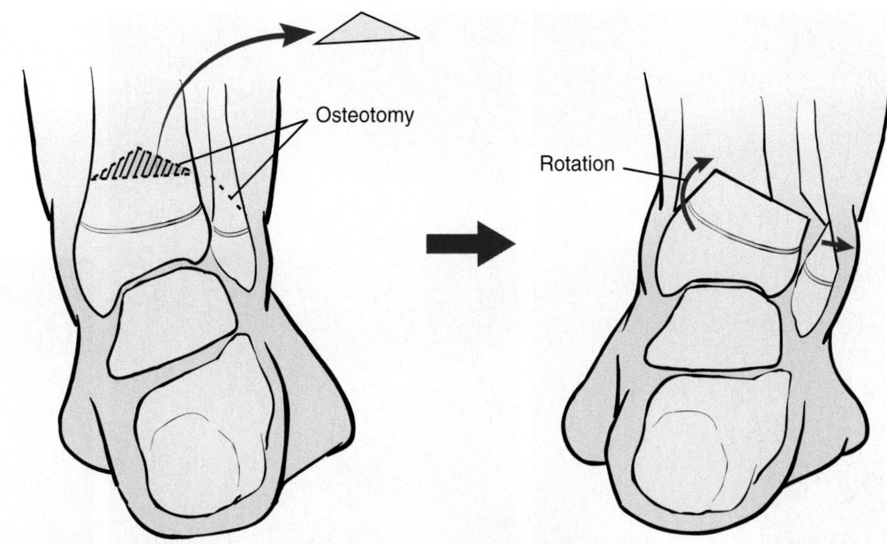

FIGURE 43–176 Wiltse-type distal tibial osteotomy for a valgus deformity.

followed by medial closure, and finally lateral closure. Medial closure occurs at approximately 13 to 14 years of age, with lateral closure beginning at 14.5 to 16 years of age; therefore, during an 18-month window patients are predisposed to this particular fracture.[110] When the distal lateral physis is still open and an external rotation force is applied to the foot, an avulsion fracture of the anterolateral distal epiphysis occurs as the inferior tibiofibular ligament pulls this fragment free (Fig. 43–177). This is a Salter-Harris type III fracture with a vertical fracture line that extends from the articular surface proximally, through the lateral physis, and out the lateral cortex (Fig. 43–178). In an older child the fracture line occurs more laterally because the physis

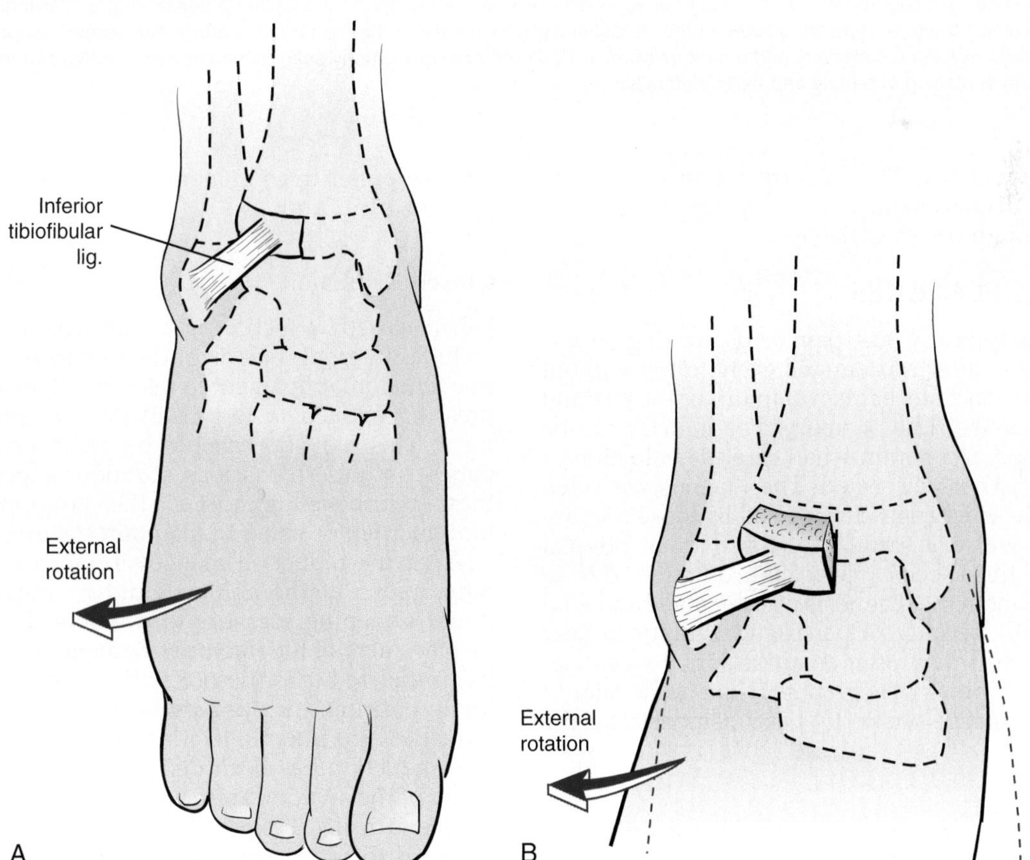

FIGURE 43–177 Mechanism of a Tillaux fracture. **A,** The inferior tibiofibular ligament travels from the distal fibula to the distal lateral tibial epiphysis. **B,** When an external rotational force is applied, the distal tibial epiphysis is avulsed.

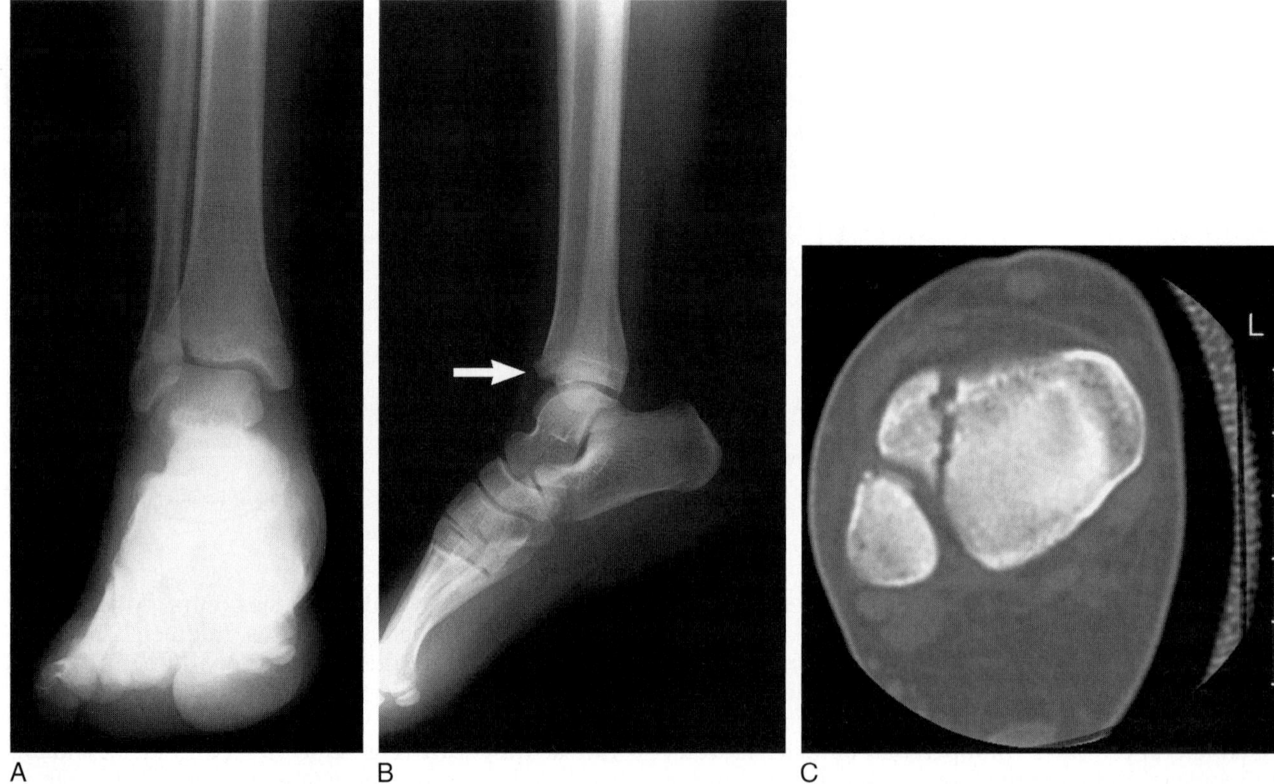

A B C

FIGURE 43–178 Radiograph of a Tillaux fracture. **A,** Anteroposterior radiograph of the ankle demonstrating a lateral distal tibial epiphyseal avulsion fracture. Note the closure of the distal tibial physis medial to the fracture. **B,** Lateral radiograph demonstrating the fracture fragment displaced superiorly and anteriorly (*arrow*). **C,** Computed tomography scan demonstrating the avulsed fragment, with the fracture line beginning anteriorly and exiting laterally.

has closed medially. The fracture fragment and the amount of displacement tend to be less in this age group, although this is variable.

CLINICAL FEATURES

The patient typically has pain and swelling in the affected ankle after a traumatic event, often without knowing the exact mechanism of injury or the position of the foot at the time of injury. The injuries can be misdiagnosed as a sprain when careful evaluation of the patient is not performed. The diagnosis is often missed in the emergency department by those who are unfamiliar with the pattern of distal tibial physeal closure and this specific injury. Letts described 5 of 26 patients in whom the diagnosis was not made and who returned only because of persistent inability to bear weight for 2 to 3 days after an ankle sprain was diagnosed.[129] The initial radiographs of the ankle should include a mortise view to best demonstrate the fracture.

TREATMENT

Treatment of these avulsion fractures has traditionally been to initially attempt closed reduction of the fracture to within 2 mm of the anatomic position. However, no studies directly support long-term good outcomes when fracture displacement of up to 2 mm is accepted, and we prefer open anatomic reduction for displacement of 1 to 2 mm.

Closed Reduction

When closed reduction is attempted, the maneuver includes internal rotation of the foot to allow the anterior tibiofibular ligament to relax, together with digital pressure applied to the distal tibial epiphyseal fragment. This reduction should be performed while the patient is under conscious sedation or general anesthesia. An above-knee cast can then be applied with the foot internally rotated to maintain fracture reduction.

After the reduction maneuver, mortise and lateral radiographs of the ankle should be obtained as an initial screening measure to evaluate the amount of displacement of the fracture fragment. If it is clear that the initial reduction is not within 2 mm of the anatomic position, the surgeon should proceed to open reduction and internal fixation of the fracture. Acceptable reduction has been defined as reduction within 2 mm of the anatomic position to prevent early degenerative arthritis. Frequently, however, fracture reduction is difficult to assess adequately, in part because the fracture fragments are obscured by the cast. A postreduction CT scan best quantifies the amount of residual fracture displacement and makes deciding whether to perform open reduction more definitive. If acceptable closed reduction is achieved, an above-knee cast should be worn for 3 to 4 weeks. It is changed to a short-leg cast, at which time the foot can be brought to a plantigrade position, for an additional 3 weeks. Serial radiographs to include a mortise view should be obtained to assess the reduction and compare it with the original one.

Open Reduction and Internal Fixation

The indications for open reduction and internal fixation are fracture displacement of more than 2 mm after an attempt at a closed reduction or a delay of more than 2 to 3 days after injury with more than 2 mm of fracture displacement. The 2 mm of fracture displacement has always been used as the threshold for performing open reduction despite the lack of long-term studies on the incidence of early degenerative arthritis and the inherent difficulty of accurately defining the amount of fracture displacement on plain radiographs. In our experience, in fractures that are displaced 2 mm or greater at the time of initial evaluation, the initial reduction attempt usually fails or an acceptable reduction is not maintained and an open procedure is necessary. Fractures with less than 2 mm of displacement can be treated by closed reduction and an above-knee cast. Some argue that only anatomic reduction of the articular surface must be achieved to prevent ankle instability, joint incongruity, and subsequent early degenerative arthritis.[213] We prefer open reduction for all Tillaux fractures that have 2 mm or more of fracture displacement because open reduction with stable fixation is a relatively small procedure that reproducibly achieves anatomic reduction of the articular surface and presumably a good long-term result.

The open reduction is performed through an anterior approach to the ankle in the interval between the extensor digitorum longus and extensor hallucis tendon to allow direct observation of the fracture fragment (Fig. 43–179). After evacuation of fracture hematoma and inspection of the articular surface of the talar dome, the foot is positioned in internal rotation and the fracture is reduced. It is important to restore the articular surface of the distal tibia anatomically, and this is best visualized directly anteriorly. In addition, the physeal fracture line should be anatomically restored to ensure that the posterior aspect of the articular surface is anatomically reduced.

After reduction, we prefer fixation with a single 4.0-mm partially threaded cancellous screw placed in an anterolateral-to-posteromedial direction (Fig. 43–180). It may be necessary to place a small Kirschner wire temporarily while the screw hole is drilled, tapped, and filled with a cancellous screw to prevent rotation as the fragment is being fixed. It is not necessary to avoid the remaining aspect of the open physis during internal fixation of these fractures because physeal closure is near completion. A short-leg non–weight-bearing cast should be worn for 4 to 6 weeks postoperatively. Percutaneous reduction plus fixation has been described for these fractures, with good results in six patients.[203]

RESULTS

The outcome of Tillaux fractures is generally very good, although no long-term follow-up studies are available. Kleiger and Mankin reported on four true Tillaux fractures, two of which needed open reduction and internal fixation to achieve adequate reduction whereas the other two underwent satisfactory closed reduction; all four fractures healed with a acceptable outcome at 1 year.[110] Letts reported on 26 patients, 8 of whom required open reduction and internal fixation with smooth Kirschner wires. There were no complications at an average follow-up of 2.5 years.[129] Dias and Giegerich reported nine cases.[60] Five patients were treated by closed reduction and casting, and four had more than 2 mm of displacement after an attempt at closed reduction and then underwent open reduction and internal fixation. All patients had full, pain-free ankle motion with a healed fracture at 18- to 36-month follow-up.[60]

Triplane Fractures

Though initially described by Marmor,[143] this fracture was best described by Lynn, who coined the term "triplane fracture" in 1972.[140] Others subsequently described similar cases in which the fracture lines occurred in the coronal, transverse, and sagittal planes.* This is a relatively rare fracture that accounts for approximately 6% to 8% of all distal tibial physeal injuries in children.[48,60,212] These injuries occur in the adolescent age group at an average age of approximately 13.5 years (range, 10 to 16 years), generally slightly younger than children with a Tillaux fracture.[48] Because the distal tibial physis closes earlier in females, on average girls with a triplane fracture are younger than boys by approximately 1 year.[67]

MECHANISM OF INJURY

The mechanism of injury is thought to be an external rotation force applied to a supinated foot. This is supported by the fact that these fractures tend to reduce, at least partially, with internal rotation of the foot, and residual deformity with incomplete reduction results in slight external rotation of the leg.[48,60,67]

The triplane fracture is so named because the fracture lines occur in three planes. The coronal fracture line begins in the physis and travels proximally through the posterior metaphysis; the sagittal fracture travels from the midjoint line to the physis and results in an anteromedial and often an anterolateral fragment; and the transverse fracture travels through the physis (Fig. 43–181). These fracture lines can result in either a two-part or a three-part triplane fracture (Fig. 43–182). In a two-part fracture, the medial fragment consists of the tibial shaft, the medial malleolus, and the anteromedial aspect of the epiphysis; the lateral fragment includes the remainder of the epiphysis and the posterior aspect of the metaphysis. In a three-part fracture the medial fragment remains the same and

*See references 48, 50, 58, 60, 67, 71, 108, 141, 169, 225, 231, 234.

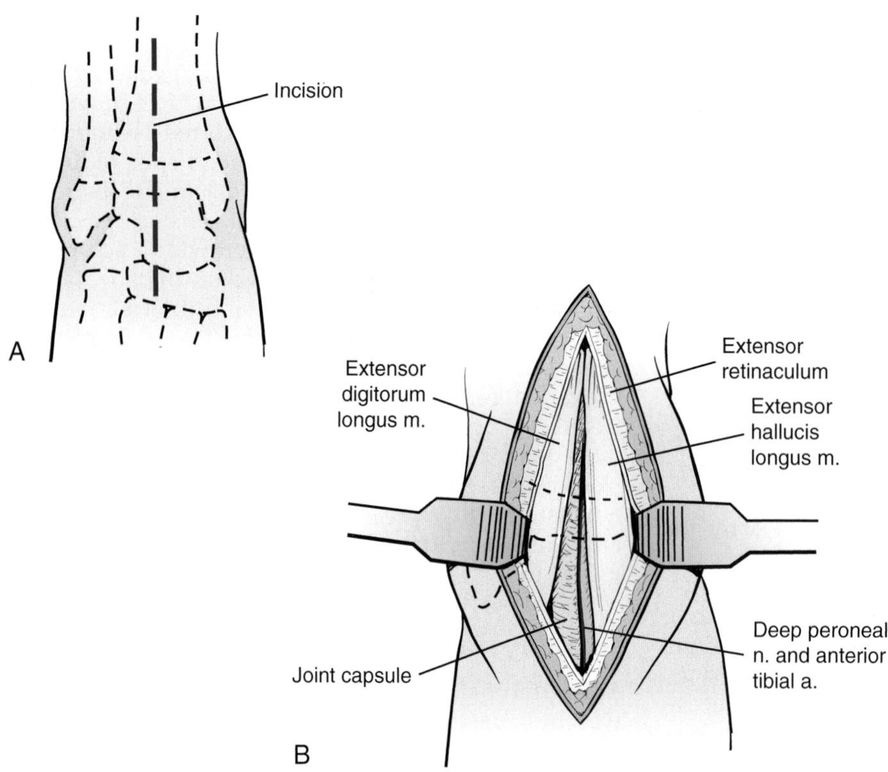

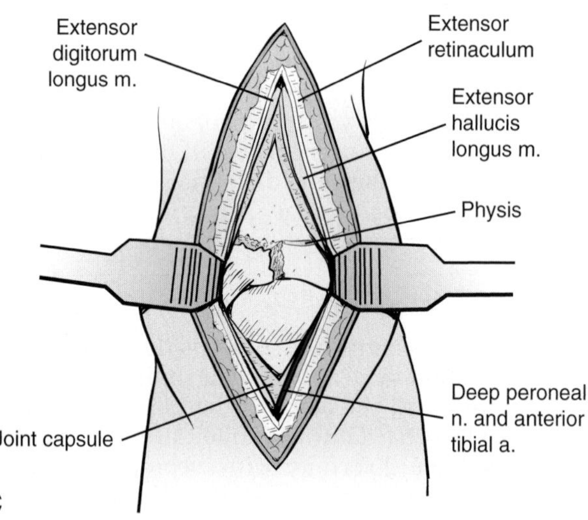

FIGURE 43–179 Anterior approach to the ankle for reduction of a Tillaux fracture. **A,** A midline anterior incision is made directly over the ankle joint. **B,** The interval between the extensor digitorum longus and the extensor hallucis longus is developed. The surgeon carefully identifies the deep peroneal nerve and anterior tibial artery. **C,** The interval is enlarged and the neurovascular bundles are retracted medially. After incision of the capsule the fracture is easily identified.

the lateral fragment is in two parts, with the rectangular anterolateral quadrant of the epiphysis being a separate fragment. Further variants of this fracture include a four-part fracture and an extra-articular triplane fracture, in which the fracture travels through the medial malleolus.[48,58,71,108,169,207,231] Cooperman and colleagues used tomography in 5 of 15 cases to demonstrate the two-part fracture: a medial fragment, which included the tibial shaft, medial malleolus, and an anteromedial fragment of the epiphysis, and a lateral fragment, which included the posterior metaphysis and the remainder of the epiphysis.[48] Dias and Giegerich reported that six of eight patients had a three-part triplane fracture and two had the two-part triplane fracture described by Cooperman.[60] In the largest series of patients reported to date, Brown and colleagues reported on 51 fractures: 8 were three-part fractures and 33 were two-part fractures.[24] An extra-articular triplane fracture or an intra-articular fracture in the non–weight-bearing zone has been described; in these cases the fracture line travels in the sagittal plane and exits through the anterior medial malleolus, the transverse fracture occurs through the physis, and the coronal fracture occurs through the posterior metaphysis of the distal tibia (Fig. 43–183).[71,207] It is important to recognize this particular variant of the triplane fracture because it can be successfully treated by closed reduction.

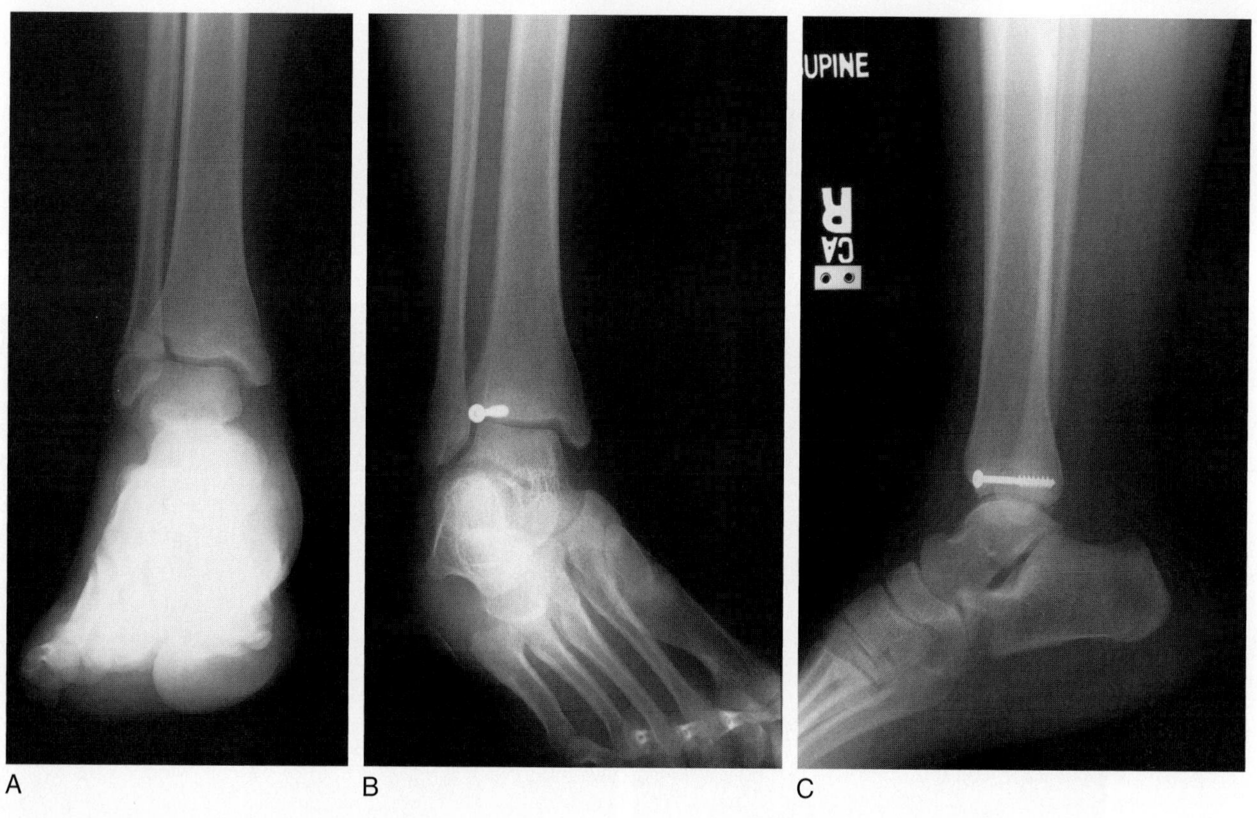

FIGURE 43–180 Open reduction and internal fixation of a Tillaux fracture. **A,** Anteroposterior radiograph. Mortise **(B)** and lateral **(C)** views after anatomic reduction with single-screw fixation.

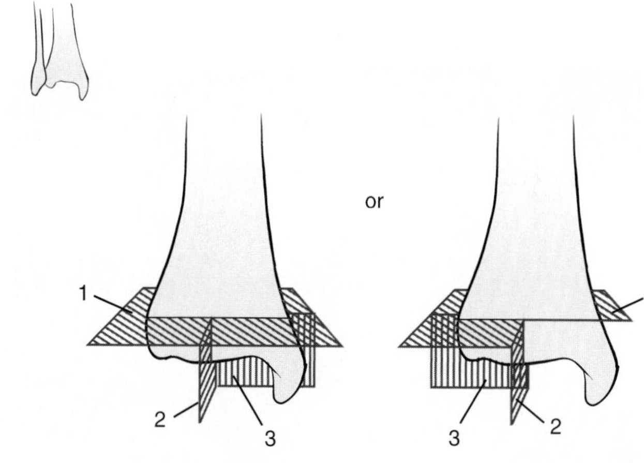

FIGURE 43–181 The triplane fracture pattern. Note the three planes in which the fracture occurs: 1, axial plane; 2, sagittal plane; 3, frontal plane.

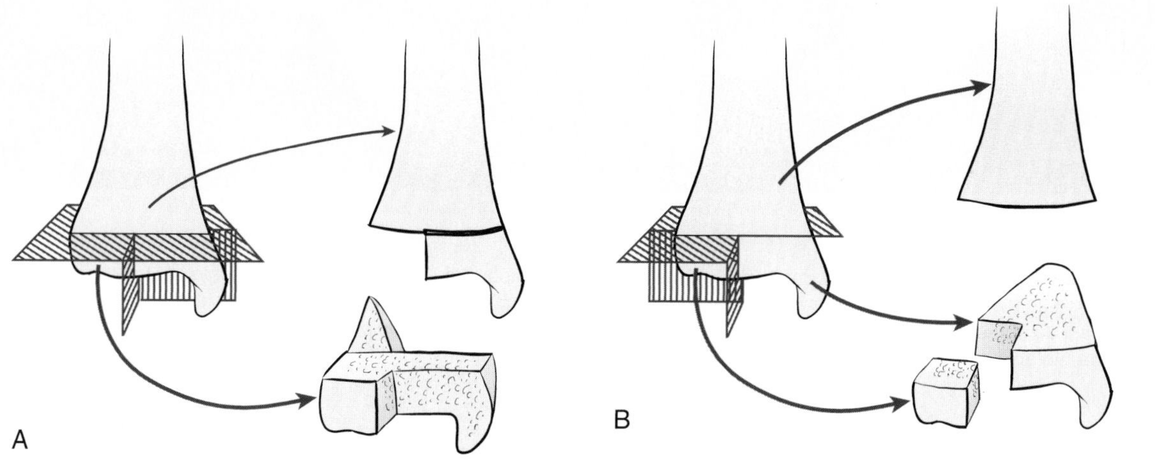

FIGURE 43–182 The triplane fracture can be two-part **(A)** or three-part **(B).**

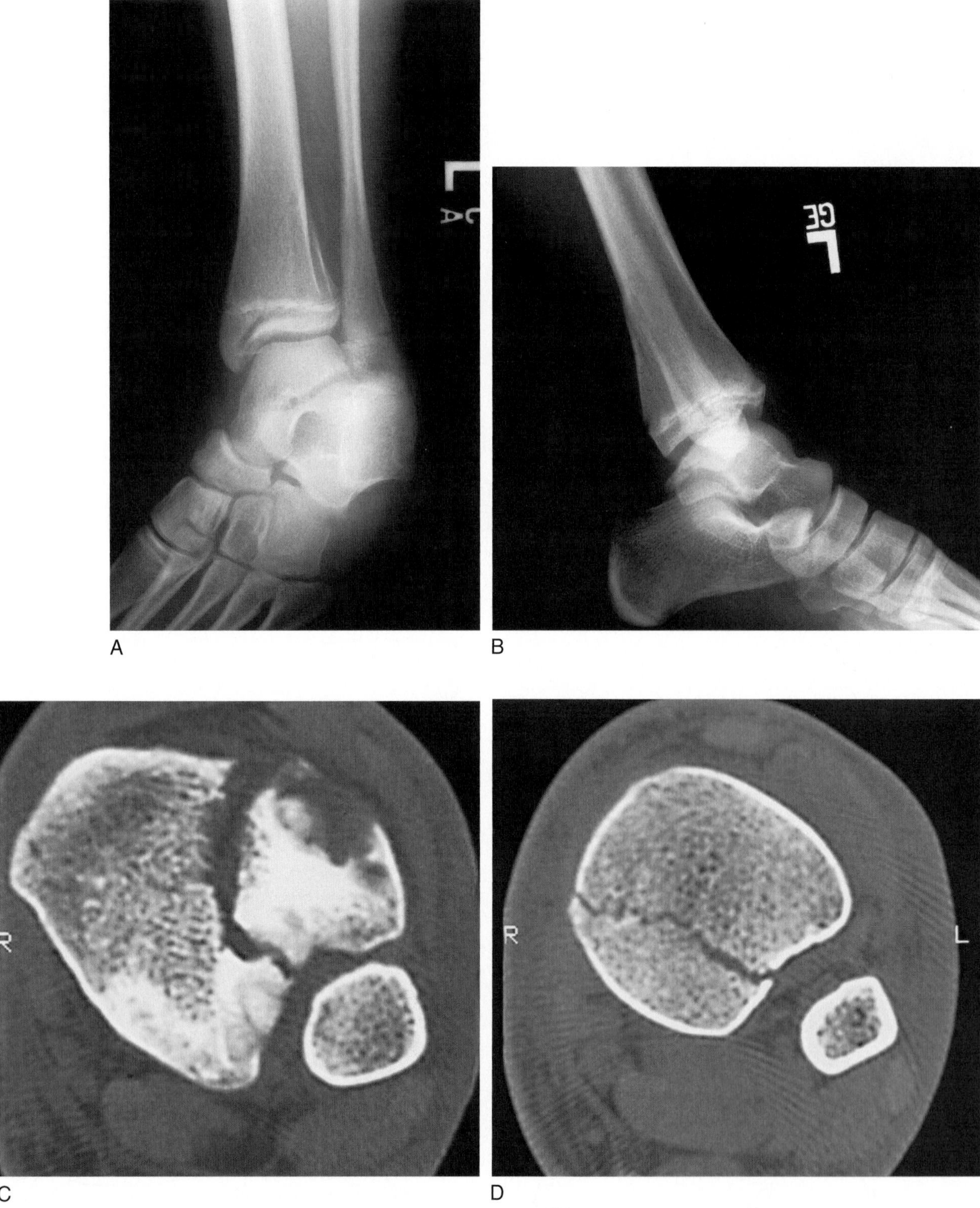

FIGURE 43–183 Three-part triplane fracture. **A,** Anteroposterior radiograph demonstrating the epiphyseal fracture, which travels in the sagittal plane. **B,** The lateral radiograph demonstrates the coronal plane metaphyseal fracture and epiphyseal fracture. **C,** Horizontal computed tomography (CT) scan showing the displaced anterolateral epiphyseal fragment. **D,** Horizontal CT scan through the metaphysis showing the mildly displaced metaphyseal fragment.

The patient is typically seen after an injury that involved twisting of the foot. Most injuries occur while the individual is participating in sports, but they may be due to a fall from a height or a twisting injury sustained while walking. Of 23 fractures, 15 occurred during sporting activities, 4 resulted from a fall from a height, 3 occurred after stepping into a hole or off a curb while walking, and 1 patient was involved in a motor vehicle accident.[67]

RADIOGRAPHIC FINDINGS

Radiographic examination of these fractures should include AP, lateral, and mortise views of the ankle because a Salter-Harris type III fracture is demonstrated on the AP radiograph and a Salter-Harris type II fracture is demonstrated on the lateral radiograph (Fig. 43–184). The vertical fracture line in the sagittal plane travels up from the articular surface, enters the physis, and extends out the physis laterally. The vertical component of the fracture line is usually in the center of the tibia, although it may be just medial to the midline and is most often displaced. Ertl and colleagues described 8 patients with less than 2 mm of displacement and 15 patients with more than 2 mm of displacement.[67] Occasionally, the fracture lines are difficult to see on plain radiographs, especially when good ankle radiographs are not obtained at the initial evaluation. The fibula is fractured in approximately 50% of all triplane fractures.[67] The mortise view better demonstrates the epiphyseal sagittal fracture line and best defines the amount of fracture displacement. Further evaluation of these fractures is best done with CT to assess the amount of articular surface step-off both before and after treatment, particularly when closed reduction is attempted (Fig. 43–185).

TREATMENT

The principal goal in the treatment of triplane fractures is to achieve anatomic reduction of the distal tibial articular surface because long-term follow-up indicates painful symptoms and early degenerative arthritis when anatomic reduction is not achieved. Ertl and colleagues reported short-term (3 years) and long-term (up to 13 years) follow-up of patients after the treatment of triplane fractures and found a significant decline in satisfactory results, especially in patients who had more than 1 mm of fracture displacement.[67] They further found that three of eight minimally displaced fractures treated by closed reduction and casting declined an outcome grade (e.g., excellent to good, good to fair) between the 3-year follow-up and the final follow-up (averaging 6 years).[67]

Closed Reduction

Most authors recommend nonoperative treatment of fractures with minimal or mild displacement (<2 mm). In these cases closed reduction can be performed with axial traction placed on the ankle and internal rotation of the foot with the patient under general anesthesia.[60] The patient is placed in a long-leg non–weight-bearing cast with the foot internally rotated for 3 to 4 weeks, followed by a short-leg cast for an additional 2 to 3 weeks. After closed reduction, lateral and mortise views should be obtained to confirm an adequate reduction. If the fracture can be satisfactorily seen on plain radiographs, residual fracture displacement of less than 2 mm is acceptable, although we prefer anatomic reduction at the time of initial reduction to allow for some mild displacement, which is likely to occur in the cast with time. In addition, one can argue that successful closed reduction in the operating room should be followed by fixation of the articular fragment with a single smooth Kirschner wire or screw to provide more secure fixation and less risk of future fracture displacement. This can be done percutaneously or through a small, 2- to 3-cm arthrotomy.

It is difficult to accurately assess such a small amount of displacement in the distal articular surface of the tibia with plain radiographs alone, so we prefer to obtain a CT scan after any closed reduction to confirm a nearly anatomic reduction. It is important to obtain serial weekly radiographs after the initial reduction to ensure that an unacceptable loss of reduction has not occurred during this period. It may also be necessary to repeat the CT study at 1 week so that open reduction and internal fixation can be performed if loss of reduction has occurred. An associated greenstick or displaced fracture of the fibula makes reduction difficult because the strong ligamentous attachments to the fibula maintain the angular deformity and the resultant shortening of the attached tibial fragment, thus making it necessary to reduce the fibular fracture before attempting any reduction of the tibia.[48]

When displacement of the fracture is more than 3 mm at the time of initial evaluation, the likelihood of achieving an acceptable reduction is low because of the energy imparted at the time of injury, soft tissue swelling, and soft tissue interposition at the fracture site. Of five fractures with displacement of more than 3 mm, no patient had a successful closed reduction, and at the time of open reduction, interposed soft tissue consisting of periosteum or the extensor hallucis longus tendon was present at the fracture site.[67]

An extra-articular triplane fracture is recognized by the two-part nature of the fracture in which the sagittal fracture exits the anterior medial malleolus, the axial fracture travels through the physis, and the coronal fracture travels through the posterior metaphysis.[71,231] These fractures can be treated by closed reduction and long-leg casting for 4 weeks, followed by short-leg casting for 2 weeks, because they are extra-articular.[71] A variant of this fracture pattern was recently described as three types of intramalleolar triplane fractures: an intra-articular fracture within the weight-bearing zone, which may require operative intervention; an intra-articular fracture outside the weight-bearing zone; and an

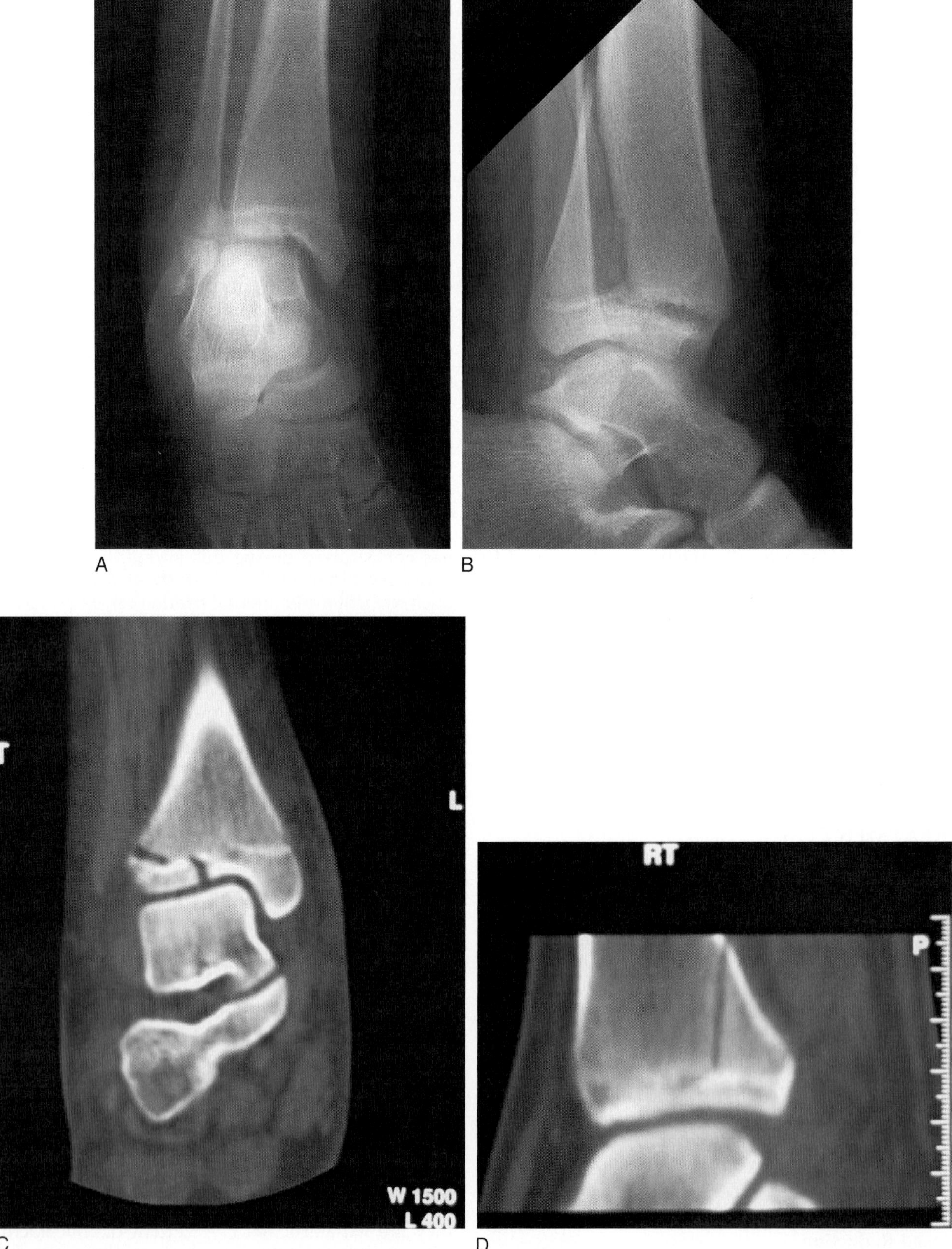

FIGURE 43–184 Typical radiographic examination of a triplane fracture. **A,** On the anteroposterior radiograph a Salter-Harris type III fracture pattern is seen. **B,** On the lateral radiograph a Salter-Harris type II fracture pattern is seen. The triplane fracture is well seen on coronal **(C)** and sagittal plane **(D)** computed tomography scans.

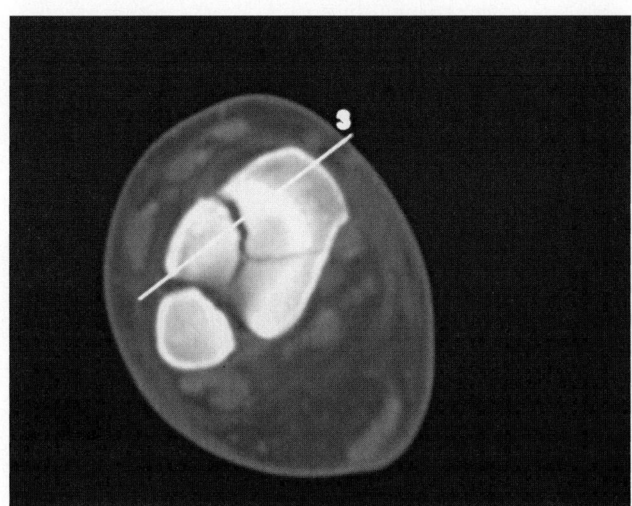

FIGURE 43–185 Computed tomography scan of a triplane fracture. Note that the fracture is similar to a Tillaux fracture in that it runs from the anterior cortex out laterally. The second fracture line seen runs in an anterior-to-posterior direction. There is minimal displacement of this fracture.

extra-articular fracture. The latter two can be treated by closed reduction.[207]

Open Reduction and Internal Fixation

The indications for open reduction and internal fixation are failure to achieve adequate reduction (to within 2 mm of the anatomic position) and a displaced fracture (>3 mm) at the time of initial evaluation. Preoperative assessment should include a thorough physical examination with special emphasis on the status of the soft tissue envelope because significant swelling can occur with these fractures and should resolve before performing an open reduction. The method of operative intervention depends on the fracture pattern and the degree of displacement. This should be assessed on plain films and CT.

When the Salter-Harris type II posterior fragment is minimally displaced or when there is a two-part fracture, anterior exposure of the ankle is the only operative incision necessary (Fig. 43–186). These fractures are not usually associated with fracture of the fibula. The fracture hematoma is removed and the fracture is reduced by internal rotation of the foot, followed by compression across the fracture site with bone reduction forceps. A small stab incision is then made over the medial malleolus, and a 4.0-mm cancellous screw is placed under fluoroscopic visualization. Cannulated systems can be used to aid in maintenance of reduction and screw placement. Arthroscopic visualization has been used in two patients with two-part fractures to allow direct visualization during hematoma evacuation and fracture reduction, with good results.[234] A short-leg cast should be worn for 4 to 6 weeks after anatomic reduction and stable internal fixation.

A displaced triplane fracture with a large displaced Salter-Harris type II metaphyseal fragment, often associated with a fibular fracture, requires a more extensive operative procedure with reduction of the fragments. The initial incision is an anterior approach to the ankle with visualization and manual displacement of the anterolateral epiphyseal fragment. Next, closed reduction of the posterior metaphyseal fragment should be attempted by direct compression and internal rotation of the foot, which can be assessed fluoroscopically. A second attempt at reduction can be made with Weber bone reduction forceps placed through a stab incision in the posterolateral aspect of the ankle, just lateral to the Achilles tendon (Fig. 43–187). If neither of these techniques is successful, open reduction with direct visualization of the fracture fragment should be performed through a posterolateral incision, lateral to the Achilles tendon, to develop the interval between the flexor hallucis longus and the peroneus brevis (Fig. 43–188). The fracture is then reduced under direct vision, held with bone reduction forceps, and internally fixed with one or two cancellous screws placed in an anterior-to-posterior direction. The fibular fracture should be temporarily reduced during the reduction maneuver for the posterior metaphyseal fragment and re-reduced if necessary after internal fixation of the posterior fragment. The last fragment to be reduced is the anterolateral epiphyseal fragment, which can be reduced under direct vision and fixed as described previously. The leg should be placed in a long-leg non–weight-bearing cast for 4 weeks, followed by a short-leg cast for an additional 2 to 3 weeks.

RESULTS

The results of treatment of triplane fractures are generally good in the short term.* Patients usually return to their preinjury level of activity without symptoms. The long-term outcome of these fractures, however, is not fully defined. The only study that has examined the relatively long-term outcome of treatment of triplane fractures noted a deterioration in successful results between the early results at 3 years and the final results (averaging just over 6 years), with pain and swelling being the most common reasons for the decline in outcome.[67] This is postulated to be due to several factors. First, it is generally accepted that less than 2 mm of fracture displacement is acceptable and leads to good results; however, three of eight patients with minimally displaced fractures at the time of injury had a deterioration in outcome between the 3- and 6-year follow-up. Second, loss of reduction may have occurred during the immobilization period of some fractures and was not assessed by the more accurate CT in these cases. Third, in some severely displaced fractures, function deteriorated over time despite anatomic reduction achieved through open reduction followed by stable internal fixation, thus suggesting significant articular cartilage damage at the time of the initial injury.

*See references 45, 48, 50, 60, 108, 111, 140, 169, 212, 225, 231.

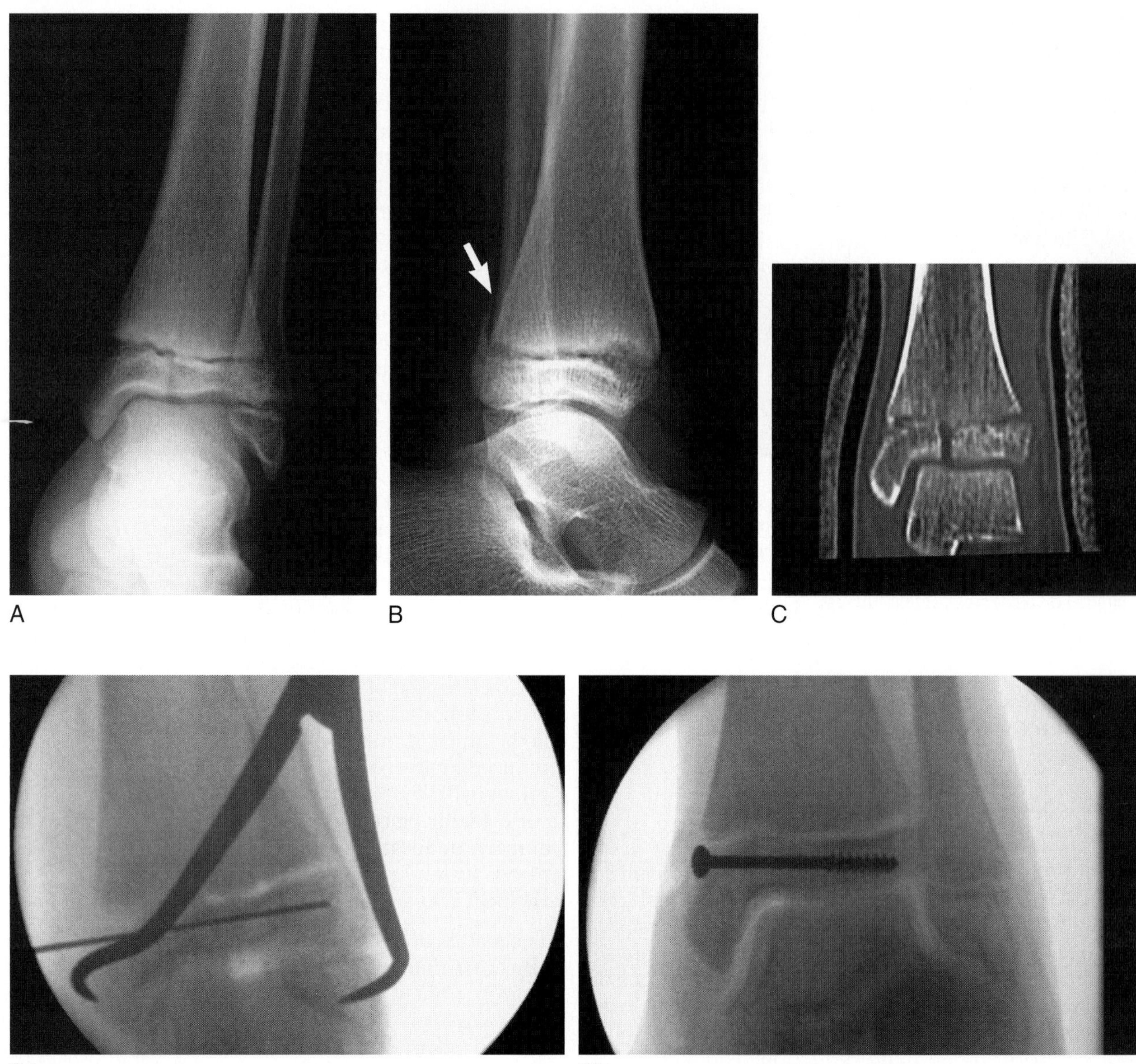

FIGURE 43–186 Open reduction and internal fixation of a triplane fracture. **A,** Anteroposterior radiograph demonstrating the Salter-Harris type III fracture pattern in the tibial epiphysis. There is approximately 4 mm of displacement. **B,** The lateral radiograph does not show an obvious Salter-Harris type II pattern. However, the Salter-Harris type II fracture pattern of the distal fibula is apparent (*arrow*). **C,** A computed tomography scan demonstrates the intra-articular fracture with displacement. **D,** Intraoperative radiographs obtained after open reduction with cannulated screw fixation. A Weber clamp was used to compress the fracture site *(left)*, which was viewed directly. The guide pin was then placed across the fracture site under fluoroscopic guidance *(right)*.

Foot

Talar Fractures

Fractures of the talus in children are very rare and account for less than 10% of all talar fractures reported in the literature. Fractures of the neck of the talus are more common and generally have a better prognosis than talar body fractures. The mechanism of injury is usually a fall from a height with a forced dorsiflexion injury at the ankle and some supination component to the injury, which results in malleolar fractures. The diagnosis is often difficult to make in a young child because of mild radiographic changes at the initial visit. Treatment of a young child is generally nonoperative, with cast immobilization resulting in good outcomes. Treatment of adolescents is similar to that of adults, with comparable results and a high risk for AVN in the displaced fracture.

ANATOMY

The talus is the transition bone between the foot and the leg. It is divided anatomically into the body, the neck, and the head. The superior dome of the talar body articulates with the distal tibial articular surface and has a quadrilateral surface that is wider anteriorly than posteriorly and is composed of the medial and lateral facets. From front to back the talar dome is convex; from side to side it is slightly concave (Fig. 43–189). The neck is relatively short and is the only surface of the talus not covered by articular cartilage, thus allowing passage of nutrient blood vessels to the body. The lateral process of the talus is a large, wedge-shaped prominence that is covered with articular cartilage. It articulates with the fibula superolaterally and with the most lateral portion of the subtalar joint inferiorly (Fig. 43–190). The distalmost end of the lateral process is the origin of the lateral talocalcaneal ligament.[88,90] The posterior region of the talus often exhibits a radiographically separate ossification center, which occurs at 11 to 13 years of age in boys and 8 to 10 years in girls and usually fuses to the talus 1 year after its appearance.[148] The inferior surface is composed of three facets that articulate with the superior aspect of the calcaneus.

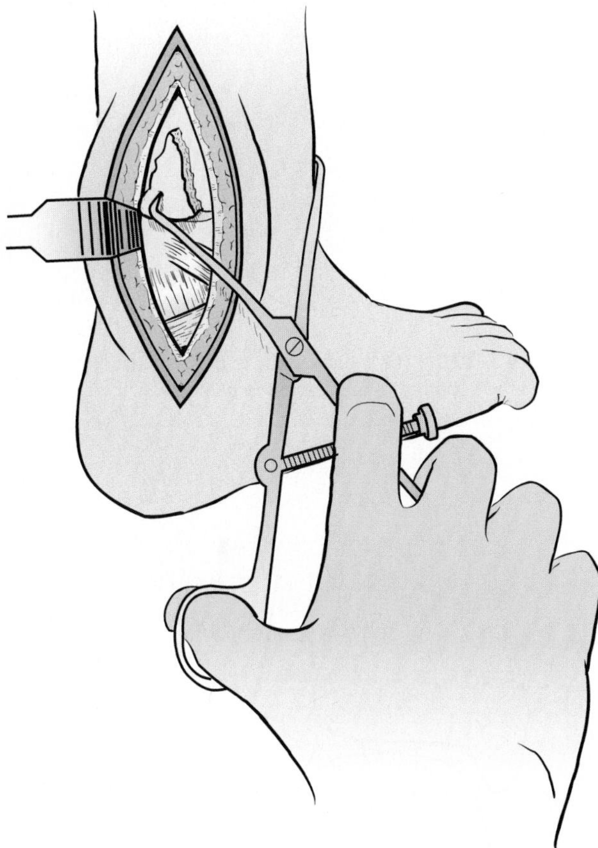

FIGURE 43–187 Reduction of a posterior metaphyseal fragmented and displaced triplane fracture. The fracture can be reduced by placing Weber bone reduction forceps directly on the posterior metaphyseal fragment and making a small stab incision in the anterior aspect of the tibia to gain reduction.

The blood supply to the talus has been well studied. It is susceptible to injury after a displaced talar neck or body fracture, with the subsequent development of AVN.[86,109,159,174,175,235] The four main sources of extraosseous blood supply are branches of the posterior tibial, anterior tibial, and peroneal arteries (Fig. 43–191). The first is the artery of the tarsal canal, which branches from the posterior tibial artery approximately 1 cm proximal to the origin of the medial and lateral plantar arteries and passes between the tendon sheaths of the flexor digitorum longus and flexor hallucis longus tendons. There it enters the tarsal canal, which is formed by the sulci of the talus and calcaneus and narrows posteromedially to anterolaterally. Branches of this artery are given off in the canal to supply the body of the talus. The second source of blood supply is the deltoid branch of the artery of the tarsal canal, which travels between the talotibial and talocalcaneal aspects of the deltoid ligament and supplies the medial periosteal surface of the body; anastomoses with the dorsalis pedis artery occur. The third major source of blood supply is the arterial branches to the dorsal neck, which arise from anastomoses between branches of the dorsalis pedis artery (extension of the anterior tibial artery). Finally, the artery of the sinus tarsi, primarily a branch of the perforating peroneal artery, supplies the lateral aspect of the talus. A rich intraosseous blood supply is present within the talus; in a simulated fracture model this blood supply becomes compromised.[174-176]

MECHANISM OF INJURY

Most talar neck fractures in children are due to falls from a height with a dorsiflexion injury of the ankle.[99,130,147] The excess dorsiflexion and axial loading

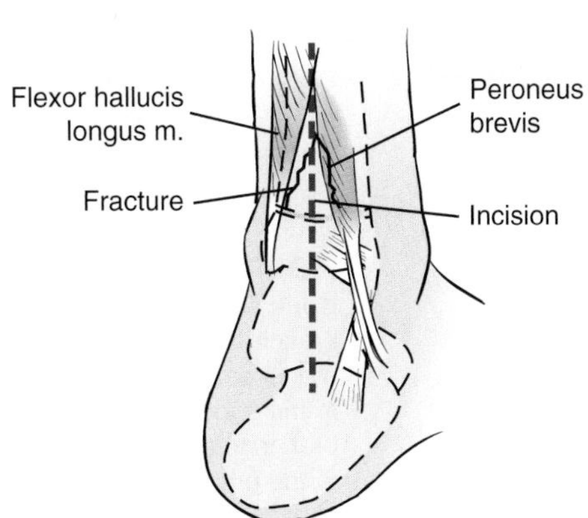

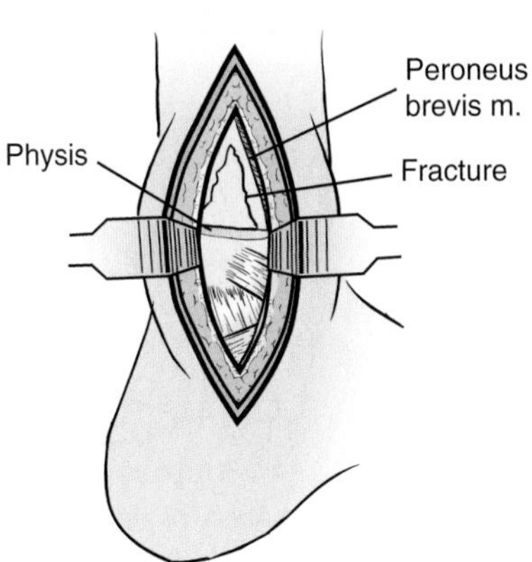

FIGURE 43–188 Approach to the posterior metaphyseal fragment in a triplane fracture. An incision is made in the posterolateral aspect of the distal end of the ankle. The interval between the peroneus brevis and the flexor hallucis longus muscles is developed. The capsule is incised and the fracture is identified.

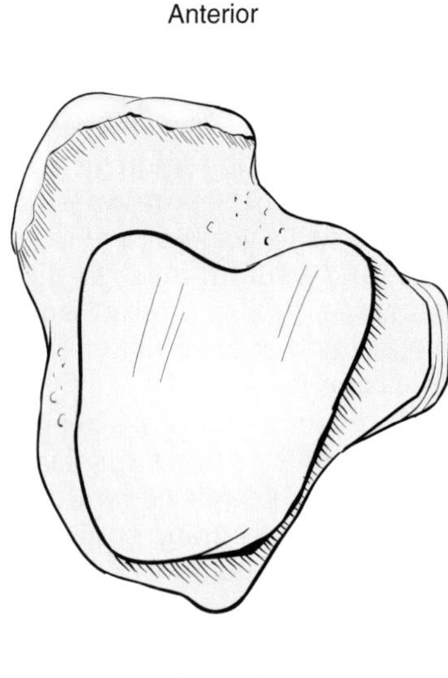

FIGURE 43–189 The superior surface of the talus. Note the greater width of the anterior dome of the talus as compared with the posterior dome.

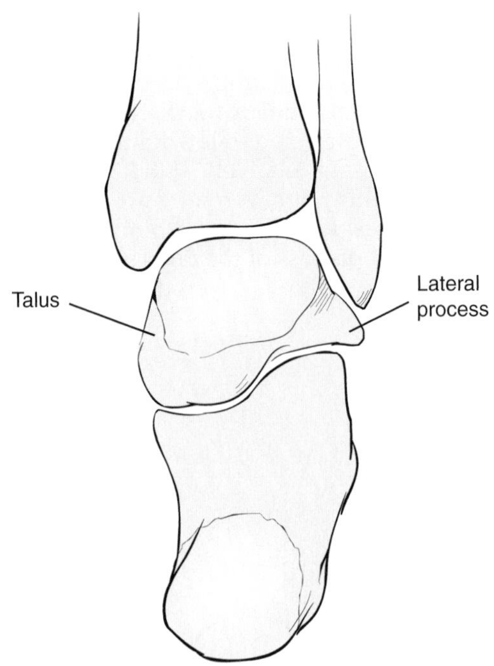

FIGURE 43–190 The lateral process of the talus. Note its articulation with both the fibula and the calcaneus.

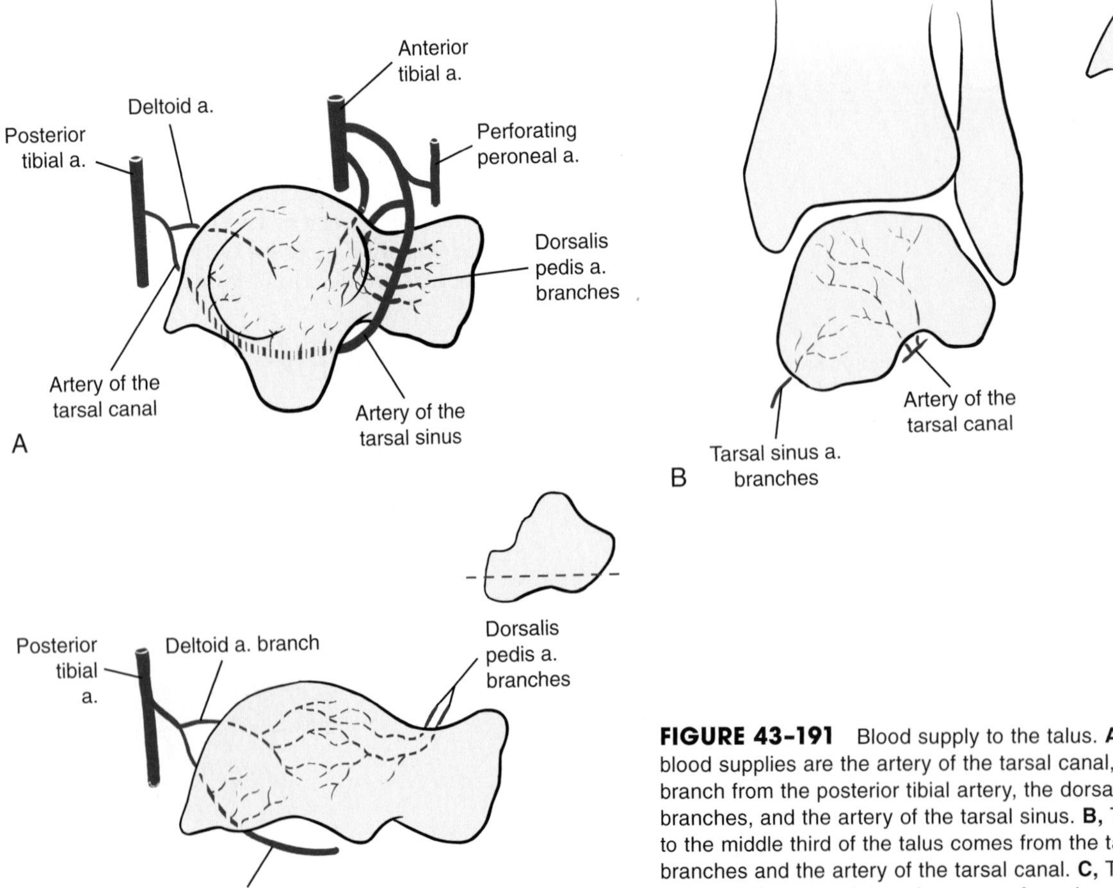

FIGURE 43–191 Blood supply to the talus. **A,** The four major blood supplies are the artery of the tarsal canal, the deltoid branch from the posterior tibial artery, the dorsalis pedis branches, and the artery of the tarsal sinus. **B,** The blood supply to the middle third of the talus comes from the tarsal sinus branches and the artery of the tarsal canal. **C,** The blood supply to the medial third of the talus comes from the artery of the tarsal canal and the deltoid and dorsalis pedis branches.

result in a dorsally directed shear force exerted against the sole of the foot while the body of the talus is fixed between the tibia and the calcaneus. The fracture line typically occurs in a vertical or slightly oblique direction between the middle and posterior subtalar facets, with displacement of the distal fragment superiorly and medially.[36] One reason that these injuries are uncommon is that high-energy force is usually necessary to produce them, estimated to be approximately twice the force needed to produce a calcaneal or navicular fracture.[177]

CLASSIFICATION

Talus fractures can be broadly divided into talar neck fractures and talar body fractures. A further division of the more common talar neck fractures was first described by Hawkins in 1970. His three-part classification was primarily based on the amount of fracture displacement and provided information on the prognosis for AVN.[89] This classification was later modified by Canale and Kelly to include a fourth type (Fig. 43–192).[36] A type I injury is an undisplaced vertical fracture of the talar neck. A type II fracture is a displaced fracture; the subtalar joint is subluxated or dislocated but the ankle joint is normal. A type III injury is similar to a type II injury, but there is subluxation or dislocation of both the ankle and subtalar joints. A type IV injury is very rare and is characterized by dislocation of the talar head from the talonavicular joint. In adults, types II and III fractures are most common and account for approximately 75% to 90% of all talar neck fractures.[36,89]

Fractures of the body of the talus were first classified in 1977 by Sneppen and colleagues,[211] whose classification was later modified by Delee[57] into a five-part classification: type I, transchondral dome fractures; type II, shear fractures; type III, posterior tubercle fractures; type IV, lateral process fractures; and type V, crush fractures (Fig. 43–193).

Children's talar fractures are probably best classified according to the age of the child, with children younger than 6 years having a better prognosis than older children.[147] Treatment of talar fractures in younger children is more often nonoperative, with generally good results, whereas talar fractures in older children are best addressed as talar fractures in adults.

CLINICAL FEATURES

A history of a fall with axial loading of the ankle, followed by pain and swelling in the area of the talus, should alert the physician to the possibility of a talus fracture. The child is usually unable to bear weight on the affected extremity, and physical examination reveals ankle effusion and pain on motion of the ankle joint, especially dorsiflexion. A patient with a displaced talar neck fracture and fractures of one or more malleoli has significant pain and massive swelling in

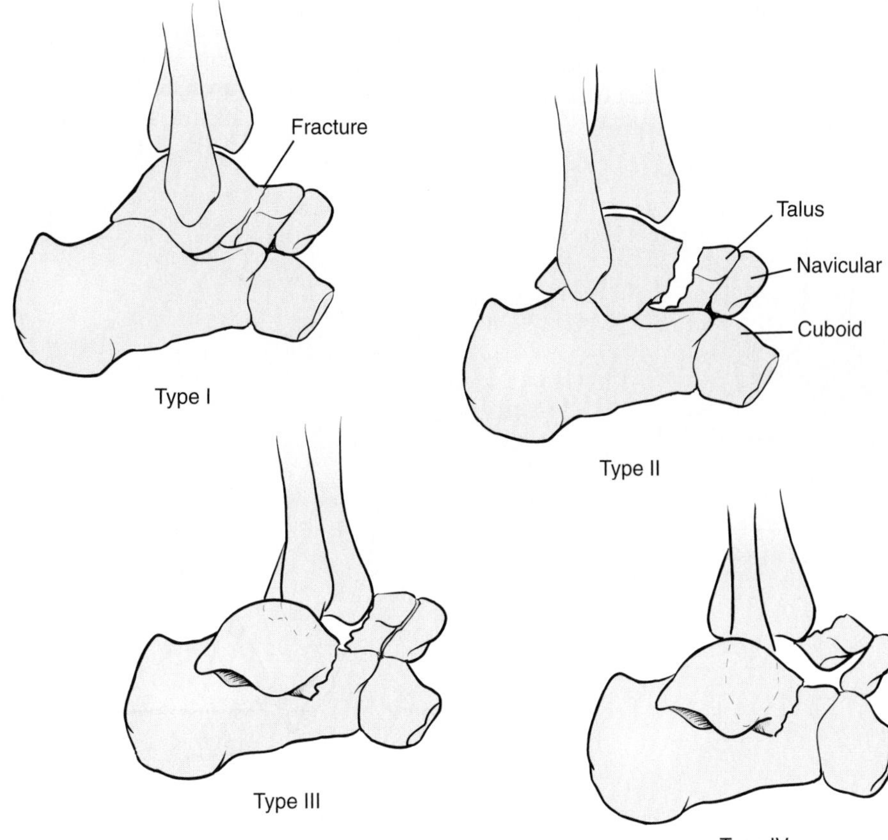

FIGURE 43-192 Classification of talar neck fractures. Type I—nondisplaced fracture. Type II—displaced fracture with subluxation or dislocation of the subtalar joint. Type III—displaced fracture with dislocation of the talar body from both the ankle and subtalar joints. Type IV—subluxation or dislocation of the talar head and dislocation of the talar body.

GOUP I

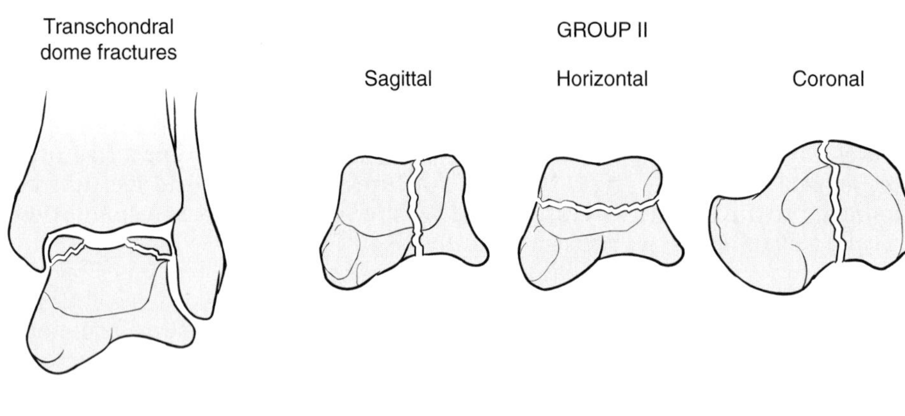

GROUP III

Posterior tubercle

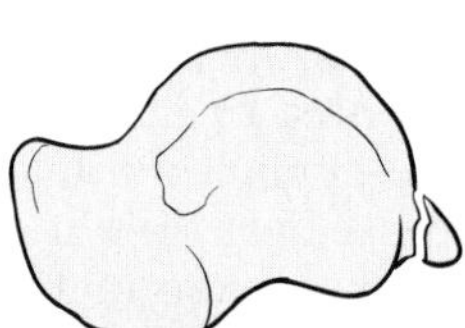

GROUP IV

Lateral process

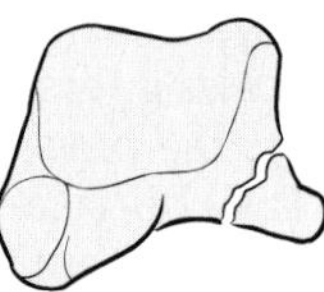

GROUP V

Crush fractures

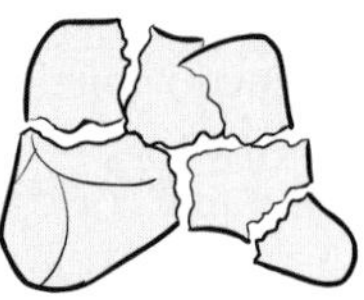

FIGURE 43–193 Classification of talar body fractures.

the region of the talus and the ankle. In a young child a talar fracture may be difficult to diagnose, especially when the talus has not fully ossified. Mazel and associates reported on 23 talar fractures in children and divided them into two groups based on the age of the patient.[147] Fractures in patients younger than 6 years were difficult to diagnose, and when the diagnosis was made, the amount of fracture displacement was often underestimated.

RADIOGRAPHIC FINDINGS

Radiographic examination should include AP, lateral, and oblique views centered at the ankle. A pronated oblique view of the talus, first described by Canale and Kelly, is an excellent view with which to see the talus (Fig. 43–194).[36] The foot is placed into equinus and pronated approximately 15 degrees, and the x-ray beam is angled 75 degrees to the horizontal. Associ-

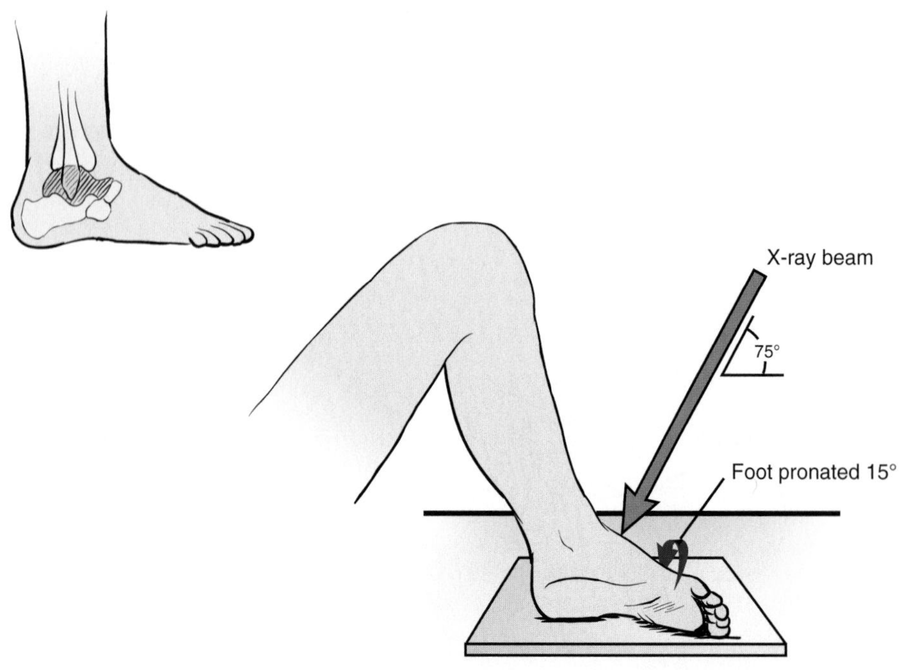

FIGURE 43–194 Positioning of the foot for an oblique radiograph to best visualize the talar neck when this fracture is suspected.

ated fractures of the medial and lateral malleoli are seen most commonly with a displaced talar fracture.[99] If a talar fracture is suspected but not confirmed on the initial radiographs, CT can be used to identify or confirm the presence of the fracture and the amount of fracture displacement.

TREATMENT

Treatment of talar fractures in children largely depends on the age of the child and the amount of fracture displacement. Most children younger than 8 years with minimally displaced fractures respond well to nonoperative treatment.[99,130,147,155]

Fractures of the Neck of the Talus

Treatment of talar neck fractures in children is solely dependent on the amount of displacement and the classification of Hawkins. The majority of talar neck fractures are undisplaced at initial evaluation (Hawkins' type I) and should be treated in a short-leg cast for 6 to 8 weeks to allow fracture consolidation. Weight bearing can be instituted when the cast is removed. In a young child with a displaced fracture but without subluxation of the ankle or subtalar joints (Hawkins' type II), an attempt at closed reduction should be made with the patient under conscious sedation or general anesthesia. The definition of acceptable reduction in children's talar neck fractures has not been established; however, we prefer to attempt gentle closed reduction of any talar neck fracture with residual angulation of greater than 15 to 20 degrees. The distal fragment is usually dorsally and often medially displaced, and therefore gentle plantar flexion and pronation of the foot should be performed to reduce the fracture. The foot may need to remain in some plantar flexion and is placed in a long-leg cast for the initial 4 weeks. The foot can then be brought up to neutral position and placed in a short-leg cast for an additional 3 to 4 weeks. If the fracture cannot be reduced to within 15 to 20 degrees on the initial attempt at closed reduction, open reduction should be performed.

Children older than 10 years with talar neck fractures should be treated as adults with these injuries. A type I fracture in an older child can generally be treated in a short-leg cast with the foot in slight plantar flexion and inversion for 6 to 8 weeks, until fracture healing has occurred. The majority of displaced fractures (Hawkins' types II and III fractures) occur in older children and should be treated as in adults, with open reduction and internal fixation. Reduction of type II fractures can often be achieved by closed methods; however, because of significant soft tissue disruption, the ability to maintain the reduction with external immobilization is poor. Early reduction with rigid internal fixation helps in reestablishing the circulation and allows early motion.

Type III injuries require open reduction and internal fixation, which is best done through a posterolateral incision to allow access to the fracture for reduction and initiation of screw placement without risking further injury to the important blood supply to the talus. When the posterior approach fails to achieve a reduction, an alternative approach is through an anteromedial incision. Care must be taken to avoid the deltoid branch of the posterior tibial artery during this approach (Fig. 43–195). The best fixation is provided by partially threaded cancellous screws placed so that they provide compression across the fracture site. The result is biomechanically strongest when the screws are placed from the posterior talus into the neck anteriorly.[146,216] In children, a single 6.5- or 4.0-mm screw works well and should be protected with a short-leg non–weight-bearing cast for 4 to 6 weeks. As in adults, these injuries have a poor prognosis despite the best of treatments. A case report describes a 10-year old girl with a type III talar neck fracture who underwent open reduction and internal fixation. The fracture healed within 3 months, but AVN developed.[171]

In a patient with a talar neck fracture, good AP and mortise radiographs of the ankle should be obtained between 6 and 8 weeks after injury to look for the Hawkins sign, which is described as subchondral atrophy of the talar dome.[89] This is a good prognostic sign that excludes the presence of AVN. When the

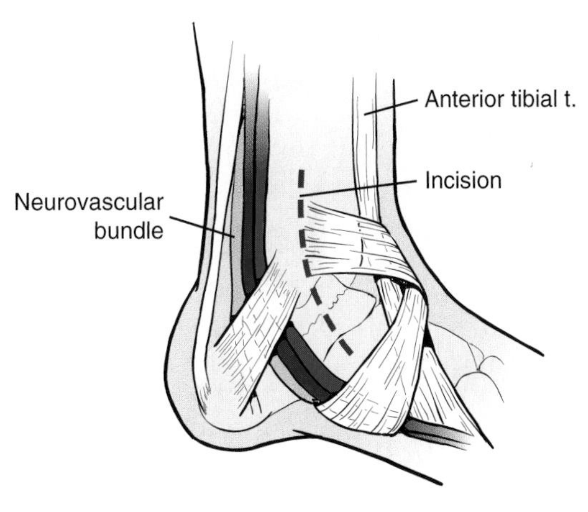

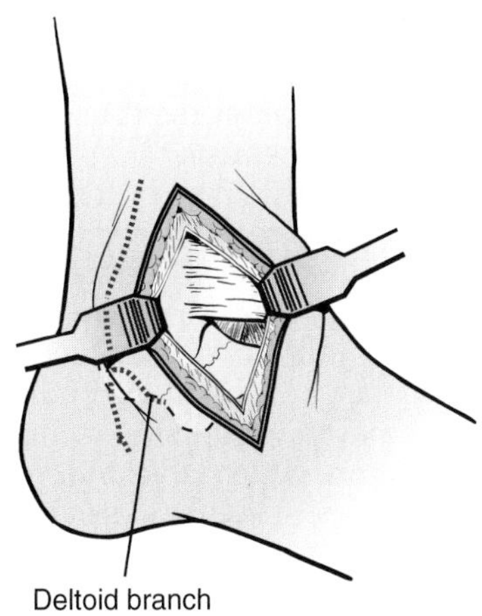

FIGURE 43–195 Anteromedial approach to the talus. A curvilinear skin incision is made just anterior to the medial malleolus. This incision is extended over the medial aspect of the midfoot. Dissection is then carried out just medial to the anterior tibialis tendon. Retraction will permit access to the fracture site and fixation of the fracture.

Hawkins sign is absent at this time, the patient should be kept non–weight bearing to prevent collapse of the talar dome.

Fractures of the Body of the Talus

Osteochondral injuries to the dome of the talus will be discussed separately. A fracture through the body of the talus is much less common than talar neck fractures in both adults and children and generally carries a worse prognosis, especially when displaced. In a series of 14 fractures in children, 4 (29%) were fractures of the talar body.[99] The majority of these fractures are undisplaced at initial evaluation and can be treated with a short-leg cast for 6 to 8 weeks, until fracture healing has occurred. Open reduction plus internal fixation is required for a displaced fracture to prevent early degenerative osteoarthritis.

Fractures of the Lateral Process

These rare injuries account for less than 1% of all ankle injuries.[157] The mechanism of injury is forced dorsiflexion and inversion of the foot.[88] The diagnosis is difficult to make, in part because it is so uncommon and in part because it is difficult to identify the fracture on radiographs on the initial visit, especially when the fracture is not displaced.[88,90] Of 13 fractures of the lateral process of the talus, 6 (46%) were missed at initial evaluation.[88] The clinician should have a high index of suspicion when there is any lateral ankle pain after an ankle injury, especially in a child who participates in athletic activities requiring quick cutting movements that stress the ankle joint. An increase in the incidence of these injuries has been seen in snowboarders over the last decade.[149,163] Treatment of these injuries depends on the amount of displacement of the fracture at the initial visit. These fractures are most commonly undisplaced and are best treated in a short-leg weight-bearing cast for 6 weeks. Fractures displaced more than 1 cm require reduction and internal fixation with a single compression screw to restore congruity of the articular surfaces.[88,90,198,228]

COMPLICATIONS

AVN is the most serious complication after a talar fracture and is well defined in the adult literature, with the incidence of this complication being directly related to the location of the fracture and the amount of fracture displacement.[36,89,155] The reported incidence of AVN with fractures of the talar neck is 0% to 10% for type I fractures, 40% to 50% for type II fractures, 80% to 90% for type III fractures, and 100% for type IV fractures.[36,89] These figures were derived in predominantly adult populations and may not reflect the true incidence of AVN in the pediatric population. In addition, newer treatment techniques, including earlier reduction with stable internal fixation of these displaced fractures, may provide improved results.[217]

The few reports in the literature on talar fractures in children offer conflicting data with respect to factors predisposing to AVN. Letts and Gibeault reported a 25% incidence of AVN in 12 patients; however, 2 of these 3 patients had undisplaced fractures that were unrecognized at the time of injury, and AVN later developed.[130] Similarly, Linhart and Hollwarth reported a 27% incidence of AVN in children, some of whom had undisplaced fractures.[133] Mazel and associates reported two of seven complete talar neck fractures in children older than 6 years in whom AVN later developed.[147] However, Jensen and colleagues reported no evidence of AVN in 11 nondisplaced fractures and 3 displaced talar fractures in children.[99]

Radiographic assessment for the Hawkins sign should be performed between 6 and 8 weeks after injury. The Hawkins sign, described as a radiolucency in the subchondral area, indicates that the body of the talus has not undergone an avascular process. If the Hawkins sign is present, there is a high likelihood that the talar body has a good blood supply and will remain viable, and the patient can begin bearing weight 6 to 8 weeks after the injury. Absence of the Hawkins sign is not considered an entirely reliable indicator that AVN will develop.[36] The patient should be kept non–weight bearing and should be reevaluated 3 months after the injury. MRI of the talus is indicated at 3 months if there is no radiographic indication of the Hawkins sign; MRI performed at that time will accurately show AVN.[91,223] It is important to use titanium implants at the time of internal fixation of displaced talar neck fractures to allow clear visualization of the talus on MRI. Though not proved to be effective, when AVN is present and fracture healing has occurred, restriction of activity is recommended in an effort to prevent collapse.

Osteochondral Fractures of the Talus

Also known as osteochondritis dissecans, an osteochondral fracture of the talus typically involves the posteromedial or anterolateral aspects of the talar dome. Although the etiology of this lesion is not completely understood, most patients recall a traumatic episode, especially those who have an anterolateral lesion. The diagnosis is based on the plain radiographic appearance or on bone scan and MRI when the initial radiographs are normal. The Berndt and Harty classification scheme is based on the radiographic nature of the injury and is used when deciding on treatment. Most children respond well to nonoperative treatment when the lesion is stable; however, operative intervention is necessary in some patients to remove or stabilize a detached fragment.

MECHANISM OF INJURY

The etiology of osteochondral fractures of the talus has been debated for many years; however, trauma appears to be the principal cause.* Berndt and Harty created osteochondral injuries of the talus in cadavers. They found that the anterolateral aspect of the talar dome impacts the medial aspect of the fibula when the dor-

*See references 4, 6, 16, 35, 92, 96, 135, 142, 178, 184, 202, 233.

siflexed foot is subjected to an inversion force. The posteromedial aspect of the talar dome is injured as it strikes the distal tibial articular surface when the plantar flexed foot is forcibly inverted and externally rotated.[16]

The link to trauma as the cause of these lesions is strongest for lesions that occur on the lateral aspect of the talus.[35,75,92,148,203] Canale and Belding reported that all 15 patients with lateral lesions had a history of trauma, whereas only 9 (64%) of 14 patients with medial lesions had a history of previous trauma[35] A review of the literature before 1985 found that 98% of patients with lateral lesions and 70% of patients with medial lesions had sustained trauma.[75] Patients seen after an acute traumatic event more often have a lateral lesion. Canale suggested that the morphology of the lateral lesions—wafer shaped and shallower than the deeper, cup-shaped lesions—is more consistent with a traumatic shearing force producing these lesions.[35]

Other factors may contribute to the development of these lesions. A familial association has been described in which more than one family member had a lesion.[3,241] In addition, lesions of the talus occur bilaterally in 5% to 10% of cases.

CLASSIFICATION

Berndt and Harty published their four-part radiographic classification of these lesions in 1959 (Fig. 43–196)[16]:

Stage I	A small subchondral trabecular compression fracture not seen radiographically
Stage II	Incomplete avulsion or separation of the fragment
Stage III	Complete avulsion without displacement
Stage IV	The fragment is detached and rotated and may be free within the joint

Because this classification is based on radiographic criteria, which may be difficult to interpret and cannot distinguish a stage I lesion, Anderson and associates modified the Berndt and Harty classification to include the associated MRI findings.[4] MRI is useful in two circumstances. The first is to identify an osteochondral injury when radiographs are normal (stage I). MRI findings consistent with an osteochondral injury were decreased signal intensity on both T1- and T2-weighted images. At times there may be increased signal on T2-weighted images because of the presence of marrow edema in a stage I lesion. The second situation in which MRI is useful is to identify a subchondral cyst in a stage II lesion, which is thought to represent areas of post-traumatic necrosis of bone followed by a cascade of host responses ultimately leading to free separation of the fragment. This finding places the lesion in the stage IIa category, which is treated by unroofing the lesion and drilling down to bleeding bone.[4] Anderson and associates found no utility of MRI in stage III and IV lesions.

Although CT is not useful in defining a Berndt and Harty stage I lesion,[186] it can be used to further define the remaining lesions.[135,233] A previously unreported lesion that has been described with the use of CT consists of a radiolucent defect, seen in 77% of cases. It is best treated by curettage and drilling.[135]

Further comparison of the radiographic classification and visualization of the lesion through the arthroscope was investigated by Pritsch and colleagues, who provided some guidelines for the treatment of these lesions.[183] The cartilage overlying the lesion was grouped into three grades: grade I indicated intact, firm, shiny cartilage; grade II cartilage was intact, but soft; and grade III indicated frayed cartilage. They reported poor correlation between the radiographic appearance of the lesion and the state of the overlying cartilage, and therefore treatment of osteochondral lesions was based on the visual appearance of the cartilage: for grade I, simple restriction of sports activities was recommended; for grade II, arthroscopic drilling was recommended; and for grade III, curettage of the lesion through the arthroscope was recommended. MRI best correlates with the arthroscopic findings and

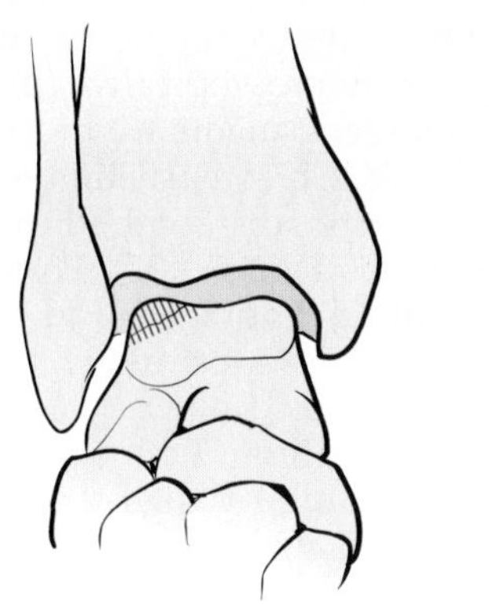
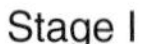

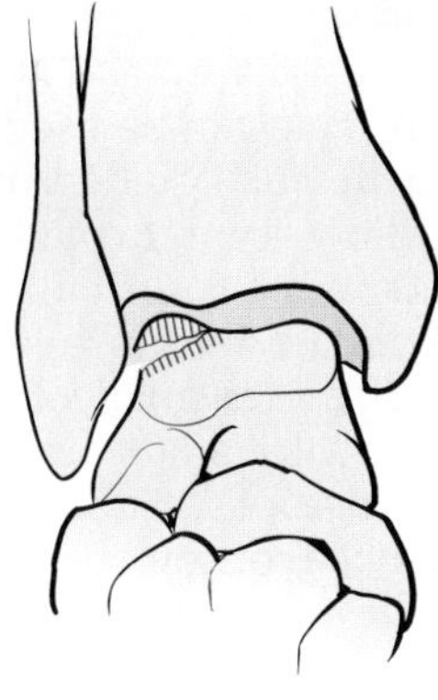

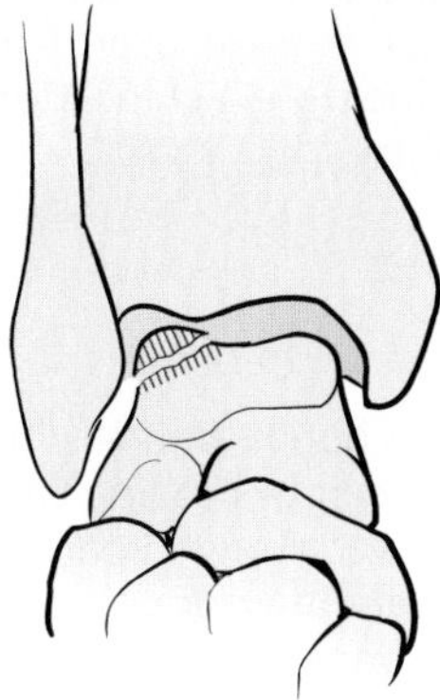

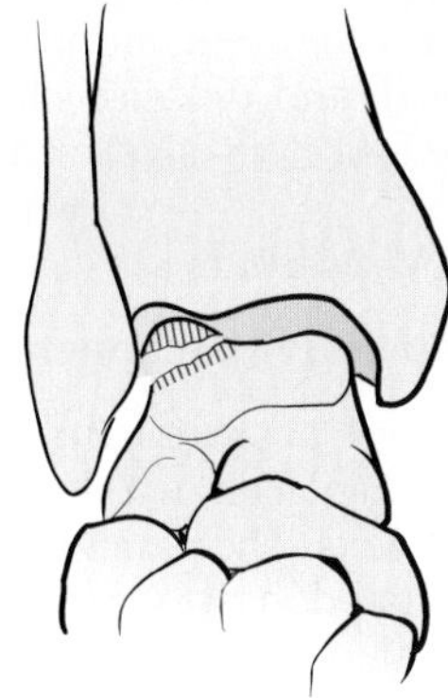

FIGURE 43–196 Berndt and Harty classification of talar osteochondral lesions. Stage I—small area of subchondral compression. Stage II—partially detached osteochondral fragment. Stage III—completely detached fragment remaining within the crater of the lesion. Stage IV—osteochondral fragment loose in the joint.

accurately predicts the stability of the fragment in 92% of cases.[59,107]

CLINICAL FEATURES

The patient is usually seen initially after an ankle injury. The evaluation can take place in the acute stage, immediately after the injury, and the diagnosis is made from the plain radiographic findings. Often, however, the patient does not seek medical attention after the acute injury but is seen at a later date with chronic ankle symptoms that have not resolved or with chronic painful symptoms without an inciting traumatic event.

The physical examination in a patient with chronic pain is often benign, without any specific findings. There may be generalized swelling in the ankle region secondary to synovitis and a joint effusion. In a stable lesion, forced dorsiflexion and inversion may cause symptoms in an anterolateral lesion, whereas a posteromedial lesion may become symptomatic when a plantar flexed foot is inverted and externally rotated at the ankle. With a loose or completely displaced fragment, passive motion of the ankle is painful.

RADIOGRAPHIC FINDINGS

The initial radiographs include AP, lateral, and mortise views of the ankle. These views should be scrutinized for evidence of an osteochondral lesion. When seen, the lesion should be classified according to the Berndt and Harty classification. Radiographs of the opposite ankle are useful to identify the rare bilateral lesions and to provide comparison views. When no radiographic lesion is seen on the initial radiographs but an osteochondral lesion is strongly suspected, further imaging studies are indicated. Anderson and colleagues diagnosed a talar osteochondral lesion in 17 (57%) of 30 patients who had been evaluated because of post-traumatic chronic instability and normal radiographs.[4]

As the next step in the evaluation of a lesion diagnosed on bone scan without radiographic changes or a type II lesion, we prefer MRI. This allows analysis of the status of the cancellous bone and evaluation for the presence of a subchondral cyst. CT is most useful in stages III and IV lesions to determine the exact location of the lesion, its size, and its stability.

TREATMENT

Nonoperative Treatment

Treatment of stage I and II lesions is nonoperative. The patient is placed in a short-leg non–weight-bearing cast for 6 weeks. The patient is then allowed weight bearing as tolerated; however, we restrict patients from strenuous athletic activities for an additional 6 weeks. Even though the concept has not been scientifically tested, the lack of load bearing may allow the talus to revascularize and permit healing of the fragment. Although many reports do not stage and size the lesion, most pediatric series report excellent results when conservative treatment is used. Bauer and colleagues reported the results in five children with an average age of 10 years at the time of treatment; in four patients the lesion healed without operative intervention, and all patients had a good or excellent result at 22-year follow-up.[13] Similarly, a 7.5-year follow-up of nonoperative treatment of stage I or II lesions demonstrated 78% good results versus only 16% good results for stage III or IV lesions.[178] Conservative treatment of stage III lesions on the medial aspect of the talus has also had good results.[35,92] Higuera and colleagues reported good results in 11 of 12 patients in whom conservative treatment was used; 7 of the patients had type III lesions.[92] They recommended initially treating all stages I to III lesions in children conservatively because good results are seen in young patients. If conservative treatment fails to produce a good clinical result or if radiographs show progression to a stage III or IV lesion, operative treatment is indicated. A delay of more than 12 months from the time of initial symptoms to operative treatment results in a worse clinical outcome.[178]

Surgical Treatment

Indications for operative intervention include lateral stage III lesions and all stage IV lesions or failure of nonoperative treatment in lesions of any stage. We prefer an arthroscopic approach to the ankle to minimize soft tissue injury while allowing good observation of the entire dome of the talus. We use anteromedial, anterolateral, and posteromedial portals and a 30-degree arthroscope.* A commercially available noninvasive ankle distracter is used to improve access to the central and posterior portions of the talar dome. The options for treatment of the specific lesion fall into three broad categories: drilling of the intact lesion, drilling and fixing the lesion with internal fixation, or curettage and drilling of the displaced lesion.

A stage II lesion with intact overlying cartilage can be drilled to promote healing and revascularization of the osteochondral fragment. Kumai and colleagues reported good results after drilling for persistently symptomatic lesions with intact cartilage. A trend toward improved results in patients with open physes was demonstrated.[114] To drill the bony bed of the osteochondral fragment, an antegrade technique for anterior lesions or a retrograde fluoroscopically guided technique can be used. In larger patients we prefer to use the tibial guide from the ACL reconstruction setup to allow accurate placement of the drill without penetration of the articular surface (Fig. 43–197). Posteromedial lesions are difficult to approach and may require transmalleolar drilling. A technique using meniscal repair instrumentation allows accurate arthroscopic localization and drilling, thus obviating the need for transmalleolar drilling.[27] Range of motion is allowed and non–weight bearing is continued for 6 weeks postoperatively.

A stage III lesion with minimal fraying of the articular cartilage can be treated in a similar fashion as

*See references 5, 10, 11, 27, 34, 44, 72, 76, 85, 116, 138, 165, 168, 183, 184, 220, 242.

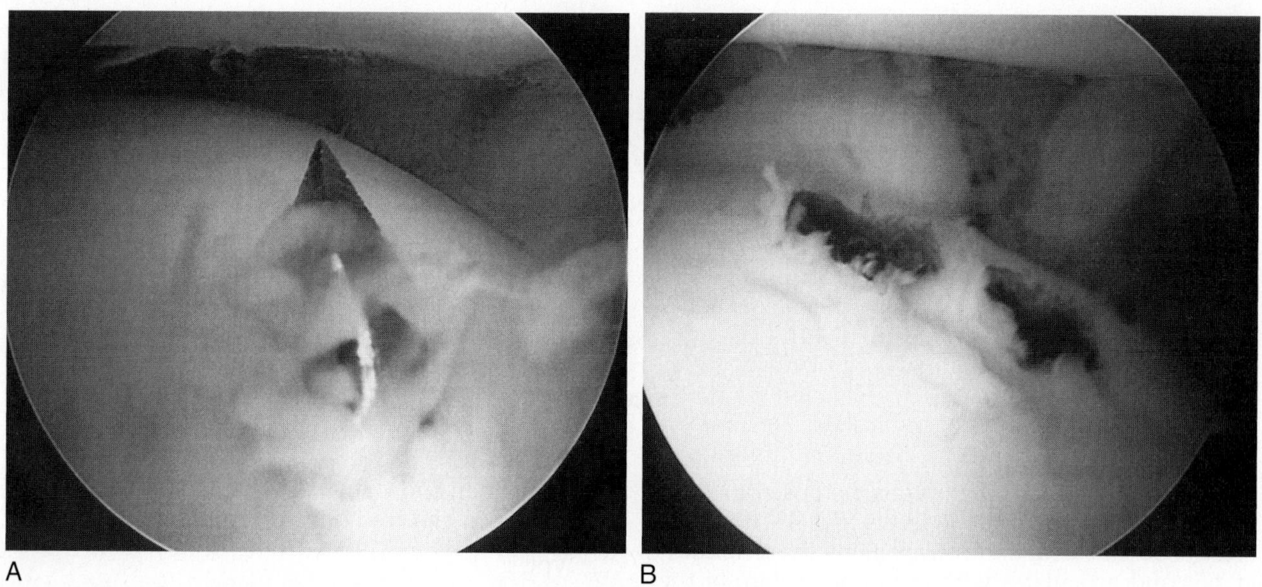

FIGURE 43-197 Arthroscopic treatment of a partially detached osteochondritis dissecans lesion. **A,** Arthroscopic view of the talar dome demonstrating the guidewire that has been used to drill retrogradely through the osteochondral lesion. **B,** Arthroscopic view of the talus from the anterolateral portal showing two bioabsorbable pins that have been placed in a loose osteochondral lesion. The pins were cut off at the joint level.

stage II lesions; however, the fragment should be stabilized with internal fixation. The ideal patient is one who has sustained an acute injury with a resulting small lesion that has good overlying articular cartilage. We prefer smooth or barbed bioabsorbable pins because they do not require removal at a later date and are not associated with tibial cartilage injury if subsequent collapse occurs. At least two pins should be placed in a divergent manner to provide optimal fragment stability. Bracing and non–weight bearing are continued for 6 to 8 weeks postoperatively, followed by gradual weight bearing until the lesion heals.

In large (>1 cm) chronic stage III lesions with frayed articular cartilage, we prefer curettage of the lesion, followed by drilling or abrading the base of the lesion. Debridement is carried out until healthy, bleeding subchondral bone is seen and continued peripherally until good articular cartilage is visible. A microfracture technique is then used. The ankle is immobilized for approximately 2 weeks and then allowed to undergo range-of-motion exercises to promote fibrocartilage formation.

An open arthrotomy can be performed; however, fairly large incisions are generally required, and medial or lateral malleolar osteotomies may be necessary to obtain good visualization and access to the osteochondral fragment.[6,26,139]

The final treatment option is bone grafting of the base of the lesion to replace the necrotic bone in the hope of stimulating more rapid healing. The articular surface is left intact, and no defect is left behind. Metal implants are not used in the talus.[82,126] We prefer bioabsorbable pins or headless compression screws. When bone grafting was compared with excision of the lesion in children with more than 2 years of follow-up, good results were seen in 83% of patients treated by bone grafting verus 50% of patients who had undergone excision.[82] Patients remain non–weight bearing in a short-leg cast for 6 weeks and are then allowed gradual motion and partial weight bearing until healing of the lesion is seen.

Calcaneal Fractures

Fractures of the calcaneus are rare in children. The usual mechanism is a fall from a height, usually a short distance in younger children and more than 10 feet in adolescents. The diagnosis in young children is often difficult to make and is frequently made only when fracture callus is seen on follow-up evaluation. Treatment is usually nonoperative, and outcomes are generally good in a young child. Operative treatment is best used in an adolescent with a displaced intra-articular fracture.

ANATOMY

The calcaneus is the largest tarsal bone in the foot. Its anatomy is designed to provide a lever arm to increase the power of the gastrocsoleus complex and to help transmit body weight to the remaining lower extremity. The posterior tuberosity is palpable as one follows the Achilles tendon inferiorly to its insertion. The inferior surface of the calcaneus extends obliquely and dorsally toward the calcaneocuboid joint. The sinus tarsi is the depression anterior and distal to the lateral malleolus and marks the lateralmost aspect of the subtalar joint. The calcaneus is irregularly shaped, with six surfaces and four articulating facets, three for the talus and one for the cuboid. On the superior surface the posterior, middle, and anterior facets lie at different angles to one another, with the sinus tarsi and the

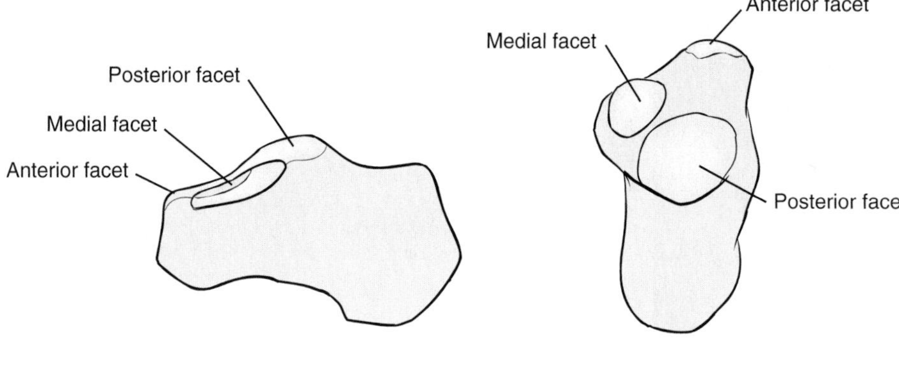

FIGURE 43–198 Articular facets of the calcaneus.

floor of the tarsal canal separating the posterior facet from the anterior and middle facets (Fig. 43–198). The posterior facet is oval and convex along the longitudinal axis and articulates with the undersurface of the talus, whereas the middle facet is concave and oval and articulates with the middle facet on the head of the talus. The sustentaculum tali projects from the medial side of the calcaneus and, together with the talus, forms the lateral boundary of the tarsal tunnel. Its inferior surface is grooved by the tendon of the flexor hallucis longus.

On a lateral radiograph in a more mature patient, Bohler's angle is formed as the angle subtended by a line from the superior point on the posterior articular surface to the superior point of the calcaneal tuberosity and a line drawn from the anterior process to the highest aspect of the posterior articular surface. This angle varies from 25 to 40 degrees and is a relative measurement of the degree of compression and deformity in calcaneal fractures. The "crucial angle" of Gissane is the angle formed by a line drawn from the sulcus calcanei to the tip of the anterior process and varies between 120 and 145 degrees. With a calcaneal fracture, the talus compresses onto the crucial angle and produces the primary fracture line in older patients.

MECHANISM OF INJURY

The mechanism of injury in the majority of calcaneal fractures is an axial load applied to the lower extremity, most often as a result of a fall from a height. The force is transmitted through the talus, which is then driven down into the calcaneus, and a fracture results. In young children the height fallen is usually less than 4 feet; in children older than 10 years the fall is usually greater than 14 feet.[238] In 56 children with calcaneal fractures, 25 (45%) were due to a fall from a height.[204] Motor vehicle accidents, lawnmower injuries, and a direct blow from an object can also result in calcaneal fractures in children.

CLASSIFICATION

The most common classification systems for calcaneal fractures in adults are the Essex-Lopresti and the Letournel classifications.[69,128] Schmidt and Weiner modified the classifications of Essex-Lopresti, Rowe,[194] and Chapman and Galway[42] to better describe the fracture types in children (Fig. 43–199):[204]

Type 1
- A—Fracture of the tuberosity or apophysis
- B—Fracture of the sustentaculum tali
- C—Fracture of the anterior process
- D—Distal inferolateral fracture
- E—Small avulsion of the body

Type 2
- A—Beak fracture
- B—Avulsion fracture of the insertion of the Achilles tendon

Type 3: Linear fracture not involving the subtalar joint

Type 4: Linear fracture involving the subtalar joint

Type 5
- A—Tongue type
- B—Joint depression type

Type 6: Any fracture with significant soft tissue injury, bone loss, and loss of insertion of the Achilles tendon

CLINICAL FEATURES

The patient is usually seen after a fall from a height and has pain in the area of the calcaneus. An older patient who falls from a height of more than 10 to 15 feet will often have significant swelling in the hindfoot area and may also have complaints corresponding to injuries to the spine and lower extremities. The physical examination should include an assessment of the foot for soft tissue swelling, a good neurologic examination, and inspection for open skin lacerations. As with any other orthopaedic injury, the patient should be thoroughly evaluated for the presence of other fractures or injuries, especially of the spine and lower extremities.

RADIOGRAPHIC FINDINGS

The radiographic examination is often difficult to interpret, especially in a young patient with a nondisplaced fracture. This may result in a missed diagnosis, which is reported to occur in 27% to 55% of cases.[97,200,204,238] When a calcaneal fracture is suspected, standard radiographic views should include lateral,

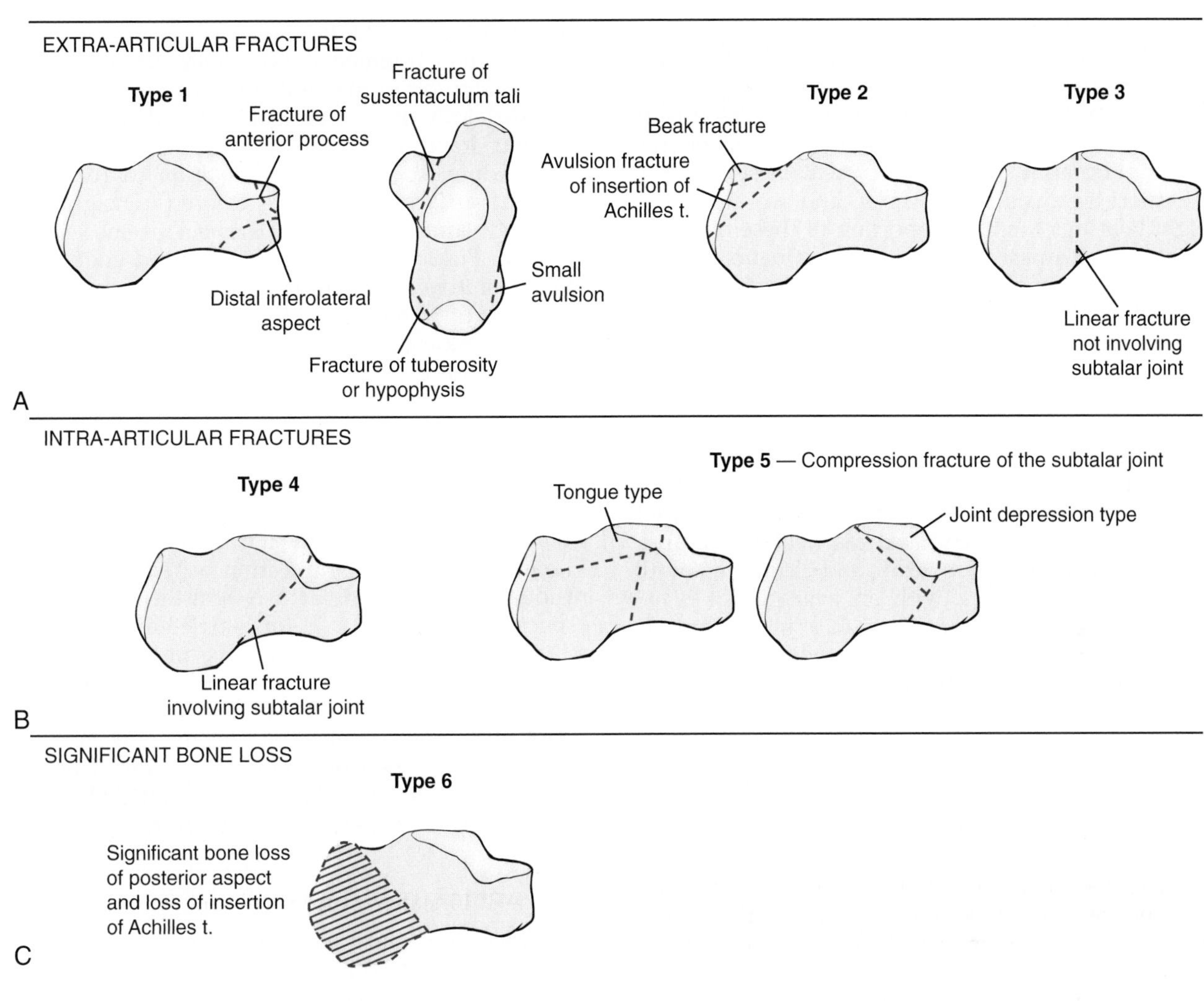

FIGURE 43-199 Classification of calcaneal fractures in children.

axial, straight dorsoplantar, and oblique dorsoplantar views.[188] Broden's views are especially useful when a fracture is suspected but not seen on the lateral or oblique views. Broden's views are obtained with the leg internally rotated 40 degrees and the x-ray beam directed 10, 20, 30, and 40 degrees toward the head and centered on the sinus tarsi.[23] These views show the posterior facet of the calcaneus from posterior to anterior as the beam is angled from 10 to 40 degrees.

For adult-type fracture patterns with intra-articular joint involvement, CT is useful for defining the fracture pattern, determining the number of intra-articular fragments, and planning treatment.[52,64,113,158,167,197] The classification system of Sanders and colleagues analyzes the posterior facet and divides the fractures into four types based on standard views:[198]

Type I Nondisplaced fractures
Type II Two-part or split fractures
Type III Three-part or split depression fractures
Type IV Four-part or highly comminuted articular fractures

This classification has prognostic value with respect to articular reduction and overall outcome. Excellent or good results are achieved in 73% of type II fractures, 70% of type III fractures, and a smaller percent of type IV fracture. CT is most useful in an older patient with an intra-articular fracture. By accurately showing the fracture pattern, it allows the surgeon to select the best treatment protocol.[167]

In a young child, radiographs may appear normal despite the presence of a calcaneal fracture. When there is high suspicion that a fracture is present, the child can be placed in a short-leg cast and radiographs repeated 2 to 3 weeks from the time of injury. An alternative is to obtain a bone scan to help define the presence of a fracture; however, the results with respect to clearly identifying the fracture are mixed,[115,214] and we prefer the former option.

TREATMENT

In general, calcaneal fractures in children are successfully treated nonoperatively by means of a short-leg cast or splint worn for 3 to 6 weeks, followed by weight bearing as tolerated.* This is especially true in children

*See references 28, 42, 46, 56, 97, 115, 145, 200, 201, 204, 222, 238.

younger than 10 years because of better healing potential and a lower incidence of intra-articular fractures in this age group.[25,41,156,201,204]

In a patient younger than 5 years, the fracture is universally undisplaced and often not seen on the initial radiographs. We prefer to treat these children with short-leg casts for 3 weeks, and we allow full weight bearing. A large proportion of these fractures are most likely missed on the initial evaluation and do well without formal treatment. Matteri and Frymoyer reported results in two of three children with missed calcaneal fractures who were younger than 3 years. Treatment of the diagnosed fracture consisted of a posterior splint for 3 weeks, with return to activity following splint removal.[145]

Children 12 years or younger have good results, even though a small proportion have displaced intra-articular fractures.[42,56,97,200,201,204,238] Schmidt and Weiner described 37 patients with extra-articular fractures, with an average age of 10 years, and 22 patients with intra-articular fractures, with an average age of 13 years.[204] In addition, the mechanism of injury imparts less energy to the calcaneus in young children because of their smaller size and because the height of the fall is generally less then 4 feet versus more than 14 feet in children older than 10 years.[238] We prefer to treat these children in short-leg non–weight-bearing casts for 4 to 6 weeks, depending on the age of the child, followed by weight bearing as tolerated.

Compared with younger children, children older than 12 years have a higher proportion of intra-articular fractures (63% versus 27%), sustain greater trauma to the extremity, and have a higher incidence of associated injuries (50% versus 20%).[204] Because the associated injuries include lumbar vertebral fractures, other lower extremity fractures, pelvic fractures, and upper extremity fractures, the treating physician should anticipate associated injuries in an older child with a calcaneal fracture, especially one involved in a motor vehicle accident, after which the incidence of associated injuries is highest.[200] Treatment of extra-articular fractures is similar to that in younger children but may include a longer period of immobilization, up to 12 weeks. Intra-articular fractures in this age group are relatively common, and the results of closed treatment of these fractures are generally good with regard to function.[56,200,201] However, most studies have short[42] or inadequate follow-up,[204] some patients do experience pain on short-term follow-up, and radiographs do demonstrate residual deformity and some evidence of early degenerative changes in the subtalar joint.[201] Brunet reported radiographic arthrosis and mild hindfoot symptoms in 2 of 19 fractures with otherwise excellent results at an average of 16 years after closed treatment.[25] Schantz and Rasmussen reported the results of a 12-year follow-up in 15 children with intra-articular calcaneal fractures that had been treated in closed fashion. Four had pain. Radiographs demonstrated an increased width of the calcaneus in nine patients, a step-off at the articular surface of the posterior facet in four, and early degenerative arthrosis in two.[201] We prefer to perform CT in an older patient with an intra-articular fracture to assess the number of intra-articular fragments and the amount of displacement or step-off of the joint surface.

A skeletally mature patient with a displaced intra-articular fracture should be treated as an adult, by open reduction and internal fixation to restore the articular surface of the joint, restore the height of the heel, and reduce the width of the heel to a more normal position. Pickle and colleagues reported good results after operative treatment in this patient subset with a follow-up of 30 months.[179] Consultation with an adult foot and ankle surgeon is advised because of the low incidence of these fractures in a typical pediatric orthopaedic practice and the complexity of the surgical procedure.[65,66,69,101,128,132,197]

COMPLICATIONS

Complications from calcaneal fractures are infrequent. The most common complication in these fractures is residual pain and early arthrosis in the subtalar joint, especially with displaced intra-articular fractures. In adult calcaneal fractures, there is an associated 10% incidence of compartment syndrome of the foot, which is treated by nine-compartment releases.[160,161] To our knowledge, compartment syndrome has not been reported in the pediatric population, but it must be evaluated for in all children, especially adolescents with displaced intra-articular fractures.

Tarsometatarsal (Lisfranc's) Fractures

This very rare injury in adults was reported in children only as individual cases[19,187] until Wiley reported a series of 18 cases in pediatric patients.[237] The diagnosis is often challenging to make because the anatomy is difficult to discern on plain radiographs and because fractures in children are usually undisplaced. Most children with these injuries can be treated with casting alone; however, closed reduction of displaced fractures, with or without internal fixation, and open reduction and internal fixation are required for displaced fractures. The results are relatively good, although some patients continue to have persistent pain in the area of a Lisfranc joint, especially if anatomic reduction is not achieved or is lost. Salvage operations for persistent discomfort include tarsometatarsal arthrodesis.

ANATOMY

The tarsometatarsal joints form articulations between the distal row of tarsals and the bases of the metatarsals: the medial three metatarsal bases articulate with their respective cuneiforms and the lateral two with the cuboid. Weak dorsal and stronger plantar tarsometatarsal ligaments connect the adjacent borders of the cuneiforms and the second and third metatarsals, the rigid keystones of the tarsometatarsal joint. The intermetatarsal ligaments provide greater strength than the dorsal and plantar ligaments do. Lisfranc's ligament travels from the second metatarsal to the first cuneiform without connections to the first cuneiform. At the base of the first and second metatarsals lies the plantar branch of the anterior tibial artery and the deep peroneal nerve.

MECHANISM OF INJURY

Three basic mechanisms have been described.[236,237] The first involves an indirect injury in which the foot sustains an impact load while in the tiptoe position (Fig. 43–200A). Most commonly this is caused by a fall from a height in which the patient lands on the foot with the toes flexed, which results in acute plantar flexion at the tarsometatarsal level. A sudden abduction moment of the foot often occurs and leads to lateral displacement of the metatarsals and fracturing at the base of the second metatarsal.

The second mechanism is a direct compression injury in which the patient is in a kneeling position and an object strikes the back of the heel and produces heel-to-toe compression (Fig. 43–200B). This injury pattern may result in lateral displacement of the second through fourth metatarsals.

The third mechanism results from the foot's being in a fixed position and sustaining a fall backward (Fig. 43–200C). The heel of the foot is the fulcrum around which the injury occurs; the injury can result in multiple fractures of the foot.[237]

In children the most common mechanism of injury was a fall from a height (56%), followed by a fall backward (22%) and heel-to-toe compression (18%).[237] In adults a large proportion of these injuries are related to motor vehicle accidents, crush injuries, and falls from heights.* Two of the pediatric patients described by Wiley had severe crushing injuries of the foot with associated tarsometatarsal fractures.[237]

CLASSIFICATION

The three-part classification of Hardcastle and colleagues,[87] a modification of the original description by Quenu and Kuss,[185] best defines these fractures, their mechanism, and their treatment (Fig. 43–201).

*See references 8, 32, 53, 162, 172, 191, 199, 221, 227, 229, 236, 239, 240.

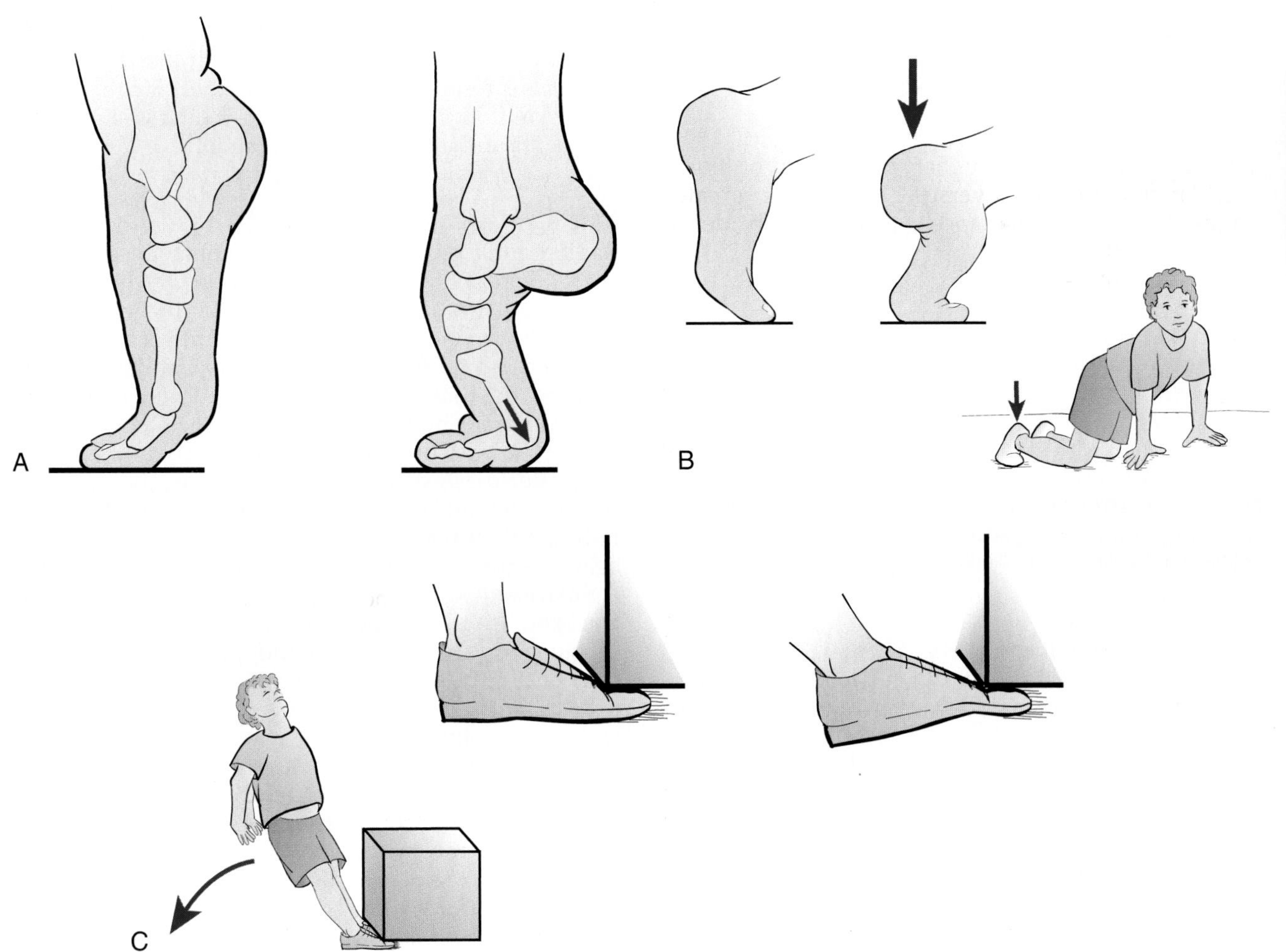

FIGURE 43–200 Mechanism of injury producing Lisfranc's fractures. **A,** Indirect injury. An impact load is applied with the foot in a tiptoe position. **B,** Direct injury pattern. While the patient is kneeling, a direct load is applied to the posterior aspect of the heel. **C,** A Lisfranc injury occurs when the patient falls backward from a fixed forefoot.

Type A
Total incongruity

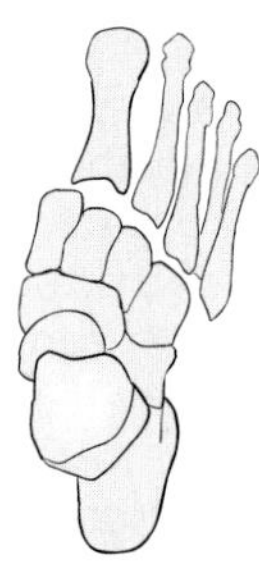

Type B
Partial incongruity

Medial
dislocation

Lateral
dislocation

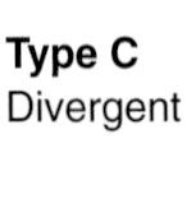

Type C
Divergent

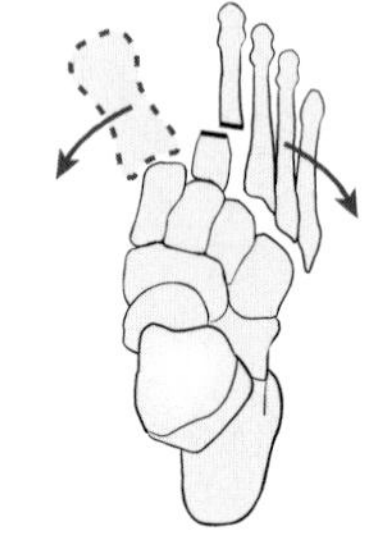

FIGURE 43–201 Classification of Lisfranc's injuries. Type A—total incongruity. Type B—partial incongruity, medial dislocation or lateral dislocation. Type C—divergent pattern.

Type A—total incongruity. There is incongruity of the entire tarsometatarsal joint in a single plane, with lateral displacement (see Fig. 43–201A).

Type B—partial incongruity. Only partial incongruity of the joint is seen, and either the medial or the lateral aspect of the foot is affected. Medial dislocation involves displacement of the first metatarsal from the first cuneiform because of disruption of Lisfranc's ligament or fracture at the base of the metatarsal, which remains attached to the ligament (see Fig. 43–201B).

Type C—divergent pattern. There may be partial or total incongruity, with the first metatarsal being displaced medially while any combination of the lateral four metatarsals may be displaced laterally (see Fig. 43–201C).

In children, the type A and C patterns are extremely rare, and the type B injury pattern usually demonstrates minimal displacement.[237] Similarly, in adults the incidence of types A, B, and C is 17%, 72%, and 10%, respectively.[172]

CLINICAL FEATURES

Diagnosis of these injuries is notoriously difficult, with as many as 20% of injuries misdiagnosed or overlooked.[31,191] The prognosis of an untreated Lisfranc fracture is generally poor. A child or adolescent will have pain in the foot and dorsal swelling, which may be localized over the dorsum of the tarsometatarsal joint. With significant trauma the entire dorsum of the foot may be swollen, and localization of the pain may be difficult. However, a mild injury with more focal swelling may allow palpation of the foot to better identify pain over the tarsometatarsal joint. Deformity of the foot is rare because the majority of injuries in children either are not displaced at the time of injury or reduce spontaneously after injury. Pain on attempted weight bearing or persistent inability to bear weight despite a normal physical examination and radiographs should raise the physician's suspicion that a tarsometatarsal injury is present. Ecchymosis on the plantar aspect of the midfoot implies trauma to the tarsometatarsal ligaments and an injury to that joint.[192]

RADIOGRAPHIC FINDINGS

Radiographs of the extremity should include AP, lateral, and oblique views of the foot. On the oblique radiograph the lateral border of the first metatarsal should be in line with the medial cuneiform, and the medial aspect of the second metatarsal should line up with the medial aspect of the middle cuneiform. A subtle Lisfranc injury is detected by visualizing a fracture at the base of the second metatarsal and a 2-mm or greater diastasis between the base of the first and second metatarsals, which can be compared with a radiograph of the opposite foot (Fig. 43–202). Weight-bearing stress views to accentuate the diastasis with comparison views of the opposite foot are helpful.[70] CT has been useful in diagnosing and defining the extent of injury in patients whose radiographs are suggestive but not confirmatory of a tarsometatarsal injury.[78,127,137] MRI can delineate ligamentous injuries of the tarsometatarsal joint in patients whose radiographs are normal. In patients with radiographs demonstrating between 0 and 2 mm of diastasis, Potter and colleagues reported 3 complete tears and 18 partial ligament tears.[181] They recommend MRI for any patient whose history or physical examination findings are suspicious for Lisfranc's injury despite normal radiographs, with operative treatment indicated in any patient with a complete or nearly complete ligamentous tear. Bone scintigraphy has been reported to be useful in diagnosis; however, it is not specific and does not accurately suggest the severity of injury.[84]

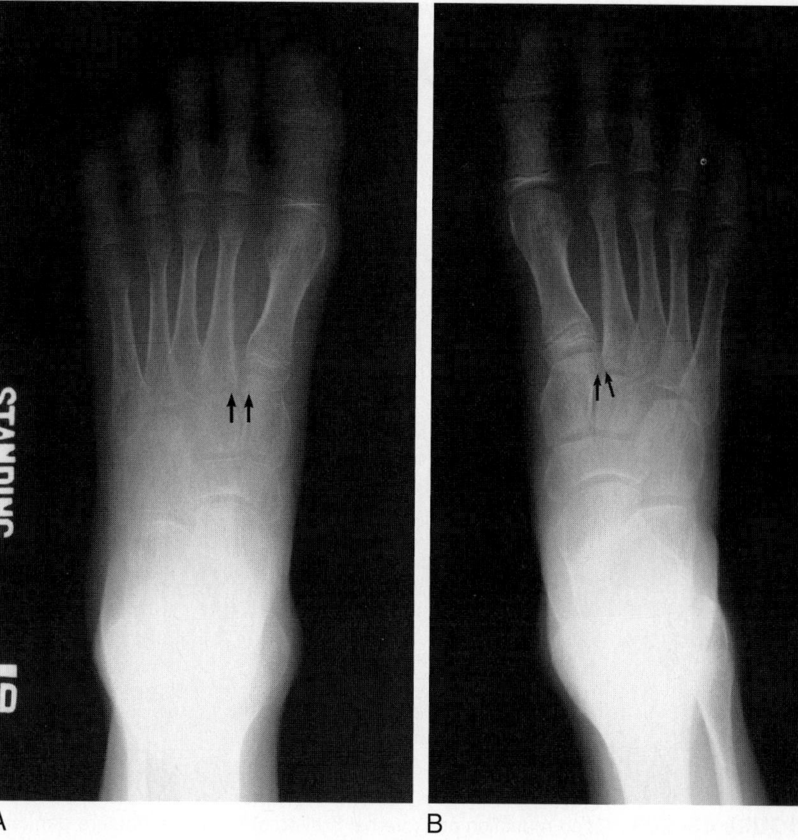

FIGURE 43-202 Lisfranc's injuries in a 10-year-girl that were sustained while performing gymnastics. **A,** Standing anteroposterior radiograph of the left foot. **B,** Comparison views of the right foot are used to identify the increased joint space in Lisfranc's joint on the left (*arrows*).

TREATMENT

The amount of displacement and the adequacy and stability of fracture reduction determine the type of treatment.

Nonoperative Treatment

The majority of tarsometatarsal fractures in children are undisplaced or displaced less than 2 mm at the time of initial evaluation and can be treated nonoperatively. When swelling is present, a bulky dressing for 2 to 3 days has been advocated to allow the soft tissue swelling to resolve.[237] This is followed by immobilization in a short-leg cast for 5 to 6 weeks. Although some recommend weight bearing in the cast, we prefer to have the patient remain non–weight bearing so that the possibility of fracture displacement is minimized.

Closed Reduction

For fractures that are displaced 2 mm or more on the initial radiographs or CT scan, we prefer to perform closed reduction under general anesthesia to obtain an anatomic reduction. Stable anatomic reduction must be achieved before the application of external immobilization. The closed reduction is performed with manual manipulation, including axial traction along the affected toes, followed by manual pressure on the dorsum of the foot when dorsal displacement is present. Adequate radiographic assessment is needed to ensure that the fracture is reduced to an anatomic position. Residual displacement of more than 1 mm is an indication for open reduction and internal fixation. The three main reasons for failure of closed reduction are interposition of the anterior tibialis tendon, incongruity of the medial cuneiform–first metatarsal articulation, and interposition of the fracture fragment in the second metatarsal–middle cuneiform joint.[18] If the fracture is reduced anatomically but is unstable, percutaneous wire fixation is required to maintain anatomic alignment of the foot. We prefer to use smooth 0.0062-inch Kirschner wires, with the most important pin traveling between the medial cuneiform and the second metatarsal and additional pins placed according to the type of fracture present. For the type A total incongruity pattern, Hardcastle and associates recommend medial and lateral pins for fixation. In the most common pattern, type B, with partial incongruity and medial dislocation, a second pin is placed between the first metatarsal and the medial cuneiform or between the first two metatarsals to stabilize the medial displacement of the first metatarsal (Fig. 43–203). For the lateral dislocation–partial incongruity pattern, lateral pins are needed. For the type C or divergent pattern, a pin construct similar to that for the medial displacement pattern can be used; however, an additional pin or pins may need to be placed from the third, fourth, or fifth metatarsals into the second or third cuneiform or the cuboid, respectively.

Open Reduction and Internal Fixation

Indications for open reduction and internal fixation are an inability to achieve anatomic closed reduction

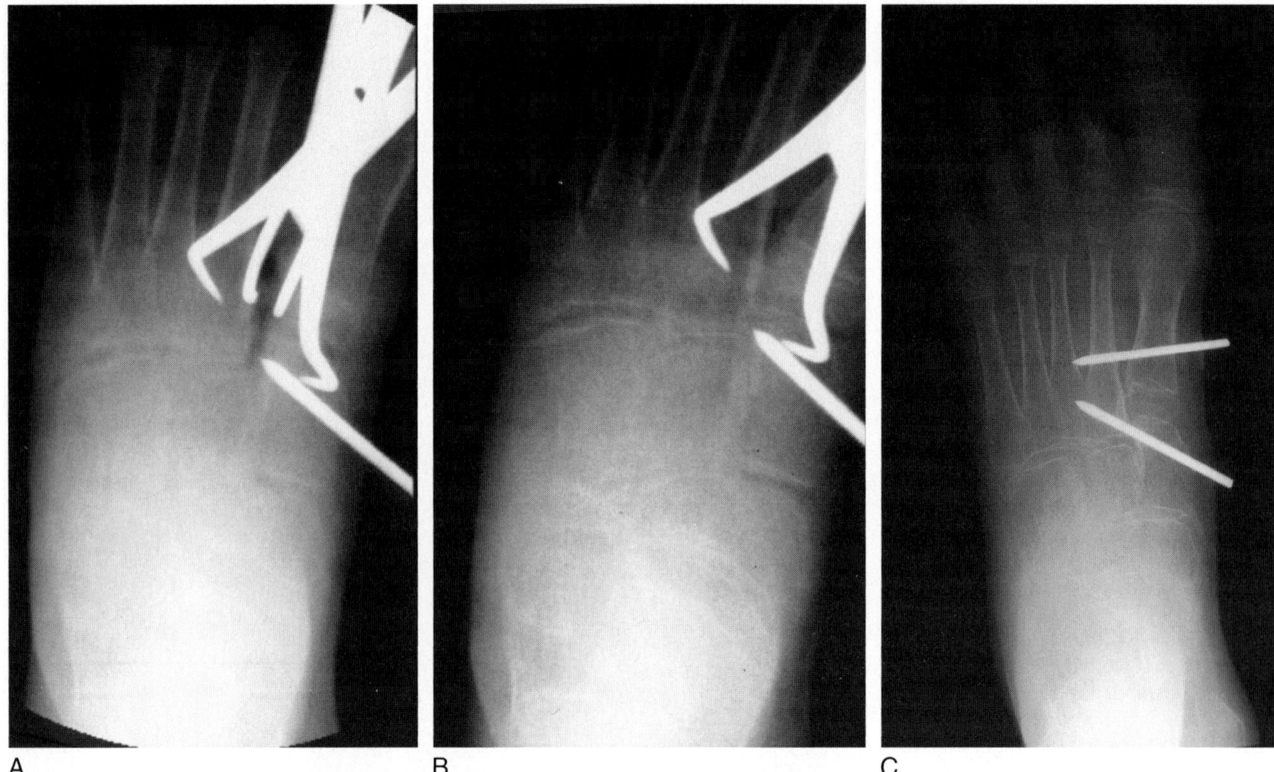

FIGURE 43–203 Open reduction and internal fixation of Lisfranc's fracture demonstrated on intraoperative radiographs. **A,** The Lisfranc joint is distracted to allow debridement of the joint in this chronic injury. **B,** Bone reduction forceps is then used to reduce the joint. **C,** The Lisfranc joint is stabilized between the first cuneiform and the second metatarsal with a threaded pin. Additional fixation is placed between the first and second metatarsals.

and chronic symptomatic injury with residual diastasis. A skeletally mature patient may best be treated similar to adults, with open reduction and internal fixation in all tarsometatarsal injuries to achieve optimal results.* One or two longitudinal incisions are made over the first–second metatarsal interspace and over the third–fourth metatarsal interspace. The injury is reduced to anatomic position under direct visualization, and percutaneous pin fixation is placed as described earlier. We prefer to leave the pins outside the skin and pull them at 6 weeks from the time of injury. In a chronic symptomatic case, treatment should consist of removal of debris from the joint, roughening of any remaining articular cartilage, and then pin fixation of the joint or joints. Open injuries are usually due to a crush injury to the foot and should be treated by thorough irrigation and debridement of the foot. Treatment of the tarsometatarsal injury should follow the aforementioned guidelines.

COMPLICATIONS

The largest series of tarsometatarsal fractures in children reported 14 of 18 patients to have excellent results without residual symptoms at short follow-up (3 and 8 months).[237] No patient required open reduction; however, four patients had discomfort at 1-year follow-up, with two having residual malreduction—one because of inability to achieve closed reduction and one whose injury was not recognized. One complication was reported: asymptomatic AVN of the second metatarsal head developed in a 16-year-old patient. Buoncristiani and colleagues reported on eight children with plantar flexion–type injuries without fractures requiring open reduction. In this series, midfoot pain and radiographic degenerative changes developed in one patient.[30] The most common complication in adults is residual pain, which may be associated with progressive flatfoot deformity or lateral impingement and is best treated by tarsometatarsal joint arthrodesis.[199,226]

*See references 7-9, 32, 53, 162, 172, 189, 191, 221, 227, 229.

Metatarsal Fractures

Fractures of the metatarsals are the most common fractures of the foot in children and account for approximately 15% of all foot injuries (Fig. 43–204).[166]

MECHANISM OF INJURY

These fractures can be due to direct trauma from an object falling onto the foot or a crush injury from a bicycle or motor vehicle running over the foot. They can also be due to indirect trauma in which the child lands on the foot with axial and torsional loads applied

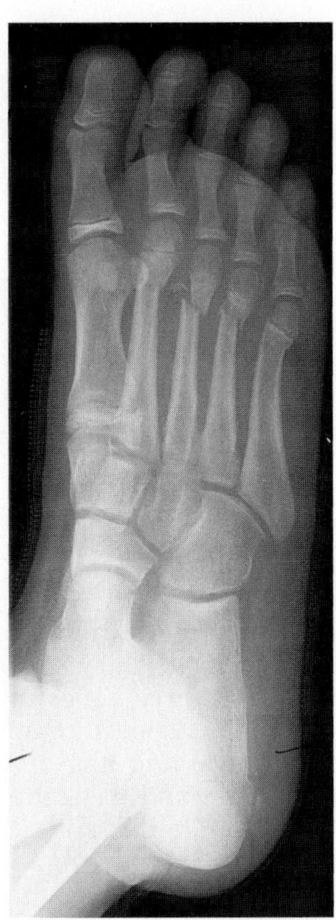

FIGURE 43–204 Radiograph of a right foot demonstrating fractures of the second, third, and fourth metatarsals.

to the midfoot. The most common fracture is fracture of the fifth metatarsal, which accounts for 45% of all metatarsal fractures in children. In a young child (<5 years) the most common fracture is fracture of the first metatarsal, whereas in children older than 10 years the most commonly fractured metatarsal is the fifth.[166] In young children the base of the first metatarsal is often fractured, manifested as a small buckle fracture. A small percentage of these fractures are missed at initial evaluation; however, fractures of the first metatarsal are especially prone to be overlooked (20% of cases).[166]

CLINICAL FEATURES

The patient usually has pain in the foot after a twisting injury or after a direct blow to the foot. The mechanism of injury is important to define because crush injuries need careful assessment of the soft tissues and evaluation for the uncommon but significant compartment syndrome. Silas and colleagues reported seven compartment syndromes of the feet in 7 children, three of whom had metatarsal fractures after a crush injury.[208] In a multiply injured child the foot fractures may seem trivial when long bone or pelvic fractures are present. However, because of the significant energy force required to produce these injuries, metatarsal fractures may be associated with severe soft tissue trauma and impending compartment syndrome, especially when hypotension is present.

RADIOGRAPHIC FINDINGS

Radiographic examination should include AP, lateral, and oblique views of the foot, with full visualization of the metatarsals and phalanges. Because the initial radiographs in a young child may not show a fracture, radiographs may have to be repeated in 2 weeks to make the diagnosis. Metatarsal neck fractures are more often due to a torsional force applied to the foot, whereas direct compression results in shaft fractures.

TREATMENT

Nonoperative Treatment

Most metatarsal fractures can be treated nonoperatively because the majority are undisplaced at initial evaluation. Soft tissue swelling of the foot is a contraindication to applying a circumferential cast at the time of initial evaluation. We prefer a short-leg posterior splint or a modification of the U-type splint with a foot plate (Fig. 43–205). The patient should keep the foot elevated for 24 to 48 hours, and the splint can then be overwrapped with fiberglass cast material in 1 week to enhance its durability. Weight bearing is allowed in the cast, which is worn for 3 to 6 weeks, depending on the age of the child and the amount of fracture displacement.

Closed Reduction

The indications for closed reduction are not fully defined. We prefer to reduce fractures that are completely displaced, especially in an older child, and fractures angled greater than 20 degrees, particularly

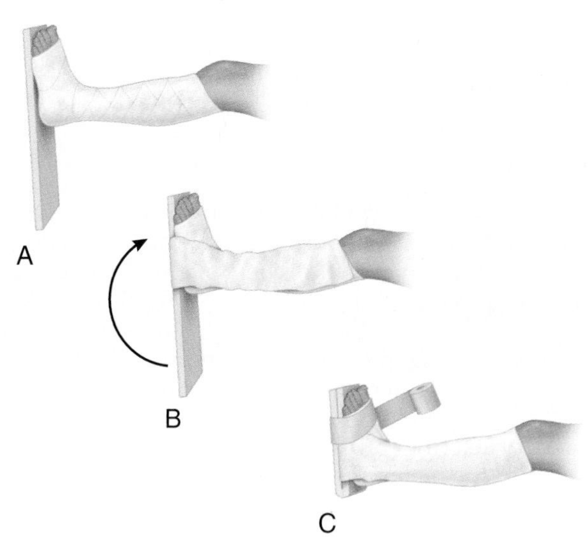

FIGURE 43–205 Construction of a short-leg splint. **A,** The leg is first wrapped with cast padding. A foot plate twice the length of the foot is then placed with the use of plaster splint material. **B,** While the foot plate is held in place, a U-slab is placed to reinforce the forefoot. **C,** The foot slab is then folded back onto itself to ensure that there is no pressure on the heel. This is then overwrapped with cast padding and a plastic bandage.

when apex-dorsal. The child should be sedated in the emergency department, and if closed reduction is difficult, finger traps can be placed on the affected toes to restore length and reduce the fracture. The foot should be placed in a short-leg plaster cast that is well molded over the dorsal and plantar aspects of the foot; however, the ankle can be left in slight plantar flexion and should be well molded to promote resolution of the foot swelling. An unreliable patient can be admitted to maintain elevation of the foot and for periodic ice pack application to the foot. If a compartment syndrome of the foot is suspected at the time of initial evaluation or subsequent to treatment, compartment pressures should be measured and a nine-compartment foot release should be performed as described by Myerson and Manoli.[160]

Open Reduction and Internal Fixation

Open reduction with internal fixation is indicated for open fractures, irreducible fractures, and fractures that cannot be maintained reduced by external immobilization in a cast. However, it is rarely necessary to perform open reduction of these fractures in children. The dorsal skin incision should be made directly over the fracture with exposure of the fracture. A Kirschner wire is then drilled antegrade through the distal fragment, followed by fracture reduction and retrograde pinning. The pin is bent, cut, and left on the plantar aspect of the skin, and the foot is immobilized in a short-leg non–weight-bearing cast for 4 to 6 weeks. The pin (or pins) can be removed at 4 to 6 weeks, depending on the age of the child, and a walking cast or a fracture boot worn for an additional 2 weeks.

Fractures of the Base of the Fifth Metatarsal

ANATOMY

The proximal fifth metatarsal can be anatomically divided into three regions: the proximal cancellous tuberosity, the more distal tuberosity, and the proximal metaphyseal-diaphyseal junction. The blood supply to the base of the fifth metatarsal is important in understanding the risk for nonunion.[38,205,210] The nutrient artery enters medially into the cortex and branches proximally and distally, with a watershed area between the proximal branch of the nutrient artery and the metaphyseal vessels (Fig. 43–206). Fractures in this watershed area are at risk for delayed union or nonunion. The proximal apophyseal growth center is usually visible radiographically at age 9 and becomes united to the diaphysis between 12 and 15 years of age. This apophyseal growth center, or the os vesalianum, can be mistaken for a fracture in children but can be differentiated by the sagittal orientation of the apophysis and the metatarsal. In contrast, the true fracture line is oriented transversely, at a right angle to the shaft of the metatarsal.

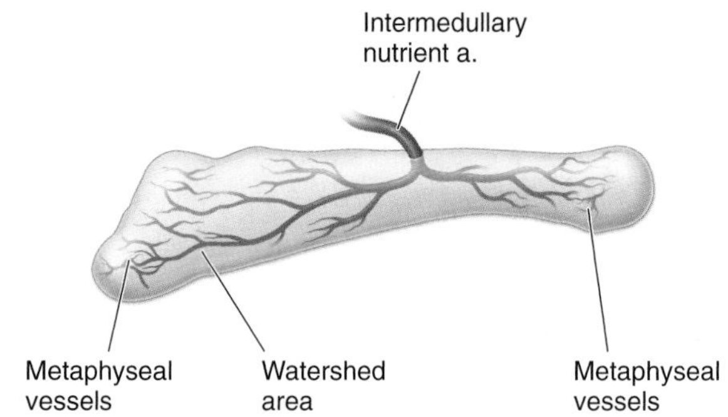

FIGURE 43-206 Blood supply of the proximal fifth metatarsal.

CLASSIFICATION

Fractures of the base of the fifth metatarsal are optimally classified according to their location, best defined by the anatomy of the three zones of the proximal metatarsal (Fig. 43–207). Zone I comprises the cancellous tuberosity, including the insertion of the peroneus brevis tendon and the calcaneometatarsal ligament of the plantar fascia; zone II is the distal aspect of the tuberosity, with dorsal and plantar ligamentous attachments to the fourth metatarsal; and zone III begins distal to the ligamentous attachments and extends to the mid-diaphyseal area. It is most important to recognize a zone 2 injury, the Jones fracture, which is prone to nonunion because of the poor blood supply.[103,124,170]

TREATMENT

Treatment of these fractures depends principally on the location of the fracture and the activity level of the patient.

Zone I Fractures

Zone I injuries are traction-type fractures in which the peroneus brevis tendon and the lateral aspect of the plantar aponeurosis are under tension, and these injuries result in avulsion of the proximal aspect of the metatarsal. Minimal treatment is needed in these patients because the outcome is universally good with healing of the fracture and full return to activities.[54] We prefer to treat these fractures in a short-leg cast or fracture boot and allow weight bearing as tolerated for

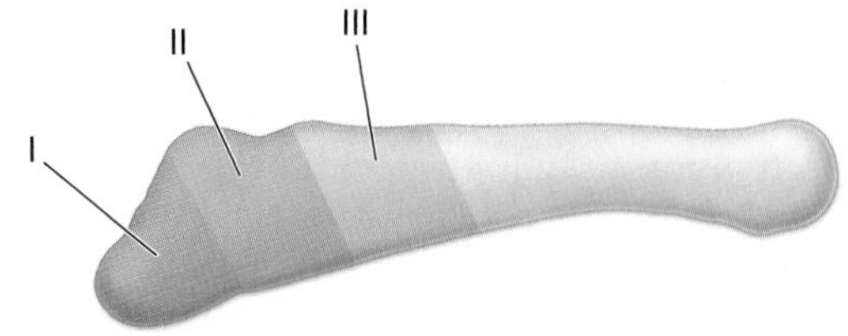

FIGURE 43-207 The three anatomic zones of the proximal fifth metatarsal.

3 to 6 weeks. Other authors have recommended a hard-soled shoe, an elastic wrap, or a functional brace, all of which have produced good results. Radiographic union generally lags behind the time to resolution of the patient's symptoms and is not a prerequisite for removal of the cast or return to activities at 3 to 4 weeks. There are reports of nonunion of these fractures, which are most often displaced more than 3 mm at the time of injury, and we prefer to immobilize these injuries in a cast for 6 weeks.[190]

Zone II Fractures

A Jones fracture is located in zone II, the proximal metaphyseal-diaphyseal junction, with the fracture line extending obliquely and proximally from the lateral cortex through the medial cortex, where articulation with the fourth metatarsal occurs. The mechanism of injury is thought to be a combination of vertical loading and coronal plane shear forces that occur at the junction of the stable proximal metaphysis, provided by ligamentous attachment to the base of the fourth metatarsal and the mobile fifth metatarsal diaphysis. It is most likely that these fractures are stress injuries that occurred before the acute event that brought the patient to the hospital.[33,49,105,124,196] These patients are generally adolescents, are most often involved in athletics, and are initially seen after a traumatic event despite having previous symptoms.

A good history is important to determine the duration of symptoms because patients with more chronic symptoms (3 to 4 months) may be more prone to nonunion. Josefsson and colleagues reported the results of a large series of patients with Jones fractures; late surgery was required in 12% of patients with acute fractures and in 50% of patients with chronic fractures when nonoperative treatment was initially used.[104]

For an acute fracture, we prefer immobilization in a short-leg cast and do not allow weight bearing for the initial 6 weeks. Serial radiographs are evaluated for evidence of fracture healing. Tenderness at the fracture site or lack of fracture callus formation at 6 weeks requires further immobilization in a short-leg non–weight-bearing cast. With evidence of fracture callus and lack of tenderness, the patient can begin protected weight bearing in a hard-soled shoe for an additional 4 weeks. Return to full activities is allowed after solid fracture union is seen radiographically (Fig. 43–208). In adults, Torg and associates reported fracture healing at 7 weeks in 14 of 15 patients treated with a short-leg non–weight-bearing cast, whereas only 4 of 10 patients who were allowed to bear weight eventually achieved union.[224]

In a chronic injury, when symptoms have been present for more than 3 months, the likelihood of fracture healing with conservative treatment is significantly decreased. In an untreated patient, at the time of initial evaluation we prefer a trial of non–weight bearing in a cast for 6 weeks in an attempt to obtain fracture healing. However, if this treatment does not result in fracture healing, we prefer intramedullary fixation with a compression screw and bone grafting (Fig. 43–209). We use the distal tibia as the site to harvest a bone graft because only a small quantity of bone is needed, the harvest site is close to the operative site, harvest at this site requires a small incision, and harvest of the distal tibia does not risk injury to the physis in a growing child. Postoperatively, the patient is allowed to bear weight, initially in a short-leg cast for 3 to 4 weeks. Use of a 4.0-mm

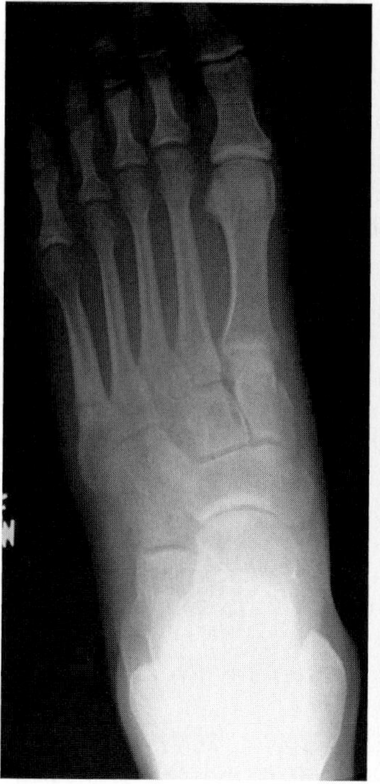
A

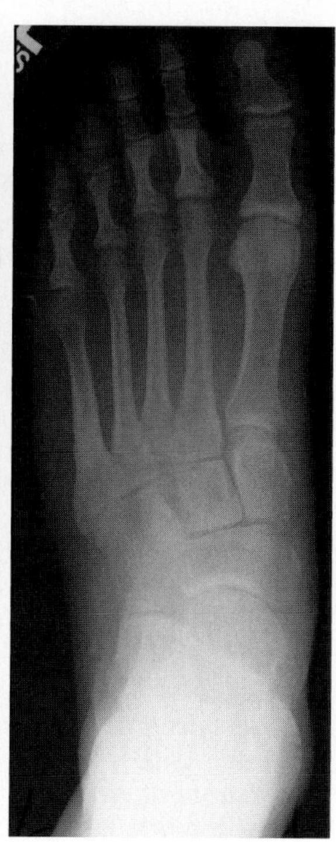
B

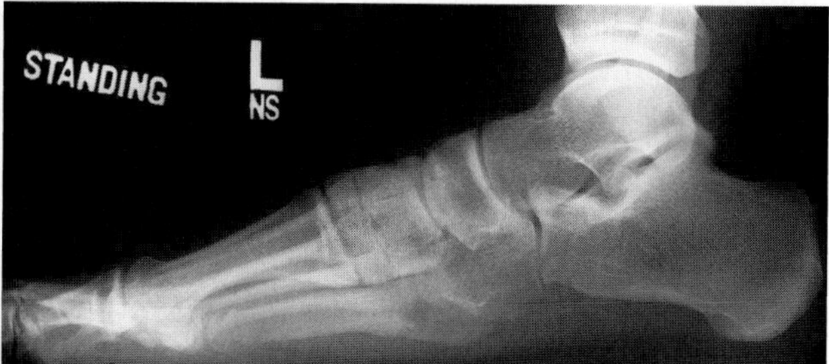

C

FIGURE 43-208 An acute zone II injury of the fifth metatarsal, the so-called Jones fracture, in a 15-year-old boy who had pain after a twisting injury while playing basketball. **A,** Injury radiograph. **B** and **C,** After 6 weeks of cast immobilization, radiographs demonstrate healing.

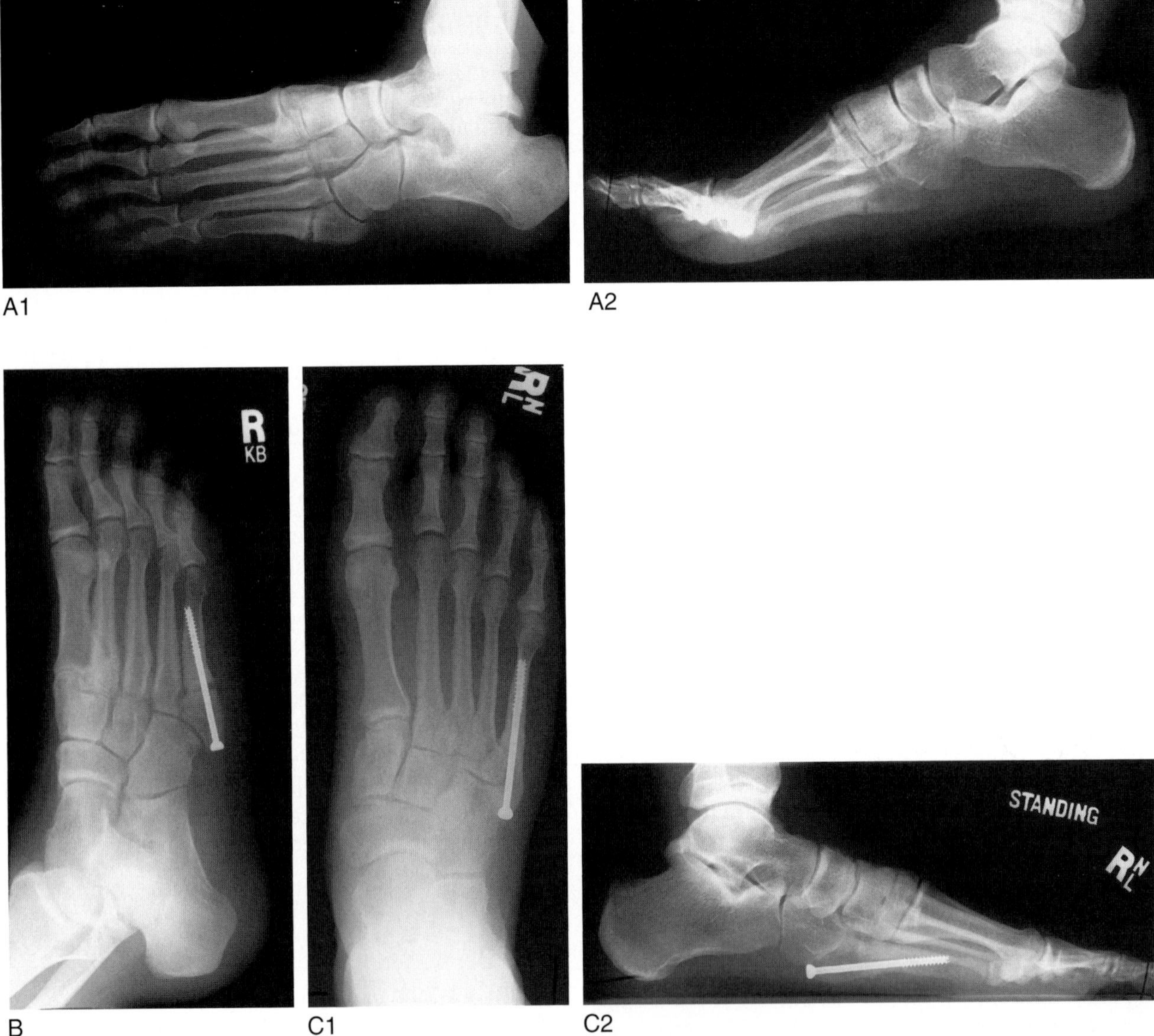

FIGURE 43-209 A chronic Jones fracture in a 16-year-old boy with a 2-year history of right foot pain. **A,** Initial radiographs. Note the chronic appearance of this Jones fracture. **B,** Postoperative radiograph after intramedullary fixation with a single screw and bone grafting of the fracture. **C,** Radiographic appearance at 3 months. The fracture has healed.

malleolar screw has been described, but a larger 6.5-mm screw may be used when the size of the metatarsal permits. The results of intramedullary screw fixation and bone grafting have been good, with few complications.[104,124,180,190,196,224]

Zone III Fractures

A zone III fracture is most often a stress fracture and usually occurs in an active athlete. Similar to a Jones fracture, an acute zone III fracture can be treated in a short-leg non–weight-bearing cast for 6 weeks, followed by protection during weight bearing for 3 to 4 weeks. An active athlete with a chronic injury or nonunion should be treated by intramedullary screw fixation with or without bone grafting.

Phalangeal Fractures

Phalangeal fractures, rare in children, are the result of direct trauma and generally require minimal treatment. The proximal phalanx is more often injured than the more distal phalanges, and injuries to the hallux are more common than injuries to the lesser toes. The mechanism is usually "stubbing" the toe or direct trauma from a falling object. These fractures may be associated with significant soft tissue injury, especially when they result from direct trauma. Open injuries are rare and most often involve the nail plate and nail bed.

Treatment of most phalangeal fractures is symptomatic, with weight bearing as tolerated in a stiff-soled shoe. In a severely displaced fracture, manual reduction may be required, followed by taping to the adjacent toe ("buddy" taping). In an older child with a displaced fracture, percutaneous pin stabilization of the fracture may be required after reduction. The pin can be removed at 6 weeks, at which time the fracture should be healed and full weight bearing is allowed. Associated nail bed injuries should be repaired and open injuries should be irrigated, debrided, and treated with intravenous antibiotics for 24 hours, followed by oral antibiotics for 5 to 7 days.

Lawnmower Injuries

Approximately 25,000 injuries occur each year from power lawnmower accidents in the United States.[2] Children are involved in approximately 20% of these injuries and account for 12% of all deaths related to lawnmowers.[55] The average age of children is between 4 and 8 years, and boys are involved more often than girls.[15,63,102,131,136,144,232] Some studies report a higher proportion of injuries in children who are passengers or operators of the lawnmower,[193,232] whereas others report a greater likelihood of injury in children bystanders.[63,136] Riding-lawnmowers are more often involved than push-mowers and generally result in more severe injury patterns.[232] Loder and colleagues reviewed amputations sustained secondary to lawnmower accidents over a 20-year period. Riding-lawnmowers engaged in reverse accounted for 39% of these amputations, and riding-mowers caused 80% of amputations overall.[134] The lower extremities are most often injured, and the majority of injuries result from direct contact with the power blades under the housing of the lawnmower. The wounds sustained from contact with the blades are of two main types, depending on the position of the child at the time of injury: the foot or toes are involved when the child is supine at the time of injury, and the plantar aspect of the foot or heel is injured when the child is prone at the time of injury.

An injured child should be assessed thoroughly and promptly to allow urgent transfer to the operating room for initial irrigation and debridement. Antibiotics should be administered in the emergency department and should achieve broad coverage with triple antibiotics consisting of a cephalosporin, an aminoglycoside, and penicillin. We prefer multiple debridements at 48-hour intervals until viable tissue is present at all wound edges, which usually requires at least three trips to the operating room.[63] VAC devices have emerged as useful tools for soft tissue management between operative procedures. VAC management may decrease the need for free tissue transfer, and Shilt and colleagues reported a trend toward a decrease in revision amputations with VAC management.[206] Significant foreign material can be forced under pressure into the soft tissue envelope, and therefore it is always preferable to repeat the irrigation and debridement procedure if there is any question about tissue viability and sterility before soft tissue closure or coverage. Bony injuries should be stabilized with standard techniques at the initial debridement. Up to 80% of these injuries require some form of ablative procedure, and attempts should be made to preserve as much length as possible and avoid transdiaphyseal amputation to prevent difficulties with overgrowth.[1,136] Although limb salvage is a natural goal after these injuries, the long-term outcome and the duration of treatment with associated complications must be objectively analyzed.

Soft tissue coverage of most lawnmower injuries can be accomplished with delayed closure or a split-thickness skin graft.[63,94,136,232] Unlike such injuries in adults, a split-thickness skin graft works extremely well for most soft tissue injuries in children, including coverage on the plantar aspect of the foot. Vosburgh and colleagues reported results in nine patients with split-thickness skin grafts applied to the heel or plantar aspect of the foot; three had no difficulty and the remaining six had minor areas of junctional hyperkeratosis.[232] It is important to obtain input from a plastic surgeon at the time of the second or third debridement to plan appropriate soft tissue coverage, especially when free flap coverage is anticipated.

The outcome in these patients is satisfactory overall and largely depends on the force imparted during the initial injury and the location of the injury.[232] Patients in whom the injury was confined to the toe and forefoot have 88% of normal function, whereas patients who sustain injuries to the posterior and plantar aspect of the foot retain 72% of normal function.[232] Similarly, Dormans and colleagues reported excellent functional outcomes in patients who sustained limited laceration-type injuries, whereas patients who sustained the more common shredding-type injury had poor results.[63]

Puncture Injuries of the Foot

Puncture injuries of the foot are common in children and most often result when a child steps on a nail.[74,230] Treatment in the emergency department should consist of tetanus toxoid administration (when appropriate) and irrigation of the entry site with saline from a large syringe and plastic angiocatheter. Such treatment can be done under local anesthesia with an ankle block or under conscious sedation. The use of antibiotics at the initial visit in the emergency department is controversial and without good scientific analysis, and we do not recommend prophylactic administration. If there is concern that the wound is severely contaminated, more formal debridement in the operating room may be necessary. *Pseudomonas* species is the most common organism cultured from children who have a puncture wound and is thought to be due to the presence of this organism in sneakers.[22,62,73,80,81,99,100,106]

Treatment is thorough surgical debridement of the soft tissues, bone and cartilage, or joint, or any combination of these tissues, followed by a 7-day course of an intravenous antibiotic.[98] *Pseudomonas* species is the most common organism and may be associated with staphylococcal infection.[98]

Complications after these injuries are relatively rare. The incidence of cellulitis after puncture wounds of the foot is reported to be close to 10%. Cellulitis can usually be treated with intravenous antibiotics but may require surgical debridement. The offending organism in cellulitis is usually *S. aureus* and not *Pseudomonas* species. Osteomyelitis is the most serious complication from this injury, producing recurrent infection, physeal arrest, and early arthritis. It is seen in up to 3% of these injuries and most often involves the metatarsals, followed by the calcaneus. Penetration of the offending object into the cartilaginous surface at the time of the initial injury is thought to be necessary to cause osteomyelitis.[74] Systemic signs are generally absent; however, the patient has continued pain and an antalgic gait. The diagnosis is often difficult to make and is best established with an initial radiograph, followed by a bone scan or MRI, or both, if necessary.

References

Ankle and Foot

1. Abraham E, Pellicore RJ, Hamilton RC, et al: Stump overgrowth in juvenile amputees. J Pediatr Orthop 1986;6:66.
2. Adler P: Ride-on Mower Hazard Analysis 1987-1990. Washington DC, Directorate for Epidemiology, 1993.
3. Anderson DV, Lyne ED: Osteochondritis dissecans of the talus: Case report on two family members. J Pediatr Orthop 1984;4:356.
4. Anderson IF, Crichton KJ, Grattan-Smith T, et al: Osteochondral fractures of the dome of the talus. J Bone Joint Surg Am 1989;71:1143.
5. Andrews JR, Previte WJ, Carson WG: Arthroscopy of the ankle: Technique and normal anatomy. Foot Ankle 1985;6:29.
6. Angermann P, Jensen P: Osteochondritis dissecans of the talus: Long-term results of surgical treatment. Foot Ankle 1989;10:161.
7. Arntz CT, Hansen ST Jr: Dislocations and fracture dislocations of the tarsometatarsal joints. Orthop Clin North Am 1987;18:105.
8. Arntz CT, Veith RG, Hansen ST Jr: Fractures and fracture-dislocations of the tarsometatarsal joint. J Bone Joint Surg Am 1988;70:173.
9. Babst R, Simmen BR, Regazzoni P: [The treatment of fresh Lisfranc dislocations and fracture-dislocations.] Z Unfallchir Versicherungsmed 1991;84:159.
10. Baker CL, Andrews JR, Ryan JB: Arthroscopic treatment of transchondral talar dome fractures. Arthroscopy 1986;2:82.
11. Barber FA, Britt BT, Ratliff HW, et al: Arthroscopic surgery of the ankle. Orthop Rev 1988;17:446.
12. Barmada A, Gaynor T, Mubarak SJ: Premature physeal closure following distal tibia physeal fractures: A new radiographic predictor. J Pediatr Orthop 2003;23:733.
13. Bauer M, Jonsson K, Linden B: Osteochondritis dissecans of the ankle. A 20-year follow-up study. J Bone Joint Surg Br 1987;69:93.
14. Benz G, Kallieris D, Seebock T, et al: Bioresorbable pins and screws in paediatric traumatology. Eur J Pediatr Surg 1994;4:103.
15. Bernardo LM, Gardner MJ: Lawn mower injuries to children in Pennsylvania, 1989 to 1993. Int J Trauma Nurs 1996;2:36.
16. Berndt AL, Harty M: Transchondral fractures (osteochondritis dissecans) of the talus. J Bone Joint Surg Am 1959;41:988.
17. Bishop P: Fractures and epiphyseal separation fractures of the ankle: A classification of 332 cases according to the mechanism of the production. Am J Rheum 1932; 28:49.
18. Blair WF: Irreducible tarsometatarsal fracture-dislocation. J Trauma 1981;21:988.
19. Bonnel F, Barthelemy M: [Injuries of Lisfranc's joint: Severe sprains, dislocations, fractures. Study of 39 personal cases and biomechanical classification.] J Chir (Paris) 1976;111:573.
20. Bostman O, Hirvensalo E, Vainionpaa S, et al: Degradable polyglycolide rods for the internal fixation of displaced bimalleolar fractures. Int Orthop 1990; 14:1.
21. Bostman O, Makela EA, Sodergard J, et al: Absorbable polyglycolide pins in internal fixation of fractures in children. J Pediatr Orthop 1993;13:242.
22. Brand RA, Black H: *Pseudomonas* osteomyelitis following puncture wounds in children. J Bone Joint Surg Am 1974;56:1637.
23. Broden B: Roentgen examination of the subtaloid joint in fractures of the calcaneus. Acta Radiol 1949; 31:85.
24. Brown SD, Kasser JR, Zurakowski D, et al: Analysis of 51 tibial triplane fractures using CT with multiplanar reconstruction. AJR Am J Roentgenol 2004;183:1489.
25. Brunet JA: Calcaneal fractures in children. Long-term results of treatment. J Bone Joint Surg Br 2000;82:211.
26. Bruns J, Rosenbach B: Osteochondritis dissecans of the talus. Comparison of results of surgical treatment in adolescents and adults. Arch Orthop Trauma Surg 1992;112:23.
27. Bryant DD 3rd, Siegel MG: Osteochondritis dissecans of the talus: A new technique for arthroscopic drilling. Arthroscopy 1993;9:238.
28. Buchanan J, Greer RB 3rd: Stress fractures in the calcaneus of a child. A case report. Clin Orthop Relat Res 1978;135:119.
29. Bucholz RW, Henry S, Henley MB: Fixation with bioabsorbable screws for the treatment of fractures of the ankle. J Bone Joint Surg Am 1994;76:319.
30. Buoncristiani AM, Manos RE, Mills WJ: Plantar-flexion tarsometatarsal joint injuries in children. J Pediatr Orthop 2001;21:324.
31. Burroughs KE, Reimer CD, Fields KB: Lisfranc injury of the foot: A commonly missed diagnosis. Am Fam Physician 1998;58:118.
32. Buzzard BM, Briggs PJ: Surgical management of acute tarsometatarsal fracture dislocation in the adult. Clin Orthop Relat Res 1998;353:125.
33. Byrd T: Jones fracture: Relearning an old injury. South Med J 1992;85:748.
34. Cameron SE: Noninvasive distraction for ankle arthroscopy. Arthroscopy 1997;13:366.
35. Canale ST, Belding RH: Osteochondral lesions of the talus. J Bone Joint Surg Am 1980;62:97.

36. Canale ST, Kelly FB Jr: Fractures of the neck of the talus. Long-term evaluation of seventy-one cases. J Bone Joint Surg Am 1978;60:143.
37. Carothers CO, Crenshaw AH: Clinical significance of a classification of epiphyseal injuries at the ankle. Am J Surg 1955;89:879.
38. Carp L: Fracture of the fifth metatarsal bone with special reference to delayed union. Ann Surg 1927;86: 308.
39. Cass JR, Peterson HA: Salter-Harris type-IV injuries of the distal tibial epiphyseal growth plate, with emphasis on those involving the medial malleolus. J Bone Joint Surg Am 1983;65:1059.
40. Caterini R, Farsetti P, Ippolito E: Long-term followup of physeal injury to the ankle. Foot Ankle 1991;11: 372.
41. Ceccarelli F, Faldini C, Piras F, et al: Surgical versus non-surgical treatment of calcaneal fractures in children: A long-term results comparative study. Foot Ankle Int 2000;21:825.
42. Chapman H, Galway H: Os calcis fractures in childhood. J Bone Joint Surg Br 1977;59:510.
43. Charlton M, Costello R, Mooney JF 3rd, et al: Ankle joint biomechanics following transepiphyseal screw fixation of the distal tibia. J Pediatr Orthop 2005;25: 635.
44. Chin TW, Mitra AK, Lim GH, et al: Arthroscopic treatment of osteochondral lesion of the talus. Ann Acad Med Singapore 1996;25:236.
45. Clement DA, Worlock PH: Triplane fracture of the distal tibia. A variant in cases with an open growth plate. J Bone Joint Surg Br 1987;69:412.
46. Cole RJ, Brown HP, Stein RE, et al: Avulsion fracture of the tuberosity of the calcaneus in children. A report of four cases and review of the literature. J Bone Joint Surg Am 1995;77:1568.
47. Cooper A: A Treatise on Dislocations and Fractures of the Joints. London, Longman, Hurst, Orme & Brown, 1822.
48. Cooperman DR, Spiegel PG, Laros GS: Tibial fractures involving the ankle in children. The so-called triplane epiphyseal fracture. J Bone Joint Surg Am 1978;60: 1040.
49. Craigen MA, Clarke NM: Bilateral 'Jones' fractures of the fifth metatarsal following relapse of talipes equinovarus. Injury 1996;27:599.
50. Crawford AH: Triplane fracture. Orthop Consult 1983;68:12.
51. Crenshaw AH: Injuries of the distal tibial epiphysis. Clin Orthop Relat Res 1965;41:98.
52. Crosby LA, Fitzgibbons T: Computerized tomography scanning of acute intra-articular fractures of the calcaneus. A new classification system. J Bone Joint Surg Am 1990;72:852.
53. Curtis MJ, Myerson M, Szura B: Tarsometatarsal joint injuries in the athlete. Am J Sports Med 1993;21:497.
54. Dameron TB Jr: Fractures and anatomical variations of the proximal portion of the fifth metatarsal. J Bone Joint Surg Am 1975;57:788.
55. David J: Deaths Related to Ride-On Mowers 1987-1990. Washington DC, US Consumer Product Safety Commission, 1993.
56. de Beer JD, Maloon S, Hudson DA: Calcaneal fractures in children. S Afr Med J 1989;76:53.
57. Delee J: Fractures and dislocations of the foot. In Mann R (ed): Surgery of the Foot. St. Louis, CV Mosby, 1986.
58. Denton JR, Fischer SJ: The medial triplane fracture: Report of an unusual injury. J Trauma 1981;21:991.
59. De Smet AA, Fisher DR, Burnstein MI, et al: Value of MR imaging in staging osteochondral lesions of the talus (osteochondritis dissecans): Results in 14 patients. AJR Am J Roentgenol 1990;154:555.
60. Dias LS, Giegerich CR: Fractures of the distal tibial epiphysis in adolescence. J Bone Joint Surg Am 1983; 65:438.
61. Dias LS, Tachdjian MO: Physeal injuries of the ankle in children: Classification. Clin Orthop Relat Res 1978;136:230.
62. Dixon RS, Sydnor CH: Puncture wound pseudomonal osteomyelitis of the foot. J Foot Ankle Surg 1993;32: 434.
63. Dormans JP, Azzoni M, Davidson RS, et al: Major lower extremity lawn mower injuries in children. J Pediatr Orthop 1995;15:78.
64. Eastwood DM, Gregg PJ, Atkins RM: Intra-articular fractures of the calcaneum. Part I: Pathological anatomy and classification. J Bone Joint Surg Br 1993;75:183.
65. Eastwood DM, Langkamer VG, Atkins RM: Intra-articular fractures of the calcaneum. Part II: Open reduction and internal fixation by the extended lateral transcalcaneal approach. J Bone Joint Surg Br 1993;75: 189.
66. Eberle C, Rhomberg P, Metzger U: [Long-term follow-up of surgically treated intra-articular calcaneus fractures.] Helv Chir Acta 1994;60:629.
67. Ertl JP, Barrack RL, Alexander AH, et al: Triplane fracture of the distal tibial epiphysis. Long-term follow-up. J Bone Joint Surg Am 1988;70:967.
68. Escalas F, Figueras JM, Merino JA: Dislocation of the peroneal tendons. Long-term results of surgical treatment. J Bone Joint Surg Am 1980;62:451.
69. Essex-Lopresti P: The mechanism, reduction technique, and results in fractures of the os calcis. Br J Surg 1952;39:395.
70. Faciszewski T, Burks RT, Manaster BJ: Subtle injuries of the Lisfranc joint. J Bone Joint Surg Am 1990;72:1519.
71. Feldman DS, Otsuka NY, Hedden DM: Extra-articular triplane fracture of the distal tibial epiphysis. J Pediatr Orthop 1995;15:479.
72. Ferkel RD, Fasulo GJ: Arthroscopic treatment of ankle injuries. Orthop Clin North Am 1994;25:17.
73. Fisher MC, Goldsmith JF, Gilligan PH: Sneakers as a source of *Pseudomonas aeruginosa* in children with osteomyelitis following puncture wounds. J Pediatr 1985;106:607.
74. Fitzgerald RH Jr, Cowan JD: Puncture wounds of the foot. Orthop Clin North Am 1975;6:965.
75. Flick AB, Gould N: Osteochondritis dissecans of the talus (transchondral fractures of the talus): Review of the literature and new surgical approach for medial dome lesions. Foot Ankle 1985;5:165.
76. Frank A, Cohen P, Beaufils P, et al: Arthroscopic treatment of osteochondral lesions of the talar dome. Arthroscopy 1989;5:57.

77. Gill G, Abbott L: Varus deformity of the ankle following injury to the distal epiphyseal cartilage of the tibia in growing children. Surg Gynecol Obstet 1941;72:659.
78. Goiney RC, Connell DG, Nichols DM: CT evaluation of tarsometatarsal fracture-dislocation injuries. AJR Am J Roentgenol 1985;144:985.
79. Grace DL: Irreducible fracture-separations of the distal tibial epiphysis. J Bone Joint Surg Br 1983;65:160.
80. Graham BS, Gregory DW: *Pseudomonas aeruginosa* causing osteomyelitis after puncture wounds of the foot. South Med J 1984;77:1228.
81. Green NE, Bruno J 3rd: *Pseudomonas* infections of the foot after puncture wounds. South Med J 1980;73:146.
82. Greenspoon J, Rosman M: Medial osteochondritis of the talus in children: Review and new surgical management. J Pediatr Orthop 1987;7:705.
83. Griffiths JD, Menelaus MB: Symptomatic ossicles of the lateral malleolus in children. J Bone Joint Surg Br 1987;69:317.
84. Groshar D, Alperson M, Mendes DG, et al: Bone scintigraphy findings in Lisfranc joint injury. Foot Ankle Int 1995;16:710.
85. Guhl JF: New techniques for arthroscopic surgery of the ankle: Preliminary report. Orthopedics 1986;9: 261.
86. Haliburton RA, Sullivan CR, Kelly PJ, et al: The extraosseous and intra-osseous blood supply of the talus. J Bone Joint Surg Am 1958;40:1115.
87. Hardcastle PH, Reschauer R, Kutscha-Lissberg E, et al: Injuries to the tarsometatarsal joint. Incidence, classification and treatment. J Bone Joint Surg Br 1982;64:349.
88. Hawkins LG: Fracture of the lateral process of the talus. J Bone Joint Surg Am 1965;47:1170.
89. Hawkins LG: Fractures of the neck of the talus. J Bone Joint Surg Am 1970;52:991.
90. Heckman JD, McLean MR: Fractures of the lateral process of the talus. Clin Orthop Relat Res 1985;199: 108.
91. Henderson RC: Posttraumatic necrosis of the talus: The Hawkins sign versus magnetic resonance imaging. J Orthop Trauma 1991;5:96.
92. Higuera J, Laguna R, Peral M, et al: Osteochondritis dissecans of the talus during childhood and adolescence. J Pediatr Orthop 1998;18:328.
93. Hirvensalo E: Fracture fixation with biodegradable rods. Forty-one cases of severe ankle fractures. Acta Orthop Scand 1989;60:601.
94. Horowitz JH, Nichter LS, Kenney JG, et al: Lawnmower injuries in children: Lower extremity reconstruction. J Trauma 1985;25:1138.
95. Hynes D, O'Brien T: Growth disturbance lines after injury of the distal tibial physis. Their significance in prognosis. J Bone Joint Surg Br 1988;70:231.
96. Iannacone WM, Dalton GP: Osteochondritis dissecans of the talus presenting as an ankle ganglion. Orthopedics 1997;20:348.
97. Inokuchi S, Usami N, Hiraishi E, et al: Calcaneal fractures in children. J Pediatr Orthop 1998;18:469.
98. Jacobs RF, McCarthy RE, Elser JM: Pseudomonas osteochondritis complicating puncture wounds of the foot in children: A 10-year evaluation. J Infect Dis 1989; 160:657.
99. Jensen I, Wester JU, Rasmussen F, et al: Prognosis of fracture of the talus in children. 21 (7-34)-year follow-up of 14 cases. Acta Orthop Scand 1994;65:398.
100. Johanson PH: *Pseudomonas* infections of the foot following puncture wounds. JAMA 1968;204:170.
101. Johnson EE, Gebhardt JS: Surgical management of calcaneal fractures using bilateral incisions and minimal internal fixation. Clin Orthop Relat Res 1993;290:117.
102. Johnstone BR, Bennett CS: Lawn mower injuries in children. Aust N Z J Surg 1989;59:713.
103. Jones R: Fracture of the base of the fifth metatarsal bone by indirect violence. Ann Surg 1902;35:697.
104. Josefsson PO, Karlsson M, Redlund-Johnell I, et al: Jones fracture. Surgical versus nonsurgical treatment. Clin Orthop Relat Res 1994;299:252.
105. Josefsson PO, Karlsson M, Redlund-Johnell I, et al: Closed treatment of Jones fracture. Good results in 40 cases after 11-26 years. Acta Orthop Scand 1994;65: 545.
106. Joseph WS, LeFrock JL: Infections complicating puncture wounds of the foot. J Foot Surg 1987;26:S30.
107. Jurgensen I, Bachmann G, Siaplaouras J, et al: [Clinical value of conventional radiology and MRI in assessing osteochondrosis dissecans stability.] Unfallchirurg 1996;99:758.
108. Karrholm J, Hansson LI, Laurin S: Computed tomography of intraarticular supination-eversion fractures of the ankle in adolescents. J Pediatr Orthop 1981;1:181.
109. Kelly PJ, Sullivan CR: Blood supply of the talus. Clin Orthop Relat Res 1963;30:37.
110. Kleiger B, Mankin HJ: Fracture of the lateral portion of the distal tibial epiphysis. J Bone Joint Surg Am 1964; 46:25.
111. Kling TF Jr: Operative treatment of ankle fractures in children. Orthop Clin North Am 1990;21:381.
112. Kling TF Jr, Bright RW, Hensinger RN: Distal tibial physeal fractures in children that may require open reduction. J Bone Joint Surg Am 1984;66:647.
113. Koval KJ, Sanders R: The radiologic evaluation of calcaneal fractures. Clin Orthop Relat Res 1993;290:41.
114. Kumai T, Takakura Y, Higashiyama I, et al: Arthroscopic drilling for the treatment of osteochondral lesions of the talus. J Bone Joint Surg Am 1999;81:1229.
115. Laliotis N, Pennie BH, Carty H, et al: Toddler's fracture of the calcaneum. Injury 1993;24:169.
116. Lamy C, Stienstra JJ: Complications in ankle arthroscopy. Clin Podiatr Med Surg 1994;11:523.
117. Langenskiöld A: Traumatic premature closure of the distal tibial epiphyseal plate. Acta Orthop Scand 1967;38:520.
118. Lapidus P: Os subtibiale: Inconstant bone over the tip of the medial malleolus. J Bone Joint Surg 1933;15:766.
119. Lauge-Hansen N: Fractures of the ankle. I. Analytic historic survey as basis of new experimental, roentgenologic, and clinical investigations. Arch Surg 1948; 56:259.
120. Lauge-Hansen N: Fractures of the ankle. II. Combined experimental-surgical and experimental-roentgenologic investigations. Arch Surg 1950;60:957.
121. Lauge-Hansen N: Fractures of the ankle. IV. Clinical use of genetic roentgen diagnosis and genetic reduction. AMA Arch Surg 1952;64:488.

122. Lauge-Hansen N: Fractures of the ankle. V. Pronation-dorsiflexion fracture. AMA Arch Surg 1953;67:813.
123. Lauge-Hansen N: Fractures of the ankle. III. Genetic roentgenologic diagnosis of fractures of the ankle. Am J Roentgenol Radium Ther Nucl Med 1954;71:456.
124. Lawrence SJ, Botte MJ: Jones' fractures and related fractures of the proximal fifth metatarsal. Foot Ankle 1993;14:358.
125. Lawson JP, Ogden JA, Sella E, et al: The painful accessory navicular. Skeletal Radiol 1984;12:250.
126. Lee CK, Mercurio C: Operative treatment of osteochondritis dissecans in situ by retrograde drilling and cancellous bone graft: A preliminary report. Clin Orthop Relat Res 1981;158:129.
127. Leenen LP, van der Werken C: Fracture-dislocations of the tarsometatarsal joint, a combined anatomical and computed tomographic study. Injury 1992;23:51.
128. Letournel E: Open treatment of acute calcaneal fractures. Clin Orthop Relat Res 1993;290:60.
129. Letts RM: The hidden adolescent ankle fracture. J Pediatr Orthop 1982;2:161.
130. Letts RM, Gibeault D: Fractures of the neck of the talus in children. Foot Ankle 1980;1:74.
131. Letts RM, Mardirosian A: Lawnmower injuries in children. Can Med Assoc J 1977;116:1151.
132. Leung KS, Yuen KM, Chan WS: Operative treatment of displaced intra-articular fractures of the calcaneum. Medium-term results. J Bone Joint Surg Br 1993;75:196.
133. Linhart WE, Hollwarth M: [Fractures of the talus in children.] Unfallchirurg 1985;88:168.
134. Loder RT, Dikos GD, Taylor DA: Long-term lower extremity prosthetic costs in children with traumatic lawnmower amputations. Arch Pediatr Adolesc Med 2004;158:1177.
135. Loomer R, Fisher C, Lloyd-Smith R, et al: Osteochondral lesions of the talus. Am J Sports Med 1993;21:13.
136. Love SM, Grogan DP, Ogden JA: Lawn-mower injuries in children. J Orthop Trauma 1988;2:94.
137. Lu J, Ebraheim NA, Skie M, et al: Radiographic and computed tomographic evaluation of Lisfranc dislocation: A cadaver study. Foot Ankle Int 1997;18:351.
138. Lundeen RO: Techniques of ankle arthroscopy. J Foot Surg 1987;26:22.
139. Ly PN, Fallat LM: Trans-chondral fractures of the talus: A review of 64 surgical cases. J Foot Ankle Surg 1993;32:352.
140. Lynn MD: The triplane distal tibial epiphyseal fracture. Clin Orthop Relat Res 1972;86:187.
141. MacNealy GA, Rogers LF, Hernandez R, et al: Injuries of the distal tibial epiphysis: Systematic radiographic evaluation. AJR Am J Roentgenol 1982;138:683.
142. Mandracchia VJ, Buddecke DE, Jr., Giesking JL: Osteochondral lesions of the talar dome. A comprehensive review with retrospective study. Clin Podiatr Med Surg 1999;16:725.
143. Marmor L: An unusual fracture of the tibial epiphysis. Clin Orthop Relat Res 1970;73:132.
144. Martin LI: Lawnmower injuries in children: Destructive and preventable. Plast Surg Nurs 1990;10:69.
145. Matteri RE, Frymoyer JW: Fracture of the calcaneus in young children. Report of three cases. J Bone Joint Surg Am 1973;55:1091.
146. Mayo K: Fractures of the talus: Principles of management and techniques of treatment. Tech Orthop 1987:42.
147. Mazel C, Rigault P, Padovani JP, et al: [Fractures of the talus in children. Apropos of 23 cases.] Rev Chir Orthop Reparatrice Appar Mot 1986;72:183.
148. McDougall A: The os trigonum. J Bone Joint Surg Br 1955;37:257.
149. McCrory P, Bladin C: Fractures of the lateral process of the talus: A clinical review. "Snowboarder's ankle." Clin J Sport Med 1996;6:124.
150. McFarland B: Traumatic arrest of the epiphyseal growth at the lower end of the tibia. Br J Surg 1931;19:78.
151. McLennan JG: Treatment of acute and chronic luxations of the peroneal tendons. Am J Sports Med 1980;8:432.
152. Michelson JD: Fractures about the ankle. J Bone Joint Surg Am 1995;77:142.
153. Michelson JD, Clarke HJ, Jinnah RH: The effect of loading on tibiotalar alignment in cadaver ankles. Foot Ankle 1990;10:280.
154. Michelson JD, Magid D, Ney DR, et al: Examination of the pathologic anatomy of ankle fractures. J Trauma 1992;32:65.
155. Mindell E, Cisek I, Kartalian G, et al: Late results of injuries to the talus: Analysis of forty cases. J Bone Joint Surg Am 1963;45:221.
156. Mora S, Thordarson DB, Zionts LE, et al: Pediatric calcaneal fractures. Foot Ankle Int 2001;22:471.
157. Mukherjee SK, Young AB: Dome fracture of the talus. A report of ten cases. J Bone Joint Surg Br 1973;55:319.
158. Mulcahy DM, McCormack DM, Stephens MM: Intra-articular calcaneal fractures: Effect of open reduction and internal fixation on the contact characteristics of the subtalar joint. Foot Ankle Int 1998;19:842.
159. Mulfinger GL, Trueta J: The blood supply of the talus. J Bone Joint Surg Br 1970;52:160.
160. Myerson M, Manoli A: Compartment syndromes of the foot after calcaneal fractures. Clin Orthop Relat Res 1993;290:142.
161. Myerson M, Quill GE Jr: Late complications of fractures of the calcaneus. J Bone Joint Surg Am 1993;75:331.
162. Myerson MS, Fisher RT, Burgess AR, et al: Fracture dislocations of the tarsometatarsal joints: End results correlated with pathology and treatment. Foot Ankle 1986;6:225.
163. Nicholas R, Hadley J, Paul C, et al: "Snowboarder's fracture": Fracture of the lateral process of the talus. J Am Board Fam Pract 1994;7:130.
164. Ogden JA, Lee J: Accessory ossification patterns and injuries of the malleoli. J Pediatr Orthop 1990;10:306.
165. Ogilvie-Harris DJ, Sarrosa EA: Arthroscopic treatment of osteochondritis dissecans of the talus. Arthroscopy 1999;15:805.
166. Owen RJ, Hickey FG, Finlay DB: A study of metatarsal fractures in children. Injury 1995;26:537.
167. Pablot SM, Daneman A, Stringer DA, et al: The value of computed tomography in the early assessment of comminuted fractures of the calcaneus: A review of three patients. J Pediatr Orthop 1985;5:435.
168. Parisien JS: Arthroscopic treatment of osteochondral lesions of the talus. Am J Sports Med 1986;14:211.

169. Peiro A, Aracil J, Martos F, et al: Triplane distal tibial epiphyseal fracture. Clin Orthop Relat Res 1981;160: 196.
170. Peltier LF: Eponymic fractures: Robert Jones and Jones's fracture. Surgery 1972;71:522.
171. Pereles TR, Koval KJ, Feldman DS: Fracture-dislocation of the neck of the talus in a ten-year-old child: A case report and review of the literature. Bull Hosp Jt Dis 1996;55:88.
172. Perez Blanco R, Rodriguez Merchan C, Canosa Sevillano R, et al: Tarsometatarsal fractures and dislocations. J Orthop Trauma 1988;2:188.
173. Peterson CA, Peterson HA: Analysis of the incidence of injuries to the epiphyseal growth plate. J Trauma 1972; 12:275.
174. Peterson L, Goldie I, Lindell D: The arterial supply of the talus. Acta Orthop Scand 1974;45:260.
175. Peterson L, Goldie IF: The arterial supply of the talus. A study on the relationship to experimental talar fractures. Acta Orthop Scand 1975;46:1026.
176. Peterson L, Goldie IF, Irstam L: Fracture of the neck of the talus. A clinical study. Acta Orthop Scand 1977; 48:696.
177. Peterson L, Romanus B, Dahlberg E: Fracture of the collum tali—an experimental study. J Biomech 1976;9: 277.
178. Pettine KA, Morrey BF: Osteochondral fractures of the talus. A long-term follow-up. J Bone Joint Surg Br 1987;69:89.
179. Pickle A, Benaroch TE, Guy P, et al: Clinical outcome of pediatric calcaneal fractures treated with open reduction and internal fixation. J Pediatr Orthop 2004; 24:178.
180. Pietropaoli MP, Wnorowski DC, Werner FW, et al: Intramedullary screw fixation of Jones fractures: a biomechanical study. Foot Ankle Int 1999;20:560.
181. Potter HG, Deland JT, Gusmer PB, et al: Magnetic resonance imaging of the Lisfranc ligament of the foot. Foot Ankle Int 1998;19:438.
182. Powell H: Extra center of ossification for the medial malleolus in children: Incidence and significance. J Bone Joint Surg Br 1961;43:107.
183. Pritsch M, Horoshovski H, Farine I: Ankle arthroscopy. Clin Orthop Relat Res 1984;184:137.
184. Pritsch M, Horoshovski H, Farine I: Arthroscopic treatment of osteochondral lesions of the talus. J Bone Joint Surg Am 1986;68:862.
185. Quenu E, Kuss G: Etude sur les luxations du metatarse (luxations metatarsotarsiennes) du diastasis entre le ler et le 2 metatarsien. Rev Chir 1909; 39:281.
186. Ragozzino A, Rossi G, Esposito S, et al: [Computed tomography of osteochondral diseases of the talus dome.] Radiol Med (Torino) 1996;92:682.
187. Rainaut JJ, Cedard C, D'Hour JP: [Tarsometatarsal luxations.] Rev Chir Orthop Reparatrice Appar Mot 1966; 52:449.
188. Rasmussen F, Schantz K: Radiologic aspects of calcaneal fractures in childhood and adolescence. Acta Radiol Diagn (Stockh) 1986;27:575.
189. Resch S, Stenstrom A: The treatment of tarsometatarsal injuries. Foot Ankle 1990;11:117.
190. Rettig AC, Shelbourne KD, Wilckens J: The surgical treatment of symptomatic nonunions of the proximal (metaphyseal) fifth metatarsal in athletes. Am J Sports Med 1992;20:50.
191. Rosenberg GA, Patterson BM: Tarsometatarsal (Lisfranc's) fracture-dislocation. Am J Orthop 1995; Suppl:7.
192. Ross G, Cronin R, Hauzenblas J, et al: Plantar ecchymosis sign: A clinical aid to diagnosis of occult Lisfranc tarsometatarsal injuries. J Orthop Trauma 1996;10:119.
193. Ross PM, Schwentker EP, Bryan H: Mutilating lawn mower injuries in children. JAMA 1976;236:480.
194. Rowe C, Sakellarides H, Freeman P, et al: Fractures of the os calcis: A long-term follow-up study of 146 patients. JAMA 1963;184:920.
195. Salter RB: Injuries of the ankle in children. Orthop Clin North Am 1974;5:147.
196. Sammarco GJ: The Jones fracture. Instr Course Lect 1993;42:201.
197. Sanders R, Gregory P: Operative treatment of intra-articular fractures of the calcaneus. Orthop Clin North Am 1995;26:203.
198. Sanders TG, Ptaszek AJ, Morrison WB: Fracture of the lateral process of the talus: Appearance at MR imaging and clinical significance. Skeletal Radiol 1999;28:236.
199. Sangeorzan BJ, Veith RG, Hansen ST Jr: Salvage of Lisfranc's tarsometatarsal joint by arthrodesis. Foot Ankle 1990;10:193.
200. Schantz K, Rasmussen F: Calcaneus fracture in the child. Acta Orthop Scand 1987;58:507.
201. Schantz K, Rasmussen F: Good prognosis after calcaneal fracture in childhood. Acta Orthop Scand 1988; 59:560.
202. Scharling M: Osteochondritis dissecans of the talus. Acta Orthop Scand 1978;49:89.
203. Schlesinger I, Wedge JH: Percutaneous reduction and fixation of displaced juvenile Tillaux fractures: A new surgical technique. J Pediatr Orthop 1993;13:389.
204. Schmidt TL, Weiner DS: Calcaneal fractures in children. An evaluation of the nature of the injury in 56 children. Clin Orthop Relat Res 1982;171:150.
205. Shereff MJ, Yang QM, Kummer FJ, et al: Vascular anatomy of the fifth metatarsal. Foot Ankle 1991; 11:350.
206. Shilt JS, Yoder JS, Manuck TA, et al: Role of vacuum-assisted closure in the treatment of pediatric lawn-mower injuries. J Pediatr Orthop 2004;24:482.
207. Shin AY, Moran ME, Wenger DR: Intramalleolar triplane fractures of the distal tibial epiphysis. J Pediatr Orthop 1997;17:352.
208. Silas SI, Herzenberg JE, Myerson MS, et al: Compartment syndrome of the foot in children. J Bone Joint Surg Am 1995;77:356.
209. Smith BG, Rand F, Jaramillo D, et al: Early MR imaging of lower-extremity physeal fracture-separations: A preliminary report. J Pediatr Orthop 1994;14:526.
210. Smith JW, Arnoczky SP, Hersh A: The intraosseous blood supply of the fifth metatarsal: Implications for proximal fracture healing. Foot Ankle 1992;13:143.
211. Sneppen O, Christensen SB, Krogsoe O, et al: Fracture of the body of the talus. Acta Orthop Scand 1977;48: 317.

212. Spiegel PG, Cooperman DR, Laros GS: Epiphyseal fractures of the distal ends of the tibia and fibula. A retrospective study of two hundred and thirty-seven cases in children. J Bone Joint Surg Am 1978;60:1046.
213. Spinella AJ, Turco VJ: Team physician #4. Avulsion fracture of the distal tibial epiphysis in skeletally immature athletes (juvenile Tillaux fracture). Orthop Rev 1988; 17:1245.
214. Starshak RJ, Simons GW, Sty JR: Occult fracture of the calcaneus—another toddler's fracture. Pediatr Radiol 1984;14:37.
215. Sucato D, Krackow K: Dislocation of the peroneal tendons: Surgical treatment. J Orthop Tech 1995;3:91.
216. Swanson TV, Bray TJ, Holmes GB Jr: Fractures of the talar neck. A mechanical study of fixation. J Bone Joint Surg Am 1992;74:544.
217. Szyszkowitz R, Reschauer R, Seggl W: Eighty-five talus fractures treated by ORIF with five to eight years of follow-up study of 69 patients. Clin Orthop Relat Res 1985;199:97.
218. Tachdjian MO: The Child's Foot. Philadelphia, WB Saunders, 1985.
219. Takakura Y, Takaoka T, Tanaka Y, et al: Results of opening-wedge osteotomy for the treatment of a post-traumatic varus deformity of the ankle. J Bone Joint Surg Am 1998;80:213.
220. Takao M, Ochi M, Shu N, et al: Bandage distraction technique for ankle arthroscopy. Foot Ankle Int 1999;20:389.
221. Tan YH, Chin TW, Mitra AK, et al: Tarsometatarsal (Lisfranc's) injuries—results of open reduction and internal fixation. Ann Acad Med Singapore 1995;24: 816.
222. Thomas HM: Calcaneal fracture in childhood. Br J Surg 1969;56:664.
223. Thordarson DB, Triffon MJ, Terk MR: Magnetic resonance imaging to detect avascular necrosis after open reduction and internal fixation of talar neck fractures. Foot Ankle Int 1996;17:742.
224. Torg JS, Balduini FC, Zelko RR, et al: Fractures of the base of the fifth metatarsal distal to the tuberosity. Classification and guidelines for non-surgical and surgical management. J Bone Joint Surg Am 1984;66:209.
225. Torg JS, Ruggiero RA: Comminuted epiphyseal fracture of the distal tibia. A case report and review of the literature. Clin Orthop Relat Res 1975;110:215.
226. Treadwell JR, Kahn MD: Lisfranc arthrodesis for chronic pain: A cannulated screw technique. J Foot Ankle Surg 1998;37:28.
227. Trillat A, Lerat JL, Leclerc P, et al: [Fracture-dislocation of the tarsometatarsal joint. Classification. Treatment. Apropos of 81 cases.] Rev Chir Orthop Reparatrice Appar Mot 1976;62:685.
228. Tucker DJ, Feder JM, Boylan JP: Fractures of the lateral process of the talus: Two case reports and a comprehensive literature review. Foot Ankle Int 1998;19:641.
229. van der Werf GJ, Tonino AJ: Tarsometatarsal fracture-dislocation. Acta Orthop Scand 1984;55:647.
230. Verdile VP, Freed HA, Gerard J: Puncture wounds to the foot. J Emerg Med 1989;7:193.
231. von Laer L: Classification, diagnosis, and treatment of transitional fractures of the distal part of the tibia. J Bone Joint Surg Am 1985;67:687.
232. Vosburgh CL, Gruel CR, Herndon WA, et al: Lawn mower injuries of the pediatric foot and ankle: Observations on prevention and management. J Pediatr Orthop 1995;15:504.
233. Wester JU, Jensen IE, Rasmussen F, et al: Osteochondral lesions of the talar dome in children. A 24 (7-36) year follow-up of 13 cases. Acta Orthop Scand 1994;65:110.
234. Whipple TL, Martin DR, McIntyre LF, et al: Arthroscopic treatment of triplane fractures of the ankle. Arthroscopy 1993;9:456.
235. Wildenauer E: Die Blutversorgung des Talus. Z Anat 1950;115:32.
236. Wiley JJ: The mechanism of tarso-metatarsal joint injuries. J Bone Joint Surg Br 1971;53:474.
237. Wiley JJ: Tarso-metatarsal joint injuries in children. J Pediatr Orthop 1981;1:255.
238. Wiley JJ, Profitt A: Fractures of the os calcis in children. Clin Orthop Relat Res 1984;188:131.
239. Wilppula E: Tarsometatarsal fracture-dislocation. Late results in 26 patients. Acta Orthop Scand 1973;44: 335.
240. Wilson DW: Injuries of the tarso-metatarsal joints. Etiology, classification and results of treatment. J Bone Joint Surg Br 1972;54:677.
241. Woods K, Harris I: Osteochondritis dissecans of the talus in identical twins. J Bone Joint Surg Br 1995; 77:331.
242. Yates CK, Grana WA: A simple distraction technique for ankle arthroscopy. Arthroscopy 1988;4:103.

Plate Index

S

T

U

V

W

Y

Z

INDEX

Note: Page numbers followed by the letter f refer to figures; those followed by the letter t refer to tables. The letter b refers to boxed material, the letter p refers to plates, and the letter V refers to video material.

A

B

C

D

E

F

G

H

J

K

L

M

N

O

P

Q

R

S

T

U

V

W

X

Y

Z